Principles of
Surgery

Seventh Edition

NOTICE

Medicine is an ever-changing science. As new research and clinical experience broaden our knowledge, changes in treatment and drug therapy are required. The editors and the publisher of this work have checked with sources believed to be reliable in their efforts to provide information that is complete and generally in accord with the standards accepted at the time of publication. However, in view of the possibility of human error or changes in medical sciences, neither the editors nor the publisher nor any other party who has been involved in the preparation or publication of this work warrants that the information contained herein is in every respect accurate or complete, and they are not responsible for any errors or omissions or for the results obtained from use of such information. Readers are encouraged to confirm the information contained herein with other sources. For example and in particular, readers are advised to check the product information sheet included in the package of each drug they plan to administer to be certain that the information contained in this book is accurate and that changes have not been made in the recommended dose or in the contraindications for administration. This recommendation is of particular importance in connection with new or infrequently used drugs.

PRINCIPLES OF SURGERY

SURGERY
SEVENTH EDITION

Editor-in-Chief

Seymour I. Schwartz, M.D.
Distinguished Alumni Professor and Chair
Department of Surgery
University of Rochester Medical Center
Rochester, New York

Associate Editors

G. Tom Shires, M.D.
Professor of Surgery
Director, Trauma Institute
University of Nevada School of Medicine
Las Vegas, Nevada

Frank C. Spencer, M.D.
Professor and Chairman
Department of Surgery
New York University Medical Center
New York, New York

John M. Daly, M.D.
Lewis Atterbury Stimson Professor and Chairman
Department of Surgery
Cornell University Medical College
New York, New York

Josef E. Fischer, M.D.
Christian R. Holmes Professor and Chairman
Department of Surgery
University of Cincinnati College of Medicine
Cincinnati, Ohio

Aubrey C. Galloway, M.D.
Professor of Surgery
Director of Surgical Research
New York University Medical Center
New York, New York

Volume 2

McGRAW-HILL
HEALTH PROFESSIONS DIVISION
New York   St. Louis   San Francisco   Auckland   Bogotá   Caracas
Lisbon   London   Madrid   Mexico City   Milan   Montreal
New Delhi   San Juan   Singapore   Sydney   Tokyo   Toronto

16/045

McGraw-Hill

A Division of The McGraw·Hill Companies

Principles of Surgery, 7/e

1234567890 DOWDOW 998

Single volume ISBN 0-07-054256-2
Two-volume ISBN 0-07-912318-X
Volume 1 ISBN 0-07-134312-1
Volume 2 ISBN 0-07-058079-0

This book was set in Times Roman by York Graphic Services, Inc. The editors were Marty Wonsiewicz and Peter McCurdy; the production supervisor was Rich Ruzycka; the cover designer was Ed Schultheis. Barb Littlewood prepared the index. R.R. Donnelley & Sons, Co. was printer and binder.

This book is printed on acid-free paper.

The illustration in the upper left of the book's cover is derived from the painting *Limb Transplantation Miracle by Saints Cosmos and Damian.* Used by permission of the Wuerttembergische Landesmuseum, Stuttgart, Germany. The image on the lower left of the cover is used courtesy of the Yale Historical Library. The figure on the lower right is from *Dis Is das Buch der Cirurgia* by Hieronymous Brunschwig. Courtesy of the National Library of Medicine, Bethesda, Maryland. The illustration on the back cover and on the part opening pages is from *An Explanation of the Fashion and Use of Three and Fifty Instruments of Chirurgery—Gathered out of Ambrosius Pareus.*

Library of Congress Cataloging-in-Publication Data
Principles of surgery/editors, Seymour I. Schwartz . . . [et al.]. —
    7th ed.
        p.   cm.
    Includes bibliographical references and index.
    ISBN 0-07-054256-2
    1. Surgery.   I. Schwartz, Seymour I.
    [DNLM: 1. Surgery. 2. Surgical Procedures, Operative.   WO
100P957 1999]
RD31.P88   1999
617—dc21
DNLM/DLC   98-28061
for Library of Congress   CIP

To students of Surgery, at all levels, in their
quest for knowledge

Contents

Contributors

James T. Adams, MD *(Chapter 33)*
Professor of Surgery
University of Rochester Medical Center

R. Peter Altman, MD *(Chapter 37)*
Rudolph N. Schullinger Professor of Surgery (Pediatric Surgery)
Columbia Presbyterian Medical Center

Kathryn D. Anderson, MD *(Chapter 37)*
Professor of Surgery (Pediatric Surgery)
University of Southern California, Los Angeles

Richard V. Anderson, MD *(Chapter 18)*
Department of Surgery
New York University Medical Center

Michael Artman, MD *(Chapter 17)*
Professor of Pediatrics, Physiology, and Neuroscience
New York University Medical Center

Stanley W. Ashley, MD *(Chapter 24)*
Associate Professor of Surgery
Harvard Medical School

Annabel Barber, MD *(Chapters 2 and 4)*
Associate Professor of Surgery
University of Nevada School of Medicine

Philip S. Barie, MD *(Chapter 32)*
Associate Professor of Surgery
Cornell University Medical College

Monica Bertagnolli, MD *(Chapter 9)*
Assistant Professor of Surgery
Cornell University Medical Center

Elisa H. Birnbaum, MD *(Chapter 26)*
Assistant Professor of Surgery
Washington University School of Medicine

Kirby I. Bland, MD *(Chapter 14)*
J. Murray Beardsley Professor and Chairman
Brown University School of Medicine

Michael F. Boland, MD *(Chapter 40)*
Department of Neurosurgery
Missouri Baptist Medical Center

Jon M. Burch, MD *(Chapter 6)*
Professor of Surgery
University of Colorado Health Sciences Center

Steve E. Calvano, PhD *(Chapter 1)*
Associate Professor of Surgery
University of Medicine and Dentistry of New Jersey—
Robert Wood Johnson Medical School

William T. Chance, MD *(Chapter 22)*
Associate Professor of Surgery
University of Cincinnati Medical Center

Joseph M. Civetta, MD *(Chapter 12)*
Professor and Head, Department of Surgery
University of Connecticut Health Sciences Center

Orlo H. Clark, MD *(Chapter 36)*
Professor and Vice Chair of Surgery
University of California, San Francisco

I. Kelman Cohen, MD *(Chapter 8)*
Professor of Surgery (Division of Plastic and
Reconstructive Surgery)
Medical College of Virginia
Virginia Commonwealth University

John J. Coleman III, MD *(Chapter 15)*
Professor of Surgery (Plastic Surgery)
Indiana University School of Medicine

Stephen B. Colvin, MD *(Chapters 17 and 19)*
Chief of Cardiothoracic Surgery
New York University Medical Center

Edward M. Copeland III, MD *(Chapter 14)*
The Edward R. Woodward Professor and Chairman of
Surgery
University of Florida College of Medicine

William T. Couldwell, MD, PhD *(Chapter 35)*
Professor and Chairman of Neurological Surgery
New York Medical College

Mary C. Crossland, BSN, RN *(Chapter 8)*
Director, Wound Healing Center
Columbia Retreat Hospital

Anthony M. D'Alessandro, MD *(Chapter 10)*
Associate Professor of Surgery
University of Wisconsin Medical School

John M. Daly, MD *(Chapters 9, 24, and 33)*
Lewis Atterbury Stimson Professor and Chairman of
Surgery
Cornell University Medical College

Jerome J. DeCosse, MD *(Chapter 9)*
Lewis Thomas University Professor
Cornell University Medical College

Mark H. Deierhoi, MD *(Chapter 10)*
Professor of Surgery
University of Alabama at Birmingham

Tom R. DeMeester, MD *(Chapter 23)*
Professor and Chairman of Surgery
University of Southern California School of Medicine,
    Los Angeles

Robert F. Diegelmann, PhD *(Chapter 8)*
Professor of Surgery (Plastic Surgery)
Medical College of Virginia
Virginia Commonwealth University

B. Mark Evers, MD *(Chapter 25)*
Chela and Jimmy Storm Distinguished Professor of
    Surgery
University of Texas Medical Branch

Denis Evoy, MD *(Chapter 24)*
Department of Surgery
Cork University Hospital, Ireland

Gary A. Fantini, MD *(Chapter 33)*
Associate Professor of Surgery
Cornell University Medical College

David R. Farley, MD *(Chapter 36)*
Assistant Professor of Surgery
Mayo Medical School

Elliott Fegelman, MD *(Chapter 11)*
Assistant Professor of Surgery
University of Cincinnati Medical Center

Josef E. Fischer, MD *(Chapters 11, 22, and 33)*
Christian R. Holmes Professor and Chairman of
    Surgery
University of Cincinnati Medical Center

James W. Fleshman, MD *(Chapter 26)*
Associate Professor of Surgery
Washington University School of Medicine

Reginald J. Franciose, MD *(Chapter 6)*
Assistant Professor of Surgery
University of Colorado Health Sciences Center

Robert D. Fry, MD *(Chapter 26)*
Professor of Colon and Rectal Surgery
Thomas Jefferson University

Aubrey C. Galloway, MD *(Chapters 17, 18 and 19)*
Professor of Surgery
New York University Medical Center

Robert J. Ginsberg, MD *(Chapter 16)*
Professor of Surgery
Cornell University Medical
Memorial Sloan-Kettering Cancer Center

Martin F. Graham, MD *(Chapter 8)*
Professor of Pediatrics, Biochemistry, and Molecular
    Biophysics
Medical College of Virginia
Virginia Commonwealth University

Richard M. Green, MD *(Chapters 20 and 21)*
Associate Professor of Surgery
University of Rochester Medical Center

Eugene A. Grossi, MD *(Chapter 18)*
Associate Professor of Surgery
New York University Medical Center

Philip C. Guzzetta, MD *(Chapter 37)*
Professor and Chairman of Pediatric Surgery
University of Texas Southwestern Medical Center

David M. Heimbach, MD *(Chapter 7)*
Professor of Surgery
University of Washington School of Medicine

Julian T. Hoff, MD *(Chapter 40)*
Professor of Neurologic Surgery
University of Michigan

Richard J. Howard, MD *(Chapter 5)*
Robert H. and Kathleen M. Axline Professor of
    Surgery
University of Florida College of Medicine

John G. Hunter, MD *(Chapter 44)*
Professor of Surgery
Emory University

William W. Hurd, MD *(Chapter 39)*
Associate Professor of Obstetrics and Gynecology
Indiana University School of Medicine

Jay Johannigman, MD *(Chapter 11)*
Assistant Professor of Surgery
University of Cincinnati Medical Center

M. J. Jurkiewicz, MD *(Chapter 43)*
Professor of Surgery (Plastic Surgery), Emeritus
Emory University School of Medicine

Munci Kalayoglu, MD *(Chapter 10)*
Professor of Surgery and Pediatrics
University of Wisconsin Medical School

Allan D. Kirk, MD, PhD *(Chapter 10)*
Senior Scientist
Naval Medical Research Institute

Orlando C. Kirton, MD *(Chapter 12)*
Associate Professor of Surgery
University of Miami School of Medicine

Stuart J. Knechtle, MD *(Chapter 10)*
Associate Professor of Surgery
University of Wisconsin Medical School

Ira J. Kodner, MD *(Chapter 26)*
Professor of Surgery
Washington University School of Medicine

Rosemary A. Kozar, MD *(Chapter 27)*
Assistant Professor of Surgery
Allegheny University of the Health Sciences

Edward Lin, DO *(Chapter 1)*
Department of Surgery
New York Hospital Medical Center

Stephen R. Lowry, MD *(Chapters 1 and 2)*
Professor and Chairman of Surgery
University of Medicine and Dentistry of New Jersey—
Robert Wood Johnson Medical School

Frederick Luchette, MD *(Chapter 22)*
Associate Professor of Surgery
University of Cincinnati Medical Center

Stephen J. Mathes, MD *(Chapter 13)*
Professor of Surgery (Plastic Surgery)
University of California, San Francisco

John D. McConnell, MD *(Chapter 38)*
Professor and Chairman of Urology
University of Texas Southwestern Medical Center

Jeffrey S. Miller, MD *(Chapter 19)*
Department of Surgery
New York University Medical Center

Ernest E. Moore, MD *(Chapter 6)*
Professor of Surgery
University of Colorado Health Sciences Center

Donald L. Morton, MD *(Chapter 9)*
Medical Director and Surgeon-in-Chief
John Wayne Cancer Institute at Saint John's Health
Center, Santa Monica, CA
Professor Emeritus
University of California, Los Angeles School of Medi-
cine

Kurt D. Newman, MD *(Chapter 37)*
Professor of Surgery and Pediatrics
George Washington University School of Medicine

Jeffrey A. Norton, MD *(Chapter 35)*
Professor and Vice Chairman of Surgery
University of California, San Francisco School of
Medicine

Michael S. Nussbaum, MD *(Chapter 22)*
Associate Professor of Surgery
University of Cincinnati Medical Center

Jon S. Odorico, MD *(Chapter 10)*
Assistant Professor of Surgery
University of Wisconsin Medical School

Kenneth Ouriel, MD *(Chapters 20 and 21)*
Associate Professor of Surgery and Radiology
University of Rochester Medical Center

Margaret S. Pearle, MD *(Chapter 38)*
Assistant Professor of Urology
University of Texas Southwestern Medical Center

Clayton A. Peimer, MD *(Chapter 42)*
Professor of Orthopaedic Surgery
School of Medicine and Biomedical Sciences
State University of New York, Buffalo

Jeffrey H. Peters, MD *(Chapter 23)*
Associate Professor of Surgery
University of California, Los Angeles School of
Medicine

Paul C. Peters, MD *(Chapter 38)*
Professor Emeritus of Urology
University of Texas Southwestern Medical Center

Thomas E. Read, MD *(Chapter 26)*
Assistant Professor of Surgery
Washington University School of Medicine

Howard A. Reber, MD *(Chapter 30)*
Professor of Surgery
University of California, Los Angeles School of
Medicine

Bruce A. Reitz, MD *(Chapter 10)*
The Norman E. Shumway Professor and Chairman of
Cardiothoracic Surgery
Stanford University School of Medicine

Robert E. Rogers, MD *(Chapter 39)*
Emeritus Professor of Obstetrics and Gynecology
Indiana University School of Medicine

Randy N. Rosier, MD *(Chapter 41)*
Professor of Orthopaedics
University of Rochester Medical Center

Joel J. Roslyn, MD *(Chapter 27)*
Alma Dea Morani Professor and Chairman of Surgery
Allegheny University of the Health Sciences

Valerie W. Rusch, MD *(Chapter 16)*
Professor of Surgery
Cornell University Medical College
Memorial Sloan-Kettering Cancer Center

Gregory P. Sadler, MD *(Chapter 36)*
Department of Surgery
Oxford University, England

Jay J. Schnitzer, MD, PhD *(Chapter 37)*
Assistant Professor of Surgery
Harvard Medical School

Seymour I. Schwartz, MD *(Chapters 3, 28, 29 and 31)*

Distinguished Alumni Professor and Chair of Surgery
University of Rochester Medical Center

G. Tom Shires, MD *(Chapters 2 and 4)*

Professor of Surgery
University of Nevada School of Medicine

G. Thomas Shires III, MD *(Chapters 2 and 4)*

Associate Professor of Surgery
University of Texas Southwestern Medical Center

Marie F. Simard, MD *(Chapter 35)*

Research Assistant Professor of Neuroendocrinology
New York Medical College

Hans W. Sollinger, MD *(Chapter 10)*

Folker O. Belzer Professor of Surgery
University of Wisconsin Medical School

Joseph Solomkin, MD *(Chapter 32)*

Professor of Surgery, Pharmacology and Cell Biophysics
University of Cincinnati Medical Center

Frank C. Spencer, MD *(Chapter 19)*

Professor and Chairman of Surgery
New York University Medical Center

Mark R. Sultan, MD *(Chapter 15)*

Assistant Professor of Surgery
Columbia-Presbyterian Medical Center

Gregory P. Sutton, MD *(Chapter 39)*

Mary Fendrich Hulman Professor of Gynecologic Oncology
Indiana University School of Medicine

James C. Thompson, MD *(Chapter 25)*

Ashbel Smith Professor of Surgery
University of Texas Medical Branch

Courtney M. Townsend, Jr., MD *(Chapter 25)*

John Woods Harris Distinguished Professor of Surgery
University of Texas Medical Branch

Jon A. van Heerden, MD *(Chapter 36)*

Fred C. Andersen Professor of Surgery
Mayo Medical School

Albert J. Varon, MD *(Chapter 12)*

Professor of Anesthesiology and Surgery
University of Miami School of Medicine

Michael P. Vezeridis, MD *(Chapter 14)*

Professor of Surgery
Brown University School of Medicine

George M. Wantz, MD *(Chapter 34)*

Clinical Professor of Surgery
Cornell University Medical College

Glenn D. Warden, MD *(Chapter 7)*

Professor of Surgery
University of Cincinnati Medical Center

Martin H. Weiss, MD *(Chapter 35)*

Professor and Chairman of Neurosurgery
University of Southern California School of Medicine, Los Angeles

Michael A. West, MD, PhD *(Chapter 32)*

Associate Professor of Surgery
University of Minnesota

Dietmar W. Wittmann, MD, PhD *(Chapter 32)*

Professor of Surgery
Medical College of Wisconsin

Robert J. Wood, MD *(Chapter 43)*

Associate Professor of Surgery (Plastic Surgery)
Emory University School of Medicine

Isaac L. Wornum, III, MD *(Chapter 8)*

Associate Professor of Surgery (Plastic Surgery)
Medical College of Virginia
Virginia Commonwealth University

Dorne R. Yager, PhD *(Chapter 8)*

Assistant Professor of Surgery (Plastic and Reconstructive Surgery), Microbiology, and Immunology
Medical College of Virginia
Virginia Commonwealth University

David M. Young, MD *(Chapter 13)*

Assistant Professor-in-Residence
University of California at San Francisco School of Medicine

David D. Yuh, MD *(Chapter 10)*

Department of Cardiothoracic Surgery
Stanford University School of Medicine

Preface

The Seventh Edition of *Principles of Surgery* completes our participation in the surgical education of an entire generation of medical students and surgical residents throughout the world. We also were pleased to have played a role in the continuing education of practicing surgeons.

Many have regarded teachers as the noblest of people; others attach that designation to healers. As one who has been privileged to serve in both roles, namely, to have provided a vehicle for educating those who will perpetuate the healing profession in the realm of Surgery, and, at the same time, to have had the opportunity to participate in relieving patients of their disease, I consider myself twice blessed.

As a surgeon I have been satisfied by successes in patient care. As a teacher, I have been literally rewarded by expressions of appreciation by our readers who have indicated that we have enhanced their education.

Thirty-two years have passed since we accepted the publisher's and our own self-generated challenge to develop a "new and modern" textbook of Surgery. The favorable reception and the text's longevity suggest that we have succeeded. As the landmark of the Seventh Edition is completed, the frustrations and toils are erased and what remains is an immeasurable sense of gratification.

Seymour I. Schwartz, M.D.
June, 1998

ACKNOWLEDGMENT

We are particularly appreciative of the efforts of Andrea Weinstein, who had an integral role in each of the processes throughout the development of this edition. John Guardiano also contributed significantly to the technical editing of the manuscript.

Preface to the First Edition

The raison d'être for a new textbook in a discipline which has been served by standard works for many years was the Editorial Board's initial conviction that a distinct need for a modern approach in the dissemination of surgical knowledge existed. As incoming chapters were reviewed, both the need and satisfaction became increasingly apparent and, at the completion, we felt a sense of excitement at having the opportunity to contribute to the education of modern and future students concerned with the care of surgical patients.

The recent explosion of factual knowledge has emphasized the need for a presentation which would provide the student an opportunity to assimilate pertinent facts in a logical fashion. This would then permit correlation, synthesis of concepts, and eventual extrapolation to specific situations. The physiologic bases for diseases are therefore emphasized and the manifestations and diagnostic studies are considered as a reflection of pathophysiology. Therapy then becomes logical in this schema and the necessity to regurgitate facts is minimized. In appreciation of the impact which Harrison's PRINCIPLES OF INTERNAL MEDICINE has had, the clinical manifestations of the disease processes are considered in detail for each area. Since the operative procedure represents the one element in the therapeutic armamentarium unique to the surgeon, the indications, important technical considerations, and complications receive appropriate emphasis. While we appreciate that a textbook cannot hope to incorporate an atlas of surgical procedures, we have provided the student a single book which will satisfy the sequential demands in the care and considerations of surgical patients.

The ultimate goal of the Editorial Board has been to collate a book which is deserving of the adjective "modern." We have therefore selected as authors dynamic and active contributors to their particular fields. The au courant concept is hopefully apparent throughout the entire work and is exemplified by appropriate emphasis on diseases of modern surgical interest, such as trauma, transplantation, and the recently appreciated importance of rehabilitation. Cardiovascular surgery is presented in keeping with the exponential strides recently achieved.

There are two major subdivisions to the text. In the first twelve chapters, subjects that transcend several organ systems are presented. The second portion of the book represents a consideration of specific organ systems and surgical specialties.

Throughout the text, the authors have addressed themselves to a sophisticated audience, regarding the medical student as a graduate student, incorporating material generally sought after by the surgeon in training and presenting information appropriate for the continuing education of the practicing surgeon. The need for a text such as we have envisioned is great and the goal admittedly high. It is our hope that this effort fulfills the expressed demands.

Seymour I. Schwartz, M.D.

CHAPTER 25

Small Intestine

B. Mark Evers, Courtney M. Townsend, Jr., and James C. Thompson

INTRODUCTION

Considered teleologically, the small bowel is the raison d'être for the entire gut. The esophagus brings food to the stomach, which prepares it for digestion. The exocrine secretions of the liver and pancreas make digestion possible. Digestion is achieved in the lumen of the small bowel, and nutrients are absorbed through the small-bowel mucosa; the colon disposes of whatever is left.

In addition to its vital function in nutrition, the small bowel has other important roles. It is the largest endocrine organ in the body. It has tremendous defenses against infection and is one of the most important, if not the most important, organs in immune defense. It is a marvel of efficiency and works so well that, excepting the proximal 3 cm of the duodenum, it is seldom afflicted with disease. We are supplied with a great excess of small bowel and can exist on less than one-half of the absorptive surface provided.

Until recently, the small intestine had been relatively inaccessible for nonoperative diagnostic procedures, compared to the stomach or colon. Several diagnostic techniques are now available for specific diseases of the small bowel. Mucosal biopsy specimens obtained with the peroral biopsy capsule are often diagnostic in diffuse mucosal diseases. Enteroclysis is a more sensitive radiographic technique than the conventional barium follow-through examination of the small bowel. Selective mesenteric angiography often is helpful in cases of discrete lesions with abnormal vascular patterns, such as neoplasms, vascular malformations, or actively bleeding lesions. Scintigraphy may be helpful in localizing sites of bleeding. Fiberoptic endoscopy of the duodenum, proximal jejunum, and distal ileum are routinely employed.

Some diseases that affect the small intestine are discussed in other chapters: intestinal obstruction (Chap 22), mesenteric vascular disease (Chap 33), diseases of the intestine in infancy and childhood (Chap 37), the intestine in trauma (Chap 6), and duodenal and gastrojejunal peptic ulcer (Chap 24).

EMBRYOLOGY

The primitive gut forms during the fourth week of fetal development. The endoderm gives rise to most of the epithelium and glands of the digestive tract. The splanchnic mesodern surrounding the endoderm gives rise to muscular connective tissue and other layers comprising the wall of the digestive tract. Early in the fourth week the duodenum begins to develop from the caudal portion of the foregut and the cranial portion of the midgut. The remainder of the small bowel is derived from the midgut. During the fifth week, the fetal gut rapidly elongates and herniates through the umbilicus (Fig. 25-1). This midgut loop has both cranial and caudal limbs; the cephalic limb develops into the distal duodenum to proximal ileum, and the caudal limb becomes the distal ileum to proximal two-thirds of the transverse colon. The juncture of the cephalic and caudal limbs is where the vitelline duct joins to the yolk sac. This duct normally becomes obliterated before birth; however, it occasionally persists as a Meckel's diverticulum. This period of midgut herniation lasts until approximately 10 weeks' gestation, after which the intestines return to the abdomen. During this period of rapid elongation and herniation the midgut rotates 90 degrees counterclockwise around an axis formed by the superior mesenteric artery. As the gut reenters the abdomen at about the tenth week, it undergoes a further 180-degree rotation, thus completing 270 degrees of rotation from the starting point. The proximal jejunum is the first portion to reenter the abdomen and occupies the left side of the abdomen, with subsequent loops lying more to the right. The cecum enters last and is located temporarily in the right upper quadrant; during the third to fifth month of fetal gestation, it descends to its normal position in the right lower quadrant. Congenital anomalies of gut malrotation and fixation can occur during this process.

The small intestine is lined with simple cuboidal epithelium during the sixth and seventh weeks of fetal gestation. The rapid epithelial proliferation may lead to occlusion of the lumen, especially in the proximal gut (particularly in the duodenum). The lumen is reestablished during weeks 9 and 10 with the formation of coalescing vacuoles that restore the patency of the lumen. Villi begin to form first in the proximal intestine at 9 weeks, proceeding caudad and eventually lining the entire gut. Differentiated crypt cells appear between the ninth and twentieth weeks of gestation. Crypt formation begins in the tenth to twelfth weeks of gestation.

This complex and regimented pattern of gut differentiation appears to be mediated by sets of genes that are characteristically turned on and off with temporal and spatial specificity during developmental transitions as the gut evolves into its adult form. This developmental pattern also appears to be dependent on interaction with the mesoderm and lamina propria, which may provide "instructive" signals for developmental progression. The epithelial cells of the gut are generated from a fixed stem-cell population localized in the lower portion of the crypts that give rise to four main cell types: absorptive enterocytes, goblet cells, enteroendocrine cells, and Paneth cells. Until recently the analysis of the factors regulating these complex developmental processes in vivo was not possible; however, elegant studies by Gordon and colleagues, using transgenic mouse techniques, have described marker systems for inferring the biologic properties of intestinal stem cells and provided direct evidence of the transcriptional regulation of spatial patterns of intestinal gene expression. Other investigators have used the intestine-specific sucrase-isomaltase and neurotensin genes as molecular models to better understand the factors regulating gut development and eventual maturation.

ANATOMY

The most impressive thing about the small bowel is its immense mucosal surface area, which is responsible for the organ's tremendously efficient digestion of food. Several layers of muscle, combined with actin and myosin components in the microstructures, provide great motility, so that not only is there great surface area, but the interface between the surface and the luminal contents presented for absorption is in constant motion as well.

Gross Anatomy

The small bowel extends from the pylorus to the cecum. The length of the small intestine depends entirely on the state of bowel activity at the time of measurement. Careful estimates provide a duodenal length of 20 cm, a jejunal length of 100 to 110 cm, and an ileal length of 150 to 160 cm. The jejunoileum extends from the peritoneal fold that supports the duodenal-jejunal junction (the ligament of Treitz) downward to the ileocecal valve. The jejunoileum is estimated to constitute 60 percent of the entire length of the gut and to be approximately 160 percent of the body height, so that the small bowel is considerably longer in a 7-ft basketball player than in a 5-ft jockey.

Generally the jejunum occupies the upper abdomen, especially on the left, and is in contact with the pancreas, spleen, colon, and left kidney and adrenal gland. Affliction of these organs may affect the jejunum; pancreatitis, for example, may cause local ileus (the "sentinel loop") of the jejunum.

The jejunum has a larger circumference and is thicker than the ileum, and it may be identified at operation because of this and also because the mesenteric vessels usually form only one or two arcades and send out long, straight vasa recta to the mesenteric border of the jejunum. In contrast, the blood supply to the ileum may have four or five separate arcades; the vasa recta are shorter, and, most important, there is usually much more fat in the mesentery of the ileum than in that of the jejunum (Fig. 25-2). The jejunal mesentery may be transparent, but mesenteric fat usually reaches all the way to the bowel in the ileum. The ileum occupies the lower abdomen, especially on the right, and the pelvis. It is smaller in diameter and somewhat more mobile.

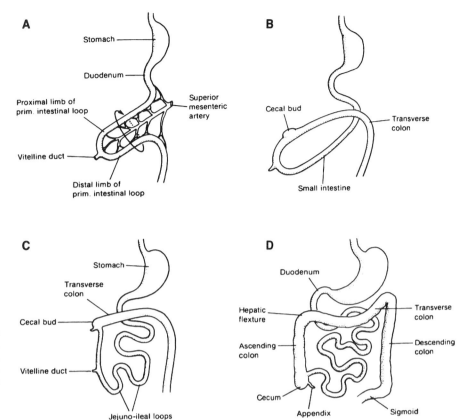

FIG. 25-1. Rotation of the intestine. *A. The intestine after a 90-degree rotation around the axis of the superior mesenteric artery, the proximal loop on the right, and the distal loop on the left. B. The intestinal loop after a further 180-degree rotation. The transverse colon passes in front of the duodenum. C. Position of the intestinal loops after reentry into the abdominal cavity. Note the elongation of the small intestine, with formation of the small intestine loops. D. Final position of the intestines after descent of the cecum into the right iliac fossa. (From: Podolsky DK, Babyatshky MW: Growth and development of the gastrointestinal tract, in Yamada T [ed]: Textbook of Gastroenterology, vol 2. Philadelphia, JB Lippincott, 1995, chap 23, with permission. [Adapted from Sadler TW [ed], Langman's Medical Embryology, 5th ed. Baltimore, Williams & Wilkins, 1985].)*

Except for the duodenum the small bowel is entirely covered with visceral peritoneum (the serosa) and is tethered only by its attachment to the mesentery, through which course arteries, veins, and lymphatics. The mesentery is obliquely attached to the posterior body wall, beginning superiorly well to the left of the second lumbar vertebra and ending obliquely downward and to the right to overlie the right sacroiliac joint. The mesentery normally is covered with glistening, nonadherent peritoneum, but after trauma (external, chemical, septic, or operative) it may become adherent to other surfaces (mesenteric, visceral, or parietal) and greatly limit bowel mobility.

Except for the proximal duodenum, which is supplied by branches of the celiac axis, the blood supply of the small bowel is entirely from the superior mesenteric artery, which is the second major branch of the infradiaphragmatic aorta. The superior mesenteric artery also supplies the appendix, cecum, and ascending and proximal transverse colon. There is an abundant collateral blood supply to the small bowel provided by the vas-

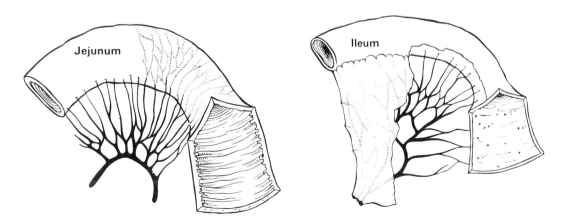

FIG. 25-2. Jejunum contrasted with ileum. In the jejunum, note the larger diameter, thicker wall, prominent plicae circulares, one or two arterial arcades, long vasa recta, and translucent (fat-free) areas at the mesenteric border. The ileum is smaller and thinner walled and has few plicae, multiple vascular arcades with short vasa recta, and abundant mesenteric fat.

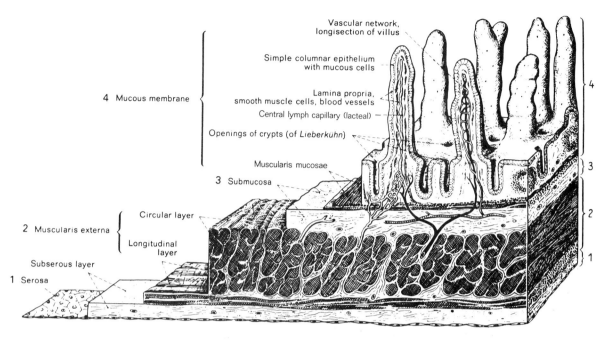

FIG. 25-3. *Layers of the small intestine. A large surface is provided by villi for the absorption of required nutriments. The solitary lymph follicles in the lamina propria of the mucous membrane are not labeled. In the stroma of both sectioned villi are shown the central chyle (lacteal) vessels or the villous capillaries. (From: Sobotta J, Figge FHJ, Hild WJ: Atlas of Human Anatomy. New York, Hafner, 1974, with permission.)*

cular arcades in the mesentery. In spite of this collateral supply, occlusion of a major branch of the superior mesenteric artery, or of the superior mesenteric artery itself, will lead to bowel death if not quickly corrected. Venous drainage of the segments of the small bowel is in parallel with the arterial supply. The superior mesenteric vein joins the splenic vein behind the neck of the pancreas to form the portal vein. The blood leaving the gut, with its relatively high oxygen content, provides a significant portion of the oxygen supply to the liver.

If the mesentery is not greatly infiltrated by fat and if there are no peritoneal adhesions, the bowel is extraordinarily mobile on its vascular tether. In some individuals jejunal segments may be sufficiently mobilized to allow anastomosis in the neck to replace the cervical esophagus.

The small bowel contains major deposits of lymphatic tissue, particularly in the Peyer's patches of the ileum. There is a rich lymphatic drainage of the entire small bowel, and this plays a major role in fat absorption. Lymphatic drainage proceeds from the mucosa through the wall of the bowel to a set of nodes adjacent to the bowel in the mesentery. Drainage continues to a group of regional nodes adjacent to the mesenteric arterial arcades and then to a group at the base of the superior mesenteric vessels. From there, lymph goes to the cisterna chyli and thence up the thoracic ducts to empty into the venous system in the neck. The lymphatics of the gut play a major role in immune defense and also in the spread of cells arising from neoplasms in the gut.

The small-bowel mucosa is characterized by transverse folds (plicae circulares, or valves or folds of Kerckring), though these are absent in the duodenal bulb and in the distal ileum. They are more prominent in the distal duodenum and the jejunum, where they may reach 1 cm in height and form interlocking transverse

ridges (see Fig. 25-2). The small-bowel mucosa has a pink, velvety appearance with a glistening surface. It usually is thicker in the jejunum than in the ileum, where there may be no folds and the surface may be entirely smooth, except for small scattered lymphatic nodules.

The innervation of the small bowel comes from both sympathetic and parasympathetic systems. Parasympathetic fibers come from the vagus and traverse the celiac ganglia. They affect secretion and motility and probably all phases of bowel activity. Vagal afferent fibers are present but apparently do not carry pain impulses. The sympathetic fibers come from the three sets of splanchnic nerves and have their ganglion cells usually in a plexus around the base of the superior mesenteric artery. Their motor impulses affect blood vessel motility and probably gut secretion and motility. Pain from the intestine is mediated through general visceral afferent fibers in the sympathetic system.

Histology

The wall of the small bowel has four layers—the serosa, the muscularis, the submucosa, and the mucosa (Fig. 25-3).

Serosa. The serosa, the outermost layer, consists of visceral peritoneum that encircles the jejunoileum but covers the duodenum only anteriorly. It consists of a single layer of flattened mesothelial cells.

Muscularis. The muscularis consists of a thin outer longitudinal layer and a thicker inner circular layer of smooth muscle. Specialized gaps in the muscle-cell membranes permit cell-to-cell communication, which facilitates the ability of the muscle layer to function as an electrical syncytium. Ganglion cells from

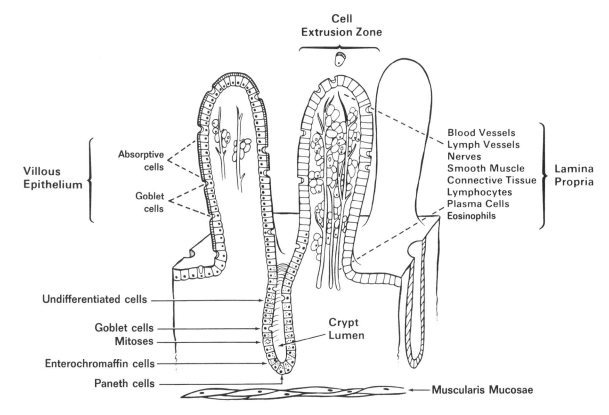

FIG. 25-4. Schematic diagram of two sectioned villi and a crypt of Lieberkühn illustrating the histologic organization of the small intestine mucosa. (Adapted and redrawn from: *Trier JS et al, in Sleisenger MH, Fordtran JS [eds]: Gastrointestinal Disease: Pathophysiology, Diagnosis, Management. Philadelphia, WB Saunders, 1983, chap 48, with permission.*)

the myenteric (Auerbach's) plexus are interposed between the two muscle layers and send fibers into both layers.

Submucosa. The submucosa is a layer of fibroelastic connective tissue containing blood vessels and nerves. It is the strongest component of the bowel wall and therefore must be included when sutures are placed through the bowel. It contains elaborate networks of lymphatics, arterioles, and venules and an extensive plexus of nerve fibers and ganglion cells (Meissner's plexus). Although frequently subdivided, the nerves from the mucosa, submucosa, and muscle layers are interconnected by small nerve fibers, and cross-connections between adrenergic and cholinergic elements have been described.

Mucosa. Looked on as a device to increase absorptive surface, the small-bowel mucosa is an architectural marvel. The gross transverse folds, the fingerlike villi protruding into the lumen of the bowel, the microvilli (brush border) covering the cells, and the glycocalyx fuzz covering the microvilli each tremendously increase the surface area exposed to luminal contents. Villi protrude 0.5 to 1 mm into the lumen; they are tallest in the distal duodenum and the proximal jejunum and become progressively shorter toward the terminal ileum.

The mucosa can be divided into three layers—the muscularis mucosae, the lamina propria, and the epithelium. The deepest of these, the muscularis mucosae, is a thin sheet of muscle separating mucosa from submucosa. The lamina propria is a continuous layer connective tissue between the epithelium and the

muscularis mucosae. It extends into the villi and around the pitlike crypts of Lieberkühn (Fig. 25-4). The lamina propria contains, additionally, a variety of cells—plasma cells, lymphocytes, mast cells, eosinophils, macrophages, fibroblasts, smooth muscle cells—and noncellular connective tissue. The lamina propria is the architectural base on which the epithelium lies, but it also has important functions of its own and apparently serves protectively to combat microorganisms that penetrate the overlying epithelium. The plasma cells are an active site of synthesis of immunoglobulins. In addition, cells in the lamina propria release various mediators (for example, cytokines, arachidonic acid metabolites, and histamine) that can modulate various cellular functions of the overlying epithelium.

The innermost mucosal layer is a continual sheet, one layer thick, of epithelial cells covering the villi and lining the crypts of Lieberkühn (see Fig. 25-4). The main functions of the crypt epithelium are cell renewal and exocrine, endocrine, water, and ion secretion; the main function of the villous epithelium is digestion and absorption. The crypts contain at least four distinct cell types: (1) goblet cells, which secrete mucus; (2) enteroendocrine cells (often called enterochromaffin or argentaffin cells in the older literature), of which there are more than ten distinct populations that produce the gastrointestinal hormones, including gastrin, secretin, cholecystokinin, somatostatin, enteroglucagon, motilin, neurotensin, and gastric inhibitory peptide; (3) Paneth cells, which secrete lysozyme, tumor necrosis factor, and the cryptidins, homologues of leukocyte defensins, and whose function is thought to be related to the host mucosal defense system; and (4) undifferentiated epithelial cells, whose function is to provide for cell renewal. The epithelium of the small intestine is a rapidly proliferating tissue in which old cells are discarded into the lumen and are replaced by newly formed cells that appear to march up from the crypt into the villus in orderly sequence. This trip takes 5 to 7 days in the proximal small bowel, but in the ileum labeled cells may travel from crypt to villous tip in 3 days.

The role of growth factors (e.g., epidermal growth factor, transforming growth factors α and β, insulinlike growth factor, and growth hormone), certain amino acids (glutamine), polyamines, prostaglandins, and gastrointestinal peptides (neurotensin, peptide YY, and glucagonlike peptide-2) in gut epithelial maturation has been the object of extensive recent investigations. All have trophic effects on the small-bowel mucosa; the precise roles, interactions, and importance have not yet been determined.

The epithelium covering the villi consists of scattered endocrine cells, goblet cells, and absorptive cells. The major known functions of the villi are digestion and absorption. These functions are carried out by the absorptive cells, tall columnar cells resting on a thin basement membrane that separates them from the lamina propria. Their luminal surface is covered by microvilli that rest on a terminal web (Fig. 25-5). The microvillar projections multiply the cell surface area exposed to the lumen by 30 times. The microvilli in turn are covered by a fuzzy coat of glycoprotein, the glycocalyx (Figs. 25-6 and 25-7). The microvilli participate actively in absorption and digestion. They contain enzymes for digestion of disaccharides and peptides, and certain cells may contain specific receptors that facilitate absorption (for example, certain ileal cells have receptors for vitamin B_{12} on their microvilli).

The plasma (or cell) membranes of the epithelial cells consist of three layers and are thicker over the microvilli than over the lateral and basal portions of the cell (see Fig. 25-6). The lateral portion of the plasma membrane also is specialized. There are tight junctions between epithelial cells that prevent communication between intercellular spaces and the lumen. Immediately underneath the tight junction is a narrow space called an intermediate junction, and beneath that is a desmosome, which provides tight attachments of adjacent membrane by binding adjacent cells together. The depths of the tight junctions are greater between adjacent absorptive cells than between adjacent undifferentiated crypt cells. The permeability of the barrier between the intestinal lumen and the space between cells may vary from one location to another.

The cytoplasm immediately beneath the microvilli consists of fine filaments known as the terminal web. This interconnects with filaments forming the core of the microvilli, which contain actin (see Fig. 25-6). Myosin also may be present at the base of the microvilli, and these contractile proteins may allow movement and contraction of the microvilli.

The processes of digestion and absorption within the epithelial cells are carried out by specific organelles (see Fig. 25-5). The mitochondria participate in intracellular oxidation and provide energy for metabolism. The lysosomal sacs contain cytotoxic substances and intracellular waste products. The endoplasmic reticulum is the main synthesizing element within the cell

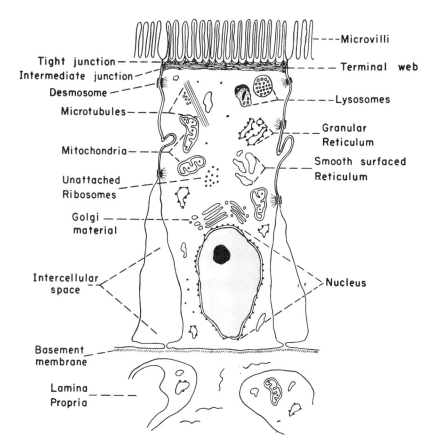

FIG. 25-5. Schematic diagram of an intestinal absorptive cell. (From: *Trier JS et al, in Sleisenger MH, Fordtran JE [eds]: Gastrointestinal Disease: Pathophysiology, Diagnosis, Management. Philadelphia, WB Saunders, 1983, chap 48, with permission.*)

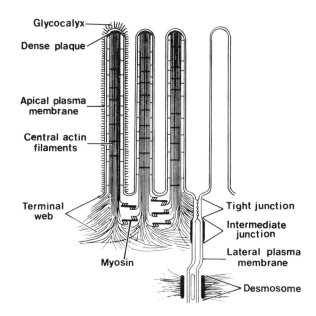

FIG. 25-6. *Schematic illustration of the specializations of the apical cytoplasm of the plasma membrane of intestinal absorptive cells. (From: Trier JS et al, in Sleisenger MH, Fordtran SJ [eds]: Gastrointestinal Disease: Pathophysiology, Diagnosis, Management. Philadelphia, WB Saunders, 1983, chap 48, with permission.)*

and appears to be responsible for at least two major processes in fat absorption, the resynthesis of triglycerides from absorbed fatty acid fragments, and the synthesis of the lipoprotein coat for chylomicrons. It is also the major synthetic site for intracellular digestive enzymes. The Golgi apparatus segregates, stores, and chemically modifies material that is absorbed and synthesized by the cell.

It may be instructive to review the path of a food element absorbed from the intestinal lumen. Initial contact is with the glycocalyx coating the microvilli, where some digestion may occur. Products of this digestion may go through the microvillous membrane, traversing the terminal web into the cytoplasm. The absorbed material may then move either laterally into the intracellular spaces or into the channels of the endoplasmic reticulum, where it may be biochemically modified and transmitted to the Golgi material, where it may be stored. Eventually the material leaves the cell by crossing either the lateral or the basal plasma (cell) membrane. It penetrates the basal lamina to enter the lamina propria, where it traverses the lymphatic or capillary endothelial cells to gain access to lymph or blood.

PHYSIOLOGY
Motility

Food is propelled through the small bowel by a complex series of muscular contractions. Motility patterns in the small bowel vary greatly between the fed and the fasting states. Pacesetter potentials, probably originating in the duodenum, initiate a series of contractions that propel food through the small bowel. These contractions are of two types—segmentation and peristalsis. Contractions of the circular muscle divide the bowel into segments that are moved to and fro over the column of bowel contents for a short distance. The contents of adjacent segments then

combine, and the process is repeated. About 40 percent of contractions are segmental. The circular muscle also initiates peristalsis, circular contractions migrating in an aboral direction, propelling intestinal contents onward. The peristaltic reflex may function independently of extrinsic nerves. Abnormal waves of powerful contractions *(peristaltic rushes)* may rapidly traverse the entire segment of small intestine during episodes of enteritis.

During the interdigestive (fasting) period between meals, the bowel is regularly swept by a series of contractions initiated by the migrating myoelectric complex (MMC). The MMC is under neural and humoral control and initiates a triphasic series of contractions; phase I is resting; in phase II intermittent contractions of moderate amplitude occur; and phase III is the activity front that consists of a brief series of high-pressure waves. The MMC in human beings is stimulated by some (but not all) fluctuating increases in serum concentrations of motilin.

Small-bowel motility is modulated by neural and humoral influences. Extrinsic nerves to the small bowel are vagal and sympathetic. Vagal fibers have two functionally different effects; one is cholinergic and excitatory, and the other is peptidergic and probably inhibitory. Sympathetic fibers from the splanchnics appear chiefly to modulate the activity of intrinsic nerves.

Although gut peptides clearly influence bowel motility, their physiologic function is uncertain, except for the role of motilin in initiating MMC activity. Gastrin, cholecystokinin, and motilin are known to stimulate muscle contraction, whereas muscle activity is inhibited by secretin and often by glucagon (Table 25-1). Cholecystokinin may be physiologically important, since ingestion of a fatty meal may stimulate peristaltic contraction.

Digestion and Absorption

Liters of water and hundreds of grams of food move across the intestinal mucosa from the lumen to the bloodstream each day. The process is remarkably efficient; nearly all food is absorbed unless protected by indigestible cellulose. There is no apparent governor; food absorption is just as efficient in the corpulent as in the starving.

Fat. Most individuals in Western Europe and North America consume 60 to 100 g of fat per day in the form of triglycerides. Fat digestion and absorption occur in the small intestine, where triglycerides are partially hydrolyzed by pancreatic lipase, which splits off the two exposed fatty acids to leave a single central fatty acid still combined with glycerol (beta monoglyceride) plus two fatty acids (Fig. 25-8). The monoglyceride and the fatty acids are poorly soluble in water but combine with bile salts to form micelles. A mixed micelle is composed of bile salts, fatty acids, and the beta monoglyceride, and may also include phospholipids, cholesterol, and fat-soluble vitamins. The micelle must traverse three diffusion barriers in the passive process of entry into the intestinal epithelial cell. These are the unstirred water layer, the mucous coat overlying the brush border, and the lipid bilayer membrane making up the brush border. The micelle may release its fatty acid and monoglyceride component in traversing these barriers. After disaggregation of the micelle, bile salts remain within the intestinal lumen to enter into the formation of other micelles, and the released fatty acids and monoglycerides traverse the plasma membrane into the epithelial cell. The major metabolic pathway within the cell is initiated by reformation of the triglyceride through the interactions of intracel-

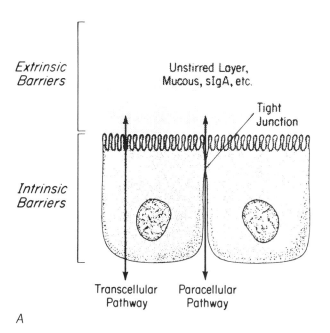

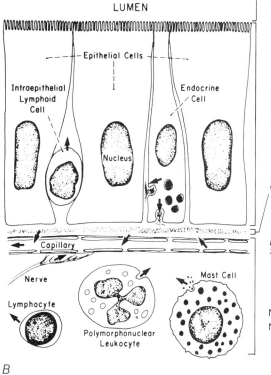

FIG. 25-7. *A. Schematic of gut epithelial barriers. B. The gut epithelium is in close proximity to factors—vascular, neural, immune—that substantially influence epithelial function. C. Schematic of the apial area of cell–cell contact: the junctional complex, which includes the important paracellular barrier, the tight junction or zonulae occludens (ZO). D. Schematic of desmosome. (From: Madara JL: Epithelia: Biologic principles of organization, in Yamada T [ed]: Textbook of Gastroenterology, vol 1. Philadelphia, JB Lippincott, 1991, chap 6, with permission.)*

lular enzymes (see Fig. 25-8) that are associated with the endoplasmic reticulum.

The triglycerides then combine with cholesterol, phospholipids, and apoproteins to form chylomicrons, which consist of an inner core containing almost all triglycerides with a membranous outer coat of phospholipids and apoproteins. The chyomicron exits the cell from the basolateral region and preferentially enters the central lacteal of the villus, where it moves to the thoracic duct. Small fatty acids with chain lengths of C_{10} and less may move directly through the cell into capillaries to flow into the portal vein. The bulk of chylomicron assimilation from the intestinal cell is via lymphatics, but some direct transfer to the portal vein may take place, particularly during periods between meals.

In one of the examples of selective sites of resorption, bile salts are resorbed into the enterohepatic circulation from the dis-

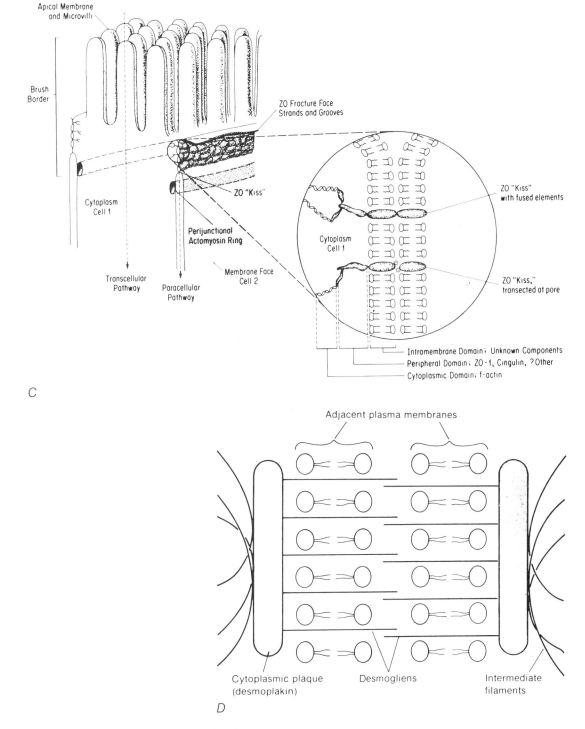

C

D

FIG. 25-7. *C, D. Continued.*

tal ileum (Table 25-2). The total bile salt pool in human beings is about 5 g, and it recirculates about six times every 24 h (the enterohepatic circulation of bile salts). Only about 0.5 g is lost in the stool every day, and this is replaced by resynthesis from cholesterol. All ingested fat is usually absorbed; the small amount appearing in the stool comes from sloughed cells and bacteria.

Protein. Protein digestion is initiated in the stomach, where gastric acid denatures proteins and proteolysis is initiated by activated pepsin. Little actual digestion takes place, however, until protein enters the duodenum and upper jejunum, where they come under the influence of pancreatic proteases. Pancreatic trypsinogen is activated by the duodenal mucosal enzyme enterokinase, and then activated trypsin further activates all proteases.

Table 25-1
Effects of Gastrointestinal Hormones on Small Bowel Motility

Gastrin — ↑[a]	Neurotensin — ↑
Cholecystokinin (CCK) — ↑[a]	Somatostatin — ↑↓[c]
Secretin — ↓[a]	Bombesin — ↑↓
Vasoactive intestinal peptide (VIP) — ↑↓	Enkephalins — ↑↓[c]
Glucagon — ↑↓[a]	Pancreatic polypeptide — ↑
Motilin — ↑[b,c]	Peptide YY (PYY) — ↓
Substance P — ↑	

↑Increased

↓Decreased

[a]Induction of fed pattern of motility from fasting

[b]Possible physiologic role

[c]Induction of migrating motor complexes

SOURCE: Adapted from Sakamoto T, Guo Y-S, Thompson JC: Motility: Gut and biliary, in Thompson JC, Greeley GH Jr, Rayford PL, Townsend CM Jr (eds): *Gastrointestinal Endocrinology.* New York, McGraw-Hill, 1987, pp 123–136.

Endopeptidases (trypsin, elastase, chymotrypsin) act on peptide bonds at the interior of the protein molecule, producing peptides that are substrates for exopeptidases (carboxypeptidases), which serially remove a single amino acid at a time from the carboxyl terminal end of the peptide. The final products are amino acids and peptides of two to six amino acid residues. The intraluminal action of pancreatic proteases is efficient and yields 70 percent short-chain peptides and 30 percent amino acids. Short peptides are optimal substrates for the peptide transport mechanism that brings dipeptides and tripeptides into the cell. Of peptides that are assimilated intact, at least 90 percent are hydrolyzed to free amino acids by cytosol peptidases before delivery to the portal venous system.

Carbohydrate. Western men and women take in about 400 g of carbohydrates a day, 60 percent as starch, 30 percent as sucrose, and 10 percent as lactose. Carbohydrates constitute about half the calories ingested in our society, but in underdeveloped countries they typically provide a much higher proportion.

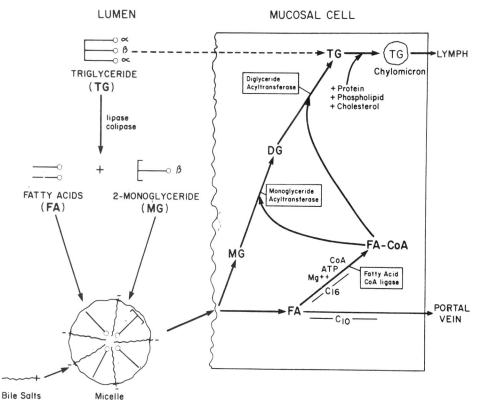

FIG. 25-8. Diagrammatic representation of fat digestion and absorption. Abbreviated structures and names are given in the figure. DG = diglyceride; C_{10} and C_{16} = carbon chain length of amino acids. (From: *Gray GM, in Sleisenger MH, Fordtran JS [eds]: Gastrointestinal Disease: Pathophysiology, Diagnosis, Management. Philadelphia, WB Saunders, 1983, chap 51, with permission.*)

Table 25-2
Differential Sites of Absorption from the Jejunoileum

Proximal	Distal
Calcium	Bile salts
Fat (absorbed mainly in jejunum)	Vitamin B$_{12}$
Folate	
Iron	

Starch is a polysaccharide consisting of long chains of glucose molecules. Amylose makes up 20 percent of starch in the diet and has an alpha glucose-to-glucose bridge. Amylopectin (80 percent of dietary starch) has branching points every 25 molecules along the straight glucose chains. Both have an alpha$_{1-4}$ glucose-linked chain. Alpha amylase attacks the alpha$_{1-4}$ linkage and converts amylose to maltotriose and maltose. Amylase converts amylopectin to shorter dextrins. Intraluminal digestion of starch in the duodenum is rapid, because of the huge amounts of pancreatic amylase, and digestion often is complete by the time the chyme enters the jejunum.

The enzyme responsible for final surface digestion is concentrated in the brush border of the luminal surface (Fig. 25-9). After dietary carbohydrate is reduced to monosaccharides by surface digestion, transport of the released hexoses (glucose, galactose, or fructose) is carried out by a specific process. Glucose and galactose are actively transported across the intestinal membrane, whereas fructose is absorbed by facilitated diffusion. The rate-limiting phenomenon for most carbohydrate absorption occurs during transport through the intestinal cell, but luminal hydrolysis of lactose is slower than its transport capacity, so surface hydrolysis of lactose is rate-limiting.

Water and Electrolytes. In addition to ingested water, salivary, gastric, biliary, pancreatic, and intestinal fluids contribute up to 8 to 10 L of water per day, and all but about 0.5 L per day is resorbed proximal to the ileocecal valve. The small bowel secretes and absorbs huge amounts of water. Net absorption is the algebraic sum of two fluxes going in opposite directions. Water may simply diffuse in or out of the cell or may be drawn through by osmotic or hydrostatic pressures. The osmotic pressures result from active transport of sodium, glucose, or amino acids into cells. Diffusion occurs through pores in plasma cell membranes. Jejunal pores are larger (7 to 9 Å) than those in the ileum (3 to 4 Å). Hypertonic solutions in the duodenum and upper jejunum are rapidly equilibrated to isotonicity by the influx of large amounts of water.

Sodium and chloride are absorbed from the small bowel by active transport, by coupling to organic solutes, and by cotransport on carriers of neutral sodium chloride. A small portion of sodium absorption in the jejunum is by active transport, but the bulk is by coupling to organic solutes. In the ileum sodium is absorbed against steep gradients and is not stimulated by glucose, galactose, or bicarbonate. Bicarbonate is absorbed by a sodium-hydrogen exchange, so that one bicarbonate ion is released into interstitial fluid for every hydrogen ion secreted. Calcium is absorbed by active transport, particularly in the duodenum and jejunum. Absorption appears to be facilitated by an

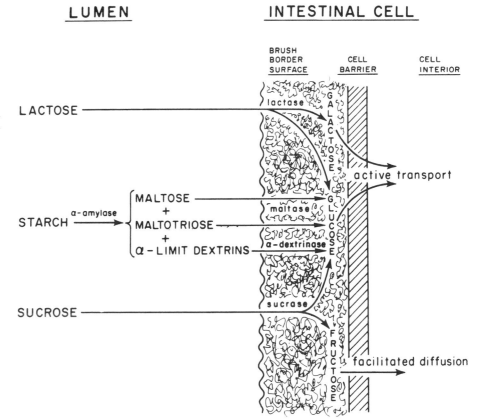

FIG. 25-9. *The digestion and absorption of carbohydrate. Note that only starch is digested in the lumen; other dietary saccharides are hydrolyzed by constitutive enzymes of the intestinal surface. The final monosaccharide products are then transported by their specific mechanisms. (From:* Gray GM, *in Sleisenger MH, Fordtran JS [eds]:* Gastrointestinal Disease: Pathophysiology, Diagnosis, Management. *Philadelphia, WB Saunders, 1983, chap 51, with permission.)*

acid environment and is enhanced by vitamin D and parathormone. Potassium appears to be absorbed by passive diffusion.

Endocrine Function

The mucosa of the small bowel is the primary source of regulatory peptides of the gut, and the muscle wall of the small bowel is rich in peptidergic nerves containing neuroendocrine peptides. Although we often call these agents hormones, they do not always function in a truly endocrine fashion; that is, the active peptides are not always discharged into blood vessels to act on some distant site. Sometimes they are discharged and act locally in a paracrine fashion (for example, bombesin [gastrin-releasing peptide] and somatostatin), or they may serve as neurotransmitters, or they may be discharged into blood vessels after nerve stimulation in a true neuroendocrine manner. We will briefly describe some of these agents.

Secretin. The discovery of secretin in 1902 gave birth to the entire field of endocrinology. Secretin is a 27–amino-acid, helical peptide that is present in specialized cells in the small-bowel mucosa and is released by acidification or by contact with bile and perhaps fat. It acts to stimulate release of water and bicarbonate from pancreatic ductal cells, and when this combination flows into the duodenal lumen the bicarbonate neutralizes gastric acid. The amount of pancreatic bicarbonate released after a meal closely approximates the amount of acid secreted by the stomach. Secretin also acts to stimulate the flow of bile and to inhibit gastrin release, gastric acid secretin, and gastrointestinal motility. Secretin has the unique ability to release gastrin from gastrinomas, and intravenous secretin is used as a diagnostic test in patients in whom the Zollinger-Ellison syndrome is suspected.

Cholecystokinin. Cholecystokinin (CCK) is released from small-bowel mucosa by contact with certain amino acids (especially tryptophan and phenylalanine) and medium- to long-chain fatty acids. In addition, the concentration of intraluminal trypsin and bile acids inversely regulates CCK release. CCK has two major actions: it stimulates contractions of the gallbladder and relaxation of the sphincter of Oddi, and it stimulates the secretion of enzymes by pancreatic acinar cells. CCK also stimulates growth of bowel mucosa and pancreas, stimulates bowel motility, and releases insulin. CCK exists in multiple molecular forms (CCK-8, CCK-33, and CCK-39, among others), and the larger forms contain the smaller ones. CCK and gastrin share the identical C-terminal tetrapeptide (Trp-Met-Asp-Phe-NH$_2$), which explains many of the similarities in their actions.

Other Peptides. Largely through the efforts of Viktor Mutt and colleagues at the Karolinska Institute, several active agents have been isolated from the mucosa of the small bowel that greatly influence physiologic activities of the gut. Of these, only *gastric inhibitory polypeptide* (GIP) has satisfied rigid criteria for hormonal status, but others will be discussed as well. GIP is a 43–amino-acid peptide member of the secretin-glucagon family that is released by fat. Although it was initially studied for its properties of inhibition of gastric secretion, later studies showed that it was a prime incretion candidate, because it greatly stimulated insulin release when levels of glucose were elevated. Glucose-stimulated release of intestinal GIP apparently solves the conundrum posed by the fact that oral ingestion of a fixed amount of glucose releases more insulin than intravenous administration of the same amount. A family of peptides reacting

with glucagon antibodies is present in small-bowel mucosa, and it has been given a variety of names. *Enteroglucagon* is a term used to designate all such gut peptides. It inhibits bowel motility. Recent findings suggest that glucagonlike peptide-2 (GLP-2), a 33–amino-acid peptide, is a potent enterotrophic factor. *Vasoactive intestinal peptide* (VIP) is a 28–amino-acid basic peptide of the secretin-glucagon family that appears to function chiefly as a neuropeptide. VIP is a potent vasodilator, and it stimulates pancreatic and intestinal secretion and inhibits gastric acid secretion. It is the chief agent in the watery diarrhea syndrome caused by pancreatic endocrine tumors. *Motilin* is a 22–amino-acid peptide widely distributed through the gut. It causes contraction of intestinal smooth muscle, including the gallbladder, and appears to be involved in the interdigestive pattern of gut motility. *Bombesin* is a 14–amino-acid peptide that was first isolated from frog skin. It has the capacity to release all gut peptides except secretin. Its mammalian equivalent, gastrin-releasing peptide, is present in small-bowel mucosa, where it probably serves as an "on" switch, regulating release of gastrointestinal hormones. *Somatostatin* is a 14–amino-acid peptide that was first isolated from the brain; it is also widely distributed in the gut, where it probably functions in a paracrine fashion as an "off" switch to inhibit gut hormone release and gastrointestinal secretion. *Neurotensin,* a 13–amino-acid peptide produced in large part by endocrine cells in the ileal mucosa, stimulates water and HCO$_3^-$ secretion from the pancreas, inhibits gastric secretion, and has trophic effects for small and large bowel mucosa. *Peptide YY* (PYY) is a 36–amino-acid peptide in the distal ileum and colon. It inhibits gastric and pancreatic secretion, has no effect on gallbladder motility, and exhibits trophic effects on small-bowel mucosa. PYY is released by perfusion of the colon with fat and may be involved in the physiologic inhibition of pancreatic secretion.

Immune Function

We ingest thousands of bacteria, parasites, and viruses every day. Only a few of these are pathogenic, but the huge surface of the small-bowel mucosa represents a massive potential portal of entry. An important component of bowel defense is the secretory immune system, which produces a special group of antibodies that resist bacterial proliferation, neutralize viruses, and minimize the penetration of enterotoxins.

The small bowel is a major source of immunoglobulin A (IgA). Cells of the lamina propria of the small intestine contain plasma cells that produce IgA. The population of cells producing IgA (the secretory immunoglobulin) is ten times greater than that producing IgG (the antibody mediating general humoral immunity).

Antigens from the intestinal lumen crossing the mucosal barrier contact M cells overlying lymphoid nodules. These cells are specialized for uptake and transport of antigen, which they convey to the underlying lymphoblasts that produce IgA. After interacting with the antigen, the lymphoblasts migrate to the regional lymph nodes, from which they enter the systemic circulation. They then are returned to the intestine, where they are widely distributed in the lamina propria (Fig. 25-10). In the lamina propria, they differentiate into plasma cells that produce a specific IgA antibody directed to the absorbed antigen. This IgA antibody traverses the epithelial cell to the lumen by means of a protein carrier (the secretory component) that not only transports the IgA but also protects it against the intracellular lyso-

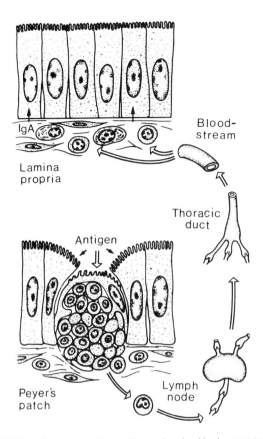

FIG. 25-10. *Schematic of the pathways involved in the secretory immune system. Lymphocytes in Peyer's patches exposed to antigens from the gut lumen migrate to regional lymph nodes and thence to the bloodstream. Circulating in the blood, they home into the lamina propria of the gut and there develop into plasma cells secreting IgA, which acquires a secretory piece in the epithelium and is released into the gut lumen. (From: Fawcett DW: A Textbook of Histology. Philadelphia, WB Saunders, 1986, with permission.)*

somes. The antibodies at the free surface of the cell collect in the glycocalyx, where they are in a strategic position to combat new antigens, preventing their attachment to the cell membrane and achieving immune exclusion.

Passage of viable bacteria from the intact gastrointestinal tract to the mesenteric lymph nodes and beyond, which has been termed *bacterial translocation,* has been implicated as a possible mechanism to explain septic complications and multiple organ system failure in burn and trauma patients. Small-intestinal mucosal integrity and function are profoundly affected by systemic injury. Cutaneous burn injury and sepsis cause early mucosal atrophy and subsequent defect in the gut mucosal barrier. This allows escape from local gut immune surveillance. One possible therapeutic strategy to prevent bacterial translocation and its systemic complications may involve stimulation of gut mucosal growth and maintenance of mucosal integrity and function during the early stages after systemic injury. Numerous gut peptides (e.g., gastrin, neurotensin, bombesin, epidermal growth factor) have trophic effects on small-intestinal mucosa; these growth factors may prove to be important in the development of therapeutic strategies for prevention of bacterial translocation. The magnitude of this problem, however, remains to be completely determined. In addition, the effects of polyamines on gastroin-

testinal growth suggest that these small polycationic substances play a central role of the regulation of intestinal cell growth and differentiation. The activity of ornithine decarboxylase (ODC), the rate-limiting enzyme in polyamine biosynthesis, is increased dramatically in instances associated with mucosal growth and repair in the duodenum and in the remaining small bowel after injury.

The exact mechanisms that maintain the epithelial integrity of the gastrointestinal tract remain largely unknown. Recent studies suggest that members of the trefoil peptide family, proteins secreted throughout the small intestine and colon in response to injury, are important in stimulating mucosal repair, since transgenic mice lacking intestinal trefoil factor demonstrated poor epithelial regeneration and mucosal healing after injury. Moreover, mice overexpressing the trefoil peptide pS2 have an increased resistance to intestinal damage.

Gut-associated lymphoid tissue (Fig. 25-11*A*) consists of the cells of the mucosal immune system located between the external environment (intestinal lumen) and the internal milieu of the host. Follicle-associated epithelial cells are located over Peyer's patch areas (in animals) or lymphoid follicles (in human beings), in which immature germinal center cells and B cells reside. Antigens from the intestinal lumen are transported through specialized epithelial cells called M cells. After being brought across the follicle-associated epithelium, the antigens come into contact with lymphocytes and macrophages. A subcompartment of T suppressor/cytotoxic lymphocytes called *intraepithelial lymphocytes* resides between absorptive epithelial cells. In animals most intraepithelial lymphocytes bear the gamma/delta T cell receptor. Within the lamina propria, mature T cells, B cells, plasma cells, and macrophages carry out cell-mediated immunologic processes, including cytokine secretion, production of IgA, and phagocytosis. Two different types of mast cells (mucosal mast cells and connective tissue mast cells) are found in the mucosa and submucosa.

Antigens within the intestinal lumen (Fig. 25-11*B*) are transported across specialized epithelial cells (M cells) into contact with underlying lymphoid cells. Antigen-induced activation of macrophages leads to secretion of interleukin-1 and activation of helper T cells, which secrete interleukin-2. Activation of intraepithelial lymphocytes and subsequent production of γ-interferon leads to enhanced production of major histocompatibility complex (MHC) class II molecules by epithelial cells. Increased numbers of MHC class II molecules on intestinal epithelial cells may lead to enhanced antigen presentation by intestinal epithelial cells, with subsequent augmentation of antigen-specific IgA antibody production. The expansion of IgM-bearing B cells is regulated by switch factors that favor the development of IgA-bearing B cells. T cells secreting interleukin-4, interleukin-5, and interleukin-6 induce the differentiation and proliferation of B cells for subsequent maturation into plasma cells, which synthesize and secrete dimeric IgA with J chain. The dimeric IgA with J chain then interacts with secretory component receptor on the basal membrane of epithelial cells for subsequent secretion into the intestinal lumen.

INFLAMMATORY DISEASES

Crohn's Disease

Background. Crohn's disease is a chronic granulomatous disease of the alimentary tract of unknown cause that is char-

Gut Associated Lymphoid Tissue

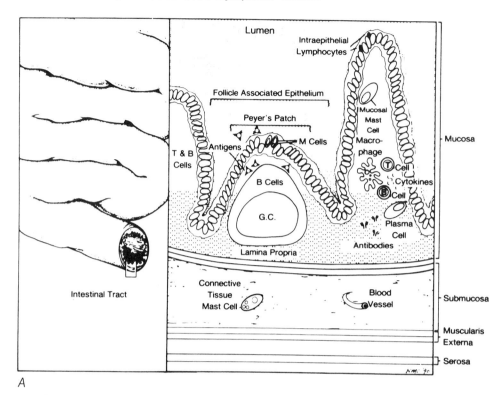

Regulation of IgA Synthesis and Secretion in the Intestine

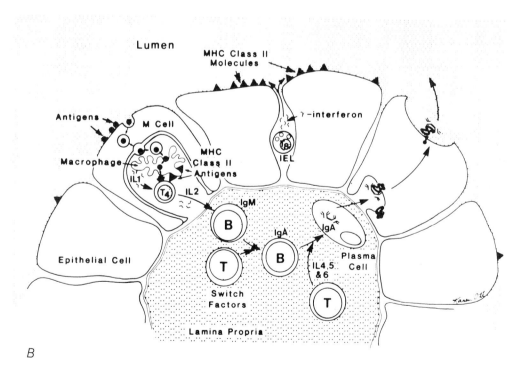

FIG. 25-11. Gut lymphoid tissue. (See text for explanation.) (From: *MacDermott RP, Stenson WF: The immune system, in Yamada T [ed]: Textbook of Gastroenterology, vol 1. Philadelphia, JB Lippincott, 1991, with permission.*)

acterized by intermittent periods of remission and exacerbation. Although earlier reports described the gross and microscopic pathologic features of this disease, it was not until the paper by Crohn, Ginsburg, and Openheimer in 1932 that the disease process was clearly and completely described. In the introduction to their landmark paper, they stated: "We proposed to describe, with pathologic and clinical details, a disease of the terminal ileum affecting mainly young adults, characterized by a subacute or chronic necrotizing and cicatrizing inflammation. The ulceration of the mucosa is accompanied by a disproportionate connective tissue reaction of the remaining walls of the involved intestine, a process which frequently leads to stenosis of the lumen of the intestine, associated with the formation of multiple fistulas."

Many different terms have been used to describe this disease process, such as regional ileitis, transmural enteritis, and granulomatous enteritis, but because of its multiple clinical appearances and because the disease is not confined to the terminal ileum, Crohn's disease has been universally accepted as its name.

Incidence and Epidemiology. Crohn's disease is the most common surgical disease of the small bowel. The annual incidence of Crohn's disease is approximately 3 to 6 cases per 100,000 of the general population, with the incidence highest in North America and northern Europe. The incidence is higher in patients in the third decade of life; however, a bimodal distribution is apparent, with a second, smaller peak in the sixth decade of life. Crohn's disease is more common in urban dwellers, and there may be a slight female predominance; some studies report an incidence approximately 20 percent higher in females, though others report a similar incidence in males and females. The risk of developing Crohn's disease is about two times higher in smokers than nonsmokers. Although Crohn's is uncommon in African blacks, blacks in the United States have rates similar to whites, suggesting that environmental influences play a role in the disease. There is a familial association, with the risk of developing Crohn's disease increased 30-fold in siblings of patients with the disease and 13-fold for all first-degree relatives.

Etiology. The cause of Crohn's disease remains unknown. Several possibilities have been suggested, including infectious, immunologic, environmental, and genetic causes.

Although controversial, proposed infectious causes that have received more than passing interest include mycobacterial infections, particularly *Mycobacterium paratuberculosis* and *M. avium.* The existence of atypical mycobacteria as a cause for Crohn's was proposed by Dalziel in 1913. Subsequent studies using the polymerase chain reaction (PCR) technique have confirmed the presence of these mycobacteria in intestinal samples of patients with Crohn's disease. Furthermore, the transplantation of intestinal samples from patients with Crohn's disease into other species has resulted in an ileitis. Koch's postulates, however, have yet to be rigorously satisfied since empirical therapy with antimicrobial agents in well-controlled clinical trials failed to ameliorate the disease process. In addition to mycobacteria, other potential sources include persistent measles virus and *Yersinia enterocolitica.*

Immunologic abnormalities that have been identified in patients with Crohn's disease have included humoral as well as cell-mediated immune reactions directed against gut cells, suggesting autoimmunity. There has been no direct correlation between these abnormalities, immunologic reactivity, and the development of Crohn's disease; therefore, these findings may represent an epiphenomenon. Other etiologic factors such as environmental and dietary factors, smoking, and psychosomatic causes have been suggested but never proved.

Genetic factors appear to have a role in the etiology of Crohn's disease, since the single strongest risk factor, by far, is having a relative with the disease. Recent European and American studies have identified a putative susceptibility locus in the centromeric region of chromosome 16 in multiply affected family members, further suggesting a genetic role in Crohn's disease. The advent of molecular biologic techniques has greatly enhanced our understanding of this disease; however, the development of an animal model (e.g., knockout mice) that simulates the findings of Crohn's disease in humans would be a great help to our understanding of this disease.

Pathology. Crohn's disease is an inflammatory disorder that is transmural in nature and associated with varying degrees of fibrosis. It can affect any portion of the gastrointestinal tract. The terminal ileum is involved in approximately 90 percent of patients with Crohn's disease; however, only about one-third of patients have small-bowel involvement alone.

Microscopic Features. The histologic features of Crohn's disease vary, but some occur with sufficient consistency to create a pattern that, though not specific, is at least characteristic of the disease. Some understanding of the pathogenesis may be gained by observing the progression of changes from early to late phases of regional enteritis.

Intense mucosal and submucosal edema may be seen microscopically before any gross changes are apparent. The earliest gross pathologic lesion is a superficial aphthous ulcer. As the disease progresses, the ulceration becomes more pronounced, and complete transmural inflammation results (Fig. 25-12A). The inflammatory reaction is characterized by extensive edema, hyperemia, lymphangiectasia, an intense infiltration of mononuclear cells and hyperplasia of lymphoid follicles. The ulcers are characteristically linear and may coalesce to produce transverse clefts and sinuses that result in the characteristic cobblestone appearance of the mucosa. Thickening and hypertrophy of the submucosa and the muscularis result in narrowing of the gut lumen; obliterative lymphangitis occurs; the bowel wall becomes thickened and edematous and quite rigid. Granulomas appear later and are found in the bowel wall and in regional lymph nodes in 60 to 70 percent of patients. These are noncaseating granulomas with Langhans' giant cells (Fig. 25-12B).

Macroscopic Features. At operation, one observes thickened, grayish pink or dull purple-red loops of bowel with areas of thick, gray-white exudate or fibrosis of the serosa. Areas of diseased bowel separated by areas of grossly normal bowel, called skip areas, are commonly encountered. A striking finding of Crohn's disease at operation is extensive fat-wrapping, caused by circumferential growth of the mesenteric fat around the wall of the bowel. The thickened bowel wall is firm, rubbery, and virtually incompressible (Fig. 25-13). The uninvolved proximal bowel often is dilated as a result of the considerable degree of obstruction in the diseased segment. Involved segments often are adherent to adjacent loops or other viscera, or several loops may be matted together into a bulky conglomerate mass. Internal fistulas are common in such adherent areas. The mesentery of the segment is characteristically greatly thickened, dull, and rubbery and contains masses of lymph nodes up to 3 or 4 cm in diameter.

Clinical Manifestations. Although Crohn's disease can occur at any age, the typical patient is a young adult, and the majority present before the age of 40 years. The onset of disease is often insidious, with a slow, protracted course. There are

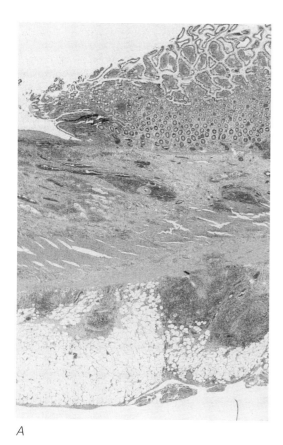

A

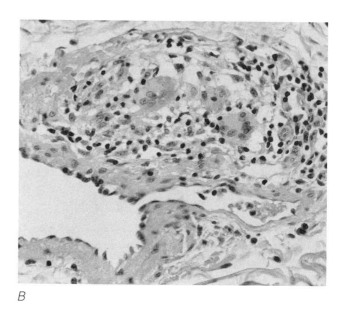

B

FIG. 25-12. *A. Photomicrograph of ileum with Crohn's disease showing transmural inflammation and fibrosis with mucosal ulceration. B. Noncaseating granuloma in ileum with Crohn's disease. (Courtesy of Brian A. West, MD.)*

symptomatic periods of abdominal pain and diarrhea interspersed with varying intervals of remission; but over time, symptomatic periods gradually become more frequent, more severe, and longer lasting. Pain (the most common symptom) usually is intermittent and cramping early in the course of the disease but may develop into persistent, dull, aching abdominal pain, most prominent in the lower abdomen. Diarrhea is the next most frequent symptom and is present, at least intermittently, in 85 percent of patients. The frequency of stools is less than in patients with ulcerative colitis, numbering two to five daily, and the stools rarely contain the mucus, pus, or blood seen in ulcerative colitis. Fever is present in about one-third of the patients, and moderate weight loss, loss of strength, and malaise, in over one-half. Frank nutritional disorders and steatorrhea are uncommon before surgical treatment.

The main intestinal complications of Crohn's disease include obstruction and perforation. The obstruction occurs as a result of chronic disease with fibrosis and progressive narrowing of the bowel lumen and can be partial or complete. Perforations can occur into the free peritoneal cavity and present as a generalized peritonitis. More commonly, however, development of fistulas and intraabdominal abscesses occurs. Fistulas can develop between the diseased bowel and any adjacent organ, such as small or large bowel, urinary bladder, vagina, or stomach, and through the skin, usually at the site of a previous laparotomy. Patients with Crohn's colitis may develop toxic megacolon, demonstrated by marked colonic dilatation, abdominal tenderness, fever, and leukocytosis. A potential intestinal complication of long-standing Crohn's disease is cancer of the affected segment of intestine, which occurs with an incidence six times greater than that

of the general population. Cancers in patients with Crohn's disease tend to be more advanced when identified and, therefore, have a worse prognosis.

Perianal disease (fissure, fistula, stricture, or abscess) is common, occurring in 25 percent of patients with small-intestinal disease, 41 percent of patients with ileocolitis, and 48 percent of patients with exclusively colonic involvement. Perianal disease is the sole presenting feature in 5 percent of patients and

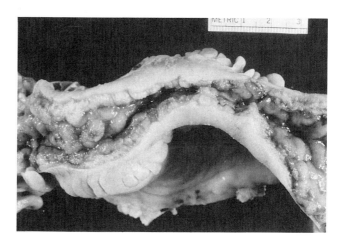

FIG. 25-13. *Terminal ileum resected for stricture secondary to Crohn's disease. A thickened bowel wall and ulcerated ileal mucosa with a cobblestone appearance is noted. (Courtesy of Brian A. West, MD.)*

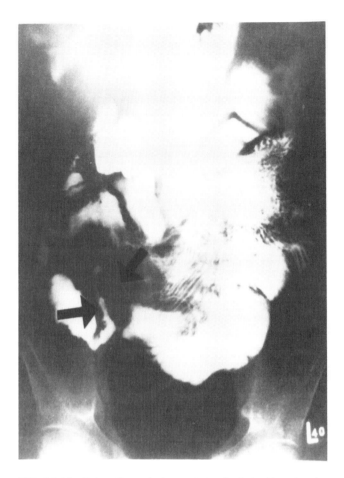

FIG. 25-14. This radiograph demonstrates Kantor's string sign (arrows). The string sign is the result of narrowing of the lumen due to mucosal ulceration, extensive thickening, and rigidity of the bowel wall.

may precede the onset of intestinal disease by months or years. Crohn's disease should be suspected in any patient with multiple, chronic, recurrent perianal fistulas. Extraintestinal manifestations of Crohn's disease occur in about 30 percent of patients and

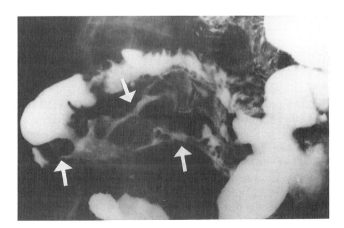

FIG. 25-15. Crohn's disease with multiple short fistulous communications between the distal loops of ileum (arrows). (Courtesy of Melvyn H. Schreiber, MD.)

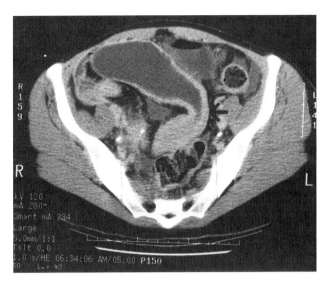

FIG. 25-16. CT scan of patient with Crohn's disease showing thickened bowel wall with obstruction (arrow) and dilated proximal bowel. (Courtesy of Melvyn H. Schreiber, MD)

include arthritis and arthralgia, uveitis and iritis, hepatitis and pericholangitis, and erythema nodosum and pyoderma gangrenosum.

Diagnosis. Patients with chronic, recurring episodes (often of long duration) of abdominal pain, diarrhea, and weight loss should be evaluated for Crohn's disease with endoscopy or radiographic studies.

When the colon is involved, sigmoidoscopy or colonoscopy reveals characteristic aphthous ulcers with granularity and a normal-appearing surrounding mucosa. With more progressive and severe disease, the ulcerations involve more and more of the bowel lumen and may be difficult to distinguish from ulcerative colitis. The presence of discrete ulcers and cobblestoning, however, particularly when discontinuous segments of bowel are involved, favors the diagnosis of Crohn's disease.

Radiographic studies of the small bowel reveal a number of findings, including a nodular contour, diffuse narrowing of the lumen, sinuses, clefts, linear ulcers, separation of bowel loops, and asymmetrical involvement of the bowel wall. A cobblestone appearance of the mucosa, composed of linear ulcers, transverse sinuses, and clefts, may be apparent. Long lengths of narrowed terminal ileum (Kantor's string sign) may be present in long-standing disease (Fig. 25-14). Fistulas between adjacent organs may be apparent (Fig. 25-15). Computed tomography may be useful to resolve diagnostic problems by ascertaining the nature of mass effects such as abscesses, separation, or displacement of segments of small intestine (Fig. 25-16).

Medical Treatment. The medical treatment of Crohn's disease is largely symptomatic and empiric and usually is followed by remissions and exacerbations until a complication that requires surgical intervention supervenes. Goals of medical therapy are relieving abdominal pain, controlling diarrhea, treating infection, and correcting any nutritional deficiencies.

Intraluminal antibiotics, particularly sulfasalazine (Azulfidine), have significant beneficial effects in certain patients. Corticosteroids, such as prednisone or the newer agent budesomide, are also useful in effecting remission of symptoms during acute exacerbations of ileitis, and a combination of sulfasalazine and steroids may be used to maintain patients for a short period after resolution of an acute inflammatory episode. Long-term maintenance therapy, with either agent alone or in combination, however, has not been shown to be of benefit in preventing recurrence of the disease. Although there have been implications of immunologic abnormalities in Crohn's disease, immunosuppressive treatment with azathioprine, 6-mercaptopurine, and cyclosporine have not been shown conclusively to be advantageous in comparison with placebo. Other immune modulators that have been tested in clinical trials with varying success include interleukin-1 receptor antagonists, monoclonal antibodies directed against helper T cells, and a diphtheria toxin–fused protein that is cytotoxic to cells that have receptors for interleukin-2. Therapies reported to be of possible benefit in early clinical trials include zileuton, a potent and specific inhibitor of the enzyme lipoxygenase that metabolizes arachidonic acid to leukotrienes, and superoxide dismutase, which blocks the toxicity of oxygen radicals; more clinical data are required before these agents can be advocated. Systemic antibiotics are valuable in the management of infectious complications but have no effect on the primary disease process and should not be considered therapeutic.

Chemically defined elemental diets and total parenteral nutrition have been touted as beneficial, even curative, in patients with acute Crohn's disease and in patients with complications such as enterocutaneous fistulas. No specific long-term benefit with any of the dietary measures has been shown; however, complete abstinence of oral intake with total parenteral nutrition may lead to temporary remission of symptoms in some patients. The provision of adequate nutrition is much more important in preparing patients for operation than it is for cure.

Surgical Treatment. *Indications.* Although medical management is certainly indicated during acute exacerbations of disease, the majority of patients with chronic Crohn's disease will require operation sometime during the course of their illness. In patients with more than 20 years of disease, the National Cooperative Crohn's Disease Study (NCCDS) has reported that the cumulative probability of operation was 78 percent. Indications for operation are limited to complications, including obstruction, abscess, fistula, free perforation, urologic complications, hemorrhage, cancer, and perianal disease. Children with Crohn's disease and resulting systemic symptoms such as growth retardation may benefit from resection. The extraintestinal complications of Crohn's disease, though not a primary indication for operation, often subside after resection of involved bowel.

General Tenets. Cure of patients with Crohn's disease is not possible by either medical or surgical therapy; therefore, operative intervention in patients with Crohn's disease should be directed to treating complications, and only the segment of bowel involved in the complicating process should be resected. Even if adjacent areas of bowel are clearly diseased, they should be ignored. Early in the history of surgical treatment of Crohn's disease, many surgeons tended toward wide resection in an attempt to effect cure. Repeated wide resections lead to the short bowel syndrome, a devastating surgical complication. In the past, the most common cause of the short bowel syndrome was repeated resections for Crohn's disease. During the past two decades or more most surgeons have accepted the view that it is not possible to surgically eradicate this disease. We have, for example, given up frozen-section study of the resected margin because we generally limit our resection to areas that are grossly involved adjacent to sites of obstruction or fistulization. We ignore microscopic evidence of involvement.

Management of Specific Problems. *Acute Ileitis.* There is a subgroup of patients with acute abdominal signs and symptoms in whom the usual preoperative diagnosis is acute appendicitis. At operation, the appendix is found to be normal, but the terminal ileum is edematous and beefy red, having a thickened mesentery with enlarged lymph nodes. The condition is acute ileitis, a self-limited disease that does not lead to subsequent development of Crohn's disease. The precise cause of acute ileitis is unknown; however, some patients have been found to have *Yersinia* or *Campylobacter* infections.

The role of appendectomy in these circumstances is less controversial now than it was in the past. In the absence of acute inflammatory involvement of the appendix or the cecum, appendectomy should be performed. This eliminates the possibility of acute appendicitis in the differential diagnosis of any subsequent abdominal complaints in these patients. In the few patients who have developed enterocutaneous fistulas after appendectomy, the fistulas originated from the ileum in all cases.

Obstruction. Intestinal obstruction is the most frequent indication for surgical therapy in most large series of patients with Crohn's disease. Obstruction in these patients often is partial, and nonoperative management is indicated initially. Operative intervention is required in instances of complete obstruction and in patients with partial obstruction that does not resolve with nonoperative management. The optimum treatment of complications of Crohn's disease is surgical resection of the involved segment with restoration of intestinal continuity (Fig. 25-17). As previously noted, the extent of resection is dictated by the extent of the complication. A short area of profound Crohn's ileitis producing partial obstruction (not involving the ileum immediately adjacent to the ileocecal valve) should be treated by local resection and primary anastomosis. It is common for the cecum and ascending colon to be involved contiguously with the terminal ileum in the disease process. In this case, the diseased bowel is removed and the ileum anastomosed to the transverse colon. No attempt should be made to dissect lymph nodes up to the origin of the ileocolic artery, since this may compromise the blood supply to uninvolved intestine. When two grossly abnormal segments of bowel have a short intervening segment of apparently normal bowel, the question arises of whether to try to save the normal "skip area." The answer depends on the length of the intervening normal segment. If it is 10 cm or longer, it probably should be saved. If it is 5 cm or shorter, it should be taken. Both areas would be excised in this instance, but each case must be individualized, and the answer will depend also on the configuration of the blood supply, the mobility of the mesentery, and other local factors. If previous resections have left the bowel critically short, we may go to great lengths to preserve small segments.

In selected patients with obstruction caused by strictures (either single or multiple), one option is to perform a stricturoplasty that effectively widens the lumen but avoids excision. Stricturoplasty is performed by making a longitudinal incision through the narrowed area of intestine followed by closure in a transverse fashion (Fig. 25-18). This technique preserves intestine and is associated with complication and recurrence rates comparable to

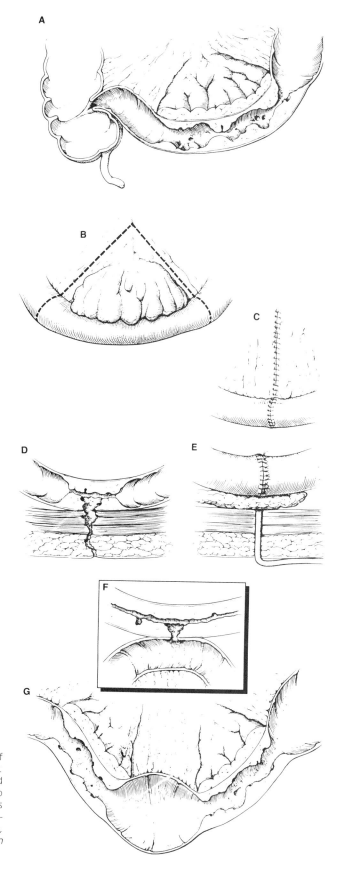

FIG. 25-17. Operative management of Crohn's ileitis. *A.* A short area of Crohn's ileitis producing partial obstruction treated by local resection. *B.* The area of excision should be confined to the most severely diseased portion, and no attempt should be made to dissect lymph nodes up to the origin of the ileocolic artery. *C.* After the grossly abnormal bowel is excised, the remaining ileum is anastomosed and the rent in the mesentery repaired. (From: *Thompson JC: Atlas of Surgery of the Stomach, Duodenum, and Small Bowel. St. Louis, Mosby–Year Book, 1992, with permission.*)

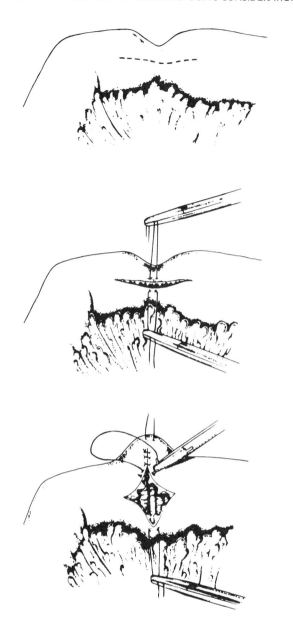

FIG. 25-18. Technique of short stricturoplasty in the manner of a Heineke-Mikulicz pyloroplasty. (From: *Alexander-Williams J, Haynes IG: Adv Surg 20:245, 1987, with permission.*)

resection. In the past, bypass procedures were commonly used, but today, bypass with exclusion is used only in elderly, poor-risk patients, in patients who have had several prior resections and can ill afford to lose any more bowel, and in patients in whom resection would necessitate entering an abscess or endangering normal structures. The reasons for this are twofold: the disease often persists in the bypassed segment with development of intraabdominal sepsis, and cancer may occur in the bypassed segment.

Fistula. Fistulas in patients with Crohn's disease usually are enteroenteral or enterocutaneous. The presence of a radiographically demonstrable enteroenteral fistula without any signs of sepsis or other complication is not in itself an indication for operation. The vast majority of patients who have radiographic demonstration of enteroenteral fistulas, however, will develop

later complications, most commonly sepsis, and will require resection of the fistula. Enterocutaneous fistulas are rarely spontaneous, but follow resections or external drainage of intraabdominal abscesses. Enterocutaneous fistulas should be managed by excising the area of grossly involved small intestine and debriding the fistulous tract through the abdominal wall from the inside. After the bowel is reanastomosed, it should be separated, if possible, from the abdominal wall with omental fat. The formation of enteroenteric or enterovesical fistulas usually involves either a previous intestinal perforation with formation of a walled-off abscess that finally perforates or the adherence of one diseased loop of bowel to another diseased loop of bowel or an adjacent normal organ. If the fistula forms between two or more adjacent loops of diseased bowel, the entire involved segment should be excised. On the other hand, if the fistula involves an adjacent normal organ, such as the bladder or the colon, only the segment of the diseased small bowel and fistulous tract should be resected, and the defect that is left in the normal organ is simply closed. The majority of patients with ileosigmoid fistulas do not require resection of the sigmoid because the disease is confined to the small bowel. If the segment of sigmoid involved in an ileosigmoid fistula is found to have Crohn's disease, it should be resected along with the segment of diseased small bowel. The extent of surgical resection in patients with Crohn's disease depends on the extent of critical involvement (Fig. 25-19).

Free Perforation. Perforation into the free peritoneal cavity is not common but occurs occasionally. Free perforation usually occurs in a diseased segment of bowel but can also occur in bowel proximal to an obstruction. The segment should be resected back to relatively good bowel on each side of the perforation, and no attempt should be made to eradicate all diseased bowel. If generalized peritonitis is present, an anastomosis should not be done, because there is a high rate of anastomotic dehiscence under these circumstances; an ileostomy should be performed until intraabdominal sepsis is controlled. Later restoration of intestinal continuity can be carried out safely.

Urologic Complications. The most common urologic complication is ureteral obstruction, which is usually due to ileocolic disease with retroperitoneal abscess. Surgical treatment of the primary intestinal disease is adequate in most patients; however, in a few instances of long-standing inflammatory disease, periureteral fibrosis may be present and require extensive ureterolysis.

Hemorrhage. Although anemia from chronic blood loss is common, life-threatening hemorrhage in patients with Crohn's disease is rare. The incidence of clinical hemorrhage is more common when Crohn's disease involves the colon rather than the small bowel, but both occur much less frequently than bleeding in patients with ulcerative colitis. When life-threatening hemorrhage occurs, the segment involved should be resected and intestinal continuity restored; arteriography may be useful to localize the bleeding before surgery.

Growth Retardation. Up to one-fourth of children with Crohn's disease have significant growth retardation, which may precede the appearance of active bowel disease. The major reason for this growth retardation appears to be nutritional sequelae that accompany Crohn's disease. In these children, in the absence of other common indications, bowel resection is indicated; resection often results in restoration of normal growth when it is performed before epiphyseal closure has occurred. As in

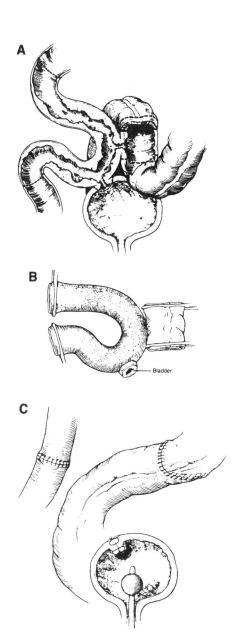

FIG. 25-19. Operative management of a complex enterocolic and enterovesical fistula secondary to Crohn's disease. *A.* This complex lesion included an enterocolic and an enterovesical fistula, with involvement of a relatively large segment of the wall of the sigmoid and a small segment of the bladder wall. The lesion was treated by excisions as indicated by the dotted lines. We decided to excise the short colonic segment because of the large area of colonic induration. *B.* The resected specimen includes the limb of ileum with adjacent involved loop of sigmoid and a rim of bladder. *C.* The anastomosed ileum and sigmoid and the repaired bladder with indwelling catheter. (From: *Thompson JC: Atlas of Surgery of the Stomach, Duodenum and Small Bowel. St. Louis, Mosby–Year Book, 1992, with permission.)*

adults, children with Crohn's disease tend to have disease of the terminal ileum and colon and can be treated with limited resection and reanastomosis. Involvement of the colon and rectum appears to be more virulent and may require proctocolectomy before restoration of growth is accomplished.

Cancer. Until recently, a causal relation between Crohn's disease and the development of cancer was not accepted. Al-

though cancer does not occur at the rate it does in patients with ulcerative colitis, a number of reports have clearly demonstrated that patients with long-standing Crohn's disease have an increased incidence of cancer. The management of these patients is the same as in any patient with cancer—that is, resection of the cancer with appropriate margins and regional lymph nodes. Patients with cancer associated with Crohn's disease tend to have a worse prognosis than those who do not have Crohn's. This can be explained in large part by the fact that many of these patients are initially managed medically and therefore present at a later time.

Anorectal Disease. Treatment of perianal disease should be conservative; wide excision of abscesses or fistulas is not indicated. Definitive fistulotomy is indicated in the majority of patients, although one must recognize that some degree of anal stenosis may occur as a result of the chronic inflammation. Fissures usually are lateral, relatively painless, large, and indolent, and they usually respond to conservative management. Abscesses should be drained, but large excisions of tissue should not be performed.

Colorectal Disease. The same principles apply to the management of Crohn's disease that is limited to the colon and rectum as to disease in the small intestine. Operative indications include a lack of response to medical management or complications of Crohn's disease. As much bowel as possible should be conserved. Procedures include segmental colectomy with colocolic anastomosis, subtotal colectomy with ileoproctostomy in a patient with mild or minimal rectal disease, and total proctocolectomy with Brooke ileostomy. Patients with a toxic megacolon should undergo colectomy, closure of the proximal rectum, and end ileostomy.

A potential problem after proctocolectomy is delayed healing of the perineal wound. Several series have reported that 25 to 60 percent of perineal wounds are open 6 months after operation. Persistent nonhealing wounds require excision with secondary closure or closure with the use of musculocutaneous flaps (most commonly gracilis or gluteus maximus flaps). Continence-preserving operations such as ileoanal-pouch anastomoses or continent ileostomies (Kock pouch) that have been used successfully in patients with ulcerative colitis are not recommended for patients with Crohn's colitis because of the high rate of recurrence of Crohn's disease in the pouch, fistulas to the anastomosis, and peripouch abscesses.

Duodenal Disease. Crohn's disease of the duodenum requiring operative intervention is rare. The primary indication for surgery in these patients is duodenal obstruction that does not respond to medical therapy. Gastrojejunostomy to bypass the disease, rather than duodenal resection, is the procedure of choice; however, strictureplasties have been performed with success in selected patients.

Prognosis. There is no medical or surgical cure for Crohn's disease. A substantial proportion of patients who have had one operation will require another operation for complications of Crohn's disease. In one study the cumulative recurrence rates were reported to be 29 percent at 5 years, 52 percent at 10 years, 64 percent at 15 years, and 84 percent at 25 years. No important differences were noted between disease location and the type of operation. Which patients will develop recurrent disease cannot be predicted. Sex, age, duration of disease, granulomas, enteral or perirectal fistulas, length of resection, length of diseased gut, and proximal resection margin have no significant influence on the rate of disease recurrence or on functional outcome. The most common site of recurrence is the small bowel proximal to the site of previous resection. Recurrence is five times more likely to involve the adjacent or remote colon in patients with ileocolitis than in patients with ileitis. Few patients with ileitis eventually require ileostomy, whereas one-third of patients with ileocolitis or colitis require permanent ileostomy.

Crohn's disease gradually recedes with advancing age. Active disease is unusual between the ages of 50 and 55 years, but gradual cicatrization on healing may cause bowel obstruction in older patients.

Tuberculous Enteritis

A resurgence in the incidence of tuberculosis has occurred in Western countries as a result of the growing AIDS epidemic, an influx of Asian immigrants, and widespread use of immunosuppressive agents after organ transplantation. Tuberculosis continues to be a significant and relatively common disease in developing countries with incidences as high as 400 to 500 people per 100,000 in some countries. Tuberculosis of the gastrointestinal tract occurs in two forms. Primary infection usually is caused by the bovine strain of *Mycobacterium tuberculosis* and results from ingesting infected milk; this now accounts for less than 10 percent of reported cases. The majority of infections occur secondarily from the swallowing of bacilli by patients with active pulmonary tuberculosis. Chemotherapy has greatly decreased the incidence of secondary tuberculous enteritis, so that it now occurs in only about 1 percent of patients with pulmonary tuberculosis.

The ileocecal region is the site of involvement in about 85 percent of patients with tuberculous enteritis, presumably because of the abundance of lymphoid tissue in this area. Three patterns of involvement are seen: hypertrophic, ulcerative, and ulcerohypertrophic.

Occasionally a hypertrophic reaction produces contracture and stenosis of the lumen of the distal ileum, which requires resection. The diagnosis is not often made preoperatively; only 50 percent of patients have evidence of active pulmonary tuberculosis; 45 percent of patients have negative skin tests. Cultures, when positive, provide a definitive answer, but results may take longer than 4 weeks. The polymerase chain reaction technique has been used successfully to differentiate tuberculosis enteritis from Crohn's disease in biopsy specimens; results may be obtained within 2 days. If the diagnosis is suspected preoperatively, chemotherapy, best given as a combination of isoniazid (100 mg three times a day) with either rifampin (600 mg daily) or ethambutol (15 mg/kg daily), should be administered for about 2 weeks before operation. If unsuspected tuberculosis is found at operation, chemotherapy should be started. In either case drugs should be continued for 1 year after the patient has become asymptomatic. Surgical therapy of hypertrophic tuberculous enteritis usually is inadvisable unless bowel obstruction from high-grade stenosis requires relief. Resection and anastomosis should be performed unless extensive disease is present; otherwise ileocolic bypass is the safer procedure.

Symptoms of the more common ulcerative form of tuberculous enteritis include alternating constipation and diarrhea associated with nonspecific crampy abdominal pain. The diagnosis sometimes is made only by radiographic intestinal examination of patients with pulmonary tuberculosis. In severe cases diarrhea is persistent, and anemia, hypoalbuminemia, and inanition are progressive. Clinical confirmation of a presumptive diagnosis may be obtained by a prompt response to antituberculous chemotherapy. Surgical therapy is contraindicated except for the rare complications of perforation, obstruction, or hemorrhage.

Typhoid Enteritis

Typhoid enteritis is an acute systemic infection of several weeks' duration caused by *Salmonella typhosa.* Hyperplasia and ulceration of Peyer's patches of the intestine occur along with mesenteric lymphadenopathy, splenomegaly, and parenchymatous changes in the liver. Confirmation of diagnosis is obtained by culturing *S. typhosa* from blood or feces or by finding a high titer of agglutinins against the O and H antigens.

Typhoid fever is still a major disease in areas of the world that have not yet attained high public health standards, but it is now rare in Western countries. The death rate, formerly about 10 percent, is now about 2 percent, in large part because of the specific antimicrobial chloramphenicol, introduced in 1948.

There is some disagreement on whether chloramphenicol remains the drug of choice, however, because of the emergence of resistant strains, high relapse rate, and risk of marrow toxicity. Trimethoprim-sulfamethoxazole has emerged as the best successor to chloramphenicol. Trimethoprim 160 mg and sulfamethoxazole 800 mg are given, either orally or parenterally, twice daily for 2 weeks. Amoxicillin also is effective and should be given intravenously or intramuscularly in doses of 1 g every 6 h for 2 weeks.

Gross hemorrhage occurs in 10 to 20 percent of hospitalized patients, even while on adequate therapy. Transfusion is indicated and usually suffices. Every effort should be made to avoid operation, since the bleeding typically is from multiple ulcers and the bowel is exceedingly friable. Rarely, laparotomy must be done for uncontrollable, life-threatening hemorrhage.

Perforation through an ulcerated Peyer's patch occurs in about 2 percent of cases. Typically it is a single perforation in the terminal ileum. Operative treatment is indicated unless the patient is moribund, since localization or walling-off of the perforation is uncommon. Simple closure of the perforation is successful in the majority of patients. With multiple perforations, which occur in about one-fourth of the patients, resection with primary anastomosis or a temporary ileostomy is preferred. The mortality rate of those with free perforation is about 10 percent.

NEOPLASMS

General Considerations

Primary neoplasms of the small bowel are rare, despite the much greater mucosal surface area and the rapidity of cell turnover of the small bowel compared to the stomach and colon. Neoplasms are 40 times more common in the colon; the reasons for this difference are unknown. Several theories have been proposed as possible explanations: rapid transit time decreases the time for contact of carcinogens with the mucosa; the local immune system of the small-bowel mucosa; the alkaline pH of the succus entericus; the absence of bacteria that might convert certain ingested products into carcinogens; and the presence of mucosal enzymes that destroy certain carcinogens.

Primary small-bowel neoplasms are either benign or malignant and may arise from any of the cells of the small bowel.

They often are asymptomatic; when symptoms occur, they usually are those of anemia or of obstruction (e.g., enteric cramping, diarrhea, distention, and obstipation). Any tumor involving the surface mucosa of the gut will bleed from time to time, and so patients present with symptoms of anemia, as do patients with colonic tumors. Benign tumors may be hamartomas, adenomas, hemangiomas, fibromas, lipomas, or leiomyomas, among others. Benign tumors usually can be excised locally. Whether or not to excise a complete segment of bowel depends on whether the tumor can be removed easily without compromising the lumen. Malignant tumors usually are adenocarcinomas, lymphomas, or leiomyosarcomas. Any kind of soft-tissue malignancy may involve the small bowel. Malignant tumors should be resected with a good margin (about 10 cm) of normal bowel on each side, along with the subtended wedge of mesentery, so as to remove local and regional lymphatics and lymph nodes.

Adenocarcinoma of the small bowel (Fig. 25-20A) is similar to colonic adenocarcinoma. Both often present as apple-core lesions that may cause blood loss and anemia; after producing constriction of the lumen, it causes cramping and intermittent diarrhea and, when the constricted lumen is ultimately plugged by enteric material, obstruction. The material causing the obtu-

rator obstruction may later be spontaneously passed, so that intermittent symptoms of obstruction and diarrhea may occur. Malignant soft-tissue tumors may appear in any form (Fig. 25-20B). Sarcomas may rarely invade the mucosa and bleed. Hamartomas or adenomas may be single or multiple (Fig. 25-20C). Benign tumors of the wall of the bowel may grow to sufficient size to cause narrowing of the lumen and even obstruction (Fig. 25-20D). Occasionally these tumors may become sufficiently large and elongated to assume a polypoid shape and may be carried along by peristalsis; sometimes they infarct and bleed. Malignant tumors should be resected with a wide margin of normal bowel and a subtended wedge of mesentery (Fig. 25-20E) in an attempt to capture any tumor in lymphatic transit. After resection an end-to-end anastomosis of the small bowel and repair of the mesentery are performed (Fig. 25-20F).

The frequencies of benign and of malignant neoplasms are reported to be equal in surgical series, and benign neoplasms far exceed malignant neoplasms in autopsy series. Malignant neoplasms (75 to 80 percent) more often produce symptoms than benign neoplasms.

Symptoms associated with small-bowel neoplasms often are vague; they include epigastric discomfort, nausea, vomiting, abdominal pain (often intermittent and colicky), diarrhea, and bleeding (often manifested as symptoms of anemia). Symptoms may be present for months or years before operation. Bleeding usually is occult; hematochezia or hematemesis may occur, although life-threatening hemorrhage is uncommon. The most common indications for operation in patients with neoplasms of the small bowel are obstruction, bleeding, and pain. The mechanism of obstruction varies, depending on whether it is caused by a benign or a malignant neoplasm. Benign neoplasms are the most common cause of intussusception in the adult, whereas malignant neoplasms commonly cause obstruction by circumferential growth or kinking of the bowel as a result of longitudinal, intramural growth.

Because of their relative infrequency and the vague symptoms they produce, the diagnosis of small-bowel neoplasms requires informed suspicion. Endoscopy is useful in evaluating the duodenum and possibly the most proximal jejunum, just beyond the ligament of Treitz. However, since most of the small bowel is not accessible to endoscopic scrutiny, barium contrast radiography usually is required. Upper gastrointestinal series with small-bowel follow-through is the single most useful diagnostic test. Enteroclysis (intubation infusion for small-bowel examination) has been promoted as a sensitive technique to demonstrate small-bowel disease. In performing enteroclysis, the tip of the nasal–small bowel tube is placed just beyond the ligament of Treitz, and dilute barium is instilled at a constant rate. The examination is complete when the barium reaches the cecum. Enteroclysis (Fig. 25-21) is superior to small-bowel follow-through for detection of small filling defects and for determination of changes in mucosal pattern; the diagnostic accuracy of enteroclysis approaches 90 percent.

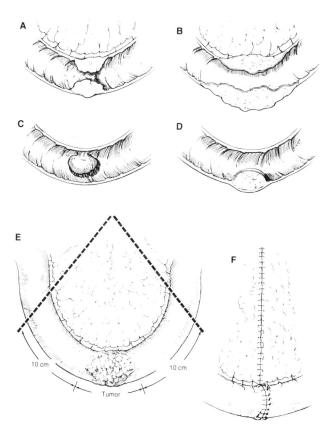

FIG. 25-20. Surgical management of adenocarcinoma of the small bowel. A. Adenocarcinoma of the small bowel producing constriction of the lumen. B. Leiomyosarcoma constricting the lumen of the small bowel. C. A solitary adenoma. D. This tumor could be a fibroma, a lipoma, or a leiomyoma. E. Malignant tumors should be resected with a wide margin of normal bowel and a subtended wedge of mesentery in an attempt to capture any tumor in lymphatic transit. F. End-to-end anastomosis of the small bowel and repair of the mesentery. (From: Thompson JC: Atlas of Surgery of the Stomach, Duodenum, and Small Bowel. St. Louis, Mosby–Year Book, 1992, with permission.)

Benign Neoplasms

Pathology. Benign tumors of the small bowel may be of epithelial or connective tissue origin. The incidence of these tumors varies, depending on whether they are reported in autopsy or clinical series. The most common lesions are adenomas, leiomyomas, and lipomas. Other benign lesions include hamartomas, fibromas, angiomas, lymphangiomas, neurofibromas, and

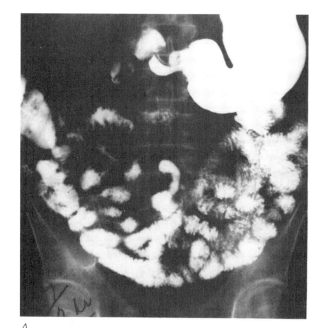

A

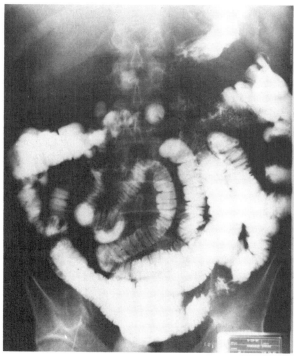

B

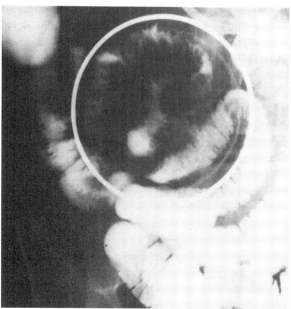

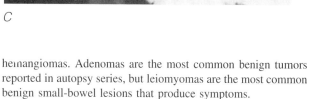

C

FIG. 25-21. Enteroclysis compared with small-bowel follow-through. *A.* An overhead view obtained 30 min after administration of barium in a small-bowel follow-through examination. Note the incomplete filling and poor distention of bowel loops. The lesion in the ileum was not found. *B.* An overhead view from an enteroclysis examination in the same patient. The entire small bowel is nicely distended, except for ileal loops in the right abdomen. Each loop is individually examined by compression. *C.* This is a compression film of the involved ileal loops. These loops exhibit thickened, irregular mucosal folds; the thickening and kinking of the bowel wall are characteristic of an infiltrating carcinoid tumor.

hemangiomas. Adenomas are the most common benign tumors reported in autopsy series, but leiomyomas are the most common benign small-bowel lesions that produce symptoms.

Clinical Manifestations. An appreciable number of small-bowel benign tumors apparently cause no serious symptoms during life and are incidental findings at autopsy. The diagnosis is delayed or missed in many patients because symptoms may be absent or vague or nonspecific until significant complications have developed. Physical examination rarely provides any clue unless intestinal obstruction is present, and radiographic studies of the small bowel and selective angiography, the only specific diagnostic aids, may fail to demonstrate an existing tumor, even if it is suspected clinically. In only about one-half of

small-bowel tumors found at operation has the correct diagnosis been made preoperatively.

The two most common clinical manifestations of small-bowel tumors are bleeding and obstruction (Fig. 25-22). Rarely, perforation of the bowel wall occurs, resulting in abscess or internal fistula formation, peritonitis, or pneumatosis cystoides intestinalis. Bleeding occurs in about one-third of patients but is rarely gross. More commonly, bleeding is occult and intermittent, producing guaiac-positive stools and iron-deficiency anemia. Leiomyomas and hemangiomas are the lesions that most often cause bleeding.

Treatment. Surgical treatment of benign tumors is nearly always indicated because of the risk of subsequent complications

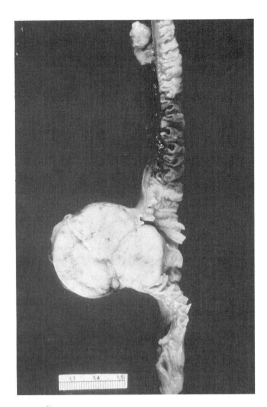

FIG. 25-22.   Resection of jejunal segment containing a large fibroma in a patient presenting with obstruction. *(Courtesy of Brian A. West, MD.)*

and because the diagnosis of benign disease cannot be made without microscopic evaluation. The complications of benign neoplasms that most often require treatment are bleeding and obstruction. Segmental resection and primary reanastomosis is most commonly used except for very small lesions that may be excised by enterotomy. The entire small bowel should be searched for other lesions, since they are often multiple.

Adenoma

Adenomas, which account for approximately 35 percent of all benign tumors, are of three primary types: true adenomas, villous adenomas, and Brunner's gland adenomas. Twenty percent of adenomas are found in the duodenum, 30 percent in the jejunum, and 50 percent in the ileum. The majority of adenomas are asymptomatic; most occur singly, and most are found incidentally at autopsy. It is rare for duodenal polyps to be sufficiently large to cause symptoms. If polyps do cause symptoms, they usually are associated with bleeding or obstruction. If symptomatic, duodenal polyps can be removed by endoscopic snare, or they may be sufficiently large to be difficult to retrieve through the pylorus. In such cases, particularly if malignancy is suspected, they may best be removed in an open operation. As a rule, the question of malignancy can be settled by endoscopic biopsy; usually the polyp can be removed endoscopically.

Villous adenomas of the small bowel are rare but do occur and are most commonly found in the duodenum. Their presence may be suspected by the characteristic "soap bubble" appearance on contrast radiography. They may attain large size (> 5 cm in diameter) and usually are found because of pain or bleeding.

Obstruction also may occur. There have been no reports of secretory diarrhea associated with villous tumors of the small bowel; however, the malignant potential of these lesions is reportedly between 35 and 55 percent.

Brunner's gland adenomas are hyperplastic proliferations of normal exocrine glands located in the submucosa of the duodenum. Brunner's gland adenomas may produce symptoms that mimic those of peptic ulcer disease, or they may cause obstruction. Diagnosis can be made by endoscopy and biopsy, and symptomatic lesions in an accessible region should be resected. There is no malignant potential for Brunner's gland adenomas, and a radical resection should not be employed.

Leiomyoma

The most common symptomatic benign lesions of the small bowel are leiomyomas. Leiomyomas are benign tumors of smooth muscle that are most common in the jejunum. They usually occur singly, although multiple tumors may occur. The incidence is equal in men and women. Two growth patterns are noted: the tumor may grow primarily intramurally and cause obstruction, or both intramural and extramural growth may occur and produce a dumbbell-shaped mass. These tumors may attain considerable size, outgrowing their blood supply, and tumor necrosis with bleeding may occur. The most common indication for operation on leiomyomas is bleeding. Angiography may provide the correct preoperative diagnosis.

Lipoma

Lipomas, most common in the ileum, are single intramural lesions, submucosal in location, and usually small. Fewer than one-third of lipomas are found at operation and, when found, usually they are the cause of obstruction, most commonly as the lead point of an intussusception. Bleeding may occur from ulceration of the overlying mucosa. Lipomas do not have malignant potential, and therefore when found incidentally, they should be removed only if the resection is simple. Pedunculated lipomas should be excised.

Hamartoma (Peutz-Jeghers Syndrome)

Hamartomas of the small bowel occur only as part of the Peutz-Jeghers syndrome, which is an inherited syndrome of mucocutaneous melanotic pigmentation and gastrointestinal polyps. The pattern of inheritance is simple mendelian dominant, with a high degree of penetrance. A single pleiotropic gene is responsible for both polyps and melanin spots. The classic pigmented lesions are small, 1- to 2-mm brown or black spots located in the circumoral region of the face, buccal mucosa, forearms, palms, soles, digits, and perianal area. The syndrome was first reported in 1921 by Peutz, and Jeghers and colleagues described it anew in 1949. Multiple pigmented lesions may be noted, or only a single buccal lesion may be present. Pigmentation appears in childhood. All cutaneous lesions may fade, leaving only buccal lesions. Polyposis with and without pigmentation has been reported. The entire jejunum and ileum are the most frequent portions of the gastrointestinal tract to be involved with multiple polyps. Fifty percent of patients may also have rectal and colonic polyps, and 25 percent may have gastric polyps. The chief point to note is that if a patient with multiple rectal, colonic, or gastric polyps is found to have hamartomas rather than adenomas, a search for small-bowel polyposis and pigmented lesions should be carried out.

The lesions are not true polyps but are hamartomas and hence are not premalignant (Fig. 25-23). However, there have been a few reported cases of malignant tumors of the gastrointestinal tract associated with Peutz-Jeghers syndrome. Some of these adenomatous and carcinomatous changes were noted in the hamartomatous polyps. It is not clear, however, whether this represents a coincidence or a true malignant transformation of this syndrome.

The most common symptom is recurrent colicky abdominal pain, caused by intermittent intussusception. Lower abdominal pain associated with palpable mass has been reported to occur in one-third of patients. Hemorrhage occurs less frequently and is most commonly manifested by insidious involvement of anemia. Acute life-threatening hemorrhage is uncommon but may occur.

Surgical therapy is required only for obstruction or persistent bleeding. The resection should be limited to the segment of bowel that is producing complications, that is, polypectomy or limited resection. Because of the widespread nature of intestinal involvement, cure is not possible and extensive resections are not indicated.

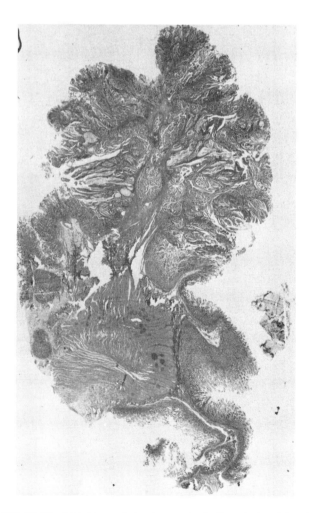

FIG. 25-23. Low-power photomicrograph of a Peutz-Jeghers jejunal polyp. Instead of one predominant cell, as seen in most intestinal polyps, these contain all cells of normal intestinal mucosa interspersed within bands of smooth muscle. They are hamartomas.

Hemangioma

Hemangiomas are developmental malformations consisting of submucosal proliferation of blood vessels. They can occur at any level of the gastrointestinal tract, and the jejunum is the most commonly affected small-bowel segment. Hemangiomas account for 3 to 4 percent of all benign tumors of the small bowel and are multiple in 60 percent of patients. Hemangiomas of the small bowel may occur as part of an inherited disorder known as Rendu-Osler-Weber disease. Besides the small bowel, hemangiomas may be present in the lung, liver, and mucous membranes. Patients with Turner's syndrome are likely also to have cavernous hemangiomas of the intestine. Most patients are symptomatic, and the most common symptom is diffuse intestinal bleeding. Diagnosis is often difficult; angiography and ^{99m}Tc–red cell scanning are the most useful diagnostic tools. If a hemangioma is localized preoperatively, resection of the involved segment of intestine is warranted. If the site is not localized preoperatively, intraoperative transillumination and palpation can be helpful.

Malignant Neoplasms

The most common malignant neoplasms of the small bowel, in approximate order of frequency, are adenocarcinomas, carcinoids, sarcomas, and lymphomas.

Clinical Manifestations. Rochlin and Longmire called attention to three distinct clinical presentations of patients with malignant small-bowel neoplasms: diarrhea, with large amounts of mucus, and tenesmus; obstruction with nausea, vomiting, and cramping abdominal pain; and chronic blood loss with anemia, weakness, guaiac-positive stools, and occasionally melena or hematochezia. As with benign neoplasms, symptoms of malignant neoplasms often are present for many months before the diagnosis is made, emphasizing their insidious nature.

Treatment. The treatment for malignant neoplasms of the small bowel is wide resection, including regional lymph nodes. This may require a radical pancreatoduodenectomy (Whipple operation) for duodenal lesions. Because of the extent of the disease at the time of operation, curative resection may not be possible. Palliative resection should be performed when possible to prevent further complications of bleeding, obstruction, and perforation. If that is not possible, however, bypass of the involved segment is an alternative that may provide worthwhile relief of symptoms. If bypass is used, the proximal end of the bypassed segment should be brought out as a mucous fistula to prevent development of a closed loop. Recent reports of an increased association of small-bowel cancers in patients with celiac sprue suggest that new intestinal complaints in these patients should be evaluated to rule out small-bowel cancer.

Prognosis. The overall survival rate for patients with malignant neoplasms of the small bowel is not good. The highest survival rates are reported for duodenal periampullary carcinomas (about 30 to 40 percent), whereas adenocarcinomas occurring elsewhere in the small bowel have a 5-year survival rate of 20 percent or less. Leiomyosarcomas of the small bowel have a 5-year survival rate of 30 to 40 percent. Radiation and chemotherapy play little role in the treatment of patients with adenocarcinomas of the small bowel. There may be some improvement in survival when radiotherapy is used in patients with sarcomas.

Determinants of survival for patients with lymphomas are the cell type and the extent of disease. Radiotherapy and chemotherapy combined with surgical excision provide the best survival rates for patients with lymphomas. Five-year survival rates have been reported to range from 10 to 50 percent, with an average of about 30 percent.

Carcinoma

Carcinomas constitute about 50 percent of the malignant tumors of the small bowel in most reported series. They are twice as common in men as in women, and the average age at diagnosis is 50 years. For unknown reasons, adenocarcinomas are more common in the duodenum and the proximal jejunum than in the remainder of the small bowel. About half of duodenal carcinomas involve the ampulla of Vater.

The carcinoma's location in the small bowel often determines the presenting symptoms. For example, periampullary adenocarcinomas are associated with intermittent jaundice, whereas carcinomas of the jejunum usually produce symptoms of mechanical small-bowel obstruction (Fig. 25-24). The presence of jaundice, often intermittent, and a guaiac-positive stool should immediately call to mind the possibility of a periampullary carcinoma.

As with carcinomas arising in other organs, survival of patients with small-bowel carcinomas is related to the stage of disease at the time of diagnosis. Diagnosis often is delayed and disease far advanced at the time of operation. The delay in diagnosis is due to a combination of factors, including lack of suspicion because of the relative rarity of the lesions, vagueness of symptoms, and absence of physical findings.

Sarcoma

Sarcomas, which arise from mesodermal tissue, constitute about 20 percent of malignant neoplasms of the small bowel. The most common sarcoma by far is the leiomyosarcoma. Leiomyosarcomas are evenly distributed throughout the small bowel. The incidence is the same for men and women, and diagnosis usually is made in the sixth decade. The most common indications for operation are bleeding and obstruction, although free perforation as a result of hemorrhagic necrosis in large tumor masses may occur. Leiomyosarcomas are spread by direct invasion of adjacent structures, by hematogenous dissemination, or by transperitoneal seeding, producing sarcomatosis. Other rare forms of sarcoma that may affect the small bowel include fibrosarcoma, angiosarcoma, liposarcoma, and Kaposi's sarcoma.

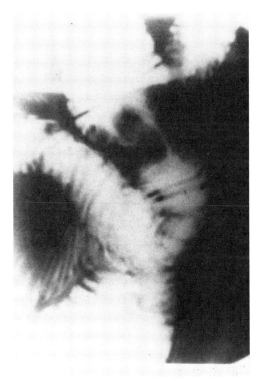

A

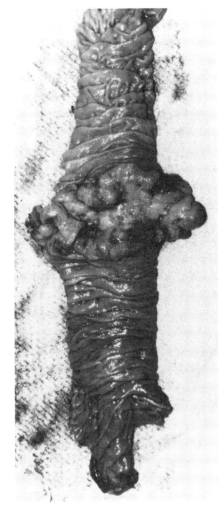

B

FIG. 25-24. Malignant tumors. *A.* Adenocarcinomas produce a typical apple-core or napkin-ring deformity of the small bowel. *B.* The excised specimen illustrates a fungating intraluminal mass that is typical of adenocarcinoma.

Table 25-3
Classification of Carcinoid Tumors

	Location	*Amines/ Hormones*	*Carcinoid Syndrome*
Foregut	Lung, stomach, pancreas, duodenum	Multihormonal, 5-HT	Frequent
Midgut	Jejunoileum	5-HT, substance P	Frequent
Hindgut	Colon, rectum	Multihormonal	Rare

Lymphoma

Lymphomas constitute 10 to 15 percent of small-bowel malignant tumors in the adult; in children under 10 years of age, they are the most common intestinal neoplasm. Lymphomas most commonly are found in the ileum, where the greatest concentration of gut-associated lymphoid tissue is present, and they may be primary or part of a generalized disease. Dawson and colleagues have devised criteria to determine whether lymphoma of the small bowel is primary. These include (1) absence of peripheral lymphadenopathy; (2) normal chest x-ray without evidence of mediastinal lymph node enlargement; (3) normal white blood cell count, total and differential; (4) at operation, the bowel lesion must predominate, and the only involved nodes are associated with the bowel lesion; and (5) absence of disease in the liver and spleen. Even when these criteria are used, one-third or more patients with lymphomatous involvement of the small bowel are found to have generalized lymphoma.

There are three syndromes of small-bowel lymphoma. *Western lymphoma* is a disease predominantly of adults, typically found in the Western Hemisphere and associated with severe malabsorption in 5 to 10 percent of patients. Another form, known as *Mediterranean lymphoma,* is a malignant form that was first noted in non-Ashkenazi Jews and Arabs in Israel and was subsequently reported in other countries and in other ethnic groups, including Hispanic Americans. Since this disease is not confined to the Mediterranean basin, the term *immunoproliferative small intestinal disease* has been used. One-third of the patients may be found to have an abnormal fragment of IgA heavy chain in their serum, which is produced by plasma cells infiltrating the small bowel. This variant is known as *heavy-chain disease.*

The third intestinal manifestation of lymphoma is childhood abdominal lymphoma. This is a group of lymphomas including American (nonendemic) Burkitt's lymphoma, undifferentiated non-Burkitt's lymphoma, and diffuse histiocytic lymphoma.

Carcinoid

Carcinoids of the small bowel arise from the enterochromaffin cells, or Kulchitsky cells, found in the crypts of Lieberkühn. These cells are also known as argentaffin cells because of their staining by silver compounds. Carcinoids may be classified by embryologic site of origin and secretory product (Table 25-3). Carcinoids of the small bowel occur with almost the same frequency as adenocarcinoma, and together they make up the preponderance of malignant neoplasms of the small bowel. Carcinoids have variable malignant potential and are composed of multipotential cells with the ability to secrete numerous humoral agents, the most prominent of which are serotonin and substance P. Although the carcinoid syndrome, characterized by episodic

attacks of cutaneous flushing, bronchospasm, diarrhea, and vasomotor collapse, occurs in fewer than 5 percent of the patients with malignant carcinoids, it is quite dramatic and has been extensively described and discussed with fascination by many authors.

The primary importance of carcinoid tumors, however, is not the carcinoid syndrome but the malignant potential of the tumors themselves. Oberndorfer coined the term *karzinoide* to indicate that this tumor is carcinomalike and to emphasize the assumed lack of malignant potential. By 1930 this concept was no longer supported, since many patients with metastatic carcinoid tumors had been reported. In 1953 and 1954 the carcinoid syndrome was described.

Pathology. Carcinoids may arise in organs derived from the foregut, midgut, and hindgut. In the gastrointestinal tract over 90 percent of carcinoids are found in three sites: the appendix is most frequently involved (46 percent), followed by the ileum (28 percent) and the rectum (17 percent), but all organs may give rise to carcinoids. Other gastrointestinal locations are listed in Table 25-4. The malignant potential (ability to metastasize) is related to location, size, depth of invasion, and growth pattern. Only about 3 percent of appendiceal carcinoids metastasize, but about 35 percent of ileal carcinoids are associated with metastasis. Seventy-five percent of gastrointestinal carcinoids are less than 1 cm in diameter; only 2 percent of this group metastasize. About 20 percent of primary tumors are 1 to 2 cm in diameter, and 50 percent of this group metastasize. Only about 5 percent are over 2 cm in diameter; 80 to 90 percent of these

Table 25-4
Distribution of Gastrointestinal Carcinoids: Incidence of Metastases and of Carcinoid Syndrome

Site	*Cases*	*Average Metastasis (%)*	*Cases of Carcinoid Syndrome*
Esophagus	1	—	0
Stomach	93	23	8
Duodenum	135	20	4
Jejunoileum	1032	34	91
Meckel's diverticulum	42	19	3
Appendix	1686	2	6
Colon	91	60	5
Rectum	592	18	1
Ovary	34	6	17
Biliary tract	10	30	0
Pancreas	2	—	1
	3718		136

SOURCE: Wilson H, Cheek RC, et al: Carcinoid tumors. *Curr Probl Surg* 4, 1970.

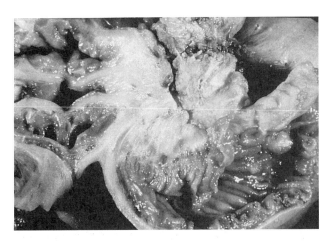

FIG. 25-25. *Carcinoid tumor of the distal ileum demonstrating the intense desmoplastic reaction and fibrosis of the bowel wall.*

metastasize. Carcinoids limited to the submucosa do not metastasize, whereas 69 percent of carcinoids involving the serosa have metastases. The histologic growth patterns appear to be related to survival and therefore have prognostic importance.

Multiple carcinoids of the small bowel occur in 30 percent of patients with carcinoid but are rare in the appendix. This tendency to multicentricity exceeds that of any other malignant neoplasm of the gastrointestinal tract. An unusual observation that is yet unexplained is the frequent coexistence of a second primary malignant neoplasm of a different histologic type; a second primary neoplasm was reported in 25 percent of patients in one large series.

Carcinoids present grossly as a slightly elevated, smooth, rounded, hard nodule, covered with normal mucosa. On cut section, they have a characteristic yellow-gray or tan appearance. Extensive fibrosis of the mesentery and of the bowel wall, caused by an intense desmoplastic reaction, may be present (Fig. 25-25). This fibrosis may produce mechanical bowel obstruction from kinking or matting of loops of small bowel together. Obstruction rarely is a result of direct tumor encroachment on the lumen of the bowel. In addition to the desmoplastic reaction, apparently produced by humoral agents elaborated by the tumor, metastases to mesenteric nodes also result in kinking and fixa-

tion by large metastatic tumor deposits. A small primary tumor associated with massive mesenteric metastases is often noted (Fig. 25-26).

Clinical Manifestations. In the absence of the malignant carcinoid syndrome, symptoms of patients with carcinoid tumors of the small bowel are similar to those of patients with small-bowel tumors of other histologic types. The most common symptoms are abdominal pain, bowel obstruction, diarrhea, and weight loss. In the majority of patients (in the absence of the malignant carcinoid syndrome), the diarrhea is a result of partial bowel obstruction rather than being secretory. Rarely, malignant carcinoid tumors of the ampulla of Vater are found in patients with disseminated neurofibromatosis (von Recklinghausen's disease).

Diagnostic Findings. Radiographic studies of the small bowel may exhibit multiple filling defects, sometimes caused by tumors but more often a result of kinking and fibrosis of the bowel, mesenteric calcifications, and fixed, rigid loops of intestine. Mesenteric vascular angiography may reveal abnormal arrangement of mesenteric arteries and narrowing of peripheral branches together with poor accumulation of contrast and poor venous drainage of the tumor area. Tumor staining during angiography may be enhanced by administration of norepinephrine. Angiography is the most sensitive diagnostic test to detect hepatic metastasis, particularly diffuse metastatic disease with fine nodular distribution. Hepatic metastases are hypervascular and intensely stained during arteriography.

Treatment. The treatment of patients with small-bowel carcinoid tumors is based on the size and the site of the tumor and the presence or absence of metastatic disease. For primary tumors less than 1 cm in diameter without evidence of regional lymph node metastasis, a segmental intestinal resection is adequate. For patients with lesions greater than 1 cm, with multiple tumors, or with regional lymph node metastasis regardless of the size of the primary tumor, wide excision of bowel and mesentery is required. Since the majority of small-bowel carcinoids are found in the ileum, wide excision usually entails a right hemicolectomy. Malignant carcinoid tumors of the duodenum may require radical pancreatoduodenectomy. When carcinoids are localized, almost all are cured by surgical resection; patients with the malignant carcinoid syndrome caused by metastatic disease

FIG. 25-26. *Mesenteric metastases from a carcinoid tumor of the small bowel.*

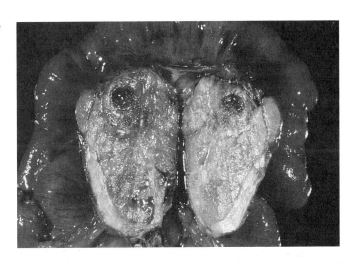

may receive significant palliation but are not cured with surgical resection.

Treatment of Carcinoid Tumors of the Appendix. Appendiceal carcinoids typically are diagnosed in patients 20 to 40 years of age, in contrast to the mean age at diagnosis of small-bowel carcinoids of 60 years. The majority of appendiceal carcinoids are located at the tip. Simple appendectomy is curative for patients with tumors less than 1 cm in diameter without gross evidence of metastasis. Because of the potential for metastasis, right hemicolectomy should be performed for tumors greater than 2 cm. Intramural lymphatic invasion, serosal involvement, or microscopic involvement of the mesoappendix associated with tumors less than 2 cm in diameter is not an indication for extensive resection.

Prognosis. The survival rate for patients with small-bowel carcinoid tumors has been reported to be 75 percent for those with tumors staged as local, 59 percent for regional tumors, and 19 percent for tumors with distant spread. The overall survival rate is 54 percent. The growth pattern of carcinoid tumors is an independent predictor of outcome. The median survival times of the various growth patterns, in decreasing order, are as follows: mixed insular plus glandular, 4.4 years; insular, 2.9 years; trabecular, 2.5 years; mixed insular plus trabecular, 2.3 years; glandular growth pattern, 0.9 years; and undifferentiated, 0.5 years.

When widespread metastatic disease precludes cure, extensive resection for palliation is indicated. Since these tumors are often indolent and slow-growing, long-term palliation often is obtained. Bypass procedures may be used in poor-risk patients with extensive disease. The overall 5-year survival rate after resection of intestinal carcinoids is about 50 percent. When "curative resection" is done, the 5-year survival rate is 70 percent. Chemotherapy has not been entirely successful; however, treatment with streptozotocin and 5-fluorouracil (5-FU) may provide significant palliation. In patients with palliative resections the 5-year survival rate is 25 percent.

Malignant Carcinoid Syndrome

This rare syndrome is widely described but rarely seen. Thirty to 70 percent of carcinoid tumors of the gut are metastatic at the time of diagnosis, but only 6 to 9 percent of patients with metastatic disease develop manifestations of the malignant carcinoid syndrome. By far the most commonly associated primary tumor is located in the small bowel, and massive hepatic replacement by metastatic tumor is usually found.

Clinical Manifestations. The syndrome is characterized by hepatomegaly, diarrhea, and flushing in 80 percent of patients, right heart valvular disease in 50 percent, and asthma in 25 percent. Malabsorption and pellagra (dementia, dermatitis, and diarrhea) are occasionally present and are thought to be caused by excessive diversion of dietary tryptophan to meet the metabolic requirements of the tumor.

Diarrhea is episodic, often occurring after meals, and is a result of elevated circulating levels of serotonin, which stimulates secretion of small-bowel fluid and electrolytes and increases intestinal motility. Some patients may present with acute abdominal symptoms, characterized by severe abdominal cramping without mechanical bowel obstruction, which has been called *carcinoid abdominal crisis.* The mechanism of this crisis is thought to be intestinal ischemia, caused by the vasoactive sub-

stances elaborated by the tumor, combined with decreased mesenteric blood supply from perivascular fibrosis.

Flushing is not temporally related to diarrhea, and, although both may be present, either may be present without the other. The lack of relationship between flushing and diarrhea suggests that these two manifestations of the syndrome are caused by different mediators. Although substance P produces all of the vasomotor phenomena associated with the flush, it has been questioned as the primary mediator. Besides serotonin and substance P, other substances that have been implicated include bradykinin and prostaglandins E and F.

Valvular heart disease is a result of irreversible endocardial fibrosis, which is similar in genesis to the fibrosis noted in the gut wall, in the retroperitoneum, and around the mesenteric blood vessels. It occurs in patients with hepatic metastases and is limited to tricuspid and pulmonary valves. The reason the lesions are restricted to the valves on the right side is that they are exposed to high levels of serotonin; the pulmonary filter deactivates serotonin, thereby preventing left-sided valvular lesions.

Asthma is due to bronchoconstriction, which may be produced by serotonin, bradykinin, or substance P. Treatment of asthma associated with carcinoid syndrome must be carried out very carefully, since the use of adrenergic drugs may cause the release of humoral agents that may cause status asthmaticus.

Although the syndrome is seen in patients with high circulating levels of serotonin and often substance P, these are probably not the only mediators of all components of the syndrome. The malignant enterochromaffin cells produce 5-hydroxytryptamine (5-HT), which is serotonin. Circulating serotonin is metabolized in the liver and in the lung to 5-hydroxyindoleacetic acid (5-HIAA), which is pharmacologically inactive. Elevated levels of 5-HIAA are seen only in patients with metastasis. However, not all patients with metastasis have increased levels of 5-HIAA. The majority of patients who exhibit malignant carcinoid syndrome have massive hepatic replacement by their metastatic disease. Tumors that bypass the hepatic filter, specifically ovarian and retroperitoneal carcinoids, may produce the syndrome in the absence of liver metastasis.

Diagnostic Findings. The diagnosis is most reliably established by repeated determinations of urinary 5-HIAA. A single determination may be normal in the presence of metastatic disease. Provocative testing to reproduce symptoms has employed injection of pentagastrin, calcium, or epinephrine. The pentagastrin test is by far the most reliable and safest provocative test. During times of testing for increased levels of 5-HIAA, the patient must avoid foods rich in serotonin, such as bananas, tomatoes, walnuts, and pineapples, and certain drugs, including phenothiazines, glycerol guaiacolate, and reserpine.

Treatment. Ideally, treatment of the carcinoid syndrome would require removal of all tumor, but this rarely is possible. Hepatic resection, however, even when known tumor is left behind, may result in significant relief of symptoms because of the removal of the mass of tumor. When resection is not possible, hepatic dearterialization or embolization of the hepatic arterial branches with chemotherapy (doxorubicin, 5-fluorouracil, cisplatin) may provide some relief. The duration of response after resection in one study was 6 months, compared to 4.8 months for hepatic artery ligation. In certain selected patients, liver transplantation may offer the hope of a longer disease-free interval; however, the long-term outcome of this radical approach is not known.

Drug therapy for prevention or relief of symptoms is directed at blockade of the effects of humoral agents elaborated by the tumor. Interferon has provided some symptomatic improvement in a small group of patients. Somatostatin-14 and its long-acting analog octreotide (Sandostatin) relieve symptoms (diarrhea and flushing) of the carcinoid syndrome in the majority of patients. Furthermore, Kvols and colleagues have found that survival is significantly prolonged in patients with carcinoid tumors treated with Sandostatin. In addition to preventing the devastating sequelae of the carcinoid syndrome, Sandostatin also may possess a direct antitumor effect. Chemotherapeutic attacks on the tumor itself have been disappointing, although streptozotocin, alone or combined with 5-fluorouracil, appears to be the most effective.

Treatment of carcinoid tumors is wide surgical resection of the small bowel and regional lymph nodes. In addition, significant palliation may be achieved with aggressive hepatic resection in patients with malignant carcinoid syndrome.

DIVERTICULAR DISEASE

Diverticula of the small bowel may be congenital or acquired. A congenital diverticulum is a true diverticulum; it is composed of all layers of the bowel wall. An acquired diverticulum is a false diverticulum; only mucosa and submucosa protrude through a defect in the muscle coat of the bowel wall. Diverticula may occur in any portion of small intestine. Duodenal diverticula are the most common acquired diverticula of the small bowel, and Meckel's diverticulum is the most common true diverticulum of the small bowel.

Duodenal Diverticula

Duodenal diverticula are common; the duodenum is the second most common site of diverticulum formation, after the colon. The true incidence of duodenal diverticula is unknown, and reported incidences vary, depending on whether they are found clinically (by x-ray, endoscopy, or operation) or at autopsy. It has been reported that 1 to 5 percent of upper gastrointestinal x-ray examinations reveal duodenal diverticula; 9 to 20 percent of upper gastrointestinal endoscopic examinations show them. In autopsy series, incidences of 10 to 20 percent are reported. More than 90 percent of these diverticula are clearly asymptomatic, and less than 5 percent will require operation because of a complication of the diverticulum itself. Duodenal diverticula occur twice as often in women as in men. They are rare in patients under 40 years of age, and the incidence increases with increasing age. Two-thirds to three-fourths of duodenal diverticula are found in a periampullary region and project from the medial wall of the duodenum (Fig. 25-27). Duodenal diverticula are clinically important for two reasons. First, they occasionally produce symptoms related to the diverticulum, including obstruction, perforation, or bleeding, and second, the presence of the diverticulum may cause recurrent pancreatitis, cholangitis, or recurrent common-duct stones after cholecystectomy.

Only those diverticula associated with the ampulla of Vater have a significant relationship to the complications of cholangitis, pancreatitis, and stone disease. In patients with these diverticula, the ampulla most often enters the duodenum at the superior margin of the diverticulum, rather than through the di-

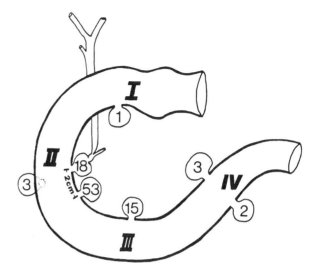

FIG. 25-27. Distribution of 95 duodenal diverticula within the four portions of the duodenum. (From: *Eggert A, Wittmann DH: Surg Gynecol Obstet 154:62, 1982, with permission.*)

verticulum itself. The mechanism proposed for the increased incidence of complications of the biliary tract is the location of the perivaterian diverticula, which may produce mechanical distortion of the common bile duct as it enters the duodenum, resulting in partial obstruction and stasis. Bile stasis allows proliferation of bacteria and subsequent formation of stones. The incidence of bacteriobilia is significantly higher in patients with perivaterian diverticula than in those with diverticula located in other parts of the duodenum. The bacteria isolated from the bile duct and from the diverticula are identical. There is also evidence that dysfunction of the choledochal sphincter is produced by the presence of diverticula. In one study of 101 patients who had undergone cholecystectomy more than 2 years earlier, a significantly higher incidence of recurrent calculi was noted in patients with diverticula than in patients without. A causal relationship of duodenal diverticula to biliary tract stones, however, has not been demonstrated. It is important not to extend indications for operation to include people with unexplained abdominal pain. Nor should retention of barium within diverticula serve by itself as an indication for operation. The important point is that the great majority of duodenal diverticula cause no trouble; they should be left alone unless they can be conclusively related to disease.

Fewer than 60 patients have been reported with intraluminal duodenal diverticula. These diverticula, which probably originate from incomplete duodenal webs, are lined both inside and out with duodenal mucosa, have a characteristic picture of a barium-filled wind sock on contrast radiography, and most often required operation because of duodenal obstruction or recurrent pancreatitis. In these diverticula the common bile duct and pancreatic duct usually enter the diverticulum, and a second orifice is present that allows drainage of the biliary-pancreatic secretions into the lumen of the gut.

Symptoms related to duodenal diverticula, in the absence of any other demonstrable disease, usually are nonspecific epigastric complaints. Bleeding, perforation, and diverticulitis all are rare. The morbidity and mortality caused by complications of diverticula are nonetheless high as a result of delay in diagnosis

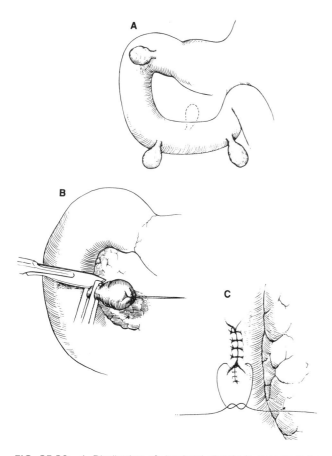

FIG. 25-28. *A. Distribution of duodenal diverticula appears to be random. Many surgeons believe that diverticula of the second part of the duodenum are more likely to cause trouble, but this may simply be because these diverticula are the most difficult to remove. B. If the diverticulum is clearly visible, it can be mobilized and traction exerted on a suture in the apex. A Kocher clamp can be placed at the base, and the diverticulum can be excised. C. The diverticulum is closed by placing a running chromic or polyglactin (Vicryl) suture back and forth behind the clamp in a basting stitch followed by inverting the suture line with interrupted 3-0 silk sutures. (From: Thompson JC: Atlas of Surgery of the Stomach, Duodenum, and Small Bowel. St. Louis, Mosby–Year Book, 1992, with permission.)*

because of the lack of suspicion of the underlying condition. Diagnosis is seldom made preoperatively.

Treatment. Treatment of complications of the diverticulum are directed toward the control of the complication. In patients who have bleeding or symptoms that are related to the duodenal diverticulum, several operative procedures have been described. The most common and most effective treatment in this situation is diverticulectomy. This is most easily accomplished by performing a wide Kocher maneuver that exposes the diverticulum (Fig. 25-28). The diverticulum then is excised, and the duodenum is closed in a transverse or a longitudinal manner, whichever produces the least amount of luminal obstruction. For diverticula embedded deep within the head of the pancreas, lateral duodenotomy is performed; the diverticulum is invaginated into the lumen and excised, and the wall is closed. An alternative method that has been described for duodenal diverticula associated with the ampulla of Vater is an extended sphincteroplasty through the common wall of the ampulla and the diverticulum.

A perforated diverticulum may cause a great deal of trouble. When found, the perforated diverticulum should be excised and the duodenum closed with a serosal patch from the jejunal loop. If the inflammation is severe, it may be necessary to divert enteric flow away from the site of the perforation, with a gastrojejunostomy or, preferably, a duodenojejunostomy if possible. It may be possible to interrupt duodenal continuity proximal to the perforated diverticulum with a row of staples. Great care should be taken if the perforation is adjacent to the papilla. In one early perforation, we were able simply to invert the diverticulum, close the duodenal wall, and reinforce this with a serosal patch.

Because of the relationship of the common bile duct and pancreatic duct in patients with intraluminal diverticula associated with the ampulla of Vater, subtotal resection of the diverticulum should be carried out to protect the entry of the biliary-pancreatic ducts. If an intraluminal diverticulum arises at a site distant from the ampulla, complete excision may be possible.

The vast majority of duodenal diverticula are asymptomatic and benign, and when they found incidentally they should not be resected.

Jejunal and Ileal Diverticula

Diverticula of the jejunum and the ileum are much less common than duodenal diverticula, with an incidence between 0.5 and 1 percent on small-bowel x-ray examination. Jejunal diverticula are more common and are larger than those in the ileum (Fig. 25-29). Multiple diverticula are more common in the jejunum and the ileum than in the duodenum. These are false diverticula that usually protrude from the mesenteric border of the bowel, and they may be overlooked at operation because they are embedded within the small-bowel mesentery. When jejunal and ileal diverticula cause trouble, the symptoms usually are from incomplete bowel obstruction, acute diverticulitis, hemorrhage, or malabsorption due to bacterial overgrowth within the diverticulum. A specific syndrome of intestinal pseudoobstruction or jejunal dyskinesia is characterized by symptoms of intermittent partial bowel obstruction. On enteroclysis, barium may be seen to pass back and forth from the intestinal lumen into the diverticulum rather than moving normally through the bowel. This

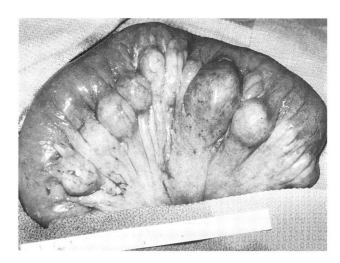

FIG. 25-29. *Multiple jejunal diverticula in an elderly patient who presented with a complete small-bowel obstruction secondary to an enterolith that became dislodged and obstructed the distal ileum.*

condition may be associated with hypertrophy and dilatation of the bowel proximal to the diverticulum. A recent study found that the condition may be associated with one of three syndromes: systemic sclerosis, visceral myopathy, or visceral neuropathy. If this condition is the only finding, resection of a large segment of jejunum containing diverticula should be avoided. Treatment of complications of obstruction, bleeding, and perforation is by intestinal resection and end-to-end anastomosis.

Obstruction also may be caused by enteroliths that form in a jejunal diverticulum and are subsequently dislodged and obstruct the distal intestine. This condition mainly occurs in the elderly and may be treated by enterotomy and removal of the enterolith. Patients with malabsorption from production of the blind loop syndrome by bacterial overgrowth within the diverticulum usually can be treated with antibiotics. Asymptomatic diverticula require no treatment.

Meckel's Diverticulum

Meckel's diverticulum, the most common true diverticulum of the gastrointestinal tract, is a congenital diverticulum that results from incomplete closure of the omphalomesenteric or vitelline duct. The usual manifestation is a relatively wide projection arising from the antimesenteric side of the ileum, generally 45 to 60 cm proximal to the ileocecal valve. Occasionally the diverticulum is merely a small bump or hillock, or it may be long and narrow (1–12 cm), but usually it is short and relatively wide (Fig. 25-30A). Various forms exist, depending on the presence or absence of communication with the umbilicus or with various stages of atrophy of the omphalomesenteric ductal connection between the ileum and the umbilical skin (variations ranging from a persistent fibrous cord to a patent fistula) (Fig. 25-30B–H). Heterotopic gastric or pancreatic tissue often is found in Meckel's diverticula. The vast majority of Meckel's diverticula are entirely benign. Trouble arises from bleeding or inflammation, which gives rise to a symptom complex usually indistinguishable from appendicitis; from perforation, usually caused by peptic ulcer from acid and pepsin secretion from ectopic gastric fundic mucosa; and from problems associated with persistence of part or all of the omphalomesenteric duct. The great majority of symptomatic Meckel's diverticula are found in childhood, and the most common symptom in childhood is bleeding. On the basis of several autopsy series, Meckel's diverticula has a reported incidence in the general population of 2 percent. In adults most Meckel's diverticula are found incidentally by radiographic examination of the small bowel. Enteroclysis usually provides an accurate diagnosis. Another technique for detection of Meckel's diverticulum in symptomatic patients is radionuclide scanning with ^{99m}Tc-pertechnetate. The basis for this is the uptake of radioisotope by the heterotopic gastric mucosa within the diverticulum. The diagnostic accuracy of this scanning technique may be increased by administration of pentagastrin (6 mg/kg subcutaneously) 15 min before the scan, which enhances the uptake of the radioisotope by the gastric mucosa. It has been shown, however, that the parietal cells do not specifically accumulate pertechnetate and are not essential for detection purposes. The scan far more useful in children than in adults.

Complications of Meckel's diverticulum in adults include intestinal obstruction, bleeding, acute diverticulitis, or the presence of a diverticulum in a hernia sac (Littre's hernia). Obstruction may be produced by one of two mechanisms. The most common is volvulus or kinking around a band running from the tip of the diverticulum to the umbilicus, abdominal wall, or mesentery. The diverticulum also may cause obstruction by intussusception. Bleeding is the second most common complication and usually is found only when there is heterotopic gastric mucosa within the diverticulum. The bleeding ulcer is found not in the diverticulum but in the ileum adjacent to the diverticulum.

Meckel's diverticulitis, which is clinically indistinguishable from appendicitis, is the third most common complication in adults. The incidence of perforation or peritonitis with Meckel's diverticulitis is about 50 percent.

A Meckel's diverticulum should be considered in the differential diagnosis of patients who present with a mechanical bowel obstruction, with low small-bowel hemorrhage, or with signs and symptoms of inflammation or peritonitis. Treatment is prompt surgical intervention, with resection of the diverticulum or resection of the segment of ileum bearing the diverticulum (Fig. 25-30I–J). Segmental intestinal resection is required for treatment of patients with bleeding, because the bleeding site usually is in the ileum adjacent to the diverticulum. Recent reports have demonstrated the feasibility and safety of laparoscopic diverticulectomy; long-term outcome with this procedure, however, are lacking.

It is generally recommended that asymptomatic diverticula found in children during laparotomy be resected; however, the treatment of an asymptomatic Meckel's diverticulum found incidentally at laparotomy in the adult patient is controversial. In a landmark paper that has greatly influenced the surgical management of the asymptomatic diverticulum, Soltero and Bill estimated that the likelihood of a Meckel's diverticulum becoming symptomatic in an adult is 2 percent or less and that morbidity from incidental removal (reported to be as high as 12 percent in some studies) far exceeds the potential for prevention of disease. From this study, the authors concluded that an asymptomatic Meckel's diverticulum in the adult should not be removed. This study has been criticized, however, since it was not a population-based analysis. An epidemiologic, population-based study by Cullen and associates has challenged the practice of ignoring an incidentally found Meckel's diverticulum. A 6.4 percent rate of developing complications from the Meckel's diverticulum was calculated to occur over a lifetime; this incidence of complications does not appear to peak during childhood as originally thought. These authors therefore recommended that an incidentally discovered Meckel's diverticulum should be removed at any age up to 80 years, as long as no additional condition (e.g., peritonitis) makes removal hazardous. The rates of short-term and long-term postoperative complications from prophylactic removal are low (approximately 2 percent), and in the Cullen series mortality was related to the primary operation or the general health of the patient and not to the diverticulectomy. Therefore, this study as well as other recent studies suggest that prophylactic diverticulectomy in selected patients may be beneficial and safer than originally reported.

MISCELLANEOUS PROBLEMS

Congenital Abnormalities

Although primarily limited to infants and children, developmental anomalies of the small intestine also may present in adulthood. In addition to Meckel's diverticulum, discussed above,

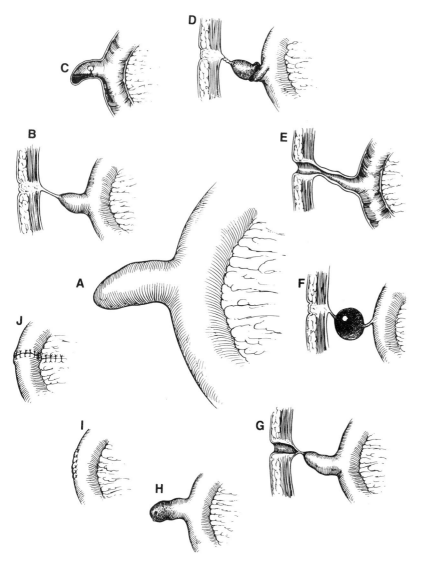

FIG. 25-30. *A.* The most common nonpathologic appearance of a Meckel's diverticulum arising bluntly from the antimesenteric border of the distal ileum. *B.* A persistent fibrous band connecting the apex of the diverticulum with the anterior abdominal wall at the umbilicus. The band should be doubly ligated and divided. *C.* Bleeding from a peptic ulcer in a Meckel's diverticulum. This is an uncommon cause of occult gastrointestinal hemorrhage (seen especially in children). The bleeding site may be localized by means of a radioisotopic scan. Treatment is excision of the diverticulum along with a small margin of ileum on each side and end-to-end anastomosis of the ileum. *D.* Rare twisting and strangulation of the diverticulum. Treatment should be partial excision of the ileum, division of the fibrous band at the anterior abdominal wall, and removal of the entire Meckel's diverticulum and persistent fibrous band. *E.* A completely patent omphalomesenteric duct leads to appearance of enteric contents at the umbilicus. This requires excision of the omphalomesenteric duct, either taking the ileal end off flush with the ileum and closing it, or dividing the ileum adjacently on each side and performing an ileoileostomy. In either case the umbilical end should be clamped and sutured and the duct excised. *F.* Cystic dilatation of the middle portion of the omphalomesenteric duct with fibrous atrophy of the duct at both ends. The cyst may become inflamed and perforate. It can be removed by double ligation of the fibrous tract, division of the tract, and removal of the cyst. *G.* A variant of a persistent attachment of the omphalomesenteric duct to the anterior abdominal wall with a persistent tract in the wall, itself opening onto the umbilicus. This should be treated by excising the Meckel's diverticulum and circumferentially excising the persistent duct through the abdominal wall, taking care to remove all mucosa, followed by closure of the ileum and closure of the abdominal wall. *H.* Inflammation of Meckel's diverticulum with a tip perforation. This will give rise to an appendicitis-like syndrome. It is best treated by local division of the ileum, being sure to carry the line of division beyond inflamed tissue, and an end-to-end ileoileostomy. *I.* The suture line after local Meckel's diverticulectomy. We usually close with a running suture of chromic or polyglactin (Vicryl) and then invert that suture line with a row of interrupted 4-0 silk sutures. *J.* A completed ileoileal anastomosis after excision of 1 to 2 cm of ileum on each side of a Meckel's diverticulum and routine two-layer end-to-end ileoileostomy. (From: *Thompson JC: Atlas of Surgery of the Stomach, Duodenum, and Small Bowel.* St. Louis, Mosby–Year Book, 1992, with permission.)

intestinal duplications and anomalies of gut rotation and fixation may be manifested in the adult.

The term *duplication* actually is a misnomer, since approximately 75 percent are enteric cysts and not true duplications. The remainder are true tubular duplications that are intimately attached to the adjacent portion of the gastrointestinal tract, possess a gastrointestinal type of mucosal lining, and may or may not communicate with the visceral lumen. Duplications occur on the mesenteric side of the intestine between the leaves of the mesentery and are most often found in the ileum. In rare instances, a duplication from the abdomen extends into the chest. Cystic lesions may present with symptoms of obstruction from extrinsic compression. Communicating tubular duplications often are lined by gastric mucosa, which may ulcerate and present with gastrointestinal hemorrhage or perforation. In addition, cancers have been reported to arise in the mucosal lining of these duplications. Treatment is surgical resection. Small tubular duplications and all cysts are excised along with overlying normal intestine; intestinal continuity is restored by end-to-end anastomosis. Long tubular duplications that would require massive small-bowel resection for complete removal are more problematic and may be treated by mucosal stripping of the duplication.

Various anomalies may occur from defects in gut rotation. Failure of the midgut to rotate results in the duodenum's descending to the right of the midline with the entire small bowel lying in the right half of the abdomen and the colon lying to the left. Patients usually are asymptomatic. Symptoms from malrotation result from the midgut's failing to rotate completely and usually occur in patients 2 months of age or less; however, symptoms of midgut volvulus occur in 10 percent of patients at a later age and present either acutely or with chronic symptoms of intermittent partial obstruction. Partial obstruction of the duodenum by peritoneal bands (Ladd's bands) may cause bilious vomiting and intermittent cramping abdominal pain. Mesocolic hernias (also referred to as paraduodenal hernias) occur when failure of proper gut fixation results in the small bowel's being trapped within the mesentery of the colon. The most common presentation is that of obstruction. Treatment for anomalies of rotation and fixation include lysis of Ladd's bands (if present), reduction of the volvulus, and repositioning of the intestine to prevent twisting.

Small-Bowel Ulcerations

The majority of ulcerations of the small bowel have definable causes, which include the following: drug-induced (enteric-coated potassium chloride tablets or corticosteroids), vascular (occlusion or vasculitis), Crohn's disease, syphilis, typhoid fever, tuberculosis, lymphoma, heterotopic gastric mucosa (Meckel's diverticulum), and ulcers associated with gastrinoma. This discussion is limited to ulcerations of the small intestine in which no causative agent can be identified.

Patients with discrete isolated ulcers of the small bowel and without any identifiable underlying disease have nonspecific ulcers. Ulcers are more common in the terminal ileum. These appear to be self-limited and do not recur after bowel resection.

These patients usually present with a single ulceration, although multiple ulcers may be present. Indications for operation are for complications of the ulcers, including perforation, bleeding, or stricture. Recurrence of ulceration in the small bowel distal to the duodenum is rare. A review of 59 patients studied from 1956 to 1979 reports the overall incidence of small-bowel ulcerations to be 4 per 100,000 new patients seen at the Mayo Clinic. These investigators noted that the yearly rate fell from 3.6 new cases per year from 1960 to 1969 to 1.2 cases per year from 1970 to 1979. They believe, despite the absence of a documented underlying cause, that the decrease in incidence was directly related to the removal of enteric-coated potassium chloride tablets from the market.

The ulcers are discrete, varying from 0.3 to 5 cm in diameter; they are sharply demarcated, and the surrounding mucosa is perfectly normal. They occur more frequently on the antimesenteric border and may be associated with fibrous scar formation, which produces the obstruction. The characteristic microscopic findings include acute granulation tissue and inflammatory cells at the base of the ulcer, local hyperplasia of the muscularis mucosae, and pyloric metaplasia of the adjacent mucosa. Varying degrees of edema and fibrosis, depending on the chronicity of the ulcer, are noted. There is no evidence of vascular disease associated with the ulcer. With time, the ulcers may increase in size, may become annular, and, with healing, may produce fibrous strictures of the intestine, which may produce obstruction.

Diagnosis is rarely if ever made before operation; the majority of patients present with complications. In the Mayo Clinic series 63 percent of patients had intermittent small-bowel obstruction, 25 percent had bleeding, and 12 percent had symptoms of acute abdominal inflammation caused by perforation. With the increasing use of enteroclysis, the diagnosis of small-bowel ulcer may be made more frequently. An asymptomatic solitary ulcer does not require treatment.

Treatment. The treatment of small-bowel ulcers depends on the complications encountered at the time of diagnosis. Mechanical bowel obstruction and bleeding should be treated by segmental resection. Although excision and primary closure of perforated ulcers has been advocated by some, high recurrence rates have been associated with this technique. The ulcerated segment of bowel should be resected.

Ingested Foreign Bodies

A great variety of objects that are capable of penetrating the wall of the gut are swallowed, usually accidentally, but sometimes intentionally by the mentally deranged. These include glass and metal fragments, pins, needles, cocktail toothpicks, fish bones, coins, whistles, toys, and broken razor blades.

Treatment is observation, since the vast majority pass without difficulty. If the object is radiopaque, progress can be followed by serial plain films. Catharsis is contraindicated.

Sharp, pointed objects such as sewing needles may penetrate the bowel wall. If abdominal pain, tenderness, fever, or leukocytosis occurs, immediate surgical removal of the offending object is indicated. Abscess or granuloma formation is the usual outcome without surgical therapy.

Small-Bowel Fistulas

The vast majority of small-bowel fistulas are a result of operation; less than 2 percent are associated with granulomatous disease of the bowel (Crohn's disease) or trauma. In some patients there are contributing factors, such as preoperative radiotherapy, intestinal obstruction, inflammatory bowel disease, mesenteric vascular disease, and intraabdominal sepsis. But in the majority, surgical misadventures are the primary cause. These include anastomotic leak, injury of bowel or blood supply at operation, laceration of bowel by wire mesh or retention sutures, and retained sponges. In addition, fistulas may result from erosion by suction catheters and by abscesses.

The major complications associated with small-bowel fistulas include sepsis, fluid and electrolyte depletion, necrosis of the skin at the site of external drainage, and malnutrition. Successful management of patients with small-bowel fistulas requires meticulous attention to detail and a logical, stepwise plan of management. One must establish controlled drainage, manage sepsis, prevent fluid and electrolyte depletion, protect the skin, and provide for adequate nutrition.

Mortality for patients with intestinal fistulas remains high (20 percent or greater), even with the use of total parenteral nutrition (TPN). Although TPN has not been shown to reduce mortality significantly, it is the single most important advance in the management of patients with enterocutaneous fistulas. Fluid, electrolyte, and nutritional status may be maintained from the time the fistula becomes apparent and throughout the time required for control of sepsis. The key to successful management of intestinal fistulas is control of sepsis and prevention of malnutrition.

Diagnosis of small-bowel fistula usually is not difficult. When the damaged area of the small bowel breaks down and discharges its contents, dissemination may occur widely in the peritoneal cavity, producing generalized peritonitis. More commonly, however, the process is more or less walled-off in the immediate area of the leak, with formation of an abscess. This usually underlies the operative incision, so that when a few skin sutures are removed to ascertain why the incision is becoming red and tender, contents of the abscess are discharged and the fistula established. The discharge initially may be purulent or bloody, but this is followed—sometimes immediately, sometimes within a day or two—by drainage of obvious small-bowel contents. If the diagnosis is in doubt, confirmation can be obtained by oral administration of a nonabsorbable marker such as charcoal or Congo red.

Small-bowel fistulas are classified according to their location and volume of daily output, since these factors dictate treatment as well as morbidity and mortality rates. In general, the more proximal the fistula in the intestine, the more serious the problem. Proximal fistulas have a greater fluid and electrolyte loss, the drainage has a greater digestive capacity, and an important (distal) segment is not available for food absorption. High-output fistulas are those that discharge 500 mL or more per 24 h. It is important, therefore, as soon as the patient's condition is stabilized, to identify the site of the fistula, to determine the extent of the associated abscess cavity by fistulogram, and to ascertain whether there is distal obstruction, since fistulas will not close in the presence of distal obstruction (Fig. 25-31). Upper gastrointestinal series with small-bowel follow-through and barium enema studies also may provide useful information.

Treatment. Control of sepsis is aided by sump suction, which provides drainage of the associated intraabdominal abscess cavity and prevents accumulation of intestinal contents. Control of fistula output is most easily accomplished by percutaneous intubation of the fistula tract. Protection of the skin around the fistulous opening is important. In the past, frequent applications of zinc oxide, aluminum paste ointment, or karaya powder were required; excoriation and destruction of skin still occurred. The advent of Stomahesive appliances used for colostomy and ileostomy bags greatly improved and facilitated pro-

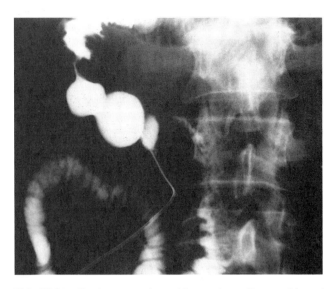

FIG. 25-31. Fistulogram performed in a patient with a small-bowel fistula. A distal obstruction is demonstrated (arrow).

tection of the skin at the site of the fistula. The Stomahesive appliance should be cut so that the opening just fits over the fistulous opening and no unprotected skin remains. The suction catheter can be brought out through the end of the bag, which is fixed firmly about the tube. This allows for collection of all the drainage and accurate quantitation of the lost volume.

The volume depletion that occurs from a proximal small-bowel fistula may present a formidable problem. Volume losses exceeding 5 L/day are not uncommon. Agents that inhibit gut motility (codeine, Lomotil, or loperamide) generally are not helpful. The hormone somatostatin is considered a general "off switch" and inhibits both intestinal secretion and motility. We and others have used a long-acting octapeptide analog of somatostatin (octreotide) in combination with TPN in the management of enterocutaneous fistulas. In most series, the overall fistula closure rate was not altered, but the analog ameliorated the problems associated with massive volume loss. Systemic antibiotics should be administered until sepsis is controlled. TPN should be instituted at the same time, because a prolonged course of inability to use the gut for nutrition is likely.

Several factors may prevent spontaneous closure of fistulas. Fistulas will not close spontaneously if there is high output (> 500 mL/24 h) or severe disruption of intestinal continuity (> 50 percent of the circumference of the bowel involved in the fistula). A fistula will not close spontaneously if it arises from a segment of bowel involved with active granulomatous disease, cancer, or radiation enteritis, if there is distal obstruction, or if there is an undrained abscess cavity. If a foreign body is in the tract, if the fistula tract is less than 2.5 cm in length, or if there is epithelialization of the tract, spontaneous closure will not occur. Radiographic investigation of the fistula by injection of water-soluble contrast material through the fistula tract should be carried out early to delineate the presence and extent of any abscess cavities and to obtain information about the length of the tract and the extent of bowel wall disruption. A diligent search by means of contrast studies for distal obstruction should be performed. CT will often reveal undrained collections of fluid.

When any of the conditions noted above are present, spontaneous closure is unlikely, and therefore management should be directed toward obtaining prompt control of sepsis, maintaining positive nitrogen balance, and early operation.

Conservative treatment for up to 3 months with TPN has been advocated by some to allow spontaneous closure of the fistula. We do not believe that the results support this approach. Fewer than 30 percent of all small-bowel fistulas will close spontaneously. In patients with low-output fistulas, particularly those located in the distal small bowel without any of the conditions that prevent spontaneous closure, a wait of up to 6 weeks may be indicated. The patient usually can wait at home. When we reviewed reported series that advocate conservative therapy for longer than 6 weeks, we found that the majority of fistulas that close spontaneously do so within 3 weeks after their appearance. After 3 weeks, if sepsis has been controlled and adequate nutritional status has been achieved, operative control of the fistula should be carried out promptly. Delay only produces delay. TPN simplifies management of patients, but it does not cure fistulas. The single most important determinant in successful treatment of fistulas is sepsis. If sepsis is not controlled, the patient will die. After sepsis has been controlled, one should not wait endlessly for a fistula to close spontaneously simply because malnutrition can be avoided by use of TPN. The proper role of TPN is prevention or treatment of malnutrition before operative closure of fistulas.

Operation is most easily accomplished by entering the previous abdominal wound. The wound should be reopened with great care to avoid needless reinjury to the bowel. The fistula tract is excised, the bowel should be completely mobilized, and the portion of bowel involved in the fistula is resected. The technique of excision and fistula closure must be precise and accurate, and all rigid or diseased bowel must be resected. Simple closure of the fistula after removing the fistula tract and minimal mobilization of the bowel almost always results in recurrence of the fistula.

If an unexpected abscess is encountered or if the bowel wall is rigid and distended over a large distance, a proximal enterostomy should be performed. Later, resection of the bowel involved in the fistula will be required for successful closure. Side-to-side bypass should not be done.

The overall mortality rate in enterocutaneous fistulas of the small bowel is greater than 20 percent. It is higher in jejunal fistulas and significantly lower in ileal fistulas. Successful treatment of the majority of patients with small-bowel fistulas requires control of sepsis, provision of adequate nutrition, and operative closure.

Pneumatosis Cystoides Intestinalis

This is an uncommon condition manifested by multiple gas-filled cysts of the gastrointestinal tract. The cysts are either submucosal or subserosal and vary in size from microscopic to several centimeters in diameter. The jejunum is most frequently involved, followed by the ileocecal region and the colon; extraintestinal structures such as mesentery, peritoneum, and the falciform ligament also may be involved. Gas cysts are associated with other lesions of the gastrointestinal tract in about 85 percent of cases. These "secondary" causes include inflammatory, obstructive, or infectious conditions of the intestine, iatrogenic conditions such as endoscopy and jejunostomy placement, ischemia, and extraintestinal diseases such as chronic obstructive pulmonary disease, diabetic enteropathy, and collagen vascular diseases. Pneumatosis not associated with other lesions (15 percent of cases) is referred to as primary pneumatosis.

Grossly, the cysts resemble cystic lymphangiomas or hydatid cysts. On section, the involved portion has a honeycomb appearance. The cysts are thin-walled and break easily. Spontaneous rupture gives rise to pneumoperitoneum.

Symptoms are nonspecific and in secondary pneumatosis may be those of the associated disease. Symptoms in primary pneumatosis, when present, resemble those of irritable bowel syndrome. The diagnosis usually is made radiographically by plain abdominal or barium studies (Fig. 25-32). Diagnosis also may be made by CT. No treatment is necessary unless one of the very rare complications supervenes, such as rectal bleeding, cyst-induced volvulus, or tension pneumoperitoneum. Prognosis in most patients is that of the underlying disease. When pneumatosis occurs in infants with necrotizing enterocolitis, it does not make the outlook any worse. The cysts may disappear spontaneously or may persist for prolonged periods without serious symptoms.

Blind Loop Syndrome

This is a rare clinical syndrome manifested by diarrhea, steatorrhea, anemia, weight loss, abdominal pain, multiple vitamin deficiencies, and neurologic disorders. The underlying cause is not a blind loop per se, but bacterial overgrowth in stagnant areas of small bowel produced by stricture, stenosis, fistulas, blind pouch, or diverticula (Table 25-5). The bacterial flora are altered in the stagnant area, both in number and in kind. Bacteria compete successfully for vitamin B_{12}, producing a systemic deficiency of B_{12} and megaloblastic anemia. Steatorrhea also occurs; bacteria in the stagnant area deconjugate bile salts, causing disruption of micellar solubilization of fats. There also may be absorptive defects of other macronutrients and micronutrients, probably caused by direct injury of the mucosal cells.

The syndrome can be confirmed by a series of laboratory investigations. First, a Schilling test (^{60}Co-labeled vitamin B_{12} absorption) is performed; this should reveal a pattern of urinary excretion of vitamin B_{12} resembling that of pernicious anemia (that is, a urinary loss of 0 to 6 percent of vitamin B_{12}, compared to the normal of 7 to 25 percent). The test is then repeated with the addition of intrinsic factor. In true pernicious anemia, the excretion should rise to normal; in the blind loop syndrome, the addition of intrinsic factor will not increase the excretion of vitamin B_{12}. Next, the patient is given a course of tetracycline for 3 to 5 days, and the Schilling test is repeated. With blind loop syndrome, absorption of ^{60}Co-labeled vitamin B_{12} returns to normal; this does not occur in the macrocytic anemia due to steatorrhea. Patients with the blind loop syndrome respond to tetracycline and parenteral vitamin B_{12} therapy. Medical treatment is not definitive but should be employed to prepare patients for operation. Surgical correction of the condition producing stagnation and blind loop syndrome effects a permanent cure and is indicated.

Radiation Enteritis

Radiation is a common adjuvant therapy in the multimodality approach to the treatment of various abdominal and pelvic cancers. Along with the beneficial effects gained by killing tumor cells, surrounding normal tissues such as the small intestine may sustain severe acute and chronic deleterious effects. The intes-

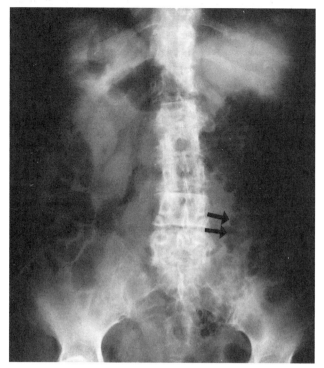

A

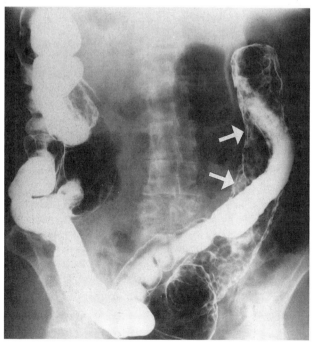

B

FIG. 25-32. *A. Plain abdominal film of a patient with pneumatosis cystoides coli demonstrating several submucosal gas cysts (arrows). B. Barium enema in the same patient, with arrows again pointing to submucosal cysts. (Courtesy of Melvyn H. Schreiber, MD.)*

tinal epithelium is the most radiosensitive tissue of the gut. The amount of radiation required to produce clinical signs of enteritis varies with the treatment regimen as well as the patient. Serious

morbidity is unusual if the total radiation dosage is less than 4,000 cGy; however, the complication rate increases when doses exceed 5,000 cGy. In addition, previous abdominal operations, preexisting vascular disease, hypertension, diabetes, and treatment with certain chemotherapeutic agents (e.g., 5-fluorouracil, doxorubicin, actinomycin D, and methotrexate) increase the likelihood of enteritis after radiation treatments.

The mucosa and the submucosal vasculature of the intestine are the most sensitive to radiation damage. With the relatively rapid turnover of the intestinal mucosa, radiation damage to this layer tends to be acute and self-limiting, with symptoms consisting mainly of diarrhea, abdominal pain, and malabsorption. Late effects of radiation are the result of damage to the small submucosal vessels, with a progressive obliterative arteritis and submucosal fibrosis, resulting eventually in thrombosis and vascular insufficiency. This injury may produce necrosis and perforation of the involved intestine, but more commonly it leads to strictures, with symptoms of obstruction, or fistula formation.

Radiation enteritis may be minimized by adjusting ports and dosages of radiation to deliver optimal treatment specifically to the tumor and not to surrounding tissues; this could be facilitated by placement of radiopaque markers, if laparotomy is performed, to delineate the area to be irradiated. Prophylactic measures to help decrease the incidence of enteritis include methods to exclude small bowel from the pelvis such as reperitonealization, omental transposition, or placement of absorbable mesh slings.

Treatment of the acute sequelae of radiation injury may be obtained by conservative measures such as the administration of antispasmodics, analgesics, and antidiarrheal agents. Agents that may prove useful in the treatment of acute sequelae include glutamine-enriched enteral formulas and the gut hormone bombesin, which ameliorates methotrexate-mediated enterocolitis in experimental animals.

Operative intervention may be required for symptomatic strictures or fistulas. Caution must be exercised when operating on patients with previously irradiated bowel, since the vascular injury may be widespread and not readily recognizable by gross inspection of the intestine; if resection and reanastomosis are performed, dehiscence of the anastomosis can occur. Extensive

Table 25-5
Clinical Conditions Predisposing to Bacterial Overgrowth in the Small Bowel

Gastric proliferation
    Achlorhydria, especially when combined with motor or anatomic
        disturbance
Small intestinal stagnation
    Anatomic
    Afferent loop of Billroth II partial gastrectomy
    Duodenal/jejunal diverticulosis
    Surgical blind loop (end-to-side anastomosis)
    Obstruction (stricture, adhesion, inflammation, cancer)
Motor
    Diabetic autonomic neuropathy
    Scleroderma
    Idiopathic intestinal pseudoobstruction
    Absence of "intestinal housekeeper"
Abnormal communication between proximal and distal gastrointestinal
    tract
Gastrocolic or jejunocolic fistula
Resection of ileocecal valve

adhesiolysis should be avoided if possible. Perforation of the intestine should be treated with resection and anastomosis; when reanastomosis is thought to be unsafe, ostomies should be created. Frozen sections and laser Doppler flowmetry have been used to assist resection and anastomosis; however, the clinical usefulness of these techniques has been debated. Obstruction caused by a rigid, fixed pelvis incorporating small intestinal loops is best treated by bypass.

Radiation enteritis is a relentless disease process reflecting widespread bowel involvement. Almost one-half of patients who survive their first laparotomy for radiation bowel injury require further surgery for ongoing bowel damage. Up to 25 percent of these patients die from radiation enteritis and complications from its management.

Short Bowel Syndrome

In the adult, emergency massive resection of the small bowel must sometimes be done when extensive gangrene precludes revascularization. Mesenteric occlusion, midgut volvulus, and traumatic disruption of the superior mesenteric vessels are the most frequent causes. Short bowel syndrome may result from such massive resections; it also may be produced by several bowel resections in patients with severe recurrent Crohn's disease. In neonates the most common cause of short bowel syndrome is necrotizing enterocolitis.

The short bowel syndrome is a group of signs and symptoms that result from a total small bowel length that is inadequate to support nutrition. The clinical hallmarks of the short bowel syndrome include diarrhea, fluid and electrolyte deficiency, and malnutrition. The small bowel has two primary functions, digestion and absorption of nutrients. Problems that result from extensive resection of the small bowel can be divided into two types: those related to the extent of small-bowel loss, and those related to the specific area of bowel removed.

Although there is considerable individual variation, resection of up to 70 percent of the small bowel usually can be tolerated if the terminal ileum and ileocecal valve are preserved. Length alone, however, is not the only determining factor of complications of small-bowel resection. For example, if the distal two-thirds of the ileum, including the ileocecal valve, is resected, significant abnormalities of absorption of bile salts and vitamin B_{12} may occur, although only 25 percent of the total length of the small bowel has been removed. Proximal bowel resection is tolerated much better than distal resection, since the ileum can adapt and increase its absorptive capacity more efficiently than the jejunum.

Digestion and absorption in the small bowel depend on the presence of brush border enzymes, an adequate number of enterocytes for absorption, and normal intestinal motility. With massive resection of the small bowel, there is reduced absorption of all nutrients, including electrolytes, water, carbohydrates, protein, fat, trace elements, and vitamins. The proximal small bowel is the primary site of absorption of iron, folate, and calcium, whereas the distal small bowel is the site of absorption of bile salts and vitamin B_{12}.

The bowel has an intrinsic capacity to adapt after small-bowel resection, and in many instances this process of intestinal adaptation effectively prevents severe complications resulting from the reduced surface area available for absorption and digestion. Any adaptive mechanism can be overwhelmed; maximum adaptation will be inadequate if too much small bowel is lost. In-

testinal adaptation is characterized by an increased absorptive surface area as a result of hyperplasia of the remaining enterocytes. The villi lengthen (but do not increase in number), more cells are produced, and there are increased cell renewal and migration to the villous tip. All this serves to produce an increase in total absorptive surface area. Although there are more cells, individual cells do not increase their life span (they must migrate farther) or their capacity to synthesize digestive enzymes or to increase absorptive processes, so the overall net increase in digestive efficacy is not great (Fig. 25-33).

The mechanisms responsible for intestinal adaptation have been studied widely in animals. Multiple factors are responsible and are required for development of successful intestinal adaptation. For unknown reasons, the ileum exhibits a much greater adaptive response than the jejunum. Luminal nutrients, trophic gut hormones, specific amino acids (e.g., glutamine), and pancreatic and biliary secretions are all required for complete adaptation to occur. In animals maintained on TPN after extensive small-bowel resection, nutrition may be maintained but intestinal adaptation does not occur. Enteral diets containing glutamine, the principal fuel used by the small intestine, have been shown to increase mucosal proliferation and gut regeneration in experimental models. In addition, dietary fiber (e.g., pectin) has been

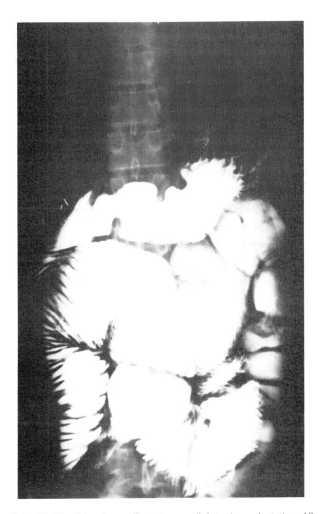

FIG. 25-33. This picture illustrates small intestine adaptation 18 months after massive bowel resection.

shown to enhance mucosal adaptation, increase stool acidity, and improve colonic water absorption. The trophic gut peptides studied most intensively in small-bowel adaptation are gastrin, CCK, secretin, neurotensin, peptide YY, and bombesin. We now know that, although hypergastrinemia is associated with the short bowel syndrome, gastrin does not play a major role in the acaptive response after resection. CCK and secretin may have direct effects on enterocyte replication; however, their primary importance in intestinal adaptation may be in stimulation of pancreaticobiliary secretions rather than in directly stimulating enterocyte proliferation. The small-bowel mucosa is a complex and highly proliferative tissue with multiple factors regulating growth. The gut hormone neurotensin appears to be one of the most potent enterotrophic factors identified to date. Administration of neurotensin stimulates small-bowel mucosal growth in rats fed a normal diet, prevents gut mucosal hypoplasia induced by feeding rats an elemental diet, and augments intestinal regeneration after small-bowel resection. Recent studies demonstrate a marked mucosal growth response by the gut-derived peptide glucagonlike peptide-2 (GLP-2), which may hold promise for patients with short bowel syndrome. Two other hormones, not derived from the gut, that have been evaluated extensively in various experimental and in limited clinical trials include growth hormone and insulinlike growth factor-1 (IGF-1). Growth hormone enhances mucosal hyperplasia in both the remnant small bowel and colon. IGF-1, which is regulated by growth hormone, increases the weight and length of the small and large intestines. Results reported recently by Byrne and colleagues using a combination of growth hormone, glutamine, and a modified diet appear promising in allowing for a reduction or elimination of TPN requirements in some refractory patients with severe short bowel syndrome and TPN dependence.

In human beings, the adaptive responses to massive resection have been found to be increased caliber of the remaining small bowel, hypertrophy of the gut wall, increased villous height, and increase numbers of enterocytes. This process often takes weeks or months to complete after small-bowel resection. With time, absorptive function increases. This increase is characterized by decreasing stool losses of water and electrolytes and increased absorption of glucose and vitamin B_{12}.

Hypergastrinemia and gastric hypersecretion occur after massive small-bowel resection and have been widely studied in experimental animals; some information has come from human subjects. Diarrhea associated with gastric hypersecretion is caused by (1) delivery of a massive volume of fluid and electrolytes to the shortened small bowel, (2) steatorrhea from failure of lipolysis by pancreatic lipase, which requires an intraluminal pH greater than 5.0 for activity (pancreatic secretion of lipase is not affected), and (3) acid enteritis. Although acid hypersecretion was at one time thought to be of prime importance in producing diarrhea after extensive small-bowel resection, both hypergastrinemia and hypersecretion of acid are transient. Acid hypersecretion is now easily managed by H_2-receptor antagonists or proton-pump blockers. Control of acid secretion controls diarrhea to a great extent during the early phase. Several operations, including vagotomy with pyloroplasty, or vagotomy with antrectomy, have been employed in treatment of the short bowel syndrome to control acid hypersecretion. Since the problem is self-limited, however, these procedures are not indicated and should not be done.

Resection of specific segments of the small bowel leads to specific problems. Resection of the distal small bowel results in diarrhea, steatorrhea, and malabsorption. Conjugated bile salts, essential for normal fat absorption, are almost totally absorbed in the distal ileum by active transport mechanisms. Resection of the ileum results in disruption of the enterohepatic circulation of bile salts and may lead to two types of diarrhea. When less than 100 cm of small bowel has been resected, excessive amounts of bile salts enter the colon and produce a chemical enteritis; this type of diarrhea has been termed *cholerheic*. The toxic effects of bile acids on colonic epithelial cells are twofold: bile salts inhibit absorption of water and electrolytes in the colon, and the injured colonic cells secrete excessive amounts of water and electrolytes. The response to decreased absorption of bile salts is increased hepatic production of bile salts, and this leads to perpetuation of diarrhea.

When more than 100 cm of ileum has been resected, the loss of bile salts is so great that hepatic synthesis cannot compensate. Furthermore, decreased intraluminal bile acids stimulate CCK release, and CCK stimulates gut motility. In addition to the direct toxic effects of bile salts on the colonic epithelium, fat malabsorption (steatorrhea) occurs. Differentiation of the two types of diarrhea associated with distal resection is important, because treatment is different. Measurement of stool fat content, vitamin B_{12} absorptive capacity, and fecal bile salt concentrations is important for accurate determination of the deficits produced. For patients who have cholerheic diarrhea, agents that bind bile acids (e.g., cholestyramine) may alleviate diarrhea. If steatorrhea is present, then medium-chain triglycerides that do not require micelle formation for absorption also should be used.

Another factor contributing to diarrhea after ileal resection is loss of the ileocecal valve. The ileocecal valve has two important actions. It prolongs intestinal transit time, and it prevents retrograde passage of colonic bacteria into the small bowel, which, if not prevented, causes bacterial enteritis.

Other complications associated with alteration of enterohepatic circulation of bile acids include gallstones and anemia. The changes in the bile salt pool produce lithogenic bile; the incidence of gallstones in patients with ileal resection is three to four times greater than in the normal population. The ileum is the specific site for transport mechanisms for intrinsic-factor—mediated vitamin B_{12} absorption, and with total ileal resection, stores of vitamin B_{12} are depleted and anemia results.

Treatment. The most important principle in the treatment of short bowel syndrome is prevention. This means that at operation, when intestinal viability is questionable, the smallest possible resections should be performed, and "second-look" operations 24 to 48 h later should be carried out to allow the ischemic bowel to demarcate. Delay may prevent unnecessary, extensive resection of bowel. In patients with Crohn's disease, the devastating complications of the short bowel syndrome have led all students of the disease to recognize that only limited resections should be performed.

After massive small-bowel resection, the program for treatment may be properly divided into early and late phases. Early on, treatment is primarily directed at the control of diarrhea, replacement of fluid and electrolytes, and the prompt institution of total parenteral nutrition. Volume losses may exceed 5 L/day, and vigorous monitoring of intake and output with adequate replacement must be carried out. Depletion of fluid volume caused by diarrhea, especially in the early phase, is often a formidable problem. Judicious use of agents that inhibit gut motility (codeine, Lomotil, loperamide) may be helpful. These drugs may cause profound ileus if used excessively, and volume lost through the gut is simply traded for volume lost through nasogastric suction. In addition, prolonged ileus with dilatation and edema of the bowel wall may result.

As intestinal adaptation progresses and gut absorption increases, the stool volume gradually decreases. Once patients have completely adapted to an oral diet, semiformed stools may appear, but these patients will likely never have the normal number or consistency of stools.

As soon as the patient has recovered from the acute phase, enteral nutrition should begin, so that intestinal adaptation may begin early and proceed successfully. The most common types of enteral diets are elemental (Vivonex, Flexical) or polymeric (Isocal, Ensure). Each presents problems with increased osmolality and may contain foodstuffs that may not be absorbed because of enzyme deficiency (for example, lactase deficiency). Milk products should be avoided, and diets should be begun at isoosmolar concentrations and with small volumes (50 mL/h), even though the full nutrient value may not be obtained. As the gut adapts, the osmolality, volume, and caloric content may be increased. As previously noted, the combination of glutamine, growth hormone, and a modified oral diet may prove efficacious at this stage. Gut hormones in combination with dietary modifications may prove to be useful in the future.

Reduction of dietary fat has long been considered to be important in the treatment of patients with the short bowel syndrome. High-carbohydrate, high-protein, low-fat diets have been prescribed. Fat has more than twice as many calories per gram as protein and carbohydrate and is important for maintenance of proper nutrition. Supplementation of the diet with 100 g or more of fat should be carried out. Often this requires the use of medium-chain triglycerides, which may be absorbed in the proximal bowel without micelle formation. Vitamins, especially fat-soluble vitamins, as well as calcium, magnesium, and zinc supplementation, also must be provided. H_2-receptor antagonists or proton-pump blockers may greatly diminish the diarrhea that is largely caused by the early, transient acid hypersecretion. Measurement of intragastric pH can be used to guide the dose of drugs required. Antacids are not useful, because they may aggravate diarrhea or bind essential ions. In no case should gastric resection or vagotomy be used for the treatment of the short bowel syndrome.

Since the dysfunction of massive small-bowel resection is caused by decreased absorptive surface and rapid transit time, most attempts at surgical treatment have been directed toward increasing the absorptive surface or slowing the intestinal transit time. The intestinal tapering and lengthening procedure, originally described by Bianchi, improves intestinal function by correcting the dilatation and ineffective peristalsis of the intestine as well as by prolonging intestinal transit time by doubling the intestinal length while preserving the mucosal surface area. Dissection is performed longitudinally on the mesenteric edge of the bowel to create a space that permits longitudinal division of the bowel with a stapling device. This procedure may be beneficial in selected patients; however, potential complications include necrosis of divided segments and anastomotic leak. Procedures to slow intestinal transit time include reversed intestinal segments, circular loops, colon interposition, and construction of valves (artificial sphincters). These procedures have received limited clinical evaluation; most reports are only anecdotal, and

the efficacy of these techniques remains questionable. In fact, some reports actually show a decreased effective functional length and an increased risk of bowel infarction with these procedures. Therapy for the short bowel syndrome may be revolutionized when small-intestine transplantation becomes a less morbid procedure. The greatest obstacles to successful bowel transplantation have been rejection and sepsis.

In summary, the present treatment of the short bowel syndrome is palliative and is directed toward control of diarrhea and prevention of dehydration and malnutrition. In the future, use of glutamine, growth factors, and gastrointestinal hormones may be useful adjuncts in certain patients; however, only with the development of successful allotransplantation of the gut will the short bowel syndrome be cured.

Intestinal Bypass

Morbid Obesity

Surgical procedures to treat morbid obesity (defined as more than 100 lb over ideal weight) have become popular because the long-term success rate of nonsurgical treatment of this condition is only 1 percent. There are two basic approaches: (1) restrict the amount of food entering the gastrointestinal tract (gastric reduction) or (2) reduce the amount of food absorbed (gut shortening). The original procedure designed to create a short-gut malabsorption syndrome, jejunocolostomy, had to be abandoned because of an unacceptable rate of complications. It was succeeded by jejunoileostomy, either end-to-side (Payne procedure) or end-to-end (Scott procedure). Many thousands of these procedures have been done in the United States. These too have been abandoned because of long-term complications, which included persistent diarrhea, profound electrolyte abnormalities, arthralgias, neurologic symptoms, enteropathies, cholelithiasis, renal disease, and hepatic failure. In addition, the long-term weight control was poor. An alternative method of operative therapy of obesity is the gastric bypass or partition. This method limits food intake by reducing the reservoir capacity of the stomach to 5 to 10 percent of normal. After a Consensus Development Conference at the National Institutes of Health in March 1991, the only procedures currently recommended for evaluation are gastric reductions.

Hyperlipidemia

Surgical bypass of a portion of the small intestine is a useful method of treating hypercholesterolemia and hypertriglyceridemia. The operation, designed by Buchwald and Varco, bypasses either the distal 200 cm or the distal one-third of the small intestine, whichever is greater (Fig. 25-34). This operation, though occasionally associated with diarrhea, does not cause significant weight loss and is not associated with the undesirable side effects of the jejunoileal bypass.

This procedure lowers serum cholesterol level through two mechanisms: the absorption of cholesterol is reduced by bypassing the usual site of absorption, and cholesterol and bile acid excretion is increased, which accelerates cholesterol turnover.

Clinical metabolic studies have demonstrated a 60 percent decrease in cholesterol absorption, a 40 percent reduction in serum cholesterol levels, and a reduction of more than 50 percent in plasma triglyceride levels. About 70 percent of patients with angina have had improvement or total remission of symptoms after this operation.

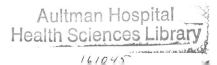

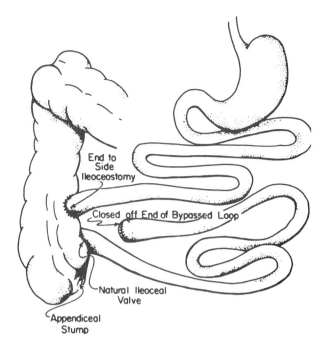

FIG. 25-34. Operative technique of partial ileal bypass. The intestine is transected 200 cm proximal to the ileocecal valve or one-third of the length of the intestine, whichever is larger. An end-to-side anastomosis is constructed between the proximal intestine and the cecum. The appendix, if still present, should be removed. The proximal end of the bypassed intestine is closed and tacked down to the anterior taenia of the cecum. The mesenteric defects are then closed. (From: Buchwald H, Varco RL et al: *Curr Probl Surg* Apr:1, 1975, with permission.)

Results have been reported from the long-term follow-up of the first group of patients studied as well as from the Program on the Surgical Control of the Hyperlipidemias (POSCH), a prospective, randomized, multicenter trial. Of the original 57 patients, partial ileal bypass produced significant sustained (longer than 20 years) reduction in total plasma cholesterol levels. Only 3.5 percent of patients required reversal of the bypass; however, 40 percent developed nephrolithiasis. These findings were confirmed in the POSCH trial. The POSCH trial data also have shown an apparent reversal of coronary artery atherosclerosis and reduction of mortality rates in some subgroups of patients. The response of the 78 women in the POSCH trial was similar to that of the group as a whole, although small numbers made statistical significance difficult to achieve. Thus, partial ileal bypass, when employed for the correction of hyperlipidemia, appears to be an effective method of lipid reduction and may result in a decrease of mortality in certain subgroups of patients.

Bibliography

Embryology

Brenner DA, Boyle WJ: Molecular and cellular biology of the small intestine. *Curr Opin Gastroenterol* 12:115, 1996.

Cheng H, Leblond CP: Origin, differentiation, and renewal of the four main epithelial cell types in the mouse small intestine. V. Unitarian theory of the origin of the four epithelial cell types. *Am J Anat* 141:537, 1974.

Evers BM: Expression of the neurotensin/neuromedin N gene in the gut: A potential model for gut differentiation, in Greeley GH Jr (ed): *Endocrinology of the Gastrointestinal System.* Totowa, NJ, Humana Press, in press.

Henning SJ, Rubin DC, et al: Ontogeny of the intestinal mucosa, in Johnson LR, Alpers DH, Christensen J, Jacobson ED, Walsh JH: *Physiology of the Gastrointestinal Tract,* 3rd ed. New York, Raven, 1994, p. 571.

Hermiston ML, Gordon JI: Use of transgenic mice to characterize the multipotent intestinal stem cell and to analyze regulation of gene expression in various epithelial cell lineages as a function of their position along the cephalocaudal and crypt-to-villus (or crypt-to-surface epithelial cuff) axes of the gut. *Dev Biol* 4:275, 1993.

Moore KL, Persaud TVN (eds): *The Developing Human: Clinically Oriented Embryology,* 5th ed. Philadelphia, WB Saunders, 1993.

Simon TC, Gordon JI: Intestinal epithelial cell differentiation: New insights from mice, flies, and nematodes. *Curr Opin Genet Dev* 5:577, 1995.

Traber PG: Differentiation of intestinal epithelial cells: Lessons from the study of intestine-specific gene expression. *J Lab Clin Med* 123:467, 1994.

Trier JS, Winter HS: Anatomy, embryology, and developmental abnormalities of the small intestine and colon, in Sleisenger MH, Fordtran JS, et al (eds): *Gastrointestinal Disease: Pathophysiology, Diagnosis, Management,* 5th ed. Philadelphia, WB Saunders, 1993, p 793.

Podolsky DK, Babyatsky MW: Growth and development of the gastrointestinal tract, in Yamada T, Alpers DH, et al (eds): *Textbook of Gastroenterology,* 2d Edition. Philadelphia, JB Lippincott, 1995, p 546.

Physiology

Brand SJ, Schmidt WE: Gastrointestinal hormones. In: Yamada T, Alpers DH, et al (eds): *Textbook of Gastroenterology,* 2d ed. Philadelphia, JB Lippincott, 1995, p 25.

Castro GA, Powell DW: The physiology of the mucosal immune system and immune-mediated responses in the gastrointestinal tract, in Johnson LR, Alpers DH, Christensen J, Jacobson ED, Walsh JH: *Physiology of the Gastrointestinal Tract,* 3d ed. New York, Raven, 1994, p 709.

Code CF (ed): *Handbook of Physiology, Section 6.* Washington, CD, American Physiological Society, 1968.

Davenport HW (ed): Intestinal secretion, in *Physiology of the Digestive Tract.* Chicago, Yearbook Medical Publishers, 1982, p 174.

Evers BM, Izukura M, et al: Differential effects of gut hormones on pancreatic and intestinal growth during administration of an elemental diet. *Ann Surg* 211:630, 1990.

Evers BM, Izukura M, et al: Neurotensin prevents intestinal mucosal hypoplasia in rats fed an elemental diet. *Dig Dis Sci* 37:426, 1992.

Fawcett DW (ed): *A Textbook of Histology,* 12th ed. New York, Chapman and Hall, 1994.

Grand RJ, Watkins JB, et al: Development of the human gastrointestinal tract: A review. *Gastroenterology* 70:790, 1976.

Hasler WL: Motility of the small intestine, in Yamada T, Alpers DH, et al (eds): *Textbook of Gastroenterology,* 2d ed. Philadelphia, JB Lippincott, 1995, p 207.

Hirsch J, Ahrens EH Jr, et al: Measurement of the human intestinal length in vivo and some causes of variation. *Gastroenterology* 31:274, 1956.

Jacobs DO, Evans DA, et al: Combined effects of glutamine and epidermal growth factor on the rat intestine. *Surgery* 104:358, 1988.

Johnson LR: Regulation of gastrointestinal mucosal growth. *Physiol Rev* 68:456, 1988.

Jones WG II, Minei JP, et al: Bacterial translocation and intestinal atrophy after thermal injury and burn wound sepsis. *Ann Surg* 211:399, 1990.

Kaunitz JD, Barrett KE, et al: Electrolyte secretion and absorption: Small intestine and colon, in Yamada T, Alpers DH, et al (eds): *Textbook of Gastroenterology,* 2d ed. Philadelphia, JB Lippincott, 1995, p 326.

Madara JL: Epithelia: Biologic principles of organization, in Yamada T, Alpers DH, et al (eds): *Textbook of Gastroenterology*, 2d ed. Philadelphia, JB Lippincott, 1995, p 141.

Madara JL, Trier JS: The functional morphology of the mucosa of the small intestine, in Johnson LR, Alpers DH, et al: *Physiology of the Gastrointestinal Tract*, 3d ed. New York, Raven, 1994, p 1577.

Merchant JL, Dickinson CJ, et al: Molecular biology of the gut: Model of gastrointestinal hormones, in Johnson LR, Alpers DH, et al: *Physiology of the Gastrointestinal Tract*, 3d ed. New York, Raven, 1994, p 295.

Podolsky DK: Peptide growth factors in the gastrointestinal tract, in Johnson LR, Alpers DH, et al: *Physiology of the Gastrointestinal Tract*, 3d ed. New York, Raven, 1994, p 129.

Sellin JH: Intestinal electrolyte absorption and secretion, in Sleisenger MH, Fordtran JS, et al (eds): *Gastrointestinal Disease: Pathophysiology, Diagnosis, Management*, 5th ed. Philadelphia, WB Saunders, 1993, p 954.

Thompson JC (ed): *Gastrointestinal Endocrinology: Receptors and Post-Receptor Mechanisms*. San Diego, Academic Press, 1990.

Thompson JC: Humoral control of gut function. *Am J Surg* 161:6, 1991.

Thompson JC, Greeley GH Jr, et al (eds): *Gastrointestinal Endocrinology*. New York, McGraw-Hill, 1987.

Turnberg LA, Riley SA: Digestion and absorption of nutrients and vitamins, in Sleisenger MH, Fordtran JS, et al (eds): *Gastrointestinal Disease: Pathophysiology, Diagnosis, Management*, 5th ed. Philadelphia, WB Saunders, 1993, p 977.

Wang JY, Johnson LR: Polyamines and ornithine decarboxylase during repair of duodenal mucosa after stress in rats. *Gastroenterology* 100:333, 1991.

Inflammatory Diseases

Ahsan N, Blanchard RL, et al: Gastrointestinal tuberculosis in renal transplantation: A case report and review. *Clin Transplant* 9:349, 1995.

Al Karawi MA, Mohamed AE, et al: Protean manifestation of gastrointestinal tuberculosis: Report on 130 patients. *J Clin Gastroenterol* 20:225, 1995.

Anand BS: Diagnosis of gastrointestinal tuberculosis. *Trop Gastroenterol* 15:179, 1994

Anand BS, Schneider FE, et al: Diagnosis of intestinal tuberculosis by polymerase chain reaction on endoscopic biopsy specimen. *Am J Gastroenterol* 89:2248, 1994.

Annibali R, Pietri P: Fistulous complications of Crohn's disease. *Int Surg* 77:19–27, 1992.

Bayless TM, Tokayer AZ, et al: Crohn's disease: Concordance for site and clinical type in affected family members—potential hereditary influences. *Gastroenterology* 111:573, 1996.

Bernstein D, Rogers A: Malignancy in Crohn's disease. *Am J Gastroenterol* 91:434, 1996.

Bitar R, Tarpley J: Intestinal perforation in typhoid fever: A historical and state-of-the-art review. *Rev Infect Dis* 7:257, 1985.

Clarridge JE III, Shawar RM, et al: Large-scale use of polymerase chain reaction for detection of *Mycobacterium tuberculosis* in a routine mycobacteriology laboratory. *J Clin Microbiol* 31:2049, 1993.

Caprilli R, Corrao G, et al: Prognostic factors for postoperative recurrence of Crohn's disease. *Dis Colon Rectum* 39:335, 1996.

Crohn BB, Ginsburg L, et al: Regional enteritis: A pathologic and clinical entity. *JAMA* 99:1323, 1932.

Dalziel TK: Chronic interstitial enteritis. *Br Med J* 2:1068, 1913.

Domej W, Wirnsberger GH, et al: Tuberculosis of the small bowel with perforation and hematogenous spread in a renal transplant recipient. *Z Gastroenterol* 31:401, 1993.

Ekbom A, Helmick C, et al: The epidemiology of inflammatory bowel disease: A large, population-based study in Sweden. *Gastroenterology* 100:350, 1991.

Elton E, Hanauer SB: Review article: The medical management of Crohn's disease. *Aliment Pharmacol Ther* 10:1, 1996.

Fazio VW, Tjandra JJ, et al: Long-term follow-up of strictureplasty in Crohn's disease. *Dis Colon Rectum* 36:355, 1993.

Gore RM, Balthazar EJ, et al: CT features of ulcerative colitis and Crohn's disease. *Am J Roentgenol* 167:3, 1996.

Griffin MG, Miner PB Jr: Conventional drug therapy in inflammatory bowel disease. *Gastroenterol Clin North Am* 24:509, 1995.

Griffiths AM, Ohlsson A, et al: Meta-analysis of enteral nutrition as a primary treatment of active Crohn's disease. *Gastroenterology* 108:1056, 1995.

Grimm IS, Friedman LS: Inflammatory bowel disease in the elderly. *Gastroenterol Clin North Am* 19:361, 1990.

Gupta V, Gupta SK, et al: Perforated typhoid enteritis in children. *Postgrad Med J* 70:19, 1994.

Hanauer SB, Schulman MI: New therapeutic approaches. *Gastroenterol Clin North Am* 24:523, 1995.

Handelsman JC, Gottlieb LM, et al: Crohn's disease as a contraindication to Kock pouch (continent ileostomy). *Dis Colon Rectum* 36:840, 1993.

Heimann TM, Greenstein AJ, et al: Prediction of early symptomatic recurrence after intestinal resection in Crohn's disease. *Ann Surg* 218:294, 1993.

Hugot J-P, Laurent-Puig P, et al: Mapping of a susceptibility locus for Crohn's disease on chromosome 16. *Nature* 379:821, 1996.

Hyman NH, Fazio VW, et al: Consequences of ileal pouch–anal anastomosis for Crohn's colitis. *Dis Colon Rectum* 34:653, 1991.

Israel EJ, Kleinman RE: Inflammatory bowel disease: Diagnosis and treatment. *Semin Gastroentol Dis* 5:95, 1994.

Khanna AK, Misra MK: Typhoid perforation of the gut. *Postgrad Med J* 60:523, 1984.

Korelitz BI: Immunosuppressive therapy of inflammatory bowel disease: A historical perspective. *Gastroenterologist* 3:141, 1995.

Lashner BA: Risk factors for small bowel cancer in Crohn's disease. *Dig Dis Sci* 37:1179, 1992.

Lashner BA: Epidemiology of inflammatory bowel disease. *Gastroenterol Clin North Am* 24:467, 1995.

Marshall JB: Tuberculosis of the gastrointestinal tract and peritoneum. *Am J Gastroenterol* 88:989, 1993.

Mekhjian HS, Switz DM, et al: Clinical features and natural history of Crohn's disease. *Gastroenterology* 77:898, 1979.

Messori A, Brignola C, et al: Effectiveness of 5-aminosalicylic acid for maintaining remission in patients with Crohn's disease: A meta-analysis. *Am J Gastroenterol* 89:692, 1994.

Michelassi F: Side-to-side isoperistaltic strictureplasty for multiple Crohn's strictures. *Dis Colon Rectum* 39:345, 1996.

Michelassi F, Balestracci T, et al: Primary and recurrent Crohn's disease: Experience with 1379 patients. *Ann Surg* 214:230, 1991.

Michelassi F, Block GE: Surgical management of Crohn's disease. *Adv Surg* 26:307, 1993.

Michelassi F, Stella M, et al: Incidence, diagnosis, and treatment of enteric and colorectal fistulae in patients with Crohn's disease. *Ann Surg* 218:660, 1993.

Mishina D, Katsel P, et al: On the etiology of Crohn disease. *Proc Natl Acad Sci USA* 93:9816, 1996.

Modigliani R: Endoscopic management of inflammatory bowel disease. *Am J Gastroenterol* 8:S53, 1994.

Ohmen JD, Yang H-Y, et al: Susceptibility locus for inflammatory bowel disease on chromosome 16 has a role in Crohn's disease, but not in ulcerative colitis. *Hum Mol Genet* 5:1679, 1996.

Orholm M, Munkholm P, et al: Familial occurrence of inflammatory bowel disease. *N Engl J Med* 324:84, 1991.

Ozuner G, Hull TL, et al: Long-term analysis of the use of transanal rectal advancement flaps for complicated anorectal/vaginal fistulas. *Dis Colon Rectum* 39:10, 1996.

Post S, Herfarth C, et al: The impact of disease pattern, surgical management, and individual surgeons on the risk for relaparotomy for recurrent Crohn's disease. *Ann Surg* 223:253, 1996.

Raab Y, Bergström R, et al: Factors influencing recurrence in Crohn's disease: An analysis of a consecutive series of 353 patients treated with primary surgery. *Dis Colon Rectum* 39:918, 1996.

Ribeiro MB, Greenstein AJ, et al: Intra-abdominal abscess in regional enteritis. *Ann Surg* 213:32, 1991.

Rieder HL, Cauthen GM, et al: Tuberculosis in the United States. *JAMA.* 262:385, 1989.

Rutgeerts P, Löfberg R, et al: A comparison of budesonide with prednisolone for active Crohn's disease. *N Engl J Med* 331:842, 1994.

Sandborn WJ: A review of immune modifier therapy for inflammatory bowel disease: Azathioprine, 6-mercaptopurine, cyclosporine, and methotrexate. *Am J Gastroenterol* 91:423, 1996.

Sartor RB: Current concepts of the etiology and pathogenesis of ulcerative colitis and Crohn's disease. *Gastroenterol Clin North Am* 24:475, 1995.

Sharif H, Alexander-Williams J: The role of stricturoplasty in Crohn's disease. *Intl Surg* 77:15, 1992.

Singleton JW: The national cooperative Crohn's disease study. *Gastroenterology* 77:825, 1979.

Small PM, Hopewell PC, et al: The epidemiology of tuberculosis in San Francisco: A population-based study using conventional and molecular methods. *N Engl J Med* 330:1709, 1994.

Snider DE Jr, Roper WL: The new tuberculosis. *N Engl J Med* 326:703, 1992.

Spencer MP, Nelson H, et al: Strictureplasty for obstructive Crohn's disease: The Mayo experience. *Mayo Clin Proc* 69:33, 1994.

Spiro HM: Alimentary tract tuberculosis, in *Clinical Gastroenterology,* 4th ed. McGraw: Marston Book Services; 1994, p 549.

Steinhart AH, McLeod RS: Medical and surgical management of perianal Crohn's disease. *Inflammatory Bowel Dis* 2:200, 1996.

Sudre P, ten Dam G, et al: Tuberculosis: A global overview of the situation today. *Bull World Health Organ* 70:149, 1992.

Telander RL: Surgical management of Crohn's disease in children. *Curr Opin Pediatr* 7:328, 1995.

Tjandra JJ, Fazio VW: Strictureplasty without concomitant resection for small bowel obstruction in Crohn's disease. *Br J Surg* 81:561, 1994.

Van Kruiningren, Ruiz HJ, et al: Experimental disease in young chickens induced by a *Mycobacterium paratuberculosis* isolate from a patient with Crohn's disease. *Can J Vet Res* 55:199, 1991.

Van Patten WN, Bargen JA, et al: Regional enteritis. *Gastroenterology* 26:347, 1954.

Venkatramani S, Boses BV, et al: Typhoid ileal perforation: A retrospective study. *Ann R Cell Surg Engl* 72:347, 1990.

Voeller G, Britt L: Surgical management of perforated Crohn's disease. *Am J Surg* 56:100, 1990.

Whelan G: Epidemiology of inflammatory bowel disease. *Med Clin North Am* 74:12, 1990.

Neoplasms

Anthony L, Johnson D, et al: Somatostatin analogue phase I trials in neuroendocrine neoplasms. *Acta Oncol* 32:217, 1993.

Ashley SW, Wells SA Jr: Tumors of the small intestine. *Sem Oncol* 15:116, 1988.

Begos DG, Kuan S, et al: Metachronous small-bowel adenocarcinoma in celiac sprue. *J Clin Gastroenterol* 20:233, 1995.

Braasch JW, Denbo HE: Tumors of the small intestine. *Surg Clin North Am* 44:791, 1964.

Ciresi DL, Scholten DJ: The continuing clinical dilemma of primary tumors of the small intestine. *Am J Surg* 61:698, 1995.

Desa LA, Bridger J, et al: Primary jejunoileal tumors: A review of 45 cases. *World J Surg* 15:81, 1991.

Dougherty MJ, Compton C, et al: Sarcomas of the gastrointestinal tract: Separation into favorable and unfavorable prognostic groups by mitotic count. *Ann Surg* 214:569, 1991.

Egan LJ, Walsh SV, et al: Celiac-associated lymphoma: A single institution experience of 30 cases in the combination chemotherapy era. *J Clin Gastroenterol* 21:123, 1995.

Evers BM, Hurlbut SC, et al: Novel therapy for the treatment of human carcinoid. *Ann Surg* 213:411, 1991.

Gerstle JT, Kauffman GL Jr, et al: The incidence, management, and outcome of patients with gastrointestinal carcinoids and second primary malignancies. *J Am Coll Surg* 180:427, 1995.

Herbsman H, Wetstein L, et al: Tumors of the small intestine. *Curr Probl Surg* 17:121, 1980.

Jeghers H, McKusick VA, et al: Generalized intestinal polyposis and melanin spots on the oral mucosa, lips, and digits. *N Engl J Med* 241:993, 1949.

Kvols LK: Therapy of the malignant carcinoid syndrome. *Endocrinol Metabol Clin North Am* 18:557, 1989.

Kvols LK, Reubi JC: Metastatic carcinoid tumors and the malignant carcinoid syndrome. *Acta Oncol* 32:1971, 1993.

Kvols LK, Reubi JC, et al: The presence of somatostatin receptors in malignant neuroendocrine tumor tissue predicts responsiveness to octreotide. *Yale J Biol Med* 65:505, 1992.

Laurent F, Drouillard J, et al: CT of small-bowel neoplasms. *Sem Ultrasound CT MRI* 16:102, 1995.

Laurent F, Raynaud M, et al: Diagnosis and categorization of small bowel neoplasms: Role of computed tomography. *Gastrointest Radiol* 16:115, 1991.

Martin IG, Aldoori MI, et al: Immunoproliferative small intestinal disease: Mediterranean lymphoma and a heavy chain disease. *Br J Surg* 81:20, 1994.

Moertel CG, Sauer WG, et al: Life history of the carcinoid tumor of the small intestine. *Cancer* 14:901, 1961.

Ng E-H, Pollock RE, et al: Prognostic factors influencing survival in gastrointestinal leiomyosarcomas: Implications for surgical management and staging. *Ann Surg* 215:68, 1992.

O'Rourke MG, Lancashire RP, et al: Lymphoma of the small intestine. *Aust N Z J Surg* 56:351, 1986.

Pearse AG, Takor TT: Neuroendocrine embryology and the APUD concept. *Clin Endocrinol* 5:229S, 1976.

Radaszkiewicz T, Dragosics B, et al: Gastrointestinal malignant lymphomas of the mucosa-associated lymphoid tissue: Factors relevant to prognosis. *Gastroenterology* 102:1628, 1992.

Rochlin DB, Longmire WP Jr: Primary tumors of the small intestine. *Surgery* 50:586, 1961.

Sellner F: Investigations on the significance of the adenoma-carcinoma sequence in the small bowel. *Cancer* 66:702, 1990.

Thompson GB, van Heerden JA, et al: Carcinoid tumors of the gastrointestinal tract: Presentation, management, and prognosis. *Surgery* 98:1054, 1985.

Thorson A, Biorck G, et al: Malignant carcinoid of the small intestine with metastases to the liver, vascular disease of the right side of the heart (pulmonary stenosis and tricuspid regurgitation without septal defects), peripheral vasomotor symptoms, broncho-construction, and an unusual type of cyanosis: A clinical pathological syndrome. *Am Heart J* 47:795, 1954.

Turowski GA, Basson MD: Primary malignant lymphoma of the intestine. *Am J Surg* 169:433, 1995.

Wilson JM, Melvin DB, et al: Primary malignancies of the small bowel: A report of 96 cases and review of the literature. *Ann Surg* 180:175, 1974.

Zollinger RM Jr: Primary neoplasms of the small intestine. *Am J Surg* 151:654, 1986.

Diverticular Disease

Alvarez OA, Mejia A, et al: Jejunal diverticulitis manifesting with abdominal wall abscess. *Am J Gastroenterol* 90:2060, 1995.

Beal SL, Walton CB, et al: Enterolith ileus resulting from small bowel diverticulosis. *Am J Gastroenterol* 82:162, 1987.

Bemelman WA, Hugenholtz E, et al: Meckel's diverticulum in Amsterdam: Experience in 136 patients. *World J Surg* 19:734, 1995.

Brain JE Jr, Stair JM: Noncolonic diverticular disease. *Surg Gynecol Obstet* 161:189, 1985.

Chendrasekhar A, Timberlake GA: Perforated jejunal diverticula: An analysis of reported cases. *Am Surg* 61:984, 1995.

Cullen JJ, Kelly KA, et al: Surgical management of Meckel's diverticulum: An epidemiologic, population-based study. *Ann Surg* 220:564, 1994.

Karoll MP, Ghahremani GG, et al: Diagnosis and management of intraluminal duodenal diverticulum. *Dig Dis Sci* 28:411, 1983.

Krishnamurthy S, Kelly MM, et al: Jejunal diverticulosis: A heterogenous disorder caused by a variety of abnormalities of smooth muscle or myenteric plexus. *Gastroenterology* 85:538, 1983.

Kusumoto H, Yoshida M, et al: Complications and diagnosis of Meckel's diverticulum in 776 patients. *Am J Surg* 164:382, 1992.

Phelan M, Kaufman H, et al: Small bowel obstruction by jejunal enterolith. *Surgery* 121:229, 1997.

Sanders LE: Laparoscopic treatment of Meckel's diverticulum: Obstruction and bleeding managed with minimal morbidity. *Surg Endosc* 9:724, 1995.

Soltero MJ, Bill AH: The natural history of Meckel's diverticulum and its relation to incidental removal: A study of 202 cases of diseased Meckel's diverticulum found in King County, Washington, over a fifteen-year period. *Am J Surg* 132:168, 1976.

Teitelbaum DH, Polley TZ Jr, et al: Laparoscopic diagnosis and excision of Meckel's diverticulum. *J Pediatr Surg* 29:495, 1994.

Tsiotos GG, Farnell MB, et al: Nonmeckelian jejunal or ileal diverticulosis: An analysis of 112 cases. *Surgery* 116:726, 1994.

Wilcox RD, Shatney CH: Surgical implications of jejunal diverticula. *South Med J* 81:1386, 1988.

Williams RA, Davidson DD, et al: Surgical problems of diverticula of the small intestine. *Surg Gynecol Obstet* 152:61, 1981.

Congenital Lesions

Andrassy RJ, Mahour GH: Malrotation of the midgut in infants and children: A 25-year review. *Arch Surg* 116:158, 1981.

Bill AH Jr: Malrotation and failures of fixation of the intestinal tract, in Holder TM, Ashcraft KW (eds): *Pediatric Surgery,* 2d ed. Philadelphia, WB Saunders, 1980.

Chavez CM, Timmis HH: Duplication cysts of the gastrointestinal tract. *Am J Surg* 110:960, 1965.

Holcomb GW III, Gheissari A, et al: Surgical management of alimentary tract duplications. *Ann Surg* 209:167, 1989.

Johnson JA III, Poole GV: Ileal duplications in adults: Presentation and treatment. *Arch Surg* 129:659, 1994.

Powell DM, Othersen HB, et al: Malrotation of the intestines in children: The effect of age on presentation and therapy. *J Pediatr Surg* 24:777, 1989.

Rescorla FJ, Shedd FJ, et al: Anomalies of intestinal rotation in childhood: Analysis of 447 cases. *Surgery* 108:710, 1990.

Snyder WH Jr, Chaffen L: Embryology and pathology of the intestinal tract: Presentation of 40 cases of malrotation. *Ann Surg* 140:368, 1954.

Tanabe ID, DiTomaso A, et al: Massive GI hemorrhage from an ileal duplication cyst in an adult. *Am J Gastroenterol* 90:504, 1995.

Wrenn EL Jr: Alimentary tract duplications, in Holder TM, Ashcraft KW (eds): *Pediatric Surgery,* 2d ed. Philadelphia, WB Saunders, 1993.

Ulcers

Boydstun JS Jr, Gaffey TA, et al: Clinicopathologic study of nonspecific ulcers of the small intestine. *Dig Dis Sci* 26:911, 1981.

Guest JL: Nonspecific ulceration of the intestine: Collective review. *Surg Gynecol Obstet* 117:409, 1963.

Kwo PY, Tremaine WJ: Nonsteroidal anti-inflammatory drug–induced enteropathy: Case discussion and review of the literature. *Mayo Clin Proc* 70:55, 1995.

Thomas WEG, Williamson RCN: Enteric ulceration and its complications. *World J Surg* 9:876, 1985.

Foreign Bodies

Decker CJ: Pica in the mentally handicapped: A 15-year surgical perspective. *Can J Surg* 36:551, 1993.

Goldman AL: Foreign bodies of the gastrointestinal tract. *Contemp Surg* 18:45, 1981.

McCanse DE, Kurchin A, et al: Gastrointestinal foreign bodies. *Am J Surg* 142:335, 1981.

Webb WA: Management of foreign bodies of the upper gastrointestinal tract: Update. *Gastrointestinal Endoscopy* 41:39, 1995.

Fistulas

Devlin HB, Elcoat C: Alimentary tract fistula: Stomatherapy techniques of management. *World J Surg* 7:489, 1983.

Hollis HW Jr, Reyna TM: A practical approach to wound care in patients with complex enterocutaneous fistulas. *Surg Gynecol Obstet* 161:178, 1985.

Lévy E, Frileux P, et al: High-output external fistulae of the small bowel: Management with continuous enteral nutrition. *Br J Surg* 76:676, 1989.

Orringer JS, Mendeloff EN, et al: Management of wounds in patients with complex enterocutaneous fistulas. *Surg Gynecol Obstet* 165:79, 1987.

Rever HA, Roberts C, et al: Management of external gastrointestinal fistulas. *Ann Surg* 188:460, 1978.

Sancho JJ, di Costanzo J, et al: Randomized double-blind placebo-controlled trial of early octreotide in patients with postoperative enterocutaneous fistula. *Br J Surg* 82:638, 1995.

Schein M, Decker GAG: Gastrointestinal fistulas associated with large abdominal wall defects: Experience with 43 patients. *Br J Surg* 77:97, 1990.

Schein M, Decker GAG: Postoperative external alimentary tract fistulas. *Am J Surg* 161:435, 1991.

Soeters PB, Ebeid AM, et al: Review of 404 patients with gastrointestinal fistulas: Impact of parenteral nutrition. *Ann Surg* 190:189, 1979.

Torres AJ, Landa JI, et al: Somatostatin in the management of gastrointestinal fistulas: A multicenter trial. *Arch Surg* 127:97, 1992.

Zera RT, Bubrick MP, et al: Enterocutaneous fistulas: Effects of total parenteral nutrition and surgery. *Dis Colon Rectum* 26:109, 1983.

Pneumatosis Cystoides Intestinalis

Cho KC, Baker SR: Extraluminal air: Diagnosis and significance. *Radiol Clin North Am* 32:829, 1994.

Ecker JA, Williams RG, et al: Pneumatosis cystoides intestinalis: Bullous emphysema of the intestine, a review of the literature. *Am J Gastroenterol* 56:125, 1971.

Hoover EL, Cole GD, et al: Avoiding laparotomy in nonsurgical pneumoperitoneum. *Am J Surg* 164:99, 1992.

Jamart J: Pneumatosis cystoides intestinalis: A statistical study of 919 cases. *Acta Hepatogastroenterol* 26:419, 1979.

Knechtle SJ, Davidoff AM, et al: Pneumatosis intestinalis: Surgical management and clinical outcome. *Ann Surg* 212:160, 1990.

Koss LG: Abdominal gas cysts (pneumatosis cystoides intestinorium hominis): An analysis with a report on a case and a critical review of the literature. *Arch Pathol* 53:523, 1952.

Lipton J, Patterson B, et al: Pneumatosis intestinalis with free air mimicking intestinal perforation in a bone marrow transplant patient. *Bone Marrow Transplant* 14:323, 1994.

North JH Jr, Nava HR: Pneumatosis intestinalis and portal venous air associated with needle catheter jejunostomy. *Am Surg* 61:1045, 1995.

Wood BJ, Kumar PN, et al: Pneumatosis intestinalis in adults with AIDS: Clinical significance and imaging findings. *Am J Roentgenol* 165:1387, 1995.

Blind Loop Syndrome

Kern L: Bacterial contamination syndrome of the small bowel. *Clin Gastroenterol* 8:397, 1979.

King CE, Toskes PP: Small intestine bacterial overgrowth. *Gastroenterology* 76:1035, 1979.

Radiation Enteritis

Choi JH, Lee HS: Effect of omental pedicle hammock in protection against radiation-induced enteropathy in patients with rectal cancer. *Dis Colon Rectum* 38:276, 1995.

Chu KU, Higashide S, et al: Bombesin improves survival from methotrexate-induced enterocolitis. *Ann Surg* 220:570, 1994.

DeCosse JJ, Rhodes RS, et al: The natural history and management of radiation-induced injury of the gastrointestinal tract. *Ann Surg* 170:369, 1970.

Delaney JP, Bonsack ME, et al: Lumenal route for intestinal radioprotection. *Am J Surg* 166:492, 1993.

Deutsch AA, Stern HS: Technique of insertion of pelvic Vicryl mesh sling to avoid postradiation enteritis. *Dis Colon Rectum* 32:628, 1989.

Galland RB, Spencer J: Surgical management of radiation enteritis. *Surgery* 99:133, 1986.

Klimberg VS, Souba WW, et al: Prophylactic glutamine protects the intestinal mucosa from radiation injury. *Cancer* 66:62, 1990.

Letschert JG: The prevention of radiation-induced small bowel complications. *Eur J Cancer* 31A:1361, 1995.

Logmans A, Trimbos JB, et al: The omentoplasty: A neglected ally in gynecologic surgery. *Eur J Obstet Gynecol Reproduct Biol* 58:167, 1995.

Logmans A, van Lent, et al: The pedicled omentoplasty, a simple and effective surgical technique to acquire a safe pelvic radiation field: Theoretical and practical aspects. *Radiother Oncol* 33:269, 1994.

Makela J, Nevasaari K, et al: Surgical treatment of intestinal radiation injury. *J Surg Oncol* 36:93, 1987.

Meri F, Hirschl RB, et al: Prevention of radiation enteritis in children, using a pelvic mesh sling. *J Pediatr Surg* 29:917, 1994.

Nussbaum ML, Campana TJ, et al: Radiation-induced intestinal injury. *Clin Plastic Surg* 20:573, 1993.

Oya M, Yao T, et al: Chronic irradiation enteritis: Its correlation with the elapsed time interval and morphological changes. *Human Pathol* 27:774, 1996.

Quastler H: The nature of intestinal radiation death. *Radiat Res* 4:303, 1956.

Smith DH, DeCosse JJ: Radiation damage to the small intestine. *World J Surg* 10:189, 1986.

Warren SL, Whipple GH: Roentgen ray intoxication. I. Unit dose over thorax negative—over abdomen lethal. Epithelium of small intestine—sensitive to x-rays. *J Exp Med* 35:187, 1922.

Short Bowel Syndrome

Asfar S, Atkison P, et al: Small bowel transplantation: A life-saving option for selected patients with intestinal failure. *Dig Dis Sci* 41:875, 1996.

Bianchi A: Intestinal loop lengthening: A technique for increasing small intestinal length. *J Pediatr Surg* 15:145, 1980.

Boeckman CR, Traylor R: Bowel lengthening for short gut syndrome. *J Pediatr Surg* 16:996, 1981.

Booth IW: Enteral nutrition as primary therapy in short bowel syndrome. *Gut* 35(1 suppl):S69, 1994.

Bristol JB, Williamson RCN: Postoperative adaptation of the small intestine. *World J Surg* 9:825, 1985.

Byrne TA: Advances in the management of patients with intestinal failure. *Transplant Proc* 28:2683, 1996.

Byrne TA, Persinger RL, et al: A new treatment for patients with short-bowel syndrome: Growth hormone, glutamine, and a modified diet. *Ann Surg* 222:243, 1995.

deMiguel E, Gomez de Segura IA, et al: Trophic effects of neurotensin in massive bowel resection in the rat. *Dig Dis Sci* 39:59, 1994.

Dowling RH, Booth CC: Functional compensation after small-bowel resection in man: Demonstration by direct measurement. *Lancet* 2:146, 1966.

Dowling RH, Booth CC: Structural and functional changes following small intestinal resection in the rat. *Clin Sci* 32:139, 1967.

Drucker DJ, Ehrlich P, et al: Induction of intestinal epithelial proliferation by glucagon-like peptide 2. *Proc Natl Acad Sci USA* 93:7911, 1996.

Galea MH, Holliday H, et al: Short-bowel syndrome: A collective review. *J Pediatr Surg* 27:592, 1992.

Georgeson KE, Breaux CW Jr: Outcome and intestinal adaptation in neonatal short-bowel syndrome. *J Pediatr Surg* 27:344, 1992.

Georgeson K, Halpin D, et al: Sequential intestinal lengthening procedures for refractory short bowel syndrome. *J Pediatric Surg* 29:316, 1994.

Gouttebel MC, Astre C, et al: Influence of N-acetylglutamine or glutamine infusion on plasma amino acid concentrations during the early phase of small-bowel adaptation in the dog. *J Parenter Enteral Nutr* 16:117, 1992.

Huskisson LJ, Brereton RJ, et al: Problems with intestinal lengthening. *J Pediatr Surg* 28:720, 1993.

Inoue Y, Copeland EM, et al: Growth hormone enhances amino acid uptake by the human small intestine. *Ann Surg* 219:715, 1994.

Izukura M, Evers BM, et al: Neurotensin augments intestinal regeneration after small bowel resection in rats. *Ann Surg* 215:520, 1992.

Kimura K, Soper RT: A new bowel elongation technique for the short-bowel syndrome using the isolated bowel segment Iowa models. *J Pediatr Surg* 28:792, 1993.

Klimberg VS, Souba WW, et al: Intestinal glutamine metabolism after massive small bowel resection. *Am J Surg* 159:27, 1990.

Koruda MJ, Rolandelli RH, et al: Harry M. Vars award. The effect of a pectin-supplemented elemental diet on intestinal adaptation to massive small bowel resection. *J Parenter Enteral Nutr* 10:343, 1986.

Roth JA, Frankel WL, et al: Pectin improves colonic function in rat short bowel syndrome. *J Surg Res* 58:240, 1995.

Souba WW, Smith RJ, et al: Glutamine metabolism by the intestinal tract. *J Parenter Enteral Nutr* 9:608, 1985.

Steeb CB, Trahair JF, et al: Prolonged administration of IGF peptides enhances growth of gastrointestinal tissues in normal rats. *Am J Physiol* 266:G1090, 1994.

Tamada H, Nezu R, et al: Alanyl glutamine–enriched total parenteral nutrition restores intestinal adaptation after either proximal or distal massive resection in rats. *J Parenter Enteral Nutr* 17:236, 1993.

Thompson JS: Management of the short bowel syndrome. *Gastroenterol Clin North Am* 23:403, 1994.

Thompson JS: Surgical considerations in the short bowel syndrome. *Surg Gynecol Obstet* 176:89, 1993.

Thompson JS, Langnas AN, et al: Surgical approach to short-bowel syndrome: Experience in a population of 160 patients. *Ann Surg* 222:600, 1995.

Todo S, Reyes J, et al: Outcome analysis of 71 clinical intestinal transplantations. *Ann Surg* 222:270, 1995.

Tzakis AG, Todo S, et al: Intestinal transplantation. *Annu Rev Med* 45:79, 1994.

Weber TR, Tracy T Jr, et al: Short-bowel syndrome in children: Quality of life in an era of improved survival. *Arch Surg* 126:841, 1991.

Williams RCN: Medical progress: Intestinal adaptation. Part 1, Structural, functional, and cytokinetic changes. Part 2, Mechanisms of control. *N Engl J Med* 298:1393, 1444, 1978.

Wilmore DW, Dudrick SJ, et al: The role of nutrition in the adaptation of the small intestine after massive resection. *Surg Gynecol Obstet* 132:673, 1971.

Windmueller HG: Glutamine utilization by the small intestine. *Adv Enzymol Relat Areas Mol Biol* 53:201, 1982.

Ziegler MM: Short bowel syndrome in infancy: Etiology and management. *Clin Perinatol* 13:163, 1986.

Intestinal Bypass

Buchwald H, Moore RB, et al: Ten years' clinical experience with partial ileal bypass in management of the hyperlipidemias. *Ann Surg* 180:384, 1974.

Terry BE: Surgical management of morbid obesity. *Bull Am Col Surg* 67:3, 1982.

Morbid Obesity

Griffen WO Jr, Bivins BA, et al: The decline and fall of the jejunoileal bypass. *Surg Gynecol Obstet* 157:301, 1983.

Grundy SM, Barondess JA, et al: Gastrointestinal surgery for severe obesity. *NIH Consensus Development Panel* 9:1, 1991.

Ravitch MM, Brolin RE: The price of weight loss by jejunoileal shunt. *Ann Surg* 190:382, 1979.

Hyperlipidemia

Buchwald H, Campos CT, et al: Women in the POSCH trial: Effects of aggressive cholesterol modification in women with coronary heart disease. *Ann Surg* 216:389, 1992.

Buchwald H, Fitch LL, et al: Perception of quality of life before and after disclosure of trial results: A report from the Program on the Surgical Control of the Hyperlipidemias (POSCH). *Controlled Clinical Trials* 14:500, 1993.

Buchwald H, Stoller DK, et al: Partial ileal bypass for hypercholesterolemia: 20- to 26-year followup of the first 57 consecutive cases. *Ann Surg* 212:318, 1990.

Buchwald H, Varco RL, et al: Effect of partial ileal bypass surgery on mortality and morbidity from coronary disease in patients with hypercholesterolemia. *N Engl J Med* 323:946, 1990.

Campos CT, Matts JP, et al: Lipid results of partial ileal bypass in patients with heterozygous, type II-A hyperlipoproteinemia. Program on the Surgical Control of Hyperlipidemias. *Surgery* 108:601, 1990.

Matts JP, Buchwald H, et al: Subgroup analyses of the major clinical endpoints in the Program on the Surgical Control of the Hyperlipidemias (POSCH): Overall mortality, atherosclerotic coronary heart disease (ACHD) mortality, and ACHD mortality or myocardial infarction. *J Clin Epidemiol* 48:389, 1995.

CHAPTER 26

Colon, Rectum, and Anus

Ira J. Kodner, Robert D. Fry, James W. Fleshman, Elisa H. Birnbaum, and Thomas E. Read

ANATOMIC CONSIDERATIONS

Embryology

The primitive gut, which is divided into the foregut, the midgut, and the hindgut, develops during the fourth week of gestation. The midgut develops into the small intestine (beginning at the entrance of the common bile duct) and the large intestine proximal to the midtransverse colon. This intestinal segment receives blood from the *superior mesenteric artery.* The hindgut develops into the large bowel distal to the midtransverse colon as well as the proximal anus and the lower urogenital tract and receives its main blood supply from the *inferior mesenteric artery.* The distal anal canal receives blood from branches of the internal pudendal artery and is ectodermal in origin (Fig. 26-1).

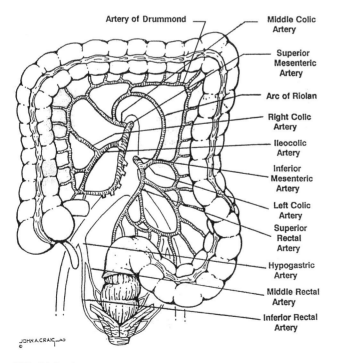

FIG. 26-1. *Arterial blood supply of colon and rectum. Note that recent studies have demonstrated that the right colic artery is a branch of the ileocolic artery in the majority of cases.*

The developing midgut migrates out of the abdominal cavity during the sixth week of pregnancy. During the ensuing 4 weeks, the midgut rotates 270° in a counterclockwise direction about the superior mesenteric artery before assuming its final anatomic position in the abdominal cavity.

The developing hindgut is terminated by the *cloaca,* which during the sixth week of development is partitioned by the anorectal septum into the ventral urogenital sinus and the dorsal rectum. The anal canal is completely formed by the end of the eighth week when the thin anal membrane ruptures. The *dentate line* in the lower anal canal marks the transition from endodermal hindgut to ectodermal tissue.

Anatomy

Colon

The colon, approximately 3 to 5 feet in length, extends from the ileum to the rectum. The terminal ileum joins the cecum on its posteromedial border at the ileocecal valve. The fold of Treves (the only antimesenteric fatty appendage on the small bowel) is located on the distal ileum just proximal to the ileocecal valve. The *cecum* projects from the antimesenteric side of the ascending colon and is a large blind pouch with no mesentery. The cecum is approximately 7.5 to 8.5 cm in diameter and is the widest portion of the colon. The colon progressively diminishes in size to the *sigmoid* colon, its narrowest portion, which is approximately 2.5 cm in diameter. This size discrepancy accounts for the frequent observation that cecal tumors can grow to be large and bulky before the onset of symptoms, whereas sigmoid tumors are symptomatic at smaller sizes. The cecum, because of its relatively large diameter, is also the most common site of colonic rupture caused by distal obstruction. This is explained by Laplace's law: Tension is directly proportional to the radius of a sphere ($T = PR$, where T is tension in the wall of the bowel, P is internal pressure, and R is the radius of the bowel).

The layers of the colon wall include mucosa, submucosa, inner circular muscle, outer longitudinal muscle, and serosa (Fig. 26-2). The longitudinal muscle is separated into three distinct bands called *teniae coli* and positioned 120° apart about the circumference of the colon. The teniae converge proximally at the appendix and disappear as distinct bands at the proximal rectum at the level of the sacral promontory. *Haustra coli* are sacculations between the teniae and are separated by crescent-shaped folds called *plicae semilunares. Appendices epiploicae* are fatty appendages attached to teniae.

The *omentum* is attached to the transverse colon on its anterosuperior edge. The ascending colon, descending colon, and posterior surface of the hepatic and splenic flexures are usually retroperitoneal, whereas the cecum, transverse colon, and sigmoid colon are intraperitoneal in location. Although volvulus is most common in the sigmoid colon, the cecum and, rarely, the transverse colon also might twist about their mesenteries because of their intraperitoneal location and relative lack of fixation.

Arterial Supply. The *superior mesenteric artery* arises from the ventral surface of the aorta just below the celiac axis (see Fig. 26-1). It passes downward behind the pancreas and crosses in front of the third portion of the duodenum. It supplies the cecum, ascending colon, and transverse colon via its ileocolic and middle colic branches. Cadaver studies have shown that the

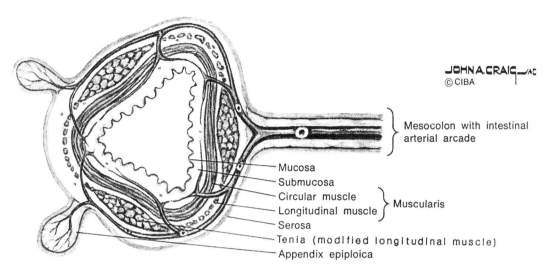

JOHN A.CRAIG_AC
©CIBA

Mesocolon with intestinal arterial arcade

Mucosa
Submucosa
Circular muscle
Longitudinal muscle } Muscularis
Serosa
Tenia (modified longitudinal muscle)
Appendix epiploica

FIG. 26-2. Anatomy of the colonic wall. (From: *Kodner U: Colostomy and ileostomy. Ciba Clinical Symposia 30:5, 1978. Copyright 1978 Ciba-Geigy Corporation. Reprinted with permission from Clinical Symposia; illustrated by John A. Craig, M.D. All rights reserved.*)

right colic artery arises from the superior mesenteric artery in fewer than 15 percent of patients. It arises from the ileocolic in 85 percent of patients. *The inferior mesenteric artery* arises from the infrarenal aorta and supplies the descending colon, sigmoid colon, and upper rectum via its left colic, sigmoidal, and superior rectal branches.

Collaterals exist between the superior and inferior mesenteric arteries in the region of the splenic flexure. The arcades of the ileocolic, right, middle, and left colic arteries are peripherally connected by a series of anastomosing vessels commonly referred to as the *marginal artery of Drummond.* The marginal artery of Drummond runs along the mesenteric border of the colon and provides the vasa recta to the colon. The *arc of Riolan* is located closer to the mesenteric root. It is an inconstant vessel that exists between the left colic branch of the inferior mesenteric artery and the middle colic branch of the superior mesenteric artery. It is frequently referred to as the *meandering mesenteric artery* because of its tortuous course, and it is best visualized when there is an occlusion of either the inferior or superior mesenteric artery.

Venous Drainage. Except for the inferior mesenteric vein, which lies adjacent to the ascending branch of the left colic artery, the veins draining the colon follow the same course as the corresponding arteries. The *inferior mesenteric vein* drains the descending colon, sigmoid colon, and proximal rectum. It runs in a retroperitoneal location to the left of the ligament of Treitz, continues behind the body of the pancreas, and enters the splenic vein. The *superior mesenteric vein* drains the cecum, ascending colon, and transverse colon and joins the splenic vein to form the portal vein.

Lymphatic Drainage. The colon is encircled by lymphatic channels located in the submucosa and the muscularis mucosae. The mucosa has rich vascular plexi but no lymphatics. For this reason, superficial cancers that do not penetrate the muscularis mucosae cannot metastasize via the lymphatic route. This segmental architecture limits longitudinal intramural extension of tumors. Circumferential extension into submucosal and se-

rosal zones results in annular lesions. Lymphatic vessels follow the arterial supply of the colon. Lymph nodes are located on the bowel wall (epicolic), along the inner margin of the bowel (paracolic), around the named mesenteric arteries (intermediate), and about the origin of the superior and inferior arteries (main).

Nerve Supply. *Sympathetic* nerves inhibit and *parasympathetic* nerves stimulate peristalsis. Sympathetic fibers to the right colon originate in the lower six thoracic segments of the spinal cord. They travel in the thoracic splanchnic nerves to the celiac plexus and then to the superior mesenteric plexus. The parasympathetic supply to the right side of the transverse colon is presumed to come from the right vagus nerve.

Sympathetic innervation of the left colon and rectum originates in the first three lumbar segments. These nerves join the preaortic plexus and become the inferior mesenteric plexus below the bifurcation of the aorta. The parasympathetic nerves to the left colon arise from the sacral nerves to form the nervi erigentes on either side of the rectum. Extensions of the sacral parasympathetics ascend through the hypogastric plexus to the area of the splenic flexure.

Rectum and Anal Canal

General Anatomy. The rectal wall consists of mucosa, submucosa, and two complete muscular layers: inner circular and outer longitudinal (Fig. 26-3). The rectum is approximately 12 to 15 cm in length and extends from the sigmoid colon to the anal canal following the curve of the sacrum (Fig. 26-4). The anterior *peritoneal reflection* is about 5 to 7.5 cm above the anus in females and 7 to 9 cm above the anus in males. The posterior peritoneal reflection is usually 12 to 15 cm above the anus. The upper third of the rectum is covered by peritoneum on its anterior and lateral surfaces. The middle third of the rectum is covered by peritoneum only on its anterior surface, and the lower third of the rectum is below the peritoneal reflection. The proximal rectum is identified as the level at which the teniae coli of the colon coalesce to form a complete layer of longitudinal muscle at approximately the level of the sacral promontory.

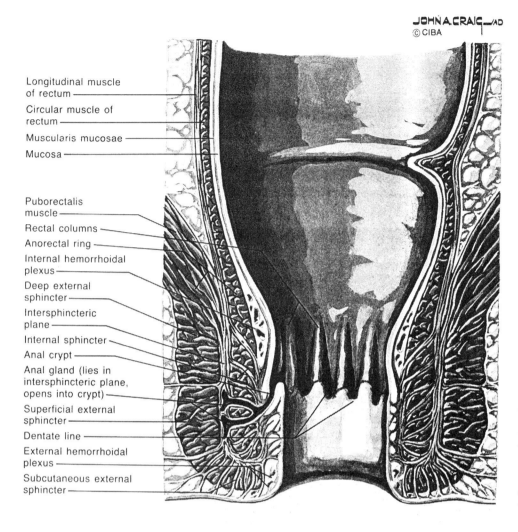

Longitudinal muscle of rectum

Circular muscle of rectum

Muscularis mucosae

Mucosa

Puborectalis muscle

Rectal columns

Anorectal ring

Internal hemorrhoidal plexus

Deep external sphincter

Intersphincteric plane

Internal sphincter

Anal crypt

Anal gland (lies in intersphincteric plane, opens into crypt)

Superficial external sphincter

Dentate line

External hemorrhoidal plexus

Subcutaneous external sphincter

JOHN A. CRAIG—AD
© CIBA

FIG. 26-3. Anorectal anatomy. (From: *Fry RD, Kodner IJ. Anorectal disorders. Ciba Clinical Symposia 37:6, 1985. Copyright 1985 Ciba-Geigy Corporation. Reprinted with permission from Clinical Symposia; illustrated by John A. Craig, M.D. All rights reserved.*)

The rectum contains three distinct curves: The proximal and distal curves are convex to the right, whereas the middle curve is convex to the left. These folds project into the lumen as the *valves of Houston.* These mucosal infoldings present some difficulty for proctoscopic examination, but they are excellent targets for mucosal biopsy because they do not contain all layers

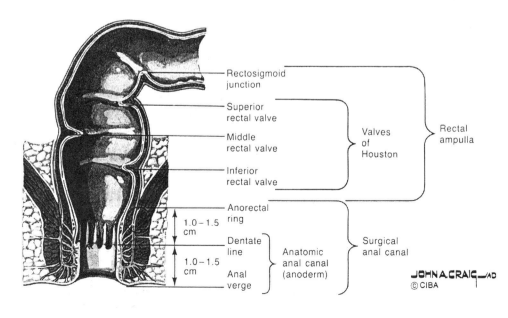

Rectosigmoid junction

Superior rectal valve

Middle rectal valve

Inferior rectal valve

Valves of Houston

Rectal ampulla

Anorectal ring

1.0–1.5 cm

Dentate line

1.0–1.5 cm

Anal verge

Anatomic anal canal (anoderm)

Surgical anal canal

JOHN A. CRAIG—AD
© CIBA

FIG. 26-4. Anatomy of anus and rectum. (From: *Fry RD, Kodner IJ. Anorectal disorders. Ciba Clinical Symposia 37:6, 1985. Copyright 1985 Ciba-Geigy Corporation. Reprinted with permission from Clinical Symposia; illustrated by John A. Craig, M.D. All rights reserved.*)

of the muscular rectal wall and the risk of perforation is therefore diminished. The middle valve of Houston roughly correlates with the level of the anterior peritoneal reflection.

Waldeyer's fascia is a dense rectosacral fascia that begins at the level of the fourth sacral body and extends anteriorly to the rectum, covering the sacrum and overlying the vessels and nerves (see Fig. 26-86E). Anterior to the extraperitoneal rectum is *Denonvilliers' fascia,* which is the rectovesical septum in men and the rectovaginal septum in women. The *lateral ligaments* of endopelvic fascia support the lower rectum but do not usually contain major blood vessels, as previously believed. Division of the lateral ligaments is thus possible without impairing the blood supply to the rectum or encountering a significant bleeding. Accessory middle hemorrhoidal arteries can be located in the lateral ligaments but are not critical to the blood supply of the rectum.

The *pelvic floor* is a musculotendinous sheet formed by the levator ani muscle and is innervated by the fourth sacral nerve (Fig. 26-5). The pubococcygeus, iliococcygeus, and puborectalis muscles make up the levator ani muscle. These are paired muscles that intertwine and act as a single unit. The line of decussation is called the *anococcygeal raphe.* The rectum, vagina, ure-

thra, and the dorsal vein of the penis pass through the levator hiatus in the pubococcygeal portion of the levator ani. During defecation, the puborectalis relaxes and the levator ani contracts, widening the levator hiatus.

The *anal canal* starts at the pelvic diaphragm and ends at the anal verge (see Fig. 26-4). It is approximately 4 cm long and normally exists as a collapsed anteroposterior slit. The *anatomic anal canal* extends from the anal verge to the dentate line. For practical purposes, however, surgeons usually define the *surgical anal canal* as extending from the anal verge to the anorectal ring, which is the circular lower (see Fig. 26-3) border of the puborectalis that is palpable by digital rectal examination. The anorectal ring is 1 to 1.5 cm above the dentate line.

The *anal verge* is the junction between anoderm and perianal skin. The anoderm is a specialized epithelium rich in nerves but devoid of secondary skin appendages (hair follicles, sebaceous glands, or sweat glands). The *dentate line* is a true mucocutaneous junction located 1 to 1.5 cm above the anal verge (see Fig. 26-3). A 6- to 12-mm transitional zone exists above the dentate line over which the squamous epithelium of the anoderm becomes cuboidal and then columnar epithelium.

The anal canal is surrounded by an internal and external sphincter, which together constitute the *anal sphincter mechanism* (see Fig. 26-5). The *internal sphincter* is a specialized continuation of the inner circular smooth muscle of the rectum. It is an involuntary muscle and is normally contracted at rest. The intersphincteric plane represents the fibrous continuation of the longitudinal smooth muscle layer of the rectum.

The *external sphincter* is a voluntary, striated muscle divided into three U-shaped loops (subcutaneous, superficial, and deep) acting as a single functional unit. It is a specialized continuation of the levator muscles of the pelvic floor, specifically of the puborectalis muscle. The *puborectalis* originates at the pubis and joins posterior to the rectum. It is normally contracted, causing an 80° angulation of the anorectal junction.

The *columns of Morgagni* consist of 8 to 14 longitudinal mucosal folds located just above the dentate line and forming the anal crypts at their distal end (see Fig. 26-3). Small rudimentary glands open into some of these crypts. The ducts of these glands penetrate the internal sphincter, and the body of the gland resides in the intersphincteric plane.

Arterial Supply. The terminal branch of the inferior mesenteric artery becomes the *superior rectal artery* as it crosses the left common iliac artery (Fig. 26-6A). It descends in the sigmoid mesocolon and bifurcates at the level of the third sacral body. The left and right branches of the superior rectal artery supply the upper and middle rectum.

The middle and inferior rectal arteries supply the lower third of the rectum. The *middle rectal arteries* arise from the internal iliac arteries, run through Denonvilliers' fascia, and enter the anterolateral aspect of the rectal wall at the level of the anorectal ring. Collaterals exist between the middle and superior rectal arteries. Preservation of the middle rectal arteries is necessary to maintain viability of the remaining rectum after proximal ligation of the inferior mesenteric artery.

The *inferior rectal arteries* are branches of the internal pudendal arteries. They traverse Alcock's canal and enter the posterolateral aspect of the ischiorectal fossa. They supply the internal and external sphincters and the lining of the anal canal and do not form collaterals with the other rectal arteries. The

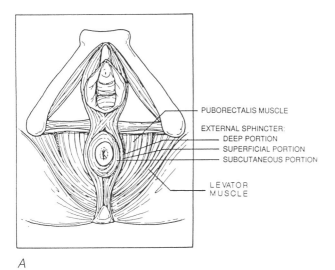

A

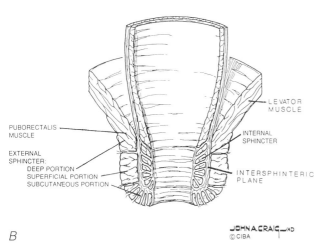

B

JOHN A. CRAIG—AD
© CIBA

FIG. 26-5. Musculature of rectum, anus, and pelvic floor. *A.* External view. *B.* Internal view. (From: *Fleshman JH, et al.: in Shackelford's Surgery of the Alimentary Tract, 1991, with permission.)*

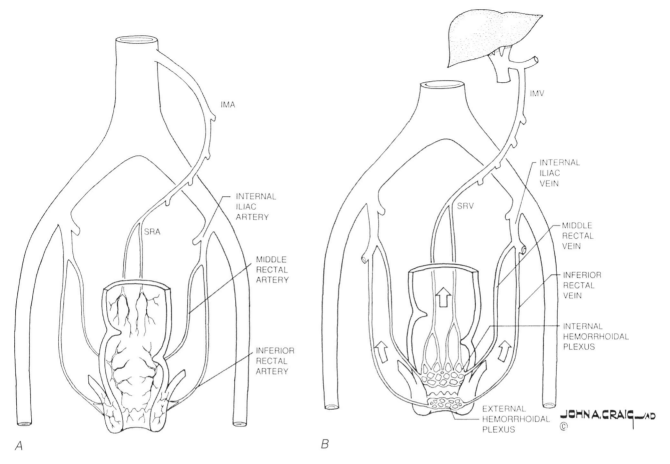

FIG. 26-6. Vascular supply of the anus and rectum. *A.* Arterial supply. *B.* Venous drainage. IMA = inferior mesenteric artery; SRA = superior rectal artery; IMV = inferior mesenteric vein; SRV = superior rectal vein. (From: *Kodner IJ, Fleshman JW, Fry RD: in Maingot's Abdominal Operations, 1989, with permission.*)

middle sacral artery arises just proximal to the aortic bifurcation and provides very little blood supply to the rectum.

Venous Drainage. The venous drainage of the rectum parallels the arterial supply and empties into both the portal and the systemic (caval) systems. The upper and middle rectum are drained by the *superior rectal vein,* which enters the portal system via the inferior mesenteric vein (see Fig. 26-6*B*). The lower rectum and upper anal canal are drained by the *middle rectal veins,* which empty into the internal iliac veins and then into the caval system. The *inferior rectal veins* drain the lower anal canal and empty into the pudendal veins, which drain into the caval system via the internal iliac veins. Low rectal tumors can thus metastasize through venous channels into both the portal and systemic venous systems.

There are three submucosal *internal hemorrhoidal complexes* located above the dentate line (see Fig. 26-3). The left lateral, right posterolateral, and right anterolateral internal hemorrhoidal veins drain into the superior rectal vein. Below the dentate line the *external hemorrhoidal veins* drain into the pudendal veins. There is communication between the internal and external plexi.

Lymphatic Drainage. The rectal lymphatic flow is segmental and circumferential and follows the same distribution as the arterial blood supply (Fig. 26-7). Lymph from the upper and middle rectum drains into the inferior mesenteric nodes. The lower rectum is drained primarily by lymphatics that follow the superior rectal artery and enter the inferior mesenteric nodes. Lymph from the lower rectum also can flow laterally along the middle and inferior rectal arteries, posteriorly along the middle sacral artery, or anteriorly through channels in the rectovesical or rectovaginal septum. These channels drain to the iliac nodes and subsequently to periaortic lymph nodes.

Lymphatics from the anal canal above the dentate line drain via the superior rectal lymphatics to the inferior mesenteric lymph nodes or laterally to the internal iliac lymph nodes. Below the dentate line, the lymphatics drain primarily to the inguinal nodes but can drain to the inferior or superior rectal lymph nodes as well.

Nerve Supply. The innervation of the rectum is shared with the urogenital organs of the pelvis and consists of both sympathetic and parasympathetic nerves (Fig. 26-8). *Sympathetic* nerves from thoracolumnar segments unite below the inferior mesenteric artery to form the *inferior mesenteric plexus.* These purely sympathetic nerves descend to the *superior hypogastric plexus* located below the aortic bifurcation. They then bifurcate and descend in the pelvis as the *hypogastric nerves.* The lower rectum, bladder, and sexual organs in both men and women re-

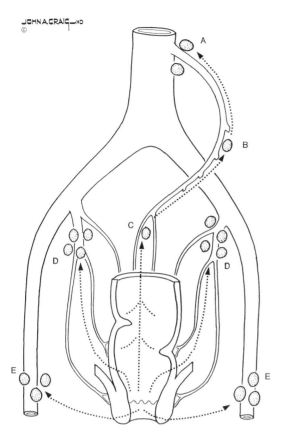

FIG. 26-7. Lymphatic drainage of the rectum and anus. A. Nodes at origin of inferior mesenteric artery. B. Nodes at origin of sigmoid branches. C. Sacral nodes. D. Internal iliac nodes. E. Inguinal nodes. (From: *Kodner U, Fleshman JW, Fry RD: in Maingot's Abdominal Operations, 1989, with permission.*)

ceive sympathetic innervation via the hypogastric nerve. Injury to the inferior mesenteric plexus can result during ligation of the inferior mesenteric artery at its origin.

Parasympathetic fibers from the second, third, and fourth sacral roots (the *nervi erigentes*) unite with the hypogastric nerves anterior and lateral to the rectum forming the *pelvic plexus,* which runs laterally in the pelvis. The periprostatic plexus arises from the pelvic plexus. Mixed fibers from these plexi innervate the rectum, internal anal sphincter, prostate, bladder, and penis. The *pudendal nerve (S2, S3, S4)* mediates sensory stimuli from the penis and clitoris via the dorsal nerve.

Both sympathetic and parasympathetic fibers are essential for penile erection. The parasympathetic fibers cause vasodilation and increased blood flow in the corpus cavernosum, resulting in an erection. The sympathetic fibers cause vasoconstriction of the penile veins and thus sustain the erection. Sympathetic nerves cause contraction of the ejaculatory ducts, seminal vesicles, and prostate and are necessary for ejaculation. Damage to the periprostatic plexus might occur during surgical dissection of the rectum. Injury to the pelvic autonomic nerves may result in bladder dysfunction, impotence, or both.

The *internal anal sphincter* is innervated by both sympathetic and parasympathetic nerves, and both are inhibitory to the sphincter. The internal sphincter has a continuous tone that decreases as rectal pressure increases. Once the rectum empties,

the internal sphincter tone rises again. The *external anal sphincter* and *levator ani muscles* are innervated by the inferior rectal branch of the internal pudendal nerve (S2, S3, S4) and the perineal branch of the fourth sacral nerve. Any distention of the rectum results in relaxation of the internal sphincter. The external sphincter can be contracted voluntarily and kept in that state for approximately 1 minute.

Below the dentate line, cutaneous sensations of heat, cold, pain, and touch are conveyed by afferent fibers of the inferior rectal and perineal branches of the pudendal nerve. Above the dentate line, a poorly defined dull sensation, experienced when the mucosa is pinched or when internal hemorrhoids are ligated, is probably mediated by parasympathetic fibers.

Resection of the sacrum with sacrifice of *sacral nerves* occasionally may be required for total resection of pelvic tumors. Sacrifice of the lower sacral nerves will lead to saddle anesthesia and possible motor weakness in the lower extremities. Preservation of at least one of the third sacral nerves is required to maintain acceptable anal continence. Near-normal continence will be maintained if the upper three sacral roots on one side are preserved along with the upper two sacral roots on the contralateral side. If all the sacral roots are destroyed unilaterally but the contralateral nerves are preserved, the patient should maintain continence. If both S3 roots are destroyed, the patient will be incontinent. The upper half of S1 is needed for stability of the spine and pelvis.

DISTURBANCES OF PHYSIOLOGY

Normal Colonic Function

The colon is much more than a receptacle and conduit for the end products of digestion. This organ absorbs water, sodium,

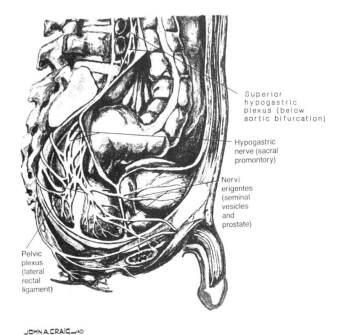

FIG. 26-8. Nerve supply of pelvic organs. (From: *Kodner U, Fry RD: Inflammatory bowel disease. Ciba Clin Symp 34:1, 1982. Copyright 1982 Ciba-Geigy Corporation. Reprinted with permission from Clinical Symposium; illustrated by John A. Craig, M.D. All rights reserved.*)

and chloride and secretes potassium, bicarbonate, and mucus; it is the site of digestion of certain carbohydrates and proteins and provides the environment for the bacterial production of vitamin K.

Water and Electrolyte Exchanges

The major absorptive function of the colon is the final regulation of water and electrolyte balance in the intestine. The colon reduces the volume of enteric contents by absorbing greater than 90 percent of the water and electrolytes presented to it. This accounts for 1 to 2 liters of fluid and 200 meq of sodium and chloride per day on average. During a 24-h period, 8 liters of fluid enters the jejunum. In healthy individuals, the small bowel absorbs about 6.5 liters and the colon 1.4 liters, leaving 0.1 liter of normal fecal water content. Under maximum conditions, the colon can absorb 5 to 6 liters of fluid a day. Only if small bowel absorption is reduced to less than 2 liters a day is colonic salvage overwhelmed, and the resulting increase in fecal water content is manifested as diarrhea.

Sodium and Potassium. In healthy persons, the colon absorbs water, sodium, and chloride while secreting potassium and bicarbonate. The colon is able to absorb sodium against very high concentration gradients, especially in the distal colon, which shares many basic cellular mechanisms of sodium and water transport with the distal convoluted tubule of the kidney (Fig. 26-9). The colon has the capacity to absorb up to 400 meq of sodium per day, and the colonic response to aldosterone stimulation may be an important compensatory mechanism during dehydration. A patient with an ileostomy loses this absorptive capacity and cannot tolerate increased sodium losses or decreased sodium intake.

Potassium transport in the colon is mainly passive, along an electrochemical gradient generated by the active transport of sodium. Potassium continues to be secreted into the lumen as long as the luminal concentration is less than 15 meq/L; however, at concentrations below this level, potassium secretion ceases and potassium absorption occurs.

Chloride and Bicarbonate. Chloride, like sodium, is actively absorbed across the colonic mucosa against a concentration gradient. Chloride and bicarbonate are exchanged at the luminal border. Chloride absorption is facilitated by an acidotic environment, and the secretion of bicarbonate is enhanced by increased concentration of luminal chloride. This becomes clinically important in patients with ureterosigmoidostomy, who may develop hyperchloremia and metabolic acidosis due to the absorption of urinary chloride accompanied by the secretion of bicarbonate into the colon.

Short-Chain Fatty Acids. Although active absorption of nutrients is minimal, the colon can passively absorb short-chain fatty acids (SCFAs) formed by intraluminal bacterial fermentation of unabsorbed carbohydrates, particularly fiber. This can account for up to 540 kcal/day of assimilated calories. The absorbed SCFAs butyrate, acetate, and propionate are the major fuel sources of the colonic epithelium. They provide the energy required for active sodium transport, and altered SCFA metabolism or SCFA deficiency may result in impaired colonic sodium absorption.

There is evidence that SCFA metabolism is impaired in patients with ulcerative colitis and that intraluminal infusion of SCFAs can be of benefit in patients with colitis. SCFAs also have been shown to be effective in treating diversion colitis

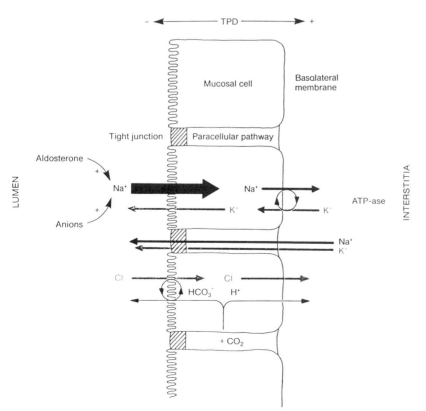

FIG. 26-9. *Basolateral membrane showing electrolyte transport across colonic epithelium. TPD=transmural potential difference. (From: Gordon PH, Nivatvongs S: 1992, p. 41, with permission.)*

(which can occur after a diverting ileostomy or colostomy), implicating colonocyte nutritional deficiency as the cause of this disorder. Elemental diets, which lack fiber, are associated with colonic mucosal atrophy.

Ammonia. Colonic bacteria degrade protein and urea to produce ammonia. Ammonium ions react with bicarbonate to form nonionized ammonia and carbon dioxide. The nonionized ammonia diffuses across the colonic mucosa and is carried to the liver through the portal vein. This absorptive process depends on bacterial degradation of protein and intraluminal pH. As the pH in the colonic lumen falls, ammonia absorption decreases.

Ammonia absorption becomes a problem in patients with severe liver disease, who are unable to metabolize ammonium. The administration of poorly absorbed broad-spectrum antibiotics, coupled with cathartics and enemas, diminishes the colonic bacterial population and decreases ammonia production. Lactulose can be administered with the rationale that its metabolism to organic acids lowers the colonic luminal pH and decreases the absorption of ammonia, and it also reduces bacterial numbers by its purgative action because it causes an osmotic diarrhea.

Diarrhea. A number of agents can stimulate fluid and electrolyte secretion in the colon, including bacteria, enterotoxins, hormones, neurotransmitters, and laxatives. The diarrhea associated with *Shigella* and *Salmonella* infection is caused by diminished absorption or increased secretion of water, sodium, and chloride. Gut hormones, particularly vasoactive intestinal polypeptide, have been shown to have significant effects on colonic absorption and secretion. Prostaglandins play a role in the pathogenesis of diarrhea associated with ulcerative colitis and several laxatives. Any sort of irritation to the colon also can cause increased secretion, such as bile salt malabsorption after terminal ileal resection and long-chain fatty acid malabsorption in steatorrhea. The induced colonic mucus and fluid are high in potassium and may result in potassium depletion in chronic cases.

Motility

Colonic motility is more difficult to study than small bowel motility because of the great regional heterogeneity in the colon and because of the intermittent and unpredictable nature of colonic contractile waves. Even the normal pattern of colonic motility remains the subject of debate. In the first decade of the twentieth century, radiologists observed three patterns of colonic contractions: retrograde movements, segmental contractions, and mass movements. More recently, electrophysiologic and manometric measurements appear to correlate with observed colonic motor contractions; however, much more research is required before the complexities of colonic motility are satisfactorily understood.

Retrograde movements were identified initially as contractile waves originating in the transverse colon and traveling toward the cecum. These contractions appear to delay the transit of material from the right colon, prolonging the exposure of luminal contents to the mucosa and thus increasing the absorption of fluid and electrolytes.

Segmental contractions are the most commonly observed motility pattern. These are localized simultaneous contractions of longitudinal and circular colonic musculature that isolate short segments of the colon. These contractions occur more frequently on the right side of the colon, but their occurrence in the sigmoid colon has been hypothesized to play a role in the formation of diverticula. This contractile activity is decreased by anticholinergic drugs and increased by food and cholinergic drugs.

The third and most infrequent type of colonic activity is the *mass movement.* This pattern is characterized by an antegrade propulsive contractile wave involving a long segment of colon. The contraction propels the colonic contents forward at the rate of 0.5 to 1.0 cm/s. These contractions are 20 to 30 s in duration and generate intracolonic pressures of 100 to 200 mmHg. They occur three or four times a day, often after arising in the morning or in the late postprandial period. Mass movements in the right colon move colonic contents to the more distal colon. A mass movement in the sigmoid colon may occur at the time of defecation.

Many factors affect colonic motility. Emotions such as hostility, anger, and resentment are associated with hypermotility, whereas anxiety and fear are associated with hypomotility. Exercise has been shown to increase segmental and peristaltic colonic activity; sleep is a colonic motility depressant. Mechanical colonic distention stimulates motility and is the basis for the effect of bulk laxatives. Nondigestible polysaccharides and cellulose derivatives absorb water and increase fecal mass, thus stimulating colonic propulsion. Fatty meals appear to have a greater stimulatory effect on colonic motility than carbohydrate or protein meals. Colonic motility is influenced by certain hormones. Glucagon and somatostatin have inhibitory effects. Cholecystokinin increases colonic motor activity and is thought to be responsible for the gastrocolic reflex (increased colonic motility during and after meals).

Neurogenic Control. Colonic motility is regulated by complex and poorly understood extrinsic and intrinsic neuronal systems. The extrinsic system consists of preganglionic parasympathetic neurons from the vagus nerve or the pelvic plexus (S2, S3, S4) and the postganglionic sympathetic neurons (T11–L2). The intrinsic (enteric) nervous system is composed of neurons residing within the colon wall. These intramural neurons communicate through extensive interconnecting plexuses. The enteric plexuses are identified by their location within the colon wall: subserosal, myenteric (Auerbach's plexus), submucosal (Meissner's plexus), and mucosal.

The enteric neurons also may be classified by function: sensory, associative, or motor. The complex interaction between these neurons can be demonstrated by a localized radial distention of the colon that activates sensory neurons. These neurons communicate through associative neurons to proximal and distal motor neurons, resulting in contraction of the colon proximal to the stimulus and simultaneous distal relaxation.

Motor neurons of the enteric nervous system may be excitatory or inhibitory. Excitatory neurons are mainly postganglionic parasympathetic cells that are located in the myenteric or submucosal plexus. Acetylcholine is the most important excitatory neurotransmitter, and its action can be blocked by atropine or scopolamine. Noncholinergic agents, such as substance P, may be released by enteric neurons and appear to have an excitatory action.

Inhibitory motor neurons of the enteric nervous system reside mainly in the myenteric plexus. These cells are noncholinergic and nonadrenergic. There is evidence that purine nucleotides such as adenosine triphosphate may be the neurotransmitters of these cells. Vasoactive inhibitory peptide (VIP) is also a very important inhibitory substance. The inhibitory neurons are involved in the coordinated propagation of colonic propulsive movements such as the mass movement.

Colonic Microflora

The human colon is sterile at birth, but within a matter of hours the intestine is colonized from the environment in an oral to anal direction. *Bacteroides*, destined to be the dominant bacteria in the colon, is first noted at about 10 days after birth. By 3 to 4 weeks after birth, the characteristic stool flora is established and persists into adult life. The large intestine harbors a dense microbial population, with bacteria accounting for approximately one-third of the dry weight of feces. Each gram of feces contains 10^{11} to 10^{12} bacteria, with anaerobic bacteria outnumbering aerobic organisms by a factor of 10^2 to 10^4. *Bacteroides* species are the most common colonic organisms, present in concentrations of 10^{11} to 10^{12} organisms per milliliter of feces. *Escherichia coli*, by comparison, is present in concentrations of 10^8 to 10^{10} organisms per milliliter.

The complex symbiotic relationship between human beings and colonic bacteria is poorly understood, but it is recognized that endogenous colonic bacteria suppress the emergence of pathogenic microorganisms, play an important role in the breakdown of carbohydrates and proteins that escape digestion in the small bowel, participate in the metabolism of numerous substances that are salvaged by the enterohepatic circulation (including bilirubin, bile acids, estrogen, and cholesterol), and produce certain beneficial elements such as vitamin K.

Colonic Gas

Nitrogen, oxygen, carbon dioxide, hydrogen, and methane make up 99 percent of all the gas in the gut. Nitrogen and oxygen are found in the atmosphere and appear in the colon via swallowing air. Hydrogen, methane, and carbon dioxide are produced by bacterial fermentation of carbohydrates and proteins in the colon. An eminent flatologist, Levitt, has shown that most patients who complain of excessive flatus have high concentrations of hydrogen and carbon dioxide in their intestinal gas. Because carbon dioxide is an end product of bacterial fermentation, therapy consists of diet manipulation to decrease the amount of ingested carbohydrate, especially lactose, wheat, and potatoes. In addition, various vegetables (particularly beans) contain undigestible carbohydrates that serve as a substrate for colonic bacterial fermentation and should be avoided by these patients.

Normal humans pass approximately 600 mL of flatus daily (ranging from 200 to 2000 mL/day). There is normally about 200 mL of gas in the intestinal tract, and the amount of detectable gas is seldom increased in patients who complain of bloating and distention. Most complaints of increased intestinal gas probably represent motility disorders instead of actual excessive production of gas.

The five predominant colonic gases (N_2, O_2, CO_2, H_2, CH_4) are odorless. Trace substances such as dimethyl sulfide and methanethiol appear to be responsible for the odor of human feces. Hydrogen and methane are combustible gases and can explode if present in the colon when electrocautery is used for polypectomy or biopsy. Adequate bowel cleansing is necessary before the use of intracolonic electrocautery. Mannitol is an inappropriate purgative under such circumstances because it is a substrate for colonic bacterial fermentation. Polyethylene glycol purgatives are not metabolized by intestinal bacteria and have not been associated with intracolonic explosions.

Disorders of Colonic Physiology

Irritable Bowel Syndrome

Irritable bowel syndrome is a disorder manifested by altered bowel habits and abdominal pain in the absence of other pathology. Patients with the diagnosis of irritable bowel syndrome have been shown to have increased slow-wave activity (3 cycles per minute) in the rectosigmoid, corresponding to increased contractile activity at the same frequency. A similar motility pattern has been noted in patients with diverticular disease, and some authors have suggested that uncoordinated smooth muscle activity followed by increased intraluminal pressure may be the underlying mechanism producing the irritable bowel syndrome and colonic diverticuli. Irritable bowel syndrome is a diagnosis of exclusion and has many different presentations. It is important to exclude organic colonic disease by the appropriate diagnostic tests. Irritable bowel syndrome is not amenable to surgical treatment.

Delayed Transit

Constipation is a symptom with numerous and diverse causes. It is difficult to formulate a precise definition of constipation, but one that is generally accepted is fewer than three stools per week while following a high-residue diet (30 g dietary fiber daily). The causes of constipation are multiple and include metabolic and endocrine disorders (hypothyroidism and hypercalcemia), faulty diet (principally inadequate intake of fiber and fluid), neurologic abnormalities (Parkinson's disease, multiple sclerosis), Hirschsprung's disease, medications (codeine, antidepressants, anticholinergics), colonic inertia, and lack of exercise. Abnormalities of pelvic floor function, such as nonrelaxation of the puborectalis muscle and intussusception of the rectum, have been implicated as important causes of constipation.

A change in bowel habits is a common presenting symptom for colorectal tumors; thus the evaluation of a patient with new-onset constipation should include colonoscopy or contrast enema plus proctoscopy. If no obstructing lesion is present, a trial of fiber supplementation and increased fluid intake relieves constipation symptoms in the majority of patients. If unsuccessful, colonic transit time can be measured. A standardized test has not been generally accepted, but the techniques used by most institutions rely on observation of the movement of ingested radiopaque markers through the intestinal tract. The patient ingests a high-fiber diet (30 g/day) and abstains from all laxatives and enemas for 48 h before and during the investigation. The markers, which are commercially available, are ingested before breakfast on the first day and then followed by radiographs, usually at days 3 and 5. If all markers are still present on the radiograph by day 3, intestinal transit time is slower than normal. Normally, at least 80 percent of markers should have passed by day 5 after ingestion, and all markers should pass by day 7. The abdominal location of the markers indicates the segment of the colon involved with the motility disorder. If a significant number of markers remain in the proximal colon for several days, total colonic inertia should be suspected; if the markers accumulate in the rectosigmoid, anorectal outlet obstruction is the likely cause of the delayed transit.

Anorectal outlet obstruction is evaluated with a variety of techniques. Defecography can demonstrate rectal intussusception and nonrelaxation of the puborectalis muscle. Cinefluoroscopy is used to obtain video images of the rectum from the lateral view during attempts to evacuate barium paste. Rectocele (anterior displacement of the posterior wall of the vagina) and enterocele (inferior displacement of the small bowel on the vagina) also can be demonstrated. Anal manometry can demonstrate absence of the normal rectoanal inhibitory reflex (relaxation of the internal anal sphincter and brief contraction of the external anal sphincter with distention of the rectum), which is suggestive of Hirschsprung's disease, and may be used as an adjunct to rectal biopsy to make this diagnosis. Inability to expel a saline-filled balloon from the rectum suggests failure of the puborectalis muscle to relax during defecation.

Slow-transit constipation (colonic inertia) is a poorly understood disorder of chronic intestinal stasis that afflicts predominantly women. This disorder is sometimes referred to as *Arbuthnot Lane's disease,* after the British surgeon who, at the beginning of the century, recommended colectomy with ileorectal anastomosis as the treatment for chronic constipation. An extreme form of colonic inertia presents as acquired megacolon, which has been seen in association with neurologic disorders and in institutionalized and psychiatric patients. These patients present with frequent fecal impaction, volvulus, and episodes of abdominal distention mimicking large bowel obstruction. The colon can attain immense proportions, filled with gas or stool. Sigmoidoscopy is often performed in these patients in an effort to reduce what appears to be a sigmoid volvulus. The instrument slips easily into the rectum, decompressing it somewhat, but significant decompression is not achieved. A water-soluble contrast enema is often diagnostic and therapeutic. Patients with chronic megacolon do not have evidence of obstruction, and the impaction may be relieved after the study. Complete evaluation includes colonic transit studies to rule out colonic inertia and defecography and anal manometry to rule out pelvic floor abnormalities.

The medical treatment of colonic inertia consists of eliminating obvious sources of constipation, encouraging proper exercise, and ensuring appropriate intake of liquids and dietary fiber. A diet containing 30 g of dietary fiber daily should be prescribed (the average American adult consumes 13 to 19 g of fiber per day). Laxatives and enemas should be avoided if possible. While laxatives are useful for occasional relief of constipation, their chronic use is counterproductive and leads to increased motility abnormalities. Medications known to cause constipation should be reduced or eliminated whenever possible.

The exact role of surgery in the treatment of colonic inertia is not clearly defined. If transit studies demonstrate total colonic inertia and appropriate medical treatment is not successful, abdominal colectomy with ileorectal anastomosis has been beneficial. Such patients are relatively rare and must be carefully selected. If the motility disorder is caused by anorectal outlet obstruction, abdominal colectomy is inappropriate; treatment should be directed toward correction of the primary problem, as described in a later section of this chapter. In rare cases where the individual is incapacitated by chronic megacolon, the only relief of symptoms may be total colectomy with construction of an ileostomy.

Colonic Pseudo-Obstruction (Ogilvie's Syndrome)

Intestinal pseudo-obstruction, a profound ileus without evidence of mechanical obstruction, was first described by Ingelfinger in 1943. The first description of the colonic variant of pseudo-obstruction is thought to be Sir Heneage Ogilvie's 1948 report of two cases associated with malignant infiltration of the celiac plexus. Colonic pseudo-obstruction is associated with neuroleptic medications, opiates, malignancy, severe metabolic illness, or any acute severe illness. Excess sympathetic tone has been postulated as the common mechanism. This concept is supported by anecdotal reports of success with epidural anesthesia, which paralyzes the sympathetic afferent and efferent nerve fibers to the colon and with neostigmine, which increases parasympathetic tone by its anticholinesterase effect.

The diagnosis of colonic pseudo-obstruction is one of exclusion; a water-soluble contrast enema or colonoscopy should be performed to exclude mechanical obstruction. Initial treatment maneuvers include nasogastric decompression, rectal tube placement, correction of metabolic disorders, and discontinuation of medications that decrease colonic motility (e.g., narcotics and anticholinergics). Evidence of rapid cecal dilatation or a cecal diameter greater than 11 to 12 cm on abdominal x-ray should prompt more aggressive intervention because of the risk of cecal ischemia, necrosis, and perforation. Colonoscopic decompression is successful initially in 70 to 90 percent of patients, with a recurrence rate of 10 to 30 percent. The majority of patients will respond to a second colonoscopic decompression. The use of long colonic tubes has not been uniformly successful. Operation is reserved for patients with persistent colonic dilatation despite colonoscopic decompression and patients with peritonitis. Cecostomy or loop colostomy are effective in relieving distention; laparotomy should be performed in patients with peritonitis, and nonviable bowel should be resected.

Volvulus

Volvulus is a twisting of an air-filled segment of bowel about its narrow mesentery, causing an obstruction that can lead to strangulation and gangrene (Fig. 26-10). Volvulus almost never occurs when the colon is filled with solid stool. The condition is classified and treated according to its location in the colon. Sigmoid, cecal, and transverse colon are the most common sites. Volvulus causes less than 10 percent of intestinal obstructions in the United States, but it has been reported as the cause of 55 percent of intestinal obstructions in parts of Iran and Russia.

Sigmoid Volvulus. Sigmoid volvulus accounts for about 90 percent of all volvulus seen in the United States. It usually occurs in older or institutionalized patients and in patients with a variety of neurologic disorders. A redundant sigmoid colon with a narrow-based mesocolon is the factor necessary for sigmoid volvulus.

Diagnosis. Patients present with complaints of abdominal pain, cramping, distention, and obstipation. Many patients give a history of previous episodes of abdominal pain and distention. Elevated white blood cell count, fever, or evidence of peritoneal irritation on physical examination suggests the presence of gangrenous bowel.

Plain abdominal radiographs may be diagnostic (Fig. 26-11). The inflated sigmoid appears as an inverted U-shaped, sausage-like loop. A dense line is often seen running downward to the point of torsion. Water-soluble contrast enema may be diagnostic

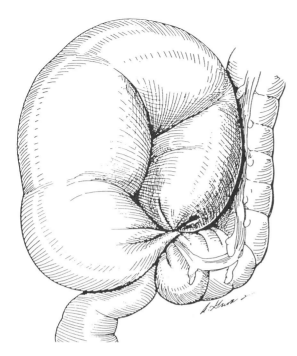

FIG. 26-10. Sigmoid volvulus. (From: *Nivatvongs S, Becker ER: Colon, rectum and anal canal, in EC James, RJ Corry, JF Perry Jr (eds): Basic Surgical Practice. Philadelphia, Hanley & Belfus, 1987, with permission.*)

but should not be performed on patients with suspected gangrene. The column of barium stops at the obstruction and tapers to a point ("bird's beak" deformity) (Fig. 26-12). Reduction of the volvulus may occur during the examination.

Treatment. If gangrene is suspected, or if the patient has signs of peritoneal irritation, reduction should not be attempted, and the patient should undergo emergency operation. If peritonitis is not present, rigid sigmoidoscopy should be performed. An attempt to reduce the volvulus by inserting a soft rectal tube through the sigmoidoscope past the point of volvulus usually results in dramatic decompression. The tube is left in place to further decompression. Flexible sigmoidoscopy or colonoscopy has been used to reduce volvulus beyond the limits of the rigid sigmoidoscope. Unsuccessful detorsion, bloody discharge, or evidence of mucosal ischemia indicates strangulation or gangrene. If this is found, sigmoidoscopy should be terminated, and the patient should undergo an emergency operation.

Recurrence rates following nonoperative reduction can be as high as 40 percent. If the volvulus is reduced successfully, the patient should be stabilized and undergo mechanical bowel preparation, followed by elective sigmoid resection. Resection with primary anastomosis is the recommended surgical treatment for sigmoid volvulus in a patient who is adequately prepared. Resection of the sigmoid colon with construction of a colostomy and Hartmann pouch is usually necessary if emergent operation is performed on unprepared bowel. All nonviable bowel must be resected, and mortality is related to the presence of gangrenous bowel.

Cecal Volvulus. Cecal volvulus is generally seen in younger patients and accounts for less than 20 percent of colonic volvulus. It is thought to be due to anomalous fixation of the

right colon to the retroperitoneum, leading to a freely mobile cecum.

Diagnosis. Abdominal pain is the most common symptom of cecal volvulus. Nausea and vomiting, obstipation, and diarrhea are also common symptoms. Clinically, the patient appears to have a small bowel obstruction, and many patients give a history of chronic intermittent symptoms.

Ninety percent of patients with cecal volvulus have a full axial volvulus; 10 percent have a cecal bascule (cecum folded on itself in an anterior cephalad direction). A plain abdominal radiograph may be diagnostic. Cecal volvulus is seen as a kidney-shaped, air-filled structure in the left upper quadrant. The convexity of the loop faces the left upper quadrant. Water-soluble contrast enema may show obstruction of the column of contrast material at the level of the volvulus. The tapered edge of the contrast material points toward the site of the torsion.

Treatment. Resection, with ileostomy and mucous fistula, is indicated if there is gangrenous bowel. The operative treatment of nongangrenous cecal volvulus is controversial. Right hemicolectomy, cecopexy, tube cecostomy, and simple detorsion have been recommended. Resection has the lowest recurrence rates (essentially zero), and primary anastomosis often can be performed safely. Suture of the right colon to the lateral peritoneal surface (cecopexy) risks the sutures pulling through the thin-

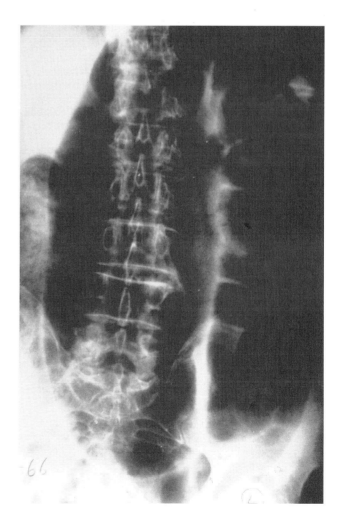

FIG. 26-11. Abdominal radiograph of sigmoid volvulus.

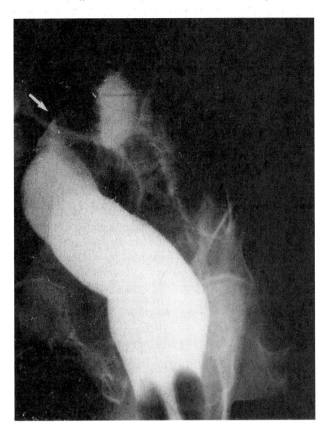

FIG. 26-12. Barium enema study of sigmoid volvulus, showing "bird's beak" deformity.

walled, distended cecum and has had variable recurrence rates. Cecostomy has been associated with abdominal wall and wound complications and persistent fecal fistula in up to 50 percent of patients and recurrence of volvulus in up to 15 percent of patients. Logic dictates that detorsion alone without fixation should lead to high recurrence rates; however, only 7 to 15 percent of patients have been reported to have recurrent volvulus. Regardless, few authors have recommended simple detorsion as adequate treatment for cecal volvulus.

Transverse Colon Volvulus. Volvulus of the transverse colon is rare because the transverse colon is normally prevented from rotation by a broad-based, short mesentery. Failure of the mesenteries to fix normally or narrowing of the mesenteric attachments, allowing a short, fixed point of attachment, may predispose the transverse colon to volvulus. Patients present with a clinical picture similar to sigmoid volvulus. Barium enema is diagnostic and reveals the point of obstruction. Successful attempts at colonoscopic detorsion have been reported. Most patients require operative detorsion with resection of the redundant transverse colon.

Diverticular Disease

General Considerations. The word *diverticulum* is used to describe an abnormal sac or pouch protruding from the wall of a hollow organ such as the colon. The term *true diverticulum* implies that the pouch is composed of all layers of the intestinal wall (true diverticula are rare), whereas a *false diverticulum* lacks a portion of the normal bowel wall. Specifically, the commonly observed diverticula of the colon consist of protrusions of mucosa through the muscular layers of the wall and are devoid of a muscular coat and thus are false diverticula.

Diverticular disease and *diverticulosis* are terms used to indicate the presence of colonic diverticula (Fig. 26-13), a condition that is rare before age 30, becomes more common with increasing age, and is present in approximately 75 percent of Americans over age 80. The variation in incidence by sex varies among reports, and a review of large series of patients fails to indicate that either men or women are more susceptible to the development of diverticula.

Diverticular disease seems to be a phenomenon of the industrial revolution and Western society. The marked increase in the prevalence of diverticulosis in England after 1910 has been attributed to the process introduced approximately 30 years earlier of roller-milling wheat flour. This advance resulted in a decreased consumption of unprocessed cereals and was accompanied by an increased consumption of sugar and meat. In the past half century, the amount of fiber consumed by individuals in North America and western Europe has declined, while the prevalence of diverticular disease has increased dramatically. Further evidence of reduced intake of fiber as a cause of diverticulosis

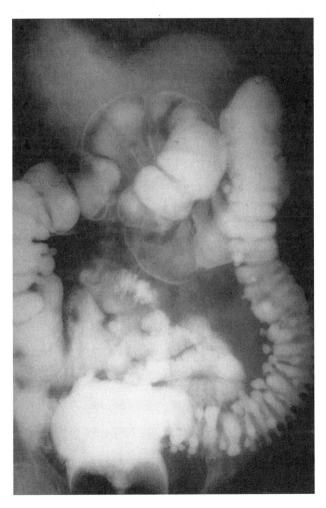

FIG. 26-13. Diverticulosis with numerous diverticula in the sigmoid colon.

is provided by the observation that the disease is almost unknown in sub-Sahara African blacks who consume a high level of dietary fiber; however, blacks in Johannesburg who consume a low-fiber diet have the same high incidence of diverticular disease as South African whites.

Etiology. The precise cause of diverticulosis is not known. Anatomic studies have demonstrated that diverticula are actually herniations of mucosa through the colon at sites where arterioles penetrate the muscular wall. These sites are located predominantly on the mesenteric side of the antimesenteric teniae. A lesser number of protrusions can occur between the antimesenteric teniae (Fig. 26-14). In some cases the artery divides, with one branch penetrating the wall at the site of a diverticulum and the other branch passing external to the muscular coat and sometimes actually being displaced over the dome of the diverticulum. This intimate association between the artery and the diverticulum is responsible for the massive hemorrhage that occasionally can complicate diverticulosis.

Another striking anatomic abnormality associated with diverticulosis is marked thickening of the affected colonic wall. This muscular abnormality seems to precede the appearance of diverticula and occurs predominantly in the sigmoid colon. Diverticula occur most often in the sigmoid, with the abnormalities being confined to the sigmoid in over half the patients with

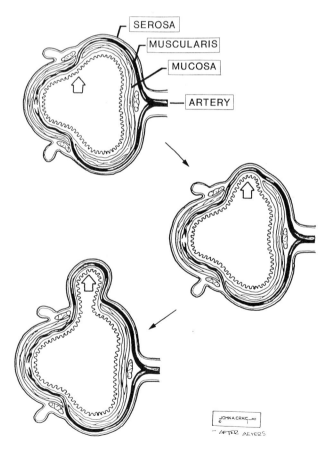

FIG. 26-14. Development of a colonic diverticulum. The mucosa protrudes through the muscular wall at the site of penetration by an arteriole. Note the close association between the artery and the diverticulum.

diverticular disease; other colonic segments (usually the descending colon) are also involved in about another 40 percent of affected patients, and the entire colon is involved in approximately 5 to 10 percent of patients.

A low-fiber diet appears to be associated with a narrow sigmoid colon. The small lumen permits segmental contractions to isolate small regions of the colon into compartments that are subjected to high pressures. Normally, the colonic pressure is only slightly above atmospheric pressure, but pressures as high as 90 mmHg can be generated in the narrow sigmoid by segmental contraction. It is presumed that repeated high-pressure contractions produce the herniation of mucosa through the colonic wall resulting in diverticula.

Diverticulitis denotes infection associated with diverticula. This term is somewhat a misnomer because the infectious process commonly associated with diverticular disease is pericolic in nature and predominantly involves the surrounding soft tissues such as mesentery or adjacent organs, in addition to the serosal surface of the colon.

Peridiverticulitis would be a more accurate descriptive term for this disease. It should be recognized that the infection is the result of a perforation of a diverticulum, leading to extravasation of feces from the lumen to the serosal surface of the colon. In most instances, the amount of fecal contamination is minute, and the body's natural defenses confine the infection. If the contamination is significant, or if the patient's response to infection is compromised, the local peritoneal defenses may be overwhelmed, and abscess formation or even generalized peritonitis can occur. Whether the perforation of the diverticulum is the result of increased colonic pressure, obstruction of the neck of the diverticulum by inspissated feces, or ischemia of the protruded mucosal sac, the end result, pericolic infection, is the same. Recognition that the cause of the abdominal infection is a perforation of a diverticulum provides a basis for understanding the signs and symptoms of the disease as well as the rationale for determining appropriate diagnostic tests and treatment.

Patients with *acute diverticulitis* usually complain of pain in the left lower abdomen. The pain may radiate to the suprapubic area, left groin, or back. An alteration in bowel habit, usually constipation or occasionally diarrhea, may be noted. Fever and chills are not unusual, and urgency or frequency of urination may be present if the inflammation is adjacent to the bladder. Rectal bleeding is distinctly unusual in the presence of diverticulitis.

The physical findings depend on the severity of the infection. The most common finding is tenderness over the left lower abdomen. If considerable inflammation is present, abdominal palpation may reveal a poorly circumscribed area of induration. A tender mass in the left lower quadrant is suggestive of a localized phlegmon or, more likely, an abscess. Occasionally, abdominal distention is caused by ileus or by partial obstruction of small bowel involved in the inflammatory process. Rectal examination may demonstrate pelvic tenderness, and a tender pelvic abscess may be palpated by rectal or vaginal examination.

A limited sigmoidoscopic examination occasionally is indicated to rule out a rectal cancer. If diverticulitis is suspected, air should not be insufflated through the sigmoidoscope because this will only distend the colon and may increase the inflammation by forcing more feces through a perforated diverticulum. Usually the sigmoidoscope cannot be advanced beyond 12 cm without undue discomfort to the patient. Fiberoptic endoscopy offers little information in the evaluation of suspected diverticulitis and carries significant risk of increasing the pericolic contamination.

Often the diagnosis of diverticulitis can be reasonably ensured based on the history and physical examination. If the diagnosis is in doubt, however, three diagnostic tests can be considered: computed tomography (CT) of the abdomen, ultrasound, and the contrast enema. The abdominal CT and ultrasound are noninvasive tests, and both can demonstrate thickened colonic wall and an associated abscess.

The CT is usually the test of choice to confirm the suspected diagnosis of diverticulitis. It reliably detects the location of the inflammation and provides valuable ancillary information such as the presence of an abscess, ureteral obstruction, or a fistula between the colon and urinary bladder (by demonstrating air in the bladder) (Fig. 26-15A). If an abscess is present, percutaneous drainage under CT guidance is a valuable therapeutic procedure.

The need for contrast enema in the evaluation of acute diverticulitis has diminished considerably since the introduction of CT scanning and ultrasound. Instilling contrast material under pressure into the colon carries the risk of spreading infection by

extravasation through the perforated diverticulum. If the infection has not been well contained by the peritoneal defenses, a localized infection may be converted to generalized peritonitis. For this reason, the use of barium should be avoided; barium combined with feces produces a more severe peritonitis than either agent as an isolated contaminant. Water-soluble contrast enemas do not carry the risk of barium-fecal peritonitis but still may result in extravasation of contrast material from the colon and spreading peritonitis. Colonic wall thickening, diverticula, fistula formation, or displacement of the colon by an abscess may be detected by contrast study. However, these findings generally can be demonstrated more safely by abdominal CT scan.

Treatment. *Uncomplicated Diverticulitis.* The treatment of diverticulitis depends on the severity of the disease. Patients with minimal symptoms or signs of inflammation can be treated on an outpatient basis with a clear liquid diet and broad-spectrum antibiotics. The antibiotics are continued for 7 to 10 days. Pain medications should be avoided. If the inflammation is so severe as to warrant analgesic administration, the patient should be hospitalized and given intravenous antibiotics. The use of morphine especially should be avoided because it increases intracolonic pressure and can aggravate the inflammatory process. Meperidine decreases intraluminal pressure and is a more appropriate analgesic.

Patients with significant signs of inflammation should be hospitalized for bowel rest, intravenous fluids, and intravenous broad-spectrum antibiotics. Nasogastric suction is usually not necessary unless the inflammation is accompanied by ileus or obstruction.

The patient's symptoms usually respond promptly to nonoperative treatment, with noticeable improvement occurring within 48 h. As the clinical situation permits, diet is resumed and investigative studies may be performed after 3 weeks. A colonoscopic examination is usually indicated, after the inflammation resolves, to evaluate the extent of diverticulosis and to rule out the presence of a cancer. A barium enema may demonstrate the extent of diverticulosis, but this is a less accurate test for identifying small polyps or malignant growths in the presence of numerous diverticula.

When a patient recovers from a simple, uncomplicated episode of diverticulitis, a high-fiber diet is recommended. Surgery is seldom indicated in such circumstances because 70 percent of patients who have recovered from one uncomplicated episode of diverticulitis will have no recurrence. However, if the patient suffers recurrent attacks of diverticulitis, surgical treatment should be considered. The chance of a subsequent attack following a second episode of diverticulitis is greater than 50 percent. Such attacks are treated similarly to the initial episode, and elective resection of the diseased colon is scheduled after the inflammation has resolved, usually 4 to 6 weeks later.

Generalized Peritonitis. Spreading generalized peritonitis may occur if the infection originating from the perforated diverticulum is not immediately localized by the normal peritoneal defenses. If the perforation remains unsealed, the entire peritoneal cavity can be contaminated, with resulting generalized fecal peritonitis. This complication is rare, but immediate surgical intervention is mandatory. Patients complain of severe abdominal pain, and there is voluntary and involuntary guarding in all abdominal quadrants. Intraperitoneal free air may be detected by abdominal x-rays, but the absence of free air does not exclude

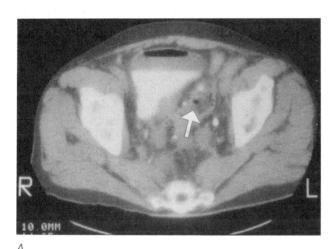

A

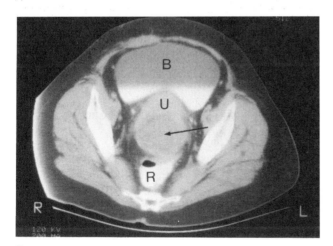

B

FIG. 26-15. *A.* CT scan of patient with sigmoid diverticulitis and a sigmoid-vesical fistula. Note phlegmon adjacent to bladder and air in bladder. *B.* Diverticulitis with a pelvic abscess. The CT scan shows an abscess (arrow) anterior to the rectum and posterior to the uterus. B=bladder; U=uterus; R=rectum.

the diagnosis. Leukocytosis with a left shift is generally observed; however, leukopenia may accompany instances of severe sepsis. Urgent celiotomy is required to control the infection. If the peritonitis is not so severe as to prohibit intestinal resection, the diseased segment of bowel containing the perforation should be resected. The distal segment of bowel should be closed or exteriorized as a mucous fistula, and the bowel proximal to the resected segment is used to construct a colostomy. Since the great majority of diverticular perforations occur in the sigmoid colon, there is seldom sufficient length of distal bowel to reach the abdominal wall as a mucous fistula. Therefore, it is usually necessary to suture or staple the distal bowel (proximal rectum) closed. This operation is frequently called *Hartmann's operation* (see Fig. 26-81) after the French surgeon, Henri Hartmann, who described it as a treatment for proximal rectal cancer in 1921. Hartmann's operation is the most common operation for the emergent treatment of diverticulitis.

If the peritonitis is so severe that resection of the perforated segment cannot be accomplished, then diversion of feces with a completely diverting colostomy constructed proximal to the perforation should be considered. This is a far less satisfactory procedure and should be avoided because the site of contamination remains in the peritoneal cavity.

Diversion of the fecal stream of the source of infection, accompanied by appropriate antibiotics and nutritional support, should permit resolution of the peritonitis. When the patient has recovered completely, usually over a period of no less than 10 weeks, the colostomy can be taken down and intestinal continuity restored with an anastomosis between the descending colon and the rectum.

Diverticulitis with Abscess. An important advance in the treatment of diverticulitis has been the development of percutaneous drainage of abdominal abscesses. A patient with an abscess that has resulted from a perforation of a diverticulum usually has pain localized to the left lower abdomen. A tender abdominal mass may be palpable, and if the abscess resides low in the pelvis, it may be palpable by digital rectal examination. Abdominal CT scan will confirm the diagnosis (see Fig. 26-15B). Either of these modalities also permits guided placement of a drain through the abdominal wall into the abscess, allowing evacuation of the purulent material. If the abscess is located low in the pelvis and cannot be approached safely through the abdominal wall, it can be drained safely into the rectum through a transanal or transvaginal approach.

These approaches are immeasurably preferable to a celiotomy, during which the abscess contents potentially could contaminate other areas of the peritoneal cavity. In such circumstances, it is usually necessary to perform Hartmann's operation, requiring the patient to have a temporary colostomy. Another option is resection of the diseased segment with primary anastomosis and proximal diverting colostomy. Percutaneous drainage of the abscess provides safe control of the infection, and an elective resection can be anticipated. At the time of elective surgery, it is usually possible to resect the diseased sigmoid colon and construct an anastomosis between the descending colon and rectum, thus avoiding a colostomy. It is mandatory to excise all abnormally thickened colon and to extend the resection to incorporate normal rectal wall. It is felt that a major cause of recurrent diverticulitis following sigmoidectomy is the failure to completely resect the abnormally thickened muscular wall at the rectosigmoid junction. It is seldom necessary to mobilize the

rectum distally beyond 2 cm below the sacral promontory to obtain normal bowel for a satisfactory anastomosis. Although diverticula may be present throughout the colon, it is not necessary to incorporate all of them in the resected specimen. Only the colon with a thickened, brittle wall needs to be excised.

Diverticulitis with Fistula. A fistula between the sigmoid colon and other organs, including bladder, vagina, small intestine, and skin, is a relatively frequent complication of diverticulitis. Diverticulitis is a more common cause of sigmoid-vesical fistula than cancer or Crohn's disease. A fistula is usually formed by an abscess that drains into an organ, establishing a tract between the source of the abscess (the perforated sigmoid diverticulum) and the secondarily involved organ. Fistulas between the sigmoid colon and the bladder are more common in men than in women because the uterus lies between the sigmoid colon and bladder in women. Women with fistulas between the sigmoid colon and bladder or vagina usually have had a previous hysterectomy. A fistula from the sigmoid colon to the skin may result from percutaneous drainage of an abscess caused by diverticulitis.

A fistula between the colon and the urinary bladder presents with recurring urinary tract infections, fecaluria, or pneumaturia. In the presence of distal urinary tract obstruction (prostatic hypertrophy in men), a sigmoid-vesical fistula may be complicated by ascending urinary tract infection and sepsis. CT most accurately confirms the fistula by demonstrating air in the bladder. A barium enema will demonstrate the presence of a fistula in fewer than 50 percent of patients, and intravenous pyelography is even less rewarding. Cystoscopy usually reveals cystitis and bullous edema in the area of the fistula.

The presence of a fistula caused by diverticulitis is seldom a cause for emergency surgical treatment. The formation of a fistula often results in improvement in the patient's condition, since it allows natural drainage of an abdominal abscess. Initial treatment should be directed toward control of any associated sepsis. Sepsis in a patient with a sigmoid-vesical fistula and distal urinary tract obstruction should be treated by relief of the obstruction (with a Foley catheter or suprapubic cystostomy) and appropriate intravenous antibiotics.

Before definitive surgical treatment, the cause of the fistula should be confirmed. The second most common cause of fistula between the sigmoid colon and the bladder is sigmoid carcinoma. Colonoscopy should be used to directly visualize the sigmoid mucosa and to exclude carcinoma, for the curative surgical treatment of sigmoid-vesical fistula caused by cancer involves obtaining wider margins of surgical resection than would be reasonable for a patient whose primary disease is diverticulitis.

After diverticulitis has been established as the cause of the fistula and sepsis has been controlled, treatment is directed toward resolution of the localized inflammation in the region of the fistula. This often can be accomplished by antibiotics administered on an outpatient basis for several weeks. Total parenteral nutrition and bowel rest, concomitant with intravenous antibiotics, have been used in some patients to permit more rapid resolution of inflammation in preparation for surgery.

The surgical treatment of a fistula caused by diverticulitis is excision of the diseased segment of the colon containing the site of perforation. We have found it helpful to place stents in the ureters by means of cystoscopy immediately prior to celiotomy. This technique facilitates identification of the ureter in an area in which the normal anatomy may be distorted or difficult to evaluate because of inflammation. Usually the fistulous tract can be interrupted surgically by blunt dissection. If the fistula involves the bladder, the defect in the bladder can be closed primarily, but unless the defect is large, this is seldom necessary. Providing adequate drainage of the bladder with a Foley catheter or suprapubic cystostomy for a week to 10 days will allow the bladder defect to heal. If the local inflammation is not severe, a one-stage operation usually can be accomplished by sigmoidectomy and anastomosis between the descending colon and rectum. If inflammation is too extensive to permit a primary anastomosis, it may be prudent to perform Hartmann's operation, as discussed previously. On some occasions it may be possible to fashion an anastomosis between the colon and rectum, but adjacent inflammation in the pelvis may be unfavorable, causing the risk of anastomotic leak to be unacceptable. In such instances, the anastomosis can be protected by a proximal transverse colostomy or ileostomy. After the patient has recovered and evaluation reveals the anastomosis to have healed satisfactorily, the proximal stoma can be closed.

On rare occasions, the infection will be so severe that sepsis cannot be controlled with the measures outlined above, and the extent of inflammation will not permit a bowel resection to be accomplished safely. In such instances, fecal diversion is mandatory, with a colostomy constructed proximal to the area of perforation and fistula.

Acquired Vascular Abnormalities

Acute lower gastrointestinal hemorrhage most commonly affects older patients. Although most episodes of bleeding stop spontaneously, between 10 and 25 percent of patients eventually will require surgery to control bleeding. The two most common causes of hemorrhage from the colon are *diverticulosis* and *angiodysplasia*. Both these disorders appear to be acquired, are rare in the young but appear with increasing frequency after age 50, and may occur simultaneously in the same individual.

Hemorrhage from Diverticular Disease. Colonic diverticula are formed at the location where the colonic arterioles penetrate the muscular wall of the bowel, and thus there is an intimate association between the arteriole and the diverticulum (Fig. 26-16). In some instances the artery is displaced over the dome of the diverticulum. With the passage of time, structural changes occur in the wall of the affected blood vessel; there are thickening of the intima and simultaneous focal attenuation of the media. These pathologic changes in arterial structure have been demonstrated in the arterioles associated with diverticula that have been observed to have been the source of hemorrhage. It appears that the vessel is prone to disruption at two sites: the dome of the diverticulum or its neck at the antimesenteric margin. Arterial disruption at either site can result in massive lower gastrointestinal hemorrhage; it is rare that diverticulosis is the cause of significant chronic bleeding. It is curious that the vascular disruption almost always occurs on the mucosal side of the artery, and the bleeding is virtually always into the colonic lumen instead of into the peritoneal cavity.

Hemorrhage from Angiodysplasia. Before the 1970s it was assumed that the great majority of cases of colonic hemorrhage were caused by bleeding from diverticula. Unexplained by this assumption was the fact that the bleeding site, when localized, was in the proximal colon most commonly, whereas

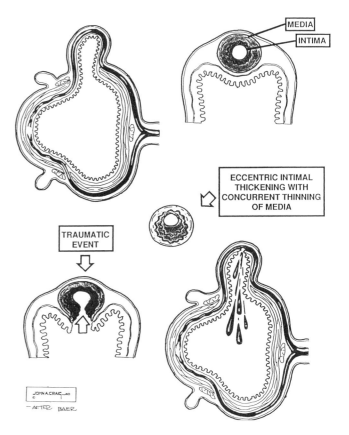

FIG. 26-16. Pathogenesis of diverticular hemorrhage.

diverticula are predominately located in the sigmoid colon. Furthermore, a significant number of patients with colonic hemorrhage had no identifiable colonic diverticula. The introduction of mesenteric arteriography provided a method of identifying the site of hemorrhage and demonstrated that a significant number of cases of colonic hemorrhage were associated not with an arteriole adjacent to a diverticulum but with a different type of vascular abnormality. Various names have been applied to this lesion, including *angiodysplasia, vascular ectasia, arteriovenous malformation,* and *angiectasia.*

It is apparently an acquired lesion, occurring more commonly with increasing age. It is rarely present in individuals under 40 years of age but becomes increasingly common after age 50, the same age group in which colonic diverticula are found. It has been suggested that the cause of colonic angiectasia is chronic, intermittent obstruction of the submucosal veins (Fig. 26-17). This is apparently caused by repeated muscular contractions of the colon that result in obstruction of the venous system. The lesions are located most commonly in the cecum; according to Laplace's law, the tension generated in the spherical cecum is greater than the tension in the remaining cylindrical colon. The lesions are not confined to the proximal colon; as many as 20 percent are found in the descending and sigmoid colon.

With the passage of time, the venules become dilated; eventually, the process extends to the precapillary sphincters, which become incompetent, forming small arterial-venous communications. Angiographic studies of this pathologic process have correlated the earliest stage of the lesion with a slowly emptying vein or a vein that contains contrast material after the dye has

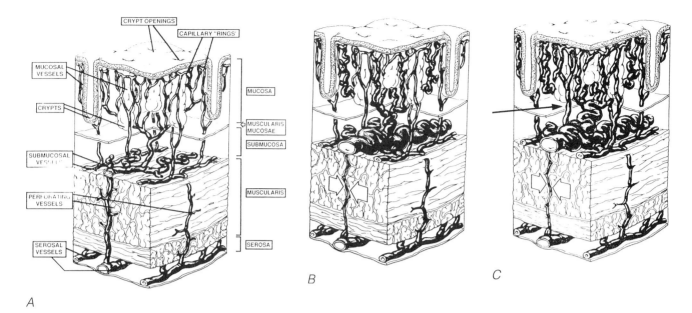

FIG. 26-17. *A. Normal colonic angioarchitecture. B. Backflow dilatation of mucosal veins. Chronic obstruction of the mural, perforating veins causes dilatation of the mucosal veins. C. Mucosal arteriovenous shunts. The precapillary sphincter in the pericrypt vasculature becomes incompetent (arrow), resulting in submucosal arteriovenous communications.*

cleared from the normal veins during the venous phase of the mesenteric angiogram. When the process becomes more advanced, dilation of a submucosal vein, a *vascular tuft,* may be recognizable by angiography. If the precapillary sphincters have become incompetent and small arterial-venous communications have developed, the angiogram will reveal the presence of an early-filling vein: a colonic vein that fills within 5 s following the injection of arterial contrast material (Fig. 26-18).

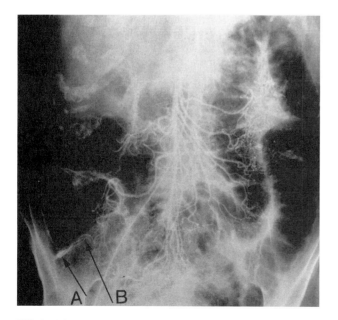

FIG. 26-18. *Mesenteric arteriogram, demonstrating vascular ectasia in the right colon; a "vascular tuft" (A) and an early-filling vein (B) can be seen.*

The more advanced lesion of dysplasia also can be identified by colonoscopy as a distinct red mucosal patch. These lesions vary in size from 2 mm to over 2 cm. Histologic study reveals tortuous, dilated capillaries in the submucosa.

Management of Massive Lower Gastrointestinal Hemorrhage. Massive lower gastrointestinal hemorrhage can be defined as bleeding distal to the ligament of Treitz that requires transfusion of more than 3 units of blood over 24 h. The causes of such bleeding are numerous, but diverticular disease and angiodysplasia are the most common causes of life-threatening colonic hemorrhage. The exact incidence of each cause is uncertain. Other causes of lower gastrointestinal hemorrhage include inflammatory bowel disease, ischemic colitis, and tumors. Anticoagulant therapy can also cause gastrointestinal bleeding. While these latter conditions are associated with some blood loss, life-threatening hemorrhage is rare. It is important to remember that gastroduodenal hemorrhage is a frequent cause of rectal bleeding, and this source should be excluded immediately by passing a nasogastric tube into the stomach and confirming the absence of blood in the stomach.

The management of the patient with lower gastrointestinal hemorrhage consists of simultaneously restoring the intravascular volume and identifying the site of the hemorrhage so that appropriate treatment can be given (Fig. 26-19). It is more important to identify the location of the bleeding point than to obtain an immediate diagnosis as to the cause of the bleeding. Lower gastrointestinal bleeding occurs most commonly in elderly patients in whom both angiodysplastic lesions and diverticula may be present. Colonic bleeding will stop spontaneously in 85 percent of patients, and the site of bleeding may be impossible to identify once the hemorrhage has stopped. Celiotomy for massive gastrointestinal hemorrhage of uncertain origin should be avoided except in the most extreme circumstances, for

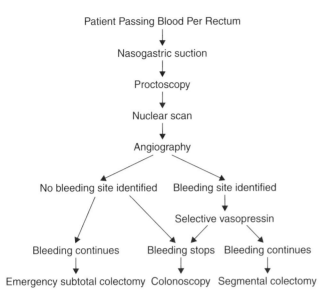

Patient Passing Blood Per Rectum

↓

Nasogastric suction

↓

Proctoscopy

↓

Nuclear scan

↓

Angiography

No bleeding site identified   Bleeding site identified

↓

Selective vasopressin

Bleeding continues   Bleeding stops   Bleeding continues

Emergency subtotal colectomy   Colonoscopy   Segmental colectomy

FIG. 26-19. Evaluation and treatment of lower gastrointestinal hemorrhage.

it is rare that the site of hemorrhage cannot be otherwise identified, and even the extreme operation of total colectomy carries the risk of leaving an unrecognized angiodysplastic lesion in the small intestine.

Blood transfusions should be administered as indicated by the clinical situation, and proctoscopy should be performed to exclude an anorectal cause. The sequence of the next diagnostic step varies somewhat among institutions but consists of nuclear imaging, mesenteric angiography, or colonoscopy. These tests are not mutually exclusive, each has advantages and disadvantages, and all depend on the expertise of the examiner.

Bleeding Scans (Scintigraphy). Nuclear scintigraphy has been reported by some investigators to be very useful in identifying a lower intestinal bleeding site, whereas others have found this approach to be unreliable and do not recommend it as a preferential test. There are two categories of nuclear scans; the first type uses substances that are cleared from the blood after being injected, whereas the second type employs nondiffusible intravascular indicators (autologous red blood cells labeled with technetium-99m). The technetium-sulfur colloid scan has the advantage of immediate availability and excellent sensitivity. Intestinal bleeding at a rate as low as 0.5 mL/min can be identified by accumulation of the isotope in the intestine at the bleeding site. The patient must be bleeding at the time the isotope is administered intravenously, however, for the label is removed from the circulatory system in about 12 min, accumulating in the liver and spleen. These sites of accumulation also may obscure a bleeding site in the region of the hepatic flexure. The autologous labeled red blood cell (RBC) scan is the scintigraphic test most commonly used in the evaluation of gastrointestinal bleeding (Fig. 26-20A). The patient's labeled RBCs remain in the circulation for as long as 24 h, permitting monitoring when the bleeding occurs intermittently. In as many as half the patients with the bleeding site identified by this technique, the location does not become evident until more than 6 h after the isotope is introduced. The labeled RBC scan can demonstrate bleeding at a rate of approximately 1 mL/min.

Mesenteric Angiography. Selective mesenteric angiography should be performed once the patient's condition is stable and hydration is adequate. A catheter is placed into the mesenteric circulation using a percutaneous approach, usually the femoral artery, and contrast material is introduced. This approach has the advantage of accurately identifying the bleeding site by visualizing the extravasation of contrast material, but bleeding must be at a rate of at least 1 mL/min for this technique to be successful (see Fig. 26-20B). Mesenteric angiography carries the distinct advantage of therapeutic options: Vasopressin can be infused through a specific mesenteric artery in an attempt to stop the bleeding by the arterial constriction and muscular contraction of the colonic wall induced by the drug. This approach will stop the bleeding in greater than 85 percent of patients in whom the bleeding site is identified. Vasopressin should not be used in patients with a history of myocardial ischemia. A variety of materials also can be introduced through the mesenteric catheter to embolize the area of bleeding. While success has been reported with this approach, intestinal ischemia is obviously a potential complication. Finally, angiographic study of the bowel may demonstrate the presence of angiodysplastic lesions. Unfortunately, these lesions are relatively common, and the mere presence of such vascular lesions, in the absence of extravasation of vascular contrast material, does not reliably indicate the source of the hemorrhage.

As implied earlier, scintigraphy and angiography are not mutually exclusive tests. If the general location of the bleeding site can be determined by scintigraphy, percutaneous arteriography can be immediately directed toward the correct vessel (superior mesenteric artery for lesions of the ascending or transverse colon, inferior mesenteric artery for sigmoid lesions), and vasopressin can be administered into the appropriate mesenteric artery.

Emergent Colonoscopy. A relatively recent approach to the patient with massive lower gastrointestinal hemorrhage has been the use of colonoscopy. The introduction of orally administered electrolyte lavage permits adequate cleansing of the colon within 2 h, and an experienced colonoscopist can reach the cecum in more than 90 percent of the patients. Colonoscopy has the advantage of providing therapeutic options if the bleeding point is identified. Vasoconstricting agents such as epinephrine can be injected at the bleeding site; vasodestructive agents such as alcohol, morrhuate sodium, or sodium tetradecyl sulfate may eradicate the lesion. Finally, thermal modalities such as laser photocoagulation, electrocoagulation, or heater probe coagulation may control the bleeding source via the colonoscope.

Celiotomy. The approaches discussed above are used to avoid an abdominal operation to control intestinal bleeding from a site that cannot be identified. Every reasonable effort should be made to identify and control the bleeding with nonoperative techniques. There will seldom be any signs that will reliably identify the cause of bleeding at the time of celiotomy. Intraoperative colonoscopy rarely may be beneficial in such circumstances, but usually the bleeding rate is too high to permit adequate visualization of the colonic lumen if emergency celiotomy has been required. In such circumstances, the small bowel should be examined carefully to exclude an obvious source of bleeding, such as lymphoma or Crohn's disease. If no specific lesion can be identified, the treatment of choice is abdominal colectomy. The decision to fashion an ileorectal anastomosis or ileostomy should be based on the patient's overall condition. The incidence

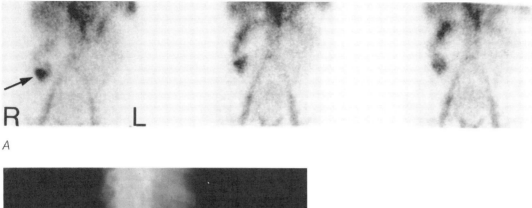

A

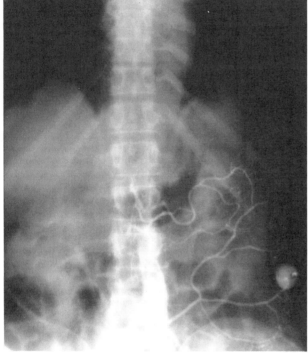

B

FIG. 26-20. *A.* Autologous-labeled red blood cell scan demonstrating a bleeding site (arrow) in the right colon at 10, 12, and 15 minutes. *B.* Selective arteriogram of inferior mesenteric artery, demonstrating bleeding site in sigmoid colon.

of recurrent bleeding after abdominal colectomy is less than 10 percent, but the mortality of such bleeding is significant, with reports ranging from 20 to 40 percent.

Ischemic Colitis. Localized ischemia of the intestine occurs most often in the colon. It may be the result of occlusion of a major mesenteric vessel by thrombosis, embolization, or iatrogenic ligation (after aortic aneurysm resection). Ischemic colitis also has been reported in patients with thromboangiitis obliterans or periarteritis nodosa. In the majority of patients, however, no specific vascular disease or underlying cause can be identified and presumably related to low blood flow. The disease occurs most commonly in the elderly, but it occasionally afflicts young adults. It has been reported to occur in women taking birth control pills.

The pathogenesis of the disease that occurs in the absence of mesenteric arterial occlusion is not well understood. The colonic mucosa becomes edematous, and colonoscopy may reveal dark, hemorrhagic mucosa with patchy ulceration. In mild cases the serosal surface of the colon appears normal, but severe cases of transmural ischemia can cause obvious gangrene of the bowel.

The disease usually presents as mild lower abdominal pain accompanied by the passage of bright red blood per rectum. Physical examination often reveals only mild abdominal tenderness, and proctoscopy reveals normal rectal mucosa with blood coming from above. The diagnosis can be made by contrast enema, which reveals submucosal hemorrhage and edema, or "thumbprinting" of the involved colonic segment. Arteriography usually does not demonstrate specific vascular abnormalities, suggesting that this is a disease of the microscopic vasculature of the bowel. The region of the splenic flexure is most commonly involved, perhaps because this is the area at the periphery of both superior and inferior mesenteric arterial blood supply; however, any area of the large intestine can be affected.

Treatment depends on the severity of the ischemia, as manifested by the patient's signs and symptoms. Patients with mild abdominal pain, minimal leukocytosis, and minimal fever should be observed closely, with the anticipation of recovery within 2 or 3 days. Follow-up colonoscopy or barium enema a few weeks later is usually normal. In some patients, however, the ischemia is more severe, with more marked abdominal pain, fever, and leukocytosis. These patients should be observed closely and treated with intravenous antibiotics. Occasionally the ischemic segment will heal with stricture formation, which may be resected electively if it causes obstructive symptoms.

A small number of patients have severe ischemia involving the full thickness of the colonic wall. This condition is characterized by signs of bowel necrosis with severe abdominal pain, peritonitis, and systemic toxicity. Immediate celiotomy is required, with resection of the ischemic intestine and proximal colostomy or ileostomy. The morbidity and mortality are high in this group of patients.

Radiation Proctocolitis. Radiation injury to the intestine is most commonly associated with pelvic irradiation for uterine or cervical cancer, but in recent years high radiation doses have been used for the treatment of prostatic and bladder cancer, as well as adjuvant or even primary treatment for selected cases of rectal malignancy. The new high-energy radiation sources deliver large doses of radiation to the viscera with sparing of the skin; thus the treating physician may not be warned of prior intestinal radiation injury.

Individual responses to radiation vary considerably, but there is a rough correlation of bowel injury with the dosage of radiation. Tissue doses of less than 4000 cGy are seldom associated with intestinal damage. Most patients will exhibit some degree of intestinal injury after exposure to 5000 cGy, and exposure to radiation in excess of 6000 cGy is associated with symptoms of radiation enterocolitis in the vast majority of patients. Factors that increase the likelihood of intestinal complications related to radiation include arteriosclerotic vascular disease, diabetes, hypertension, advanced age, and adhesions from previous abdominal operations that fix the bowel in the pelvis.

Radiation injury to the intestine is manifested in early and late stages. During radiation therapy the proliferating intestinal epithelial cells are affected, and the mucosa becomes edematous and hyperemic. Acute ulceration may occur if reepithelialization is significantly impaired. After therapy is completed, the mucosa usually heals, although the villi are shortened. Patients having radiation to the intestine often have nausea and vomiting, cramping abdominal pain, and diarrhea during the course of treatment. Tenesmus and rectal bleeding may occur during high levels of pelvic irradiation. Usually these symptoms can be managed symptomatically, but sometimes the radiation dosage must be decreased or treatment interrupted until the symptoms subside.

The late stages of intestinal radiation injury occur from weeks to years following completion of radiation therapy and are the manifestations of a progressive vasculitis affecting the arterioles of the submucosa. This radiation arteritis is characterized by thickening of the arteriole wall with subsequent microvascular thrombosis. This chronic ischemic process is associated with thickening and fibrosis of the intestinal wall and ulceration of the mucosa. Progressive ischemia can result in stricture formation, intestinal perforation, or abscess and fistula formation. The rectum is by far the most common site of involvement because of its location in close proximity to the uterus, cervix, and prostate.

Radiation proctitis is associated with tenesmus and bleeding. These symptoms may occur from months to years after completion of therapy and are the result of mucosal ulceration secondary to radiation endarteritis and ischemia. The symptoms often can be managed symptomatically with stool softeners, topical 5-aminosalicylic acid preparations, and occasionally, corticosteroid enemas. Should these measures fail, topical application of 10% formalin to the affected mucosa has been very efficacious. On rare occasions, a proximal colostomy is required for severe tenesmus or bleeding. It is extremely rare for proctectomy to be necessary to control symptoms.

Rectal stricture following pelvic radiation may cause symptoms of colonic obstruction. Recurrent cancer should be excluded by careful endoscopic evaluation and biopsies of suspected radiation-induced rectal strictures. If gentle dilation does not relieve the obstructive symptoms, diverting colostomy may be necessary.

Radiation-induced rectovaginal fistula most commonly occurs in women who have been treated for carcinoma of the uterine cervix. The fistula usually occurs within 2 years after completion of radiation therapy, but it may occur decades later. Patients usually note bleeding and rectal pain in the weeks preceding the passage of stool and gas through the vagina. A rectal stricture is often associated with the rectovaginal fistula, and occasionally there is also a concomitant fistula between the urinary bladder and vagina.

A proximal colostomy is invariably required to relieve the symptoms of radiation-induced rectovaginal fistula. It is mandatory to exclude recurrent carcinoma as the cause of the fistula, a diagnosis that is at times difficult and may require examination under anesthesia. If cancer is excluded and the patient's health is satisfactory, consideration should be given to treating the fistula by resecting the involved rectum and restoring continuity by low colorectal anastomosis or, more commonly, by coloanal anastomosis. Local excision and closure of the fistula are rarely successful, even when preceded by a diverting colostomy. Bricker has advocated repair of rectovaginal fistula caused by radiation using a technique of reconstructing the anterior rectal wall with nonirradiated sigmoid colon brought down as a fold-over patch graft. All these approaches to repair a complicated radiation-induced fistula require protection by a temporary colostomy or ileostomy. Often the entire pelvis is "frozen" with radiation-injured structures, including multiple loops of small intestine. In this situation, complete fecal diversion with a colostomy should be the definitive treatment, avoiding injury to the irradiated small intestine, which has limited healing capability.

Normal Function of Anorectum

The rectum functions mostly as a storage capacitance vessel. The rectum has very little peristaltic function of its own and relies on external pressure to empty. The outer longitudinal muscle is thick and has some contractility but has lost the organization of the teniae found on the colon. The rectum has a normal manometric resting pressure of approximately 10 mmHg, mostly due to intraperitoneal pressure and resting muscle tone. Conditions such as Crohn's disease or radiation injury cause the rectum to lose its natural compliance. This loss of compliance and capacitance is occasionally incapacitating to the patient.

The normal rectum can hold 650 to 1200 mL of liquid. A rectum that holds more than 1500 mL can be classified as a megarectum. The normal daily volume of stool eliminated by the rectum ranges from 250 to 750 mL of formed feces.

The anal sphincter mechanism is the other component of defecation and continence. Its anatomy and innervation have been described previously (see Fig. 26-5). The external sphincter fibers are responsible for 20 percent of the resting pressure and 100 percent of generated squeeze pressure. The internal sphincter provides 80 percent of anal resting pressure. Both the internal and external sphincter muscles are contracted at rest.

Defecation and continence are coordinated mechanisms. *Continence* can be described as controlled elimination of the rectal contents at a socially acceptable time and place. The coordination of rectal emptying and sphincter contraction and relaxation is very complex, and there are numerous abnormalities that occur.

Defecation can be divided into four components. The first is movement of feces into the rectal vault or capacitance organ. A mass peristaltic wave in the proximal colon and sigmoid colon occurs two or three times per day to pass solid substance into the rectum. The gastrocolic reflex is a well-known phenomenon that results in colonic mass peristaltic movement after distention of the stomach, probably hormonally mediated.

The second component of defecation is the *rectal-anal inhibitory reflex* or *sampling reflex*. Distention of the rectum results in involuntary relaxation of the internal anal sphincter and allows sensation of the rectal contents at the transitional zone. The sampling reflex has been shown by ambulatory manometry to occur frequently throughout the day and night.

The third component of defecation is voluntary relaxation of the external sphincter mechanism. Voluntary relaxation of the pelvic floor, puborectalis muscle, and external sphincter allows the rectal contents to be pushed farther into the anal canal and expelled. The relaxation of the sphincter mechanism is actually a failure to contract rather than an active relaxation, because the mechanism is paradoxically contracted when the rest of the individual is relaxed, yet continent (Fig. 26-21).

The fourth component of defecation is the voluntary increase of intraabdominal pressure, using the diaphragm and abdominal wall muscles. This increase in pressure serves to propel the rectal contents through the anal canal and accomplish defecation.

The passage of flatus also requires coordination of multiple factors. The sensation of gas at the transitional zone and in the anoderm informs the individual that gas is present to be eliminated. If the situation is such that full evacuation of the rectum is not possible but elimination of gas is desired, a voluntary contraction of the pelvic floor including the puborectalis and external sphincter muscles occurs to prevent loss of solid rectal contents. With an increase in abdominal pressure and a coordinated relaxation of some of the external sphincter, selective passage of flatus may be accomplished. During defecation, the gaseous contents of the rectum will be expelled with the solid contents without discrimination. This mechanism of discrimination appears to be learned. Patients eventually can pass flatus selectively even after the rectum has been removed and replaced by a reservoir of ileum for diseases such as ulcerative colitis and familial adenomatous polyposis.

Continence, or the control of rectal contents, requires an adequate rectal capacity and normal compliance. It may be difficult

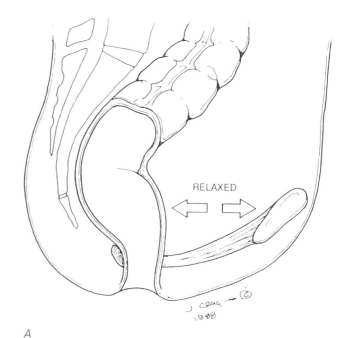

A

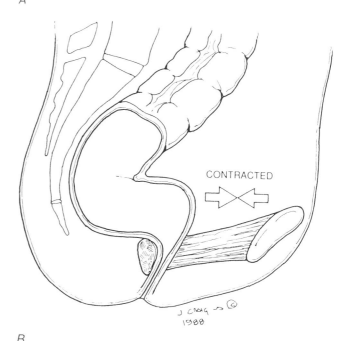

B

FIG. 26-21. Mechanism of normal defecation: The puborectalis muscle maintains the anorectal angle. *A.* Relaxation and straightening of the anorectal angle during defecation. *B.* Contraction and sharpening of the anorectal angle to maintain continence. (From: *Fleshman JW, et al: in Shackelford's Surgery of the Alimentary Tract, 1991, with permission.*)

to retain rectal contents in conditions such as Crohn's disease, in which the rectum becomes a rigid tube rather than a soft distensible bag, even if the external and internal sphincter mechanisms work properly. Adequate sensation at the transitional cell zone is required to coordinate pelvic pressure and sphincter tone during the sampling reflex. The external sphincter is most responsible for the fine control of solid, liquid, and gas. The puborectalis muscle has been proposed as the mainstay of the sphincter mechanism and is probably responsible for the control of solid stool. The internal sphincter may be responsible for fine control of gas on the basis of the sampling reflex and constantly provides resting pressure to prevent release of flatus. The pudendal nerves provide both the sensory afferents of the anal canal and the motor efferents to the voluntary muscles of the anal canal.

Dysfunction of Anorectum
Incontinence

Anal incontinence can be defined as the inability to control elimination of rectal contents. Incontinence can be categorized as either constant or intermittent. It also can be characterized by the type of material that the anal canal is unable to control. Incontinence to solid, liquid, and gas is complete incontinence. Incontinence to liquid and gas and incontinence to gas only represent degrees of partial incontinence.

Etiology. Anal incontinence can be caused by mechanical or neurogenic defects in the anal sphincter mechanism. *Mechanical defects* result from trauma to the anal sphincter mechanism. The most common cause of sphincter trauma is obstetric injury during vaginal delivery. The true incidence of anal incontinence after vaginal delivery is unknown, but there is an increased likelihood of incontinence after a midline episiotomy or a perineal tear that extends into the rectum (fourth degree), after multiple vaginal deliveries with midline episiotomies, after infection of an episiotomy repair, and after prolonged labor followed by traumatic vaginal delivery.

The treatment of cryptogenic abscess/fistula disease of the anal canal by fistulotomy also can cause anal incontinence. A fistulotomy performed through a significant amount of external sphincter, in the anterior quadrant, often causes incontinence. This is especially true in women because continence depends on one thin band of anterior external sphincter muscle.

Some systemic diseases also can cause mechanical malfunction of the anal sphincter and result in incontinence. Scleroderma, for example, produces a progressive sclerosis and fibrosis of the muscle and nerve endings and prevents normal function. The internal sphincter is known to become dense, spastic, and occasionally stenotic. The external sphincter may fail to function voluntarily, resulting in total incontinence.

Neurogenic causes for anal incontinence include isolated pudendal nerve injury as well as systemic neurologic disease. Stretch or trauma to the pudendal nerve during prolonged labor at childbirth has been documented to cause partially reversible pudendal nerve injury. Lifelong straining to have a bowel movement has only recently been recognized as a cause of pudendal nerve injury. The pudendal nerve is stretched over the ischial spine as the perineum descends during straining to eliminate the rectal contents. This form of neurogenic incontinence occurs most commonly in elderly women and has been called *idiopathic fecal incontinence.* Systemic diseases may affect selected nerves (e.g., multiple sclerosis) or may cause diffuse damage that affects all nerves and eventually causes incontinence by its effect on the pudendal system (e.g., diabetic neuropathy).

Other causes of anal incontinence that are unrelated to anal sphincter malfunction include severe diarrhea, fecal impaction with overflow incontinence, irritable bowel syndrome, radiation proctitis and fibrosis, inflammatory bowel disease of the rectum, and tumors of the distal colon and rectum.

Physiologic Evaluation of Disordered Anorectal Function. The visual and digital rectal examination remains very important in the evaluation of a patient with anal incontinence. The perineal body is often thin in the setting of incontinence after obstetric trauma. There is usually a scar present when this is the source of the injury. Occasionally fistulous tracts or fistulotomy scars will be evident. An estimate of the resting tone and squeeze pressure can be obtained from the digital rectal examination.

Anal manometry measures the resting pressure, the squeeze pressure, the sphincter length, and the minimal sensory volume of the rectum. Maximal rectal tolerance also can be measured. There are various techniques for performing anal manometry. Normal resting pressure is usually reported as 40 to 80 mmHg. The maximal squeeze pressure generated by the external sphincter is 80 to 160 mmHg, which is twice the normal resting pressure. The average sphincter length of 3 cm is based on measurement of the high-pressure zone of the anal canal. The sphincter is shorter anteriorly where the puborectalis muscle does not complete the circle of fibers at the upper extent of the anal canal. The entire sphincter mechanism is shorter in women than in men. Normal minimal sensory volume is less than 10 mL of air instilled into a latex balloon placed within the rectum just above the anal canal. Resting *rectal* pressure is normally 10 mmHg (Fig. 26-22).

The measurement of the pudendal nerve *terminal motor latency* uses a stimulating electrode on the tip of a gloved finger that is placed over the ischial spine to stimulate the pudendal nerve. The resulting contraction of the external sphincter muscle is detected by means of a recording electrode at the base of the same finger. Normal pudendal nerve terminal motor latency is 2.0 ms, and it has been shown to increase with age, after childbirth, after prolonged excessive straining with perineal descent, and in systemic diseases such as diabetes and multiple sclerosis.

Nerve injury to the sphincter mechanism also can be determined by the electromyographic measurement of single-fiber density of the external sphincter muscle. This uses a thin bipolar needle with a $250-\mu m$ recording surface on the side of the needle. Motor unit potentials from a bundle of muscles innervated by a single terminal branch of the pudendal nerve are recorded. The external sphincter and puborectalis muscle maintain a constant resting tone, with spontaneous motor unit potentials documented in the muscle at rest. Injury to a terminal branch of a nerve is demonstrated by a multiphasic reinnervation pattern. As more muscle bundles are reinnervated, the average fiber density in numerous samplings may increase beyond the normal limits, also indicating nerve injury. Surgical correction of a mechanical defect in the muscle will not be successful if the innervation is severely impaired. Electromyographic techniques are also used to "map" the anal sphincter for viable, contracting motor units to document the extent and site of mechanical injury.

Transrectal ultrasound is as accurate as needle electromyography for sphincter mapping and is better tolerated by patients. A 360° 10-mHz probe can image the puborectalis, external anal sphincter, and internal anal sphincter and identify defects in these muscles.

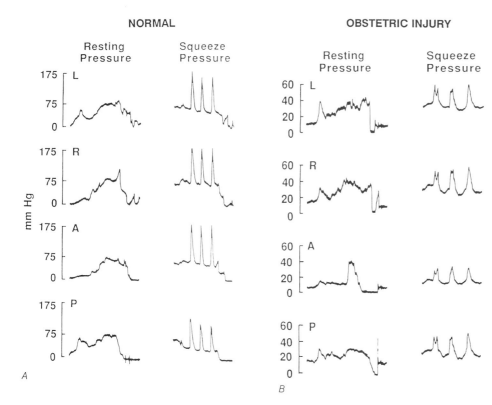

FIG. 26-22. *Anal manometry. A. Normal sphincter pressures: resting pressure and maximal squeeze pressure. (From: Fleshman JW, et al: in Shackelford's Surgery of the Alimentary Tract, 1991, with permission.) B. Abnormal sphincter pressure pattern due to obstetric injury.*

Surgical Correction. If a patient has a minor defect demonstrated by anal manometry or has not responded completely to anal sphincter reconstruction, muscle/sensory retraining may be helpful using biofeedback techniques to improve anal continence. The majority of mechanical problems in the anal sphincter can be corrected by restoring the circular integrity of the sphincter mechanism. The technique most commonly used is the overlapping muscle repair (Fig. 26-23). In a patient with a defect in the circular fibers of the external and internal sphincters, the muscle can be mobilized and the ends of the scar and muscle brought together, in overlapping or end-to-end configuration, to complete the circular ring of the anal sphincter. The normal sphincter length is restored in the anterior quadrant, which may in itself provide a barrier to leakage of liquid and gas.

Extensive injury to the muscles and nerves of the anal sphincter may preclude simple muscle repair. In such cases, some success has been reported from use of the gracilis or gluteal muscle to create an encirclement of the anus; the degree of true continence that this provides is still questioned. Studies are evaluating the use of implantable pacemakers to drive the denervated external sphincter muscle or a transferred muscle, such as the gracilis or gluteus. These techniques are usually reserved for complete denervation of the anal canal or for severe mechanical injury in a patient who wishes to avoid a colostomy. The complicated process of diagnosing and treating anal incontinence is summarized in Fig. 26-24.

Obstructed Defecation

Obstructed defecation or pelvic floor outlet obstruction is a disorder of the anorectum resulting from nonrelaxation of the puborectalis muscle, or internal intussusception of the rectum, these disorders being the major components of a spectrum of disturbances known as *pelvic floor abnormalities,* the end stage of which is complete rectal prolapse.

Anal stenosis is a rare cause of obstructed defecation that results in thin, frequent stools, abdominal bloating, and dilatation of the large intestine. The most common cause of anal stenosis is scarring after anal operation such as an improperly performed circumferential Whitehead hemorrhoidectomy. Other causes of anal stenosis include chronic laxative abuse (particularly mineral oil), radiation injury, recurrent anal ulcer, Crohn's disease, trauma, and anal tumors. Occasionally anal stenosis will respond to dilation. The so-called Whitehead deformity includes a scarred stenosis of the anal canal and an ectropion of mucosa that is pulled from the rectum onto the perineal skin. Both anal ectropion and stenosis can be corrected by advancing a full-thickness pedicled flap of skin into the circumferential scar (Fig. 26-25). The success of this procedure depends on the presence of normal tissue surrounding the obstructing scar.

Nonrelaxation of the puborectalis muscle is a functional disorder in which a normal muscle displays abnormal function or control. Patients complain of straining, incomplete evacuation, need for digital maneuvers to eliminate the rectal content, and anal or pelvic pain. The diagnosis of nonrelaxing puborectalis muscle as a cause of constipation symptoms relies on the documentation of normal colonic transit to the rectum. A persistent image of the puborectalis muscle distorting the posterior rectum is seen on defecography (Fig. 26-26). Defecography is accomplished by instilling methylcellulose-thickened barium into the rectum. Video cinefluoroscopy is used to record a lateral image of the rectum while the patient strains in the sitting position. The inability to expel an air-filled latex balloon from the rectum while sitting on a toilet may be a more accurate means of documenting nonrelaxation (or paradoxical contraction) of the pu-

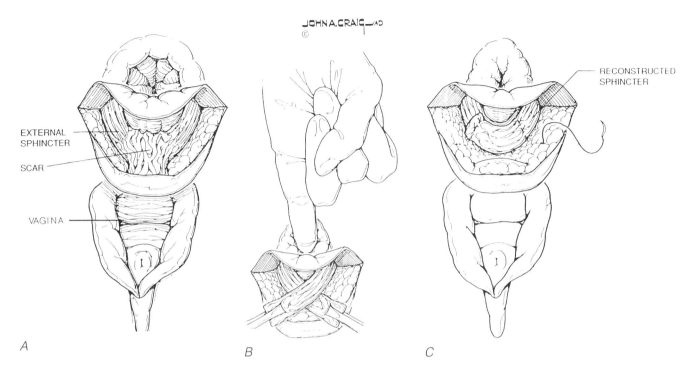

JOHN A. CRAIG AD ©

EXTERNAL
SPHINCTER

SCAR

VAGINA

RECONSTRUCTED
SPHINCTER

A   B   C

FIG. 26-23. Anal sphincter muscle repair. *A.* Rectal flap is created and sphincter muscles are isolated. *B.* Muscles are overlapped around a 15-mm rubber dilator or fingertip. *C.* Muscle components are sutured in place and perineal body repaired. (From: *Fleshman JW, et al: in Shackelford's Surgery of the Alimentary Tract, 1991, with permission.*)

borectalis. The treatment of this problem is nonoperative. Biofeedback is the most effective method for teaching the patient the cognitive aspects of defecation.

Internal intussusception (or internal prolapse of the rectum) is another cause of outlet obstruction. This condition accompanies laxity of the rectal fixation at the sacrum (Fig. 26-27) and

FIG. 26-24. Evaluation and management of anal incontinence.

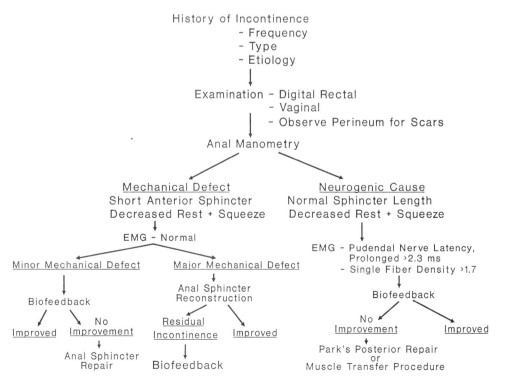

History of Incontinence
- Frequency
- Type
- Etiology

Examination - Digital Rectal
- Vaginal
- Observe Perineum for Scars

Anal Manometry

<u>Mechanical Defect</u>
Short Anterior Sphincter
Decreased Rest + Squeeze

<u>Neurogenic Cause</u>
Normal Sphincter Length
Decreased Rest + Squeeze

EMG - Normal

EMG - Pudendal Nerve Latency,
Prolonged >2.3 ms
- Single Fiber Density >1.7

<u>Minor Mechanical Defect</u>

<u>Major Mechanical Defect</u>

Biofeedback

Anal Sphincter
Reconstruction

Biofeedback

<u>Improved</u>   No
<u>Improvement</u>

<u>Residual
Incontinence</u>   <u>Improved</u>

No
<u>Improvement</u>   <u>Improved</u>

Anal Sphincter
Repair

Biofeedback

Park's Posterior Repair
or
Muscle Transfer Procedure

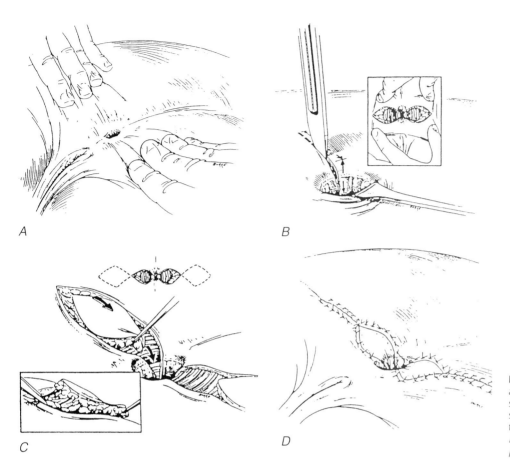

FIG. 26-25. Surgical treatment of anal stricture or stenosis. *A.* Anal stenosis. *B.* Release of anal stenosis. *C.* Flap design and mobilization. *D.* Inset of flaps. (From: *Caplin DA, Kodner IJ: 1986, with permission.*)

will be discussed in more detail later. The intestine telescoping into itself causes partial obstruction to defecation while simultaneously contributing to a feeling of rectal fullness and a need to defecate.

Other Associated Problems. *Proctalgia fugax,* or the *levator muscle syndrome,* is spasm of the anal sphincter, which causes pain, often at night. The puborectalis muscle goes into spasm and typically awakens the patient. The pain usually lasts only a few minutes and can be relieved by heat, dilation, or muscle relaxants. It may be stress-related and has been associated with the irritable bowel syndrome or a past history of migraine headaches. Other causes of anal pain such as abscess, foreign body, or cancer should be excluded before this diagnosis can be confirmed.

Fecal impaction and *stercoral ulceration* are occasionally seen in patients with outlet obstruction due to nonrelaxing puborectalis or internal intussusception. The symptoms of bleeding and rectal fullness are treated by regulation of the bowel habits and periodic emptying of the rectum with a bowel regimen consisting of enemas, increased fiber, and stool softeners.

Descending perineum syndrome was in the past thought to be a primary process. It is now known to be the result of chronic straining at defecation. The primary process is, therefore, chronic constipation, disordered defecation, or intussusception. Descending perineum syndrome causes stretching of the pudendal nerve, which leads to neurogenic weakening of the external sphincter and puborectalis muscle, which eventually can lead to anal incontinence.

Rectocele is the result of weakened muscle and soft tissue between the rectum and the vagina after years of straining to defecate. The bulge, or rectocele (see Fig. 26-26*B*), occurs in the posterior vaginal wall and in severe cases may even cause protrusion of tissue through the vagina. Symptoms are similar to those of other types of obstructed defecation, and the patient may need to put a finger in the vagina and push the rectum posteriorly in order for it to empty. A rectocele is a signal that a basic problem exists in the rectum or mechanism of defecation. Repair of a rectocele without correction of internal intussusception or outlet obstruction is seldom successful, and recurrence is common in such circumstances.

Psychological Profile of an Outlet Obstruction Patient. Psychological abnormality has never been clearly documented as the cause of disordered defecation, but many patients with constipation have been found by psychological evaluation to have depression, somatization disorder, and an extreme need to control. Patients with nonrelaxing puborectalis have similar findings. These patients also seem to exhibit a cancer fear, which is alleviated when they find that their work-up is normal. It is prudent to obtain a psychological profile on these patients before considering biofeedback or surgery.

Physiologic Evaluation of Disordered Defecation (Pelvic Floor Abnormality). Disordered defecation or pelvic floor abnormality is a complex problem. An overlap in symptoms between causes may result in a diagnostic dilemma unless a well-planned evaluation has been performed (Fig. 26-28). *De-*

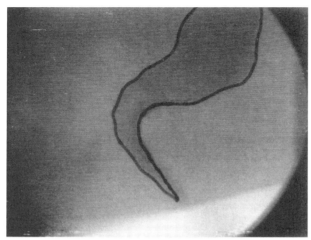

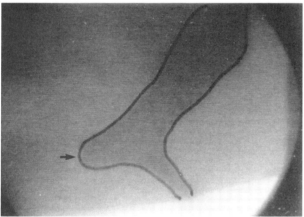

FIG. 26-26. Defecography during straining to empty the rectum. (*Top*) Paradoxical nonrelaxation of the sphincter mechanism as the patient strains. (*Bottom*) Puborectalis relaxes appropriately on straining, but rectocele (arrow) forms anteriorly. (From: *Kodner U, Fry RD, Fleshman JW: Surgery Annual, 1992, with permission.*)

fecography uses cinefluoroscopy from a lateral position as the patient attempts to empty thickened barium while sitting on a commode. The features of a *normal defecogram* include fixation of the posterior rectum to the curve of the sacrum, rapid rectal emptying with straining, and appropriate relaxation of the puborectalis muscle. Abnormal findings are observed when the rectum moves from the sacrum during straining, when it displays excessive mobility from the sacral curve, and when it forms a funnel configuration (complete intussusception) (Fig. 26-29).

Complete rectal prolapse also can be documented by defecography. Obstructed defecation is suggested if the puborectalis does not relax during attempted defecation (see Fig. 26-26*A*).

Colonic *transit time,* as described previously, is important in differentiating colonic from anorectal malfunction in patients with disordered defecation. Outlet obstruction may exist with normal colonic transit to the rectum. Colonic transit studies will show markers within the rectum after the fifth day because the rectum does not empty normally.

Anal manometry rarely has a role in the evaluation of disordered defecation. Its main use in this context is to document the presence of a normal rectal-anal inhibitory reflex to rule out Hirschsprung's disease as the cause of constipation. *Megarectum*

is an acquired problem thought to be a result of failure to respond to the normal signals for defecation and can result in an abnormal rectoanal inhibitory reflex. Manometry also shows an increase in the maximal tolerable rectal volume in patients with megarectum.

Balloon expulsion recently has been found to be helpful in establishing the diagnosis of nonrelaxing puborectalis muscle as the cause for disordered defecation. Defecography often reveals a persistent puborectalis shadow and poor relaxation of the sphincter during efforts to evacuate the rectum; however, many of these patients are able to empty their rectum at other times. The overdiagnosis of nonrelaxing puborectalis muscle can be avoided by performing a balloon expulsion test. The inability to pass a 60-mL inflated latex balloon in a private bathroom, sitting on a toilet, seems to be an accurate means of documenting the absence of the normal coordination of muscle function required for defecation.

Therapeutic Options for the Treatment of Disordered Defecation. Nonrelaxation of the puborectalis muscle has been treated with limited transection of the puborectalis muscle itself, an approach that initially was reported to cause improvement in some patients with outlet obstruction; long-term follow-up revealed that almost all patients treated with the operation develop incontinence with very little improvement in symptoms. The most consistent improvement in patients with nonrelaxing puborectalis muscle has come via the use of biofeedback. Several series have now documented a long-term improvement using behavioral modification techniques to retrain the patient to relax the pelvic floor during straining to defecate.

The anatomic abnormalities associated with internal intussusception can be corrected surgically. Retrorectal sacral fixation straightens the rectum and fixes the bowel to the sacrum, eliminating the abnormal mobility (Fig. 26-30*A*). Unfortunately, this operation often fails to relieve the symptoms of disordered defecation. Success has been reported with low anterior resection of the rectum (Fig. 26-30*B*), but more data concerning long-term results are needed. Most of the patients with internal intussusception as a cause of outlet obstruction respond well to medical management, once the cause of symptoms has been clearly diagnosed. Only those with the most severe problems and impending pudendal nerve damage should be considered for operative correction. It is important to remember that if an outlet obstruction is not corrected before other causes of constipation are treated, the method of treating the constipation will fail. Even the use of abdominal colectomy for severe constipation due to colonic inertia has failed if outlet obstruction is a major component of the problem.

Abnormal Rectal Fixation

Internal Intussusception. Internal intussusception has already been described as a cause of outlet obstruction. It is also possible that a nonrelaxing puborectalis muscle induces internal intussusception from prolonged, aberrant straining at defecation. It is further thought that internal intussusception is a precursor to complete rectal prolapse. There seems to be an increased incidence of intussusception of the rectum with aging, connective tissue disorders, and irritable bowel syndrome. Internal intussusception is also now known to be the cause of the *solitary rectal ulcer.* The ulcer develops as the lead point of the intussuscepting

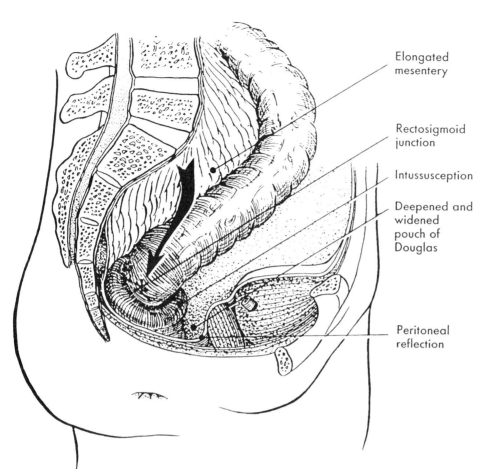

Elongated
mesentery

Rectosigmoid
junction

Intussusception

Deepened and
widened
pouch of
Douglas

Peritoneal
reflection

FIG. 26-27. Anatomy of the pelvic floor abnormality: internal intussusception of the rectum. (From: *Hoffman MJ, Kodner IJ, et al: 1984, with permission.*)

tissue becomes chronically ischemic and traumatized. If the ulcer heals, glands may be trapped in the deep tissues, causing the lesion of *colitis cystica profunda,* large glandular lakes within the mucosal and submucosal tissue in the area of the solitary rectal ulcer. Colitis cystica profunda is characterized by the presence of localized or diffuse submucosal cysts and may be mis-

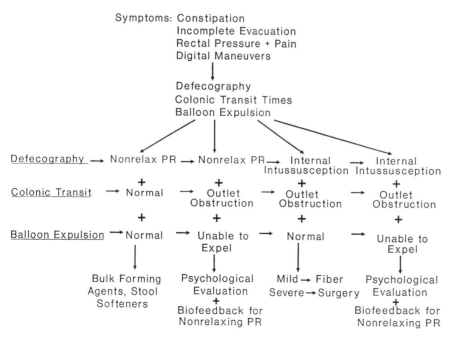

FIG. 26-28. Evaluation and management of disordered defecation.

Symptoms: Constipation
Incomplete Evacuation
Rectal Pressure + Pain
Digital Maneuvers

Defecography
Colonic Transit Times
Balloon Expulsion

Defecography	Nonrelax PR	Nonrelax PR	Internal Intussusception	Internal Intussusception
	+	+	+	+
Colonic Transit	Normal	Outlet Obstruction	Outlet Obstruction	Outlet Obstruction
	+	+	+	+
Balloon Expulsion	Normal	Unable to Expel	Normal	Unable to Expel
	Bulk Forming Agents, Stool Softeners	Psychological Evaluation + Biofeedback for Nonrelaxing PR	Mild → Fiber Severe → Surgery	Psychological Evaluation + Biofeedback for Nonrelaxing PR

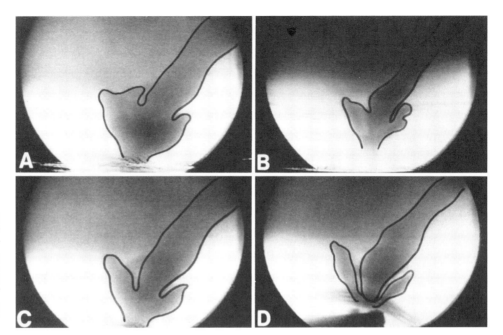

FIG. 26-29. Defecogram showing progressive outlet obstruction due to the pelvic floor abnormality of internal intussusception on straining. *A.* Funnel forms in midrectum. *B, C, and D.* The funnel descends to plug the anal canal and cause outlet obstruction. (From: *Kodner IJ, Fry RD, Fleshman JW: Surgery Annual, 1992, with permission.*)

taken for rectal cancer, resulting in inappropriate resection. It may be found in association with several different clinical conditions, including radiation injury, postoperative changes, adenomatous polyps, malignant growth, or inflammatory bowel disease. Patients may have symptoms of mucous discharge, rectal bleeding, or tenesmus. Feelings of rectal fullness or incomplete evacuation are common patient complaints. Colonoscopy or barium enema should be performed to rule out malignant growth, and the patient should be evaluated for rectal prolapse or intussusception by defecography. Spontaneous resolution can occur but is rare. Colitis cystica profunda associated with rectal prolapse is treated by correcting the rectal prolapse.

The majority of patients with internal intussusception respond to increased bulk in their diet, stool softeners, and glycerine suppositories or small enemas to stimulate rectal emptying. Indications for surgical correction of internal intussusception include symptoms severe enough to change the patient's life despite maximal medical and psychological therapy, chronic bleeding from a solitary rectal ulcer, or impending anal incontinence because of the descending perineum and subsequent stretch injury to the pudendal nerve.

Rectal Prolapse. *Rectal prolapse* is the protrusion of the full thickness of rectum and occasionally sigmoid through the anus. Rectal prolapse may be the long-term result of outlet obstruction or internal intussusception of the rectum. There is an increased incidence in elderly women and institutionalized patients treated with constipating psychotropic drugs. There is also an increased incidence of prolapse in women who have had hysterectomy and in spinal cord–injured patients who require routine use of laxatives to maintain bowel function. Surprisingly, there is not an increased incidence of rectal prolapse in women who have had multiple vaginal deliveries.

The symptoms of rectal prolapse include anorectal pain, bleeding, mucous discharge, and incontinence. Some patients will be hesitant to describe the large bolus of protruding tissue and will instead present with symptoms of mucous discharge or progressive incontinence. As the condition progresses, spontaneous reduction may not occur, and manual replacement of the prolapsed rectum becomes necessary. In severe instances, the prolapsed tissue becomes too edematous to replace, and necrosis of the prolapsed segment may occur. Sometimes the patient is unable to demonstrate the prolapse in the physician's office, and defecography is required to reveal increased mobility from the sacrum, marked intussusception, and finally protrusion of the rectum through the anal canal. Occasionally, a solitary rectal ulcer is seen at the lead point of the prolapse. It is important to differentiate rectal prolapse from prolapsing internal and mixed hemorrhoids. In hemorrhoidal disease, there will be a deep groove between the areas of prolapsing tissue as opposed to the concentric rings on the mucosa seen on the rectal prolapse. It is a significant mistake to perform a hemorrhoidectomy when the problem is really complete rectal prolapse.

Complete evaluation of the patient with rectal prolapse should include colonoscopy or air-contrast barium enema to fully evaluate the colon and rule out the presence of a malignant growth that might be serving as the lead point for the prolapse. Anal manometry and electromyography are helpful in evaluating sphincter function in patients with rectal prolapse in order to choose the appropriate corrective procedure.

Therapeutic options in the treatment of rectal prolapse can be divided into three groups (see Fig. 26-30). The first group, patients with full rectal prolapse and normal sphincter function, should be considered for a low anterior resection or retrorectal sacral fixation. If constipation is a significant factor, or if the patient is found to have a very redundant sigmoid colon, low anterior resection with fixation of the lateral rectal ligaments is probably a better choice of procedure. Any operation for rectal prolapse must include full mobilization of the rectum, preceding fixation of the rectum, to prevent forward motion and avoid distal prolapse. Excellent functional results should be anticipated for this group of patients.

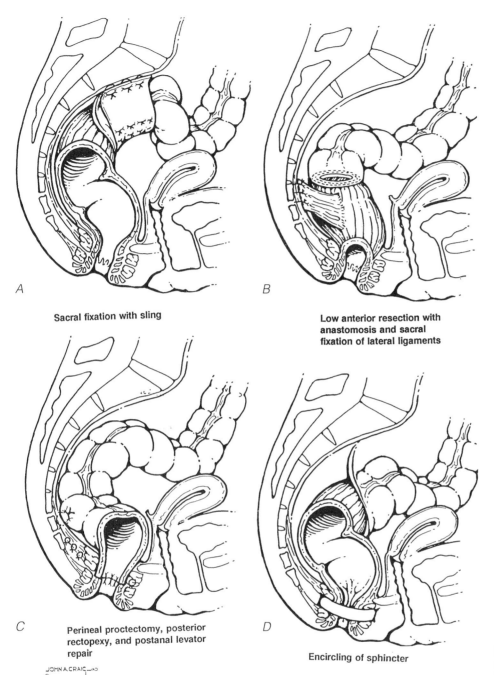

A

Sacral fixation with sling

B

Low anterior resection with anastomosis and sacral fixation of lateral ligaments

C

Perineal proctectomy, posterior rectopexy, and postanal levator repair

JOHN A. CRAIG—AD

D

Encircling of sphincter

FIG. 26-30. Surgical techniques for correction of pelvic floor abnormalities.

The second group of patients has full rectal prolapse and incontinence. Most patients recover sphincter function after repair of the prolapse (60 to 70 percent), but it is difficult to predict which of these patients would tolerate a low resection of the rectum. These patients should be treated by retrorectal sacral rectopexy using a synthetic sling via an abdominal approach or by a perineal proctectomy combined with rectopexy and a posterior sphincter-enhancing procedure (see Fig. 26-30C). Of patients having surgical correction of rectal prolapse, 30 percent will not recover fecal continence. This is true especially in patients with documented neurogenic incontinence who have prolonged pudendal nerve latency. These patients may be helped by the "posterior repair" of the anal canal using the technique described by Sir Alan Parks. The external sphincter and puborectalis sling are brought together posteriorly to elongate the anal canal, to decrease the anal opening, and to add bulk to the posterior aspect of the canal. In some cases continence is further improved by reconstruction of the anterior aspect of the sphincter as well as posteriorly. This technique has been combined with a perineal proctectomy to correct rectal prolapse and associated anal incontinence.

The third group of patients consists of those at extremely high operative risk or elderly individuals with incontinence and prolapse who have a very short life expectancy. These patients may be considered for an anal encircling procedure (see Fig. 26-30D). The original procedure used a silver wire (Thiersch procedure)

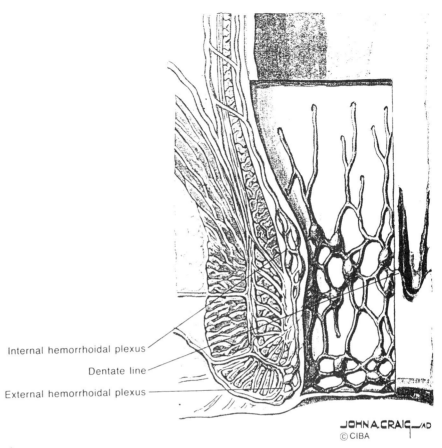

Internal hemorrhoidal plexus

Dentate line

External hemorrhoidal plexus

JOHN A. CRAIG—AD
©CIBA

A

placed in the ischiorectal fat around the external sphincter mechanism. The wire served to cause obstruction of the anal outlet and to compress the sphincter mechanism. Currently, the encircling procedure is performed with a band of soft synthetic mesh, a silicone tube, or a gracilis muscle graft to the anal canal. The majority of these patients require laxatives or enemas to avoid fecal impaction. The complications of this procedure include erosion of the encircling band and infection. This is obviously not the first choice of treatment for rectal prolapse and is used less frequently because the combined perineal proctectomy procedure is available for use in elderly patients under spinal or epidural anesthesia.

Hemorrhoids

Pathophysiology. Hemorrhoidal tissue is normally found at the distal end of the rectum within the anal canal (Fig. 26-31*A*). These vascular and connective tissue cushions are usually found in the right anterolateral and posterolateral positions and the left lateral position. Internal hemorrhoids are above the dentate line (see Fig. 26-31*B*); external hemorrhoids are the vascular complexes under the anoderm of the anal canal (see Fig. 26-31*C*).

The pathophysiology of symptomatic hemorrhoids is related to engorgement of the vascular pedicles in the hemorrhoidal complexes, which then dilate, stretch, and cause the cushions to enlarge. The vascular complexes engorge as pressure is applied to the pelvic floor during straining, lifting, or standing. Bleeding

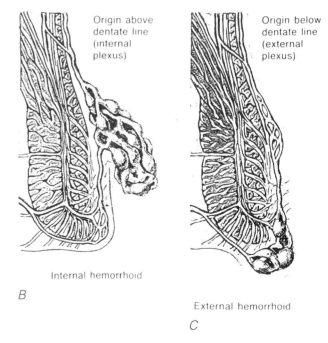

Origin above dentate line (internal plexus)

Origin below dentate line (external plexus)

Internal hemorrhoid

External hemorrhoid

B

C

FIG. 26-31. Hemorrhoids. (From: *Fry RD, Kodner U: Anorectal disorders. Ciba Clin Symp 37:6, 1985, with permission.*)

occurs from local trauma to the hemorrhoidal complex, usually during defecation. Hard stools, prolonged straining, increased abdominal pressure, and prolonged lack of support to the pelvic floor all combine to increase the likelihood that abnormal hemorrhoidal tissue will develop.

Internal hemorrhoids, which are covered by mucosa, typically bleed or prolapse but do not cause pain. Patients complain of rectal fullness, mucous discharge, and bright red blood dripping into the toilet or on the toilet paper. Occasionally, internal hemorrhoids will incarcerate within the outer ring of the anal canal and develop thrombosis and necrosis. Internal hemorrhoids can be classified as follows: First-degree hemorrhoids bleed; second-degree hemorrhoids bleed and prolapse but reduce spontaneously; third-degree hemorrhoids bleed and prolapse and require manual reduction; and fourth-degree hemorrhoids bleed and incarcerate and cannot be reduced.

External hemorrhoids beneath the anal skin can become enlarged over time as a result of dilatation or repeated thrombosis. The overlying skin may stretch to develop a skin tag, which prevents adequate hygiene. Occasionally, a clot within an external hemorrhoid will cause severe pain and may bleed if the clot erodes through the overlying skin. It is rare for an internal hemorrhoid to cause pain unless it becomes incarcerated and thrombosed. External hemorrhoids usually cause pain even after a small thrombosis because they are beneath richly innervated skin.

The symptoms of hemorrhoids are limited, and caution must be used not to misdiagnose other anorectal problems as hemorrhoids (Table 26-1). Defecography is helpful when symptoms of rectal prolapse or obstructed defecation exist, and sigmoidoscopy, colonoscopy, or contrast enema identifies malignant growths or inflammatory bowel disease.

Treatment. *Medical Therapy.* The majority of bleeding first- and second-degree hemorrhoids respond to the addition of dietary fiber (e.g., psyllium) or stool softeners and avoidance of straining or prolonged sitting on the commode. It is important to counsel the patient to ingest an appropriate amount of water with the fiber. The goal is to produce soft stool that is easy to pass. Failure of medical therapy is an indication for mechanical intervention, e.g., elastic ligation, excision, etc. of second-degree hemorrhoids. Surgery rarely is indicated for the bleeding of first-degree hemorrhoids.

Elastic Ligation. Elastic ligation of second- and third-degree internal hemorrhoids, 1 to 2 cm above the dentate line, is very effective for control of bleeding and prolapse. The tissue is grasped and pulled into the cylinder of a rubber-band applier, and the rubber bands are placed at the base of the hemorrhoidal tissue (Fig. 26-32). The tissue necroses, sloughs, and leaves a scar in the area of the vascular pedicle, which prevents further prolapse of tissue or bleeding. Care is taken to avoid placement of the bands on the transitional zone or anoderm, both of which are richly innervated with pain fibers. One also must avoid placement of the rubber bands on the deep internal sphincter muscle, since symptoms of spasm may become so severe that urinary retention may result. The majority of patients can tolerate a single-quadrant ligation in the office every 2 weeks. If symptoms are severe or the patient has significant external hemorrhoids and other anorectal problems, three quadrants may be banded in the operating room under local anesthesia.

Severe sepsis has been reported after ligation of hemorrhoids in immunocompromised patients or patients with pelvic floor abnormalities in whom the full thickness of the distal prolapsing rectum has been ligated. This life-threatening complication is heralded by inordinate pain, fever, and urinary retention within 12 h of ligation. The incidence of urinary retention after a single ligation should be less than 1 percent. Urinary retention after multiple ligations may be as high as 10 to 20 percent. The septic patient requires intravenous antibiotic coverage for gram-negative and anaerobic organisms, removal of the rubber bands, and hospitalization.

Normally, the rubber bands fall off with the necrotic tissue after 7 to 10 days. Bleeding may occur, but it is usually minimal. One percent of patients develops significant hemorrhage, which may require cautery or suture ligation of the bleeding site. Nonsteroidal anti-inflammatory drugs or aspirin taken during the 7 to 10 days after banding may increase the incidence of bleeding when the bands and tissue slough.

Photocoagulation. This is a very simple technique by which heat causes necrosis fibrosis of the vascular pedicle in several areas within the anal canal to achieve the same result as elastic ligation on smaller pedicles, but larger hemorrhoids require another form of treatment.

Sclerosis. A mixture of 5% phenol and almond oil developed at St. Mark's Hospital in London may be used to stop bleeding from first- and second-degree hemorrhoids. The mixture is injected through a spinal needle into the submucosa at the base of each hemorrhoid to raise a bleb of mucosa. The depth and amount of sclerosing agent are critical to avoid slough of the entire anal mucosa. Minimizing the amount of IV fluids given during an operation decreases the rate of this complication. Other complications include allergic reaction, local infection, and prostatitis. Many surgeons believe that if tissue can be treated by sclerosis, it probably should not have surgical treatment at all.

Table 26-1
Anal Symptoms Mistakenly Attributed to Hemorrhoids

Symptoms	Cause
1. Pain and bleeding after bowel movement	Ulcer/fissure disease
2. Forceful straining to have bowel movement	Pelvic floor abnormality
3. Blood mixed with stool	Neoplasm
4. Drainage of pus during or after bowel movement	Abscess/fistula, inflammatory bowel disease
5. Constant moisture	Condyloma acuminatum
6. Mucous drainage and incontinence	Rectal prolapse
7. Anal pain with no physical findings	Caution: possible psychiatric disorder

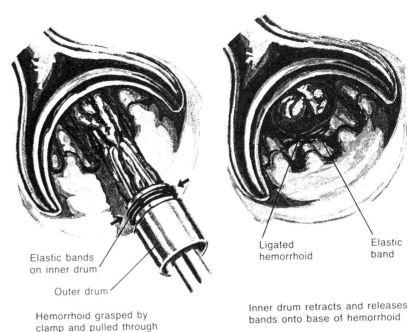

Elastic bands
on inner drum

Outer drum

Hemorrhoid grasped by
clamp and pulled through
drums of instrument

Ligated
hemorrhoid

Elastic
band

Inner drum retracts and releases
bands onto base of hemorrhoid

JOHN A. CRAIG—AD
© CIBA

FIG. 26-32. Elastic ligation technique for internal hemorrhoids. (From: *Fry RD, Kodner IJ: Anorectal disorders. Ciba Clin Symp 37:6, 1985, with permission.*)

Cryosurgery and Direct-Current Coagulation. Hemorrhoidal tissue can be coagulated by freezing with liquid N_2 or a CO_2 probe. Because frozen tissue undergoes liquefication necrosis and there is poor control of the depth of freezing, the majority of surgeons avoid using this technique. Patients also complain of profuse, foul-smelling seropurulent discharge.

Direct-current coagulation requires approximately 10 min per site to coagulate the hemorrhoidal cushion. The resulting scar prevents prolapse and further bleeding of first-, second-, and some third-degree internal hemorrhoids. The technique is simply another means of treating internal hemorrhoids in the outpatient or office setting.

Excisional Hemorrhoidectomy. The excision of hemorrhoids should be limited to large third- and fourth-degree hemorrhoids that cannot be treated on an outpatient basis, mixed hemorrhoids with an external anoderm component that are not amenable to ligation, and acutely thrombosed, incarcerated hemorrhoids with severe pain and impending gangrene. Patients on anticoagulant medication are also better treated with closed, excisional hemorrhoidectomy rather than elastic ligation because of the risk of excessive bleeding when the necrotic tissue sloughs. There are numerous techniques for excising hemorrhoids. All of them are best done with the patient in the prone, flexed position. The closed technique uses either a laser, scalpel, scissors, or cautery to elliptically incise the pedicles of the hemorrhoid cushion, including the external and internal components (Fig. 26-33). The incision avoids the underlying internal sphincter muscle as the vascular cushion is dissected from the surface of the muscle. The mucosal defect is then closed after the vascular pedicle is secured with the suture.

Urinary retention is the most common complication after excisional hemorrhoidectomy and has been reported in 10 to 50 percent of patients. Minimizing the amount of IV fluids given during an operation decreases the rate of this complication. Other complications include bleeding, infection, fecal impaction, and sphincter injury. Many of the complications can be prevented by proper use of analgesia to avoid pain and straining to urinate or defecate in the immediate postoperative period. Significant bleeding after hemorrhoidectomy must be managed by complete visualization of the operative site and cautery or suture ligature of the bleeding tissue. This requires adequate anesthesia, usually a spinal or epidural. Anal stenosis is a long-term complication following circumferential excision of the anoderm and dentate line during an improperly performed Whitehead procedure. Excision of the dentate line and anoderm causes circumferential scarring at the new mucocutaneous junction. The result is eversion of rectal mucosa to form ectropion and stenosis of the anal canal. This *Whitehead deformity* often requires an island advancement flap procedure in which normal skin is inserted into the anal canal to relieve the ectropion and the stenosis (see Fig. 26-25).

Acute thrombosis and incarceration of mixed hemorrhoids can be treated conservatively with bed rest and stool softeners or with excisional hemorrhoidectomy after injecting local anesthesia and reducing the edematous rectal tissue. Epinephrine and sometimes hyaluronidase may be added to the local anesthetic agent to decrease swelling and allow the tissue to reduce. A standard three-quadrant excisional hemorrhoidectomy is safe in this setting and should not cause anal stricture and sphincter injury if performed carefully.

Excision of Thrombosed External Hemorrhoid. A patient seen in the office or emergency department with an acutely thrombosed external hemorrhoid may obtain relief by excision of the acutely thrombosed tissue. This is performed with local anesthesia, and the wound is usually left open. Merely incising the hemorrhoid and expressing the clot carries a significant risk of recurrence of the thrombosis and bleeding. The patient who is seen more than 48 h after thrombosis of a hemorrhoid is best

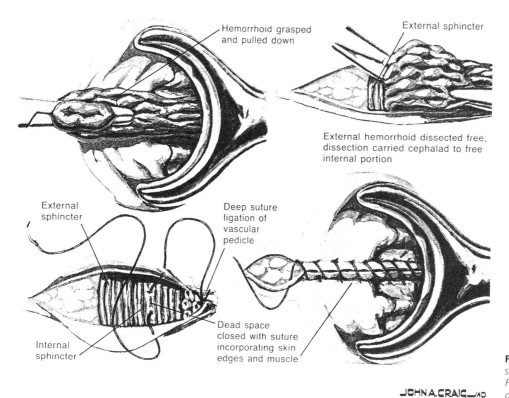

Hemorrhoid grasped and pulled down

External sphincter

External hemorrhoid dissected free; dissection carried cephalad to free internal portion

External sphincter

Deep suture ligation of vascular pedicle

Internal sphincter

Dead space closed with suture incorporating skin edges and muscle

JOHN A. CRAIG—AD
© CIBA

FIG. 26-33. Technique of excisional hemorrhoidectomy. (From: *Fry RD, Kodner IJ: Anorectal disorders. Ciba Clin Symp 37:6, 1985, with permission.*)

treated conservatively with warm soaks, an increase in fiber in the diet, and stool-softening agents.

Prevention. The majority of hemorrhoids occur because of a patient's poor bowel habits. It is important to stress the use of fiber and water in the diet, the avoidance of straining, and the cessation of sitting on the toilet for long periods of time. Symptomatic hemorrhoids can recur despite surgical treatment if these instructions are disregarded.

Anal Fissure/Anal Ulcer

General Principles. The very common problem of anal fissure was first described in 1829 by Recamier, who recommended stretching the anal sphincter to treat the condition. An *anal fissure* is a split in the anoderm, usually in either the posterior or anterior midline just distal to the dentate line (Fig. 26-34*A*). Ninety percent of all fissures occur posteriorly and 10 percent anteriorly. Less than 1 percent of patients will be found to have a fissure in both the anterior and posterior positions. The very characteristic symptoms of the fissure or ulcer include tearing pain on defecation, blood on the toilet paper or stool, and, rarely, blood in the toilet bowl. Patients also may complain of a perineal or perirectal ache or spasm for several hours after defecation.

The cause of the anal fissure has been postulated to be a hard bowel movement or prolonged diarrhea with stretching of the anal canal to cause a split in the anoderm. Increased anal sphincter pressure has been documented on anal manometry in patients with an anal fissure. However, patients in the general population with increased anal pressure have not been found to be at high risk for developing an anal fissure. Fissures may result from

ischemia, since anodermal blood flow in the posterior midline less than in other segments of the anal canal, and increased anal pressure correlates with reduced blood flow to this area. The pain and irritation of the fissure result in spasm of the underlying internal sphincter muscle, which then fails to relax during defecation, resulting in further tearing of the anoderm and deepening of the fissure to form an anal ulcer. The presence of this anal ulcer implies a chronic fissure and is accompanied by an external skin tag and a hypertrophied anal papilla in its most mature form (see Fig. 26-34*B*). The white fibers of the internal sphincter are found at the base of the ulcer.

Crohn's disease or tuberculosis of the anal canal should be suspected when the fissure or ulcer is in an atypical position. Anal disease is the first manifestation in 10 percent of patients with Crohn's disease. Patients with anal tuberculosis will have a prior history of pulmonary tuberculosis or a concomitant infection. Anal cancer may present as a painless ulcer, but it is usually associated with a mass and persists despite treatment. It is important to biopsy all nonhealing ulcers for this reason. Occasionally, abscess/fistula disease, cytomegalovirus, herpes, or *Chlamydia* infection, or syphilis will mimic some of the features of fissure and ulcer disease.

Diagnosis and Management. The diagnosis is made by visual inspection to identify either the fissure or the ulcer complex at the dentate line. Digital examination can be very painful but, if possible, will reveal not only the ulcer but also the characteristic spasm and hypertrophy of the underlying internal sphincter muscle. Medical treatment of the fissure and ulcer relies primarily on stool softeners and the addition of bulk to the diet. Almost 90 percent of simple anal fissures will heal with

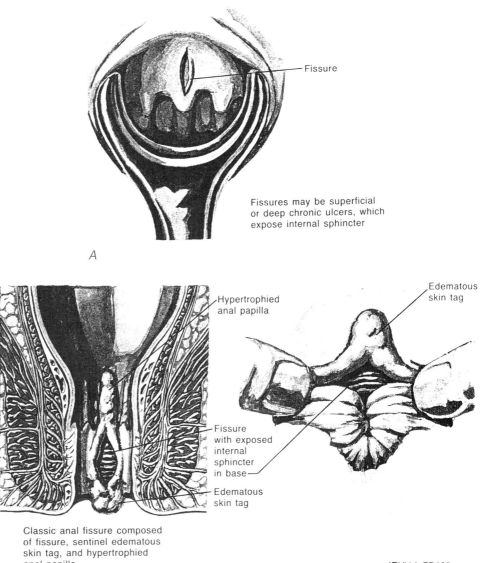

Fissure

Fissures may be superficial or deep chronic ulcers, which expose internal sphincter

A

Hypertrophied anal papilla

Edematous skin tag

Fissure with exposed internal sphincter in base

Edematous skin tag

Classic anal fissure composed of fissure, sentinel edematous skin tag, and hypertrophied anal papilla

FIG. 26-34. *A.* Anal fissure. *B.* Anal ulcer. (From: *Fry RD, Kodner U: Anorectal disorders. Ciba Clinl Symp 37:6, 1985, with permission.*)

B

JOHN A.CRAIG—AD
© CIBA

simple medical therapy. Stool softeners and bulk, as well as warm sitz baths, will relieve symptoms and produce healing in 60 to 80 percent of patients with a second episode. Topical nitroglycerin 0.2% to 0.5% (a nitric oxide donor) has been used to relax the anal sphincter and has achieved healing of anal fissures in 80 percent of a small series of patients. Botulin toxin injection also has been used to effect transient paralysis of the anal sphincter and promote healing in some patients with anal fissure. Only after the fissure has been shown to be chronic is operation considered.

Surgical Management. The surgical methods of treating fissure and ulcer disease include stretching or dividing the internal sphincter. The four-finger stretch produces uncontrolled fracturing of the internal sphincter even though it may give initial relief of symptoms. Approximately 40 percent of patients

treated this way develop recurrence, and a significant proportion are partially incontinent. The lateral internal anal sphincterotomy is considered the procedure of choice by most surgeons. A success rate of 90 to 95 percent is reported after lateral sphincterotomy for a chronic anal fissure or ulcer. Recurrence rates usually are below 10 percent, and minor incontinence, such as leakage of mucus and gas, is reported in less than 10 percent of the patients. The sphincterotomy is usually performed in the posterior lateral anus. The distal third of the internal sphincter is hypertrophied and presents a distinct, palpable band. If this hypertrophied band is not present, another cause of the ulcer should be considered. An open or closed sphincterotomy will give similar results, and each has its proponents (Fig. 26-35). The procedure is performed with the patient in the prone, flexed position, usually with local anesthesia; it is almost always performed on an outpatient basis.

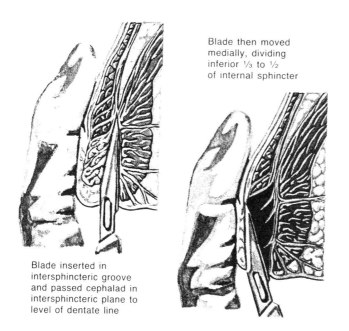

Blade then moved medially, dividing inferior ⅓ to ½ of internal sphincter

Blade inserted in intersphincteric groove and passed cephalad in intersphincteric plane to level of dentate line

A

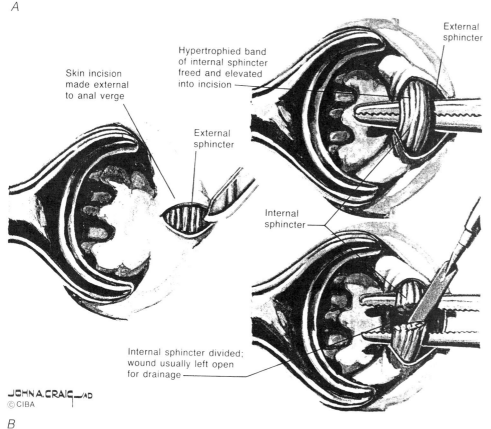

Skin incision made external to anal verge

Hypertrophied band of internal sphincter freed and elevated into incision

External sphincter

External sphincter

Internal sphincter

Internal sphincter divided; wound usually left open for drainage

JOHN A. CRAIG AD
© CIBA

B

FIG. 26-35. Lateral internal sphincterotomy. *A.* Closed technique. *B.* Open technique. (From: *Fry RD, Kodner IJ: Anorectal disorders. Ciba Clinl Symp 37:6, 1985, with permission.*)

INFECTIONS

Colitis

Pseudomembranous Colitis

Pseudomembranous colitis presents as an acute diarrheal syndrome in patients who are undergoing or have recently completed antibiotic therapy. Antibiotics alter the normal colonic bacterial population, permitting an overgrowth of the pathogen *Clostridium difficile.* This bacterium elaborates two separate exotoxins, a cytopathic toxin and an enteropathic toxin. The cytopathic toxin can be fortuitously neutralized by a cross-reaction with the antitoxin to *C. sordellii,* providing the basis for the tissue culture assay to detect the presence of *C. difficile.* If the cytopathic effects of *C. difficile* can be demonstrated by tissue culture and that effect is eliminated by culture with *C. sordellii* antitoxin, the diagnosis of *C. difficile* infection is presumed. A latex fixation test has been reported to successfully detect the cytopathic toxin. The assay should be performed within 24 h of collection of the stool. The toxin is moderately heat labile and deteriorates rapidly.

C. difficile colitis is usually preceded by the administration of antibiotics, and in as many as one-fourth of the patients the antibiotic has been discontinued before the development of diarrhea. Symptoms may appear as long as 6 weeks after antibiotic therapy. Virtually all antibiotics have been associated with the subsequent development of *C. difficile* colitis, but clindamycin, ampicillin, and the cephalosporins are most commonly implicated. There also is a contagious risk to this disease, with cross-infection occurring in hospitals and nursing homes. For this reason, isolation precautions should be used for patients with *C. difficile* colitis.

The clinical syndrome of this infection varies widely from mild, self-limited diarrhea to severe, invasive colitis associated with megacolon and perforation. When the disease is suspected, the implicated antibiotic should be stopped immediately. Proctoscopy or colonoscopy is a useful measure to detect pseudomembranes, and stool should be sent for toxin assay. Usually mild disease is self-limited. For more severe symptoms, including abdominal pain, fever, and leukocytosis, the patient should be admitted to the hospital for observation and intravenous hydration. Metronidazole is the antibiotic of choice and is usually prescribed in a dosage of 250 to 500 mg orally four times a day for 10 days. Vancomycin (125 mg orally four times a day for 10 days) is also effective, but it is much more expensive. In patients in whom oral therapy is not possible, intravenous metronidazole may be used. Intravenous vancomycin does not achieve therapeutic concentrations in the colon, however, and has no role in this setting. Cholestyramine has been recommended because it binds the toxin and renders it ineffective; however, the resin also may bind the therapeutic antibiotic, rendering it ineffective.

Most patients respond rapidly to the aforementioned treatment. Unfortunately, the recurrence rate is at least 20 percent, but these patients generally respond well to retreatment. Rarely, the disease becomes fulminant and fails to respond to appropriate antibiotic treatment; should the disease progress to a fulminant stage with toxic dilatation of the colon, abdominal colectomy with ileostomy may be necessary.

Amebic Colitis

Amebiasis is an infectious disease caused by the protozoan *Entamoeba histolytica* that infects primarily the colon but may involve other organs (usually the liver) secondarily. In the United States, amebiasis is usually thought to be a tropical disease, to be considered only if the patient has traveled abroad. However, it has been estimated that at least 5 percent of the untraveled population of the United States is infected with *E. histolytica*. The disease is transmitted by the fecal-oral route, which may include sexual contact, contamination of the water supply, and fecal soilage in day-care centers or institutions for the retarded.

E. histolytica exists in the human colon in two forms: the trophozoite and the cyst. The latter is the infective form that is ingested, causing colonization. The majority of patients infected with the protozoa remain asymptomatic carriers. However, the cysts may transform to invasive *trophozoites* at any time, and

the contributing factors leading to the emergence of virulence are not understood. The pathologic lesions of invasive amebiasis are small ulcers that may occur throughout the colon but most commonly affect the cecum. The ulcers may be covered with a yellow exudate. As the disease progresses, the ulcers may grow to more than 2 cm in diameter, with edges of undermined mucosa and necrotic tissue filling the ulcer base. The intervening mucosa may appear completely normal. In rare circumstances the ulcer may perforate, causing fulminant peritonitis. On histologic section, the amebae can be detected at the edge of the ulcer.

The clinical spectrum of amebiasis varies greatly from asymptomatic carriers to acute illness with bloody diarrhea resembling fulminant ulcerative colitis. On rare occasions the disease can cause toxic dilatation of the colon, and emergency colectomy is lifesaving. It is important to distinguish this disease from ulcerative colitis or Crohn's disease; the steroids often prescribed for the latter diseases are contraindicated in patients with amebiasis because immunologic suppression can lead to lethal dissemination of the disease. Microscopic examination of fresh stool specimens will reveal trophozoites in 90 percent of patients with symptomatic invasive amebiasis. Sigmoidoscopy is occasionally helpful if the ulcers are located in the distal bowel; however, these lesions more commonly occur in the cecum. Appropriate stool cultures should be taken to distinguish this disease from infectious bacterial colitis.

Metronidazole is the recommended treatment for invasive amebiasis. This medication, however, might be ineffective against organisms within the bowel lumen and in carriers. Iodoquinol (diiodohydroxyquin) is recommended as an accompanying medication to eliminate luminal organisms.

An uncommon complication of amebic infection that is of interest to surgeons is the *ameboma*, a mass of inflammatory tissue that may cause colonic narrowing and be confused with a carcinoma (Fig. 26-36). Colonoscopy may help in establishing the exact nature of the lesion. This lesion occurs most commonly in the cecum and is difficult to diagnose because the parasite is usually not present in the stools. The indirect hemagglutination

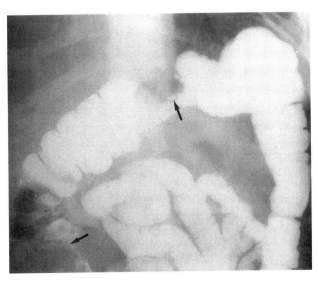

FIG. 26-36. Mass lesions (arrows) in the cecum and transverse colon that mimic cancer but proved to be amebomas.

test is usually positive in patients with an ameboma, and this test should be done if a lesion is suspicious or if there is a history of previous amebic infection. If the diagnosis is established, these patients should be treated with the antibiotics previously described. If the lesion does not resolve with antibiotic treatment, operation should be performed under cover of antiamebic therapy.

Actinomycosis

Actinomycosis is an uncommon bacterial infection caused by the gram-positive anaerobic or microaerophilic bacterium *Actinomyces israelii*. This organism formerly was misclassified as a fungus; but the species is closer to a bacterium than it is to a fungus. Clinical disease is characterized by chronic inflammatory induration and sinus formation. The organism is a normal resident of the mouth, and the cervicofacial area is the most frequently involved site, followed by thoracic and abdominal involvement.

Abdominal infection most frequently involves the cecal area, usually following appendectomy. An indurated, firm pericecal mass may develop, and, if untreated, the condition progresses to formation of indolent sinuses extending to the abdominal skin.

The diagnosis of actinomycosis should be suspected if an indolent mass or chronic sinus follows an appendectomy. The organisms make *sulfur granules,* which are actually tiny bacterial colonies consisting of a central core of intertwined branching filaments, with club-shaped bodies at the periphery, held together by a polysaccharide protein. These colonies create a sunburst pattern recognized microscopically, from which the organism derives its name. While sulfur granules are highly suggestive of *Actinomyces,* they are neither a consistent finding nor pathognomonic; *Nocardia, Streptomyces, Actinobacillus,* and *Staphylococcus* may form similar granules. Diagnosis can be confirmed by aerobic and anaerobic cultures. The microbiology laboratory should be alerted to the possible diagnosis of actinomycosis, since it often takes up to a week to isolate the organism in anaerobic culture.

Treatment consists of adequate surgical drainage and antibiotics. Penicillin and tetracycline are both effective; antifungal agents are not effective.

Neutropenic Enterocolitis

Neutropenic enterocolitis occurs most often in patients with acute myelogenous leukemia receiving high-dose cytosine arabinoside chemotherapy, but it may be seen in patients with other types of leukemia or in association with other types of chemotherapy. The syndrome is characterized by sepsis, abdominal pain and tenderness, and neutropenia. High fever, watery or bloody diarrhea, and abdominal distention are common. Tenderness is often localized to the right lower abdominal quadrant, and abdominal x-rays may show partial small bowel obstruction, thickened irregular mucosal folds, a dilated cecum, and air within the bowel wall. CT examination may reveal an edematous cecum with inflammation of the adjacent soft tissues and air in the cecal wall.

The pathogenesis of the syndrome and its proclivity to affect the cecum are not clear. It has been suggested that leukemic infiltrates in the colonic wall become necrotic after chemotherapy, resulting in ulceration of the mucosa and sepsis. Other theories include mucosal hemorrhage accompanying thrombocytopenia causing mucosal disruption and subsequent sepsis or

ischemia caused by stasis of the enteric vessels resulting in mucosal necrosis and ulceration.

Treatment consists of complete bowel rest with total parenteral nutrition and intravenous broad-spectrum antibiotics. If the sepsis cannot be controlled, or if colonic perforation occurs, operative intervention will be necessary. In such circumstances, all necrotic bowel must be removed, and the viable limbs of the bowel must be exteriorized as an ileostomy and mucous fistula. It has been suggested that elective right hemicolectomy may be indicated to prevent recurrence in patients who have recovered from neutropenic colitis and require additional chemotherapy.

Cytomegalovirus Colitis

Cytomegalovirus (CMV) infects approximately 90 percent of patients with the acquired immune deficiency syndrome (AIDS) during the course of their illness. It appears to be more commonly associated with homosexuals infected with the human immunodeficiency virus (HIV I). The infection can involve numerous organs, including the lungs, eyes, brain, liver, adrenal glands, intestinal tract, and anus. CMV colitis may occur in up to 10 percent of patients with AIDS and is the most common reason for emergency abdominal operations in this group of patients.

The virus causes mucosal ulceration and submucosal hemorrhage, and symptoms include diarrhea, rectal bleeding, fever, and weight loss. Biopsy will reveal CMV inclusions and inflammation.

Dihydroxypropoxymethyl guanine (DHPG, or ganciclovir) is the drug of choice. If the disease progresses to toxic megacolon or perforation, emergency colectomy is mandatory. Emergency colectomy also might be required for massive colonic hemorrhage. Anastomosis is seldom advisable under such circumstances, and ileostomy is almost always necessary. The prognosis is very poor; fewer than half of patients are alive at 6 months.

Chagas' Disease

Chagas' disease is endemic in Central and South America and is a frequent cause of acquired megacolon in these regions. Infection with the protozoan *Trypanosoma cruzi* results in destruction of Auerbach's myenteric plexus followed by intramural fibrosis. Although various lengths of colon may be affected, the rectum is the site most frequently involved. Loss of normal propulsive ability causes a functional obstruction and results in a proximal megacolon.

Conservative therapy may be possible in patients with mild symptoms. Complications of severe constipation, fecal impaction, or volvulus require resection of the involved colon and rectum. Sigmoidectomy, left colectomy, and subtotal colectomy all have high recurrence rates because the dyskinetic rectum is preserved. Abdominoperineal endoanal pull-through resection with delayed colorectal anastomosis or the Duhamel procedure are the techniques of choice.

Infections of Anorectum

Anorectal Abscess and Fistula

Cryptoglandular Abscess. There are several potential spaces around the anorectum that are ordinarily filled with fat and areolar tissue (Fig. 26-37).

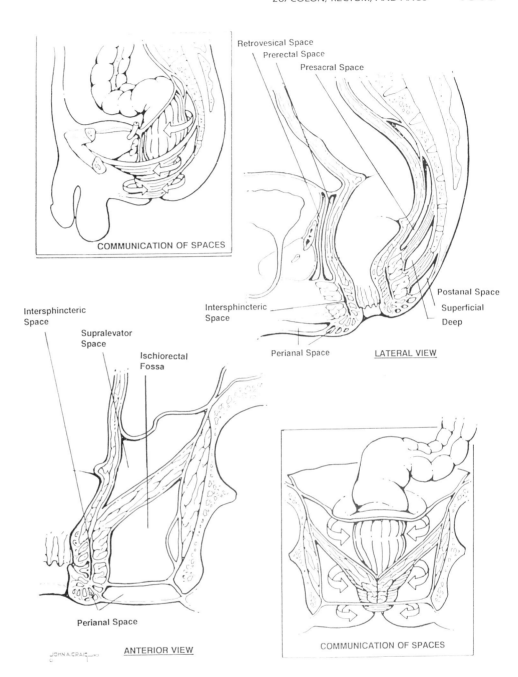

FIG. 26-37. Perirectal spaces.

Pathophysiology. The *perianal space* surrounds the anus and becomes continuous with the fat of the buttocks. The *intersphincteric space* separates the internal and external sphincters. It is continuous with the perianal space and extends cephalad into the rectal wall. Lateral and posterior to the anus is the pyramidal *ischiorectal space.* It is found below the levator ani and bound medially by the external sphincter, laterally by the ischium, and inferiorly by the transverse septum. This space contains the inferior rectal vessels and lymphatics. The two ischiorectal fossae connect posteriorly above the external sphincter forming the *deep postanal space* between the levator ani and the anococcygeal ligament. An abscess in one ischiorectal fossa can infect the other via the deep postanal space, creating a "horseshoe" abscess. The *supralevator spaces* lie above the levator ani

on either side of the rectum. These spaces communicate with each other posteriorly.

The majority of anorectal suppurative disease results from infections of the anal glands (cryptoglandular) (Fig. 26-38) and is usually due to a mixture of fecal and cutaneous flora. The glands are found in the intersphincteric plane, traverse the internal sphincter, and empty into the anal crypts in the anal canal at the level of the dentate line. Not all crypts contain glandular openings. These common infections should not be confused with anorectal manifestations of Crohn's disease, pilonidal disease, hidradenitis suppurativa, or the rarer tuberculosis or actinomycosis. The *acute* phase of cryptoglandular disease results in formation of an abscess. If the abscess drains and an infected tract persists, the process enters the *chronic* phase of fistula-in-ano.

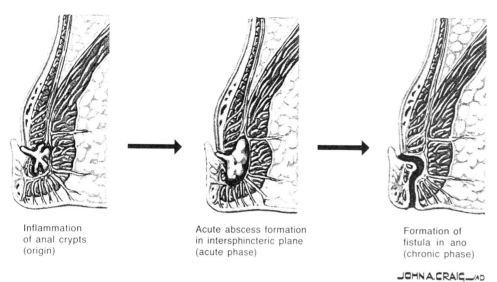

Inflammation
of anal crypts
(origin)

Acute abscess formation
in intersphincteric plane
(acute phase)

Formation of
fistula in ano
(chronic phase)

JOHN A. CRAIG ᴀᴅ
ⒸCIBA

FIG. 26-38. Cryptoglandular origin theory of anorectal abscess and fistula-in-ano. (From: *Fry RD, Kodner U: Anorectal disorders. Ciba Clin Symp 37:6, 1985, with permission.*)

Diagnosis. Severe anal pain is the most frequent presenting complaint. Walking, coughing, or straining can aggravate the pain. A palpable mass is often detected by inspection of the perianal area or by digital examination of the rectum. Occasionally patients present with fever, urinary retention, or life-threatening sepsis.

Infection of an anal gland initially results in the formation of an abscess in the intersphincteric plane (Fig. 26-39). As the abscess enlarges, it spreads in one of several directions. A *perianal abscess* is the most common manifestation. It forms when pus spreads downward between the two sphincters and presents as a tender, erythematous bulge at the anal verge. If the pus penetrates the external sphincter below the level of the puborectalis and expands into the ischiorectal fossa, an *ischiorectal abscess* is formed. A *supralevator abscess* is formed when an intersphincteric or ischiorectal abscess expands upward. Pus is found above the levators, lateral to the rectum, and below the peritoneal reflection. These abscesses can become quite large, are seldom visible, and are palpated by digital rectal examination as a bulge above the puborectalis. These abscesses are uncommon, accounting for less than 5 percent of patients with anorectal abcesses.

Treatment. Perirectal abcesses should be treated by drainage as soon as a diagnosis is established. It is not necessary to delay operation to allow erythema or purulence to develop. Antibiotics are not indicated unless there is extensive cellulitis or the patient is immunocompromised, has diabetes, or has valvular heart disease. In this group of patients, expeditious treatment is critical, because the infection can spread rapidly and become life-threatening. Usually the abscess can be localized by digital examination. If an indurated area is all that is found, examination under anesthesia and needle localization are indicated. Once adequate anesthesia has been obtained, proctosigmoidoscopy should be performed to rule out other anorectal disease.

An *intersphincteric abscess* is treated by an internal sphincterotomy. The sphincterotomy drains the abscess and destroys the infected crypt. *Perianal* and *ischiorectal abscesses* are treated by drainage through an incision in the perianal skin overlying the abscess. The abscess must be drained completely, either by excising an adequate amount of overlying skin or by

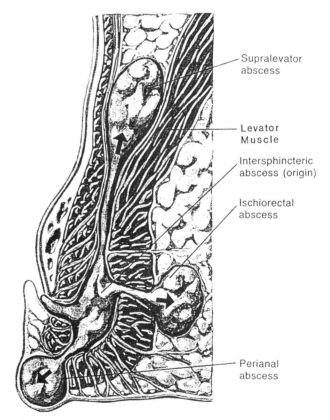

Supralevator
abscess

Levator
Muscle

Intersphincteric
abscess (origin)

Ischiorectal
abscess

Perianal
abscess

Upward extension of acute inflammation
results in supralevator abscess; lateral
in ischiorectal abscess; and downward
in perianal abscess

JOHN A. CRAIG ᴀᴅ
ⒸCIBA

FIG. 26-39. Classification of abscesses of the anorectum. (From: *Fry RD, Kodner U: Anorectal disorders. Ciba Clinl Symp 37:6, 1985, with permission.*)

inserting a mushroom catheter into the abscess cavity. After the acute phase has resolved, the mushroom catheter may be injected with dilute methylene blue or povidone-iodine. If there is no evidence of a fistula (the presence of an internal opening), the catheter is removed. If a fistula is present, it should be treated as described below. *Supralevator abscesses* should be drained transanally by incising the rectal wall overlying the abscess. A supralevator abscess should not be drained externally or through the ischiorectal fossa; this may cause a supralevator fistula that will seldom heal without a colostomy for diversion of feces (Fig. 26-40).

Drainage alone results in cure for 50 percent of patients. The other 50 percent develop an anal fistula with persistent symptoms of local infection. If only skin pathogens are cultured from an anorectal abscess, there is a decreased incidence of fistula formation. This is probably because such an abscess originates from the skin instead of from an anal crypt. The majority of the recurrences are in patients with ischiorectal abscesses. Although an argument can be made to do a primary fistulotomy at the time of incision and drainage, it is not always possible to find the internal opening in the setting of acute inflammation. Unless the internal opening can be clearly identified, it is probably preferable to treat ischiorectal abscesses by incision and drainage, because a complicated fistulotomy may result in injury to the anal sphincter.

The immunocompromised patient may present with anal pain but no evidence of a fluctuant mass because of the paucity of white blood cells. These patients should be examined under anesthesia. In such circumstances, a painful indurated area should be drained even if no purulence is found. The tissue should be biopsied (to exclude a leukemic infiltrate) and cultured (to aid in selection of antibiotics).

Necrotizing Anorectal Infections. *Pathophysiology.* Necrotizing anorectal infections (nonclostridial and streptococcal cellulitis, clostridial gangrene, and Fournier's gangrene) are perianal and perineal infections caused by either a monobacterial or mixed synergistic flora. The source of infection may be anorectal or urogenital.

Diagnosis. Examination of the perineum may reveal only limited necrosis of skin overlying crepitant tissue, but extensive tissue necrosis may be rapidly progressing in the deeper tissue. Many patients present with systemic toxicity. Most patients have an underlying chronic systemic disease. Cultures may reveal the causative organism, but surgical therapy should not be delayed while waiting for results.

Treatment. Early recognition and aggressive surgical debridement are important. Excision of all nonviable perineal and perianal tissue is required. Antibiotics are an adjunct to adequate surgical therapy. Orchiectomy is seldom necessary because the blood supply to the testicles is different from that to the scrotum and penile skin. Colostomy may be required to decrease fecal contamination or if the anal sphincters are destroyed by the infective process. Hyperbaric oxygen has been used for clostridial infections but should not interfere with or delay adequate debridement of devitalized tissue. Early diagnosis and treatment are necessary for a successful outcome; the mortality is approximately 50 percent.

Fistula-in-Ano. *Pathophysiology.* Acute infection of the anal crypt leads to an anorectal abscess; an anal fistula represents the chronic form of this infection (Fig. 26-41). The fistula con-

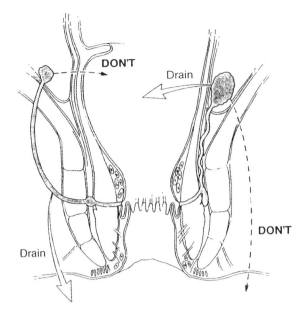

FIG. 26-40. Drainage of a supralevator abscess. (From: *Gordon PH, Nivatvongs S: 1992, with permission.*)

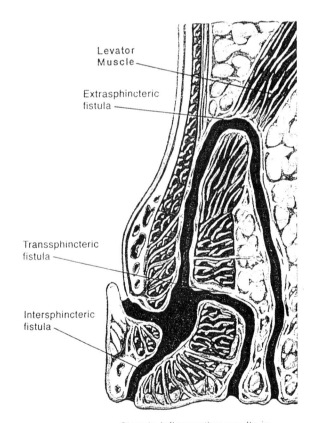

Levator Muscle

Extrasphincteric fistula

Transsphincteric fistula

Intersphincteric fistula

Chronic inflammation results in communication of abscess sites with surface, causing fistulas

JOHN A. CRAIG_AD
© CIBA

FIG. 26-41. Classification of anorectal fistulas. (From: *Fry RD, Kodner U: Anorectal disorders. Ciba Clinl Symp 37:6, 1985, with permission.*)

sists of the infected crypt and a tract extending to the site of drainage. It is therefore important to drain an abscess as close to the anus as possible to avoid the formation of a long fistulous tract. Fistulas also may be secondary to infections due to trauma, fissures, tuberculosis, Crohn's disease, carcinoma, radiation, actinomycosis, and *Chlamydia* infection.

Diagnosis. Patients present with persistent purulent drainage from the external and internal openings of the fistula. An indurated tract is often palpable. The internal opening is usually detectable by anoscope examination. Goodsall's rule can be used as a guide in determining the location of the internal opening (Fig. 26-42). It states that if the anus is bisected by a transverse line, external openings anterior to the line will connect to an internal opening by a short, direct fistulous tract. External openings posterior to this line join tracts that curve toward an internal opening in the posterior midline. An exception to this rule occurs if an anterior external opening is greater than 3 cm from the anal margin. These fistulas are more likely to have an internal opening in the posterior midline.

Treatment. The mainstay of treatment for anal fistula is eradication of sepsis with preservation of anorectal function. A simple fistula is treated by *fistulotomy* (opening the fistulous tract), curettage or cautery of the tract, and healing by secondary intention. *Fistulectomy* (complete excision of the fistulous tract) is not indicated because the magnitude of tissue loss associated with the procedure increases the risk of compromise to sphincter function.

An anal fistula that results from a drained ischiorectal abscess is usually a *transsphincteric fistula*, crossing both the internal and external sphincters. Incising the tract results in an internal sphincterotomy as well as division of a portion of the external sphincter. Continence usually will be maintained if the puborectalis muscle is not divided.

Horseshoe fistulas usually have an internal opening in the posterior midline of the anus and may extend anteriorly and laterally to one or both ischiorectal spaces by way of the deep postanal space (see Fig. 26-37). Incision and drainage of horseshoe abscesses are associated with a high recurrence rate. Adequate treatment of a horseshoe abscess requires incision and drainage of the postanal space and counterdrainage of the lateral ischiorectal spaces through separate incisions (Fig. 26-43).

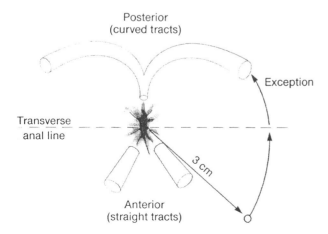

FIG. 26-42. Goodsall's rule of managing fistula-in-ano. (From: *Gordon PH, Nivatvongs S: 1992, with permission.*)

Counterdrainage is maintained until the incision over the deep postanal space is healed. This method is preferable to a fisulotomy, which would require a long skin incision to unroof the entire tract. High, complicated fistulas should not be treated by fistulotomy because of the risk of significant sphincter damage. A *seton* (see Fig. 26-57) used in this situation acts as a drain for the primary tract, but use of the seton to transect the muscle carries a significant risk of incontinence. Primary drainage followed by an endorectal sliding flap has been used to treat complicated anterior fistulas without impairment of the sphincter. This method, a modification of the technique used to treat rectovaginal fistulas (Fig. 26-44), removes the involved crypt and closes the internal opening with a sliding endorectal flap. The fistulous tract is counterdrained, and the drain is removed after the endorectal flap has healed.

Untreated fistulas may cause chronic intermittent infections, episodes of sepsis, rare cases of carcinoma, and, occasionally, death. The use of a seton is associated with an incontinence rate of 17 percent, which is increased to 39 to 63 percent after the tract is laid open at a second stage. Therefore, our technique has been to establish drainage of the primary abscess to control the sepsis. Anorectal function is preserved, and an endorectal sliding flap is used to close the internal opening. The technique is the same as will be described for rectovaginal fistula, except for the perineal counterdrain.

Rectovaginal Fistula

Pathophysiology. A *rectovaginal fistula* is a communication between the rectum, proximal to the dentate line, and the vagina. These fistulas are classified by their location. The rectal opening in a *low rectovaginal fistula* is close to the dentate line with the vaginal opening just inside the fourchette. The vaginal opening in a *high rectovaginal fistula* is near the cervix, and the opening of a *midrectovaginal fistula* is between the high and low locations.

The cause varies with the location of the fistula. Low rectovaginal fistulas are commonly caused by obstetric injuries (especially midline episiotomies that become infected), foreign body penetration of the rectum, or Crohn's disease. Midrectovaginal fistulas may result from extension of an undrained ischiorectal abscess, Crohn's disease, surgical excision or fulguration of an anterior rectal tumor, radiation injury, or extensive childbirth trauma. High rectovaginal fistulas are caused by Crohn's disease, radiation injury, operative injury, and diverticulitis. These septic processes are more prone to occur through the vaginal cuff after hysterectomy. Diverticulitis may cause a colovaginal fistula. Carcinoma of the rectum, cervix, or vagina also may result in a rectovaginal fistula at any level.

Diagnosis. Patients describe the very characteristic symptoms of passing gas and stool through the vagina and report varying degrees of continence. Diagnosis is usually evident on anoscopic or vaginal examination. A barium enema or vaginogram may reveal the fistula. Sometimes the history is characteristic, but the site cannot be identified. In such circumstances, administration of a dilute methylene blue enema may stain a tampon placed in the vagina, confirming the presence of a fistula.

Treatment. The treatment of a rectovaginal fistula depends on its cause, location, and the condition of the adjacent tissue.

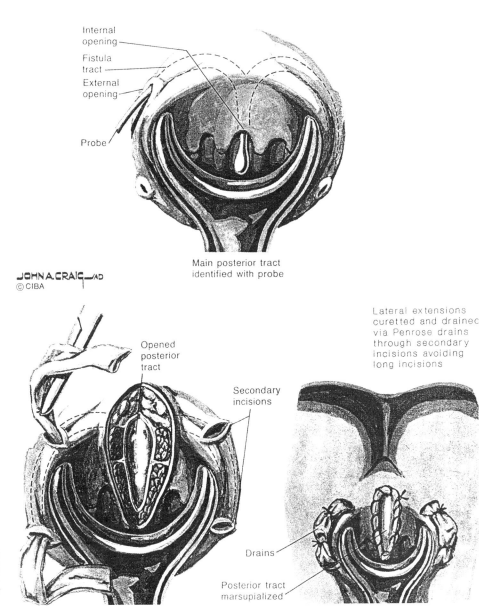

Internal opening

Fistula tract

External opening

Probe

Main posterior tract identified with probe

JOHN A. CRAIG AD
© CIBA

Opened posterior tract

Secondary incisions

Lateral extensions curetted and drained via Penrose drains through secondary incisions avoiding long incisions

Drains

Posterior tract marsupialized

FIG. 26-43. Surgical management of horseshoe abscess/fistula. (From: *Fry RD, Kodner IJ: Anorectal disorders. Ciba Clin Symp 37:6, 1985, with permission.*)

If the fistula is caused by a cryptoglandular abscess, appropriate drainage of the infection may result in spontaneous closure of the fistula. Fistulas resulting from obstetric injury may heal spontaneously, and it is wise to wait at least 3 months before attempting surgical repair. This also allows the acute inflammatory reaction to resolve.

Low and midrectovaginal fistulas are best treated by an endorectal advancement flap (see Fig. 26-44). If a sphincter injury is also present, it may be repaired simultaneously. A protecting colostomy is not necessary, but full bowel preparation and systemic antibiotics are important, because infection is the major source of failure of the repair. Treatment of a high rectovaginal fistula requires a transabdominal approach, allowing resection of the diseased tissue that caused the fistula.

Fistulas caused by Crohn's disease, radiation injury, or cancer almost never heal spontaneously. Intensive medical treatment and conservative local drainage procedures establish adequate drainage of abscesses and preserve the anal sphincter in patients with perianal Crohn's disease. Local sliding endorectal flaps for Crohn's fistulas in which the sepsis has been controlled and the disease is in remission have been used with good results, as will be described in the section on Crohn's disease. Proctectomy may be required for patients with severe perineal Crohn's disease unresponsive to local anorectal surgical procedures or for patients with extensive destruction of the rectum.

Rectovaginal fistulas due to pelvic radiation are seldom amenable to transanal repair because the tissue is permanently damaged. Tissue repairs constructed with irradiated bowel are doomed to fail. Biopsy of the fistulous tract is mandatory in patients with a history of cancer or radiation therapy. It is sometimes very difficult to clinically differentiate radiation injury from recurrent cancer.

Pilonidal Disease

Pathophysiology. *Pilonidal disease* consists of a hair-containing sinus or abscess that involves the skin and subcutaneous

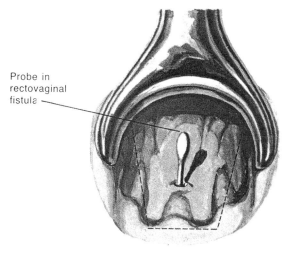

Probe in
rectovaginal
fistula

1. Rectovaginal fistula
identified by probe;
flap outlined

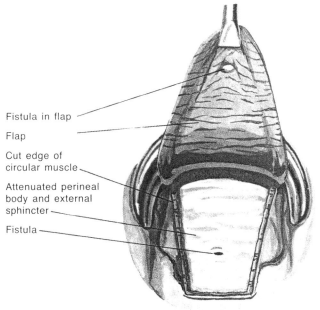

Fistula in flap

Flap

Cut edge of
circular muscle

Attenuated perineal
body and external
sphincter

Fistula

2.

Advancement flap of rectal
mucosa, submucosa, and
circular muscle elevated
from rectal wall

JOHN A. CRAIG _AD
©CIBA

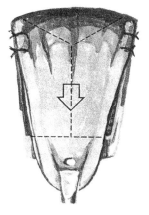

Flap advanced over reconstructed
perineal body; redundant portion
with fistula excised

3.

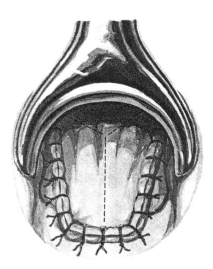

4.

Flap sutured in position
with interrupted sutures

FIG. 26-44. Advancement flap repair of rectovaginal fistula. (From: *Fry RD, Kodner IJ: Anorectal disorders. Ciba Clin Symp 37:6, 1985, with permission.*)

tissues in the postsacral intergluteal region. The cause of the disease is not clear; it may be a congenital or an acquired condition. Most investigators believe that the condition is due to ingrown hair. Pilonidal disease can occur in any age group but is most prevalent from adolescence to the third decade, with a male predominance. The sinus is superficial to the periosteum of the sacrum and may be single or have multiple extensions.

An external orifice is not always visible but is usually in the midline approximately 5 cm from the anus. The soft tissues surrounding the sinus exhibit acute and chronic inflammation. Patients present with complaints of pain, swelling, and purulent drainage when these sinuses become acutely infected. Once an acute episode has resolved, the patient rarely remains asymptomatic; recurrent infections are common.

Diagnosis. Pilonidal disease is confirmed as the cause of an abscess when the typical midline pits are identified in association with the inflammatory process. Adequate anal examination should rule out an anal fistula as the source of the abscess.

Treatment. There are numerous treatments reported in the literature, all with imperfect results. Incision, drainage, and curettage with secondary healing constitute the simplest method of treatment and are used for acute abscesses and chronic sinus tracts. This method often can be performed with local anesthesia on an outpatient basis. All hair must be removed, and the wound must be kept clean and shaved until complete healing occurs. Complete excision and secondary healing leave a large open wound and are associated with a prolonged healing time. Excision and primary closure are often successful for small sinuses but are complicated in extensive disease. Excision of the sinus followed by a Z-plasty to obliterate the intergluteal cleft has been used in some centers with low recurrence rates. The Z-plasty also serves to eliminate complicated recurrent pilonidal disease.

Hidradenitis Suppurativa

Hidradenitis suppurativa is an infection of the cutaneous apocrine sweat glands. Infected glands rupture and form subcutaneous sinus tracts. The infection spreads by direct extension and can spread to the perineum, labia, and scrotum. The perianal skin can become a network of superficial abscesses and sinuses. This infection may mimic complicated anal fistula disease but stops at the anal verge because there are no apocrine glands in the anal canal.

The diagnosis is made by clinical appearance. The glands are destroyed by the inflammation resulting from their rupture; thus there are no specific histologic identifying features. Abscesses are initially treated by wide incision, including resection of the severely indurated, infected skin that overlies the infected tracts. A colostomy is almost never indicated. Recurrence is frequent, and any recurrent infections are best incised early in the process.

Pruritus Ani

Diagnosis and Pathophysiology. *Pruritus ani* (severe perianal itching) is a symptom complex that may be caused by a number of factors but often must be classified as idiopathic because a specific etiologic agent cannot be discovered.

Patients complain of perianal itching that is often worse at night. Many have tried numerous over-the-counter medications to relieve their discomfort. A special problem occurs when products containing local anesthetic agents cause contact dermatitis and magnification of the original symptoms. A careful history and physical examination should identify any obvious causes.

The appearance of the perianal skin varies. The skin may appear normal, or it may be erythematous and weeping serum from numerous excoriations. Chronic pruritus ani is characterized by thickened, leathery, white skin.

Pinworms (*Enterobius vermicularis*) are the most common cause of perianal itching in children and may be transmitted to other family members. The worms come out of the anus at night and deposit eggs on the perianal skin, causing intense nocturnal pruritus. The diagnosis is confirmed by swabbing the perianal skin with cellophane tape and examining it under the microscope to identify the *Enterobius* eggs.

Common anal lesions (prolapsing hemorrhoids, villous tumors of the rectum, and rectal prolapse) often cause excessive

moisture in the perianal region. This moisture causes irritation and itching of the perianal skin.

Dietary habits, cleansing habits, or a combination of the two are common causes of pruritus. Overzealous, as well as careless, cleaning of the perianal skin can lead to itching. Frequent application of topical ointments keeps the area moist, causing further irritation.

Treatment. The treatment of pruritus ani is directed at the cause. Hemorrhoids, villous adenomas, and rectal prolapse should be specifically treated as discussed in this chapter. Piperazine citrate is the curative treatment for pinworms. Patients must be instructed that frequent washing and topical ointments should be avoided. The perianal area should be kept as dry as possible, and scratching should be avoided. Short term course of topical steroids is likely to provide symptomatic relief. Coffee, tea, cola, beer, chocolate, and tomatoes all can induce perianal itching, and abstaining from these foods, as well as use of proper anal hygiene, for about 2 weeks should alleviate most of the symptoms. It is, however, very common for the symptoms to recur and require reinstitution of the treatment regimen.

Proctitis

Proctitis and *anusitis* are nonspecific entities characterized by inflammation of various degrees within the anus or rectum. The differential diagnosis can be complex and includes infection, inflammatory bowel disease, and various forms of trauma.

Inflammatory Proctitis. Ulcerative colitis always involves the rectum as well as variable amounts of colon. There is a specific, mild form that involves only the rectum and is referred to as *ulcerative proctitis.* Ninety percent of these patients respond to medical management and never go on to have involvement of the colon. Patients with Crohn's disease also may have isolated rectal involvement, making the differentiation between the two difficult at times.

Diagnosis. The diagnosis may be suggested by a good history. Rectal bleeding or discharge, diarrhea, and tenesmus are common presenting symptoms. Endoscopy reveals an inflamed and friable rectal mucosa and biopsy will verify the diagnosis. The remainder of the colonic mucosa may have a normal appearance.

Treatment. The initial treatment consists of steroid retention enemas given over a course of 2 weeks. A short course of oral steroids may be considered in patients who do not respond to the enemas, with the dose being tapered over 4 to 6 weeks. Sulfasalazine may be given orally or its active ingredient, 5-aminosalicylic acid (5-ASA), may be administered as retention enemas or suppositories. Dietary measures to decrease the frequency of bowel movements, such as avoidance of milk, fruit, and fiber, and the addition of bulk-forming agents such as psyllium products may be beneficial, as well as antimotility agents such as loperamide.

Radiation Proctitis. Another cause of proctitis is radiation injury. An accurate history usually reveals the diagnosis. Early symptoms are diarrhea, rectal bleeding or discharge, tenesmus, rectal pain, and incontinence. Late symptoms appear several months to years after irradiation. Bleeding is the most common late symptom, but rectal strictures and fistulas to the bladder or vagina can develop. Examination reveals telangiectasia and friable mucosa.

Treatment. Bulk-forming agents, antispasmodics, and antidiarrheal medications are used initially. Steroid or 5-ASA retention enemas or suppositories may be helpful. Laser coagulation of bleeding telangiectasias may be required to control bleeding. Topical application of 10% formalin may be helpful in patients with persistent bleeding. Rarely, the rectum will be so badly injured that intestinal diversion is necessary.

Sexually Transmitted Disease

The differential diagnosis of proctitis and especially anusitis must include the spectrum of sexually transmitted diseases are common in individuals who practice anal intercourse.

Gonococcal Proctitis. Anorectal gonorrhea is caused by *Neisseria gonorrhoeae,* an intracellular gram-negative diplococcus. It is associated with anal intercourse, and vaginal discharge can transfer the disease to the rectum in women. Initially, patients are asymptomatic or present with rectal bleeding or discharge. Perianal excoriation, painful defecation, and fistulas also may occur. Proctoscopy reveals edematous and friable mucosa and a purulent exudate. The diagnosis should be established by cultures of anus, vagina, urethra, and pharynx, since these areas are also frequently infected.

Intramuscular procaine penicillin G with oral probenecid is the treatment of choice. Penicillinase-producing *N. gonorrhoeae* requires treatment with spectinomycin or ceftriaxone and tetracycline. Follow-up examination and cultures are necessary to avoid inadequate treatment. Sexual partners also should be evaluated.

Anorectal Syphilis. There is a rising incidence of syphilis in the Western Hemisphere. The causative organism is the spirochete *Treponema pallidum.* After an incubation period of up to 8 weeks, the primary lesion (chancre) is found at the site of inoculation. Syphilitic chancres are usually asymptomatic and can easily go unrecognized. Ulcers, proctitis, pseudotumors, and condylomata lata also may be found. Condylomata lata are the lesions of secondary syphilis and are highly contagious. They are hypertrophic papules found in areas of warmth, moisture, and friction.

Dark-field examination of exudate may reveal the spirochetes. The rapid plasma reagin (RPR) test and Venereal Disease Research Laboratory (VDRL) slide test are nonspecific screening tests that become positive 1 to 3 weeks after the appearance of the primary chancre. These tests are positive in 75 percent of patients with primary syphilis. Both the RPR and VDRL tests remain positive for long periods even after treatment. The fluorescent treponemal antibody-absorption test (FTA-ABS) is more specific and sensitive but is also more expensive. Syphilis is treated with benzathine penicillin G or erythromycin.

Chlamydia trachomatis. *Chlamydia trachomatis* is an obligate intracellular parasite that causes chlamydial proctitis and lymphogranuloma venereum (LGV). Chlamydial proctitis is associated with anal intercourse or may spread via the lymphatics in the rectovaginal septum in women. The infection may be asymptomatic, or the patient may complain of anal pain, pruritus, rectal bleeding, or rectal discharge.

The primary lesion of LGV is a small shallow ulcer that often is not noticeable. Inguinal adenopathy develops and can form large matted nodes. If left untreated, the patient could develop hemorrhagic proctitis and late rectal strictures. The LGV complement fixation test or the microimmunofluorescent antibody titer confirm the diagnosis. Tissue cultures can be used to isolate the organism.

Tetracycline (or doxycycline) is the treatment of choice, but erythromycin may be used as an alternative. Antibiotics should be continued for 14 to 21 days. Rectal strictures may be dilated early in the disease. Complete obstruction is rare and requires colostomy.

Chancroid. Chancroid, caused by *Haemophilus ducreyi,* is a disease manifested by soft, multiple lesions that are very painful and bleed easily. Multiple lesions may develop as a result of autoinoculation and are often seen in the perineum and around the anus. Inguinal adenopathy is a common finding. Lymph nodes become fluctuant and rupture through the skin, causing draining sinuses. Treatment is with erythromycin or trimethoprim-sulfamethoxazole.

Herpes Proctitis. Herpes proctitis is caused primarily by type II herpes simplex virus, although the type I virus can cause the same symptoms. The virus is transmitted by direct mucosal contact. Patients present with tenesmus, anal pain, rectal bleeding, discharge, and perianal ulcerations. The pain may be so intense that the patient is reluctant to have a bowel movement. Fever and malaise are frequently present.

The anorectal lesions appear 3 to 7 days after sexual contact. The primary lesions are clusters of vesicles that rupture, coalesce, and form painful ulcers. The ulcers become infected secondarily. These lesions tend to recur, and the recurrent form is usually less painful than the original. The disease is contagious while the lesions are present. Diagnosis is made by viral cultures of vesicular fluid or biopsies.

There is no cure; treatment is symptomatic. Oral acyclovir reduces the frequency and duration of recurrent episodes and reduces virus shedding, but acyclovir does not prevent recurrences and does not alter the long-term natural history of the disease.

Condylomata Acuminata. Condylomata acuminata are warts that occur in the anorectal and urogenital regions, caused by infection with the human papillomavirus. In developed countries, genital warts are now the most common viral sexually transmitted disease, estimated to be three times more common than genital herpes. Anal intercourse is the most common means of transmission of anorectal warts, and there is a high association with other sexually transmitted diseases. Although condylomata are found more commonly in homosexual men, heterosexual men and women can be infected. This virus is autoinoculable and has an incubation period that can be as long as 1 year; both factors account for frequent treatment failures.

Diagnosis. Most patients present after noticing the visible perianal growths. Pruritus, anal discharge, bleeding, and pain are occasionally present. The diagnosis is usually obvious because of the characteristic appearance of the warts. Anoscopy and proctosigmoidoscopy should be performed on all patients because condylomata may be found within the anal canal. Tests for other venereal diseases, e.g., HIV and hepatitis B are indicated. Condylomata lata associated with secondary syphilis are usually smoother, flatter, and lighter in color and can occur simultaneously with condylomata acuminata.

Treatment. There are numerous treatments for condylomata acuminata. Evaluation of treatment efficacy is complicated by occasional spontaneous regression of lesions, reinfection, and lack of prospective, randomized, controlled trials. Bichloroacetic acid and 25% podophyllin application are the two most common treatments performed in the office setting. These treatments are satisfactory only if the warts are small and few in number. Weekly evaluation and treatment are necessary until all the warts are gone.

Excision and electrocoagulation under local anesthesia are effective treatment for the patient with a large number of warts. The warts are destroyed using the cautery; care is taken to preserve the adjacent skin and anoderm. The smoke generated from the procedure contains viable organisms and should be thoroughly evacuated. Carbon dioxide lasers have been used to eradicate condylomata but have been shown to be associated with a slightly higher recurrence rate. Small lesions can be treated using local anesthesia; larger lesions require regional or general anesthesia. Immunotherapy with an autogenous vaccine and intralesional injection of interferon have had variable results. All treatments for condylomata have been associated with recurrence rates up to 70 percent.

Malignancy. There appears to be an association between the human papillomaviruses 16, 18, and 31 and carcinomas of the anal and genital tracts. Malignant degeneration to squamous carcinoma has been reported with increasing frequency in anal condylomata. Immunosuppression, most commonly encountered today with HIV disease, appears to confer additional risk. Resected condylomata specimens should be examined microscopically, and recurrent or persistent condylomata should be submitted for histologic examination. The incidence and rate of malignant transformation are unknown. Radical surgical removal of the rectum has been the usual treatment for these cancers but is associated with a high recurrence rate. Combined chemoradiation has been reported to shrink large lesions, making them surgically curable. The choices of treatment for anal cancer will be discussed later.

Giant condylomata acuminata (Buschke-Lowenstein tumors) involving the perianal region may appear to be histologically benign but exhibit malignant behavior. They are thought to represent a low-grade, well-differentiated variant of conventional squamous cell carcinoma. These tumors do not respond to conservative therapy, and radical surgical excision offers the only hope for cure or adequate palliation.

Acquired Immune Deficiency Syndrome (AIDS).

Acquired immune deficiency syndrome (AIDS) has been associated with numerous gastrointestinal complications. Tumors such as Kaposi's sarcoma and non-Hodgkin's lymphoma, as well as infections with fungi, viruses, atypical bacteria, and protozoa, can involve the entire gastrointestinal tract in immunosuppressed patients. Heterosexuals with AIDS get fewer anorectal infections and malignancies than homosexual men with AIDS.

Kaposi's sarcoma is the most common malignant tumor in AIDS patients. The lesions may appear as small telangiectasias or larger purple nodules; their color is due to extravasation of blood. The skin is the most frequently affected site, but the gastrointestinal tract may be involved as well. These lesions are often multiple and may occur anywhere along the gastrointestinal tract. Usually patients are asymptomatic, but the lesions can cause hemorrhage or obstruction. Diagnosis is made by the endoscopic appearance of the lesions, and biopsies for histologic confirmation should be taken. These lesions are submucosal, and superficial biopsies are often nondiagnostic; deeper biopsies are necessary, and although the lesions have a vascular appearance, they rarely bleed after biopsy. Therapy is palliative and may require chemotherapy with an agent such as vincristine or vinblastine. Surgery is seldom indicated. If surgery is required for complications such as persistent hemorrhage, obstruction, or intussusception, only the involved section of bowel should be resected.

Lymphoma is found with increased frequency in patients with immune deficiencies, particularly in patients with AIDS. Most are non-Hodgkin's B-cell lymphomas, which are highly aggressive, and multiple organ involvement is common. Rectal involvement is rare but has been reported in homosexual men and should be considered in the differential diagnosis of anorectal masses in this population. Patients present with fever and perirectal masses. The lesions should be biopsied for diagnosis. Chemoradiation is the treatment of choice, but the response rate in patients with AIDS is poor. Surgical resection or bypass may be necessary for obstructing or perforating gastrointestinal lymphomas.

CMV is ubiquitous in the homosexual AIDS population. CMV ileocolitis is the most common intestinal infection in patients with AIDS. Patients frequently present with diarrhea, melena or hematochezia, fever, and weight loss. Examination reveals diffuse ulceration that can occur anywhere along the gastrointestinal tract. Biopsies of the ulcers show CMV inclusion bodies. The diagnosis is confirmed by viral culture of biopsy specimens or antigen assay of washings taken from ulcers. Resection may be required for the complications of bleeding or perforation. The mortality is high.

Infections with *Campylobacter, Shigella, Mycobacterium avium-intracellulare, Cryptosporidium, Isospora belli, Entamoeba histolytica,* and *Giardia lamblia* may cause enterocolitis or intractable diarrhea in patients with AIDS. Many patients present with persistent diarrhea, lower abdominal cramping, and, occasionally, bloody stools. Anoscopic and sigmoidoscopic findings may range from normal-appearing mucosa to friable ulcerations. Diagnosis is based on special stool cultures, examination of fresh stool specimen for ova and parasites, and biopsies of ulcers sent for histologic examination. Treatment is directed at a causative agent, and surgery is rarely necessary.

Sexually transmitted anorectal diseases are common in AIDS patients, including gonorrhea, syphilis, chlamydia, herpes simplex, and papillomavirus infection. Anorectal disease in AIDS patients has been approached with nihilism in the past because of reports of high morbidity and mortality postoperatively and because of short overall survival from AIDS. However, now that new drug treatments are increasing the life expectancy in AIDS patients, it becomes more important to diagnose and aggressively treat anorectal disease to avoid disabling complications.

INFLAMMATORY BOWEL DISEASE

General Considerations

The term *inflammatory bowel disease* encompasses two major entities: *ulcerative colitis* and *Crohn's disease.* There are several synonyms for each of these diseases. Ulcerative colitis is also referred to as *mucosal ulcerative colitis* and *idiopathic ulcerative colitis.* Crohn's disease is also called *segmental colitis, regional enteritis, regional ileitis, terminal ileitis, granulomatous colitis,* or *transmural colitis.*

Ulcerative colitis is an inflammatory process involving the colonic mucosa, characterized by alterations in bowel function and symptoms of intestinal inflammation. The most frequent sign of ulcerative colitis is hematochezia, the passage of red blood from the rectum. The presence of abdominal pain, fever, and weight loss depends on the severity of the inflammation (Table 26-2). Ulcerative colitis has been recognized since the nineteenth century, when it was reported in several London hospitals.

Crohn's disease was first described as "chronic interstitial enteritis" by the Scottish surgeon Dalziel in 1913, but the description of the clinical entity "regional ileitis" in 1932 by Crohn, Ginsberg, and Oppenheimer from Mt. Sinai Hospital in New York led to widespread recognition of the disease involving the ileum. Subsequently, Lockhart-Mummery and Morson reported the colonic involvement by transmural inflammation, distinguishing the entity from ulcerative colitis. It is now recognized that Crohn's disease can occur anywhere in the gastrointestinal tract, from mouth to anus, and that the extraintestinal manifestations of the disease may precede those of the intestine.

The annual incidence of both diseases in western Europe and North America increased up to 1970 and has since stabilized or decreased. While men more frequently have ulcerative colitis and women more frequently have Crohn's disease, genetic and environmental factors seem to be important etiologic considerations. Other factors under investigation include smoking, oral contraceptives, alcohol, refined sugar, infectious diseases, and Jewish heritage. A defect in immune regulation in the gastrointestinal tract, in either an initiating or a perpetuating role, is also being investigated. Some observations implicate gut-associated lymphoid tissue in the pathobiology of both ulcerative colitis and Crohn's disease, for example, the granuloma in Crohn's disease (indicative of T-cell-mediated immunity), the lymphoid infiltrate resembling an Arthus reaction in ulcerative colitis, the presence of extraintestinal manifestations of inflammatory bowel disease (IBD) in other immunologically mediated diseases, and

IBD patients displaying hypergammaglobulinemia and autoantibody production as seen in an immunologically activated state.

Recent studies focus on a fundamental defect of mucosal immune regulation leading to immunologic hyperactivation rather than on a direct autoimmune assault on a specific target cell, the focus of earlier studies. This fundamental defect, leading to uncontrolled immune reaction to environmental agents and antigens, can cause an unregulated immune response, including lymphocyte proliferation, cytokine release, secondary recruitment of auxiliary effector cells, excessive neutrophil products (especially leukotriene B_4 and reactive oxygen metabolites), and ultimately, tissue injury (Fig. 26-45). The actual tissue damage probably reflects a nonspecific "innocent bystander" injury.

Crohn's disease and ulcerative colitis appear closely related; when the disease exists in the colon, 15 percent of cases cannot be clearly differentiated (Table 26-3). Distinguishing Crohn's colitis from ulcerative colitis carries therapeutic significance: There is a significant recurrence of disease involving the small intestine in patients with Crohn's disease treated by colectomy, whereas such recurrence is rare in patients with ulcerative colitis. The two entities are similar because they are both characterized by exacerbations and remissions of intestinal inflammation. Each also has a chronic phase. Ulcerative colitis is a disease of the mucosa that is limited to the colon and rectum. Crohn's disease, on the other hand, can involve any part of the gastrointestinal tract; this chapter will deal mainly with its involvement of the large intestine.

The symptoms also overlap and generally consist of those which would be caused by inflammation of the intestine, the specifics varying with the depth of the inflammation and the location along the intestinal tract (see Table 26-2). Many diagnostic modalities may be used to differentiate and define the extent of the disease as well as the degree of inflammation. These include contrast studies of the intestine, endoscopic evaluation, CT, magnetic resonance imaging (MRI), ultrasonography, and special nuclear scans (Table 26-4).

The tissue changes of ulcerative colitis are depicted in Fig. 26-46, which shows the progression from superficial, homogeneous ulceration and purulent discharge, to the intense inflammatory reaction resulting in edema and pseudopolyp formation, to the chronic changes of a flattened, potentially dysplastic lining of the large intestine. The disease generally involves only the mucosal layer of the large intestine. Crohn's disease, as depicted in Fig. 26-47, shows the early phase of the disease to involve only isolated areas of the mucosa in the form of aphthoid ulcers. As the activity of the disease progresses, deep ulceration and inflammation extend through the full thickness of the intestine, with thickening of the intestinal wall. It is this full-thickness destruction of tissue that results in the eventual perforation of the intestine, leading to many of the complications of Crohn's disease. In the chronic phase of Crohn's disease, the intestinal wall is thickened, fibrotic, and nondistensible, causing symptoms of intestinal obstruction. In all phases of the disease there may be areas of normal mucosa that are spared the inflammatory process; in contrast, ulcerative colitis is a more homogeneous inflammatory process.

Both ulcerative colitis and Crohn's disease have systemic manifestations contributing to the hypothesis that there is some type of autoimmune phenomenon involved in the causation of IBD (Table 26-5).

Table 26-2
Inflammatory Bowel Disease: Signs and Symptoms

	Crohn's Disease	Ulcerative Colitis
Symptoms		
Diarrhea	+++	+++
Rectal bleeding	+	+++
Tenesmus	0	+++
Abdominal pain	+++	+
Fever	++	+
Vomiting	+++	0
Weight loss	+++	+
Signs		
Perianal disease	+++	0
Abdominal mass	+++	0
Malnutrition	+++	+

SOURCE: Ogorek CP, et al: 1992. Elsevier Science Publishing, New York, with permission.

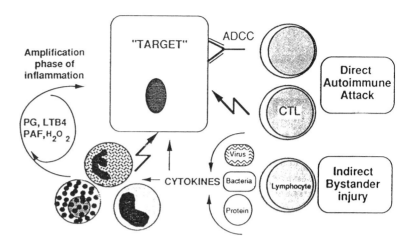

FIG. 26-45. Potential immunologic mechanisms leading to tissue injury in inflammatory bowel disease. These include a direct autoimmune attack on a putative target, such as the epithelial cell, through antibody-dependent cellular cytotoxicity (ADCC) or cytotoxic T lymphocytes (CTL). Alternatively, tissue injury may occur as an "indirect" or "innocent bystander" effect caused by mucosal T-cell hyperactivation. In addition to the direct effects of T-cell-derived cytokines on the epithelium and local immune system, persistent or excessive cytokine release may lead to recruitment of auxiliary effectors such as neutrophils. Neutrophil products, particularly leukotriene B₄ (LTB₄) and reactive oxygen metabolites, amplify the inflammatory response and injure the local microenvironment. PG = prostaglandin; PAF = platelet-activating factor. (From: *Shanahan F, Targan SR: 1992, with permission.*)

The gross as well as the radiologic appearance of the intestine in the two diseases is depicted in Fig. 26-48. Ulcerative colitis is characterized by an intestinal wall of normal caliber with severe inflammatory changes of the mucosa and a normal-appearing mesentery. In Crohn's disease, the intestine is markedly thickened, as is the adjacent mesentery, with enlargement of the mesenteric lymph nodes. The serosal surface of the intestine is inflamed, and the fat takes on a strange configuration of enveloping the intestine ("fat wrapping"). Ulcerative colitis appears in contrast radiography as homogeneous ulceration with mucosal edema, on the other hand, chronic Crohn's disease is characterized by segmental narrowing with thickening of the loops of intestine involved.

A better understanding of the differentiation of the two diseases can be accomplished by looking at the effect of the two diseases as they involve the colon (Table 26-6). Ulcerative colitis always involves the rectum and may extend, in continuity, to the more proximal colon; Crohn's disease has a segmental distribution with areas of normal bowel located between diseased segments. Rectal bleeding occurs in both diseases but is usually more of a problem in ulcerative colitis. The distinction between rectal and anal involvement is an important differentiating fea-

Table 26-3

Morphologic Features Most Useful in Distinguishing Ulcerative Colitis from Crohn's Disease

Suggestive of Crohn's disease
    Focal inflammation in the mucosa
    Ileal involvement
    Linear or fissuring ulcers
    Rectal sparing
    Right-sided predominance
Highly suggestive of Crohn's disease
    Discontinuous segmental involvement
    Aphthoid ulcers
Virtually pathognomonic of Crohn's disease
    Sarcoid granulomas
    Transmural inflammation with lymphoid nodules
    Fistulas (at sites other than anus)

SOURCE: Owen DA: 1992. Elsevier Science Publishing, New York, with permission.

Table 26-4

Endoscopic Differentiation Between Chronic Ulcerative Colitis and Crohn's Disease

	Chronic Ulcerative Colitis	Crohn's Disease
Early findings	Edema, confluent erythema, rectal involvement	Rectal sparing, perianal disease, aphthous ulceration
Moderate changes	Granularity, contact bleeding	Linear ulcers, coblestoning, skip lesions
Late changes	Discrete ulcers, pus	Contact bleeding, confluent ulcers, strictures, mucosal bridging

SOURCE: Kozarek RA: Elsevier Science Publishing, 1992. New York, with permission.

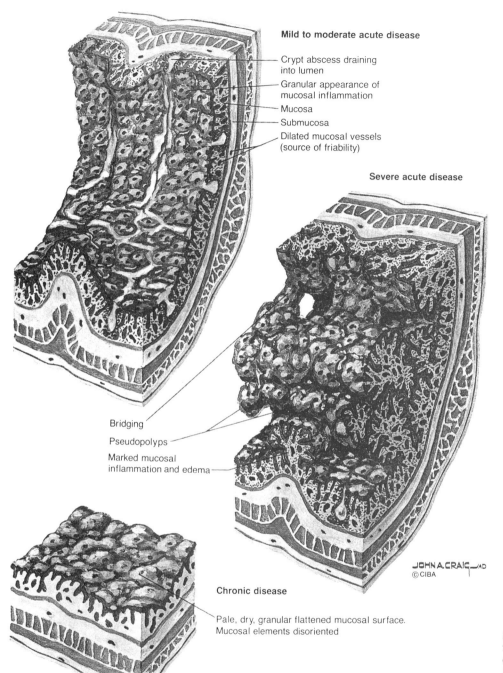

Mild to moderate acute disease

Crypt abscess draining
into lumen

Granular appearance of
mucosal inflammation

Mucosa

Submucosa

Dilated mucosal vessels
(source of friability)

Severe acute disease

Bridging

Pseudopolyps

Marked mucosal
inflammation and edema

Chronic disease

Pale, dry, granular flattened mucosal surface.
Mucosal elements disoriented

JOHN A. CRAIG AD
© CIBA

FIG. 26-46. Progression of inflammatory process in ulcerative colitis. (From: *Kodner U, Fry RD: Inflammatory bowel disease. Ciba Clin Symp 34:1, 1982, with permission.*)

ture. In patients with ulcerative colitis, the rectum is always involved; only 50 percent of patients with Crohn's colitis will have rectal involvement. Anal disease, on the other hand, is highly suggestive of Crohn's disease. Anal fistulas are rare in patients with ulcerative colitis but are found frequently in patients with Crohn's disease.

Mucosal ulceration exists in both diseases, but the ulcers are more irregular and in a continuous distribution with ulcerative colitis, as opposed to being linear with transverse fissures (cobblestone appearance) in Crohn's disease. Strictures occur rarely in ulcerative colitis; when they do, they are often indicative of cancer. On the other hand, benign stricture formation is a characteristic of Crohn's disease. Ulcerative colitis is considered a premalignant condition. While there is an increased risk of large bowel cancer in patients with Crohn's disease, the risk is less than that of ulcerative colitis. Toxic dilatation, or more appropriately, fulminant colitis, occurs in both diseases. In patients with fulminant ulcerative colitis, the inflamed colon can dilate, presenting the clinical situation termed *toxic megacolon*. Severe inflammation can cause colonic perforation in patients with

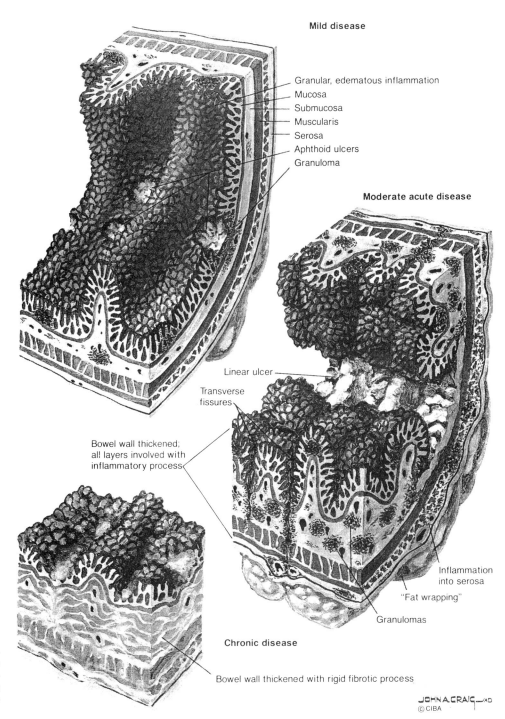

FIG. 26-47. Progression of inflammatory process in Crohn's disease. (From: *Kodner U, Fry RD: Inflammatory bowel disease. Ciba Clin Symp 34:1, 1982, with permission.*)

Crohn's disease, but because of fibrosis and thickening, dilatation is less frequently a component of the severe colonic involvement.

Each of the diseases can present with variable intensity, and the clinical management depends on the activity of the disease. In some cases, there can be rapid progression to the fulminant phase. Management of the patient with IBD requires knowledge of the *acuity* of the disease as well as the geographic *distribution* within the intestinal tract. *Mildly active* Crohn's disease consists of mucosal aphthoid ulcers; mildly active ulcerative colitis con-

sists of mucosal edema and friability. These subtle changes are sometimes difficult to recognize by endoscopy. As the activity progresses to the *moderately severe* form, Crohn's disease is characterized by thickening of the intestinal wall, deep linear ulceration of the mucosa, edema of the bowel wall, wrapping of fat about the serosa, mesenteric thickening, and enlarged mesenteric lymph nodes. In moderately severe ulcerative colitis, there is progression of the mucosal disease with more purulent discharge, diffuse ulceration, and bleeding. As the diseases enter their *severe acute* inflammatory phase, Crohn's disease is char-

Table 26-5
Extraintestinal Nonhepatic Manifestations of Idiopathic Inflammatory Bowel Disease

Musculoskeleton
    Ankylosing spondylitis and sacroiliitis
    Peripheral arthritis
    Pelvic osteomyelitis
Skin and mouth
    Erythema nodosum
    Pyoderma gangrenosum
    Aphthous stomatitis
Eye
    Uveitis (iritis)
    Episcleritis
Blood and vascular system
    Anemia (iron loss, vitamin B_{12} or folate deficiency, hemolytic)
    Thrombocytosis
    Leukocytosis
    Hypercoagulable state
Kidneys and genitourinary tract
    Nephrolithiasis
    Obstructive uropathy
    Fistulas to genitourinary tract
Other
    Bronchopulmonary vasculitis
    Pleurocarditis

SOURCE: O'Brien J: 1992. Elsevier Science Publishing, New York, with permission.

acterized by deep ulceration of the bowel wall, increased serosal fat wrapping, and extension of the inflammatory process beyond the wall of the intestine, resulting in a phlegmon or abscess. Ulcerative colitis, on the other hand, is associated with the formation of pseudopolyps with severe fluid, electrolyte, and sometimes blood loss from the intense inflammatory process involving the mucosal surface of the colon and rectum.

The *chronic phase* of both diseases is depicted in Fig. 26-49. In ulcerative colitis, the mucosa takes on a dry, granular appearance, and the colon is markedly contracted, as seen in the radiograph. The colon loses its distensibility, and in this phase, where most of the lining of the intestine looks abnormal by endoscopy, the identification of malignant change becomes important. Crohn's disease, in its chronic phase, is characterized by intense fibrosis of the intestinal wall without acute mucosal inflammatory changes. If the rectum is involved, the loss of the reservoir function results in intolerably frequent, and often difficult to control, bowel movements, to the point where patients can be incapacitated with the chronic form of the disease and yet not have any acute inflammatory changes. Steroids and immunosuppressive medications will have little effect on this chronic, fibrotic state.

The two diseases are also similar in the use of antibiotics, anti-inflammatory agents, and immunosuppressive drugs in their management. Medical therapy is summarized in Table 26-7.

Ulcerative Colitis

Indications for Surgery

The indications for surgery in the treatment of ulcerative colitis include *active disease unresponsive to medical therapy, risk of cancer,* and *severe bleeding.* Because only the large intestine is involved, a proctocolectomy should cure the patient of intes-

tinal disease. Patients requiring operation because of active disease usually have extensive edema and ulceration of the intestine; fluid, electrolyte, and blood loss; and sometimes dilatation of the colon with possible perforation (Table 26-8). These patients with *toxic colitis* or *toxic megacolon* must be treated aggressively with bowel rest, antibiotics, and corticosteroids. Should their clinical situation deteriorate, they should have emergency abdominal colectomy or, if walled-off perforation is encountered, a diverting loop ileostomy combined with a decompressing colostomy, as described for fulminant Crohn's colitis. Barium enema, antidiarrheal agents, and morphine should be avoided because they might intensify the colonic dilatation. Careful observation of the patient is more important than serial radiographs of the abdomen looking for an arbitrary limit to cecal dilatation as an indication for surgery.

The patient at risk for cancer usually has had total colonic involvement for a period of at least 10 years. Studies have shown a 10 percent incidence of cancer in patients with such chronic disease. The risk of cancer in ulcerative colitis is related to the extent of colonic mucosal involvement and to the duration of the disease but apparently not to the intensity of the inflammation. Unfortunately, some patients who had childhood ulcerative colitis that became quiescent develop colon cancer in early adult life. The cancer risk was not recognized because the disease was in long-term remission. Such a colon at risk for developing malignant changes is illustrated in Fig. 26-49. Before the advent of colonoscopy, it was observed that almost all patients who developed cancer of the colon manifested changes of mucosal dysplasia that could be detected by sigmoidoscopy and biopsy of the rectum. It was this finding that led to a cancer surveillance plan for patients with chronic ulcerative colitis. Now colonoscopic evaluation of the entire large intestine is possible, and a plan for organized surveillance of patients with chronic ulcerative colitis has been developed, as illustrated in Fig. 26-50.

Colonoscopic surveillance has been recommended by the American Society of Gastrointestinal Endoscopy after 7 years of disease in patients with pancolitis and after 10 years of disease in patients with left-sided colitis. Colonoscopy and biopsy for dysplasia should be performed every 1 or 2 years in these patients. If severe dysplasia is identified, surgical removal of the colon and rectum is indicated. The surveillance regimen includes random segmental biopsies and biopsies of any suspicious lesions. Random biopsies are necessary because malignant growths that occur in ulcerative colitis are frequently of the endophytic, rather than exophytic, type of cancer and are difficult to detect with the colonoscope (Fig. 26-51). Colon cancer in patients with ulcerative colitis is a major exception to the concept of polyp–cancer sequence, i.e., the cancer may arise in a flat mucosal surface. The pathologic determination of *dysplasia* is often difficult because the early changes of dysplasia are subtle, and dysplasia cannot be diagnosed in the presence of active inflammation.

Surgical Management

The characteristic inflammation of ulcerative colitis is confined to the mucosa of the large bowel. Complete excision of the large intestine is curative in this disease (unlike in Crohn's colitis, which carries a significant risk of recurrent disease following excision of involved intestine). These characteristics provide the rationale for sphincter-saving reconstructive procedures as treatment for ulcerative colitis. Since the disease is confined

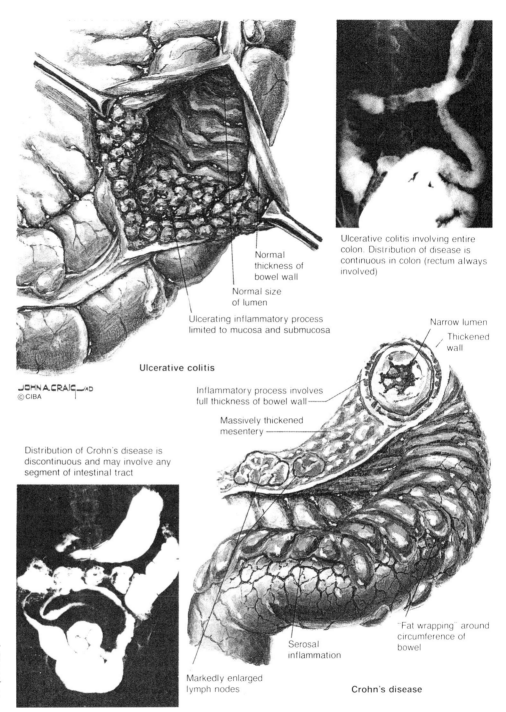

Normal
thickness of
bowel wall

Normal size
of lumen

Ulcerating inflammatory process
limited to mucosa and submucosa

Ulcerative colitis involving entire
colon. Distribution of disease is
continuous in colon (rectum always
involved)

Ulcerative colitis

JOHN A. CRAIG AD
© CIBA

Distribution of Crohn's disease is
discontinuous and may involve any
segment of intestinal tract

Narrow lumen

Thickened
wall

Inflammatory process involves
full thickness of bowel wall

Massively thickened
mesentery

"Fat wrapping" around
circumference of
bowel

Serosal
inflammation

Markedly enlarged
lymph nodes

Crohn's disease

FIG. 26-48. Differentiating features of ulcerative colitis and Crohn's disease. (From: *Kodner IJ, Fry RD: Inflammatory bowel disease. Ciba Clin Symp 34:1, 1982, with permission.*)

to the mucosa, the rectal sphincters can be preserved; since the disease does not involve the small intestine, a reservoir can be fashioned from the ileum that can serve as a substitute for the excised rectum. If the anal sphincter cannot be preserved, a "continent ileal reservoir" can be constructed (Table 26-9). The ileorectal anastomosis or any other procedure that leaves the rectum in situ carries the risk of recurrence of inflammation as well as the risk of subsequent cancer. The surgical options are illustrated in Fig. 26-52.

The current preference is to give a patient the choice for a sphincter-preserving operation as long as the individual can tolerate the increased magnitude of the surgery and has a demonstrated adequate anal sphincter function. It is most important that the patient not have Crohn's disease. In a few patients, this distinction is difficult to make, and a subset of patients has been recognized as having "indeterminate colitis." The patients treated by a sphincter-preserving operation have an increased risk of complications at the ileoanal anastomosis and have an increased risk of requiring resection of the pouch because of subsequent complications. Total colectomy with ileal pouch–anal anastomosis also requires, in most cases, a temporary ileostomy, making this a two-stage procedure. Patients who have an impaired

Table 26-6
Inflammatory Disease of Colon

	Ulcerative Colitis	Crohn's Colitis
Usual location	Rectum, left colon	Anywhere
Rectal bleeding	Common, continuous	Uncommon, intermittent
Rectal involvement	Almost always	Approx. 50%
Fistulas	Rare	Common
Ulcers	Shaggy, irregular, continuous distribution	Linear with transverse fissures ("cobblestone")
Bowel stricture	Rare (suspect carcinoma)	Common
Carcinoma	Increased incidence	Increased incidence
Toxic dilatation of colon	Occurs in both	

anal sphincter or those who do not wish to accept the increased risk of the reconstructive procedure should be treated by total proctocolectomy and ileostomy. If the surgeon treating a patient with fulminant colitis is unfamiliar with the sphincter-saving procedures, an abdominal colectomy with closure of the rectum allows the patient to recover from the life-threatening colitis. Subsequently, this patient can be referred to an institution where the more complex reconstructive procedure can be accomplished.

The use of the continent ileostomy or Kock pouch (see Table 26-9) has decreased since the advent of the new ileal pouch–anal anastomotic procedures and probably should be offered only to patients with ulcerative colitis who have permanent ileostomies that cannot be maintained properly because of severe skin allergies or to patients who have been treated by total proctocolectomy but desire a form of continence. The only advantage of the continent ileostomy is avoidance of the need to wear a permanent appliance. It requires intubation six to eight times a day to empty the pouch. There is also the risk of delayed complications related to the loss of the nipple valve created by intussusception of the ileum.

The preferred sphincter-saving operation for a patient with ulcerative colitis is total proctocolectomy with preservation of the anal sphincters, construction of an ileal reservoir, and anastomosis of the reservoir to the anus (Fig. 26-53A,B). This removes the distal disease (some current forms of the operation leave a small amount of distal rectum at the anastomosis), maintains transanal defecation with reasonable continence, and provides a satisfactory quality of life without a permanent ileostomy. The main disadvantages of the procedure are frequent bowel movements (approximately five to seven per day), nocturnal fecal soilage (occasional in 55 percent of patients), and "pouchitis" (usually a transient inflammation of the pouch that responds to metronidazole).

The details of this operation include excision of the entire colon and proximal rectum, but only the diseased mucosa of the distal rectum and proximal anal canal is removed. Three centimeters of rectal muscularis, the pelvic floor, and the entire anal sphincter mechanism are preserved. Then 30 cm of terminal ileum is fashioned into a neorectum using either a J or S configuration (J is simpler; S has larger capacity and reaches the anus with less difficulty). Intestinal continuity is restored by connecting the pouch to the anal canal at the dentate line. A temporary ileostomy allows healing of the pouch and anastomosis and protects the patient from sepsis should an anastomotic leak

occur. After 2 or 3 months, integrity of the pouch, anastomosis, and sphincter mechanism is evaluated; if all is well, the ileostomy is closed, restoring intestinal continuity. The first 3 months after ileostomy closure can be difficult because of the frequent need to pass stool. The pouch capacity increases with time, and the need to empty the pouch can be reduced to an average of four or five times per day.

None of the surgical procedures for ulcerative colitis should prevent completion of normal pregnancy in women who have been cured of the disease. Even normal vaginal delivery is a possibility after any of the resective or restorative procedures.

Crohn's Disease

General Considerations

The diagnosis of Crohn's disease usually takes longer to establish than that for ulcerative colitis, possibly because of the nonspecific nature of the symptoms: diarrhea, abdominal pain, weight loss, and anal disease. The mean time from onset of symptoms to diagnosis is approximately 35 months.

Surgery for Crohn's disease is indicated only for the management of complications, not for cure of the disease, since recurrence is common. Surgery for Crohn's disease is preferably done as an elective procedure rather than waiting until severe complications make urgent surgical intervention necessary, increasing the risk of postoperative complications. The choice of surgical management for Crohn's disease must take into account the geographic distribution of the disease within the intestinal tract and the nature and severity of the complication requiring surgery.

The intensity of activity of the Crohn's disease may determine the type of complication that occurs and may affect the prognosis, including risk and rate of recurrence. Crohn's disease may be considered to have two phases of activity. The *acute* inflammatory process consists of intense inflammation of the involved intestine, deep ulceration into the bowel wall with possible perforation, phlegmon, or abscess, and adherent loops of bowel not involved with the primary disease. The *chronic* fibrotic phase of the disease exists for a longer period and results in narrowing and stricture formation. Any adjacent organs may be involved by the inflammatory process. Hydronephrosis of the right kidney can result from ileocolonic Crohn's disease causing partial occlusion of the ureter. The condition is relieved when the Crohn's disease is resected.

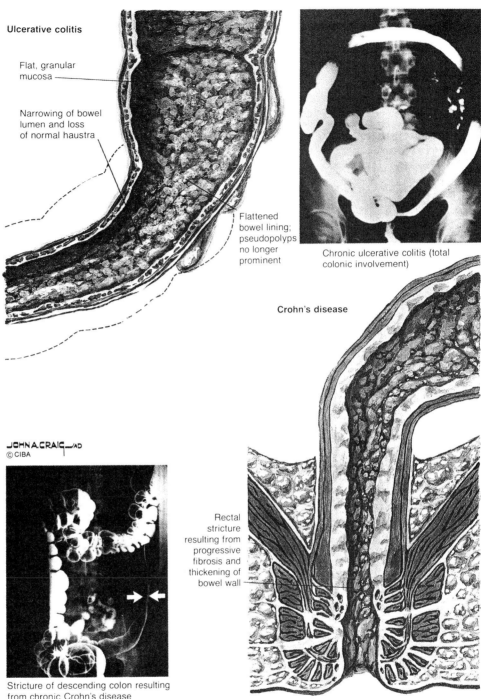

Ulcerative colitis

Flat, granular mucosa

Narrowing of bowel lumen and loss of normal haustra

Flattened bowel lining; pseudopolyps no longer prominent

Chronic ulcerative colitis (total colonic involvement)

Crohn's disease

Rectal stricture resulting from progressive fibrosis and thickening of bowel wall

JOHN A. CRAIG—AD
© CIBA

Stricture of descending colon resulting from chronic Crohn's disease

FIG. 26-49. Chronic inflammatory bowel disease. (From: *Kodner IJ, Fry RD: Inflammatory bowel disease. Ciba Clin Symp 34:1, 1982, with permission.*)

The surgeon should prepare the patient adequately so that a single operation will suffice to correct the complication requiring treatment. This often involves the use of anti-inflammatory medications, antibiotics, complete bowel rest (including parenteral nutritional support), and when indicated, percutaneous drainage of abscesses. The nutritional fitness of the patient undergoing surgical treatment probably contributes more to a favorable outcome than most other variables. By careful preoperative management, the surgeon can avoid operating on a phlegmon with resulting injury to normal, uninvolved intestine with the risk of postoperative disruption of the anastomosis and subsequent fis-

tula formation leading to the eventual creation of a short bowel syndrome.

Surgical Management

Surgical management of Crohn's disease involves resection of the diseased segment of intestine responsible for the complications requiring operation. The extent of resection usually encompasses intestine that is grossly involved with the disease. Recurrence of disease is not reduced by obtaining wide margins of uninvolved intestine or by verifying normal margins by frozen-section histology. The uninvolved margin of resection usu-

Table 26-7
The Medical Therapy of Ulcerative Colitis and Crohn's Disease

Sulfasalazine Indications
Ulcerative colitis
    Mild to moderate active disease
    Maintenance of remission
Crohn's disease
    Mild to moderate active disease
      (colitis > ileitis)
    Maintenance of remission not established
    No effect on postoperative recurrence
Pregnancy and nursing
    No adverse effect on pregnancy
    No teratogenicity
    No kernicterus
Metronidazole
Indications
    Crohn's ileocolitis and colitis
    ? Crohn's ileitis alone
    Perineal Crohn's disease
    Not effective in active ulcerative colitis
Toxic effects
    Nausea
    Anorexia
    Furry tongue, metallic taste
    Monilial infections
    Peripheral neuropathy
    ? Risk of malignancy

Corticosteroid Indications
Topical
    Proctitis and left-sided colitis
Oral
    Mild to moderate active ulcerative colitis and
      Crohn's disease
    No role as maintenance therapy
Parenteral
    Severe or toxic ulcerative colitis or Crohn's
      disease
Immunosuppressive Agents
Indications
    Ulcerative colitis
      Steroid sparing
      Refractory disease
    Crohn's disease
      Steroid sparing
      Fistulas
      Refractory disease
      Perineal disease
      Maintenance of remission
Toxic effects
    Rash and fever
    Bone marrow depression
    Pancreatitis
    Hepatitis
    ? Risk of malignancy
    ? Teratogenicity

SOURCE: Peppercorn MA: *The Medical Therapy of Ulcerative Colitis and Crohn's Disease.* New York, Elsevier Science Publishing, 1992, with permission.

ally can be detected by demonstrating a normal margin at the mesenteric-intestinal border. It is not necessary to include a large segment of mesentery in the resected tissue. If normal-appearing bowel remains after resection and there is not significant intra-abdominal infection, intestinal continuity can be restored by primary anastomosis. Should there be significant intraabdominal infection or intestine that is so severely inflamed that it cannot be removed safely, an intestinal stoma fashioned from bowel proximal to the inflamed intestine will allow the patient to resume eating and taking medication until the inflammatory process resolves and definitive surgical resection can be accomplished.

The symptoms requiring surgical resection depend on the geographic distribution of the disease.

Ileocolonic Crohn's Disease. As shown in Table 26-10, ileocolonic Crohn's disease presents with internal fistula and abscess formation as often as it does with intestinal obstruction. Here the surgical principle of draining an abscess and allowing a phlegmon to resolve becomes critically important. The timing of operation should be such that sepsis is controlled by total bowel rest and percutaneous drainage of abscesses before definitive resection is carried out. Usually intraabdominal abscesses associated with ileocolonic Crohn's disease can be drained percutaneously with the aid of guidance by CT. This allows definitive surgery after the inflammation has resolved, avoiding injury

Table 26-8
Criteria of Severity of Ulcerative Colitis

	Mild	*Moderate*	*Severe*
Stool frequency/24 h	<4	4–6	>6
Pulse (beats/min)	<90	90–100	>100
Hematocrit (%)	Normal	30–40	<30
Weight loss (%)	None	1–10	>10
Temperature (°C)	Normal	37.2–38.1	>38.1
ESR*(mm/h)	Normal	20–30	>30
Albumin (g/liter)	Normal	30–35	<30

*ESR = erythrocyte sedimentation rate

SOURCE: Kodner IJ, Fry RD, Fleshman JW: *Curr Opin Gastroenterol* 6:1990, Current Science, Ltd. with permission.

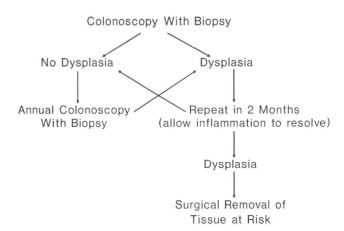

FIG. 26-50. Surveillance for extensive, chronic (8–10 years), mucosal ulcerative colitis.

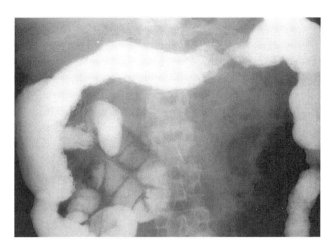

FIG. 26-51. Endophytic cancer of the transverse colon, typical of ulcerative colitis.

to noninvolved small intestine and other intraabdominal structures that may be involved secondarily by the inflammatory process. Drainage of such abscesses can lead to fistula formation because of the factors summarized in Table 26-11. For this reason, abscesses should be drained from locations on the abdominal wall that would be amenable to application of an appliance, as used for an intestinal stoma. This allows containment of the output even if it should be of high volume and potentially damaging to the abdominal skin.

Colonic Crohn's Disease. Patients with colonic Crohn's disease often require operation after a shorter duration of symptoms than is usual for patients with small intestinal or ileocolonic disease (see Table 26-10B). Colonic perforation can occur in patients with Crohn's disease and toxic colitis without the dilatation of the colon that is seen in patients with toxic ulcerative colitis. This is probably due to the thickening of the colonic wall,

which prevents dilatation; thus the term *toxic megacolon* is not usually appropriately applied in Crohn's colitis. The prognosis and risk of recurrence for Crohn's colitis depend significantly on the presence of simultaneous involvement of the small intestine. The surgical management depends somewhat on the presence and severity of rectal involvement. The risk of recurrence in Crohn's disease prohibits the use of the more sophisticated sphincter-preserving procedures described for ulcerative colitis and sometimes for familial polyposis.

The choices of surgical procedure for Crohn's colitis include abdominal-perineal proctocolectomy with a permanent end ileostomy, total abdominal colectomy with an end ileostomy (with retention of the rectal segment as a Hartmann's pouch), and total abdominal colectomy with ileorectal anastomosis (sometimes protected with a proximal loop ileostomy). The specific choice of surgical procedure is governed by the condition of the rectum and anal sphincter, as well as by the patient's metabolic and emotional status. The latter becomes an important factor because this disease, which frequently involves young adults, should not result in construction of a permanent stoma unless the individual can participate in the decision. A permanent ileostomy presents a change in body image; and although it can be life-preserving, the choice of a permanent stoma should be made by the patient, not by the parents or the physician. Since an ileostomy is not truly permanent until the rectum is removed, significant effort should be made to retain the rectum and preserve the hope of restoration until the patient realizes that the ileostomy is tolerable; the diseased rectum can interfere with long-term health and normal life activity. Recent reports indicate that the retained rectum, even for Crohn's disease, is at some increased risk of developing cancer. Therefore, surveillance of the rectal stump by regular endoscopy is necessary.

The patient presenting with *acute, catastrophic* Crohn's disease is so ill that urgent operation is often necessary. These patients should be managed as previously described for toxic ulcerative colitis. Intense medical treatment, including intravenous hyperalimentation and antibiotics, should be instituted.

Table 26-9
Comparison of Three Operations as Treatment for Ulcerative Colitis

1. *Proctocolectomy with Brooke ileostomy*

Advantages	Curative; one operation	
Disadvantages	Incontinence; external ileostomy appliances; need to empty 4–8 times per day	
Complications	Stoma revision	10%–25%
	Perineal wound problems	10%–25%
	Small bowel obstruction	10%–20%
	Bladder dysfunction	Minimal
	Sexual dysfunction	Minimal
Contraindications	None	

2. *Colectomy with ileorectal anastomosis*

Advantages	Sphincter unchanged; evacuation 2–4 times per day; no stoma, no bladder or sexual dysfunction
Disadvantages	Not curative; cancer risk persists; protectomy for cancer of disease in 5%–50%
Complications	Small bowel obstruction in 10%–20%; anastomotic leak with disease
Contraindications	Sphincter incontinence; severe rectal disease; rectal dysplasia; rectal cancer

3. *Total proctocolectomy with ileoanal anastomosis with pouch*

Advantages	Curative; continent
Disadvantages	Failure 10%; need to evacuate 4–8 times per day
Complications	Pouch fistulas; sepsis; stenosis; small bowel obstruction in 10%–20%; pouchitis; bladder dysfunction minimal; sexual dysfunction minimal; anal excoriation
Contraindications	Crohn's disease; diarrhea; rectal cancer in distal half

SOURCE: Kodner IJ, Fry RD, Fleshman JW: *Curr Opin Gastroenterol* 6:1990, Current Science, Ltd., with permission.

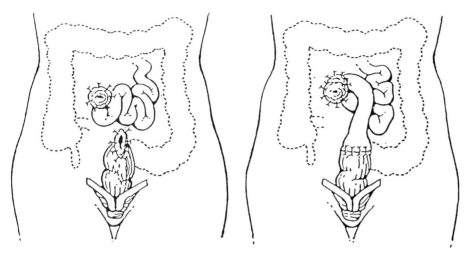

Abdominal colectomy and ileostomy
(rectum undisturbed)

Abdominal colectomy with
ileal-rectal anastomosis
(temporary ileostomy)

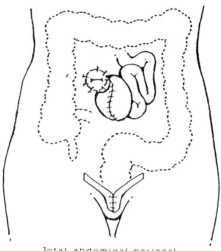

Total abdominal perineal
proctocolectomy with Koch
pouch (continent ileostomy)

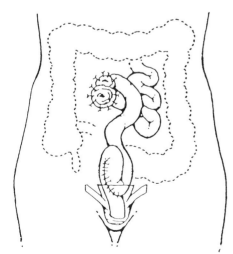

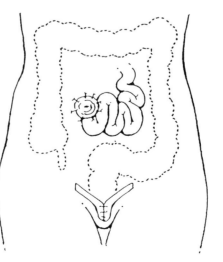

Total abdominal colectomy,
mucosal proctectomy, ileal
pouch anal anastomosis
(temporary ileostomy)

Total abdominal perineal
proctocolectomy (permanent
ileostomy)

FIG. 26-52. Surgical management of ulcerative colitis.

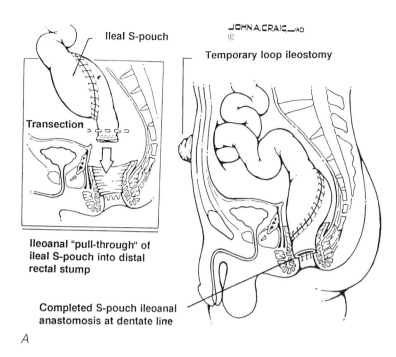

JOHN A. CRAIG. AD
©

Ileal S-pouch

Temporary loop ileostomy

Transection

Ileoanal "pull-through" of
ileal S-pouch into distal
rectal stump

Completed S-pouch ileoanal
anastomosis at dentate line

A

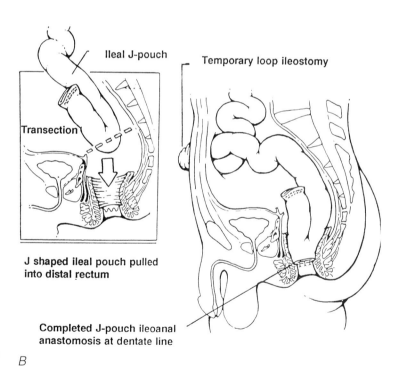

Ileal J-pouch

Temporary loop ileostomy

Transection

J shaped ileal pouch pulled
into distal rectum

Completed J-pouch ileoanal
anastomosis at dentate line

FIG. 26-53. *Ileoanal "pull-through" procedure. A. S-pouch.*
B. J-pouch.   *B*

Some patients revert to a more stable condition, but others require urgent surgical treatment. If peritoneal signs and the general status of the patient do not improve rapidly, operation is required. A site should be marked preoperatively for a possible ileostomy and, if the colon is massively dilated, for a possible decompressing transverse colostomy as well. Sigmoidoscopy should be done in the operating room, after induction of anesthesia, to determine the status of rectal disease.

At the time of operation, if a severely diseased intact colon is found, it should be removed along with any involved terminal ileum. If the rectum is uninvolved and the patient is stable, consideration can be given to constructing an ileorectal anastomosis. If the status of the rectum is questionable, an ileorectal anastomosis can be performed but should be protected with a proximal loop ileostomy. If the rectum is significantly diseased, it should be left in place, the colon removed, and an end ileostomy established. Once the patient achieves an adequate level of postoperative health and nutrition, the rectum can either be excised or incorporated in an ileorectal anastomosis. If the rectum is severely diseased, it is safer to make a formal mucous fistula than

Table 26-10
Indications for Surgical Treatment of Crohn's Disease

A. *Ileocolonic* Crohn's disease	
Internal fistulas and abscess	38%
Intestinal obstruction	37%
Perianal fistulas	15%
Poor response to medical therapy	6%
B. *Colonic* Crohn's disease	
Internal fistulas and abscesses	25%
Perianal disease	23%
Severe disease with poor response to medical therapy	21%
Toxic megacolon	19%
Intestinal obstruction	12%

SOURCE: Kodner IJ, Fry RD, Fleshman JW: Elsevier Science Publishing, New York, 1992, with permission.

to close the end of the rectum and leave it in place. This mucous fistula decreases the risk of rectal perforation. If a severely diseased colon with free perforation is found at the time of exploration, colectomy is necessary, but no anastomosis should be made. The abdominal cavity should be irrigated, and an end ileostomy should be constructed with the rectum left in place.

In rare situations, exploration will reveal a sealed-off perforation of the colon, usually in the region of the splenic flexure, with a tense, thin-walled colon. Resection in this situation is unsafe; the surgeon should treat this with a loop ileostomy and a "blowhole" decompressing colostomy, as described by the late Rupert Turnbull and his colleagues. This operation requires both diversion and decompression; neither component should be used by itself.

In a patient with *long-standing colonic Crohn's disease,* especially with severe anal or rectal involvement, a single-stage proctocolectomy and ileostomy may be done. The proctectomy should be done differently from that performed for cancer in order to preserve normal sexual function (Figs. 26-54 and 26-55).

Rarely, a colonic stricture can form in an isolated segment of Crohn's disease, causing obstructive symptoms. Resection of such a segment should be considered if the obstructive symptoms are significant. Colonoscopic dilation of strictures has been described in situations where surveillance of the proximal colon was not possible. Since the colon has no critical physiologic function, stricturoplasty to retain a colonic segment is seldom indicated; involved segments should be resected and intestinal continuity restored. Complete colectomy is the better procedure for extensive colonic disease.

Rectal Crohn's Disease. Crohn's disease can involve the rectum or the anus, either separately or simultaneously. It is critical to differentiate these anatomic distributions of Crohn's dis-

Table 26-11
Factors Preventing Spontaneous Closure of Fistulas

1. Distal obstruction
2. Loss of bowel continuity
3. Presence of intervening abscess
4. Infiltration of fistulous tract with cancer, Crohn's disease, or foreign material
5. Fusion of bowel mucosa with skin

ease. If a patient with rectal Crohn's disease has severe bleeding and tenesmus that cannot be relieved by medical management (including bowel rest with total parenteral nutrition), consideration should be given to removal of the rectum or at least temporary diversion with a colostomy or an ileostomy. Once the rectum has become so fibrotic that it has lost its reservoir function (see Fig. 26-49), proctectomy should be considered because of intolerably frequent, and sometimes poorly controlled, bowel movements. In the rare situation where only the rectum is involved with Crohn's disease, a completely diverting colostomy may allow the rectum to regain its functional capacity. This is especially important in the patient who has had previous small-bowel resections, when it becomes more important to preserve the water-absorbing capacity of the right colon. An end colostomy also may be considered for patients with colonic sparing but severe destructive anal or perineal Crohn's disease. In such cases, diversion may be needed to control sepsis or anal incontinence. If a colostomy is done in a patient with Crohn's disease, it should be constructed as a protruding spigot similar to that of an ileostomy.

The proctectomy in a patient with Crohn's disease should be performed by confining the rectal dissection to the immediate proximity of the rectum (see Figs. 26-54 and 26-55), but any fistulous tracts extending to the perineum should be radically debrided.

Certain precautions must be taken during proctectomy for IBD. The nerves to the genitalia and the urinary bladder lie in close approximation to the rectum (see Fig. 26-8). There is a significant incidence of injury to these nerves when a proctectomy is done for cancer, because some of the surrounding tissue must be included in the resection. For IBD, however, the dissection of the rectum need not involve adjacent tissue, and the dissection should be precisely on the rectal wall.

Another complication of removal of the rectum for IBD is nonhealing of the perineal wound, usually more of a problem in Crohn's disease than in ulcerative colitis. This can be avoided by preserving the external sphincter and levator muscles. The operation involves removal of the rectum from the perineal field and secure closure of the musculature, accompanied by drainage of the pelvis from above, as depicted in Fig. 26-55.

Another complication of proctectomy occurs in women when the ovaries, which are normally intraperitoneal structures, fall into the space formed by removal of the rectum. The peritoneum may reconstitute in a fashion that excludes the ovaries from the peritoneal cavity, in effect making them extraperitoneal organs (Fig. 26-56A). As ovulation occurs, large cystic structures can form in the pelvis, and the woman obviously has reduced fertility. This situation can be avoided by simply suturing the ovaries out of the pelvis after the rectum is removed (see Fig. 26-56B).

Anal and Perineal Crohn's Disease. Involvement of the anus occurs in 35 percent of all patients with Crohn's disease at some time during the course of their illness. Four percent of patients present with only anal disease as the first manifestation of Crohn's, but all go on to have other intestinal involvement. It is important to recognize the possibility of anal disease being secondary to the presence of Crohn's, because the surgical treatment should be much less radical than for non-Crohn's-related anal disease. Procedures such as excisional hemorrhoidectomy and extensive fistulotomy should be avoided because of the necessity of preserving anal sphincter function in a patient with

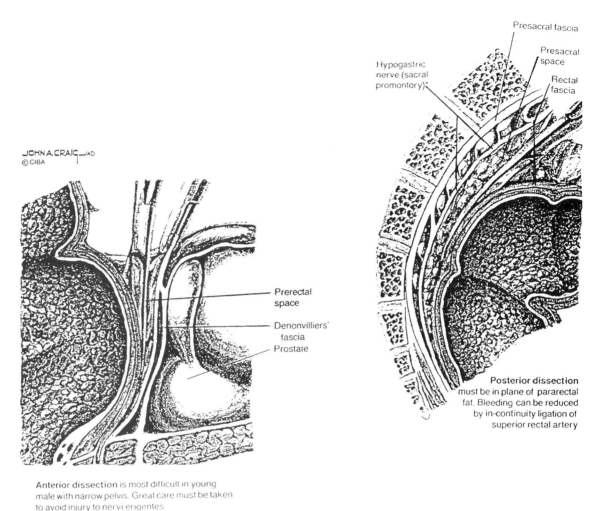

JOHN A.CRAIG—AD
©CIBA

Hypogastric nerve (sacral promontory)

Presacral fascia

Presacral space

Rectal fascia

Prerectal space

Denonvilliers' fascia

Prostate

Posterior dissection must be in plane of pararectal fat. Bleeding can be reduced by in-continuity ligation of superior rectal artery

Anterior dissection is most difficult in young male with narrow pelvis. Great care must be taken to avoid injury to nervi erigentes

Abdominal dissection of rectum is taken circumferentially to level of levator muscles to facilitate perineal phase of procedure

FIG. 26-54. Surgical removal of rectum for inflammatory bowel disease: abdominal phase. (From: *Kodner U, Fry RD: Inflammatory bowel disease. Ciba Clin Symp 34:1, 1982, with permission.*)

inflammatory bowel disease who is prone to have diarrhea and loss of rectal capacity. Of particular importance is preservation of the anterior aspect of the sphincter mechanism in a woman, in whom continuity of the sphincter muscle is maintained by only one band of external striated muscle. Through the use of conservative and often prolonged and tedious management of anal and perineal disease, very few patients with Crohn's disease require proctectomy because of the anal-perineal disease. This is especially important as more effective medical management becomes available. Conservative surgical drainage of septic processes and the use of intensive medical treatment allow preservation of the rectum and anal sphincter function and in many instances allow the Crohn's disease to go into remission so that the source of the sepsis can be resolved to one small internal opening, which can be closed with the endoanal sliding flap advancement technique (see Fig. 26-44). The medications most advantageous for treating anorectal Crohn's disease include (see Table 26-7) the antibiotic metronidazole, the anti-inflammatory

agents 5-aminosalicylic acid and cortisone (by enema or suppository), and such immunosuppressive agents as azathioprine (Imuran), 6-mercaptopurine (6-MP), and cyclosporine. The longterm effectiveness of the agents is difficult to evaluate because of the intermittent nature of the disease. This conservative management is not possible when severe destruction of the rectum exists. These patients often require eventual proctectomy because the loss of the reservoir capacity of the rectum is intolerable.

Anal Crohn's disease should be suspected when a patient presents with inflamed edematous tags (mistaken for external hemorrhoids), anal or perineal fistulas, or abscesses (Fig. 26-57). Often there are multiple abnormalities and poor healing after minor anal surgical procedures. Management of such a patient should begin with examination under anesthesia, including sigmoidoscopy, to determine the presence of disease within the rectum. The edematous skin tags can be removed if they are causing symptoms. This tissue has been shown to serve as a rich source

A. Dissection carried out in intersphincteric plane, preserving levators and external sphincters

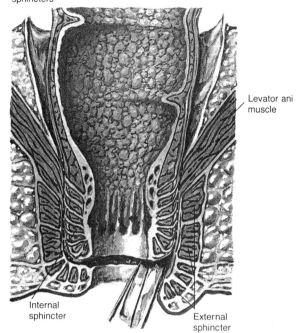

Levator ani muscle

Internal sphincter

External sphincter

B. Perineal wound closed in layers, with skin left open. Pelvis drained from above by sump system irrigation

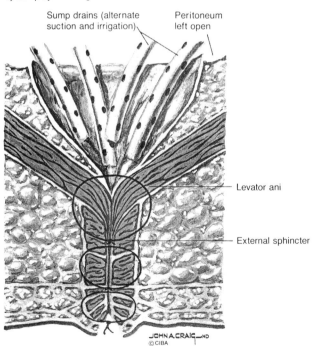

Sump drains (alternate suction and irrigation)

Peritoneum left open

Levator ani

External sphincter

JOHN A. CRAIG —MD
©CIBA

FIG. 26-55. Surgical removal of rectum for inflammatory bowel disease: perineal phase. (From: *Kodner IJ, Fry RD: Inflammatory bowel disease. Ciba Clin Symp 34:1, 1982, with permission.*)

for *granulomas,* which can help confirm the diagnosis of Crohn's disease. The objective of treatment then becomes the management and control of septic processes, in anticipation of

medical treatment to put the Crohn's disease into remission. This can be accomplished with mushroom-tipped catheters or unroofing of abscesses and with the use of setons to provide drainage of fistulous tracts. A superficial fistulotomy can be performed if the external sphincter mechanism is not involved. Special care must be observed for preservation of the anterior component of the sphincter mechanism in women. These conservative and tedious drainage processes may go on for years in an attempt to preserve the rectum. As part of this preservation, evaluation of the sphincter mechanism should be carried out, including manometry and electromyography. Intestinal continuity should never be restored to a poorly functioning anorectum or to one that is extensively destroyed. Such patients would do better with resection and a good intestinal stoma.

Outcome of Surgical Treatment of Crohn's Disease. The incidence of the need for operation and the development of recurrence in the postoperative period for a large series of patients with Crohn's disease, followed over a long period of time at the Cleveland Clinic Foundation, can be seen in Table 26-12. After the immediate perioperative period, the

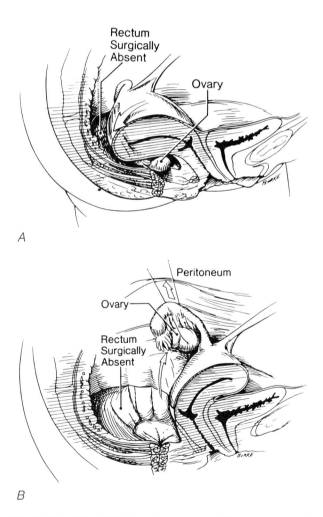

Rectum Surgically Absent

Ovary

A

Peritoneum

Ovary

Rectum Surgically Absent

B

FIG. 26-56. The entrapped ovary syndrome (A) occurs when the ovary falls into the retroperitoneal space after proctectomy and (B) is eliminated by the simple surgical technique of fixing the ovary to the lateral abdominal wall. (From: *Matthews JM, et al: 1986, with permission.*)

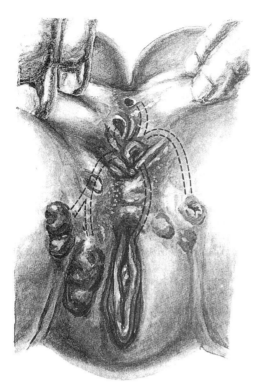

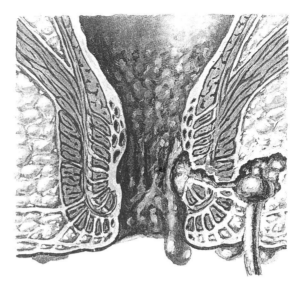

Abscess drained by
placing small mushroom
catheter as close to
anus as possible to
avoid subsequent long
fistula tract

Unusually located (often multiple) anal
fistulas, abscesses, ulcers and edematous
hemorrhoidal skin tags

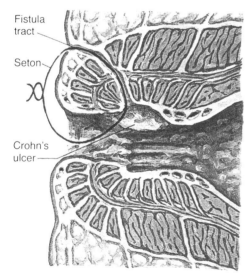

Fistula
tract

Seton

Crohn's
ulcer

JOHN A. CRAIG—AD
© CIBA

Seton left in place between internal
and external openings to prevent
abscess formation and further
destruction of sphincter mechanism

FIG. 26-57. Appearance and management of anorectal Crohn's disease.
(From: *Kodner U, Fry RD: Inflammatory bowel disease. Ciba Clin Symp 34:1,
1982, with permission.*)

major complication of Crohn's disease is the high rate of recurrence. Its true incidence can only be discovered by long-term observation of a large, carefully defined population. This series, originally reported by Farmer, attributed the risk of recurrence to the *pattern of initial presentation* of Crohn's disease within the intestinal tract, suggesting that ileocolonic Crohn's disease

had a higher recurrence rate. After 15 years, the rates of recurrence, based on patterns of presentation, converged. Thus the reliance on disease distribution to predict recurrence was no longer useful. Their series showed, in addition, that the rate of recurrence seemed to be biphasic, with the slope of the recurrence curve improving 8 years after surgery, suggesting that the

Table 26-12
Outcome of Surgical Treatment of Crohn's Disease*

	Initial Surgery Required	Subsequent Surgery Required	
		1st Recurrence	2nd Recurrence
Ileocolon	92%	53%	35%
Small intestine	66%	44%	38%
Colon/anorectum	58%	45%	34%

*Cleveland Clinic Series. Mean follow-up 13 years.

SOURCE: Kodner IJ, Fry RD, Fleshman JW: Elsevier Science Publishing, New York, 1992, with permission.

longer the patient lives without recurrence, the less likelihood there is of the disease presenting itself again. Both Farmer and Sachar, from another institution, presented statistics to indicate that the *severity* of the presenting symptoms was perhaps a better predictor of risk for severe complications and early, frequent recurrence of disease. Perforation and intense inflammatory changes as presenting symptoms, including severe anal or perineal disease, carried a much higher likelihood of postoperative recurrence than more indolent symptoms such as obstruction. We also have seen a more rapid as well as increased incidence of recurrence and a more severe intensity of disease in the African American population. Although Crohn's disease was initially said to exist primarily in the Jewish population and to spare blacks, we found that not only did African-Americans acquire Crohn's disease, but also a higher percentage required operation. There was also an increased requirement for second operations, and all of them had extraintestinal manifestations of Crohn's disease. Recent studies have suggested a relationship between the rate of recurrence and the immunologic status of the patient, showing a lower and slower recurrence rate in patients with ileocolonic resections who had the immunosuppressive effect of preoperative blood transfusions. The interpretation of this clinical finding is still not clear.

An important principle to which one must adhere is that the need for surgical management of a complication of Crohn's disease should not be ignored because of the risk of recurrence. In addition, the fact that one operation for resection of Crohn's disease is necessary does not increase the subsequent need for further surgery, nor does it mandate the eventual creation of a short bowel syndrome.

Ileostomy Construction and Management. An ileostomy can be constructed with different configurations, depending on the goal to be accomplished by its construction. A permanent ileostomy is usually constructed with the end of the ileum, and enough of the mesentery is preserved to allow adequate vascularization (Fig. 26-58). The stoma is everted on itself to prevent the serious problem of "ileostomy dysfunction" that historically led to severe fluid and electrolyte imbalance due to partial obstruction of the small intestine. This technique of eversion was described by Brooke and by Crile and Turnbull in 1954. A *loop* of ileum also may be used for construction of a stoma (Fig. 26-59). This leaves the mesentery intact and is usually constructed on a temporary basis to protect distal, precarious anastomoses or the new restorative procedures for maintaining anal continence, although these latter procedures are not indicated in patients with Crohn's disease because of the risk of recurrence.

A loop ileostomy can be constructed with the bowel in continuity or separated (Fig. 26-60).

The techniques of ileostomy construction are based on the fact that the output from an ileostomy is relatively high in volume, liquid in consistency, and contains active proteolytic enzymes. Thus a properly constructed ileostomy must be situated precisely on the abdominal wall at a site chosen carefully preoperatively with the patient in various positions (Fig. 26-61). The abdominal incision performed on patients for IBD should always preserve the right lower quadrant skin, even if the possibility of an ileostomy seems remote at the time of the operation. The ileostomy stoma must be constructed with a protruding spigot configuration to allow an appliance to seal perfectly to the skin (Fig. 26-62). An ileostomy stoma must have adequate blood supply, a goal not easy to accomplish, especially in the obese patient.

An individual with a well-constructed and properly located ileostomy should be able to empty the appliance four to six times a day and should not need to have complete change of the appliance more often than every 4 or 5 days. Neither belts nor supporting straps should be necessary, and the ostomate should be able to perform all routine activities (Table 26-13). The only true disability caused by a properly constructed ileostomy is a change in body image.

Long-term management of an ileostomy includes provision of adequate fluid replacement in hot weather, because the individual is at risk for rapid dehydration during periods of intense physical activity. Oral electrolyte-containing solutions are beneficial for this purpose. The ileostomy patient also should be advised to have available antidiarrheal agents for control of episodes of high output from the stoma. Large quantities of fibrous foods should be avoided, because they can cause blockage of the intestinal stoma (Fig. 26-63). If this occurs, the patient must be seen in the emergency room, where the ileostomy can be irrigated through a #24 Foley catheter inserted just below the fascia with 3 mL of saline in the balloon. Then 50 mL of warm saline is used to irrigate the stoma. The diagnosis of food blockage can be confirmed by the passage of particles of food after each irrigation. These patients often require intravenous fluids and nasogastric decompression to alleviate the severe cramps and dehydration that result from these episodes of small-intestinal obstruction. If the obstruction is not diagnosed as due to food blockage, other causes should be sought, and a water-soluble contrast study should be performed through the intestinal stoma. This can serve as a therapeutic as well as a diagnostic modality because of the cathartic action of the contrast solution. Digital inspection of an ileostomy is inappropriate, because the stoma is smaller than that of a colostomy, and insertion of a finger may be injurious.

A patient with a properly constructed ileostomy should have a normal life expectancy, assuming no malignant growth existed at the time of initial operation, and should anticipate no restrictions of normal life activity, with the exception of the extra time needed to provide meticulous care of the intestinal stoma.

NEOPLASTIC DISEASE

Etiology

Although the exact cause of colon and rectal cancer is not known precisely, recent laboratory work has provided a veritable explo-

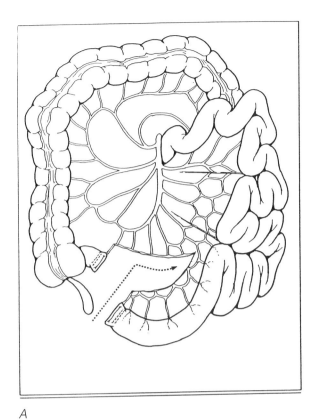

A

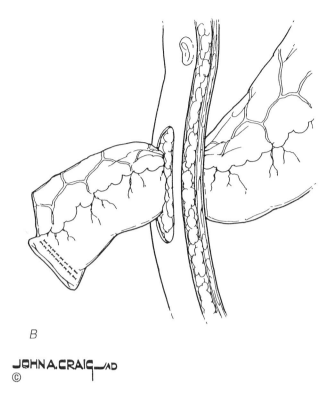

B

JOHN A. CRAIG AD
©

THREE POINT SUTURES
(FULL THICKNESS ILEUM-
ILEAL SEROSA - DERMIS)

C

FIG. 26-58. Construction of an end ileostomy. *A.* The distal arcade of vessels and some mesentery are preserved on the segment to be used for ileostomy construction. *B.* The closed ileum is pulled through the abdominal wall to a length of 6 cm. *C.* The spigot configuration is achieved by placing sutures to include the full thickness of the intestine, the seromuscular layer at the base of the stoma, and the dermis. (From: *Kodner IJ, et al: in MacDermott RP, et al: 1992, with permission.*)

sion in the understanding of the molecular basis of colorectal carcinogenesis. These advances have significantly altered many concepts about the development of cancer of the large bowel, and studies at the molecular level promise to radically alter colorectal cancer screening, diagnosis, treatment, and prognostication in the coming years. It is now recognized that colorectal cancer is a genetic disease, meaning that the cause of the uncontrolled proliferation of cells that we recognize as carcinoma resides in abnormalities or alterations in the genetic code. These genetic mutations may be in the germ line, in which case the disease is inherited, or somatic mutations in the genes may occur, which would result in the type of cancer that we usually have referred to as *sporadic*.

Genetic Predisposition

It has been estimated that approximately 10 to 15 percent of colorectal cancer is familial and that 1 person in 200 may carry high-risk alleles of the genes causing inherited colorectal cancer. It also is estimated that the same genes may be involved in as many as 15 percent of sporadic cancers.

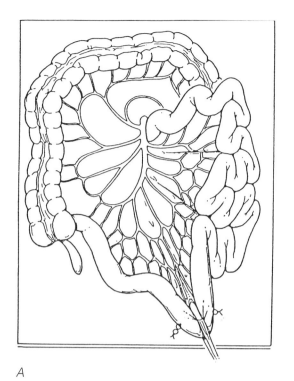

A

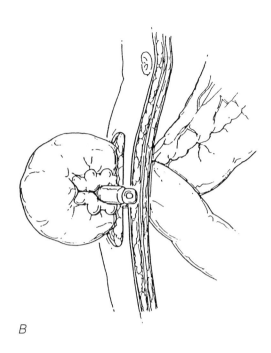

B

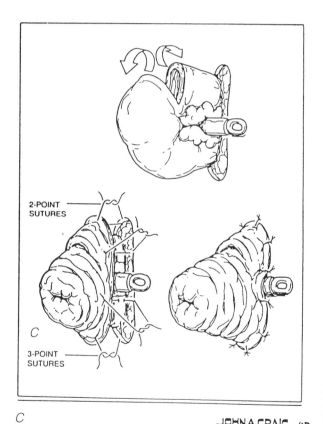

C

JOHN A. CRAIG — AD
©

FIG. 26-59. Construction of a loop ileostomy. *A.* Tracheostomy tape is placed at the segment for the intended ileostomy with sutures to identify proximal and distal limbs. *B.* The tape is replaced by a plastic rod. *C.* The spigot configuration is completed. (From: *Kodner U, et al: in MacDermott RP, et al: 1992, with permission.*)

Familial Adenomatous Polyposis. *Pathophysiology and Diagnosis.* Familial adenomatous polyposis (FAP) is the prototypical hereditary polyposis syndrome. It is an autosomal dominant disorder diagnosed when a patient has more than 100 adenomatous polyps in the large bowel or when a member of an FAP family has any number of colonic adenomas detected.

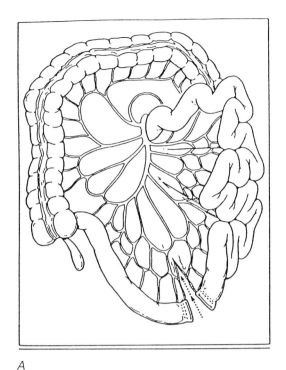

A

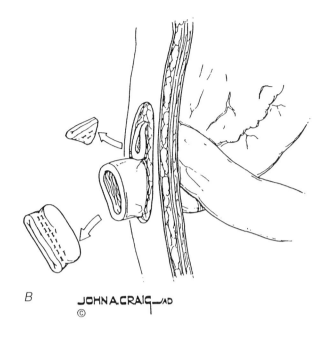

B

JOHN A. CRAIG—AD
©

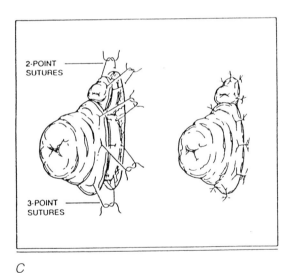

C

FIG. 26-60. Construction of a separated loop ileostomy. *A.* The distal ileum, but very little of the mesentery, is transected, using a linear-cutting staple device, in preparation for constructing the ileostomy. *B.* The entire staple line of the proximal component and a corner of the distal component are excised. *C.* The functioning spigot and nonfunctioning recessive opening are completed. (From: *Kodner IJ, et al: in MacDermott RP, et al: 1992, with permission.*)

FAP includes a spectrum of syndromes formerly defined by various extraintestinal manifestations. FAP also includes Gardner's syndrome (epidermal inclusion cysts, osteomas of bone, and colonic polyps) and Turcot's syndrome (colonic polyps and brain tumors). The genetic defect responsible for adenomatous polyposis has been detected on chromosome 5, near the q21 locus. The gene has been called the APC (adenomatous polyposis coli) gene. FAP occurs in anywhere from 1 in 8000 to 1 in 29,000 individuals. The common expression of the syndrome is the presence of multiple polyps in the colon and the associated extraintestinal manifestations, including epidermoid cysts, desmoid tumors in the abdomen, osteomas of the bones, and brain tumors (usually gliomas or medulloblastomas). The gene expression occurs in 100 percent of patients with the defect. Autosomal dominance results in expression in 50 percent of offspring. Between 10 and 20 percent of all patients with FAP appear to harbor the genetic defect as a result of spontaneous mutation. All patients with the defective gene will develop cancer of the colon if left untreated. The average age of discovery of a new patient with FAP is 29 years. The average age of a patient who is newly discovered to have colorectal cancer related to FAP is 39 years.

Two rare variants of FAP include *attenuated adenomatous polyposis coli* (AAPC) and *hereditary flat adenoma syndrome* (HFAS). AAPC patients have relatively few polyps but retain a high risk of colorectal cancer. Patients with HFAS develop small adenomas (usually less than 100) that are frequently dysplastic and prone to malignant transformation. One interesting marker for FAP is congenital hypertrophy of the retinal pigmented ep-

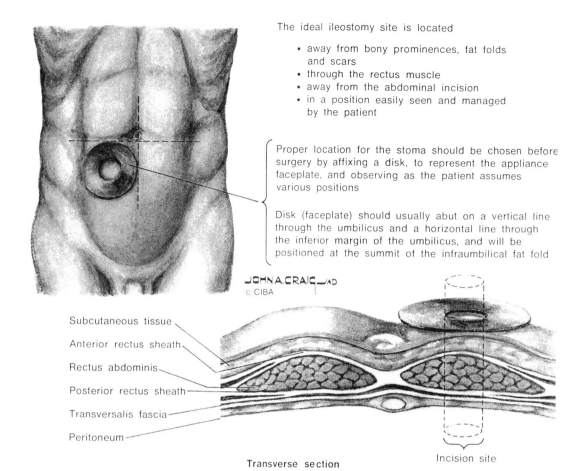

The ideal ileostomy site is located

- away from bony prominences, fat folds and scars
- through the rectus muscle
- away from the abdominal incision
- in a position easily seen and managed by the patient

Proper location for the stoma should be chosen before surgery by affixing a disk, to represent the appliance faceplate, and observing as the patient assumes various positions

Disk (faceplate) should usually abut on a vertical line through the umbilicus and a horizontal line through the inferior margin of the umbilicus, and will be positioned at the summit of the infraumbilical fat fold

JOHN A. CRAIG AD
c. CIBA

Subcutaneous tissue
Anterior rectus sheath
Rectus abdominis
Posterior rectus sheath
Transversalis fascia
Peritoneum

Transverse section

Incision site

FIG. 26-61. Location for ileostomy. (From: *Kodner U: Colostomy and ileostomy. Ciba Clin Symp 30:5, 1978. Copyright 1978. Ciba-Geigy Corporation. Reprinted with permission from Clinical Symposia; illustrated by John A. Craig, M.D. All rights reserved.*)

ithelium (CHRPE), which is seen on indirect ophthalmoscopy in approximately 70 to 80 percent of FAP patients.

Our understanding of the genetic basis for colorectal cancer has resulted in clinical applications for screening of patients in FAP kindreds by DNA analysis for the APC gene or its products in peripheral blood leukocytes. This test, which requires only venipuncture, has obvious advantages over the standard screening, which consists of an annual endoscopy. This is particularly useful for young patients for whom screening is indicated. A single negative blood test, showing the noninheritance of a mutated APC gene, suggests that the individual will not develop polyposis and may not require intensive screening. This depends on the genetic defect's being clearly identified by testing the blood of known involved members of the family. It is believed that occasional surveillance colonoscopy is still indicated.

Upper endoscopy should be used to screen for gastric and duodenal adenomas beginning at age 30, even though such polyps have been found in patients under 20 years of age. Prior to the development of genetic screening for the APC gene, young children were screened by ophthalmoscopic examination. If the patients were found to have an area of retinal pigmentation, the chances of developing colonic polyps approached 100 percent.

DNA analysis probably will replace the need for such screening procedures.

Surgical Management. Appropriate treatment for patients with FAP is removal of all colonic and rectal mucosa. Total proctocolectomy with permanent ileostomy accomplishes this goal, but the development of sphincter-saving procedures has virtually eliminated this operation as an acceptable form of therapy, unless the patient should have already developed a cancer of the distal rectum before operative treatment.

Total proctocolectomy with ileal reservoir and ileoanal anastomosis is the most commonly recommended operation for patients with FAP. The procedure must include a mucosectomy to the level of the dentate line to remove all mucosa at risk. Patients who undergo this procedure for FAP have a better functional result than patients similarly treated for ulcerative colitis, in that the incidence of inflammation in the ileal pouch (pouchitis) is much less in patients with familial polyposis. An alternative approach, total abdominal colectomy with ileorectal anastomosis, has been used successfully by several institutions. This latter approach was used extensively before the development of the technique of ileal pouch–anal anastomosis. The disadvantage of subtotal colectomy is that the precancerous rectum remains in

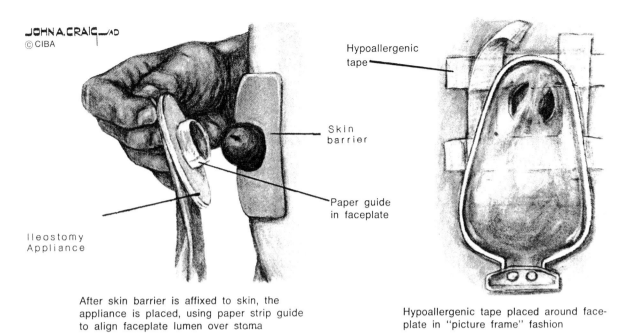

Hypoallergenic
tape

Skin
barrier

Paper guide
in faceplate

Ileostomy
Appliance

After skin barrier is affixed to skin, the
appliance is placed, using paper strip guide
to align faceplate lumen over stoma

Hypoallergenic tape placed around faceplate in "picture frame" fashion

FIG. 26-62. Components of ileostomy appliance. (From: *Kodner U: Colostomy and ileostomy. Ciba Clin Symp 30:5, 1978. Ciba-Geigy Corporation. Reprinted with permission from Clinical Symposia; illustrated by John A. Craig, M.D. All rights reserved.*)

situ, and repeated endoscopic procedures are needed every 6 months to detect and eradicate (by fulguration or snare excision) any adenomatous polyps that appear in the rectum. The early fears of unacceptable incontinence, intractable diarrhea, and impotence in men that might accompany proctocolectomy with ileal pouch–anal anastomosis, thus making subtotal colectomy with ileorectal anastomosis the preferred procedure, have not been confirmed.

FAP patients treated by proctocolectomy of any type remain at risk of death from upper gastrointestinal cancer. In one series this risk was greater than the risk of death from cancer in the residual rectum after total abdominal colectomy and ileorectal anastomosis. These patients require continued periodic surveillance by gastroduodenoscopy.

Extracolonic Manifestations. Some patients with FAP develop epidermoid cysts, osteomas, desmoids, and upper gastrointestinal neoplasms (Gardner's syndrome). The epidermoid

cysts require no treatment unless they become symptomatic or cause significant cosmetic deformities. It is extremely rare for osteosarcomas to arise from osteomas in patients with FAP. The intraabdominal *desmoid* is probably the only incapacitating, lethal extraintestinal manifestation. After surgical procedures, dense fibrous tissue forms in the mesentery of the small intestine and encroaches on the vascular supply, tethers the small intestine, and causes obstruction or ischemia. Treatment has been attempted with chemotherapy, radiation, tamoxifen, and sulindac. Operative therapy is completely inadequate and should be reserved only for decompression of obstruction or to relieve incapacitating symptoms. Sulindac has been reported to cause tumor regression in some patients with desmoid tumors.

Upper gastrointestinal neoplasms in patients with FAP (Gardner's syndrome) include duodenal or ampullary adenomas, which are premalignant, and hyperplastic fundic polyps in the stomach, which do not become malignant. The current recom-

Table 26-13
Return to Preillness Activities*

| | Ileostomates | | | Colostomates |
| | Cancer (329 patients) % | Ulcerative Colitis (4360 patients) % | Crohn's Disease (1088 patients) % | Cancer (5739 patients) % |
Activity				
Household	79	89	90	79
Vocation	56	70	65	43
Social	85	92	90	83
Sexual	52	77	75	41

*Based on figures from United Ostomy Association Ostomy Data Registry.

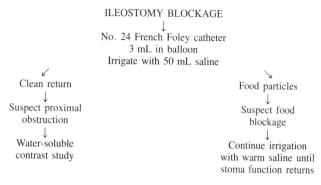

FIG. 26-63. *Management of the patient who presents with cessation of ileostomy function and symptoms of intestinal obstruction. (From: Kodner IJ: in Fazio VW: 1989, with permission.)*

mendation is for upper gastrointestinal surveillance after the age of 30 and endoscopic polypectomy, if possible, to remove all large adenomas within the duodenum. If an ampullary cancer is discovered at an early stage, pancreatoduodenectomy (Whipple procedure) is indicated.

Turcot's syndrome (colonic polyps and intracranial gliomas or medulloblastomas) is very rare, with only 50 patients reported in the literature. Patients with Turcot's syndrome usually die at an early age, before developing colonic polyposis and before having children.

Hereditary Nonpolyposis Colorectal Cancer. Aldred S. Warthin first recognized an increased incidence of cancer in certain families in 1913. One family characterized by Warthin became the prototype of cancer families. This family was afflicted by an excess of uterine and gastric cancers. The family was evaluated four times in the past 80 years, and a predominance of colorectal cancers has been detected in family members. A half century after Warthin's observations, Henry Lynch collected data that accurately characterized these cancer-prone families. Colorectal cancer is the most predominant cancer in this syndrome, but it is not associated with multiple polyps, which characterize familial polyposis. For this reason, the syndrome was named *hereditary nonpolyposis colorectal cancer* (HNPCC). In 1984 the terms *Lynch syndrome I and II* were proposed to indicate two apparently distinct clinical presentations. In Lynch syndrome I, the cancer usually occurs in the proximal colon, is site-specific within an affected family, and is the only type of tumor these patients develop. Lynch syndrome II is characterized by development of colorectal, endometrial, gastric, upper urinary tract, ovarian, and other types of cancer.

There are no phenotypic markers for HNPCC, so a standard clinical definition of the syndrome is necessary. The most widely accepted definition uses the *Amsterdam criteria,* which require (1) at least three relatives with histologically verified colorectal cancer, one of which is a first-degree relative of another, (2) involvement of a least two generations, and (3) at least one colorectal cancer diagnosed before the age of 50 years. HNPCC is characterized by an autosomal dominant inheritance pattern, an early age of colorectal cancer development, a predominance of right-sided cancers, and a tendency toward the development of synchronous and metachronous cancers.

Molecular scientists recognized widespread genetic instability in most cancers studied in patients with HNPCC, and for this reason, a DNA "mutator" gene was suspected as playing a carcinogenic role. The particular genetic instability in tumors from patients with HNPCC is characterized by variations in length of "microsatellite" DNA, which are short repetitive DNA sequences located throughout the genome. While microsatellites vary in length among individuals (a fact used in forensic DNA "fingerprinting"), they should be the same in all cells from a single individual. HNPCC tumors have microsatellites that differ in length from the normal cells of the same individual, indicating a loss of fidelity in DNA repair. This defect in the DNA repair process has been referred to as a *replication error* (RER). To date, four mismatch repair genes have been identified, and these are responsible for the majority of, but not all, HNPCC cancers. These genes are *hMSH2*, located on chromosome 2p; *hMLH1*, located on chromosome 3p; *hPMS1*, on chromosome 2q; and *hPMS2* on chromosome 7p.

The cancers that arise in patients with HNPCC are more often poorly differentiated and mucin-producing than sporadic colorectal cancer. "Signet ring" cancers are also more common in HNPCC tumors. Despite these findings, which are usually associated with a poor prognosis, the prognosis for patients with HNPCC is more favorable than that of patients with sporadic colorectal cancer of the same pathologic stage. Approximately 20 percent of HNPCC patients with colon cancer will have a synchronous cancer, and about 25 percent will develop a metachronous cancer of the remaining colon. It is recommended that patients with this syndrome be treated with subtotal colectomy.

Colorectal cancers arising in HNPCC patients develop through a typical adenoma-carcinoma progression. The hypermutable cancer may accelerate the time frame in which malignancy occurs. The optimal intervals for surveillance in this disease have not yet been ascertained. Because most of the tumors will occur in the proximal colon, flexible sigmoidoscopy is not an effective screening approach. A 3-year interval of screening significantly reduces the incidence of colorectal cancer, but surveillance intervals of 1 or 2 years may be more appropriate for this syndrome. There has been no significant study on the impact of any diagnostic screening to prevent the development of upper gastrointestinal tract cancers or gynecologic cancers.

Assays undoubtedly will become available that identify mismatch repair gene mutations in suspected HNPCC kindreds. This advance will be of practical and theoretical importance: practical, to identify gene carriers in a given HNPCC kindred, and theoretical, because HNPCC kindreds are currently defined by family history alone, which may be incomplete or misleading. Individuals may carry the disease trait but not fulfill the current clinical criteria. Future definitions of HNPCC will be based on genetic analysis rather than on family history alone.

Acquired Somatic Defects. The chromosome defect in FAP is a germ cell line defect and is present from birth. The majority of patients with colorectal cancer have no inherited component, and the initiating genetic mutation that causes neoplastic growth occurs in a single cell or in a group of mucosal cells. These tumors are not inherited, but there may be a familial predisposition to their development. Lynch has shown that the risk for developing colorectal cancer is increased threefold to ninefold if one or more first-degree relatives have had colorectal cancer.

Available evidence suggests that adenomas of the colon develop after such a gene mutation. The adenomatous tissue contains crypt cells with atypical genetic expression. Tumor formation may be the result of more than one mutation. A *somatic* mutation, associated with an *inherited* mutation, may be expressed as the adenoma or tumor progresses. The inherited mutation is felt to be tumorigenic but may not be expressed or detectable in the tumor. Fearon and Vogelstein have proposed that, once the adenoma has developed, a second mutation may be required to change the adenoma to a cancer. A progression of mutations actually can occur in the course of the development of a malignancy. Oncogenes function by initiating events that result in abnormal cellular growth and the development of tumors. For example, the *ras* gene family has been found in 50 percent of colorectal cancers and in adenomas larger than 1 cm, but it has been found in less than 10 percent of adenomas smaller than 1 cm.

As a tumor develops, subsequent mutation can result in the deletion of suppressor genes. This loss usually occurs on chromosomes 17, 18, and 5. For example, the p53 gene is absent from chromosome 17 in 85 percent of colorectal cancers. The chromosome 5 MCC gene (mutated colorectal cancer) is found in some tumors in patients with nonpolyposis cancers. The chromosome 18 DCC gene (deleted in colorectal cancer) is found in more than 70 percent of colorectal cancers. These mutations are postulated to affect cell-to-cell relationships in all tumors and thereby also affect the development of metastases.

Fearon and Vogelstein have proposed a model for genetic changes leading to colorectal cancer (Fig. 26-64). First, a mutational *activation* is initiated by oncogenes. This mutational activation is accompanied by a mutational *inactivation* of multiple suppressor genes. The mutations allow uncontrolled growth in varying degrees. More mutations are required for the development of cancer than for the development of benign polyps. The progression of cellular changes from normal mucosa to adenoma to cancer could be related to a progression of mutations over time.

Environmental Factors

Diet. Diet has been proposed as a significant etiologic factor in the development of colorectal cancer. Fats have been suggested to be toxic to the colonic mucosa. Diets high in oleic acid (found in olive oil, coconut oil, and fish oil) cause no increase in cancer in animals. The monounsaturated fatty acids (omega-3 and omega-6 fatty acids) appear to be less carcinogenic than polyunsaturated or saturated fats. Epidemiologic studies of populations that consume less than 5 percent of their diet as fat have shown a lower incidence of colorectal cancer, whereas those having diets with 20 percent of their fat as either corn oil or safflower oil have an increase in cancer. Therefore, it appears that unsaturated animal fats and highly saturated vegetable oils may cause some event to occur in the colonic mucosa that stimulates the development of colorectal cancer.

Some studies suggest that certain elements of the diet protect against the development of neoplasia. Selenium, dithiothiones, thioethers, terpenes, and carotenoids might act as "anticarcinogens" by reducing free oxygen radicals in the colon at the mucosal surface. An increase in dietary fiber may lower the incidence of cancer in patients who have a high-fat diet. An increase in fat, however, can negate the beneficial effect of the fiber. A high-fiber, low-fat diet has been described as better protection

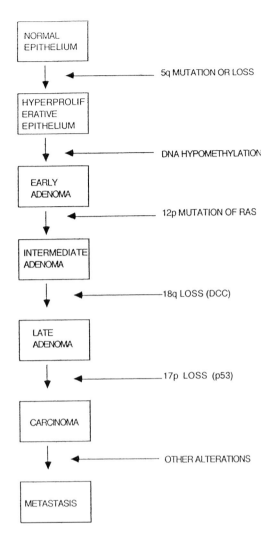

FIG. 26-64. A genetic model for colorectal tumorigenesis. Tumorigenesis proceeds through a series of genetic alterations involving oncogenes (*ras*) and tumor suppressor genes (particularly those on chromosomes 5q, 17p, and 18q). Allelic deletions of chromosome 17p and 18q usually occur at a later stage of tumorigenesis than do deletions of chromosome 5q or *ras* gene mutations. However, the order of these changes is not invariant, and accumulation of these changes, rather than their order with respect to one another, seems most important. Tumors continue to progress once carcinomas have formed, and the accumulated loss of suppressor genes on additional chromosomes correlates with the ability of the carcinomas to metastasize and cause death. (From: *Fearon ER, Vogelstein B: 1990. Copyright by Cell Press, with permission.*)

against neoplasia than a fat-free diet. An increase in bulk also tends to dilute carcinogens, shorten colonic transit time, and as a result, decrease the growth of harmful bacteria. So far, controlled trials have shown little relationship between dietary fiber and colon cancer, but the studies used a relatively low dose of fiber.

The National Research Council established interim guidelines for diet recommendations in 1982 until definitive studies could be performed. These recommendations included

1. Decrease fat in the diet from 40 to 30 percent of total calories.
2. Increase consumption of fiber-containing foods.
3. Limit salt-cured, pickled, and smoked foods.

4. Limit food additives shown to be potential carcinogens.
5. Establish research protocols for detection of mutagens in foods.
6. Limit alcohol consumption.

Epidemiologic studies indicate that diet has a role in the development of colon cancer. People in less-industrialized nations are noted to have a low incidence of colorectal cancers. These people have fewer processed foods and more natural fiber in their diets. People from these countries who immigrate to the industrialized United States or United Kingdom acquire the high risk of colon cancer found in these countries.

Exposure to Carcinogens. No clear relationship has been established between specific carcinogens and colorectal cancer, but potential agents currently under investigation include bile acids (such as chenodeoxycholic acid), food additives, alcohol, and ionizing radiation. Each of these may function as a promoter of mutational changes in the colonic mucosa, but none has been clearly shown to have a carcinogenic effect. Oxygen free radicals, which are unstable by-products of oxygen metabolism, may serve as promoters or chemical stimulants to the development of altered gene expressions. This is not a true carcinogenic effect but the creation of a "milieu" that predisposes to the development of mutations.

Premalignant Conditions

Ulcerative Colitis. The overall incidence of neoplasia in patients with pancolitis is 1 percent per year after 10 years; so the cumulative risk of a cancer is 10 percent by 20 years' duration of disease. Dysplasia identified in the colonic mucosa by repeated colonoscopic biopsies has been shown to be a precursor of cancer. The cancers tend to be more advanced because they are difficult to detect at an early stage. Approximately 35 percent are Dukes' C or D lesions. There is a controversy over the implication of adenomatous polyps found in patients with chronic ulcerative colitis. The question arises as to whether this represents dysplasia and is an indication for total colectomy or whether this is a benign polyp arising from inflamed mucosa.

The most effective method for preventing colon cancer in patients with ulcerative colitis is to remove the colon once dysplasia has been identified. The risk of cancer in the presence of dysplasia is approximately 30 percent.

Crohn's Disease. The overall incidence of cancer occurring in patients with Crohn's disease is approximately 7 percent over 20 years. Most of the intestinal cancers were found in the excluded segments of patients treated by segmental bypass. This procedure is no longer recommended because of a 20 percent incidence of adenocarcinoma and persistent disease in these bypassed segments. Patients with colonic strictures have a slightly higher incidence of adenocarcinoma at the site of the fibrotic narrowing. Reports of adenocarcinoma arising at the site of stricturoplasty in the small intestine have made it apparent that there is a risk of adenocarcinoma in these lesions. For this reason, a biopsy of the intestinal wall should be performed at the time of stricturoplasty. There also have been reports of squamous cell cancer and adenocarcinoma arising in chronic fistulas (especially of the anus and perineum) in patients with Crohn's disease. Overall, the risk for neoplasia in patients with Crohn's disease is only slightly higher than that of the general population and is certainly lower than in patients with ulcerative colitis or familial adenomatous polyposis.

Detection

Tests for Occult Blood

A colorless phenol in guaiac gum is converted to a blue quinone by oxidation. The reaction relies on the presence of a peroxidase catalyst. Oxidation is accomplished by the addition of hydrogen peroxide in the presence of a catalyst, such as hemoglobin. Unfortunately, there are other catalysts in the diet. Careful elimination of some of these products may be necessary to improve the accuracy of the test. Red meat, some vegetables, and other intrinsic peroxidases may cause the reaction in the absence of hemoglobin. The guaiac occult blood test will detect 20 mg of hemoglobin per gram of stool or 20 mL/day.

An immunofluorescent test for occult blood relies on the conversion of hemoglobin to fluorescent porphyrins and detects between 5 and 10 mg of hemoglobin per gram of stool. The false-positive rate is prohibitively high.

There are inherent problems in using the detection of occult blood as a screening test for colorectal cancer. Other sources of bleeding may produce positive tests, or the test may be too sensitive for blood. Cancers might bleed only intermittently or not at all, and the occult blood test may be falsely negative. Test processing, dietary manipulation, ingestion of gastrointestinal irritants (aspirin), the number of tests, and the interval of testing all affect the accuracy of the occult blood screening process.

There have been numerous uncontrolled studies of occult blood testing for screening populations for colorectal cancer. These reports usually show 2 to 6 percent positive tests. The positive predictive value for cancer in these studies has been 2 to 5 percent, and the positive predictive values for a polyp in these studies has been close to 20 percent. Cancer has been detected in 0.03 to 0.2 percent of all tested subjects, and polyps have been found in 0.6 percent.

The results of screening 46,000 individuals for occult blood using the guaiac test revealed a sensitivity of 89.3 percent, a specificity of 92.7 percent, and a positive predictive value for cancer of 2.5 percent. Long-term follow-up results from a University of Minnesota study showed an increase in more advanced lesions B and C in the control group, which translates to a decrease in mortality for the screened group. The cost-effectiveness of the test for occult blood as a screening tool is questionable. False-positive tests result in expensive evaluations to rule out real disease. False-negative tests result in patients presenting with a more advanced lesion that ultimately may cause more expensive, radical treatment.

Diagnosis

Rectal Examination. The digital rectal examination can reach approximately 8 cm above the dentate line. It was long believed that 50 percent of colorectal cancers were within the reach of the finger. It has been shown that almost 50 percent of all colorectal cancers and polyps will occur proximal to the splenic flexure. The digital rectal examination remains an important tool in the detection of colorectal cancer and should not be abandoned. Twenty percent of colorectal cancers can be palpated and their degree of fixation to surrounding tissue evaluated.

Proctosigmoidoscopy. Rigid proctosigmoidoscopy uses a lighted tube 2 cm in diameter and 20 to 25 cm long. The examination usually reaches 20 to 25 cm from the dentate line, but the acute angulation of the rectosigmoid junction can prevent complete insertion of the instrument. This examination should detect 20 to 25 percent of colorectal tumors. Rigid proctosigmoidoscopy is safe and effective for screening low-risk adults under 40 years of age when combined with evaluation of the stool for occult blood. The endoscopist must remember to follow the contour of the rectum, advancing the scope only when the lumen can be seen. An enema is sometimes used to prep the patient before the examination.

Flexible Sigmoidoscopy. The flexible sigmoidoscope is a fiberoptic or video scope that measures 60 cm in length and should reach the proximal left colon or even the splenic flexure in most patients (and will identify 50 percent of colorectal cancers). The patient does not need a complete bowel prep because the left colon can be cleansed by one or two small enemas. The flexible sigmoidoscope should not be used for therapeutic polypectomy, cautery, and the like, except in special circumstances, such as after an ileorectal anastomosis. Polypectomy or biopsy using electrocautery in unprepped colon can be disastrous if an explosion of colonic methane gas occurs or perforation allows leakage of feces into the peritoneal cavity.

Flexible sigmoidoscopy every 5 years beginning at age 50 is the current endoscopic screening method recommended for asymptomatic persons at average risk for colorectal carcinoma. An adenomatous polyp found on flexible sigmoidoscopy is an indication for colonoscopy, because even small (<10 mm) adenomas in the distal colon are associated with aggressive neoplasms in the proximal colon in 6 to 10 percent of patients.

Contrast Studies. The most commonly used contrast study to detect colorectal cancer is the air-contrast barium enema. An air-contrast (double-contrast) barium enema has been found to be 90 percent sensitive in detecting polyps larger than 1 cm. The air-contrast barium enema, in conjunction with the flexible sigmoidoscope, has been suggested as a cost-effective alternative to colonoscopy for patients who do not tolerate colonoscopy or for use on an alternating basis with colonoscopy for long-term follow-up in patients who have had a previous polyp or cancer excised. The risk of perforation of the colon by barium enema is low (less than 0.02 percent). If perforation is a possibility, water-soluble contrast should be used rather than barium. Barium peritonitis is a disastrous complication that causes severe infection and subsequent intraperitoneal fibrosis. The patient usually requires an emergency operation to clear the barium from the abdomen and construction of a colostomy to protect the repair of the perforation. Water-soluble contrast material unfortunately does not provide the necessary detail for detecting small colonic mucosal lesions.

Colonoscopy. Colonoscopy allows visualization of the mucosa of the entire colon and rectum and usually the terminal ileum. Colonoscopy originally depended on flexible fiberoptics as the source of the imaging. New technology has allowed a video camera to be placed at the tip of the flexible colonoscope, allowing greater flexibility and better resolution of image. The standard colonoscope is 160 cm in length. Colonoscopy is the most accurate method of detecting polyps less than 1 cm in diameter. It also allows biopsy, polypectomy, control of hemorrhage, and dilation of strictures. Adequate colonoscopy includes good patient compliance, good bowel preparation, patient sedation in most cases, and monitoring of vital signs and blood oxygenation. Colonoscopy is a safe procedure, and major com-

plications (including bleeding, anesthetic complications, and perforation) should occur in less than 0.2 percent of patients. Colonoscopy is useful in the diagnosis and management of inflammatory bowel disease, nonacute diverticulitis, sigmoid volvulus, gastrointestinal bleeding, nontoxic megacolon, colonic foreign body, colonic strictures, neoplastic disease, and unexplained diarrhea.

Complications after colonoscopy are more frequent after therapeutic colonoscopy (polypectomy, stricture dilation, control of hemorrhage) than after diagnostic colonoscopy. The most common complications of diagnostic or therapeutic colonoscopy are related to the use of conscious sedation. The most common major complication after therapeutic colonoscopy is hemorrhage after polypectomy (up to 3 percent). Postpolypectomy hemorrhage may occur immediately, in which case local measures are appropriate for control (epinephrine injection at bleeding site, electrocautery, resnaring polyp stalk). Management of delayed hemorrhage requires colonoscopy or angiography if the patient is bleeding massively. The source is usually arterial when the eschar separates from the polypectomy site. The majority of patients stop bleeding spontaneously, but colonoscopic measures or vasopressin via arteriogram catheter may be required if bleeding persists. Perforation is the most common major complication after diagnostic colonoscopy and is associated with free intraperitoneal air, abdominal pain, and variable degrees of peritoneal signs depending on the contamination of the abdominal cavity. A patient who develops free air without peritonitis and minimal contamination of the abdomen may be observed closely and treated with bowel rest, antibiotics, and intravenous fluids. The presence of (or progression to) diffuse peritonitis indicates the need for exploration. Depending on the size of the perforation, degree of contamination, and status of the patient, the patient may be treated with colectomy with primary anastomosis (plus or minus proximal diverting stoma), colectomy with colostomy and mucous fistula or Hartmann stump, or debridement and closure of the perforation.

Imaging Techniques. As technology progresses, more sophisticated imaging techniques are becoming available. CT, MRI, positron-emission tomographic (PET) scan, and transrectal ultrasonography are specific imaging techniques and not screening tests. They are important in the evaluation, staging, and follow-up of patients with colorectal cancer. They are used to evaluate primary cancers and their potential metastases to adjacent or distant organs.

Computed Tomography. Computed tomography (CT) allows preoperative evaluation of the abdominal cavity in patients with colorectal cancer. The CT scan can identify metastases to the liver, adrenal gland, ovary, lymph nodes, and other organs in the pelvis, and it can verify the integrity of the urinary tract because intravenous contrast material is excreted by the kidney. The CT scan is useful in searching for recurrent or residual cancer in patients with an elevated carcinoembryonic antigen (CEA) level after surgery for colorectal cancer. A combined angiogram and CT scan with dynamic imaging (scan during arterial injection of contrast material) is useful to evaluate the vascular anatomy of the liver and to accurately identify all possible metastases in the liver. The sensitivity of the angio-CT is approximately 95 percent.

The CT scan plays a special role in patients with rectal cancer because of the difficulty in staging the lesion preoperatively.

Treatment options other than total rectal excision are available for selected patients with favorable lesions, as will be discussed in the section on rectal cancer. Sphincter-saving operations and local therapy may be appropriate if the tumor has not invaded deeply or metastasized to regional lymph nodes. Pelvic CT scanning documents rectal wall invasion by the tumor with a 60 to 90 percent accuracy and detects lymph nodes larger than 1 cm in 75 percent of patients.

Magnetic Resonance Imaging. Magnetic resonance imaging (MRI) is a relatively new technique for evaluating colorectal cancer. Axial and sagittal views can be used to detail anatomy. T_1- and T_2-weighted images facilitate the differentiation of cancer from normal tissue and fibrotic scar. A coil placed in the rectum allows enlarged, detailed images of the rectum that may facilitate staging of rectal cancer. MRI is a lengthy study that requires the patient to lie quietly in a small tunnel, causing patients with claustrophobia to dislike the technique. The test does not require the use of contrast material. Early experience suggests that MRI offers little or no advantages over CT in the preoperative evaluation of patients with colorectal cancer. MRI is more specific for tumor in the liver than CT scanning and is frequently used to clarify a questionable lesion seen on CT scan. Because it is more sensitive than the CT scan, it is also used to identify other liver metastases when a liver resection is contemplated.

Positron-Emission Tomography. Positron-emission tomography (PET) is still investigational but eventually may be most helpful in evaluating recurrent tumor in the pelvis where scar formation is very dense. The PET scan detects differences in tissue metabolism using an injected substrate, fluorodeoxyglucose. Scar and recurrent tumor appear essentially the same on CT. The PET scan, however, will show an increase in metabolism in an area of cancer. Positron emission is greatest in hypermetabolic tissue such as tumors.

The major advantage of the PET scan may be to identify extrahepatic or intraperitoneal disease before performing a liver resection for metastasis or wide radical resection of local recurrence. This reduces unnecessary surgery and improves the selection of patients who will benefit from resection of recurrent or metastatic disease (Fig. 26-65).

Transrectal Ultrasound. Transrectal ultrasonography or endosonography of the rectum is useful for staging rectal cancer. There is no radiation risk, and the procedure takes little time and can be directed to the upper rectum using a modified proctoscope. The ultrasound image allows clear delineation of the layers of the rectal wall and, as a result, a very accurate definition of the depth of invasion of the tumor into the bowel wall: Stage T1=limited to mucosa and submucosa; Stage T2=limited to muscularis propria; Stage T3=through the entire bowel wall (Fig. 26-66). The most important aspect of staging is the identification of those lesions which invade through the bowel wall into surrounding fat. Ultrasonography easily detects small lymph nodes, but the positive predictive value for cancer is only 50 percent for those under 1 cm. Larger lymph nodes (>1 cm) seen on ultrasonography have a 70 percent positive predictive value for cancer. It is difficult to perform endosonography in a patient with an obstructing lesion because the rectal probe cannot pass beyond the lesion. Endosonography of a rectal cancer also may reveal invasion of the tumor into adjacent prostate, sacrum, or vagina (Stage T4).

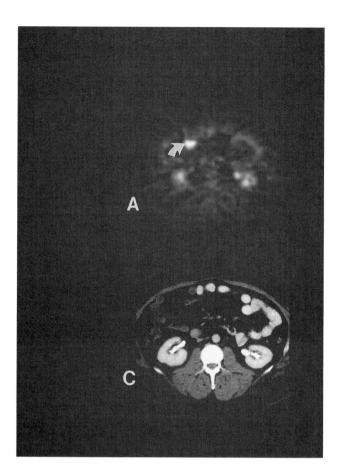

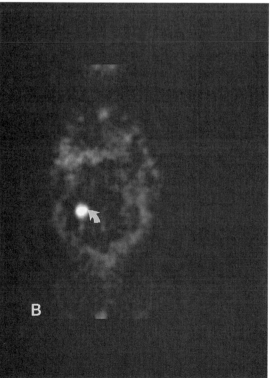

FIG. 26-65. *A* and *B.* Positron-emission tomographic transaxial image at the level of the midkidneys and whole-body coronal image demonstrate focal accumulation of 2-[¹⁸]-fluoro-2-deoxy-d-glucose in the midabdomen (arrows) consistent with unsuspected peritoneal metastases in a 48-year-old man with rising plasma CEA level 19 months following resection of sigmoid cancer. *C.* Transaxial CT image (at the same level as A) demonstrates no abnormality. Histologic confirmation of recurrent carcinoma was obtained at laparotomy.

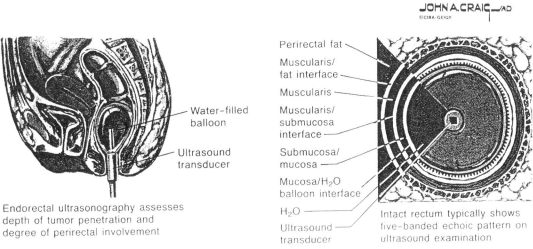

JOHN A.CRAIG—AD
©CIBA-GEIGY

Water-filled balloon

Ultrasound transducer

Endorectal ultrasonography assesses depth of tumor penetration and degree of perirectal involvement

A

Perirectal fat
Muscularis/ fat interface
Muscularis
Muscularis/ submucosa interface
Submucosa/ mucosa
Mucosa/H_2O balloon interface
H_2O
Ultrasound transducer

Intact rectum typically shows five-banded echoic pattern on ultrasound examination

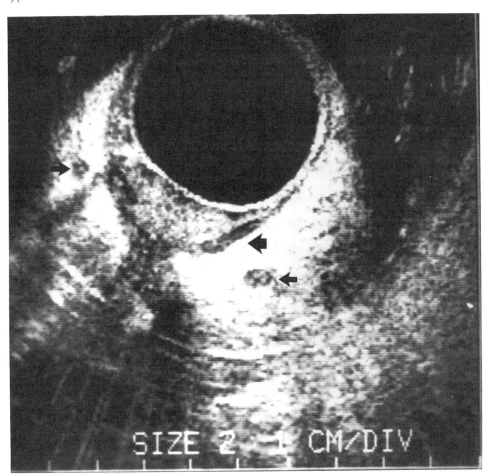

B

FIG. 26-66. *A.* Endorectal ultrasonography. (From: *Fry RD, Fleshman JW, Kodner IJ: Cancer of colon and rectum. Ciba Clin Symp 41:5, 1989. Copyright 1989 Ciba-Geigy Corporation. Reprinted with permission from Clinical Symposia; illustrated by John A. Craig, M.D. All rights reserved.) B.* Ultrasound of an invasive cancer (large arrow) with suspicious nodes (small arrows).

Endoluminal Ultrasound. Colonoscopic ultrasound evaluation of a colonic lesion is available. The small side-scanning transducer is placed on the colonoscope tip. The planar view allows determination of depth of invasion, attachment to adjacent structures, and spread to close mesenteric lymph nodes by tumors in the colon. The usefulness of such information is un-

clear at present because treatment is determined by the portion of the colon involved rather than depth of invasion.

Ultrasound-guided biopsy of the lymph nodes or extraluminal tumor in the pelvis is possible with newer ultrasound equipment. This has the benefit of documenting local recurrence of tumor in the pelvis in patients after previous sphincter-sparing resections of a rectal cancer. Patients who have tumor present in lymph nodes at the time of diagnosis of a rectal cancer are not candidates for local treatment.

Monoclonal Antibodies. Hybridoma techniques have allowed the development of a library of monoclonal antibodies to colorectal cancer. There are two types of monoclonal antibodies: one that recognizes CEA and the other that recognizes cell membrane features of colon cancer. Monoclonal antibodies tagged with a radioactive isotope allow tumor imaging. Therapeutic destruction of rectal or colonic cancer using this technology may be possible in the future.

Surveillance

Screening. Screening must be differentiated from evaluating patients who are at high risk for developing colorectal cancer. Screening programs are aimed at the general population. Cost-effectiveness, reliability, ability to follow up on findings, and a reduced mortality in the screened population are factors to consider when evaluating a screening program. *Sensitivity* of the screening method is based on the *true positives* in the population and is often difficult to prove. *Specificity* is determined by the *true negatives,* which are defined by a negative test. This also is difficult to evaluate because lengthy follow-up is necessary.

Even though screening is an excellent idea, there are limitations. The ideal situation might indeed be to perform colonoscopy on the entire population and remove all polyps to prevent the occurrence of colorectal cancer. This obviously is impractical because of the inordinately high expense, tremendous amount of time involved, and risk of complications of colonoscopy. The medical community has defined *high-risk* groups and is focusing its attention on these groups in order to reduce the incidence of cancer and to improve the cost-benefit and risk-benefit ratios for its patients. Traits of high-risk individuals are listed in Table 26-14.

Recommendations. The summary of recommendations of the US Preventive Services Task Force (USPSTF) is as follows: Screening for colorectal cancer is recommended for all persons aged 50 and older with annual fecal occult blood testing (FOBT), or signoidoscopy (periodically unspecified), or both.

There is sufficient evidence to determine which of these screening methods is preferable or whether the combination of FOBT and sigmoidoscopy produces greater benefits than does either test alone.

There is also insufficient evidence to recommend for or against routine screening with digital rectal examination, barium enema, or colonoscopy, although recommendations against such screening in average-risk persons may be made on other grounds. Persons with a family history of hereditary syndromes associated with a high risk of colon cancer should be referred for diagnosis and management.

Colonoscopy is recommended for blood in the stool, a past history of adenomatous polyps, a positive family history of colorectal cancer, a history of ulcerative colitis or FAP, or an adenomatous polyp found on flexible or rigid sigmoidoscopy. The last recommendation is based on the fact that about 30 percent of patients with a rectosigmoid adenoma will have synchronous neoplasms elsewhere in the colon.

High-Risk Individuals. *Previous Neoplasia.* Metachronous neoplasms, polyps or cancer, have been reported in 40 to 50 percent of patients with a primary colorectal cancer. Cancer has developed in 2 to 5 percent of these patients. The risk of subsequent cancer in patients who have had an adenomatous polyp removed varies from 2.7 to 7.7 times that of the general population. The risk of cancer is increased by polyp number, polyp size, and the presence of villous architecture in the polyp. The National Polyp Study reported that 32 percent of patients who had adenomatous polyps removed via colonoscopic polypectomy were found to have metachronous neoplasms at colonoscopy 3 years later. In addition, colonoscopic polypectomy resulted in a lower-than-expected incidence of colorectal cancer in these patients, suggesting that routine surveillance may reduce the incidence of metachronous cancer. The influence of surveillance on survival is unknown. Patients who have had resection of a cancer or a polyp should have routine surveillance.

The following are guidelines for surveillance after resection of a colorectal cancer. These recommendations may vary depending on the number of polyps, the ease of the examination, and the age of the patient (Fig. 26-67). The plan can be summarized as follows:

1. Colonoscopy in the perioperative period to remove all synchronous polyps and detect synchronous cancers.
2. Colonoscopy 1 year after surgery to check for missed synchronous lesions and to detect any new lesions. Colonoscopy can be repeated yearly until no further lesions are identified.
3. Colonoscopy 3 years after a negative 1-year examination.
4. Colonoscopy every 5 years after a negative 3-year examination.

A similar surveillance strategy can be used after colonoscopic removal of adenomatous polyps, with the exception that the first follow-up colonoscopy can be performed 3 years after polypectomy.

Family History. There is a significantly increased risk of cancer in individuals with a family history of colorectal cancer. This risk depends on the number of first-degree relatives who have had cancer. This information should be used to begin earlier screening with colonoscopy of the group at risk. Patients who are members of families with FAP and Lynch syndromes also should have routine surveillance. The National Polyp Study also has demonstrated an increased risk of colorectal cancer in individuals whose first-degree relatives have adenomatous polyps.

It is very common for young patients (under 40 years) with colorectal cancer to have first-degree relatives with colon cancer (89 percent) and to be part of an HNPCC family (18 percent). Therefore, it is advisable for family members of young patients with colon cancer to be screened with colonoscopy at an early age (25 years old).

Table 26-14
High Risk for Colorectal Cancer

1. Age over 50 years
2. Premalignant condition:
   a. Ulcerative colitis longer than 10 years
   b. Crohn's disease with stricture
   c. Familial adenomatous polyposis
   d. Hereditary nonpolyposis colon cancer syndrome
   e. Previous history of colon polyps
3. Family history of colorectal cancer or polyps

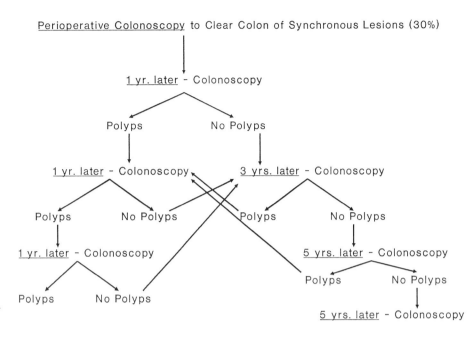

FIG. 26-67. *Surveillance plan for metachronous neoplasia of the colon.*

Hereditary Nonpolyposis Colon Cancer. HNPCC is an autosomal dominant disease that carries a 50 percent risk of cancer in family members. Metachronous colon cancer is also possible in affected individuals. The appropriate screening or surveillance protocol for these individuals is not known. Genetic testing for microsatellite instability as an indicator of errors in mismatch repair is not adequate because a large proportion of tumors in patients without HNPCC have microsatellite instability. The use of white blood cell mutational analysis in family members of patients with HNPCC is under investigation. Recommendations for individuals with HNPCC include total abdominal colectomy and ileorectal anastomosis with yearly screening of the residual rectum. Family members in HNPCC families should have colonoscopy every 2 years beginning at age 18 or at least 5 years before the age at diagnosis of the youngest family member with cancer. Mutational analysis eventually may be used to detect one of the at least four defects (MSH2, MLH1, PMS1, PMS2) in the mismatch repair genes on chromosomes 2 and 3 in individuals at risk for cancer. The need for prophylactic colectomy rather than continuous surveillance colonoscopy has not been established.

Ulcerative Colitis. Patients with ulcerative colitis for longer than 10 years should be examined by colonoscopy and biopsies for dysplasia, as discussed previously, with treatment based on the fact that the cancer risk in the setting of severe dysplasia is 30 percent (see Fig. 26-50).

Polyps

Hamartoma

Peutz-Jeghers Syndrome. The combination of hamartomatous polyps of smooth muscles and mucocutaneous pigmentation was first described in 1896 by Hutchinson. The existence of *familial* hamartomatous polyps originally was described by Peutz and then again in 1949 in a follow-up article by Jeghers. The syndrome consists of pigmentation, produced by melanin in the mucocutaneous areas, and of hamartomas of intestinal smooth muscle throughout the gastrointestinal tract. This is an autosomal dominant syndrome and carries with it a well-documented risk of cancer in the breast, cervix, ovary, fallopian tubes, thyroid, lung, skin (basal cell), gallbladder, pancreas, testicle, and bile ducts. An overall risk of 2 to 13 percent for developing intestinal cancer arising in the stomach, small intestine, and colon has been documented in these patients.

Symptoms of the hamartomas include bleeding or intestinal obstruction secondary to intussusception. Treatment includes removing any polyp that is larger than 1.5 cm, even if asymptomatic. If a surgeon is forced to operate for symptoms, every effort should be made to completely clear the polyps with intraoperative endoscopy and polypectomy. Cancer, if present, is usually found in the mucosa overlying or adjacent to the hamartoma. After an operation to remove the polyps, colonoscopy is recommended every other year to survey for recurrence of colonic polyps. Patients also should undergo periodic screening for breast, cervix, testicle, ovary, upper gastrointestinal, and pancreatic cancers.

Juvenile Polyposis. *Juvenile polyposis* was first described by Verse in 1908. The familial inheritance of these polyps was reported by Veale at St. Mark's Hospital in 1966. Juvenile polyps occur as cystic dilatations of glandular structures within the fibroblastic stroma of the lamina propria. Juvenile polyps usually cause symptoms of gastrointestinal bleeding or obstruction due to intussusception, with the polyp as the lead point. These complications require surgical or endoscopic removal of the polyp. There are varying patterns of occurrence of juvenile polyps. Approximately 1 percent of all infants have a single juvenile polyp discovered in infancy. A second peak incidence is seen at 25 years of age. The most common cause of gastrointestinal bleeding in a child is a juvenile polyp. There has been no malignant potential documented for these isolated juvenile polyps.

Isolated polyps are best treated with polypectomy, primarily for establishing the correct diagnosis. No other treatment is indicated. Autoamputation of the polyp often causes the initial bleeding. Once the bleeding has stopped, no further treatment is necessary.

Multiple polyposis coli (diffuse juvenile polyps) is an autosomal dominant syndrome with high penetrance that carries an increased risk of cancer in the gastrointestinal tract and in other nongastrointestinal tissues. The syndrome usually causes bleeding, obstruction due to intussusception, or malnutrition due to excessive protein loss. Diffuse juvenile polyposis occurs in less than 1 percent of patients with juvenile polyps and may carry an even higher risk of cancer when mixed or heterogeneous types of polyps are present (polyps of both adenomatous and juvenile types). Adenomas have been documented on juvenile polyps as well as in adjacent mucosa. The malignant potential has been estimated at approximately 10 percent in patients with the multiple polyposis coli type of juvenile polyposis and is even higher in patients with the diffuse variety. As in the other polyposis syndromes, the risk of cancer appears to increase with the duration of the disease and the age of the patient.

The multiple juvenile polyposis syndrome requires colonoscopic polypectomy in patients with a few colonic polyps because of the possibility of bleeding, intussusception, and a low but real incidence of adenomatous change. In patients with this condition, it is sometimes best to perform an abdominal colectomy with ileorectal anastomosis and to continue to screen the rectum. The entire colonic and rectal mucosa should be removed in patients with the diffuse form of juvenile polyposis and an ileal reservoir constructed with ileal pouch–anal anastomosis.

Hyperplastic Polyps. *Hyperplastic polyps* are common in the colon. They have been estimated to be 10 times more common than adenomas. Their typical histologic findings consist of epithelial dysmaturation and hyperplasia. They are usually less than 5 mm in diameter and show a thickened mucosa without atypia. There is usually no evidence of adenomatous change. They are associated with an increase in myofibrils and T cells in the lamina propria. The clinical significance of hyperplastic polyps continues to be the subject of some debate, but most studies indicate that they are not premalignant lesions and are not associated with adenomatous change elsewhere in the colon. *Serrated* or *mixed polyps* have a combination of hyperplasia and adenoma. These polyps have been associated with the development of cancer.

Hyperplastic polyps tend to increase in incidence with age. There is also a rare inherited syndrome of hyperplastic polyposis in which larger hyperplastic polyps occur in young adults. Hyperplastic polyps can be biopsied, destroyed, or removed during colonoscopy.

Other Lesions. There are several other less well-known and rare hamartomatous syndromes. *Cowden's syndrome* is an autosomal dominant defect that includes hamartomas of all three embryonal cell layers. Tricholemmomas, breast cancer, thyroid disease, and gastrointestinal polyps with occasional gastrointestinal cancers are typical of the syndrome. Treatment is based on symptoms. Polyps should be removed, and the patient should be screened for other cancers.

Cronkhite-Canada syndrome is typified by nonfamilial juvenile polyps with other epidermal changes but no evidence of malignancies. The polyps should be removed only if they cause symptoms.

The *Ruvalcaba-Myhre-Smith syndrome* includes developmental abnormalities, microcephaly, and juvenile polyps. It is a very rare syndrome that occurs in males, and to date, no cancers have been documented. The polyps should be removed when symptomatic, and other members of the family should be screened.

Adenoma

Pathology. The *adenoma,* or *adenomatous polyp,* of the colon or rectum is a benign neoplasm. It represents proliferation and unrestricted cell division in a well-circumscribed area of glandular epithelium within the colonic mucosa. The surface is usually rounded and lumpy, like a raspberry, or flat and velvety with a shaggy appearance. Polyps can exist in a pedunculated (with a stalk), sessile (flat), or semisessile (raised) form. Each of these macroscopic forms may have similar histologic adenomatous appearances of the epithelium and the same cytology. The histologic architecture of the polyps may vary from branched tubular glands, to fingerlike, elongated villi, to villous configuration.

Polyps are classified as *tubular adenoma, tubulovillous adenoma,* or *villous adenoma* depending on the predominant pattern. In general, 65 to 80 percent of all adenomatous polyps removed are tubular adenomas, 10 to 25 percent are tubulovillous, and only 5 to 10 percent are pure villous adenomas. Tubular adenomas usually are pedunculated, and villous adenomas usually are sessile. However, all types of histologic characteristics can be found in each type of polyp. Incompletely differentiated epithelial cells are found along the fingerlike villi. The degree of differentiation decreases as the polyp becomes more like a cancer. The term *severe atypia* is now accepted for the finding of a malignancy in the epithelium of a polyp that has not invaded the muscularis mucosae of the bowel. Such lesions previously were referred to as *carcinoma in situ.*

Polyp-Cancer Sequence. It is generally accepted that a benign adenoma has been the precursor to a colorectal cancer in the majority of patients. However, Shimoda has shown that cancers also may arise de novo in nonadenomatous mucosa. These flat cancers usually are advanced and seem to have arisen as intramucosal cancers with no evidence of preceding polyp formation. This finding is consistent with a rapid progression of the genetic changes postulated by Fearon and Vogelstein as a polyp changes to a cancer (Fig. 26-68).

The evidence for the existence of an adenoma-carcinoma sequence includes the following:

1. Polypectomy has been shown to decrease the incidence of cancer. Patients with small adenomas have a 2.3 times increased risk of cancer after polypectomies as compared with an 8-fold increase in the risk of cancer in patients who do not undergo polypectomy.
2. Colonic adenomas are observed more frequently in patients with cancer. Nearly 30 percent of all patients with a colorectal cancer also will have a synchronous polyp.
3. Larger adenomas are found to contain cancer and severe dysplasia more often than are smaller polyps. Sixty percent of adenomas larger than 2 cm are villous adenomas. Villous adenomas have a 40 percent risk of containing a cancer, as compared to a 22 percent risk of cancer in tubulovillous adenomas and a 5 percent risk of cancer in tubular adenomas; however, the size of the polyp seems to be more important than the histologic features. The risk of a cancer in a villous adenoma, tubulovillous adenoma, or tubular adenoma larger than 2 cm is 53, 46, and 35 percent, respectively.

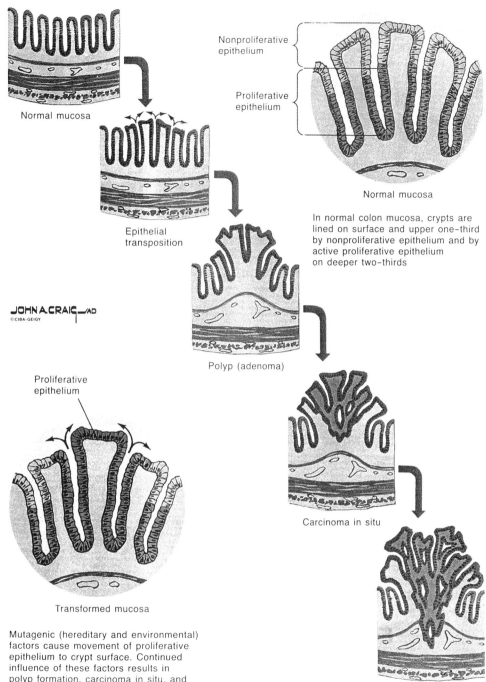

Nonproliferative epithelium

Proliferative epithelium

Normal mucosa

In normal colon mucosa, crypts are lined on surface and upper one-third by nonproliferative epithelium and by active proliferative epithelium on deeper two-thirds

Normal mucosa

Epithelial transposition

Polyp (adenoma)

Carcinoma in situ

JOHN A.CRAIG—AD
©CIBA-GEIGY

Proliferative epithelium

Transformed mucosa

Invasive cancer

FIG. 26-68. Polyp-cancer sequence. (From: *Fry RD, Fleshman JW, Kodner IJ: Cancer of colon and rectum. Ciba Clin Symp 41:5, with permission.*)

Mutagenic (hereditary and environmental) factors cause movement of proliferative epithelium to crypt surface. Continued influence of these factors results in polyp formation, carcinoma in situ, and eventually invasive cancer

4. Severe dysplasia has been shown to progress to cancer in polyps. The differentiation between carcinoma in situ and invasive cancer relies on the depth of invasion of the dysplastic area. Invasion beneath the muscularis mucosae defines invasive adenocarcinoma in a polyp because the cancer cells at this depth have access to the vascular and lymphatic systems.

5. Residual adenomatous tissue is found in the majority of invasive cancers. This is presumptive evidence that the cancer has arisen within the polyp and has progressed to replace the majority of the polyp.

6. Patients with familial adenomatous polyposis (>100 polyps) develop cancer 100 percent of the time if the colon is not removed. The adenomas of FAP are histologically the same as sporadic adenomas.

7. There is a high prevalence of adenomas in populations with a high rate of cancer. This seems to indicate that the polyp is a precursor or a necessary factor in the development of cancer.

8. It has been shown that the presence of an adenoma places a patient at a lifetime risk for the development of cancer.

9. The peak incidence for the discovery of colonic polyps is at 50 years of age. The peak incidence for the development of cancer is at 60 years of age. This would indicate that there is a 10-year time span for the conversion of the adenomatous polyps to cancer. Investigators at the Mayo Clinic reported that a polyp larger than 1 cm has a cancer risk of 2.5 percent in 5 years, 8 percent in 10 years, and 24 percent in 20 years.

The adenoma-carcinoma sequence suggests that colonic mucosa progresses through stages to the final development of an invasive cancer. Normal epithelium is stimulated by some event to allow undifferentiated dividing cells to leave the crypts and move to the surface of the villi. Continued proliferation of these cells on the surface of the mucosa results in a polyp or adenoma. As proliferation continues, the glands begin to resemble normal tissue less and less. Eventually this disorganized growth crosses the muscularis mucosae barrier and becomes invasive cancer.

Treatment

Pedunculated Polyps. Pedunculated polyps have a stalk that is usually less than 1.5 cm in diameter. Colonoscopic polypectomy is the best treatment for most pedunculated polyps. The cautery snare is placed at a point on the stalk to adequately remove the polyp with a clear margin from the head but distant enough to avoid thermal injury to the colonic wall at the base of the stalk. It is also important to avoid transmission of electric current via the head of the polyp to the opposite wall of the colon. Complete removal and retrieval of the polyp are essential for histologic diagnosis (Fig. 26-69).

Semisessile Polyps. Semisessile polyps have a broad pedicle, larger than 1.5 cm. These polyps usually can be removed in piecemeal fashion if they do not have a malignant appearance. Bites of 0.5 to 1.5 cm are taken with the cautery snare until the stalk is seen. It is important to mark the area with 0.1 mL of India ink as a tattoo in the mucosa to facilitate repeat colonoscopic examination or surgical removal of the same site.

Sessile Polyps. Sessile polyps larger than 2 cm usually can be removed in piecemeal fashion also (Fig. 26-70). Small, 0.5- to 1.5-cm bites are taken to avoid burning the full thickness of bowel. A lower current also helps to avoid full-thickness burning. A "second look" colonoscopy and polypectomy is necessary if residual tissue is left behind as in the semisessile lesion.

Colectomy. Cancer in the head of a polyp may be treated by colonoscopic polypectomy (Fig. 26-71). Colectomy must be performed when the cancer within the head of the polyp has unfavorable features. Because the incidence of nodal metastases in these patients varies widely (1 to 25 percent in different series), various characteristics of excised polyps have been examined to improve the estimation of this risk, including level of invasion of the malignant process into the polyp; local invasion of lymphatic, vascular, and neural tissues; degree of differentiation of the malignant cells; and DNA ploidy. If the neoplasm is limited to the mucosa or invades only the head of a pedunculated polyp, the risk of lymph node metastasis is small (0 to 3 percent), and patients may be considered for close follow-up rather than resection. If the carcinoma reaches the base of the polyp, or if the lesion is sessile, then the risk of lymphatic spread may be as high as 10 to 27 percent. Intermediate lesions that invade only the neck or the stalk of the polyp are rarely associated with lymph node metastases unless the lesion is poorly differentiated or there is lymphovascular invasion. According to Nivatvongs, the finding of lymphatic or vascular invasion, poorly differentiated adenocarcinoma, or cancer close to the resection line of the stalk indicates the need for colonic resection. The risk of local recurrence is at least 10 percent, and the risk of spread of cancer to lymph nodes is approximately 10 percent in these patients. It should be noted that if a patient does not undergo resection, colonoscopic follow-up may not detect per-

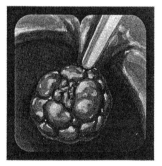

Snare resection of
pedunculated polyp

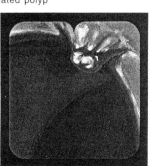

Postoperative view
of colon

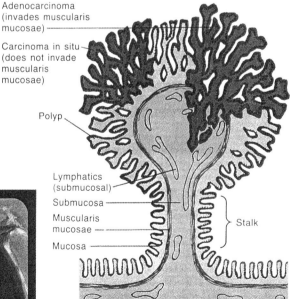

Adenocarcinoma
(invades muscularis
mucosae)

Carcinoma in situ
(does not invade
muscularis
mucosae)

Polyp

Lymphatics
(submucosal)

Submucosa

Muscularis
mucosae

Mucosa

Stalk

FIG. 26-69. Pedunculated polyp. (From: *Fry RD, Fleshman JW, Kodner U: Cancer of colon and rectum. Ciba Clin Symp 41:5, 1989, with permission.*)

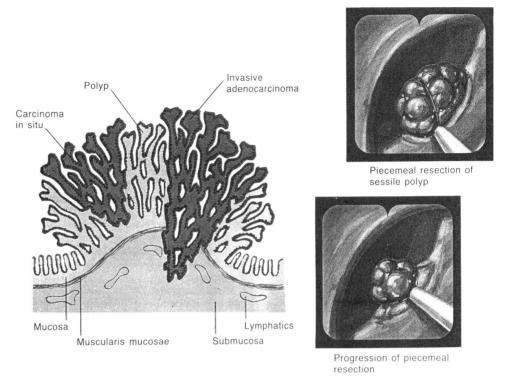

FIG. 26-70. Sessile polyp. (From: Fry RD, Fleshman JW, Kodner IJ: Cancer of colon and rectum. Ciba Clin Symp 41:5, 1989, with permission.)

JOHN A. CRAIG—AD
© CIBA-GEIGY

sistent or recurrent tumor because the lesion may reside outside the lumen of the bowel. Each case must be individualized, taking into consideration the life expectancy, operative risk, and personal philosophy of the patient.

A sessile polyp, by definition, has no stalk, and the submucosa is immediately adjacent to the muscularis propria. The invasion of the cancer through the muscularis mucosae into the submucosa puts the patient at high risk for local recurrence and spread of cancer to regional lymph nodes. A fold of adjacent mucosa is occasionally confused as the pedicle of a sessile polyp. Therefore, even if completely excised, the sessile polyp with an invasive carcinoma requires colectomy for complete cure. Laparoscopic colectomy may be a less invasive approach to managing polyps that are benign in appearance and have no obvious cancer present on biopsy analysis but are too large to be removed colonoscopically.

FIG. 26-71. Management of polyps.

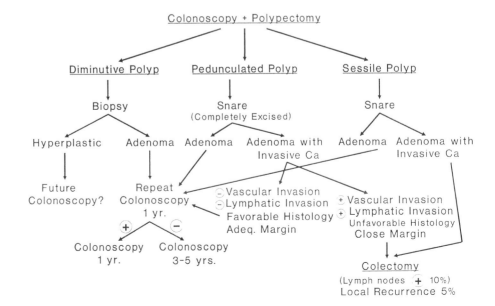

Villous Adenoma of the Rectum

Villous adenomas of the rectum are typically flat, velvety, and soft sessile polyps within the rectum. They occasionally present with watery diarrhea and hypokalemia. The finding of a large (>4 cm) villous adenoma in the rectum, with areas of induration, indicates a very high risk for cancer (90 percent). Transrectal ultrasonography of the villous lesion is helpful to determine the thickness of the lesion. Ultrasonography, however, is unable to distinguish between carcinoma in situ and invasive cancer. Because of the risk of sampling error in these large, exuberant lesions, the only adequate biopsy is complete excision, preferably transanally if possible. If cancer is present, the patient should be treated with appropriate resection. The transanal excision should include adequate peripheral margins for complete cure if cancer is present. It is helpful to inject the submucosal layer with epinephrine both to raise the lesion from the underlying muscle and to reduce blood loss. The defect should be closed with suture to provide primary healing and to mark the site. There is a high risk of recurrence if inadequate excision is performed.

Occasionally, a villous tumor will cover the entire mucosal surface of the distal rectum. If the polyp appears to be benign, a coloanal anastomosis after distal mucosal proctectomy and full-thickness proximal proctectomy are the preferred treatment. The coloanal anastomosis allows preservation of the anal sphincter and removes all the mucosa at risk in the rectum. It is important to document by frozen section the absence of cancer in this situation unless the tumor is well above the anal canal and there is very little risk of invasion into the levator or external sphincter muscles.

The use of a colonic J-pouch in selected individuals may improve their function after a coloanal anastomosis. The terminal 10 to 15 cm of the left colon are folded into a J, and the intervening septum is divided and the two limbs stapled together with a linear-cutting gastrointestinal anastomosing stapler introduced through a hole in the apex of the J. The coloanal anastomosis is then performed using an end-to-end intraluminal circular stapler or a hand-sewn anastomosis to the anal canal mucosa. A protecting loop ileostomy is usually placed if there is concern for the anastomotic integrity for any reason.

Thermal ablation of the villous adenoma has been used in some patients in whom local excision is not possible. The disadvantages of thermal ablation include the risk of undiagnosed cancer or cancer developing in the base of a repeatedly cauterized, scarred segment. If the villous adenoma recurs after several laser treatments, the patient should be referred for surgical treatment.

In the past, transsphincteric (York-Mason) and transsacral (Kraske) approaches to the rectum were used to remove villous adenomas and allow sphincter preservation. These methods are currently used infrequently because the coloanal anastomosis and low stapled anastomotic techniques allow preservation of anorectal function and appear to be more effective in treatment of the disease.

Colon Cancer

Incidence

Cancer of the colon and rectum is the most common cancer of the gastrointestinal tract. In women, colorectal cancer is second only to breast cancer as a cause of cancer-related death. In men, it is the third most common lethal cancer, preceded by carcinoma of the lung and prostate. The incidence of this malignant tumor increased in the United States during the first part of this century but has stabilized over the past four decades.

It is estimated that approximately 131,000 new cases of colorectal cancer (94,000 colon and 37,000 rectal) will develop in the United States in 1997, and approximately 58,300 patients will die of the disease. Rectal cancer is slightly more common in men, whereas there is a slight predominance of colon cancer in women. An American has approximately a 5 percent probability of developing colorectal cancer during a 70-year life span. Most cases of colorectal cancer are diagnosed in patients over the age of 50, and the incidence of the disease rises steadily after that age. Despite the clear relationship with aging, colorectal cancer is not strictly a disease of the elderly; between 6 and 8 percent of cases occur in individuals under the age of 40. The onset of familial and hereditary forms of the disease occurs at a much earlier age, typically around the third decade.

Signs and Symptoms

The signs and symptoms of colorectal cancer are varied and nonspecific. The symptoms that most often prompt patients to seek medical attention include rectal bleeding, a change in bowel habits, and abdominal pain. Whether a patient has any noticeable symptoms or what form the symptoms take depends somewhat on the location of the tumor and the extent of disease.

Subacute Presentation. Tumors in the *right colon* typically do not cause changes in bowel habits (although large, mucus-secreting tumors may cause diarrhea). Patients might notice dark or tarry stools, but more often these tumors cause truly occult bleeding, which is not detected by the patient. Such chronic blood loss may cause iron-deficiency anemia, with resulting fatigue, dizziness, or palpitations. When a postmenopausal woman or an adult man develops iron-deficiency anemia, colorectal cancer should be suspected and appropriate diagnostic studies performed. Because the bleeding associated with colon tumors tends to be intermittent, negative tests for occult blood in the feces do not rule out the presence of a large-bowel cancer.

Lower abdominal pain is more often associated with tumors located in the narrower left colon. The pain is of a cramping nature and may be relieved by bowel movements. These patients are more likely to notice a change in bowel habits and the passage of bright red blood.

Less common nonacute symptoms of large-bowel cancer include weight loss and fever. About 50 percent of patients who have other symptoms also report a loss of body weight, but weight loss is almost never the sole manifestation of a colorectal tumor. Fever is an unusual presenting symptom. Septicemia is rare but can occur with any stage of large-bowel tumor; *Streptococcus bovis* bacteremia is highly suggestive of colorectal carcinoma.

Rarely, colon cancer will present as the lead point of colonic intussusception in an adult. In all adults who are found to have obstruction or partial obstruction because of intussusception, a colonoscopy or air-contrast barium enema is warranted to rule out a colon cancer.

Acute Presentation. A significant proportion of patients are first seen with acute symptoms reflecting obstruction or perforation of the large bowel. Colonic obstruction is highly suggestive of cancer, particularly in older patients. Complete ob-

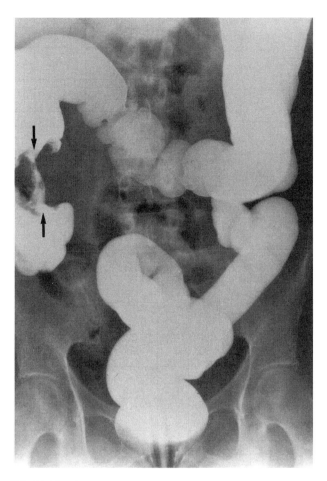

FIG. 26-72. *Barium enema demonstrating a cancer ("apple-core" lesion) of the right colon (arrows).*

struction occurs in less than 10 percent of patients with colorectal cancer, but it is an emergency that requires immediate diagnosis and surgical treatment. Ideally, this surgical emergency could be avoided by early recognition of changes in bowel habits. Patients with complete obstruction complain of inability to pass flatus or feces, cramping abdominal pain, and abdominal distention. Examination reveals a distended, tympanitic abdomen; occasionally the obstructing tumor can be palpated as an abdominal mass.

If the obstruction is not relieved and the colon continues to distend, the pressure in the intestinal wall can exceed the capillary pressure, and oxygenated blood will not reach the bowel wall, resulting in ischemia and necrosis. In such situations the patient will complain of severe abdominal pain, and abdominal examination will reveal rebound tenderness and decreased or absent bowel sounds. If not treated immediately, the necrosis will progress to perforation with fecal peritonitis and sepsis.

The large bowel also can perforate at the tumor site, probably because a transmural tumor loses its blood supply and becomes necrotic. Such cases are easily mistaken for acute diverticulitis, and the inflammatory process may be confined to the site of the perforation; however, in some cases a perforation may not be contained, resulting in generalized peritonitis. In rare cases, perforation into an adjacent organ (usually the bladder or vagina)

occurs and is manifested by pneumaturia, fecaluria, or feculent vaginal drainage.

Unfortunately, the first signs of colon cancer may be caused by metastatic disease. Massive liver metastases may cause pruritus and jaundice. Ascites, enlarged ovaries, and scattered deposits in the lungs detected by a chest radiograph can be caused by an otherwise asymptomatic colon cancer. Treatment is rarely beneficial in such advanced disease.

Diagnosis and Evaluation

In patients with symptoms suggestive of colon cancer, the definitive diagnosis is usually established by endoscopy (flexible sigmoidoscopy or colonoscopy) or barium enema. Other tests are necessary to evaluate the extent of disease and search for metastases.

Barium studies of the colon may demonstrate the primary lesion (Fig. 26-72) and reveal a synchronous cancer elsewhere in the colon (which occurs in 3 to 5 percent of patients). Dietary restrictions and cathartics usually are necessary to prepare the patient for barium enema. However, if acute colonic obstruction is suspected and plain films of the abdomen reveal dilated colon, water-soluble contrast study may be obtained with no preparation, to reveal the location and nature of the obstructing lesion.

Colonoscopy is currently the most accurate and complete examination of the large bowel. Colonoscopy and barium enema studies should be regarded as complementary to each other. The purpose of a *complete* colon and rectal evaluation for patients with large-bowel cancer is to rule out synchronous carcinomas and polyps.

A chest x-ray should be taken routinely to rule out pulmonary metastasis. CT of the abdomen is being used increasingly to assess the extent of invasion of the primary tumor and to search for intraabdominal metastatic disease.

Elevated liver function test results, including alkaline phosphatase, lactate dehydrogenase, bilirubin, and transaminase enzyme determinations, can suggest liver metastases. These tests are useful in the postoperative follow-up and, if elevated, can suggest the need for CT scan to search for hepatic metastases.

The serum level of CEA is important in the evaluation of patients with colorectal cancer. This antigen, a glycoprotein, is present in embryonic and fetal tissue and in colorectal cancers but is absent in normal adult colonic mucosa. In patients with cancer that has not penetrated the bowel wall, the serum CEA level is usually not elevated. The test is somewhat nonspecific, since it can be elevated in patients with tumors of the lung, breast, stomach, or pancreas. Levels also may be elevated in smokers and in patients with cirrhosis, pancreatitis, renal failure, and ulcerative colitis. Thus the test is not useful for screening.

An elevated CEA level does have a high correlation with tumor recurrence and with the presence of metastases from colorectal cancer. If the CEA level is elevated before operation, the recurrence rate is higher, regardless of the disease stage. Postoperative CEA levels may indicate the completeness of surgical resection or the presence of occult metastases. A rising CEA titer after treatment may indicate a recurrence, before clinical disease becomes evident. When used alone, the CEA assay is 70 percent accurate in predicting the development of liver metastases within 1 year; in combination with CT scans, accuracy increases to up to 90 percent.

Surgical Treatment

Preoperative Bowel Preparation. Wound infection and intraabdominal abscess formerly were common problems following colorectal surgery. The primary source of infection was the endogenous bacteria in the bowel lumen, with *E. coli* being the most common aerobic species and *Bacteroides fragilis* the most common anaerobic organism involved in septic complications. The large bowel cannot be sterilized prior to surgery, and colorectal operations are classified as "clean-contaminated" procedures by the American National Research Council; operations during which the large bowel is opened virtually always expose the operative field to colonic bacteria. Accordingly, steps must be taken before the operation to reduce the bacterial population as much as possible. The preoperative preparation generally includes two components: *mechanical cleansing* and *antibiotic administration.*

There is no absolute consensus regarding appropriate mechanical bowel preparation. A decade ago the most common method was a 3-day regimen consisting of a low-residue or liquid diet combined with laxatives (magnesium citrate or castor oil) and enemas. This approach was time-consuming, was often hampered by incomplete patient compliance, and severely restricted the patient's caloric intake for 3 days before major surgery. Other approaches are used more commonly today, including mono- and dibasic sodium phosphate purgatives and whole-gut lavage with polyethylene glycol (Golytely or Colyte).

A commonly used bowel preparation today is an isotonic lavage solution containing polyethylene glycol (PEG) in a balanced salt solution. PEG also acts as an osmotic purgative, but it does not serve as a culture medium for bacteria and is not associated with the production of explosive colonic gas. With this method of cleansing, the patient may have a light meal at lunch and clear liquids the evening before surgery. To achieve adequate cleansing of the colon, an average of 4 L of PEG solution must be ingested within 4 h. The solution can be drunk or instilled through a small nasogastric tube. This method has been associated with less fluid retention than saline lavage but is still somewhat uncomfortable for the patient. Metoclopramide may be given one-half hour before starting the lavage to reduce nausea.

Mono- and dibasic sodium phosphate acts as a purgative when given in adequate volume (45 mL) and accompanied by large volumes (24 oz) of clear liquids. Two doses (noon and 6 p.m.) the day prior to surgery are adequate to achieve a complete mechanical bowel preparation. Patients with renal failure or severe hypertension on sodium restriction should be given this preparation cautiously because hypocalcemia, hyperphosphatemia, hypernatremia, and acidosis may occur. Patients with severe congenital megacolon may develop hypernatremic dehydration. Fleet's phospha soda and clear liquids has become a preferred alternative to whole-gut irrigation and is better tolerated than high-volume preparations, with equal results in bowel cleansing.

Mechanical bowel preparation will reduce the absolute number of colonic bacteria, but the bacterial concentration in the lumen seems unaffected, and the postoperative wound infection rate without antimicrobial use remains unacceptably high (between 30 and 60 percent). Reduction of colonic bacterial concentration can be achieved by oral or intravenous antibiotic preparations, and there is no consensus concerning the ideal preparation. Most surgeons use a combination of oral antibiotics

(neomycin plus erythromycin, 1 g each at 1 p.m., 2 p.m., and 11 p.m. the day before operation or 0.5 g of neomycin instead of erythromycin) and an intravenous broad-spectrum antibiotic administered immediately before the operation. The timing of the administration of antibiotics is important; the postoperative infection rate can be reduced to well below 10 percent with proper bowel cleansing and preoperative antibiotic administration, but postoperative antibiotics do not appear to be effective.

Operative Technique: Colon Carcinoma. The objective in the treatment of carcinoma of the colon is to remove the cancerous segment of bowel, the mesentery containing its lymphatic drainage, and any organ that has been directly invaded by the tumor. Since lymphatic channels of the colon accompany the main arterial supply, the length of the bowel resected depends on which vessels are supplying the segment containing the cancer (Fig. 26-73). Surgical techniques that minimize the risk of intraoperative spillage of tumor cells are essential. The arterial supply to the uninvolved intestine must be preserved so that intestinal continuity can be restored by anastomosis.

During the operation, the peritoneal cavity is carefully explored, and the liver is examined to identify any unsuspected metastases. The intestine is encircled with ties, proximal and distal to the tumor, to prevent intraluminal spread of cancer cells during manipulation of the bowel. The main segmental artery

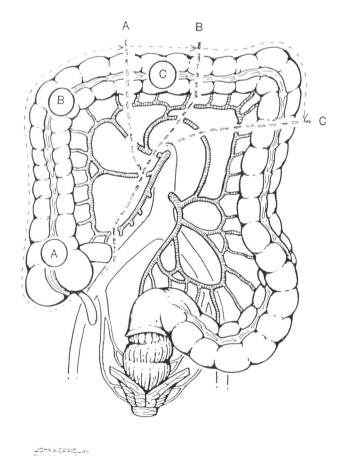

FIG. 26-73. *Surgical management of proximal colon cancer: extent of distal resection relative to tumor location (O=location of cancer; ----- = extent of distal resection).*

supplying the cancerous segment of bowel is ligated and divided, allowing resection of the mesentery in continuity with the bowel. If the tumor is adherent to or invading adjacent organs such as the small bowel, ovaries, uterus, or kidney, an en bloc resection should be performed if technically feasible. Adhesions between the tumor and contiguous organs are often inflammatory, but this cannot be determined before resection. If the adhesions prove to be cancerous and they are merely divided instead of removed by an en bloc resection, the chance for cure will be lost. If all tumor cannot be removed, a palliative colon resection is generally indicated to relieve symptoms and prevent future obstruction and bleeding from the primary tumor. In the rare situation of a nonresectable tumor, a bypass operation should be considered to relieve or prevent intestinal obstruction. If multiple colon carcinomas are present, or if a colon carcinoma is associated with multiple neoplastic polyps, a subtotal colectomy (total abdominal colectomy) with ileorectal anastomosis should be considered.

Carcinoma of the right colon is treated by right hemicolectomy, which includes excision of approximately 10 cm of terminal ileum. The ileocolic artery, right colic artery, and right branch of the middle colic artery are ligated and divided, and an anastomosis is fashioned between the ileum and the left transverse colon. The anastomosis can be either hand-sewn or achieved by stapling instruments.

Carcinoma of the hepatic flexure or the right transverse colon is treated by extending the hemicolectomy to include the middle colic artery along with its left branch (see Fig. 26-73).

Carcinoma of the midtransverse colon is treated by extending the hemicolectomy even farther and performing the anastomosis between the ileum and the proximal descending colon. An alternative, in this situation, is to ligate only the middle colic artery and excise the transverse colon, making an anastomosis between the ascending and descending colon.

In a similar fashion, the surgical treatment of left colon cancer incorporates resection of the arteries and accompanying mesentery, as shown in Fig. 26-74.

The resected specimen should be inspected immediately by a pathologist to assess the surgical margins. A 5-cm margin of normal bowel on either side of the tumor is ideal; however, margins as small as 2 cm from the tumor edge may be satisfactory if adequate mesentery is resected with the specimen. Wider margins are required for a poorly differentiated or anaplastic carcinoma. While the anastomosis can be fashioned by either hand-sewn or stapling techniques, it is essential that the bowel edges be meticulously approximated to form a lumen of adequate size, that there be no tension on the anastomosis, and that the blood supply to both sides of the anastomosis is adequate.

The functional results after colectomy vary according to the segment of colon resected. The right colon absorbs approximately 1000 mL of fluid delivered from the terminal ileum. After a right colectomy, the stool generally is softer, and 750 mL/ day is passed rather than 250 mL. A left colectomy or sigmoid colectomy generally results in several small stools per day but the same volume as before surgery. Patients who require a total abdominal colectomy with ileorectal anastomosis will experience 4 to 10 bowel movements per day immediately after their operation from 1000 mL of ileal contents entering the rectum during a 24-h period. Over time this will decrease as the ileum compensates for loss of the right colon and begins absorbing bile salts and more water. Younger patients tolerate removal of

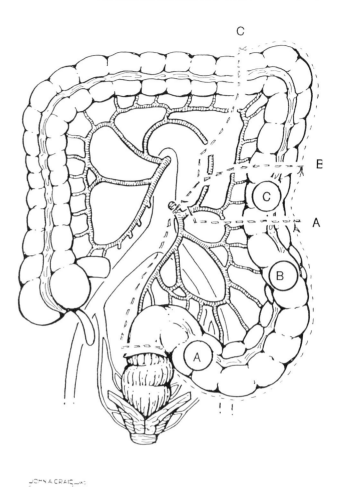

FIG. 26-74. *Surgical management of distal colon cancer: extent of proximal resection relative to tumor location (O=location of cancer; - - - - = proximal extent of distal resection).*

the colon better than the elderly, but this option should not be withheld from older patients.

Laparoscopic colectomy has been described for all types of colorectal disease. The first cases were reported in 1991, and since that time, numerous reports have entered the literature. Several large series have documented the safety and potential efficacy of this technique in the management of colorectal disease, including cancer. Randomized control trials have not confirmed these findings, and the use of laparoscopic colectomy in the treatment of cancer is controversial. Laparoscopic techniques such as laparoscopic segmental colectomy, abdominoperineal resection, rectopexy, ostomy construction and takedown, and small-bowel resection can provide earlier recovery (shorter postoperative ileus and hospital stay) and less pain for most patients regardless of the reason for operation. Laparoscopic colectomy requires advanced skill, thorough knowledge of intraabdominal anatomy, and an ability to recognize structures from unusual angles and perspectives. The same principles of surgical technique that guarantee a good outcome for open operations apply to laparoscopic procedures.

Emergency Operations. *Obstruction.* When a colon or rectal cancer causes complete obstruction, immediate surgical treatment is necessary. Obstructing cancer of the right or transverse colon usually can be treated by resection and primary anastomosis. The entire colon proximal to the obstruction should be resected, and the terminal ileum then should be anastomosed to the remaining normal colon. In such cases, diversion by proximal ileostomy is rarely needed.

Obstruction by a left-sided cancer presents a more difficult problem. If the obstruction is only partial, with feces and gas present in the rectum, it may be possible to proceed with preoperative cleansing of the colon as described earlier. However, when radiography reveals a distended colon with no air in the rectum, the obstruction is complete, and emergency surgical treatment is mandatory. Water-soluble contrast should be performed to confirm the presence of an obstruction and to determine its exact location.

The appropriate surgical procedure depends on the location of the obstruction, the initial surgical findings, and the surgeon's experience and judgment. The current trend is toward immediate resection of the lesion. However, if the colon is extensively dilated and the patient's condition unstable, it may be appropriate to relieve the obstruction by a colostomy placed proximal to the lesion (described in the section on rectal cancer). After the patient's condition has stabilized, the bowel can be properly prepared and the obstructing lesion resected at a later time. If the surgeon feels that it is possible to resect the lesion, several options are available, including the following:

1. Primary resection without anastomosis, bringing the proximal end of the colon to the abdominal wall as a colostomy and the distal end to a separate location on the abdominal wall as a mucous fistula. If the tumor is located so far distally that the distal end of colon cannot be exteriorized, the Hartmann procedure is used.
2. Primary resection with anastomosis. Anastomosis between two segments of unprepared bowel is associated with an anastomotic dehiscence rate above 20 percent. There has been interest in cleansing the proximal bowel at the time of emergency celiotomy by the technique of intraoperative colonic lavage. A catheter is inserted into the cecum through an appendicostomy, and several liters of saline solution are instilled. The solution washes out the bowel contents through a large-bore catheter (or sterile anesthesia tubing) that has been placed in the colon proximal to the cancer. The cancerous segment of bowel, including the site of insertion of the evacuating tubing, is then excised, and an anastomosis is fashioned using the prepared, cleansed colon.
3. Primary resection with anastomosis and proximal protective colostomy or ileostomy.
4. Subtotal colectomy with ileosigmoidostomy. This approach is particularly suited for treating obstructing lesions of the sigmoid colon. The procedure requires more dissection and takes longer than segmental resection, but it eliminates the problem of synchronous polyps or cancers and removes the entire obstructed distended segment. In addition, the excellent blood supply of the ileum helps to ensure that the anastomosis is secure and reduces the risk of anastomotic leakage.

Perforation. Cancer causing a perforation of the colonic wall represents a life-threatening surgical emergency. The diagnosis may not be obvious before celiotomy because the clinical picture can mimic a perforated peptic ulcer or diverticulitis with generalized peritonitis. Thorough exploration of the peritoneal cavity is mandatory. Often, it can be difficult to distinguish an inflammatory pelvic mass caused by diverticulitis from that caused by a perforated sigmoid colon cancer.

There are fewer surgical options for treating a perforated colon cancer than for an obstructing cancer. The goal of operation is to remove the diseased, perforated segment of bowel. It may

be possible to fashion an anastomosis; however, an anastomosis of unprepared bowel fashioned in a contaminated field should always be protected by proximal colostomy or ileostomy. The temporary diverting stoma can be closed about 10 weeks after the emergency operation.

An alternative is to resect the perforated segment and exteriorize the proximal and distal limbs as described above (or to use Hartmann's operation for more distal lesions). After the patient has recovered from the initial surgery, intestinal continuity can be restored.

After the perforated segment has been resected, the peritoneal cavity should be thoroughly irrigated with saline solution to remove all visible contamination, and intravenous antibiotics should be continued postoperatively.

Every effort should be made to perform a curative operation for obstructing or perforated cancers. The prognosis is somewhat poorer for these patients, but the 5-year survival rate approaches 30 percent in patients with no obvious metastases who are treated by immediate resection of the lesion.

Staging and Prognosis

In the absence of obvious metastatic disease, the precise stage of colorectal cancer can be determined only after surgical resection and histopathologic analysis. Unlike other solid tumors, the size of the primary lesion has little influence on prognosis of colon cancer. The factors that are most closely related to outcome are (1) the depth of tumor penetration into the bowel wall, (2) the involvement of regional lymph nodes, and (3) the presence of distant metastases. Numerous staging systems have been developed over the past several decades, but the system proposed by Dukes in 1932 for description of rectal cancer has continued to be used widely because of its simplicity (Fig. 26-75). The classification scheme proposed by Dukes concerned only rectal cancer and recognized three stages; however, the most often used variant of this system recognizes a fourth stage (distant metastases) and has been extended to include colon cancers. This system fails to include important prognostic information such as vascular invasion, perineural invasion, histologic differentiation, or DNA content of tumor cells. Nevertheless, the simplicity of the Dukes classification system and its consistent correlation with prognosis suggest that it will continue to be in use for some time.

The American College of Surgeons' Commission on Cancer has urged adoption of the TNM (tumor-node-metastasis) staging system (Fig. 26-76). This system separately identifies the depth of invasion of the tumor (T), the regional lymph node status (N), and the presence of distant metastases (M):

Primary Tumor (T)

TX—Primary tumor cannot be assessed.
T0—No evidence of primary tumor.
T1—Tumor invades submucosa.
T2—Tumor invades muscularis propria.
T3—Tumor invades through the muscularis propria into the subserosa or into nonperitonealized pericolic or perirectal tissues.
T4—Tumor perforates the visceral peritoneum or directly invades other organs or structures.

Regional Lymph Nodes (N)

NX—Regional lymph nodes cannot be assessed.
N0—No regional lymph node metastasis.
N1—Metastasis in 1 to 3 pericolic or perirectal lymph nodes.

The TNM system provides more detailed pathologic information and can be converted easily to the simpler Dukes system. Stage I is equivalent to Dukes' Stage A, Stage II to Dukes' Stage B, Stage III to Dukes' Stage C, and Stage IV to Dukes' Stage D.

The 5-year survival rates clearly demonstrate the prognostic importance of disease staging. The best outcome is associated with Stage I disease, with more than 90 percent of patients surviving at 5 years. For Stage II disease, this figure drops to between 60 and 80 percent, and for patients with lymph node metastasis (Stage III), 5-year survival rates range from 20 to 50 percent. When distant metastases are present, fewer than 5 percent of patients survive for 5 years.

For all but Stage IV disease, survival rates have improved since the 1940s and 1950s. Whether this improvement is attributable to diagnostic or treatment advances is not clear. More thorough and precise staging procedures may now be responsible for eliminating or reducing the misclassification of patients, which can artificially and adversely affect the observed response to treatment.

Other disease factors that have a negative prognostic influence include poor histologic differentiation of the tumor (mucin-producing tumors and "signet ring" cell tumors have a poorer prognosis) (Fig. 26-77), venous or perineural invasion by the cancer, bowel perforation, elevated CEA level, and aneuploid nuclei.

Adjuvant Chemotherapy

Colorectal carcinoma has been resistant to most chemotherapeutic agents. However, chemotherapy following extirpation of all detectable disease is theoretically appealing because effective agents should have an advantage if the tumor burden is minimal. Chemotherapy is most effective when the burden of carcinoma is smallest and the fraction of malignant cells in growth phase is highest. Recently, there have been indications that the combination of 5-fluorouracil (5-FU) and levamisole or 5-FU and leucovorin is associated with increased survival when administered postoperatively to selected patients with no apparent residual disease (*adjuvant chemotherapy*).

A large intergroup clinical trial examined the effect of levamisole alone, levamisole with 5-FU, and observation only in patients with resected colon carcinoma. Levamisole alone produced no significant effect, but the combination of 5-FU and levamisole improved disease-free survival rate and overall survival rates compared with surgery alone in patients with Stage III colon cancer. Therapy with 5-FU and levamisole reduced the risk of cancer recurrence by 39 percent, cancer-related deaths by 32 percent, and the overall death rate by 31 percent in these patients. There was no survival benefit in patients with Stage II disease who received chemotherapy. A combination of 5-FU and leucovorin has improved survival rates in patients with Stage III colon cancer.

The role of adjuvant chemotherapy for rectal cancer is less well defined. Variation in surgical technique, particularly with regard to the extent of mesorectal excision and the use of pre- or postoperative radiation, makes comparison of available data difficult. The few prospective, randomized trials evaluating postoperative adjuvant chemotherapy suggest that there may be a modest survival advantage in treating Stage II and Stage III rectal cancer.

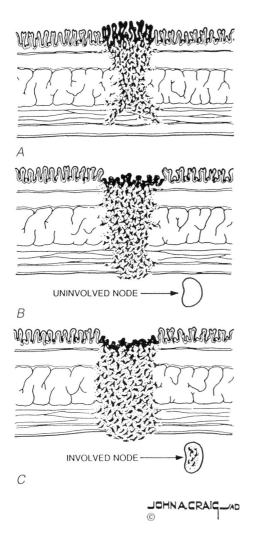

FIG. 26-75. Dukes' histologic classification system for rectal cancer. *A.* Cancer growth limited to the wall of the rectum. *B.* Cancer growth extended through the wall of the bowel, but not involving adjacent lymph nodes. *C.* Cancer metastatic to regional lymph nodes. (From: *Kodner IJ, Fleshman JW, Fry RD: Anal and rectal cancer: Principles of management, in Maingot's Abdominal Operations, 1989, with permission.*)

N2—Metastasis in 4 or more pericolic or perirectal lymph nodes.
N3—Metastasis in any lymph node along the course of a named vascular trunk.

Distant Metastasis (M)

MX—Presence of distant metastasis cannot be assessed.
M0—No distant metastasis.
M1—Distant metastasis.

The stage of the TNM system is as follows:

Stage I	T1	N0	M0
	T2	N0	M0
Stage II	T3	N0	M0
	T4	N0	M0
Stage III	Any T	N1	M0
	Any T	N2,N3	M0
Stage IV	Any T	Any N	M1

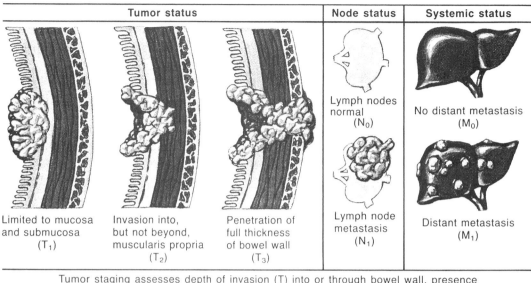

Tumor status			Node status	Systemic status

Limited to mucosa and submucosa (T_1)

Invasion into, but not beyond, muscularis propria (T_2)

Penetration of full thickness of bowel wall (T_3)

Lymph nodes normal (N_0)

No distant metastasis (M_0)

Lymph node metastasis (N_1)

Distant metastasis (M_1)

Tumor staging assesses depth of invasion (T) into or through bowel wall, presence or absence of lymph node (N) and distant organ metastasis (M)

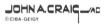
JOHN A. CRAIG___AD
©CIBA-GEIGY

FIG. 26-76. TNM staging system for colorectal cancer. (From: *Fry RD, Fleshman JW, Kodner IJ: Cancer of colon and rectum. Ciba Clin Symp 41:5, 1989, with permission.*)

Long-Term Follow-Up

There is some controversy about the frequency of follow-up examinations for tumor recurrence in patients treated for colorectal cancer. Some physicians have adopted a nihilistic approach (because of poor prognosis once recurrent cancer is detected) and recommend that once a patient is discharged following surgery, further treatment should be given only if symptoms of recurrent disease develop.

A small group of patients, however, definitely benefit from detection and aggressive treatment of recurrent cancer. About 70 percent of recurrent cancers become detectable within 2 years of initial treatment and 90 percent within 4 years. Patients who have been treated successfully for colon or rectal cancer have a higher incidence of metachronous colorectal cancer, and early detection and treatment of these cancers can improve the prognosis for these patients. This fact alone should provide sufficient rationale for long-term follow-up of all patients treated for colorectal cancer.

Follow-up evaluation may include physical examination, sigmoidoscopy, colonoscopy, liver function tests, CEA assay, chest radiography, barium enema, liver scan, CT, and MRI.

Physical examinations following surgical treatment for colorectal cancer may assuage both patient and physician, but they are of little value in the early detection of recurrent disease. By the time a recurrent cancer has become palpable by abdominal examination, it is invariably unresectable.

Sigmoidoscopy is of some value when following patients treated with low anterior resection and anastomosis for rectal or sigmoid cancer because it allows direct inspection of the anastomosis. *Colonoscopy* is most useful for the detection of metachronous polyps or cancers in patients with previously treated colorectal cancer.

Both *liver function tests* and *CEA assay* can indicate the presence of liver metastases from colorectal cancer. A significant elevation of any of the liver function tests or a rising CEA level calls for a CT scan of the abdomen and a chest radiograph.

The principles of managing metastatic disease are similar for cancer of the colon and the rectum and are discussed in the following section on rectal cancer.

Rectal Cancer

Pathophysiology

As with colon cancer, the vast majority of malignant neoplasms of the rectum are adenocarcinomas. The significant premalignant conditions such as adenomatous and villous polyps, familial adenomatous polyposis, and ulcerative colitis are also the same. Adenocarcinomas of the rectum must be differentiated from squamous cell cancer of the anal canal because the management is entirely different. Malignant melanoma rarely can be found in the rectum, and its management again differs from that of adenocarcinoma. The prognosis of rectal malignant melanoma is so poor that wide resective surgery is not always indicated.

Rectal cancer is considered separately from colon cancer because of its anatomic location and configuration. Because the rectum resides within the confines of the pelvis, wide excision of the cancer and surrounding structures (as is possible with colon cancer) is usually impossible. The proximity of the rectum to the anal sphincter mechanism also creates unique problems of management. In order to achieve a curative distal margin beyond the cancer, a surgeon must consider the risk of injury to the sphincter mechanism. If the sphincter cannot be preserved to function perfectly, it should be removed. It is this need to remove the sphincter mechanism that results in the need for a

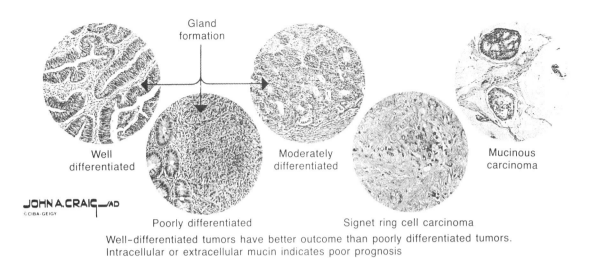

FIG. 26-77. Histology of colorectal cancer. (From: *Fry RD, Fleshman JW, Kodner U: Cancer of colon and rectum. Ciba Clin Symp 41:5, 1989, with permission.*)

colostomy, and it is wrong to jeopardize cure of a cancer to avoid a colostomy. The details of colostomy construction and care will be described later, but it is critically important for the patient to understand that a colostomy is usually constructed because of the anatomic location of the cancer, not its severity. Most patients assume that the need for a colostomy indicates a hopelessly incurable cancer.

Rectal cancer also requires special consideration because the innervation of the urogenital system lies in close proximity, as in fact do the organs of the urogenital tract (see Fig. 26-8). There is a high rate of impotence in men from radical treatment of rectal cancer, and we are reminded that accurate definitions of sexual dysfunction in women are lacking. The relationship of the rectum to the genitourinary system can be of supreme importance in determining the surgical procedure itself; the posterior wall of the vagina can be resected in continuity with an invasive rectal cancer, but a cancer invading the prostate or bladder base in a man requires a much more extensive and complicated procedure. The rectum also requires special consideration because it has a dual arterial blood supply (see Fig. 26-6), and the lymphatic channels of cancer metastasis follow the routes of the arterial system (see Fig. 26-7). The primary physiologic function of the rectum is to serve as a reservoir for fecal material, which can be stored until the individual chooses to empty it. Any disturbance of the reservoir or continence mechanism can result in significant handicap to the individual. This consideration is of prime importance in determining the treatment of rectal cancer. It is because of the distensible nature of the rectal reservoir that cancers can grow to considerable size before causing any symptoms. This fact makes screening for rectal, as well as colon, cancers mandatory. The organ is accessible, and asymptomatic (more curable) cancers should be sought by routine screening or surveillance, especially in individuals known to be at significant risk.

Perhaps the most unique aspect of the anatomy of the rectum is its easy accessibility. The anus allows access to the rectum with several therapeutic and diagnostic modalities, including the physician's finger. This easy access has resulted in consideration of tumor treatment less than the radical resective procedures that

often require removal of the rectum and anus, necessitating construction of a colostomy.

These unique features of the rectum must be considered for the screening, diagnosis, and treatment of patients known to have or suspected of having rectal cancer. One must consider the *local* factors related to the rectum itself. The next level of consideration involves the relationship of the cancer to the structures *adjacent* to the rectum such as lymph nodes, sphincter mechanism, and surrounding organs. Perhaps the most important prognostic consideration lies in the status of the cancer with respect to *distant* metastasis. Rectal cancer can spread through the lymphatics of the mesenteric or iliac system. It can metastasize to the liver via the portal venous system or to the lungs, or rarely to the brain or bones, via other hematogenous routes.

Diagnosis and Classification

The important aspects of complete evaluation of rectal cancer are related to the *local, regional,* and *systemic* manifestation of the cancer (Fig. 26-78).

Local Aspects. *Local evaluation* of a rectal cancer helps determine the proper modality of management and gives some insight into the prognosis of the cancer. Careful digital rectal examination must be performed to evaluate size, fixation, and ulceration of the cancer, as well as any suggestion of extension of the cancer to pararectal lymph nodes or adjacent organs. The rectal cancer needs to be visualized by the surgeon using a rigid sigmoidoscope, adequate biopsy taken, degree of fixation to surrounding tissue evaluated, risk of obstruction predicted, size and ulceration of lesion determined, and distance from the distal edge of the tumor to the dentate line measured carefully. Flexible fiberoptic instruments are not totally reliable because only tiny biopsies can be taken, and the flexibility of the instrument can give a false sense of security relative to the distance between the cancer and the mucocutaneous junction (dentate line). It is this distance that ultimately determines if a surgeon can preserve the anal sphincter mechanism.

Cancers that have an adequate "clinical" classification system allow the treating physicians to securely plan a course of treat-

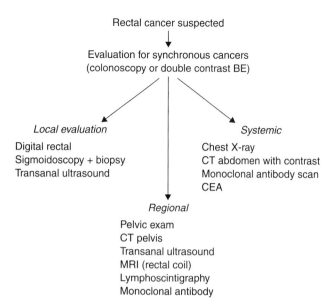

FIG. 26-78. *Evaluation of suspected rectal cancer.*

ment before operation. So far this cannot be fully accomplished with rectal cancer because the important variables either have not been defined completely or cannot be determined before initiating treatment. The previously noted classification systems (see Figs. 26-75 and 26-76) describe the depth of cancer invasion and the status of cancer spread to surrounding lymph nodes. This is a "histologic" classification that requires removal of the rectum and pararectal tissue before its application.

The biologic behavior of rectal cancer cannot be predicted by its location or size. Poorly differentiated cancers have a worse long-term prognosis than those which are well differentiated. Some very aggressive histologic patterns such as "signet ring" cell and mucinous cancers carry an especially poor prognosis. Attempts are being made to further predict the biologic aggressiveness of rectal cancers by analysis of the DNA from biopsies of the cancers (see Fig. 26-77). These biologic predictors become important when local, nonresective techniques are described for small, favorable-appearing cancers. If the cancers that look favorable but have aggressive biologic behavior can be identified, they should be treated by nothing less than radical resection.

The *depth of invasion* of a rectal cancer is known to be an important variable. In order for a rectal cancer to be classified as "invasive," it must extend at least into the muscularis mucosae, for at this level it has access to the vascular and lymphatic systems, and metastasis becomes a possibility. Morson showed long ago that even a small, mobile cancer, confined to the rectal wall but extending into the muscularis mucosae, will have a 10 percent incidence of metastasis to pararectal lymph nodes. A major, unfulfilled challenge in evaluating rectal cancer is the pretreatment determination of lymph node involvement by cancer.

The depth of cancer invasion can be determined accurately by use of *transanal ultrasonography* (see Fig. 26-65). Each layer of the rectal wall can be identified and its penetration by cancer described. Although lymph nodes can be visualized by ultrasonography, the presence of cancer within these nodes cannot be

accurately predicted. CT scanning of the rectum has been extremely helpful in evaluation of the cancer itself, but nuclear magnetic resonance imaging, especially with the use of newly available transrectally positioned coils, should be very helpful in predicting depth of invasion and involvement of lymph nodes and other pararectal structures by the primary cancer. Sometimes transanal excisional biopsy of an entire small lesion is helpful for determining depth of invasion, but this will not define lymph node involvement.

The advantages of these accurate descriptions of the cancer become evident when the treatment is chosen and decisions must be made regarding extent of operation and use of adjuvant modalities such as chemotherapy or radiation therapy.

Regional Aspects. Regional evaluation of pararectal structures involves transanal ultrasound and CT scanning or MRI, as just described, plus some special considerations. A major factor early in the evaluation of a patient with rectal cancer involves determination of the possibility and extent of resectability. After a cancer grows through the wall of the rectum, it can invade any of the surrounding structures. This is usually determined by evaluation of the *fixation* or tethering of the tumor to these structures. This makes complete examination of these structures necessary. A woman should have a complete pelvic examination with care to determine if the tumor is suspected of invading the vagina or has spread to the ovaries. In a man, evaluation of extension into the prostate or bladder is important. This could require transanal ultrasonography, CT scanning, MRI, or even cystoscopy and biopsy.

It is suspected that the extent of fixation of the tumor is an important predictor of prognosis. It is also a major factor in determining the need for adjuvant radiation therapy, sometimes coupled with chemotherapy. Even if the cancer shrinks with preoperative adjuvant therapy, consideration must be given to resection of the involved structures originally suspected of invasion by the cancer. The performance of very extensive resective procedures must be tempered by the patient's age and general health. The determination of extent of fixation of the cancer is complicated by the fact that many invasive cancers are surrounded by an intense inflammatory reaction that creates the sensation of fixation rather than actual invasion by the cancer.

The surgeon also should know the status of the upper urinary tract. If, for example, one of the ureters is involved with the invasive cancer, a determination should be made before operation that the contralateral kidney is functioning. Specific plans may need to be made for a urologist to deal with the bladder and ureter at the time of surgery. Our own preference is to use intravenous contrast material at the time of CT scanning for liver metastases to evaluate kidney size and function, as well as position and possible involvement of the ureters.

One of the most frustrating aspects of regional evaluation of rectal cancer is the inability to determine cancer involvement of the adjacent, or regional, lymph nodes. This one fact would be most helpful in determining need for adjuvant treatment preoperatively. CT and transanal ultrasound, as well as distal palpation, have allowed determination of the presence of enlarged nodes but have not been helpful in determining presence of cancer within these nodes. There is hope that improved MRI techniques, use of monoclonal antibodies, and perhaps PET scanning will be helpful in this important aspect of staging. Most studies have shown the involvement of lymph nodes in the resected specimen to be the most influential predictor of prognosis. Recently, more credence is being placed on the involvement of the "tangential" margin of resection (Fig. 26-79). This is the peripheral margin, including the extent of clearance of the cancer from surrounding tissue. Interestingly, this margin is not reported by the pathologist unless special effort is made to "ink" the tissue immediately after the resection. A great deal of discussion exists in the surgical literature over what represents an adequate distal margin, the range being 2 to 5 cm. This is based on studies to evaluate the extent of microscopic spread of cancer distal to the palpable edge of the tumor. What difference does it make if the distal margin is 2 or 5 cm when the tangential margin is minimal or nonexistent? Many surgeons believe that this nonreported regional margin is the major cause of local recurrence of rectal cancer. Although the cure of rectal cancer can be very high, the cure of locally recurrent rectal cancer is exceedingly small and often requires devastatingly radical surgery. Thus the complicated evaluation of regional spread is critical.

Distant Spread. Determination of distant spread of rectal cancer is important because these patients generally are considered to be incurable. The knowledge of metastasis to the liver or lungs may significantly modify the surgical management of the primary cancer. Routine evaluation for distant metastatic disease consists of a chest radiograph, determination of CEA level, and a contrast-enhanced CT scan of the upper and lower abdomen. The latter also allows evaluation of the urinary tract, as described previously. Suspicious lesions in the liver may need further evaluation by MRI or angio-CT. CT also will help in determining metastasis to the ovaries or dissemination within the peritoneal cavity. Rectal cancer rarely metastasizes to the bones or to the brain, and in the absence of symptoms, these two areas are not included in routine surveillance. The liver must be involved extensively with cancer before liver function tests become abnormal, and most authors find limited use in these tests. PET scanning is extremely sensitive in its ability to detect metastatic or recurrent tumor and is often helpful in planning treatment.

Surgical Treatment

General Principles. The surgical treatment of rectal cancer should accomplish complete removal of the cancer and involved regional tissue. The resection should encompass an adequate margin around all facets of the cancer, not just the usually reported distal margin. The extent and timing of the surgery must be planned carefully, including partial or complete resection of surrounding structures. Because most of the rectum resides within the confines of the bones of the pelvis, the technical accomplishment of an anastomosis can be difficult. This difficulty has resulted in a history of significant complications with the colorectal anastomosis and many suggestions for avoiding serious complications, including the use of temporary, protecting intestinal stomas. The ability to construct low anastomoses, deep within the pelvis, has improved in recent years with the advent of the intraluminal surgical stapling instruments. This has markedly reduced the need for abdominal perineal resection without reducing the level of local control of the rectal cancer (Fig. 26-80 and Table 26-15).

Basic principles of cancer surgery should be used, in that dissection of the rectum and surrounding tissue must be accomplished first, and then consideration should be given to restoration of intestinal continuity (Fig. 26-81). Intestinal continuity should be restored ("low anterior resection") only if the anastomosis can be performed with an excellent blood supply and no tension. In addition, the sphincter muscle must function adequately. It is a disservice to accomplish a heroically low anastomosis in an elderly person, only to leave her or him with impaired continence. After all, an opening of the colon without sphincter control is a "colostomy," and a person is much better served to have a well-positioned, well-constructed colostomy on the abdominal wall rather than in the perineal area, which is inaccessible and incapable of having secure coverage by an appliance.

If anal sphincter function cannot be preserved, or if the cancer is so low that the sphincter or anus must be encompassed in the resection, the entire rectum must be removed and egress of feces accomplished by construction of a permanent colostomy (Fig. 26-82). The operation is performed by mobilization of the left colon and rectum through a laparotomy or celiotomy, with dissection of the distal rectum from the perineum, and is referred to as an *abdominal-perineal,* or *AP, resection.* The precise terminology is an *abdominal-perineal proctosigmoidectomy.*

Preparation of a patient for resection of a rectal cancer should include antibiotics and mechanical bowel preparation, as described for colonic cancer, plus a few special considerations. The patient should always have potential colostomy sites identified and marked on the abdominal wall before surgery (Fig. 26-83). This should be done even if an anastomosis is anticipated, because unexpected problems can be encountered at the time of surgery, and a colostomy might be required. An unpredicted colostomy is made worse by having it in a poor location. End colostomies are usually constructed of the distal descending (not sigmoid) colon and are located in the left lower quadrant of the abdomen or in the midline, sometimes at the umbilicus. The site is chosen as illustrated in Fig. 26-83. The patient is marked in the supine position and then asked to sit and move about. The site of the stoma should be accessible to the patient for care and on the summit of a fold of fat, not in a crease or on a scar or bony prominence. Any position off the midline should bring the stoma through the body of the rectus muscle. A low anastomosis is sometimes protected with a temporary loop ileostomy, and for this reason, it is advantageous to mark the right lower quadrant before surgery (see Fig. 26-61). The best sites are marked with ink, and the next day, in the operating room, the sites are identified by scratching the skin with a needle.

The operation is performed with general anesthesia, sometimes supplemented with epidural anesthesia; the latter provides perfect relaxation and may facilitate a lower dissection of the rectum and anastomosis. It is not unusual for blood transfusion to be required during or immediately after the procedure, and preparation should be made well in advance, especially if "directed donors" are involved. If the cancer is suspected of involving the bladder or ureter, or if there has been previous pelvic surgery, cystoscopy and placement of ureteral catheters after induction of anesthesia can be extremely helpful. This does not preclude injury to the ureter but usually makes its intraoperative identification and preservation easier.

A patient who is to have surgical resection of the rectum should be positioned on the operating table so that a sterile field can be prepared for access to the perineum, as well as to the abdomen (Fig. 26-84). This allows mobilization of the left colon and rectum from above and passage of anastomotic stapling in-

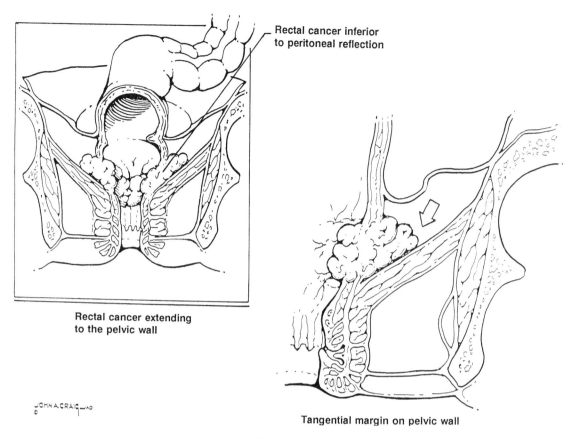

Rectal cancer extending
to the pelvic wall

Rectal cancer inferior
to peritoneal reflection

Tangential margin on pelvic wall

FIG. 26-79. Tangential margins in rectal cancer.

struments or removal of the rectum from below. Before the operation is started, a Foley catheter is placed in the bladder, a nasogastric tube in the stomach, and a #34 mushroom-tipped catheter in the rectum. Irrigation of the rectum with saline solution is accomplished through the rectal catheter; and when the effluent is clear, approximately 100 mL of povidone-iodine solution is instilled in the rectum.

The abdomen is opened through a midline incision, and exploration is carried out, looking for other intraabdominal problems, especially the presence of metastatic disease to the peritoneum, the ovaries, or the liver. Small liver metastases, especially on the surface of the liver, may have been missed by CT scan. Any suspicious lesions should be biopsied and undergo frozen-section examination while the operation proceeds. The liver is most accurately evaluated for metastatic disease by use of intraoperative ultrasonography.

The entire left colon is then mobilized on its mesentery, using the embryonic fusion plane (white line of Toldt) between the mesentery and the fat of the lateral pelvic wall (Fig. 26-85A,B). When this is done properly, the ureter and genital vessels can be identified and reflected posteriorally. Especially if low anastomosis is a possibility, full mobilization of the splenic flexure of the colon may be helpful.

The inferior mesenteric artery is ligated at the aorta (see Fig. 26-85C). This is done not so much to enhance the cure of the cancer as to allow better mobilization of the descending colon and to clearly define the parameters of the distal dissection. This is the first of five potential injury points to the innervation nec-

essary for normal sexual function (Fig. 26-86C). The mesentery is then incised to the junction of the descending and sigmoid

MAJOR RESECTIONS

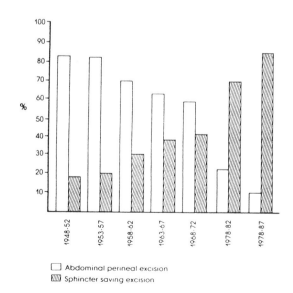

□ Abdominal perineal excision
▨ Sphincter saving excision

FIG. 26-80. Trends in surgery for rectal carcinoma, 1948–1988 (From: *Hackford AW: 1990, with permission.*)

Table 26-15
Recurrence Rates for Abdominal Perineal Resection vs. Low Anterior Resection

Author	Abdominal Perineal Resection		Low Anterior Resection	
	No.	Recurrence Rate	No.	Recurrence Rate
Morson	1238	8.3%	177	7.9%
Deddish/Stearns	236	14.4%	65	9.2%
Williams/Johnson	83	8.0%	71	11.0%
Heimann et al.	118	17.0%	202	16.0%
Goligher et al.	26	23.0%	105	8.6%
Lasson et al.	49	37.0%	40	35.0%
Floyd et al..	5	20.0%	16	56.0%
Glenn/McSherry	422	21.0%	163	13.0%
Williams et al.	33	18.8%	100	13.6%
Heald/Ryall			115	2.6%
TOTAL	2210	12.85%	1054	12.33%

SOURCE: Hackford AW: The extent of major resections for rectal cancer. *Semin Colon Rectal Surg* 1:16, 1990, with permission.

colon. The ascending left colic artery and the inferior mesenteric vein will be transected as this is done (see Fig. 26-85*C*). If the need for further mobility is anticipated, the inferior mesenteric vein should be transected a second time at the peripheral margin of the duodenum (see Fig. 26-85*D*). This will allow the descending colon, with its blood supply through collaterals from the superior mesenteric artery, to be placed deep within the pelvis without tension.

The bowel is then transected at the junction of the descending and sigmoid colon. The proximal component is protected for construction of an anastomosis or a colostomy. If an anastomosis is anticipated, preparation can be made for using the stapling instrument by inserting a purse-string suture (see Fig. 26-84).

The distal dissection of the rectum is then completed (see Fig. 26-86), first posteriorly between the presacral fascia and the enveloping fascia of the rectum (the second and third nerve injury points), then laterally with transection of the "lateral liga-ments" (the fourth nerve injury point), and finally anteriorly with care taken to avoid the seminal vesicles or vagina (the fifth nerve injury point). During this dissection, the rectum rises out of the pelvis. Before beginning the anterior dissection, the surgeon may irrigate the rectum from above with 40% ethanol in an attempt to lessen the chance of implanting viable tumor cells should the rectum be entered during the difficult anterior dissection. The extent of the distal dissection is then determined by the location of the cancer, aiming for a margin 3 to 5 cm beyond the palpable edge of the tumor. If the cancer cannot be palpated, sigmoid-oscopy should be performed to precisely locate the cancer and an adequate transection site marked from the abdominal aspect. The dissection can be extended to within the levator muscles. The rectum can be transected with a linear stapling instrument in anticipation of a double-stapled anastomosis (Fig. 26-87). If anastomosis is not possible, the rectum can be removed from below by a second operating team (Fig. 26-88), or the abdominal part of the procedure can be completed, including colostomy construction, the patient turned to the prone-flexed position, and the rectum removed by perineal dissection.

If the rectum and sphincter mechanism are completely re-moved, a permanent colostomy must be constructed using the prepared distal descending colon. If an anastomosis is con-structed but is of questionable security (suspect blood supply, tension, or surrounding sepsis), a protecting loop colostomy or ileostomy, of a temporary nature, can be constructed. This should occur only rarely, because any problems should be cor-rected before completing the operation. A leaked colorectal anas-tomosis, even with a temporary colostomy, is a serious problem and is better avoided by correcting the cause for concern.

A special situation is created when a *coloanal anastomosis* is considered (see Fig. 26-81). This involves stripping the distal rectal mucosa and constructing an anastomosis between descend-ing colon and anus, similar to the technique of ileal pouch–anal anastomosis used after colectomy and mucosal proctectomy for mucosal ulcerative colitis or familial polyposis. In fact, some centers are describing construction of a colonic J-pouch as part of the "coloanal" procedure. If a coloanal anastomosis is con-structed, it should be protected with a temporary proximal di-verting colostomy or, preferably, a protecting loop ileostomy. Some surgeons find limited use for the coloanal anastomosis

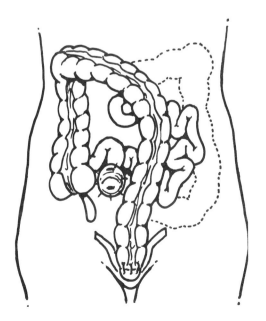

FIG. 26-81. Options in the surgical management of rectal cancer.

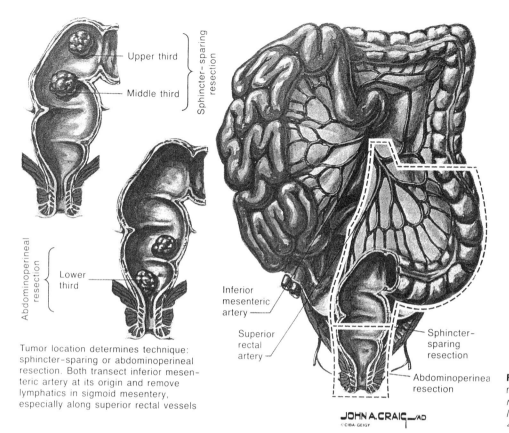

Tumor location determines technique: sphincter–sparing or abdominoperineal resection. Both transect inferior mesenteric artery at its origin and remove lymphatics in sigmoid mesentery, especially along superior rectal vessels

FIG. 26-82. Surgical resection of rectal cancer. (From: *Fry RD, Fleshman JW, Kodner IJ: Cancer of colon and rectum. Ciba Clin Symp 41:5, 1989, with permission.*)

because removing only the mucosa is not adequate treatment for an invasive cancer. The coloanal procedure is an excellent, albeit complex, procedure for benign neoplasms, such as "carpet-type" villous adenomas, and for management of radiation-induced rectal injury, where normal well-vascularized tissue can be pulled through the radiation-damaged rectum.

The *Hartmann resection* is a compromise type of resection used occasionally for rectal cancer (see Fig. 26-81). It involves resection of the rectum and/or sigmoid colon and construction of an end colostomy, but it avoids anastomosis and perineal dissection of the distal rectum and perineum. This procedure is used most often for treating sigmoid diverticulitis, but it can be used for management of rectal cancer if there has been too much obstruction or sepsis to allow a safe anastomosis. It is also useful for the elderly or severely unstable patient in whom an adequate distal margin can be accomplished but anastomosis is inappropriate because the procedure should not be prolonged or because the sphincter may not function adequately for a very low anastomosis. If there is no reason to anticipate distal obstruction of the rectal segment, the proximal end can be closed and allowed to reside within the peritoneal cavity. If there is an anal stricture or any other possible distal obstruction, a mucous fistula should be constructed of the distal rectum.

When the Hartmann procedure is done, it is usually anticipated to be a temporary situation with ultimate construction of a colorectal anastomosis to restore intestinal continuity. This eventual anastomosis is sometimes not safe or possible, so the Hartmann procedure becomes the definitive procedure. For this reason, the stoma site should be chosen carefully, because these "temporary" colostomies can become "permanent."

Metastatic Disease. The management of metastatic disease from rectal cancer is the same as that for colon cancer. Suspicious lesions on or within the liver should have biopsies taken early during the operative procedure and frozen-section evaluation completed. If a small number of easily resectable lesions exist, they can be removed with some margin, once the rectal cancer has been definitely managed. If many lesions exist, biopsy should be taken to help plan subsequent treatment. If massive replacement of the liver exists, management of the primary cancer may need to be modified. Such patients have an extremely limited life expectancy, and the now "palliative" procedure should do just that: provide relief of symptoms with as little morbidity as possible. This may mean only a colostomy without attempted resection of a "fixed" cancer, or it may mean resection with a "short" distal margin to eliminate the need for a colostomy during the few remaining months of life.

If the patient can have adequate resection of local and regional aspects of the rectal cancer, significant cures are being reported with liver resection when there are fewer than four lesions and both lobes of the liver are not involved. This is determined by repeat evaluation of the liver after the patient has recovered from treatment of the primary lesion. Most oncologists will treat diffuse hepatic involvement with systemic chemotherapy, although some prefer to wait until symptoms occur. The delivery of chemotherapeutic agents directly to the liver via the portal vein or the hepatic artery has been described, but no reports have yet shown a favorable ratio of treatment benefits versus morbidity of this modality of treatment.

Metastases to the lung, the second most common site of metastasis from colorectal cancer, are also managed by resection if

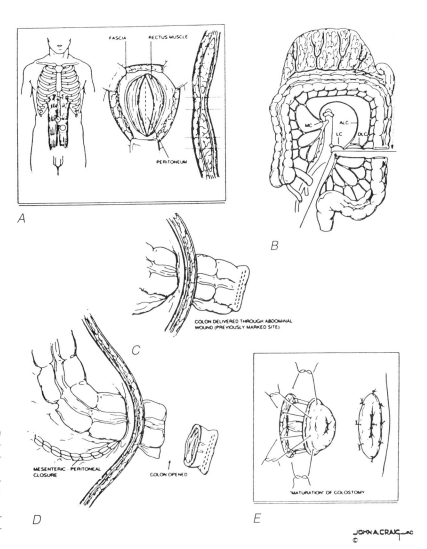

FIG. 26-83. Construction of an end colostomy. *A.* Selection of stoma location and technique of incision of the abdominal wall at the colostomy site. *B.* Technique of colonic mobilization and provision of adequate blood supply for the colostomy. *C, D,* and *E.* Final stages of constructing a "mature" end colostomy. Arterial blood supply: MC=middle colic; LC=left colic; ALC=ascending left colic; DLC= descending left colic. (From: *Kodner LJ, Fry RD, Fleshman JW: Current options in the management of rectal cancer. Adv Surg 24:1, 1991, with permission.*)

the primary site can be considered "cured" and the lesions within the lung appear to have the potential for "cure" by resection.

Complications. Complications resulting from the surgical management of rectal cancer overlap with those of any major abdominal procedure, including sepsis, myocardial infarction, bleeding, pulmonary embolus, and wound problems.

There are some specific problems related to rectal cancer. One is risk of injury to sexual function. The sites of these injuries have been described. It is not known precisely how to avoid these injuries and still do an adequate cancer operation. There is at least a 50 percent incidence of significant impotence in men following resection of the rectum for cancer. For this reason, it is critical to discuss the situation with the patient before surgery and to record the pretreatment status of sexual function. It is prudent to include this risk of sexual impairment as part of a preoperative informed-consent note. This and mention of the possible need for a colostomy are the two most important elements of such a note for the patient with rectal cancer.

If a man is rendered impotent by treatment of a rectal cancer, it is advisable to wait a year before seeking consultation for implantation of some type of penile prosthetic device. The wait

is important to be sure that the malignant growth has been cleared from the pelvis and to give the patient a chance to overcome functional and psychological impediments to normal sexual function that can result from pelvic surgery and the change in body image caused by the colostomy.

Leakage from colorectal anastomosis has been reported in up to 20 percent of cases using current techniques. This complication can be decreased by constructing the anastomosis with well-vascularized bowel under no tension and by draining the pelvis from above. It is suspected that most "leaks" are due to sepsis in the pelvis that dissects into the anastomosis rather than to primary defects in the anastomosis. Young, muscular men have a higher incidence of anastomotic leaks. This may be due to the technical difficulty of operating within a muscular pelvis, or it may be due to the power of their sphincter mechanism, which acts as a postoperative obstruction and stresses the anastomosis. Such patients should have dilation of the anal sphincter in the operating room, at the conclusion of the procedure, and every few days in the postoperative period, until normal intestinal function returns.

A leaked colorectal anastomosis usually presents between 4 and 7 days postoperatively. The symptoms range from mild tem-

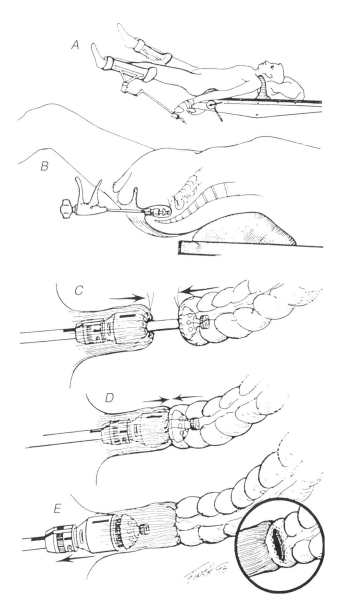

FIG. 26-84. *Technique of anastomosis using intraluminal stapler. A. Patient's legs put in stirrups for exposure of perineum. B. Insertion of stapler into rectal stump. C. Purse-string suture on rectum tied over cartridge on the shaft. Purse-string suture on the colon tied over the anvil. D. Anvil brought down to meet cartridge. E. Staple gun fired and withdrawn. (From: Goldberg SM, Gordon PH, Nivatvongs S: Essentials of Anorectal Surgery. Philadelphia, Lippincott, 1980, with permission.)*

perature elevation, to fecal fistula in the wound, to diffuse peritonitis. When such a problem is suspected, feeding is discontinued and radiologic studies are performed, at first supine and upright films of the abdomen and chest looking for extraluminal gas. CT scan can be helpful to show abscess formation, inflammation, or extraluminal gas, and a water-soluble contrast study can demonstrate the actual leak. Barium should be avoided because leakage of barium (especially mixed with stool) creates a severely destructive form of peritonitis.

The management of a leaking colorectal anastomosis depends on the severity of the problem. The majority cause minimal symptoms of sepsis and are demonstrated only with water-soluble contrast studies of the rectum. Antibiotics and bowel rest usually suffice for treatment. If the leakage has caused an abscess that drains into the rectum or a fistula that drains to the wound, the patient should be placed on antibiotics, complete bowel rest, and total parenteral nutrition for at least 2 weeks. If a large leak is demonstrated, or if the patient has symptoms of diffuse peritonitis, laparotomy should be performed with the intention of constructing a completely diverting colostomy with mucous fistula, or a loop ileostomy. Rarely the anastomosis is taken down and the proximal component used for the colostomy, but the anastomosis should never be reconstructed in the face of significant sepsis. It is important to drain the area of sepsis with the drain placed external to the rectum. Drains placed through the rectal wall perpetuate the fistula.

A special problem can occur intraoperatively during the performance of the rectal dissection: massive venous bleeding from the presacral space. This type of bleeding has been notoriously difficult to control because it actually comes from venous structures within the bone. The older control maneuvers of ligating the iliac vessels are ineffective and may be hazardous. The specimen should be removed and the pelvis packed for 24 to 48 h, or, preferably, a surgical metal "tack" should be driven into the sacrum to compress the venous space.

Malfunction of the urinary system, mainly urinary retention, is also common after resection of the rectum. This is especially true in men, in whom prostatic hypertrophy may coexist. The perineal dissection of the rectum comes very close to the membranous urethra. Foley catheters should be left in place at least 1 week after proctectomy. If urinary symptoms exist preoperatively, urologic consultation should be obtained. Sometimes a patient must be discharged from the hospital with an indwelling urinary catheter or have prostatic resection performed before discharge. Women also may have problems with bladder function postoperatively. The other problem is distortion of the vagina, which impairs sexual function in the postoperative period.

Obstructing Rectal Cancer. Obstructing rectal cancer causes a special problem because it forces the surgeon to operate on intestine that cannot be prepared, and it precludes the use of such adjuvant measures as preoperative radiation therapy. The cancers frequently are at an advanced stage and are fixed to adjacent structures; the patient may be medically compromised by the obstructed intestine as well as by the cancer. The general principles are the same as those discussed previously for obstructing cancer of the left colon.

The simplest and safest way of handling an obstructing rectal cancer is to do a limited laparotomy and construct a *decompressing* transverse colostomy (Fig. 26-89). Ileostomy may not be sufficient for decompression because a competent ileocecal valve may prevent reflux of colonic contents to the ileum. This can be done through a small upper midline incision directly over the dilated colon. The choice of location for the incision and the stoma can be aided by a preoperative x-ray of the abdomen with a coin placed at the umbilicus. Either a loop colostomy (over a small supporting rod) or "blowhole" colostomy (using only one wall of a massively dilated colon) can be constructed (Fig. 26-90). Construction of a decompressing colostomy allows subsequent complete evaluation of the patient and elective resection of the rectal cancer. If adjuvant preoperative treatment is not elected, the definitive resection can be done during the same

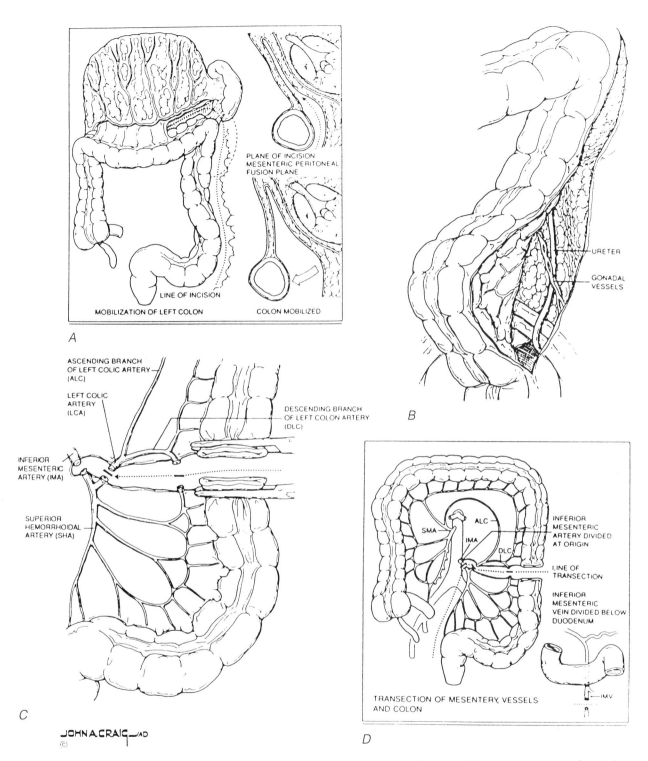

FIG. 26-85. Mobilization of the left colon. *A.* Incision line around left colon and avascular fusion plane between mesentery and retroperitoneum. *B.* Left colon reflected medially, exposing retroperitoneum. *C.* Inferior mesenteric artery divided close to aorta. Arcade of Riolan is preserved, and left colon and mesentery are divided at junction of descending and sigmoid colon. *D.* Proximal transection of inferior mesenteric vein for extra mobility. (From: *Fry RD, Fleshman JW, Kodner U: Sphincter-saving procedures for rectal cancer, in Maingot's Abdominal Operations, 1989, with permission.*)

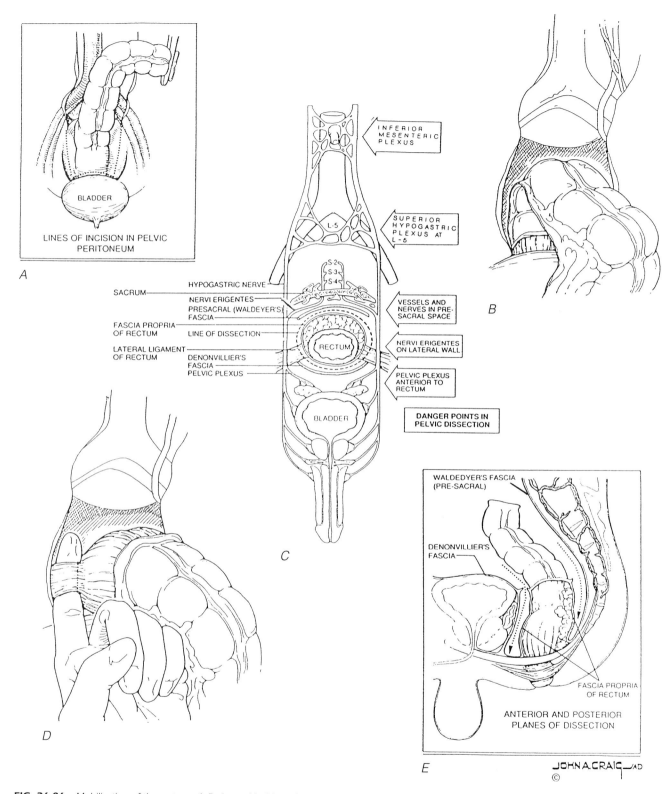

FIG. 26-86. Mobilization of the rectum. *A.* Peritoneal incision of the pelvis. *B.* Rectum reflected anteriorly and posterior avascular plane entered between presacral fascia of Waldeyer and fascia propria of rectum. *C.* Pelvic autonomic nerves and points of injury. *D.* Division of lateral stalks. *E.* Projected line of dissection in pelvis—vertical plane (From: *Kodner IJ, Fry RD, Fleshman JW: Current options in the management of rectal cancer. Adv Surg 24:1, 1991, with permission.*)

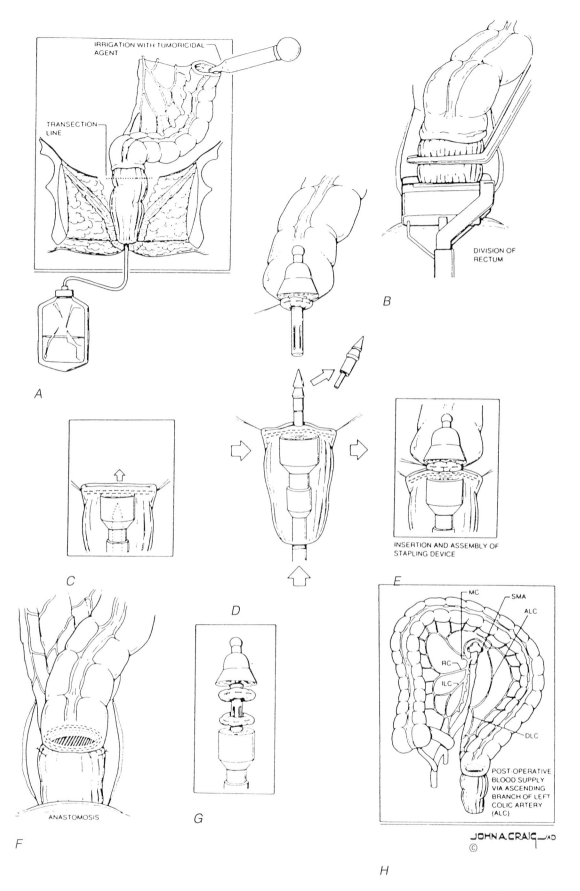

FIG. 26-87. Colorectal anastomosis: double-staple technique. *A.* Irrigation of rectum with tumoricidal agent. *B.* Transection of the distal rectum with linear stapler. *C.* Stay sutures placed in corners of rectal staple line and stapling instrument penetrating through staple line. *D.* Descending colon purse-string suture is tied around shaft of anvil; trocar is removed before reconnecting anvil to shaft. *E.* Instrument reconnected, reapproximated, and fired. *F.* Completed anastomosis. *G.* Inner doughnuts containing purse-string sutures and center of staple line. *H.* Completed low anterior resection. (From: *Kodner U, Fry RD, Fleshman JW: Current options in the management of rectal cancer. Adv Surg 24:1, 1991, with permission.*)

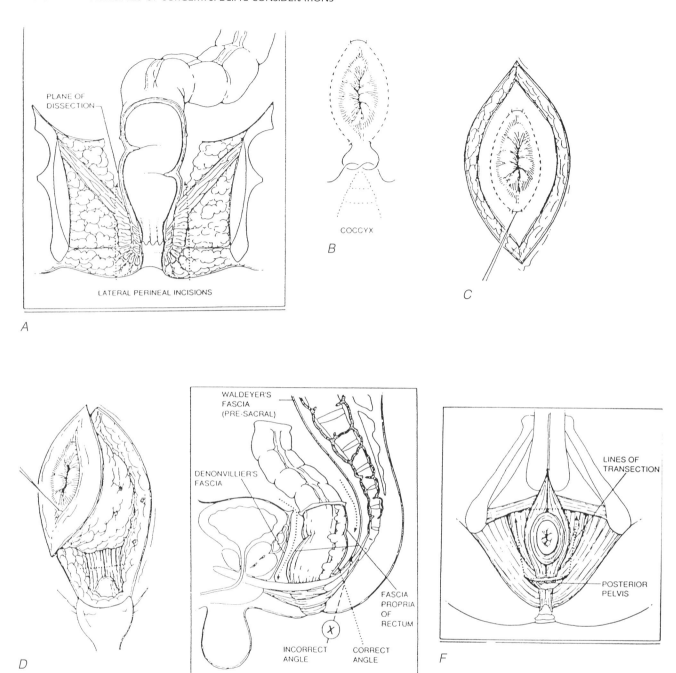

FIG. 26-88. Perineal dissection: two-team synchronous approach. *A.* Projected lines of pelvic floor re-section—vertical plane. *B, C,* and *D.* Anal closure, perineal incision, and dissection. Incision line in front of coccyx through anococcygeal ligament. *E.* Planes of pelvic dissection and posterior plane of entry into pelvis through pelvic floor. *F.* Projected lines of pelvic floor transection. *G.* Lateral transection of levator ani muscle. *H.* Completion of anterior dissection and removal of the rectum through the perineal wound. *I.* Pelvic floor closed and drains in place. (From: *Fleshman JW, Kodner IJ, Fry RD: Total proctectomy for malignancy, in Maingot's Abdominal Operations, 1989, with permission.*)

hospitalization. If adjuvant therapy is chosen, the patient can be discharged from the hospital and the definitive, elective resection performed weeks or months after the decompressing procedure. The major disadvantage of the staged procedure with initial colonic decompression is the inability to explore the entire abdom-inal cavity at the time of decompression. This may carry some risk in the patient with a "competent" ileal-cecal valve, pre-venting decompression of the obstruction into the small intestine. Such patients may have massive cecal dilatation and be at some risk of necrosis of the cecal wall.

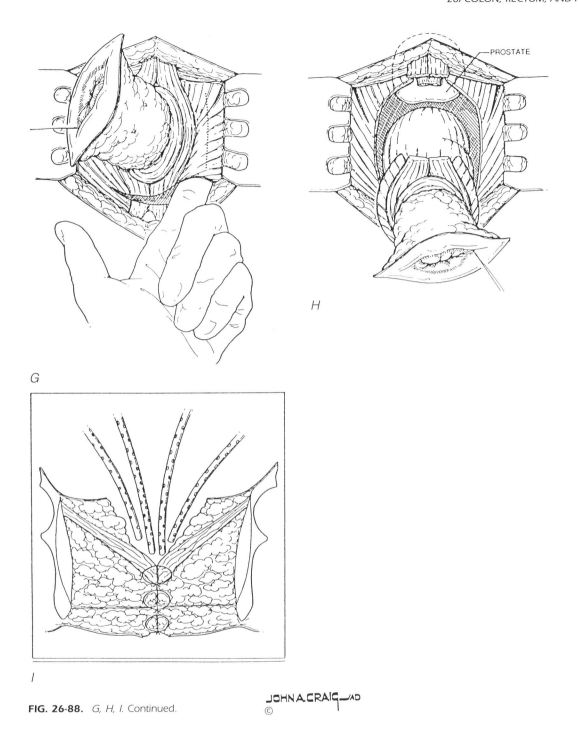

PROSTATE

H

G

I

JOHN A. CRAIG—AD
©

FIG. 26-88. *G, H, I. Continued.*

Some surgeons who operate for obstructing rectal cancer prefer to resect the cancer, using a Hartmann resection, as described previously. Others prefer to resect the cancer and all the dilated abdominal colon, allowing construction of an ileal-rectal anastomosis (see Fig. 26-81), which can be done safely when the cancer and dilated colon are removed. This type of anastomosis causes some, but usually not significant, increase in the number of daily bowel movements.

One also can resect an obstructing rectal cancer, construct an anastomosis, allow the bowel to decompress through the connection, and then protect the anastomosis with a temporary transverse colostomy or loop ileostomy, as described previously.

Colostomy Construction and Management. The construction of a colostomy is sometimes needed in the management of rectal cancer. The indications for its use have already been described, but it is important to emphasize several points. A colostomy is an opening of the colon to the abdominal wall, without the benefit of a sphincter to control the timing of its emptying. The need for a colostomy is determined more by the location of the cancer than by its severity. This is important for patients to understand, since they usually assume, as does all of our society, that the need for a colostomy indicates incurability of the cancer. In years past, this was in fact the case. Until Miles popularized the safe surgical removal of the rectum by the ab-

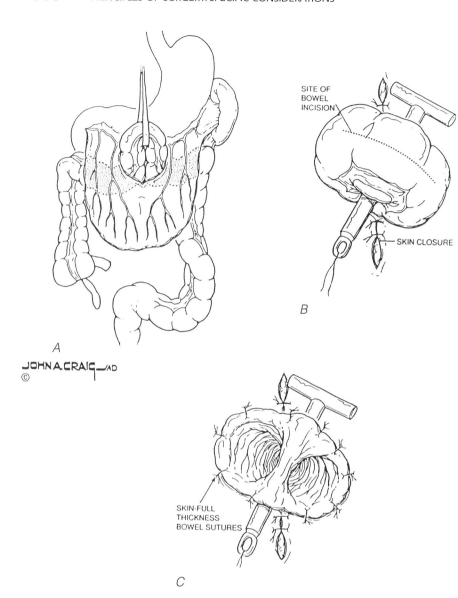

FIG. 26-89. Construction of a loop transverse colostomy. *A.* Tracheostomy tape is used to pull the loop of colon through the incision. *B* and *C.* The loop of colon is opened over a supporting rod and is sutured to the skin of the abdominal wall. (From: *Kodner U, et al: Intestinal stomas, in Maingot's Abdominal Operations, 1989, with permission.*)

dominal-perineal approach, most cancers continued to grow until they obstructed as late-stage lesions, and a colostomy was required to prolong a life complicated by the misery of uncontrolled growth of a rectal cancer within the pelvis. As explained previously, colostomies are also used to protect distal complicated anastomoses or perforations or to decompress a colon that is dilated because of distal obstruction. A loop ileostomy has been used increasingly to accomplish the same goal. Its construction does not require colonic dissection or any manipulation of the blood supply to the colorectal anastomosis. Its closure can be performed easily without involving the colon or its vessels.

The function and care of a colostomy are determined by the physiologic differences between the proximal and distal colon. The proximal colon functions to absorb water from the material that passes to it from the ileum. Its contents are liquid, and its peristaltic motion is frequent and irregular. The distal colon acts as a reservoir to allow fecal material to accumulate until it can be expelled. Its content is solid or semisolid, and its peristaltic motion is powerful and infrequent.

Although the functional aspects are important, colostomy construction is better defined by the surgeon according to the required *objective of the stoma* rather than its location. A surgeon must decide if a *decompressing* or a *diverting* stoma is required.

A *decompressing* colostomy is constructed to relieve the colonic distention caused by distal obstruction. A transverse loop colostomy is the most frequently employed stoma of this type (see Fig. 26-89). It is made by bringing a loop of colon to the abdominal wall and suspending it over a small supporting rod. If the colon is too massively dilated to bring through the abdominal wall, only one wall of the colon is used to form a so-called blowhole colostomy (see Fig. 26-90). The technique can be used for a dilated cecum as well, but this results in a stoma that is difficult to manage. Studies have shown that a well-constructed loop transverse colostomy also will provide *diversion* for as long as 6 weeks. After that time, the posterior wall of the colon falls below the abdominal wall, and fecal material can pass into the distal segment.

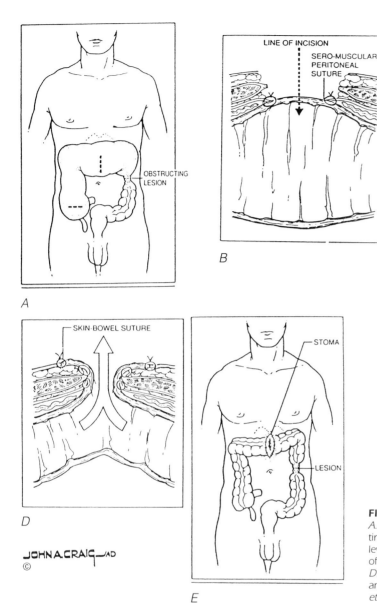

FIG. 26-90. Construction of "blowhole" cecostomy or colostomy. *A.* The incision is located over the most dilated aspect of the intestine. *B.* Placement of the quarantine sutures. *C.* Details of the second level of quarantine sutures between fascia and seromuscular layer of colonic wall (should be completed before the bowel is opened). *D.* The stoma is completed by placement of sutures between skin and colonic wall. *E.* Completed blowhole stoma. (From: *Kodner IJ, et al: Intestinal stomas, in Maingot's Abdominal Operations, 1989, with permission.*)

If complete diversion is required because of distal perforation of the intestine, a loop colostomy is inadequate. Complete diversion can be guaranteed only if the colon is divided, with construction of an end colostomy and mucous fistula.

All colostomies are opened primarily in the operating room, and full thickness of the intestine is sutured to full thickness of skin. This "maturation" of the colostomy allows immediate application of an appliance and avoids subsequent stricture of the stoma, a condition that causes significant difficulty for the patient, requiring ineffective dilation of the stoma and eventual revision. The construction of a colostomy by suspending a dilated loop of colon over a large glass supporting rod and opening it 24 to 48 h later should be relegated to history.

Any patient with abdominal trauma, diverticulitis, or a cancer anywhere in the left colon or rectum should have potential colostomy and ileostomy sites marked preoperatively, as described previously, and the possible need for a stoma should be discussed. For the patients who have a high probability of needing a stoma, more definitive preoperative preparation is made. They and their close family are given information about the stoma and its function, if possible by an enterostomal therapy nurse or other nurse who works closely with surgeons and their ostomy patients. If possible, a visit is arranged with another person who has had successful construction of a similar stoma. This visit can be arranged through the United Ostomy Association, a well-organized volunteer group made up of people who have had ostomy surgery.

The immediate *postoperative care* of the colostomy involves observation for viability and infection and application of an appliance. Supporting rods are removed after 1 week in most patients. Colostomies initially become edematous and then shrink considerably, requiring adjustment in the size of the appliance opening. If a colostomy becomes necrotic because of inadequate blood supply, gentle evaluation must be made into the lumen of the stoma. Necrosis deep in the abdominal wall requires laparotomy and reconstruction of the stoma. More superficial necrosis will be tolerated but usually results in eventual stricture of the stoma.

A patient with an end colostomy and a preoperative regular bowel habit may elect to "control" the colostomy with an *irrigation* regimen. This takes advantage of the infrequent, mass peristaltic motions of the left colon that can be stimulated by distending the distal colon with irrigation solution—the same effect as an enema in the rectum. These patients can begin small-volume irrigation (250 to 500 mL of saline solution or warm water) on the fifth postoperative day and increase to the normal 1000-mL irrigating volume. An individual who irrigates an end colostomy successfully often will not wear an appliance over the stoma but at most a small cover with a pad to absorb mucous and a charcoal filter to control odor.

The long-term care of a colostomy depends on the type of stoma and individual preference. A transverse colostomy requires constant wearing of an appliance that must be emptied multiple times during the day. An end colostomy on the left side can be irrigated or controlled with diet and medication, or it can be left alone to function with an appliance in place. Colostomy problems are usually related to a poor location of the stoma that makes sealing an appliance difficult and the control of gas and odor impossible. Since the colostomy has no sphincter, gas passes without control. Colostomy patients therefore must be observant of gas-forming foods and should have available medications to slow intestinal function during social occasions.

Bleeding and obstructive symptoms should be evaluated for proximal sources, especially synchronous or metachronous cancer. A person with rectal cancer is at increased risk of developing additional cancers. Surveillance endoscopy should be performed through the colostomy just as it would be through the anus. Colostomies can become blocked by impaction just as a rectum does, and the presenting symptoms may be frequent passage of liquid stool around an obstructing bolus. This should be considered before prescribing antidiarrheal agents to a patient having "diarrhea" from the colostomy.

Colostomy stricture usually results from a stoma opened in a delayed fashion in which serositis developed or from a poorly vascularized colostomy. An initially huge stoma can stricture down to a tiny, incapacitating opening. The stenosis is always at skin level, prevents irrigation, and can be the source of enormous difficulty for the patient. These strictures can be corrected easily by excising the scarred skin and resuturing well-vascularized bowel to the skin (Fig. 26-91).

Adjuvant Therapy for Rectal Cancer. The overall 5-year survival rate of rectal cancer has been no better than 50 percent in many series. Death results from distant metastatic disease or, perhaps more significantly, from recurrent disease in the pelvis. Local recurrence in the pelvis is usually reported to be between 20 and 30 percent. This pelvic recurrence is the source of severe misery and suffering. Local recurrence happens because the ability to do wide resection of the rectal cancer and surrounding tissue is limited by the confines of the pelvis. Adjuvant radiation therapy has been advocated to control tumor spread to the periphery of the margins of resection (Fig. 26-92). Some prefer to apply this postoperatively when the adequacy of cancer resection is in doubt. Others prefer to use the radiation therapy preoperatively to destroy the cancer at the periphery before surgical dissection is performed. Our statistics have shown a very low incidence of local recurrence and a high 5-year sur-

vival rate with preoperative radiation therapy (Table 26-16). Two treatment regimens were used: The shorter course is used when tumor shrinkage is not required. The biologic dose of radiation is highly dependent on the timing of administration, so 2000 cGy administered in 5 days is not very different from 4500 cGy delivery over a 5-week period. In the longer regimen, there is a 7-week waiting period after completion of radiation therapy to allow resolution of all radiation-induced inflammatory changes and to permit surgery before the fibrotic phase of radiation injury begins.

There is little complication resulting from the use of preoperative radiation therapy, whereas many have seen serious problems with the use of postoperative radiation therapy. This is usually caused by injury to the small intestine, which becomes fixed in the pelvis after surgery (see Fig. 26-92). The major disadvantage of preoperative radiation therapy is that some favorable lesions, not needing adjuvant radiation therapy, will be included. In some series, these favorable but invasive cancers have always been treated with something less than surgical resection, as will be explained shortly.

Some institutions use a compromise referred to as the "sandwich" technique, in which a short course of radiation therapy is given preoperatively, with an additional postoperative dosage used if the pathology of the cancer is unfavorable. Because of the low risk and good results from the preoperative regimens, we have not seen the need for the "sandwich" technique. A modern schema for the utilization of adjuvant radiation therapy in the management of rectal cancer is summarized in Table 26-17.

Currently, systemic adjuvant chemotherapy is used to improve long-term survival by reducing the incidence of distant metastatic disease and to improve local disease control as a radiosensitizer in combination with external-beam radiotherapy. Data from large trials indicate that patients with Stage II and Stage III rectal carcinomas achieve a modest survival benefit from adjuvant chemotherapy. Preliminary evidence suggests that combined-modality treatment with 5-fluorouracil-based chemotherapy in conjunction with radiation therapy provides additional survival benefit. Decreased local recurrence rates with chemoradiation therapy also suggest that 5-fluorouracil acts, in part, as a radiosensitizer. Another local benefit of chemoradiation therapy is its ability to downstage locally advanced rectal cancers (as demonstrated by transrectal ultrasonography) when given preoperatively, which may render a tumor resectable. Trials are underway to further define the role of chemoradiation in the treatment of rectal carcinoma.

Nonresectional Therapy

So far we have described only radical resection for invasive rectal cancer, yet it has long been known that some cancers are detected in their early phase, before onset of regional extension. In these cases, patients could be cured by effective local destruction of the tumor (Table 26-18). Adequate local palliation also becomes an issue in patients with widespread metastatic disease and a severely limited life expectancy.

Identifying the cancer appropriate for something less than resection is made difficult because no adequate clinical staging system exists for rectal cancer in the pretreatment state. Morson warned that even small presumed Dukes' A lesions will have spread to regional lymph nodes 10 percent of the time. New diagnostic modalities described previously, such as transanal ul-

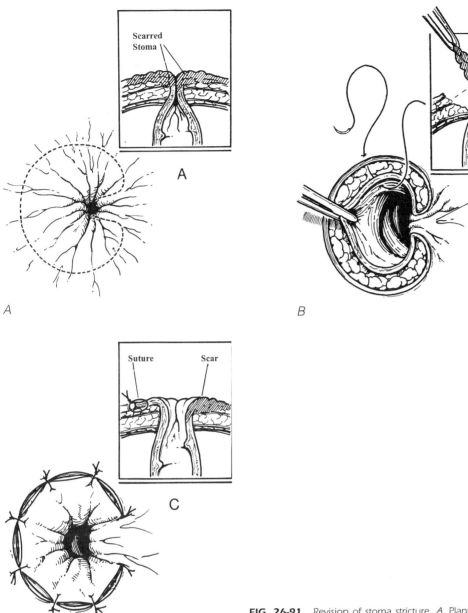

FIG. 26-91. Revision of stoma stricture. A. Planned line of excision. B. Scar mobilized and excised. C. Maturation of new stoma.

trasound, CT scanning, MRI, monoclonal antibody, nuclear scan, and PET scanning, and accurate tumor markers of biologic activity should soon allow more accurate selection of favorable yet invasive rectal cancer that is amenable to treatment by something less than radical proctectomy.

These cancers have been treated by local excision, excision and deep electrocoagulation, and most recently, *endocavitary radiation* (Fig. 26-93). This latter technique applies high-dose, superficial, low-voltage radiation directly to the cancer. This accurately directed high dosage avoids injury to normal surrounding tissue, the dose-limiting factor of external radiation treatment.

We have advanced from excision and deep coagulation of these favorable but invasive cancers, to endocavitary radiation, and finally, to external combined with endocavitary radiation treatment. We have had good results with selected cancers but

have learned that initially "aggressive" cancers require resection, even in high-risk patients and those with metastatic disease. The future probably will show that external radiation, combined with any adequate form of local destruction, will constitute adequate, definitive treatment for some rectal cancers. Endocavity radiation is not available in all centers.

Incurable Cancer

The management of hepatic and pulmonary metastases has been described previously. The question arises as to what to do with the rectal cancer itself in the patient who presents with incurable, massive metastatic disease. If the life expectancy is longer than 6 months, it is probably appropriate to give 4500 cGy external radiation (perhaps combined with systemic chemotherapy) to shrink the tumor and then to perform a palliative resection. This takes away a significant amount of "out-of-hos-

Treatment field

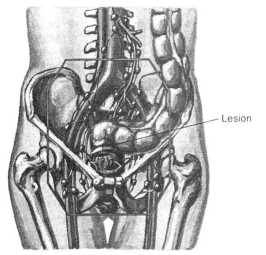

Anterior and posterior radiation
portals designed to encompass lesion
and primary lymphatic drainage zones

Lesion

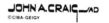
JOHN A. CRAIG—AD
©CIBA-GEIGY

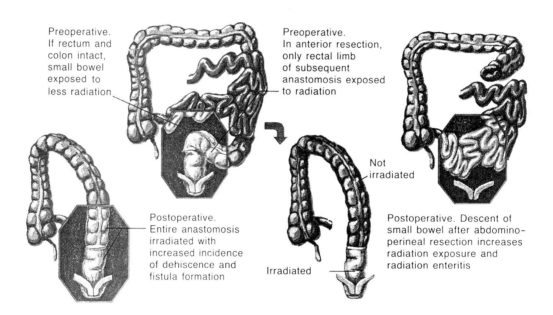

Preoperative.
If rectum and
colon intact,
small bowel
exposed to
less radiation

Preoperative.
In anterior resection,
only rectal limb
of subsequent
anastomosis exposed
to radiation

Not
irradiated

Postoperative.
Entire anastomosis
irradiated with
increased incidence
of dehiscence and
fistula formation

Irradiated

Postoperative. Descent of
small bowel after abdominoperineal resection increases
radiation exposure and
radiation enteritis

Frequency of radiation complications increases with postoperative
radiation therapy as compared to preoperative radiation

FIG. 26-92. Preoperative or postoperative radiation therapy. (From: *Fry RD, Fleshman JW, Kodner IJ: Cancer of colon and rectum. Ciba Clin Symp 41:5, 1989, with permission.*)

pital" time from the patient whose time has become precious, but it is clearly the best form of palliation, even if it requires a colostomy. An alternative recently described is to give a course of external radiation, with or without chemotherapy, and maintain a lumen through the cancer by laser destruction, dilation, or stenting of the tumor, thus avoiding resective surgery and the need for a colostomy. This choice must be used in highly selected patients. Since both plans start with external radiation therapy, the ultimate choice of treatment can be delayed until

response to the external radiation is observed. It also allows the surgeon to better understand the patient, his or her desires, and his or her general state of health during the process.

Recurrent Cancer

A special and complicated problem exists for local recurrence of rectal cancer. It had been thought previously that the cancers recurred at the distal margin of the anastomosis and grew into the lumen. This surely happens with an inadequate margin, but

Table 26-16
Survival and Local Recurrence of Rectal Cancer Treated by Preoperative Radiation and Surgical Resection

Results	No. of Patients = 112	
	2000 cGY Plus Surgery	4500 cGy Plus Surgery
5-yr survival	81%	73%
5-yr survival (excluding initially incurable lesions)	85%	86%
Local recurrence	0	1.8%

SOURCE: Kodner IJ, Fry RD, Fleshman JW: Current options in the management of rectal cancer, in Cameron JL: 1990, with permission.

most surgeons in the field now believe that there is residual cancer on the pelvic wall at the time of initial resection. It takes approximately 18 months for this cancer to grow large enough to present through the anastomosis. These cancers, by their nature, are fixed to the pelvic wall and surrounding viscera. They cause significant symptoms of pain secondary to sacral nerve roots, obstruction of the ureters, or rectal obstruction after low anterior resection are difficult to palliate and almost impossible to cure. This low salvage for locally recurrent rectal cancer has been the major impetus for investigating adjuvant modalities of treatment, such as preoperative radiation therapy.

Locally recurrent disease can be detected by biopsy after a low anterior resection and in women through the vagina after an abdominal-perineal resection. A more difficult problem exists in men after an abdominal-perineal resection, when no orifice exists to allow access to the suspicious area. Any postoperative patient with symptoms in the pelvis or a rising CEA titer should be suspected of recurrent disease. PET scanning is becoming most helpful in the diagnosis of these patients. Once the suspicious area is identified, CT-guided biopsy becomes helpful in confirming the diagnosis.

Once the diagnosis is made, therapy must be planned carefully. External radiation usually combined with chemotherapy is especially important if it has not been used before. The tissue damage from radiation is cumulative, and repeat courses are im-

Table 26-17
Comprehensive Plan for Management of Invasive Rectal Cancer

Tumor Status	Recommended Therapy
Favorable (yet invasive)	4500 cGy external + local destruction of cancer
Suspected transmural invasion Nonfixed, favorable histology	2000 cGy external over 5 days + immediate surgery
Suspected transmural invasion Fixed, unfavorable histology	4500 cGy external over 5 weeks + delayed surgery
Poor operative risk	4500 cGy external + reevaluation

SOURCE: Kodner IJ, Fry RD, Fleshman JW: Colorectal tumors, in Cameron JL: 1992, with permission.

Table 26-18
Techniques of Local Treatment of Rectal Cancer

1. Excision
   a. Transanal
   b. Transsacral
   c. Transsphincteric
2. Electrocoagulation
3. Contact radiotherapy
4. Cryotherapy
5. Laser vaporization

SOURCE: Fazio VW: 1991, with permission.

possible. Resection should be planned to include all involved organs, such as vagina, bladder, sacrum, or adherent small intestine. Preoperative cystoscopy with biopsy and careful pelvic examination are mandatory. Removal of the rectum and urinary bladder with surrounding lymphatic tissue is called a *pelvic exenteration* (Fig. 26-94). This requires the patient to have two permanent stomas, one for feces and one for urine. Some but not all of the sacrum can be removed, as described previously in the section on anatomy.

Consideration has been given to intraoperative radiation therapy to the tumor using a linear accelerator; this requires a combined operating room–radiation therapy suite, and the results so far have not been favorable. Techniques are being described for implanting high-dose afterload radiation therapy catheters to the areas suspicious for unclear margins.

Despite such heroic measures, the palliation and salvage rate of recurrent rectal cancer is very low (10 to 20 percent). The mode of death from locally recurrent rectal cancer involves much more intense suffering than that which results from the progressive malnutrition of distant metastatic disease. For these reasons, it is important that a surgeon managing rectal cancer know all the management options and that the first therapy applied be the best "curative" procedure for a given patient.

Other Rectal Tumors

Lymphoma. Most gastrointestinal lymphomas represent metastatic disease. Primary, non-Hodgkin's, colonic lymphomas account for approximately 10 percent of all gastrointestinal lymphomas. The gastrointestinal tract is a common site of HIV-associated non-Hodgkin's lymphomas. For the diagnosis of primary lymphoma of the gastrointestinal tract to be made, there should be no palpable peripheral adenopathy, no involvement of the liver or spleen, a normal white blood cell count, and no involvement of other sites. The cecum and rectum are the most common sites of colonic involvement.

Lymphoma of the intestinal tract may appear as annular thickening, bulky exophytic growth, or thickened dilatations of the bowel wall. The cut surface has the appearance of "fish flesh." Colonic lymphomas are classified by cell type and in order of frequency are histiocytic, lymphocytic, mixed cell, and Hodgkin's diseases.

Diagnosis. Patients are typically 50 to 60 years old, with colonic lymphoma more common in men and rectal involvement more common in women. Abdominal or rectal pain, altered bowel habits, weight loss, and rectal bleeding are the most common presenting symptoms. Approximately 20 percent of patients will present with obstructive symptoms.

Excision

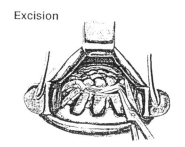

Contraindications

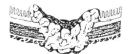

Endophytic ulcerated, undifferentiated lesion
(>3 cm diameter) with radial penetration located
more than 12 cm above anal verge

Fulguration

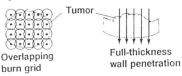

Overlapping
burn grid

Full-thickness
wall penetration

Indications

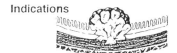

Exophytic, well-differentiated intramural lesion
(<3 cm diameter) located less than 12 cm above
anal verge

Endocavitary radiation

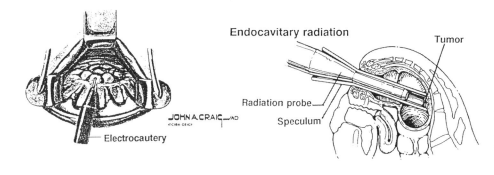

Electrocautery

FIG. 26-93. Local therapy for rectal cancer. (From: *Fry RD, Fleshman JW, Kodner U: Cancer of colon and rectum. Ciba Clin Symp 41:5, 1989, with permission.*)

An accurate history and physical examination with complete blood work, chest x-ray, barium enema, abdominal CT scan, and bone marrow biopsy are used for preoperative staging. Most rectal lymphomas are palpable by digital examination or visible by biopsy through a sigmoidoscope. Patients with colonic lymphoma may have tender, palpable abdominal masses. Barium enema examination may reveal multiple lesions consisting of filling defects and infiltrating or ulcerating lesions. The appearance of a lymphoma on barium enema examination can be similar to that of a carcinoma. The lesions often are submucosal; consequently, superficial colonoscopic biopsies are not diagnostic. CT scan may help to characterize primary colonic lymphomas and to identify tumor spread or invasion.

Treatment. Complete excision is the treatment of choice for these tumors. Resection of primary gastrointestinal lymphomas permits accurate staging, better local control of the tumor, and decreased complications of bleeding and perforation. Liver and lymph node biopsies, as well as splenectomies, have been recommended for complete operative staging.

Postoperative radiation therapy and chemotherapy are given according to the stage of the tumor. Radiation therapy is indicated for palliation of unresectable disease and in cases when the surgical resection is not complete. Chemotherapy is recommended for treatment of systemic disease.

Prognosis depends on the stage at diagnosis. The 5-year survival rate following curative resection is 50 percent. The best prognosis exists in patients with intraluminal lymphomas less than 5 cm in diameter with no lymph node metastases. Patients with AIDS and those with widespread disease have a poor prognosis.

Retrorectal Tumors. *Pathophysiology.* The retrorectal space is bound anteriorly by the rectum, posteriorly by the presacral fascia, superiorly by the peritoneal reflection, inferiorly by the rectosacral fascia, and laterally by the lateral ligaments, ureters, and iliac vessels (see Fig. 26-37). More than 50 percent of these lesions are congenital (Table 26-19). The remainder are classified as neurogenic, osseous, or miscellaneous lesions. Inflammatory lesions and metastatic carcinoma also should be considered in the differential diagnosis of lesions in this space. Malignancy is more common in lesions found in the postnatal pediatric population than in adults. In the adult population, 10 percent of cystic lesions are malignant, whereas solid lesions have a 60 percent malignancy rate.

Developmental cysts constitute the majority of congenital lesions and may arise from any of the germ cell layers. Dermoid and epidermoid cysts are benign lesions that have an ectodermal origin. When these cysts communicate with the skin surface, a postanal dimple is found. These cysts can become infected and may be misdiagnosed as a fistula-in-ano. Enterogenous cysts are endodermal in origin and are benign, thin-walled, and lined by columnar epithelium. They are usually asymptomatic, but they have a tendency to become infected. Teratomas are true neoplasms and contain tissue from each germ cell layer. They are

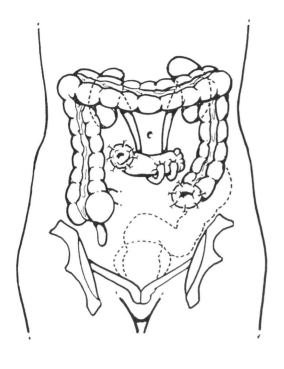

JOHN A.CRAIG—AD
©

FIG. 26-94. Pelvic exenteration.

more common in women and are considered tumors of infancy and childhood. Teratomas are uncommon in adults, but when they occur, 30 percent become malignant.

Chordomas are the most common malignant tumors found in this region and are believed to arise from remnants of the notochord. These cancers are slow-growing, invasive lesions that destroy adjacent bone. Plain radiographs show the expansion and destruction of bone, trabeculation, and calcification.

Anterior sacral *meningoceles* contain cerebrospinal fluid. Patients present with headaches, often associated with constipation and low back pain. The "scimitar" sign (a sacrum with a rounded, concave border without bony destruction) is the pathognomonic x-ray appearance of anterior sacral meningoceles. Meningitis can occur, and aspiration of these lesions should be avoided to prevent this complication.

Diagnosis. Many patients are symptom-free and the tumor is found on routine pelvic or rectal examination. Symptomatic patients with retrorectal tumors often complain of postural pain in the lower back, perianal, or rectal region, with the pain often referred to the legs or buttocks. Other complaints include recurrent infections, constipation, diarrhea, urinary symptoms, or obstructed labor. More than 90 percent of these lesions are palpable by digital rectal examination.

Plain x-ray or CT scans are used to confirm the diagnosis and to aid in surgical planning. CT scans help to define the limits of the lesion and to determine whether it is cystic or solid. Bony destruction indicates malignancy. Barium enema will show anterior displacement of the rectum. Myelograms may be indicated if central nervous system involvement is suspected. Biopsy is not recommended if the lesion is deemed operable because tu-

mor seeding along biopsy tracts and septic complications after needle biopsies have been reported.

Treatment. Surgical resection is the treatment of choice, even in asymptomatic patients, because of the risk that the lesion may become infected, cause dystocia, be malignant, or have malignant potential. The abdominal approach is recommended for high retrorectal and extraspinal neurogenic lesions. The posterior (transsacral) approach is recommended for low lesions and infected cysts. For large lesions, an abdominal-sacral approach has been most useful. The coccyx needs to be removed to gain better exposure and to decrease the risk of recurrence, since it is frequently the source of the cysts. If needle biopsy was performed, the tract must be included in the resection to prevent tumor implantation in the needle tract. En bloc resections of sacrum, neural structures, and rectum are sometimes needed for curative resection of chordomas. Anterior sacral meningoceles can be treated by posterior laminectomy, anterior transabdominal, or a combination anteroposterior approach.

Benign tumors and cysts have a good prognosis and are treated adequately by surgical excision. Chordomas have a high local recurrence rate. They are slow-growing tumors, and 10-year survival rates vary from 20 to 70 percent. High-dose radiotherapy may provide palliation in inoperable or inadequately resected chordomas. Chemotherapy has no role in the management of tumors in this region.

Colonic Carcinoid. Carcinoid tumors arise from neuroectodermal tissue. In the gastrointestinal tract they originate in

Table 26-19
Differential Diagnosis of Retrorectal Tumors and Cysts

Congenital
Developmental cysts (epidermoid, dermoid, and mucus-secreting cysts; teratoma)
Chordoma
Teratocarcinoma
Adrenal rest tumor
Anterior sacral meningocele
Duplication of rectum
Inflammatory
Foreign body granuloma
Perineal abscess
Internal fistula
Pelvirectal abscess
Chronic infectious granuloma
Neurogenic
Neurofibroma and sarcoma
Neurilemmoma
Ependymoma
Ganglioneuroma
Neurofibrosarcoma
Osseous
Osteoma
Osteogenic sarcoma
Simple bone cyst, sacrum
Ewing's tumor
Chondromyxosarcoma
Aneurysmal bone cyst
Giant cell tumor
Miscellaneous
Metastatic neoplasm
Saroma
Other benign soft tissue neoplasms

SOURCE: Gordon PH, Nivatvongs S (eds): *Principles and Practices of Surgery for the Colon, Rectum and Anus.* St Louis, Quality Medical Publishers, with permission.

the enterochromaffin cells at the base of the crypts of Lieber-kühn. These cells contain neurosecretory granules and are part of the amine precursor uptake and decarboxylation (APUD) system. Approximately 2 percent of gastrointestinal carcinoids occur in the colon and 15 percent in the rectum. Colonic carcinoids occur most frequently in the cecum, followed by the transverse and sigmoid colon. The male-to-female ratio is equal, and the peak incidence is in the sixth to seventh decades of life. There is a high incidence of synchronous or metachronous lesions in patients with colonic or rectal carcinoids.

Diagnosis. Colonic carcinoids smaller than 1 cm are usually asymptomatic and almost never malignant. They are submucosal and rarely seen on barium enema examination or colonoscopy. They are usually found incidentally during operation for other disease.

Because most midgut and hindgut carcinoids are clinically silent, the diagnosis is often made late in the course of the disease. Symptomatic colonic carcinoids are often bulky, advanced lesions. Many patients present with weight loss, anorexia, abdominal discomfort, and occasionally a palpable mass. Barium enema may reveal polypoid or circumferential lesions, simulating findings seen with adenocarcinomas. Carcinoid tumors evoke a desmoplastic reaction that may distort surrounding tissues. Less than 5 percent of colonic carcinoids cause the carcinoid syndrome; if the syndrome is present, it usually indicates liver metastases.

Invasive malignancy correlates with size of the lesions. Lesions smaller than 2 cm rarely metastasize, but symptomatic carcinoids larger than 2 cm are usually aggressive malignancies. Eighty percent of patients with lesions larger than 2 cm have metastases at the time of diagnosis, 45 percent have local spread, and 38 percent have distant metastases, with the liver being the most common site of distant spread.

Lesions greater than 2 cm that have invaded the muscularis propria or show positive nodes have a very poor prognosis. Median survival for these lesions is less than 12 months. The overall 5-year survival rate for colonic carcinoid is less than 50 percent.

Treatment. Small lesions found incidentally during exploration may be removed by wedge or segmental resection. Local excision can be curative for lesions less than 2 cm discovered before invasion of the muscularis propria, if lymph nodes are negative. The surgical treatment for larger lesions with no liver metastasis is similar to that for colonic adenocarcinoma. Single liver metastases should be resected. Resection of the primary tumor can be palliative in patients with otherwise incurable metastatic disease. There is evidence that α-interferon used in the treatment of malignant carcinoids resulted in decreased symptoms and stabilization of disease. Somatostatin has been used for management of symptomatic carcinoid syndrome. The prognosis of patients with colonic carcinoids is worse than that of patients with carcinoids of the rectum or appendix.

Rectal Carcinoid. *Diagnosis.* Rectal carcinoids are yellow-gray submucosal nodules covered by intact mucosa. They are usually small and asymptomatic and may be seen on proctosigmoidoscopy. Larger lesions can ulcerate, causing rectal bleeding and pain. Malignancy correlates with the size of the lesion and is based on invasion into the muscularis propria, not histologic differentiation. There is a 4 percent chance of malignancy in lesions smaller than 2 cm, but it is unsafe to assume solely on the basis of its size that a lesion is benign. More than

60 percent of rectal carcinoids larger than 2 cm have liver metastases, and 90 percent have local lymph node metastases at the time of diagnosis.

Treatment. Transanal excision is indicated for small, asymptomatic rectal lesions. The depth of invasion should be evaluated, and a more extensive cancer operation should be performed for those lesions with invasion of the muscularis propria. Malignant lesions should be treated by anterior resection or abdominal perineal resection. Radical surgery, however, has not been beneficial for rectal carcinoids with evidence of distant metastatic disease. The 5-year survival rate among persons with no metastases is 92 percent. The 5-year survival rate is 44 percent if there are local lymph node metastases and less than 10 percent if distant metastases are present.

Composite Carcinoid-Carcinomas. Composite carcinoid-carcinomas (adenocarcinoids) are uncommon tumors that have histologic features of both carcinoid and adenocarcinoma. Neoplastic change involving a common precursor cell is more likely than coincidental malignant change of two mature cell types.

These tumors behave more like adenocarcinomas than carcinoids. They have been reported in various locations along the gastrointestinal tract; 80 percent are found in the appendix and 10 percent in the colon and rectum. Metastases to regional lymph nodes are found in 69 percent and to the liver in 23 percent of patients at the time of diagnosis.

Surgical treatment should be planned as if the lesions were adenocarcinomas. Somatostatin may control symptoms by preventing release of pharmacologically active tumor products.

Anal Neoplasms

Tumors of the Anal Margin

Squamous Cell Carcinoma. A major consideration in managing anal cancers involves the precise anatomic location of the lesion. Squamous cancer of the skin at the anal *margin* behaves similarly to other cutaneous squamous cell cancers, whereas squamous (or transitional) cancer of the anal *canal* is a high-grade cancer with significant risk of metastasis and death.

Squamous cell carcinomas of the anal margin arise between the dentate line and the outer limit of perianal skin (defined as 5 cm from the anal verge). These tumors are well-differentiated keratinizing lesions similar to squamous carcinoma of the skin.

Diagnosis. These cancers are more common in men. Patients frequently present with complaints of a palpable mass, bleeding, itching, pain, or tenesmus. The lesions have rolled, everted edges and a central ulceration. Associated anal condylomata or chronic fistula-in-ano may be found in up to 15 percent of patients. Any chronic, nonhealing ulceration in the perianal area should be biopsied to rule out squamous carcinoma. These cancers are slow-growing and metastasize late, and most patients present 12 to 24 months after the onset of symptoms.

Treatment. Small lesions are treated by wide local excision with a 2-cm margin. Combined chemotherapy and radiation have been used successfully to induce regression of large lesions. Abdominal-perineal resection should be reserved for patients with fecal incontinence and those who develop local recurrence after conservative treatment. Synchronous metastases to the inguinal nodes occur in 8 to 40 percent of patients and are treated by inguinal node dissection once positive nodes have been identified. Lesions less than 5 cm have a better prognosis, and the overall 5-year survival rate is 60 to 80 percent.

Basal Cell Carcinoma. Basal cell carcinoma is a rare tumor of the anal margin and behaves like basal cell carcinoma elsewhere on the skin. It is more common in men and presents as a lesion with raised edges and central ulceration. Basal cell carcinoma is treated by wide local excision with adequate margins and primary closure or skin grafting. Large lesions may require abdominal-perineal resection. Although these cancers rarely metastasize, there is a 30 percent local recurrence rate. Recurrences are treated by reexcision.

Bowen's Disease. Bowen's disease is an intraepidermal squamous cell carcinoma (carcinoma in situ) that is a rare, slow-growing cancer. It usually presents in the elderly but has been reported in association with anal condyloma in young, sexually active patients.

Diagnosis. Patients often complain of perianal itching, burning, or bleeding. Many lesions go unnoticed but may be found incidentally during histologic examination of tissues removed during minor anal procedures. Discrete, erythematous, scaly plaques are found on examination. Lesions may have the appearance of eczema or chronic irritation due to pruritus ani.

The presence of ulceration may indicate the development of an invasive carcinoma. Less than 10 percent of untreated lesions go on to develop invasive squamous cell carcinoma, and 35 percent of these develop metastases. Associated malignancies have been reported in the past with high percentage of patients with Bowen's disease, but recent studies have proved this to be incorrect.

Treatment. Treatment consists of wide local excision with adequate margins, as determined by frozen section. Multiple biopsies in all four quadrants of the perineal skin are then taken to ensure complete resection. Skin grafts may be necessary for coverage if the excision is extensive. Recurrent lesions, without invasion, can be treated by reexcision.

Paget's Disease. Extramammary, perianal Paget's disease is a rare pathologic entity. It arises from the intraepidermal portion of the apocrine glands. Paget's disease is frequently but not always associated with an underlying carcinoma. If left untreated, adenocarcinoma of the apocrine glands may develop after a long preinvasive phase.

Diagnosis. Patients usually are 60 to 70 years old, and there is a female predominance. Severe, intractable pruritus is characteristic of this disease. Examination reveals an erythematous, eczematous rash. Diagnosis often is delayed because lesions frequently are treated with a variety of topical medications without success before biopsy. A biopsy should be obtained from any nonhealing, pruritic anal lesion in order to exclude this diagnosis. Histologic examination reveals Paget cells, which are large pale cells with eccentric nuclei. A detailed physical examination and complete evaluation of the gastrointestinal tract should be performed; patients with extramammary Paget's disease are at increased risk of developing noncontiguous malignancies.

Treatment. Wide local excision with clear margins, confirmed by frozen section, and with multiple biopsies of the perianal skin is the treatment of choice. Abdominal-perineal resection may be necessary for the very few advanced lesions associated with invasive carcinoma. Lymph node dissection is indicated only for patients with proven positive inguinal nodes.

The most frequent sites of metastatic disease are the inguinal and pelvic lymph nodes, followed by liver, bone, lung, brain, bladder, prostate, and adrenal glands. Patients with metastatic disease do poorly despite aggressive treatment.

Anal Canal Cancer

Epidermoid Carcinoma. The cloacogenic or transitional zone of the anal canal is located 6 to 12 mm above the dentate line. Carcinomas of this area may be referred to as *nonkeratinizing squamous, basaloid, cloacogenic,* or *transitional.* Basaloid carcinomas have the characteristic histologic appearance of palisading nuclei. Squamous carcinomas in this region are generally nonkeratinizing. Although these cancers have different histologic features, they exhibit similar biologic behavior and are grouped together as epidermoid carcinomas of the anal canal.

Diagnosis. These cancers are more common in women. Many patients have only minor symptoms and are often erroneously diagnosed as having benign anorectal disorders. These lesions can present as an indurated, bleeding mass that may itch or cause discomfort; however, some patients present with a painless mass lesion.

Digital rectal examination reveals the size, location, and degree of fixation of these tumors. Proctosigmoidoscopy verifies the exact location of the tumor relative to the dentate line. Biopsies of the mass are necessary for diagnosis. Evaluation of the remainder of the colon should be done with colonoscopy or barium enema. Examination of both inguinal regions determines if there is any suspicious nodal enlargement, and a chest radiograph and CT scan of the liver are performed to search for distant metastatic disease.

Between 30 and 40 percent of these patients have metastatic disease at the time of diagnosis. The risk of metastasis increases with the depth of invasion, the size of lesion, and the histologic grade of the lesion. When located below the dentate line, these cancers metastasize to the inguinal nodes. Those above the dentate line will spread to the superior rectal, internal pudendal, hypogastric, or obturator lymph nodes. The most common site of distant metastatic disease is the liver.

Treatment. Small, early, node-negative lesions that are confined to the submucosa may be treated by local excision. The treatment for larger, more deeply invasive lesions has changed in the past two decades. In the past, abdominal-perineal resection was the standard treatment for squamous carcinoma of the anal canal. Local recurrence after abdominal-perineal resection was 25 to 50 percent, and the 5-year survival rate ranged from 50 to 70 percent.

Radiation therapy along with surgical treatment for residual disease has been used successfully. A 5-year survival rate of 79 percent has been reported, but there is a high complication rate associated with the high doses of radiation used for treatment.

In 1972, Nigro began using combined chemoradiation in an effort to reduce the radiation dose necessary to adequately treat these tumors. In his initial protocol, 3000 cGy external radiation, combined with 5-fluorouracil and mitomycin C, was followed by abdominal-perineal removal of the rectum. No residual carcinoma was found in 60 to 90 percent of patients, and the protocol was modified to reserve surgery for those patients with residual disease after chemoradiation.

Simultaneous chemoradiation is the preferred method of treatment for squamous carcinoma of the anus (Table 26-20). Local recurrence is 15 percent and is treated by abdominal-per-

Table 26-20
Chemoradiation Therapy for Squamous Cancer of Anal Canal

External Radiation
3000 rad (30 Gy) to the primary tumor, pelvic, and inguinal nodes;
start: day 1 (200 rad/day)
Systemic Chemotherapy
A. 5-FU 1000 mg/m^2 per 24 h as a continuous infusion for 4 days;
start: day 1
B. Mitomycin C: 15 mg/m^2 intravenous bolus; start: day 1 *only*
C. 5-FU: repeat 4-day infusion; start: day 28

SOURCE: Nigro ND: Multidisciplinary management of cancer of the anus. *World J Surg* 11:1987, with permission.

ineal resection. Treatment toxicity is increased for those patients with a history of pelvic surgery and those patients requiring abdominal-perineal resection after chemoradiation. Several salvage chemoradiation protocols have been used with variable success. Negative prognostic factors include the presence of involved nodes, lesions greater than 5 cm, and invasion of contiguous organs other than the rectum and skin. The overall 5-year survival rate is 83 percent, and as expected, patients with visceral metastases have a poor prognosis.

The presence of involved inguinal lymph nodes at the time of diagnosis of the primary carcinoma is a bad prognostic sign. Involved inguinal nodes are included in the radiation field, but lymph node dissection is reserved only for patients with positive nodes after chemoradiation. There is no indication for prophylactic lymph node dissection.

Squamous cell carcinoma has been reported in the chronic perineal wounds and sinus tracts seen in Crohn's disease. Malignancy should be considered in any patient with continuous anal pain or a nonhealing perineal wound. Biopsy of such sinus tracts is mandatory and may be diagnostic.

Adenocarcinoma. Adenocarcinoma of the anal canal is usually the distal extension of a primary rectal cancer. It may rarely arise from the columnar epithelium of the anal glands or within a long-standing anorectal fistula. Patients complain of perianal pain, swelling, and frequently have an abscess or fistula-in-ano. Abdominal-perineal resection is indicated in these carcinomas, sometimes after preoperative radiation therapy. Many of these patients have distant metastases at the time of diagnosis, and the long-term outlook is poor.

Melanoma. Melanoma represents 1 to 3 percent of anal canal cancers. It is the third most common site for melanoma, following the skin and the eye. The majority arise from the epidermoid lining of the anal canal adjacent to the dentate line. They spread submucosally, and by the time they cause symptoms, the extent of invasion is usually beyond surgical cure.

Diagnosis. The average age at presentation is between the fifth and sixth decades of life, the male-to-female ratio is equal, and the majority of patients reported in the literature are Caucasian.

Patients commonly present with bleeding, pain, or an anal mass. They may complain of alteration in bowel habits and are often misdiagnosed as having a thrombosed hemorrhoid. Most melanomas in this region are nonpigmented or lightly pigmented polypoid lesions.

Metastases occur via lymphatic and hematogenous routes, with lymphatic spread to the mesenteric nodes being more common than to inguinal nodes. Thirty-eight percent of patients have metastatic disease at the time of diagnosis, with lung, liver, and bone the most frequent sites of hematogenous spread.

Treatment. There has been no difference in survival in patients treated by wide local excision or abdominal-perineal resection; however, the radical resection is more effective for control of local disease and is the only procedure that removes clinically undetected lymph nodes.

Prophylactic lymph node dissection is of no value, and therapeutic lymph node dissection is advised only for those patients with positive inguinal nodes. Current chemotherapy has been ineffective. Overall 5-year survival rate is less than 20 percent, with few reported long-term survivors. Five-year survival rates in patients with lesions larger than 1.6 mm have not been reported.

PSYCHIATRIC DISORDERS

Many psychiatric disorders include symptoms of anorectal pathology as manifestations of the psychiatric disease. Surgeons must be aware of this and limit surgical therapy to specifically diagnosed surgically remediable problems. It is a serious error to operate for severe anorectal symptoms without definite findings of a primary disease process. For example, there has been extensive work seeking a psychiatric basis for the irritable bowel syndrome.

Patients who present with severe constipation or pelvic floor malfunction (such as nonrelaxation of the anal sphincter mechanism) have been shown to have a high incidence of psychological abnormalities, but no specific psychiatric diagnosis has been consistent.

The problem of unexplained anal pain is a difficult diagnostic dilemma. One must consider psychological overlay in most patients who continue to complain of anal pain despite no abnormal findings on examination. The full evaluation of these patients must include physical examination, CT scan, defecography, anal manometry, and electromyography. Cancer, inflammation, abscess, and nerve root compression are all considered possibilities. If the pain persists despite a negative evaluation, one must consider a psychological causation and refer the patient for behavioral evaluation. It is possible that spasm of the levator floor and the proctalgia fugax syndrome are related to stress, much as are migraine headaches. For these patients, treatment of the underlying problem is appropriate after cancer and other surgical problems are eliminated as possibilities.

Bibliography

General References
Allan RN, Rhodes JM, et al (eds): *Inflammatory Bowel Diseases.* New York, Churchill-Livingstone, 1997.
Bayless TM (ed): *Current Therapy in Gastroenterology and Liver Disease—3.* Philadelphia, BC Decker, 1990.
Beck, DE (ed): *Handbook of Colorectal Surgery.* St Louis, Quality Medical Publishing, 1997.
Corman ML: *Colon and Rectal Surgery,* 3d ed. Philadephia, Lippincott, 1993.
Fazio VW (ed): *Current Therapy in Colon and Rectal Surgery.* Philadelphia, BC Decker, 1990.

Fielding LP, Goldberg SM (eds): Surgery of the colon, rectum and anus, in Rob C, Smith R (eds): *Rob and Smith's Operative Surgery,* 5th ed. Oxford, UK, Butterworth-Heinemann, 1993.

Gordon PH, Nivatvongs S: *Principles and Practice of Surgery for the Colon, Rectum, and Anus.* St Louis, Quality Medical Publishing, 1992.

Hicks TC, Beck DE, et al (eds.): *Complications of Colon and Rectal Surgery.* Baltimore, Williams & Wilkins, 1996.

Keighley MRB, Williams NS (eds): *Surgery of the Anus, Rectum, and Colon.* London, WB Saunders, 1993.

Kodner IJ, Fry RD, Roe JP (eds): *Colon, Rectal and Anal Surgery:Current Techniques and Controversies.* St Louis, Mosby, 1985.

Mazier WP, Levien DH, et al (eds): *Surgery of the Colon, Rectum, and Anus.* Philadelphia, WB Saunders, 1995.

Wilmore DW, Brennan MF, et al (eds): *Care of the Surgical Patient.* New York, Scientific American Press, 1989.

Zinner MJ, Schwartz SI, Ellis H (eds): *Maingot's Abdominal Operations,* 10th ed. Norwalk, CT, Appleton & Lange, 1997.

Zuidema GD (ed): *Shackelford's Surgery of the Alimentary Tract,* 4th ed. Philadelphia, WB Saunders, 1996.

Anatomic Considerations

Boxall TA, Smart PJG, et al: The blood supply of the distal segment of the rectum in anterior resection. *Br J Surg* 50:399, 1962.

Church JM, Raudkivi PJ, et al: The surgical anatomy of the rectum—A review with particular relevance to the hazards of rectal mobilisation. *Int J Colorectal Dis* 2:158, 1987.

Duthie HL, Gairns FW: Sensory nerve-endings and sensation in the anal region of man. *Br J Surg* 47:38, 1960.

Fry RD, et al: Diseases of the anus, in ME Copeland et al (eds): *Current Practice of Surgery.* New York, Churchill-Livingstone, 1992.

Garcia-Ruiz A, Milsom JW, et al: Right colonic arterial anatomy: Implications for laparoscopic surgery. *Dis Colon Rectum* 39:906, 1996.

Gunterberg B, Kewenter J, et al: Anorectal function after major resections of the sacrum with bilateral or unilateral sacrifice of sacral nerves. *Br J Surg* 63:546, 1976.

Longo WE, Ballantyne GH, et al: The colon, anorectum, and spinal cord patient: A review of the functional alterations of the denervated hindgut. *Dis Colon Rectum* 32:261, 1989.

Moore KL: *The Developing Human: Clinically Oriented Embryology,* 4th ed. Philadelphia, WB Saunders, 1988.

Sonneland J, Anson BJ, et al: Surgical anatomy of the arterial supply to the colon from the superior mesenteric artery based on a study of 600 specimens. *Surg Gynecol Obstet* 106:385, 1958.

Disturbances of Physiology

Altemeier WA, Culbertson WR, et al: Nineteen years' experience with the one-stage perineal repair of rectal prolapse. *Ann Surg* 173:993, 1971.

Ballantyne GH, Brandner MD, et al: Volvulus of the colon: Incidence and mortality. *Ann Surg* 202:83, 1985.

Bartolo DC, Read NW, et al: Differences in anal sphincter function and clinical presentation in patients with pelvic floor descent. *Gastroenterology* 85:68, 1983.

Benn PL, Wolff BG, Ilstrup DM: Level of anastomosis and recurrent colonic diverticulitis. *Am J Surg* 151:269, 1986.

Bricker EM: Repair of postirradiation damage to colorectum: A progress report. *Ann Surg* 193:555, 1981.

Brodân B, Snellman B: Procidentia of the rectum studied with cineradiography: A contribution to the discussion of causative mechanism. *Dis Colon Rectum* 11:330, 1968.

Camilleri M, Thompson G, et al. Clinical management of intractable constipation. *Ann Intern Med* 121:520, 1994.

Caplin DA, Kodner IJ: Repair of anal stricture and mucosal ectropion by simple flap procedures. *Dis Colon Rectum* 29:92, 1986.

Chapman M, Grahn M, et al. Butyrate oxidation is impaired in the colonic mucosa of sufferers of quiescent ulcerative colitis. *Gut* 35:73, 1994.

Clausen M, Mortensen P. Kinetic studies on the metabolism of short chain fatty acids and glucose by isolated rat colonocytes. *Gastroenterology* 108:423, 1994.

Finlay IG, Carter DC: A comparison of emergency resection and staged management in perforated diverticular disease. *Dis Colon Rectum* 30:929, 1987.

Fleshman JW, Dreznik Z, et al: Anal sphincter repair for obstetric injury: Manometric evaluation of functional results. *Dis Colon Rectum* 34:1061, 1991.

Fleshman JW, Dreznik Z, et al: Outpatient protocol for biofeedback therapy of pelvic floor outlet obstruction. *Dis Colon Rectum* 35:1, 1992.

Fleshman JW, et al: Anal incontinence, in GD Zuidema (ed): *Shackelford's Surgery of the Alimentary Tract,* 3d ed. Philadelphia, WB Saunders, 1991.

Fleshman JW, Fry RD, et al: Surgical management of constipation, in *Anorectal Disorders: Balliere's Clinical Gastroenterology.* London, WB Saunders, 1992.

Fleshman JW, Kuijpers HC: Pelvic floor abnormalities and disordered defecation, in MJ Zinner, SI Schwartz, H Ellis (eds): *Maingot's Abdominal Operations,* 10th ed. Norwalk, CT, Appleton & Lange, 1997, p 1417.

Fleshman JW, Peters WR, et al: Anal sphincter reconstruction: anterior overlapping muscle repair. *Dis Colon Rectum* 34:739, 1991.

Fry RD, Fleshman JW, Kodner IJ: Abdominal colectomy with ileorectal anastomosis. *South Med J* 77:711, 1984.

Fry RD, Kodner IJ: Anorectal disorders. *Clin Symp* 37:2, 1985.

Fry RD. Benign diseases of the anorectum, in MJ Zinner, SI Schwartz, H Ellis (eds): *Maingot's Abdominal Operations,* 10th ed. Norwalk, CT, Appleton & Lange, 1997, p 1437.

Hackford AW, Schoetz DJ Jr, et al: Surgical management of complicated diverticulitis: The Lahey Clinic experience, 1967–1982. *Dis Colon Rectum* 28:317, 1985.

Hackford AW, Welch HF: Retroperitoneal infection: II. Etiology, diagnosis, and treatment. *Complications Surg* 10:46, 1991.

Harig J, Soergel K, et al: Treatment of diversion colitis with short chain fatty acid irrigation. *N Engl J Med* 320:23, 1989.

Henry MM, Swash M (eds): *Coloproctology and the Pelvic Floor: Pathophysiology and Management,* 2d ed. London, Butterworth, 1992.

Hertz A, Newton A: The normal movements of the colon in man. *J Physiol (Lond)* 45:57, 1913.

Hoffman MJ, Kodner IJ, et al: Internal intussusception of the rectum: Diagnosis and surgical management. *Dis Colon Rectum* 27:435, 1984.

Ingelfinger E: The diagnosis of sprue in nontropical cases. *N Engl J Med* 228:180, 1943.

Jones IT, Fazio VW: Colonic volvulus: Etiology and management. *Dig Dis* 7:203, 1989.

Kirsh GM, Hampel N, et al: Diagnosis and management of vesicoenteric fistulas. *Surg Gynecol Obstet* 173:91, 1991.

Kissmeyer-Nielsen P, Mortensen F, et al: Transmural trophic effect of short chain fatty acid infusions on atrophic, defunctioned rat colon. *Dis Colon Rectum* 38:946, 1995.

Kodner IJ, Fry RD, Fleshman JW: Rectal prolapse and other pelvic floor abnormalities: Current state of the art as related to physiologic studies and surgical alternatives. *Surg Ann* 24:157, 1992.

Lee J, Taylor B, Singleton B: Epidural anesthesia for acute pseudo-obstruction of the colon (Ogilvie's syndrome). *Dis Colon Rectum* 31:686, 1988.

Levitt M. Intestinal gas production—Recent advances in flatology. *N Engl J Med* 302:1474, 1980.

Lund JN, Scholefield JH: A randomized, prospective, double-blind, placebo-controlled trial of glyceryl trinitrate ointment in treatment of anal fissure. *Lancet* 349:11, 1997.

Marshak RH, Janowitz HD, Present DH: Granulomatous colitis in association with diverticula. *N Engl J Med* 283:1080, 1970.

Mathai V, Seow-Choen F: Endoluminal formalin therapy for haemorrhagic radiation. *Br J Surg* 82:190, 1995.

Meyers MA, Volberg F, et al: The angioarchitecture of colonic diverticula. *Radiology* 108:249, 1973.

Morris J, Stellato TA, et al: The utility of computed tomography in colonic diverticulitis. *Ann Surg* 204:128, 1986.

Murray JJ, Schoetz DJ Jr, et al: Intraoperative colonic lavage and primary anastomosis in nonelective colon resection. *Dis Colon Rectum* 34:527, 1991.

Ogilvie H. Large intestinal colic due to sympathetic deprivation: A new clinical syndrome. *Br Med J* 2:671, 1948.

Ouriel K, Schwartz SI: Diverticular disease in the young patient. *Surg Gynecol Obstet* 156:1, 1983.

Painter N, Truelove S, et al: Segmentation and the localization of intraluminal pressures in the human colon, with special reference to the pathogenesis of colonic diverticula. *Gastroenterology* 49:169, 1965.

Painter NS, Burkitt DP: Diverticular disease of the colon: A deficiency disease of Western civilization. *Br Med J* 2:450, 1971.

Parks AG, Percy JP: Resection and sutured colo-anal anastomosis for rectal carcinoma. *Br J Surg* 69:301, 1982.

Rabinovici R, Simansky DA, et al: Cecal volvulus. *Dis Colon Rectum* 33:765, 1990.

Rao PN, Knox R, et al: Management of colovesical fistula. *Br J Surg* 74: 362, 1987.

Ripstein CB: Procidentia: Definitive corrective surgery. *Dis Colon Rectum* 15:334, 1972.

Roediger W: The colonic epithelium in ulcerative colitis: An energy-deficient disease? *Lancet* 2:712, 1980.

Roediger W: The starved colon—Diminished mucosal nutrition, diminished absorption, and colitis. *Dis Colon Rectum* 33:858, 1990.

Saclarides TJ, King DG, et al: Formalin instillation for refractory radiation-induced hemorrhagic proctitis: Report of 16 patients. *Dis Colon Rectum* 39:196, 1996.

Senagore A, MacKeigan J, et al: Short-chain fatty acid enemas: A cost-effective alternative in the treatment of nonspecific proctosigmoiditis. *Dis Colon Rectum* 35:923, 1992.

Shemesh EI, Kodner IJ, et al: Severe complication of rubber band ligation of internal hemorrhoids. *Dis Colon Rectum* 30:199, 1987.

Snape W, Carlson G, et al: Evidence that abnormal myoelectrical activity produces colonic motor dysfunction in the irritable bowel syndrome. *Gastroenterology* 72:383, 1977.

Stephenson B, Morgan A, Wheeler M: Parasympathomimetics in Ogilvie's syndrome (letter). *Dis Colon Rectum* 37:289, 1994.

Trotman IF, Misiewica JJ: Sigmoid motility in diverticular disease and the irritable bowel syndrome. *Gut* 29:218, 1988.

Tyau ES, Prystowsky JB, et al: Acute diverticulitis: A complicated problem in the immunocompromised patient. *Arch Surg* 126:855, 1991.

Vernia P, Gnaedinger A, et al: Organic anions and the diarrhea of inflammatory bowel disease. *Dig Dis Sci* 33:1353, 1988.

Walker WA, Rothenberger DA, et al: Morbidity of internal sphincterotomy for anal fissure and stenosis. *Dis Colon Rectum* 28:832, 1985.

Watts JD, Rothenberger DA, et al: The management of procidentia: 30 years' experience. *Dis Colon Rectum* 28:96, 1985.

Wilson RG, Smith AN, Macintyre IMC: Complications of diverticular disease and non-steroidal anti-inflammatory drugs: A prospective study. *Br J Surg* 77:1103, 1990.

Infections

Ferenczy A, Mitao M, et al: Latent papillomavirus and recurring genital warts. *N Engl J Med* 313:784, 1985.

Gal AA, Meyer PR, et al: Papillomavirus antigens in anorectal condyloma and carcinoma in homosexual men. *JAMA* 257:337, 1987.

Goodsall DH, Miles WE: Classic articles in colonic and rectal surgery: Diseases of the anus and rectum. *Dis Colon Rectum* 25:262, 1982.

Grissom R, Snyder TE: Colovaginal fistula secondary to diverticular disease. *Dis Colon Rectum* 34:1043, 1991.

Hook EW: Syphilis and HIV infection. *J Infect Dis* 160:530, 1989.

Lee MH, Waxman M, et al: Primary malignant lymphoma of the anorectum in homosexual men. *Dis Colon Rectum* 29:413, 1986.

Parks AG: Pathogenesis and treatment of fistula-in-ano. *Br Med J* 1:463, 1961.

Parks AG, Gordon PH, et al: A classification of fistula-in-ano. *Br J Surg* 63:1, 1976.

Pearl RK, Andrews JK, et al: Role of the seton in the mangement of anorectal fistulas. *Dis Colon Rectum* 36:573, 1993.

Prasad ML, Read DR, et al: Supralevator abscess: Diagnosis and treatment. *Dis Colon Rectum* 24:456, 1981.

Sanders LLJ, Harrison HR, et al: Treatment of sexually transmitted chlamydial infections. *JAMA* 255:1750, 1986.

Schmid GP, Sanders LLJ, et al: Chancroid in the United States: Reestablishment of an old disease. *JAMA* 258:3265, 1987.

Shemesh EI, Kodner IJ, et al: Endorectal sliding flap repair of complicated anterior anoperineal fistulas. *Dis Colon Rectum* 31:22, 1988.

Smith LE, Henrichs D, et al: Prospective studies on the etiology and treatment of pruritus ani. *Dis Colon Rectum* 25:358, 1982.

Wexner SD: Sexually transmitted diseases of the colon, rectum, and anus: The challenge of the nineties. *Dis Colon Rectum* 33:1048, 1990.

Wise WE Jr, Aguilar PS, et al: Surgical treatment of low rectovaginal fistulas. *Dis Colon Rectum* 34:271, 1991.

Inflammatory Bowel Disease

Becker JM, McGrath KM, et al: Late functional adaptation after colectomy, mucosal proctectomy, and ileal pouch–anal anastomosis. *Surgery* 110:718, 1991.

Braslow L: Pouchitis and extraintestinal manifestations of inflammatory bowel disease after ileal pouch–anal anastomosis. *Ann Surg* 213:371, 1991.

Carter FM, McLeod RS, et al: Subtotal colectomy for ulcerative colitis: Complications related to the rectal remnant. *Dis Colon Rectum* 34:1005, 1991.

Chambers TJ, Morson BC: The granuloma in Crohn's disease. *Gut* 20:269, 1979.

Crile G Jr, Turnbull RB Jr: Mechanism and prevention of ileostomy dysfunction. *Ann Surg* 140:459, 1954.

De Silva HJ, De Angelis CP, et al: Clinical and functional outcome after restorative proctocolectomy. *Br J Surg* 78:1039, 1991.

Deutsch AA, McLeod RS, et al: Results of the pelvic-pouch procedure in patients with Crohn's disease. *Dis Colon Rectum* 34:475, 1991.

Farmer RG, Hawk WA, et al: Clinical patterns in Crohn's disease: A statistical study of 615 cases. *Gastroenterology* 68:627, 1975.

Farmer RG, Hawk WA, et al: Indications for surgery in Crohn's disease: Analysis of 500 cases. *Gastroenterology* 71:245, 1976.

Farmer RG, Whelan G, et al: Long-term follow-up of patients with Crohn's disease: Relationship between the clinical pattern and prognosis. *Gastroenterology* 88:1818, 1985.

Fazio VW, Galandiuk S, et al: Strictureplasty in Crohn's disease. *Ann Surg* 210:621, 1989.

Fleshman JW, Cohen Z, et al: The ileal reservoir and ileoanal anastomosis procedure: Factors affecting technical and functional outcome. *Dis Colon Rectum* 31:10, 1988.

Fleshman JW, Lewis MG: Complications and quality of life after stoma surgery: A review of 16,740 patients in the UOA data registry. *Semin Colon Rectal Surg* 2:65, 1991.

Fry RD, Shemesh EI, et al: Techniques and results in the management of anal and perianal Crohn's disease. *Surg Gynecol Obstet* 168:42, 1989.

Galandiuk S, Pemberton JH, et al: Delayed ileal pouch–anal anastomosis: Complications and functional results. *Dis Colon Rectum* 34:755, 1991.

Galandiuk S, Wolff BG, et al: Ileal pouch–anal anastomosis without ileostomy. *Dis Colon Rectum* 34:870, 1991.

Goldman CD, Kodner IJ, et al: Clinical and operative experience with non-Caucasian patients with Crohn's disease. *Dis Colon Rectum* 29:317, 1986.

Hamilton SR, Reese J, et al: The role of resection margin frozen section in the surgical management of Crohn's disease. *Surg Gynecol Obstet* 160:57, 1985.

Harling H, Hegnhoj J, et al: Fate of the rectum after colectomy and ileostomy for Crohn's colitis. *Dis Colon Rectum* 34:931, 1991.

Harper PH, Fazio VW, et al: The long-term outcome in Crohn's disease. *Dis Colon Rectum* 30:174, 1987.

Helzer JE: Psychiatric aspects of inflammatory bowel disease, in IJ Kodner et al (eds): *Colon, Rectal and Anal Surgery:Current Techniques and Controversies.* St Louis, Mosby, 1985, p 329.

Hyman NH, Fazio VW, et al: Consequences of ileal pouch-anal anastomosis for Crohn's colitis. *Dis Colon Rectum* 34:653, 1991.

Kelly KA: Anal sphincter-saving operations for chronic ulcerative colitis. *Am J Surg* 163:5, 1992.

Kodner IJ: Colostomy and ileostomy. *Clin Symp* 30:1, 1978.

Kodner IJ: Stoma complications, in VW Fazio (ed): *Current Therapy in Colon and Rectal Surgery.* Philadelphia, BC Decker, 1989, p 420.

Kodner IJ, et al: Surgical management of Crohn's disease, in RP MacDermott et al (eds): *Inflammatory Bowel Disease.* New York, Elsevier Science Publishing, 1992, p 615.

Kodner IJ, Fry RD: Inflammatory bowel disease. *Clin Symp* 34:3, 1982.

Kodner IJ, Fry RD, et al: The surgical management of inflammatory bowel disease. *Curr Opin Gastroenterol* 6:547, 1990.

Koltun WA, Schoetz DJ Jr, et al: Indeterminate colitis predisposes to perineal complications after ileal pouch–anal anastomosis. *Dis Colon Rectum* 34:857, 1991.

Kotanagi H, Kramer K, et al: Do microscopic abnormalities at resection margins correlate with increased anastomotic recurrence in Crohn's disease? Retrospective analysis of 100 cases. *Dis Colon Rectum* 34:909, 1991.

Kozarek RA: Endoscopy in inflammatory bowel disease, in RP MacDermott, WF Stenson (eds): *Current Topics in Gastroenterology Series:Inflammatory Bowel Disease.* New York, Elsevier Science Publishing, 1992.

Levin B, Lennard-Jones J, et al: Surveillance of patients with chronic ulcerative colitis. *Bull WHO* 69:121, 1991

Liss JL: Management of psychiatric problems in patients with inflammatory bowel disease and ostomy patients, in IJ Kodner et al (eds): *Colon, Rectal and Anal Surgery: Current Techniques and Controversies.* St Louis, Mosby, 1985, p 336.

Lock MR, Farmer RG, et al: Recurrence and reoperation for Crohn's disease: The role of disease location in prognosis. *N Engl J Med* 304:1586, 1981.

Matthews JM, Kodner IJ, et al: Entrapped ovary syndrome. *Dis Colon Rectum* 29:341, 1986.

McMullen K, Hicks TC, et al: Complications associated with ileal pouch–anal anastomosis. *World J Surg* 15:763, 1991.

Monsen U, Bernell O, et al: Prevalence of inflammatory bowel disease among relatives of patients with Crohn's disease. *Scand J Gastroenterol* 26:302, 1991.

Nelson H, Dozois RR, et al: The effect of pregnancy and delivery on the ileal pouch–anal anastomosis functions. *Dis Colon Rectum* 32:384, 1989.

O'Brien J: Extraintestinal manifestations of inflammatory bowel disease, in RP MacDermott, WF Stenson (eds): *Current Topics in Gastroenterology Series: Inflammatory Bowel Disease.* New York, Elsevier Science Publishing, 1992.

Ogorek CP, Caroline DF, Fisher RS: Presentation, evaluation, and natural history of inflammatory bowel disease, in RP MacDermott, WF Stensen (eds): *Current Topics in Gastroenterology Series: Inflammatory Bowel Disease.* New York, Elsevier Science Publishing, 1992.

Owen DA: Pathology of inflammatory bowel disease, in RP MacDermott, WF Stenson (eds): *Current Topics in Gastroenterology Series: Inflammatory Bowel Disease.* New York, Elsevier Science Publishing, 1992.

Pemberton JH, Phillips SF, et al: Quality of life after Brooke ileostomy and ileal pouch–anal anastomosis: Comparison of performance status. *Ann Surg* 209:620, 1989.

Peters WR, Fry RD, et al: Multiple blood transfusions reduce the recurrence rate of Crohn's disease. *Dis Colon Rectum* 32:749, 1989.

Prasad ML, Pearl RK, et al: End-loop colostomy. *Surg Gynecol Obstet* 158:380, 1984.

Riddell RH, Goldman H, et al: Dysplasia in inflammatory bowel disease: Standardized classification with provisional clinical applications. *Hum Pathol* 14:931, 1983.

Riddell RH, Shove DC, et al: Precancer in ulcerative colitis. *Major Probl Pathol* 10:95, 1978.

Savoca PE, Ballantyne GH, et al: Gastrointestinal malignancies in Crohn's disease: A 20-year experience. *Dis Colon Rectum* 33:7, 1990.

Senay E, Sachar DB, et al: Small bowel carcinoma in Crohn's disease: Distinguishing features and risk factors. *Cancer* 63:360, 1989.

Shanahan F, Targan SR: Mechanisms of tissue injury in inflammatory bowel disease, in RP MacDermott, WF Stenson (eds): *Inflammatory Bowel Disease.* New York, Elsevier Science Publishing, 1992.

Shemesh EI, Kodner IJ, et al: Endorectal sliding flap repair of complicated anterior anoperineal fistulas. *Dis Colon Rectum* 31:22, 1988.

Shiloni E, Coronado E, et al: Role of total parenteral nutrition in the treatment of Crohn's disease. *Am J Surg* 157:180, 1989.

Siminovitch JM, Fazio VW: Ureteral obstruction secondary to Crohn's disease: A need for ureterolysis? *Am J Surg* 139:95, 1980.

Sitzmann JV, Converse RL Jr, et al: Favorable response to parenteral nutrition and medical therapy in Crohn's colitis: A report of 38 patients comparing severe Crohn's and ulcerative colitis. *Gastroenterology* 99:1647, 1990.

Turnbull RB, Hawk WA, et al: Surgical treatment of toxic megacolon: Ileostomy and colostomy to prepare patients for colectomy. *Am J Surg* 122:325, 1971.

Turnbull RB, Weakley FL: *Atlas of Intestinal Stomas.* St Louis, Mosby, 1967.

VA TPN Cooperative Study Group: Perioperative total parenteral nutrition in surgical patients. *N Engl J Med* 325:525, 1991.

Wexner SD, James K, et al: The double-stapled ileal reservoir and ileoanal anastomosis: A prospective review of sphincter function and clinical outcome. *Dis Colon Rectum* 34:487, 1991.

Neoplastic Disease

Atkin WS, Morson BC, et al: Long-term risk of colorectal cancer after excision of rectosigmoid adenomas. *N Engl J Med* 326:658, 1992.

Brady LW, Markoe AM, et al: The present and future role of monoclonal antibodies in the management of cancer. *Front Radiat Ther Oncol* 24:247, 1990.

Church JM, Fazio VW, et al. Quality of life after prophylactic colectomy and ileorectal anastomosis in patients with familial adenomatous polyposis. *Dis Colon Rectum* 39:1404, 1996.

Fearon ER: The genetics of colorectal tumor development: The emerging picture and clinical implications. *Semin Colon Rectal Surg* 2:253, 1991.

Fearon ER, Vogelstein B: A genetic model for colorectal tumorigenesis. *Cell* 61:759, 1990.

Fishel R, Lescoe MK, et al: The human mutator gene homologue MSH2 and its association with hereditary nonpolyposis colon cancer. *Cell* 75:1027, 1993 (published erratum appears in *Cell* 77:167, 1994).

Fitzgibbons RJJ, Lynch HT, et al: Recognition and treatment of patients with hereditary nonpolyposis colon cancer (Lynch syndromes I and II). *Ann Surg* 206:289, 1987.

Fleshman JW, Fry RD, et al: Laparoscopic-assisted and minilaparotomy approaches to colorectal diseases are similar in early outcome. *Dis Colon Rectum* 1996;39:15-22.

Fleshman JW, Fry RD, et al: Nonneoplastic polyposis syndrome. *Semin Colon Rectal Surg* 2:277, 1992.

Fleshman JW, Nelson H, et al: Clinical Outcomes of Surgical Therapy (COST) Study Group: Early results of laparoscopic surgery for colorectal cancer. Retrospective analysis of 372 patients treated by Clinical Outcomes of Surgical Therapy (COST) Study Group. *Dis Colon Rectum* 39:S53, 1996.

Fozard JB, Dixon MF: Colonoscopic surveillance in ulcerative colitis—Dysplasia through the looking glass. *Gut* 30:285, 1989.

Frommer D: Cleansing ability and tolerance of three bowel preparations for colonoscopy. *Dis Colon Rectum* 40:100, 1997.

Fry RD: Surgery for colorectal polyps, in VW Fazio (ed): *Current Therapy in Colon and Rectal Surgery.* Philadelphia, BC Decker, 1990, p 277.

Fry RD, Kodner IJ: Anorectal disorders. *Clin Symp* 37:2, 1985.

Granowska M, Britton KE: Radiolabelled monoclonal antibodies in oncology: II. Clinical applications in diagnosis. *Nucl Med Commun* 2:83, 1991.

Greenstein AJ, Sachar DB, et al: Cancer in universal and left-sided ulcerative colitis: Factors determining risk. *Gastroenterology* 77:290, 1979.

Griffin TW, Brill AB, et al: Initial clinical study of indium-111-labeled clone 110 anticarcinoembryonic antigen antibody in patients with colorectal cancer. *J Clin Oncol* 9:631, 1991.

Guillem JG, Bastar AL, et al. Clustering of colorectal cancer in families of probands under 40 years of age. *Dis Colon Rectum* 39:1004, 1996.

Haggitt RC, Glotzbach RE, et al: Prognostic factors in colorectal carcinomas arising in adenomas: Implications for lesions removed by endoscopic polypectomy. *Gastroenterology* 89:328, 1985.

Hardcastle JD, Chamberlain JO, et al. Randomized controlled trial of faecal-occult-blood screening for colorectal cancer. *Lancet* 348:1472, 1996.

Helfand M, Marton KI, et al: History of visible rectal bleeding in a primary care population: Initial assessment and 10-year follow-up. *JAMA* 277:44, 1997.

Hollstein M, Sidransky D, et al: p53 mutations in human cancers. *Science* 253:49, 1991.

Jass JR: Nature and clinical significance of colorectal hyperplastic polyp. *Semin Colon Rectal Surg* 2:246, 1991.

Jass JR, Stewart SM, et al: Screening for hereditary nonpolyposis colorectal cancer in New Zealand. *Eur J Gastroenterol Heptol* 4:523, 1992.

Kinzler KW, Nilbert MC, et al: Identification of FAP locus genes from chromosome 5q21. *Science* 253:661, 1991.

Kronborg O, Fenger C, et al: Randomized study of screening for colorectal cancer with faecal-occult-blood-test. *Lancet* 348:1467, 1996.

Lange MK, Martin EW Jr: Monoclonal antibodies in imaging and therapy of colorectal cancer. *World J Surg* 15:617, 1991.

Lynch HT, Smyrk TC, et al: Genetics, natural history, tumor spectrum, and pathology of hereditary nonpolyposis colorectal cancer: An updated review. *Gastroenterology* 104:1535, 1993.

Lynch HT, et al: Hereditary nonpolyposis colon cancer, in VW Fazio (ed): *Current Therapy in Colon and Rectal Surgery.* Philadelphia, BC Decker, 1990, p 288.

Madoff RD: Colorectal cancer genetics. *Bull Am Coll Surg* 81:26, 1996.

Mandel JS, Bond JH, et al: Sensitivity, specificity, and positive predictivity of the Hemoccult test in screening for colorectal cancers. The University of Minnesota's Colon Cancer Control Study. *Gastroenterology* 97:597, 1989.

Marra G, Boladn CR: Review: Hereditary nonpolyposis colorectal cancer: The syndrome, the genes, and historical perspectives. *J Natl Cancer Inst* 87:1114, 1995.

Meling GI, Rognum TO, et al: Association between DNA ploidy pattern and cellular atypia in colorectal carcinomas: A new clinical application of DNA flow cytometric study. *Cancer* 67:1642, 1991.

Nivatvongs S: Endoscopic treatment of colorectal polyps, in VW Fazio (ed): *Current Therapy in Colon and Rectal Surgery.* Philadelphia, BC Decker, 1990, p 280.

O'Brien MJ, Winawer SJ, et al: The National Polyp Study: Patient and polyp characteristics associated with high-grade dysplasia in colorectal adenomas. *Gastroenterology* 98:371, 1990.

Opelka FG, Hicks TC: Management of malignant polyps. *Semin Colon Rectal Surg* 2:296, 1991.

Philpott GW, Siegel BA, et al: Initial clinical study of a new indium-labeled anti-colorectal carcinoma antibody (MAv 1A3) in patients with advanced colorectal cancer. *Proc Soc Nucl Med* 32:1054, 1991.

Pollard CW, Nivatvongs S, et al: The fate of patients following polypectomy alone for polyps containing invasive carcinoma. *Dis Colon Rectum* 35:933, 1992.

Poulard JB, Shatz B, et al: Preoperative tattooing of polypectomy site. *Endoscopy* 17:84, 1985.

Read TE, Read JD, Butterly LF: Importance of adenomas 5 mm or less in diameter that are detected by sigmoidoscopy. *N Engl J Med* 336:8, 1997.

Rosen L, Abel ME, et al: Practice parameters for the detection of colorectal neoplasms—Supporting documentation. *Dis Colon Rectum* 35:389, 1992.

Selby JV, Friedman GD, et al: A case-control study of screening sigmoidoscopy and mortality from colorectal cancer. *N Engl J Med* 326:653, 1992.

Wexner SD, Jagelman DG: Familial polyposis syndromes. *Semin Colon Rectal Surg* 2:269, 1991.

Winawer SJ, St John J, et al: Screening of average-risk individuals for colorectal cancer. WHO Collaborating Centre for the Prevention of Colorectal Cancer. *Bull WHO* 68:505, 1990.

Winawer SF, Zauber AG, et al: Randomized comparison of surveillance intervals after colonoscopic removal of newly diagnosed adenomatous polyps. The National Polyp Study Workgroup. *N Engl J Med* 328:901, 1993.

Winawer SF, Zauber AG, et al: Prevention of colorectal cancer by colonoscopic polypectomy. The National Polyp Study Workgroup. *N Engl J Med* 329:1977, 1993.

Winawer SF, Zauber AG, et al: Risk of colorectal cancer in the families of patients with adenomatous polyps. The National Polyp Study Workgroup. *N Engl J Med* 334:82, 1996.

Colorectal Cancer

Advanced Colorectal Cancer Meta-analysis Project: Modulation of fluorouracil by leucovorin in patients with advanced colorectal cancer: Evidence in terms of response rates. *J Clin Oncol* 10:896, 1992.

Agranovich AL, Anderson GH, et al: Carcinoid tumor of the gastrointestinal tract: Prognostic factors and disease outcome. *J Surg Oncol* 47:45, 1991.

Amato A, Pescatori M, et al: Local recurrence following abdominoperineal excision and anterior resection for rectal carcinoma. *Dis Colon Rectum* 34:317, 1991.

Auger MJ, Allan NC: Primary ileocecal lymphoma: A study of 22 patients. *Cancer* 65:358, 1990.

Beart RW: Prevention and management of recurrent rectal cancer. *World J Surg* 15:589, 1991.

Brunetaud JM, Maunoury V, et al: Palliative treatment of rectosigmoid carcinoma by laser endoscopic photoablation. *Gastroenterology* 92:663, 1987.

Brunschwig A, Barber HR: Pelvic exenteration combined with resection of segments of bony pelvis. *Surgery* 65:417, 1969.

Cohen AM, Enker WE, et al: Proctectomy and coloanal reconstruction for rectal cancer. *Dis Colon Rectum* 33:40, 1990.

Crile G, Turnbull RB: The role of electrocoagulation in the treatment of carcinoma of the rectum. *Surg Gynecol Obstet* 135:391, 1972.

Daneker GW JR, Carlson GW, et al: Endoscopic laser recanalization is effective for prevention and treatment of obstruction in sigmoid and rectal cancer. *Arch Surg* 126:1348, 1991.

De Lange EE, Fechner RE, et al: Rectal carcinoma treated by preoperative irradiation: MR imaging and histopathologic correlation. *AJR* 158:287, 1992.

Devine RM, Beart RW Jr, et al: Malignant lymphoma of the rectum. *Dis Colon Rectum* 29:821, 1986.

Dukes CE: Cancer of the rectum: an analysis of 1000 cases. *J Pathol Bacteriol* 50:527, 1940.

Dukes CE: The surgical pathology of rectal cancer. *J Clin Pathol* 2:95, 1949.

Dukes CE, Bussey HJR: The spread of rectal cancer and its effect on prognosis. *Br J Cancer* 12:309, 1958.

Ellis LM, Mendenhall WM, et al: Local excision and radiation therapy for early rectal cancer. *Am Surg* 54:217, 1988.

Erlichman C, Fine S, et al: A randomized trial of fluorouracil and folinic acid in patients with metastatic colorectal carcinoma. *J Clin Oncol* 6:469, 1988.

Evans DB, Shumate CR, et al: Use of Dexon mesh for abdominal partitioning above the peritoneal reflection. *Dis Colon Rectum* 34:833, 1991.

Fazio VW: Curative local therapy of rectal cancer. *Int J Color Dis* 6:66, 1991.

Fearon ER, Vogelstein B: A genetic model for colorectal tumorigenesis. *Cell* 61:759, 1990.

Fleshman JW, Kodner IJ, et al: Accuracy of transrectal ultrasound in predicting pathologic stage of rectal cancer after preoperative irradiation. *Dis Colon Rectum* 35:823, 1992.

Fisher B, Wolmark N, et al: Postoperative adjuvant chemotherapy or radiation therapy for rectal cancer: Results from NSABP Protocol R-01. *J Natl Cancer Inst* 80:21, 1988.

Fry RD, Fleshman JW, et al: Cancer of colon and rectum. *Clin Symp* 41:2, 1989.

Fry RD, Shemesh EI, et al: Perforation of the rectum and sigmoid colon during barium-enema examination: Management and prevention. *Dis Colon Rectum* 32:759, 1989.

Gastrointestinal Tumor Study Group: Prolongation of the disease-free interval in surgically resected rectal cancer. *N Engl J Med* 312:1465, 1985.

Gerard A, Berrod JL, et al: Interim analysis of a phase III study on preoperative radiation therapy in resectable rectal carcinoma. Trial of the Gastrointestinal Tract Cancer Cooperative Group of the European Organization for Research on Treatment of Cancer (EORTC). *Cancer* 55:2373, 1985.

Goligher JC, Graham NG, et al: Anastomotic dehiscence after anterior resection of rectum and sigmoid. *Br J Surg* 57:109, 1970.

Grinnell RS: Distal intramural spread of carcinoma of the rectum and rectosigmoid. *Surg Gynecol Obstet* 99:421, 1954.

Hackford AW: The extent of major resections for rectal cancer. *Semin Colon Rectal Surg* 1:16, 1990.

Heald RJ: The "holy plane" of rectal surgery. *J R Soc Med* 81:503, 1988.

Heald RJ, Husband EM, et al: The mesorectum in rectal cancer surgery—The clue to pelvic recurrence? *Br J Surg* 69:613, 1982.

Hildebrandt U, Feifel G: Preoperative staging of rectal cancer by intrarectal ultrasound. *Dis Colon Rectum* 28:42, 1985.

Horn A, Dahl O, et al: Venous and neural invasion as predictors of recurrence in rectal adenocarcinoma. *Dis Colon Rectum* 34:798, 1991.

Jao SW, Beart RWJ, et al: Retrorectal tumors: Mayo Clinic experience, 1960–1979. *Dis Colon Rectum* 28:644, 1985.

Kashtan H, Papa MZ, et al: Use of photodynamic therapy in the palliation of massive advanced rectal cancer: Phase I/II study. *Dis Colon Rectum* 34:600, 1991.

Kligerman MM, Urdaneta N, et al: Preoperative irradiation of rectosigmoid carcinoma including its regional lymph nodes. *AJR* 114:498, 1972.

Kodner IJ: Colostomy and ileostomy. *Clin Symp* 30:1, 1978.

Kodner IJ: Rectal cancer, in MJ Zinner, SI Schwartz, H Ellis (eds): *Maingot's Abdominal Operations,* 10th ed. Norwalk, CT, Appleton & Lange, 1997, p 1455.

Kodner IJ, Fry RD, et al: Current options in the management of rectal cancer. *Adv Surg* 24:1, 1991.

Kodner IJ, Fry RD, Fleshman JW: Current options in the management of rectal cancer. *Adv Surg* 24:1, 1991.

Kodner IJ, Fry RD, Roe JP (eds): *Colon and Rectal and Anal Surgery: Current Techniques and Controversies.* St Louis, Mosby, 1985.

Kodner IJ, Shemesh EI, et al: Preoperative irradiation for rectal cancer: Improved local control and long-term survival. *Ann Surg* 209:194, 1989.

Kraybill WG, Lopez MJ, et al: Total pelvic exenteration as a therapeutic option in advanced malignant disease of the pelvis. *Surg Gynecol Obstet* 166:259, 1988.

Krook JE, Moertel CG, et al: Effective surgical adjuvant therapy for high-risk rectal carcinoma. *N Engl J Med* 324:709, 1991.

Laurie JA, Moertel CG, et al: Surgical adjuvant therapy of large-bowel carcinoma: an evaluation of levamisole and the combination of levamisole and fluorouracil. The North Central Cancer Treatment Group and the Mayo Clinic. *J Clin Oncol* 7:1447, 1989.

Levendoglu H, Cox CA, et al: Composite (adenocarcinoid) tumors of the gastrointestinal tract. *Dig Dis Sci* 35:519, 1990.

Martin EWJ, Minton JP, et al: CEA-directed second-look surgery in the asymptomatic patient after primary resection of colorectal carcinoma. *Ann Surg* 202:310, 1985.

McAnena OJ, Heald RJ, et al: Operative and functional results of total mesorectal excision with ultra-low anterior resection in the management of carcinoma of the lower one-third of the rectum. *Surg Gynecol Obstet* 170:517, 1990.

Meade PG, Blatchford GJ, et al: Preoperative chemoradiation downstages locally advanced ultrasound-staged rectal cancer. *Am J Surg* 170: 609, 1995.

Mendenhall WM, Million RR, et al: Initially unresectable rectal adenocarcinoma treated with preoperative irradiation and surgery. *Ann Surg* 205:41, 1987.

Miles WE: A method of performing abdomino-perineal excision for carcinoma of the rectum and of the terminal portion of the pelvic colon. *Lancet* 2:1812, 1908.

Minsky BD, Cohen AM, et al: Radiation therapy for unresectable rectal cancer. *Int J Radiat Oncol Biol Phys* 21:1283, 1991.

Moertel CG, Fleming TR, et al: Intergroup study of fluorouracil plus levamisole as adjuvant therapy for stage II/Dukes' B2 colon cancer. *J Clin Oncol* 13:2936, 1995.

Moertel CG, Fleming TR, et al: Levamisole and fluorouracil for adjuvant therapy of resected colon carcinoma. *N Engl J Med* 322:352, 1990.

Morson BC: Factors influencing the prognosis of early cancer of the rectum. *Proc R Soc Med* 59:607, 1966.

Morson BC, Bussey HJ, et al: Policy of local excision for early cancer of the colorectum. *Gut* 18:1045, 1977.

Myerson R, Walz B, et al: Endocavitary radiation therapy for rectal carcinoma: Results with and without external beam endocurietherapy/hyperthermia. *Oncology* 5:195, 1989.

Myerson RJ, Zusag TW, et al: Adjunctive radiation therapy for rectal carcinoma. *Am J Clin Oncol* 15:102, 1992.

Naunheim KS, Zeitels J, et al: Rectal carcinoid tumors: Treatment and prognosis. *Surgery* 94:670, 1983.

NIH Consensus Conference: Adjuvant therapy for patients with colon and rectal cancer. *JAMA* 264:1444, 1990.

Palmer JG, Scholefield JH, et al: Oswald Vaughan Lloyd-Davies, 1905–1987: Lithotomy-Trendelenburg position for resection of rectum and lower pelvic colon (classical article). Anal cancer and human papillomaviruses. *Dis Colon Rectum* 32:1016, 1989.

Papillon J: Intracavitary irradiation of early rectal cancer for cure: A series of 186 cases. *Cancer* 36:696, 1975.

Papillon J: New prospects in the conservative treatment of rectal cancer. *Dis Colon Rectum* 27:695, 1984.

Parks AG, Percy JP: Resection and sutured colo-anal anastomosis for rectal carcinoma. *Br J Surg* 69:301, 1982.

Petrelli N, Douglass HO, et al: The modulation of fluorouracil with leucovorin in metastatic colorectal carcinoma: A prospective, randomized phase III trial. *J Clin Oncol* 67:257, 1989.

Pollett WG, Nicholls RJ: The relationship between the extent of distal clearance and survival and local recurrence rates after curative anterior resection for carcinoma of the rectum. *Ann Surg* 198:159, 1983.

Rhoads JE, Schwegman CW: Surgical techniques: One-stage combined abdominoperineal resection of the rectum (Miles) performed by two surgical teams. *Surgery* 58:600, 1965.

Rich T, Gunderson LL, et al: Patterns of recurrence of rectal cancer after potentially curative surgery. *Cancer* 52:1317, 1983.

Santangelo ML, Romano G, et al: Sexual function after resection for rectal cancer. *Am J Surg* 154:502, 1987.

Sauven P, Ridge JA, et al: Anorectal carcinoid tumors: Is aggressive surgery warranted? *Ann Surg* 211:67, 1990.

Schild SE, Martenson JAJ, et al: Postoperative adjuvant therapy of rectal cancer: An analysis of disease control, survival, and prognostic factors. *Int J Radiat Oncol Biol Phys* 17:55, 1989.

Schoetz DJ Jr: *Controversies in the Management of Rectal Cancer.* Philadelphia, WB Saunders, 1990.

Steele G, Bleday R, et al: A prospective evaluation of hepatic resection for colorectal carcinoma metastases to the liver. Gastrointestinal Tumor Study Group Protocol 6584. *J Clin Oncol* 9:1105, 1991.

Steele G Jr: Combined-modality therapy for rectal carcinoma—The time has come. *N Engl J Med* 324:764, 1991.

Stockholm Rectal Cancer Study Group: Preoperative short-term radiation therapy in operable rectal carcinoma: A prospective, randomized trial. *Cancer* 66:49, 1990.

Stolfi VM, Milsom JW, et al: Newly designed occluder pin for presacral hemorrhage. *Dis Colon Rectum* 35:166, 1992.

Tomoda H, Furusawa M, et al: A rectal carcinoid tumor of less than 1 cm in diameter with lymph node metastasis: A case report and a review of the literature. *Jpn J Surg* 20:468, 1990.

Uhlig BE, Johnson RL: Presacral tumors and cysts in adults. *Dis Colon Rectum* 18:581, 1975.

United States Preventive Services Task Force: Guide to clinical services. Washington, DC, Department of Health and Human Services, 2d ed, 1995.

Vahrson H, Haas R, et al: Primary HDR afterloading brachytherapy of inoperable rectal cancer. *Sonderb Strahlenther Onkol* 82:278, 1988.

Van den Heule B, Taylor CR, et al: Presentation of malignant lymphoma in the rectum. *Cancer* 49:2602, 1982.

Vasen HF, Mecklin JP, Khan PM, et al: The International Collaborative Group on Hereditary Non-Polyposis Colorectal Cancer (ICG-HNPCC). *Dis Colon Rectum* 34:424, 1991.

Waizer A, Powsner E, et al: Prospective comparative study of magnetic resonance imaging versus transrectal ultrasound for preoperative staging and follow-up of rectal cancer: Preliminary report. *Dis Colon Rectum* 34:1068, 1991.

Wang QY, Shi WJ, et al: New concepts in severe presacral hemorrhage during proctectomy. *Arch Surg* 120:1013, 1985.

Warneke J, Petrelli NJ, et al: Local recurrence after sphincter-saving resection for rectal adenocarcinoma. *Am J Surg* 158:3, 1989.

Weingrad DN, DeCosse JJ, et al: Primary gastrointestinal lymphoma: A 30-year review. *Cancer* 49:1258, 1982.

Wilking N, Petrelli NJ, et al: Surgical resection of pulmonary metastases from colorectal adenocarcinoma. *Dis Colon Rectum* 28:562, 1985.

Willett CG, Shellito PC, et al: Intraoperative electron beam radiation therapy for recurrent locally advanced rectal or rectosigmoid carcinoma. *Cancer* 67:1504, 1991.

Williams NS, Dixon MF, et al: Reappraisal of the 5 centimetre rule of distal excision for carcinoma of the rectum: A study of distal intramural spread and of patients' survival. *Br J Surg* 70:150, 1983.

Wolmark N, Fisher B: An analysis of survival and treatment failure following abdominoperineal and sphincter-saving resection in Dukes' B and C rectal carcinoma. *Ann Surg* 204:480, 1986.

Anal Neoplasms

Arbesman H, Ransohoff DF: Is Bowen's disease a predictor for the development of internal malignancy? A methodological critique of the literature. *JAMA* 257:516, 1987.

Beck DE, Fazio VW: Perianal Paget's disease. *Dis Colon Rectum* 30:263, 1987.

Birnbaum EB, Myerson RJ: Carcinoma of the anus, in MJ Zinner, SI Schwartz, H Ellis (eds): *Maingot's Abdominal Operations,* 10th ed. Norwalk, CT, Appleton & Lange, 1997, p 1503.

Cooper PH, Mills SE, et al: Malignant melanoma of the anus: Report of 12 patients and analysis of 255 additional cases. *Dis Colon Rectum* 25:693, 1982.

Gordon PH: Squamous-cell carcinoma of the anal canal. *Surg Clin North Am* 68:1391, 1988.

Jensen SL, Hagen K, et al: Long-term prognosis after radical treatment for squamous-cell carcinoma of the anal canal and anal margin. *Dis Colon Rectum* 31:273, 1988.

Nigro ND: An evaluation of combined therapy for squamous cell cancer of the anal canal. *Dis Colon Rectum* 27:763, 1984.

Nigro ND: Multidisciplinary management of cancer of the anus. *World J Surg* 11:446, 1987.

Wexner SD, Milsom JW, et al: The demographics of anal cancers are changing: Identification of a high-risk population. *Dis Colon Rectum* 30:942, 1987.

White WB, Schneiderman H, et al: Basal cell carcinoma of the anus: Clinical and pathological distinction from cloacogenic carcinoma. *J Clin Gastroenterol* 6:441, 1984.

CHAPTER 27

The Appendix

Rosemary A. Kozar and Joel J. Roslyn

ANATOMY AND FUNCTION

The appendix first becomes visible during embryologic development in the eighth week of life as a protuberance off the terminal portion of the cecum. During both antenatal and postnatal development, the growth rate of the cecum exceeds that of the appendix, displacing the appendix medially toward the ileocecal valve. The relationship of the base of the appendix to the cecum remains constant, whereas the tip can be found in a retrocecal, pelvic, subcecal, preileal, or right pericolic position. These anatomic considerations have significant clinical importance in the context of acute appendicitis. The three taenia coli converge at the junction of the cecum with the appendix and can be a useful landmark to identify the appendix. The appendix can vary in length from less than 1 to greater than 30 cm; most appendices are 6 to 9 cm in length. Appendiceal absence, duplication, and diverticula have all been described.

For many years, the appendix was erroneously viewed as a vestigial organ with no known function. It is now well recognized that the appendix is an immunologic organ which actively participates in the secretion of immunoglobulins, particularly IgA. Though the appendix is an integral component of the gut-associated lymphoid tissue (GALT) system, its function is not essential and appendectomy has not been associated with any predisposition to sepsis or any other manifestation of immune compromise. Lymphoid tissue first appears in the appendix about 2 weeks after birth. The amount of lymphoid tissue increases throughout puberty, remains steady for the next decade, and then begins a steady decrease with age. After the age of 60, virtually no lymphoid tissue remains within the appendix and complete obliteration of the appendiceal lumen is common.

INFLAMMATION OF THE APPENDIX

Acute Appendicitis

Historical Background. There is evidence in the literature that alchemists and physicians in the 1500s recognized the existence of a clinical entity associated with severe inflammation of the cecal region, known as "perityphlitis." Although the first successful appendectomy was reported in 1736, it was not until 1886 that Reginald Fitz helped establish the role of surgical removal of the inflamed appendix as curative therapy for this disease, which was once thought to be fatal. In 1889, Charles McBurney presented his classic report before the New York Surgical Society on the importance of early operative intervention for acute appendicitis in which he described the point of maximal abdominal tenderness to be determined by the pressure of one finger placed one-third of the distance between the anterior superior iliac spine and the umbilicus. Five years later he devised the muscle-splitting incision which today bears his name.

Incidence. Appendicitis remains one of the most common acute surgical diseases. The incidence of acute appendicitis roughly parallels that of lymphoid development, with the peak incidence in early adulthood. Appendicitis occurs more frequently in males especially at the time of puberty. A review of over 2000 patients with appendicitis demonstrated an overall 1.3:1 male predominance.

A decline from 100 cases per 100,000 population to 52 cases per 100,000 population was demonstrated over a study period from 1975 to 1991. This degree of change does not seem to be explained by improved diagnosis, and the explanation for this phenomenon remains elusive. Currently, 84 percent of all appendectomies are performed for acute pathology. The rate of normal appendectomy averages 16 percent, with females comprising 68 percent of those patients found to have a normal appendix at exploration.

Etiology and Pathogenesis. Obstruction of the lumen is the dominant causal factor in acute appendicitis. Fecaliths are the usual cause of appendiceal obstruction. Less common are hypertrophy of lymphoid tissue; inspissated barium from previous x-ray studies; vegetable and fruit seeds; and intestinal worms, particularly ascarids.

The frequency of obstruction rises with the severity of the inflammatory process. Fecaliths are found in about 40 percent of cases of simple acute appendicitis, about 65 percent of cases of gangrenous appendicitis without rupture, and about 90 percent of cases of gangrenous appendicitis with rupture.

The probable sequence of events following occlusion of the lumen is as follows. A closed-loop obstruction is produced by the proximal block, and continuing normal secretion of the appendiceal mucosa rapidly produces distention. The luminal capacity of the normal appendix is only about 0.1 mL—there is no real lumen. Secretion of as little as 0.5 mL distal to a block raises the intraluminal pressure to about 60 cmH$_2$O. The human being is one of the few animals with an appendix capable of secreting at pressures high enough to lead to gangrene and perforation. Distention stimulates nerve endings of visceral afferent pain fibers, producing vague, dull, diffuse pain in the mid-abdomen or lower epigastrium. Peristalsis is also stimulated by the rather sudden distention, so that some cramping may be superimposed on the visceral pain early in the course of appendicitis.

Distention continues, not only from continued mucosal secretion, but also from rapid multiplication of the resident bacteria of the appendix. As pressure in the organ increases, venous pressure is exceeded. Capillaries and venules are occluded, but arteriolar inflow continues, resulting in engorgement and vascular congestion. Distension of this magnitude usually causes reflex nausea and vomiting, and the diffuse visceral pain becomes more severe. The inflammatory process soon involves the serosa of the appendix and in turn parietal peritoneum in the region, producing the characteristic shift in pain to the right lower quadrant.

The mucosa of the gastrointestinal tract, including the appendix, is very susceptible to impairment of blood supply. Thus its integrity is compromised early in the process, allowing bacterial invasion of the deeper coats. As progressive distention encroaches on the arteriolar pressure, the area with the poorest blood supply suffers most: ellipsoidal infarcts develop in the antimesenteric border. As distention, bacterial invasion, compromise of vascular supply, and infarction progress, perforation occurs, usually through one of the infarcted areas on the antimesenteric border.

This sequence is not inevitable; some episodes of acute appendicitis apparently subside spontaneously. Many patients who are found at operation to have acute appendicitis give a history of previous similar but less severe attacks of right lower quadrant pain. Pathologic examination of the appendices removed from these patients often reveals thickening and scarring, suggesting old healed acute inflammation.

Bacteriology. A variety of anaerobes, aerobes, or facultative bacteria have been cultured from peritoneal fluid, abscess contents, and appendiceal tissue in patients with gangrenous or perforated appendicitis. An average of 10 different organisms were recovered per specimen. Bacteroides fragilis and Escherichia coli were isolated from almost all specimens. Other frequent isolates were Peptostreptococcus (80 percent), Pseudomonas (40 percent), Bacteroides splanchnicus (40 percent), and Lactobacillus (37 percent).

A quantitative bacteriologic study of the appendix wall of children showed no significant differences between the flora of normal and of acutely inflamed appendices. Bacteroides, *E. coli*, and streptococci were the most common organisms isolated.

Cytomegalovirus-associated appendicitis has been reported in a patient with acquired immunodeficiency syndrome.

Clinical Manifestations. *Symptoms.* Abdominal pain is the prime symptom of acute appendicitis. Classically the pain is initially diffusely centered in the lower epigastrium or umbilical area, is moderately severe, and is steady, sometimes with intermittent cramping superimposed. After a period varying from 1 to 12 h, but usually within 4 to 6 h, the pain localizes in the right lower quadrant. This classic pain sequence, though usual, is not invariable. In some patients the pain of appendicitis begins in the right lower quadrant and remains there. Variations in the anatomic location of the appendix account for many of the variations in the principal locus of the somatic phase of the pain. For example, a long appendix with the inflamed tip in the left lower quadrant causes pain in that area; a rectrocecal appendix may cause principally flank or back pain; a pelvic appendix, principally suprapubic pain; and a retroileal appendix may cause testicular pain, presumably from irritation of the spermatic artery and ureter. Malrotation is also responsible for puzzling pain patterns. The visceral component is in the normal location, but the somatic component is felt in that part of the abdomen where the cecum has been arrested in rotation.

Anorexia nearly always accompanies appendicitis. It is so constant that the diagnosis should be questioned if the patient is not anorectic. Vomiting occurs in about 75 percent of patients, but is not prominent or prolonged, and most patients vomit only once or twice.

Most patients give a history of obstipation from before the onset of abdominal pain, and many feel that defecation would relieve their abdominal pain. However, diarrhea occurs in some patients, particularly children, so that the pattern of bowel function is of little differential diagnostic value.

The sequence of symptom appearance has great differential diagnostic significance. In over 95 percent of patients with acute appendicitis, anorexia is the first symptom, followed by abdominal pain, which is followed in turn by vomiting (if vomiting occurs). If vomiting precedes the onset of pain, the diagnosis should be questioned.

Signs. Physical findings are determined principally by the anatomic position of the inflamed appendix as well as by whether the organ has already ruptured when the patient is first examined.

Vital signs are not changed very much by uncomplicated appendicitis. Temperature elevation is rarely more than 1°C; the pulse rate is normal or slightly elevated. Changes of greater magnitude usually mean that a complication has occurred or that another diagnosis should be considered.

Patients with appendicitis usually prefer to lie supine, with the thighs, particularly the right thigh, drawn up, because any motion increases pain. If asked to move, they do so slowly and gingerly.

The classic right lower quadrant physical signs are present when the inflamed appendix lies in the anterior position. Tenderness is often maximal at or near the point described by McBurney as being "located exactly between an inch and a half and two inches from the anterior spinous process of the ileum on a straight line drawn from that process to the umbilicus." Direct rebound tenderness is usually present, and referred or indirect rebound tenderness is frequently present, and the tenderness is felt maximally in the right lower quadrant, indicating peritoneal irritation. Rovsing's sign—pain in the right lower quadrant when palpatory pressure is exerted in the left lower quadrant—also indicates the site of peritoneal irritation. Cutaneous hyperesthesia in the area supplied by the spinal nerves on the right at T10, T11, and T12 frequently but not always accompanies acute appendicitis. In patients with obvious appendicitis, this sign is superfluous, but in some early cases it may be the first positive sign. It is elicited either by needle prick or, better, by gently picking up the skin between the forefinger and thumb. This ordinarily is not unpleasant but is painful in areas of cutaneous hyperesthesia.

Muscular resistance to palpation of the abdominal wall roughly parallels the severity of the inflammatory process. Early in the disease, resistance, if present, consists mainly of voluntary guarding. As peritoneal irritation progresses, muscle spasm increases and becomes largely involuntary—true reflex rigidity as opposed to voluntary guarding.

Variations in the position of the inflamed appendix produce variations from the usual in physical findings. With a retrocecal appendix, the anterior abdominal findings are less striking, and tenderness may be most marked in the flank. When the inflamed appendix hangs into the pelvis, abdominal findings may be entirely absent, and the diagnosis may be missed unless the rectum is examined. As the examining finger exerts pressure on the peritoneum of the cul-de-sac of Douglas, pain is felt in the suprapubic area as well as locally. Signs of localized muscle irritation may also be present. The psoas sign indicates an irritative focus in proximity to that muscle. The test is performed by having patients lie on their left side; the examiner then slowly extends the right thigh, thus stretching the iliopsoas muscle. The test is positive if extension produces pain. Similarly, a positive obturator sign of hypogastric pain on stretching the obturator internus indicates irritation at that locus. The test is performed by passive internal rotation of the flexed right thigh with the patient supine.

Laboratory Findings. Mild leukocytosis, ranging from 10,000 to 18,000/mm³, is usually present in patients with acute, uncomplicated appendicitis and is often accompanied by a moderate polymorphonuclear predominance. If a normal white blood cell count with no left shift is present, the diagnosis of acute appendicitis should be reconsidered. It is unusual for the white blood cell count to be greater than 18,000/mm³ in uncomplicated appendicitis. White blood cell counts above this level raise the possibility of a perforated appendix with or without an abscess. Urinalysis can be useful to rule out the urinary tract as the source of infection. Although several white or red blood cells can be present from ureteral or bladder irritation as a result of an inflamed appendix, bacteriuria in a catheterized urine specimen will not be seen with acute appendicitis.

Plain films of the abdomen, although frequently obtained as part of the general evaluation of a patient with an acute abdomen, are rarely helpful in diagnosing acute appendicitis, although they can be of significant benefit in ruling out additional pathology. In patients with acute appendicitis, one often sees an abnormal bowel gas pattern, which is a nonspecific finding. The presence of a fecalith is rarely noted on plain films, but when present is highly suggestive of the diagnosis. A chest x-ray is sometimes indicated to rule out referred pain from a right lower lobe pneumonic process.

Graded compression sonography has been suggested as an accurate way to establish the diagnosis of appendicitis. The appendix is identified as a blind-ending, nonperistaltic bowel loop originating from the cecum. With maximal compression, the diameter of the appendix is measured in the anteroposterior dimension. A scan is considered positive if a noncompressible appendix 6 mm or greater in the anteroposterior direction is demonstrated (Fig. 27-1). The presence of an appendicolith establishes the diagnosis. Sonographic demonstration of a normal appendix, which is an easily compressible blind-ending tubular structure measuring 5 mm or less, excludes the diagnosis of acute appendicitis. The study is considered negative if the appendix is not visualized and there is no pericecal fluid or mass. When the diagnosis of acute appendicitis is excluded by sonography, a brief survey of the remainder of the abdominal cavity should be performed to establish an alternative diagnosis. In females of childbearing age, the pelvic organs must be adequately visualized either transabdominally or by endovaginal examination in order to exclude gynecologic pathology as a possible cause of acute abdominal pain. The sonographic diagnosis of acute appendicitis has a reported sensitivity of 78 to 96 percent and a specificity of 85 to 98 percent. Sonography is similarly effective in children and pregnant women, although its application is somewhat limited in late pregnancy.

Sonography has definite limitations and results are user-dependent. A false-positive scan can occur in the presence of periappendicitis from surrounding inflammation, a dilated fallopian tube can be mistaken for an inflamed appendix, inspissated stool can mimic an appendicolith, and, in obese patients, the appendix may not be compressible not because of an acutely inflamed appendix but because of overlying fat. False-negative sonograms can occur if appendicitis is confined to the appendiceal tip, the cecum is retrocecal in location, the appendix is markedly enlarged and mistaken for small bowel, or if the appendix is perforated and therefore compressible.

Additional radiographic techniques include computed tomography, barium enema, and radioisotope-labeled leukocyte scans. Although CT has been reported to be as, or more, accurate than sonography, it is significantly more expensive. Because of the cost and added radiation exposure, CT should be used primarily when an appendiceal abscess is suspected to ascertain the feasibility of percutaneous drainage. Diagnosis based on barium enema depends on the nonspecific findings of extrinsic mass effect on the cecum and nonfilling of the appendix, and is associated with an accuracy ranging from 50 to 84 percent. Radiographic evaluation of patients with suspected appendicitis should be reserved for patients in whom the diagnosis is in doubt and should not delay, or substitute for, prompt operative intervention when clinically indicated.

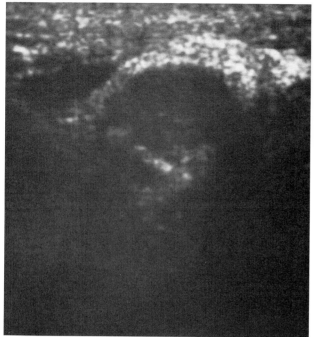

A

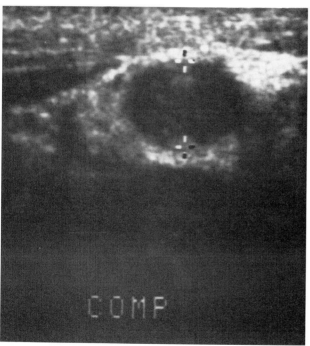

B

FIG. 27-1. Sonogram of a 10-year-old female who presented with nausea, vomiting, and abdominal pain. The appendix measured 10.0 mm in maximal anteroposterior diameter in both the noncompression (A) and compression (B) views.

Laparoscopy can serve as both a diagnostic and therapeutic maneuver for patients with acute abdominal pain and suspected acute appendicitis. Laparoscopy is probably most useful for the evaluation of females with lower abdominal complaints, since appendectomy is performed on a normal appendix in as many

as 30 to 40 percent of such patients. Differentiating acute gynecologic pathology from acute appendicitis is easily accomplished using the laparoscope.

Appendiceal Rupture

Immediate appendectomy has long been the recommended treatment of acute appendicitis because of the known progression to rupture. A study on the natural history of appendicitis demonstrated a rate of 14 percent normal, 70 percent inflamed, and 16 percent perforated appendices. This study suggested that delays in presentation were responsible for the majority of perforated appendices. There is no accurate way of determining when and if an appendix will rupture prior to resolution of the inflammatory process. Although it has been suggested that observation and antibiotic therapy alone may be an appropriate treatment for acute appendicitis, nonoperative treatment risks the morbidity and mortality associated with a ruptured appendix.

Appendiceal rupture occurs most frequently distal to the point of luminal obstruction along the antimesenteric border of the appendix. Rupture should be suspected in the presence of fever greater than 39°C (102°F) and a white blood cell count greater than 18,000/mm^3. In the majority of cases rupture is contained and patients display localized rebound tenderness. Generalized peritonitis will be present if the walling-off process is ineffective in containing the rupture.

In 2 to 6 percent of cases, an ill-defined mass will be detected on physical examination. This could represent a phlegmon, which is matted loops of bowel adherent to the adjacent inflamed appendix, or a periappendiceal abscess. Patients who present with a mass have a longer duration of symptoms, usually at least 5 to 7 days. The ability to distinguish acute, uncomplicated appendicitis from perforation on the basis of clinical findings is often difficult, but it is important to make the distinction since their treatment differs. CT scan may be very beneficial in guiding therapy. Phlegmons and small abscesses can be treated conservatively with intravenous antibiotics; well-localized abscesses may be managed with percutaneous drainage; and complex abscesses should be considered for surgical drainage. If operative drainage is required, it should be performed using an extraperitoneal approach, with appendectomy reserved for cases in which the appendix is easily accessible. Interval appendectomy performed at least 6 weeks following the acute event has classically been recommended for all patients treated either nonoperatively or with simple drainage of an abscess. The reported incidence of recurrent appendicitis in patients not undergoing interval appendectomy ranges from 0 to 37 percent, and is highest during the first year. Because a perforated cecal carcinoma can be mistaken for an appendiceal abscess, all patients over the age of 50 years should undergo either barium enema or colonoscopic examination prior to interval appendectomy.

Differential Diagnosis. The differential diagnosis of acute appendicitis is essentially the diagnosis of the "acute abdomen" (see Chap. 22). This is because clinical manifestations are not specific for a given disease but are specific for disturbance of a physiologic function or functions. Thus an essentially identical clinical picture can result from a wide variety of acute processes within or near the peritoneal cavity that produce the same alterations of function as acute appendicitis.

Accuracy of preoperative diagnosis should be about 85 percent. If it is consistently less, some unnecessary operations are probably being done, and a more rigorous preoperative differential diagnosis is in order. On the other hand, an accuracy consistently greater than 90 percent should also cause concern, since this may mean that some patients with atypical but bona fide acute appendicitis are being "observed" when they should have prompt surgical intervention. The Haller group has shown, however, that this is not invariably true. Before their study, the perforation rate at the hospital where the study took place was 26.7 percent, and acute appendicitis was found at 80 percent of the operations. By a policy of intensive in-hospital observation when the diagnosis of appendicitis was unclear, the group raised the rate of acute appendicitis found at operation to 94 percent, while the perforation rate remained unchanged at 27.5 percent.

There are a few conditions in which operation is contraindicated, but in general the disease processes that are confused with appendicitis are also surgical problems or, if not, are not made worse by surgical intervention. The more frequent error is to make a preoperative diagnosis of acute appendicitis only to find some other condition (or nothing) at operation; much less frequently, acute appendicitis is found after a preoperative diagnosis of another condition. The most common erroneous preoperative diagnoses—accounting for more than 75 percent—in descending order of frequency are acute mesenteric lymphadenitis, no organic pathologic condition, acute pelvic inflammatory disease, twisted ovarian cyst or ruptured graafian follicle, and acute gastroenteritis.

Differential diagnosis of appendicitis depends upon three major factors: the anatomic location of the inflamed appendix; the stage of the process, that is, whether simple or ruptured; and the age and sex of the patient.

Acute Mesenteric Adenitis. This is the disease most often confused with acute appendicitis in children. Almost invariably an upper respiratory infection is present or has recently subsided. The pain is usually less or more diffuse, and tenderness is not as sharply localized as in appendicitis. Voluntary guarding is sometimes present, but true rigidity is rare. Generalized lymphadenopathy may be noted. Laboratory procedures are of little help in arriving at the correct diagnosis, although a relative lymphocytosis, when present, suggests mesenteric adenitis. Observation for several hours is in order if the diagnosis of mesenteric adenitis seems likely, since mesenteric adenitis is a self-limited disease, but if the differentiation remains in doubt, immediate operation is the only safe course.

Acute Gastroenteritis. This is very common in childhood but can usually be easily differentiated from appendicitis. Viral gastroenteritis, an acute self-limited infection of diverse causes, is characterized by profuse watery diarrhea, nausea, and vomiting. Hyperperistaltic abdominal cramps precede the watery stools. The abdomen is relaxed between cramps, and there are no localizing signs. Laboratory values are normal.

Salmonella gastroenteritis results from ingestion of contaminated food. Abdominal findings are usually similar to those in viral gastroenteritis, but in some cases the abdominal pain is intense, localized, and associated with rebound tenderness. Chills and fever are common. The leukocyte count is usually normal. The causative organisms can be isolated from essentially 100 percent of patients, but culturing may take too long to help the clinician in making a timely differential diagnosis in cases of abdominal pain. Similar attacks in other persons eating the same food as the patient greatly strengthen the presumptive diagnosis of salmonella gastroenteritis.

Typhoid fever is now a rare disease. This probably accounts for the frequency of missed diagnosis—it is rarely seen and rarely thought of. The onset is less acute than in appendicitis, with a prodrome of several days. Differentiation is usually possible because of the prostration, maculopapular rash, inappropriate bradycardia, and leukopenia. Diagnosis is confirmed by culture of Salmonella typhosa from stool or blood. Intestinal perforation, usually in the lower ileum, develops in about 1 percent of cases and requires immediate surgical therapy.

Diseases of the Male. Diseases of males must be considered in differential diagnosis of appendicitis, including torsion of the testis and acute epididymitis, since epigastric pain may overshadow local symptoms early in these diseases. Seminal vesiculitis may also mimic appendicitis but can be diagnosed by palpating the enlarged, tender seminal vesicle on rectal examination.

Meckel's Diverticulitis. This causes a clinical picture very similar to that of acute appendicitis. Preoperative differentiation is academic and unnecessary, since Meckel's diverticulitis is associated with the same complications as appendicitis and requires the same treatment—prompt surgical intervention. Diverticulectomy can nearly always be done through a McBurney incision, extended if necessary. If the base of the diverticulum is broad, so that removal would compromise the lumen of the ileum, then resection of the segment of ileum bearing the diverticulum with end-to-end anastomosis is done.

Intussusception. In contrast to Meckel's diverticulitis, it is extremely important to differentiate intussusception from acute appendicitis, because the treatment is quite different. The age of the patients is important: appendicitis is very uncommon under age 2, whereas nearly all idiopathic intussusceptions occur under age 2. Intussusception occurs typically in a well-nourished infant who is suddenly doubled up by apparent colicky pain. Between attacks of pain the infant appears quite well. After several hours, the patient usually passes a bloody mucoid stool. A sausage-shaped mass may be palpable in the right lower quadrant. Later, as the intussusception progresses distad, the right lower quadrant feels abnormally empty. The preferred treatment of intussusception, if seen before signs of peritonitis supervene, is reduction by barium enema, but treatment of acute appendicitis by barium enema may be catastrophic.

Regional Enteritis. The manifestations of acute regional enteritis—fever, right lower quadrant pain and tenderness, and leukocytosis—often simulate acute appendicitis. Diarrhea and the infrequency of anorexia, nausea, and vomiting favor a diagnosis of enteritis but are not sufficient to exclude acute appendicitis without celiotomy. In an appreciable percentage of patients with chronic regional enteritis, the diagnosis has been first made at the time of operation for presumed acute appendicitis. Acute ileitis should be distinguished from Crohn's disease. In the face of an acutely inflamed distal ileum with no cecal involvement and a normal appendix, appendectomy is indicated. Progression to Crohn's ileitis is uncommon.

Perforated Peptic Ulcer. Perforated peptic ulcer closely simulates appendicitis if the spilled gastroduodenal contents gravitate down the right gutter to the cecal area and if the perforation spontaneously seals fairly soon, thus minimizing upper abdominal findings.

Other Lesions. Diverticulitis or perforating carcinoma of the cecum or of that portion of the sigmoid that lies on the right side may be impossible to distinguish from appendicitis. Extensive diagnostic studies in an attempt to make a preoperative differentiation are not warranted.

Epiploic Appendagitis. Epiploic appendagitis probably results from infarction of the appendage(s) secondary to torsion. Symptoms may be minimal, or there may be continuous abdominal pain in an area corresponding to the contour of the colon, lasting several days. Pain shift is unusual, and there is no diagnostic sequence of symptoms. The patient does not look ill, nausea and vomiting are unusual, and appetite is commonly unaffected. Localized tenderness over the site is usual and is often marked on rebound but without rigidity. In 25 percent of reported cases, pain has persisted or recurred until the infarcted epiploic appendages were removed.

Urinary Tract Infection. Acute pyelonephritis, on the right side particularly, may mimic a retroileal acute appendicitis. Chills, right costovertebral angle tenderness, pus cells, and particularly bacteria in the urine usually suffice to differentiate the two.

Ureteral Stone. If the calculus is lodged near the appendix, it may simulate a retrocecal appendicitis. Pain referred to the labia, scrotum, or penis; hematuria; and/or absence of fever or leukocytosis suggest stone. Pyelography usually confirms the diagnosis.

Primary Peritonitis. Primary peritonitis rarely mimics simple acute appendicitis but presents a picture very similar to diffuse peritonitis secondary to a ruptured appendix. The diagnosis is made by peritoneal aspiration. If nothing but cocci are seen on the Gram's-stained smear, peritonitis is primary and treated medically; if the flora are mixed, secondary peritonitis is indicated.

Henoch-Schönlein Purpura. This syndrome usually occurs 2 to 3 weeks after a streptococcal infection. Abdominal pain may be prominent, but joint pains, purpura, and nephritis are nearly always present also.

Yersiniosis. Human infection with Yersinia enterocolitica or *Y. pseudotuberculosis* is probably transmitted through food contaminated by feces or urine. Yersinia infections cause a variety of clinical syndromes, including mesenteric adenitis, ileitis, colitis, and acute appendicitis. Many of the infections are mild and self-limited, but some lead to a systemic septic course with a high fatality rate if untreated. The organisms are usually sensitive to tetracyclines, streptomycin, ampicillin, and kanamycin. A preoperative suspicion of the diagnosis should not delay operative intervention, since appendicitis caused by Yersinia cannot be clinically distinguished from appendicitis of other causation. About 6 percent of cases of mesenteric adenitis and 5 percent of cases of acute appendicitis are caused by Yersinia infection.

Campylobacter jejuni causes diarrhea and pain that mimics the pain of appendicitis. The organism can be cultured from stool.

Gynecologic Disorders. The rate of erroneous diagnosis of acute appendicitis is highest in young adult females. Rates of appendectomy being performed on a normal appendix of 32 to 45 percent have been reported in women 15 to 45 years old. Diseases of the female internal generative organs that may be erroneously diagnosed as appendicitis are, in approximate descending order of frequency, pelvic inflammatory disease, ruptured graafian follicle, twisted ovarian cyst or tumor, endomet-riosis, and ruptured ectopic pregnancy. Laparoscopy plays a significant role in establishing the diagnosis.

Pelvic Inflammatory Disease. The infection is usually bilateral but if confined to the right tube may mimic acute appendicitis. Nausea and vomiting are nearly always present in patients with appendicitis, but only in approximately half of those with pelvic inflammatory disease. The greatest value of these symptoms for establishing a diagnosis of pelvic inflammatory disease is their absence. Pain and tenderness are usually lower, and motion of the cervix is exquisitely painful. Intracellular diplococci may be demonstrable on smear of the purulent vaginal discharge. The ratio of appendicitis to pelvic inflammatory disease is low in the early phase of the menstrual cycle and high during the luteal phase. The clinical use of all the above-mentioned distinctions has resulted in a reduction of the incidence of negative findings on laparotomy in young women to 15 percent.

Ruptured Graafian Follicle. Not uncommonly, ovulation results in the spill of sufficient blood and follicular fluid to produce brief, mild lower abdominal pain. If the fluid is unusually copious and from the right ovary, appendicitis may be simulated. Pain and tenderness are rather diffuse. Leukocytosis and fever are minimal or absent. Since this pain occurs at the midpoint of the menstrual cycle, it is often called mittelschmerz.

Other Diseases. Diseases not mentioned in the previous sections that occur in patients of all ages and both sexes and that must be considered in the differential diagnosis of appendicitis are foreign body perforations of the bowel; closed-loop intestinal obstruction; mesenteric vascular occlusion; pleuritis of the right lower chest; acute cholecystitis; acute pancreatitis; hematoma of the abdominal wall; and numerous conditions too rare to mention.

Appendicitis in the Young. The establishment of a diagnosis of acute appendicitis in the young is even more difficult than in the adult. The inability of young children to give an accurate history, diagnostic delays by both parents and physicians, and the frequency of gastrointestinal upset in children are all contributing factors. The more rapid progression to rupture and the inability of the underdeveloped greater omentum to contain a rupture lead to significant morbidity rates in children. In a study of 1366 specimens from pediatric patients undergoing appendectomies, histologic analysis revealed 12 percent normal appendices, 68 percent nonperforated appendices, and 20 percent perforated appendices. Children under 8 years old had a twofold increase in the rate of perforation as compared to older children. The incidence of major complications was related to rupture, with an incidence of 1.2 percent in simple appendicitis compared to 6.4 percent in perforated appendicitis. The treatment regimen for perforated appendicitis generally includes immediate appendectomy, antibiotic irrigation of the peritoneal cavity, transperitoneal drainage through the wound, and a 10-day antibiotic treatment regimen. Laparoscopic appendectomy has also been shown to be safe and effective in children.

Appendicitis in the Elderly. Although the incidence of appendicitis in the elderly is lower than in younger patients, the morbidity and mortality are significantly increased in this patient population. Delays in diagnosis, a more rapid progression to perforation, and concomitant disease are all contributing factors. The diagnosis of appendicitis may be more subtle and less typical than in younger individuals, and a high index of suspicion needs to be maintained. In patients over 80 years old, perforation rates of 49 percent and mortality rates of 21 percent have been cited.

Appendicitis During Pregnancy. Appendicitis is the most frequently encountered extrauterine disease requiring surgical treatment during pregnancy. The incidence is approximately 1 in 2000 pregnancies. Acute appendicitis can occur at any time during pregnancy but is more frequent during the first two trimesters. As fetal gestation progresses, the diagnosis of appendicitis becomes more difficult as the appendix is displaced laterally and superiorly (Fig. 27-2). Nausea and vomiting after the first trimester or new-onset nausea and vomiting should raise the consideration of appendicitis. Abdominal pain and tenderness will be present, although rebound and guarding are less frequent due to laxity of the abdominal wall. Elevation of the white blood cell count above the normal pregnancy levels of 15,000 to 20,000/mm^3 with a predominance of polymorphonuclear cells is usually present. When the diagnosis is in doubt, abdominal ultrasound may be beneficial. Laparoscopy may be indicated in equivocal cases, especially early in pregnancy. The performance of any operation during pregnancy carries a risk of premature labor of 10 to 15 percent, and the risk is similar for both negative laparotomy and appendectomy for simple appendicitis. The most significant factor associated with both fetal and maternal death is appendiceal perforation. Fetal mortality increases from 3 to 5

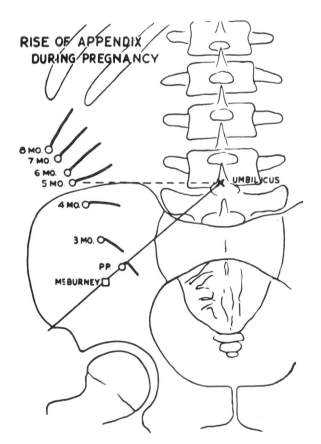

FIG. 27-2. Changes in position and direction of appendix during pregnancy. PP = postpartum. (From: Baer JL, Reis RA, Arens RA: Appendicitis in pregnancy. JAMA 98: 1359, ©1932, American Medical Association, with permission.)

percent with early appendicitis to 20 percent with perforation. The suspicion of appendicitis during pregnancy should prompt rapid diagnosis and surgical intervention.

Appendicitis in Patients with AIDS or HIV Infection. The cause of appendicitis in HIV-positive patients and patients with AIDS is similar to the cause of appendicitis in the general population. In some cases, however, an underlying opportunistic infection, usually secondary to cytomegalovirus or Kaposi's sarcoma, may be responsible for the development of appendiceal inflammation. Although the clinical presentation of appendicitis in patients who have AIDS or are HIV-positive does not differ significantly from patients without AIDS or HIV infection, the leukocytosis usually noted in acute appendicitis may not be present. Cytomegalovirus enteritis and tuberculosis or lymphoma involving the distal ileum can mimic appendicitis. Diagnostic laparoscopy can be helpful, with laparoscopic appendectomy being indicated when an inflamed appendix is found. If appendectomy is performed prior to perforation, there is no increase in morbidity or mortality.

Treatment. Despite the advent of more sophisticated diagnostic modalities, the importance of early operative intervention should not be minimized. Once the decision to operate for presumed acute appendicitis has been made, the patient should be prepared for the operating room. Adequate hydration should be insured, electrolyte abnormalities corrected, and preexisting cardiac, pulmonary, and renal conditions should be addressed. Many trials have demonstrated the efficacy of preoperative antibiotics in lowering the infectious complications in appendicitis. It is common practice by most surgeons to routinely administer antibiotics to all patients with suspected appendicitis. If simple acute appendicitis is encountered, there is no benefit in extending antibiotic coverage beyond 24 h. If perforated or gangrenous appendicitis is found, antibiotics are continued until the patient is afebrile and has a normal white blood cell count. For intra-abdominal infections of gastrointestinal tract origin of mild to moderate severity, the Surgical Infection Society has recommended single-agent therapy with cefoxitin, cefotetan, or ticarcillin-clavulanic acid. For more severe infections, single-agent therapy with carbapenems or combination therapy with a third-generation cephalosporin, monobactam, or aminoglycoside, plus anaerobic coverage with clindamycin and metronidazole, is indicated.

Open Appendectomy (Fig. 27-3). Most surgeons employ either a McBurney (oblique) or Rocky-Davis (transverse) right lower quadrant muscle-splitting incision in patients with suspected appendicitis. The incision should be centered over the point of maximal tenderness or a palpable mass. If an abscess is suspected, a laterally placed incision is imperative to avoid generalized contamination of the peritoneal cavity. If the diagnosis is in doubt, a lower midline incision is recommended by some to allow a more extensive examination of the peritoneal cavity.

Several techniques can be used to locate the appendix. Since the cecum is usually visible within the incision, the convergence of the taeniae can be followed to the base of the appendix. A sweeping laterial to medial motion can aid in delivering the appendiceal tip into the operative field. Occasionally limited mobilization of the cecum is needed to aid in adequate visualization. Once identified, the appendix is mobilized by dividing the mesoappendix, taking care to ligate the appendiceal artery securely.

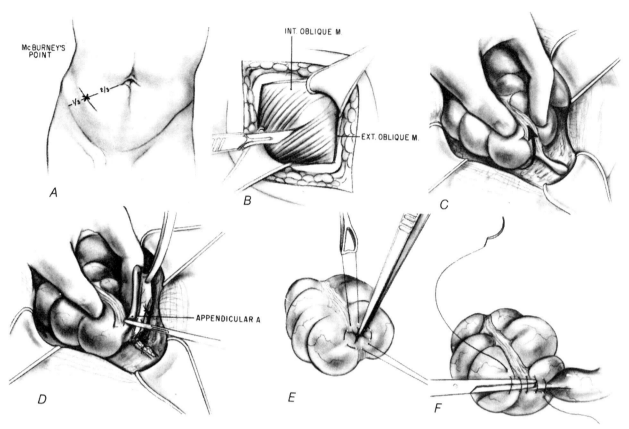

FIG. 27-3. Appendectomy. *A.* McBurney incision passing through McBurney's point, which is located one-third of the distance from the anterior superior iliac spine to the umbilicus. *B.* The incision has been carried through skin and subcutaneous tissue and has divided the aponeurosis of the external oblique muscle in the course of its fibers. The internal oblique muscle is being separated in the direction of its fibers. *C.* The peritoneum has been incised and the peritoneal cavity entered. The appendix is delivered into the wound by rotation of the cecum up and out. *D.* The vessels within the mesoappendix have been doubly ligated and transected with particular attention directed toward the appendicular artery. A crushing clamp is applied to the base of the appendix and then moved distad (to dotted line), so that a ligature may be placed in the resulting groove. *E.* The stump of the appendix may or may not be tied with a ligature. It is customary to invert the stump and place a purse-string suture through the seromuscular layers of the cecum. *F.* An alternative method of inverting the appendiceal stump is demonstrated with a continuous seromuscular suture. A Z suture can also be used to achieve this end.

The appendiceal stump can be managed by simple ligation or by ligation and inversion with either a purse-string or Z stitch as tradition dictates. As long as the stump is clearly viable and the base of the cecum not involved with the inflammatory process, the stump can be safely ligated with a nonabsorbable suture. The mucosa is frequently obliterated to avoid the development of a mucocele. The peritoneal cavity is irrigated and the wound closed in layers. If perforation or gangrene is found, the skin and subcutaneous tissue should be left open and allowed to heal by secondary intent or be closed in 4 to 5 days as a delayed primary closure. In children, who generally have little subcutaneous fat, primary wound closure has not led to an increased incidence of wound infection.

If appendicitis is not found, a methodical search for an alternative diagnosis must be performed. The cecum and mesentery should first be inspected. Next, the small bowel is examined in a retrograde fashion beginning at the ileocecal valve. In females, special attention should be paid to the pelvic organs. An attempt is also made to examine the upper abdominal contents. Perito-

neal fluid should be sent for Gram's stain and culture. If purulent fluid is encountered, it is imperative that the source be identified. A medial extension of the incision (Fowler-Weir), with division of the anterior and posterior rectus sheath, is acceptable if further evaluation of the lower abdomen is indicated. If upper abdominal pathology is encountered, the right lower quadrant incision is closed and an appropriate upper midline incision performed.

Laparoscopy. Laparoscopy has emerged as a new technique for both the diagnosis and treatment of acute appendicitis. Laparoscopy can be of enormous assistance in the evaluation of young women of childbearing age in whom acute appendicitis is suspected. Laparoscopic appendectomy may be preferable in obese patients who would require a large incision for the open approach or in individuals who are particularly concerned about cosmesis. There are a number of theoretical advantages for the laparoscopic approach over the traditional open operation described over 100 years ago. These include decreased incidence of wound infection, less pain for the patient, reduced hospitalization, and a more rapid return to employment. The data have not demonstrated any significant economic benefit to laparoscopic appendectomy for the general population. Both operative time and supply costs are increased while duration of hospital stay is not significantly shortened. Nonetheless, laparoscopic appendectomy has been demonstrated to be a safe and effective treatment. Recently reported prospective randomized trials comparing open and laparoscopic techniques (Table 27-1) indicate that operative time is generally greater using the laparoscopic approach, but the time between the operation and return to activity, and the rate of wound infection, are decreased.

The superiority of laparoscopic appendectomy over the conventional approach continues to be an issue of some debate. Laparoscopy's most important role is in diagnostic evaluation of young females whose symptoms are not the classical symptoms of appendicitis and in patients in whom the diagnosis remains in question. It does provide visualization the entire abdominal cavity, unlike the limited exposure provided by a right lower quadrant incision. For properly trained personnel, laparoscopic appendectomy may be appropriate for most cases of appendicitis, with a conversion rate of approximately 10 percent, mostly in patients with ruptured appendices.

The principles behind laparoscopic appendectomies are similar to those for other laparoscopic procedures (Fig. 27-4). All patients should have an indwelling urinary catheter and nasogastric tube inserted prior to trochar insertion. The surgeon frequently stands to the patient's left with the video monitor at the foot of the table, or to the patient's right. Pneumoperitoneum is established and a 10-mm trochar cannula is inserted through the umbilicus. A 10-mm forward-viewing laparoscope is placed through the cannula and the peritoneal cavity is inspected. Next, a 10-mm trochar is introduced into the suprapubic region in the midline and additional 5-mm ports placed in either the right upper or lower quadrant. Exposure is facilitated by placing the patient in the Trendelenburg position, right side up. Generally the cecum is easily visualized and the appendix easily identified. Gentle traction can be applied to the mesoappendix by retracting the tip of the appendix with an atraumatic grasper placed through the right upper quadrant trochar. The mesoappendix is divided with a stapling device or by using electrocautery for dissection and clips or a ligating loop to secure the appendiceal artery. Division of the mesoappendix should be done as close to the appendix as possible. After the base of the appendix is adequately exposed, two ligating loops are placed proximally and one distally over the base. The appendix is divided with scissors

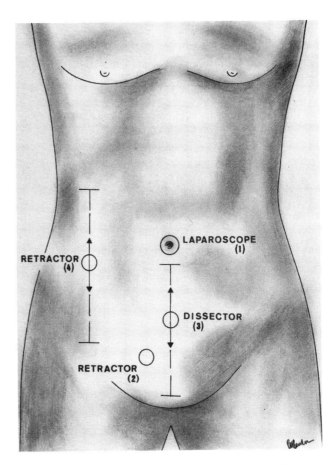

FIG. 27-4. Location of laparoscopic ports for laparoscopic appendectomy. *(From: Modified from Geis WP, Miller CE, et al, 1992, with permission)*.

or electrocauterization. Alternatively, the appendix could be divided using a stapling device. Invagination of the appendiceal stump is not routinely performed. The appendix is removed via the suprapubic trocar site.

The role of laparoscopic appendectomy for removal of the normal appendix has not been well defined. As for an open procedure, an appendectomy should be considered in patients explored for right lower quadrant pain with no identifiable pathol-

Table 27-1
Prospective Randomized Trials Comparing Open Versus Laparoscopic Appendectomy

Author	#Patients O/L	Operation Time (minutes) O/L	Length of Stay (days) O/L	Return to Activity (days) O/L	Wound Infection (%) O/L
Frazee	37/38	65/87*	2.8/2	25/14*	8/5
Hanson	72/79	40/63*	3/3	14/7*	11/2*
Kum	57/52	40/43	4/3	30/17*	9/0*
Mompean	100/100	46/51	6/4.8*	—	7/1*
Tate	70/70	47/70*	3.6/3.5	—	14/10
Attwood	32/30	51/61	3.8/2.5*	16/10*	3/0

*p < 0.05.

O = open; L = laparoscopic.

ogy. Complication rates of 1 to 3 percent have been reported under these circumstances. If the appendix is normal, the same thorough search for an alternative diagnosis should be performed as with an open procedure.

Prognosis. *Mortality.* The mortality from appendicitis in the United States has steadily decreased from a rate of 9.9 per 100,000 in 1939 to 0.2 per 100,000 in 1986. Among the factors responsible are the significantly decreasing incidence of appendicitis; better diagnosis and treatment, attributable to the now-available antibiotics, intravenous fluids, blood, and plasma; and a higher percentage of patients receiving definitive treatment before rupture.

Principal factors in mortality are (1) whether rupture occurs before surgical treatment and (2) the age of the patient. The overall mortality rate in unruptured acute appendicitis is a little higher than the rate for a general anesthetic, which is 0.06 percent. The overall mortality rate in ruptured acute appendicitis is about 3 percent—a 30-fold increase. The mortality rate of ruptured appendicitis in the elderly is about 15 percent—a fivefold increase from the overall rate.

Death is usually attributable to uncontrolled sepsis—peritonitis, intraabdominal abscesses, or gram-negative septicemia. Sepsis may impose metabolic demands of such magnitude on the cardiovascular or respiratory systems that they cannot be met, in which case cardiac or respiratory insufficiency is the direct cause of death. Pulmonary embolism continues to account for some deaths. Aspiration causing the patient to drown in his or her own vomitus is a significant cause of death in the older age group.

Morbidity. Morbidity rates parallel mortality rates, being precipitously increased by rupture of the appendix and to a lesser extent by old age. In one report, complications occurred in 3 percent of patients with nonperforated appendicitis and in 47 percent of patients with perforations. Most of the serious early complications are septic and include abscess and wound infection. Wound infection is common but is nearly always confined to the subcutaneous tissues and promptly responds to wound drainage, which is accomplished by reopening the skin incision. Wound infection predisposes to wound dehiscence also. The type of incision is relevant; complete dehiscence rarely occurs in a McBurney incision. The efficacy of systemic antibiotics in reducing the incidence of wound infections has not been agreed on. But a significant reduction in morbidity has been shown in patients receiving metronidazole or the combination of systemic clindamycin and topical ampicillin.

The incidence of intraabdominal abscesses secondary to peritoneal contamination from gangrenous or perforated appendicitis has decreased markedly since the introduction of potent antibiotics. The sites of predilection for abscesses are the appendiceal fossa, pouch of Douglas, subhepatic space, and between loops of intestine. The latter are usually multiple. Transrectal drainage is preferred for an abscess that bulges into the rectum.

Fecal fistula is an annoying but not particularly dangerous complication of appendectomy that may be caused by sloughing of that portion of the cecum inside a constricting purse-string suture, by the ligature's slipping off a tied but not inverted appendiceal stump, or by necrosis from an abscess encroaching on the cecum.

Intestinal obstruction, initially paralytic but sometimes progressing to mechanical obstruction, may occur with slowly resolving peritonitis with loculated abscesses and exuberant adhesion formation.

Late complications are quite uncommon. Adhesive band intestinal obstruction after appendectomy does occur but much less frequently than after pelvic surgical therapy. The incidence of inguinal hernia is three times greater in patients who have had an appendectomy. Incisional hernia is like wound dehiscence in that infection predisposes to it, it rarely occurs in a McBurney incision, and it is not uncommon in a lower right paramedian incision.

TUMORS

Appendiceal malignancies are rare, occurring in 0.5 percent of all appendectomies. The tumors are usually discovered at the time of laparotomy either as an incidental finding or in association with acute inflammation of the appendix. In a recent review of over 2000 appendectomy specimens, histologic confirmation of appendiceal neoplasms included carcinoid (0.27 percent), adenocarcinoma (0.14 percent), malignant mucocele (0.005 percent), and lymphoma (0.005 percent).

Carcinoid

The finding of a firm, yellow, bulbar mass in the appendix should raise the suspicion of an appendiceal carcinoid. The appendix is the most common site of gastrointestinal carcinoid followed by the small bowel and rectum. Carcinoid syndrome is rarely associated with appendiceal carcinoid unless widespread metastases are present, which occurs in 2.9 percent of cases. Symptoms attributable directly to the carcinoid are rare, though the tumor can occasionally obstruct the appendiceal lumen much like a fecalith and result in acute appendicitis.

The majority of carcinoids are located in the tip of the appendix. Malignant potential is related to size, with tumors less than 2 cm rarely resulting in extension outside of the appendix. In one report, 78 percent of appendiceal carcinoids were less than 1 cm, 17 percent were 1 to 2 cm, and only 5 percent were greater than 2 cm. Treatment rarely requires more than simple appendectomy. For tumors less than 2 cm with extension into the mesoappendix, and for all tumors greater than 2 cm, a right hemicolectomy should be performed.

Adenocarcinoma

Primary adenocarcinoma of the appendix is a rare neoplasm of three major histologic subtypes: mucinous adenocarcinoma, colonic adenocarcinoma, and adenocarcinoid. The most common mode of presentation for appendiceal carcinoma is that of acute appendicitis. Patients may also present with ascites or a palpable mass, or the neoplasm may be discovered during an operative procedure for an unrelated cause. The recommended treatment for all patients with adenocarcinoma of the appendix is a formal right hemicolectomy. Appendiceal adenocarcinomas have a propensity for early perforation, though not clearly associated with a worsened prognosis. The presence of pseudomyxoma peritonei secondary to mucinous adenocarcinoma does not adversely affect prognosis. Overall 5-year survival is 55 percent and varies with stage and grade. Patients with appendiceal adenocarcinoma are at significant risk for both synchronous and metachronous neoplasms, approximately half of which will originate from the gastrointestinal tract.

Mucocele

An appendiceal mucocele leads to progressive enlargement of the appendix from the intraluminal accumulation of a mucoid substance. Mucoceles are of four histologic types, and the type dictates the course of the disease and prognosis: retention cysts, mucosal hyperplasia, cystadenomas, and cystadenocarcinomas. A mucocele of benign etiology is adequately treated by a simple appendectomy.

In a small percentage of patients, the mucocele occurs along with gelatinous ascites known as pseudomyxoma peritonei. Pseudomyxoma peritonei can be associated with either ovarian or appendiceal mucinous tumors, usually of a malignant nature. When pseudomyxoma peritonei is present, survival is significantly decreased probably due to the association with the ascites and malignancy. The initial surgical procedure should include cytoreductive surgery along with a right hemicolectomy for cystadenocarcinoma of the appendix and bilateral oophorectomy, hysterectomy, and appendectomy for ovarian cystadenocarcinoma. A recent review found that even with aggressive surgical treatment, there is a 57 percent incidence of local recurrence of pseudomyxoma peritonei from an appendiceal primary site. Once a recurrence is detected, death usually ensues from progressive bowel obstruction and renal failure. Adjuvant therapy including radiation and intraperitoneal and systemic chemotherapy has been recommended, but its efficacy and role are unclear.

Bibliography

Anatomy and Function

Buschard K, Kjaeldgaard A: Investigation and analysis of the position, fixation, length and embryology of the vermiform appendix. *Acta Chir Scand* 139:293, 1973.

Fitz R: Persistent omphalo-mesenteric remains: Their importance in the causation of intestinal duplication, cyst formation and obstruction. *Am J Med Sci* 88:30, 1884.

Skandalakis JE, Gray SW, Ricketts R: The colon and rectum, in Skandalakis JE, Gray SW (eds): *Embryology for Surgeons.* Baltimore, Williams & Wilkins, 1994, p 242.

Wakeley CPG: The position of the vermiform appendix as ascertained by an analysis of 10,000 cases. *J Anat Physiol* 67:277, 1993.

Inflammation

Amyand C: Of an inguinal rupture with a pin in the appendix caeci encrusted with stone: Some observations on wounds in the guts. *Philosoph Trans R Soc Lond* 39:329, 1736.

Arnbjornsson E: Invagination of the appendiceal stump for the reduction of peritoneal bacterial contamination. *Curr Surg* 42:184, 1985.

Attwood SEA, Hill ADK, et al: A prospective randomized trial of laparoscopic versus open appendectomy. *Surgery* 112:497, 1992.

Bailey LE, Finley RK Jr, et al: Acute appendicitis during pregnancy. *Am Surg* 52:218, 1986.

Balthazar EJ, Birnbaum BA, Yee J, et al: Acute appendicitis: CT and US correlation in 100 patients. *J Radiol* 190:31, 1994.

Baron EJ, Bennion R, Thompson J, et al: A microbiological comparison between acute and complicated appendicitis. *Clin Infect Dis* 14:227, 1992.

Bauer T, Vennits B, et al: Antibiotic prophylaxis in acute nonperforated appendicitis. The Danish multicenter study group III. *Ann Surg* 209:307, 1989.

Bennion RS, Baron EJ, et al: The bacteriology of gangrenous and perforated appendicitis revisited. *Ann Surg* 211:165, 1990.

Bennis RS, Thompson JE Jr, et al: The role of Yersinia enterocolitica in appendicitis in the southwestern United States. *Am Surg* 57:766, 1991.

Binderow SR, Shaked AA: Acute appendicitis in patients with AIDS/HIV infection. *Am J Surg* 162:9, 1991.

Blair NP, Bugis SP, Turner LJ, et al: Review of the pathologic diagnoses of 2,216 appendectomy specimens. *Am J Surg* 165:618, 1993.

Bohnen JM, Solomkin JS, Dellinger EP, et al: Guidelines for clinical care: Anti-infective agents for intra-abdominal infection. A Surgical Infection Society policy statement. *Arch Surg* 127:83, discussion 89, 1992.

Busuttil RW, Davidson RK, et al: Effect of prophylactic antibiotics in acute nonperforated appendicitis: A prospective, randomized, double-blind clinical study. *Ann Surg* 194:502, 1981.

Crady SK, Jones JS, Wyn T, et al: Clinical validity of ultrasound in children with suspected appendicitis. *Ann Emerg Med* 22:1125, 1993.

Droegemueller W: Upper genital tract infections, In Herbst AL, Mishell DR, Stenchever MW, Droegemueller W (eds): *Comprehensive Gynecology,* 2d ed. St. Louis, Mosby Year Book, 1992, p 691.

Fallon WF, Newman JS, Fallon GL, et al: The surgical management of intra-abdominal inflammatory conditions during pregnancy. *Surg Clin North Am* 75:1, 1995.

Fitz RH: Perforating inflammation of the vermiform appendix: With special reference to its early diagnosis and treatment. *Trans Assoc Am Physicians* 1:107, 1886.

Frazee RC, Roberts JW, Symmonds RE, et al: A prospective randomized trial comparing open versus laparoscopic appendectomy. *Ann Surg* 219:725, 1994.

Gamal R, Moore TC: Appendicitis in children aged 13 years and younger. *Am J Surg* 159:589, 1990.

Geis WP, Miller CE, et al: Laparoscopic appendectomy for acute appendicitis: rationale and technical aspects. *Contemp Surg* 40:13, 1992.

Ghonei EA, Valla JS, Limonne B, et al: Laparoscopic appendectomy in children: Report of 1379 cases. *J Pediatr Surg* 29:786, 1994.

Guidry SP, Poole GV: The anatomy of appendicitis. *Am Surg* 60:68, 1994.

Harrison LE, French TS, Caushaj PF: Appendectomy, in Ballantyne GH, Leahy PF, Modlin M (eds): *Laparoscopic Surgery.* Philadelphia, W. B. Saunders, 1994, p 215.

Horattas MC, Guyton DP, Wu D: A reappraisal of appendicitis in the elderly. *Am J Surg* 160:291, 1990.

Jeffrey RB, Jain KA, Nghiem HV: Sonographic diagnosis of acute appendicitis: Interpretive pitfalls. *Am J Roentgenol* 162:55, 1994.

Kum CIK, Ngoi SS, Goh PMY, et al: Randomized controlled trial comparing laparoscopic and open appendicectomy. *Br J Surg* 80:1599, 1993.

Lin J, Bleiweiss IJ, et al: Cytomegalovirus-associated appendicitis in a patient with the acquired immunodeficiency syndrome. *Am J Med* 89:377, 1990.

McBurney C: Experience with early operative interference in cases of disease of the vermiform appendix. *NY State Med J* 50:676, 1889.

McBurney C: The incision made in the abdominal wall in cases of appendicitis. *Ann Surg* 20:38, 1894.

Miranda R, Johnston AD, O'Leary JP: Incidental appendectomy: Frequency of pathologic abnormalities. *Am Surg* 46:355, 1980.

Lo Cy, Chu KW: Acute diverticulitis of the right colon. *Am J Surg* 171:244, 1996.

Lund DP, Murphy EU: Management of perforated appendicitis in children: A decade of aggressive treatment. *J Pediatr Surg* 29:1130, 1994.

McCahy P: Continuing fall in the incidence of acute appendicitis. *Ann R Coll Surg Engl* 76:282, 1994.

McCahill LE, Pellegrini CA, Wiggins T, et al: A clinical outcome and cost analysis of laparoscopic versus open appendectomy. *Am J Surg* 171:533, 1996.

Mompean LA, Campos RR, Paricio PP, et al: Laparoscopic versus open appendicectomy: A prospective assessment. *Br J Surg* 81:133, 1994.

Mueller GP, Williams RA: Surgical infections in AIDS patients. *Am J Surg* 169:5A, 1995.

Nitecki S, Assalia A, Schein M: Contemporary management of appendiceal mass. *Br J Surg* 80:18, 1993.

Ooms HW, Koumans RK, et al: Ultrasonography in the diagnosis of acute appendicitis. *Br J Surg* 78:315, 1991.

Paajanen H, Kettunen J, Kostiainen S: Emergency appendectomies in patients over 80 years. *Am Surg* 60:12, 1994.

Pearl RH, Hale DA, Molloy M, et al: Pediatric appendectomy. *J Pediatr Surg* 30:173, 1995.

Rioux M: Sonographic detection of the normal and abnormal appendix. *Am J Roentgenol* 158:773, 1992.

Rothrock SG, Green SM, Dobson M, et al: Misdiagnosis of appendicitis in nonpregnant women of childbearing age. *J Emerg Med* 13:1, 1995.

Rutkow IM: The nineteenth century. in Rutkow IM (ed.): *Surgery: An Illustrated History.* St. Louis, Mosby Year Book, 1993, p 489.

Tamir IL, Bongard FS, Klein SR: Acute appendicitis in the pregnant patient. *Am J Surg* 160:571, 1990.

Tate JJT, Dawson JW, et al: Laparoscopic versus open appendicectomy: Prospective randomized trial. *Lancet* 342:633, 1993.

Temple CL, Huchcroft SA, Temple WJ: The natural history of appendicitis in adults. *Ann Surg* 221:278, 1995.

White J, Santillana M, Haller JA Jr: Intensive inhospital observation: A safe way to decrease unnecessary appendectomy. *Am Surg* 41:793, 1975.

Yacoe ME, Jeffrey RB: Sonography of appendicitis and diverticulitis. *Radiol Clin North Am* 32:5, 1994.

Tumors

Aranha GV, Reyes CV: Primary epithelial tumors of the appendix and a reappraisal of the appendiceal "mucocele." *Dis Colon Rectum* 22:472, 1979.

Bak M, Asschenfeldt P: Adenocarcinoid of the vermiform appendix: A clinicopathologic study of 20 cases. *Dis Colon Rectum* 31:605, 1988.

Deans, GT, Spence RAJ: Neoplastic lesions of the appendix. *Br J Surg* 82:299, 1995.

Landen S, Bertrand C, et al: Appendiceal mucoceles and pseudomyxoma peritonei. *Surg Gynecol Obstet* 175:401, 1992.

Lyss AP: Appendiceal malignancies. *Semin Oncol* 15:129, 1988.

Nitecki S, Wolff B, et al: The natural history of surgically treated primary adenocarcinoma of the appendix. *Ann Surg* 219:51, 1994.

Roggo A, Wood W, Ottinger L: Carcinoid tumors of the appendix. *Ann Surg* 217:385, 1993.

Syracuse DC, Perzin KH, et al: Carcinoid tumors of the appendix: Mesoappendiceal extension and nodal metastases. *Ann Surg* 190:58, 1979.

Wertheim I, Fleischhacker D, McLachlin C, et al: Pseudomyxoma peritonei: A review of 23 cases. *Gynecology* 84:1, 1994.

Young RH, Gilks CB, Scully RE: Mucinous tumors of the appendix associated with mucinous tumors of the ovary and pseudomyxoma peritonei. A clinicopathological analysis of the 22 cases supporting an origin in the appendix. *Am J Surg Pathol* 15:415, 1991.

CHAPTER 28

Liver

Seymour I. Schwartz

ANATOMY

The liver constitutes approximately one-fiftieth of total body weight. Its size reflects the complexity of its functions. True

division into right and left lobes (hemilivers) is in line with the fossa for the inferior vena cava posteriorly and the gallbladder fossa anteroinferiorly (Cantlie's line) (Fig. 28-1). Based on the distribution of the intrahepatic branches of the hepatic artery, portal vein, and bile ducts, the right lobe is divided into an anterior section and a posterior section, and the left lobe is divided into a medial section and a lateral section. Couinad proposed a functional division of the liver related to the hepatic venous drainage (Fig. 28-2). The liver is divided into two "livers" (lobes) by the portal scissura in which the middle hepatic vein courses. The right lobe is divided into two "sectors" by the right hepatic vein. The right posterolateral "sector" contains segment VI anteriorly and segment VII posteriorly. The right anterolateral "sector" contains segment V anteriorly and segment VIII posteriorly. The left lobe is divided by a line containing the left

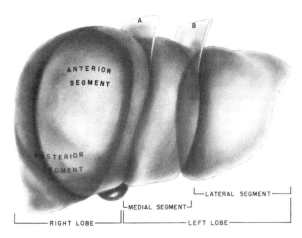

FIG. 28-1. Lobar and segmental divisions of the liver. *A.* Lobar fissure. *B.* Left segmental fissure. A right segmental fissure divides the right lobe into its anterior and posterior segments. (From: *Schwartz, 1964, with permission.*)

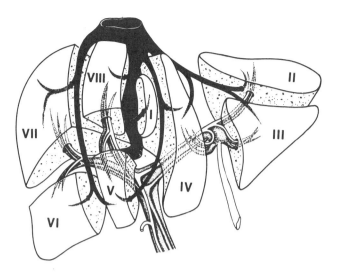

FIG. 28-2. *The functional division of the liver and the segments according to Couinaud's nomenclature. (From: Bismuth, 1982, with permission.)*

hepatic vein. The left anterior sector is divided by the umbilical fissure into segment IV, the anterior part of which is the quadrate lobe, segment III, which is the anterior part of the left lobe. The posterior portion is segment II. The dorsal segment I, in regard to its vascularization, is independent of the portal division and the three main hepatic veins (Fig. 28-3).

Biliary Drainage. Each sector is drained by a major segmental duct formed by the confluence of subsegmental draining structures. The anterior and posterior sectoral ducts in the right lobe join to form the right hepatic duct, while the medial and lateral segmental ducts in the left lobe terminate in the left hepatic duct, which joins the right duct to form a common hepatic duct in the porta hepatis. This lies anteriorly in relation to other structures in the area.

Blood Supply. The afferent blood supply to the liver arises from two sources: (1) the hepatic artery, which carries oxygenated blood and accounts for approximately 25 percent of hepatic blood flow, and (2) the portal vein, which accounts for approximately 75 percent of hepatic blood flow and drains the splanchnic circulation. The common hepatic artery originates from the celiac axis and, after contributing the gastroduodenal and right gastric artery, ascends in the hepatoduodenal ligament to the left of the common bile duct and anterior in the portal vein. It bifurcates into a right and left branch to the left of the line dividing the right and left lobes. The major right hepatic artery originates from the superior mesenteric artery in 17 percent of people. This vessel usually courses to the liver in the hepatoduodenal ligament to the right of the common duct and anterior to the portal vein. Intrahepatic anastomoses between the right and left hepatic arteries do not occur. The cystic artery is usually an extrahepatic branch of the right hepatic artery.

The portal venous system contains no valves (Fig. 28-4). It returns to the liver the blood that the celiac, superior mesenteric, and inferior mesenteric arteries supply to the gastrointestinal tract, pancreas, and spleen. The vessel is formed behind the pan-

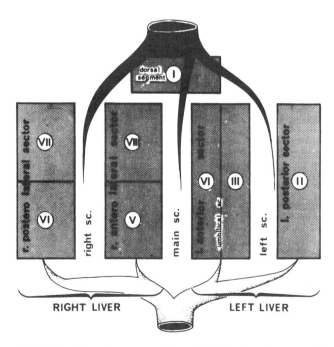

FIG. 28-3. *Schematic representation of the functional anatomy of the liver; three main hepatic veins divide the liver into four sectors, each of them receiving a portal pedicle; hepatic veins and portal pedicles are intertwined as the fingers of the two hands. (From: Bismuth, 1982, with permission.)*

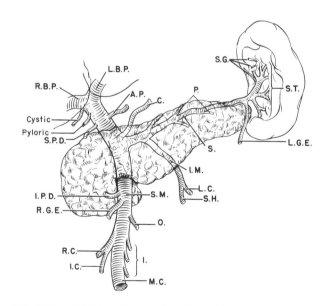

FIG. 28-4. *Anatomy of the extrahepatic portal venous system, anterior aspect. The termination of each vein is shown as it was encountered most frequently in 92 dissections. The pancreas is represented by the shaded area. A.P., accessory pancreatic vein; C., coronary vein; Cystic, cystic vein; I., intestinal veins; I.C., ileocolic vein; I.M., inferior mesenteric vein; I.P.D., inferior pancreaticoduodenal vein; L., liver; L.B.P., left branch of portal vein; L.C., left colic vein; L.G.E., left gastroepiploic vein; M.C., middle colic vein; O., omental vein; P., pancreatic veins; Pyloric, pyloric vein; R.C., right colic vein; R.G.E., right gastroepiploic vein; R.B.P., right branch of portal vein; S., splenic vein; S.G., short gastric veins; S.H., superior hemorrhoidal vein; S.M., superior mesenteric vein; S.P.D., superior pancreaticoduodenal vein; S.T., splenic trunks. (From: Douglass BE, et al: The anatomy of the portal vein and its tributaries. Surg Gynecol Obstet 91:562, 1950, with permission.)*

creas, at the level of L_1 to L_2, by the confluence of the superior mesenteric and splenic veins and, at times, the inferior mesenteric vein. The portal vein resides posteriorly in relation to the hepatic artery and bile duct in the hepatoduodenal ligament but, in rare instances, is located anterior to the pancreas and first portion of the duodenum, in which circumstance it is frequently associated with a partial or complete situs inversus and is subject to injury during cholecystectomy or gastrectomy. In the porta hepatis, the vein divides into two branches, which course to each lobe. The average length of the main portal vein is 6.5 cm, and the average diameter is 0.8 cm.

The hepatic venous system (Fig. 28-5) begins in the liver lobules as a central vein into which the sinusoids empty. The central veins unite to form sublobular veins, which in turn fuse to form collecting veins. The collecting veins gradually increase in size by joining other large intrahepatic collecting channels, which coalesce to form the three major hepatic veins. The hepatic venous tributaries are intersectoral in position. The major hepatic veins are classified as right, left, and middle. The right hepatic vein drains the entire posterior portion as well as the superior area of the anterior portion of the right lobe. The left hepatic vein drains the entire area to the left of the umbilical fissure. The inferior areas of the medial and anterior portions of the two lobes are drained by the middle vein. In human beings there are no valves in the hepatic venous system. Total hepatic blood flow can be measured by means of hepatic vein catheterization and use of the Fick principle. The average value is 1500 mL/min/1.73 m^2 of body surface.

LIVER FUNCTION

The liver consists of four physiologic-anatomic units that are interrelated:

1. The circulatory system. A dual blood supply nourishes the liver and acts as a vehicle for material absorbed from the intestinal tract to be utilized in the metabolic pool. Blood vessels are accompanied by lymphatics and nerve fibers that contribute to the regulation of blood flow and intrasinusoidal pressure.
2. Biliary passages. These serve as channels of exit for materials secreted by liver cells, including bilirubin, cholesterol, and detoxified drugs.

This system originates with the Golgi apparatus adjacent to the microvilli of the bile canaliculi and eventually terminates in the common bile duct.

3. The reticuloendothelial system. This system has 60 percent of its cellular elements in the liver and includes the phagocytic Kupffer cells and endothelial cells.
4. The functioning liver cells (hepatocytes), which are capable of wide variation of activity. The metabolic pool in the liver serves the needs of the entire body. The cell performs both anabolic and catabolic activities, secretes, and stores. The large amount of energies required for these transformations result from the conversion of adenosine triphosphate (ATP) to adenosine diphosphate (ADP). A second source is the aerobic oxygenation in the metabolic pool via the tricarboxylic acid cycle of Krebs.

Function Tests

The so-called liver function tests (Table 28-1) evaluate liver activity by assessing the degree of functional impairment. They do not provide a pathologic diagnosis, and the extreme functional reserve of the organ occasionally produces normal results in the face of significant lesions. Many of these tests do not measure a specific function of the liver, and other organ systems may be implicated. False-positive results for each of the tests are found in about 10 percent of hospital controls. False-negative tests also occur in about 10 percent of most tests.

Proteins. Hepatic cells are responsible for the synthesis of albumin, fibrinogen, prothrombin, and other factors involved in blood clotting. A reduction of serum albumin is one of the most accurate reflections of the extent of liver disease and the effects of medical therapy. Because the half-life of albumin is 21 days, impairment of hepatic synthesis must be present for over 3 weeks before abnormalities are noted. The correlation between total protein and disease of the liver is not as close as that between the serum albumin level and liver disease, since albumin is produced only by hepatic cells and a reduction is frequently compensated for by an increase in the level of globulin.

Carbohydrates and Lipids. Glycogenesis, glycogen storage, glycogenolysis, and the conversion of galactose into

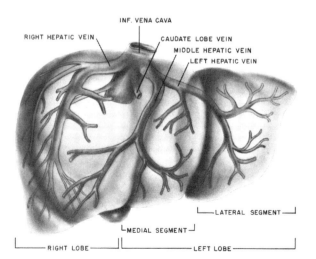

FIG. 28-5. *Prevailing pattern of drainage of hepatic veins in the human liver. (From: Schwartz, 1964, with permission.)*

Table 28-1
Normal Values for Hepatic "Function" Tests

Test	Normal Value
Serum albumin	3.5–4.6 g/dL
Total protein	6.0–7.4 g/dL
Cholesterol	135–300 mg/dL
Alkaline phosphatase	24–100 IU/dL
Serum glutamic oxalacetic transaminase (AST)	10–36 units/dL
Serum glutamic pyruvic transaminase (ALT)	10–48 units/dL
Gamma glutamyl transferase (GGT)	0–48 units/dL males 4–26 units/dL females
Lactic acid dehydrogenase (LDH)	180–225 units/dL
Prothrombin time	90–100% of laboratory control
Fibrinogen	200–400 mg/dL
Blood "ammonia"	10–63 µg/dL
Serum bilirubin	
Total	Less than 1.4 mg/dL
Direct	Less than 0.3 mg/dL
Indirect	Less than 1.1 mg/dL
Urinary bilirubin	0

glucose all represent hepatic functions. Hypoglycemia is a rare accompaniment of extensive hepatic disease, but the amelioration of diabetes in patients with hemochromatosis is considered an indication of neoplastic change. The more common effect of hepatic disease is a deficiency of glycogenesis with resulting hyperglycemia. A hepatic enzyme system is responsible for the conversion of galactose into glucose, and abnormal galactose tolerance tests are seen in hepatitis and active cirrhosis. In rare instances, a familial deficiency in this enzyme system accounts for spontaneous galactosemia accompanied by an obstructive type of jaundice that appears after the first week of life and subsides when lactose is removed from the diet.

Synthesis of both phospholipid and cholesterol takes place in the liver, and the latter serves as a standard for the determination of lipid metabolism. The liver is the major organ involved in the synthesis, esterification, and excretion of cholesterol. In the presence of parenchymal damage, both the total cholesterol and percentage of esterified fraction decrease. Biliary obstruction results in a rise in cholesterol, and the most pronounced elevations are noted with primary biliary cirrhosis and the cholangiolitis accompanying toxic reactions to phenothiazine derivatives.

Enzymes. The three enzymes that achieve abnormal serum levels in hepatic disease and have been studied widely are alkaline phosphatase, serum glutamic oxalacetic transaminase (SGOT), and serum glutamic pyruvic transaminase (SGPT). SGOT is present in the liver, myocardium, skeletal muscles, kidney, and pancreas. Cellular damage in any of the above-mentioned tissues results in elevation of the serum level. In reference to the liver, the most marked increases accompany acute cellular damage regardless of cause, and extremely high levels are noted in patients with hepatitis. SGOT is only moderately increased in cirrhosis and biliary obstruction. SGPT is more particularly applicable to the evaluation of liver disease, since the hepatic content greatly exceeds myocardial concentration. Elevations accompany acute hepatocellular damage. Lactic acid dehydrogenase (LDH) levels also may be elevated.

Serum alkaline phosphatase provides an elevation of the patency of the bile channels at all levels, intrahepatic and extrahepatic. Elevation is demonstrated in 94 percent of patients with obstruction of the extrahepatic biliary tract due to neoplasm and 76 percent of those in whom the obstruction is caused by calculi. Intrahepatic biliary obstruction and cholestasis also cause a rise in the enzyme level. In the presence of space-occupying lesions such as metastases, primary hepatic carcinoma, and abscesses, the alkaline phosphatase level is also increased. The overall correlation between metastatic carcinoma of the liver and an elevated enzyme level is as high as 92 percent. Sixty percent of patients with primary hepatic carcinoma also demonstrate a significant increase. Granulomatous and infiltrative lesions such as sarcoidosis, tuberculosis, and lymphoma are irregularly associated with mild to moderate increases in the alkaline phosphatase. Elevation of the serum level of this enzyme is also associated with diseases that have as a common denominator increased osteoblastic activity. 5'-Nucleotidase is a phosphatase that catalyzes hydrolysis of nucleotides. Levels are elevated in hepatobiliary disease.

Dye Excretion. The hepatic removal of dyes from the circulation depends on hepatic blood flow, hepatocellular function, and biliary excretion. The presence of jaundice produces a disproportionate indocyanine green or sulfobromophthalein (Brom-

sulphalein) retention, and fever, shock, hemorrhage, and recent surgical treatment may all result in increased levels. An increased retention is associated with acute cellular damage and is also noted in patients with cirrhosis, carcinoma, and chronic passive congestion. Since the rate of disappearance from the blood is constant, hepatic blood flow can be determined by injecting the dye at a rate that will maintain a constant blood level and applying Fick's principle to the blood removed from a catheterized hepatic vein. An intestinal xenon technique has been shown to provide an accurate method of measuring portal vein and total hepatic blood flow. Determination of the fecal excretion of the radioactive material has been applied to the differential diagnosis of obstructive jaundice, particularly in the establishment of the diagnosis of congenital atresia of the bile ducts, in which case HIDA or DISIDA fails to appear in the stool.

Coagulation Factors. In liver disease, multiple coagulation defects may occur. Two mechanisms contribute to the deficiency of coagulation factors: (1) in obstructive jaundice, the bile source required for the absorption of the fat-soluble vitamin K results in a decreased synthesis of prothrombin, and (2) hepatocellular dysfunction is accompanied by an inability of the liver to synthesize prothrombin. Abnormal values for prothrombin time have been noted in a variety of hepatic diseases with parenchymal damage, and determination is particularly applicable in the evaluation of patients undergoing liver biopsy or surgical procedures. An increase in prothrombin time subsequent to the injection of parenteral vitamin K is used as an indication of hepatic function and suggests obstructive jaundice. Decreases in factors V, VII, and IX and fibrinogen also have been noted in hepatic disease. Cirrhosis also has been associated with an increased fibrinolysis due to defective synthesis of fibrinolytic inhibitors and delayed removal of plasminogen activators.

Quantitative Tests. Maximal rate of urea synthesis after an oral challenge with casein or an intravenous bolus of amino acids provides an assessment of hepatic function, as does the determination of galactose elimination capacity.

Bile Pigment Metabolism. See the section Jaundice in Chap. 22.

SPECIAL STUDIES

Needle Biopsy of the Liver. This is the one preoperative study that provides a pathologic diagnosis. It depends on an area of tissue measuring 1 to 4 cm in length and containing approximately 5 to 20 lobules representing a general anatomic change. Close to 100 percent accuracy has been demonstrated for both posthepatitic and postnecrotic cirrhosis. Intrahepatic cholestasis, hepatitis, and cellular degeneration resulting from toxicity are all diffuse lesions and readily diagnosed. Focal lesions, such as neoplasms, granulomas, and abscesses, may be missed, but the correlation between needle biopsy and operative and autopsy findings is high. In the case of focal nodular hyperplasia, a needle biopsy often reports normal structure made up of normal hepatocytes and fails to diagnose the lesion because the classic central scar is missed. Occasionally, exsanguination has been reported, particularly in patients with hemangioma, and pain, pneumothorax, hemorrhage, and bile peritonitis are the complications to be considered. If hemangioma is a considered diagnosis, needle biopsy is contraindicated.

Ultrasonography, Computed Tomography, Magnetic Resonance Imaging, and Scintigrams. Preoperative ultrasonography (US) has its highest yield in defining hepatic abscesses, cystic lesions, and most hemangiomas. Intraoperative US detects lesions unidentified by preoperative studies and demonstrates the intraparenchymal vascular anatomy, thus facilitating resection. US and duplex scanning can determine the patency of a portasystemic shunt noninvasively.

Computed tomography (CT) is used with or without vascular enhancement. Intravenous contrast material improves the diagnostic yield over plain CT, but the best results in definition of parenchymal lesions are obtained with intraarterial infusion scans. A catheter is placed in the common hepatic artery, and the scan is taken while the artery is infused. The tumor lights up. The catheter is then positioned in the superior mesenteric artery, and a scan is taken while it is infused and again during the venous phase. Lesions present as radiolucencies. For most lesions, CT provides the best results.

Magnetic resonance imaging (MRI) is particularly applicable for assessing vascular lesions. The T_2 phase provides a characteristic demonstration of a hemangioma. Scintillation scanning also can detect intrahepatic focal lesions. Using tagged red cells or technetium (^{99m}Tc)-sulfur colloid, the diagnosis of hemangioma can be established.

A prospective analysis of laboratory tests and imaging studies has shown greater than 65 percent accuracy in the detection of hepatic lesions. No combination of laboratory tests increased this accuracy. If the laboratory tests were used with one of the imaging studies, the accuracy was increased to 76 percent. The use of all the liver imaging tests and laboratory tests lowers the accuracy and needlessly increases the expense.

Angiography. Since hepatic tumors, both primary and metastatic, depend on an arterial circulation, unusual vascular patterns are also detected by injection of the hepatic artery with radiopaque material. Unusual arrangements of the arteries and "tumor staining," analogous to that found in cerebral and osseous neoplasms, may be noted. Angiography also demonstrates extrahepatic vascular anatomy and provides a "road map" for the surgeon. Angiography is currently used less frequently.

Measurements of Portal Pressure and Evaluation of Portal Circulation. See Portal Hypertension later in this chapter.

TRAUMA

(See Chap. 6, Trauma.)

HEPATIC ABSCESSES

Hepatic abscesses are related to two distinct groups of pathogens, pyogenic bacteria and *Entamoeba histolytica.* Distinctive features in the clinical manifestations and therapy of these two variations necessitate separate consideration.

Pyogenic Abscesses

Incidence. The lesion is present in 0.36 percent of autopsies. The highest percentage of cases occur in the sixth and seventh decades, and there is no predilection for either sex.

Etiology. Pyogenic abscesses of the liver result from (1) ascending biliary infection, (2) hematogenous spread via the portal venous system, (3) generalized septicemia with involvement of the liver by way of the hepatic arterial circulation, (4) direct extension from intraperitoneal infection, or (5) other causes, including hepatic trauma. Recently, the most frequent antecedent cause has been cholangitis secondary to calculi or carcinoma in the extrahepatic biliary duct system. In one series, over 80 percent of patients with a pyogenic liver abscess had an underlying hepatobiliary or pancreatic cancer. The second most common cause is related to generalized septicemia, while the portal venous route of infection has decreased in importance. Pylephlebitis occurs in 0.05 percent of cases of acute appendicitis and 3 percent of patients with perforated appendicitis. No segment of the intestine drained by the portal venous system can be excluded as a possible cause, and the incidence associated with acute diverticulitis is as high as that of appendicitis. There is an increased incidence in immunocompromised patients. There has been an increase in the percentage in which no cause is apparent. These account for about 20 percent of cases.

Cultures are positive in over 90 percent of cases in which they were obtained. *Escherichia coli, Klebsiella,* and *Streptococcus* are the organisms most commonly isolated. *Staphylococcus* and *Pseudomonas* are occurring more frequently, and mixed bacterial and fungal abscesses are noted in about 25 percent of patients.

Pyogenic abscesses may be solitary, multiple, and multilocular. Single and multiple abscesses occur with equal frequency. When a single abscess is present, it is usually located in the right lobe.

Clinical Manifestations. Since most pyogenic hepatic abscesses are secondary to other significant infections, it is difficult to delineate a pathognomonic symptom. Fever is the most common symptom, and a "picket fence" configuration of the temperature chart generally has been noted. Fever is frequently accompanied by chills, profuse sweating, nausea, vomiting, and anorexia. Pain is a late symptom and is more common with large, solitary abscesses. Liver enlargement is noted in 30 to 60 percent of cases. Hepatic tenderness is present in half the patients. Jaundice is related to the causative pathology.

Diagnostic Studies. Leukocytosis with white blood cell counts ranging between 18,000 and 20,000/mm^3 is usual. Half the patients are anemic. Positive blood cultures are demonstrated in approximately 40 percent of patients, the most significant yields accompanying abscesses secondary to systemic septicemia. Liver function tests are not diagnostic, but elevation of the alkaline phosphatase level is the most frequent abnormality. Hypoalbuminemia is inconsistent. Characteristically, radiographs reveal an elevation and immobility or restriction of motion of the right leaf of the diaphragm. There is also obliteration of the right cardiophrenic angle on the posteroanterior chest film and the anterior costophrenic angle on the lateral film. Abscesses produced by gas-forming microorganisms are associated with air-fluid levels in the liver. The CT is the most accurate radiographic study (over 90 percent) as contrasted with ultrasound (80 percent) and radionuclide (70 percent) (Figs. 28-6 and 28-7).

Treatment. This is based on appropriate antibiotic therapy combined with drainage in selected cases. Intravenous antibiotics are usually administered for 2 weeks, followed by 1 month of

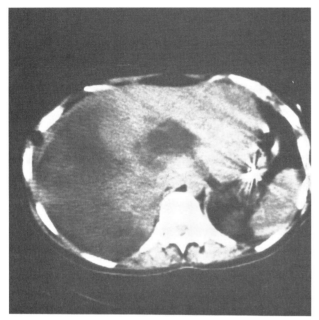

A

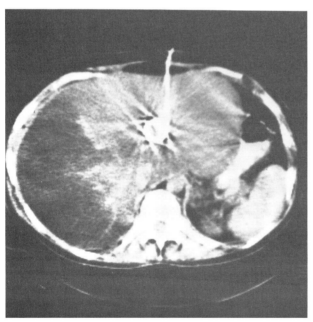

B

FIG. 28-6. *A. Hepatic abscess located in medial segment of left lobe. B. Abscess drained extrasonographically with pigtailed catheter.*

oral therapy. The abscesses may be drained percutaneously under US or CT control. Several series have reported success rates of 80 percent using this technique. Equivalent results have been reported for percutaneous and surgical drainage. The route of surgical access depends on the position of the abscess and may be transthoracic or transabdominal (Figs. 28-8 and 28-9). Because of the availability of antibacterial agents, transperitoneal drainage is no longer associated with prohibitive morbidity or mortality. In a small group of patients with multiple abscesses

confined to a lobe, treatment is best managed by resection (Fig. 28-10).

Prognosis and Complications. Percutaneous and surgical drainage have been associated with mortality rates ranging from 7.5 to 20 percent. With multiple abscesses, the rate is significantly increased. The likelihood of death for patients treated with antibiotics alone is approximately 50 percent.

Amebic Abscesses

Incidence. *E. histolytica* has been found wherever surveys have been made on the human population from northern Canada to the Straits of Magellan. Amebic abscess of the liver is a disease of the middle-aged adult and predominates in males with a 9:1 ratio. The concept of racial immunity is invalid.

Pathology. Amebas reach the liver by way of the portal venous system from a focus of ulceration in the bowel wall. Hepatic involvement is usually a large, single abscess containing liquefied material with a characteristic reddish brown "anchovy paste" fluid. The lesions are usually single and occur in the right lobe of the liver, either near the dome or on the inferior surface in juxtaposition to the hepatic flexure. The wall is only a few millimeters thick and consists of granulation tissue with little or no fibrosis. Microscopically, three zones are recognized: a necrotic center, a middle zone with destruction of parenchymal cells, and an outer zone of relatively normal hepatic tissue in which amebas may be demonstrated.

Clinical Manifestations. Abscesses become evident when they cause generalized systemic disturbances coupled with symptoms and signs of hepatic involvement. The chief complaints are fever and liver pain. Pain is present in 88 percent of patients, and the pattern is related to the location of the hepatic abscess. With pain and tenderness over the right lower intercostal spaces, there may be associated bulging and pitting edema of the subcutaneous tissue. Superior surface abscesses result in pain referred to the right shoulder, whereas abscesses in the bare area, which have no contact with the serosal surface, are latent as far as pain is concerned. Left lobe abscesses present as a painful epigastric swelling.

Fever accompanied by chills and sweating is present in over three-quarters of patients, but the temperature does not reach the levels resulting from pyogenic abscesses unless there is secondary infection. One-third to one-half of adults offer a history of antecedent diarrhea, whereas in children grossly bloody, mucous stool occurs more frequently. Tender hepatomegaly is an almost constant feature. Clinical jaundice is relatively rare.

Diagnostic Studies. Patients with acute disease show no anemia but an appreciable degree of leukocytosis, whereas those with prolonged illness have anemia with less marked leukocytosis. Amebas are found in the stool of only 15 percent of cases collected from the literature. Liver function tests are not helpful in establishing the diagnosis. The indirect hemagglutination test is almost always positive. Radiographic findings are similar to those described for pyogenic abscesses. Scintillography, US, and angiography also have helped to localize the lesion.

Diagnosis is frequently established by aspiration of the abscess cavity, a relatively innocuous procedure. Although the "anchovy paste" aspirate is considered pathognomonic, the abscess content may be creamy white, even though there is no secondary

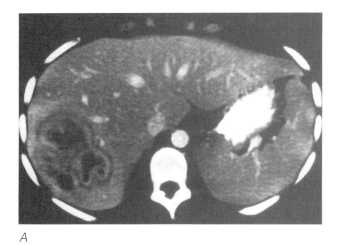

A

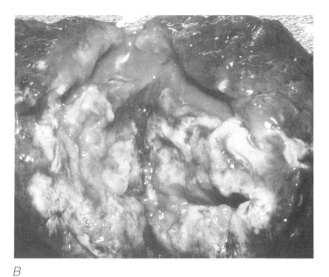

B

FIG. 28-7. *A. CT scan of patient with multiple abcesses originating from Crohn's disease of the small intestine. B. Specimen containing abscesses from right hepatic lobectomy.*

bacterial infection. Amebic trophozoites are demonstrated in the aspirate of fewer than one-third of patients.

Complications. The most common complication is secondary infection, which occurs in approximately 22 percent of patients. Rupture of the amebic abscess accounts for the next most common group of complications. The direction of rupture is reproduced in Fig. 28-11. Pleuropulmonary complications occur in 20 percent of patients. This is usually the result of direct extension of the hepatic process. The most serious route of rupture is into the pericardial cavity, and this is usually secondary to extension of an abscess in the left lobe. Rupture into the peritoneal cavity or into an intraabdominal viscus occurs in 6 to 9 percent of the patients.

Treatment. This consists of administration of amebicidal drugs combined with aspiration or surgical drainage when indicated. The initial approach is usually conservative and directed toward eradicating the parasite from the intestinal tract, liver, and abscess itself. In general, the patient is not considered for surgical treatment until the intestinal phase is controlled. Metronidazole, which acts in both the hepatic and intestinal sites, has replaced emetine and chloroquine. Both the hepatic and intestinal infections generally have been cured by 400 mg three times a day for 4 days, occasionally combined with closed aspiration. In endemic areas, most patients are managed with drugs alone and rarely require aspiration. A single dose of 2.5 g combined with aspiration also has had dramatic results.

Surgical Procedures. The indications for aspiration are (1) the persistence of clinical manifestations following a course of amebicidal drugs, (2) clinical or radiographic evidence of a hepatic abscess, and (3) absence of findings that would suggest secondary infection of a liver abscess. Drug therapy should be instituted several days prior to aspiration. In most instances, aspiration is not required, and the abscess will be resolved by the medication. There is no indication for injection of any drug directly into the abscess cavity. In the absence of localizing signs, the preferred route for percutaneous drainage is through the ninth or tenth interspace between the anterior and posterior axillary

lines. Once an abscess has been demonstrated to be secondarily infected, open drainage is the treatment of choice.

Prognosis. This depends on the relative virulence of the organism and the resistance of the host, the stage of infection, the multiplicity of abscesses, and the presence of complications. In uncomplicated cases, the mortality rate is less than 5 percent, whereas with complications a 43 percent mortality has been reported.

CYSTS AND BENIGN TUMORS

Nonparasitic Cysts

These lesions may be single, multiple, diffuse, localized, unilocular, or multilocular. They include (1) blood and degenerative cysts, (2) dermoid cysts, (3) lymphatic cysts, (4) endothelial cysts, (5) retention cysts, consisting of (a) solitary retention cysts and (b) multiple retention cysts (polycystic disease), and (6) proliferative cysts (cystadenomas). Autopsy incidences of approximately 0.15 percent have been reported. One percent of CT scans reveal intrahepatic cysts. The clinically apparent nonparasitic solitary cysts occur more frequently in women in the fourth, fifth, and sixth decades, at an average age of 52 years. Polycystic hepatic disease also occurs much more frequently in women.

Pathology. Solitary nonparasitic cysts are usually located in the right lobe of the liver. The cyst content is a clear, watery material, and characteristically, the cysts have a low internal pressure, in contrast to the high tension in parasitic cysts. Occasionally, the fluid is yellowish brown, suggesting necrosis of adjacent parenchyma. Polycystic disease of the liver has a honeycomb appearance with multiple cavities, and the lesions commonly are distributed throughout the entire liver. At times, however, one lobe, more frequently the right, is preferentially involved. Unlike the solitary nonparasitic cyst, polycystic disease of the liver (Fig. 28-12) frequently is associated with cystic involvement of other organs; 51.6 percent of polycystic livers are associated with polycystic kidneys. Conversely, the inci-

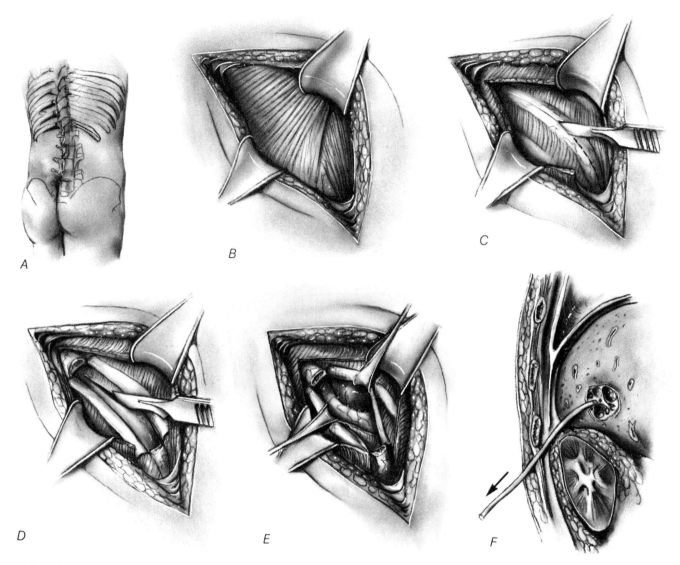

FIG. 28-8. *Extraserous transthoracic drainage. A. Incision is made posteriorly over right twelfth rib. B. Latissimus dorsi muscle exposed. C. Periosteum of twelfth rib incised. D. Twelfth rib removed subperiosteally and bed incised. E. Diaphragm is detached and peritoneum is reflected from the inferior surface of diaphragm. F. Schematic drawing of position of drain. (From: Schwartz, 1964, with permission.)*

dence of hepatic cysts in patients with known polycystic renal disease varies between 19 and 34 percent. Polycystic livers have been implicated as a rare cause of portal hypertension and also have been associated with atresia of the bile ducts, cholangitis, and hemangiomas.

Traumatic cysts are usually single, are filled with bile, and contain no epithelial lining. Cystadenomas are grossly smooth, encapsulated, and lobular and contain a mucoid material. They are lined by a proliferative columnar epithelium.

Clinical Manifestations. Both solitary and polycystic lesions grow slowly and are relatively asymptomatic. A painless right upper quadrant mass is the most frequent complaint, and when symptoms occur, they are usually related to pressure on adjacent viscera, such as early satiety. Acute abdominal pain may accompany the complications of torsion, intracystic hem-

orrhage, or intraperitoneal rupture. Physical examination may reveal the mass, and the kidneys may be palpable. Jaundice is rare. Liver function tests usually demonstrate no abnormality. Scintillography, CT scan, US, and arteriography have been used to define the intrahepatic position of the mass, and peritoneoscopy may be diagnostic (Fig. 28-13).

Treatment. Asymptomatic solitary nonparasitic cysts and polycystic disease of the liver require no treatment. Large, solitary symptomatic cysts usually can be managed electively unless there is rupture, intracystic hemorrhage, or torsion. Patients have been managed successfully with radiographically controlled percutaneous catheter drainage, at times reinforced with injection of a sclerosing solution such as alcohol. This procedure is frequently associated with recurrence. Permanent resolution can be effected by a simple operation in which the cyst is widely un-

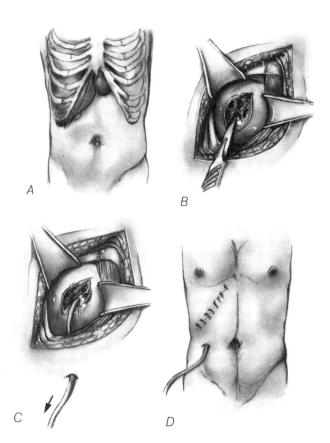

FIG. 28-9. *Transabdominal drainage. A. Subcostal incision. B. Peritoneum has been entered and abscess incised. C. Drain is positioned in abscess and brought out through the stab wound. D. Closure of wound and position of stab wound. (From: Schwartz, 1964, with permission.)*

roofed back to its junction with normal hepatic parenchyma. This can be accomplished laparoscopically. In the case of significant intracystic bleeding, cystectomy might be required. Internal drainage into the intestine is indicated only if there is erosion into a major hepatic duct that cannot be repaired.

In patients with significant symptoms attributed to the mass effect of polycystic liver, palliation can be achieved by nonanatomic resection and wide fenestration of the larger cysts.

Prognosis. The prognosis of polycystic disease is essentially that of the accompanying renal disease. Hepatic failure, jaundice, and the manifestations of portal hypertension are rare. The mortality rate for surgically treated nonparasitic cysts of the liver approaches zero.

Hydatid Cysts

Hydatid disease *(echinococcosis)* is characterized by worldwide distribution and frequent hepatic involvement. The incidence among human beings depends on the incidence in intermediate hosts, including sheep, pigs, and cattle. The southern half of South America, Iceland, Australia, New Zealand, and southern parts of Africa are regarded as intensive endemic areas. Most cases reported in the United States have occurred in immigrants from Greece and Italy.

Pathology. The most common unilocular hydatid cyst is caused by *Echinococcus granulosus,* whereas the alveolar type is caused by *E. multilocularis.* Approximately 70 percent of hydatid cysts are located in the liver, and in one-quarter to one-third of these cases there are multiple cysts. The right lobe is affected in 85 percent of patients. Cysts are usually superficial and are composed of a two-layer laminated wall, an inner germinative membrane, and an outer adventitia. The two membranes are in close contact with each other but are not linked. The fluid in the hydatid cyst has a high pressure of approximately 300 mL of water and is colorless, opalescent, and slightly alkaline. Inside the main hydatid vesicle, daughter cysts are usually found. Extension is commonly into the peritoneal cavity, but progressive intrahepatic expansion may result in the replacement of liver parenchyma.

In contrast to the unilocular hydatid cysts, the alveolar hydatid is a growth without a capsule and with a tendency toward multiple metastases. As growth progresses, the center becomes necrotic, and the periphery invades the blood vessels and lymph channels. The causative agent of this lesion is found more frequently in the colder regions of Alaska, Russia, and the Alps.

Complications. Intrabiliary rupture represents the most common complication and occurs in 5 to 10 percent of cases. Suppuration, the second most common complication, is caused by bacteria from the biliary tract. The formation of the purulent material results in death of the parasite and conversion into a pyogenic abscess. Intraperitoneal rupture results in the showering of hydatid fluid, brood capsules, and scolices into the peritoneum, leading to transient peritoneal irritation of varying intensity. Usually, the reproductive elements survive and initiate the formation of new cysts *(secondary echinococcosis of the peritoneum).* Cysts located in the superior portion of the liver tend to grow craniad into the pleural cavity and become intrathoracic. These can be differentiated from primary pulmonary cysts by the presence of daughter cysts and bile pigments. Empyema and bronchopleural fistula must result.

Clinical Manifestations. Patients with simple or uncomplicated multivesicular cysts are usually asymptomatic. When symptoms occur, they are caused by pressure on adjacent organs. Abdominal pain and tenderness are the most common complaints, followed by a palpable mass. A tumor, which is palpable in 70 percent of the patients, or diffuse hepatic enlargement in a patient who has lived in an endemic region is cause for suspicion. The so-called hydatid thrill and fremitus are quite rare. Jaundice and ascites are uncommon. With secondary infection, tender hepatomegaly, chills, and spiking temperatures occur. Urticaria and erythema offer evidence of a generalized anaphylactic reaction. With biliary rupture, the classic triad of biliary colic, jaundice, and urticaria may be noted. Vomiting with passage of hydatid membranes in the emesis *(hydatidemesia)* and passage of membranes in the stool *(hydatidenteria)* also may occur. The complication of intraperitoneal rupture is heralded by abdominal pain and signs of anaphylactic shock. Intrathoracic rupture is associated with shoulder pain and cough initially productive of a frothy blood-stained fluid that subsequently becomes stained with bile. Membranes are intermittently expectorated in 80 percent of these patients.

Diagnostic Studies. Radiographically, an unruptured cyst presents as a round, reticulated, calcified shadow in the liver

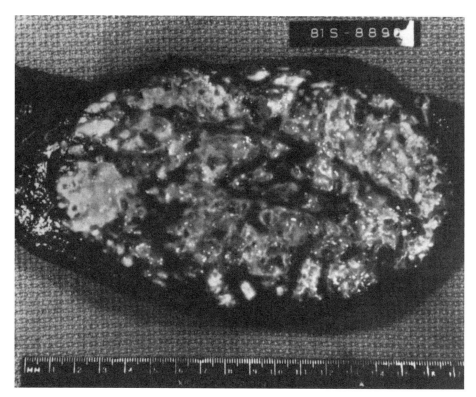

FIG. 28-10. The specimen was 1950 g. The greater part was made up of large yellow-green grumous material that replaced the parenchyma. There also was a significant amount of thick yellowish green fluid. On histologic examination there were areas of extensive necrosis and fibrosis, and a diagnosis of multilocular abscess was made. The drainage material grew coagulase-negative *Staphylococcus* and diphtheroid.

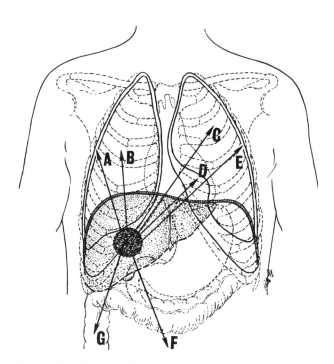

FIG. 28-11. Directions of rupture in 44 cases of amebic liver abscess: *A.* 8 cases, right pleural cavity. *B.* 13 cases, right lung. *C.* 4 cases left lung. *D.* 7 cases, pericardium. *E.* 1 case, left pleural cavity. *F.* 10 cases, peritoneal cavity. *G.* 1 case, colon. (After: *Lamont. Q J Med 27:389, 1958, with permission.*)

(Fig. 28-14). Secondary infection with gas-producing organisms might be confused with daughter cysts. With intrabiliary rupture, gas is noted in the remaining cyst cavity. CT scans furnish useful information and correlate well with operative findings (Fig. 28-15). Eosinophilia is the least reliable of immunologic responses, being present in only 25 percent of all patients. The indirect agglutination test is positive in about 85 percent of patients; the complement fixation test is slightly less sensitive. This reaction becomes negative 2 to 6 months after removal of the cyst. Casoni's skin test is positive in approximately 90 percent of patients, and the reaction can be obtained years after surgical removal of the cyst or after the parasite has died.

Treatment. Small calcified cysts in patients with negative serologic test results need no treatment. Treatment is surgical, since there is no response to drug administration. Therapy consists of removal of the cyst contents without contaminating the patient, followed by appropriate management of any remaining cavity. Since the hydatid fluid is under high tension, evacuation and sterilization are carried out initially with a scolicidal agent such as hibitane, alcohol, or hypertonic saline. Following evacuation and irrigation, primary closure may effect cure. External drainage and marsupialization are accompanied by high complication rates and prolonged drainage. Removal of the parasite is accomplished by excision of the hydatid vesicle using the natural cleavage plane that exists between the germinative layer and adventitia. Omentoplasty provides a method of managing the cavity successfully (Fig. 28-16). Total removal of the cysts, including the adventitial layer, also may be performed. Partial hepatectomy with controlled hepatic resection has been advised for larger and multiple cysts. Marsupialization and partial hepatectomy are the alternatives for large or injected cysts. In uncom-

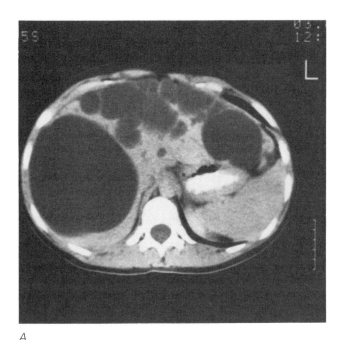

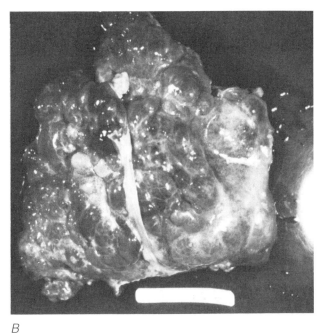

A   *B*

FIG. 28-12. *A. CT scan of polycystic liver demonstrating large cyst in right lobe and multiple cysts throughout the right lobe. B. Specimen of resected polycystic left lobe of liver. Right cyst was unroofed.*

plicated cases, the results of surgical treatment are excellent, and the postoperative mortality is less than 5 percent. With intrabiliary rupture, marsupialization should be accompanied by drainage of the bile duct if there is associated obstruction. Rupture into the peritoneal cavity is treated by laparotomy and thorough cleansing, although it is frequently impossible to prevent secondary contamination. Intrathoracic rupture generally can be controlled by evacuating and draining the hepatic cysts. Alveolar disease of the liver was inevitably fatal, but more recently, satisfactory results have been obtained with extensive hepatic resection.

Benign Tumors

Hamartoma. Hamartomas are composed of tissues normally present in the organ but arranged in a disorderly fashion. The lesions vary from minute nodules to large tumors and are rarely of clinical significance. Large mesenchymal hamartomas have presented as rapidly growing abdominal masses in infants

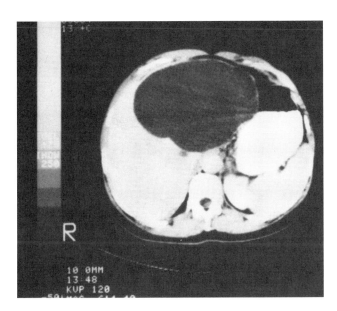

FIG. 28-13. CT scan demonstrating solitary, nonparasitic cyst of left lobe of liver.

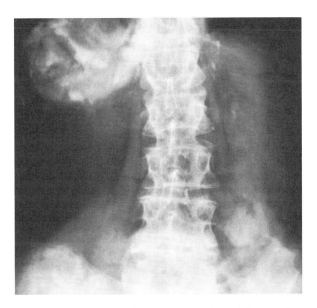

FIG. 28-14. Hydatid cyst of liver, demonstrating calcification. (From: *Schwartz, 1964, with permission.*)

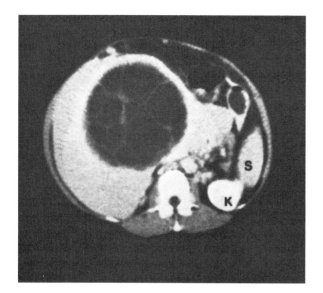

FIG. 28-15. *CT scan showing large echinococcus cyst with multiple septa.*

the potential for bleeding and malignant transformation, along with the current safety of removing the lesions, favors routine resection. Deaths associated with elective resections are rare; an 8 percent mortality is reported for emergency resection. The lesions are readily identified by their pale yellow color and homogeneous appearance. They often can be removed by enucleation with a narrow rim of normal hepatic parenchyma. Because

and children. US and CT are the most useful diagnostic tests. Grossly, the tumors are firm, nodular, and located immediately beneath the surface of the liver, and they may be solitary or multiple. They are generally well encapsulated and often cystic. With lesions of clinical significance, surgical excision is generally indicated. Deeply located lesions should be left alone after histologic diagnosis has been established because they do not grow rapidly and do not undergo malignant transformation.

Adenoma. Hepatic adenoma is a benign tumor that was rarely noted before the introduction of oral contraceptives in the 1960s. In an accumulation of data from many series, more than 60 percent of patients were exposed only to mestranol; an additional 20 percent of patients were exposed to a product that included mestranol. More than half the patients used oral contraceptives continuously for durations longer than 5 years; lesions have become manifest even after discontinuation of the drug. These lesions also develop during pregnancy, in patients with diabetes mellitus or glycogen storage disease, and rarely, as adenomatosis, which is defined as more than 10 adenomas in an otherwise normal hepatic parenchyma. Adenomatosis occurs with equal frequency in men and women.

In patients who were contraceptive users, hepatic adenomas tend to be larger and have higher rates of intratumoral and intraperitoneal hemorrhage. Bleeding also has occurred during pregnancy. Transformation of the adenomas into hepatocellular carcinoma has been documented; this occurs more frequently in patients with adenomatosis.

The diagnosis typically is made in women of childbearing age. Eighty percent are symptomatic, with pain or mass effect generally related to intratumoral or intraperitoneal bleeding. The latter may cause shock. The hepatic lesion usually can be identified by US or CT (Fig. 28-17). At times, a small lesion is not detected, but the diagnosis is suggested by a subglissonian hematoma. Percutaneous biopsy is contraindicated because it is associated with a high risk of bleeding.

Although regression and disappearance of hepatic adenomas have been reported after the discontinuation of contraceptives,

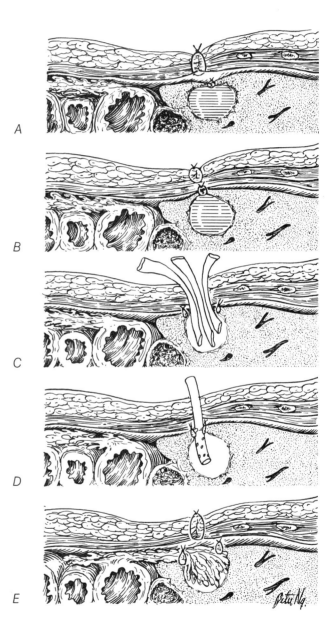

FIG. 28-16. *Methods of handling residual hepatic cavity. A. Suture without drainage (capsulorrhaphy). Cavity is filled with sterile saline solution, and adventitia is closed without drainage. B. Same as A but peripheral peritoneum of anterior abdominal wall is sutured to periphery of capsule to facilitate extraperitoneal drainage of secondary infection, if one arises. C. Marsupialization. Edges of cavity are sutured to abdominal wall, and several drains are inserted into depths of wound. D. Variant of marsupialization. Catheter is inserted into cavity, and closed drainage is used. E. Omentoplasty. Omentum is used to fill remaining cavity and is sutured to periphery of fibrous capsule. Vascular omental pedicle absorbs effusion. (From: Schwartz, 1964, with permission.)*

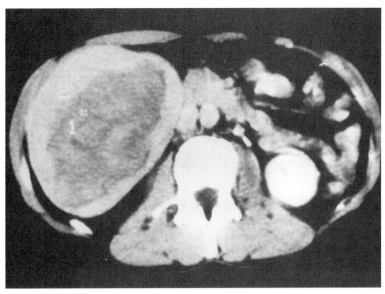

A

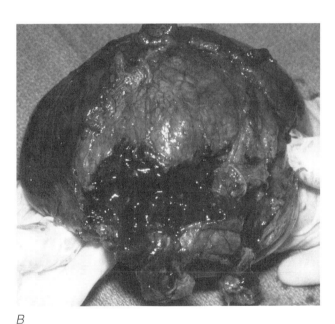

B

FIG. 28-17. *A. Dynamic CT scan revealing a large hemangioma of the right lobe of the liver and involving the medial segment of the left lobe. B. Arteriogram of lesion depicted in A showing classic laking effect of a hemangioma.*

of the diffuse nature of adenomatosis and its potential for malignancy, transplantation has been used.

Focal Nodular Hyperplasia (FNH). This is a benign lesion that usually occurs in women of reproductive age. Many believe that it is neither a neoplasm nor a hamartoma but a reaction to injury or a hyperplastic response to a preexisting spider-like vascular malformation. There is no consistent relationship to oral contraceptive use. US and CT frequently fail to define the lesion because it is isodense. The angiogram demonstrates a typical sunburst, hypervascular pattern. The patients are almost always asymptomatic, and the lesions frequently are detected at celiotomy. Spontaneous bleeding rarely occurs. The cut surfaces are tan and demonstrate a characteristic central stellate scar. To make a histologic diagnosis, a deep biopsy is necessary to define the scar because the hepatic cell structure is

otherwise normal (Fig. 28-18). FNH was regarded as a possible precursor to fibrolamellar carcinoma, but unlike the latter, it contains no neurotensin. Resection is occasionally indicated for significant pain ascribed to the lesion and rarely for spontaneous rupture.

Hemangioma. Hemangioma is the most common nodule in the liver, and the liver is the internal organ most frequently affected with this lesion. The tumor occurs five times more frequently in women than in men. These are occasionally associated with FNH and cysts of the liver and pancreas. Malignant degeneration does not occur. The hemangioma must be distinguished from hemangioendothelioma or diffuse hemangiomatosis. The latter consists of widespread multicentric lesions accompanied by vascular involvement of the skin and occurs in children with clinical manifestations in the first week of life.

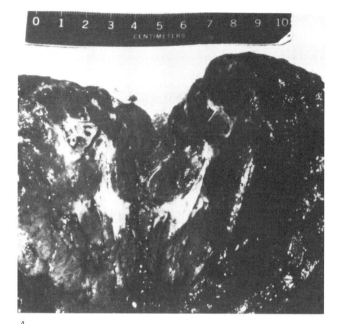

A

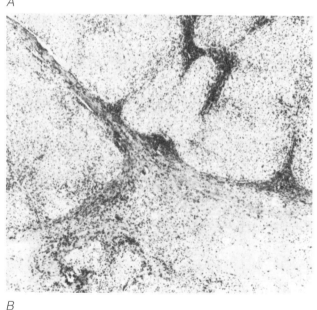

B

FIG. 28-18. *A.* Focal nodular hyperplasia gross specimen. *B.* Microscopy demonstrated normal parenchymal cells surrounding large scar. (From: *Gutierrez and Schwartz, 1984, with permission.*)

Most lesions are detected radiographically, are less than 5 cm in diameter, and are asymptomatic. Larger lesions can be painful and palpable. Platelet trapping in giant hemangiomas can result in thrombocytopenia. Growth of the lesions as a consequence of pregnancy or estrogen therapy has been varied. Most small lesions followed ultrasonographically during pregnancy grow minimally, but occasionally, significant increases in size occur. Rupture of a hemangioma is a rare event. In infants, large hemangiomas often are associated with high-output cardiac failure.

Hemangiomas can present a characteristic pattern on US and CT (Fig. 28-19A). The diagnosis can be made on a T_2-weighted

MRI or scintigram with ^{99m}Tc-labeled red blood cells. The arteriogram demonstrates pooling in small peripheral vessels (Fig. 28-19B). Percutaneous biopsy often provides the histologic diagnosis but is rarely indicated because it is associated with the complication of bleeding.

In infants with high-output congestive heart failure, supportive therapy, at times with the addition of steroids, is effective, and the lesion regresses. In rare cases, hepatic artery embolization or ligation may be required to reverse cardiac failure. In adults, most hepatic hemangiomas should not be excised. Even

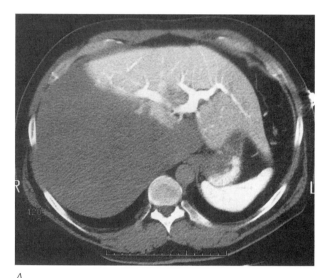

A

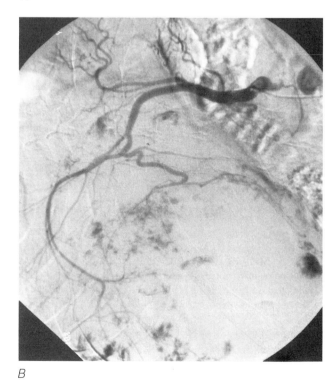

B

FIG. 28-19. *A.* Celiac angiogram demonstrating typical pooling of radiopaque throughout right lobe of liver. *B.* Infusion CT scan showing large, centrally located hemangioma of liver containing several organized clots. (From: *Schwartz and Husser, 1987, with permission.*)

large lesions followed for long periods show no notable increase in size or clinical manifestations. The potential for rupture is minimal and should not constitute an indication for excision. Pain, mass effect, significant growth, platelet trapping, and early rupture are indications for surgical excision. Few reports have documented reduction in size with radiation therapy, and hepatic arterial ligation is rarely effective in adults. Resection is the therapy of choice when indicated. Large lesions may necessitate anatomic resection, but enucleation is often feasible.

MALIGNANT TUMORS

Primary Carcinoma

Incidence. Although the disease is rare in people of western Europe and North America, primary carcinoma is remarkably common among the aboriginal inhabitants of Africa and in many parts of Asia. Postmortem rates in the United States average 0.27 percent, whereas in Africa the postmortem rate is 1.1 percent, hepatic carcinomas representing 17 to 53 percent of all cancers. In some Asian countries, the autopsy incidence is 2.5 percent.

Primary carcinoma of the liver occurs with greater frequency in males. In whites it is rare before age 40, whereas in Africans and Asians the affliction usually occurs before age 40. American blacks do not exhibit a predisposition toward the disease. By contrast, a higher incidence is present in Chinese subjects even after they have changed their habitation. In children, the first appearance of the neoplasm is usually before age 2, and primary carcinoma of the liver represents the most common carcinoma in the first few years of life. Hepatoblastoma usually affects children less than 2 years old; the male-to-female ratio is 6:1. This lesion also occurs in adults. Fibrolamellar carcinoma, a variant of hepatocellular carcinoma, has a propensity for adolescents and young adults, with an equal sex incidence.

Etiology. A number of etiologic factors have been implicated. Aflatoxins of the mold *Aspergillus flavus* contaminate the diet in African and Asian communities with a high incidence of hepatocellular carcinoma. Low protein intake and consequent kwashiorkor also may be factors. Just as almost every type of experimentally induced cirrhosis may be followed by carcinoma of the liver, so a definite association between cirrhosis and primary carcinoma has been noted in human beings. Postnecrotic cirrhosis is the type most commonly preceding hepatocellular carcinoma; cirrhosis is present in 60 percent of patients. Serologic markers for hepatitis B virus or antibodies to hepatitis C virus are detected in most patients with hepatocellular carcinoma in endemic areas. Hepatic malignant tumors occur in 4.5 percent of cirrhotic patients, and the incidence is increased in patients with hemochromatosis. Parasite infestation with the liver fluke *Clonorchis sinensis* has been considered a factor in the development of cholangiocarcinoma, but this is open to question. There is no increased risk for hepatic carcinoma following infectious hepatitis that does not progress to cirrhosis. In the pediatric age group, the tumor is rarely related to cirrhosis. Another factor associated with hepatocellular carcinoma is aberrant α_1-antitrypsin-piZ.

Pathology. Liver cell (*hepatocellular*) carcinoma is the most common type; the tumor cells resemble the parenchymal cell. Bile duct carcinoma (*cholangiocarcinoma*) is apparently derived from bile duct epithelium. *Hepatoblastoma* represents an immature variant of hepatocellular carcinoma.

Grossly, each of these types may present as a single, large nodule, as extensive nodularity, or as a diffuse permeation throughout the organ. The anatomic distribution of fibrolamellar carcinoma is unusual in that 75 percent present as solitary, large left lobe tumors. They have a prominent central scar. The hepatocellular carcinomas have a trabecular structure, and vascularity is a prominent feature. These lesions frequently invade branches of the portal vein and occasionally the hepatic veins. The formation of giant cells is a feature of hepatocellular carcinoma and aids in distinguishing this lesion from secondary carcinoma of the liver. Fibrolamellar carcinoma is characterized by eosinophilic hepatocytes and abundant fibrous stroma arranged in parallel bands around tumor cells. The cell type of bile duct carcinoma is columnar, and its microscopic appearance may be impossible to distinguish from that of carcinoma of the gallbladder or extrahepatic biliary duct system. Bile is never seen in the acini or the cells, whereas mucus formation is common.

Hepatic tumors extend by four methods:

1. Centrifugal growth, which indicates nodular expansion leading to compression of the surrounding hepatic tissue.
2. Parasinusoidal extension, which refers to tumor invasion into the surrounding parenchyma, either through the parasinusoidal spaces or through the sinusoids themselves.
3. Venous spread or extension of tumor from small branches of the portal system in a retrograde fashion into larger branches and eventually into the portal vein. Invasion of hepatic vein tributaries is less common but may extend up to the inferior vena cava or right atrium.
4. Distant metastases, the result of invasion of lymph channels and vascular systems. The most frequently involved locations are regional lymph nodes and lungs.

Metastases occur in 48 to 73 percent of patients.

Clinical Manifestations. Weight loss and weakness occur in 80 percent of patients, whereas abdominal pain is present in half (75 percent of patients with fibrolamellar carcinoma). The pain is usually dull and persistent, but dramatic sudden onset may occur in patients with intraperitoneal hemorrhage secondary to rupture of a necrotic nodule or erosion of a blood vessel. Manifestations of portal hypertension, such as bleeding varices, are infrequent but foreboding symptoms.

The liver is almost always enlarged but not tender. Splenic enlargement is present in one-third of patients, as are other signs of portal hypertension. The incidence of jaundice varies from 20 to 58 percent. Ascites develops in one-half to three-quarters of patients. A rapid increase in the symptoms and signs associated with cirrhosis or hemachromatosis is highly suggestive of superimposed hepatic carcinoma. In these patients, the amelioration of diabetes and occasional hypoglycemic intervals also indicate neoplastic change.

In over half of pediatric patients, the first evidence is an abdominal mass. Hemihypertrophy and sexual precocity occur in an occasional pediatric patient with hepatoblastoma.

Diagnostic Studies. The most consistently altered liver function test is the alkaline phosphatase determination. The serum bilirubin level is usually normal; 5'-nucleotidase is usually elevated.

The demonstration of alpha-fetoprotein (AFP) in the serum by immunodiffusion, immunoelectrophoresis, and immunoassay techniques is useful in the differential diagnosis and epidemiologic studies. This protein is normally present in the fetus but disappears a few weeks after birth. Positive AFP tests are noted in about 75 percent of Africans but in only 30 percent of patients in the United States and Europe. False-positive results occur with embryonic tumors of the ovary and testis. Resection of the tumor converts the test to "negative"; recurrence may be detected by the reappearance of AFP in the serum.

Selective hepatic arteriography has been used to demonstrate an arterial pattern within the tumor, characterized by pooling and increased vascularity (Fig. 28-20). Scintillation scanning also may identify the space-occupying lesion within the liver, but CT and MRI are more sensitive. Percutaneous needle biopsy can provide a definitive diagnosis. US is particularly helpful in differentiating cystic from solid tumors. Intraoperative US has added an important surgical refinement and permitted more limited resections.

Treatment. The only curative therapy for hepatocellular carcinoma is surgical excision. In most instances, this entails a lobectomy, but with an appreciation of segmental anatomy, lesser "anatomic" resections are being performed more frequently. A major resection is compromised by cirrhosis because of increased vascularity, increased morbidity, and an inability for the cirrhotic liver to regenerate. The use of intraoperative US has permitted limited resections particularly in cirrhotic patients. Limited resections, including segmentectomies and bisegmentectomies, have achieved success in cirrhotic patients. Resection has resulted in survival rates of over 40 percent in patients with small, unifocal, well-differentiated tumors without vascular invasion. Transarterial chemoembolization using gelatin sponges, iodized oil, and chemotherapeutic agents has achieved 1-, 2-, and 5-year survival rates of 51, 24, and 6 percent, respectively, while decreasing the tumor size in almost a third of patients. Unresectable hepatocellular carcinomas may be converted to resectable lesions with combined radiation chemotherapy. Percutaneous Ethanol injection has resulted in the disappearance of tumors less than 4.5 cm in diameter. Cryosurgery, using an intraoperatively placed probe that delivers liquid nitrogen, also has effected tumor necrosis and destruction. Transplantation and resection yield equivalent 5-year survival rates of approximately 50 percent, but the recurrent rate is lower in patients who were transplanted. Transplantation achieved the best results in patients with small uninodular or binodular lesions. Resection of extrahepatic recurrences of hepatocellular carcinomas has resulted in several 5-year survivals.

In the case of hepatoblastoma, particularly in children, lesions often deemed not resectable can be converted into resectable tumors that have potential for cure. A combination of preoperative chemotherapy followed by resection resulted in a cure rate of 90 percent in children.

Prognosis. The outlook for untreated primary carcinoma of the liver is extremely poor, and the duration of the disease is rarely longer than 4 months from the time of onset of symptoms. Death is the result of cachexia, hepatic failure, sequelae or portal vein thrombosis, intraperitoneal hemorrhage, and metastases. In

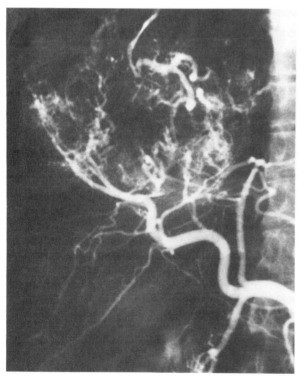

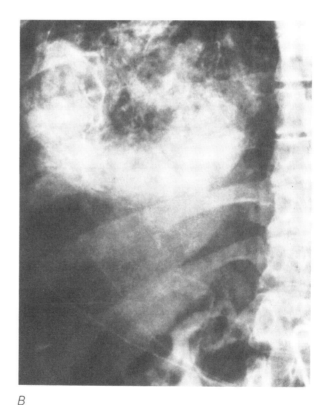

A   *B*

FIG. 28-20. *A. Hepatic arteriogram showing a 13 × 14 cm hypervascular mass in the superior portion of the right lobe of the liver supplied by vessels from the right and medial branches of the left hepatic artery. B. A lucent center within this mass represented either central necrosis or hemorrhage. (From: Gutierrez and Schwartz, 1984, with permission.)*

the Mayo Clinic experience, the 5-year survival after curative resection of a primary hepatic malignancy was 27 percent. Cholangiocarcinoma, nodal metastases, cirrhosis, hypocalcemia, and increased alkaline phosphatase level and prothrombin time were associated with decreased survival. In Pittsburgh, the 5-year survival was 32 percent, with a more favorable prognosis noted for patients with fibrolamellar carcinoma. Similar survival rates were achieved with partial hepatic resection and by hepatectomy and orthotopic transplantation. In children under age 2 with hepatoblastoma, 21 of 27 who survived operation were alive and well with no evidence of disease for a mean of 53 months. By contrast, in children with hepatocellular carcinoma, the prognosis is poorer. Most tumors are not resectable, and 5-year cures are anecdotal.

Other Primary Neoplasms

The three major lesions are sarcoma, mesenchymoma, and infantile hemangioendothelioma. All hepatic mesenchymal lesions are considered malignant. Angiosarcoma is the most common primary sarcoma of the liver. Exposure to vinyl chloride and Thorotrast injection have been implicated as etiologic factors.

Angiosarcoma is characterized by a short illness, jaundice, and coma progressing rapidly to death. Infantile hemangioendotheliomas occur in children under the age of 5 and are associated with skin lesions and cardiac failure secondary to arteriovenous shunts within the tumor. Although most of these pediatric lesions are fatal, spontaneous regression has been recorded, as has success with partial hepatectomy.

Metastatic Neoplasms

Metastatic neoplasms represent the most common malignant tumors of the liver. The relative proportion of primary to secondary neoplasms is estimated to be 1:20, and there is no statistical difference between those with and those without cirrhosis. The liver is second only to regional lymph nodes as a site of metastases for tumors, and 25 to 50 percent of all patients dying of cancer have been found to have hepatic metastases. Fifty percent of patients with gastrointestinal tumors have hepatic metastases when autopsied.

Metastatic neoplasms reach the liver by four routes: (1) portal venous circulation, (2) lymphatic spread, (3) hepatic arterial system, and (4) direct extension.

Metastases appear in the liver at varying times in relation to primary lesions: (1) Precocious metastasis is evident when the primary lesion is not suspected (carcinoid of the ileum). (2) Synchronous metastases occur when the hepatic neoplasm is detected at the same time as the primary lesion. (3) Metachronous metastasis is one in which appearance is delayed following the successful removal of a primary tumor (ocular melanoma). The growth pattern of the metastatic tumor is frequently more rapid than the original lesion, and the mitotic count of metastatic hepatic neoplasms has been shown to be five times greater than that of the extrahepatic primary lesion.

Clinical Manifestations. Symptoms referable to the liver are present in 67 percent of patients with proven metastases. These include hepatic pain, ascites, jaundice, anorexia, and weight loss. On examination, hepatic nodularity is apparent in half the patients, and a friction rub is audible in 10 percent. Jaundice, ascites, and the signs of portal hypertension are present in approximately one-quarter to one-third of patients. With car-

cinoid tumors, hepatic metastases are of major importance in the pathogenesis of the flushing syndrome.

Diagnostic Studies. The alkaline phosphatase level is increased in over 80 percent of patients. The SGOT level is elevated in approximately two-thirds of patients, but the serum AFP determination is negative. The carcinoembryonic antigen (CEA) level may provide a marker for metastatic colon carcinoma. Enhanced CT, particularly that performed with selective arterial infusion via the hepatic artery, is the most sensitive means of defining intrahepatic metastases. MRI, scintigraphy, and arteriography also have been used. In the case of patients who have undergone resection of colorectal carcinomas, surveillance generally relies on sequential determinations of the CEA level. If elevation occurs, CT is performed. Intraoperative US has aided in the definition of resectable lesions.

Treatment. Surgical treatment of hepatic metastases should be considered only if (1) control of the primary tumor is accomplished or anticipated, (2) there are no systemic or intraabdominal metastases, (3) the patient's condition will tolerate the major operative procedure, and (4) the extent of hepatic involvement is such that resection and total extirpation of the metastasis is feasible. Resection of segments of the liver containing metastases has effected reasonable long-term survival without recurrence for patients with primaries in the colon and rectum and for those with Wilms' tumor. Rare survivors have been reported for other primaries.

A metastasis noted during a colon resection should be removed at that time if it is readily removable without anticipated blood loss. However, if it appears that a major hepatic resection will be required, the operation is delayed for months and is preceded by CT scan and angiography to assess resectability. Although 20 percent of patients with colorectal cancer have hepatic metastasis, only one-quarter of these are potentially resectable; half of these, in turn, have other metastases that would negate the value of resection.

A multi-institutional study of hepatic resection for colorectal metastases reported a 5-year actuarial survival of 33 percent and a 5-year actuarial disease-free survival of 21 percent. Single metastases and unilobar disease were associated with improved survival. Hepatic resection of greater than four metastatic lesions rarely was associated with prolonged survival. Forty percent of patients with recurrent disease after hepatic resection for metastatic colorectal tumors initially have only liver metastases. Reresection is followed by long-term survival in about one-third of carefully selected patients. Bismuth and associates have treated patients with colorectal hepatic metastases that were initially considered to be unresectable with doxorubicin, and this resulted in regression to a size that permitted resection. Cure rates equivalent to series of more favorable patients were achieved.

An implantable refillable pump has been used to intraarterially infuse floxuridine and other chemotherapeutic agents, but most series could demonstrate no improvement in survival or reduction in toxicity compared with intravenous administration of the drugs.

Patients with Wilms' tumor metastatic to the liver frequently can be cured by hepatic resection and adjuvant chemotherapy and radiation therapy. Resection of metastases from occular melanoma, breast, stomach, uterus, cervix, ovary, and renal carcinomas rarely has achieved a cure (Table 28-2).

Table 28-2
Hepatic Resection Non-Colorectal Non-Neuroendocrine Metastases

	No. of Cases	No. of 5-Year Survivals
Gastric	17	1
Esophageal	4	0
Pancreas and periampullary	13	0
Wilms' tumor	16	6
Renal	13	4
Adrenocortical	8	2
Ovarian	10	1
Cervical and endometrial	8	1
Uterine leiomyosarcoma	5	0
Vaginal	1	0
Breast	22	2
Melanoma	19	2*

*1 died of disease later

Palliative cytoreductive surgical measures are indicated for marked pain associated with hepatic neoplasm and for the excision of metastases in patients with the flushing syndrome of carcinoid tumor. Resection of the major portion of the hepatic metastases (debulking procedure), even if residual tumor remains, has resulted in significant symptomatic improvement and reduction of the 5-hydroxyindoleacetic acid levels to normal. These subjective and objective changes have persisted for several years. Dearterialization and radiographically controlled embolization have achieved similar results.

HEPATIC RESECTION

The indications for hepatic resection include (1) trauma with resulting devascularization of hepatic tissue, (2) cysts, (3) granulomas, (4) primary neoplasms of the liver, and (5) secondary malignant tumors that involve the liver either by direct extension or as metastatic lesions.

Removal of up to 80 percent of the liver is compatible with life. Following excision of this amount, patients maintain normal blood ammonia levels and normal prothrombin times. Fibrinogen production is insignificantly impaired; clinical jaundice is a transient phenomenon. Following major resections, by the fifth postoperative day 95 percent of patients show clinical improvement in function, with the bilirubin and alkaline phosphatase levels returning to normal by the end of the third week. The most profound changes are noted in the serum albumin, which, by the third week, is usually restored to normal.

Regeneration results from marked hypertrophy of the remaining tissue. The remaining portion of the liver responds as rapidly and completely after second and third partial hepatectomies as after an initial insult. There is experimental evidence for hepatotropic substances in portal venous blood. Insulin may represent the major anabolic factor. Very little restoration occurs after partial hepatectomy of the cirrhotic liver.

Management of the Patient. Preoperative therapy is directed at maintaining optimal liver function and correcting any defects that may be present. A diet high in calories, proteins, and carbohydrates is utilized, and the administration of albumin may be required to achieve normal levels. Vitamin K is given routinely until a normal prothrombin time results. In the presence of jaundice, other fat-soluble vitamins are added. Fresh-frozen plasma will rapidly replenish coagulation factors. Since many patients have a reduced hematocrit, transfusion with fresh whole blood rich in platelets and coagulation factors is indicated. Major hepatic resection is attended by a prohibitive mortality rate in the patient with sulfobromophthalein retention greater than 35 percent, a serum albumin level lower than 2.0 g, and an increased prothrombin time that does not respond to parenteral vitamin K.

Postoperatively, infusion of 10% glucose is continued until the patient maintains an adequate oral intake to obviate severe hypoglycemia, which has been reported. Following more intensive resections, daily administration of 25 to 50 g albumin is usually required for 7 to 10 days to maintain the serum level above 3 g/dL. Antibiotics are administered prophylactically. Analgesics and hypnotics that are detoxified by the liver are used only sparingly. Intraabdominal abscess formation and sepsis are the most common complications of major hepatic resection, occurring in 20 to 30 percent of cases. Subphrenic abscesses usually can be managed with percutaneous drainage.

Operative Procedures. *Control of Bleeding.* This may be accomplished by (1) ligation or compression of blood vessels within the substance of the remaining liver segment, (2) efforts directed at the raw surface, including cautery and argon beam coagulation, and (3) control of the main blood vessels entering the porta hepatis.

Omental grafts, peritoneal grafts, Gelfoam, micronized collagen, and rapidly polymerizing adhesives have been applied to the raw surface as local hemostatic agents. Compression of the main vessels entering the liver facilitates the demonstration of bleeding sites along the raw surface. The hepatic artery and portal vein may be compressed for over an hour without affecting hepatic structure or function.

In order to obviate uncontrollable bleeding, total vascular occlusion can be helpful for lesions located close to the major hepatic veins and the inferior vena cava. After a vascular clamp is applied to the hepatoduodenal ligament, the vena cava above and below the liver is occluded. If the patient is loaded with fluids, 1 hour of total occlusion can be tolerated.

Techniques of Resection. On the basis of new concepts of segmental anatomy, the following classification of hepatic resection is applicable (Fig. 28-21): (1) *Subsegmental,* or *wedge, resection* is removal of an area of the liver that is less than a segment and without an anatomic dissection plane. (2) *Left lateral segmentectomy* ("left lobectomy" in the old nomenclature) is excision of the liver mass to the left of the left segmental fissure along an anatomic plane. (3) *Left medial segmentectomy* is resection between the main interlobar fissure and the left segmental fissure. (4) *Left lobectomy* ("left hepatectomy") is excision of all hepatic tissue to the left of the main lobar fissure. (5) *Right lobectomy* ("right hepatectomy") is removal of the liver to the right of the main lobar fissure. (6) *Extended right lobectomy* is excision of the entire lobe plus the medial segment of the left lobe *(trisegmentectomy),* i.e., excision of all tissue to the right of the umbilical fossa, fossa for the ligamentum venosum, and the ligamentum teres.

Based on portal distribution, Couinaud has defined eight hepatic segments (see Fig. 28-2). Segmental resection of one or two contiguous segments can be performed by a transparenchy-

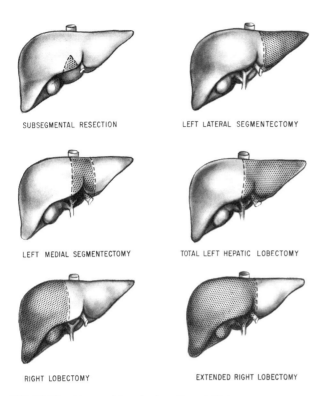

SUBSEGMENTAL RESECTION

LEFT LATERAL SEGMENTECTOMY

LEFT MEDIAL SEGMENTECTOMY

TOTAL LEFT HEPATIC LOBECTOMY

RIGHT LOBECTOMY

EXTENDED RIGHT LOBECTOMY

FIG. 28-21. Nomenclature for hepatic resection.

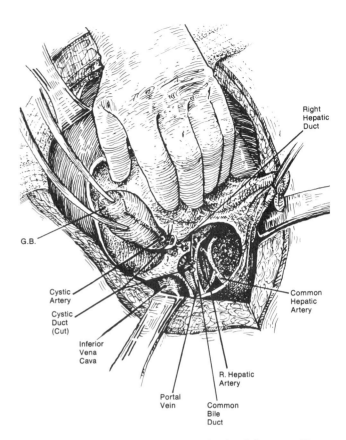

FIG. 28-23. Dissection of the hepatoduodenal ligament. (From: *Schwartz, 1981, with permission.*)

matous approach following the anatomic scissura to the vascular pedicle (Fig. 28-22).

The liver is mobilized initially by dividing the appropriate ligamentous attachments, i.e., ligamentum teres, falciform, and triangular and coronary ligaments. Dissection of the porta hepatis identifies the branches of the hepatic artery, portal vein, and biliary duct system supplying the segment or lobe to be removed (Fig. 28-23). These are individually temporarily occluded. By rotating the liver, the hepatic veins may be isolated at their junc-

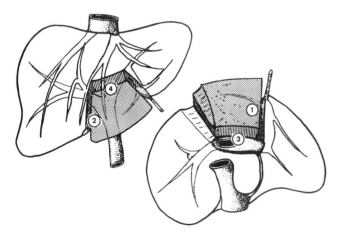

FIG. 28-22. Anterior segmentectomy IV or resection of the quadrate lobe. The different steps of the technique: (1) opening of the umbilical fissure, (2) opening of the anterior part of the main scissura, (3) ligation of the portal pedicles entering the posterior part of the quadrate lobe, and (4) transverse transection of the parenchyma. (From: *Bismuth, 1982, with permission.*)

tions with the inferior vena cava and ligated (Fig. 28-24). Glisson's capsule is then incised along the surgical plane (Fig. 28-25*A*), and the cleavage plane of the hepatic parenchyma itself is best established by means of a scalpel handle or finger to permit exposure of the larger ducts and vessels, which may be individually clamped and ligated as they are encountered. This incision is continued posteriorly until the major hepatic vein or veins are identified (Fig. 28-25*B*), double ligated, and transected. The specimen is removed. The previously occluded structures in the porta hepatis are unclamped, and if bleeding or biliary drainage from the raw surface persists, the appropriate structure is ligated. The remaining raw surface may be covered with omentum. The blood flow to and from the remaining segments of the liver must be preserved carefully.

The majority of lobar resections, even right lobe resections, can be carried out transabdominally, and it is not necessary to proceed along the outlined sequence of events for surgical excision. Finger fracture is employed for trauma but is also applied in many instances for tumor. The sequence is summarized in Fig. 28-26. One can reduce the blood flow into the liver by temporarily cross-clamping the hepatoduodenal ligament; this procedure can be carried out for 60 min using a vascular clamp intermittently. Glisson's capsule is then incised anteroinferiorly, and the incision is carried down to the region of the porta hepatis. The vessels in the porta hepatis are then picked up in the parenchyma as they enter the liver. The parenchymal dissection is continued along anatomic planes, picking up vessels and ducts as they traverse the liver, until the hepatic venous structures are

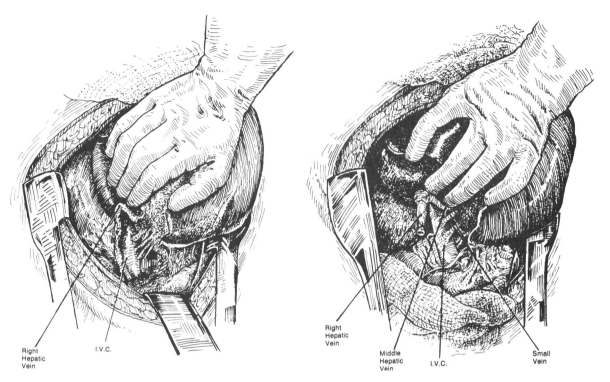

FIG. 28-24. Dissection and ligation of hepatic veins draining right lobe of liver. (From: *Schwartz, 1981, with permission.*)

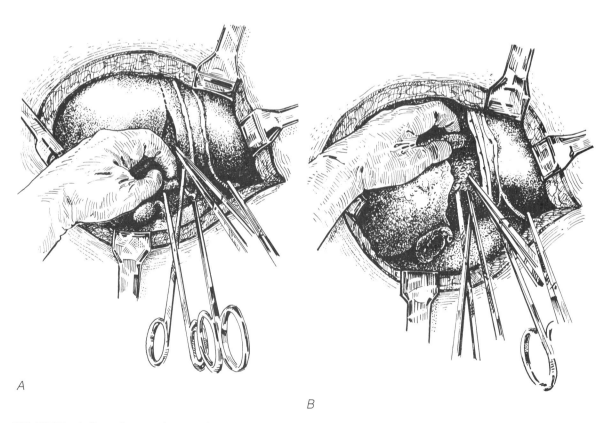

A

B

FIG. 28-25. *A.* Finger fracture of anteroinferior portion of the liver to isolate portal structures. *B.* Intra-parenchymal isolation of hepatic vein. (From: *Schwartz, 1981, with permission.*)

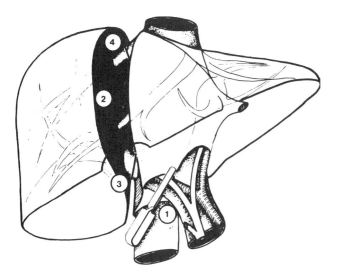

FIG. 28-26. Sequence of events: (1) temporary occlusion of structures in hepatoduodenal ligation, (2) anterior parenchymal dissection, (3) parenchymal dissection of portal structures, and (4) parenchymal dissection of hepatic vein. (From: *Bismuth, 1982, with permission.*)

also picked up in the hepatic parenchyma. Intraoperative US is helpful in locating the intraparenchymal major vessels. The operative time is significantly reduced by this technique, and blood loss is only moderately increased. An ultrasonic disruption of the parenchyma can be used to isolate vessels as they traverse the resection plane. Trisegmentectomy necessitates anatomic dissection in order to avoid interrupting veins from the remaining segment.

PORTAL HYPERTENSION

Hypertension with the portal vein and its tributaries may accompany hepatic disease or disturbance in the anatomy of the extrahepatic vascular system. As a consequence of this elevated pressure, congestion of collateral pathways is established and may be manifested by esophagogastric varices, ascites, hypersplenism, or encephalopathy.

Etiology. The etiologic factors implicated in portal hypertension are listed in Table 28-3. Increased hepatopetal flow is an infrequent cause of portal hypertension. Hepatic arterial-portal venous fistula has been reported rarely, and the diagnosis can be established by CT, MRI, or angiography. Successful treatment has been effected by ligation of the hepatic artery or by direct closure of the fistula through an arteriotomy. Splenic arteriovenous fistula is also a relatively uncommon lesion. This has a predilection for women between the ages of 20 and 50 and may become asymptomatic during pregnancy. Calcification in the left upper quadrant is suggestive, and aortography may be diagnostic. Resection of the fistula or splenic artery and splenectomy are therapeutic.

An increase in forward blood flow in the portal venous system also has been proposed as the cause of portal hypertension in patients with tropical splenomegaly and myeloid metaplasia. In patients with increased hepatopetal flow related to splenomegaly, splenectomy alone may be therapeutic.

Since the hepatic veins constitute the sole efferent vascular drainage of the liver, obstruction or increased pressure within these vessels or their radicals results in an increased sinusoidal and portal pressure. This outflow obstruction (Budd-Chiari) syndrome is associated most frequently with an endophlebitis of the hepatic veins, which may be isolated or part of a generalized thrombophlebitis process. A web in the suprahepatic vena cava has been reported to cause the syndrome in Japanese people.

The clinical picture depends on the rapidity and degree of venous obstruction. With sudden and complete obstruction, the presentation is that of an abdominal catastrophe with severe abdominal pain, nausea, vomiting, and rapid enlargement of the abdomen by ascites. This rarely occurs. More commonly, obstruction to the hepatic venous system appears to be gradual and is associated with mild to moderate abdominal discomfort and ascites. Patients should be evaluated with an inferior vena cavagram to demonstrate occluded hepatic veins. If liver biopsy defines advanced cirrhosis, transplantation should be considered. If cirrhosis is absent, a mesenteric systemic venous shunt is the treatment of choice. A peritoneovenous shunt has provided temporary relief. Definitive treatment demands a side-to-side portal systemic anastomosis, since the portal vein must act as an efferent hepatic conduit. If the inferior vena cava is obstructed, a mesenteric-atrial shunt with a conduit may be required. In some patients, the manifestations have disappeared spontaneously.

Portal hypertension secondary to impaired flow in the extrahepatic portal venous system is unique in that the hypertension usually is not complicated by hepatocellular dysfunction. Congenital atresia or hypoplasia, as an extension of the obliterative process of the umbilical vein and ductus venosus, is rare. More commonly, there is a cavernomatous transformation of the portal vein that probably represents organization and recanalization of thrombi within the vessel. The most common etiologic factor in the development of extrahepatic portal venous obstruction in childhood may be some form of infection. Bacteria may be trans-

Table 28-3
Etiology of Portal Hypertension

Increased hepatopetal flow without obstruction
    Hepatic arterial-portal venous fistula
    Splenic arteriovenous fistula
    Intrasplenic origin
Extrahepatic outflow obstruction
    Budd-Chiari syndrome
    Failure of right side of heart
Obstruction of extrahepatic portal venous system
    Congenital obstruction
    Cavernomatous transformation of portal vein
    Infection
    Trauma
    Extrinsic compression
Intrahepatic obstruction
    Nutritional cirrhosis
    Postnecrotic cirrhosis
    Biliary cirrhosis
    Other diseases with hepatic fibrosis
        Hemochromatosis
        Wilson's disease
        Congenital hepatic fibrosis
    Infiltrative lesions
    Venoocclusive diseases
        Senecio poisoning
        Schistosomiasis

mitted via a patent umbilical vein, but a history of neonatal omphalitis is rarely obtainable.

Extrahepatic obstruction also may be secondary to trauma and extrinsic compression caused by adhesions, inflammatory processes, and tumors. Isolated splenic vein thrombosis, usually a consequence of alcoholic pancreatitis, may cause esophagogastric varices. In this case, splenectomy cures the portal hypertension.

The overwhelming majority of cases of portal hypertension are related to an intrahepatic obstruction. This accounts for over 90 percent of patients with portal hypertension in most large series. A number of hepatic diseases have been implicated, but no single explanation of pathogenesis has proved totally satisfactory. The pathogenetic factors include (1) hepatic fibrosis with compression of portal venules, (2) compression by regenerative nodules, (3) increased arterial blood flow, (4) fatty infiltration and acute inflammation, and (5) intrahepatic vascular obstruction. The hepatic diseases associated with portal hypertension include nutritional cirrhosis, postnecrotic cirrhosis, schistosomiasis, biliary cirrhosis, hemochromatosis, Wilson's disease (hepatolenticular degeneration), congenital hepatic fibrosis, and infiltrative lesions.

Nutritional cirrhosis is the most common and has a worldwide distribution. In Western countries it is frequently associated with chronic alcoholism. As is true with all intrahepatic lesions, with the exception of congenital hepatic fibrosis and schistosomiasis, the major resistance to the flow of portal blood is located on the hepatic venous side of the sinusoid (postsinusoidal). Postnecrotic cirrhosis accounts for 5 to 12 percent of cases and represents progression of an acute viral hepatitis or toxic hepatic injury. Frequently, a history of viral infection is not obtainable. In the Orient, in most cases cirrhosis is a consequence of hepatitis. Both hepatitis B and C have been indicted. Biliary cirrhosis may be due to extrahepatic obstructions and secondary cirrhosis or to a primary hepatic lesion. Advanced portal cirrhosis is an almost invariable feature of hemochromatosis. Wilson's disease is characterized by alteration of hepatic function and structure and by mental deterioration. Congenital hepatic fibrosis may be related to dilatation of the intrahepatic bile ducts. It is usually an autosomal recessive disease. Clinical features include gross enlargement and firm consistency of the liver, accompanied by manifestations of portal hypertension and cholangitis. Hepatic function is not disturbed. As hepatic infestation with *Schistosoma mansoni* results in presinusoidal obstruction, there is no impairment of hepatic function until late in the course of the disease.

Pathophysiology. Portal hypertension refers to an elevated pressure within the portal venous system. This pressure reflects a dynamic, constantly fluctuating force. In addition to diurnal fluctuations, the pressure varies with changes of position, phases of respiration, and intraabdominal pressure. The normal portal pressure is less than 250 mmH$_2$O, with a mean value of 215 mmH$_2$O.

Portal pressure can be assessed by a variety of techniques. During an operative procedure, cannulation of an omental vein or the portal vein itself provides a direct recording. The pressure also can be determined by occlusive catheterization of the hepatic venule. This procedure is analogous to determination of pulmonary capillary pressure, in that it is based on the assumption that the occluding catheter creates a static column of blood

extending from the hepatic vein to the junction of the hepatic arterial and portal venous streams as they converge in the sinusoidal bed. The procedure is carried out by cardiac catheterization technique and is particularly valuable in the diagnosis of extrahepatic portal obstruction. In this situation, the presinusoidal obstruction is associated with a normal occlusive hepatic venule pressure and an elevated splenic pulp pressure.

In all instances of portal hypertension, splenic pulp pressure is elevated. Intrasplenic pressure is essentially uniform throughout the pulp and is unrelated to the size of the organ. The pressure is usually 2 to 6 mmHg higher than the pressure within the portal vein per se, a function of the direction of venous flow. Splenic pulp manometry is carried out under local anesthesia but is contraindicated in patients with a bleeding tendency, thrombocytopenia, or severe jaundice.

Splenoportography or the venous phase of celiac and superior mesenteric angiography defines the pathologic features of the portal circulation. The studies provide a demonstration of collateral veins, particularly esophagogastric varices. They also provide graphic demonstration of the site of obstruction, i.e., intrahepatic or extrahepatic. Under normal circumstances, no collaterals are visualized and a good arborization is noted in the liver (Fig. 28-27). Whenever collaterals are apparent, the diagnosis of portal hypertension is suggested. Usually one can define the coronary vein contributing to esophageal varices by this technique (Fig. 28-28).

The umbilical vein also has been used to outline the portal system. In 80 percent of these cases, the obliterated vein can be isolated and dilated to permit passage of a catheter and injection of radiopaque material into the left portal vein. The portal and hepatic veins also can be visualized by percutaneous transhepatic cannulation.

Pathologic Anatomy. The collateral vessels (Fig. 28-29) that become functional in cases of portal hypertension are classified in two groups:

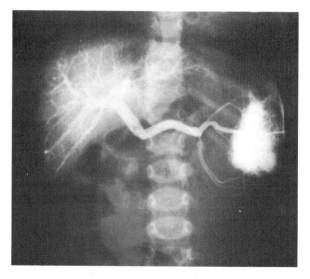

FIG. 28-27. Normal splenoportogram. Note size of injection in spleen and diffusion of radiopaque material through organ. Main splenic vein and two hilar veins are visualized. Portal vein, major branches, and intrahepatic arborization can be seen. No collateral veins are present. Note radiolucency at junction of splenic and superior mesenteric veins. (From: *Schwartz, 1964, with permission.*)

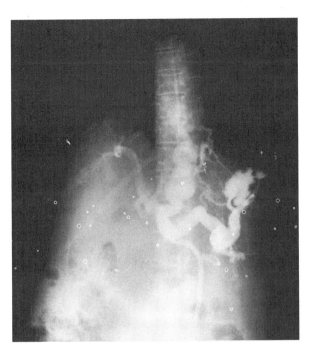

FIG. 28-28. Splenoportogram: portal hypertension secondary to intrahepatic obstruction. Note large tortuous coronary vein and inferior mesenteric vein. Intrahepatic arborization is minimal. (From: *Schwartz, 1964, with permission.*)

1. Hepatopetal circulation occurs only when the intrahepatic vasculature is normal and obstruction is limited to the portal vein. In this situation, the accessory veins of Sappey, the deep cystic veins, the epiploic veins, the hepatocolic and hepatorenal veins, the diaphragmatic veins, and the veins of the suspensory ligaments carry a limited amount of portal venous blood to the liver.
2. Hepatofugal flow is the type most commonly provided by the collateral circulation.

The vessels of the hepatofugal circulation include

1. The coronary vein, which courses to the esophageal veins and then to the azygos and hemiazygos veins with eventual termination in the superior vena cava.
2. The superior hemorrhoidal veins, which communicate by way of the hemorrhoidal plexus with hemorrhoidal branches of the middle and inferior hemorrhoidal veins and ultimately drain into the inferior vena cava.
3. The umbilical and paraumbilical veins, which communicate with superficial veins of the abdominal wall and anastomose freely with the superior and inferior epigastric veins. Dilatation occurs in 22 percent of patients with portal cirrhosis, and the advanced stage is known as the *caput medusae*. The cephalad portion of the obliterated umbilical vein may remain patent in adult life or become recanalized, contributing to the Cruveilhier-Baumgarten syndrome.
4. Retroperitoneally, the veins of Retzius, which form an anastomosis between the mesenteric and peritoneal veins and empty directly into the inferior vena cava.

In general, the collateral circulation does not effectively decompress the portal system, and the amount of blood shunted is relatively insignificant. Assuming the cross-sectional diameter of the normal portal vein to be 2 cm, then, according to Poiseuille's law, over 4000 collateral veins 0.5 cm in diameter will be needed to provide equivalent flow. The highest values of portal pressure are recorded in the group in which collateralization is more marked. In rare instances, spontaneous portal systemic shunts have effectively decompressed the portal system.

Esophagogastric Varices

As the veins become engorged, vessels in the submucosal plexus of the esophagus increase in size and become dilated. In the later stages, the overlying submucosa may disappear, and the walls of the vein actually may form a lining of the esophagus. The submucosal veins in the fundus and subfundal regions of the stomach also become varicose. Gastric varices occur predominantly in the cardiac end of the stomach but also have been found along the lesser curvature. Varices also have been demonstrated in the duodenum and ileum.

Although the presence of esophagogastric varices is, in itself, of minor consequence, rupture and bleeding from these vessels constitute the most alarming and serious complication of portal

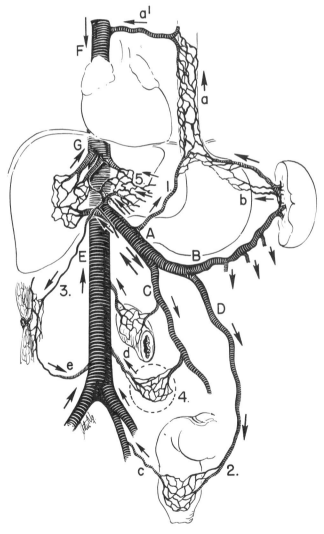

FIG. 28-29. Collateral circulation: 1, coronary vein; 2, superior hemorrhoidal veins; 3, paraumbilical veins; 4, veins of Retzius; 5, veins of Sappey; A, portal vein; B, splenic vein; C, superior mesenteric vein; D, inferior mesenteric vein; E, inferior vena cava, F, superior vena cava; G, hepatic veins; a, esophageal veins; a¹, azygos system; b, vasa brevia; c, middle and inferior hemorrhoidal veins; d, intestinal; e, epigastric veins. (From: *Schwartz, 1964, with permission.*)

hypertension. The varices are almost always associated with portal hypertension but infrequently have occurred in patients with normal pressure. Over 90 percent of adult patients demonstrate intrahepatic disease, whereas in childhood the varices are usually related to extrahepatic portal obstruction. Precipitation of the bleeding episode has been ascribed to two factors: increased pressure within the varix and ulceration secondary to esophagitis. Regurgitation of gastric juice into the esophagus has been implicated, and ulcers of the esophagus have been demonstrated in 25 percent of nonintubated and 50 percent of intubated patients. The frequency and severity of bleeding also are related to the degree of hepatocellular dysfunction.

Natural Course. Bleeding is to be anticipated in approximately 30 percent of cirrhotic patients with demonstrable varices. The elapsed time from the diagnosis of varices to the first hemorrhage varies between 1 and 187 weeks. Almost all hemorrhages occur within 2 years of the initial observation. It is difficult to predict bleeding in a patient with known varices. A prospective multicenter study using univariate analysis of endoscopic variables was able to identify patients at high risk. Etiology is a prime consideration. Varices secondary to extrahepatic portal obstruction must be considered separately, since it is rare for these patients to die of hemorrhage. By contrast, the mortality risk of repeated hemorrhage in patients with esophageal varices secondary to cirrhosis is extremely high. Approximately 70 percent of these patients die within 1 year of the first hemorrhage. Sixty percent of cirrhotic patients who have hemorrhaged once rebleed massively within 1 year.

Prophylactic sclerotherapy, propranalol, and a combination of the two modalities were of no benefit in preventing bleeding from varices in patients with alcoholic cirrhosis. A prophylactic shunt is not advised for a patient with varices that have not bled, since one cannot predict which patients will bleed; the survival is not improved, and encephalopathy may be induced. A cooperative Japanese study group has presented data suggesting that a prophylactic devascularization procedure or selective shunt can prevent bleeding without leading to a significant increase in mortality or morbidity in Child's A and B patients. There is also evidence of improved survival with prophylactic nondecompressive devasularizing procedures.

Acute Bleeding. In children, massive hematemesis almost always emanates from bleeding varices. Acute hemorrhage is usually the first manifestation of portal hypertension in children. Seventy percent of patients experience their first bleeding episode before age 7, and almost 90 percent hemorrhage before age 10.

In the adult, bleeding varices comprise one-quarter to one-third of cases of massive upper gastrointestinal tract bleeding. In cirrhotic patients, varices are the source of bleeding in approximately 50 percent, whereas gastritis is implicated in 30 percent and duodenal ulcers in 9 percent. It is now believed that peptic ulcer does not occur more frequently in cirrhotic patients. Correlation of the lesion with the severity of bleeding reveals that in the majority of cases bleeding from varices is severe hemorrhage, whereas bleeding from gastritis involves only mild to moderate blood loss.

Since the management of bleeding varices differs significantly from that of bleeding due to other causes, it is important to establish a diagnosis on an emergency basis. Physical examination may reveal the stigmata of cirrhosis. Splenomegaly is

particularly suggestive of portal hypertension. Tests of hepatic function have been used but do not have uniform reliability. Barium swallow has a significantly high percentage of false-negative results. In a series of patients with proved varices, radiographic demonstration was present in only half. Celiac or superior mesenteric arteriography will rule out an arterial bleeding site, and the venous phase of the arteriogram will demonstrate collateral venous circulation. Bleeding from a varix is not visualized. Esophageal balloon tamponade has been used as a diagnostic measure, but varices are controlled in only two-thirds of the patients, and moreover, peptic ulcer may stop bleeding after the gastric balloon is inflated. Esophagoscopy represents the single most reliable technique, since it alone defines the bleeding point. On the other hand, esophagoscopy may fail to reveal varices because of variations in transvariceal blood flow. In addition, there is a significant observer variation in the endoscopic evaluation of varices.

Treatment. The therapeutic regimen is directed at promptly controlling bleeding without further disturbing an already impaired hepatic function. Rapid control is critical in order to avoid the injurious effects of shock on hepatic function as well as the toxic effects of absorption of blood from the gastrointestinal tract. The therapeutic approaches may be divided into nonoperative and operative methods that directly approach the bleeding site and techniques that act indirectly by decreasing portal pressure (Table 28-4).

Balloon tamponade has reduced the mortality and morbidity from bleeding varices in good-risk patients, particularly those in whom the varices were secondary to extrahepatic portal hypertension or compensated cirrhosis. Little change has been noted in the mortality rate for poor-risk patients, and reports have indicated failure to control hemorrhage in 25 to 55 percent of patients. Increasing awareness of the complications associated with this technique, including aspiration, asphyxiation, and ulceration at the site of the tamponade, has reduced its use. Either a four-lumen tube should be used or a small nasogastric tube should be positioned proximal to the esophageal balloon to provide suction and prevent aspiration.

Endoscopic injection of a sclerosing solution into varices also has controlled bleeding successfully. In a large series, bleeding

Table 28-4
Control of Acute Bleeding

Nonoperative
    Direct: control of bleeding site
        Tamponade
        Esophagoscopic injection of sclerosing solution
        Esophagoscopic banding
    Indirect: reduction of portal pressure
        Vasopressin
        Propranolol
        Somatostatin
        Paracentesis
        TIPS (transjugular intrahepatic portal-systemic shunt)
Operative
    Direct control of bleeding site
        Transesophageal ligation/esophageal transection
        Devascularization (Sugiura)
        Gastroesophageal resection: colon or jejunum interposition
    Indirect: reduction of variceal pressure
        Portal-systemic shunt

was controlled in 93 percent of patients. There are significant risk factors associated with sclerotherapy. Endoscopic ligation of esophageal varices has resulted in control of bleeding equivalent to that of sclerotherapy, with fewer complications.

Drug therapy to reduce portal hypertension has employed surgical vasopressin, which acts by constricting the splanchnic arterial circulation and consequently reducing portal pressure and flow by approximately 40 percent. The drug is contraindicated in patients with angina, since generalized vasoconstriction results. Effective control has accompanied direct infusion of vasopressin, 0.2 unit/mL per minute. Isoproterenol may be given simultaneously to reduce the hemodynamic hazards of vasopressin related to its potential effect on the cardiac output. Somatostatin has been proved as effective as vasopressin in controlling acute bleeding and has less significant side effects. Paracentesis in a patient with bleeding varices and tense ascites will reduce portal pressure immediately.

Transjugular intrahepatic portal-systemic shunts (TIPS) using a self-expanding stent have reduced the portal-systemic gradient to about 10 mmHg and successfully stopped bleeding from esophagogastric varices. The procedure can be performed successfully in over 90 percent of patients. TIPS is followed by variceal rebleeding in 10 to 20 percent of patients. The incidence of shunt dysfunction ranges between 15 to 60 percent over a 6- to 12-month period. In the vast majority of cases, patency can be reestablished. TIPS is particularly applicable to control bleeding in patients with minimal hepatic reserve, in whom a transplant is indicated. The procedure obviates a portacaval shunt that compromises the transplant operation.

Surgical therapy includes transesophageal ligation and emergency portal-systemic shunt. The results of transesophageal ligation have improved significantly with stapling techniques, and results better than those with sclerotherapy have been reported. Devascularization procedures such as the Sugiura procedure have had variable success. Success rates from Western nations have not matched the Japanese success.

A more liberal use of emergency portacaval shunts to stop bleeding has been advised for the cirrhotic patients whose bleeding cannot be controlled by nonoperative measures. Emergency portal-systemic shunt remains an important option for selected patients with acute variceal bleeding. Recent experience of emergency shunt performed on 400 unselected patients within 8 h of initial contact indicated survival rates of 85, 78, and 71 percent at 30 days, 5 years, and 10 years, respectively. In most series, the mortality rate for patients with Child's class C disease remains high. The base figure that serves as a frame of reference for comparison is the mortality for patients with bleeding varices not subjected to emergency portacaval shunts, and this ranges between 66 and 73 percent. There is little question that an effective portal-systemic decompressive procedure almost always stops bleeding. No significance could be attributed to the presence or absence of jaundice, but ascites, when present, was associated with a marked reduction of survival rate.

In the pediatric age group and in adults with extrahepatic portal venous obstruction and normal liver function, despite the fact that the bleeding is often alarming, spontaneous cessation almost always occurs, and esophageal tamponade or vasopressin is rarely necessary. Hospitalization, bed rest, blood replacement, and sedation almost always suffice for patients with bleeding secondary to extrahepatic portal obstruction.

The majority of patients with acute bleeding varices is not in shock at the time of admission to the hospital, although the hematocrit is often reduced, and blood replacement may be necessary. Frozen red blood cells and fresh-frozen plasma should be employed for transfusing cirrhotic patients. This provides the clotting factors that are frequently diminished in the presence of hepatic disease and avoids the increased ammonia content and diminished platelet and prothrombin supply characteristic of old blood. There is a linearly progressive daily increment of 35 μg/dL ammonia nitrogen in banked blood, which can be responsible for exogenous hepatic coma. Therapy directed at preventing hyperammonemia and hepatic coma consists primarily of removing blood from the gastrointestinal tract. Catharsis, gastric lavage, and enemas are employed. If vasopressin has been administered, it will induce intestinal motility and effect a catharsis. A reduction in intestinal bacterial flora also contributes to the prevention of coma, and nonabsorbable antibiotic therapy is used to accomplish this.

Prevention of Recurrent Hemorrhage. Sclerotherapy has been used to eradicate varices subsequent to a major bleeding episode. This has been achieved in 80 to 90 percent of patients with an average of five injection sessions over a 9-month period. Endoscopic banding provides equivalent results. Somatostatin has been administered after bleeding was controlled initially by sclerotherapy to obviate future bleeding episodes.

The case for surgical intervention is based on the precept that a patient who has bled from esophageal varices is likely to rebleed and that subsequent bleeding episodes are associated with a higher mortality than an elective operative procedure.

Opinions differ about the role of decompressive procedures in children and in adults with portal hypertension due to extrahepatic portal venous thrombosis. Some children can be treated satisfactorily and safely without operation despite repeated episodes of variceal bleeding. The results of operation in terms of survival are significantly more encouraging in this population than in adults. Therefore, many series have suggested an aggressive approach in children with recurrent bleeding episodes. Central or distal splenorenal shunt or an anastomosis between the inferior vena cava and the superior mesenteric vein is applicable to this group of patients. The incidence of postoperative encephalopathy has been negligible. Devascularization operations such as the Sugiura procedure also have been used for these patients.

Presinusoidal obstruction (hepatic fibrosis, extrahepatic portal venous thrombosis, schistosomiasis) is characterized by portal hypertension and may be associated with normal hepatic function. In patients with hepatic fibrosis and extrahepatic portal venous obstruction, the results are gratifying; the surgical procedure generally will prevent subsequent bleeding and provide the patient with an essentially normal life expectancy. The patients with schistosomiasis are a unique group in that they are extremely liable to postshunt encephalopathy. A selective splenorenal shunt or devascularization procedure is the preferred operation.

Postsinusoidal portal hypertension is invariably complicated by impaired hepatic function. The role of decompressive procedures is least well defined for this group of cirrhotic patients. An elective procedure should be considered when the presence of an active intrahepatic process such as hyaline necrosis or acute fatty infiltration has been ruled out. Ascites that fails to respond to medical therapy, a prothrombin time that remains prolonged following parenteral administration of vitamin K, a serum bilirubin level above 3 mg/dL, a sulfobromophthalein retention greater than 20 percent, and a serum albumin level less than 2.5 g/dL are all associated with a poor postoperative prognosis. In these patients there is immediate deterioration following portacaval shunting, but this is actually no greater than after other operations of comparable severity. Child's criteria and other assessments of hepatic function are not completely predictive and relate only to the immediate postoperative course.

In patients with end-stage liver disease and marked hepatocellular dysfunction, after the bleeding had been controlled with sclerotherapy or TIPS, orthotopic liver transplantation often is appropriate.

Ascites

Etiology. The mechanisms contributing to the formation of ascites are complex and incompletely understood. Portal hypertension is regarded as a contributory but minor factor, since there is no correlation between the degree of portal hypertension and the extent of ascites. Ascites is not a usual accompaniment of extrahepatic portal venous obstruction but has been noted occasionally. Impairment of hepatic venous outflow with subsequent congestion of the liver is accompanied by an increase in the size of lymphatic vessels and increased production of the hepatic lymph that extravasates through the capsule of the liver into the peritoneal cavity. In clinical cirrhosis, there is an increase in the size of hepatic channels and an augmented flow of thoracic duct lymph. Two distinct patterns of intrahepatic vasculature have been correlated with the presence or absence of ascites. With irreversible ascites, there is an absolute decrease in the hepatic venous bed and a concomitant increase in both the portal venous and hepatic arterial beds. By contrast, when cirrhosis is unaccompanied by ascites, there is a deficit in all vascular systems.

Reduced serum osmotic pressure related to hypoalbuminemia does exert some influence. The response of patients to albumin infusion is variable, and the reduced osmotic pressure may represent the result rather than the cause of fluid accumulation. The most profound biochemical change that accompanies the formation of ascites is the retention of sodium and water. There is evidence that adrenocortical hormone is a factor in the renal retention of sodium, and higher concentrations of antidiuretic substances have been noted in the urine of patients with cirrhosis and ascites.

Treatment. Bed rest reduces the functional demand on the liver. A diet high in calories with an excess of carbohydrates and proteins, supplemented by vitamins, is directed toward improving hepatic function, while low sodium (10 to 20 meq daily) intake is essential. Fluid is usually not restricted, and potassium supplements are provided routinely to treat the potassium depletion that accompanies the formation of ascites.

Chlorothiazide is usually used to initiate diuretic therapy, and approximately two-thirds of patients will respond to this medication. Potassium supplements are required. The aldosterone antagonists are employed for patients with incipient hepatic coma. Abdominal paracentesis as an initial procedure has diagnostic value, but repeated procedures are contraindicated because they deplete the body of protein and contribute to the development of systemic hyponatremia. Furosemide (Lasix) is the most fre-

quently used drug. In some refractory cases, ethacrynic acid will help.

Emphasis on the importance of obstruction of hepatic venous outflow led to the proposal of side-to-side portacaval shunts as a method of therapy. These procedures were based on the hypothesis of providing a second outflow tract, with the portal vein acting as a hepatofugal conduit. At present, the operation is limited to patients with Budd-Chiari syndrome and to those patients who cannot be managed on a strict low-sodium diet and diuretic therapy, an unusual circumstance. Peritoneal venous shunts of the Leveen and Denver types have effectively controlled medically intractable ascites. The peritoneovenous shunt provides greater relief of ascites in a shorter period of time than does intensive medical therapy; also, ascites recurs more rapidly in medically treated patients. Improvement may be related to increased creatinine clearance and normalization of renin activity and aldosterone levels. Adverse consequence of the procedures include disseminated intravascular coagulopathy and initiation of variceal bleeding. Persistent patency of any peritoneal venous shunt is difficult to achieve.

Umbilical herniorrhaphy in a cirrhotic patient with marked ascites presents a significant risk, with hazards of leakage of ascitic fluid, infection, necrosis of the abdominal wall, and variceal bleeding due to interruption of collateral veins.

Hypersplenism

Splenomegaly, with engorgement of the vascular spaces, frequently accompanies portal hypertension. There is little correlation between the size of the spleen and the degree of hypertension. When hematologic abnormalities occur, they have been related to sequestration and destruction of the circulating cells by immune mechanisms mediated by the enlarged spleen or secretion by the hyperactive spleen of a substance that inhibits bone marrow activity. Patients may demonstrate reduction of any or all of the cellular elements of blood. The usual criteria for hypersplenism are a white blood cell count below 4000/mm^3 and a platelet count below 100,000/mm^3. Schistosomal fibrosis frequently induces hypersplenism.

No correlation exists between degree of anemia or leukopenia and the 5-year survival rate in patients. Splenectomy is rarely indicated and does not permanently reduce portal pressure. Removal of the spleen negates the possibility of performing a selective shunt. Decompression of the portal venous system is rarely indicated for treatment of hypersplenism alone. Significant hypersplenism in a patient undergoing elective surgical treatment for bleeding varices favors a splenorenal anastomosis, but both portacaval anastomosis and selective splenorenal shunt have been accompanied by reduction of the spleen and correction of the hypersplenism in about two-thirds of patients.

Encephalopathy and Coma

The development of neuropsychiatric symptoms and signs is related to natural and surgically created portal-systemic shunts and is identified by the term *portal-systemic encephalopathy*. This rarely occurs in patients with obstruction of the extrahepatic portal venous system without hepatocellular dysfunction. The neuropsychiatric syndrome usually is associated with cirrhosis and occurs in patients with marked hepatic dysfunction. Postshunt encephalopathy rarely occurs in patients with extrahepatic portal obstruction unaccompanied by hepatic dysfunction. Operative procedures that decompress the portal system also have been associated with varying incidences of encephalopathy in cirrhotic patients. With splenorenal anastomoses, the syndrome is demonstrated in 5 to 19 percent, whereas it has been reported in 11 to 38 percent following a portacaval anastomosis. The Warren distal splenorenal shunt has been associated with a reduced incidence of postoperative encephalopathy compared with portacaval and mesocaval shunts.

Hepatic coma has been related to hyperammonemia and ammonia intoxication. Both exogenous and endogenous sources contribute to the blood ammonia level. Dietary protein is the usual source of intestinal ammonia. In patients who bleed, blood within the intestinal tract is also converted into ammonia by bacteria. In the patient with hepatic disease, the ammonia formed within the intestine is carried to the liver but, because of hepatic dysfunction, cannot enter the Krebs-Henseleit (ornithine-citrulline-arginine) cycle. Endogenous urea produced within the gastrointestinal tract also represents an important source of ammonia, and gastric ammonia production from urea is a significant factor in patients with azotemia and cirrhosis. There was less deterioration of maximum urea synthesis following a selective splenorenal shunt than after total shunts.

In the cirrhotic patient with portal hypertension, the two factors implicated in the disturbed ammonia metabolism are impairment of hepatocellular function and portal-systemic collateralization. The blood ammonia level is also raised by increased ammonia production by the kidneys and by muscles that are actively contracting during delirium tremens.

The neuropsychiatric manifestations involve the state of consciousness, motor activity, and deep tendon reflexes. These have been divided into three stages: delirium, stupor, and coma. In the early stages there are mental confusion and exaggerated reflexes. The characteristic "liver flap" may be elicited. In the second stage there is an accentuation of muscular hypertonicity, to the extent of rigidity, and in the final stage there is complete flaccidity. The electroencephalogram is a sensitive indicator of portal-systemic encephalopathy, and the changes antedate clinical manifestations. Blood ammonia level does not define precisely the nature of material measured by standard tests. In patients with hepatic coma, the concentration of ammonia in the blood has correlated well with clinical progress in over 90 percent of patients. An elevated level, over 125 μg/dL, is usually associated with the clinical features of hepatic coma. Treatment with antibiotics negates the value of the test.

Treatment. Treatment is directed at (1) reducing nitrogenous material within the intestinal tract, (2) reducing the production of ammonia from the nitrogenous material, and (3) increasing ammonia metabolism. Since ammonia is an end product of protein metabolism, dietary protein must be reduced drastically to 50 g daily or less. Glucose is included in the diet, since it inhibits ammonia production by bacteria. Gastrointestinal hemorrhage frequently precipitates portal-systemic encephalopathy, with blood acting as a course of ammonia. A major factor in the prophylaxis of hepatic coma is prompt control of active bleeding. Potassium supplements are administered, particularly in patients who are receiving thiazide diuretics, because the rise in blood ammonia that accompanies diuresis has been related to hypokalemia.

The protein substrate on which bacteria can act may be reduced initially by using cathartics and enemas to purge the gastrointestinal tract. If active bleeding has occurred, infused va-

sopressin plays a dual role in temporarily stopping the bleeding as well as stimulating motility and evacuation of the intestine. Bacteria within the bowel are reduced by administering nonabsorbable antibiotics such as neomycin or kanamycin. In the presence of renal disease, kanamycin is preferred because there is less associated renal toxicity. For patients with severe renal impairment, chlortetracycline is more appropriate because it is not excreted primarily by the kidneys. Lactulose acts as a mild cathartic, and the products of its oxidation by bacteria include lactic and acetic acids, which lower the colonic pH and interfere with ammonia transfer across colonic mucosa. This drug has produced encouraging results in the treatment of hepatic encephalopathy.

Since the colon is the site of most ammonia absorption into the portal circulation, partial colectomy has been suggested as treatment of intractable encephalopathy but has not been effective.

Surgery of Portal Hypertension

The surgical therapy of portal hypertension may be divided into two major categories (1) procedures that directly attack a manifestation of portal hypertension, such as bleeding varices or ascites; and (2) procedures aimed at decreasing the portal hypertension and/or portal venous flow (Table 28-5).

Transesophageal Ligation of Varices and Esophageal Transection. Using either a transthoracic or transabdominal approach, transesophageal ligation of varices and esophageal transection have been directed at controlling bleeding varices. The end-to-end stapler has facilitated the procedure. The procedures do provide temporary control, particularly in children

Table 28-5
Operative Procedures

Control of manifestation
  Bleeding varices
    Ligation of varices
      Transthoracic
      Transabdominal
    Transection procedures
      Gastric
      Esophageal (stapler)
      Esophageal, with paraesophageal devascularization
    Resection of varix-bearing area-esophagogastrectomy
      Roux-en-Y
      Jejunal interposition
      Colonic interposition
      Reversed gastric tube
  Ascites
    Peritoneal cavity-venous shunt
Reduction of portal pressure and flow
  Splenectomy
  Portacaval shunt
    End-to-side
      End-to-side shunt with arterialization of the portal vein stump
    Side-to-side
    H graft
  Splenorenal shunt
    End-to-end
    End-to-side
    Distal (selective)
  Superior mesenteric-inferior vena cava shunt
    Side-to-end
    H graft

with extrahepatic portal block who are too small to be considered for splenorenal anastomosis.

Technique. Transthoracic ligation (Fig. 28-30) is performed through the eighth left intercostal space. The lower esophagus is freed, but the esophageal hiatus of the diaphragm is not disturbed. An umbilical tape is tightened around the esophagus just above the hiatus to minimize bleeding. A 7-cm longitudinal incision is made through all layers, and three tortuous columns of veins, coursing longitudinally and communicating with one another, are obliterated with continuous locking sutures of 3-0 chromic catgut. The esophagotomy is closed in two layers with interrupted silk sutures, and the edges of the defect in the mediastinal pleura are reapproximated. Direct ligation of varices can be performed transabdominally.

For transection of the esophagus, the peritoneal cavity is entered, and the esophagogastric junction is exposed. The lower 3 cm of the esophagus is mobilized, and care is taken to avoid the vagus nerves. The periesophageal veins are ligated. A high vertical incision is made in the anterior wall of the stomach, and the stapler is inserted, using the largest-size cartridge possible. The esophagus is tied over the center rod 2 cm above the gastric junction. The instrument is fired, resulting in simultaneous transection and reanastomosis of the esophagus (Fig. 28-31).

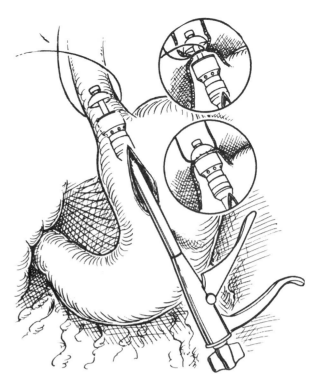

FIG. 28-31. The stapler is introduced and the esophagus securely tied over the center rod 2 cm above the gastric junction. The instrument gap is closed and the trigger fired, completing the simultaneous transection and reanastomosis. (From: *Wexler MJ: Treatment of bleeding esophageal varices by transabdominal esophageal transection with the EEA stapling instrument. Surgery 88:406, 1980, with permission.*)

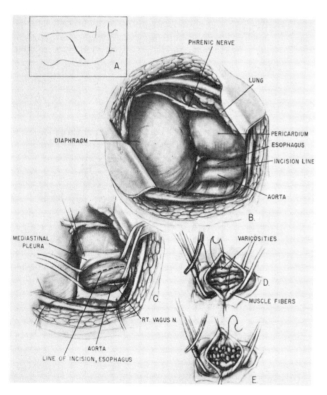

FIG. 28-30. *Transthoracic transesophageal ligation. A. Left eighth intercostal space incision. Patient in right lateral decubitus position. B. Pulmonary ligament has been divided to permit retraction of lung, and line of incision in mediastinal pleura is outlined. C. Mediastinal pleura is incised, esophagus is mobilized, and line of incision in esophagus is outlined. D. Umbilical tape is tightened around esophagus just above hiatus to minimize bleeding, and edges of esophageal incision are retracted by stay sutures. E. The tortuous columns of esophageal veins are obliterated with continuous locked suture of 3-0 chromic catgut swaged on an atraumatic needle. (From: Schwartz, 1964, with permission.)*

Esophageal Transection with Paraesophageal Devascularization. This procedure was introduced by Sugiura (Fig. 28-32), who found the perioperative mortality to be about 7 percent in elective cases and 25 percent in emergency cases. Hepatic function is not compromised, and postoperative encephalopathy does not occur. Unfortunately, American studies have not duplicated the Oriental results. The initial and late mortality rates were high, and over half the patients rebled. At least one Western report indicates that better results are achieved with a modified Sugiura procedure compared with portal-systemic results, citing better survival and a lower incidence of encephalopathy accompanied by only a slight increase in recurrent bleeding. However, the consensus is that best results are effected by a shunt. The procedure consists of esophageal transection and paraesophagogastric devascularization, splenectomy, and either selective vagotomy with pyloroplasty or highly selective vagotomy without pyloroplasty.

Procedures for Reduction of Portal Pressure. The operations directed at portal hypertension are based on the consideration that any reduction in portal pressure should decrease the potential for bleeding from varices. Splenectomy is effective only when portal hypertension is due to splenic vein thrombosis or increased flow, as in the massive splenomegaly of myeloproliferative disorders. Reduction of portal pressure by diffuse shunts between a high-pressure portal venous system and low-pressure systemic circulation was attempted. These procedures included omentopexy, posterior mediastinal packing, and trans-

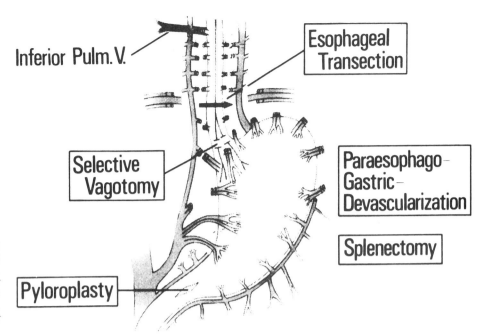

FIG. 28-32. Illustration of esophageal transection with paraesophagogastric devascularization (Sugiura procedure). (From: *Sugiura M, Futagawa S: Further evaluation of the Sugiura procedure in the treatment of esophageal varices. Arch Surg 112:1317, 1977; copyright 1977, American Medical Association.*)

position of the spleen into the thoracic cavity. Application of Poiseuille's law would suggest that any diffuse shunting would be less effective than a major portal-systemic shunt.

Functionally, portal-systemic shunts have been categorized as either totally or partially diverting portal venous flow away from the liver and also as decompressing or failing to decompress intrahepatic venous hypertension (Fig. 28-33). The end-to-side portacaval shunt prevents blood from reaching the liver by providing complete drainage of the splanchnic venous circulation to the vena cava. The associated alteration of hepatic blood flow is extremely variable, ranging from an increase of 34 percent to a decrease of 53 percent. This shunt also prevents the portal vein

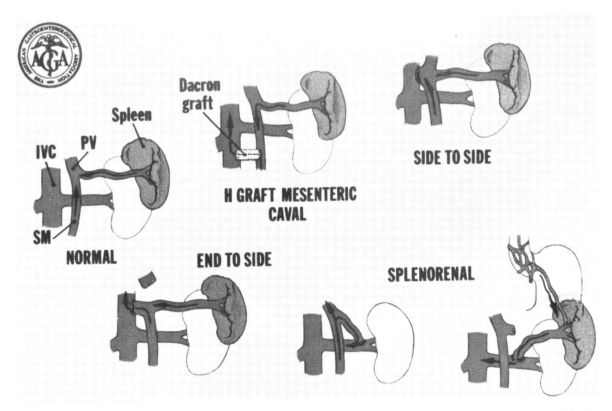

FIG. 28-33. Surgical portacaval shunts.

from serving as an efferent conduit from the liver. It has been shown that following the end-to-side shunt, the wedged hepatic vein pressure declines. Proponents of the end-to-side shunt have indicated this as the best method of preventing recurrent bleeding from varices, since it most completely decompresses the portal venous system's splanchnic circulation. In refutation, it has been shown that end-to-side and side-to-side portacaval shunts demonstrate equal flow and equivalent reductions of portal pressure.

The idea that the side-to-side portacaval shunt provides the liver with portal venous flow is erroneous in most circumstances. Injection of radioisotope into the distal portal vein results in minimal recovery in the portal vein cephalad to a side-to-side anastomosis. A variant of the side-to-side portacaval shunt uses a small-diameter (8 to 10 mm) portacaval H graft. Patients who maintained portal perfusion postoperatively had improved survival.

Accumulated evidence indicates that the side-to-side portacaval shunt converts the cephalad portion of the portal vein to an outflow from the liver. This is an important feature in patients with Budd-Chiari syndrome. Whether decompression of sinusoidal hypertension is greater with the side-to-side shunt than with the end-to-side shunt has not been defined. There is also concern as to whether the portal vein is beneficial or harmful as an efferent conduit because of a possible siphon effect that may reduce the blood available to the hepatic cell.

The classic end-to-side splenorenal shunt using the central end of the splenic vein also prevents the flow of portal venous blood to the liver if it adequately performs its prescribed function of decompressing esophagogastric varices. The other functional side-to-side shunts, including the end-to-side inferior vena cava–superior mesenteric artery shunt and the interposition of an H graft between these vessels, do not maintain hepatic perfusion with portal venous blood.

The distal splenorenal shunt proposed by Warren and associates is the one procedure that can be classified as truly selective because it decompresses esophagogastric varices while maintaining portal hypertension within the portal veins and hepatic sinusoids. Portal perfusion has been demonstrated in over 90 percent of patients with selective distal splenorenal shunts; the total hepatic blood flow has been shown to be unchanged, while the splenic venous circulation and esophagogastric veins have been reasonably decompressed. Angiographic and other studies have demonstrated that the distal splenorenal shunt loses its selectivity a few months after the operation. Prospective, randomized trials comparing the distal splenorenal shunt with nonselective (portacaval or mesocaval) shunts demonstrate no difference in survival, postoperative complications, or ascites. It is generally believed that the selective shunt is associated with a lower incidence of encephalopathy.

Selection of Procedure. Before a major shunt is performed, the presence of portal hypertension should be defined manometrically. Infrahepatic vena caval pressure should be measured to rule out caval hypertension that would interfere with splanchnic venous decompression. A splenoportogram or a selective superior mesenteric arteriogram with a venous phase should be obtained to determine the status of the major veins. Portal vein thrombosis occurs as a complication in approximately 2 percent of patients with portal cirrhosis. However, lack of visualization of the portal vein in and of itself does not establish this diagnosis, and collateral veins of Sappey must be visualized. If a

selective or central splenorenal shunt is being considered, the anatomy of the left renal vein and its relation to the splenic vein should be identified.

Estimations of hepatic blood flow are fraught with errors in interpretation, particularly in cirrhotic patients. Pressure determinations and differentials within the portal venous system, measurements of the estimated hepatic blood flow, and splenoportographic findings did not approximate true flow, and these findings could not be related to the subsequent development of postshunt encephalopathy. The increase in hepatic arterial flow subsequent to the creation of a portacaval shunt has offered a hemodynamic correlate with the patient's prognosis.

The end-to-side portacaval shunt is the procedure most commonly performed, since it is technically easiest and has been associated with the lowest incidence of thrombosis. The presence of a large caudate lobe is less compromising to this procedure than to a side-to-side shunt. For some patients with extensive adhesions from previous operative procedures in the right upper quadrant, splenorenal and mesocaval shunts are preferred. Thrombosis with or without recanalization of the portal vein (cavernomatous transformation) generally precludes a portacaval anastomosis. The Budd-Chiari syndrome, related to endophlebitis of the hepatic veins, dictates a side-to-side shunt to decompress the liver.

In reference to the factor of ascites as a determinant of the decompressive procedure, in one series 39 percent of patients with end-to-side shunts who had preoperative ascites experienced postoperative relief; in 12 percent ascites appeared after the shunt, while all patients with side-to-side shunts and ascites had permanent relief. The splenorenal shunt, which is a functional side-to-side shunt, failed to relieve ascites in 12 percent of patients, and ascites appeared after the shunt in 16 percent. It is therefore thought that ascites per se cannot be considered a significant factor in determining the shunt to be performed. Some series have indicated that the selective splenorenal shunt is not ascitogenic.

Similarly, whether previous encephalopathy and the presence of asterixis are important determinants of the type of shunt has not been resolved. In general, the selective splenorenal shunt is associated with a lower incidence of encephalopathy than other decompressive procedures, but patients with minimal hepatocellular dysfunction rarely develop encephalopathy regardless of the shunt used; devascularization operations rarely cause encephalopathy. Another consideration in shunt selection is the anticipation of performing an orthoptic transplant on the patient in the future. In this circumstance, it is preferable to perform a distal splenorenal shunt.

Selection of Patients. Ascites that failed to respond to medical therapy, a prothrombin time that remained prolonged after parenteral administration of vitamin K, serum albumin level less than 3 g/dL, serum bilirubin level greater than 1 mg/dL, and sulfobromophthalein retention greater than 10 percent are all associated with poor postoperative prognosis. Child divided patients into three groups, including those with good hepatic function (A), those with moderate hepatic function (B), and those with advanced disease and poor reserve (C). In group A are patients with a serum bilirubin level below 2 mg/dL, albumin level above 3.5 g/dL, no ascites, no neurologic disorders, and excellent nutrition. Patients in group B have bilirubin levels between 2 and 3 mg/dL, albumin levels between 3 and 3.5 g/dL, easily controlled ascites, minimum neurologic disorder, and good nutrition. In the C group, the bilirubin level is above 3 mg/dL, the albumin level is below 3 g/dL, and the ascites is poorly controlled, with advanced coma and wasting. Operative mortality following portacaval shunts in group A was zero, in group B was 9 percent, and in group C was 53 percent. There is general agreement that hepatic function is more important than the type of shunt in determining prognosis.

Portacaval Shunt Technique. This shunt (Fig. 28-34) generally is performed through a subcostal incision, but in the presence of extreme hepatomegaly or obesity, a thoracoabdominal approach may be used. The liver is retracted craniad, and a Kocher maneuver is performed to permit mobilization of the duodenum. Dissection is begun in the hepatoduodenal ligament, and the portal vein, which resides posteriorly in relation to the common bile duct, is dissected free along the entire course. Attention is then directed to dissection of the inferior vena cava. The incision in the retroperitoneum is extended, and the anterior and lateral aspects of the inferior vena cava are exposed from the renal veins to the point where the vessel passes retrohepatically. Atraumatic clamps are applied to the portal vein just above its

FIG. 28-34. End-to-side portacaval shunt technique. *A.* Subcostal transabdominal incision. *B.* Thoracoabdominal incision over ninth intercostal space. *C.* Line of incision for Kocher maneuver. Initial dissection of hepatoduodenal ligament, with isolation and retraction of common bile duct and exposure of portal vein. *D.* Completion of dissection of portal vein, with demonstration of bifurcation in porta hepatis. Dissection of retroperitoneum to clear inferior vena cava. *E.* Technique for end-to-side anastomosis. Note partially occluding clamp on anteromedial aspect of inferior vena cava. Atraumatic clamps are applied to proximal and distal portions of portal vein. *F.* An ellipse has been removed from inferior vena cava. This should measure one and one-half times diameter of portal vein. Portal vein has been transected. *G.* Distal end of portal vein has been oversewn with continuous silk sutures. (This may be handled by ligature and transfixion ligature.) Portal vein has been approximated to stoma of inferior vena cava. Two stay sutures are initially tied, and posterior layer is in place. *H.* Placement of posterior layer of sutures is facilitated by passing cranial suture into lumen of portal vein and continuing this suture to caudal limb of portal vein, where it is then passed to outside and tied. *I.* Closure of anterior row is accomplished with interrupted horizontal mattress sutures. (A continuous suture also may be employed.) *J.* Completed anastomosis. (From: *Schwartz, 1964, with permission.*)

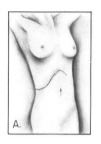
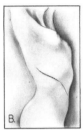

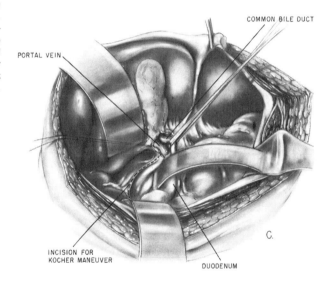

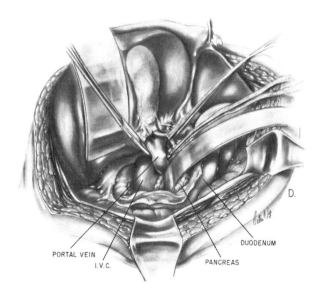

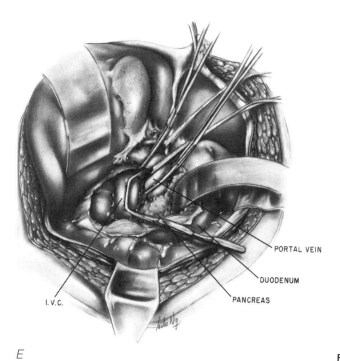

E

FIG. 28-34. *E.* Continued.

FIG. 28-34. *F–J.* Continued.

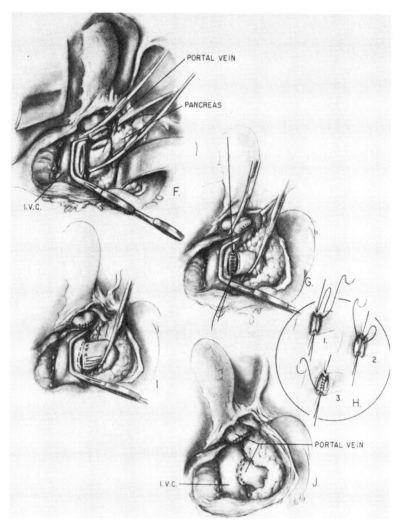

origin and just below its bifurcation, after which the vein is transected as far craniad as possible. The hepatic end is either ligated or oversewn. A sidearm, nonocclusive clamp is positioned along the anterior aspect of the inferior vena cava, and an incision is made in the inferior vena cava wall. This should be approximately one and one half times as long as the diameter of the portal vein. Employing vascular suture techniques, an anastomosis is made between the portal vein and the side of the inferior vena cava, utilizing a continuous suture that is interrupted at the two ends. Following mobilization of the portal vein and inferior vena cava, a side-to-side shunt may be performed. After the anastomosis is completed, the clamp is removed from the inferior vena cava, and then the clamp occluding the portal vein is removed. Pressure should be recorded directly from the portal vein.

Central Splenorenal Shunt. In the cirrhotic patient with postsinusoidal obstruction, the splenorenal anastomosis is not as hemodynamically efficient as the portacaval shunt and is associated with a higher incidence of recurrent bleeding. Proponents of this procedure indicate that in their experience the prevention of recurrent bleeding is similar to that resulting from a portacaval shunt, and the incidence of portal-systemic encephalopathy and persistent hypersplenism is reduced. The operation is generally employed in patients with obstruction of the extrahepatic portal venous system in which the portal vein is not available for shunting. In the pediatric age group, it is preferable to postpone this procedure until the child is 10 years old and the splenic vein is large enough to maintain its patency.

Technique (Fig. 28-35). An oblique subcostal incision or thoracoabdominal approach may be used. The transverse colon and splenic flexure are mobilized and retracted caudad, and the short gastric vessels are doubly ligated and transected. The splenophrenic splenorenal ligaments are then transected, and dissection is continued in the hilus until an ultimate pedicle of splenic artery and vein remains. The splenic vein is freed as it courses along the pancreas. The posterior peritoneum is incised just medial to the hilus of the kidney, and the left renal artery and vein are dissected free. Tapes are passed around the main renal vein and the major branches in the hilus of the kidney. Traction on these tapes establishes control of bleeding and minimizes the number of clamps interfering with the anastomosis. The splenic artery is double ligated and transected, and an atraumatic clamp is applied to the central end of the splenic vein. The splenic vein is then transected as close to the hilus of the spleen as possible and brought down to an appropriate site on the anterosuperior aspect of the renal vein. The renal artery is occluded temporarily with a bulldog clamp, and an incision is made in the renal vein. An end-to-side anastomosis is performed by initially securing two stay sutures and completing the posterior layer as a continuous suture. Anastomosis of the anterior layer is accomplished with either horizontal mattress sutures or a continuous suture.

Superior Mesenteric Vein-Inferior Vena Cava Shunt. This operation is generally used for patients with extrahepatic vein obstruction and is particularly applicable to the patient in whom a previous splenorenal shunt failed or to a small child in whom a splenorenal anastomosis is doomed to failure because of the size of the splenic vein. The operation is also advised for patients with cirrhosis if there is associated thrombosis of the portal vein or extensive scarring in the right upper quadrant that

precludes safe dissection of the portal vein or marked enlargement of the caudate lobe of the liver.

Interruption of the inferior cava, which is required for the end-to-side shunt, results in venous stasis in the lower extremity, and in the immediate postoperative period the foot of the bed must be elevated to reduce potential edema. The procedure is well tolerated by young patients, in whom postoperative chronic dependent edema of the legs is uncommon. In older patients, any edema may be readily controlled with elastic stockings.

Technique (Fig. 28-36). The peritoneal cavity is entered through a midline or right paramedian incision extending from the xiphoid process to well below the umbilicus. Upward traction on the transverse colon exposes the superior mesenteric vessels. The peritoneum is incised in the region of the superior mesenteric arterial pulse, and the superior mesenteric vein is identified and dissected free. The lateral reflection of the ascending colon is then incised along its entire length to permit medial displacement of the transverse and ascending colons and medial reflection of the ascending mesocolon. This exposes the inferior vena cava and the third portion of the duodenum. The inferior vena cava is mobilized from its origin up to the entrance of the right renal vein. The paired lumbar veins are ligated and transected. After the entire inferior vena cava has been freed, vascular clamps are applied immediately below the renal veins and at the junction of the iliac veins. The inferior vena cava is transected as far distal as possible, and the caudal stump is ligated. The right iliac vein may be left attached to the vena cava to achieve greater length. A "window" is created in the mesentery of the small intestine between the ileocolic vessels and the origin of the main ideal trunk to permit approximation of the end of the inferior vena cava to the right posterolateral aspect of the superior mesenteric vein. The anastomosis between the inferior vena cava and the superior mesenteric vein is usually performed proximal to the right colic vein, utilizing a continuous arterial suture interrupted at both ends.

Decompression is more commonly accomplished by the construction of an H graft using a 19- to 22-mm prosthesis interposed between the superior mesenteric vein and the inferior vena cava (Fig. 28-37). A high incidence of immediate and long-term thrombosis of the graft has been reported from some institutions, but this is not uniform.

Selective Splenorenal Shunt. The indications for the selective distal splenorenal shunt include a substantial portal venous flow to the liver, favorable anatomic features related to the site and patency of the splenic vein and the site and size of the left renal vein, and satisfactory liver function in the absence of marked ascites.

Technique. The operative procedure is shown in schematic fashion in Fig. 28-38. Decompression is effected through the short gastric vessels in the spleen. The spleen is not removed, and the distal or splenic side of the splenic vein is used for an anastomosis to the left renal vein. This technique can be modified by transecting the left renal vein close to the hilus of the kidney, turning and anastomosing the caval side of the renal vein to the side of the splenic vein, and ligating the splenic vein close to the confluence with the superior mesenteric vein. Included in the procedure is ligation of the coronary vein and devascularization of the stomach by ligating all vessels with the exception of the right gastric artery and the short gastric veins. Both Inokuchi and Warren have devised modifications of splenopancreatic disconnection to prevent future portal malcirculation.

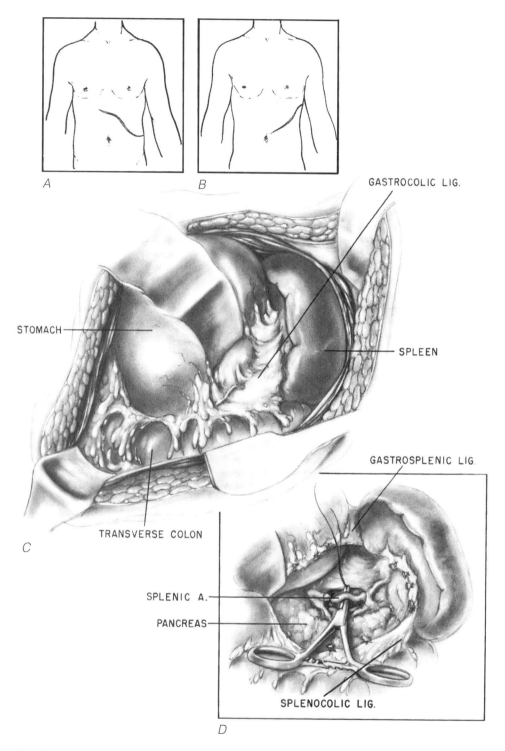

FIG. 28-35. Splenorenal anastomosis. *A.* Subcostal transabdominal incision. *B.* Thoracoabdominal incision overlying ninth intercostal space. *C.* Retraction of stomach medially. *D.* Vasae breviae have been transected. Splenic artery is ligated. Gastrosplenic and splenocolic ligament are to be transected. *E.* Spleen is mobilized so that an ultimate pedicle of splenic vein remains. *F.* Retroperitoneum has been incised, and tapes are placed around renal artery and renal vein. *G.* Tapes are placed around major tributaries of renal vein within hilus of kidney and around main renal vein. Renal artery is occluded with bulldog clamp, and traction is applied to tapes around renal vein to secure control. An ellipse is then removed from anterosuperior aspect of renal vein. This should be one and one-half times diameter of splenic vein. Vascular clamp has been applied to splenic vein, and spleen is removed; as long a segment of splenic vein as possible is retained. *H.* Splenic vein is brought down and anastomosed to stoma that has been created in main renal vein. Occlusive tapes have been removed from splenic vein and renal artery. (From: *Schwartz, 1964, with permission.*)

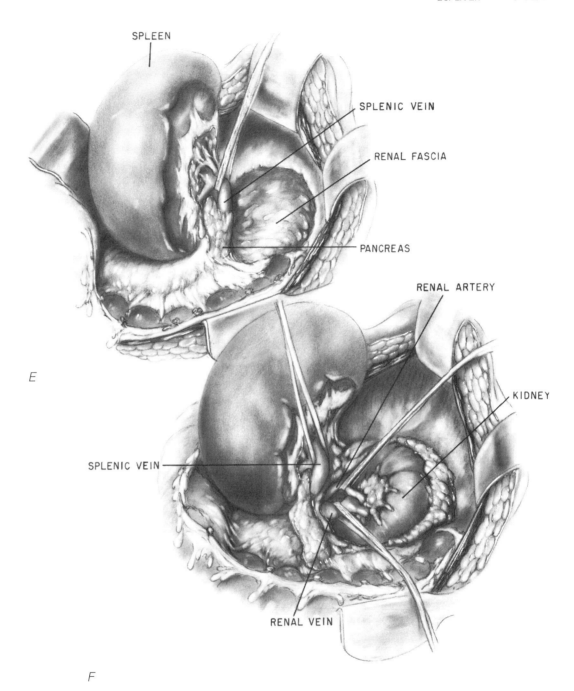

SPLEEN

SPLENIC VEIN

RENAL FASCIA

PANCREAS

RENAL ARTERY

KIDNEY

SPLENIC VEIN

RENAL VEIN

E

F

FIG. 28-35. *E–F.* Continued.

Complications of Portal-Systemic Shunts. The complications uniquely associated with portal-systemic shunting procedures occur intraoperatively or during the postoperative period. The intraoperative complications include bleeding and a nonshuntable situation, whereas the postoperative complications include rebleeding, hepatic failure, changes in cardiorespiratory dynamics, the hepatorenal syndrome, and delayed complications of hemosiderosis, peptic ulcer, and portal-systemic encephalopathy.

The complication of intraoperative bleeding can be reduced by correction of coagulation defects and by continuing the infusion of vasopressin during the operative procedure. A non-shuntable situation may be related to extension of cavernomatous transformation of the portal vein to involve the superior mesenteric vein and the splenic vein. In these patients, the so-called makeshift shunt, using large collaterals, is generally doomed to failure. The circumstance of caval hypertension caused by hypertrophy and nodularity of the caudate lobe encroaching on the infrahepatic vena cava has been referred to previously. Attempts have been made to shunt between the superior mesenteric vein and the atrium.

Early postoperative bleeding is usually related to thrombosis of a reconstructed shunt. This can be defined by splenoportography in the case of a portacaval shunt. The rapid onset of ascites

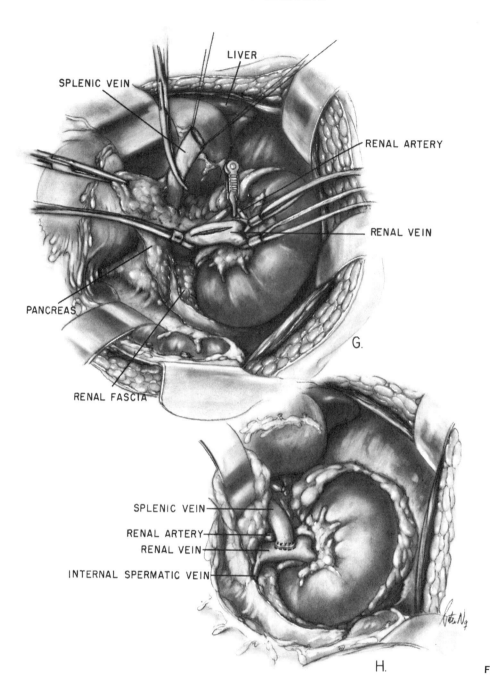

FIG. 28-35. *G–H.* Continued.

during the early postoperative period may be managed by restriction of sodium intake and the administration of diuretic agents. In this circumstance, the early institution of a peritoneal-venous shunt has provided dramatic relief. Renal failure following a portal-systemic shunt is not predictable, and treatment consists of supportive measures. The early postoperative development of hepatic coma is an ominous sign.

Portacaval Shunt for Glycogen Storage Disease and Hypercholesterolemia

In 1963, Starzl and associates performed a portacaval transposition on an 8-year-old child with type III glycogen storage disease, which resulted in resumption of weight gain and growth rate. Since then, several investigators have reported clinical improvement following an end-to-side portacaval shunt in children with type I glycogen storage disease in which the enzyme glucose 6-phosphatase is deficient or absent. Intravenous hyperalimentation for 2 to 3 weeks prior to surgery is advised to reduce liver size, restore bleeding time to normal, correct acidosis and hypoglycemia, and promote a favorable outcome of the shunting procedure. Children who have undergone diversion of portal flow have shown no evidence of encephalopathy. Portacaval shunts also have been applied with success to a few patients with homozygous hypercholesterolemia and to an occasional patient with heterozygous type 2 hypercholesterolemia.

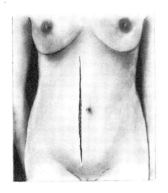

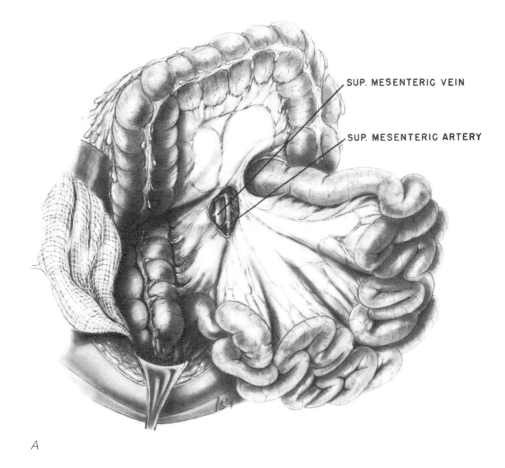

SUP. MESENTERIC VEIN

SUP. MESENTERIC ARTERY

A

FIG. 28-36. Superior mesenteric-inferior vena cava shunt, right route. *A. Insert:* Right paramedian incision. Traction applied to transverse colon exposes superior mesenteric artery and vein. Peritoneum over vessels has been incised. Right side of superior mesenteric vein is dissected carefully to preserve colic branches. *B.* Lateral reflection of ascending colon has been incised, and colon is reflected medially. This has exposed inferior vena cava and third portion of duodenum. Inferior vena cava is mobilized from convergence of two common iliac veins up to entrance of right renal vein. In course of this dissection, paired lumbar veins are ligated in continuity and transected. *C.* Inferior vena cava has been transected. Stay sutures are inserted into adventitia of proximal vena cava, to be used for traction and orientation. Window has been created in small intestinal mesentery between ileocolic vessels and origin of main ileal trunk. *D.* Distal end of inferior vena cava has been oversewn. Proximal inferior vena cava is passed anterior to third portion of duodenum and through window in mesentery. Anastomosis is made between end of inferior vena cava and right posterolateral aspect of superior mesenteric vein. (From: *Schwartz, 1964, with permission.*)

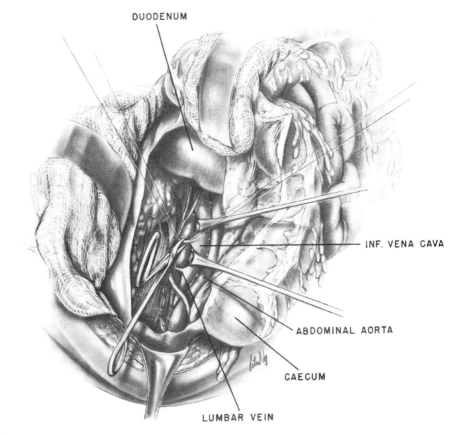

DUODENUM

INF. VENA CAVA

ABDOMINAL AORTA

CAECUM

LUMBAR VEIN

B

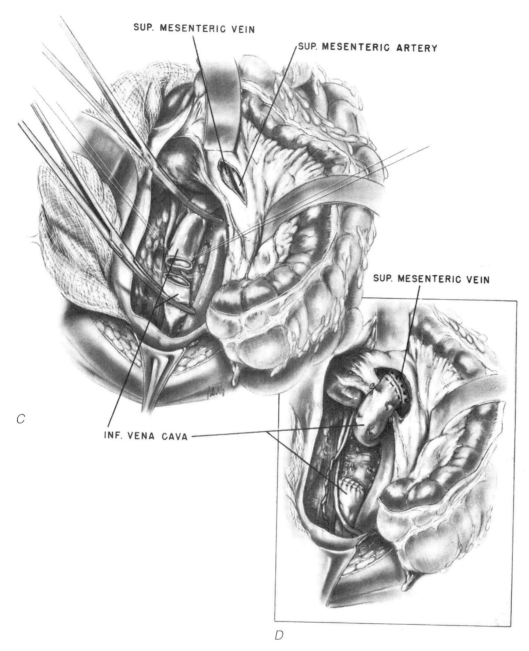

SUP. MESENTERIC VEIN

SUP. MESENTERIC ARTERY

SUP. MESENTERIC VEIN

C

INF. VENA CAVA

D

FIG. 28-36. *C–D.* Continued.

FULMINANT HEPATIC FAILURE

Fulminant hepatic failure refers to the clinical syndrome characterized by sudden, severe impairment of hepatic function generally as a consequence of massive necrosis of liver cells. In most instances, the cause is acute hepatitis of viral origin. Massive necrosis and dysfunction have been reported with Reye's syndrome, as a rarity in pregnancy, and following exposure to a variety of drugs. Circulatory necrosis of hepatic cells has been reported following vasopressor therapy and following the inadvertent intraarterial infusion of vasopressin into the hepatic artery.

General supportive therapy is directed at reducing hyperammonemia. A number of intercessions are all aimed at removing so-called noxious elements from the affected patient and preserving life long enough for the liver to regenerate sufficiently. Included in this category are hemodialysis and peritoneal dialysis, exchange transfusion, plasmapheresis, asanguineous hypothermic total-body perfusion, ex vivo perfusion of a liver of the same or different species, and cross-circulation with a human being or a subhuman primate. Orthotopic liver transplantation has led to the survival of several moribund patients and is now the treatment of choice.

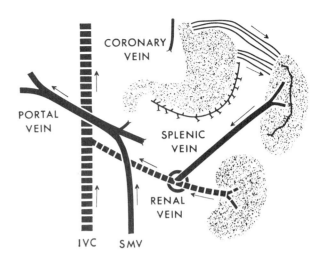

FIG. 28-38. Diagrammatic illustration of the selective distal spleno-renal shunt. Note coronary vein ligation and gastric devascularization that protects the vasa brevia and other collateral vessels from esophagus and diaphragm. (From: *Salam AA, Warren WD, et al: Hemodynamic contrasts between selective and total portal systemic decompression. Ann Surg 173:827, 1971, with permission.*)

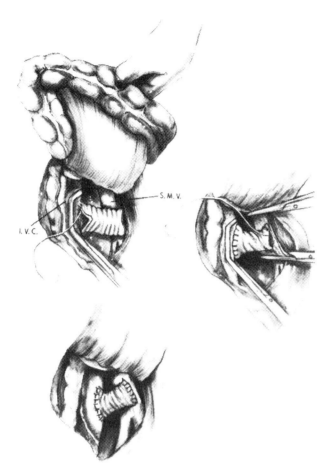

FIG. 28-37. H graft (interposition mesocaval shunt). The transverse colon is elevated, and the superior mesenteric vein is dissected free at the route of the small bowel mesentery. A partially occlusive clamp is applied to the infrarenal vena cava, and an anastomosis is made between the vena cava and a 19- to 22-mm Dacron prosthesis. Occlusive clamps are then placed on the superior mesenteric vein, and the graft is anastomosed in an end-to-side fashion to the superior mesenteric vein. Heparinization is unnecessary.

Patients in fulminant hepatic failure who are categorized at the comatose level with spasticity have a mortality of between 85 and 90 percent; this approaches 100 percent when the flaccidity stage is reached. The effect of any form of therapy is difficult to evaluate because spontaneous recovery occurs in 10 to 20 percent of patients.

Bibliography

General

Foster JH, Berman MM: *Solid Liver Tumors.* Philadelphia, Saunders, 1977.

Schwartz SI: *Surgical Diseases of the Liver.* New York, McGraw-Hill, 1964.

Sherlock S: *Diseases of the Liver and Biliary System,* 6th ed. Oxford, Blackwell Scientific Publications, 1981.

Anatomy

Bismuth H: Surgical anatomy and anatomical surgery of the liver. *World J Surg* 6:2, 1982.

Couinaud C: *Controlled Hepatectomies and Exposure of the Intrahepatic Bile Ducts.* Paris, C Couinaud, 1981.

Special Studies

Castaing D, Emond J, et al: Utility of operative ultrasound in the surgical management of the liver tumors. *Ann Surg* 204:600, 1986.

Kemeny MM, Sugarbaker PH, et al: A prospective analysis of laboratory tests and imaging studies to detect hepatic lesions. *Ann Surg* 195:163, 1982.

Hepatic Abscesses

Branum GD, Tyson GS, et al: Hepatic abscess: Changes in etiology, diagnosis, and management. *Ann Surg* 212:655, 1990.

Donovan AJ, Yellin AE, Ralls PW: Hepatic abscess. *World J Surg* 15:162, 1991.

Gerzof SG, Johnson WC, et al: Intrahepatic pyogenic abscesses: Treatment by percutaneous drainage. *Am J Surg* 149:487, 1985.

Huang CJ, Pitt HA, et al: Pyogenic hepatic abscess. *Ann Surg* 223:600, 1996.

Johnson RD, Mueller PR, et al: Percutaneous drainage of pyogenic liver abscesses. *AJR* 144:463, 1985.

Klatchko BA, Schwartz SI: Diagnostic and therapeutic approaches to pyogenic abscess of the liver. *Surg Gynecol Obstet* 168:332. 1989.

McDonald AP, Howard RJ: Pyogenic liver abscess. *World J Surg* 4:369, 1980.

Robert JH, Mirescu D, et al: Critical review of the treatment of pyogenic hepatic abscess. *Surg Gynecol Obstet* 174:97, 1992.

Cysts and Benign Tumors

Baer HU, Dennison AR, et al: Enucleation of giant hemangiomas of the liver: Technical and pathologic aspects of a neglected procedure. *Ann Surg* 216:673, 1992.

Baum JK, Brockstein JJ, et al: Possible association between benign hepatomas and oral contraceptives. *Lancet* 2:926, 1973.

Belli L, del Favero E, et al: Resection virus pericystectomy in the treatment of hydatidosis of the liver. *Am J Surg* 145:239, 1983.

Brady MS, Coit DG: Focal nodular hyperplasia of the liver. *Surg Gynecol Obstet* 171:377, 1990.

DeMaioribus CA, Lally KP, et al: Mesenchymal hamartoma of the liver: A 35-year review. *Arch Surg* 125:598, 1990.

Edmondson HA, Reynolds TB, et al: Regression of liver cell adenomas associated with oral contraceptives. *Ann Intern Med* 86:180, 1977.

Farges O, Daradkeh S, Bismuth H: Cavernous hemangiomas of the liver: Are there any indications for resection? *Wold J Surg* 19:19, 1995

Ker CG, Chen JS, et al: Laparoscopic fenestration for a giant liver cyst. *Endoscopy* 26:754, 1994.

Kerlin P, Davis GL, et al: Hepatic adenoma and focal nodular hyperplasia: Clinical, pathologic, and radiologic features. *Gastroenterology* 84:994, 1983.

Kuo PC, Lewis WD, Jenkins RL: Treatment of giant hemangiomas of the liver by enucleation. *JACS* 178:49, 1994.

Langer JC, Rose DB, et al: Diagnosis and management of hydatid disease of the liver: A 15-year North American experience. *Ann Surg* 199:412, 1984.

Leese T, Farges O, Bismuth H: Liver cell adenomas: A 12-year surgical experience from a specialist hepato-biliary unit. *Ann Surg* 208:558, 1988.

Libutti SK, Starker PM: Laparoscopic resection of a nonparasitic liver cyst. *Surg Endosc* 8:1105, 1994.

Moazam F, Rodgers BM, et al: Hepatic artery ligation for hepatic hemangiomatosis of infancy. *J Pediatr Surg* 18:120, 1983.

Moreno González E, Rico Selas P, et al: Results of surgical treatment of hepatic hydatidosis: Current therapeutic modifications. *World J Surg* 15:254, 1991.

Nagorney DM: Benign hepatic tumors: focal nodular hyperplasia and hepatocellular adenoma. *World J Surg* 19:12, 1995.

Newman KD, Torress VE, et al: Treatment of highly symptomatic polycystic liver disease: Preliminary experience with a combined hepatic resection-fenestration procedure. *Ann Surg* 212:30, 1990.

Schwartz SI, Husser WC: Cavernous hemangioma of the liver. *Ann Surg* 205:456, 1987.

Shortell CK, Schwartz SI: Hepatic adenoma and focal nodular hyperplasia. *Surg Gynecol Obstet* 173:426, 1991.

Stanley P, Geer GD, et al: Infantile hepatic hemangiomas: Clinical features, radiologic investigations, and treatment of 20 patients. *Cancer* 64:936, 1989.

Vauthey JN, Maddern GJ, Blumgart LH: Adult polycystic disease of the liver. *Br J Surg* 78:524, 1991.

Yamagata M, Kanematsu T, et al: Management of hemangioma of the liver: Comparison of results between surgery and observation. *Br J Surg* 78:1223, 1991.

Malignant Tumors

Bismuth H, Chiche L, et al: Liver resection versus transplantation for hepatocellular carcinoma in cirrhotic patients. *Ann Surg* 218:145, 1993.

Bismuth H, Adam R, et al: Resection of nonresectable liver metastases from colorectal cancer after neoadjuvant chemotherapy. *Ann Surg* 224:509, 1996.

Chang E, Schneider PD, et al: A prospective randomized trial of regional versus sytemic continuous 5-fluorodeoxyuridine chemotherapy in the treatment of colorectal liver metastases. *Ann Surg* 206:685, 1987.

Craig JR, Peters RL, et al: Fibrolamellar carcinoma of the liver. *Cancer* 46:372, 1980.

Doci R, Gennari L, et al: One hundred patients with hepatic metastases from colorectal cancer treated by resection: Analysis of prognostic determinants. *Br J Surg* 78:797, 1991.

Farmer DG, Rosove MH, et al: Current treatment modalities for hepatocellular carcinoma. *Ann Surg* 219:236, 1994.

Griffith KD, Sugarbaker PH, Chang AE: Repeat hepatic resections for colorectal metastases. *Surgery* 107:101, 1990.

Gutierrez O, Schwartz SI: *Diagnostic Atlas of Hepatic Lesions.* New York, McGraw-Hill, 1984.

Huguet C, Bona S, et al: Repeat hepatic resection for primary and metastatic carcinoma of the liver. *Surg Gynecol Obstet* 171:398, 1990.

Iwatsuki S, Startzl TE, et al: Hepatic resection versus transplantation for hepatocellular carcinoma. *Ann Surg* 214:221, 1991.

Kanematsu T, Takenaka K, et al: Limited hepatic resection effective for selected cirrhotic patients with primary liver cancer. *Ann Surg* 199:51, 1984.

Kemeny M, Goldberg D, et al: Results of a prospective randomized trial of continuous regional chemotherapy and hepatic resection as treatment of hepatic metastases from colorectal primaries. *Cancer* 57:492, 1986.

King DR, Ortega J, et al: The surgical management of children with incompletely resected hepatic cancer is facilitated by intensive chemotherapy. *J Pediatr Surg* 26:1074, 1991.

Lee NW, Wond J, Ong GB: The surgical management of primary carcinoma of the liver. *World J Surg* 6:66, 1982.

Lo CM, Lai EC, et al: Resection for extrahepatic recurrence of hepatocellular carcinoma. *Br J Surg* 81:1029, 1994.

Locker GY, Doroshow JH, et al: The clinical features of hepatic angiosarcoma: A report of four cases and a review of the English literature. *Medicine* 58:48, 1979.

McEntee GP, Nagorney DM, et al: Cytoreductive hepatic surgery for neuroendocrine tumors. *Surgery* 108:1091, 1990.

Maton PN, Camilleri M, et al: Role of hepatic arterial embolization in carcinoid syndrome. *Br Med J* 287:932, 1983.

Mazzaferro V, Regalia E, et al: Liver transplantation for the treatment of small hepatocellular carcinomas in patients with cirrhosis. *N Engl J Med* 334:693, 1996.

Nagorney DM, Adson MA, et al: Fibrolamellar hepatoma. *Am J Surg* 149:113, 1985.

Nagorney DM, vanHeerden JA, et al: Primary hepatic malignancy: Surgical management and determinants of survival. *Surgery* 106:740, 1989.

Nagasue N, Yukaya H, et al: Clinical experience with 118 hepatic resections for hepatocellular carcinoma. *Surgery* 99:694, 1986.

Ni Y-H, Chang M-H, et al: Hepatocellular carcinoma in childhood: Clinical manifestations and prognosis. *Cancer* 68:1737, 1991.

Paquet KJ, Koussouris P, et al: Limited hepatic resection for selected cirrhotic patients with hepatocellular or cholangiocellular carcinoma: A prospective study. *Br J Surg* 78:459, 1991.

Registry of Hepatic Matastases: Resection of the liver for colorectal carcinoma metastases: A multi-institutional study of indications for resection. *Surgery* 103:278, 1988.

Schwartz SI: Hepatic resection for noncolorectal nonneuroendocrine metastases. *World J Surg* 19:72, 1995.

Schwartz SI, Jones LS, et al: Assessment of treatment of intrahepatic malignancies using chemotherapy via an implantable pump. *Ann Surg* 201:560, 1985.

Sitzman JV, Abrams R: Improved survival for hepatocellular cancer with combination surgery and multimodality treatment. *Ann Surg* 217:149, 1993.

Stone MD, Cady B, et al: Surgical therapy for recurrent liver metastases from colorectal cancer. *Arch Surg* 125:718, 1990.

Tartter PI, Slater G, et al: Screening for liver metastases from colorectal cancer with carcinoembryonic antigen and alkaline phosphatase. *Ann Surg* 193:357, 1981.

Vauthey JN, Klimstra D, et al: Factors affecting long-term outcome after hepatic resection for hepatocellular carcinoma. *Am J Surg* 169:28, 1995.

Hepatic Resection

Bismuth H, Denneson AR: Segmental liver resection. *Adv Surg* 26:189, 1993.

Bismuth H, Castaing D, Garden OJ: Major hepatic resection under total vascular exclusion. *Ann Surg* 210:13, 1989.

Bismuth H, Houssin D, Castaing D: Major and minor segmentectomies "reglees" in liver surgery. *World J Surg* 6:10, 1982.

Couinaud C: *Controlled Hepatectomies and Exposure of the Intrahepatic Bile Ducts: Anatomical and Technical Study.* Paris, C Couinaud, 1981.

Schwartz SI: Liver resection. *Mod Tech Surg* 10:1, 1981.

Starzl TE, Bell RH, et al: Hepatic trisegmentectomy and other liver resections. *Surg Gynecol Obstet* 141:429, 1975.

Portal Hypertension

Borgonovo G, Costantini M, et al: Comparison of a modified Sugiura procedure with portal systemic shunt for prevention of recurrent variceal bleeding in cirrhosis. *Surgery* 119:214, 1996.

Burroughs AK, Hamilton G, et al: A comparison of sclerotherapy with staple transection of the esophagus for the emergency control of bleeding from esophageal varices. *N Engl J Med* 321:857, 1989.

Capussotti L, Vergara V, et al: A critical appraisal of the small-diameter portacaval H graft. *Am J Surg* 170:10, 1995.

Collins JC, Rypins EB, Sarfeh IJ: Narrow-diameter portacaval shunts for management of variceal bleeding. *World J Surg* 18:211, 1994.

Crecelius SA, Soulen MC: Transjugular intrahepatic portosystemic shunts for portal hypertension. *Gastroenterol Clin North Am* 24:201, 1995.

Dowling JB: Ten years' experience with mesocaval grafts. *Surg Gynecol Obstet* 149:518, 1979.

Fulenwider JT, Smith RB III, et al: Peritoneovenous shunts: Lessons learned from an eight-year experience with 70 patients. *Arch Surg* 119:1133, 1984.

Garrett KO, Reilly JJ Jr, et al: Bleeding esophageal varices: Treatment by sclerotherapy and liver transplantation. *Surgery* 104:819, 1988.

Goff JS, Reveille RM, Stiegmann GV: Three years experience with endoscopic varicel ligation for treatment of bleeding varices. *Endoscopy* 24:401, 1992.

Grauer S, Schwartz SI: Extrahepatic portal hypertension: Retrospective analysis. *Ann Surg* 189:566, 1979.

Halff G, Todo S, et al: Liver transplantation for the Budd-Chiari syndrome. *Ann Surg* 211:43, 1990.

Hashizume M, Kitano S, et al: Endoscopic injection sclerotherapy for 1000 patients with esophageal varices: A nine-year prospective study. *Hepatology* 15:69, 1992.

Henderson JM: The role of distal splenorenal shunt for long-term management of variceal bleeding. *World J Surg* 18:205, 1994.

Inokuchi K: Present status of surgical treatment of esophageal varices in Japan: A nationwide survey of 3588 patients. *World J Surg* 9:171, 1985.

Jalan R, Redhead DN, Hayes PC: Transjugular intrahepatic portasystemic stent-shunt in the treatment of variceal hemorrhage. *Br J Surg* 82:1158, 1995.

Jenkins SA, Shields R, et al: The management of gastrointestinal haemorrhage by somatostatin after apparently successful endoscopic injection sclerotherapy for bleeding oesophageal varices. *J Hepatol* 12:296, 1991.

Johnson WC, Nabseth DC, et al: Bleeding esophageal varices: Treatment with vasopressin, transhepatic embolization and selective splenorenal shunting. *Ann Surg* 195:393, 1982.

Kerlan RK Jr, LaBerge JM, et al: Transjugular intrahepatic portosystemic shunts: Current status. *AJR* 164:1059, 1995.

Klein AS, Sitzmann JV, et al: Current management of the Budd-Chiari syndrome. *Ann Surg* 212:144, 1990.

Langer B, Taylor BR, et al: Further report of a prospective randomized trial comparing distal splenorenal shunt with end-to-side portacaval shunt: An analysis of encephalopathy, survival, and quality of life. *Gastroenterology* 88:424, 1985.

McKee RF, Garden OJ, Carter DC: Injection sclerotherapy for bleeding varices: Risk factors and complications. *Br J Surg* 78:1098, 1991.

Madras PN: Portacaval shunt for familial heterozygous hypercholesterolemia. *Surg Gynecol Obstet* 152:187, 1981.

Millikan WJ, Warren WD, et al: The Emory prospective randomized trial: Selective versus nonselective shunt to control variceal bleeding: Ten-year follow-up. *Ann Surg* 201:712, 1985.

Mosimann R, Marquis C, et al: Long-term follow-up after a distal splenorenal shunt procedure: A clinical and hemodynamic study. *Am J Surg* 145:253, 1983.

Nakao K, Adachi S, et al: Radical operation for Budd-Chiari syndrome associated with obstruction of the inferior vena cava: Report of six patients. *J Cardiovasc Surg* 25:216, 1984.

The North Italian Endoscopic Club for the Study and Treatment of Esophageal Varicies: Prediction of the first variceal hemorrhage in patients with cirrhosis of the liver and esophageal varices: A prospective multicenter study. *N Engl J Med* 319:983, 1988.

Orloff MJ: Emergency shunt for variceal bleeding. *JACS* 181:386, 1995.

Orloff MJ, Girard B: Long term results of treatment of Budd-Chiari syndrome by side to side portacaval shunt. *Surg Gynecol Obstet* 168:33, 1989.

Orloff MJ, Orloff MS, Rambotti M: Treatment of bleeding esophagogastric varices due to extrahepatic portal hypertension: Results of portal-systemic shunts during 35 years. *J Pediatr Surg* 29:142, 1994.

Orozco H, Takahashi T, et al: The Sugiura procedure for patients with hemorrhagic portal hypertension secondary to extrahepatic portal vein thrombosis. *Surg Gynecol Obstet* 173:45, 1991.

The PROVA Study Group: Prophylaxis of first hemorrhage from esophageal varices by sclerotherapy, propranolol or both in cirrhotic patients: A randomized multicenter trial. *Hepatology* 14:1016, 1991.

Raia S, Mies S, et al: Surgical treatment of portal hypertension in schistosomiasis. *World J Surg* 8:738, 1984.

Resnick RK, Langer BR, et al: Results and hemodynamic changes after interposition mesocaval shunt. *Surgery* 95:275, 1984.

Rikkers LF, Jin G: Emergency shunt: Role in the present management of variceal bleeding. *Arch Surg* 130:472, 1995.

Ringe B, Lang H, et al: Role of liver transplantation in management of esophageal variceal hemorrhage. *World J Surg* 18:233, 1994.

Salam AA, Warren WD, Tyras DH: Splenic vein thrombosis: Diagnosable and curable form of portal hypertension. *Surgery* 74:961, 1973.

Santangelo WC, Dueno MI, et al: Prophylactic sclerotherapy of large esophageal varices. *N Engl J Med* 318:814, 1988.

Schwartz SI: Complications or portal-systemic shunting procedures, in Beebe H (ed): *Complications of Vascular Disease*. Philadelphia, Lippincott, 1973.

Spence RAJ, Johnston GW: Results in 100 consecutive patients with stapled esophageal transection for varices. *Surg Gynecol Obstet* 160:323, 1985.

Spina GP, Santambrogio R, et al: Emergency portosystemic shunt in patients with variceal bleeding. *Surg Gynecol Obstet* 171:456, 1990.

Stanley MM, Ochi S, et al: Peritoneovenous shunting as compared with medical treatment in patients with alcoholic cirrhosis and massive ascites. *N Engl J Med* 321:1989.

Steigmann GV, Goff JS, et al: Endoscopic sclerotherapy as compared with endoscopic ligation for bleeding esophageal varices. *N Engl J Med* 326:1527, 1992.

Sugiura M, Futagawa S: Esophageal transection with paraesophagogastric devascularizations (the Sugiura procedure) in the treatment of esophageal varices. *World J Surg* 8:673, 1984.

Terblanche J, Kahn D, Bornman PC: Long-term injection sclerotherapy treatment for esophageal varices: A 10-year prospective evaluation. *Ann Surg* 210:725, 1989.

Triger DR, Smart HL, et al: Prophylactic sclerotherapy for esophageal varices: Long-term results of a single-center trial. *Hepatology* 13:117, 1991.

Warren WD: Splenopancreatic disconnection. *Ann Surg* 204:346, 1986.

Glycogen Storage Disease and Hypercholesterolemia

Folkman J, Philippart A, et al: Portacaval shunt for glycogen storage disease: Value of prolonged intravenous hyperalimentation before surgery. *Surgery* 72:306, 1972.

Starzl TE, Putnam CW: Portacaval shunt and hyperlipemia. *Arch Surg* 113:71, 1978.

CHAPTER 29

Gallbladder and Extrahepatic Biliary System

Seymour I. Schwartz

ANATOMY

Duct System. The extrahepatic biliary system begins with the hepatic ducts and ends at the stoma of the common bile duct in the duodenum. The right hepatic duct is formed by the intrahepatic confluence of dorsocaudal and ventrocranial branches. The former enters with a sharp curve, which accounts for the fact that calculi are less common in this segment. The left hepatic duct is longer than the right and has a greater propensity for dilatation as a consequence of distal obstruction. The two ducts join to form a common hepatic duct that is 3 to 4 cm in length. It is then joined at an acute angle by the cystic duct to form the common bile duct (Fig. 29-1).

The common bile duct is approximately 8 to 11.5 cm in length and 6 to 10 mm in diameter. The upper portion is situated in the free edge of the lesser omentum, to the right of the hepatic artery and anterior to the portal vein. The middle third of the common duct curves to the right behind the first portion of the duodenum, where it diverges from the portal vein and hepatic arteries. The lower third of the common bile duct curves more to the right behind the head of the pancreas, which it grooves, and enters the duodenum at the hepatopancreatic ampulla (of Vater), where it is frequently joined by the pancreatic duct. The portions of the duct are referred to according to their relationship to intestinal viscera–*suprapancreatic, intrapancreatic,* and *intraduodenal.*

The union of the bile duct and the main pancreatic duct follows one of three patterns. The structures may: (1) unite outside the duodenum and traverse the duodenal wall and papilla as a single duct; (2) join within the duodenal wall and have a short, common, terminal portion; or (3) exit independently into the duodenum. Separate orifices have been demonstrated in 29 per-

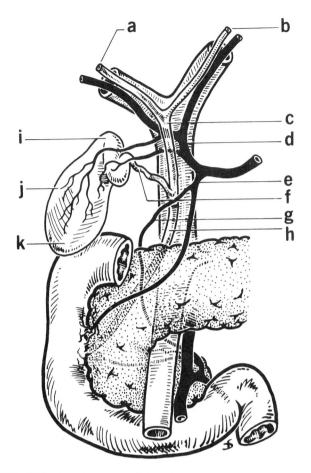

FIG. 29-1. *Anterior aspect of the biliary anatomy. a. right hepatic duct, b. left hepatic duct, c. common hepatic duct, d. hepatic artery, e. gastroduodenal artery, f. cystic duct, g. retroduodenal artery, h. common bile duct, i. neck of the gallbladder, j. body of the gallbladder, k. fundus of the gallbladder. Note particularly the situation of the hepatic bile duct confluence anterior to the right branch of the portal vein, the posterior course of the cystic artery behind the common hepatic duct and the relationship of the neck of the gallbladder to the right branch of the hepatic artery.*

cent of autopsy specimens, and injection into cadavers reveals reflux from the common bile duct into the pancreatic duct in 54 percent. Radiographically, reflux from the common bile duct into the pancreatic duct is present in about 16 percent of cases. The sphincter of Oddi surrounds the common bile duct at the ampulla of Vater. This provides control of the flow of bile and, in some cases, pancreatic juice. An ampullary sphincter that is present in one-third of adults may produce a common channel for the terminal common and pancreatic ducts.

Gallbladder. The gallbladder is located in the bed of the liver in line with that organ's anatomic division into right and left lobes. It is a pear-shaped organ with an average capacity of 50 mL and is divided into four anatomic portions: the fundus, the corpus or body, the infundibulum, and the neck. The fundus is the rounded, blind end that normally extends beyond the liver's margin. It may be unusually kinked and present the appearance of a "phrygian cap." It contains most of the smooth muscle of the organ, in contrast to the corpus or body, which is the major storage area and contains most of the elastic tissue.

The body tapers into the neck, which is funnel-shaped and connects with the cystic duct. The neck usually follows a gentle curve, the convexity of which may be distended into a dilatation known as the infundibulum, or Hartmann's pouch.

The wall of the gallbladder is made up of smooth muscle and fibrous tissue, and the lumen is lined with a high columnar epithelium that contains cholesterol and fat globules. The mucus secreted into the gallbladder originates in the tubular alveolar glands in the globular cells of the mucosa lining the infundibulum and neck.

The gallbladder is supplied by the cystic artery, which normally originates from the right hepatic artery behind the cystic duct. It is approximately 2 mm in diameter and courses above the cystic duct for a variable distance, until it passes down the peritoneal surface of the gallbladder and branches. Venous return is carried through small veins, which enter directly into the liver from the gallbladder, and a large cystic vein, which carries blood back to the right portal vein. Lymph flows directly from the gallbladder to the liver and drains into several nodes along the surface of the portal vein. The nerves of the gallbladder arise from the celiac plexus and lie along the hepatic artery. Motor nerves are made up of vagus fibers mixed with postganglionic fibers from the celiac ganglion. The preganglionic sympathetic level is at T8 and T9. Sensory supply is provided by fibers in the sympathetic nerves coursing to the celiac plexus through the posterior root ganglion at T8 and T9 on the right side.

The gallbladder is connected with the common duct system via the cystic duct, which joins the common hepatic duct at an acute angle. The segment of the cystic duct adjacent to the gallbladder bears a variable number of mucosal folds that have been referred to as the "valves of Heister" but do not have any valvular function. Immediately behind the cystic duct resides the right branch of the hepatic artery. The length of the cystic duct is highly variable, though the average is around 4 cm. Variations of the cystic duct and its point of union with the common hepatic duct are surgically important (Fig. 29-2). The cystic duct may run parallel to the common hepatic duct and actually be adherent to it. It may be extremely long and unite with the hepatic duct at the duodenum. It may be absent or very short and have a high (cephalad) union with the hepatic duct, in some cases joining the right hepatic duct instead. The cystic duct may spiral anteriorly or posteriorly in relation to the common hepatic duct and join it on the left side. Congenital biliary atresia is discussed in Chap. 37.

Anomalies

The classic description of the extrahepatic biliary passages and their arteries applies in only about one-third of patients. There are surgically important anomalies in the gallbladder's position and form, and even its number (Fig. 29-3). Isolated congenital absence of the gallbladder is extremely rare; autopsy incidences of 0.03 percent have been reported. Before the diagnosis is made, the presence of an intrahepatic vesicle or left-sided organ must be ruled out. Duplication of the gallbladder with two separate cavities and two separate cystic ducts has an incidence of approximately 1 in 4000. The accessory gallbladder may be situated on the left side, and its cystic duct may empty into the left hepatic duct rather than the common duct. Pathologic processes such as cholelithiasis and cholecystitis may involve one organ while the other is spared.

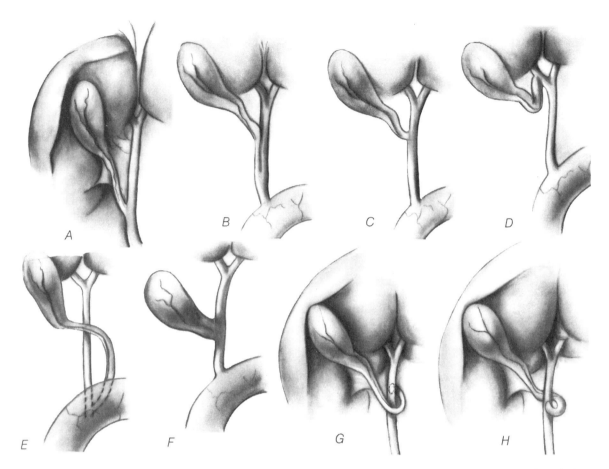

FIG. 29-2. Variations of the cystic duct. *A.* Low junction between cystic duct and common hepatic duct. *B.* Cystic duct adherent to common hepatic duct. *C.* High junction between cystic and common hepatic duct. *D.* Cystic duct drains into right hepatic duct. *E.* Long cystic duct that joins common hepatic duct behind duodenum. *F.* Absence of cystic duct. *G.* Cystic duct crosses anterior to common hepatic duct and joins it posteriorly. *H.* Cystic duct courses posteriorly to common hepatic duct and joins it anteriorly. (After: *Hollinshead WH: Anatomy for Surgeons, vol 2. New York, Hoeber Medical Division, Harper & Row, 1956, with permission.*)

The gallbladder may be found in a variety of anomalous positions. The so-called "floating gallbladder" occurs when there is an increase in the peritoneal investment. The organ may be completely invested by peritoneum with no mesentery. In other instances, the gallbladder may be suspended from the liver by a complete mesentery, or the neck may have a mesentery in which

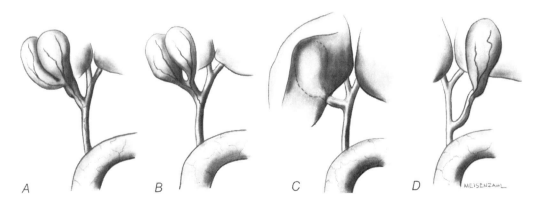

FIG. 29-3. Anomalies of the gallbladder. *A.* Double gallbladder with single cystic duct. *B.* Bilobed gallbladder. *C.* Intrahepatic gallbladder. *D.* Left-sided gallbladder.

the cystic artery lies, while the fundus and body are free. This condition occurs in about 5 percent of patients and predisposes to torsion and resulting gangrene or perforation of the viscus. A left-sided gallbladder with the cystic duct entering directly into the left hepatic duct or common duct is extremely rare, as is the situation known as *retrodisplacement*, in which the fundus extends backward in the free margin of the gastrohepatic omentum. The gallbladder may also be totally intrahepatic, a situation that occurs in many animals. In human beings, the partial or complete intrahepatic gallbladder is associated with an increased incidence of cholelithiasis.

Anomalies of the cystic duct were described earlier (see Fig. 29-2). Accessory hepatic ducts are present in approximately 15 percent of cases. Large ducts are usually single and drain a portion of the right lobe of the liver joining the right hepatic duct, common hepatic duct, or infundibulum of the gallbladder. Small ducts (of Luschka) may drain directly from the liver into the body of the gallbladder. When these ducts go unrecognized and are not ligated or clipped at cholecystectomy, an accumulation of bile (biloma) may occur in the subhepatic area.

Anomalies of the hepatic artery and the cystic artery are present in about 50 percent of cases (Fig. 29-4). A large accessory left hepatic artery, originating from the left gastric artery, occurs in about 5 percent of cases. In about 20 percent of cases, the right hepatic artery originates from the superior mesenteric artery, and in about 5 percent of cases there are two hepatic arteries: one originating from the common hepatic and other from the superior mesenteric artery. The right hepatic artery is vulnerable during surgical procedures, particularly when it parallels the cystic duct and is adherent to it or when it resides in the mesentery of the gallbladder. A "caterpillar hump" right hepatic artery may be mistaken for the cystic artery. The right hepatic artery may course anteriorly to the common duct. In 10 percent of cases, the cystic artery originates from the left hepatic artery or from the junction of the left or right hepatic arteries with the common hepatic artery. In about 15 percent of cases, the cystic artery passes in front of the common hepatic duct, rather than to the right of or posterior to this duct. Double cystic arteries occur in about 25 percent of cases, and they may both arise from the right hepatic artery, or one may have another origin.

Cystic Disease of the Extrahepatic Biliary Tract (Choledochal Cyst)

Congenital cystic abnormalities may occur throughout the entire biliary system, i.e., from intrahepatic biliary radicles to the terminal common duct. Intrahepatic cystic dilatation is discussed in Chap. 28. Choledochal cysts are discussed in Chap. 37. There are three major varieties (Fig. 29-5): cystic dilatation involving the entire common bile duct and common hepatic duct with the cystic duct entering the choledochal cyst; a small cyst usually localized to the distal common bile duct; and diffuse fusiform dilatation of the common bile duct.

Congenital biliary atresia is discussed in Chap. 37.

PHYSIOLOGY

Bile Formation. The normal adult with an intact hepatic circulation and consuming an average diet produces within the liver 250 to 1000 mL bile per day. This is, in large part, an active process that takes place within the hepatocytes and is dependent on a supply of oxygen. The secretion of bile is respon-

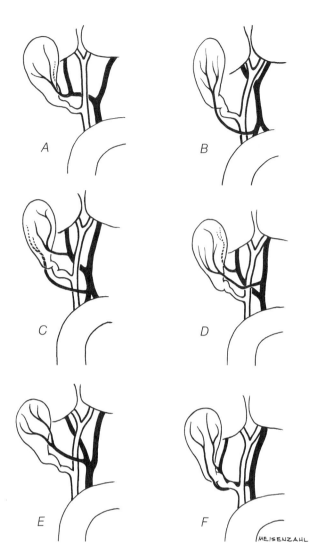

FIG. 29-4. Anomalies of the arteries to the gallbladder. *A.* Cystic artery arises from right hepatic artery in 95 percent of cases. *B.* Cystic artery arises from gastroduodenal artery. *C.* Two cystic arteries, one arising from right hepatic artery and the other from common hepatic artery. *D.* Two cystic arteries; anomalous one arises from left hepatic artery and crosses common hepatic duct anteriorly. *E.* Cystic artery arises from right hepatic artery, but courses anterior to common hepatic duct. *F.* Two cystic arteries arising from right hepatic artery. Right hepatic artery is adherent to cystic duct and neck of gallbladder. Posterior cystic artery is very short (a common finding).

sive to neurogenic, humoral, and chemical control. Vagal stimulation increases secretion, whereas splanchnic nerve stimulation results in decreased bile flow, probably related to vasoconstriction. The release of secretin from the duodenum after the stimulus of hydrochloric acid, breakdown products of proteins, and fatty acids increases bile flow and the production of an alkaline solution by the canaliculi. Bile salts are also choleretic and augment bile secretion by the liver.

The active transport of bile acids from the hepatocytes into the canaliculi creates an osmotic gradient that causes water to diffuse into those canaliculi. In addition, there is a "bile acid-independent" active transport of electrolytes and other solutes

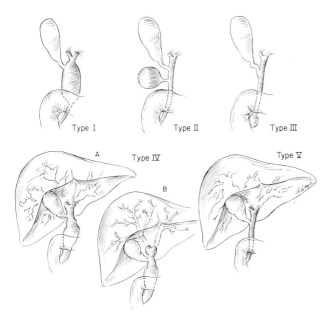

FIG. 29-5. *Classification of choledochal cysts. Type I, cystic dilatation of the common bile duct; Type II, single bile duct diverticulum; Type III, cystic dilatation of the intraduodenal portion of the bile duct (choledochocele); Type IV-A, combination of extrahepatic and intrahepatic cysts; Type IV-B, multiple cysts within the extrahepatic ducts; Type V, multiple diffuse dilatations of the intrahepatic ducts, Caroli's disease.*

into the canaliculi with consequent passive diffusion of water and solutes.

Composition of Bile. The main constituents of bile are water, electrolytes, bile salts, proteins, lipids, and bile pigments. Sodium, potassium, calcium, and chloride have the same concentration in bile as in extracellular fluid or plasma. As secretion increases, there is an increase in the concentration of bicarbonate and in pH, and a slight increase in chloride. The pH of hepatic bile is usually neutral or slightly alkaline and varies with diet; an increase in protein shifts the pH to the acidic side.

Cholesterol and phospholipids are synthesized in the liver. The rate of cholesterol synthesis, subject to a negative feedback mechanism, is inhibited by high cholesterol intake. Bile acids, produced endogenously or taken orally, reduce cholesterol synthesis and increase cholesterol absorption from the intestine. The synthesis of phospholipids is also regulated by bile acids. The concentrations of cholesterol and phospholipids are both lower in hepatic bile than in plasma.

The principal bile acids, cholic and deoxycholic acids, are synthesized from cholesterol within the liver; they are conjugated there with taurine and glycine and act within the bile as anions that are balanced by sodium. The concentration of these salts within liver bile is 10 to 20 mEq/L. Proteins are present in bile in lesser concentrations than in plasma, with the exception of mucoproteins and lipoproteins that are not present in plasma. Liver bile also contains unesterified cholesterol, lecithin, and neutral fats.

The color of the bile secreted by the liver is related to the presence of the pigment bilirubin diglucuronide, which is the metabolic product of the breakdown of hemoglobin and is present in bile in concentrations 100 times greater than in plasma. After this pigment has been acted upon by bacteria within the

intestine and converted into urobilinogen, a small fraction of the urobilinogen is absorbed and secreted into the bile.

Gallbladder Function. The gallbladder provides storage and concentration of bile. The selective absorption of sodium, chloride, and water results in a concentration of bile salts, bile pigments, and cholesterol ten times higher than in liver bile. The gallbladder mucosa has the greatest absorptive power per unit area of any structure in the body. This rapid absorption prevents a rise in pressure within the biliary system under normal circumstances. The absorption of fluid by the gallbladder is driven by an energy-dependent active transport of sodium and a consequent passive transport of water.

Secretion of mucus, approximately at the rate of 20 mL/h, protects the mucosa from the lytic action of bile and facilitates the passage of bile through the cystic duct. This mucus makes up the colorless, "white bile" present in hydrops of the gallbladder resulting from obstruction of the cystic duct. The gallbladder also secretes calcium in the presence of inflammation or obstruction of the cystic duct.

Motor Activity. The passage of bile into the duodenum involves the coordinated contraction of the gallbladder and relaxation of the sphincter of Oddi. Some bile flows from the gallbladder continuously and there are rhythmic contractions occurring two to six times per minute and mediating pressures less than 30 mmH$_2$O. The gallbladder's emptying, however, is mainly a response to the ingestion of food and the release of cholecystokinin (CCK) by the duodenum. CCK also relaxes the terminal bile duct, the sphincter of Oddi, and the duodenum. After the intravenous injection of CCK, the gallbladder is two-thirds evacuated within 30 min. CCK exerts its contractile effects mainly through action directly on the gallbladder smooth muscle cells, but also via interaction with cholinergic nerves. There is a feedback inhibition of CCK secretion by bile acids and proteases. Somatostatin has a direct inhibitory action against CCK-induced gallbladder contraction.

The vagus nerve stimulates contraction of the gallbladder, and splanchnic sympathetic stimulation is inhibitory to its motor activity. Although vagotomy for duodenal ulcer increases the size and volume of the gallbladder, the rate of emptying is unchanged. Parasympathomimetic drugs contract the gallbladder, whereas atropine leads to relaxation. Magnesium sulfate is a potent evacuator of the gallbladder. Emptying of the gallbladder takes place 30 min after ingestion of a fatty meal. There is an increased risk of gallbladder disease in patients on prolonged total parenteral nutrition (TPN) because of the lack of intestinal stimulus and consequent stasis of bile within the organ.

Gallbladder filling occurs when the pressure in the bile duct is greater than that within the gallbladder. This is correlated with reduced CCK levels but is also affected by vasoactive intestinal polypeptide (VIP), pancreatic polypeptide (PP), and peptide YY (PYY).

The common bile duct can be shown to have waves of peristalsis. During starvation, the sphincter of Oddi maintains an intraductal pressure that approximates the maximal expulsive pressure of the gallbladder, i.e., 30 cmH$_2$O, thereby preventing emptying. During the interdigestive periods, the hormone motilin regulates sphincteric pressure to allow continuous flow of small amounts of bile into the duodenum. After the ingestion of food, the sphincteric pressure is reduced to 10 cmH$_2$O. When pressure within the extrahepatic bile ducts is greater than 36 cmH_2O, secretion of bile is suppressed.

Biliary dyskinesia lacks objective findings. The term has been used to describe disturbances of biliary tract motility that occur in the absence of anatomic changes. It has been applied as a primary condition and as a complication of biliary tract surgery. Pain has been noted to occur after the ingestion of fatty foods and the injection of CCK at the time that contraction of the gallbladder is induced. Biliary tract pain has also been ascribed to spasm of the sphincter of Oddi. The concept of hyperplastic cholecystosis, characterized by hyperconcentration and excessive emptying of the gallbladder manifest on a cholecystogram, is questionable, but cholecystectomy has been reported to be curative in symptomatic patients.

Enterohepatic Circulation. After the bile enters the duodenum, over 80 percent of the conjugated bile acids are absorbed in the terminal ileum, and the remainder is deconjugated by bacterial activity and absorbed in the colon. Eventually, almost 95 percent of the bile acid pool is absorbed and returns via the portal venous system to the liver. Only 5 percent is excreted in the stool, thereby permitting a relatively small pool of bile acids to have maximal effectiveness. A negative feedback mechanism regulates the hepatic synthesis of bile acids. When the distal ileum has been resected, there is usually adaptation, but occasionally the lack of a feedback mechanism persists and causes significant diarrhea.

DIAGNOSIS OF BILIARY TRACT DISEASE

(See also Jaundice in Chap. 22.)

Radiologic Studies

Abdominal Ultrasonography. Ultrasound imaging is the most widely applied diagnostic technique for biliary tract disease in elective and emergent situations. It provides anatomic and pathologic information with great flexibility and portability, and at low cost. The technique may be limited by obesity and large amounts of intestinal gas. Ultrasonography employs a high-frequency vibration in which alternate compression and rarefaction waves travel through the tissue and are reflected off of tissues or items that differ in acoustic impedance. The reflected portion of the sound beam returns to a transducer to create an image. There is variability in the quality of images, and the technique is operator dependent. The gallbladder is readily imaged because echo-free bile contrasts with the organ's wall and the liver parenchyma. The intrahepatic and extrahepatic major bile ducts are also defined. Calculi can be demonstrated in more than 95 percent of cases in which they are present. The discrimination of ductal dilatation has an accuracy of 90 percent.

Ultrasonography is the most cost effective and reliable method for demonstrating gallstones. They appear as reflective foci within the gallbladder or ducts and cast acoustic shadows (Fig. 29-6). A stone impacted in the gallbladder neck or cystic duct may be difficult to detect because the walls themselves return strong echoes. Ultrasonography has been used to guide lithotripsy.

Ultrasound imaging also provides diagnostic information for acute and chronic cholecystitis. The characteristic signs include edema and thickening of the gallbladder wall, occasionally gas in the wall, and absence of visualization of the organ. Thickening

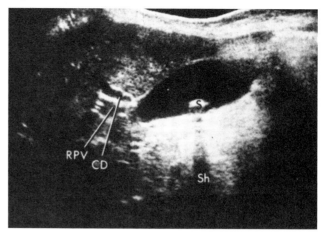

A

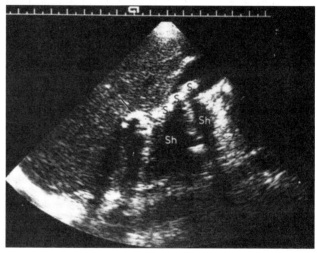

B

FIG. 29-6. *Gallstones. Echogenic foci in the gallbladder with acoustic shadowing are the characteristic ultrasound appearance of gallstones, whether solitary (A) or multiple (B). Note the stone (arrow) in the neck of the gallbladder in B. (CD = common duct, S = stone, Sh = acoustic shadow, RPV = portal vein. (From: Cosgrove DO: Ultrasound in surgery of the liver and biliary tract, in Blumgart LH (ed): Surgery of the Liver and Biliary Tract, vol 2. Churchill Livingstone, New York, 1994, chap 15, p 212.)*

and edema of the wall is particularly useful in establishing the diagnosis of acalculous cholecystitis when they are coupled with tenderness over the organ evoked by pressure of the ultrasound probe. Ultrasonography also can establish the diagnoses of hydrops, porcelain gallbladder, adenomas, and carcinomas.

Ultrasound is the first radiologic step in the evaluation of jaundice because it provides a sensitive method for detecting intrahepatic and extrahepatic ductal dilatation. The level of obstruction can be defined by tracing the dilatation down to a point or termination. It can distinguish between intraductal calculi and tumors as the causative agent. Postoperatively it readily defines bilomas and subhepatic abscesses.

Abdominal Radiography. Plain x-ray films of the abdomen are of limited value in assessing patients with gallstones or with jaundice. Supine and upright films of the abdomen may be useful in excluding other causes of abdominal pain, such as a perforated viscus or a bowel obstruction. The presence of significant amounts of calcium within gallstones, which occurs in 15 to 20 percent of patients, causes stones to appear as opacified objects located in the right upper quadrant on plain x-ray films (Fig. 29-7). There are a number of unusual circumstances in which complications from gallstones may be suggested by specific radiographic findings. The presence of gas within the biliary tree outlining its anatomy occurs in patients with a cholecystenteric fistula (abnormal communication between the gallbladder and duodenum, which typically occurs as a consequence of chronic cholecystitis). Opacification of the gallbladder, or of parts of it, occurs in patients with a "porcelain" gallbladder. Gas bubbles may be present in the wall of the gallbladder in patients with emphysematous cholecystitis (infection secondary to anaerobic, gas-producing organisms).

Oral Cholecystography.

Oral cholecystography, a relatively simple and effective test for diagnosing gallstones, was introduced by Graham and Cole in 1924. While this test may permit visualization of gallstones within the gallbladder, the critical function that is assessed is the absorptive ability of the gallbladder. A radiopaque iodine containing halogenated dye is orally ingested by the patient. The dye is first absorbed by the gastrointestinal tract and extracted in the liver. The liver excretes the dye into the biliary ductular system, and the dye then passes through the cystic duct into the gallbladder. Ultimately, if the gallbladder has normal mucosal function, the dye becomes concentrated through the physiologic absorption of water and solutes. A "positive" study—one suggestive of gallstones or gallbladder pathology—occurs when stones are noted as filling defects in a visualized, opacified gallbladder (Fig. 29-8) or when the dye is not adequately concentrated and the gallbladder cannot be visualized. When nonvisualization occurs, a second, double dose of contrast medium is frequently administered. Although the accuracy of this modality has been reported to be as high as

95 percent, a number of important limitations have reduced its use. False positives may occur when patients have been noncompliant or have been unable to ingest the tablets because of nausea and emesis or general medical conditions; when the tablets have not been absorbed through the gastrointestinal tract or have not been excreted into the biliary tract as a result of hepatic dysfunction; or when there is some technical problem with the equipment. Oral cholecystography has been largely replaced by the development and refinement of abdominal ultrasonography.

Computed Tomography and Magnetic Resonance Imaging.

Computed tomography (CT) is used to assess biliary dilatation and calculi (Fig. 29-9), but because both can be studied more readily by ultrasound imaging, CT is not routinely performed. CT is inferior to ultrasonography for the detection of stones. The major application of CT is to define the course and status of the extrahepatic biliary tree and adjacent structures. Intravenous contrast enhancement of the biliary tract is mandatory in this study. Use of CT is an integral part of the differential diagnosis of obstructive jaundice. Magnetic resonance imaging currently has little application in biliary disease. With the introduction of new contrast agents, its applicability may be expanded.

Biliary Scintigraphy.

After technetium 99m-labeled derivatives of iminodiacetic acid (HIDA) are injected intravenously, they are cleared by the Kupffer's cells in the liver and excreted in the bile. Normally, after injection, peak activity is detected in the liver in 10 min, and the biliary ducts can be identified shortly thereafter. The gallbladder is visualized within 60 min in fasting subjects (Fig. 29-10). The test is particularly applicable when the diagnosis of acute cholecystitis is being considered. Evidence of cystic duct obstruction, as indicated by nonvisualization of the gallbladder, is highly diagnostic. The isotopic visualization of the gallbladder essentially precludes the diagnosis. The accuracy of the test in diagnosing acute cholecystitis is about 97 percent.

Percutaneous Transhepatic Cholangiography (PTC).

With fluoroscopic guidance, a small needle is introduced under local anesthesia through the abdominal wall and into the substance of the liver. After position in a bile duct has been confirmed, a guide wire is introduced and a catheter can be placed. PTC facilitates diagnosis by providing a cholangiogram and permits therapeutic intervention, as necessary, based on the clinical situation. The technique has little role in the management of patients with uncomplicated gallstone disease, but it has been particularly useful for patients with more complex biliary problems, including strictures and tumors (Fig. 29-11). PTC is the preferred approach for patients in whom ultrasonography demonstrates intrahepatic ductal dilatation and no extra hepatic ductal dilatation, e.g., Klatskin's tumor at the confluence of the right and left hepatic ducts. As with any invasive procedure, there are potential risks: bleeding, cholangitis, bile leak, and other catheter-related problems. Hematobilia occurs often but is usually self-limiting and of little consequence.

Endoscopic Retrograde Cholangiopancreatography (ERCP).

Using a side-viewing endoscope, the biliary tract and pancreatic duct can be intubated and visualized. This procedure is generally performed with the patient under light intravenous

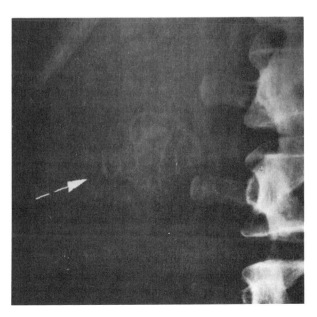

FIG. 29-7. *Routine abdominal x-ray demonstrating radiopaque biliary calculi in gallbladder.*

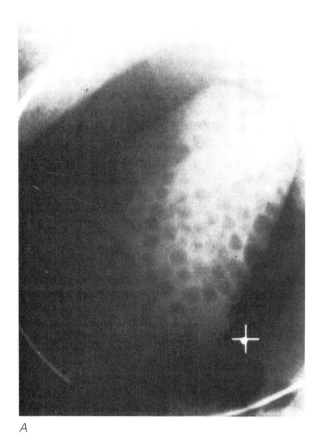

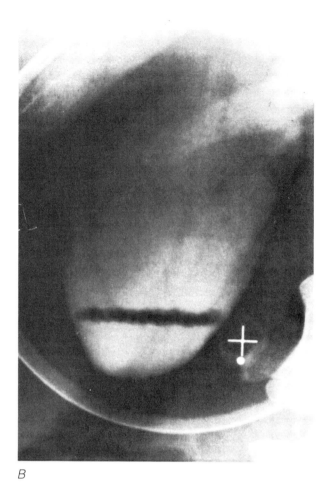

A

B

FIG. 29-8. Multiple gallbladder stones. *A.* With the patient supine, the stones are seen scattered throughout the gallbladder. *B.* With the patient upright and a horizontal x-ray beam, the stones are in a dense layer *(arrow)*, floating in a partially contrast-filled gallbladder. (From: *Skucas J: Diagnostic and interventional radiology, in Schwartz SI, Ellis H (eds): Maingot's Abdominal Operations. Norwalk, CT, Appelton-Century-Crofts, 1985, pp 68–69, with permission.*)

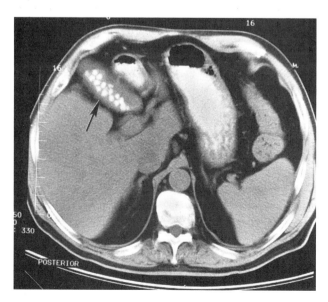

FIG. 29-9. CT scan of abdomen. Arrow points to gallbladder filled with calcified gallstones.

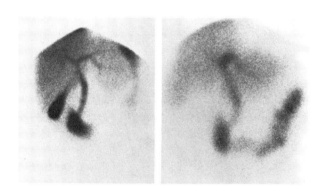

FIG. 29-10. HIDA scan of biliary tract. *Left:* Normal, with visualization of gallbladder, hepatic ducts, and common bile ducts, and second portion of the duodenum. *Right:* Acute cholecystitis with visualization of the common bile duct and second and third portions of the duodenum. The gallbladder did not appear in the scan.

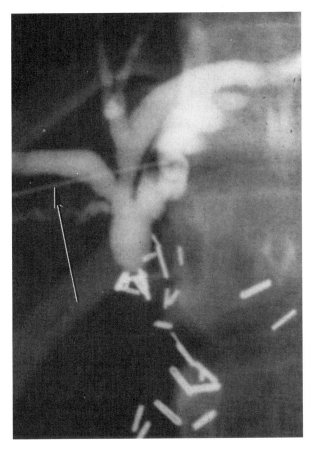

FIG. 29-11. *Percutaneous transhepatic cholangiogram. Arrow points to transhepatic needle that has been inserted percutaneously. This patient has an iatrogenic stricture of the common bile duct.*

sedation. Advantages of ERCP include direct visualization of the ampullary region and direct access to the distal bile duct, which facilitates diagnosis and therapeutic intervention. This test is generally not required when dealing with patients who have benign gallbladder disease, though it has been of enormous benefit for patients with common bile duct disease (benign and malignant). This is particularly true for the evaluation and treatment of patients with obstructive jaundice when there is dilatation of the common duct or gallbladder (Fig. 29-12).

Choledochoscopy. Rigid and flexible choledochoscopes inserted into the supraduodenal common duct to visualize the lumen of the extrahepatic ducts have been used to determine the presence or absence of calculi; an accuracy of over 90 percent has been reported. The technique is used as an adjunct to operative cholangiography when the common duct is explored. Choledochoscopy can also aid in the removal of stones and bile duct tumors, and in inspecting and obtaining biopsy samples from stenoses.

TRAUMA

Penetrating and Nonpenetrating Injuries of the Gallbladder

Injuries of the gallbladder are uncommon, occurring in 2 to 8 percent of patients with major abdominal trauma. Penetrating

injuries are usually caused by gunshot wounds or stab wounds; they also occur rarely during a needle biopsy procedure of the liver. Nonpenetrating injuries are extremely rare. Fewer than 100 cases have been reported, and in only 20 percent was the trauma isolated to the gallbladder.

The types of traumatic injuries to the gallbladder include contusion, avulsion, laceration, rupture, and traumatic cholecystitis. Contusion is difficult to verify but may be associated with vague or temporary symptoms that require no specific therapy. The contused area may undergo necrosis and perforate. Avulsion of the gallbladder from its liver bed occurs as a result of nonpenetrating injury. When the gallbladder's attachments are torn the organ usually hangs by its neck but may be attached only by the cystic duct and artery. Volvulus of the gallbladder may result. Traumatic cholecystectomy, in which the cystic duct, cystic artery, and gallbladder attachments are transected, has been reported. Laceration is the most common type of injury following penetrating wounds but also may result from blunt trauma. Delayed rupture of the gallbladder can occur days to weeks following injury. Traumatic cholecystitis is an unusual condition that occurs as a result of blunt trauma. Bleeding into the gallbladder, from injury of the gallbladder or of the liver, precipitates cholecystitis and sometimes gangrene of the gallbladder. The retained blood may clot and block the cystic duct, in which case the patient presents with the manifestations of hematobilia, including intermittent jaundice, colicky pain, hematemesis, and melena.

Effects of Intraperitoneal Bile. The effects of extravasation of bile into the peritoneal cavity depend on whether or

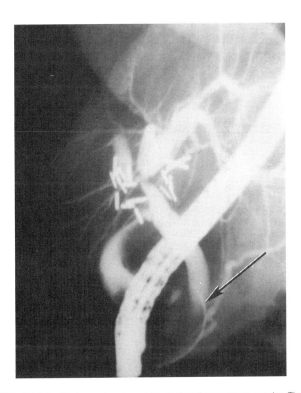

FIG. 29-12. *Endoscopic retrograde cholangiopancreatography. The arrow points to the ERCP catheter inserted in the common bile duct. This patient has an iatrogenic stricture of the common bile duct.*

not the bile is infected. When infected bile escapes into the peritoneal cavity, a fulminating and often fatal peritonitis results. When bile is sterile, however, it is well tolerated and results in a chemical peritonitis that may be relatively mild. In the majority of gallbladder injuries, the organ is normal and the bile is sterile. The fact that sterile bile is relatively innocuous is borne out by the very low mortality rate associated with nonpenetrating wounds of the gallbladder. Continuous leakage of noninfected bile, however, is not innocuous. The extravasated bile may produce ascites or become encysted, and extensive chemical peritonitis causes an outpouring of fluid into the peritoneal cavity from the general circulation that may result in shock. There is also some evidence that large amounts of bile salts may be toxic.

Clinical Manifestations. Bile leakage through the penetrating wound suggests the possibility of damage to the biliary system, but duodenal laceration may have a similar manifestation. With blunt trauma, manifestations may be delayed for 36 h or more, in part because typically there are other serious injuries that mask injury of the biliary tract, and sterile bile itself causes only minimal symptoms. The presence of severe shock and pain in the right upper quadrant or lower part of the right side of the chest should raise clinical suspicion of gallbladder injury. The manifestations of bacterial peritonitis may ensue, or if the bile leakage is minimal, the patient may appear to recover but subsequently develop ascites or an intraperitoneal cyst. The finding of bile-stained fluid during diagnostic paracentesis is suggestive, but a negative tap does not exclude gallbladder injury. In most instances the diagnosis is made at celiotomy, emphasizing the need for careful examination of the biliary system after abdominal trauma.

Treatment. The injured gallbladder has been successfully treated by simple suture of the laceration, cholecystostomy, and cholecystectomy. In general, it is preferable to remove the traumatized gallbladder. Cholecystectomy is usually quite easy to perform, since the gallbladder is rarely diseased, and it must be performed if the gallbladder has been avulsed or the cystic artery torn. In the severely ill patient, cholecystostomy may be used for treatment of the extensive laceration or traumatic cholecystitis in order to reduce the time of operative procedure and avoid injury to the common duct. Prognosis is directly related to the incidence of associated injuries.

Injury of the Extrahepatic Bile Ducts

Rare cases of solitary penetrating wounds involving the bile duct have been reported, but there is usually associated trauma to other viscera. Approximately 120 cases of traumatic rupture of the extrahepatic bile duct have been reported, and in 20 cases complete transection occurred. The clinical manifestations are similar to those described for gallbladder injury.

Treatment consists initially of meticulous exploration, particularly if injury to the gallbladder has been excluded and bile has been demonstrated retroperitoneally or within the peritoneal cavity. A Kocher maneuver should be performed to rule out perforation of the common duct behind the duodenum. The presence of hematoma in this region should raise the surgeon's suspicions. Tangential injuries may be treated by primary repair. Complete transection of the common hepatic duct or the common bile duct (e.g., by a penetrating knife wound) may be treated by debridement and an end-to-end anastomosis over a T

tube, which should be left in place for several weeks. In most cases of complete transection and injuries caused by blunt trauma, however, the proximal end of the duct should be anastomosed to a Roux-en-Y limb of jejunum. The patient should be placed on an appropriate regimen of antibiotics.

Operative Injury of the Bile Ducts

The great majority of injuries of the extrahepatic biliary duct system are iatrogenic, occurring in the course of laparoscopic or open cholecystectomy. In over 70 percent of cases, the cholecystectomy had apparently been carried out without incident.

Diagnosis. In approximately 15 percent of the cases, ductal injuries are recognized and treated at the time of operation. The remaining 85 percent become manifest by either increasing obstructive jaundice or profuse and persistent drainage of bile through a fistula. Jaundice usually becomes manifest in 2 to 3 days, but in some instances it does not develop for weeks. It may be continuous or intermittent; if intermittent, it is frequently accompanied by attacks of chills and fever, suggesting ascending cholangitis. Hepatomegaly almost always accompanies jaundice if it has been persistent for several weeks, and splenomegaly also may occur if secondary biliary cirrhosis has evolved. Some patients do not display the signs or symptoms of partial or complete blockage until months or years after surgical treatment. Blockage in such cases is the result of increasing fibrosis and narrowing of the channel or of repeated episodes of cholangitis, which in turn leads to fibrosis. ERCP or PTC most clearly defines the site of obstruction or leak.

Treatment. Patients with jaundice or persistent fistula require a vigorous preoperative regimen that includes a high-protein, low-fat diet and intravenous administration of fat-soluble vitamins, particularly vitamin K. Concomitant portal hypertension with bleeding varices may preclude repair of the common duct; the portal hypertension is usually best treated by a splenorenal shunt because of extensive scarring in the right upper quadrant.

Operative Approach. Injury of the bile duct recognized during surgical operation should be corrected with an immediate reconstructive procedure. Restoration of the continuity of the duct with an end-to-end anastomosis over a T tube may be feasible after a sharp transection, but stricture develops in about half the cases. Direct anastomosis is usually impractical for acute injuries and chronic strictures where the proximal end of the duct should be anastomosed to a Roux-en-Y of jejunum. A mucosa-to-mucosa approximation provides the best long-term results. If this is not feasible, a lateral-lateral anastomosis between the left hepatic duct and a Roux-en-Y limb of jejunum (Hepp-Soupault) is preferable to the Smith transhepatic mucosal pull-through technique. The Longmire operation, with transection of the left lobe of the liver and anastomosis of the jejunum to a large intrahepatic bile duct, has been associated with discouraging results.

The operative mortality of patients with chronic stricture is reported to be 3 to 5 percent. A satisfactory result is obtained in about 70 percent of patients after one or more operative procedures. If the patient is symptom-free 4 years after reconstruction, the cure is almost always permanent.

GALLSTONES

Composition. The major elements involved in the formation of gallstones are cholesterol, bile pigment, and calcium. Other constituents include iron, phosphorus, carbonates, proteins, carbohydrates, mucus, and cellular debris. In Western cultures, most stones are made up of the three major elements and have a particularly high content of cholesterol, averaging 71 percent. Pure cholesterol stones are uncommon, usually large with smooth surfaces, and solitary. Bilirubin pigment stones are also uncommon, with a characteristic smooth, glistening, green or black surface. The pigment stones may be "pure" or consist of calcium bilirubinate. The "pure" pigment stones are usually associated with hemolytic jaundice or situations in which the bile is abnormally concentrated. Increased red blood cell destruction after cardiac valve replacement has resulted in production of gallstones. Calcium bilirubinate stones are prevalent in Asia, where they constitute 30 to 40 percent of all gallstones.

Formation. Gallstones form as a result of solids settling out of solution. The solubility of cholesterol depends on the concentrations of conjugated bile salts, phospholipids, and cholesterol in bile. Lecithin is the predominant phospholipid in bile, and, although insoluble in aqueous solutions, it is dissolved by bile salts in micelles. Cholesterol is also insoluble in aqueous solution but becomes soluble when incorporated into the lecithin-bile salt micelle. By plotting the percentages of cholesterol, lecithin, and bile salts on triangular coordinates (Fig. 29-13), the limits of micellar liquid in which bile is less than saturated with cholesterol may be defined. Above these limits, the bile is either a supersaturated liquid or a two-phase system of liquid bile and solid crystalline cholesterol.

Perhaps no more than 30 percent of biliary cholesterol is transported in micelles, and of that the majority is carried in a vesicular form. These vesicles are made up of lipid bilayers similar to those found in cell membranes. The vesicles are able to solubilize more cholesterol than are micelles, and the stability of these structures is believed to be the key determinant of cholesterol saturation and precipitation. Current theory suggests that there is an equilibrium between the physicochemical phases of these vesicles such that the formation of liquid crystals may or may not result in actual gallstones. When crystals achieve macroscopic size during a period of entrapment in the gallbladder, gallstones form. The basic secretory defect in nonobese patients is decreased bile salt and phospholipid secretion. Conversely, in obese subjects cholesterol secretion is greatly increased without any reduction in bile salt or phospholipid secretion.

Nucleation is the process by which cholesterol monohydrate crystals form and aggregate. The time required for nucleation is shorter in patients with gallstones than in those without stones. Specific heat-labile glycoproteins within cholesterol-saturated bile induce vesicular aggregation and consequent stone growth. Factors that have been implicated in the formation and precipitation of cholesterol include constitutional elements, bacteria, fungi, reflux of intestinal and pancreatic fluid, hormones, and bile stasis. Constitutional elements are best exemplified in the Pima Indians, of whom 70 percent of females by age thirty and 70 percent of males by age sixty have gallstones. The Masai of Kenya, in contrast, do not have gallstones. Evidence in favor of infection as a cause includes the isolation of such organisms as *Escherichia coli*, *Salmonella typhi*, and *Streptococcus* species from gallbladder walls and from the center of stones in a high percentage of cases, and the demonstration of slow-growing actinomycetes recovered from over half the stones examined in one series. Given that gallstones develop in the absence of infection or inflammation, infection appears not to be a universal factor. In Asians, concretions are known to form about liver flukes and other parasites within the bile ducts.

The reflux factor receives support from the findings of pancreatic enzymes in the gallbladders of patients with cholelithiasis. Trypsin disturbs colloidal balance, and pancreatic phospholipase A can convert lecithin into toxic lysolecithin. Hormones have been implicated in a unproved correlation between calculi and parity, diabetes, hyperthyroidism, and the predominance in females.

Stasis, which includes temporary cessation of bile flow into the intestine and stagnation in the gallbladder, has also been assigned a major role in stone formation. Temporary bile stasis may be due to functional disorders or to a mechanical blockage in the region of the choledochoduodenal junction or the gallbladder. The interruption of bile flow to the intestine is associated with an interruption in enterohepatic circulation, which in turn is accompanied by a decrease in the output of bile salts and phospholipids, reducing the solubility of cholesterol. When more than 20 percent of bile is diverted, the bile salt pool cannot be maintained. Bile salt secretion is also diminished by reduction of the distal third of the intestine, explaining the development of stones in patients with ileal resection or disease. Cholecystectomy causes a greater fraction of the bile salt pool to cycle around the enterohepatic circulation, thereby increasing bile salt and phospholipid secretion.

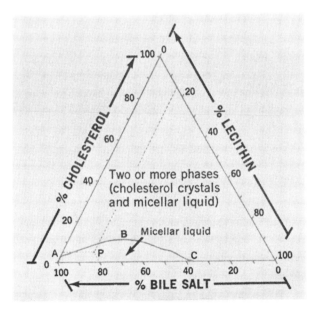

FIG. 29-13. Three major components of bile (bile salts, lecithin, and cholesterol) plotted on triangular coordinates. Point *P* represents bile consisting of 80 mol percent bile salt, 5 percent cholesterol, and 15 percent lecithin. Line *ABC* represents the maximal solubility of cholesterol in varying mixtures of bile salt and lecithin. Because point *P* falls below line *ABC* and within the zone of a single phase of micellar liquid, this bile is less than saturated with cholesterol. Bile with a composition that would place it above line *ABC* would contain excess cholesterol in supersaturated or precipitated form. (After: *Small DM: Gallstones. N Engl J Med 279:588, 1968, with permission.*)

Solubility has been investigated as a possible regimen to prevent the development of stones in patients at risk as well as to dissolve stones already formed. Chenodeoxycholic acid and ursodeoxycholic acid, which replenish the bile acid pool and reduce cholesterol synthesis and secretion, administered to potential stone formers may return supersaturated bile to its normal composition, preventing stone formation. In one series the drug was administered for 2 years; complete dissolution of radiolucent stones occurred in 13.5 percent of patients. Partial dissolution occurred in 41 percent. The effects were more frequent in women, in thin patients, and in patients with serum cholesterol levels greater than 227 mg/dL. Clinically significant hepatotoxicity was rare.

The direct instillation into the gallbladder of agents that are capable of dissolving cholesterol gallstones has become a reality largely as a result of advances in interventional radiologic technology. Although experience is limited, infusion of a potent cholesterol solvent, methyl-*tert*-butyl ether (MTBE), into the gallbladder via a percutaneously placed catheter has been shown to be effective in selected patients in achieving gallstone dissolution. This procedure is invasive and is therefore associated with some specific risks, including hemorrhage and catheter-related and drug-regulated problems. The major disadvantage of this technology is the high recurrence rate, which approaches 50 percent at 5 years. Lithotripsy has successfully fragmented biliary calculi but generally is not regarded as appropriate therapy because a diseased organ remains to form new stones and the flushing effected by normal bile flow is not equivalent to that of urinary flow.

Pigment stones can be further classified as either "brown" or "black" stones. Brown stones have a characteristic appearance and consistency and are typically found in Asia. These stones presumably occur as a result of infection and are quite similar to primary bile duct stones. Black stones, by contrast, typically are not associated with infected bile. These stones are found in patients with hemolytic disorders or cirrhosis. Altered solubilization of unconjugated bilirubin with precipitation of calcium bilirubinate and insoluble salts is presumed to be the common final pathway for the formation of all pigment stones, regardless of the clinical setting.

Asymptomatic Gallstones

The liberal use of cholecystography and ultrasonography has resulted in the diagnosis of calculi in patients without symptoms referable to the biliary tract. In several large series of asymptomatic patients with gallstones who were followed without surgical treatment, symptoms developed in 50 percent, and serious complications occurred in 20 percent. By contrast, McSherry and associates reported that only 10 percent of patients developed symptoms during a mean 5-year follow-up. Similarly, Gracie and Ransohoff reported a 15-year cumulative probability of developing symptoms of 18 percent for 123 patients with asymptomatic gallstones, and no deaths from gallbladder disease.

The relationship of cholelithiasis and carcinoma of the gallbladder is also of some significance. A review of several series showed that the incidence of calculi in cancer of the gallbladder ranged from 65 to 100 percent, with a mean of 90 percent. Conversely, the incidence of cancer of the gallbladder in patients with symptomatic gallstones ranged from 1 to 15 percent, with a mean of 4.5 percent. Comfort and associates reported no carcinoma among 112 patients with asymptomatic cholelithiasis.

In general, patients with asymptomatic gallstones should not be treated. Dyspepsia, eructations, and flatulence are not regarded as specific symptoms. With the advent of laparoscopic cholecystectomy, the number of cholecystectomies performed has increased. Cholecystectomy for asymptomatic stones may be appropriate for elderly patients with diabetes and for individuals who will be isolated from medical care for an extended period.

Cystic Duct Obstruction

Temporary obstruction to the outflow of bile from the gallbladder is responsible for the most common manifestation of calculous disease, which is biliary colic. This consists of the intermittent spasmodic pain in the right upper quadrant, often radiating to the shoulder or scapula, and precipitated by a fatty or fried meal. The attacks are self-limiting but have a tendency to recur in an unpredictable manner. Significant temperature elevation or leukocytosis are uncommon. The bilirubin and alkaline phosphatase levels are normal or slightly elevated because of an inflammatory process, and hyperamylasemia may be present. The treatment is cholecystectomy, preferably by the laparoscopic approach, and is best performed during that hospitalization but not as an emergent procedure.

Calculi, usually of the cholesterol type, may become impacted in the cystic duct or the neck of the gallbladder, resulting in what is called *hydrops of the gallbladder*. The bile is absorbed, and the gallbladder becomes filled and distended with mucinous material. The gallbladder is generally palpable and tender, and the impacted stone with the resulting edema may encroach on the common duct and cause mild jaundice. Although hydrops may persist with few consequences, early cholecystectomy is generally indicated to avoid the complications of biliary tract infection, empyema, or perforation of the gallbladder. In questionable cases, isotopic scanning of the gallbladder following intravenous CCK can define cystic obstruction or patency.

Choledocholithiasis

Common duct stones may be single or multiple and are found in 4 to 12 percent of cases subjected to cholecystectomy. Most common duct calculi are formed within the gallbladder and migrate down the cystic duct into the common bile duct. Less commonly, stones are thought to form within the ducts. These are classified as *primary stones*, in contradistinction to the *secondary stones* formed in the gallbladder. Primary stones are usually soft, nonfaceted, yellowish brown, and friable. In patients infected with tropical parasites such as *Clonorchis sinensis* and in the Asian population of the Far East, stones may form within the hepatic ducts or the common bile duct itself. Although small stones may pass via the common duct into the duodenum, the distal duct with its narrow lumen (2 to 3 mm) and thick wall frequently obstructs their passage. Edema, spasm, or fibrosis of the distal duct secondary to irritation by the calculi contribute to biliary obstruction. Both extrahepatic and intrahepatic bile ducts become dilated, and there is evidence of laking in the biliary radicles of the liver. There is also thickening of the duct walls and inflammatory cell infiltration. Chronic biliary obstruction may cause secondary biliary cirrhosis with bile thrombi, bile duct proliferation, and fibrosis of the portal tracts. Also associated with chronic obstruction is the development of infection within the bile duct, giving rise to ascending cholangitis and occasionally extending up to the liver, resulting in hepatic abscesses. The offending organism is almost always *E. coli.*

Gallstone pancreatitis is generally associated with the presence or passage of common bile duct stones. The best evidence for this is the frequency with which stones can be found if the stool is filtered at the time of an attack. The frequency with which stones are found in the common duct varies from 1 percent to 70 percent, depending on the time of the operation. At the time of exploration, the pancreas may appear entirely normal, or it may demonstrate edema and rarely necrosis (necrotizing pancreatitis).

Clinical Manifestations. The manifestations of calculi within the common duct are variable. Stones may be present within the extrahepatic duct system for many years without causing symptoms. Characteristically, the symptom complex consists of colicky pain in the right upper quadrant radiating to the right shoulder with intermittent jaundice accompanied by pale stools and dark urine. Biliary obstruction is usually chronic and incomplete but may be acute or complete. If obstruction is complete, jaundice progresses but is rarely intense. In contrast to patients with neoplastic obstruction of the common bile duct or the ampulla of Vater, the gallbladder is usually not distended because of associated inflammation (Courvoisier's law). Liver function tests demonstrate the pattern of obstructive jaundice, and the alkaline phosphatase level usually becomes elevated earlier and remains abnormal for longer periods than the serum bilirubin level. The prothrombin time is frequently prolonged because the absorption of vitamin K is dependent on bile entering the intestine, but a normal level can usually be achieved with parenteral vitamin K. Tests of hepatocellular function generally have normal results. In patients with ascending cholangitis, Charcot's intermittent fever accompanied by abdominal pain and jaundice is characteristic. The diagnosis may be established by ERCP or PTC.

Treatment. The indications for the removal of common duct stones are: (1) their presence as defined preoperatively in a symptomatic patient or by palpation or cholangiographically at the time of operation; (2) a dilated extrahepatic duct; (3) jaundice; (4) recurrent chills and fevers suggestive of cholangitis; and (5) gallstone pancreatitis.

Common duct stones can be removed by ERCP, and the performance of an adequate destruction of the sphincter of Oddi will permit stones that were not extracted or form at a later date to pass into the duodenum without obstruction in the extrahepatic ducts. In a patient undergoing an elective cholecystectomy in whom common duct stones are thought to be present, a preoperative ERCP and sphincterotomy can be followed by laparoscopic cholecystectomy. In some elderly patients ERCP and sphincterotomy have constituted definitive treatment and the gallbladder was not removed.

If common duct stones are detected during laparoscopic cholangiogram, they can be removed by subsequent ERCP or during the procedure by trans-cystic duct retrieval or pushing them into the duodenum. Alternatively, the common duct can be opened, the stones extracted, and a T tube inserted. If common duct stones are suspected or detected during open cholecystectomy, the same alternatives apply. The use of the choledochoscope and ureteral baskets facilitates the procedure. In the patient population as a whole, concomitant choledochostomy at the time of cholecystectomy increases the operative mortality by less than 1

percent. In addition, in the face of dilated common duct and multiple stones, a choledochoduodenostomy can provide definitive treatment.

Retained Common Duct Stones. If stones are noted to be present when a T-tube cholangiogram is performed postoperatively (Fig. 29-14), several approaches can be entertained. Small stones, particularly those located in the branches of the hepatic duct, may be disregarded; the majority will remain asymptomatic, and for those that do generate symptoms operative extraction is not associated with significantly increased morbidity. Another approach employs either flushing or chemical dissolution. Capmul 8210, a mono-octanoin, is the agent of choice. The use of heparin, 250,000 units in a 250-mL solution infused every 8 h for 5 days, has been successful.

The mechanical extraction of the retained stone can be performed under radiographic control. Mazzariello reported a 96 percent success rate for 1086 cases, and Burhenne and associates reported a 91 percent success rate for 612 patients managed at 38 hospitals, with no deaths and no significant complications. The T tube is generally left in place for at least 4 weeks after the operation; it is then extracted and a polyethylene catheter is used to instill radiopaque material into the common duct. A Dormia basket is then advanced through the catheter to entrap the stone (Fig. 29-15).

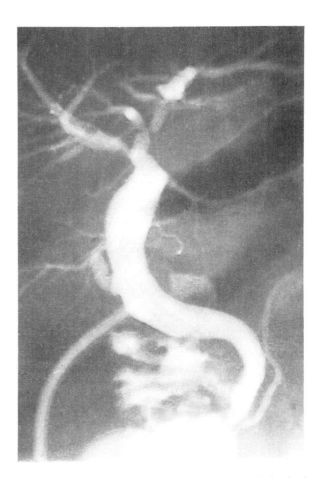

FIG. 29-14. T-tube cholangiogram demonstrating calculus in the right hepatic duct. (From: *Skucas J, Spataro RF (eds): Radiology of the Acute Abdomen. New York, Churchill Livingstone, 1986, Fig. 9-30, with permission.)*

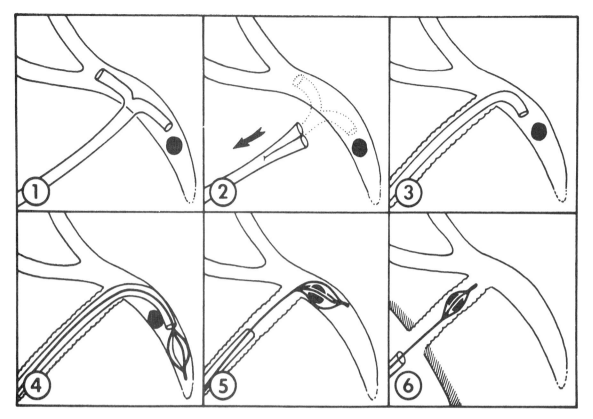

FIG. 29-15. Technical steps for retained common duct stone extraction. *1.* A repeat T-tube cholangiogram is obtained on the day of stone extraction 4 to 5 weeks after choledochotomy. *2.* After the location of the retained stone has been ascertained, the T tube is withdrawn. *3.* Using the sinus tract of the T tube, the steerable catheter is guided into the bile duct, and its movable tip is advanced beyond the retained stone. *4.* The basket is inserted through the steerable catheter, the catheter is withdrawn, and the basket is opened. *5.* The open basket is withdrawn in order to engage the stone. The basket is only retracted—it is never advanced outside the enclosure of the steerable catheter. *6.* The stone is extracted through the drain tract. (After: *Burhenne HJ: Radium therapy and nuclear medicine. Am J Roentgenol 117:388, 1973, with permission.)*

The most commonly used approach is transduodenal papillotomy with extraction of the stone under endoscopic visualization (Fig. 29-16). The success rate for extraction or spontaneous passage after this procedure was 86 percent for 731 collected cases. A complication rate of 7 percent was noted, but two-thirds of complications were treated conservatively. The mortality rate related to the technique was 1.25 percent. Operative intervention is indicated in some cases if there is evidence of obstruction or cholangitis, or if nonoperative methods fail.

Some calculi remain within the liver and may cause irreversible damage. The most common location is a left main hepatic duct that forms a cisterna, and successful treatment is best achieved in this circumstance by resection of the left lobe of the liver. In occasional patients with recurrent hepatic duct stones, a Roux-en-Y limb can be anastomosed to the hepatic duct (usually the left main duct) and positioned so that it can be entered under radiographic guidance to permit stone extraction.

Biliary Enteric Fistula and Gallstone Ileus

A stone in the ampulla of the gallbladder (Hartmann's pouch) can encroach upon and erode the common bile duct. This is known as Mirizzi's syndrome. Operative management depends on the extent to which the common duct has been compromised.

If there is only a pressure effect, cholecystectomy is sufficient. If the common duct segment is partially or completely destroyed, a reconstructive procedure is mandated and may require a Roux-en-Y limb anastomosis to the proximal normal duct. When biliary enteric fistulas develop, they usually run between the gallbladder and the duodenum, but 15 percent are cholecystocolic fistulas. Mechanical obstruction of the gastrointestinal tract caused by gallstones is a relatively infrequent occurrence. Gallstone ileus causes 1 to 2 percent of mechanical small-intestine obstructions; the mortality rate is less than 10 percent.

Since cholelithiasis occurs three to six times more commonly in the female than in the male, a higher incidence of gallstone ileus in the female is to be anticipated. Preponderance in the female is actually higher than one would expect, and in several series all patients were female. It is characteristically a disease of the aged, with an average age of sixty-four, and is unusual under the age of fifty.

The process usually begins with formation of the stone within the gallbladder, but cases have been reported in which the gallbladder was not present, having been removed several years prior to the intestinal obstruction. After the gallstone has left the gallbladder, it may obstruct the alimentary tract in one of two ways. Typically, *intraluminal obstruction* is produced by the en-

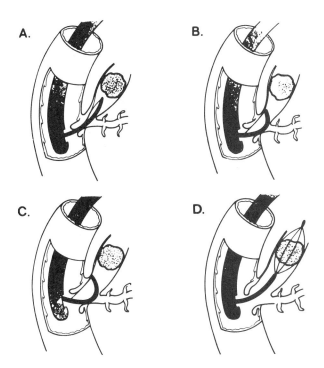

FIG. 29-16. *Steps in endoscopic sphincterotomy. A. Sphincterotome is inserted in closed position into common bile duct. B. Proximal part of bent wire appears just outside papilla. C. Current is applied for cutting sphincter. D. Extraction of stone through opened papilla. (After: Safrany L: Transduodenal endoscopic sphincterectomy and extraction of bile duct stones. World J Surg 2:457, 1978, with permission.)*

trance of the stone into the gastrointestinal tract. Rarely, the stone enters the peritoneal cavity, causing kinking or inflammation and *extrinsic obstruction* of the intestine. The stone may enter the duodenum via the common duct, but this is unusual, and almost always the offending calculus enters through a cholecystenteric fistula. The fistulous tract may connect the gallbladder with the stomach, duodenum, jejunum, ileum, or colon. In addition, internal biliary fistulas may communicate with the pleural or pericardial cavities, tracheobronchial tree, pregnant uterus, ovarian cyst, renal pelvis, and urinary bladder. In a series of 176 fistulas caused by gallstones, the duodenum was involved in 101, the colon in 33, the stomach in 7, and multiple sites in 11.

The fistula probably originates with a stone obstructing the cystic duct, acute cholecystitis, empyema, and the formation of adhesions between the gallbladder and adjacent viscera. Perforation then occurs between the intimately adherent organs, and the stone traverses the fistula. The cholecystenteric fistula then frequently closes, and only a fibrous remnant remains. Having entered the alimentary tract, the gallstone, which is usually single, may be vomited or passed spontaneously via the rectum. The size of the stone is important, since stones smaller than 2 to 3 cm usually pass. When obstruction occurs, the site is usually at the terminal ileum, which is the narrowest portion of the small intestine. Of 154 cases, the duodenum was obstructed in 6, the jejunum in 14, the proximal ileum in 6, the middle ileum in 31, the terminal ileum in 88, the colon in 3, and the rectum in 2. When a gallstone blocks the small intestine, the morbid anatomic and physiologic effects of a mechanical obstruction obtain.

There are very large losses of fluid into the intestine. Edema, ulceration, or necrosis of the bowel may occur, and perforation may result.

Clinical Manifestations. A past history suggestive of cholelithiasis is present in 50 to 75 percent of patients. Symptoms of acute cholecystitis immediately preceding the onset of gallstone ileus occur in one-quarter to one-third of the cases. A history of jaundice is present in about 10 percent of the cases. Occasionally, there may be an initial episode of pain suggestive of biliary colic, but major pain is usually not experienced until the intestinal colic results. There is associated cramping, nausea, and vomiting, which may be intermittent. When complete small intestinal obstruction occurs, the vomiting increases and obstipation results. Vomiting is present in almost 100 percent, cramps in 90 percent, distention in 90 percent, obstipation in 78 percent, and feculent vomiting in 67 percent. Serum electrolyte levels reveal the pattern of lower intestinal obstruction with marked hypochloremia, hyponatremia, hypokalemia, and an elevated carbonate level.

The correct preoperative diagnosis is infrequently made, ranging between 13 and 30 percent in several series. The usual diagnosis is that of intestinal obstruction of unknown cause. Radiologic examination may be diagnostic if gas is demonstrated within the biliary tract (Fig. 29-17). Flat, upright, and lateral films plus spot films over the liver are indicated if the diagnosis is considered. The plain x-ray film reveals the pattern of small-intestine obstruction, and a stone is visualized in less than 20 percent of the cases. The diagnosis has also been based on the migration of a previously observed radiopaque gallstone.

Treatment. Biliary enteric fistulas are managed by cholecystectomy and closure by primary repair of the intestinal opening. The patient with gallstone ileus often requires fluid and

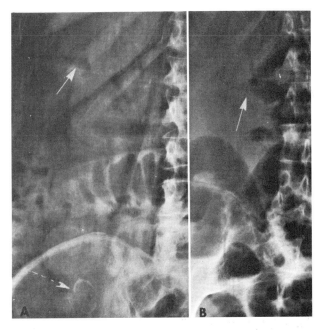

FIG. 29-17. *Gallstone ileus. A. Radiopaque calculus present in right lower quadrant; suggestion of gas in biliary tract within liver. B. Demonstration of gas in intrahepatic biliary system.*

electrolyte replacement in order to correct deficiency, and a nasogastric tube is used to decompress the stomach. Definitive therapy consists of locating the stone or stones, enterotomy proximal to the stone, and removal of the offending calculi with closure of the intestine. The recurrence rate of gallstone ileus is 5 to 9 percent, and it is important to palpate the entire small intestine, gallbladder, and common duct for retained stones, particularly if the obstructing stone is faceted. Either concomitant or planned interval cholecystectomy and closure of the fistula, if patent, is indicated, since recurrent symptoms or complications develop in one-third of the patients. Carcinoma of the gallbladder has also been present or developed 5 to 16 years after removal of the obstructing gallstone. Performance of concomitant cholecystectomy is determined by the patient's general condition. Many of these patients are extremely ill and depleted, and prolongation of the operative procedure may be contraindicated.

INFLAMMATORY AND OTHER BENIGN LESIONS

Acute Cholecystitis

Acute cholecystitis is usually associated with an obstruction of the neck of the gallbladder or cystic duct caused by stones impacted in Hartmann's pouch. Direct pressure of the calculus on the mucosa results in ischemia, necrosis, and ulceration with swelling, edema, and impairment of venous return. These processes in turn increase and extend the intensity of the inflammation. The ulceration may be so extensive that the mucosa is frequently hard to define on microscopic examination, and segmented leukocytes are found infiltrating all layers. The results of necrosis are perforation with pericholecystic abscess formation, fistulization, or bile peritonitis. In the past, acute cholecystitis secondary to systemic infection occurred most commonly with typhoid fever, but this is now rare. A bacterial cause has been proposed and positive bile cultures have been noted in 60 percent of patients. *E. coli*, *Klebsiella* species, streptococci, *Enterobacter aerogenes*, salmonellae, and clostridia have all been implicated.

Acute cholecystitis, caused by generalized sepsis or by stasis or impaction of a calculus, may occur while the patient is recovering from trauma or an operation. Among other causes of acute cholecystitis are the vascular effects of collagen disease, terminal states of hypertensive vascular disease, and thrombosis of the main cystic artery. Acute cholecystitis in which the gallbladder is devoid of stones is known as acalculous cholecystitis. Less than 1 percent of acutely inflamed gallbladders contain a malignant tumor that may play a role in causing obstruction. The incidences of common duct calculi are similar in acute and in chronic cholecystitis, averaging 7 to 15 percent.

Clinical Manifestations. Most attacks of acute cholecystitis occur in patients who give a history compatible with chronic cholecystitis and cholelithiasis. Acute cholecystitis can occur at any age, but the greatest incidence is between the fourth and eighth decades, and patients over the age of sixty comprise between one-quarter and one-third of the group. Caucasians are afflicted more frequently than blacks, and women more than men.

The onset of acute symptoms is frequently related to a vigorous attempt of the gallbladder to empty its contents, usually after a heavy, fatty, or fried meal. Moderate to severe pain is experienced in the right upper quadrant and epigastrium and may radiate to the back in the region of the angle of the scapula or in the interscapular area. The patient is often febrile, and vomiting may be severe. Tenderness, usually along the right costal margin, often associated with rebound tenderness and spasm, is characteristic. The gallbladder may be palpable, or a palpable mass in the region may be the result of omentum wrapped around the gallbladder. Mild icterus may be present and may be caused by calculi within the ampulla and edema encroaching on the common duct. Moderate to marked jaundice, particularly with a serum bilirubin level greater than 6 mg/dL, suggests the presence of associated choledocholithiasis but can occur with isolated cholecystitis.

The differential diagnosis includes perforation or penetration of peptic ulcer, appendicitis, pancreatitis, hepatitis, myocardial ischemia or infarction, pneumonia, pleurisy, and herpes zoster involving an intercostal nerve.

The hemogram usually demonstrates leukocytosis with a shift to the left. Radiographs of the chest and abdomen are indicated to rule out pneumonia. A radiopaque calculus is noted in less than 20 percent of cases. The serum bilirubin level may determine the presence of common duct obstruction. Although an elevated amylase level is generally regarded as evidence of acute pancreatitis, levels as high as 1000 Somogyi units have been associated with acute cholecystitis uncomplicated by pancreatitis. To rule out myocardial ischemia, an electrocardiogram should be performed on any patient over the age of forty-five being considered for surgical treatment. Acute cholecystitis may be responsible for some electrocardiographic changes. Oral cholecystography is of limited value because of impaired absorption of dye. An ultrasonogram may demonstrate calculi and/or a thickened wall of the gallbladder and is the diagnostic procedure of choice. Radionuclide scanning with DISIDA (diisopropyl iminodiacetic acid) or PIPIDA (N-para-isopropyl-acetanilide-iminodiacetic acid) is the most effective diagnostic study in this situation.

Treatment. There have been conflicting opinions on the management of acute cholecystitis, particularly on the optimal time for surgical intervention. For the purposes of discussion, early operation is defined as one performed within 72 h after the onset of symptoms; intermediate operation is one carried out between 72 h and the cessation of clinical manifestations; delayed operative management permits the acute inflammatory process to subside; and scheduled elective surgery is performed after an interval of 6 weeks to 3 months. Most surgeons now favor early operation, i.e., with 24 to 48 h. The mortality rate for emergent cholecystectomy ranges from 0 to 5 percent. In the majority of cases, laparoscopic cholecystectomy is successful, but the incidence of conversion to open cholecystectomy is greater in this group of patients when compared to those without acute inflammation. In rare instances of extremely ill patients, cholecystostomy under local anesthesia is applicable.

Emphysematous Cholecystitis. Emphysematous cholecystitis is a rare form of acute, usually gangrenous, cholecystitis, associated with the presence of gas in the gallbladder (Fig. 29-18). Unlike ordinary acute cholecystitis, which is more prevalent among women, emphysematous cholecystitis is more often found in men, with incidences of 75 percent for males and 25 percent for females. Pathogenesis is related to acute inflammation of the gallbladder, which often begins aseptically, compli-

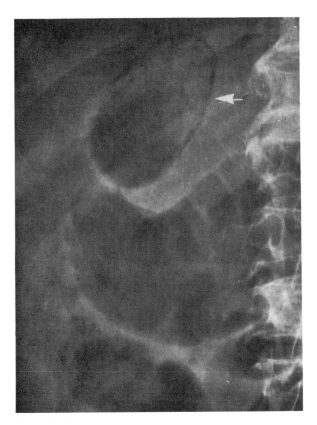

FIG. 29-18. Emphysematous cholecystitis. Gallbladder is visible as a gas-filled organ.

cated by a secondary infection with gas-forming bacilli. These may reach the gallbladder by bile ducts, bloodstream, or lymphatic channels and grow in an anaerobic environment. The clinical manifestations are similar to those of acute cholecystitis. In approximately half the patients, a history of previous gallbladder attacks can be elicited. Cholelithiasis is also present in half the patients, who are frequently diabetic.

The diagnosis is usually made on the basis of radiographs that show a globular, gas-filled shadow in the region of the gallbladder. Later, intramural or submucosal gas may appear, and gas may also appear in the pericholecystic area, denoting extension of the pathologic process outside the confines of the gallbladder. The treatment of choice is early operation, since the incidence of free perforation is reported to be 40 to 60 percent. Cholecystectomy is indicated, but if it is not feasible, cholecystostomy should be performed. In 9 percent of cases, choledocholithiasis is present, and exploration of the common duct may be required. Although positive bile cultures are found in only half the cases, antibiotics directed toward the clostridial and coliform organisms are indicated. The mortality rate is significantly greater than that for nonemphysematous cholecystitis.

Chronic Cholecystitis

Chronic inflammation of the gallbladder is generally associated with cholelithiasis and consists of round cell infiltration and fibrosis of the wall. Buried crypts of mucosa (Rokitansky-Aschoff sinuses) may be seen dipping into the mucosa (Fig. 29-19). Obstruction by gallstones of the neck of the cystic duct may pro-

duce a mucocele of the gallbladder (hydrops). The bile is initially sterile but may be secondarily infected with coliform bacilli, *Klebsiella* species, streptococci, and occasionally clostridia or *Salmonella typhi*. Secondary effects of cholecystitis include obstruction of the common duct, cholangitis, perforation of the gallbladder with formation of a pericholecystic abscess or a cholecystenteric fistula, bile peritonitis, and pancreatitis. There may be associated carcinoma of the gallbladder.

Clinical Manifestations. The patients generally present with moderate intermittent abdominal pain in the right upper quadrant and epigastrium, occasionally radiating to the scapula and interscapular region. There is usually a history of intolerance of fatty or fried foods, and the patient may have noted intermittent nausea and anorexia. If the patient is not experiencing acute pain, there may be no diagnostic findings on physical examination. Occasionally tenderness is elicited over the gallbladder. Diagnosis is usually established by ultrasound scanning or an oral cholecystogram, which demonstrates either the absence of filling of the gallbladder or the presence of stones.

Hyperplastic Cholecystoses. Hyperplastic cholecystoses are characterized by the proliferation of normal tissue elements. The two most common of these lesions are cholesterolosis and adenomyomatosis. In patients with cholesterolosis there is evidence of cholesterol deposition within the epithelial cells of the lamina propria. The bile of these patients contains significantly more cholesterol than that of normal adults, and the abnormality pre-

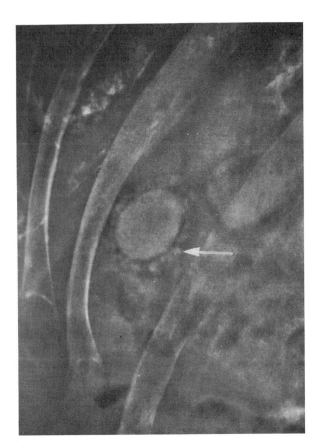

FIG. 29-19. Rokitansky-Aschoff sinuses presenting as a halo effect, a finding present in chronic cholecystitis.

sumably arises from some aberration in cholesterol transport and absorption by the gallbladder epithelium. The deposition of cholesterol within the wall gives rise to the gross description·of the "strawberry gallbladder." Adenomyomatosis is characterized by hyperplasia of the muscle and mucosa of the gallbladder. Malignant degeneration is unusual, and it is unclear whether these disorders can truly be the source of symptoms. Cholecystectomy should be offered to these patients only if warranted by symptoms.

Treatment. The treatment of chronic cholecystitis and cholelithiasis is cholecystectomy, and the results are usually excellent. Laparoscopic cholecystectomy is the procedure of choice. Early cholecystectomy is particularly important for the diabetic patient. Operative mortality of less than 1 percent has been reported for large series. Seventy-five percent of patients undergoing cholecystectomy for cholelithiasis are completely relieved of all preoperative symptoms, and the remaining 25 percent have only mild symptoms that are apparently unrelated to the biliary system.

Acalculous Cholecystitis

Acute and chronic inflammatory disease of the gallbladder can occur without stones. Acute acalculous cholecystitis frequently is a complication of burns, sepsis, multiple system failure, cardiovascular disease, diabetes, prolonged illness, or a major operation.

The incidence of chronic acalculous cholecystitis is difficult to establish. It is present in over 50 percent of children and 35 percent of Nigerians with gallbladder disease, and the accepted incidence of adults in the United States is less than 5 percent of cases of cholecystitis. Possible causes include (1) anatomic conditions such as kinking, fibrosis, and obstruction of the cystic duct by tumor or anomalous vessels; (2) thrombosis of major blood vessels, producing ischemia and gangrene; (3) spasm or fibrosis of the sphincter of Oddi in patients with a "common channel" with or without associated pancreatitis; (4) systemic diseases such as diabetes mellitus and collagen diseases; (5) specific infections such as typhoid fever, actinomycosis, and parasitic infestation; and (6) scarlet fever and a wide variety of febrile illnesses in young children. The DISIDA or PIPIDA scan and the ultrasound scan are occasionally normal in these patients, but characteristically the ultrasound demonstrates thickening of the wall. Percutaneous cholecystostomy has been used successfully (80 percent) for diagnosis and treatment of acalculous cholecystitis.

Treatment. Cholecystectomy is preferable, but in one series the patient's condition mandated cholecystostomy in 14 of 16 cases. In children with acute febrile illness, cholecystostomy has been particularly effective, and subsequent cholecystectomy has not been required in many of these patients.

Cholangitis

Infection within the biliary duct system is most frequently associated with choledocholithiasis but also has accompanied choledochal cysts and carcinoma of the bile duct, and has followed sphincteroplasty. Infection and inflammatory changes may extend up the duct system into the liver and give rise to multiple hepatic abscesses. Clinically, the condition is characterized by intermittent fever, upper abdominal pain, exacerbation of jaundice, pruritus, and at times rigor.

In patients with common duct stones in whom there is ascending cholangitis, a broad-spectrum antibiotic directed particularly at *E. coli*, which is the most common offending organism, should be given for several days before surgical treatment. Antibiotics usually control the infection, but if the patient's temperature does not fall, surgical drainage should not be delayed. This can be accomplished percutaneously by the transduodenal or transhepatic routes or operatively.

Acute Suppurative Cholangitis. Suppurative cholangitis, in which there is gross pus within the biliary tract, constitutes one of the most urgent causes for laparotomy in patients with obstructive jaundice. The condition was first described in 1877 by Charcot, who suggested a diagnostic triad of jaundice, chills and fever, and pain in the right upper quadrant. To these, Reynolds and Dargan added shock and central nervous system depression as specific identifying features of the condition.

The disease occurs almost exclusively in patients over 70 years of age. All patients are febrile, and a majority are jaundiced. Hypotension, confusion, or lethargy occurs in about 20 percent of cases. A white blood cell count of less than 12,000/ mm^3 has been reported in over half the patients, probably related to the age and lack of marrow response. Bilirubin, SGOT, and alkaline phosphatase levels are characteristically elevated, but the serum amylase level is usually normal. The correct diagnosis has been made in less than one-third of the patients. Patients have been managed emergently by establishing initial drainage via ERCP or PTC followed by definitive operation.

At operation, all patients demonstrate gross distention of the common bile duct, with frank pus, frequently under considerable pressure, and choledocholithiasis or a tumor obstructing the distal bile duct. If the gallbladder is present, it is invariably distended and inflamed. Spontaneous perforation of the bile ducts has been reported. Surgical treatment is directed at rapid decompression of the duct system and is combined with large doses of antibiotics, particularly those that achieve high levels in the bile. In a review of the literature, it was reported that all patients who were not operated on died, and mortality following drainage or surgical procedures ranged from zero to 88 percent, averaging 33 percent.

Cholangiohepatitis

Cholangiohepatitis, which is also known as recurrent pyogenic cholangitis, is found almost exclusively among the Chinese, with the largest number of cases seen among Cantonese living in the Pearl River delta in China. In Hong Kong it is the most commonly encountered disease of the biliary passages and is the third most common abdominal surgical emergency after appendicitis and perforated ulcer. It has also been encountered in Great Britain, in Australia, and in the Chinese population in the United States. Cholangiohepatitis occurs most frequently in the third and fourth decades but has been reported at all ages and occurs with equal frequency among men and women.

The etiology of cholangiohepatitis is summarized in Fig. 29-20. The pyogenic element probably originates from the bowel and is caused by *E. coli*, *Klebsiella* species, *Bacteroides* species, or *Enterococcus faecalis*. In most instances, positive cultures are obtainable from the bile and the portal venous blood. The Chinese liver fluke, *C. sinensis*, was thought to be an important contributing factor. Other factors that have been implicated as

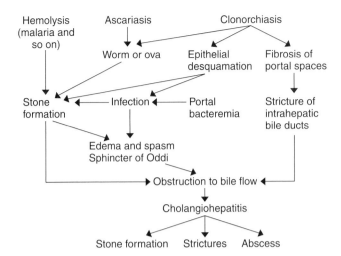

FIG. 29-20. *Schema of etiologic factors implicated in cholangiohepatitis. (After: Stock FE, Fung JHY: Oriental cholangiohepatitis, in Smith R, Sherlock S (eds): Surgery of the Gallbladder and Bile Ducts. London, Butterworth, 1964, with permission.)*

contributing causes of cholangiohepatitis include ascariasis and hemolysis associated with malaria.

Pathology. The gallbladder wall is thickened but not grossly inflamed. The common bile duct is also usually grossly distended and contains large stones. The stones are produced by precipitation of bile pigments, desquamation of epithelium, and products of inflammation; the nucleus of the stone may contain an adult *Clonorchis* worm, an ovum, or an ascarid. Acute or hemorrhagic pancreatitis occurs in less than 1 percent of cases. The most marked changes occur in the liver, where the intrahepatic bile ducts are both dilated and constricted. Inflammatory changes are present in the periductal tissue and may progress to frank abscess formation.

Clinical Manifestations. In highly endemic areas, cholangiohepatitis is the first consideration in patients with jaundice, pain, and pyrexia. Pain is usually located in the right upper quadrant and epigastrium and may be colicky or constant. In most acute attacks there is fever accompanied by chills and rigors, and 50 percent of the patients are jaundiced, while the remainder have an elevation of the serum bilirubin level. Recurrence of symptoms is one of the most characteristic features of the disease.

Most patients appear to be in a toxic condition, with temperatures up to 40°C. There is tenderness and guarding in the right upper quadrant. The white blood cell count is usually about 15,000/mm^3, and the serum bilirubin level is generally above 2 mg/dL, with accompanying bilirubinuria. There may be evidence of impairment of hepatocellular function. In the majority of cases calculi are not demonstrable on routine x-ray films. An occasional finding of significance is the presence of gas in the biliary tree, which may be due to a secondary gas-forming organism or a fistula between the duct and duodenum. ERCP or PTC may establish the diagnosis. Manifestations of portal hypertension may be present.

Treatment. Patients are generally prepared with antibiotics. Surgical therapy, however, should not be delayed for the

patient who is jaundiced and has pain and pyrexia. The operation consists of removal of the stones and debris from the extrahepatic bile ducts followed by establishment of open drainage between the involved ducts and intestine, usually with a Roux-en-Y limb. Anchoring the Roux-en-Y limb to the anterior abdominal wall facilitates subsequent repeated dilatation and stone extractions.

If large hepatic abscesses are noted, drainage should be performed. Left hepatic lobectomy has been carried out on occasion, when there has been gross dilatation of the ducts and abscess formation in the left lobe while the right was apparently normal.

The prognosis is generally guarded, since recurrence is not uncommon. In one study, common duct exploration, transhepatic intubation, and hepatotomy were associated with recurrence rates of 24, 37, and 75 percent, respectively. Hepatic resection had a failure rate of only 4 percent, and none of the patients had recurrent stones. In advanced cases, particularly with multiple abscesses, the prognosis is poor, and the patient eventually succumbs to liver failure, septicemia, or cholangiocarcinoma.

Sclerosing Cholangitis

Sclerosing cholangitis is an uncommon disease that involves all or part of the extrahepatic biliary duct system and often affects the intrahepatic biliary radicals as well. The disease has also been called *obliterative cholangitis* and *stenosing cholangitis*, in reference to a progressive thickening of the bile duct walls encroaching upon the lumen. It may be associated with gallstones, but several series have been presented in which there were no stones in the gallbladder or the common duct. A significant number of cases have been associated with ulcerative colitis, Crohn's disease, Riedel's struma, retroperitoneal fibrosis, and porphyria cutanea tarda.

The cause of sclerosing cholangitis is unknown. Histologic sections in several cases failed to reveal any granulomatous lesion, metaplasia, or neoplasia. In several series, none of the patients had previous surgical treatment, and therefore local trauma was excluded as an etiologic agent; irritation of the common duct by passage of calculi is unlikely given that there are usually no stones present in either the common duct or the gallbladder. It has been suggested that the disease may be caused by local response to viral infection, since a relative lymphocytosis with atypical lymphocytes has been noted. Immune response and collagen disease have also been considered as possible causes. A positive cellular immune response to biliary antigens has been demonstrated. The disease has been noted in patients with HIV infection.

Pathology. Grossly, there is diffuse thickening of the wall of the extrahepatic biliary tract and sometimes of the intrahepatic ducts, with a concomitant encroachment on the lumen, resulting in marked luminal narrowing. The duct system may be completely involved, or the hepatic ducts may be spared and the disease restricted to the entire length of the common duct. The gallbladder is usually not involved, but the lymph nodes in the region of the common duct and foramen of Winslow are usually markedly enlarged and succulent. Microscopic analyses of the affected duct show that the walls are as much as eight times thicker than normal. The areas of inflammation and fibrosis are in the submucosal and subserosal portions, with an edematous field between them. The mucosa is intact throughout. Biopsy examination of the liver may reveal bile stasis or, in long-standing cases, biliary cirrhosis. The histologic evaluation is critical, since it is difficult to differentiate this disease from sclerosing carcinoma of the bile ducts.

Clinical Manifestations. The diagnosis is to be considered in patients (particularly middle-aged men) with a clinical and laboratory picture of extrahepatic jaundice. Jaundice is usually associated with intermittent pain in the right upper quadrant, nausea, vomiting, and occasionally chills and fever. In long-standing cases with biliary cirrhosis, the manifestations of portal hypertension, such as bleeding varices and ascites, may be apparent. The diagnosis has been established by ERCP. At operation a dense inflammatory reaction in the region of the gallbladder and gastrohepatic ligament is noted. Palpation of the duct reveals a cordlike structure that may feel like a thrombosed blood vessel, but the wall of the common duct is obviously thickened and cuts with difficulty. The edges of the incision characteristically pout out. Usually only a fine probe or small Bakes dilator can be inserted into the lumen. Cholangiography may vividly demonstrate the extensive narrowing of the lumen (Fig. 29-21).

Treatment. The appropriate management of sclerosing cholangitis remains unclear. No drug therapy has achieved consistent, or even usual, success.

The asymptomatic anicteric patient is not treated and is not studied with repeated cholangiograms if jaundice or cholangitis does not develop. The pruritic and icteric patient is treated for

4 to 6 weeks with prednisone; if there is no improvement, or if cholangitis is present or develops, an operation is performed with a preoperative cholangiogram as a guide. If there is minimal intrahepatic involvement and dilatation of a segment of the common duct or common hepatic duct proximal to marked stenosis, the stenotic segment is excised as a biopsy section to rule out cholangiocarcinoma, and a direct mucosa-to-mucosa anastomosis is effected between the dilated segment of duct and a Roux-en-Y limb of jejunum, preferably without a stent. Stricture of the confluence of the hepatic ducts is managed by excision of the distal ducts for pathologic evaluation and anastomosis of the hepatic ducts to the Roux-en-Y limb of jejunum by the mucosa-to-mucosa technique. If the hepatic ducts are sufficiently dilated, no stent is used. If these ducts are small, transhepatic stents are used, but no attempt is made to dilate intrahepatic ducts.

Data from several large centers suggest that selected patients with primarily extrahepatic disease can be successfully managed with hepaticojejunostomy and long-term stenting. In patients with more diffuse or advanced parenchymal disease, hepatic transplantation has become the procedure of choice. The role of transplantation might be extended as we begin to understand more fully the risk of cholangiocarcinoma developing in patients with sclerosing cholangitis.

Fibrosis or Stenosis of the Sphincter of Oddi

In 1884 Langenbuch, only 2 years after reporting the first successful removal of a gallbladder, suggested transduodenal division of the "diverticulum" of Vater in cases of cicatricial stenosis for chronic inflammation. In 1901 Opie called attention to the "common channel" theory as the cause of pancreatitis, and in 1913 Archibald suggested sphincteroplasty as the treatment for pancreatitis.

The pathogenesis of fibrosis or stenosis of the sphincter of Oddi and the papilla of Vater is not fully understood. Long-standing spasm may play an important role, and infection of the biliary tract or pancreas has also been implicated. Irritation from stones within the common duct may also lead to fibrosis. In a series of 50 patients in whom sphincteroplasty was performed because a small Bakes dilator could not be passed through the sphincter of Oddi, biopsy analysis revealed no abnormalities in 18, while 18 showed inflammatory infiltration, 17 had minimal fibrosis, and 2 had diffuse fibrosis. No definite correlation could be found between the various manifestations of biliary tract disease and the histologic changes.

Clinical Manifestations. The main symptom of fibrosis or stenosis of the sphincter of Oddi is abdominal pain, usually colicky and frequently associated with nausea and vomiting. The pain begins in the right upper quadrant and radiates to the shoulder, and it may be intermittent. Over half the patients give a history of intermittent jaundice, and many indicate that they have had previous cholecystectomy without relief of symptoms.

Treatment. The diagnosis is generally made when there is difficulty in passing a No. 3 Bakes dilator through the ampulla of Vater. Cholangiography and pressure studies on the common bile duct have theoretical application. If a 3-mm dilator cannot be easily passed through the ampulla, a transduodenal exploration should be carried out. Thomas and associates compared the results of transduodenal sphincteroplasty and choledochoduodenostomy in 30 patients with stenosis or stricture of the sphinc-

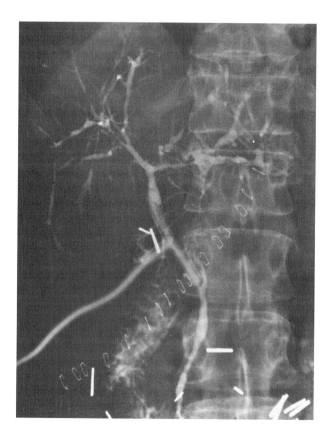

FIG. 29-21. *Sclerosing cholangitis T-tube cholangiogram showing severe sclerosing cholangitis, giving the appearance of a pruned tree.*

ter. The procedures were equally and highly effective, and neither was associated with a significant incidence of subsequent cholangitis. Sphincteroplasty is preferable if the common duct is small, and a transduodenal approach is indicated if an ampullary tumor is suspected. Endoscopic papillotomy has been used successfully, particularly in Europe, where the disorder is more frequently diagnosed.

Papillitis

In 1926 DelValle first described a benign inflammatory and fibrous process of the ampulla of Vater and indicated that it was a factor in producing stenosis. It was postulated that acute and subacute inflammatory changes occur and that stenosis is the final and irreversible result of these changes. Acosta and Nardi have presented 61 cases of papillitis, 21 of which were chronic ulcerative papillitis, 20 chronic sclerosing papillitis, 15 chronic granulomatous papillitis, and 5 chronic adenomatous papillitis. The acute stage, which is characterized by edema, papillary dilatation, hemorrhage, and infiltration, may be reversible, whereas sclerosing papillitis and chronic granulomatous papillitis are considered irreversible in view of their inevitable evolution into scar tissue.

The clinical and pathologic features associated with papillitis include the postcholecystectomy syndrome in 30 percent, dilatation of the common duct in 50 percent, biliary disease without stones in 25 percent, obstructive jaundice in 60 percent, pancreatitis in 70 percent, and liver damage in 25 percent. There has been no correlation between the specific clinical syndromes and the pathologic changes. A pancreatic evocative test, using morphine-neostigmine or secretin-CCK, has been used. Elevation of at least one serum pancreatic enzyme level by a factor of four over the normal level, coupled with reproduction of the patient's pain, is considered a positive test result. The efficacy of this test has been disputed. Since the majority of patients with papillitis have irreversible lesions, sphincteroplasty is generally employed.

TUMORS

Carcinoma of the Gallbladder

Carcinoma of the gallbladder accounts for 2 to 4 percent of gastrointestinal malignancies. Its occurrence in random autopsy series is about 0.4 percent, and approximately 1 percent of patients undergoing biliary tract operations have carcinoma either as an anticipated diagnosis or found incidentally.

Etiology. Approximately 90 percent of patients with carcinoma of the gallbladder have cholelithiasis, but the pathogenesis has not been defined. There is also an association with polypoid lesions of the gallbladder. Areas of dysplasia have been noted in juxtaposition to larger (greater than 2.5 cm) stones and in adenomas. Malignant changes have been noted more frequently in polypoid lesions greater than 10 mm. The calcified "porcelain" gallbladder is associated with a 20 percent incidence of gallbladder carcinoma.

Pathology. Approximately 80 percent of the tumors are adenocarcinomas (75 percent of these are scirrhous, 15 percent polypoid, and 10 percent mucoid). Squamous carcinomas, adenoacanthomas, and melanomas occur rarely. The routes of metastasis include spread along the lymphatics to the choledochal, peripancreatic, and periduodenal nodes. There is often localized invasion of vessels within the wall of the gallbladder, and the tumor frequently extends transmurally into the parenchyma of the liver. When metastases are present, the liver is involved in two-thirds of patients, the regional lymph nodes in about one-half, and the omentum, duodenum, colon, or porta hepatis in about one-fourth. Early reports suggest more frequent and rapid recurrences of carcinomas of the gallbladder after laparoscopic cholecystectomy. By 1995, 15 cases of trocar-site metastases from unsuspected gallbladder carcinoma following laparoscopic cholecystectomy were reported.

Clinical Manifestations. Signs and symptoms of carcinoma of the gallbladder are generally indistinguishable from those associated with cholecystitis and cholelithiasis. These include abdominal discomfort, right upper quadrant pain, nausea, vomiting, and weight loss. Half the patients are jaundiced, and two-thirds of those with clinical manifestations have a palpable mass. Laboratory findings are not diagnostic. Ultrasound or CT scan may suggest the diagnosis.

Treatment. Most long-term survivors are patients who underwent cholecystectomy for cholelithiasis and in whom the malignancy was an incidental finding. The management of these patients is controversial. There is some suggestion that T2 or more advanced tumors have a better prognosis if a radical second procedure, which includes lymphadenectomy and partial hepatic resection for lesions located adjacent to the liver, is performed. For lesions that are apparent at operation, removal of the hepatoduodenal nodes, resection of segment IV/V or extended right hepatectomy and, in some cases, pancreaticoduodenectomy has been reported to improve survival. By contrast, other reports have indicated that there has been no improvement associated with these procedures. Some groups have reported that adjuvant radiation therapy or chemotherapy improves survival.

Prognosis. Large cumulative series report 5-year survival rates of 5 percent. The overwhelming majority of survivors are in the group that had incidentally diagnosed tumors. T1 lesions have a 5-year survival rate of approximately 100 percent. T2 lesions have a survival rate of 40 percent when subjected to the more radical operations. In some series, no difference was noted when node-negative and node-positive patients were compared.

Bile Duct Carcinoma

Pathology. The autopsy incidence of bile duct carcinoma is about 0.3 percent. Unlike gallbladder carcinomas, bile duct tumors occur more frequently in men. There is no evidence that bile duct stones have a role, and the relationship between the tumors and sclerosing cholangitis remains ill-defined. Approximately two-thirds of the lesions are located in the proximal ducts, often at the confluence of the right and left main hepatic ducts (Klatskin tumors). The tumors are generally small but involve the whole thickness of the duct, growing in a scirrhous concentric manner and resulting in ductal obstruction. The proximal lesions often extend into the hepatic parenchyma. Rarely, the ductal tumors are polypoid tumors, which are associated with a more favorable prognosis, as is the case with carcinomas of the ampulla of Vater.

Ductal lesions are cholangiocarcinomas of the adenocarcinoma type. Most tumors are well differentiated and associated with a marked fibrous reaction. Perineural involvement is common. Intraoperative frozen-section diagnosis is often difficult.

The liver and regional lymph nodes are the most frequent sites of metastasis. The incidence of metastasis at operation is 50 percent. In some cases multicentric ductal tumors have been reported.

Clinical Manifestations. Characteristically, patients present with the recent onset of jaundice, acholic stools, and dark urine. The jaundice is often preceded by pruritus. Almost all patients have had significant weight loss associated with loss of appetite. Half the patients have abdominal pain; cholangitis may result from the obstruction. The gallbladder is palpable in one-third of the patients who have distal lesions and is not felt with proximal tumors.

The laboratory findings are compatible with the diagnosis of obstructive jaundice with elevation of the bilirubin and alkaline phosphatase and mild increase of the transaminases. Increased level of carcinoembryonic antigen (CEA) can be detected in the bile. Ultrasound scanning demonstrates intrahepatic ductal dilatation and distention of the extrahepatic ducts proximal to the point of obstruction. CT scanning will also define the extent and location of ductal dilatation; it rarely demonstrates the tumor itself. Precise demonstration of the site of obstruction is achieved by PTC or ERCP. In the face of isolated intrahepatic ductal dilatation, the former is preferable, and when there is evidence of distention of the gallbladder or extrahepatic ducts, ERCP is more rewarding (Fig. 29-22).

Treatment. Treatment is directed at resecting the tumor, if possible, or palliation by relieving the obstruction. Cure can be achieved only by surgical removal of the lesion, while palliation can be effected by operation, radiologic intervention, or endoscopic decompression. Curative resection generally entails removal of the common duct and the common hepatic duct up to and sometimes including the confluence of the right and left hepatic ducts, followed by anastomosis of the proximal dilated system to a Roux-en-Y limb of small intestine (Fig. 29-23). The resectability of proximal tumors is about 20 percent, and the cure rate remains under 15 percent. If a proximal lesion extends into the liver parenchyma, varying amounts of the liver are removed en bloc, and proximal intrahepatic ducts are anastomosed to the intestine (Fig. 29-24). Orthotopic liver transplants have been performed for intrahepatic tumors with some long-term survivors. The cure of distal bile duct tumors has been improved by radical lymphadenectomy and pancreaticoduodenectomy (Whipple procedure).

Surgical palliation is performed by anastomosing the dilatated ductal system proximal to the point of obstruction to the limb of intestine. In more proximal lesions, this can be achieved by using the extrahepatic portion of the left main hepatic duct (Fig. 29-25). Transection of the liver to the left of the falciform ligament and anastomosing the intestine to the dilated hepatic duct (Longmire procedure) rarely provides long-term relief of jaundice. Using PTC or ERCP, a stent can be passed through the tumor to provide drainage of the dilated ducts. These require

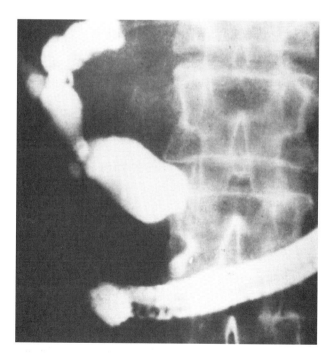

FIG. 29-22. Carcinoma of the pancreas. There is an irregular stricture of the common bile duct, with marked dilatation of the intrahepatic and common bile ducts proximal to the stricture. The pancreatic duct is completely blocked. The tumor precluded obtaining a simultaneous pancreatogram. (From: *Shapiro H: Endoscopic retrograde cholangiography, in Way LW, Pellegrini CA (eds): Gallbladder and Bile Ducts. Philadelphia, WB Saunders, 1987, chap 11, p 197, with permission.*)

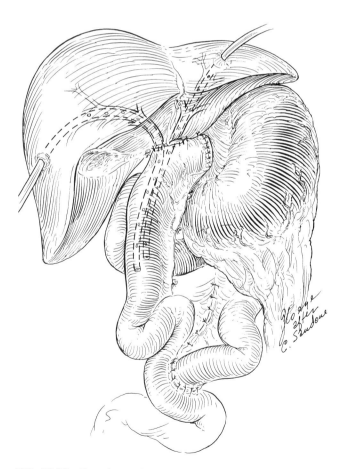

FIG. 29-23. Resection and reconstruction of hilar bile duct tumor. The entire extrahepatic biliary tree is resected with the tumor, and the reconstruction is done with a Roux-en-Y limb of jejunum. The hepaticojejunostomy reconstruction is performed over bilateral transhepatic Silastic catheters.

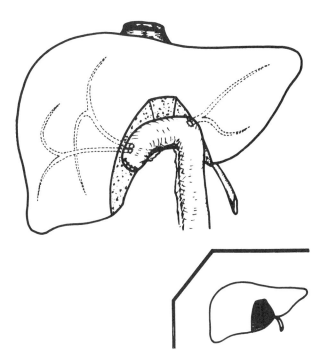

FIG. 29-24. Diagram of the resection of the main hepatic duct junction and segment IV. After resection of segment IV, performed to obtain adequate exposure of the hilus of the liver, en bloc excision of the entire major hepatic duct junction, gallbladder, cystic duct, and common bile duct was done, followed by anastomosis of a Roux-en-Y jejunal loop. The right hepatic ducts, divided proximal to a secondary junction, were inserted into the jejunal loop in a "double-barreled" manner, and the left hepatic duct was inserted directly into the loop. (From: *Launois B, Campion J-P, et al: Carcinoma of the hepatic hilus. Ann Surg 190:151, 1979, with permission.*)

frequent changes. Effort should be directed to providing drainage into the intestine rather than externally because external drainage of bile prevents an enterohepatic circulation and is accompanied by loss of appetite. There have been conflicting reports regarding the efficacy of adjuvant radiotherapy and chemotherapy for either cure or palliation.

OPERATIONS OF THE BILIARY TRACT

Perioperative Considerations. Prophylactic antibiotics are not indicated for patients undergoing elective cholecystectomy unless there are specific risk factors. These include jaundice, common duct stones, diabetes, and age greater than 65 years. Interventional procedures such as PTC or ERCP, especially in patients with biliary tract obstruction, should be covered with prophylactic antibiotic therapy. The antibiotic usually is selected with the assumption that the most likely involved organisms are *E. coli, Klebsiella* species, and enterococci. A second-generation cephalosporin is appropriate. The drug is administered before the operation or intervention, and two subsequent doses are given at 6-h intervals.

Preoperative decompression of the proximal distended ducts in patients with obstructive jaundice does not significantly improve the outcome and has been associated with an increased incidence of complications. Short-term drainage may be indicated as a bridge to an operation in a patient with cholangitis

and sepsis. The preoperative placement of catheters transhepatically may facilitate dissection of proximal tumors, and they can be left in place as stents that traverse anastomoses.

Cholecystostomy

Cholecystostomy accomplishes decompression and drainage of the distended, hydropic, or purulent gallbladder. It is particularly applicable if the patient's general condition is such that it precludes prolonged anesthesia, since the operation may be performed under local anesthesia. It is also performed in cases in which marked inflammatory reaction obscures the anatomic relation of critical structures. Cholecystostomy may be a definitive procedure, particularly if a postoperative tube cholangiogram is normal.

Technique (Fig. 29-26). A circumferential purse-string suture is placed in the fundus of the gallbladder, and a small incision is made through the serosa within the suture. A trocar is inserted into the lumen of the gallbladder, which is then decompressed. After the gallbladder has been emptied, a stone forceps may be introduced to the junction of the ampulla and cystic duct, and obstructing calculi may be removed. A mushroom or Foley catheter is inserted into the lumen of the gallbladder, and a second purse-string suture is placed concentrically to the first one. The sutures are tied, inverting the serosa. Unless a small, oblique incision was used initially, the drainage tube should be brought out through a stab wound.

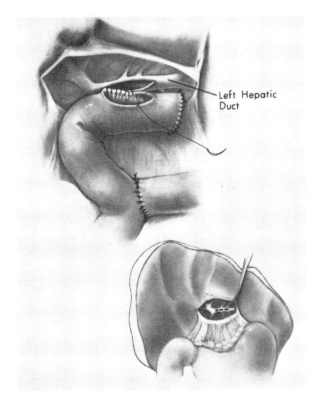

FIG. 29-25. Hepp-Couinaud procedure. Lower illustration demonstrates detachment of tissue in the hilus of the liver in order to visualize the left hepatic duct, which is incised longitudinally. Upper illustration demonstrates side-to-side anastomosis between the main left hepatic duct and a defunctionalized (Roux-en-Y) limb of jejunum.

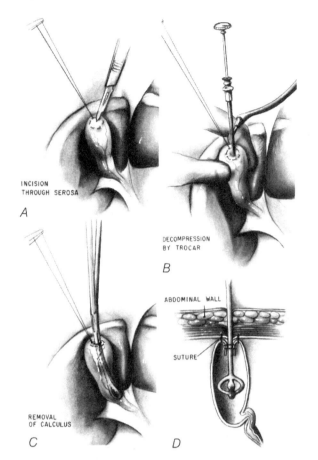

FIG. 29-26. *Cholecystostomy. A. Placement of purse-string suture in fundus of gallbladder, and incision through serosa. B. Trocar decompression. C. Removal of calculus from ampulla. D. Sagittal section demonstrating two concentric purse-string sutures, intraluminal catheter, and suturing of serosa of gallbladder to peritoneum.*

If the fundus of the gallbladder is necrotic, the gangrenous portion should be excised and the remainder of the gallbladder closed around the catheter, using purse-string sutures.

Open Cholecystectomy

A principal aim of open cholecystectomy is to avoid injury to the common duct close to its junction with the common bile duct to obviate a long cystic duct remnant. A more conservative approach toward elective cholecystectomy is indicated for cirrhotic patients. If an operation is performed, increased bleeding should be anticipated; extensive intrahepatic dissection should be avoided. Intraoperative infusion of vasopressin and an antifibrinolytic agent should be considered.

Technique (Fig. 29-27). The gallbladder may be approached through an oblique right upper quadrant incision (Kocher or Courvoisier), through a vertical right paramedian incision, or through the upper midline. There are frequently adhesions between the gallbladder, particularly the ampulla, and the duodenum and colon. These should be lysed by sharp dissection. By applying traction laterally to the ampulla and retracting the duodenum medially, the veil of peritoneum running from ampulla to hepatoduodenal ligament may be accentuated and incised. The cystic duct is identified and a silk ligature passed

around it. Traction is applied to the ligature to prevent passage of a stone down the cystic duct during dissection of the gallbladder. Dissection is continued craniad in this peritoneal fold, and the cystic artery is identified. The course of this artery to the gallbladder should be demonstrated to avoid ligating the right hepatic artery. The cystic artery should be doubly ligated and transected. If bleeding occurs from the cystic artery, it is best controlled by applying pressure on the hepatic artery within the hepatoduodenal ligament. The artery is compressed between the index finger, which is inserted into the foramen of Winslow, and the thumb anteriorly. The peritoneum overlying the gallbladder is then incised close to the liver, and dissection is begun from the fundus of the gallbladder down to an ultimate pedicle of cystic duct. During this dissection, blood vessels coursing from the liver may require ligation, and the gallbladder bed should be inspected for large draining ducts, which should also be ligated. Attention is then directed toward visualization of the junction of the cystic duct and the common duct. The cystic duct is transected and ligated 3 to 5 mm from the common bile duct. It is not necessary to close the bed of the gallbladder. A drain may be brought out from the hepatorenal pouch, which is the most dependent portion of the upper abdomen with the patient in the supine positon, via a separate stab wound if there is any concern that blood will accumulate or if there is marked pericholecystic inflammation and edema. Several series have shown that in the absence of specific indications, drainage is not required.

This method is directed at facilitating demonstration of the junction between the cystic duct and the common bile duct. The gallbladder may also be removed in the so-called retrograde fashion, in which the cystic duct is ligated close to the junction with the common duct as the initial part of the procedure. Then, after the cystic duct and artery have been transected, dissection is begun from the cystic duct and continued outward toward the fundus (Fig. 29-28).

Laparoscopic Cholecystectomy

The application of minimally invasive surgical techniques to removal of the gallbladder has emerged as the preferred way of treating symptomatic gallstone disease. Although a subcostal incision is avoided, these operations should be viewed with the same respect for surgical principles as are the open procedures. Trocars are introduced after the instillation of a pneumoperitoneum, and the gallbladder and liver can be retracted so as to provide optimal visualization. It is essential that the ductal structures be carefully identified before division. Because of the nature of this procedure, bleeding is a particularly worrisome problem and should be guarded against. This procedure begins by retracting the gallbladder up over the edge of the liver so as to facilitate exposure of the triangle of Calot (Fig. 29-29). The cystic duct and artery are then identified, and ductal anatomy is confirmed. Operative cholangiography can be used to selectively define anatomy as well as to search for common bile duct stones. The cystic duct is then divided. The gallbladder is dissected from this area up toward the fundus. Before complete separation of the gallbladder from the liver bed, the gallbladder fossa should be carefully inspected for bleeding. After this has been managed, the gallbladder is carefully withdrawn through one of the ports and the pneumoperitoneum released. As with open cholecystectomy, bile duct injury and hemorrhage can and should be avoided.

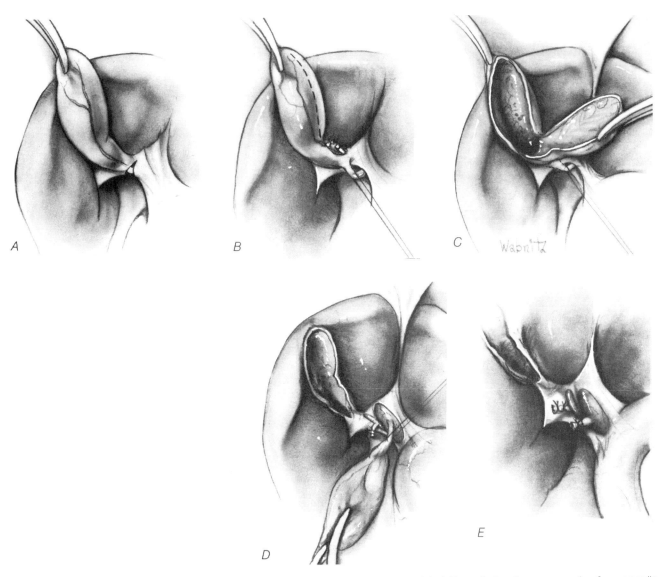

FIG. 29-27. Cholecystectomy (preferred approach). *A.* The veil of peritoneum coursing from ampulla to hepatoduodenal ligament is transected, and the cystic duct is identified. *B.* A ligature is passed around the cystic duct, and traction is applied to prevent passage of calculi from the gallbladder into the common duct during the course of subsequent dissection. Dissection is continued along the same fold of peritoneum, and the cystic artery is double ligated and transected. An incision is made in the peritoneum overlying the gallbladder. *C.* The gallbladder is removed from its bed, and if large vessels or bile ducts are encountered, they are ligated. Dissection continues from the fundus toward the junction between the cystic duct and the common bile duct. *D.* The ultimate pedicle of the cystic ducts is established, and the junction between cystic duct and common bile duct is defined. *E.* The cystic duct is ligated and transfixed and then transected approximately 3 mm from its junction with the common bile duct.

Operations of the Extrahepatic Bile Duct

Exploration for Choledocholithiasis (Fig. 29-30). Exploration for choledocholithiasis is indicated when ductal stones have been identified by palpation or cholangiography or when the cause of obstruction has not been defined. The procedure is often facilitated by performing a Kocher maneuver (freeing the lateral and posterior attachments of the second portion of the duodenum). Common duct dissection can be facilitated by traction on the cystic duct. After the anterior aspect of the duct has been visualized, aspiration of bile with a fine needle provides confirmation. After a fixation suture has been placed laterally and medially and traction applied, a vertical incision is made between these through the anterior wall. A choledochoscope can be introduced at this time to visualize the lumen and determine whether any stones are present.

Ductal stones can be removed by irrigation, balloon-tipped catheters, scoops, or forceps. These procedures should be applied initially to the distal common duct and subsequently proximally to each of the main hepatic ducts. After the stones have been removed, a No. 3 Bakes dilator is passed into the duodenum and the tip is visualized through the anterior wall. When the duct is clear of stones, a T tube is inserted into the duct. The limbs of the T tube should be short so that the distal limb does not pass

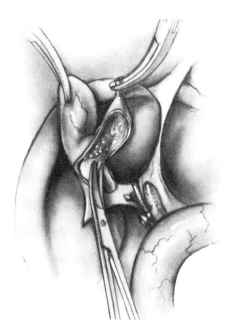

FIG. 29-28. *Retrograde dissection of the gallbladder. After the cystic duct has been identified, its junction with the common bile duct is defined and the cystic duct is transected. The cystic duct is also double ligated and transected, and the gallbladder is removed from its bed with dissection progressing from the cystic duct and ampulla outward toward the fundus.*

through the ampulla, and the proximal limb does not obstruct either of the hepatic ducts. The incision in the duct is closed around the long limb of the tube, and saline is injected to demonstrate the absence of leaks. A completion cholangiogram confirms the absence of stones and the passage of dye into the duodenum. The latter can be facilitated by the injection of glucagon. The T tube should be brought out through a stab

wound. A postoperative cholangiogram is performed about 1 week postoperatively, and if absence of stones and clear passage of opaque medium into the duodenum are demonstrated, the tube is removed.

The common duct can be explored and cleared of stones laparoscopically (see Chap. 44).

Transduodenal Sphincteroplasty (Fig. 29-31). Division of the sphincter of Oddi is occasionally indicated for a stone impacted at the ampulla, a stricture, or a functional disorder. The procedure is also applicable for multiple or recurrent ductal stones. A generous Kocher maneuver should be performed initially, followed by a longitudinal anterior duodenotomy. The passage of a Bakes dilator or cathether down the duct facilitates identification of the sphincter, which should be incised at the 11-o'clock position to avoid damaging the pancreatic duct. A pie-shaped segment is removed from the sphincter and the duodenal and ductal mucosa are coapted with fine absorbable sutures. A T tube is inserted into the common duct, and the duodenotomy is closed either longitudinally or horizontally, with care being taken not to compromise the lumen.

Choledochoduodenostomy (Fig. 29-32). This procedure is applicable to patients with multiple common duct stones to obviate the use of a T tube. The sine qua non for the performance of this procedure is a dilated common duct. A Kocher maneuver is performed to relieve any tension on the anastomosis. The distal common duct is incised longitudinally, as is the anterior portion of the duodenum, and a one-layer, large-diameter anastomosis is made.

Choledochojejunostomy (Roux-en-Y) (see Fig. 29-23). Although an occasional transection of the common duct with a sharp instrument can be repaired by end-to-end anastomosis over a T tube, most ductal injuries and strictures are preferably repaired with choledochojejunostomy or, more often, a hepaticojejunostomy, using a 45-cm defunctionalized Roux-en-Y limb of

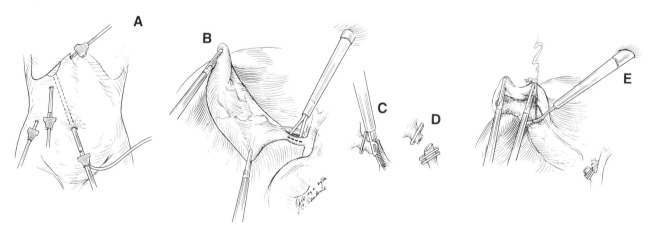

FIG. 29-29. *Laparoscopic cholecystectomy. A. The peritoneal cavity has been insufflated with CO_2 and four trocars placed. The central trocar in the periumbilical area will hold the laparoscope attached to a video system for viewing the intraabdominal manipulation. B. The cystic duct and cystic artery are bluntly dissected in the triangle of Calot. C. After the cystic duct is identified, a catheter is placed in it to perform a cholangiogram. This is done for two purposes: to identify any calculi in the common bile duct, and to clarify the anatomy in the region. D. Once this is done, the cystic duct is divided. E. With the cystic artery and cystic duct divided, the gallbladder is then removed from the gallbladder fossa using cautery. Once the gallbladder is free of the gallbladder fossa, it is removed through one of the large port sites.*

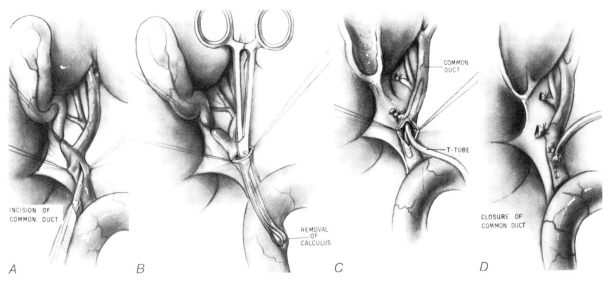

FIG. 29-30. Exploration of the common bile duct. *A.* A ligature has been placed around the cystic duct to prevent the passage of stones from the gallbladder into the common duct. After the common bile duct has been identified by dissection and aspiration, two stay sutures are placed on either side. A longitudinal incision is made in the common duct. *B.* The duct is explored with stone forceps and scoops and irrigated in both directions, i.e., toward liver and toward ampulla of Vater. Before a T tube is inserted, a No. 3 Bakes dilator should pass readily into the duodenum. *C.* An ellipse is removed from the junction of the horizontal and vertical limbs of the T tube, and the T tube is inserted into the common duct via a choledochostomy. The distal limb of the T tube should be short and should not pass through the ampulla of Vater. The proximal limb should also be short and positioned so that it does not obstruct either of the hepatic ducts. *D.* The choledochostomy is closed tightly around the T tube, which is irrigated to demonstrate the absence of leakage.

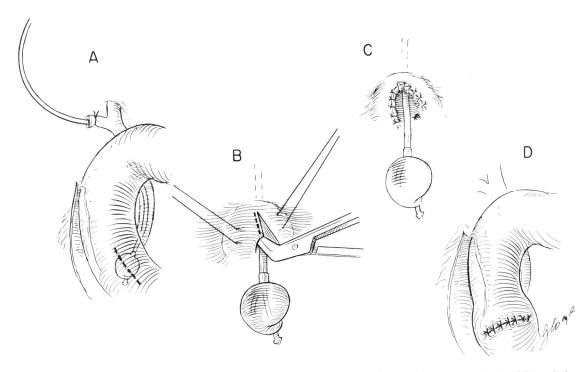

FIG. 29-31. Transduodenal sphincteroplasty. *A.* A biliary balloon-tipped catheter is placed through the common duct or through the cystic duct stump to clearly identify the location of the ampulla of Vater in the duodenum. *B.* The duodenum is opened longitudinally, and the balloon-tipped catheter is used to guide the sphincterotomy. The incision is made at the 11-o'clock position and along the lines of the balloon catheter. *C.* The mucosa of the duodenum is opened and then reapproximated with sutures. Note the opening of the pancreatic duct at its usual location. *D.* The duodenotomy is closed transversely. If the common duct has not been opened, then no T tube need be placed. However, if a common duct is open, then a T tube should be placed.

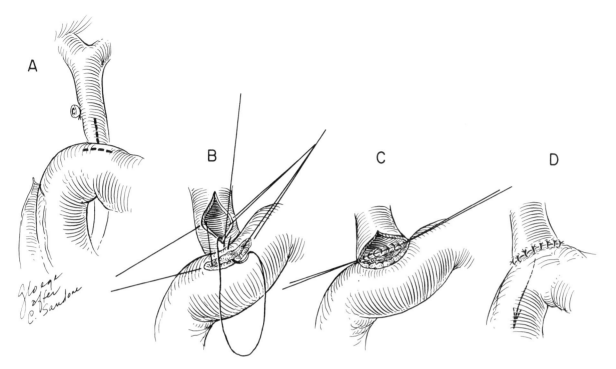

FIG. 29-32. Choledochoduodenostomy. *A. The distal common bile duct is opened longitudinally, as is the duodenum, in preparation for side-to-side anastomosis. B. Interrupted sutures are placed between the common bile duct and the duodenum. C. The interrupted sutures can have knots on the outside (as shown) or can be done with absorbable sutures and knots on the inside of the duct. D. A completed choledochoduodenostomy showing the wide stoma between the duodenum and the common bile duct.*

jejunum to obviate reflux of intestinal contents into the biliary tree. A precise mucosa-to-mucosa anastomosis should be performed using the antimesenteric side of the jejunum with interrupted absorbable sutures. In most instances, a stent is not necessary.

Bibliography

General

Blumgart LH (ed): *Surgery of the Liver and Biliary Tract*, 2d ed. London, Churchill Livingstone, 1988.

Way LW, Pellegrini CA (ed): *Surgery of the Gallbladder and Bile Ducts.* Philadelphia, WB Saunders, 1987.

Anatomy

Benson EA, Page RE: A practical reappraisal of the anatomy of the extrahepatic bile ducts and arteries. *Br J Surg* 63:853, 1976.

Boyden EA: The anatomy of the choledochoduodenal junction in man. *Surg Gynecol Obstet* 104:641, 1957.

Linder HH, Green RB: Embryology and surgical anatomy of the extrahepatic biliary tract. *Surg Clin North Am* 44:1273, 1964.

Michels NA: *Blood Supply and Anatomy of the Upper Abdominal Organs.* Philadelphia, Lippincott, 1955.

Physiology

Ahrendt SA, Magnussen TH, et al: Effect of cholecystectomy on gallbladder bile composition. *Dig Dis Sci* 37(8):1232, 1992.

Conter RL, Roslyn JJ, Taylor IL: The effects of peptide YY on gallbladder motility. *Am J Physiol* 252:G736, 1987.

Fudim-Levin E, Bor A, et al: Cholesterol precipitation from cholesterol-supersaturated bile models. *Biochimica et Biophysica Acta* 1259(1):23, 1995.

Grace PA, Poston GJ, Williamson RCN: Biliary motility. *Gut* 31:571, 1990.

Green GM: Feedback inhibition of cholecystokinin secretion by bile acids and pancreatic proteases. *Ann NY Acad Sci* 713:167, 1994.

Grider JR, Makhlouf GM: Distinct receptors for cholecystokinin and gastrin on muscle cells of stomach and gallbladder. *Am J Physiol* 259:G184, 1990.

Halpern Z, Dudley MA, et al: Vesicle aggregation in model systems of super-saturated bile: Relation to crystal nucleating and lipid composition of the vesicular phase. *J Lipid Res* 27:295, 1986.

Holzbach RT: Current concepts of cholesterol transport and crystal formation in human bile. *Hepatology* 12:26S, 1990.

Muller EL, Grace PA, et al: The influence of motilin and cholecystokinin on sphincter of Oddi and duodenal pressures in the prairie dog. *Am J Physiol* 253:G679, 1987.

O'Grady SM, Wolters PJ: Sodium and chloride transport across the isolated porcine gallbladder. *Am J Physiol* 257:G45, 1989.

Richter HM III: Physiologic consequences of vagotomy and gastric resection. *Gastroenterol Clin North Am* 23(2):193, 1994.

Thimister PW, Hopman WP, et al: Role of intraduodenal proteases in plasma cholecystokinin and pancreaticobiliary responses to protein and amino acids. *Gastroenterology* 110(2):567, 1996.

Tierney S, Pitt HA, et al: Physiology and pathophysiology of gallbladder motility. *Surg Clin North Am* 73(6):1267, 1993.

Vhlahcevic ZR, Heuman DM, Hyleman PB: Regulation of bile acid synthesis. *Hepatology* 13:590, 1991.

Yu P, DePetris G, et al: Cholecystokinin-coupled intracellular signaling in human gallbladder muscle. *Gastroenterology* 106(3):763, 1994.

Diagnosis

Blankenberg F, Wirth R, et al: Computed tomography as an adjunct to ultrasound in the diagnosis of acute acalculous cholecystitis. *Gastrointest Radiol* 16:149, 1991.

Cooperberg PL, Burhenne HJ: Real-time ultrasonography: Diagnostic technique of choice in calculous gallbladder disease. *N Engl J Med* 302:1277, 1980.

Gibbons CP, Griffiths GJ, Cormack A: The role of percutaneous transhepatic cholangiography and grey-scale ultrasound in the investigation and treatment of bile duct obstruction. *Br J Surg* 70:494, 1983.

Hricak H, Gilly RA, et al: Nuclear magnetic resonance imaging of the gallbladder. *Radiology* 147:481, 1983.

Lang IM, Martin DF: Gallbladder function after endoscopic sphincterotomy: A dynamic ultrasound assessment. *Br J Radiol* 66(787):585, 1993.

Lo LD, Vogelzang RL, et al: Percutaneous cholecystostomy for the diagnosis and treatment of acute calculous and acalculous cholecystitis. *J Vasc Interv Radiol* 6(4):629, 1995.

Rattner DW, Warshaw AL: Impact of choledochoscopy on the management of choledocholithiasis: Experience with 499 common duct explorations at the Massachusetts General Hospital. *Ann Surg* 194:76, 1981.

Robinson BL, Donohe JH, et al: Selective operative cholangiography. Appropriate management for laparoscopic cholecystectomy. *Arch Surg* 130(6):625, 1995.

Suarez CA, Block F, et al: Role of HIDA/PIPIDA scanning in diagnosing cystic duct obstruction. *Ann Surg* 191:391, 1980.

White TT, Waisman H, et al: Radiomanometry, flow rates, and cholangiography in the evaluation of common bile duct disease. *Am J Surg* 123:73, 1972.

Gallstones

Bailey RW, Zucker KA, et al: Laparoscopic cholecystectomy: Experience with 375 consecutive patients. *Ann Surg* 214:531, 1991.

Berci G, Morgenstern L: Laparoscopic management of common bile duct stones: A multi-institutional SAGES study. Society of American Gastrointestinal Endoscopic Surgeons. *Surg Endosc* 8(10):1168, 1994.

Burhenne HJ: Complications of nonoperative extraction of retained common duct stones. *Am J Surg* 131:260, 1976.

Burnstein MJ, Ilson RG, et al: Evidence for a potent nucleating factor in the gallbladder bile of patients with cholesterol gallstones. *Gastroenterology* 85:801, 1983.

Comfort MW, Gray HK, Wilson JM: Silent gallstones: 10 to 20 year follow-up study of 112. *Ann Surg* 128:931, 1948.

Frazee RC, Roberts J, et al: Combined laparoscopic and endoscopic management of cholelithiasis and choledocholithiasis. *Am J Surg* 166(6):702, 1993.

Friedman GD: Natural history of asymptomatic and symptomatic gallstones. *Am J Surg* 165(4):399, 1993.

Gleeson D, Ruppin DC, et al: Final outcome of ursodeoxycholic acid treatment in 126 patients with radiolucent gallstones. *Q J Med* 76:711, 1990.

Gracie WA, Ransohoff DF: The natural history of silent gallstones: The innocent gallstone is not a myth. *N Engl J Med* 307:798, 1982.

Holzbach RT, Kibe A, et al: Biliary proteins: Unique inhibitors of cholesterol crystal nucleation in human gallbladder bile. *J Clin Invest* 73:35, 1984.

Hunter JG, Soper NJ: Laparoscopic management of bile duct stones (Review). *Surg Clin North Am* 72(5):1077, 1992.

Inoue K, Fuchigami A, et al: Gallbladder sludge and stone formation in relation to contractile function after gastrectomy: A prospective study. *Ann Surg* 215(1):19, 1992.

Jarvinen HJ, Hastbacka J: Early cholecystectomy for acute cholecystitis: A prospective randomized study. *Ann Surg* 191:501, 1980.

Kaufman M, Weissberg D, et al: Cholecystostomy as a definitive operation. *Surg Gynecol Obstet* 170:533, 1990.

Maher JW, Summers RW, et al: Early results of combined electrohydraulic shock-wave lithotripsy and oral litholytic therapy of gallbladder stones at the University of Iowa. *Surgery* 108:648, 1990.

Mazzariello RM: A fourteen-year experience with nonoperative instrument extraction of retained bile duct stones. *World J Surg* 2:447, 1978.

McSherry CK, Festenberg H, et al: The natural history of diagnosed gallstone disease in symptomatic and asymptomatic disease. *Ann Surg* 202:59, 1985.

Panis Y, Fagniez PL, et al: Long-term results of choledochoduodenostomy versus choledochojejunostomy for choledocholithiasis. The French Association for Surgical Research. *Surg Gynecol Obstet* 177(1):33, 1993.

Pellegrini CA: Surgery for gallstone pancreatitis. *Am J Surg* 165(4):515, 1993.

Reiss R, Nudelman I, et al: Changing trends in surgery for acute cholecystitis. *World J Surg* 14:567, 1990.

Reisner RM, Cohen JR: Gallstone ileus: A review of 1001 reported cases. *Am Surg* 60:441, 1994.

Schoenfield LJ, Lachin JM, et al: Chenodiol (chenodeoxycholic acid) for dissolution of gallstones: The National Cooperative Gallstone Study: A controlled trial of efficacy and safety. *Ann Intern Med* 95:257, 1981.

Stewart L, Smith AL, et al: Pigment gallstones form as a composite of bacterial microcolonies and pigment solids. *Ann Surg* 206:242, 1987.

Tang E, Stain SC, et al: Timing of laparoscopic surgery in gallstone pancreatitis. *Arch Surg* 130(5):496, 1995.

Thistle JL, Nelson PE, May GR: Dissolution of cholesterol gallbladder stones by methyl-tert-butyl ether administered by percutaneous transhepatic catheter. *N Engl J Med* 320:633, 1989.

Tompkins RK: Surgical management of bile duct stones. *Surg Clin North Am* 70:1329, 1990.

Inflammatory and Other Benign Lesions

Acosta J, Nardi GL: Papillitis of the ampulla of Vater. *Arch Surg* 92:354, 1966.

Bender JS, Zenilman ME: Immediate laparoscopic cholecystectomy as definitive therapy for acute cholecystitis. *Surg Endosc* 9(10):108, 1995.

Cameron JL, Pitt HA, et al: Resection of hepatic duct bifurcation and transhepatic stenting for sclerosing cholangitis. *Ann Surg* 207:614, 1988.

Cangemi JR, Wiesner RH, et al: Effect of proctocolectomy for chronic ulcerative colitis on the natural history of primary sclerosing cholangitis. *Gastroenterology* 96:790, 1989.

Choi TK, Wong J: Partial hepatectomy for intrahepatic stones. *World J Surg* 10:281, 1986.

Farges O, Malassagne B, et al: Primary sclerosing cholangitis: Liver transplantation or biliary surgery. *Surgery* 117(2):146, 1995.

Himal HS, Lindsay T: Ascending cholangitis: Surgery versus endoscopic or percutaneous drainage. *Surgery* 108:629, 1990.

Lipsett PA, Pitt HA: Acute cholangitis. *Surg Clin North Am* 70:1297, 1990.

Martin FM, Braasch JW: Primary sclerosing cholangitis. *Curr Probl Surg* 29(3):133, 1992.

Matsumoto Y, Fujii H, et al: Biliary strictures as a cause of primary intrahepatic bile duct stones. *World J Surg* 10:867, 1986.

Moody FG, Calabuig R, et al: Stenosis of the sphincter of Oddi. *Surg Clin North Am* 70:1341, 1990.

Pitt HA, Kaufman SL, et al: Benign postoperative biliary strictures: Operate or dilate? *Ann Surg* 210:417, 1989.

Roslyn JJ, Tompkins RK: Reoperation for biliary strictures. *Surg Clin North Am* 71:109, 1991.

Sinanan MN: Acute cholangitis. *Infect Dis Clin North Am* 6(3):571, 1992.

Wiesner RH: Current concepts in primary sclerosing cholangitis. *Mayo Clin Proc* 69(10):969, 1994.

Tumors

Abi-Rached B, Neugut AI: Diagnostic and management issues in gallbladder carcinoma. *Oncology* 9(1):19, 1995.

Bloechle C, Izbicki JR, et al: Is radical surgery in locally advanced gallbladder carcinoma justified? *Am J Gastroenterol* 90(12):2195, 1995.

Blumgart LH, Hadjis NS, et al: Surgical approaches to cholangiocarcinoma at confluence of hepatic ducts. *Lancet* 1:66, 1984.

Cameron JL, Pitt HA, et al: Management of proximal cholangiocarcinomas by surgical resection and radiotherapy. *Ann Surg* 159:91, 1990.

Copher JC, Rogers JJ, et al: Trocar-site metastasis following laparoscopic cholecystectomy for unsuspected carcinoma of the gallbladder: Case report and review of the literature. *Surg Endosc* 9(3):348, 1995.

Cubertafond P, Gainant A, et al: Surgical treatment of 724 carcinomas of the gallbladder: Results of the French Surgical Association Survey. *Ann Surg* 219(3):275, 1994.

Houry S, Schlienger M, et al: Gallbladder carcinoma: Role of radiation therapy. *Br J Surg* 76:448, 1989.

Langer JC, Langer B, et al: Carcinoma of the extrahepatic bile ducts: Results of an aggressive surgical approach. *Surgery* 98:752, 1985.

Nakamura S, Nishiyama R, et al: Hepatopancreatoduodenectomy for advanced gallbladder carcinoma. *Arch Surg* 129(6):625, 1994.

Nakeeb A, Lipsett PA, et al: Biliary carcinoembryonic antigen levels are a marker for cholangiocarcinoma. *Am J Surg* 171(1):147, 1996.

Onoyama H, Yamamoto M, et al: Extended cholecystectomy for carcinoma of the gallbladder. *World J Surg* 19(5):758, 1995.

Pichlmayr R, Ringe B, et al: Radical resection and liver grafting as the main components of surgical strategy in the treatment of proximal bile duct cancer. *World J Surg* 12:68, 1988.

Reding R, Buard JL, et al: Surgical management of 552 carcinomas of the extrahepatic bile ducts (gallbladder and periampullary tumors excluded). Result of the French Surgical Association Survey. *Ann Surg* 212:236, 1991.

Shirai Y, Yoshida K, et al: Radical surgery for gallbladder carcinoma: Long-term results. *Ann Surg* 216(5):565, 1992.

Tompkins RK, Saunders K, et al: Changing patterns in diagnosis and management of bile duct cancer. *Ann Surg* 211:614, 1990.

Principles of Biliary Tract Surgery

Dubois F, Berthelot G, et al: Coelioscopic cholecystectomy: Experience with 2006 cases. *World J Surg* 19(5):748, 1995.

Fried GM, Barkun JS, et al: Factors determining conversion to laparotomy in patients undergoing laparoscopic cholecystectomy. *Am J Surg* 167(1):35, 1994.

Grace PA, Qureshi A, et al: Selective cholangiography in laparoscopic cholecystectomy. *Br J Surg* 80(2):244, 1993.

Jatzko GR, Lisborg PH, et al: Multivariate comparison of complications after laparoscopic cholecystectomy and open cholecystectomy. *Ann Surg* 221(4):381, 1995.

Miles RH, Carballo RE, et al: Laparoscopy: The preferred method of cholecystectomy in the morbidly obese. *Surgery* 112(4):818, 1992.

Pitt HA, Gomes AS, et al: Does preoperative percutaneous biliary drainage reduce operative risk or increase hospital cost? *Ann Surg* 201:545, 1985.

Targarona EM, Garau J, et al: Single-dose antibiotic prophylaxis in patients at high risk for infection in biliary surgery: A prospective and randomized study comparing cefonicid with mezlocillin. *Surgery* 107:327, 1990.

Taylor AM, Li MK: Laparoscopic management of complications following laparoscopic cholecystectomy. *Aust N Z J Surg* 64(12):827, 1994.

CHAPTER 30

Pancreas

Howard A. Reber

ANATOMY

The pancreas lies almost transversely in the retroperitoneum, behind the stomach, between the duodenum on the right and the spleen on the left. It is arbitrarily divided into a head with its uncinate process, a neck, a body, and a tail. The *head* of the pancreas lies at the level of the second lumbar vertebra near the midline. The posterior surface of the head rests next to the me- dial border of the right kidney, on the right renal vessels, and the inferior vena cava (Fig. 30-1). The *uncinate process* extends posterior and to the left of the head of the gland, behind the portal vein and the superior mesenteric vessels. The *neck* of the pancreas, which joins the head with the body of the gland, is anterior to the superior mesenteric vessels and portal vein.

The portal vein is formed by the confluence of the superior mesenteric and splenic veins. There are usually no tributaries between the anterior surface of the superior mesenteric and portal veins and the posterior surface of the neck. Thus, during resection of the head of the pancreas, the two can be separated safely by blunt dissection, and the neck may be transected.

The *body* of the pancreas lies at the level of the first lumbar vertebra and begins at the left border of the superior mesenteric vein. The posterior surface is in contact with the aorta, the left adrenal gland and kidney, the left renal vessels, and the splenic artery and vein, which run along its superior border. The *tail* of the pancreas lies at the level of the twelfth thoracic vertebra, and its tip usually reaches the hilus of the spleen.

Bile and Pancreatic Ducts. The common bile duct passes posterior to the head of the pancreas on its way to the duodenum and is partially or completely covered by the pancreas in over 70 percent of cases. The duct enters the duodenal wall and runs within it for about 1.5 cm. The main pancreatic duct (*Wirsung*) arises in the tail of the pancreas and enters the duodenal wall caudal to the bile duct. The two ducts usually lie side by side for several millimeters before they join as a common channel. The single pancreaticobiliary duct enters the duodenal lumen on the papilla of Vater, located on the posteromedial wall of the second portion of the duodenum, at the level of the second or third lumbar vertebra. The *ampulla of Vater* is a dilatation of the common pancreaticobiliary channel within the papilla and is distal to the junction of the two ducts. An ampulla is present in about 90 percent of cases, and it usually is quite short (5 mm or less). In 10 percent of people, the individual ducts empty sepa-

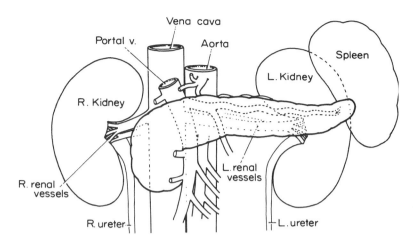

FIG. 30-1. Pancreatic anatomy, showing the relationship of the pancreas to the kidneys, spleen, and major vessels. (From: *Skandalakis JE, Gray SW, et al: Anatomical complications of pancreatic surgery. Contemp Surg 15(5,6):17, 1979, with permission.)*

rately into the duodenum, and there is no ampulla. When a common channel exists, it may be important in the pathogenesis of gallstone pancreatitis because a calculus could lodge in the ampulla and obstruct the ducts.

The accessory pancreatic duct (*Santorini*) usually drains the anterior and superior portions of the head of the pancreas. In 60 percent of cases, it enters the duodenum about 2 cm cranial and slightly anterior to the papilla of Vater, through the minor papilla. Because the accessory duct often communicates with the duct of Wirsung, drainage can occur through either the minor or major papilla. The minor papilla is always found distal to the point where the gastroduodenal artery crosses posterior to the duodenum. To avoid injury to the accessory pancreatic duct during gastrectomy, dissection of the duodenum should not progress past the artery.

Numerous variations of ductal anatomy occur, but only *pancreas divisum,* which occurs in up to 10 percent of normal people, occasionally may cause disease. Pancreas divisum occurs when the embryologic dorsal and ventral pancreatic ducts do not fuse, and the main pancreatic duct empties through the minor papilla (Fig. 30-2). In this case, only the duct draining the uncinate process empties through the papilla of Vater. In some people with pancreas divisum, pancreatitis may occur as a result of relative obstruction to the outflow of pancreatic juice through a minor papilla not normally required to handle such a large volume.

In adults, the main pancreatic duct is about 3 to 4 mm in diameter in the head of the pancreas, 2 to 3 mm in the body, and 1 to 2 mm in the tail. Some dilatation occurs normally with aging, and a diameter of 5 to 6 mm may be normal in patients age 70. Nevertheless, ductal dilatation is more commonly an indication of disease and implies ductal obstruction.

Blood Supply (Fig. 30-3). The blood supply to the head of the gland comes from the superior pancreaticoduodenal *artery,* which arises from the gastroduodenal artery and divides into anterior and posterior branches. These form collaterals with branches of the inferior pancreaticoduodenal artery, which arise from the superior mesenteric artery. The dorsal pancreatic artery usually arises from the proximal 2 cm of the splenic artery and, after supplying some branches to the head, passes to the left to supply the body and tail of the gland. There it is called the transverse pancreatic artery. Numerous branches from the sple-

nic artery anastomose with the transverse artery and also supply the body and tail. Variations of the arterial supply are common, although most are not important to the surgeon. In the most common significant variation (25 percent of cases), the right hepatic artery originates from the superior mesenteric instead of from the common hepatic artery. The right hepatic artery may then pass through the substance of the pancreas, usually the uncinate process, where it can be injured during pancreatic resection. It continues posterior to the portal vein and often along the

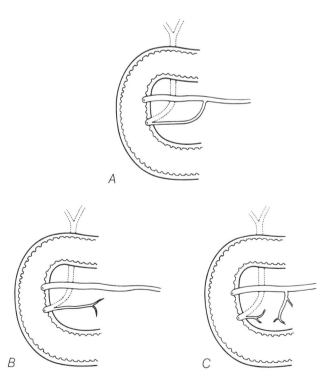

FIG. 30-2. *A.* Normal arrangement of ducts, present in about 60 percent of cases. *B* and *C.* Pancreas divisum: The principal drainage of the pancreas is through the minor papilla. This occurs in about 10 percent of cases. (From: *Skandalakis JE, Gray SW, et al: Anatomical complications of pancreatic surgery. Contemp Surg 15(5,6):17, 1979, with permission.)*

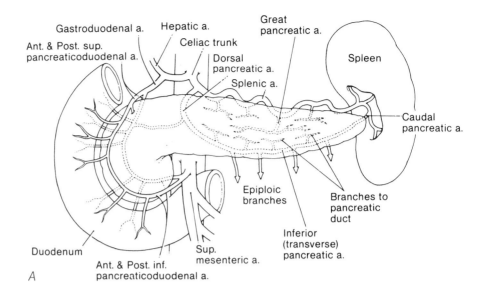

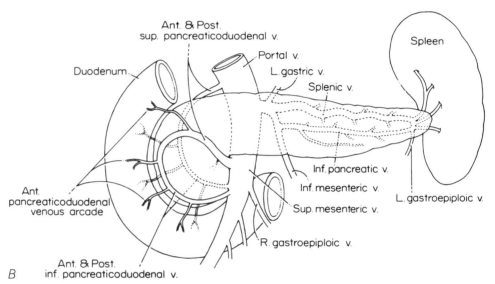

FIG. 30-3. Pancreatic blood supply. *A.* Arterial supply. *B.* Venous drainage. (From: *Skandalakis JE, Gray SW, et al: Anatomical complications of pancreatic surgery. Contemp Surg 15(5,6):17, 1979, with permission.)*

right side of the common bile duct. Some surgeons perform preoperative arteriography before pancreatic resection to forewarn themselves of such anomalies.

The head of the pancreas is drained by *veins* that parallel the arteries. The superior pancreaticoduodenal, right gastroepiploic, and a colic vein join to form a major gastrocolic trunk on the anterior surface of the head. This trunk empties into the superior mesenteric vein just before it passes under the neck of the pancreas and may be a useful anatomic landmark to identify the vessel during pancreatic surgery. The trunk may be ligated without consequence when a pancreatectomy is performed. Another fairly constant unnamed vein drains the posterior portion of the head of the pancreas and empties into the anterior aspect or right side of the portal vein at the superior margin of the gland. Additional delicate veins also empty into the right side of the superior mesenteric and portal veins directly from the pancreas. These can only be seen during resection of the head of the gland and must be ligated carefully. Venous drainage of the body and tail of the pancreas is directly to the splenic vein and through the inferior pancreatic vein to the inferior or superior mesenteric veins.

Lymphatics. Lymphatic drainage of the pancreas is rich and, in general, follows venous drainage in all directions. The *superior* nodes, located along the superior border of the pancreas, collect lymph from the anterior and superior upper half of the gland. The *inferior* nodes, along the inferior margin of the head and body, drain the anterior and posterior lower half. *Anterior* nodes drain the anterior surface of the head of the pancreas. They are located beneath the pylorus, anteriorly in the groove between the pancreas and duodenum, and the root of the mesentery of the transverse colon. *Posterior* nodes drain the posterior surface of the head. They are found posteriorly in the groove between the pancreas and duodenum, along the common bile duct, the aorta as high as the origin of the celiac axis artery, and at the origin of the superior mesenteric artery. *Splenic* nodes drain the tail of the pancreas. Lymphatic drainage is important in regard to the spread of pancreatic cancer, which arises most commonly in the head of the gland. Most patients with cancer already have nodal metastases at the time of diagnosis, usually involving several of the groups mentioned, except for the splenic. Any curative procedure must eradicate the involved nodes as well as the primary tumor.

Nerves. The pancreas receives sympathetic fibers by way of the splanchnic nerves and parasympathetic innervation by way of the vagus nerves (celiac division of the posterior vagus trunk). In general, the nerves follow the blood vessels and pancreatic ducts as they travel to the pancreatic acini. The splanchnic nerves also carry visceral afferent pain fibers that pass through the celiac plexus and ganglia. It is not known whether afferent fibers of the vagus are involved in pancreatic pain. Because pancreatic cancer and chronic pancreatitis are often accompanied by significant pain, efforts to relieve it sometimes include destruction of the celiac ganglia, with variable success.

PHYSIOLOGY

Exocrine Function

The pancreas secretes 1 to 2 L/day of a clear, watery, alkaline (pH 8.0-8.3) liquid that contains more than 20 different digestive enzymes. This electrolyte-rich juice is isosmotic with plasma and is secreted chiefly by the centroacinar cells and those cells which make up the walls of the smaller pancreatic ducts in response to secretin. The principal cations of this juice are sodium and potassium, which are always present in concentrations similar to those found in plasma (the sum of the two is approximately 165 mmol/L). The concentrations of the principal anions (bicarbonate and chloride) vary. When the stimulus to secrete is minimal, the chloride concentration is high (e.g., 110 mmol/L) and that of bicarbonate low (e.g., 50 mmol/L). When the secretory stimulus is maximal, the bicarbonate concentration rises (to approximately 140 mmol/L), and the chloride concentration falls (to ~20 mmol/L). The secretion of bicarbonate at such high concentrations requires active transport. In part, the reciprocal relationship of the two anions is achieved by the passive exchange of intraductal bicarbonate for interstitial chloride. This exchange occurs as the juice flows through the larger pancreatic ducts on its way to the duodenum. At slower flow rates, there is more opportunity for exchange to take place, and more bicarbonate is lost. The alkaline pancreatic juice helps to neutralize gastric acid in the duodenum and provides the optimal pH for the activity of the pancreatic digestive enzymes.

The digestive enzymes are synthesized and stored in the pancreatic acinar cells and are released in response to cholecystokinin (CCK) and vagal cholinergic stimulation. Pancreatic enzymes are proteolytic (e.g., trypsin, chymotrypsin, carboxypeptidase, ribonuclease, deoxyribonuclease, and elastase), lipolytic (lipase, colipase, and phospholipase A_2), and amylolytic (amylase). Although lipase and amylase are secreted in their active forms, the proteolytic enzymes and phospholipase A_2 are secreted as inactive "zymogens." Activation of trypsinogen to trypsin occurs when the zymogen is exposed to the duodenal enzyme enterokinase. Trypsin then converts the other zymogens to their active forms. In the intestine, the proteolytic enzymes digest proteins into peptides, lipase breaks fats into glycerol and fatty acids, phospholipase A_2 catalyzes the conversion of biliary lecithin to lysolecithin, and amylase converts starch to disaccharides and dextrins.

Enzyme synthesis occurs on polysomes attached to the rough endoplasmic reticulum, following which the newly formed enzymes migrate through various subcellular compartments and end up as zymogen granules, which are stored. Lysosomal enzymes, which degrade unneeded intracellular constituents, are also synthesized by a similar process. They are segregated from the digestive enzymes and stored separately in other subcellular structures called *lysosomes*. Secretory stimulation results in fusion of the zymogen granule membrane with the apical (luminal) membrane of the acinar cell, and the enzymes are discharged into the duct. There is experimental evidence that the lysosomal enzymes (e.g., cathepsin B) could activate trypsinogen inside the cell if the two ever came into contact. Thus segregation of the lysosomal enzymes from the inactive digestive enzymes may be important to prevent the cellular injury that might follow enzyme activation. Such abnormal intracellular enzyme activation seems to be the cause of pancreatitis in several experimental animal models, although it is unknown whether this can occur in human beings.

Regulation of Secretion. Pancreatic secretion is under complex neurohormonal control. Ductal fluid and bicarbonate are secreted chiefly in response to the hormone secretin, which is released from the mucosa of the duodenum and proximal small bowel in response to acid in the bowel lumen. Bicarbonate secretion is triggered when the pH of the duodenal lumen falls below 4.5. Acinar enzyme secretion is stimulated both by vagal cholinergic discharge and by the hormone CCK. CCK is released from the proximal small bowel by fatty acids, oligopeptides, and some amino acids.

Pancreatic secretion has been divided artificially into cephalic, gastric, and intestinal phases. The *cephalic* phase begins with the sight, smell, and anticipation of food. Although mostly enzymes are secreted, some bicarbonate is also produced. Enzymes are released by vagal cholinergic pathways; vasoactive intestinal polypeptide (VIP), which is structurally related to secretin, may cause the bicarbonate response. The *gastric* phase begins when food enters the stomach. Gastric distention, as well as the exposure of the stomach mucosa to nutrients (e.g., peptides), causes primarily an enzyme-rich pancreatic secretion. This effect is blocked by atropine or truncal vagotomy and probably involves a gastropancreatic vagovagal reflex. The *intestinal* phase begins when the chyme empties into the duodenum. This phase is important for the maintenance of enzyme output as gastric distention diminishes. Gastric acid is also responsible for pancreatic bicarbonate secretion. When the buffering effect of the food is lost, the duodenal pH begins to fall, and secretin is released. The mechanisms responsible for this phase are both neural and hormonal, involving both stimulatory (e.g., secretin, CCK, gastrin-releasing peptide [GRP], bombesin, neurotensin, VIP) and inhibitory (e.g., pancreatic polypeptide [PP], calcitonin-gene-related peptide [CGRP], peptide YY [PYY], neuropeptide Y [NPY], somatostatin) effects on the pancreas. In addition to these inhibitory effects, there is also evidence for a negative feedback mechanism for pancreatic secretion. The presence of pancreatic proteases and bile within the duodenum appears to inhibit the release of CCK. Thus pancreaticobiliary diversion from the intestine is characterized by elevated plasma CCK levels and stimulation of pancreatic secretion. This may have some clinical relevance in patients with chronic pancreatitis who are sometimes treated with large amounts of oral pancreatic enzymes in an effort to inhibit pancreatic secretion.

The quantity of pancreatic enzymes that is secreted in response to a meal is almost 90 percent in excess of what is actually needed for normal digestion. Thus patients develop symptoms of malabsorption only when secretion falls to about 10 percent or less of normal. Pancreatic insufficiency can result from blockage of the main pancreatic duct, which prevents the enzymes from entering the intestine (e.g., pancreatic cancer), from destruction of the pancreatic secretory parenchyma (e.g., chronic pancreatitis), and from surgical procedures that remove the pancreas or result in poor mixing of the gastric chyme with the pancreatic secretions (e.g., partial gastrectomy with gastrojejunostomy). Pancreatic insufficiency affects fat absorption much more than protein or carbohydrate absorption because protein digestion is aided by gastric pepsin and small bowel brush border enzymes and carbohydrate digestion by salivary amylase. Moreover, fat malabsorption causes troublesome diarrhea, while malabsorption of protein and carbohydrate is generally asymptomatic. On a diet containing 100 g of fat a day, normal subjects excrete 5 to 7 g/day of fat in the feces (i.e., 5 to 7 percent fat malabsorption is normal). A total pancreatectomy causes 70 percent fat malabsorption; partial pancreatic resections may not cause any malabsorption, providing that the pancreatic remnant is normal. Vitamin malabsorption is rarely a problem, since water-soluble B vitamins are absorbed throughout the small intestine, and fat-soluble vitamins do not require pancreatic enzymes for absorption. Vitamin B_{12} malabsorption occurs in some patients but is rarely a significant problem. Therefore, vitamin B_{12} replacement is unnecessary.

Because complete correction of malabsorption is not possible, the goal of treatment of pancreatic exocrine insufficiency is to eliminate the diarrhea that the steatorrhea provokes. At least 5 to 10 percent of the normal amount of enzymes must be delivered to the duodenum at the same time as the gastric chyme in order for this goal to be achieved. This represents about 30,000 units of lipase for each meal, which can be given either throughout the meal or as a single dose at the beginning. A number of different enzyme preparations are available; the least expensive and most effective one should be chosen. Because lipase is inactivated below pH 4.0 and gastroduodenal pH may fall below this level, enzyme therapy may be ineffective if gastric acidity is high.

Patients should be instructed to begin a diet consisting of 4 meals per day and a minimum of 3000 kcal/day. The diet should contain at least 400 g of carbohydrate, 100 to 150 g of protein, and moderate amounts of fat (25 g/meal). If the enzymes eliminate the diarrhea, the fat in the diet can be liberalized until symptoms recur and then maintained just below that level. If the enzymes do not eliminate the symptoms, fat should be restricted further to 50 to 75 g/day. If the diarrhea still persists, H_2 blockers should be added to decrease gastric acidity. If this is still not effective, the H_2 blockers should be stopped, and an enteric-coated enzyme preparation may be tried. In this form, these enzymes are coated with a protective polymer that resists acid and dissolves only above pH 5.0. Thus lipase is more likely to be delivered to the duodenum in its active form.

Endocrine Function

The islets of Langerhans constitute 1 to 2 percent of the pancreatic mass, but they receive about 20 percent of the total pancreatic blood flow. They are dispersed throughout the pancreatic parenchyma, but some of the hormone-secreting cells are concentrated in specific areas. The insulin-secreting cells are evenly distributed and are usually localized in the core of each islet, where they form 60 to 80 percent of the cells. They are surrounded peripherally by a mantle of other cells that are specialized to secrete glucagon (15 to 20 percent of the islet cells), somatostatin (5 to 10 percent), or pancreatic polypeptide (15 to 20 percent). These last cells are found chiefly in the islets of the head of the pancreas. The glucagon cells occur chiefly in the body and tail of the gland.

Insulin. Insulin is a 51-amino-acid peptide (MW 5734 Da) that consists of two polypeptide chains. It is synthesized by the beta cells by means of a precursor, proinsulin. Insulin lowers blood glucose concentration by enhancing glucose uptake by all the body cells, promoting glycogenesis and inhibiting gluconeogenesis. It also stimulates lipogenesis, inhibits lipolysis, and enhances protein synthesis. Although the factors that govern insulin secretion are multiple and complex, the most important is an elevation of the extracellular blood glucose concentration. Other substrates, including amino acids (e.g., arginine) and fatty acids, also stimulate insulin release. The primary sites of action of the hormone are the liver, muscle, and fat cells.

Glucagon. Glucagon is a single-chain 29-amino-acid peptide (MW 3483 Da) formed in the alpha cells of the islets. It increases blood glucose by causing hepatic glycogenolysis and gluconeogenesis. Thus the effects of glucagon counterbalance those of insulin. Glucagon also relaxes and dilates smooth muscle such as the stomach, duodenum, and sphincter of Oddi. The hormone is released by a low blood glucose concentration, amino acids, catecholamines (e.g., during stress), sympathetic nervous discharge, and CCK. Insulin and hyperglycemia suppress glucagon release.

Somatostatin. Somatostatin is a tetradecapeptide (MW 1637 Da) arising in the delta cells of the islets. Both oral and intravenous nutrients stimulate somatostatin secretion, and both neural and hormonal mechanisms may be involved. The hormone inhibits the release of insulin, and in turn, its own release is inhibited by insulin. It may act as an important local paracrine regulator of glucose homeostasis. Somatostatin has a wide spectrum of activities, most of which are inhibitory. These include suppression of the release of gastrin, secretin, VIP, PP, gastric acid, pepsin, pancreatic enzymes, and glucagon. Somatostatin also inhibits intestinal, biliary, and gastric motility.

Pancreatic Polypeptide. Pancreatic polypeptide (PP) is a 36-amino-acid peptide (MW 4200 Da) arising in the PP cells. Orally ingested protein, vagal cholinergic stimulation, and hypoglycemia are all potent stimulants for the release of PP. PP itself inhibits pancreatic exocrine secretion.

The endocrine pancreas influences the synthesis and secretion of pancreatic enzymes from the exocrine parenchyma. At least in part, this is the result of an *islet-acinar portal system* in which the blood that first perfuses the islets collects into a vascular network that surrounds the acini before draining out of the gland. Thus the acini are exposed to higher concentrations of the islet hormones than are the peripheral tissues of the body. This may be important clinically. For example, insulin activates amylase gene expression and amylase synthesis in acinar cells and regulates their sensitivity to CCK. This could explain why about 40 percent of patients with type I diabetes have some impairment in exocrine pancreatic function. Up to 70 percent of patients with chronic pancreatitis also develop diabetes.

CONGENITAL ANOMALIES

Annular Pancreas. Annular pancreas is formed by a thin band of normal pancreatic tissue that completely encircles the second portion of the duodenum and is continuous with the head of the pancreas anteriorly and posteriorly. It is probably the result of abnormal rotation and fusion of the ventral pancreatic primordium during the second month of fetal life. Forty percent of infants with annular pancreas have associated duodenal stenosis or atresia. Symptoms of duodenal obstruction (gastric distention and vomiting) occur in about one-third of cases in the first week of life and about one-half of cases in the first year. The rest are asymptomatic until adulthood, when abdominal pain, nausea, and vomiting may occur. Some cases, however, probably never cause problems and remain undiagnosed. There is no gender predilection in infancy, although adult patients are more often males. The diagnosis may be suspected when an upper gastrointestinal series shows obstruction of the second portion of the duodenum, but it can only be confirmed by direct inspection at surgery. In adults, duodenal narrowing from chronic ulcer disease also must be considered in the differential diagnosis. The treatment is duodenojejunostomy or gastrojejunostomy, either of which bypasses the obstruction. The obstructing pancreatic ring must not be simply divided because this may not relieve the obstruction, and pancreatic fistula can result.

Pancreatic Cysts. Congenital cysts of the pancreas are rare but are increasingly likely to be diagnosed at any age on abdominal CT scans for unrelated disease. If they are single, they may require surgery to distinguish them from a pseudocyst or a cystic neoplasm. Congenital cysts have an epithelial lining; pseudocysts do not. The diagnosis of benign polycystic disease of the pancreas may be possible from the CT image of multiple cysts of various sizes involving the entire pancreas, especially when cysts are also present in other organs (e.g., kidneys, liver, cerebellum, as in von Hippel-Lindau disease). In the absence of symptoms or serious concern that the cysts are neoplastic, surgery may be unnecessary.

Ectopic Pancreas. Ectopic pancreas usually occurs in the stomach or duodenum but has been found in Meckel's diverticulum, the colon, the appendix, and elsewhere. The tissue usually functions and contains islets in about one-third of cases. The condition is usually asymptomatic. However, if symptoms occur, they may simulate duodenal ulcer, appendicitis, intestinal obstruction, etc., depending on the site. Treatment is surgical, and the diagnosis may be suspected from the characteristic gross appearance. The lesions are submucosal, firm, yellowish nodules with a visible central umbilication.

PANCREATITIS

Acute pancreatitis is a nonbacterial inflammation of the pancreas caused by the activation, interstitial liberation, and the digestion of the gland by its own enzymes. It is characterized clinically by acute abdominal pain, elevated concentrations of pancreatic enzymes in blood, and an increase in the amount of pancreatic enzymes excreted in urine. There may be just a single episode of pancreatitis, or several episodes may recur. In the United States, the most common cause of acute pancreatitis is cholelithiasis.

During a mild attack, the morphologic changes are characterized by pancreatic and peripancreatic edema and fat necrosis, but pancreatic necrosis is absent. This is often referred to as *edematous pancreatitis.* The mild form may turn into a severe form (or the episode may be severe from the beginning). In its severe form, extensive pancreatic and peripancreatic fat necrosis, pancreatic parenchymal necrosis, and hemorrhage into and around the pancreas are evident. This form of the disease is often referred to as *necrotizing pancreatitis.* During such an episode of acute inflammation, both the exocrine and endocrine functions of the gland are impaired for some weeks or even months. If the cause (e.g., cholelithiasis) and any complications (e.g., a pseudocyst) of the pancreatitis are eliminated, the pancreas usually returns to normal. Some scarring may persist after a severe attack, but both exocrine and endocrine functions are normal, and there is little, if any, histologic abnormality evident. Even multiple attacks of acute pancreatitis rarely lead to chronic pancreatitis.

Chronic pancreatitis is characterized clinically by recurrent, acute episodes of abdominal pain indistinguishable from those of acute pancreatitis. For several years or more, patients may be asymptomatic in between episodes that typically occur two or three times a year. In most cases the pain-free intervals shorten, and pain eventually may become constant. As the disease progresses, pancreatic function becomes impaired. The exocrine insufficiency is manifested as steatorrhea and malabsorption. The endocrine insufficiency causes diabetes, often requiring insulin for its management. An unusual form of chronic pancreatitis occurring in about 5 percent of cases is not associated with pain. The principal clinical manifestation of the disease in these patients is pancreatic functional insufficiency. In the United States, the most common cause of chronic pancreatitis is alcoholism. Morphologically, chronic pancreatitis is characterized by a permanent and usually progressive destruction of pancreatic parenchyma. The acinar cells are destroyed first, replaced by dense fibrous scar tissue. Eventually, the islet cells are also damaged by this sclerotic process. Often the main pancreatic duct is dilated, sometimes with focal areas of narrowing along its length. Intraductal protein plugs and/or calculi are common. Both acute and chronic inflammatory cells are present, as well as edema and focal necrosis. Cysts and pseudocysts occur frequently.

A distinct morphologic form of chronic pancreatitis is *obstructive chronic pancreatitis.* Here the ductal system is moderately dilated proximal to the obstruction, which is most often caused by a tumor or scar from a previous injury. In the obstructed part of the pancreas, there is uniform, diffuse atrophy and fibrosis of the acinar parenchyma. Calculi and intraductal protein plugs are unusual.

In chronic pancreatitis (unlike acute pancreatitis), the morphologic changes in the pancreas are irreversible and often progressive, even if the cause (e.g., alcoholism) is removed. This usually leads to permanent functional impairment as more and more acinar and islet cell mass is destroyed. The only exception is obstructive chronic pancreatitis. Here there does seem to be some improvement both morphologically and functionally when the obstruction is relieved.

The terms *recurrent acute* and *recurrent* or *relapsing chronic pancreatitis* are obsolescent. They referred to repetitive episodes of pancreatic inflammation in patients with either of the two forms of the disease.

Etiology. *Gallstone pancreatitis* accounts for about 40 percent of all cases of pancreatitis and about 90 percent of cases of acute pancreatitis in the United States. Eradication of the gallstone disease prevents further attacks of pancreatitis. The etiologic mechanism probably involves the transient obstruction of the pancreatic duct by a gallstone in the common bile duct at the ampulla of Vater. Gallstones are recoverable in the feces of over 90 percent of patients within 10 days of an attack, suggesting that the obstruction is brief and that most such stones pass into the duodenum. The usual age at onset is the middle to late forties, with women more commonly affected than men.

Alcoholic pancreatitis accounts for 40 percent of all cases of pancreatitis and about 75 percent of cases of chronic pancreatitis in the United States. In some cases, an episode of binge drinking may precipitate an attack typical of acute pancreatitis. This usually occurs in a patient who is a chronic alcoholic, in whom the pancreas has probably already been permanently damaged by alcohol even though other evidence of pancreatic disease is absent (e.g., pancreatic exocrine insufficiency, diabetes). In other cases, the presentation is less acute. Patients may present with chronic abdominal and/or back pain, often with steatorrhea and diabetes from pancreatic exocrine and endocrine insufficiency. Pancreatic calcifications are found in at least one-third of patients. Weight loss is common, since food often aggravates the pain and intake is voluntarily restricted. The patients may be addicted to the narcotics necessary for pain relief. The usual age at onset is the midthirties, with men more commonly affected than women.

Alcoholic pancreatitis generally is diagnosed after patients have consumed alcohol for at least 2 years and usually between 6 to 10 years. It probably makes no difference whether the ethanol is consumed as wine, beer, or spirits, but the daily consumption averages 100 to 150 g/day. There is evidence that the diet of alcoholic patients who develop pancreatitis is richer in fat and protein than the diets of other alcoholics who do not. It is estimated that about 10 to 15 percent of individuals who consume such large amounts of alcohol eventually develop pancreatitis; a similar number develop cirrhosis of the liver. The factors that govern individual susceptibility to each are unknown.

Early studies suggested that ethanol caused pancreatitis by inducing spasm of the sphincter of Oddi, thereby creating an obstruction to the outflow of pancreatic juice. Experimentally, secretion in the face of similar obstruction has caused acute pancreatitis, but this cannot be the full explanation. Ethanol is also a cellular metabolic poison, and it has deleterious effects on the synthesis and secretion of digestive enzymes by the pancreatic acinar cells. This causes an increase in the concentration of enzyme protein in pancreatic juice and the eventual precipitation of this protein in the pancreatic ducts. Calcium, normally soluble in pancreatic juice, may then precipitate within the matrix of these protein plugs. This creates multiple points of ductal obstruction randomly scattered throughout the pancreas. Further damage follows continued secretion in the face of this widespread obstruction. Ethanol also increases the permeability of the pancreatic ducts. This allows pancreatic enzymes, normally contained within the ducts, to leak out into the surrounding tissue.

If the enzymes are active, damage to the pancreas results. There is recent evidence that acute ethanol ingestion markedly but transiently depresses pancreatic blood flow. Thus cellular damage could be provoked by ischemia. Table 30-1 lists the common causes of acute pancreatitis.

Hypercalcemic states, most commonly hyperparathyroidism, may cause acute and chronic pancreatitis. The mechanism is unclear, but hypercalcemia may favor the intraductal precipitation of calcium stones, which are seen in up to half these patients. Calcium also influences the activation of certain pancreatic enzymes and a variety of acinar cell synthetic and secretory events. Acute hypercalcemia increases the permeability of pancreatic ducts, perhaps allowing enzymes to leak from them and damage the tissue.

Hyperlipidemia, especially that associated with elevated chylomicrons and very low density lipoproteins, may be a cause of acute pancreatitis. The mechanism may involve the release by pancreatic lipase of large amounts of toxic fatty acids in the pancreatic capillary circulation. Vascular endothelial damage might cause sludging of red blood cells, stasis, and pancreatic ischemic injury and inflammation. Hyperlipidemia also can occur transiently during an attack of pancreatitis, usually in alcoholics. In such patients, it is not thought to play an etiologic role.

Hyperlipidemia as a cause of pancreatitis should be recognized for two reasons. First, because the elevated serum lipid level interferes with the chemical determination of amylase, the serum amylase level in these patients with acute pancreatitis is often reported as "normal." The appearance of a milky white (lactescent) serum in a patient with acute abdominal pain, however, should alert the clinician to the correct diagnosis. Because the lipid is not excreted in the urine, the finding of a high urinary amylase excretion may still be diagnostic in this setting. Second, dietary or pharmacologic control of the hyperlipidemia minimizes the chances of recurrent episodes of pancreatitis.

Hereditary pancreatitis is transmitted as a mendelian dominant trait. At least one form is due to a mutation in the gene for trypsinogen, which may interfere with the normal protective mechanism by which active trypsin is degraded. Trypsin could then digest the pancreas, producing pancreatitis. The condition is rare, although over 250 patients have been reported. Symptoms typical of acute pancreatitis appear in most patients between the ages of 12 and 14 years. Relentless progression of the process is usual, with recurrent attacks of acute inflammation.

Table 30-1
Etiologies of Acute Pancreatitis

Biliary tract disease (e.g., cholelithiasis)
Alcohol
Drugs
Trauma
Hyperparathyroidism (elevated calcium)
Malnutrition (protein-calorie)
Hyperlipidemia
Pancreatic duct obstruction (e.g., pancreas divisum)
Duodenal obstruction
Infection
Ischemia
Hereditary
Scorpion venom

Eventually, many patients develop the typical manifestations of chronic pancreatitis, including calcifications (32 percent), diabetes (19 percent), and steatorrhea from exocrine insufficiency (15 percent). As in patients with chronic pancreatitis from other causes, an increased incidence of pancreatic cancer has been noted. In most of the reported cases where endoscopic retrograde cholangiopancreatography (ERCP) has been performed, the pancreatic ducts have been dilated.

Protein deficiency in children with severe protein-calorie malnutrition may cause kwashiorkor and a specific type of chronic pancreatitis. Treatment with adequate diet rapidly restores pancreatic function to normal, provided that parenchymal fibrosis is not too extensive. Pancreatic calcification is absent, and episodes of abdominal pain are infrequent. Another variety of chronic pancreatitis, possibly related to malnutrition, occurs only in certain tropical and subtropical countries (e.g., Nigeria). It begins in childhood and in most cases is associated with abdominal pain, pancreatic calcification, steatorrhea, and diabetes. The pancreatic ducts are usually dilated and obstructed. Adequate nutrition does not reverse the process.

Postoperative (iatrogenic) pancreatitis occurs after a variety of procedures in proximity to the pancreas, and the causes are usually obvious. They include direct injury to the gland (e.g., pancreatic biopsy, pancreatic resection) or obstruction of the pancreatic duct (e.g., the placement of a long-arm T-tube through the sphincter of Oddi into the duodenum or forceful dilation of the sphincter of Oddi to a diameter of more than 5 mm during common duct exploration). For this reason, these latter two procedures are no longer done. Pancreatitis also occasionally follows endoscopic sphincterotomy or surgical sphincteroplasty.

Sometimes the operation is distant from the pancreas, and there is no obvious explanation. For example, pancreatitis complicates up to 5 percent of cases of heart surgery that require cardiopulmonary bypass. It has been suggested that impaired pancreatic perfusion may damage the pancreas in this setting.

Pancreatitis can follow Billroth II gastrectomy if the afferent limb of the jejunum becomes obstructed. In this case, pancreatic juice and bile accumulate in the limb and may reflux into the pancreatic duct under pressure.

Drugs are an uncommon but important cause of acute pancreatitis. Those most commonly incriminated include steroids, azathioprine, 6-mercaptopurine, thiazide diuretics, furosemide, sulfonamides, tetracycline, and estrogens (which produce pancreatitis by inducing hypertriglyceridemia).

Duct obstruction of brief duration may cause acute pancreatitis, but when it is persistent over months or years, it is a recognized cause of chronic pancreatitis. Unlike other forms of chronic pancreatitis, some morphologic and functional recovery of the pancreas can occur if the obstruction is removed. Of course, when the process is advanced, significant recovery is not possible. Obstruction occurs in a variety of clinical settings.

Chronic pancreatitis has been reported in patients with severe *strictures* at the point where fusion of the ventral and dorsal pancreatic ducts occurs during fetal life. Strictures also occur in other areas of the main duct and are probably due to scarring after trauma or acute pancreatitis from any cause.

Pancreas divisum has been most commonly associated with recurrent episodes of acute pancreatitis in young adulthood, but chronic pancreatitis may occur when the outflow obstruction is severe and persistent over a period of years. In patients with acute pancreatitis and pancreas divisum, therapy directed toward relief of obstruction at the minor papilla may be effective. However, once chronic pancreatitis is established, surgical treatment should consist of pancreatic resection or drainage.

Chronic *inflammation of the papilla of Vater* with obstruction of the duct of Wirsung is rare. In most cases the inflammation is probably caused by the passage of common duct stones through the papilla. In others there is no apparent explanation. There are probably some cases of chronic pancreatitis that are secondary to the outflow obstruction caused by this process. Nevertheless, the clinician must be extremely cautious about attributing chronic pancreatitis to this entity. In any case, as with pancreas divisum, treatment of chronic pancreatitis directed toward relief of the papillary obstruction is ineffective.

Miscellaneous additional causes of pancreatitis exist. They include acute pancreatitis that follows scorpion (*Tityus trinitatis*) venom poisoning, various infectious agents (mumps, group B Coxsackie viruses, herpes simplex, mononucleosis), and exposure to anticholinesterase insecticides.

Idiopathic pancreatitis still accounts for 15 to 20 percent of the total, suggesting that a number of other causes are still obscure. About one-third of patients with no obvious cause for their episodes of acute pancreatitis eventually will be found to have cholelithiasis. Thus, to avoid overlooking a treatable condition, an extensive search for the cause always must be made before the designation *idiopathic* is applied.

Pathogenesis. Acute pancreatitis is thought to result from enzymatic digestion of the gland by its own enzymes, although the mechanism(s) by which enzyme activation occurs in humans remains unknown. The pathogenesis of pancreatitis is best discussed within the framework of various theories that attempt to relate experimental observations to known clinical characteristics of the disease.

Obstruction-Secretion. Ligation of the pancreatic duct in animals results in edema of the pancreas that may resemble mild acute edematous pancreatitis in humans. It is self-limited, however, and generally resolves within a week; over several months the acinar tissue is replaced by fibrous scar. Partial duct obstruction, along with stimulation of pancreatic secretion, produces a more severe pancreatic inflammation. These observations may be relevant to biliary pancreatitis, when a gallstone obstructs the pancreatic duct during pancreatic secretion. Acute alcoholic pancreatitis also may have a similar mechanism. Alcohol in the stomach stimulates the secretion of gastric acid, which enters the duodenum and releases secretin. This, in turn, stimulates the pancreas to secrete. Alcohol also causes spasm of the sphincter of Oddi, which would obstruct the flow of pancreatic juice. This theory does not explain the mechanism by which the pancreatic enzymes become activated to begin the autodigestive process.

Common Channel Theory. In two patients who died from acute pancreatitis, Opie (1901) observed at autopsy that a gallstone was lodged in the ampulla of Vater, obstructing the bile and pancreatic ducts and creating a common channel between them. He suggested that bile reflux through the channel into the pancreatic duct was the cause of the pancreatitis. This hypothesis continues to be debated. It is known that infected bile that contains deconjugated bile salts and bile incubated with pancreatic juice that contains lysolecithin injure the lining of the pancreatic ducts. Their permeability is increased so that pancreatic enzymes can leak from them into the surrounding pancreatic parenchyma. This could initiate pancreatitis. On the other hand, fresh bile is apparently innocuous to the ducts. Moreover, in 90 percent of people the common channel may be too short to allow for bile reflux in the presence of an obstructing gallstone.

Duodenal Reflux. Reflux of duodenal contents through the papilla of Vater into the pancreatic duct causes pancreatitis in experimental animals. The rare case of pancreatitis that occurs after a Billroth II gastrectomy with obstruction of the afferent loop probably has a similar causation. This theory is attractive because it explains pancreatic enzyme activation, since duodenal enterokinase would gain access to the pancreatic duct. Nevertheless, normal mechanisms inherent in the duodenal wall and sphincter of Oddi efficiently prevent reflux, and there is no direct evidence that this mechanism accounts for pancreatitis in humans.

Increased Pancreatic Duct Permeability. Animal experiments have shown that a variety of conditions can increase the permeability of the pancreatic ducts so that pancreatic enzymes, normally contained within the ducts, can leak out. These include the acute ingestion of ethanol, direct exposure of the duct to deconjugated bile salts, pancreatic secretion against an obstruction, and acute hypercalcemia. If those enzymes have been activated, they cause acute pancreatitis. Nevertheless, there is no direct evidence that this occurs in human pancreatitis, and it is unknown how enzyme activation might occur.

Enzyme Autoactivation. In experimental animals, intrapancreatic autoactivation of trypsinogen occurs, and pancreatitis develops when pancreatic secretion is stimulated by supramaximal doses of cerulein or when animals are fed a choline-deficient diet supplemented with ethionine. These observations may be important because they offer a novel explanation for enzyme activation that does not require exposure to duodenal enterokinase. However, there is no evidence that enzyme autoactivation occurs in human pancreatitis, and there is no apparent connection between these experimental models and the human disease.

Presently we have only an incomplete understanding of the pathogenesis of pancreatitis. The diverse causes of the disease suggest that any of a number of inciting factors may result in injury to the gland and that the pancreas responds in a limited fashion. Biliary pancreatitis is associated with *acute* inflammation and almost certainly follows transient obstruction of the pancreatic duct by a gallstone. It is unknown whether bile reflux, elevated ductal pressures, or other factors are important. Alcoholic pancreatitis is associated with *chronic* inflammation, although acute inflammatory episodes do occur. The chronic changes are due to the toxic effects of ethanol on the acinar secretory cells and probably to widespread ductal obstruction from protein plugs.

Acute Pancreatitis

Clinical Manifestations. The typical attack of acute pancreatitis begins with severe and persistent epigastric or upper abdominal pain that often radiates through to the back. Frequently it follows the ingestion of a large meal and is associated with nausea and persistent vomiting and retching. The findings are the same regardless of the causation, even if the event represents an episode of acute pancreatic inflammation in a patient with chronic pancreatitis.

The pain is of variable intensity and may be less severe with edematous pancreatitis compared with the necrotizing form of the disease. Examination of the abdomen reveals tenderness most marked in the epigastrium but sometimes present through-

out. The bowel sounds are decreased or absent. Usually there are no masses palpable; when one is present, it most often represents a swollen pancreas (phlegmon), pseudocyst, or abscess. With necrotizing pancreatitis, the abdomen may be distended with intraperitoneal fluid. The temperature is only mildly elevated (100 to 101°F) in uncomplicated cases. There may be evidence of a pleural effusion, especially on the left side.

When the disease is more severe, the patient also may exhibit signs of profound fluid losses from sequestration of edema fluid and/or blood in the peripancreatic retroperitoneal spaces or in the peritoneal cavity (ascites). Severe dehydration, tachycardia, and hypotension may be present. In about 1 percent of patients, a bluish color is evident around the umbilicus (Cullen's sign) or in the flanks (Grey Turner's sign). This represents blood that has dissected to those areas from the retroperitoneum near the pancreas in patients with necrotizing pancreatitis.

Although the clinical presentation often suggests the correct diagnosis, and the laboratory findings usually confirm it, it is important to stress that *acute pancreatitis is a diagnosis of exclusion.* Other acute upper abdominal conditions (e.g., perforated peptic ulcer, acute cholecystitis, gangrenous small bowel obstruction) must be considered in every patient. If doubt remains, a laparotomy may be indicated for diagnosis (<5 percent of patients), since the diseases with which acute pancreatitis is most likely to be confused are often lethal if not treated surgically.

Diagnostic Studies. The hematocrit may be elevated because of dehydration or low as a result of pancreatic or retroperitoneal blood loss in necrotizing pancreatitis. In the absence of suppurative complications, white blood cell counts over 12,000/mm³ are unusual. Liver function tests are usually normal, but mild elevations of the serum bilirubin concentration (<2 mg/dL) may be seen. This is probably due to partial obstruction of the intrapancreatic portion of the common bile duct by the swollen head of the pancreas. Ultrasound examination may reveal evidence of pancreatic and peripancreatic edema or fluid collections. CT scans may indicate similar changes. Nevertheless, these latter two studies are not commonly needed to diagnose pancreatitis. Their main value is in the diagnosis and management of complications of the disease.

The most widely used tests to diagnose acute pancreatitis depend on the release of various pancreatic enzymes from the inflamed gland. The serum *amylase* concentration rises to more than 2.5 times normal within 6 h of the onset of an acute episode and usually remains elevated for several days. Values above 1000 I.U./dL are characteristic (but not diagnostic) of biliary pancreatitis; lower values are typical for acute alcoholic pancreatitis. The level of the serum amylase concentration does not correlate with the severity of the episode of pancreatitis.

There are several reasons why a patient with acute pancreatitis may have a normal serum amylase concentration: (1) The urinary clearance of amylase increases shortly after the onset of pancreatic inflammation. Thus the serum concentration may fall to normal because more is excreted in the urine. For this reason, the urinary excretion of amylase is often measured as well. Excretion of more than 5000 I.U./24 h is abnormal. (2) In patients with hyperlipidemia and pancreatitis, the chemical determination of amylase is interfered with by the lipid. Serum amylase values are usually falsely normal in this setting. Urinary amylase measurement is still accurate and is usually elevated, however. (3) In patients with chronic pancreatitis who have suffered significant destruction of pancreatic parenchyma, there may be insufficient amylase released to raise the serum concentration above normal, even with an episode of acute inflammation. Pancreatic fibrosis also may limit the permeability of the gland and its capillaries, so absorption of amylase into the blood is restricted.

It is important to recognize that the serum amylase concentration and the urinary amylase excretion both may be increased in patients without pancreatitis. Examples are patients with perforated duodenal ulcer, gangrenous cholecystitis, small bowel obstruction, and other acute intraabdominal inflammatory conditions. This probably occurs because the pancreatic amylase leaks directly into the peritoneal cavity (e.g., perforated viscus) or translocates through the inflamed and permeable bowel wall and is absorbed into the blood.

The usual laboratory assay measures amylase isoenzymes from both pancreatic (p-type amylase) and salivary or other (s-type amylase) sources. Thus serum amylase elevations in some patients without pancreatic disease may be due to excessive s-type amylase alone. Examples are salivary or ovarian tumors, chronic sialadenitis, and liver disease. Macroamylasemia is another condition in which the serum amylase concentration is elevated but the pancreas is normal. In this abnormality, the amylase molecules (usually s-type) exist in the serum as large macromolecular aggregates whose effective size and molecular mass are much greater than the normal amylase molecule's ($\sim$55,000 Da). These macromolecules are too large for glomerular filtration and excretion by the kidney, so their serum concentration increases. Urinary excretion of amylase is low. The identification of both macroamylasemia and s-type amylase can be made by electrophoretic analysis of the serum. This should be done when the serum amylase concentration is high and the clinical picture is inconsistent with the diagnosis of pancreatitis.

Other pancreatic enzymes also have been measured in an effort to improve the diagnostic accuracy of serum amylase determinations. The greatest experience has been with serum *lipase,* which appears to be more reliable than amylase to diagnose acute pancreatitis. This is probably because the pancreas is the main source of lipase in the blood. Nevertheless, the test is still not used widely because the older method for lipase determination was cumbersome and time-consuming. A new technique that is rapid and simple may increase its utility. Radioimmunoassay kits are now available for the rapid determination of serum *trypsin* and *elastase* concentrations, and these also appear to be sensitive markers of pancreatic inflammation. To date, they have been used mostly in research protocols.

Radiologic studies are not used commonly to diagnose acute pancreatitis, but certain nonspecific abnormalities are often present. The most frequent finding on a plain abdominal film is the dilatation of an isolated loop of intestine (duodenum, jejunum, or transverse colon) adjacent to the pancreas (*sentinel loop*). A gas-filled ascending and right transverse colon that stops abruptly in the middle or left transverse colon (*colon cutoff sign*) is due to colonic spasm near the inflamed pancreas. An upper gastrointestinal series may show a widened duodenal loop or a swollen ampulla of Vater because of edema in the head of the pancreas. Calcification in the pancreas itself signifies the presence of chronic pancreatitis but does not prove the presence of acute inflammation. Chest films may reveal pleural effusions, more common on the left side.

In patients with biliary pancreatitis, a plain abdominal film may show radiopaque gallstones in the region of the gallbladder.

However, the best way to confirm the presence of gallstones when biliary pancreatitis is suspected is with *ultrasound* (US) examination. Ultrasound also may reveal an edematous, swollen pancreas, peripancreatic fluid collections, or pseudocysts. Serial US examinations may be useful to follow the clinical course of patients with protracted or complicated pancreatitis or pseudocysts. In about 20 percent of cases of acute pancreatitis, US examination of the pancreas is technically unsatisfactory because of the presence of overlying bowel gas.

A *CT scan* of the pancreas should be obtained in all patients with acute pancreatitis whose illness has not begun to resolve within 2 or 3 days or whenever complications are suspected. Possible findings include a normal pancreas, pancreatic edema, a mass of inflamed peripancreatic tissue and pancreas (phlegmon), pancreatic and/or peripancreatic fluid collections (acute pseudocysts), or abscess. Extension of the inflammation from the area of the pancreas to other tissue planes (retrocolic, perinephric) may be evident and implies a more serious prognosis. The adequacy of pancreatic perfusion also can be estimated if the CT is done first without and then with intravenous contrast material, which must be injected rapidly as a bolus. A viable pancreas "enhances" as the contrast material flows through it; lack of enhancement suggests necrosis of that part of the pancreas (Fig. 30-4). This technique represents a major advance in the diagnosis and management of complicated acute pancreatitis, since patients with significant pancreatic necrosis (>50 percent of the pancreas) are more likely to develop pancreatic infection and to require surgical intervention. If infection is suspected, a percutaneous ("skinny") needle can be introduced into collections of fluid, especially near poorly perfused pancreatic tissue, using CT or US as a guide. The aspirated material should be sent for Gram stain and bacterial and fungal culture. Proof of infection is an indication for laparotomy and surgical drainage.

Prognostic Signs. Early identification of patients who are at increased risk for the development of serious complications of pancreatitis allows them to be managed more aggressively, which may decrease the mortality rate. Three different approaches have been used: (1) Specific biochemical markers have been sought that discriminate between edematous and necrotizing pancreatitis, since the latter is known to have a higher rate of complications. For example, in necrotizing pancreatitis, the serum level of α_2-macroglobulin (which binds trypsin) falls, and the levels of α_1-protease inhibitor and complement (C3 and C4) increase. So far the best discrimination between edematous and necrotizing pancreatitis has been achieved with serum C-reactive protein, a nonspecific acute-phase reactant that is elevated in the latter. C-reactive protein is still not widely used outside the research setting, however. (2) Multiple biochemical and/or physiologic measurements have been made during the first several days after hospital admission, which, taken together, have prognostic value. Ranson developed a series of different criteria for the severity of acute pancreatitis (Table 30-2). Modifications of these criteria exist, but Ranson's original ones are still used most widely. The APACHE II scoring system also has been applied recently to patients with acute pancreatitis and appears to have prognostic significance as well. (3) Contrast-enhanced CT scan provides the most objective information about the extent of the inflammatory process, the degree of pancreatic necrosis, and the presence of infection, all of which affect the treatment and the prognosis. Because it is an invasive and expensive test, however,

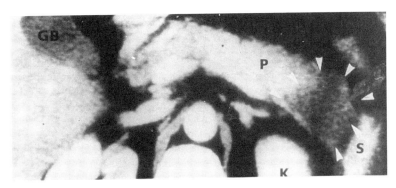

A

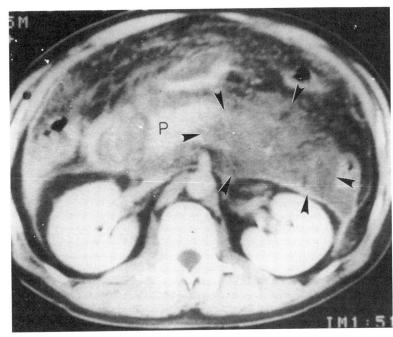

B

FIG. 30-4. Contrast-enhanced abdominal CT scans in two patients with acute pancreatitis. *A.* The head and body of the pancreas (P) opacify with the injection of intravenous contrast material. The poorly perfused tail (*arrowheads*) does not. The kidney (K) and spleen (S) are also shown. *(Kindly provided by Professor Hans Beger, University of Ulm.) B.* In this patient, only the head of the pancreas (P) opacifies; the rest of the gland is poorly perfused. At operation, the body and tail of the pancreas were necrotic and infected. They were debrided and drained.

Table 30-2
Ranson's Prognostic Criteria for Acute Pancreatitis
Morbidity and Mortality Rates Correlate with the Number of Criteria Present: 0–2 = 2% mortality; 3–4 = 15% mortality; 5–6 = 40% mortality; 7–8 = 100% mortality

Present on admission:
  Age >55 years
  White blood cell count >16,000/μL
  Blood glucose >200 mg/dL
  Serum lactate dehydrogenase >350 I.U./L
  SGOT (AST) >250 I.U./dL
Developing during first 48 h:
  Hematocrit fall >10%
  Blood urea nitrogen increase >8 mg/dL
  Serum Ca^{2+} <8 mg/dL
  Arterial P$_{O_2}$ <60 mmHg
  Base deficit <4 mEq/L
  Estimated fluid sequestration >600 mL

it is not done on all patients who are admitted with the disease. It should be done on patients who appear to be at higher risk based on any of the preceding prognostic criteria (e.g., >3 Ranson signs), those whose illness is not resolving within 2 or 3 days of admission, or for any other reason if a complication is suspected.

Treatment. *Medical Treatment.* The treatment of uncomplicated acute pancreatitis is medical and is directed primarily toward the restoration of fluid and electrolyte balance and the avoidance of secretory stimulation of the pancreas. *Nasogastric suction* should be instituted in most patients, except those with mild disease unassociated with significant vomiting or pain. All oral intake should be withheld until the ileus has resolved and pain is absent. The enzyme abnormalities usually have returned to normal by that time. For unclear reasons, the serum enzymes sometimes remain elevated even though the patient is asymptomatic. The resumption of oral intake is usually tolerated in these circumstances. Occasionally, symptoms will recur when oral intake is resumed. When this occurs, another period of fasting is indicated.

Fluid requirements may be considerable, since large volumes can be sequestered in the retroperitoneum adjacent to the pancreas. The amount of crystalloid and colloid (albumin, blood) given should be sufficient to maintain an adequate hematocrit, circulating blood volume, and urine output. It should be stressed that the most important aspect of early resuscitation is adequate and aggressive fluid replacement. Renal failure from inadequate replacement is a frequent finding in patients who die from this disease. Moreover, the pancreatitis itself may progress from the impaired pancreatic perfusion that can accompany the shock state. Electrolyte derangements may be present if vomiting has been significant and dehydration is severe. A hypokalemic, hypochloremic, metabolic alkalosis is most common. Hypocalcemia may occur in patients with severe pancreatitis. It must be treated urgently with parenteral calcium because it predisposes to cardiac arrhythmias. The prognosis appears to be related to the degree of hypocalcemia and the ease with which it is corrected. Hypomagnesemia is also common, particularly in alcoholic patients, and the magnesium should be replaced. About 30 percent of patients with acute pancreatitis develop arterial hypoxemia (Pa_{O_2} <70 mmHg) and require supplemental O_2 by mask. Because the onset of this is often insidious and may precede any changes on the chest film, it is prudent to determine arterial blood gases every 12 h for the first several days after admission to the hospital in most patients and longer in those who appear to have more serious disease. An occasional patient may develop adult respiratory distress syndrome (ARDS) and require endotracheal intubation and mechanical ventilation. Table 30-3 lists the changes in cardiovascular function in acute pancreatitis, and Table 30-4 lists the changes in respiratory function.

A number of drugs have been shown to exert no beneficial effect in patients with acute pancreatitis. These include antibiotics (which should be used only to treat specific suppurative complications), anticholinergics, gastric acid antisecretory agents, glucagon, somatostatin, and inhibitors of proteolytic enzymes (e.g., Trasylol). Parenteral nutrition has no specific beneficial effect on the course of pancreatitis. It should be used, as in any other patient, when oral intake must be withheld for prolonged periods and enteral nutrition is not possible. Elemental diets introduced by tube into the small intestine do not avoid pancreatic stimulation.

Peritoneal lavage has been used in patients with severe acute pancreatitis and intraperitoneal fluid to remove toxins and various metabolites from the peritoneal cavity and minimize their systemic absorption. Although controlled trials failed to show that this decreased mortality rates, there was some evidence that the incidence of cardiopulmonary complications was lessened. For this reason, and because there are many anecdotal reports where patients rapidly improved during lavage therapy, it is still done. The usual indication is severe pancreatitis that fails to show significant clinical improvement after several days of intensive therapy by more conventional means. The technique requires the insertion of a peritoneal lavage catheter and the rapid infusion and withdrawal of lactated Ringer's solution (1 to 2 L/h) for 2 to 3 days or longer. If a response is seen, it is usually during the first 6 to 8 h. If no improvement occurs, surgery may be required.

Biliary pancreatitis is caused by a gallstone that obstructs the pancreatic and bile ducts. In the majority of cases, the gallstone dislodges spontaneously and usually passes into the intestine.

Table 30-3

Changes in Cardiovascular Function in Acute Pancreatitis

Depressed myocardial contractility
Decreased left ventricular stroke work
Decreased systemic vascular resistance
Decreased tissue perfusion
Electrocardiogram abnormalities
ST-segment and T-wave changes

When this happens, the patient's clinical course begins to improve, and the episode is generally short-lived. If the stone remains impacted, the attack of pancreatitis may become severe and refractory to the usual treatment. Impaction should be suspected when a patient with pancreatitis is known to have gallstones, when the serum bilirubin concentration is elevated more than 4 mg/dL, when the alkaline phosphatase level is elevated, and when the clinical course does not improve within 24 to 36 h. If a skilled endoscopist is available, ERCP with *endoscopic sphincterotomy* to remove the stone may abort the attack. Otherwise, surgical removal of the impacted stone is indicated.

Surgical Treatment. Surgery is contraindicated in uncomplicated acute pancreatitis. Surgery is occasionally performed in patients with abdominal pain in whom the diagnosis is unclear, and the patient is found to have acute pancreatitis. If the pancreatitis is mild to moderate in severity and gallstones are present, a cholecystectomy should be done, and an operative cholangiogram should be obtained. Common duct stones should be removed. The pancreas should not be disturbed. For severe pancreatitis, the biliary tree should be drained if stones are present (cholecystostomy), but cholecystectomy probably should not be done. The common duct should be decompressed with a T-tube if stones are present, and if a stone is impacted at the ampulla of Vater, it should be removed. It is unclear whether drains should be placed to the area of the pancreas; many surgeons would not do this, thinking that the foreign body might predispose to infection. If necrotic pancreas or peripancreatic tissue is found, it should be debrided and drained widely.

In most patients with biliary pancreatitis, the diagnosis is obvious without the need for operation, and the pancreatitis resolves within 2 or 3 days. In these patients, cholecystectomy should be performed during the same hospitalization, usually 4 to 6 days after the original admission. The older practice of discharging the patient and delaying cholecystectomy for 6 weeks was associated with a 60 to 80 percent incidence of recurrence of pancreatitis. On the other hand, patients with severe episodes of biliary pancreatitis should be discharged once they

Table 30-4

Changes in Respiratory Function in Acute Pancreatitis

Decreased ventilation
   Vital capacity
   FEV_1/FVC
Decreased efficiency of gas exchange
   Carbon monoxide diffusing capacity
      Decreased oxygen-carrying capacity of hemoglobin

have recovered, and cholecystectomy should be deferred for at least 6 weeks. By this time, the inflammation has subsided and the operation can be done without increased risk.

Complications. Severe episodes of acute pancreatitis may be associated with both systemic and local complications. *Systemic complications* include respiratory insufficiency with ARDS, renal failure, and depressed myocardial function. To some extent, this multiple organ failure may be due to secondary pancreatic infection and the systemic effects of sepsis, as seen in other disorders. Bacterial translocation and absorption of endotoxin from adjacent inflamed colon may be important. There is also evidence that systemic absorption of pancreatic proteases, phospholipase A_2, and inflammatory cytokines such as interleukin-1, interleukin-6, and tumor necrosis factor, and other noxious agents released from the inflamed pancreas may contribute. This is the rationale for peritoneal lavage: to remove the putative toxins. Inadequate fluid resuscitation accounts for some cases of renal failure. The treatment of multiple organ failure in this setting is no different from that in any other. Resistance to maximal treatment may justify surgical intervention to debride and drain the pancreas, although pancreatic infection is the usual indication.

Local complications include the development of pancreatic or peripancreatic infection and pseudocyst formation. Pseudocysts will be discussed in a separate section. Septic complications are best divided into infection of pancreatic necrosis and pancreatic abscess. *Infected pancreatic necrosis* occurs in at least 40 percent of patients with severe acute pancreatitis and necrosis of more than 50 percent of the pancreas (demonstrated by CT scan). Infection is difficult to recognize clinically. Even with sterile necrosis, patients may appear septic, with high fever, leukocytosis, and abdominal tenderness. Sterile necrosis in a stable patient should be managed expectantly, without surgical intervention. If gas bubbles (presumed to originate from bacterial fermentation) are seen on the CT image, infection is certain, and surgery should be undertaken (Fig. 30-5). Nevertheless, percutaneous aspiration with Gram stain and culture of the involved material is usually required to prove the presence of infection. Infected pancreatic necrosis is most often diagnosed during the second week of an episode of pancreatitis. The organisms are usually a mixed flora including *Escherichia coli, Bacteroides, Staphylococcus, Candida albicans,* etc., so broad-spectrum antibiotics should be used. Antibiotics, however, are only adjunctive. Surgical drainage is necessary for definitive management. Percutaneous drainage is almost always inadequate, since the material is thick and contains particulate debris that rapidly clogs the narrow lumen of these tubes. At operation, the infected necrotic material should be debrided widely and the involved areas drained to the outside with large sump drains or packed open. Postoperatively, peritoneal lavage may be useful to mechanically remove additional devitalized tissue. Reoperation to drain recurrent or persistent infection is required in at least *one-fifth* of these patients. Associated complications such as fistulas from the bowel or pancreas or bleeding from the retroperitoneal structures are common. The overall mortality rate varies from 10 to 35 percent. Table 30-5 lists the indications for surgery in severe acute pancreatitis.

The decision to operate on a patient with severe acute pancreatitis is often difficult and requires mature clinical judgment. Those indications which are widely accepted include (1) for dif-

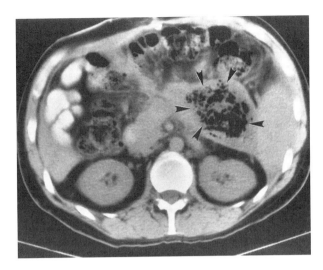

FIG. 30-5. Abdominal CT scan in a patient with acute pancreatitis and infection in the lesser sac in the region of the body and tail of the pancreas. Infection is indicated by the presence of intraperitoneal gas bubbles (*arrowheads*).

ferential diagnosis when the surgeon is concerned that the symptoms are due to a disease other than pancreatitis for which operation is mandatory, (2) in persistent and severe biliary pancreatitis when an obstructing gallstone that cannot be removed endoscopically is lodged at the ampulla of Vater, (3) in the presence of infected pancreatic necrosis, and (4) to drain a pancreatic abscess if percutaneous drainage is not adequate. Other indications that are less well defined are (1) the presence of sterile pancreatic necrosis involving more than half the pancreas and (2) when the pancreatitis persists or the patient's condition deteriorates despite maximal medical therapy. Some less common indications for operation in these patients (e.g., peritonitis, hemorrhage, biliary obstruction, duodenal obstruction, etc.) have been omitted because the need for operation is generally more *apparent*.

Pancreatic abscesses are localized collections of pus in or near the pancreas and are confined by a capsule. They are usually diagnosed later than infected necrosis, about 3 to 4 weeks after the onset of the attack. Although systemic evidence of toxicity is often less, the patients may appear quite septic. CT scans reveal a fluid collection that may be indistinguishable from a pseudocyst. As with infected necrosis, gas bubbles in the fluid prove infection, but aspiration of the fluid with Gram stain and culture is usually required for the diagnosis. If the fluid is thin in consistency and there is little particulate matter in it, percutaneous drainage may be adequate treatment. Open surgical drainage is indicated if the material is thick, if rapid improve-

Table 30-5
Indications for Surgery in Severe Acute Pancreatitis

Accepted	Controversial
Differential diagnosis	>50% Sterile pancreatic necrosis
Persistent biliary pancreatitis	Stable but persistent disease
Infected pancreatic necrosis	Deterioration in clinical course
Pancreatic abscess	Organ system failure

ment does not occur after percutaneous drainage, or if there is CT evidence of considerable surrounding tissue necrosis in addition to the abscess. The mortality rate is about 20 percent.

Prognosis. The mortality rate for all patients with acute pancreatitis is approximately 10 percent. Necrotizing pancreatitis associated with infection has a mortality rate of about 35 percent, although there is some evidence that earlier diagnosis of infection and aggressive surgical intervention may lower this figure.

Chronic Pancreatitis

Clinical Manifestations. In 95 percent of patients with chronic pancreatitis, the principal symptom is *abdominal pain.* It is usually located in the epigastrium and is described as cramping, boring, or aching. In more than half the cases, it is also felt in the back. During an episode of acute inflammation, the pain is similar to that felt by patients suffering attacks of acute pancreatitis. In between such episodes, patients have recurrent pain that may last from a few days to several weeks, separated initially by several months or more. Typically the pain-free intervals become shorter and the painful attacks last longer so that pain eventually occurs every day. When the disease is so far advanced that most of the exocrine function is lost, about one-third of patients experience spontaneous pain relief. Another 10 to 20 percent have temporary remissions of pain that last 1 to 3 years. Some pain relief is typically obtained when the patients sit with the knees flexed and a pillow pressed to the abdomen. Most require analgesic drugs and many become addicted to narcotics. Assessment of the severity of pain is often difficult because many of these patients are addicted to alcohol and/or narcotics and have unstable personalities. Consequently, secondary gain may lead to an exaggeration of symptoms. The mechanism of the pain is uncertain, although it may be related to elevated duct and pancreatic tissue pressures and impaired parenchymal blood flow, a kind of compartment syndrome. Table 30-6 lists the potential causes of pain in chronic pancreatitis.

Variable *weight loss* occurs in 75 percent of patients with chronic pancreatitis because food usually aggravates the pain, and thus intake is voluntarily restricted. Significant weight loss from malabsorption is less common. Nevertheless, patients may complain of bulky, offensive, fatty or oily stools.

About two-thirds of patients with chronic pancreatitis have abnormal glucose tolerance, and half of these have *diabetes mellitus.* In these patients some degree of malabsorption is also present, since exocrine and endocrine insufficiency usually develop concurrently. The diabetes is usually easily controlled with insulin, but hypoglycemia may be a problem in alcoholics with irregular eating habits.

Table 30-6
Potential Causes of Pain in Chronic Pancreatitis

Pancreatic ductal hypertension
Inflammation of the intrapancreatic nerves
Loss of the protective perineural sheath in pancreatic nerves
Pancreatic ischemia
Pseudocysts
Pancreatic and peripancreatic infection
Biliary obstruction
Cholangitis
Duodenal obstruction

As a rule, most patients with chronic pancreatitis have failed to adapt to the stresses of society and have inadequate personalities. The additional stresses created by the disease often result in depression and anxiety. These personality traits are important in evaluating these patients, as well as in choosing specific types of therapy.

In most patients with chronic pancreatitis there are few physical findings. There may be some epigastric tenderness, some evidence of weight loss, and occasionally jaundice. If a mass is palpable, it is most likely a pancreatic pseudocyst.

Diagnostic Studies. These are not especially helpful in the diagnosis of chronic pancreatitis. About two-thirds of patients with alcoholic pancreatitis have abnormal liver function. Mild elevations of serum concentrations of bilirubin (2 to 4 mg/dL), alkaline phosphatase, and serum glutamic-oxaloacetic transaminase (SGOT) and mild depression of serum albumin concentration may occur. Pancreatic exocrine function is impaired in almost all patients, but there is a wide range of normal values for bicarbonate and enzyme secretion and volume flow in response to secretory hormones. Thus mild abnormalities may not be apparent. Pancreatic function tests are rarely indicated in patients with overt pancreatic disease (chronic pancreatitis or pancreatic cancer). Although these tests would confirm the presence of pancreatic insufficiency, they (1) rarely influence therapeutic decisions and (2) cannot distinguish between pancreatitis and cancer. They are of greater value in patients with vague complaints in whom the presence of pancreatic disease is suspected but for which no direct evidence exists. In these patients, these tests are 90 percent sensitive in detecting functional abnormalities. Thus a normal test along with one or two other studies that are also normal (e.g., ERCP or CT scan) reliably rules out pancreatic disease.

In 30 to 50 percent of patients with chronic pancreatitis, plain x-rays of the abdomen reveal pancreatic calcifications (Fig. 30-6). When calcifications are present, the diagnosis of chronic pancreatitis is certain even if there is no clinical evidence. With early chronic pancreatitis, and even in some patients with advanced disease, ductal abnormalities demonstrated by ERCP may be minimal. In the majority of patients with advanced disease, the main duct may be dilated up to 1 cm or more in diameter with intermittent points of obstruction (Fig. 30-7). Strictures, cysts, and ductal calculi may be seen. The common bile duct is also opacified by this technique, and distortion of its anatomy is evident. Chronic pancreatitis characteristically produces angulation of the distal common duct with a smooth, tapered narrowing of its intrapancreatic portion (Fig. 30-8). Generally, all patients with chronic pancreatitis who are being considered for operation should undergo ERCP examination. The study provides critical information about ductal anatomy. Patients with dilated ducts are candidates for drainage procedures; those who do not have ductal dilatation may require pancreatic resection (Fig. 30-9). Occasionally, it is impossible to obtain a preoperative ERCP. In these cases, a pancreatogram can be done at operation by puncturing the duct directly through the anterior surface of the gland.

CT scans also provide useful information. When the duct is grossly dilated, it usually can be seen running the length of the gland (Fig. 30-10). Pseudocysts and cystic communications with the ductal system are evident. Biliary dilatation and the level of bile duct obstruction are defined. CT scans provide the most

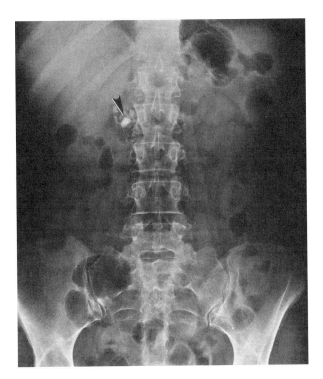

FIG. 30-6. Plain film with pancreatic calcifications (*arrowhead*).

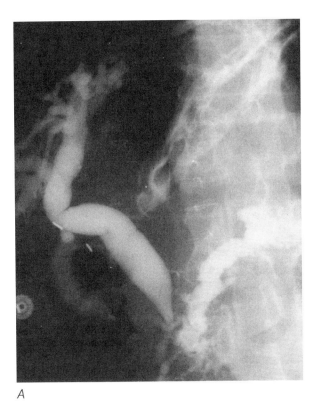

A

precise information about the size and configuration of the pancreas, information that is useful in decisions regarding possible pancreatic resection.

Differential Diagnosis. The diagnosis of chronic pancreatitis is usually straightforward. Most patients are chronic alcoholics with recurring episodes of abdominal pain, diabetes,

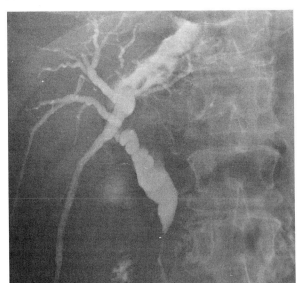

B

FIG. 30-8. ERCP in patients with chronic pancreatitis. *A.* The common bile duct is compressed by the fibrotic pancreas in the head of the gland and is dilated proximal to the obstruction. The patient was jaundiced. *B.* The smooth, tapered narrowing typical of common bile duct compression from chronic pancreatitis is evident. The bile duct is dilated proximally.

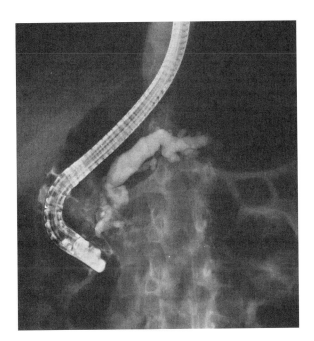

FIG. 30-7. ERCP in a patient with chronic pancreatitis. The duct is dilated to more than 1 cm in diameter and contains multiple strictures.

weight loss, pancreatic calcifications, and some evidence of malabsorption. Occasionally, the distinction between chronic pancreatitis and pancreatic cancer may be difficult. This may occur when there is no previous history of pancreatitis, when the patient presents with jaundice and pain is not a prominent part of

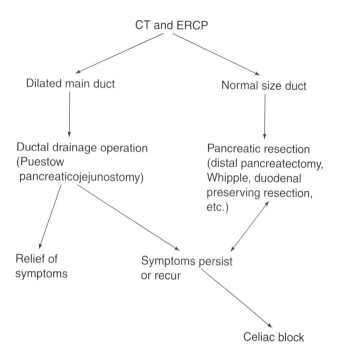

FIG. 30-9. *Algorithm for the surgical management of patients with chronic pancreatitis.*

the picture, or when weight loss is significant. In such circumstances, surgery may be necessary to make the diagnosis.

Complications. The principal complications of chronic pancreatitis are pseudocyst formation, diabetes mellitus, and malnutrition. *Jaundice* is seen sometime during the course of the disease in up to one-third of patients. This is most often the result of transient obstruction of the intrapancreatic portion of the common bile duct during an episode of acute pancreatic inflammation. It subsides when the acute process resolves. As many as 10 percent of patients develop persistent *common duct obstruction* from fibrous constriction of the duct in the head of

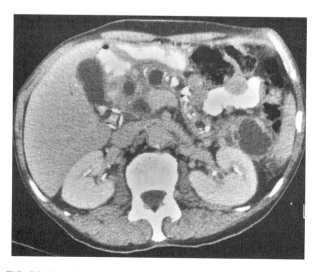

FIG. 30-10. *CT scan in a patient with chronic pancreatitis. The pancreatic duct is dilated and contains multiple calcifications. In addition, a pseudocyst is seen near the tail of the pancreas.*

the gland. The obstruction is almost never complete, which is different from the obstruction caused by pancreatic cancer. *Duodenal* or *colonic obstruction* occurs in less than 1 percent of patients with chronic pancreatitis and is caused by the inflammation in the adjacent pancreas with subsequent scarring. Gastrojejunostomy is effective in the former case, resection of the involved segment of colon in the latter.

Medical Treatment. The medical treatment of an episode of acute pancreatic inflammation is the same as the treatment of any bout of acute pancreatitis. In patients with *diabetes* from chronic pancreatitis, ketoacidosis is rare, even if blood glucose levels are quite high. Even small amounts of insulin may induce a profound hypoglycemia. This is probably due to concurrent glucagon deficiency. Thus the patient must be instructed thoroughly on the dangers of hypoglycemia, its symptoms, and management. Mild elevations in blood sugar do not require treatment, but fasting elevations in excess of 250 mg/dL should be managed with insulin. Frequently, only 20 to 30 units a day is required. Rigid control of blood sugar is not advisable. Oral agents are almost never successful.

The medical management of *pain* in patients with chronic pancreatitis should include the cessation of all alcohol intake. As many as 50 percent of patients experience some pain relief when they stop drinking. Pancreatic secretion itself may exacerbate the pain. For this reason, patients have been treated with somatostatin analogues, which effectively suppress secretory activity. Efficacy is as yet unproven, but even if the pain is relieved, long-term administration of these drugs is impractical because they can only be given parenterally, they are expensive, and they have significant side effects (e.g., gallstones).

The analgesic management of these patients should begin with small doses of oral medications such as codeine derivatives, either alone or combined with acetaminophen. If more potent narcotic analgesics are required, especially for prolonged periods, serious consideration must be given to surgical pain relief. All too often these patients are denied surgical treatment until after they have become addicted to narcotics and are severely disturbed psychologically as a result of living with constant pain.

Surgical Treatment. The most common indication for surgery is persistent severe pain, although a variety of other complications may require operative intervention (Table 30-7). The indications for surgery for pain relief are impossible to state in precise terms. When the pain interferes substantially with the quality of life, surgery should be considered. Pertinent considerations include obvious effects on health and well-being such as weight loss and nutritional status, need for frequent hospitalization, inability to maintain employment, psychiatric manifes-

Table 30-7
Indications for Surgery in Chronic Pancreatitis

Pain
Common bile duct obstruction
Duodenal obstruction
Colon obstruction
Pseudocyst
Suspicion of pancreatic cancer
Splenic vein obstruction with left-sided portal hypertension
Portal vein obstruction with portal hypertension

tations (usually depression), deterioration of family life, and narcotic addiction.

All patients who are being evaluated for possible surgical intervention should undergo an abdominal CT scan and an ERCP, in addition to the standard preoperative assessment for a major abdominal procedure. Psychiatric evaluation is also appropriate in many patients. Information from these studies helps with decisions about the type of surgical procedure that may be indicated.

There are two categories of operations for the relief of pain in patients with chronic pancreatitis. The first are drainage operations, which attempt to drain more adequately a dilated ductal system that is presumed to be obstructed. The second are the pancreatic resection operations, which remove diseased pancreatic tissue, usually in situations where the pancreatic ducts are normal or narrowed in size. Sphincterotomy or sphincteroplasty of the sphincter of Oddi has no place as the primary treatment of pain in patients with this disease.

Drainage Procedures. When the diameter of the main pancreatic duct in the head and body of the pancreas increases to 7 mm or more, a *lateral pancreaticojejunostomy* (the *Puestow procedure*) is technically feasible (Fig. 30-11). The duct is opened throughout the length of the pancreas and anastomosed side to side to a Roux-en-Y limb of jejunum. Immediate pain relief is likely in 80 to 90 percent, but pain recurs unpredictably in 25 to 50 percent of patients after 5 years. In some patients, recurrence of pain may be due to stenosis of the pancreaticojejunal anastomosis. This can be proved by ERCP. Reconstruction of the anastomosis may then be beneficial. In the majority of cases, there is no apparent cause for the recurrence of pain, and pancreatic resection must be considered. If the Puestow operation is done in a pancreas with a normal-sized duct, both short- and long-term results are unsatisfactory, perhaps because the anastomosis strictures close in most cases.

The operative mortality of longitudinal pancreaticojejunostomy is about 4 percent, and the morbidity is minimal. Because almost no pancreas is resected, the procedure rarely results in diabetes. Nevertheless, a number of patients eventually will require insulin, since destruction of the pancreas probably continues. Although pancreatic enzymes can now empty freely through the pancreaticojejunostomy, there is rarely any clinical improvement in the degree of malabsorption. However, patients may gain weight because eating no longer produces pain, and therefore, they eat more.

Pancreatic Resections. Pancreatic resection should be considered for pain relief when the pancreatic duct is narrow or normal in diameter, when a previous pancreaticojejunostomy has failed, or when the pathologic changes in the pancreas particularly involve one part of the gland and the rest is less diseased. The standard *Whipple pancreaticoduodenectomy* (the operation usually done for pancreatic cancer) may be indicated when most of the disease involves the head of the pancreas (Fig. 30-12). A modification of this operation is the pancreaticoduodenectomy with preservation of the stomach and pylorus (Fig. 30-13). The theoretical advantage of this procedure is that it preserves gastric function and avoids some of the nutritional disturbances that may follow the standard pancreaticoduodenectomy. *Ninety-five percent distal pancreatectomy* entails removal of the spleen and all the pancreas except for a thin rim of tissue that lies within the C loop of the duodenum. Because the spleen is sacrificed and all the patients require insulin after this operation, it is not

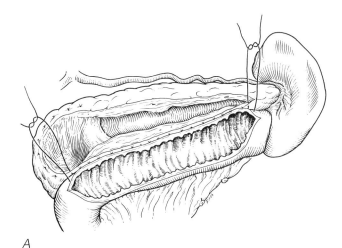

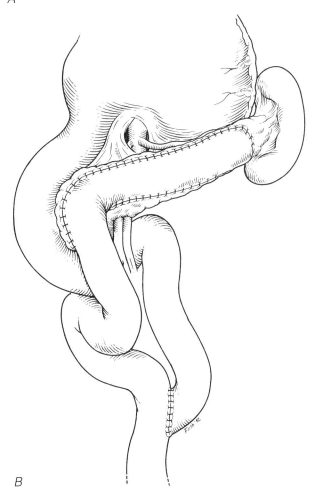

FIG. 30-11. Longitudinal pancreaticojejunostomy (Puestow procedure). *A.* The pancreatic duct has been opened longitudinally throughout the length of the pancreas, and additional pancreatic tissue has been removed from the head of the gland in order to remove calcifications and establish adequate drainage. The anastomosis to a Roux-en-Y segment of jejunum is begun. *B.* The anastomosis is complete and gastrointestinal continuity has been restored.

done frequently. Today, *total pancreatectomy* is performed rarely because of the uniform requirement for insulin and the significant alterations in digestive and absorptive functions that

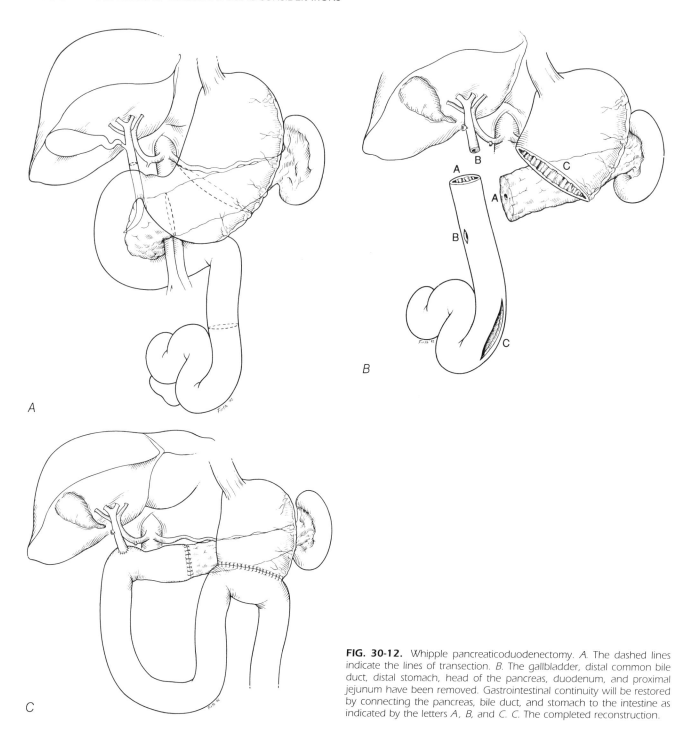

FIG. 30-12. Whipple pancreaticoduodenectomy. *A.* The dashed lines indicate the lines of transection. *B.* The gallbladder, distal common bile duct, distal stomach, head of the pancreas, duodenum, and proximal jejunum have been removed. Gastrointestinal continuity will be restored by connecting the pancreas, bile duct, and stomach to the intestine as indicated by the letters *A, B,* and *C. C.* The completed reconstruction.

follow. A new operation, in which the head of the pancreas is resected but the entire duodenum is preserved, may be preferred to the Whipple procedure in those patients in whom the head of the pancreas is the major focus of disease. The theoretical advantages of this procedure include the preservation of gastroduodenal and biliary continuity and function and a low likelihood of the development of diabetes, since most of the pancreas is preserved.

The mortality rate of the various pancreatic resection operations is less than 5 percent. The significant drawback associated with major pancreatic resections is the creation of the diabetic state, which is often difficult to control. For this reason, such procedures should not be done in unreliable alcoholic patients who may be addicted to narcotics. Pain is relieved in 80 to 90 percent of patients in the first several years after these operations, and even after 5 years, about 80 percent continue to be pain-free. Tables 30-8 through 30-10 list late results, mortality rates, and long-term pain relief of pancreaticoduodenectomy for chronic pancreatitis in various hands.

Nonsurgical *destruction of the celiac ganglia* may have a place in the management of patients with severe pain from chronic pancreatitis. In those in whom the surgeon and gastro-

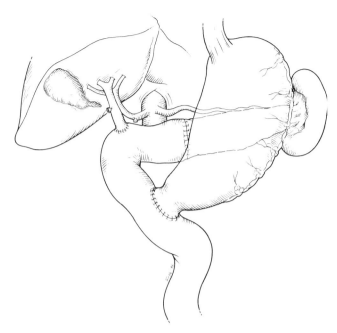

FIG. 30-13. Pylorus-preserving Whipple pancreaticoduodenectomy. The entire stomach and pylorus are preserved, and gastrointestinal continuity is restored as shown.

enterologist wish to avoid or delay pancreatic resection, percutaneous injection of the ganglia with absolute ethanol may provide some relief for a period of time. Consultation with an anesthesiologist interested in pain management may be helpful. Although permanent pain relief is unusual with this technique, a limited period of improvement may be useful for patient and physician alike, resulting in a better rapport and a better understanding of the patient's commitment to a treatment program. In a few cases, spontaneous improvement in the pain may even occur.

Pancreatic Transplantation. In an effort to avoid diabetes, autografts of the body and tail of the pancreas have been done in a small number of patients who were subjected to total or near-total pancreatectomy. Success has been limited, and more experience is required before this approach can be recommended widely.

Prognosis. In patients with alcoholic chronic pancreatitis, life expectancy is reduced by 10 to 15 years, and the mean age at death is approximately 50 years. The principal causes of death include upper respiratory malignancies (most patients are heavy

Table 30-8
Late Results (6 mos–16 years) after Pancreaticoduodenectomy in 79 Evaluable Patients

Pain-free (occasional pain)	79% (15%)
Increase in weight	77%
Returned to work	66%
Exocrine insufficiency	24%
Endocrine insufficiency	12%
Operative and hospital mortality	0.9%
Late mortality	11%

SOURCE: Modified from: Trede M, 1990, with permission.

Table 30-9
Operative Mortality Rates of Pancreaticoduodenectomy for Chronic Pancreatitis (1987–1990)

Authors	Number of Patients	Deaths
Gall	289	3 (1%)
Kohler et al.	24	3 (12%)
Morel et al.	20	0
Rossi et al.	73	2 (3%)
Williamson et al.	6	0
Stone et al.	15	0
Mannell et al.	10	0
Howard	30	0
TOTAL	467	8 (1.7%)

SOURCE: Modified from Howard JM, 1998, with permission.

cigarette smokers), malnutrition, complications of diabetes, and suicide. Abuse of ethanol and/or drugs is often contributory.

PSEUDOCYSTS

Pancreatic pseudocysts are localized collections of fluid with high concentrations of pancreatic enzymes. They occur usually as a complication of pancreatitis, although some occur after trauma. Pseudocysts are located either within the pancreatic parenchyma or in one of the potential spaces that separate the gland from the adjacent abdominal viscera. Most of the time they are found in the lesser peritoneal sac behind the stomach, but they also may occur at great distances from the pancreas (e.g., neck, mediastinum, pelvis). They are called *pseudocysts* because, unlike congenital cysts or cystic neoplasms, they lack a true epithelial lining.

The pathogenesis of pseudocysts depends on the clinical setting in which they develop. During an attack of acute pancreatitis, fluid extravasates from the pancreas, where it becomes walled off by surrounding structures and fails to reabsorb as the inflammation resolves. In patients with chronic pancreatitis, ductal strictures or stones may obstruct the pancreatic duct or its branches and produce localized ductal dilatations. These areas coalesce and lose their epithelial lining as they enlarge to form a pseudocyst. Some pseudocysts follow trauma and are the result of either pancreatitis or ductal disruption with direct leakage of fluid from the gland. Occasionally, pseudocysts form after the pancreas is injured during splenectomy.

Ethanol abuse and biliary tract disease account for most of the cases, with men outnumbering women 2:1 in most series. The average age at diagnosis is 45 years. About one-third of pseudocysts are located in the head and two-thirds in the body or tail of the gland. Multiple cysts occur in 20 percent of patients.

Clinical Manifestations. Pseudocysts should be suspected when a patient with acute pancreatitis fails to recover after 5 to 7 days of treatment or, after some improvement, begins to deteriorate again. In patients with chronic pancreatitis, there is often no acute episode to herald the appearance of the cyst. Instead, the patient may complain of abdominal pain or symptoms that reflect compression of an adjacent viscus by the cyst. Nausea, vomiting, and weight loss may reflect duodenal or gastric outlet obstruction from a pseudocyst. Jaundice may be present if the cyst compresses the common bile duct.

Table 30-10
Long-Term Relief of Pain after Pancreaticoduodenectomy for Chronic Pancreatitis

Authors	Number of Patients	Follow-up (percentages)	Good	Fair	Failure
Rossi et al.	33	5	61	18	21
Williamson et al.	6	3.5	66.6	16.6	16.6
Gauthier-Benoit and Perissat	237	3.8	65	—	—
Stone et al.	15	6	53	27	20
Mannell et al.	9	10	100	0	0
Kohler et al.	24	—	61	—	—
Gall	289	8	65	—	—
Howard	17	5–15	94	—	6

SOURCE: Modified from Howard JM, 1998, with permission.

Diagnostic Studies. Ultrasound (US) and CT scanning are the most useful tests to diagnose pseudocysts. However, CT scans are more sensitive and specific than US and have the additional advantages of superior resolution and more precise localization (Fig. 30-14). Moreover, bowel gas, obesity, and displacement of intraabdominal structures from prior surgery may impair US images. The main disadvantages of CT are the relatively high cost compared with US and exposure to ionizing radiation. CT scan should be used for the initial evaluation of patients suspected of having pseudocysts; US should be reserved for follow-up examinations.

ERCP also has been used before surgery to provide anatomic information about pseudocysts, but it should not be done routinely. ERCP is indicated in jaundiced patients to differentiate between common bile duct compression by the cyst and a stricture of the intrapancreatic portion of the common duct caused by a fibrotic pancreas. In the former case, cyst drainage alone would relieve the jaundice, whereas in the latter instance, a biliary bypass procedure to relieve the biliary obstruction also would be required. Because it may introduce bacteria into a previously sterile cyst, ERCP should be performed only when cyst drainage is to be done within 24 h.

Complications. The most feared complications of pseudocyst are hemorrhage, rupture, and infection. Hemorrhage occurs in approximately 6 percent of patients, rupture into the gastrointestinal tract or peritoneal cavity in 7 percent, and infection in 14 percent. Other complications include obstruction of the gastrointestinal tract (duodenum or stomach) in 3 percent and common bile duct obstruction in 6 percent.

Hemorrhage, from erosion of pseudocysts into major blood vessels (e.g., splenic or gastroduodenal arteries), may be massive. Arteriography is the initial diagnostic procedure of choice if the patient is stable. It offers the opportunity for selective

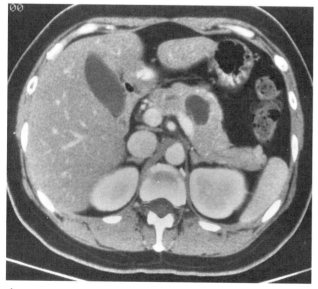

A

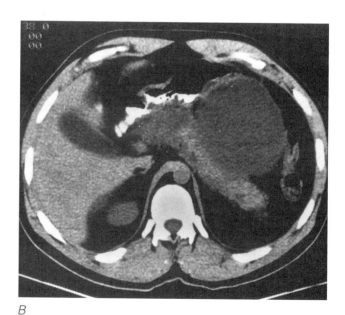

B

FIG. 30-14. *CT scans in patients with pseudocysts. A. A traumatic pseudocyst is seen within the body of the pancreas. The patient had sustained blunt abdominal trauma 1 month before but had few symptoms and was not explored at the time. B. A large pseudocyst has developed in association with an episode of acute pancreatitis. The patient was unable to eat because the cyst compressed and obstructed the stomach. The pseudocyst was drained internally into the stomach (pseudocystgastrostomy).*

embolization to plug the bleeding vessel. This may be definitive or, by temporarily stopping the hemorrhage, allow resuscitation of a critically ill patient and permit surgery to proceed on an urgent rather than emergency basis. Frequently, blood loss may be so rapid that it precludes diagnostic procedures and requires emergency operation. Both the cyst and the bleeding vessel should be excised, if possible. Even with aggressive surgical management, the mortality rate is at least 30 percent.

If the pseudocyst *ruptures* freely into the peritoneal cavity, the patient may develop symptoms and signs of acute peritonitis. Treatment of free rupture requires urgent operation with irrigation of the peritoneal cavity and usually external drainage of the cyst. Free rupture of a pseudocyst is a serious complication; the mortality rate is approximately 15 percent. Rupture into the gastrointestinal tract may produce vomiting or diarrhea but is usually not a surgical emergency.

Pseudocyst *infection* may occur in the early weeks after cyst formation as a complication of an episode of severe acute pancreatitis. Pseudocyst infection must be distinguished from infected pancreatic necrosis. Less commonly, superinfection of a mature cyst is heralded by fever and leukocytosis in a patient who has not been acutely ill. In either case, infection can be proved by percutaneous drainage of the cyst under US or CT guidance, with Gram stain and culture of the fluid. Infected pseudocysts may resolve permanently with percutaneous drainage for a week or so. However, if percutaneous drainage does not produce prompt clinical improvement, surgery is required.

Treatment. Pseudocysts that develop in patients with chronic pancreatitis are unlikely to resolve spontaneously and may be viewed as mature from the time of discovery. About 40 percent of acute pseudocysts (those which develop during an episode of acute pancreatitis) will disappear spontaneously as the pancreatitis resolves, however. If mature pseudocysts are asymptomatic and are less than 5 cm in diameter, they probably require no treatment, since serious complications generally occur in cysts that are larger. These patients should be followed and the cysts reevaluated at 3- to 6-month intervals with US. The onset of symptoms, growth in the size of the cyst, or development of a complication demands intervention.

Surgery. The three types of surgical procedures used to treat pseudocysts are resection, external drainage, and internal drainage. Elective surgery should be delayed until the pseudocyst is mature, i.e., until the wall is firm enough to hold sutures. This requires 4 to 6 weeks for cysts that arise during acute pancreatitis. For cysts that arise during chronic pancreatitis, no wait is necessary. At operation, the interior of the cyst should be inspected for evidence of tumor, and a biopsy of the cyst wall should be obtained to exclude a cystic neoplasm (e.g., cystadenocarcinoma). *Resection* is the preferred method of treatment but is usually possible only for cysts in the tail of the gland, when the head and body are normal or minimally changed (e.g., traumatic pseudocysts). *External drainage* is preferred when the cyst wall is not sufficiently thickened to allow anastomosis to the gut lumen. A large-bore tube is sewn into the cyst lumen, and the other end is brought out through the abdominal wall. Pancreatic fistulas complicate about 20 percent of external drainage operations and usually close within a few months. Fistulas and recurrent cysts are more common when the cyst communicates with the pancreatic duct. *Internal drainage,* in which the cyst is anastomosed to a Roux-en-Y limb of jejunum (cystojejunos-

tomy), to the posterior wall of the stomach (cystogastrostomy), or to the duodenum (cystoduodenostomy), is the most frequently used operation for pseudocysts. Dependent drainage by cystogastrostomy is preferred for collections adjacent to the stomach, whereas cystojejunostomy can be done for cysts in any location. Obliteration of the cyst cavity usually follows internal drainage within a few weeks. Patients recover rapidly and are usually eating within a week. Infected pseudocysts adherent to the stomach can be drained by cystogastrostomy. Otherwise, drainage should be external because the suture line of a Roux-en-Y cystojejunostomy may not heal in an infected surgical field.

Mature pseudocysts also may be treated nonsurgically, but these techniques are still being evaluated. External drainage may be established with a narrow-lumen catheter placed percutaneously via US or CT guidance. Successful obliteration is claimed in as many as 80 percent of cases; if the cyst persists, surgery should be performed. Nonsurgical management is contraindicated in patients with cyst rupture or hemorrhage or when adjacent vascular structures preclude a percutaneous approach. In addition, if there is ever concern that the "pseudocyst" may actually represent a cystic neoplasm, surgery is required. This should be considered if there is no history of pancreatitis, septations are seen within the cyst on CT scan, or cyst calcifications are present. If any of these features are present, suspicion that the cyst represents a neoplasm should be high. Strong consideration should be given to surgical intervention rather than nonoperative management (e.g., percutaneous drainage). Table 30-11 lists the characteristics of cystic neoplasms of the pancreas.

Prognosis. Pancreatic pseudocysts recur at a rate of approximately 10 percent, although most of these probably are new cysts that arise from recurrent episodes of pancreatitis. After external drainage, the rate is approximately 20 percent. Even when pseudocysts do not recur, many patients experience chronic pain, a manifestation of underlying chronic pancreatitis.

Pancreatic Ascites

Ascites may occur when pancreatic secretions collect within the abdomen following disruption of the pancreatic duct or when a pseudocyst continuously leaks into the abdomen. A leak into the retroperitoneum may track some distance from its source, and the fluid collection may appear in the mediastinum, pleural space (pancreatic pleural effusion), or groin. Most patients are male alcoholics with chronic pancreatitis, although ascites also may occur following pancreatic trauma. Symptoms of a distinct episode of acute pancreatitis rarely precede pancreatic ascites. Pa-

Table 30-11
Characteristics of Cystic Neoplasms of the Pancreas versus Pseudocysts

No history of pancreatitis
Internal septa and/or solid intracystic components seen on CT scan
Calcification within the cyst or its wall
Recurrence or persistence of the cyst after treatment of any sort (i.e., surgical or nonsurgical)
If any of these features are present, suspicion that the cyst represents a neoplasm should be high.
Strong consideration should be given to surgical intervention, rather than nonoperative management (e.g., percutaneous drainage).

tients usually present with increasing abdominal girth, weight loss, and muscle wasting. Although the presentation can be confused with cirrhosis, abdominal paracentesis is diagnostic. The combination of high protein content (>3 g/100 mL) and amylase concentration in the ascitic fluid greater than the serum amylase concentration is pathognomonic. The initial therapy should consist of parenteral nutrition, especially if malnutrition is severe. A somatostatin analogue to suppress pancreatic secretions also may be useful. In some cases, the ascites resolves with this treatment, which should continue for 10 to 14 days. If the ascites persists, operation is indicated and should be preceded by endoscopic retrograde pancreatography to show the site of the ductal disruption. If it is located in the distal pancreas, distal pancreatectomy may be appropriate. If the leak is located in the head or body of the gland, internal drainage using a Roux-en-Y limb of jejunum is preferable. The success rate is approximately 85 percent, but in patients who are severely debilitated, postoperative morbidity is considerable.

TUMORS OF THE PANCREAS

Ductal Adenocarcinoma

In the United States, cancer of the exocrine pancreas is the fourth leading cause of cancer death in men and the fifth in women. Each year, about 28,000 cases will be diagnosed, and almost as many patients will die of advanced disease. Ductal adenocarcinoma of the pancreas accounts for approximately 90 percent of exocrine tumors, and it is a characteristically aggressive lesion. At the time of diagnosis, the tumor is confined to the pancreas in fewer than 10 percent of patients, 40 percent have locally advanced disease, and over 50 percent have distant spread. More than 95 percent of patients eventually die of their disease, and even after resection for attempted cure, the median length of survival is only 18 to 20 months.

Clinical Manifestations. Pancreatic cancer occurs in the head of the pancreas in 75 percent of cases and in the body and tail of the gland in the rest. This distinction is important because lesions of the head, close to the bile duct, may produce obstructive jaundice when they are still small and curable. Indeed, biliary obstruction, in the absence of other symptoms, is associated with a better prognosis. Painless jaundice alone (13 percent) is uncommon, however. About 75 percent of patients with carcinoma of the head of the pancreas present with *obstructive jaundice, weight loss* (average 20 pounds), and deep-seated *abdominal pain.* The jaundice is usually unrelenting but fluctuates in about 10 percent of patients. Cholangitis is uncommon (10 percent). Jaundice may be accompanied by pruritus. When back pain occurs (25 percent), it is associated with a worse prognosis, and it implies retroperitoneal invasion by the tumor. The sudden onset of diabetes mellitus is noted in about 20 percent of patients. Body and tail tumors almost always produce symptoms late and are usually far advanced at the time of diagnosis. Very few are resectable, and the prognosis is particularly grim.

Physical examination and routine laboratory tests are primarily of value in supporting the diagnosis of obstructive jaundice and in detecting very advanced disease. Hepatomegaly, present in 65 percent of patients, is a nonspecific finding. Although it can indicate liver metastases, the liver also may enlarge as a result of bile duct obstruction alone. A palpable abdominal mass

(10 percent) and ascites (5 percent) suggest advanced disease. *Courvoisier's sign,* a distended and palpable gallbladder in the jaundiced patient, suggests malignant obstruction. It is present in only 25 percent of patients.

Diagnostic Studies. The total bilirubin level tends to be greater with malignant obstruction compared with benign causes such as choledocholithiasis (e.g., mean levels of 15 versus 5 mg/dL). Serum amylase elevations are uncommon (5 percent) in patients with pancreatic cancer.

A number of screening tests for pancreatic cancer have been investigated. Ideally, such a test would be inexpensive, abnormal early in the course of the disease when it was still curable (high sensitivity), and normal in other conditions (high specificity). Of the many *serum markers* that have been evaluated (CEA, POA, GT-II, CA 19-9, DU-PAN-2), the results with CA 19-9 have been the most encouraging. However, even CA 19-9, a monoclonal antibody to the Lewis blood group antigen, has a sensitivity of only 80 percent. The smallest lesions and presumably those most amenable to cure are least likely to be detected. Gastric, colorectal, and other carcinomas also may be associated with elevations in CA 19-9, so the specificity is only about 90 percent.

The diagnostic approach to pancreatic cancer varies depending on whether the patient presents with obstructive jaundice or other symptoms. In those with jaundice, the clinician's attention is directed rapidly toward an assessment of the biliary tree. An abdominal CT scan, perhaps preceded by a US examination, is generally performed early in the evaluation. ERCP also may be done. The presumptive diagnosis usually can be arrived at within several days. In patients without jaundice, where the complaints are weight loss, pain, or other nonspecific problems, a number of other studies may precede a CT scan and/or ERCP examination. Nevertheless, in both groups, CT and ERCP have become the mainstay for diagnosis of this disease.

Ultrasound. US is relatively inexpensive and has a sensitivity of 70 percent and a specificity of 95 percent for the diagnosis of pancreatic cancer. However, the examination is unsatisfactory because of body habitus or overlying bowel gas in 20 percent of patients. When it demonstrates dilated intrahepatic and extrahepatic biliary radicles, it confirms the presence of extrahepatic biliary obstruction. US also helps to identify gallstones as a cause of obstruction.

Computed Tomography. Spiral CT has a sensitivity of 85 percent and a specificity of 95 percent for the diagnosis of pancreatic cancer. Lesions larger than 2 cm are usually detectable (Fig. 30-15). More reliable than US, CT visualizes the entire pancreas and also provides some information about resectability (e.g., liver metastases and major vascular involvement may be detected). Nodal enlargement may reflect metastases, but nodes smaller than 1 to 2 cm may be missed altogether, and inflammatory changes in nodes cannot be distinguished from neoplastic ones. About 20 percent of metastatic liver lesions are overlooked.

Endoscopic Retrograde Cholangiopancreatography. ERCP has a sensitivity of 95 percent but a specificity of only 85 percent. This is due to the difficulty in distinguishing between cancer and chronic pancreatitis. The study can be performed successfully in over 90 percent of patients and detects some tumors that are not visualized by CT.

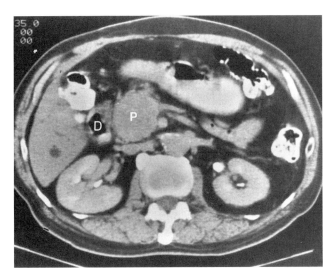

FIG. 30-15. CT scan in a patient with carcinoma of the head of the pancreas. The mass is evident (P). The duodenum (D) is shown as well.

The characteristic finding that suggests the diagnosis of pancreatic cancer is a constriction of both the pancreatic and bile ducts in the head of the gland. This is the so-called double-duct sign (Fig. 30-16). However, ERCP is superfluous in some patients. If the patient has a typical history for pancreatic cancer and a mass in the head of the pancreas is seen on CT scan that is consistent with the diagnosis, ERCP is not needed. During ERCP, cytologic study of cells obtained directly from the pancreatic duct may reveal cancer in up to 80 percent of cases. It also may be possible to determine the origin of a periampullary tumor (pancreatic versus duodenal, ampullary, or bile duct) with this technique. Therapeutic ERCP also permits endoscopic stent placement. Although this is not indicated for preoperative biliary decompression, it provides effective palliation of the jaundice for certain patients who may not need an operation.

Fine-Needle Aspiration. Preoperative fine-needle aspiration (FNA) for cytologic examination can be obtained percutaneously under CT or US guidance. The technique has a sensitivity of about 85 percent and a specificity of almost 100 percent. *However, the clinician must remember that a negative FNA never reliably eliminates the possibility that cancer is present.* FNA is justified when the knowledge that the diagnosis is pancreatic cancer will unquestionably alter the patient's management. For example, a patient with cancer of the body of the pancreas and retroperitoneal extension of tumor seen on CT scan is not likely to benefit from operation. Proof of the diagnosis by FNA would avert the need for operative biopsy and permit the use of other palliative measures (radiotherapy, chemotherapy, celiac ganglion injection, etc.) (Fig. 30-17). The routine use of FNA for patients with a mass in the head of the pancreas and obstructive jaundice is unnecessary.

Laparoscopy. Laparoscopy has been used to stage patients with pancreatic cancer. At least 20 percent of patients with no evidence of metastases from the preceding tests have small lesions evident on the liver surface, omentum, or peritoneum that can be seen laparoscopically. Such documentation of unresectability could be helpful in the patient with a body or tail lesion who would not benefit from surgery. It has no value in the patient who requires surgical bypass for relief of jaundice and gastric outlet obstruction.

Magnetic Resonance Imaging. MRI appears to offer no advantage over CT scan.

Upper Gastrointestinal Series. An upper gastrointestinal (UGI) series may show displacement of the stomach and widening of the duodenal C loop, but these are relatively late changes and are usually detectable on CT examination. A UGI series may be of some value to assess gastric outlet obstruction

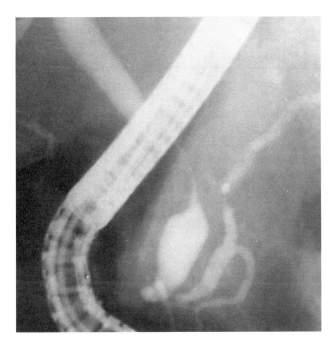

FIG. 30-16. ERCP in a patient with carcinoma of the head of the pancreas. Compression of both the common bile duct and the pancreatic duct by the cancer (the double-duct sign) is seen.

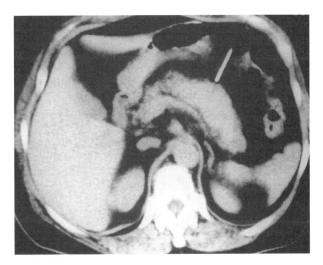

FIG. 30-17. CT scan in a patient with carcinoma of the body of the pancreas. A fine needle has been inserted into the tumor to obtain cells for cytologic examination. In this patient, cytologic proof of the diagnosis was obtained, avoiding the need for operation.

but is not performed routinely in the absence of specific indications.

Percutaneous Transhepatic Cholangiography. Percutaneous transhepatic cholangiography (PTC) permits visualization of the proximal biliary tree in patients with ductal obstruction who cannot be studied from below with ERCP. Although PTC is the preferred method for proximal bile duct tumors (e.g., Klatskin tumors), ERCP provides more diagnostic information and is better for periampullary lesions.

Angiography. This study is not performed for diagnosis but may provide information about resectability of the cancer. Rarely, complete occlusion of the celiac, hepatic, and/or superior mesenteric arteries or the portal vein suggests that the lesion is unresectable. More commonly, distortion of the vessels is seen, which is more difficult to interpret. The sensitivity and specificity of angiography to determine resectability are each 70 percent. Preoperative recognition of such vascular anomalies as a right hepatic artery arising from the superior mesenteric artery (25 percent of patients) can facilitate their preservation at surgery. Nevertheless, such anomalies also can be determined at the time of operation. Since modern spiral CT provides similar information, most surgeons do not routinely perform angiography.

Summary. An *algorithm* for the *management* of the patient with suspected cancer is presented in Fig. 30-18. Spiral CT scan provides the best overall initial assessment and may be the only test required. If the history and clinical picture suggest pancreatic cancer and CT reveals a mass in the head of the pancreas without evidence of unresectability, laparotomy may be undertaken without additional studies. Exploration provides the best means of confirming resectability; and even if resection is not possible, most patients will benefit from biliary and gastric bypass. If the CT suggests hepatic or peritoneal metastases or vascular invasion that precludes resection, percutaneous FNA may be appropriate if a positive biopsy will avoid an operation. If the biopsy

is negative, laparoscopy should be the next step. In some patients with a general medical condition that makes operation too risky, no further evaluation may be necessary. Age alone is not a contraindication to major pancreatic resection. Endoscopically placed biliary stents effectively relieve biliary obstruction and are an alternative to surgical biliary bypass in patients who do not undergo operation.

If the mass involves the body and tail of the gland, usually there is evidence of metastatic disease or local spread. Since these patients seldom benefit from palliative operations, percutaneous FNA is often indicated to provide a tissue diagnosis before initiating adjuvant therapy. Occasionally, these tumors appear resectable or the biopsy is negative or equivocal. In these cases, laparoscopy for further assessment may be reasonable. The patient should undergo laparotomy under the same anesthetic if the attempted biopsy is unsuccessful or the lesion appears resectable.

If the patient with suspected pancreatic cancer has a normal or nondiagnostic CT, ERCP is indicated. If both the CT and ERCP are normal, pancreatic cancer is an extremely unlikely cause of the symptoms that are being evaluated.

Differential Diagnosis. The other periampullary neoplasms (carcinoma of the ampulla of Vater, distal common bile duct, or duodenum) also may present with abdominal pain, weight loss, and obstructive jaundice. While the preoperative studies may suggest the correct diagnosis, sometimes this is possible only at operation. Occasionally it is not apparent even at that time, and the pathologist may have to determine the true origin of the neoplasm. This element of diagnostic uncertainty is acceptable because the treatment (pancreaticoduodenectomy) is the same for each of these lesions. Chronic pancreatitis also can be confused with pancreatic cancer, and it may be impossible to distinguish between the two even at operation. Nevertheless, pancreaticoduodenectomy is an acceptable treatment for this as well.

Treatment. Pancreatic resection for pancreatic cancer is appropriate only if all evidence of gross tumor can be removed with a standard resection, i.e., if cure is considered possible. Resection for palliation is not commonly done. In the absence of evidence of distant metastases (e.g., to the liver, peritoneal surfaces, distant lymph nodes), resectability usually depends on whether the tumor has grown to involve adjacent major vascular structures. These structures are the superior mesenteric and portal veins and the superior mesenteric and hepatic arteries. The vena cava also may be involved. Because the pancreas is so close to the portal vein and superior mesenteric vessels, and because of the propensity of pancreatic cancer to spread early to adjacent structures, only about 20 percent of tumors of the head are resectable at the time of exploration. Fewer than 5 percent of tumors of the body and tail can be removed.

In some patients, the diagnosis has already been determined preoperatively by FNA or other technique. If this is not the case, most surgeons will try to establish a tissue diagnosis at an early stage of the operation. When the cancer has extended to the surface of the gland, a simple "shave" biopsy of the lesion is safe and reliable. If the lesion is located deep within the pancreas, a needle biopsy or FNA is preferred. For cancers in the head of the pancreas, the needle is often inserted into the gland through the duodenum so that if a pancreatic fistula develops, it will drain into the bowel rather than leak into the peritoneal

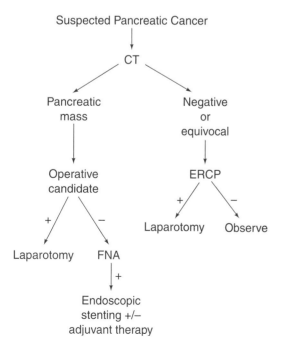

FIG. 30-18. *Algorithm for the workup of patient with suspected pancreatic cancer.*

cavity. Although these techniques are accurate and reasonably safe, they are often inconclusive with the small deep-seated lesions that are most likely to be cured by resection. This occurs because the tumor is surrounded by a zone of chronic inflammation and may be missed altogether when the needle is inserted. Thus most experienced pancreatic surgeons are willing to perform a pancreaticoduodenectomy on the basis of clinical inferences, drawn preoperatively and at operation, that suggest the diagnosis of cancer. Biopsy proof is not required.

Pancreaticoduodenectomy (Whipple Resection). This is the most commonly performed operation for carcinoma of the pancreatic head (see Fig. 30-12). It includes resection of the distal stomach, gallbladder, common bile duct, head of the pancreas, duodenum, proximal jejunum, and regional lymphatics. Truncal vagotomy used to be done to reduce the risk of marginal ulceration, but it is done infrequently today. Instead, many patients are managed with acid antisecretory agents. Restoration of gastrointestinal continuity requires pancreaticojejunostomy, choledochojejunostomy, and gastrojejunostomy. The operative mortality rate in expert hands is less than 5 percent. When death occurs, it is most often due to complications such as postoperative pancreatic or biliary fistula, hemorrhage, and infection.

Pylorus Preservation. About a third of all pancreatic surgeons in the United States now perform a modification of the Whipple procedure in which the stomach and pylorus are preserved (see Fig. 30-13). This operation is preferred by some because it is believed that it avoids the undesirable nutritional sequelae (i.e., weight loss, dumping syndrome, diarrhea) that may follow the standard Whipple procedure. Although the lymphatic dissection is less radical than with the standard operation, there is no evidence as yet that it is associated with a lower survival rate.

In the United States, the 5-year survival rate in all patients who have undergone pancreatic resection for pancreatic cancer is approximately 10 percent. In those patients without lymph node involvement, the 5-year survival rate is about 35 percent.

Total Pancreatectomy. A number of more extensive procedures have been proposed to improve the cure rates associated with the Whipple operation. To date, none has proved more effective. One of the proposed procedures is *total pancreatectomy*. The rationale for this procedure included the observation that in 30 to 40 percent of pancreatic cancer patients, the tumor was multicentric and would not be removed completely by a Whipple resection. However, most series of total pancreatectomy showed no evidence of increased survival, and recent studies have suggested that concerns regarding multifocal disease were unwarranted. However, it may still be appropriate when tumor is present at the planned site of transection of the pancreas or when the gland is too soft to permit a satisfactory anastomosis to the jejunum.

Extended Whipple Resections. These operations involve wider soft tissue and lymph node dissections than the standard Whipple and include resections of the superior mesenteric vessels and portal vein when they are involved with tumor. Some retrospective data have suggested a better outcome with this aggressive approach. Nevertheless, these operations are best done within the framework of an experimental protocol, since the morbidity is greater and increased efficacy has not been proven.

Palliative Operations. Surgical palliation in patients with cancer of the head of the pancreas is directed toward relief of obstructive jaundice, gastric outlet obstruction, and pain. Patients with body and tail lesions are less likely to have jaundice or duodenal obstruction, but pain is often significant. Nonoperative techniques for pain relief are preferred.

At some time in the course of the disease, obstructive jaundice develops in about 70 percent of patients with pancreatic cancer. Cholecystojejunostomy and choledochojejunostomy are both safe and are the procedures of choice to relieve the biliary obstruction (Fig. 30-19). If the gallbladder is chosen for the anastomosis, the surgeon must be certain that the cystic duct is patent and enters the common bile duct away from the tumor. An intraoperative cholangiogram may be necessary to confirm this. Roux-en-Y jejunostomy theoretically is better than simple loop reconstruction because it prevents reflux of intestinal contents into the biliary tree and secondary cholangitis. Since most of these patients die within 7 or 8 months, this is rarely a concern, and the simpler loop reconstruction is usually done. Jaundice is relieved in 85 to 90 percent of patients. When it is not, it is usually because of irreversible hepatic parenchymal damage from high bilirubin levels and long-standing obstruction.

For patients in poor general medical condition or in whom the tumor is known to be unresectable, nonoperative palliation of obstructive jaundice is preferred. Percutaneous or endoscopically placed plastic biliary stents are each effective, but the latter are better accepted by patients. The major problem with either technique is stent occlusion, associated with recurrent jaundice and sepsis. This requires stent replacement every 3 to 4 months in up to two-thirds of patients. Metal stents have a larger diameter and may last longer.

About one-third of patients with cancer of the head of the pancreas eventually develop gastric outlet obstruction, which is treated effectively by a gastrojejunostomy (Fig. 30-20). If obstruction is not present at the time of initial exploration and biliary bypass, there is some debate about whether gastrojejunostomy should be done prophylactically. Because it is difficult to predict which patients will obstruct later in the course of their disease, and it does not appear to increase the operative morbidity or mortality rates, many surgeons do perform gastrojejunostomy in patients who are expected to survive more than a few months.

Pain is a symptom in up to 80 percent of patients with pancreatic cancer, and its severity and persistence correlate well with the stage of the disease. This problem is managed best by chemical destruction of the celiac nerves, achieved by percutaneous injection of 50% ethanol into the region of the ganglia under CT guidance. This also can be done at operation. Adequate pain relief is possible in up to 80 percent of patients, although it often recurs. Celiac injection can be repeated if needed.

Adjuvant Therapy. Neither radiation nor chemotherapy given singly is effective. Radiotherapy combined with 5-fluorouracil given as a radiosensitizer has been shown to increase survival in both patients with resectable and those with unresectable disease.

Prognosis. Most patients with pancreatic cancer die within 1 year of the time that the diagnosis is made (Table 30-12). In patients with carcinoma of the head of the pancreas who have undergone resection, prognosis is related to whether lymph node metastases have already occurred. In patients with positive nodes, the 5-year survival rate is less than 10 percent; in those patients without nodal involvement, the 5-year survival rate is approximately 35 percent.

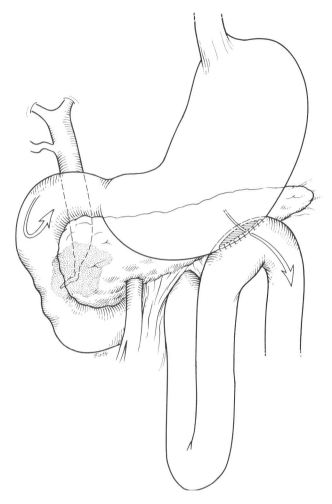

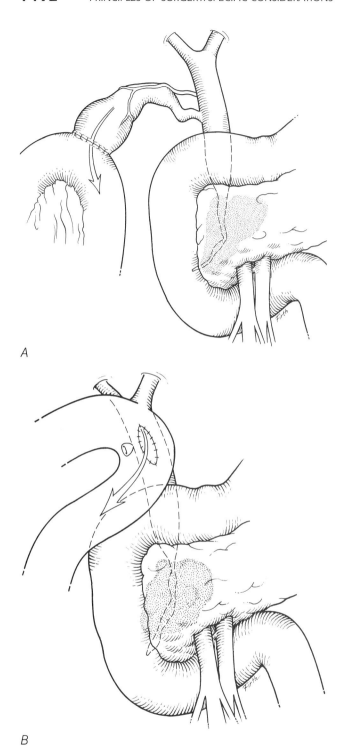

FIG. 30-20. *Gastric contents are unable to pass through the duodenum, which is narrowed and distorted by the tumor. A gastrojejunostomy bypasses this obstruction.*

sent in almost all patients because of the location of the lesion near the bile duct. Jaundice may fluctuate because as pieces of the tumor slough into the duodenal lumen, the degree of obstruction of the bile duct varies. The stools often contain occult blood from the ulcerating neoplasm. The lesion is visible by endoscopy if it extends into the duodenal lumen, and a tissue diagnosis can be obtained easily by biopsy. If the neoplasm resides entirely within the ampulla, the diagnosis of ampullary neoplasm may

FIG. 30-19. *The tumor obstructs the intrapancreatic portion of the common bile duct. The obstruction may be bypassed by (A) a cholecystojejunostomy or (B) a choledochojejunostomy.*

Carcinoma of the Ampulla of Vater

About 10 percent of periampullary cancers arise from the ampulla of Vater. These tumors produce symptoms that are similar to those seen in pancreatic cancer, although weight loss and pain are less prominent. Obstructive jaundice occurs early and is pre-

Table 30-12
Prognosis of Periampullary Tumors

Site	5-Year Survival Rate, %
Pancreas	10
Ampulla of Vater	35
Duodenum	30
Bile duct	15
After pancreaticoduodenectomy, the 5-year survival rate for pancreatic cancer without lymph node metastases is 35%. Rates as high as 50% have been reported.	

not be possible. It may be suspected if the ERCP or CT scan suggests that the obstruction is at the most distal point in the bile duct. Sometimes it may not be possible to distinguish an ampullary tumor from one that arises from the head of the pancreas, even at the time of operation. Because these tumors grow more slowly and tend to remain localized longer than pancreatic cancers, many more are resectable for cure. The treatment consists of pancreaticoduodenectomy, and the 5-year survival rate is 35 to 40 percent. Occasionally, in patients who are not candidates for the Whipple resection, local excision of the tumor through a duodenotomy may be indicated.

Cystic Neoplasms

Approximately 90 percent of primary malignant neoplasms of the nonendocrine pancreas are carcinomas of duct cell origin. Several types of cystic neoplasms also occur that may be confused with pseudocysts.

Papillary-cystic neoplasm of the pancreas is a rare lesion that occurs almost exclusively in women under 25 years of age. It is often large and may present as a hemorrhagic cystic tumor in the body or tail of the gland. Although it can be locally invasive, metastases are unusual, and resection is generally curative. *Serous (microcystic) cystadenomas* are the most common benign neoplasm of the exocrine pancreas, and they occur with equal distribution throughout the gland. Histologically, they appear as numerous, small cysts lined by flattened cuboidal epithelial cells. The cell cytoplasm contains glycogen but no mucin. The cystic spaces are filled with a serous material. The tumor has been likened to the cut surface of the lung, with multiple epithelium-lined cystic spaces analogous to alveoli. *Mucinous cystadenomas* are premalignant lesions that often evolve into *cystadenocarcinomas,* which are frankly malignant tumors. These are most common in the body or tail of the pancreas and are often quite large (e.g., 10 to 20 cm) when diagnosed. Most patients are women (8:1). The cellular lining consists of mucin-producing columnar epithelial cells. They take the form of papillary projections into the lumen of the cyst, giving it an irregular appearance.

Manifestations. The most common symptom of any of these tumors is vague abdominal discomfort. Obstructive jaundice occurs in fewer than 10 percent of patients. Anorexia, weight loss, and weakness may occur, particularly with cystadenocarcinoma. Radiographic studies may reveal calcification within the cyst (at least 10 percent of patients), which is an uncommon finding with pseudocysts. Barium studies of the stomach and duodenum may reveal displacement by the tumor mass. Angiography characteristically reveals hypervascularity, and arteriovenous shunting is frequently observed. The hypervascularity differentiates these cystic tumors from pseudocysts and the usual type of ductal adenocarcinoma, both of which are hypovascular. US and CT demonstrate multicystic tumors, sometimes with solid components.

Treatment. Surgery is usually indicated because of the concern that a cyst may be malignant and to manage symptoms that may be present. At operation, the diagnosis of malignancy may be difficult. Benign serous cystadenomas typically have a honeycombed appearance on cut section. They may contain hundreds of small cystic spaces that vary in diameter from a few millimeters to a centimeter. These lesions apparently have no malignant potential, but they should be excised if it can be done safely. They should *not* be drained internally. Both the benign and malignant neoplasms may be unilocular or multilocular. The most characteristic feature of the malignant cystadenocarcinoma is the viscid mucinous fluid it contains. This fluid has the gross appearance of raw egg white and can be strung like egg white for 6 to 12 in. between the instrument and the tumor. Examination of a frozen section is helpful but is not reliable in distinguishing benign from malignant stages unless it shows frank carcinoma or papillary projections, which are almost synonymous with malignancy. Whether or not overt malignancy is present, these macrocystic lesions should be excised, since there is a high likelihood that they will become malignant. During the resection of neoplastic cysts, efforts should be made to remove the tumor intact (rupture may disseminate cells). In order to be certain of the diagnosis in patients with presumed pseudocysts, a frozen-section diagnosis should always be obtained on a portion of the cyst wall before proceeding with internal drainage.

Prognosis. Cystadenocarcinomas have a better prognosis than the usual adenocarcinomas of the pancreas. Although precise statistics are unavailable because of the rarity of the lesions, resection of apparently localized tumors probably cures about two-thirds of patients.

Islet Cell Neoplasms

Insulinoma

Insulinoma arises from the beta cells and is the most common islet cell neoplasm. It produces insulin, and the symptoms are all related to hypoglycemia. The tumors may occur at any age and are found equally distributed throughout the pancreas. About 80 percent are solitary and benign, and about 40 percent are less than 1 cm in diameter. Fifteen percent are malignant, and metastases are usually evident at the time of diagnosis. Fewer than 5 percent of insulinomas are associated with the multiple endocrine adenopathies (MEA I) syndrome; these are usually multiple and are distributed throughout the pancreas.

Clinical Manifestations. Symptoms related to cerebral glucose deprivation include bizarre behavior, memory lapse, and unconsciousness. Some patients have been mistakenly diagnosed with psychiatric or neurologic illness. Symptoms related to sympathetic discharge include palpitations, nervousness, sweating, and tachycardia. Many patients gain significant weight because symptoms are produced by fasting; consequently, they eat excessively to avoid this. The classic diagnostic criteria (*Whipple's triad*) are usually present. These include (1) hypoglycemic symptoms produced by fasting, (2) blood glucose concentration below 50 mg/dL during symptomatic episodes, and (3) relief of the symptoms during intravenous administration of glucose.

Diagnostic Studies. The most useful diagnostic test, and the one indicated in most patients, is the demonstration of fasting hypoglycemia in the face of inappropriately high levels of insulin in the serum. The patient is fasted, and blood samples are obtained every 6 h for blood glucose and insulin measurements. The fast is continued until hypoglycemia or symptoms appear or for a maximum of 72 h. By 48 h, over 95 percent of the tumors have been diagnosed. If hypoglycemia has not developed after 70 h, the patient should be exercised for the final 2 h. Although the insulin levels are not always elevated in patients with insulinoma, they will be high relative to the blood glucose concentration. A ratio of plasma insulin to glucose greater than 0.3 is diagnostic. Proinsulin, which constitutes more than 25 percent of total insulin in about 85 percent of patients with islet cell tumors, also should be measured. Very high proinsulin levels (>50 percent) suggest that the insulinoma is malignant.

Provocative tests using a variety of drugs that stimulate the release of insulin (e.g., tolbutamide, leucine, arginine) have been used in some patients, but they are diagnostic in only 50 percent of patients and are rarely indicated. A calcium infusion provocative test also may be of value.

Differential Diagnosis. Fasting hypoglycemia occurs with some nonpancreatic tumors as well, and the clinical picture may be identical with that seen with insulinoma. Plasma insulin levels are normal, however. In most cases, the nonpancreatic tumors are large and are readily detected with various diagnostic studies. The majority are of mesenchymal origin (e.g., hemangiopericytoma, fibrosarcoma) and are located in the abdomen or thorax, although hepatoma, adrenocortical carcinoma, and a number of other lesions also can produce hypoglycemia. The principal mechanisms by which these tumors produce hypoglycemia are (1) secretion by the tumor of somatomedins (insulin-like peptides that mediate the effects of growth hormone), which can be measured by specific radioimmunoassay, and (2) inhibition of gluconeogenesis or glycogenolysis. Surreptitious self-administration of insulin is also seen, most often by individuals who have access to insulin in their job. Insulin antibodies are usually detectable in the serum if these individuals have been taking injections for at least 2 months. Circulating C-peptide levels are normal in these patients but usually are elevated in patients with insulinoma.

Treatment. Surgery should be undertaken promptly, since the tumor may be malignant and, with repeated attacks of hypoglycemia, permanent cerebral damage may occur.

Surgical Therapy. Because 10 to 20 percent of the tumors are not easily identified at operation, preoperative localization studies are helpful. CT scans are usually obtained, but the majority of lesions are not seen because of their small size. Selective angiography demonstrates the tumor in about 50 percent of patients. Percutaneous transhepatic venous catheterization allows sampling of blood draining from the pancreas at multiple sites along the splenic and portal veins. Insulin is measured in the samples, and the point where the insulin concentration rises sharply indicates the location of the tumor. If patients are receiving diazoxide, it should be discontinued for at least a week prior to operation because of the reported association with hypotension on induction of anesthesia.

At operation, the entire pancreas must be fully mobilized and carefully palpated to find the tumor. Intraoperative US also should be done. If the tumor is found, it should be enucleated if it is superficial. If it is deeply situated, it should be removed as part of a partial pancreatectomy. Tumors in the head of the gland can nearly always be enucleated, so a pancreaticoduodenectomy is not often indicated. If the tumor cannot be found, and the results of venous sampling studies suggest its location, that portion of the pancreas should be resected. Under these circumstances, a Whipple resection may be appropriate if these studies indicate that the tumor is in the head of the gland. If no such localizing information is available, it is common practice to remove the distal half of the pancreas and have a pathologist

slice the specimen into thin sections to look for the tumor. If it is found, the operation is concluded. If not, more is removed until an 80 percent distal pancreatectomy has been done. Since the tumors are evenly distributed, this confers an 80 percent probability of cure.

For islet cell hyperplasia, nesidioblastosis, or multiple benign adenomas, distal subtotal pancreatectomy is indicated to sufficiently decrease insulin levels so that medical management can be more effective. For malignant insulinomas, both resection of the primary tumor and debulking of metastases are warranted if technically feasible and safe.

Medical Therapy. Frequent feedings supplemented with a slowly absorbed form of carbohydrate such as cornstarch may be helpful, but usually patients require treatment with diazoxide, which suppresses the release of insulin. Fewer than two-thirds of patients are controlled successfully with this agent, and many develop significant adverse reactions that include hirsutism and salt and water retention. For incurable islet cell tumors, streptozocin appears to increase survival, with 60 percent of patients living an additional 2 years. Toxicity of the drug is considerable, however, so streptozocin is not used routinely as an adjuvant to surgical therapy.

Gastrinoma (Zollinger-Ellison Syndrome)

The principal manifestations of the Zollinger-Ellison syndrome are due to gastric acid hypersecretion caused by excessive gastrin production by the tumor. Although the normal pancreas does not contain gastrin-producing cells, most gastrinomas arise in the pancreas. The others are found chiefly in the duodenum. In the pancreas, about 60 percent of gastrinomas are non-beta islet cell carcinomas, 25 percent are solitary adenomas, and 10 percent are microadenomas or hyperplasia. About 5 percent of gastrinomas occur in the first or second part of the duodenum. One-quarter of gastrinomas are associated with the multiple endocrine neoplasia type I (MEN I) syndrome, in which case the tumors are usually multiple and benign. Those without MEN I (sporadic gastrinomas) are more often single and malignant. The diagnosis of malignancy requires the histologic demonstration of blood vessel invasion or the finding of metastatic disease, since the cellular characteristics of benign and malignant lesions are similar. Even when malignancy is present, the tumors are often slow-growing and compatible with a long survival, however. Thus the principal threat to life is the severe peptic ulcer diathesis that the hypergastrinemia provokes, and this is the main focus of therapy.

Clinical Manifestations. Symptoms of gastrinoma are chiefly those of gastric acid hypersecretion: severe, refractory peptic ulcer disease and, often, diarrhea. The diarrhea results from fat malabsorption, since the excessive quantities of gastric acid destroy pancreatic lipase. In addition, the acid damages the small bowel mucosa, and the intestine is overwhelmed with large volumes of gastric and pancreatic secretions. About 5 percent of patients present with diarrhea alone. The diagnosis should be suspected when (1) patients present with ulcer disease that is refractory to the usual forms of acid antisecretory therapy (antacids and H_2-receptor antagonists), (2) patients present with multiple ulcers or ulcers in unusual locations (e.g., third-fourth portion of duodenum, proximal jejunum), and (3) ulcers recur after surgical procedures that would normally cure the ulcer diathesis.

Diagnostic Studies. The diagnosis of gastrinoma requires the demonstration of fasting hypergastrinemia (>200 pg/mL of blood) in the face of gastric acid hypersecretion (basal acid output >15 mEq/h with an intact stomach or >5 mEq/h after ulcer surgery). Most patients with gastrinoma have serum gastrin values that exceed 500 pg/mL, and some are as high as 10,000 pg/mL. When the serum gastrin level is in the range 200 to 500 pg/mL, however, a secretin provocative test is usually done to confirm the diagnosis. Following 2 units/kg secretin (bolus, I.V.), a rise in the serum gastrin level of 200 pg/mL within 15 min or a doubling of the fasting gastrin level is diagnostic. An upper gastrointestinal series will reveal the ulcers, and in the stomach, prominent rugal folds and excessive luminal secretions are often seen. The duodenum and small bowel may be hyperactive, with edema in the bowel wall and accelerated transit time. A CT scan should be done in all patients, and it often shows the tumor. If not, angiography with portal venous sampling to find "hot spots" of gastrin may be helpful.

Differential Diagnosis. The differential diagnosis of gastrinoma includes gastric outlet obstruction, retained antrum after a Billroth II gastrectomy, and antral G cell hyperplasia, all of which are characterized by hypergastrinemia and acid hypersecretion. In these conditions, the secretin test is negative.

Treatment. *Medical Treatment.* The medical treatment of gastrinoma is directed at control of the acid hypersecretion. Although H$_2$-blocking agents (cimetidine, ranitidine) may be effective, because of its long duration of action, omeprazole (a proton pump blocker) is the drug of choice. The dose should be adjusted to keep the H$^+$ output less than 5 mEq during the hour preceding the next dose. Over 90 percent of patients are adequately controlled in this fashion. In patients with malignant gastrinoma, a combination of streptozocin and fluorouracil, with or without doxorubicin, may be effective.

Surgical Treatment. All patients with sporadic gastrinoma should undergo surgical exploration, unless there is evidence of extensive metastatic disease. Because patients with gastrinoma and MEN I syndrome have multiple small pancreatic tumors that cannot all be resected, surgery is generally not indicated (Fig. 30-21).

At operation, if the tumor is found in the pancreas, it should be enucleated if possible. If not, a distal pancreatectomy may be required. Pancreaticoduodenectomy is rarely indicated. Ninety percent of the tumors are found in the triangle defined by the junction of the cystic and common bile ducts, the junction of the second and third portions of the duodenum, and the junction of the neck and the body of the pancreas ("gastrinoma triangle"). US may be useful to detect small lesions deep within the substance of the gland. Intraoperative endoscopy to transilluminate the duodenal wall may help to find duodenal tumors that otherwise would escape attention. These tumors are often very small. Resection of lymph nodes that contain gastrinoma appears to have cured some patients of the syndrome, with serum gastrin concentrations returning to normal. In about a third of patients, the tumor is never identified at operation.

Total gastrectomy should be done in patients whose ulcer disease is refractory to medical therapy and who are unable to undergo resection of the tumor because of multiple hepatic metastases or the MEN I syndrome.

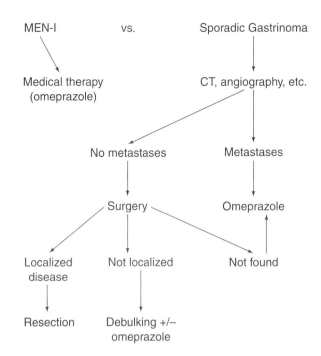

FIG. 30-21. *Algorithm for the management of a patient with gastrinoma.*

VIPoma (Verner-Morrison Syndrome; WDHA Syndrome: Watery Diarrhea, Hypokalemia, and Achlorhydria; Pancreatic Cholera)

Eighty to ninety percent of cases of WDHA syndrome are caused by an islet cell tumor of the pancreas that secretes VIP. The rest are associated with tumors in extrapancreatic sites such as the retroperitoneal sympathetic chain and the adrenal medulla.

Clinical Manifestations. The syndrome is characterized by a profuse watery diarrhea that contains large quantities of potassium, resulting hypokalemia (often 2 to 3 mEq/L), and profound weakness. Some gastric acid secretion is present in about half the patients; in the rest it is absent. Stool volume can be as great as 10 L/day but averages about 5 L/day during acute episodes. It contains over 300 mEq potassium (20 to 25 times normal) and resembles dilute tea. The diarrhea is "secretory" in nature; it persists during fasting and does not respond to antidiarrheal agents. Severe metabolic acidosis is common from loss of bicarbonate in the stool. Many patients are hypercalcemic, perhaps because the tumor also secretes a parathormone-like substance. Abnormal glucose tolerance may be the result of hypokalemia and altered sensitivity to insulin. Flushing is a prominent feature in about 15 percent of patients, usually in association with a bout of diarrhea. Up to 50 percent of the pancreatic tumors are malignant, and 75 percent of those have already metastasized by the time of diagnosis.

Diagnostic Studies. Patients with severe diarrhea must be studied carefully before attributing the cause to VIPoma. Chronic laxative abuse is the most common explanation. The specific diagnosis requires the demonstration of elevated fasting plasma VIP concentration by radioimmunoassay; plasma VIP levels are normal in other diarrheal states. Plasma PP and prostaglandin levels also should be measured, since some people with the syndrome have had elevations in the level of these substances, while VIP levels were normal. CT scan and then angiography should be used to localize the tumor. Transhepatic portal and splenic venous sampling also may be helpful.

Treatment. The immediate goal of management is the correction of dehydration and electrolyte abnormalities, especially hypokalemia. Once the diagnosis is suspected, a trial of somatostatin is indicated. This should control the diarrhea during the preoperative preparation and performance of the diagnostic studies. At operation, the tumor should be resected, and if metastases are present, they should be debulked. Plasma VIP concentrations should return to normal if all the tumor has been removed. If no pancreatic tumor is identified, the adrenal glands and sympathetic chains should be explored. If no tumor is found anywhere, a distal 80 percent pancreatectomy should be performed. In some patients with diffuse islet cell hyperplasia, symptoms have improved with this strategy.

In patients with inoperable or metastatic malignant tumors in whom complete resection is not possible, streptozocin alone or in combination with 5-fluorouracil may be effective. Almost all tumors respond initially, and a few long-term remissions have been noted. Renal function must be monitored carefully when streptozocin is used; selective arterial administration of the drug is preferred when renal function is impaired. In patients for whom no definitive therapy is possible, symptomatic relief has been reported with several agents, including high-dose steroids, trifluoperazine, and somatostatin. The tumors appear to be radioresistant.

Patients with benign tumors are cured by surgical excision. The average survival rate for patients with malignant tumors is approximately 1 year.

Glucagonoma

These tumors arise from α_2 cells in the islets. They produce a distinctive syndrome consisting of a migratory necrolytic dermatitis usually involving the legs and perineum, weight loss, stomatitis, hypoaminoacidemia, anemia, and mild diabetes mellitus. Visual scotomata may occur. An increased tendency to venous thrombosis and pulmonary emboli also has been reported. The condition is more common in women, and the age range is 20 to 70 years. The diagnosis is confirmed by demonstrating elevated plasma glucagon levels. The tumor should be localized with CT scans and arteriography, if necessary. About 25 percent of glucagonomas are benign. The majority are malignant and have metastasized by the time of diagnosis, however. The most common sites are the liver, lymph nodes, adrenal gland, or vertebrae. A few cases of the syndrome have been due to islet cell hyperplasia.

Treatment. Surgical excision of the primary tumor and debulking of metastases are indicated. Oral zinc supplements may improve the dermatitis. Somatostatin has been reported to return serum glucagon and amino acid levels to normal, clear the rash, and promote weight gain. Streptozocin and dacarbazine are the most effective chemotherapeutic agents.

Somatostatinoma

Somatostatin-producing tumors of the islet cells are characterized by mild diabetes mellitus, malabsorption and diarrhea, and dilatation of the gallbladder, often with cholelithiasis.

Weight loss also may be prominent. Most of the tumors are located in the head of the pancreas and are malignant, with metastases to the liver at the time of exploration. CT scan usually shows a mass in the pancreas, with evidence of spread to the liver. The plasma levels of somatostatin are elevated, confirming the diagnosis.

The clinical manifestations are the result of the physiologic actions of the peptide. Inhibition of insulin release produces the diabetic state. Because glucagon release is also suppressed, the diabetes is easy to control. Cholelithiasis results from inhibition of gallbladder motility. Decreased biliary and pancreatic secretions probably cause the malabsorption.

Surgery may be indicated if the disease appears to be localized. More often, chemotherapy with streptozocin, dacarbazine, doxorubicin, etc. is the only treatment possible.

Miscellaneous Neoplasms

Because the pancreatic islets are part of the APUD (*a*mine *p*recursor *u*ptake and *d*ecarboxylation) system, they retain the potential to produce a variety of neoplasms with multiple secretory products. For example, MEN I syndrome (Werner's syndrome) is a syndrome complex associated with tumors or hyperplasia in two or more of the endocrine glands. It involves the pancreas (81 percent), parathyroid (87 percent), pituitary (65 percent), and less frequently, the adrenal cortex (38 percent) and thyroid glands (19 percent). When the pancreas is involved, it usually becomes evident clinically later than does the parathyroid disorder (hyperparathyroidism is diagnosed in most patients before 40 years of age). In the pancreas, gastrinomas are most common, followed by insulinomas. Less often, the pancreatic tumors may secrete VIP, glucagon, pancreatic polypeptide, calcitonin, or 5-hydroxytryptophan (carcinoid-islet cell tumor). MEN I syndrome is present in about 25 percent of patients with gastrinoma and about 4 percent of all patients with insulinoma. Whatever the predominant cell type, the tumors are usually multicentric.

TRAUMA

Because of its protected retroperitoneal position, pancreatic injury only occurs with deep penetrating wounds or blunt trauma of significant force. Injury to the pancreas must be considered, however, in all patients who sustain injury to the upper abdomen. The diagnostic approach varies with the mechanism of injury. With penetrating trauma, almost all patients are operated on, and the diagnosis of pancreatic injury is made at the time of exploration. The diagnosis of blunt injury requires a high degree of clinical suspicion, since there may be few symptoms during the initial phases of management. In the first several days, the majority of patients will eventually develop epigastric and/or back pain, nausea, vomiting, ileus, and tenderness to abdominal palpation. Although the serum amylase concentration may be normal early, it eventually becomes elevated in 80 percent of patients. An elevated amylase level by itself is generally not an indication for surgical exploration, however. The decision to operate should be supported by evidence from physical examination or CT scan. CT may show fluid in the area of the pancreas or pancreatic ductal or parenchymal disruption. Because significant pancreatic injury may be missed by CT, it should be used primarily in patients in whom there is suspicion of injury, and operation is planned only if test results are positive. Diagnostic peritoneal lavage may be valuable, since many patients with pancreatic injury also have associated visceral injury that will result in a positive lavage.

Minor contusions and lacerations of the pancreas without evidence of ductal injury require only the control of hemorrhage and external drainage. Deeper lacerations or crush injuries with ductal injury and/or devitalization of the gland are best managed by distal resection of the injured gland and external drainage. Injuries to the head of the gland with significant damage to the duodenum and adjacent structures occasionally require a pancreaticoduodenectomy. However, even the majority of injuries to this area can be managed more conservatively.

Pancreatic trauma is associated with significant morbidity (e.g., pancreatic fistula in 10 percent and infection) and a mortality rate of about 20 percent. Most deaths are due to massive hemorrhage from erosion of adjacent vessels.

Bibliography

Anatomy

Skandalakis JKE, Gray SW, et al: Surgical anatomy of the pancreas, in Howard JM, Jordan GL, Reber HA (eds): *Surgical Diseases of the Pancreas.* Philadelphia, Lea & Febiger, 1987, pp 11-36.

Physiology

Adler G, Nelson DK, et al: Neurohumoral control of human pancreatic exocrine secretion. *Pancreas* 10:1, 1995.

Doty JE, Fink AS, Meyer JH: Alterations in digestive function caused by pancreatic disease. *Surg Clin North Am* 69:447, 1989.

Go VLW, DiMagno EP, et al (eds): *The Pancreas: Biology, Pathobiology, and Diseases,* 2d ed. New York, Raven Press, 1993, p 1176.

Schonfeld JV, Goebell H, Muller MK: The islet-acinar axis of the pancreas. *Int J Pancreatol* 16:131, 1994.

Acute Pancreatitis

Bassi C: Infected pancreatic necrosis. *Int J Pancreatol* 16:1, 1994.

Bradley EL III: Open packing for infected pancreatic necrosis, in Beger HG, Buchler M, Maltfertheiner P (eds): *Standards in Pancreatic Surgery.* Berlin, Springer, 1993, pp 220-232.

Bradley EL III, Allen K: A prospective longitudinal study of observation versus surgical intervention in the management of necrotizing pancreatitis. *Am J Surg* 161:19, 1991.

Buchler M, Uhl W, et al: Necrotizing pancreatitis: necrosectomy and closed continuous lavage of the lesser sac: The Ulm experience, in Beger HG, Buchler M, Maltfertheiner P (eds): *Standards in Pancreatic Surgery.* Berlin, Springer, 1993, pp 191-202.

Carr-Locke DL: Acute gallstone pancreatitis and endoscopic therapy (review). *Endoscopy* 22:180, 1990.

Fan ST, Lai ECS: Early treatment of acute biliary pancreatitis by endoscopic papillotomy. *N Engl J Med* 328:228, 1993.

Freeny PC: Incremental dynamic bolus computed tomography of acute pancreatitis. *Int J Pancreatol* 13:147, 1993.

Heath DI, Cruickshank A, et al: Role of interleukin-6 in mediating the acute phase protein response and potential as an early means of severity assessment in acute pancreatitis. *Gut* 34:41, 1993.

Isenmann R, Buchler MW, et al: Antibiotics in acute pancreatitis. *Dig Surg* 13:365, 1996.

Kloppel G, Maillet B: Pathology of acute and chronic pancreatitis. *Pancreas* 8:659, 1993.

Lerch MM, Adler G: Experimental animal models of acute pancreatitis. *Int J Pancreatol* 15:159, 1994.

McFadden DW, Reber HA: Indications for surgery in severe pancreatitis: State of the art. *Int J Pancreatol* 15:83, 1994.

Maltfertheiner P, Dominguez-Munoz JE: Prognostic factors in acute pancreatitis. *Int J Pancreatol* 14:1, 1993.

Parenti DM, Steinberg W, Kang P: Infectious causes of acute pancreatitis. *Pancreas* 13:356, 1994.

Pederzoli P, Bassi C, et al: A randomized multicenter clinical trial of antibiotic prophylaxis of septic complications in acute necrotizing pancreatitis with imipenem. *Surg Gynecol Obstet* 176:480, 1993.

Sherman S, Lehman GA. ERCP and endoscopic sphincterotomy-induced pancreatitis. *Pancreas* 6:350, 1991.

Steer ML: Classification and pathogenesis of pancreatitis. *Surg Clin North Am* 69:467, 1989.

Steer ML: How and where does acute pancreatitis begin? *Arch Surg* 127:1350, 1992.

Steinberg WM: Predictors of severity of acute pancreatitis. *Gastroenterol Clin North Am* 19:849, 1990.

Warshaw AL, Simeone JF, et al: Evaluation and treatment of the dominant dorsal duct syndrome (pancreas divisum redefined). *Am J Surg* 159:59, 1990.

Whitcomb DC, Gorry MC, et al: Hereditary pancreatitis is caused by a mutation in the cationic trypsinogen gene. *Nature Genet* 14:141, 1996.

Widdison AL, Karanjia ND, Reber HA: Antimicrobial treatment of pancreatic infection in acute pancreatitis. *Br J Surg* 811:886, 1994.

Wilson C, Heath DI, Imrie CW: Prediction of outcome in acute pancreatitis: A comparative study of APACHE II clinical assessment and multiple factors scoring systems. *Br J Surg* 77:1260, 1990.

Chronic Pancreatitis

Balthazar EJ, Chako AC: Computed tomography of pancreatic masses. *Am J Gastroenterol* 85:343, 1990.

Bockman DE, Buchler M, et al: Analysis of nerves in chronic pancreatitis. *Gastroenterology* 94:1459, 1988.

Buchler MW, Friess H, et al (eds): Surgical treatment of chronic pancreatitis: New standards. *Dig Surg* 13, 1996.

Carr-Locke DL: Endoscopic procedures in the treatment of pancreatic pain. *Acta Chir Scand* 156:293, 1990.

Gebhart C: Surgical treatment of pain in chronic pancreatitis: Role of the Whipple procedure. *Acta Chir Scand* 156:303, 1990.

Grace PA, Pitt HA, Longmire WP: Pylorus-preserving pancreaticoduodenectomy: An overview. *Br J Surg* 77:968, 1990.

Howard JM: Surgical treatment of chronic pancreatitis, in Howard JM, Jordan GL, Reber HA (eds): *Surgical Diseases of the Pancreas.* Philadelphia, Lea & Febiger, 1987, pp 496-521.

Howard JM, Zhang Z: Pancreaticoduodenectomy (Whipple's resection) in the treatment of chronic pancreatitis. *World J Surg* 14:77, 1990.

Ihse I, Gasslander T: Surgical treatment of pain in chronic pancreatitis: Role of pancreaticojejunostomy. *Acta Chir Scand* 156:299, 1990.

Karanjia ND, Singh SM, et al: Pancreatic ductal and interstitial pressures in chronic pancreatitis. *Dig Dis Sci* 37:268, 1992.

Karanjia ND, Widdison AL, et al: Compartment syndrome in experimental chronic obstructive pancreatitis: Effect of decompressing the main pancreatic duct. *Br J Surg* 81:259, 1994.

Kozarek RA, Traverso LW: Endotherapy for chronic pancreatitis. *Int J Pancreatol* 19:93, 1996.

Lankisch PG: Function tests in the diagnosis of chronic pancreatitis. *Int J Pancreatol* 14:9, 1993.

Layer P, Holtmann G: Pancreatic enzymes in chronic pancreatitis. *Int J Pancreatol* 15:1, 1994.

Malcynski JT, Iwanow IC, et al: Severe pancreatitis: Determinants of mortality in a tertiary referral center. *Arch Surg* 131:242, 1996.

Nealon WH, Thompson JC: Progressive loss of pancreatic function in chronic pancreatitis is delayed by main pancreatic duct decompression: A longitudinal prospective analysis of the modified Puestow procedure. *Ann Surg* 217:466, 1993.

Rattner DW, Fernandez-del Castillo C, et al: Pitfalls of distal pancreatectomy for relief of pain in chronic pancreatitis. *Am J Surg* 171:142, 1996.

Reber H: Chronic pancreatitis: Etiology, diagnosis and pathology, in Howard JM, Jordan GL, Reber HA (eds): *Surgical Diseases of the Pancreas.* Philadelphia, Lea & Febiger, 1987, pp 475-495.

Reber HA, Karanjia ND, et al: Pancreatic blood flow in cats with chronic pancreatitis. *Gastroenterology* 103:652, 1992.

Rossi RL, Soeldner JS, et al: Long term results of pancreatic resection and segmental pancreatic autotransplantation for chronic pancreatitis. *Am J Surg* 159:51, 1990.

Sarles H, Bernard JP, Gullo L: Pathogenesis and epidemiology of chronic pancreatitis. *Gut* 31:629, 1990.

Pseudocysts, Ascites, and Fistulas

Howard JM: Cysts of the pancreas, in Howard JM, Jordan GL, Reber HA (eds): *Surgical Diseases of the Pancreas.* Philadelphia, Lea & Febiger, 1987, pp 539-563.

Liguory C, Lefebvre JF, Vitale GC: Endoscopic drainage of pancreatic pseudocysts. *Can J Gastroenterol* 4:568, 1990.

Maringhini A, Ciambra M, et al: Ascites, pleural, and pericardial effusions in acute pancreatitis: A prospective study of incidence, natural history, and prognostic role. *Dig Dis Sci* 41:848, 1996.

Trede M, Carter DC (eds): *Surgery of the Pancreas.* Edinburgh, Churchill-Livingstone, 1993, pp 433–442.

van Sonnenberg E, Wittich GR, et al: Percutaneous drainage of infected and noninfected pancreatic pseudocysts: Experience in 101 cases. *Radiology* 170:757, 1989.

Vitas GJ, Sarr MG: Selected management of pancreatic pseudocysts: Operative versus expectant management. *Surgery* 111:123, 1992.

Walt AJ, Bouwman DL, et al: The impact of technology on the management of pancreatic pseudocyst. *Arch Surg* 125:759, 1990.

Yeo CJ, Bastidas JA, et al: The natural history of pancreatic pseudocysts documented by computed tomography. *Surg Gynecol Obstet* 170:411, 1990.

Yeo CJ. Pancreatic pseudocysts, ascites, and fistulas. *Curr Opin Gen Surg* 31:173, 1994.

Pancreatic Cancer

Alvarez C, Livingston EH, et al: Cost benefit analysis of workup for pancreatic cancer. *Am J Surg* 165:53, 1993.

Beger HG, Buchler MW, Schoenberg MH (eds): *Cancer of the Pancreas.* Ulm, Germany, University Press, 1996, p 493.

Brennan MF, Moccia RD, et al: Management of adenocarcinoma of the body and tail of the pancreas. *Ann Surg* 223:506, 1996.

Brugge WR: The role of endoscopic ultrasound in pancreatic disorders. *Int J Pancreatol* 20:1, 1996.

Buchler M, Friess H, et al: Role of octreotide in the prevention of postoperative complications following pancreatic resection. *Am J Surg* 163:125, 1992.

Caldas C, Kern SE. K-*ras* mutation and pancreatic adenocarcinoma. *Int J Pancreatol* 18:1, 1995.

Cameron JL, Crist DW, et al: Factors influencing survival after pancreaticoduodenectomy for pancreatic cancer. *Am J Surg* 161:120, 1991.

Cameron JL, Pitt HA, et al. One hundred forty-five consecutive pancreatoduodenectomies without mortality. *Ann Surg* 217:430, 1993.

Conlon KC, Klimstra DS, et al: Long-term survival after curative resection for pancreatic ductal adenocarcinoma. *Ann Surg* 223:273, 1996.

Conlon KC, Klimstra DS, et al: Long-term survival after curative resection for pancreatic ductal adenocarcinoma: Clinicopathologic analysis of 5-year survivors. *Ann Surg* 223:272, 1996.

Cullinan S, Moertel CG, et al: A phase III trial on the therapy of advanced pancreatic carcinoma: Evaluations of the Mallinson regimen and combined 5-fluorouracil, doxorubicin, and cisplatin. *Cancer* 65:2207, 1990.

Dresler CM, Fortner JG, et al: Metabolic consequences of (regional) total pancreatectomy. *Ann Surg* 214:131, 1991.

Fietkau R, Sauer R: Future prospects of radiotherapy in pancreatic cancer. *Eur J Surg Oncol* 17:201, 1991.

Gattani AM, Mandeli J, et al: Tumor markers in patients with pancreatic carcinoma. *Cancer* 78:57, 1996.

Geer RJ, Brennan MF: Resection of pancreatic adenocarcinoma: prognostic indicators for survival. *Am J Surg* 165:68, 1993.

Gordon TA, Burleyson GP, et al: The effects of regionalization on cost and outcome for one general high-risk surgical procedure. *Ann Surg* 221:43, 1995.

Griffin JF, Smalley SR, et al: Patterns of failure after curative resection of pancreatic carcinoma. *Cancer* 66:56, 1990.

Hyoty MK, Nordback IH: Biliary stent or surgical bypass in unresectable pancreatic cancer with obstructive jaundice. *Acta Chir Scand* 156:391, 1990.

Klapdor R: Perspectives in chemotherapy of pancreatic cancer. *Eur J Surg Oncol* 17:153, 1991.

Kloppel G, Maillet B: Histological typing of pancreatic and periampullary carcinoma. *Eur J Surg Oncol* 17:139, 1991.

Lillemoe KD, Cameron JL, et al: Pancreaticoduodenectomy: Does it have a role in the palliation of pancreatic cancer? *Ann Surg* 223:718, 1996.

Livingston EH, Reber HA: Treatment of pancreatic carcinoma. *Curr Opin Gen Surg* 30:294, 1993.

Lowenfels AB, Maisonneuve P, et al: Pancreatitis and the risk of pancreatic cancer. *N Engl J Med* 328:1433, 1993.

Niederau C, Grendell JH: Diagnosis of pancreatic carcinoma: Imaging techniques and tumor markers. *Pancreas* 7:66, 1992.

Patel AG, Toyama MT, et al: Standard vs pylorus-preserving Whipple resection: Is it any better? *Arch Surg* 130:838, 1995.

Poston GJ, Gillespie J, Guillou PJ: Biology of pancreatic cancer. *Gut* 32:800, 1991.

Rosch T, Braig C, et al: Staging of pancreatic and ampullary carcinoma by endoscopic ultrasonography: Comparison with conventional sonography, computed tomography, and angiography. *Gastroenterology* 102:188, 1992.

Seydel HG, Stablein DM, et al: Hyperfractionated radiation and chemotherapy for unresectable localized adenocarcinoma of the pancreas: The Gastrointestinal Tumor Study Group experience. *Cancer* 65:1478, 1990.

Singh SM, Longmire WP Jr, Reber HA: Surgical palliation for pancreatic cancer: The UCLA experience. *Ann Surg* 212:132, 1990.

Spencer MP, Sarr MG, Nagorney DM: Radical pancreatectomy for pancreatic cancer in the elderly: Is it safe and justified? *Ann Surg* 212:140, 1990.

Steinberg W: The clinical utility of the CA 19-9 tumor-associated antigen. *Am J Gastroenterol* 85:350, 1990.

Trede M, Schwall G, Saeger HD: Survival after pancreatoduodenectomy: 118 consecutive resections without an operative mortality. *Ann Surg* 211:447, 1990.

Tsuchiya R, Tsunoda T, Yamaguchi T: Operation of choice for resectable carcinoma of the head of the pancreas. *Int J Pancreatol* 6:295, 1990.

Warshaw AL, Compton CC, et al: Cystic tumors in the pancreas: New clinical, radiologic, and pathologic observations in 67 patients. *Ann Surg* 212:432, 1990.

Zinner MJ, Shurbaji MS, Cameron JL: Solid and papillary epithelial neoplasms of the pancreas. *Surgery* 108:475, 1990.

Islet Cell Neoplasms

Delacore R, Cheung LY, Freisen SR: Outcome of lymph node involvement in patients with the Zollinger-Ellison syndrome. *Ann Surg* 208:291, 1988.

Delvalle J, Yamada T: Secretory tumors of the pancreas, in Sleisinger MH, Fordtran JS (eds): *Gastrointestinal Disease: Pathophysiology, Diagnosis, Management,* 4th ed. Philadelphia, WB Saunders, 1989, pp 1884-1896.

Doherty GM, Norton JA: Preoperative and intraoperative localization of gastrinomas. *Probl Gen Surg* 7:521, 1990.

Frucht H, Norton JA, et al: Detection of duodenal gastrinomas by operative endoscopic transillumination: A prospective study. *Gastroenterology* 99:1622, 1990.

Howard TJ, Passaro E Jr: Gastrinoma: New medical and surgical approaches. *Surg Clin North Am* 69:667, 1989.

Konomi K, Chijiwa K, et al: Pancreatic somatostatinoma: A case report and review of the literature. *J Surg Oncol* 43:259, 1990.

McArthur KE, Collen MJ, Maton PN: Omeprazole: Effective convenient therapy for Zollinger-Ellison syndrome. *Gastroenterology* 88:939, 1985.

Moertel CG, Lefkopoulo M, et al: Streptozocin-doxorubicin, streptozocin-fluorouracil, or chlorozotocin in the treatment of advanced islet-cell carcinoma. *N Engl J Med* 326:519, 1992.

Mozell E, Stenzel P, et al: Functional endocrine tumors of the pancreas: Clinical presentation, diagnosis, and treatment. *Curr Probl Surg* 27:303, 1990.

Norton JA, Shawker TH, et al: Localization and surgical treatment of occult insulinomas. *Ann Surg* 212:615, 1990.

Prinz RA. Localization of gastrinomas. *Int J Pancreatol* 19:79, 1996.

Rosin RD: Endocrine pancreatic tumors, in Schwartz SI, Ellis H (eds): *Maingot's Abdominal Operations,* 9th ed. New York, Appleton & Lange, 1989, pp 1619–1632.

Vinayek R, Frucht H, et al: Intravenous omeprazole in patients with Zollinger-Ellison syndrome undergoing surgery. *Gastroenterology* 99:10, 1990.

Wermers RA, Fatourechi V, et al: The glucagonoma syndrome: Clinical and pathologic features in 21 patients. *Medicine* 75:53, 1996.

Trauma

Chandler C, Waxman K: Demonstration of pancreatic ductal integrity by endoscopic retrograde pancreatography allows conservative surgical management. *J Trauma* 40:466, 1996.

Degiannis E, Levy RD, et al: Gunshot injuries of the head of the pancreas: Conservative approach. *World J Surg* 20:68, 1996.

Emmick RH, Petersen SR: Evaluation of pancreatic injury after blunt abdominal trauma. *Ann Emerg Med* 27:658, 1996.

Jordan GL Jr: Pancreatic trauma, in Howard JM, Jordan GL, Reber HA (eds): *Surgical Diseases of the Pancreas.* Philadelphia, Lea & Febiger, 1987, pp 875-897.

Spleen

Seymour I. Schwartz

ANATOMY

The spleen arises by mesenchymal differentiation along the left side of the dorsal mesogastrium in the 8-mm embryo. The weight of the spleen in the healthy adult ranges between 75 and 100 g, decreasing somewhat with age. The organ is located in the left upper quadrant, having a superior relationship to the undersurface of the left leaf of the diaphragm and protected anteriorly, laterally, and posteriorly by the lower portion of the rib cage. Its position is maintained by several suspensory ligaments, the major ones being the splenophrenic, splenorenal, splenocolic, and gastrosplenic ligaments. The gastrosplenic ligament normally contains the short gastric vessels, while the remaining ligaments are generally avascular, except in patients with portal hypertension, when collateral veins become apparent. Arterial blood enters the spleen via the splenic artery, a branch of the celiac artery. The major venous drainage courses through the splenic vein, which joins the superior mesenteric vein to form the portal vein.

Accessory spleens have been reported in 14 to 30 percent of patients, with a higher incidence occurring in patients operated on for hematologic disorders. These accessory organs, which receive their vascular supply from the splenic artery, are present, in decreasing order of frequency, in the hilus of the spleen, the gastrosplenic and splenocolic ligaments, the gastrocolic ligament, the splenorenal ligament, and the greater omentum (Fig. 31-1). They also may occur in the pelvis of the female, and functioning splenic tissue has been removed from the scrotum in juxtaposition to the left testicle.

The spleen consists of a capsule that is normally 1 to 2 mm thick and trabeculae that enclose the pulp. The pulp itself has conventionally been divided into three zones: white, marginal, and red. Peripheral to the white pulp is the marginal zone, which contains end arteries arising from the central artery and from the penicillary arteries. The marginal zone contains lymphocytes, macrophages, and some red cells that have exited the terminal arteries. The marginal zone contains the marginal sinus, which filters material from the white pulp. Locally produced immunoglobulins enter this sinus and course to the peripheral circulation. Peripheral to the marginal zone is the red pulp, which consists of cords and sinuses that contain cellular elements of blood in transit.

Blood brought to the spleen via the splenic arteries courses through branches, the trabecular arteries, that leave the trabeculae and enter the white pulp as central arteries (Fig. 31-2). These central arteries give off at right angles numerous arterioles, some of which terminate in the white pulp. The perpendicularity contributes to a skimming effect by which plasma exits while most red cells pass to the red pulp. Other branches cross the white pulp and end in the marginal zone or in the red pulp

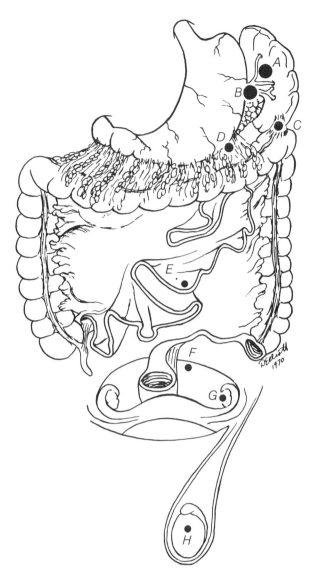

FIG. 31-1. Location of accessory3 spleens. *A.* Splenic hilus. *B.* Along splenic vessels; tail of pancreas. *C.* Splenocolic ligament. *D.* Greater omentum; perirenal regions. *E.* Mesentery. *F.* Presacral region. *G.* Adnexal region. *H.* Peritesticular region. (From: *Schwartz SI, Adams JT, Bauman AW: Splenectomy for hematologic disorders. Curr Probl Surg, May 1971. Copyright 1971, Chicago, Year Book Medical Publishers. Used by permission.*)

itself. The branch of the central artery that terminates in the red pulp, known as the "artery of the pulp," breaks up into many branches. Within the red pulp, the blood is collected in splenic sinuses. These large, thin-walled venous spaces drain into the pulp veins, which in turn drain into the trabecular veins and then into the main splenic veins to enter the portal circulation. Thus splenic pulp pressure reflects pressure throughout the portal venous system. The tissue between the splenic sinuses is a reticular, connective tissue meshwork that appears as cords on histologic section, and hence is designated the "splenic cords." At points of passage from cords to sinuses, deformability and flexibility are demanded of the red blood cells so that they can squeeze through. Although these fenestrations are of small diameter (0.5 to 5.0 mm), they are traversed by normal red cells, which easily adjust to these dimensions. Under normal condi-

tions, 10 percent of red cells pass from terminal arterioles through arteriovenous connections; 90 percent of cells course from terminal arterioles into pulp cords and into splenic sinuses after traversing the cordal-sinus wall apertures. The total splenic blood flow averages 300 mL/min.

PHYSIOLOGY AND PATHOPHYSIOLOGY (Fig. 31-3)

Galen is credited with the phrase "The spleen is an organ full of mystery." During the fifth to eighth month of fetal life, the spleen contributes actively to the production of both red cells and white cells that enter the circulation. This function does not continue in the normal adult. The role of the spleen in the immunologic processes of the body is discussed in Chap. 10. The splenic function that is the focus of surgical attention is related to the organ's reticuloendothelial tissue, which contributes to the removal of cellular elements from the circulating blood. Normally, cells pass through the spleen rapidly, but in the presence of splenomegaly and other disease states, the flow patterns become circuitous, contain more obstacles, and result in pooling of cells within the cords.

Abnormal and aged erythrocytes, abnormal granulocytes, normal and abnormal platelets, and cellular debris may be cleared by the spleen, which apparently is capable of discriminating between these and normal cellular components. In the normal adult, the spleen is the most important site of selective erythrocyte sequestration, and during its 120-day life cycle, the red cell spends an estimated minimum of 2 days within the spleen.

The action of the spleen that results in the pathologic reduction of circulating cellular elements of blood has been attributed to two possible mechanisms: (1) excessive splenic destruction of cellular elements, and (2) splenic production of an antibody that results in the destruction of cells within the circulating blood. Overactivity of splenic function leading to accelerated removal of any or all of the circulating cellular elements of the blood with resultant anemia, leukopenia, or thrombocytopenia, alone or in combination, is referred to as *hypersplenism*.

The normal adult spleen contains about 25 mL of red blood cells, but relatively few of these are removed during a single passage through the organ. The spleen is capable of removing nuclear remnants (Howell-Jolly bodies) from circulating erythrocytes. The postsplenectomy blood smear is characterized by the presence of circulating erythrocytes with Howell-Jolly bodies and Pappenheimer bodies (siderotic granules that stain with Wright's stain) as a result of the loss of the pitting function of the spleen.

During the course of a day, approximately 20 mL of aged red blood cells are removed. Aging changes the biophysical properties of the red cell, making splenic entrapment of red cells that have circulated for 105 to 120 days more likely. Delay in splenic transit of aged or abnormal cells can lead to further cell injury because of the relatively hypoxic, acidotic, and substrate-(glucose-) deprived environment that is present in congested splenic red pulp cords. These environmental conditions lead to further physical and chemical deterioration of the erythrocyte, making it more susceptible to phagocytosis by splenic macrophages and reticuloendothelial cells or to intrasinusoidal disintegration. The central event in cytolysis may be the fall in cellular adenosine triphosphate (ATP) to very low levels and the

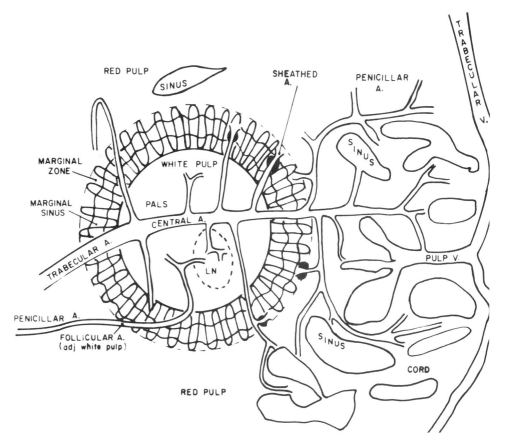

FIG. 31-2. Diagram illustrating splenic compartments and potential vascular supply routes. Symbols: A = artery or arteriole; V = vein; LN = lymphatic nodule, which may include germinal center; PALS = periarterial lymphatic sheath. (From: *Barnhart MI, Lusher JM: Structural physiology of the human spleen. Am J Pediatr Hematol Oncol 1:311, 1979, with permission.*)

loss of vital cellular functions dependent on ATP, such as sodium and calcium efflux, priming of glycolysis, and maintenance of membrane integrity. To what extent repeated passages through the spleen contribute to normal red cell aging is not certain, but evidence that the red cell loses surface area with aging, combined with the ability of the spleen to remove bits of red cell with surgical precision, raises this possibility. On the other hand, a normal red cell life span in splenectomized subjects suggests that red cell aging occurs independently of splenic presence and at approximately the normal rate. A variety of erythrocytes altered by intrinsic factors (membrane, hemoglobin, or enzymic abnormalities) or extrinsic factors (antibody and nonantibody injury) may be prematurely removed by the spleen. Severely damaged cells may be removed by the reticuloendothelial system at a variety of sites. Minimally altered erythrocytes may require the specific rigors of the splenic circulation for premature destruction and therefore may have normal or near-normal survival after splenic removal.

The neutrophil is removed from the circulation with a half-life of about 6 h. Although the role of the spleen in the destruction of neutrophils under normal conditions is not well quantified, in some hypersplenic states the spleen's role is augmented, with resulting neutropenia. This augmented removal can occur because of splenic enlargement and sequestration of granulocytes or because of enhanced splenic removal of altered granulocytes, as seen in immune neutropenias.

The platelet (thrombocyte), under normal circumstances, survives about 10 days in the circulation. One-third of the total platelet pool is normally sequestered in the spleen, but the role of the spleen in the final removal of normal platelets has not

been precisely defined. With splenomegaly, a larger proportion of platelets is sequestered in the spleen (up to 80 percent), and this and accelerated platelet destruction in the spleen account for thrombocytopenia. Increased sequestration and destruction of platelets occur in the absence of splenomegaly in patients with idiopathic thrombocytopenic purpura (ITP) as a consequence of immunologic alteration of the platelets. In thrombotic thrombocytopenic purpura (TTP), platelets are sequestered in the spleen because of encroachment of the vascular lumen by increased subendothelial collagen.

Splenectomy results in an increase in platelets, which at times reach levels greater than 1,000,000 mm³. Postsplenectomy thrombocytosis is usually transient but may persist. This is particularly notable in congenital hemolytic states that do not re-

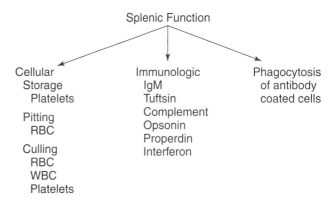

FIG. 31-3. Splenic function.

spond well to splenectomy. In these circumstances, continued hemolysis in the absence of the splenic removal mechanism can lead to persistent, extreme thrombocytosis and intravenous thrombosis.

DIAGNOSTIC CONSIDERATIONS

Evaluation of Size. Normally the spleen is not palpable on abdominal examination, but the organ may be felt in about 2 percent of healthy adults. In healthy subjects, no significant dullness is elicited by percussion over the spleen either anteriorly or laterally. As the organ enlarges, dullness may be detected at the level of the ninth intercostal space in the left anterior axillary line, especially on expiration. Thereafter, it becomes first percussible and then palpable below the left costal margin. With increasing splenomegaly, notching may be palpable on the anteromedial surface, distinguishing the spleen from other abdominal masses.

Routine radiologic examination of the abdomen usually provides an accurate estimate of the size of the spleen. Although splenomegaly may be suggested by medial or caudad displacement of the stomach bubble, frequently accompanied by caudad displacement of air in the splenic flexure of the colon, the organ's outline can often be clearly demarcated in the left upper quadrant, corroborating enlargement. Computed tomography (CT) and magnetic resonance imaging (MRI) depict the spleen and define abnormalities in size, shape, and parenchymal pathology, i.e., cyst, abscess (Fig. 31-4), or tumor. Radioisotopic scanning with ^{99m}Tc-sulfur colloid also defines the organ; vascular shunts that allow blood to bypass splenic phagocytes interfere with the procedure.

Evaluation of Function. The functional abnormality of hypersplenism may be manifested by a reduction in the number of red cells, neutrophils, or platelets in the peripheral blood. An increase in the rate of red cell destruction will always result in a compensatory rise in the rate of production unless disease of the marrow coexists. The hallmark of increased red cell turnover

(hemolysis) is reticulocytosis in the absence of blood loss. Other tests such as measurement of the plasma bilirubin, haptoglobin, and hemoglobin levels are less sensitive and are dependent on the rate and sites of hemolysis as well as on liver function, and are therefore only of adjunctive value.

Reduced red blood cell survival in patients with hemolytic anemia may be more precisely demonstrated by measuring the disappearance of blood radioactivity after the patient's erythrocytes are labeled with $Na_2{}^{51}CrO_4$. With this technique, the normal half-life of the red cells is about 30 days (i.e., 50 percent of the cells remain in the circulation at that time). A half-life of 15 days or less indicates significantly increased hemolysis. The spleen's role in a hemolytic anemia may be assessed by determining the relative uptakes of ^{51}Cr-tagged erythrocytes by the spleen and the liver. A spleen-liver ratio greater than 2:1 indicates significant preferential splenic sequestration and anticipates a beneficial effect of splenectomy.

Radioisotopic labeling also has been used to evaluate the survival of neutrophils and platelets. There is no clinically practical method of assessing the decreased longevity of neutrophils or of measuring the role of the spleen in the destruction of these cells. Platelet destruction in the spleen is such a common mechanism in thrombocytopenia that radioisotopic studies are not often done if the bone marrow aspirate indicates an abundance of megakaryocytes, suggesting adequate platelet production.

RUPTURE OF THE SPLEEN (see Chap. 6)

HEMATOLOGIC DISORDERS FOR WHICH SPLENECTOMY IS THERAPEUTIC

In 1887 Sir Spencer Wells operated on a patient with the preoperative diagnosis of a uterine fibroid, but instead he noted a "wandering spleen," which he removed. The patient later proved to have hereditary spherocytosis; thus the first surgical cure of a hematologic disorder was inadvertent and became manifest postoperatively when the patient's anemia and chronic jaundice disappeared. Micheli is generally given credit for introducing the

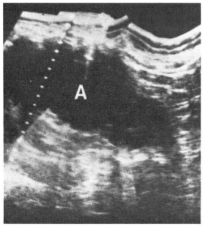
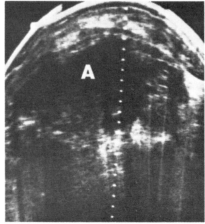
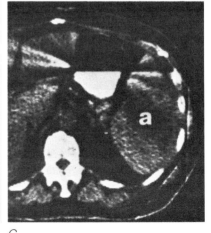

A   *B*   *C*

FIG. 31-4. Splenic abscess. *A.* Coronal sonogram of spleen. Large irregular anechoic area (A) containing a few internal scattered echoes due to debris. *B.* Transverse axial sonogram of spleen demonstrates abscess (A). *C.* CT scan at corresponding level. Abscess (a) is area of diminished attenuation in center of spleen. Lesion was drained percutaneously. (From: *Pawar S, Kay CJ, et al: Sonography of splenic abscess. AJR 138:259, 1982, with permission.*)

concept of splenectomy as treatment for hemolytic anemia in an article published in 1911. Kaznelson, as a medical student in Prague, proposed to Schloffer, a professor of surgery, splenectomy to treat idiopathic thrombocytopenic purpura in a 36-year-old woman. The case, and the successful elevation of the platelet count to above-normal levels, was reported four weeks after the procedure in 1916.

Hemolytic Anemias

Hemolytic anemias include a broad spectrum of disorders in which there is accelerated destruction of mature red blood cells. The congenital anemias are due to an intrinsic abnormality of the erythrocytes, and the acquired anemias are related to an extracorpuscular factor acting on an intrinsically normal cell. In both types of disorder, the reduced red blood cell survival may be demonstrated by measuring the disappearance of the patient's radioactive erythrocytes (labeled with ^{51}Cr), and the spleen's role may be evaluated by determining the relative uptakes of this radioactivity by the spleen and liver.

Hereditary Spherocytosis. Hereditary spherocytosis is transmitted as an autosomal dominant trait and is the most common of the symptomatic familial hemolytic anemias. Ovalocytosis and stomatocytosis usually exist as harmless traits, but occasionally, when these forms constitute 50 to 90 percent of the red cell population, clinical manifestations indistinguishable from those noted with hereditary spherocytosis may occur. The fundamental abnormality stems from a defective erythrocyte membrane that causes the cell to be smaller than normal, unusually thick, and almost spherical. These cells also demonstrate increased osmotic fragility, i.e., lysis occurs at a higher concentration of sodium chloride than normal. The role of the spleen in this disorder is related to the inability of the spherocytic cells to pass through the splenic pulp. The cells that escape from the spleen are more susceptible to trapping and disintegration during each successive passage, until cell loss ensues. The precise pathogenesis of the cell injury may be related to a decreased availability of red cell ATP in the environment of the spleen, combined with a cell membrane that has been shown in in vitro studies to be more susceptible to reduction in ATP levels.

The salient clinical features of the disease are anemia, reticulocytosis, jaundice, and splenomegaly. It is unusual for the anemia to be extremely severe, and the jaundice usually parallels the severity of the anemia. Periodic and sudden increases in the intensity of the anemia and jaundice may occur, and rare fatal crises have been reported. Cholelithiasis with gallstones of the pigmented variety has been reported in 30 to 60 percent of patients but is rare in children under the age of ten. Leg ulcers are uncommon specific manifestations.

Diagnosis is generally established by peripheral blood smear analysis, which demonstrates that more than 60 percent of the red blood cells are spherocyte-shaped with a mean diameter less than normal and a thickness greater than normal. Increased osmotic fragility of the red blood cells provides diagnostic confirmation, but this test is rarely performed.

Splenectomy is the sole therapy for hereditary spherocytosis and ovalocytosis. It is generally recommended that the operation be delayed until the fourth year of life. Intractable leg ulcers associated with hereditary spherocytosis mandate early splenectomy because they heal only after the spleen has been removed. The results of splenectomy as a method of correcting anemia

and preventing hemolysis have been uniformly good. Although the inherent membrane abnormality persists and the spherocytosis and increased osmotic fragility of the cells are not altered, in vivo hemolysis virtually ceases, and following removal of the spleen, the erythrocytes achieve a normal life span and the jaundice, if present, disappears. It is appropriate to perform an oral cholecystogram or ultrasonogram prior to splenectomy, and the gallbladder should always be examined at the time of operation. If gallstones are present, the gallbladder should be removed during the operation.

Thalassemia. Thalassemia (Mediterranean anemia) is transmitted as a dominant trait and primarily derives from a defect in hemoglobin synthesis. The development of intracellular precipitates (Heinz bodies) contributes to premature red cell destruction. The disease is classified as alpha, beta, and gamma types, determined by the specific defect in synthesis rate of the peptide chain. In the United States, most thalassemia patients are of southern European origin and suffer from beta thalassemia, i.e., a quantitative reduction in the rate of beta chain synthesis, resulting in a decrease in hemoglobin A (Hb-A). Thalassemia occurs in two major degrees of severity: homozygous thalassemia (thalassemia major), a severe disorder in which the affected child receives a gene for thalassemia from each parent, and heterozygous thalassemia (thalassemia minor), a mild disorder in which the affected child receives a gene from only one parent. Gradations of thalassemia range from heterozygous thalassemia (minor), often not detected until examination of the blood for an unrelated problem, to homozygous thalassemia, a severe, chronic anemia, with icterus, splenomegaly, and death early in life. In thalassemia minor, Hb-A$_2$ is always increased, and slight increases in Hb-F occur in 50 percent of patients. In both types of thalassemia, the hemoglobin-deficient cells are small, thin, and misshapen. The cells appear washed out and have a characteristic resistance to osmotic lysis.

The clinical manifestations of thalassemia major usually occur in the first year of life and consist of pallor, retarded body growth, and enlargement of the head. Intractable leg ulcers may be noted, intercurrent infections are common, and gallstones are reported in about one-fourth of patients. The manifestations of thalassemia minor may vary. Most patients with thalassemia minor lead normal lives, but some patients have a more severe expression of their disease (referred to as thalassemia intermedia) and generally present with signs and symptoms attributable to mild anemia, chronic mild jaundice, and moderate splenomegaly.

The diagnosis of thalassemia major is established by the peripheral blood smear, which reveals hypochromic, microcytic anemia with markedly distorted red cells of various sizes and shapes. Nucleated red cells, or "target cells," are invariably present, and the reticulocyte count is elevated, as is the white cell count. The characteristic feature of the disease is the persistence of Hb-F and reduction of Hb-A levels, demonstrated by the alkali denaturation study. It is important that both parents have evidence of thalassemia minor.

Treatment is indicated only for symptomatic patients. Transfusions are usually required at regular intervals, but as most patients accommodate to low hemoglobin levels, the transfusions should be directed at maintaining the hemoglobin level at 10 g/dL. Although splenectomy does not influence the basic hematologic disorder, it may reduce both the hemolytic process and the transfusion requirements. Marked splenomegaly and/or symptomatic repeated splenic infarction also constitute indications for splenectomy. A postoperative complication rate of 43 percent following splenectomy in thalassemia is contrasted with 3 percent in patients undergoing splenectomy for other reasons; overall, however, the benefit-to-risk ratio favors splenectomy when indications are present.

Hereditary Hemolytic Anemia with Enzyme Deficiency. Included in this category are (1) enzyme deficiencies in anaerobic glycolytic pathways, the prototype of which is pyruvate-kinase (PK) deficiency, and (2) enzyme deficiencies in the hexose monophosphate shunt, the prototype of which is glucose-6-phosphate (G-6-PD) deficiency. These deficiencies render the cells susceptible to increased hemolysis. Splenic enlargement occurs more frequently with PK deficiency, and the spleen is rarely enlarged in patients with G-6-PD deficiency. Specific enzyme assays are employed to define the deficiency.

The majority of patients maintain hemoglobins greater than 8 g/dL, are asymptomatic, and do not require therapy. With significant anemia, blood transfusions are indicated, and the transfused cells survive normally. ^{51}Cr-tagged red cell studies are not predictive of results with a high enough degree of accuracy to be useful. In severe cases of PK deficiency, splenectomy may be worthwhile. In patients with this disorder postoperative thrombocytosis with consequent hepatic, portal, or inferior vena caval thrombosis may occur if the hemolytic rate is unabated. Splenectomy is not indicated for patients with G-6-PD deficiency.

Hereditary High Red Cell Phosphatidylcholine Anemia (HPCHA). When patients with HPCHA have undergone splenectomy, the anemia worsens and the hemolysis is unchanged.

Sickle Cell Disease. Sickle cell anemia is a hereditary hemolytic anemia seen predominantly in blacks and characterized by the presence of sickle- and crescent-shaped erythrocytes. In this hereditary hemoglobinopathy, the normal Hb-A is replaced by the abnormal form of hemoglobin, sickle hemoglobin (Hb-S). Hb-F is usually mildly increased. Combinations of Hb-S with other hemoglobin variants also occur as a result of an abnormal trait inherited from each parent, e.g., Hb-S/Hb-C or Hb-S/thalassemia.

Under conditions of reduced oxygen tension, Hb-S molecules undergo crystallization within the red cell, which elongates and distorts the cell. The sickling phenomenon occurs more readily with higher percentages of Hb-S, with a reduced pH, and under conditions of circulatory stasis that tend to exaggerate hemoglobin deoxygenation. The sickle cells themselves contribute to increased blood viscosity and circulatory stasis, thus establishing a vicious cycle. The primary consequence of this stagnation is thrombosis, which leads to ischemia, necrosis, and organ fibrosis.

The role of the spleen in this disorder is not clear. Early in the course of the disease, splenomegaly occurs, but following varying intervals in most patients, the spleen undergoes infarction and marked contraction with eventual autosplenectomy.

Although the sickle cell trait occurs in approximately 9 percent of the black population, the majority are asymptomatic. However, sickle cell anemia has been observed in 0.3 to 1.3 percent of blacks, who often show remarkable adaptation to the state of chronic anemia and jaundice. This adaptive state may be interrupted at intervals by acute symptoms or crises that are related to vascular occlusion. Depending on the vessels involved, the patient may have bone or joint pain, hematuria, priapism, neurologic manifestations, or ulcers over the malleoli. Abdominal pain and cramps due to visceral stasis are frequent, simulating an acute surgical abdomen. Thrombosis of the splenic vessels may result in the unusual complication of splenic abscess, manifested by splenomegaly, splenic pain, and fever. Many patients with sickle cell anemia die in the first decade of life, but a few survive to the fifth decade. Death may be the result of intercurrent infections or cardiac or renal failure.

The diagnosis is established by the presence of anemia, characteristic sickle cells on peripheral blood smear analysis, hemoglobin electrophoresis showing 80 percent or more Hb-S, and the presence of the trait in both parents. Leukocytosis is often noted, and the platelet count is frequently elevated. There may be modest elevation of the serum bilirubin, and cholelithiasis is a frequent accompaniment.

For most patients only palliative treatment is possible. Sodium cyanate will prevent sickling of Hb-S. Transfusions may be required to maintain adequate hemoglobin levels. Adequate hydration and partial exchange transfusion may help during a crisis. Splenectomy may benefit patients with marked hypersplenism or splenic abscesses. In the circumstance of splenic abscess, incision and drainage of the abscess cavity within the parenchyma of the spleen may be necessary, since removal of the organ is hindered by marked inflammatory and adhesive processes. Splenectomy may be of benefit in a very few patients in whom acute splenic sequestration of red cells can be demonstrated, although the operation does not affect the sickling process. A report on forty-six children who underwent splenectomy for hypersplenism and fourteen patients operated on for acute splenic sequestration with a median follow-up of 6 years noted that two patients died of overwhelming sepsis; neither received prophylaxis, and neither pneumococcal septicemia nor meningitis was confirmed.

Idiopathic Autoimmune Hemolytic Anemia. This is a disorder in which the life span of a presumably normal erythrocyte is shortened when exposed to an endogenous hemolytic mechanism. The causation has not been defined, but an autoimmune process appears to be fundamental. In such patients, antibodies reacting with the patient's normal red cells have been defined, and there is evidence that the spleen may serve as a source of antibody. Both "warm" and "cold" antibodies have been described. Some "warm" antibodies have Rh specificity. Most of these antibodies are hemagglutinins rather than hemolysins. It is believed that the reticuloendothelial system traps and destroys the immunologically altered cells. Sequestration occurs primarily in the spleen. By binding the F_c portion of the IgG molecule to the corresponding macrophage surface F_c receptor, the spherocytes become more rigid and more sensitive to destruction in the splenic circulation.

Although autoimmune hemolytic anemia may be encountered at any age, it occurs more frequently after the age of fifty and twice as often in females. Mild jaundice is often present. The spleen is palpably enlarged in half the cases, and gallstones have been demonstrated in a quarter of the cases. The extent of anemia varies, and hemoglobinuria and tubular necrosis have been reported in severe cases. In this circumstance, the prognosis is serious, as the mortality rate is 40 to 50 percent.

The diagnosis of hemolysis is made by demonstrating anemia and reticulocytosis accompanied by the products of red cell destruction in the blood, urine, and stool. The bone marrow is hypercellular with a predominance of erythroid precursors. A distinguishing feature of the disease is the demonstration by direct Coombs' test of an autoantibody on the patient's red cells.

In some patients the disorder tends to run an acute, self-limited course, and no treatment is necessary. If the anemia becomes severe, corticosteroids or blood transfusions may be required. In the "warm" antibody immune hemolytic anemias, splenectomy should be considered (1) if steroids have been ineffective, (2) if excessive doses of steroids are required to maintain remission, (3) if toxic manifestations of steroids become apparent, and (4) if steroids are contraindicated for other reasons. Excessive splenic sequestration of ^{51}Cr-tagged red cells offers a guide for the selection of patients who may respond to splenectomy. A favorable response is to be anticipated in about 80 percent of selected splenectomized patients. Patients without prominent spleen-liver sequestration ratios may respond to splenectomy. Late relapses may occur in splenectomized patients.

Idiopathic Thrombocytopenic Purpura

Idiopathic thrombocytopenic purpura (immune thrombocytopenic purpura) (ITP) is an acquired disorder caused by the destruction of platelets exposed to circulating IgG antiplatelet factors. The spleen is the source of these factors. It is also the major site for sequestering sensitized platelets. The term ITP should be reserved for a hemorrhagic disorder characterized by a subnormal platelet count in the presence of bone marrow containing normal or increased megakaryocytes and in the absence of any systemic disease or history of ingestion of drugs capable of inducing thrombocytopenia.

Female patients outnumber males at a ratio of 3:1. The most common presenting signs are petechiae and/or ecchymoses. ITP occurs in some patients who are HIV positive or who have acquired immunodeficiency syndrome (AIDS). In the majority of patients these signs are accompanied by one or several other symptoms, including, in order of frequency, bleeding gums, vaginal bleeding, gastrointestinal bleeding, and hematuria. In some patients the clinical manifestations take an almost cyclic course with exacerbations occurring at the time of menses. The incidence of central nervous system bleeding ranges between 1 and 2 percent and usually occurs early in the course of the disease. The spleen is rarely palpable, and its enlargement should evoke suspicion of the presence of another disease causing thrombocytopenia.

The characteristic laboratory findings include a platelet count generally reduced to 50,000 mm[3] or less and in some patients approaching zero. Associated with reduced platelet count, the bleeding time may be prolonged, but the clotting time remains normal. There is usually no significant anemia or leukopenia. When ITP is accompanied by an autoimmune hemolytic anemia it is known as Evans's syndrome. Platelet survival time following the transfusion of ^{51}Cr-labeled normal platelets is short, but this test is not necessary for establishing the diagnosis of ITP. Bone marrow examination reveals either a normal or an elevated megakaryocyte count with or without a relative increase in small forms. Qualitative changes in the megakaryocytes are characterized by degranulation of the cytoplasm, rounding of cytoplasmic

edges, the disappearance of the usual pseudopodia containing granule-free platelets, and a varying degree of vacuolization of the cytoplasm.

Acute ITP has an excellent prognosis in children under the age of sixteen; approximately 80 percent of these patients will make a complete and permanent recovery without specific therapy. Much of the discussion regarding therapy for ITP centers on the relative values and disadvantages of steroid therapy and splenectomy. In most series, the results achieved by splenectomy are significantly more impressive than are the responses to steroids (Fig. 31-5). Between 75 and 85 percent of the total number of patients subjected to splenectomy respond permanently and require no further steroid therapy. The same rates are reported for patients with systemic lupus erythematosus and AIDS. No reliable predictive factors for satisfactory response to splenectomy have been uncovered. Opinions differ regarding a correlation between an initial response to steroid therapy and the efficacy of splenectomy. In most patients the platelet count rises to over 100,000 mm[3] in 7 days. Rarely, return to normal levels may take months. Even in patients in whom the platelet count does not return to normal levels, recurrent petechiae or bleeding episodes are rare. A long-term follow-up of splenectomized patients does not support the contention that disseminated lupus erythematosus develops after this procedure.

The generally accepted protocol for managing patients with diagnosed ITP includes an initial 6-week to 2-month period of steroid therapy. Infusions of high doses of intravenous γ-globulin and plasmapheresis have been used with limited permanent success. If the patient does not respond with elevation of the platelet count, splenectomy is performed. If the patient does respond, the steroid therapy is tapered off, and if thrombocytopenia recurs, splenectomy is carried out. The same criteria pertain to patients with AIDS or HIV positivity. Any manifestation suggestive of intracranial bleeding demands emergency splenectomy. In one series, five of six patients with ITP and life-threatening intracranial bleeding were saved by splenectomy.

For patients with platelet counts approaching zero, platelet packs should be available for the operative procedure but should not be administered preoperatively. Platelet transfusion is re-

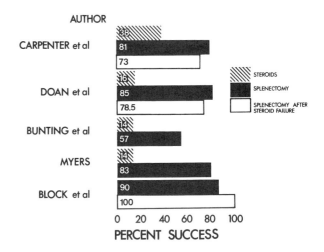

FIG. 31-5. Idiopathic thrombocytopenic purpura. Comparative responses to steroids and splenectomy. (From: *Schwartz SI, Adams JT, Bauman AW: Splenectomy for hematologic disorders. Curr Probl Surg, May 1971. Copyright 1971, Chicago, Year Book Medical Publishers. Used by permission.*)

served for patients who continue bleeding after removal of the spleen. Occasional patients in whom signs of the disease recurred months or years following splenectomy have achieved permanent cure following removal of an accessory spleen, the presence of which may be defined by technetium scan.

Systemic Lupus Erythematosus (SLE). Refractory cytopenias associated with SLE may respond to splenectomy. The platelet count returns to normal in about two-thirds of patients, the hematocrit level increases 20 percent or more, and the white cell count returns to normal in almost all patients with SLE following splenectomy.

Thrombotic Thrombocytopenic Purpura

Although thrombotic thrombocytopenic purpura (TTP) is a disease of arterioles and capillaries, there are significant accompanying hematologic changes for which the response to splenectomy may be striking. The causation has not been precisely defined, but immune mechanisms have been suggested. Approximately 5 percent of reported cases occurred during pregnancy. TTP in pregnancy must be distinguished from an idiopathic thrombocytopenia that may develop in the third trimester because this state is reversed by termination of the pregnancy. Histologically there is widespread occlusion of multiple arterioles and capillaries by hyaline membranes, with minimal inflammatory change and limited infarction.

The pentad of clinical features of virtually all cases of TTP consists of fever, purpura, hemolytic anemia, neurologic manifestations, and signs of renal disease. The pertinent laboratory findings include anemia with reticulocytosis, thrombocytopenia, and leukocytosis, sometimes accompanied by an elevated serum bilirubin level, proteinuria, hematuria, casts, or azotemia. The peripheral blood smear reveals pleomorphic, normochromic red cells that are fragmented and distorted. The degree of thrombocytopenia varies during the course of the illness, but a profound decrease in platelet count often develops within hours of onset. The bone marrow usually reveals erythroid and myeloid hyperplasia with a normal or increased number of megakaryocytes.

In the majority of cases, the disease has a rapid onset, fulminant course, and fatal outcome usually due to intracerebral hemorrhage or renal failure. Repeated plasmapheresis usually reverses the process, but in occasional cases in which no response is effected, splenectomy coupled with high-dosage steroids has resulted in cure.

Secondary Hypersplenism

Pancytopenia, thrombocytopenia, and leukopenia or anemia may occur whenever there is splenomegaly or splenic congestion. Splenomegaly with engorgement of the vascular spaces accompanies portal hypertension, resulting in accelerated destruction of the circulating cells within the spleen. The clinical manifestations of thrombocytopenia, i.e., petechiae and spontaneous bleeding, are extremely uncommon in patients with portal hypertension. As no correlation exists between the degree of anemia, leukopenia, or thrombocytopenia and the long-term survival of patients with cirrhosis, hypersplenism per se is not an indication for splenectomy in a patient with portal hypertension. Percutaneous transfemoral embolization of the splenic arterial circulation has been performed in some of these patients. Although splenic hyperfunction was controlled, the development of painful

infarction of the spleen and septic splenitis suggests that such an approach has limited value. The more common surgical situation entails the patient with bleeding esophagogastric varices accompanied by significant secondary thrombocytopenia. In the experience of Child and Turcotte with more than 300 shunts, it was necessary to perform only one splenectomy for persistent, clinically significant hypersplenism. Thrombocytopenia is generally improved by a portacaval shunt, and in the few instances in which the platelet count does not return to normal, complications are rarely attributable to thrombocytopenia. Splenectomy alone should not be performed in a patient with portal hypertension and secondary hypersplenism as there is no long-term effect on the elevated portal pressure. In the rare circumstance that splenectomy is required for a severe degree of hypersplenism in such a patient, it should be combined with a splenorenal shunt to decompress the portal circulation.

Myeloproliferative Disorders

Myeloid metaplasia is a panproliferative process manifested by increased connective tissue proliferation of the bone marrow, liver, spleen, and lymph nodes and simultaneous proliferation of hemopoietic elements in the liver, spleen, and long bones. The disease is closely related to polycythemia vera, myelogenous leukemia, and idiopathic thrombocytosis. The causation remains unclear. The spleen may be markedly enlarged, and portal hypertension has been described in some patients, due either to hepatic fibrosis of sufficient degree to be obstructive to the portal circulation or to increased forward blood flow through the splenoportal system in the absence of hepatic involvement.

Clinical manifestations generally become apparent in middle-aged and older adults. The presenting symptoms usually are related to anemia and increasing splenomegaly. Symptoms related to the spleen include the intermittent pain of splenic infarction, generalized abdominal discomfort, and a feeling of fullness after meals. Other symptoms include spontaneous bleeding, secondary infection, bone pain, pruritus, hypermetabolism, and complications associated with hyperuricemia. The most common physical findings are pallor and splenomegaly. Hepatomegaly is present in about three-quarters of the patients.

The laboratory hallmark of myeloid metaplasia is in the peripheral blood smear. The red cells are characterized by fragmentation and immature forms and poikilocytosis with numerous teardrop and elongated shapes. Characteristically, the patients have anemia of the normochromic type. The white blood cell count is under 50,000 mm^3 in the majority of the patients but may reach extremely high levels. Immature myeloid cells are found in the peripheral smear. The platelet counts are normal in about one-quarter of the patients, thrombocytopenia is present in about one-third, and marked thrombocytopenia is present in 5 percent. Thrombocytosis with a platelet count over 1,000,000 mm^3 is observed in one-quarter of the patients. The platelets are frequently enlarged and bizarre in appearance. The leukocyte alkaline phosphatase is usually high, and hyperuricemia is frequently present. Radiographs of the bone demonstrate increased density in approximately 50 percent of the patients, particularly in the pelvic region. Marrow biopsy sections show varying degrees of bone marrow replacement by fibrous tissue interposed with small foci of megakaryocytes, erythropoiesis, and myeloid cells.

Treatment is generally directed at the anemia and splenomegaly. It usually consists of transfusions, hormones, chemotherapy, and radiotherapy. Male hormone preparations may be of value in patients with anemia due to marrow failure. Alkylating agents may be effective in reducing splenic size and transfusion requirements as well as for patients whose predominant clinical problem is hypermetabolism. Busulfan is the most commonly used alkylating agent, but cyclophosphamide may also be used in thrombocytopenic subjects since it is less likely to suppress platelet production. Since patients with myelofibrosis are very sensitive to chemotherapy, such agents must be used very cautiously.

Although splenectomy does not alter the general course of the disorder, the procedure is indicated for control of anemia and thrombocytopenia, and for symptoms attributable to splenomegaly. Prolonged partial thromboplastin time, abnormal prothrombin consumption, prothrombin time, and bleeding time are usually normalized by splenectomy. Thrombocytopenia associated with sufficiently reduced megakaryocytes to contraindicate chemotherapy is also a frequent indication for splenectomy, as is the large spleen that causes digestive difficulties or is symptomatic because of multiple infarctions despite chemotherapy and/or local irradiation. In patients with esophagogastric varices portal pressures should be determined before and after splenectomy. In most instances splenectomy alone will effect significant reduction in pressure, causing varices to decrease in size or disappear and obviating the need for a concomitant splenorenal or portacaval shunt.

The old concept that splenectomy resulted in the removal of a significant hemopoietic element has been disproved. Mortality and morbidity rates for patients with myeloid metaplasia undergoing splenectomy are higher than those reported for other hematologic disorders. Splenectomy in patients with myeloid metaplasia is associated with an operative mortality of 13 percent, a morbidity rate of nearly 45 percent, and a late morbidity rate of 16 percent. Postoperative thrombocytosis and/or thrombosis of the splenic vein extending into the portal and mesenteric vein occurs more commonly in these patients. The complication is characterized by intractable ascites, hepatic failure, and renal failure that is often not noted until a week after the operation. The incidence of this complication can be reduced by correction of a thrombocytotic state, if present, preoperatively using alkylating agents and by the use of drugs to prevent platelet aggregation and clotting during the perioperative period.

Hodgkin's Disease, Lymphomas, and Leukemias

Chemotherapy and/or radiation therapy is the standard approach to treatment of these disorders.

In Hodgkin's disease, non-Hodgkin's lymphoma, and chronic lymphocytic leukemia (CLL), splenectomy has improved cytopenia in over 75 percent of cases. In these patients, palliative splenectomy should be performed before the platelet count is excessively low or there are marked clinical abnormalities. Splenectomy may allow patients to begin or maintain chemotherapy. Palliative splenectomy may be indicated for symptomatic splenomegaly.

Hairy cell leukemia, or reticuloendotheliosis, is characterized by malignant cells with filamentous cytoplasmic projections. Patients without symptomatic splenomegaly and few "hairy" cells in the circulating blood do well without any treatment. Patients who live 4 years after the diagnosis has been established have a favorable long-term prognosis and do not require splenectomy. When hairy cell leukemia is accompanied by problems caused by neutropenia, thrombocytopenia, and anemia, splenectomy is effective therapy. A complete response occurs in two-thirds to three-quarters of patients, and a partial response is effected in another 20 percent. The 5-year survival rate has been reported as 61 to 76 percent. The response to splenectomy is unrelated to the weight of the spleen. Survival is not related to the hematologic response to splenectomy. Failures are managed with steroids and chemotherapeutic agents.

Staging of Hodgkin's Disease and Non-Hodgkin's Lymphoma

The diagnosis of Hodgkin's disease is generally established by histologic evaluation of a clinically suspect area of lymphadenopathy or splenomegaly. Demonstration of the typical, large, multinuclear cell, the Sternberg-Reed cell, is regarded as essential for the diagnosis. These cells, however, do not form the bulk of the tumor. Four major histologic types have been defined: lymphocyte predominance, nodular sclerosis, mixed cellularity, and lymphocyte depletion. Survival with Hodgkin's disease is related in part to the histologic type and also to the distribution of disease and the presence or absence of specific symptoms. Stage I disease is defined as limited to one anatomic region; Stage II disease is limited to two or more contiguous or noncontiguous regions on the same side of the diaphragm; Stage III disease refers to disease on both sides of the diaphragm with involvement limited to lymph nodes, spleen, and Waldeyer's ring; and Stage IV refers to involvement of the bone marrow, lung, liver, skin, gastrointestinal tract, and any organ or tissue other than the lymph nodes or Waldeyer's ring.

The indications for surgical staging of Hodgkin's disease have decreased significantly in recent years because of greater reliance on CT scans and the more liberal use of chemotherapy, which negates the need to determine the presence of infradiaphragmatic involvement. Currently the indications for surgical staging focus on Stage I patients in whom the disease is apparently limited to one anatomic region, and on Stage II patients in whom the disease is detected in two regions above the diaphragm and the pathology demonstrates nodular sclerosis.

The staging procedure begins with obtaining a wedge biopsy specimen of the liver before retractors are applied and cause confusing white blood cell migration. Splenectomy is then carried out, followed by removal of representative retroperitoneal, mesenteric, and hepatoduodenal nodes. An iliac marrow biopsy procedure is usually included. Surgical staging was found to upgrade the clinical stage in 27 to 36 percent of cases and to decrease it in 7 to 15 percent, for a total alteration of 42 percent. Current consensus is that surgical staging is not indicated for patients with non-Hodgkin's lymphoma. In these patients the combination of CT scans, marrow biopsy, and laparoscopically directed nodal and liver biopsies offers a reasonable alternative to diagnostic celiotomy.

Miscellaneous Diseases

Felty's Syndrome. The triad of rheumatoid arthritis, splenomegaly, and neutropenia is referred to as Felty's syndrome. Mild anemia and/or thrombocytopenia has been noted in some cases, and gastric achlorhydria is common. An antibody specifically directed against neutrophil nuclei is nearly always demonstrable by fluorescent stains. Corticosteroids and splenectomy have been used to reverse the neutropenia in order to reduce susceptibility to infection. The response to steroids is usually not long-lasting, but the hematologic effects of splenectomy generally are excellent. Splenectomy in these patients should be reserved for neutropenic patients who have serious or recurrent infections, patients who require transfusions for anemia, patients with profound thrombocytopenia, and patients with intractable leg ulcers. There is a sharp rise in the total number of leukocytes in the first 24 h, reaching a peak at about the third postoperative day. Although relative neutropenia may persist, the neutrophilic response to infection in the postsplenectomy state becomes normal. The clinical course of the arthritis is rarely altered.

Sarcoidosis. This disease affects young adults. There are few constitutional symptoms, and fever is unusual, although night sweats have been noted. Cough and shortness of breath may attend mediastinal or pulmonary involvement. Skin lesions appear in about 50 percent of patients, and generalized lymphadenopathy is frequent. Involvement of the liver and spleen may produce hepatomegaly and splenomegaly in about 25 percent of patients. About 20 percent of the patients with splenomegaly develop manifestations of hypersplenism, particularly thrombocytopenic purpura. Hemolytic anemia, neutropenia, pancytopenia, and spontaneous splenic rupture have all been observed.

There is no specific treatment, and spontaneous recovery can be anticipated in the majority of cases. Splenectomy should be considered for patients with splenomegaly when there are complications of hypersplenism, since the operation has been almost uniformly followed by correction of the hematologic abnormality.

Gaucher's Disease. This is a familial disorder characterized by abnormal storage or retention of glycolipid cerebrosides in reticuloendothelial cells. Proliferation and enlargement of these cells produce enlargement of the spleen, liver, and lymph nodes. The disease is generally discovered in childhood but may become evident either early in infancy or late in adult life.

The sole clinical manifestation may be awareness of a progressively enlarging abdominal mass, primarily due to splenomegaly and, to a lesser extent, to hepatomegaly. Yellowish-brown pigmentation of the head and extremities occurs in 45 to 75 percent of cases. Bone pain and pathologic fracture may develop in long-standing cases. Many patients develop the hematologic manifestations of hypersplenism as a result of excessive sequestration of formed blood elements. Moderate to severe thrombocytopenia and normocytic anemia are almost always present, and often there is mild leukopenia. In the patients with hypersplenism, splenectomy almost uniformly has been beneficial in correcting the hematologic disorder, but there is no evidence that the operation influences the course of the basic disease. Partial splenectomy has been performed in children for symptomatic splenomegaly and hypersplenism to obviate development of overwhelming postsplenectomy infection (OPSI); 400 to 3800 g of tissue has been removed without complication. There has been no OPSI and no postoperative increase in accumulation of beta-glucocerebroside in the liver or bones. All children had an improved growth rate and hematologic picture.

Erythropoietic Porphyria. This is a congenital disorder of erythrocyte pyrrole metabolism that is transmitted as a recessive trait and characterized by the excessive deposition of porphyrins in the tissues. In the skin this results in pronounced photosensitization and severe bullous dermatitis. Premature red cell destruction within the spleen contributes to severe anemia. When the disease is complicated by hemolysis or splenomegaly, splenectomy is followed by marked improvement in the anemia and decreased concentrations of porphyrins in the red cells, bone marrow, and urine.

Systemic Mast Cell Disease (SMCD). This disorder is manifested by urticaria pigmentosa and mast cell infiltration of the skin, bone marrow, or gastrointestinal tract. In patients with aggressive disease, including lymphadenopathic mastocytosis and eosinophilia and severe thrombocytopenia, splenectomy may be beneficial, extending survival and improving the ability to tolerate chemotherapy.

OTHER LESIONS

Ectopic Spleen. This unusual condition, also known as wandering spleen, is ascribed to lengthening of the splenic ligaments, which results in extreme mobility of the organ so that the spleen of normal size may be palpable in the lower abdomen or in the pelvis. In some cases, acute torsion of the pedicle occurs, necessitating surgical intervention. Adult women are more frequently affected but males predominate in the thirty-five recorded pediatric cases. Elective splenopexy, wrapping the spleen in Dexon mesh and tacking it to the diaphragm and retroperitoneum in its normal position, is indicated to preserve the organ and prevent acute torsion.

Cysts and Tumors. Cysts of the spleen are unusual. Parasitic cysts are usually due to echinococcal involvement, while the nonparasitic cysts may be categorized as dermoid, epidermoid, epithelial, and pseudocysts. Pseudocysts occur after occult rupture of the spleen caused by trauma. Symptomatic parasitic cysts of the spleen are best managed by splenectomy. Large symptomatic nonparasitic cysts may be widely unroofed to assure permanent cure. This can be performed laparoscopically. Asymptomatic pseudocysts do not require operation but should be followed ultrasonographically to rule out significant expansion.

Primary malignant tumors of the spleen are usually sarcomatous. Primary splenic non-Hodgkin's lymphoma is a rarity which has an excellent prognosis following splenectomy. Autopsy series have refuted the concept that metastases to the spleen are rare. Exploration for undiagnosed splenomegaly rarely reveals unsuspected metastatic deposit in the absence of known generalized metastases but may establish the diagnosis of a hematologic malignancy.

Abscesses. Splenic abscess is an uncommon cause of abdominal sepsis. Primary splenic abscesses occur much more often in the tropics, where they are frequently related to thrombosis of the splenic vessels with infarction in patients with sickle cell anemia. Pyogenic splenic abscesses have been reported with increasing frequency in intravenous drug abusers. Clinical manifestations include fever, chills, splenomegaly, and left upper quadrant tenderness. Diagnosis may be established by ultrasound or CT scan (Fig. 31-6). Removal of the spleen is the operation of choice, but some patients have been treated with splenotomy and drainage when there were gross adhesions or the condition of the patient did not permit splenectomy. Splenic fungal abscesses have developed in immunosuppressed patients and in patients taking steroids or chemotherapeutic agents. Many of these patients have been on systemic antibiotics, and intestinal colonization with *Candida* developed. In some cases the ab-

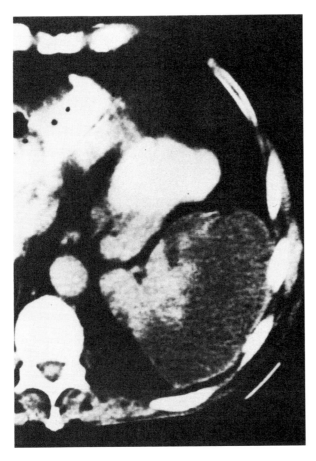

FIG. 31-6. Initial CT scan at the level of the spleen. There is a large low-density area in the spleen containing tiny gas pockets indicative of splenic abscess. *(Courtesy of Robert M. Lerner, Department of Radiology, University of Rochester Medical Center.)*

scesses resolved with treatment with antifungal drugs, but more often success has been achieved when the drugs were combined with splenectomy.

SPLENECTOMY

When elective splenectomy is performed for hematologic disorders, specific considerations arise. Patients with malignant lymphoma and leukemia may develop cryoglobulinemia, and therefore the blood should be administered at room temperature. For patients with thalassemia and, more particularly, acquired hemolytic anemia, typing and crossmatching may be difficult, and sufficient time should be allotted during the preoperative period to accumulate the blood that may be required during the operation. For patients with marked immune thrombocytopenia (ITP), platelet packs are not administered preoperatively, since the platelets are rapidly destroyed by the spleen and thus are not very effective. A nasogastric tube is inserted after endotracheal intubation to decompress the stomach and to facilitate handling of the short gastric veins.

Technique. Although the midline incision is preferred for exposure of a ruptured spleen, either a left subcostal incision or a midline incision may be used for elective resection. The spleen is mobilized initially by dividing the ligamentous attachments, which are usually avascular but may contain large vessels in

patients with secondary hypersplenism and myeloid metaplasia (Fig. 31-7*A*). The short gastric vessels are then doubly ligated and transected (Fig. 31-7*B*), with care being taken not to traumatize the stomach itself. If compromise of blood supply to the fundic portion of the greater curvature of the stomach is a concern, enfolding of this area should be performed to prevent the development of a gastric fistula. Finally, dissection of the splenic hilus with individual ligation and division of the splenic artery and vein is performed (Fig. 31-7*C*). During the course of hilar dissection, care should be taken to avoid injury to the tail of the pancreas in order to avoid pseudocyst formation. The technique of initial ligation of the splenic artery by exposure through the gastrosplenic omentum has been used in cases of hypersplenism and splenomegaly. Preoperative occlusion of the splenic artery using steel coils placed selectively in the splenic artery under radiographic control has achieved the same end.

Whenever splenectomy is performed for a hematologic disorder, a careful search should be made for accessory spleens. The splenic bed is not drained routinely, but drains are used in patients with myeloid metaplasia if there is a question of continued oozing from distended collateral veins.

Partial Splenectomy. This procedure is particularly applicable in children with Type I Gaucher's disease to minimize the risk of postsplenectomy sepsis. After transection of the ligamentous attachment to permit complete mobilization of the organ, the hilar vessels to the segment to be removed are ligated and divided. The demarcation of the devascularized segment defines the line for transection; at least 30 percent of the spleen should be preserved (Fig. 31-7*D*). Bleeding from the raw surface is controlled by cauterization, argon coagulation, or fibrin glue. The omentum can be used to cover the remaining raw surface.

Postoperative Course and Complications. Following splenectomy, characteristic changes in blood composition occur. Howell-Jolly bodies are present in almost all patients, and siderocytes are common. Generally, leukocytosis and increased platelet counts are observed. In patients with marked thrombocytopenia, the platelet count often returns to normal within 2 days, but peak levels may not be reached for 2 weeks. The white blood cell count usually is elevated the first day and may remain persistently elevated for several months. The most frequent complication is that of left lower lobe atelectasis. Other complications include subphrenic hematoma and abscess, injury to the pancreas causing fistula, or pancreatitis. Excessively elevated platelet counts, particularly in patients with myeloid metaplasia, and increased platelet adhesiveness have been reported. Although these factors have been implicated in the greater incidence of thrombophlebitis following splenectomy, many series can show no good correlation between these complications and the platelet counts. In patients with hereditary hemolytic anemia and associated red cell enzyme deficiency, postoperative thrombocytosis may lead to hepatic, portal, or caval thrombosis, particularly if the hemolytic rate is unabated by splenectomy.

There has been increasing concern regarding infection and sepsis in splenectomized patients. In a large review Singer reported that deaths from sepsis in splenectomized patients were 200 times as frequent as in the population at large. Fulminant postsplenectomy infection is very rare following removal of a traumatized spleen, but the incidence of pneumonia, septicemia, and meningitis was reported to be 166 times greater in patients who had undergone splenectomy for trauma than is expected for

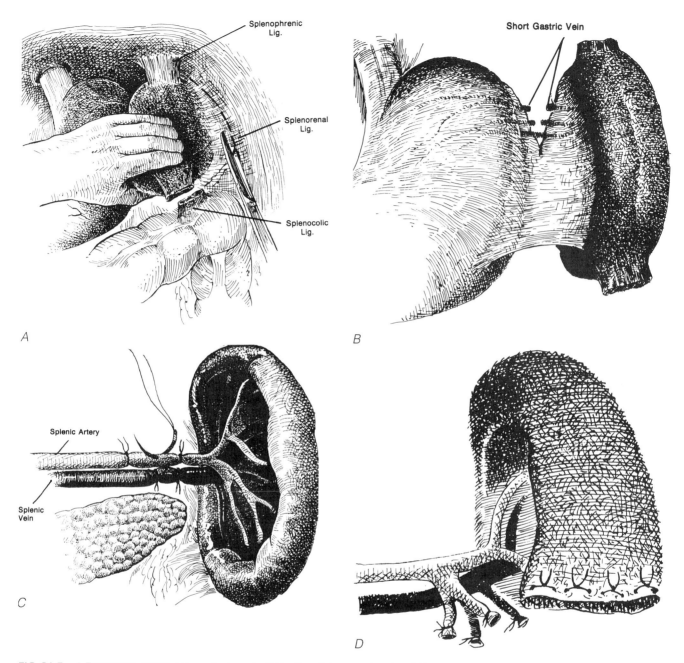

FIG. 31-7. *A.* Transection of ligamentous attachments. *B.* Ligation of short gastric veins. *C.* Management of hilus. *D.* Partial resection. (Adapted from: *Schwartz SI: Modern Technics in Surgery; Abdominal Surgery, Armonk, NY, Futura Publishing Co., 1980, chap 5, with permission.*)

the normal population. No neutrophil defect or impairment of serum opsonin or chemotactic activity could be demonstrated after splenectomy for trauma. When the risk of infection in childhood Hodgkin's disease was assessed in 181 consecutive, previously untreated patients, the episode did not correlate with splenectomy alone, but appeared to be related more to the treatment with chemotherapy and radiotherapy. In a series of 221 patients with hematologic disease, late postsplenectomy pulmonary infection was seen in eight patients; all but one were receiving immunosuppressive therapy or had advanced malignant disease.

Splenectomy results in a variety of immunologic defects, including a poor response to intravenous immunization with par-

ticulate antigens, a deficiency in phagocytosis-promoting peptide, decreased serum IgM, and decreased properdin. The organisms most frequently isolated from septic splenectomized children are those of diplococcus pneumonia and *Haemophilus influenzae*. It is therefore reasonable to delay splenectomy for hematologic disorders in very young children, especially those under the age of 2 years, to attempt to preserve the traumatized spleen in the pediatric patient and to maintain patients with at-risk diseases on long-term oral antibiotic therapy.

All patients undergoing splenectomy should receive, as prophylaxis, pneumococcus vaccine and a vaccine against *H. influenzae*, if available. Vaccination is best performed about 10 days before elective splenectomy and preoperatively in traumatized patients in whom splenectomy is anticipated, but should be performed postoperatively if preoperative vaccination was neglected. Equivalent response to pneumococcal antigens has been demonstrated for patients vaccinated after splenectomy compared with those vaccinated with the spleen in place. All children whose spleens have been removed should receive penicillin until the age of eighteen. The patients with diseases associated with high infection rates, such as thalassemia, sickle cell anemia, and autoimmune hemolytic anemia and thrombocytopenia, should not be denied splenectomy but should be kept under close surveillance postoperatively.

Bibliography

Anatomy and Physiology

Skandalakis PN, Colborn GL, et al: The surgical anatomy of the spleen. *Surg Clin North Am* 73:747, 1993.

Schwartz SI: Physiology of the spleen and the role of splenectomy in hematologic disorders, in Condon RE, DeCosse J (eds): *Surgical Care II.* Philadelphia, Lea & Febiger, 1985, chap 6, pp 118, 118–125.

Diagnostic Considerations

Freeman JL, Jafri SZ, et al: CT of congenital and acquired abnormalities of the spleen. *Radiographics* 13:597, 1993.

Pawar S, Kay CJ, et al: Sonography of splenic abscess. *AJR* 138:259, 1982.

Hematologic Disorders

Adler A, Stutzman L, et al: Splenectomy for hematologic depression in lymphocytic lymphoma and leukemia. *Cancer* 35:521, 1975.

Akwari OE, Itani KMF, et al: Splenectomy for primary and recurrent immune thrombocytopenic purpura (ITP): Current criteria for patient selection and results. *Ann Surg* 206:529, 1987.

Benbassat J, Gilon D, Penchas S: The choice between splenectomy and medical treatment in patients with advanced agnogenic myeloid metaplasia. *Am J Hematol* 33:128, 1990.

Brenner B, Nagler A, et al: Splenectomy in agnogenic myeloid metaplasia and postpolycythemic myeloid metaplasia: A study of 34 cases. *Arch Intern Med* 148:2501, 1988.

Coon WW: Splenectomy for splenomegaly and secondary hypersplenism. *World J Surg* 9:437, 1985.

Coon WW: Splenectomy for idiopathic thrombocytopenic purpura. *Surg Gynecol Obstet* 164:225, 1987.

Coon WW: Splenectomy for cytopenias associated with systemic lupus erythematosus. *Am J Surg* 155:391, 1988.

Delpero JR, Houvenaeghel G, et al: Splenectomy for hypersplenism in chronic lymphocytic leukaemia and malignant non-Hodgkin's lymphoma. *Br J Surg* 77:443, 1990.

Emond AM, Morais P, et al: Role of splenectomy in homozygous sickle cell disease in childhood. *Lancet* 1:88, 1984.

Friedman B, Darling G, et al: Splenectomy in the management of systemic mast cell disease. *Surgery* 107:94, 1990.

Golomb HM, Vardiman JW: Response to splenectomy in 65 patients with hairy cell leukemia: Evaluation of spleen weight and bone marrow involvement. *Blood* 61:349, 1983.

Gordon DH, Schaffner D, et al: Postsplenectomy thrombocytosis: Its association with mesenteric, portal, and/or renal thrombosis in patients with myeloproliferative disorders. *Arch Surg* 113:713, 1978.

Hollenberg JP, Subak LL, Ferry JJ Jr: Cost-effectiveness of splenectomy versus intravenous gamma globulin in treatment of chronic immune thrombocytopenic purpura in childhood. *J Pediatr* 112:530, 1988.

Jacobs P, King HS, et al: Splenectomy as primary treatment for hairy cell leukaemia. *Br J Surg* 74:1169, 1987.

Morgenstern L, Verham R, et al: Subtotal splenectomy for Gaucher's disease: A follow-up study. *Am Surg* 59:860, 1993.

Otsuka A, Sugihara T, Yawata Y: No beneficial effect of splenectomy in hereditary high red cell membrane phosphatidylcholine hemolytic anemia: Clinical and membrane studies of 20 patients. *Am J Hematol* 34:8, 1990.

Pinna AD, Argiolu F, et al: Indications and results for splenectomy for beta thalassemia in two hundred and twenty-one pediatric patients. *Surg Gynecol Obstet* 167:109, 1988.

Rudowski WJ: Accessory spleens: Clinical significance with particular reference to the recurrence of idiopathic thrombocytopenic purpura. *World J Surg* 9:422, 1985.

Schlinkert RT, Mann D: Laparoscopic splenectomy offers advantages in selected patients with immune thrombocytopenic purpura. *Am J Surg* 170:624, 1995.

Schneider PA, Abrams DI, et al: Immunodeficiency-associated thrombocytopenic purpura (IDTP): Response to splenectomy. *Arch Surg* 122:1175, 1987.

Schneider PA, Rayner AA, et al: The role of splenectomy in multimodality treatment of thrombotic thrombocytopenic purpura. *Ann Surg* 202:318, 1985.

Schwartz SI: Myeloproliferative disorders. *Ann Surg* 182:464, 1975.

Schwartz SI: Splenectomy for thrombocytopenia. *World J Surg* 9:416, 1985.

Schwartz SI: Role of splenectomy in hematologic disorders. *World J Surg* 20:1156, 1996.

Schwartz SI, Cooper RA Jr: Surgery in the diagnosis and treatment of Hodgkin's disease, in *Advances in Surgery.* Chicago, Year Book Medical Publishers, 1972, vol 6.

Taylor MA, Kaplan HS, Nelsen TS: Staging laparotomy with splenectomy for Hodgkin's disease: The Stanford experience. *World J Surg* 9:449, 1985.

Tyler DS, Shaunak S, et al: HIV-1-associated thrombocytopenia: The role of splenectomy. *Ann Surg* 211:211, 1990.

Van Norman AS, Nagorney DM: Splenectomy for hairy cell leukemia: A clinical review of 63 patients. *Cancer* 57:644, 1986.

VerHeyden CN, Beart RW, et al: Accessory splenectomy in management of recurrent idiopathic thrombocytopenic purpura. *Mayo Clin Proc* 53:442, 1978.

Wanachiwanawin W, Piankijagum A, et al: Emergency splenectomy in adult idiopathic thrombocytopenic purpura: A report of seven cases. *Arch Intern Med* 149:217, 1989.

Other Lesions

Allen KB, Andrews G: Pediatric wandering spleen—the case for splenopexy: Review of 35 reported cases in the literature. *J Pediatr Surg* 24:432, 1989.

Helton WS, Carrico CJ, et al: Diagnosis and treatment of splenic fungal abscesses in the immune-suppressed patient. *Arch Surg* 121:580, 1986.

Kehoe J, Straus DJ: Primary lymphoma of the spleen: Clinical features and outcome after splenectomy. *Cancer* 62:1433, 1988.

Nallathambi MN, Ivatury RR, et al: Pyogenic splenic abscess in intravenous drug addiction. *Am Surg* 53:342, 1987.

Rubin M, Yampolski I, et al: Partial splenectomy in Gaucher's disease. *J Pediatr Surg* 21:125, 1986.

Splenectomy

Boxer MA, Braun J, et al: Thromboembolic risk of postsplenectomy thrombocytosis. *Arch Surg* 113:808, 1978.

Cadiere GB, Verroken R, et al: Operative strategy in laparoscopic splenectomy. *J Am Coll Surg* 179:668, 1994.

Emmermann A, Zornig C, et al: Laparoscopic splenectomy: Techniques and results in a series of 27 cases. *Surg Endosc* 9:924, 1995.

Guzzetta PC, Ruley EJ, et al: Elective subtotal splenectomy: Indications and results in 33 patients. *Ann Surg* 211:34, 1990.

Singer DB: Postsplenectomy sepsis, in *Perspectives in Pediatric Pathology.* Chicago, Year Book Medical Publishers, 1973, vol 1, pp 285–311.

CHAPTER 32

Intraabdominal Infections

Joseph S. Solomkin, Dietmar W. Wittman, Michael A. West, and Philip S. Barie

INTRODUCTION

Intraabdominal infections are commonly encountered in surgical practice and represent an important problem in decision-making, operative technique, and perioperative management. Improvements in supportive care, diagnostic methods, anti-infective therapy, and interventional techniques have resulted in improved outcomes, decreased mortality, and a decreased incidence of recurrent abscess. Despite state-of-the-art care, infections result in considerable morbidity and mortality because of activation of local and systemic inflammatory responses.

Prompt and effective decision making is critical; delay in treatment for intraabdominal infection risks physiologic deterioration and increased mortality. Diagnostic uncertainty must be balanced against the risk of treatment delay. The precise nature of the operative procedure is a critical determinant of outcome and must be tailored to the pathology encountered.

The patient with findings suggestive of infection, typically with unexplained ileus, in whom no source of nosocomial infection can be identified by routine investigations represents a major diagnostic problem. In patients who have recently undergone abdominal operation, a concern for abscesses is often sufficient to lead to empiric treatment. Such an approach can result in overlooking less common causes of infection, bowel ischemia, pseudomembranous colitis, or pancreatitis.

STRUCTURE AND FUNCTION OF THE PERITONEAL CAVITY

Mesothelium. The total area of the peritoneum is approximately 1.8 m². It is formed by a single layer of mesothelial cells with an underlying supporting layer of highly vascularized loose connective tissue. The mesothelial cells contain microvilli 1.5 to 3.0 μm in length, which greatly increase the surface area of the mesothelial cells. The relative density of microvilli differs throughout the peritoneal cavity. Tight intra-mesothelial cell

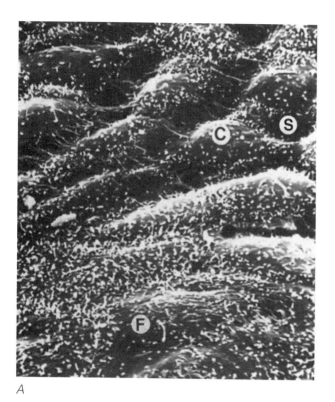

A

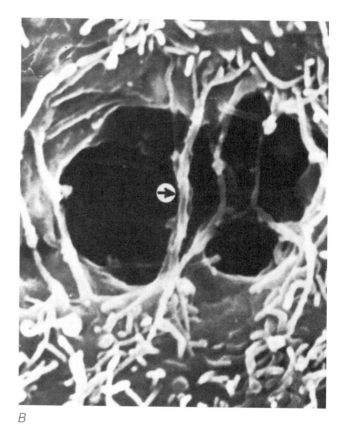

B

FIG. 32-1. *A.* There are two kinds of cells, cuboidal cells (C) and flattened cells (F), on the peritoneum of the muscular portion of the diaphragm. Stomata (S) are detected among cuboidal cells (× 1650). (Source: *JJ Chang: Study on the ultrastructure of the peritoneal stomata in humans. Acta Anatomica 141:26–30, 1991, with permission.*) *B.* There are some filamentous projections *(arrow)* across the stoma, which is a deep pore on the tendinous portion of the diaphragmatic peritoneum (× 8300). (Source: *JJ Chang, Acta Anatomica 141:26–30, 1991, with permission.*) *C.* Diagram of a typical stoma and underlying channel linking the peritoneal cavity with the lumen of a lymphatic lacuna. Lacunar mesothelial cells forming the stoma and flaplike endothelial processes that bridge the channel contain actin filaments. Where lacunar mesothelial cells and lacunar endothelial cells meet, their apposed plasma membranes lack junctional specializations. Both types of cell lack a basement membrane. The connective tissue adjacent to the channel contains abundant microfibrils. A pseudopod of a fibroblast contacts an endothelial cell. (Source: *Tsilibary EC, Wissig SL: American Journal of Anatomy 180:195, 1987, with permission.*)

junctions generally connect these cells, although there also are large intercellular gaps, sometimes as large as 500 angstroms, between these lining cells. Alterations in mesothelial cell metabolism and cellular swelling may influence diffusion across this cell layer.

Mesothelial cells are organized into two discrete populations: cuboidal cells and flattened cells. Gaps (stomata) between neighboring cells of the peritoneal mesothelium are found only among cuboidal cells. Peritonitis increases the width of these stomata. Beneath the mesothelial cells is a basement membrane of loose collagen fibers, which offers little resistance to diffusion of molecules smaller than 30 kD. The basement membrane overlies a complex connective tissue layer that includes collagen and other connective tissue proteins, elastic fibers, fibroblasts, adipose cells, endothelial cells, mast cells, eosinophils, macrophages, and lymphocytes (Fig. 32-1). The capillaries branch and ramify within the peritoneal lining layer. In addition, there is a rich lymphatic network.

Peritoneal fluid is secreted by the peritoneal serosa and has the properties of lymph. Diaphragmatic lymphatic channels provide a means for the entry of peritoneal fluid (and any bacteria and proinflammatory mediators) through the thoracic duct into the venous circulation. Inspiration decreases intrathoracic pressure relative to intraabdominal pressure, creating a pressure gradient favoring fluid movement out of the abdomen. Intravascular entry of proinflammatory substances produces many of the hemodynamic and respiratory findings of severe sepsis. Positive-pressure ventilation likely attenuates this process but has not been well studied as a therapeutic maneuver.

Anatomy. The peritoneal cavity encompasses the potential space defined by the mesothelial serous membrane and extends superiorly from the diaphragm to the pelvis in its most caudad extent (Figs. 32-2 and 32-3). Anteriorly the peritoneal cavity reflects onto the posterior aspect of the anterior abdominal musculature. Posteriorly the peritoneal lining lies superficial to the

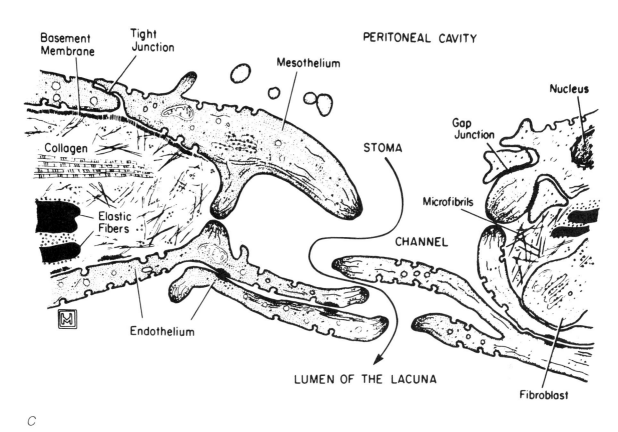

C

FIG. 32-1. Continued.

retroperitoneal viscera, including the aorta, vena cava, ureters, and kidneys. The anterior and posterior peritoneal layers are described collectively as the parietal peritoneum. The visceral peritoneum represents the mesothelial lining cells that are reflected onto the surface of the viscera, including the stomach, small bowel, spleen, liver, gallbladder, ovaries, uterus, and portions of the bladder, colon, and pancreas. The peritoneum covering the intestine is the serosa of the bowel. The peritoneum also lines the lesser sac, which communicates with the remainder of the peritoneal cavity via the epiploic foramen (foramen of Winslow). In women the peritoneal lining is reflected onto the fallopian tubes, which communicate through the open fimbriated ends with the uterus and vagina.

The visceral peritoneal lining of the liver and spleen (the "capsules") are thicker and can be detached from the underlying organ parenchyma, whereas the visceral lining of the bowel is thin and intimately attached to the lamina muscularis mucosae.

The parietal peritoneum is thicker than the visceral peritoneum and contains a richer capillary network that ramifies extensively within the peritoneal lining. This vascular supply allows the parietal peritoneum to be readily dissected free from deeper structures without altering its viability.

The retroperitoneum, which contains a subfascial plane extending from the pelvis to the posterior pharynx, is located deep to the posterior peritoneal lining. In some types of intraabdominal infection, once the inflammatory process penetrates the serosal lining, it is possible for it to spread laterally, caudad, or cephalad with relative ease.

Under normal circumstances the peritoneal cavity is largely a potential space, as only a thin film of fluid separates the parietal and visceral layers. This fluid layer serves as a lubricant, allowing the abdominal viscera to slide freely within the peritoneal cavity. The capacity of this space is illustrated during peritoneal dialysis, as 2 to 3 L of fluid are instilled into the peritoneal cavity without any patient discomfort. Inflammation of the immense surface area of the peritoneal mesothelium can result in massive fluid shifts. For example, an increase in thickness of the peritoneal lining of 1 mm will sequester around 1.8 L of fluid. Peritonitis thus may be regarded as requiring the resuscitation equivalent of an 80 percent burn.

Compartmentalization of the peritoneal cavity by various ligaments and retroperitoneal attachments creates several recesses into which fluid or exudate may pool (see Fig. 32-3).

Inframesocolic Spaces. The area below the transverse mesocolon is subdivided into several gutters, or watersheds, by the ascending and descending colon, the root of the mesentery, and the pelvic mesosigmoid. The *right lateral paracolic gutter* lies between the cecum and ascending colon and the right lateral abdominal wall. The drainage pathway of the right lateral paracolic gutter is in a superior direction when the patient is in the supine position, since the superior portion of this sulcus lies on a more posterior plane than the inferior portion. The right lateral paracolic gutter continues superiorly to the region behind the right lobe of the liver and anterior to the right kidney as the hepatorenal pouch. The hepatorenal pouch communicates through the foramen of Winslow with the lesser sac.

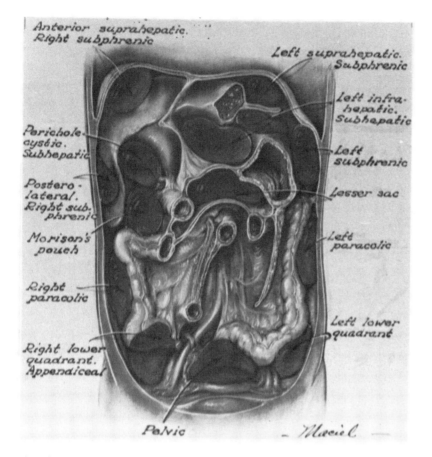

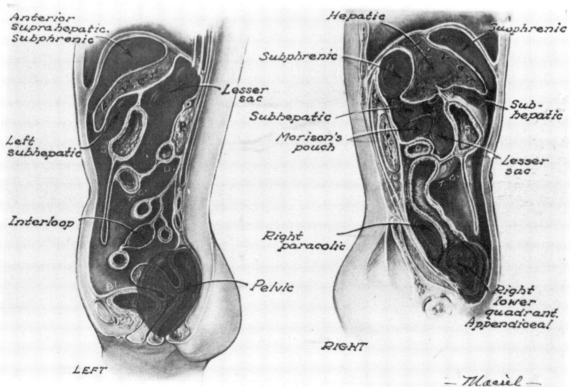

FIG. 32-2. Anterior and left and right sagittal views of the peritoneal cavity demonstrating the anatomic locations of various intraperitoneal abscesses, such as right lower quadrant, subphrenic, subhepatic, pelvic, lesser sac, interloop, Morison's pouch, right paracolic, and left paracolic. (From: *Altemeier WA, Culbertson WR, et al: Intra-abdominal sepsis. Adv Surg 5:305, 1961, with permission.*)

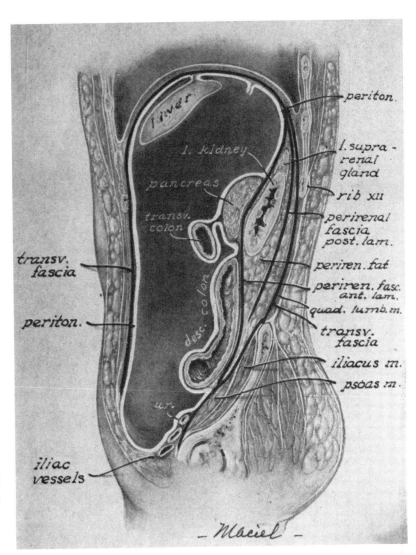

FIG. 32-3. Left sagittal drawing of the compartments of the retroperitoneal space in this area and its relationship to the contiguous viscera. Note that the anterior and posterior layers of the renal fascia are fused superiorly but open inferiorly, favoring the spread of infections inferiorly. (From: *Altemeier WA, Retroperitoneal abscess. Arch Surg 83:512, 1961, with permission.*)

Between the mesentery and the cecum and ascending colon is the *right medial paracolic gutter.* This recess is limited inferiorly by the junction of the mesentery and the jejunum and ileum, where the mesentery meets with the cecum, and superiorly by the transverse mesocolon. The drainage from the right medial paracolic gutter occurs in a superior direction, passing above the root of the mesentery into the *left medial paracolic gutter.* The left medial paracolic gutter is limited by the transverse mesocolon above, by the root of the mesentery on the right, and by the descending and sigmoid colon on the left. Drainage from the left medial paracolic gutter is downward into the pelvis. The *left lateral paracolic gutter* extends superiorly from the phrenicocolic ligament to the sigmoid colon inferiorly and from the descending colon on the right to the left lateral abdominal wall. Fluids in the left lateral paracolic gutter tend to remain there.

Supramesocolic Spaces. With the patient in the supine position, drainage on the right tends to flow superiorly toward the right subphrenic area. This area in turn is divided into two portions, a right and a left, by the falciform ligament, which extends from the anterior abdominal wall and inferior surface of the diaphragm to the anterosuperior surface of the liver. The right

subphrenic space is further subdivided by the right lobe of the liver into a suprahepatic portion and an infrahepatic portion. The left subphrenic area is divided by the left lobe of the liver and the horizontally placed stomach and lesser omentum. There are two major subdivisions of this space. The larger area lies anterior to the stomach, the spleen, and the left lobe of the liver and is limited by the diaphragm and the abdominal wall anteriorly. The smaller area, the lesser sac, lies behind the stomach and lesser omentum.

With the body in the supine position, the most dependent recess is in the pelvis. In the upper abdomen, the posterosuperior extension of the subhepatic space known as Morison's pouch also collects fluid in recumbent individuals. Morison's pouch connects via the foramen of Winslow (bounded by the free border of the gastrohepatic omentum and the posterior parietal peritoneum) to the lesser sac, which is the largest recess in the peritoneal cavity. Because of the limited communication of the lesser sac to the main peritoneal cavity, abscesses in the lesser sac may not produce physical signs on examination of the anterior abdominal wall. The left subhepatic and subphrenic spaces communicate freely around the small lateral left hepatic lobe. The falciform ligament limits communication between the right and left subphrenic spaces. This may explain the clinical observation that fewer than 15 percent of subphrenic abscesses are bilateral.

Innervation. Innervation of the peritoneal lining figures prominently in clinical recognition of intraabdominal infections. There are some nerve fibers within the visceral peritoneum, but they are much less numerous than those in the parietal peritoneum. They arise from the visceral structures beneath the mesothelial lining. Stretching of the visceral peritoneum produces nausea and poorly localized pain. Most intraperitoneal visceral structures arise from the embryologic foregut, and, accordingly, their nerve supply arises from the visceral branches of the vagus nerve. Pain usually is localized to the dermatome distribution of the associated visceral organ (Table 32-1). For example, the gallbladder arises from the upper thoracic dermatomes; hence, with stretching of the visceral peritoneum overlying the gallbladder, pain is initially perceived as arising in the epigastrium and right upper back. When the inflammatory process also involves the adjacent diaphragmatic structures, pain also may be perceived in the neck or shoulder because the diaphragm arises from and is innervated by the cervical dermatomes. Visceral peritoneal irritation, usually from distention of a hollow viscus, causes dull, poorly localized, often periumbilical, and often crampy pain. Visceral structures are generally completely insensitive to surgical transection, cauterization, heat, cold, or pinching.

The nerve supply of the parietal peritoneum, the somatic afferents, arises from branches of cutaneous nerves in the anterior abdominal wall. In contrast to the visceral peritoneum, the parietal peritoneum is exquisitely pain sensitive to stretch as well as light touch and cutting, particularly anteriorly. Pain arising from irritation of the parietal peritoneum can usually be very precisely localized by patients and is the basis for the clinical findings of "peritoneal signs." Anterior parietal peritoneal pain may be associated with tenderness and involuntary muscle spasm (guarding). "Rebound tenderness" can sometimes be elicited from the taut peritoneum even in the absence of inflammation, such as in ileus. Irritation of the peripheral diaphragmatic peritoneum is perceived as pain in the adjacent body wall, whereas central irritation manifests itself as ipsilateral shoulder pain. Diaphragmatic irritation may arise not only from direct involvement by adjacent inflammation but also from the movement of infected fluid into the subphrenic spaces.

The blood and lymphatic supply of the peritoneum generally follow the distribution of the innervation. The blood supply of the visceral peritoneum arises from the ajdacent visceral organ.

PHYSIOLOGY OF THE PERITONEUM

Peritoneal Fluid Exchange. The mesothelial lining cells of the peritoneum secrete serous fluid that circulates within the peritoneal cavity. The peritoneal cavity normally contains 50 to 100 mL of fluid with solute concentrations nearly identical to that of plasma. The protein content of peritoneal fluid is somewhat less than that of plasma, about 3 g/dL. Fluid is absorbed by the peritoneal mesothelial lining cells and subdiaphragmatic lymphatics. Mesothelial cells also absorb solutes by the continuous process of endocytosis. Exchange of solutes across the peritoneal lining is the basis for peritoneal dialysis. Most solutes with a molecular weight less than 30 kD traverse the mesothelial lining with relative ease. Splanchnic blood flow and factors that alter membrane permeability affect the efficiency of fluid exchange. Peritoneal permeability is markedly increased by intraperitoneal inflammation.

Peritoneal Fluid Movement. The routes of normal fluid movement within the peritoneum have been defined by injection of water-soluble contrast material into normal individuals. The right paracolic gutter is the main conduit between the upper and lower peritoneal cavities, because the left gutter is obstructed by the phrenicocolic and splenorenal ligaments. Fluid introduced into the right upper quadrant gravitates inferiorly via the subhepatic space into the right subphrenic space. From there it may travel inferiorly into the pelvis via the right gutter before returning to the upper abdomen. Because of the obstruction on the left, fluid from the left upper quadrant migrates into the left subphrenic space. Fluid introduced into the lower abdomen gravitates first to the pelvis, and thereafter ascends, even with the patient in the upright position, into the subhepatic and subphrenic spaces.

Two primary forces govern the movement of fluid within the peritoneal cavity: gravity and the negative pressure created beneath the diaphragm with each normal respiratory cycle. Fluid flux within the peritoneal cavity is dramatically altered by the presence of adhesions, fibrin, paralytic ileus, or mechanical ventilation. Movement of fluid into the pelvis was in the past an important component of the surgical treatment of intraabdominal infections. Earlier generations of surgeons routinely positioned patients in Fowler's position—almost a sitting position—to facilitate dependent movement of purulent material and formation of a pelvic abscess, which could then be drained transrectally without laparotomy. Today the Fowler position is seldom used and pelvic abscesses are relatively rare. Intraabdominal abscesses are most frequently encountered beneath the liver or diaphragm and between loops of bowel.

Subphrenic purulent fluid collections occur because a relatively negative pressure is created beneath the diaphragm with each exhalation. Intraperitoneal pressure measurements show that the pressure is lowest beneath the diaphragm during expiration. The diaphragm raises during exhalation, producing a transiently larger space in the upper abdomen. As the volume increases the pressure decreases. Lower pressures are encountered whether patients are breathing spontaneously or on mechanical ventilation. With positive-pressure mechanical ventilation there

Table 32-1
Dermatome Origin of the Innervation of Intraabdominal Structures

Organ/Structure	Dermatome Innervation
Esophagus	Vagus (brainstem)
Stomach	T5–7
Small intestine	T8–10
Colon	T10–L1
Liver	T6–8
Gallbladder	T6–8
Uterus	T10–L1
Kidney	T10–L1
Bladder	S2–4
Diaphragm	C4–8

C = cervical; L = lumbar; T = thoracic; S = sacral.

is a significantly impaired capacity of the peritoneal cavity to clear particulate debris.

Peritoneal Response to Injury

Peritoneal Injury and Repair. Any inflammatory event in the peritoneal cavity results in local peritoneal irritation with loss of regional mesothelial cells. The defect in the mesothelial lining is repaired by "metastasis" of nearby mesothelial lining cells. Peritoneal defects heal everywhere simultaneously. A large peritoneal defect heals in the same amount of time as a small defect, usually 3 to 5 days. This process is rapid and usually reconstitutes the peritoneal continuity without adhesion formation. The origin of the migrating mesothelial cells remains obscure; they may arise from submesothelial stem cells.

Adhesion Formation. Fibrin polymerization occurs when platelets and fibrin come into contact with the exposed basement membrane, an automatic accompaniment of intraperitoneal inflammation. Normally, well-oxygenated intact mesothelial cells produce plasminogen activator, which lyses the fibrin clots that form after acute injury. In experimental wounds fibrinolytic activity has been found to be minimal 3 days after injury, before reconstitution of the mesothelial integrity. Fibrinolytic activity increases to supranormal levels 8 days after injury. With hypoxia the fibrous adhesions are invaded by fibroblasts and there is stimulation of angiogenesis and collagen synthesis. Fully developed fibrous adhesions are seen at 10 days and become maximal 2 to 3 weeks after peritoneal injury. This explains the difficulty of reoperation 2 to 4 weeks after an acute insult. With time, fibrous adhesions undergo remodeling and usually become progressively attenuated. In patients with intraabdominal soiling complications, such as patients with enterocutaneous fistulas, mortality is 20 percent in operations performed between 10 and 120 days but 10 percent before 10 days and after 120 days.

Host Defense Against Intraabdominal Infection

The three major intraperitoneal defense mechanisms are (1) mechanical clearance of bacteria via lymphatics, (2) phagocytic killing of bacteria by immune cells, and (3) mechanical sequestration. Experimentally, bacterial clearance occurs rapidly, before influx of phagocytic cells. Particulate material within the peritoneal cavity is cleared through stomata that overlie large lymphatic channels (lacunae) on the subdiaphragmatic surface. Diaphragmatic movement with respiration produces influx of fluid into the lacunae with exhalation, and respiratory contraction empties the lacunae into the thoracic duct and ultimately the left subclavian vein. Bacteria (1 to 2 μm) and red blood cells (7 to 8 μm) readily pass through the stomata (8 to 12 μm) into the thoracic duct and thence into the central venous blood. This rapid access of bacterial products to the systemic circulation explains why patients who develop an acute gastrointestinal perforation often present with rigors and fever.

PATHOPHYSIOLOGY OF THE LOCAL AND SYSTEMIC RESPONSE TO INTRAABDOMINAL INFECTIONS

The cellular defense mechanisms of the peritoneal cavity help to explain the specific pattern of response. Elements of these defenses include resident peritoneal macrophages and large recruitable pools of circulating neutrophils and monocytes, cell types

that participate in abscess formation. Ingestion of microorganisms by these cells may result in secretion of a variety of proinflammatory molecules that generate the systemic response (Table 32-2).

The peritoneal host defense system also serves to localize and contain bacterial contamination. Hyperemia and exudation of fluid follow activation of immune cells (macrophages, and probably mast cells) and sloughing of peritoneal mesothelium. Histamine and other permeability-increasing substances mediate this response. Several events favor the deposition of fibrin, including the activation of mesothelial and macrophage-mediated procoagulant activity acting on fibrinogen in reactive peritoneal fluid, coupled with the loss of plasminogen activator from mesothelial cells. The combined effect is the deposition of fibrinous exudates that serve to wall off and trap bacteria. Ileus and adhesion formation accentuate the process, but extensive loculation may impede immune cell migration to sites of infection.

The defense system's recognition that microorganisms are present within the peritoneal cavity occurs primarily through phagocytosis of the microorganisms by resident peritoneal macrophages. This results in activation of the local macrophages, with secretion of proinflammatory signaling molecules that recruit from a large circulating pool of phagocytes.

Cells Involved in the Inflammatory Response in the Peritoneal Cavity. At least four major cell types play key roles in the inflammatory response. These include resident as well as recruited macrophages, mesothelial cells, adjacent capillary endothelial cells, and recruited neutrophils. While the macrophage has been traditionally considered the first line of cellular defense, developments in our understanding of cytokines and the immunologic functions of mesothelial cells suggest that the inflammatory response is actually initiated by interactions between these two cell types. It has been suggested that the mesothelial cell could even be considered an immune cell, if this designation were not dependent on its lineage. The first step in the response to contamination is probably induced by a host response to mi-

Table 32-2
Mediators Released After Intraabdominal Injury or Infection

Mediator	Action
Tumor necrosis factor (TNF)	Amplifies inflammatory response
	Increased vascular permeability
	Endothelial adherence for PMNs
	Primes PMNs for phagocytosis
Interleukin (IL)-1	Endothelial PMN adherence
	Enhances release of IL-2
	Amplifies acute inflammatory response
	Lymphocyte activation
IL-8	PMN chemotaxis
Histamine	Increased vascular permeability
	Leukocyte activation
Complement	Bacterial destruction
	PMN chemotaxis (C5a, C3a)
	Bacterial opsonization (C3b)
Platelet-activating factor (PAF)	Activates PMNs
	Activates macrophages
	Endothelial PMN adherence
	Potent vasoconstrictor

C = complement; PMN = polymorphonuclear leukocyte.

crobial cell products. In the case of gram-negative organisms, this is most likely lipopolysaccharide (LPS). For gram-positive organisms, the cell wall product teichoic acid and specific cell wall glycans induce a macrophage response. Lipopolysaccharide, present on gram-negative organisms, interacts with monocytes and other cell types, including subpopulations of neutrophils via the CD14 receptor. Interaction with the CD14 receptor is mediated by lipopolysaccharide binding protein (LBP), and leads to macrophage activation, with subsequent production of tumor necrosis factor-α (TNF-α), interleukin (IL)-1, IL-6, IL-8, granulocyte-macrophage colony-stimulating factor (GM-CSF), prostaglandin E_2 (PGE$_2$), and nitric oxide. LPS is a very potent immunomodulator, with concentrations in the few-picograms-per-milliliter range inducing near maximal responses from human cells.

Macrophages. Macrophages, including resident peritoneal macrophages and those recruited from the circulation, serve as an early line of cellular defense and coordinate the inflammatory response. Macrophage products include IL-1, IL-6, IL-8, IL-10, IL-12, TNF-α, GM-CSF, granulocyte colony-stimulating factor (G-CSF), monocyte chemoattractant protein-1 (MCP-1), monocyte inflammatory protein α (MIP-α), and several eicosanoids. These molecules recruit and activate mesothelial cells as secretors of inflammatory molecules. Mechanisms of macrophage microbicidal activity and associated parenchymal injury include the respiratory burst and release of proteolytic enzymes into intracellular vesicles and into the extracellular space. These enzymes include plasminogen activator, collagenase, elastase, gelatinase, acid phosphatase, and cathepsin D.

Mesothelial Cells. Macrophage secretion products and microbes and their products activate and injure mesothelial cells. This mesothelial injury is a prominent feature of most types of inflammation. In response to these products mesothelial cells produce a variety of inflammatory molecules that recruit additional cells to the peritoneal cavity and activate them there. Mesothelial cells secrete IL-8, a neutrophil chemoattractant and activator. Macrophage-secreted components of complement, upon activation, also recruit neutrophils and monocytes. Mesothelial cells also express various adhesion molecules that promote leukocyte–mesothelial cell adherence.

Neutrophils. Neutrophils are the key effector cells in the inflammatory response and are responsible for the parenchymal destruction seen in inflammation. Neutrophils possess an array of granular enzymes that are capable of digesting basement and interstitial proteins, facilitating directed migration and allowing for digestion of injured tissue. Neutrophil-derived proteases also can degrade a variety of functionally important molecules found at sites of inflammation, including immunoglobulins and intermediates of the kinin, complement, fibrinolytic, and clotting cascades. Neutrophil azurophilic granules also contain the cationic antibacterial protein bactericidal permeability increasing (BPI) factor. BPI factor has sequence homology with lipopolysaccharide-binding protein and binds to the lipid A portion of lipopolysaccharide, preventing its interaction with the CD14 receptor and thereby inhibiting its toxic effects. BPI factor is also specifically cytotoxic to gram-negative bacteria. Neutrophil microbicidal activity and cytotoxicity are in part determined by a nicotinamide adenine dinucleotide phosphate (NADPH) oxidase, which produces reactive oxygen intermediates. NADPH oxidase, a membrane-bound enzyme, produces reactive oxygen species such as hydrogen peroxide. Neutrophils also secrete TNF-α,

IL-1, and IL-8, which activate cells and recruit additional neutrophils to sites of inflammation; in turn, they are highly responsive to TNF-α, IL-1β, IL-6, and IL-8.

Host defense systems have an obligatory requirement for molecular oxygen to enable the humoral and cellular immune systems to function optimally. Normally, after opsonization a microorganism is phagocytosed by a neutrophil. The phagosome containing the bacteria then fuses with lysosomal granules within the neutrophils. In the presence of molecular oxygen, toxic oxygen radicals, such as hydrogen peroxide or superoxide, are generated, which result in lysis of bacteria. In the presence of devitalized tissue and in many shock states, delivery of oxygen to the neutrophils is inadequate. In these instances, even though phagocytosis may occur, bacteria may not be destroyed and infection develops or persists.

Endothelial Cells. Macrophage, neutrophil, and mesothelial cell products also injure the closely approximated endothelial cell lining and can thereby increase movement of mediators into the vascular space. It is only upon activation or injury, mediated by TNF-α, IL-1, or oxygen radicals, that the endothelial cells secrete inflammatory molecules, which enhance leukocyte-endothelial adhesion and leukocyte transendothelial cell migration. Thus activation of the vascular endothelium is a key mechanism of inflammation.

Endothelial cells produce a variety of adhesion molecules, including members of the selectin and immunoglobulin families, that mediate leukocyte trafficking to sites of inflammation. Endothelial cells also produce IL-8 and platelet-activating factor (PAF), which localize on the endothelial surface in association with various extracellular-matrix proteins. Endothelial cell-associated IL-8 and PAF contribute to the arrest of neutrophil locomotion and also activate them. IL-8 also is thought to mediate neutrophil emigration from the vasculature, in part by forming a chemotactic gradient from the luminal side to the basal side of the endothelium.

Other Cells. Additional cell types also are recruited in the acute inflammatory response. Platelet activation and adherence to sites of injury results in the formation of platelet plugs. During activation, platelets release several preformed molecules into the area of evolving inflammation, including platelet basic protein and its proteolytic derivative neutrophil-activating peptide 2 (NAP-2), a neutrophil chemoattractant. Platelets also produce PAF, tumor growth factor β (TGF-β), prostaglandins, thromboxane A$_2$ (TXA$_2$), lipoxin A$_4$ (LXA$_4$), and nitric oxide, which can modulate the inflammatory response. Vascular smooth muscle cells and fibroblasts also can release cytokines that can modulate the immune response. Additionally, T and B cells participate in the specific inflammatory response by recognition of antigens presented by monocytes, epithelial cells, and endothelial cells.

Mechanisms of Cell Recruitment to Sites of Injury: The Chemokines and Other Chemoattractants

Nonchemokine Chemoattractants. An early epithelial and endothelial event is contraction of these cells, allowing the influx of several important classes of molecules, including components of the complement system. The complement system is a series of proteins whose ordered polymerization results in activation of the coagulation system, the release of inflammatory molecules, recruitment of leukocytes (C5a), opsonization of microorganisms (C3b), and induction of microbial and host cell lysis (membrane attack complex). Released C5a also induces polymorphonuclear cell activation, adherence, and aggregation. C5a can induce the production of TNF-α, IL-1, and IL-6 by monocytes. In the lung C5a increases vascular resistance and induces hypoxemia. Complement also synergistically enhances the effects of TNFα in producing hemorrhagic necrosis.

Other chemoattractants recruit cells to the peritoneal cavity, including leukotriene B$_4$ (LTB$_4$), formyl-methionyl-leucyl-phenylalanine (FMLP), and platelet activating factor (PAF). LTB$_4$ is generated by macrophages (and other cells) in response to such stimuli as LPS. LTB$_4$ is chemotactic for neutrophils and increases neutrophil adhesion to endothelium. It also promotes IL-1, IL-6, TNF-α, and H$_2$O$_2$ production by monocytes. Additionally, LTB$_4$ increases vascular permeability. FMLP is derived from bacterial cell walls and induces neutrophil and monocyte chemotaxis, degranulation, superoxide production, and phagocytosis. PAF, released by neutrophils, monocytes, platelets, and endothelial cells, also stimulates macrophage and neutrophil chemotaxis. PAF also enhances superoxide production by neutrophils at the endothelial surface, increases endothelial permeability, alters vascular reactivity, enhances platelet aggregation, and stimulates production of eicosanoids. PAF release from endothelial cells can be induced by TNF, IL-1, LPS, thrombin, phorbol myristate acetate, histamine, leukotrienes, and reactive oxygen species.

Chemokines. Chemokines, or chemotactic cytokines, are the key mediators of leukocyte recruitment to sites of inflammation. Two broad categories of chemokines are the CXC chemokines and the CC chemokines, where "C" refers to the location of cysteine residues in the molecules.

CXC Chemokines. Important cytokines in this category include IL-8, NAP-2, and melanoma growth stimulatory activity/growth related oncogene (MGSA/GRO). IL-8 is an 8-kD protein that is produced by macrophages, mesothelial epithelial cells, neutrophils, endothelial cells, fibroblasts, T cells, and hepatocytes. IL-8 and, to a variable extent, NAP-2 and GRO induce neutrophil chemotaxis, prime neutrophils for enhanced superoxide production, modulate adhesion molecule expression, and enhance transendothelial migration. IL-8 also has some chemotactic activity on lymphocytes.

Several studies have identified elevated plasma levels of IL-8 in various patient groups. However, IL-8 is only functional when bound to matrix and cell surface proteins. Free IL-8 is bound by circulating autoantibodies and to a low-specificity erythrocyte receptor, the Duffy antigen, which may serve as a clearing mechanism. The cell surface-IL-8 interaction is dependent on specific heparin molecules, which provide a high degree of specificity to the response. Heparin sulfate proteoglycan chains self-associate and bind to various extracellular matrix proteins, growth factors, and cell surface enzymes. Heparinase activity releases growth factors from their heparin sulfate storage sites in the extracellular matrix, providing a mechanism for the induction of migration of diverse cell types in normal or pathologic situations. Neutrophils themselves possess and secrete heparinases.

GROα is secreted by endothelial cells, monocytes, and fibroblasts after stimulation with LPS, IL-1, or TNF-α. NAP-2 is derived from cleavage of a platelet secretory product, platelet basic protein. Macrophages and neutrophils can cleave it from its precursors, and NAP-2 serves to modify subsequent neutrophil function.

CC Chemokines. The second set of chemokines, CC chemokines, include monocyte inflammatory protein (MIP), monocyte chemoattractant protein (MCP), and RANTES. MCP-1 is a 76 AA polypeptide, produced by monocytes, endothelial cells, lymphocytes, and fibroblasts, that induces monocyte chemotaxis and activation. Mononuclear phagocyte-derived MIP-1α is chemotactic for T cells and monocytes. MIP-1 is produced by monocytes, lymphocytes, and fibroblasts and mediates both T cell chemotaxis and adhesion. RANTES is induced by TNFα and IL-1 in lung epithelial cells and is chemotactic for T lymphocytes.

Leukocyte–Endothelial Cell Adhesion and Emigration from the Vasculature.

Binding of the recruited leukocyte to the endothelial cell, emigration from the vasculature and into the parenchyma, and subsequent activation are mediated via a series of adhesion molecules. These include members of the immunoglobulin (intercellular adhesion molecule, ICAM), integrin, and selectin families. A well-accepted model of neutrophil adhesion to endothelium involves at least three sequential events.

Selectin-Mediated Leukocyte Rolling. The first stage, rolling, occurs constantly and involves the transition of the leukocyte from the circulating state, in which it is moving in the center of the vessel, to a slower rolling state, in which it is tumbling along the wall of the capillary or venule. Rolling leukocytes may adhere firmly or may detach and rejoin the mainstream of flowing blood. The prevailing wall sheer rate in postcapillary venules determines in part the level of leukocyte rolling and of firm adhesion and dictates the contact area between rolling leukocytes and the endothelial cell surface.

Rolling involves the selectins, which are calcium-dependent glycoprotein receptors that have a common molecular structure. The selectins are named after the cell type on which they are primarily found: E-selectin (endothelial cell), P-selectin (platelet), and L-selectin (leukocyte). L-selectin mediates rolling in part by presenting neutrophil carbohydrate ligands to the endothelial E- and P-selectins. E-selectin (endothelial leukocyte adhesion molecule-1, ELAM-1) is found exclusively on endothelial cells activated by TNF-α, IL-1, LPS, interferon-γ, and substance P. It allows endothelial cells to bind to neutrophils, monocytes, and certain memory T cells. L-selectin is expressed by neutrophils and monocytes as well as certain populations of lymphocytes, natural killer (NK) cells, and hematopoietic progenitor cells. It is concentrated on the microvilli projections of unstimulated neutrophils. Rolling also allows neutrophils to pick up endothelial-borne chemical signals such as IL-8 and PAF, which then promote integrin-mediated adhesion and subsequent migration of neutrophils.

Integrin-Mediated Leukocyte Activation and Transendothelial Migration. The second event in neutrophil–endothelial cell adhesion is activation, mediated by chemotactic agents that are released from or are attached to the endothelium. Leukocyte surface expression of the β_2 integrin CD11B/CD18 integrin is increased. This activation enables the third stage of firm adhesion and transendothelial migration to occur by promoting the function of integrin adhesion molecules on the leukocyte surface.

Subsequent neutrophil transmigration to the extravascular space involves adherence via other leukocyte integrins.

Cytokines in the Systemic Response to Infection. Liver dysfunction is common during the course of intraabdominal infection and occasionally progresses to fatal hepatic failure. There is considerable evidence that various macrophage products, including IL-1, IL-6, and TNF-γ, substantially alter hepatocyte function. Aside from conversion of hepatic synthetic function to acute phase reactants, serum chemistry studies reveal evidence of ductal epithelial cytotoxicity, including elevated levels of alkaline phosphatase and bilirubin. The large number of fixed tissue phagocytes (Kupffer cells) in the liver capable of responding to endotoxin absorbed from systemic or mesenteric blood vessels represents a potentially important source of cytokines and other hepatocyte regulatory substances, although portal endotoxemia has not been detected in humans.

BACTERIOLOGY OF PERITONITIS AND INTRAABDOMINAL INFECTION

Normal Bowel Flora. The vast majority of the bacteria in the colon are anaerobic species that, so far as is known, contribute little to clinical intraabdominal infection. The most common bacteria isolated in clinical infections are *Escherichia coli* and *Enterobacter, Klebsiella,* and *Pseudomonas* species (Table 32-3), which make up less than 0.1 percent of the normal colonic flora. Even the most common anaerobic pathogen, *Bacteroides fragilis,* accounts for only 1 percent of the colonic flora. The presence of large numbers of nonpathogenic bacteria provides a measure of protection to the host by suppressing the growth of potentially pathogenic bacteria. Overgrowth of pathogenic gram-negative aerobic bacteria is commonly seen after treatment with broad-spectrum antibiotics. Many of these bacteria are associated with nosocomial infections that are much more difficult to eradicate.

Effect of Level of Gastrointestinal Perforation. The morbidity and mortality of intraabdominal infections vary dramatically with the level of gastrointestinal tract perforation, because the number and type of microorganisms vary throughout the gastrointestinal tract. Under normal circumstances the stomach contains fewer than 10^3 bacteria per cubic millimeter, largely because of the action of hydrochloric acid and the very low pH in the stomach. When patients receive H_2-receptor blockers and proton-pump inhibitors that raise gastric pH, the number of bacteria rapidly approaches the levels seen in the proximal small bowel. The number of bacteria per cubic millimeter increases with distance down the gastrointestinal tract. In the proximal small bowel there are approximately 10^4 to 10^5 bacteria/mm^3, whereas the terminal ileum contains more than 10^9/mm^3. The highest absolute numbers of bacteria are found in the colon, where there are between 10^{10} and 10^{12} bacteria/mm^3.

The type of bacteria changes with distance down the gastrointestinal tract as well. In the upper gastrointestinal tract facultative gram-negative aerobic bacteria predominate, whereas the colon contains many more anaerobic than aerobic bacteria. In the colon, gram-negative and gram-positive anaerobic bacteria are present, along with facultative aerobes. The number of species of bacteria isolated also is highest in the colon, with more than 500 species of bacteria and fungi.

Virulence Factors. Virulence factors provide pathogenic bacteria with a selective advantage in that they thwart normal host defense mechanisms by impairing opsonization or phagocytosis. In other cases, extracellular products such as coagulase and catalase are secreted by *Staphylococcus aureus.* In the case of *B. fragilis,* the presence of a polysaccharide capsule is strongly associated with abscess formation. In experimental studies, the injection of a component of the polysaccharide capsule is as efficient as the entire bacteria for causing abscesses.

Microbial Adherence to Peritoneum. Microbial colonization of the peritoneal mesothelial surface is a rapid phenomenon after penetration injury of the distal bowel. Bacteria adherent to the peritoneum are resistant to removal by peritoneal lavage, in contrast to the bacteria present in peritoneal fluid, which are significantly decreased after lavage. Enterobacteriaceae (aerobic *E. coli* and similar organisms) rapidly colonize serosal mesothelium and become the predominant flora within 4 h after induction of peritonitis. After 8 h, the *B. fragilis* group is the predominant organism adherent to the peritoneum and is unaffected by extended saline lavage.

Antimicrobial lavage produces an immediate but transitory decrease in the numbers of bacteria; the microbial population exceeds prelavage levels 24 h later. This favors reexploration at 24-h intervals when operative management of intraabdominal infection is done by staged abdominal repair.

Role of Aerobic and Anaerobic Bacteria. Among aerobic bacteria, gram-negative species of the Enterobacteriaceae family (particularly *E. coli*) and the *Klebsiella* and *Enterobacter*

Table 32-3
Bacteria Commonly Encountered in Intraabdominal Infections

Facultative Gram-negative Bacilli	Obligate Anaerobes	Facultative Gram-positive Cocci
Escherichia coli	*Bacteroides fragilis*	Enterococci
Klebsiella species	*Bacteroides* species	*Staphylococcus* species
Proteus species	*Fusobacterium* species	*Streptococcus* species
Enterobacter species	*Clostridium* species	
Morganella morganii	*Peptococcus* species	
Other enteric gram-negative bacilli	*Pepostreptococcus* species	
Aerobic gram-negative bacilli	*Lactobacillus* species	
Pseudomonas aeruginosa		

SOURCE: From Solomkin JS, Moulton JS: Diagnosis and management of intraabdominal sepsis, in Rippe JM, Irwin RS, Fink MP, Cerra FB (eds): *Intensive Care Medicine,* 3d ed, Boston, Little, Brown, 1996. Used by permission.

genera predominate. Among anaerobic bacteria the most common isolates are *Bacteroides* species. In experimental models that have been reported, when pure cultures of *E. coli* were injected into animals, peritonitis developed in all animals, with a high incidence of *E. coli* bacteremia and significant mortality. Injection with *E. coli* alone did not result in any intraabdominal abscesses, which are usually seen in patients who survive the diffuse inflammatory phase of peritonitis. By contrast, when *B. fragilis* was injected, there was almost no mortality, and very few *B. fragilis* were recovered from the bloodstream, but the incidence of intraabdominal abscesses was almost 100 percent. Injection of the combination of *E. coli* and *B. fragilis* resulted in a picture similar to that seen in human patients, with significant mortality and intraabdominal abscesses in most survivors.

The LPS present on the surface of gram-negative organisms, including those of the Enterobacteriaceae family, is a key virulence mechanism, because it interacts with a broad range of human cell types to induce an inflammatory response. The initial response includes thrombosis, restricting blood supply to an area of contamination. An influx of cells that are profoundly cytotoxic, both for the bacteria and resident tissue, follows. These responses reduce the numbers of organisms needed to establish an infection, a paradoxical consequence of the inflammatory response. This paradox may be explicable if the inflammatory response is a means of generating abscesses with subsequent extrusion to an external surface.

Microbial Synergy. The consequences of synergy are most evident in necrotizing soft tissue infections. Characteristic histologic findings include extensive local thrombosis and dense growth of microorganisms responding only to wide excision with normal tissue. Synergistic interactions between anaerobes, most notably *B. fragilis,* and endotoxin-bearing gram-negative organisms suppress local host defense mechanisms and facilitate the establishment of infection. *B. fragilis* produces a capsular polysaccharide that interferes with complement activation and inhibits leukocyte function. Delivery of phagocytes to the site of infection is restricted, permitting a more rapid rate of bacterial growth.

Aerobic bacteria lower the oxidation-reduction potential, thus favoring the growth of anaerobic bacteria. Anaerobic bacteria elaborate short-chain fatty acids that interfere with neutrophil function. Either type of bacteria may enhance the growth of other bacteria by provision of nutrient factors or destruction of antibiotics. High concentrations of bacteria inhibit the ability of most antimicrobial agents to function optimally. Extracellular products such as proteases facilitate bacterial invasion.

Host Effects on Bacterial Growth. The host neurohumoral response to infection may enhance bacterial growth in that gram-negative bacterial growth is dramatically enhanced by physiologic concentrations of norepinephrine, an effect mediated by a receptorlike mechanism within the bacteria. Some bacterial pathogens may have evolved mechanisms to exploit the inflammatory milieu. This may partially explain the well-known effect of traumatic injury on enhancing the lethality of intraabdominal infection.

Adjuvant Substances. The inoculum of bacteria needed to establish experimental infections is much less if subjects simultaneously are inoculated with adjuvant substances. Adjuvants increase bacterial virulence or interfere with host defenses. In

Table 32-4
Adjuvant Substances for Intraabdominal Infection

Factor	Effect
Blood	Nutritive effect on bacterial growth, Hgb toxic to WBCs
Fibrin	Impairs PMN chemotaxis, sequesters bacteria
Fluid	Impairs phagocytosis, dilutes opsonins
Bile	Lysis of host leukocytes
Urine	Opsonin deficient
Chyle	Opsonin deficient
Pancreatic fluid	Opsonin deficient
Platelets	Impair bacterial clearance, perhaps secondary to physical obstruction of diaphragmatic lymph channels

Hgb = hemoglobin; PMN = polymorphonuclear leukocyte; WBC = white blood cell.

gastrointestinal perforation, a surgical procedure, or trauma, the bacterial inoculum is invariably accompanied by adjuvant substances (Table 32-4).

Clinically, the most important adjuvant substance is blood. Hemoglobin, fibrin, and platelets in blood all impair peritoneal defenses. Hemoglobin decreases the median lethal dose of bacteria in standard rodent models of peritonitis by five orders of magnitude. Hemoglobin increases bacterial growth rates, perhaps because of the liberation of iron, an essential growth factor for *E. coli.* Iron may depress neutrophil migration and phagocytic function. Stroma-free hemoglobin is directly toxic to neutrophils as well. Platelets impair clearance of bacteria from the peritoneal cavity, presumably by physical obstruction of the diaphragmatic lymphatic channels. Fibrin promotes bacterial trapping and abscess formation but may impede the ability of neutrophils to reach the bacteria. Fibrinolytic agents instilled intraperitoneally in experimental animals were found to lyse clots and prevent abscess formation but were associated with higher bacteremia rates and higher lethality.

Other substances that may gain access to the peritoneal cavity during infection include bile salts, gastric mucin, pancreatic secretions, urine, and chyle. Bile salts aid in digestion of lipids because of their detergent action. Bile salt also can result in destruction of leukocytes and impaired host defense. Some bacteria may be digested by bile salts, but others, for example, *Enterococcus fecalis,* can readily grow in media that is 40 percent bile salts—which is the basis of the most common microbiologic test to identify *E. fecalis.* Pancreatic secretions contain proenzymes that can become activated by bacterial infection, resulting in tissue digestion and increased bacterial invasion.

Foreign Materials. Foreign materials may play an important role in the pathogenesis of infection. Microorganisms adherent to foreign materials are far more difficult for phagocytes to kill, and the foreign body may itself induce an inflammatory reaction, reducing the inoculum needed to establish infection. Foreign materials that play a role in the pathogenesis of abdominal infections may be macroscopic or microscopic (Table 32-5). Macroscopic foreign bodies such as drains, suture material, microscopic fragments of cotton gauze sponges shed from laparotomy pads, and hemostatic agents such as collagen or cellulose potentiate infection. Microscopic foreign materials include talc, barium sulfate, necrotic tissue, and fecal material. Some foreign

Table 32-5
Foreign Bodies That May Enhance Intraabdominal Infection

Macroscopic Foreign Material
Surgical drains
Suture material
Laparotomy sponges
Hemostatic pads/powders
Surgical clips
Prosthetic implants

Microscopic Foreign Materials
Barium sulfate
Clothing fibers (can be introduced during penetrating trauma)
Fecal material
Necrotic tissue
Talcum powder or other surgical glove powders (less likely with modern corn starch)

materials may be directly toxic to neutrophils. Mucin and fiber can activate complement. Nylon, including the nylon in sutures, can cause neutrophil degranulation and impairment of oxidative microbial killing. Barium sulfate, a particularly virulent adjuvant, produces its own acute inflammatory insult. The combination of barium and feces is more lethal than either alone. The chemical injury to the peritoneum by barium increases its permeability. Free barium activates the coagulation system by way of the intrinsic pathway, resulting in severe fibrinous peritonitis that carries a mortality of 53 percent even when surgically controlled.

EVOLUTION OF INTRAABDOMINAL INFECTION

Peritoneal Contamination. When peritoneal injury is accompanied by bacterial contamination, degranulation of peritoneal mast cells dramatically increases the permeability of peritoneal endothelial and mesothelial cells. The resultant exudation of protein-rich fluid contains complement, opsonins, and fibrinogen. Increased vascular permeability also results in a significant fluid influx into the peritoneal cavity. This fluid comes at the expense of depleted intravascular volume, resulting in hypotension.

The systemic response to peritonitis includes the release of catecholamines, glucocorticoids, aldosterone, and vasopressin (antidiuretic hormone). These responses, combined with hypovolemia from the copious fluid sequestration within the peritoneum, can create hemodynamic instability with hypotension, reduced cardiac index, increased peripheral resistance, and increased peripheral oxygen consumption. The patient may manifest the hyperdynamic hemodynamic picture of septic (distributive) shock, i.e., increased cardiac output, decreased peripheral resistance, and decreased arteriovenous oxygen difference. Fluid resuscitation may change the patient's condition from a hypodynamic to a hyperdynamic state.

After a free perforation into the intestinal cavity, the contaminating bacteria migrate with the peritoneal fluid to the subdiaphragmatic area, where large numbers are cleared into the systemic circulation via the subdiaphragmatic lymphatic "pump." The bacteria empty into the systemic circulation through the thoracic duct and into the left subclavian vein within 6 min of inoculation. More than 90 percent of circulating bacteria are cleared by phagocytosis in the reticuloendothelial system, particularly hepatic Kupffer cells.

Concept of the Decisive Period. After peritoneal contamination the ultimate outcome, resolution, or establishment of infection becomes a race between bacterial multiplication and bacterial destruction by the host defenses. Resident peritoneal macrophages are the initial leukocytic cell on the scene capable of phagocytosing bacteria. Normal peritoneal fluid contains less than 300 cells/mm^3, with more than 50 percent macrophages, 40 percent lymphocytes, and 5 to 10 percent mast cells or eosinophils. During the first 1 to 2 h after bacterial contamination, macrophages and mast cells are the only phagocytic host defense cells in the peritoneal cavity. Macrophages are capable of phagocytosis on the peritoneal surface even without prior opsonization. Bacterial opsonization, with IgG or C3b, improves phagocytic efficiency. Prompt clinical recognition and appropriate treatment can drastically shift this dichotomy. Miles and Burke suggested the concept of a "decisive period" for bacterial infection. This period refers to the time required for bacterial numbers in fluid or tissue to exceed 10^5/mm^3 (or per gram of tissue) and establish an infection. Surgeons must deal with the infection before bacterial numbers reach these levels or remove the focus of infection so that after operation the residual numbers of bacteria are less than 10^5/mm^3 (Fig. 32-4).

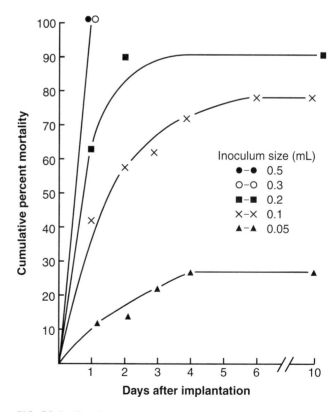

FIG. 32-4. Experimental (rat) model indicating cumulative percentage mortality with varying inoculum size of human fecal material in the peritoneal cavity. (From: *Nichols RL, et al, Peritonitis and intraabdominal abscess: An experimental model for the evaluation of human disease. J Surg Res 25:129, 1979, with permission.*)

CARE FOR PATIENTS WITH INTRAABDOMINAL INFECTIONS

Diagnosis of Intraabdominal Infection

The history and physical examination of patients with a suspected intraabdominal infection are pivotal in defining the need for and urgency of intervention and the use of diagnostic techniques. A brief history should determine how long the patient has been ill; whether fever or chills are present; whether pain is present, and if so where it is located, what its character is (crampy, dull, burning, etc.), whether it has changed location, character, or intensity, and whether it is associated with anorexia, vomiting, or ileus. A pertinent past medical history, including recent hospitalizations, medications, chronic disease diagnoses, and prior operations, is important.

Stretching of the visceral peritoneum produces nausea and poorly localized pain. Most intraperitoneal visceral structures arise from the embryologic foregut, and, accordingly their nerve supply arises from the visceral branches of the vagus nerve. Pain usually is localized to the dermatome distribution of the associated visceral organ. For example, the gallbladder arises from the upper thoracic dermatomes; hence, stretching of the visceral peritoneum overlying the gallbladder produces epigastric and right upper back pain. When the inflammatory process involves the adjacent diaphragmatic structures, pain may be perceived in the neck or shoulder (fourth cervical nerve), because the diaphragm arises from the embryologic cervical dermatomes.

Visceral peritoneal irritation, usually from distention of a hollow viscus, causes dull, poorly localized, often periumbilical, and often crampy pain. Visceral structures are generally completely insensitive to surgical transection, cauterization, heat, cold, or pinching. Most symptoms result from inflammation of the visceral peritoneum, which receives afferent innervation only from the autonomic nervous system and is relatively insensitive. Visceral afferent nerves respond primarily to traction or distention, but less well to pressure, and are not capable of mediating pain and temperature sensation. Hence stimuli are perceived as poorly localized, dull discomfort.

The root of the small bowel mesentery and the biliary tree are relatively better innervated than the rest of the visceral peritoneum, accounting for more intense and better localized responses to stimulation of these areas. The term *biliary colic* refers to the sensation transduced by visceral afferents from an overdistended gallbladder undergoing muscular spasm because of an obstructing stone. The small bowel itself is not well innervated, and so stimulation of its visceral afferents produces only a vague, dull ache in the midabdomen. Stimulation of the colonic afferents results in a similar dull pain located in the lower abdomen. Pain may start abruptly with a perforation when a highly irritating agent such as pancreatic or gastric juice diffusely inflames the somatic nerve endings of the parietal peritoneum.

A good example of the effects of the dual mechanism of pain perception is in the progression of symptoms in the development of acute appendicitis. Initially inflammation of the appendix is projected via autonomic nerve fibers to the region of the umbilicus and epigastrium, with symptoms of diffuse epigastric pain, nausea, and vomiting. As the somatic pathways of the parietal peritoneum and adjacent structures become involved, the pain seems to "migrate" from the epigastrium and umbilicus to the right lower abdomen and to grow in intensity, and then to localize at McBurney's point. When fully developed, pain in parietal peritonitis is steady, unrelenting, burning, and aggravated by motion, and usually it is most intense in the region of the most advanced peritoneal inflammation.

Assessment of Hemodynamic and Respiratory Status. There are two potential causes of hypotension in patients with intraabdominal infection. Fluid loss occurs through a variable combination of decreased intake, increased respiratory fluid losses from the tachypnea accompanying fever, and intraabdominal fluid sequestration. The extent of fluid sequestration that accompanies infection is a result of both the local peritoneal response and the diffuse capillary leak that accompanies major sepsis. Hypotension also may be caused by the cardiac and vascular dysfunction that is part of septic shock.

Immediate differentiation between these two distinct entities may not be straightforward. Hypotensive patients should receive boluses of 500 mL lactated Ringer's solution until an adequate blood pressure response occurs. If 3 L have been given and a sustained blood pressure response has not occurred, particularly in an elderly patient, a pulmonary artery catheter should be placed to determine hemodynamic function and to monitor fluid and pressor therapy.

Physical Examination. In addition to a review of the vital signs, the general appearance of the patient, including tachypnea or labored breathing, agitation, or evidence of dehydration, should be carefully noted. Each part of the examination should be explained to the patient before it is performed, with reassurances that it will not be painful. The scleras and conjunctivae may reveal icterus or pallor. The chest should be percussed and auscultated to rule out pneumonia, particularly of the lower lobes, which may produce the abdominal findings. In a hypotensive patient, rolling the patient from side to side rather than sitting him or her up is appropriate. A cardiac examination should rule out congestive failure or valvular disease, since aggressive fluid therapy may be required and because acute congestive failure with hepatic distention and capsular stretching may produce abdominal pain.

Inspection and Auscultation. The abdomen should be inspected for distention and any scars noted. The patient should be assured at this point that the examination will cause minimal discomfort but is needed to determine the need for diagnostic measures and therapy. The patient is asked to point with one finger to the area of most severe pain in the abdomen. Auscultation is begun in the quadrant diagonally opposite to this point. Auscultation is performed to simply determine whether bowel sounds are diminished, normoactive (determined according to when the patient last ate), or hyperactive. Hyperactive bowel sounds suggest an obstructive element either as a primary disease process or as part of a localized inflammatory process. Often an inflammatory focus is partially walled off by adherent small bowel. A local ileus occurs, resulting in a functional obstruction. Abdominal distention is a result of concomitant ileus or ascites. Hyperresonance caused by accumulating gas in the distended intestines usually can be demonstrated by percussion. As inflammation spreads, small-bowel sounds disappear and the abdomen becomes nearly silent.

Palpation. The parietal peritoneum is innervated by somatic and visceral afferent nerves and is quite sensitive. The anterior parietal peritoneum is the most sensitive, and the pelvic peritoneum the least sensitive. The ability to localize an inflammatory stimulus affecting the parietal peritoneum, particularly of the anterior abdominal wall, underlies much of our ability to diagnose acute intraabdominal infection.

In addition to the perception of pain as localized tenderness, local inflammation adjacent to the parietal peritoneum leads initially to protective voluntary muscular guarding. If the inflammatory process continues, reflex muscular spasm of the anterior abdominal wall occurs, progressing to various degrees of rigidity. Gentle palpation of the abdomen, the last step in the examination, is intended to determine whether the pain-producing intraabdominal process has resulted in parietal peritoneal inflammation. Palpation starts at the quadrant most removed from the identified point of maximal pain. The purpose of abdominal palpation is to confirm the location of maximal tenderness and the resting tone in various portions of the anterior abdominal wall. To do this, the examiner begins in a part of the abdomen that is asymptomatic and gently presses until the tone of the underlying musculature is determined. In patients with acute peritonitis, a rigid abdomen will be found with no substantial differences from one quadrant to another. For patients with localized tenderness, and a localized increase in abdominal wall tone, voluntary versus involuntary guarding must be distinguished.

Rigidity of the abdominal muscles is produced by voluntary guarding initially and also by reflex muscle spasm. Reflex muscle spasm can become so severe that boardlike abdominal rigidity is produced and the abdominal wall may become scaphoid, as is typically seen after chemical peritonitis caused by peptic ulcer perforation.

Rectal and Vaginal Examinations. Rectal and vaginal examinations are essential to locate the extent of tenderness and whether a pelvic mass or pouch of Douglas abscess is present. Vaginal examination of the cervix may provide clues to the origin of the inflammatory process.

Laboratory and Other Tests. Leukocytosis is common in acute intraabdominal infection, but the total leukocyte count taken alone without a differential count can be very misleading. A leukocyte count of more than 25,000/mm^3 or leukopenia with fewer than 4,000/mm^3 are both associated with higher mortality. The differential count provides evidence of the presence of acute inflammation by showing relative lymphopenia and moderate-to-marked leftward shift, even if the leukocyte count is normal or subnormal.

Plain radiographs of the abdomen may reveal free air, a uniform indicator of visceral perforation in the absence of recent prior intervention. Free air may be visible on an upright abdominal or lateral decubitus film if a ruptured hollow viscus is the cause of peritonitis. Air beneath the diaphragm may be noted on radiographs of the chest if the patient remains in an upright position for 5 min or more before the film is made. Other findings from plain radiographs that support the diagnosis of intraabdominal infection include intestinal pneumatosis, bowel obstruction, and a mass effect. There are rare benign causes of pneumatosis. More dramatic but less common findings are air in the portal vein or extraluminal gas collections indicative of an abscess; these radiographic signs are sufficiently specific to justify immediate intervention.

The radiologic picture of intraabdominal infection otherwise mimics that of paralytic ileus. Inflammatory exudate and edema

of the intestinal wall produce widening of the space between adjacent bowel loops on a plain film of the abdomen. Peritoneal fat lines and the retroperitoneal psoas shadow may be obliterated because of edema. The fat lines in the pelvis may be obliterated, suggesting fluid in the pelvis.

Preoperative Preparation

Acute perforations of the gastrointestinal tract with peritonitis mandate initial treatment in an intensive care environment. In addition, patients with serious intraabdominal infections often require intervention to control infection.

Perforations of the upper gastrointestinal tract cause impressive physical findings of peritonitis but rarely manifest evidence of septic shock. Conversely, perforations of the colon result in massive bacterial contamination and are accompanied by hypotension. In either setting, progressive clinical deterioration will continue until soiling of the peritoneal cavity is terminated. This puts important temporal limits on resuscitation prior to operative intervention. Patients with acute perforations of the gastrointestinal tract should be sufficiently resuscitated to survive the induction of anesthesia, but resuscitation should continue during operation. Rapid volume loading will counter the vasodilatory effects of anesthetics. More refined parameters of completed resuscitation, such as maximization of cardiac output or oxygen delivery, should await the completion of successful intervention.

In addition to intravascular volume loading, other maneuvers are of value in protecting patients from intraoperative hypotension. Infusing low doses of dopamine improves renal blood flow and reduces the incidence of acute renal failure. Positive end-expiratory pressure (PEEP) should be used sparingly, as it decreases venous return and can compromise cardiac output. High inspired oxygen concentrations maintain adequate arterial oxygen saturation until intravascular volume has been satisfactorily restored.

Preoperative preparation of patients with peritonitis involves fluid resuscitation, administration of antibiotics and oxygen, nasogastric intubation, urinary catheterization, and monitoring of vital signs and biochemical and hemodynamic data. Major metabolic derangements and fluid deficits should be corrected before operation, although an inordinate delay is deleterious to outcome. Oxygen is administered to correct the mild hypoxemia in patients with peritonitis secondary to intrapulmonary shunting and the mechanical impairment of pulmonary ventilation by the distended, tender abdomen. Assessment of respiratory function should include apparent tidal volume and work of breathing. If impairment is suspected, ventilatory volume and arterial blood gases should be measured. Ventilatory support should be initiated whenever any of the following is present: (1) inability to maintain adequate alveolar ventilation as evidenced by a Pa_{CO_2} of 50 mmHg or greater; (2) hypoxemia, with a Pa_{O_2} below 60 mmHg and a fraction of inspired oxygen of 1.0; or (3) shallow, rapid respirations, muscle fatigue, or the use of accessory muscles of respiration.

Vital signs—temperature, blood pressure, pulse rate, respiration rate—are continuously recorded. Preoperative biochemical evaluation should include measurement of serum levels of electrolytes, creatinine, glucose, bilirubin, and alkaline phosphatase, and a urinalysis.

Nasogastric intubation is performed to evacuate the stomach, to prevent further vomiting, and to reduce accumulation of additional air in the paralyzed bowel. Urinary catheterization is used to record initial bladder urine volume and to monitor subsequent urinary output. Renal dysfunction requires early corrective measures. Patients with peritonitis develop renal failure as a result of hypovolemic shock, septic shock, increased intraabdominal pressure, and nephrotoxic drugs such as the aminoglycosides. Diuretics are used but may be toxic to tubular cells. If there is cardiopulmonary dysfunction, a Swan-Ganz catheter allows measurement of pulmonary capillary wedge and pulmonary artery pressures, systemic vascular resistance, and cardiac output as indices for pharmacologic intervention.

Once a decision to operate has been made, pain should be relieved with potent narcotics. Morphine is preferred, and should be given intravenously in doses of 1 to 3 mg, repeated every 20 to 30 min or even more frequently, to maintain comfort. Small intravenous doses of morphine are safer than the traditional larger intramuscular doses, particularly in unstable patients whose absorption of intramuscular medication may be unpredictable and variable.

Administration of pharmacologic doses of steroids to septic patients has been advocated in the past, but controlled trials have not shown this treatment to be efficacious. Recent clinical studies support the concept that large doses of steroids may delay mortality in sepsis, particularly if given before the onset of shock or very soon after, but they do not alter the eventual outcome. Steroids are not recommended in the management of bacterial peritonitis.

Patients with hyperthermia or hypothermia should have their temperature corrected toward normal before operation. Administration of acetaminophen is often effective in reducing fever. If not, or if the patient is hypothermic, a cooling or warming mattress should be used.

MANAGEMENT OF DIFFUSE PERITONITIS

The history and physical examination usually are sufficient to make the diagnosis, and no further testing is necessary. Even if infection spreads diffusely throughout the peritoneal cavity, if the source is controlled by early surgical intervention, peritonitis usually responds to vigorous antibiotic and supportive therapy. On the other hand, death nearly always follows continued peritoneal soiling.

Operative management of peritonitis involves immediate evacuation of all purulent collections, with particular attention to subphrenic, subhepatic, interloop, and pelvic collections. The perforated bowel should be resected. Evidence has accumulated from studies of several decades of mortality rates following surgical treatment of perforated diverticulitis that resection with end colostomy significantly decreases acute mortality as compared to transverse loop colostomy and drainage. Primary anastomosis is not recommended in the face of purulent peritonitis; in one study, mortality from primary anastomosis was 23 percent, with most deaths attributed to anastomotic leakage. Controversies in the operative management of peritonitis focus primarily on wound closure techniques and scheduled relaparotomies. Patients with diffuse peritonitis secondary to colonic perforation or anastomotic dehiscence typically develop abdominal wall edema as part of a generalized syndrome of increased capillary permeability. This syndrome is exacerbated by the aggressive restoration of intravascular and extravascular volume. Under these circumstances, primary closure of the abdominal incision may be difficult or even unwise, as increased intraabdominal pressure

can result in compression of mesenteric and renal veins, leading in some instances to acute renal failure or bowel necrosis. A fascial prosthesis prevents an overly tight closure. A variety of materials have been employed, including Marlex, Silastic, and polytetrafluoroethylene (PTFE). Each material has its own virtues and problems. Impermeable materials can exacerbate peritonitis and should be used only if a relaparotomy is planned.

Recurrent abscesses and persistent peritonitis largely account for the high mortality in patients with diffuse peritonitis. A continued septic state with renal and/or hepatic dysfunction should raise suspicion of diffuse peritonitis, but there is little satisfaction with current approaches for operative management. A variety of mechanical approaches have been proposed to reduce mortality, generally based on the notion that failure of host defense mechanisms of the peritoneal cavity leads to persistent infection. Planned relaparotomy at present seems most attractive. Patients treated in this fashion undergo standard operative management of their infection, but the fascia is not closed; instead, a prosthetic material is sewn to the fascia as a temporary closure, and at intervals of 24 to 48 h the mesh is opened and the peritoneal cavity debrided and irrigated. Early reports were quite positive, but used historical controls. More recent reports have not found that survival is substantially improved or that the incidence of late abscess formation is reduced. Occasional fistulas have occurred.

We have used planned relaparotomy in conjunction with prosthetic fascial closure for a relatively small number of patients with septic shock and colon-derived peritonitis. The obvious benefits are absence of intraabdominal and wound tension and the ability to obtain sequential microbiologic data to guide antimicrobial therapy. Once the prosthetic mesh is in place, relaparotomy is performed on a scheduled basis, or as dictated by the patient's clinical course and adjunctive tests, particularly computed tomography. The latter, more conservative approach seems worthwhile for patients who recover from their initial episode of shock and who do not manifest progressive organ failure. In such patients, abdominal wall and visceral edema typically resolves over the first week, at which time definitive closure of the abdomen is performed.

Management of Specific Forms of Peritonitis

Perforation of the Stomach and Duodenum. Infection after peptic ulcer perforation presents acutely; the patient is commonly able to give the exact time at which the perforation occurred. This form of peritonitis is initially chemical, but with time it becomes infected. The patient usually seeks help early because of the severe pain, and operative repair often is possible before significant bacterial overgrowth has occurred. The proper management is simple closure of the perforation; some authors have recommended definitive treatment of the ulcer disease in addition if the perforation is less than 12 h old. Parietal cell vagotomy and a Graham patch of the perforation is favored by many.

Small-Bowel Perforation. Infection after small-bowel perforation falls into two categories. In the first, bowel obstruction is present, so that ileus precedes peritonitis. Colic and other features of bowel obstruction are the presenting signs and symptoms, gradually changing to those of localized or diffuse peritonitis, with fever and leukocytosis after perforation. In the second form, bowel wall necrosis as a result of inflammation or impaired vascular supply leads to perforation. Peritonitis may be diagnosed at a late stage because of the lack of initial symptoms, and hence mortality rates can exceed 50 percent.

Colon Perforation. About 20 percent of cases of peritonitis have their origin in the colon. More than half of these are due to inflammatory disease such as diverticulitis and other forms of colitis. The remaining cases are due to perforation proximal to or at stenosis caused by luminal bowel obstruction (tumor) or external bowel obstruction such as incarcerated hernia, intussusception, and volvulus. In colonic obstruction, the colon distends proximally and ruptures as a result of either increased intraluminal pressure or diminished vascular supply to one segment. A malignant growth usually does not cause peritonitis directly but may lead to bowel obstruction with either perforation of dilated segments or bowel ischemia, and/or bacterial migration through the necrotic bowel wall. Carcinoma of the colon, if the ileocecal valve is competent, may lead to diffuse fecal peritonitis as a result of rupture of the cecum or ascending colon.

A ventral midline incision is preferred, as it is quick to open and close and allows easy exploration of the entire abdomen, especially in cases in which the organ source of peritonitis is not clear. Complete control of the source of infection is essential for therapeutic success. The elimination of the infectious source or focus reduces the infectious inoculum to a magnitude that is treatable successfully by antibiotic therapy coupled with active intrinsic host defense mechanisms. When the infectious focus cannot be adequately controlled, the prognosis is poor.

Peritonitis of Genitourinary Origin. Ruptured perinephric abscess and ruptured chronic cystitis after radiation therapy for female reproductive tract cancer can cause peritonitis. A colon anastomosis should be avoided in peritonitis associated with a urine leak. Pelvic peritonitis due to sexually transmitted infection is common in young women; usually there is acute, severe lower abdominal pain, typically just cephalad to the inguinal creases. The condition is diagnosed by Gram stain of cervical discharge. Treatment with antimicrobials is successful in most cases, and operation is reserved for the occasional patient with persisting tubo-ovarian abscess.

Postoperative Peritonitis. Postoperative peritonitis is usually the result of an anastomotic leak and is often discovered only after some delay, typically between the fifth and seventh postoperative day. Delay contributes to a high mortality rate. After duodenal operations, the high mortality of leakage is explained by the fact that the duodenum is fixed in the retroperitoneum and cannot be exteriorized, and the source of infection often cannot be adequately controlled or closed. Consequently, infective material and proteolytic enzymes continue to soil the peritoneal cavity, sustaining the infection. Drainage, controlled fistula formation, exteriorization, repair, or resection and reanastomosis are performed as indicated.

Peritonitis After Trauma. Peritonitis may develop after blunt trauma in patients who have unrecognized intraabdominal injuries such as a ruptured mesentery with loss of the vascular supply to the small or large bowel, or a frank unrecognized bowel perforation. This type of intraabdominal infection usually is severe because the diagnosis is delayed or masked by other injuries elsewhere in the body, particularly head injury. Management in such instances is no different from that of other forms of peritonitis.

Patients suffering penetrating trauma, typically gunshot wound or stab wound, usually are operated on, and the wound is repaired or controlled immediately; these injuries lead to peritonitis only when the initial repair leaks. Perforation of a bacteria-containing hollow viscus by blunt trauma is less frequent but more of a clinical diagnostic problem since symptoms can be masked by pain from the injury. Contamination of the abdominal cavity seen after penetrating abdominal trauma is usually not considered an intraabdominal infection. Only one-third of patients with penetrating trauma to the colon actually sustain documented contamination of the peritoneal cavity.

Cleaning the Abdominal Cavity

Various approaches to cleaning the abdominal cavity include suction, swabbing, lavage, radical debridement, and postoperative irrigation. There is broad agreement about the utility of suction and swabbing to remove pus and necrotic material, followed by local irrigation/lavage and limited debridement—measures typically used in every case. Controversy remains over the efficacy of high-volume lavage, radical debridement, and postoperative irrigation.

Intraoperative High-Volume Lavage. This treatment involves extensive intraoperative lavage of the entire abdominal cavity. Initially, 1 to 1.5 L of physiologic saline or Ringer's solution is placed into the abdominal cavity. The viscera are manipulated so that the fluid reaches all parts of the abdominal cavity to wash out pus, feces, and necrotic material, and then the fluid is suctioned away. This procedure is repeated until the suctioned fluid runs repetitively clear. The total volume of lavage should be at least equal to the estimated volume of the peritoneal cavity, which in adults is 8 to 12 L.

Povidone-Iodine. This should not be used in peritoneal lavage fluid. Iodine is highly toxic to the mesothelial cells of the peritoneum and it kills the phagocytic cells needed to clear bacteria. In animal experiments, use of povidone-iodine increases mortality, and in a controlled clinical trial the outcome with povidone-iodine was worse than with saline.

Radical Debridement. This is a poorly defined technique because it is almost impossible, without causing significant bleeding, to radically debride all necrotic tissue in intraabdominal infections, including intraabdominal abscesses. This may be one explanation for there being no significant outcome advantage in using radical debridement over other techniques. Surgical judgment is the critical element, since the drawbacks of radical debridement must be balanced against the fact that bacteria may be trapped in fibrin, and that necrotic tissue is an excellent medium for bacterial growth. Removal of such foci is the primary goal of the operative procedure, but given the adjuvant effect of hemoglobin, the procedure should not cause additional intraperitoneal hemorrhage.

Continuous Postoperative Irrigation. Four to six Tenckhoff catheters are placed in the abdominal cavity and irrigation fluid infused for 1 h. The abdominal cavity is drained, and the cycle is repeated. The drains often occlude, and there is no way to ensure that all diseased areas of the abdominal cavity are lavaged. Drains also may erode into the intestine to cause new complications. Controlled studies comparing continuous postoperative irrigation to standard therapy have yielded differing results, and in general the numbers of cases examined are small and do not permit any firm conclusions about efficacy.

OTHER FORMS OF PERITONITIS (Table 32-6)

Primary Peritonitis. Primary peritonitis is an inflammation of the peritoneum from a suspected extraperitoneal source, often via hematogenous spread. It occurs in children and in adults and can be a life-threatening illness, particularly in patients with cirrhosis. The spectrum of bacteria causing this syndrome and the population primarily affected have changed over recent decades. Spontaneous bacterial peritonitis is now more common in adults than in children and shows no differential sex incidence. Children with nephrosis, formerly the group most commonly affected, have been replaced by adults with cirrhosis or systemic lupus erythematosus.

Spontaneous peritonitis in adults is seen most commonly in patients with ascites and is a monomicrobial infection (i.e., only a single species of bacteria is present), in contrast to the polymicrobial infection of typical suppurative (secondary) peritonitis. Although pneumococci formerly were the most frequent infecting organisms at all ages, coliforms now are the chief pathogens in adults, accounting for 70 percent of infections, with *E. coli* being the most common isolate. Gram-positive cocci account for

Table 32-6
Classification of Intraabdominal Infections

I. Primary Peritonitis
  A. Spontaneous peritonitis in children
  B. Spontaneous peritonitis in adults
  C. Peritonitis in patients with CAPD
  D. Tuberculous and other granulomatous peritonitis
  E. Other forms
II. Secondary Peritonitis
  A. Acute perforation peritonitis (acute suppurative peritonitis)
    1. Gastrointestinal tract perforation
    2. Bowel wall necrosis (intestinal ischemia)
    3. Pelvic peritonitis
    4. Other forms
  B. Postoperative peritonitis
    1. Anastomotic leak
    2. Leak of a simple suture
    3. Blind loop leak
    4. Other iatrogenic leaks
  C. Posttraumatic peritonitis
    1. Peritonitis after blunt abdominal trauma
    2. Peritonitis after penetrating abdominal trauma
    3. Other forms
III. Tertiary Peritonitis
  A. Peritonitis without evidence for pathogens
  B. Peritonitis with fungi
  C. Peritonitis with low-grade pathogenic bacteria
IV. Other Forms of Peritonitis
  A. Aseptic/sterile peritonitis
  B. Granulomatous peritonitis
  C. Drug-related peritonitis
  D. Periodic peritonitis
  E. Lead peritonitis
  F. Hyperlipidemic peritonitis
  G. Porphyric peritonitis
  H. Foreign-body peritonitis
  I. Talc peritonitis
V. Intraabdominal Abscess
  A. Associated with primary peritonitis
  B. Associated with secondary peritonitis

10 to 20 percent of cases, and anaerobes are seen in 6 to 10 percent. In children the common pathogens are hemolytic streptococci and pneumococci. Two peaks of incidence are characteristic, one in the neonatal period and the other at age four to five. There may be a history of previous ear or upper respiratory infection. Children with nephrotic syndrome and systemic lupus erythematosus are disproportionately affected.

The route by which bacteria are transmitted to the peritoneal cavity is not known. The hypothesis of transmural migration of bacteria from the intestine is supported by the presence of endotoxin in ascitic fluid and blood in many cirrhotic patients with decompensation, even though the bacteria themselves are not present in the ascitic fluid and patients have no clinical evidence of peritonitis. The frequent clinical association of spontaneous peritonitis with urinary tract infection harboring the same organisms, and cases of simultaneous spontaneous pulmonary empyema and pericarditis associated with spontaneous peritonitis, favor the hypothesis that transmission is hematogenous.

Clinical symptoms usually are of short duration in children; onset is more insidious in ascitic adults. Most patients complain of abdominal pain and distention; vomiting, lethargy, and fever are more prominent in children. Diarrhea is typical in neonates but seldom seen in adults. Bowel sounds are variable. Free air usually is not seen on abdominal radiographs. The clinical picture may be nonspecific.

Paracentesis is the most useful diagnostic test. Fluid is examined for neutrophil cell count and pH; a Gram stain should be done and a specimen sent for culture. The neutrophil cell count has the highest sensitivity and specificity in making the diagnosis; a neutrophil count greater than 250 cells/mm^3 is positive. Studies of ascitic fluid in patients with suspected spontaneous peritonitis have shown that a wide arterial–fluid pH gradient also correlates with a positive diagnosis. Ascitic fluid pH is low in spontaneous bacterial peritonitis, while in sterile ascitic fluid the pH is the same as in serum. In only one-third of patients with positive fluid cultures are organisms seen on a stain of centrifuged peritoneal fluid, which is a reflection of the low concentration of bacteria in many cases of primary bacterial peritonitis. If the stain shows only gram-positive cocci, spontaneous peritonitis is strongly suggested. If a mixed flora of gram-positive and gram-negative bacteria is present, intestinal perforation is more likely and exploratory laparotomy is necessary. The presence of only gram-negative bacteria on the stain is consistent with either primary or secondary bacterial peritonitis.

When the diagnosis of spontaneous bacterial peritonitis is confirmed, antibiotic therapy should be started and the patient initially managed nonoperatively. Usually a cephalosporin or ampicillin-sulbactam is appropriate, since 90 percent of the organisms causing spontaneous peritonitis are sensitive to these antibiotics.

Peritonitis Related to Peritoneal Dialysis. Peritonitis is the dominant complication of continuous ambulatory peritoneal dialysis (CAPD) in patients with end-stage renal disease. Peritonitis occurs more frequently with CAPD than with intermittent peritoneal dialysis. Catheter-related infection is the most common mechanism, with no correlation with catheter location. Other causes of peritonitis in CAPD patients are tunnel infections and cuff extrusion. The bacteriology and treatment of dialysis-related peritonitis are considerably different from those of patients with other types of peritoneal infections. The incidence of dialysis-related peritonitis varies from center to center, but an overall average of 1.3 episodes per patient per year is estimated. In contrast to other causes of intraabdominal infection, dialysis-related peritonitis usually is caused by a single organism, and fungal infections are more common in this group. Two-thirds of patients with positive cultures have a gram-positive coccus as the causative organism, usually *Staph. aureus* or *Staph. epidermidis*. Gram-negative bacteria usually are found only in patients with recurring episodes of peritonitis, which may reflect antibiotic administration for prior episodes. Patients with dialysis-related peritonitis rarely have a positive blood culture, in contrast to patients with other causes of peritonitis. Anaerobes rarely are recovered. The presence of anaerobes or a mixed flora suggests intestinal perforation or other intraabdominal disease (e.g., diverticulitis or cholecystitis). Yeasts and tubercle bacilli are rare. Culture-negative peritonitis in dialysis patients ranges from 10 to 27 percent. *Pseudomonas aeruginosa* has been reported to cause around 3 percent of cases and generally cannot be cured by antibiotic therapy alone; the dialysis catheter must be removed in these patients.

Turbidity of the dialysate is the earliest sign, and the only finding in one-fourth of cases. If accompanied by abdominal pain or fever, prompt diagnostic laboratory studies and therapy are required. The diagnosis is established when any of the following is present: (1) positive culture from the peritoneal fluid; (2) a cloudy dialysate effluent; and (3) clinical signs of peritonitis. The stain of dialysis effluent is frequently negative in dialysis catheter-related peritonitis. Attention to sterile technique, use of topical povidone-iodine about the catheter wound, and use of sterile dialysate prepackaged in plastic bags all reduce the incidence of infection.

The initial treatment of dialysis-related peritonitis is administration of antibiotics and heparin in the dialysate as well as an increase in the dwell time of dialysate fluid. The indications for catheter removal include persistence of peritonitis after 4 to 5 days of treatment, the presence of fungal or tuberculous peritonitis, fecal peritonitis, or a severe skin infection at the catheter site.

Patients with a chronically implanted peritoneal catheter may develop sclerosing peritonitis, with a reported incidence of 1 to 6 percent. The cause is unknown, although a relationship with antecedent infection is possible. Affected patients usually have had frequent previous bouts of peritonitis. Treatment is directed at such complications as bowel obstruction.

A related form of peritonitis, due to infection of a ventriculoperitoneal shunt, exhibits clinical signs and symptoms similar to those of peritoneal dialysis catheter peritonitis. Peritonitis should be suspected in any patient having such a shunt who develops any abdominal symptoms.

Tuberculous Peritonitis. Tuberculous peritonitis, formerly frequently fatal as a manifestation of uncontrolled generalized tuberculosis, now is undergoing a renaissance in Europe and North America because of the increasing prevalence of acquired immunodeficiency syndrome (AIDS) due to human immunodeficiency virus (HIV) infection and of other immunocompromised states. It has always been a serious problem in India, Southeast Asia, Africa, and Latin America. Some cases are the result of reactivation of latent peritoneal tuberculosis established by hematogenous spread from a pulmonary focus during an earlier episode of acute disease. The tubercle bacillus presumably gains entry to the peritoneal cavity transmurally from diseased bowel, from the fallopian tube in tuberculous salpingitis, from the kidney in nephritis, or from some other distant source. Clinically, most patients lack an obvious source; however, a primary focus can be identified in all patients at autopsy. Patients usually have a positive tuberculin skin test.

Clinical Manifestations. Clinically, tuberculous peritonitis is insidious, presenting with fever, anorexia, weakness, and weight loss. Some ascites almost always is present, and more than half of affected patients have dull, diffuse abdominal pain.

In the past the disease was classified into "moist" and "dry" phases. The moist phase refers to the early, subacute stage with fever, ascites, abdominal pain, and weakness. Ascites is progressive and may become massive. The dry form presents later without ascites, following resolution, during which dense adhesions are formed. On examination, the abdomen is somewhat tender, but the classically described "doughy abdomen" is rarely seen today. Clinical manifestations of generalized tuberculous infection are seen in about one-third of patients and include anorexia, weight loss, and night sweats.

Diagnosis. A peritoneal fluid tap will show mostly lymphocytes. Tubercle bacilli can be retrieved from ascitic fluid 80 percent of the time if more than 1 L of fluid is cultured. The ascitic fluid has an increased protein concentration, lymphocytic pleocytosis, and a glucose concentration below 30 mg/dL. If the fluid tap analysis does not establish the diagnosis, peritoneoscopy and direct biopsy of the peritoneum are recommended. On laparoscopy, the appearance of tuberculous peritonitis includes stalactite-like fibrinous masses hanging from the parietal peritoneum in the lower part of the abdomen. A directed, percutaneous needle biopsy specimen of a granulomatous lesion as well as samples of peritoneal fluid for direct smear examination and injection into a guinea pig should be obtained. As a last resort, exploratory laparotomy may establish the diagnosis. At laparotomy a peritoneal biopsy should be taken; the placement of drains or exteriorization of bowel should be avoided.

Treatment. Treatment is administration of antituberculous drugs. Given reports in recent years of resistance to commonly used tuberculostatic drugs, triple antituberculous drug therapy is instituted early in the course of the disease, generally with good results. Therapy should be continued for at least 2 years after the patient becomes asymptomatic. Tuberculous peritonitis may heal with formation of dense fibrous adhesions; treatment with prednisone during the initial few months of antituberculous drug therapy may reduce adhesion formation and subsequent obstruction.

Operation should be reserved for diagnosis if needle biopsy fails, or for the treatment of such complications as fecal fistula. Because tuberculous peritonitis heals with formation of dense fibrous adhesions, patients with this disease are prone to developing an intestinal obstruction.

Typhoid Perforation. Typhoid perforation usually is seen in the third week of infection with *Salmonella typhi* in patients with acute disease. The disease is rarely seen in Europe or North America but is endemic in regions with poor hygienic conditions and water contamination, such as India, Pakistan, and countries in South America and Africa. Typhoid bacilli are thought to penetrate the Peyer's patches of the intestine wall, mainly in the distal ileum. These collections of lymphoid cells hypertrophy, leading to hemorrhage and then perforation.

Perforation often is not appreciated in an already severely diseased patient, and it is superinfection resulting from leakage of intestinal bacteria that leads to the full-blown picture of suppurative bacterial peritonitis. Treatment consists of closure of the punched-out lesions and evacuation of pus from the peritoneal cavity. Staged abdominal repair may be indicated if abdominal toilet is incomplete during the first operation. Trimethoprim-sulfamethoxazole is the treatment of choice for uncomplicated typhoid, but in patients with peritonitis cefotaxime plus metronidazole is preferable.

Amebic Perforation. *Entamoeba histolytica* infection of the intestine usually causes a dysentery-like illness, but sometimes liver abscess or perforation of the large bowel occurs. Liver abscesses also can perforate secondarily and cause diffuse peritonitis. The clinical picture is that of bacterial peritonitis. Treatment consists of resection of the diseased bowel segment with anastomosis, application of the general principles of treating peritonitis, and the administration of metronidazole in combination with a third-generation cephalosporin.

Aseptic/Sterile Peritonitis. This form of peritonitis develops from irritant material (talc or foreign bodies) that has gained entry to the peritoneal cavity. Aseptic peritonitis can be caused by a variety of substances. They all act as adjuvants when secondary bacterial contamination occurs, promoting proliferation of microorganisms and transition to suppurative peritonitis. The soilage initially is sterile or nearly so, which distinguishes chemical peritonitis at onset from suppurative peritonitis. In chemical peritonitis following peptic ulcer perforation, cultures are initially sterile, but as time progresses, positive cultures are recovered. After 24 h, all cultures are positive and the patient has developed suppurative peritonitis. A similar shift from initially aseptic to bacterially infected peritonitis can occur with all forms of chemical peritonitis.

Foreign-Body Peritonitis. Foreign bodies may be deposited in the peritoneal cavity during operations (sponge or instrument inadvertently left behind) or may result from penetrating injuries or perforation of the intestines following ingestion. A larger foreign body can lead to the formation of an abscess in the presence of bacteria, but otherwise foreign bodies are sealed off and encapsulated.

Periodic Peritonitis. Recurrent episodes of abdominal pain, fever, and leukocytosis occur in certain population groups in and around the Levant, notably in Armenians, Jews, and Arabs. The disease appears to be familial. The major point for the surgeon is that laparotomy is not required in these episodes. Laparotomy is often performed for the first episode, since an acute intraabdominal process requiring surgical cure cannot be ruled out. At operation, the peritoneal surfaces may be inflamed and there is free fluid, but no bacteria. The appendix should be removed even if normal to eliminate the possibility of acute appendicitis in the differential diagnosis of future episodes. Colchicine is effective in preventing recurrent attacks, and a favorable response to chronic administration of colchicine is a definitive diagnostic test.

Drug-Related Peritonitis. Administration of isoniazid and erythromycin estolate have been reported to cause acute abdominal symptoms mimicking peritonitis, but not development of true peritonitis. A number of cases have been reported in which beta-blocking drugs have resulted in striking thickening of the visceral peritoneum. The most frequent clinical presentation is as a typical small-bowel obstruction, often subtle at onset, associated with weight loss and with an abdominal mass on physical examination. The operative findings are striking: the whole small bowel usually is caught up in a thick sac, which sometimes can be lifted as a single mass from the peritoneal cavity. The agglomeration of the small bowel produces the mass that is palpable preoperatively.

Lead Peritonitis. Lead peritonitis has the same clinical picture as acute intermittent porphyria. It is associated with lead intoxication (occurring in painters, smelter workers, pica in children), and a careful history will lead to the correct diagnosis. Unlike true intraabdominal infection, in this disorder sudden stretching of the peritoneum by rebound palpation usually does not cause peritoneal irritation and guarding.

Hyperlipemic Peritonitis. Abdominal pain mimicking peritonitis may be seen in patients with type I and type V hyperlipoproteinemia, a group of heterogeneous disorders resulting from increased concentration of chylomicrons or very-low-density lipoproteins in the blood. These disorders usually lead to pancreatitis. If erroneously operated on during early stages, the abdominal cavity is found to be full of chylous milky material. A careful family history will clarify the differential diagnosis.

Porphyric Peritonitis. This is a condition of perceived abdominal pain rather than an inflammation of the peritoneum. It is seen in patients with acute intermittent porphyria, who suffer from acute attacks that cause nervous system damage, especially to the autonomic system. The pain may be localized or general and is often accompanied by vomiting and constipation. It may be colicky or constant and is associated with abdominal tenderness. With low-grade fever and mild leukocytosis the disorder further imitates intraabdominal infection. The diagnosis is established by the demonstration of porphobilinogen in the Watson-Schwartz test.

Talc Peritonitis. Peritoneal inflammation, exudation and formation of pseudotumors (chronic inflammatory omental tumors), and formation of dense adhesions may follow contamination of the peritoneal cavity by glove lubricants (talc, lycopodium, mineral oil, cornstarch, rice starch) or by cellulose fibers from disposable gauze pads, drapes, and gowns. The reaction, particularly that to rice starch, is largely a hypersensitivity response.

The clinical features include migratory abdominal pain, fever, physical signs of peritonitis, and, often, the presence of an abdominal mass, all developing within 3 weeks after an otherwise uncomplicated abdominal operation. The surgical wound may appear normal or may be moderately indurated. Plain abdominal films are nonspecific. The total white blood cell count is normal; eosinophilia of 4 to 9 percent may be present.

When the diagnosis remains unclear, laparoscopy may be helpful. If talc peritonitis is recognized, reoperation may be avoided and corticosteroids or nonsteroidal anti-inflammatory agents administered. Eventually the peritonitis resolves. If laparotomy is undertaken because the diagnosis is obscure, a thickened peritoneum studded with white nodules is found. Histologically, nodules that contain starch granules are doubly refractive under polarized light and are surrounded by granulomatous foreign-body inflammation.

The cornerstone of management of this problem is prevention. Talc should not be used in glove manufacture or as a glove lubricant. Current techniques of wiping and washing gloves do not remove all the starch; nonetheless, gloves should be washed or wiped before gloved hands are put into the peritoneal cavity, and care should be taken to avoid spillage of glove contents should a glove be torn during an operation. Sodium bicarbonate has been used successfully as a gloving agent, but it requires special sterilization measures. Silicones also have been suggested.

Tertiary Peritonitis. Patients in whom peritonitis and sepsis initially have been controlled operatively and in whom bacteria have been eliminated by successful antibiotic therapy may progress to tertiary peritonitis, a state in which host defense systems produce a syndrome of continued systemic inflammation.

The clinical picture is one mimicking occult sepsis, as manifested by a hyperdynamic cardiovascular state, low-grade fever, and general hypermetabolism. The patient has the clinical picture of sepsis without the presence of a focus of infection. Such patients sometimes are subjected to laparotomy in an attempt to provide drainage of anticipated recurrent or residual collections of infected fluid. On operation no pathogens are present. Empiric anti-infective therapy is of no value.

DIAGNOSTIC IMAGING FOR SUSPECTED INTRAABDOMINAL INFECTIONS

In the absence of physical findings of diffuse peritonitis, diagnostic imaging with computed tomography (CT) or ultrasonography should be routinely performed in seriously ill patients with suspected intraabdominal infection. The urgency of investigation is dictated by the degree of hemodynamic instability present. Most patients should be evaluated within hours of presentation. Interventional radiology has replaced operative treatment for many localized processes, including diverticular abscesses.

CT is the single best modality for fully evaluating the extent of disease. Ultrasonography is also quite versatile and has the added advantage of being portable, allowing certain procedures to be performed at bedside. Ultrasonography is limited by bowel gas, body habitus, and a lower sensitivity for retroperitoneal processes and parenchymal infection. Usually the choice of modality is based on the experience and preference of the interventional radiologist.

When feasible, nonoperative (i.e., percutaneous) drainage of purulent collections is preferable to open surgical intervention, because of the initial deterioration that almost always occurs after operative manipulation in the presence of intraabdominal infection. The exact basis for this is unclear, but a substantial proportion of patients undergoing emergency operation for intraabdominal infection suffer acute hemodynamic compromise in the early postoperative period. When used for appropriate indications, percutaneous abscess drainage (PAD) is at least as effective as operation and is associated with less morbidity. Percutaneous drainage of an intraabdominal abscess usually is successful if the following criteria are met: (1) there is a well-established, unilocular fluid collection; (2) a safe percutaneous route of access is available; this often means that the abscess is adjacent to the body wall; (3) joint evaluation by a surgeon and a radiologist is done so that correct judgments and decisions are

made; and (4) there is immediate operative backup available in case of failure or complications.

OPERATIVE MANAGEMENT OF ABSCESSES

The indications for open surgical drainage are failure of percutaneous drainage, inability to safely drain percutaneously, the presence of a pancreatic or carcinomatous abscess, an association with a high-output bowel fistula, the involvement of the lesser sac, or the presence of multiple, isolated interloop abscesses. Additionally, exploration and open drainage are undertaken whenever the presence of an abscess is suspected clinically but cannot be localized by CT or ultrasonography. Abscesses in the pelvis usually are drained directly through the rectum or vagina, obviating the need for either percutaneous drainage or an abdominal procedure.

If the abscess is in contact with the abdominal wall or the diaphragm, a direct and, when possible, extraperitoneal approach is preferred. Subphrenic abscesses on either side and right subhepatic abscesses are best approached via the lateral extraserous route. A left subphrenic abscess also can be drained posteriorly through the bed of the twelfth rib. The point at which the abscess is encountered during dissection is usually much deeper than expected.

A lesser sac abscess is approached directly via an upper abdominal incision. Drains are placed dependently; sump-suction drains are frequently helpful. Interloop abscesses are explored through a midabdominal incision. Each abscess cavity is thoroughly debrided, but drains are not generally used. If exploration of the abdomen is being done to find an occult abscess, a midline approach is more efficient, but a transverse incision may be better tolerated. The initial exploration should be limited to the area either above or below the transverse colon and mesocolon, the choice depending on clinical suspicion of the origin of infection.

Confirmation of the presence of pus is obtained by needle aspiration. It is essential to obtain specimens of the abscess content for stain, aerobic and anaerobic culture, and sensitivity studies. All of the abscess contents should be evacuated by suction. The cavity should be thoroughly explored digitally and all loculations within it broken down to create a single residual space. The cavity is irrigated and debrided of nonviable tissue. Multiple drains then should be brought from the abscess cavity to the exterior as directly and dependently as possible. If the abscess cavity is particularly large, or if thorough dependent drainage cannot be established, sump-suction drains should be employed in addition.

After percutaneous or open drainage of an abscess, the drains are left in place until external drainage stops or is clear. The drainage tract should then be irrigated and a sinogram obtained to verify collapse of the cavity before the drains are moved. It may take 2 to 3 weeks for a large cavity to become small enough to permit drains to be slowly advanced, allowing the drainage tract to seal as they are withdrawn.

Left Subphrenic Abscess. Formerly uncommon, these are now the most common variety of upper abdominal abscess after peritonitis or leakage from a viscus. Left subphrenic abscess also follows splenectomy, particularly when the splenic fossa is drained, and also is a consequence of pancreatitis. Unlike the subdiaphragmatic space on the right, which is divided by the liver into suprahepatic and subhepatic spaces, on the left side all these spaces are contiguous. The physical signs are costal tenderness on the left, sometimes pain in the shoulder (Kehr's sign), the presence of a left pleural effusion, and limitation of diaphragmatic motion noted by physical examination or radiography.

Lesser Sac Abscess. Technically the lesser sac abscess is a variety of left subhepatic-subphrenic abscess, since the lesser peritoneal sac anatomically is a portion of the left subhepatic space. However, the anatomic features of this abscess—and the surgical maneuvers required for drainage—are distinctly different. Lesser sac abscess is an unusual complication of diseases of the stomach, duodenum, and pancreas. The most common cause is a pancreatic abscess or a secondarily contaminated pancreatic pseudocyst that involves the lesser sac by direct extension. Perforation of a gastric ulcer or, less commonly, of a duodenal ulcer, and occasionally rupture of an ulcerating malignant gastric tumor, also may result in formation of a lesser sac abscess.

Diagnosis of a lesser sac abscess can be difficult, since much of this space is overlapped anteriorly by the left lobe of the liver. Tenderness to palpation in the midepigastrium usually is present but is a nonspecific sign. Ultrasonography is a most useful diagnostic test. Radiographic studies may show displacement of the stomach; occasionally plain radiographs show fine gas bubbles within the lesser sac, indicative of the presence of purulent material.

Lesser sac abscess has been associated with a poorer prognosis than abscesses located in other portions of the abdominal cavity. This abscess must be drained adequately; the location often dictates the use of suction drains; dependent drainage may not be easily established.

Right Subphrenic Abscess. The right subphrenic space is a potential space between the liver and the diaphragm, above the posterior attachments of the coronary and triangular ligaments to the diaphragm and posterior body wall, and extending anteriorly to the costal margin. Because the potential space is so limited in the vertical dimension, a right subphrenic abscess tends to be localized to only a portion of the total potential space, loculating either anteriorly or posteriorly. Abscesses within this space are most frequently secondary to rupture of a hepatic abscess and sometimes to operations on the stomach or duodenum.

Signs and symptoms of a right subphrenic abscess may be quite minimal. Pain is occasionally reported in the upper part of the abdomen or the lower part of the chest, sometimes referred to the back or to the right shoulder. Chest radiographs show a pleural effusion or platelike atelectasis in the right lower lung in 90 percent of patients, and the diaphragm is elevated and shows reduced motion on inspiration in sniffing or physical examination in two-thirds of patients. An air fluid level can be demonstrated in about one-fourth of those affected and establishes the diagnosis. An abscess in the right subphrenic space cannot be drained through a posterior approach unless the route of drainage transgresses the pleural space, a step that is not desirable.

Right Subhepatic Abscess. The right subhepatic space lies under the liver, bounded inferiorly by the hepatic flexure and the transverse mesocolon, medially by the duodenum and the hepatoduodenal ligament, and laterally by the body wall. The most posterior (deepest) part of this space is Morison's pouch.

A gastric procedure, especially an emergency operation for complications of ulcer disease, is the most common antecedent event. Biliary tract procedures are second in etiologic frequency. Appendicitis has declined in importance and accounts for only 8 percent of right subhepatic abscesses. Complications of colonic surgery are increasing in importance. A right subhepatic abscess usually produces some tenderness in the right upper quadrant, and the patient may complain of pain, particularly exacerbated by coughing or similar activities that produce visceral motion in the region.

Interloop Abscess. Interloop abscesses often are multiple abscesses that arise as loculations between loops of bowel, mesentery, abdominal wall, and omentum. The transverse mesocolon acts as a barrier to superior extension so that interloop abscesses usually do not involve the upper part of the abdomen. They are commonly associated with a simultaneous abscess in the pelvis.

There are no reliable symptoms or signs. A huge abscess containing more than 1 L of pus may occur without any significant physical findings. Occasionally an interloop abscess may produce a palpable, enlarging abdominal mass. The possible presence of an interloop abscess must be suspected if there has been a preceding episode of peritonitis with incomplete clinical resolution. Occasionally abdominal films show edema in the wall of loops of bowel involved in the loculation or separation or fixation of involved structures. CT examination is the most reliable diagnostic tool.

Halasz emphasized the serious problem of failure to recognize synchronous or multiple abscesses and recommended transperitoneal exploration as preferable to more limited exploration. In his series of 43 patients, one-fourth had synchronous abscesses elsewhere in the abdomen. Failure to find and drain the concomitant abscess resulted in therapeutic failure. Today, with CT diagnosis to demonstrate whether the multiple loculations are interconnected or separate, a choice between percutaneous and open drainage is more easily made. If the multiple pockets do not interconnect, open drainage is preferable; otherwise, initial percutaneous drainage is preferred.

Pelvic Abscess. This form of abscess most often follows a ruptured colonic diverticulum, pelvic inflammatory disease, ruptured appendix, or drainage into the pelvis during resolution of generalized peritonitis. Unless the abscess involves the anterior abdominal wall, few symptoms or physical signs are present on examination of the abdomen. The patient may complain only of poorly localized, dull, lower abdominal pain. Irritation of the urinary system and the rectum produces symptoms of urgency and frequency or diarrhea and tenesmus.

A localized purulent collection in the pelvis is easy to diagnose. The abscess usually can be palpated directly by rectal or vaginal examination. The typical pelvic abscess bulges as a tender mass into the anterior rectal wall. In general, pelvic inflammatory masses involving the fallopian tubes do not bulge into the rectum and tend to become less tender and to resolve over serial examinations, whereas a true pelvic abscess tends to enlarge and finally to rupture.

Pelvic drainage should be accomplished, whenever possible, directly through the rectum or vagina. Drainage should be delayed until formation of the pyogenic membrane has effectively excluded the small bowel and other intraabdominal viscera. Readiness for drainage is apparent when the most prominent aspect of the abscess presenting vaginally or rectally begins to soften. Using a speculum or anoscope, the abscess should be exposed and the presence of pus confirmed by needle aspiration. The needle is left in place as a guide; sharp incision with a knife is preferred to blunt digital entry into the abscess cavity. To ensure continued drainage and obliteration of the cavity, daily dilation of the tract digitally or with an instrument should be done until the cavity becomes obliterated. Alternatively, a Penrose drain may be placed under direct vision.

Retroperitoneal Abscess. Abscesses within the retroperitoneal spaces are not common. An abscess located in the upper retroperitoneum usually is secondary to infection of the pancreas. Retroperitoneal abscesses in other locations may be caused by primary or secondary infections of the kidneys, ureters, or colon, or by osteomyelitis of the spine, or they may be secondary to trauma. They are usually insidious in onset, thereby causing a delay in diagnosis and therapy. Commonly fever is present and there is tenderness over the involved site.

CT is helpful in defining the anatomic location and the extent of the abscess. Treatment consists of intravenous antibiotic therapy and surgical drainage, preferably via an extraperitoneal approach. Percutaneous catheter drainage with CT or ultrasound guidance may be attempted and serves as a temporizing measure in patients who are poor candidates for prompt open surgical drainage. Despite aggressive therapy, overall mortality remains higher than 50 percent in the presence of multiple organ system failure.

Percutaneous Drainage Procedures for Intraabdominal Abscesses

Percutaneous abscess drainage (PAD) and open operative intervention are best viewed as complementary rather than competitive techniques. There are many situations for which PAD is the definitive procedure of choice, others for which surgery alone is indicated, and some for which both techniques are applicable, alone or in conjunction. Inflammation may present as a phlegmon (viable inflamed tissue), a liquefied abscess, infected necrotic (nonviable) tissue, or a combination. Liquefied abscesses are drainable, whereas phlegmonous or necrotic tissue is not. Decisions regarding which modality to employ are largely based on CT findings and require experience, clinical judgment, and careful consideration of underlying and coexistent disease processes. Close cooperation between the surgeon, the interventional radiologist, and other physicians involved in the patient's care is mandatory. Specific indications for PAD have expanded significantly over the past decade and now include many conditions previously thought undrainable, such as multiple or multiloculated abscesses, abscesses with enteric communication, and infected hematomas.

The basic requirements for PAD include a safe route of percutaneous access and the presence of a fluid collection of drainable consistency. Bleeding dyscrasias are a relative contraindication. It is generally possible to distinguish drainable fluid from phlegmonous or necrotic tissue using a combination of imaging and fine-needle aspiration. Not all fluid collections require drainage, although it is generally required for infected collections and for sterile collections that cause symptoms because of their mass. The determination of whether drainage is required is made on a case-by-case basis. A *cure* is achieved when the abscess is resolved by the drainage procedure. *Temporization* refers to resolution of an abscess and clinical improvement, with operative intervention needed to treat the underlying cause. *Palliation* refers to improvement in the patient's condition as a result of abscess drainage.

The possibility of underlying neoplastic disease must be considered in enteric perforation, especially in the elderly. Significant soft-tissue thickening of the bowel wall, especially if localized and noncircumferential, should raise the possibility of underlying tumor, as should the demonstration of potential metastatic disease such as adenopathy or liver lesions. A "target" appearance, with circumferential low-attenuation submucosal thickening sandwiched between the enhancing mucosa and submucosa, is likely to be specific for inflammatory disease. To fully exclude the possibility of neoplasia, follow-up imaging is used to verify resolution of the abscess, or confirmatory tests such as barium studies or endoscopy may be performed.

Technical Aspects. Imaging permits precise localization and characterization of disease, appropriate access route planning, and, after drainage, immediate assessment of whether the procedure was successful. Imaging also is needed for adequate follow-up to identify any problems and to gauge outcome. The drainage route should not cross a sterile fluid collection or other infected space, because of the risk of cross-contamination. Crossing the pleural space for thoracic and upper abdominal drainage carries the risk of empyema formation. Collections in the upper abdomen thus often require an angled subcostal or low intercostal approach. It is acceptable to cross the peritoneal space in order to drain an extraperitoneal abscess. Placement of a catheter through the small bowel or colon should always be avoided. Transgastric drainage of lesser sac pseudocysts has been advocated by some authors and appears to be safe, although this approach remains controversial. Lesser sac collections also can be approached transhepatically through the left lobe of the liver, although traversing solid organs should be avoided whenever possible. It is important to be aware of and to avoid major vascular structures.

In most cases drainage is performed after fine-needle (18–22 gauge) aspiration, with the aspirate being used to document infection and to gauge the viscosity of the fluid. Immediate Gram stain of the fluid is useful to determine the need for drainage. In some situations single-step aspiration of the fluid may suffice, without the need for tube placement. Examples include clearly aseptic collections, small abscesses (2 to 3 cm) into which tube placement would be difficult, and relatively nonviscous collections that can be completely evacuated. For most collections, a drain should be placed to ensure complete evacuation and to minimize the chances of recurrence. The aspiration needle can be used for placement of a guide wire or as a guide for tandem insertion of the drain. Antimicrobial therapy should be initiated before the drainage procedure to minimize any infectious complications of contaminating sterile tissue and the systemic consequences of drainage.

A wide variety of techniques and equipment are available for catheter placement, the majority falling into two categories. The *trocar technique* involves the one-step insertion of a catheter that is loaded coaxially onto a stiffening cannula and needle. This is the technically simpler approach and is applicable to most superficial and large collections. The *Seldinger technique* is preferable for deep abscesses with difficult access, for drainages whose access route crosses exceptionally firm tissue, and for placement of catheters larger than 14F. A needle is first inserted into the collection. A guide wire is then passed through the needle, and the needle is withdrawn. The tract is sequentially dilated over the guide wire until it is possible to insert the catheter.

A variety of catheters are available for percutaneous insertion. The choice of catheter size is determined primarily by the viscosity of the fluid to be drained. In the majority of cases, 8F to 12F drains are sufficient. Larger drains may be needed for collections containing debris or higher-viscosity fluid, although the likelihood of success decreases. If needed, larger drains can be placed by exchange over a guide wire. There is no absolute limit on the number of drains that can be placed. While most abscesses can be drained with a single catheter, there should be no hesitation in placing as many drains as are needed to effectively evacuate the abscess(es).

After catheter placement, the cavity should be evacuated as completely as possible and irrigated with saline or antibiotic solution until the fluid is clear. Initial manipulation of the catheter(s) and irrigation should be done as gently as possible to minimize the induction of bacteremia. Immediate imaging determines the need for repositioning of the catheter, for placing a larger-bore catheter, or for placing additional drains. For cavities that are completely evacuated at the initial drainage and for which there are no abnormal communications to viscera, simple gravity drainage generally suffices. For larger or more viscous collections and for those with ongoing output from fistulous connections, suction drainage with sump catheters is more effective, although success is less likely. Thoracic drains always should be placed with water-seal suction.

Proper catheter management after the initial placement is a critical determinant of success and requires the interventional radiologist to remain an active member of the management team. Drains should be checked regularly (at least daily) to monitor the volume and nature of the output, to ensure adequate function and clinical response, and to recognize early and quickly correct any catheter-related problems. Periodic irrigation of the drains, once or several times per day, with sterile saline solution is recommended. In general, irrigation with proteolytic agents (e.g., acetylcysteine) or antibiotics is of no value, although fibrinolytic agents may be useful for evacuation of fibrinous or hemorrhagic collections. There is no standard protocol for follow-up imaging. Serial imaging studies and catheter injections are frequently used to monitor progress and identify problems. Occasionally it is necessary to replace or reposition tubes or to add additional catheters. The need for follow-up imaging studies should be determined on a case-by-case basis by monitoring clinical progress and drainage output.

Catheters should be removed when criteria for abscess resolution are met. The clinical criteria of success include the resolution of symptoms and of indicators of infection (fever, leukocytosis). The catheter-related criteria include a decrease in daily drainage to less than 10 mL and a change in the character of the drainage from purulent to serous. Radiographic criteria include verification of abscess resolution and of closure of any fistulous communications. If catheters are maintained until these criteria are satisfied, the likelihood of recurrence of the abscess will be minimized. Although some authorities recommend gradual catheter removal over several days, we usually remove the drain in one step and have had no significant problems with recurrence. For sterile fluid collections, the drain should be removed as soon as possible, generally within 24 to 48 h, to minimize the risk of superinfection.

Causes of Failure. A number of factors are consistently identified as causes of PAD failure. Prominent among these are fluid that is too viscous for drainage, or the presence of phlegmonous or necrotic debris. Technical modifications such as increasing the drain size and using irrigation can salvage some of these procedures. When phlegmonous or necrotic tissue is recognized on follow-up imaging studies, attempts at PAD may be ended in favor of open drainage, or the goals and expected outcome for PAD may be revised. Multiloculated collections and multiple abscesses are another cause of failure that can be minimized by using an adequate number of catheters along with mechanical disruption of adhesions with a guide wire. Fistulous communications, either unrecognized or persistent, are yet another potential cause of failure, as is drainage of a necrotic tumor mistaken for an abscess in imaging studies. Recognition of a significant soft-tissue component, maintenance of a high index of suspicion, and the use of percutaneous biopsies can minimize the risk of failing to appreciate the presence of tumor. Suspicious fluid also may be sent for cytologic examination. The success rate for PAD tends to be lower in immunocompromised patients. Lambiase and associates reported a cure rate of 53 percent in immunocompromised patients (including those with alcoholism, AIDS, diabetes, renal failure, or steroid use) as compared to 73 percent in immunocompetent patients.

MANAGEMENT OF SPECIFIC INTRAABDOMINAL INFECTIONS

In cases with abscesses complicating diverticulitis, PAD usually permits stabilization and allows time to prepare the patient optimally for operative therapy. Subsequent operation is required in most patients and is generally simplified to a one-step procedure. In some patients who remain asymptomatic after drainage, such as those with other, ultimately fatal diseases, subsequent colectomy may be avoided. It is important to perform follow-up radiographic studies to exclude the possibility of a perforated neoplasm. Percutaneous drainage for abscesses complicating Crohn's disease is less successful. Patients without fistulous communications to the bowel are usually cured by PAD, whereas those with fistulas generally require bowel resection. Among patients requiring operation, initial PAD usually leads to significant clinical improvement.

Low pelvic abscesses in contact with the rectum or vagina may be treated surgically by incision and drainage through these organs. The same approach can be taken using ultrasound guidance, and recent advances in endoluminal ultrasound techniques have facilitated such procedures. Ultrasound-guided transrectal and transvaginal drainage are effective and well tolerated. Good results also have been achieved in the management of tubo-ovarian abscesses complicating pelvic inflammatory disease that are refractory to medical management. In many such cases the need for hysterectomy and oophorectomy has been obviated.

The distributions of bacterial isolates in clinical intraabdominal infections as reported in several studies are listed in Table 32-7.

Infections Complicating Acute Pancreatitis. Acute necrotizing pancreatitis is the antecedent cause of pancreatic abscess in the majority of cases. Secondary infection of a pancreatic pseudocyst and abdominal trauma with pancreatic injury are other important causes. Abdominal pain, nausea, vomiting, dis-

Table 32-7
Bacterial Isolates from Intraoperative Cultures in Clinical Intraabdominal Infection

	% of Patients with Organism			
Organism	Gorbach 1974	Stone 1975	Solomkin 1990	Mosdell 1991
Gram-negative Aerobes				
Escherichia coli	61	67	58	69
Enterobacter/Klebsiella sp.	37	32	39	23
Proteus sp.	22	28	6	3
Pseudomonas aeruginosa	17	20	15	19
Gram-positive Aerobes				
Staphylococcus sp.	34	6	11	11
Anaerobes				
Bacteroides fragilis	26	34	23	45
Other Bacteroides sp.	58	51	21	
Fusobacterium sp.	14	8	6	5
Peptostreptococcus sp.	26	14	7	16
Enterococcus sp.	4	23	23	11

tention, and absent bowel sounds are frequently present. Abdominal tenderness and fever with a temperature higher than 39°C also are commonly present.

Pancreatic abscesses are polymicrobial in nature, the common organisms being aerobic representatives of the fecal flora, predominantly E. coli and aerobic hemolytic streptococci. Staphylococci usually are not involved in a primary pancreatic abscess but are frequently recovered in abscesses that follow abdominal exploration in the presence of pancreatitis.

Percutaneous drainage has a high failure rate with pancreatic abscesses, and therefore open surgical drainage is preferred. The approach is transperitoneal above the transverse mesocolon and involves radical debridement of all necrotic tissues, followed by irrigation with saline and placement of large-bore sump-suction drains. Reexploration with further debridement is frequently needed, and the staged abdominal approach has been helpful.

Infections superimposed on acute pancreatitis are among the most difficult intraabdominal infections to manage, and no consistently successful approach exists for lesser sac collections with pancreatic necrosis. Current surgical therapy consists of repetitive scheduled debridement at 48-h intervals.

For pancreatic debridement, a bilateral subcostal (chevron) or transverse incision is used to stay superior to the transverse mesocolon and avoid exposure of the small bowel. The lesser sac is entered and the stomach and colon retracted cephalad and caudad, respectively. Blunt dissection is used to remove necrotic pancreas and to open loculated abscesses. The pancreatic bed is irrigated and often packed with gauze. The value of using packing material has not been established by clinical studies and probably has little merit. Foreign material incites an inflammatory response and prolongs the time needed to clear the infection. Failure to remove packing within 48 h results in recurrent fever and other findings of infection. The use of topical antibiotic solutions is not recommended since parenteral antibiotics penetrate sites of inflammation well and topical solutions may produce unwanted adverse systemic effects.

Three or four reexplorations suffice to remove necrotic tissue and produce a granulating wound. After the final reexploration

prosthetic material used to facilitate abdominal reentry should be removed and the fascia closed. Patients should be monitored closely for evidence of recurrent infection and undergo CT scanning if infection is suspected.

For localized (acute or chronic) fluid collections, percutaneous drainage is successful in most cases. Fistulous communications to the pancreatic duct are commonly present but may be difficult to detect radiographically. To minimize the risk of recurrence with pancreatic fluid collections, it is especially important to verify complete cessation of drainage (< 25 mL/day) before the drains are removed. Endoscopic retrograde cholangiopancreatography (ERCP) is valuable in determining patency of the pancreatic duct, since fistulas associated with obstruction are unlikely to heal and generally require operation.

CT is the imaging tool of choice for localizing and characterizing complications of acute pancreatitis, and fine-needle aspiration is invaluable in determining and evaluating infection. Percutaneous drainage is a therapeutic option for evacuation of infected fluid but is not capable of removing infected necrotic tissue. Percutaneous drainage can be used to temporize and allow for a delayed definitive necrosectomy. Factors that would militate against this approach include the presence of multiple small lesser sac abscesses or concern about erosion of the inflammatory mass into the colon or major blood vessels. Two recent series detailing the use of PAD for severe complicated pancreatitis reported success rates of only 37 and 47 percent. Although the fluid collections associated with pancreatitis usually can be drained percutaneously, operation is required for debridement of infected necrotic tissue. Drainage of central collections (in the pancreatic bed and lesser sac) is less often successful than is drainage of peripheral collections because of the frequent presence of phlegmon and necrosis in the central regions.

A combination of percutaneous drainage and surgical debridement is used for infections complicating pancreatitis. One possible approach that has already been mentioned is to perform PAD initially, followed by operation for necrosectomy. This carries the risk of unduly delaying definitive surgical therapy in critically ill patients. A preferable approach is to perform early surgical debridement of the central necrotic tissues and to use PAD, if needed, for peripheral or residual fluid collections. Antimicrobial chemotherapy for patients with infections complicating pancreatitis should be guided by cultures of specimens from the pancreatic bed. Often patients are sequentially infected with gram-negative enteric flora, then gram-positive methicillin-resistant organisms, and finally Candida species.

Intraabdominal Infections in Postoperative Patients. Postoperative peritonitis generally is a consequence of anastomotic dehiscence. This is a highly lethal condition, in part because it often is diagnosed late because of reluctance to entertain the possibility of a suture-line leak. This diagnosis should be considered in any patient with signs of sepsis who has undergone a gastrointestinal anastomosis. Typical findings of diffuse abdominal tenderness may be masked by incisional pain. Because laparotomy itself introduces free air into the abdominal cavity, pneumoperitoneum is a nonspecific finding in patients during the first few days after celiotomy. Ultrasonography or CT will reveal peritoneal fluid, which, if present, should lead to ultrasound-guided aspiration for diagnostic purposes. A stain that reveals white blood cells or bacteria is an indication for immediate laparotomy. Surgical treatment should include resection and reanastomosis in the absence of purulence (small bowel) or end colostomy (colon). Postoperative abscesses are managed as detailed above.

Fistulas. Intestinal fistulas present some of the more difficult diagnostic and therapeutic problems following intraabdominal operation. The most common source is the small intestine, followed by colon, stomach, duodenum, biliary tract, and pancreas. The initial finding in most patients is occult sepsis, and the systemic response is caused by the inflammation surrounding the nascent fistula. Radiographic evaluation commonly suggests an abscess.

Abscesses with fistulous communication to the alimentary canal, biliary tree, or pancreatic duct represent a special problem for percutaneous drainage. Fistulas are loosely characterized as high-output (more than 500 mL/day) or low-output (less than 200 mL/day). Low-output fistulas may be managed with PAD, but most fistulas require sump drainage.

In several series an average of only 26 percent (range 17 to 40 percent) of fistulas were identified at the time of initial drainage. Presumably the abnormal communication is initially occluded with debris, or adequate maneuvers to uncover the leak are not performed, in the interest of minimizing tissue manipulation. A sudden change in the character of drainage or persistent output greater than 50 mL/day should alert the clinician to the presence of a fistula. Injection of contrast medium into the drainage catheter provides accurate imaging; other contrast studies (upper gastrointestinal contrast study, barium enema, ERCP, or radionuclide biliary scan) are less likely to be useful.

A catheter should be placed as close as possible to the site of leakage, using additional catheters as needed for abscess drainage. Suction drainage should be used to gain control of the leak. Slowly withdrawing the drain may promote tract closure after drainage stops. Some authors recommend a trial of capping the drain before removal, followed by imaging, to exclude fluid reaccumulation.

In five reported series the success rate of PAD with fistulas ranged from 67 to 85 percent. For a significant number of patients who were not cured, the procedure served to temporize, simplifying subsequent surgery to cure the underlying disease. When the involved bowel or duct is otherwise normal, as commonly occurs with postoperative fistulas, the vast majority of drainage procedures are successful. The presence of active underlying inflammatory disease (e.g., Crohn's disease, diverticulitis), ischemia, or neoplasia is associated with a higher rate of failure, and temporization in these cases is often a more reasonable goal. Downstream obstruction must be excluded, as this invariably prevents closure of the fistula. Maintenance of nutrition (intestinal tube feeding or parenteral nutrition) is a critical determinant of success. Some low-volume distal colonic fistulas can be managed by elemental diets.

If possible, enteric nutrition should be provided through catheters placed distal to the fistula, but it can also be given proximal to the fistula if there are 4 feet of bowel between the feeding tube and the fistula. For high-output fistulas, parenteral nutrition is often required. Somatostatin appears useful in the management of patients with pancreatic and biliary fistulas, but not enteric fistulas.

ANTIMICROBIAL THERAPY FOR INTRAABDOMINAL INFECTIONS

The goals of antibiotic therapy for intraabdominal infections that will be treated by either percutaneous or operative intervention are to hasten the elimination of infecting microorganisms and thereby shorten the clinical manifestations of infection and minimize the risk of recurrent intraabdominal infection. Since the surgical wound is heavily contaminated by the infecting microorganisms, effective antimicrobial therapy should be begun prior to operation. Necrotizing fasciitis and other forms of extension of infection to the surgical wound represent catastrophic failures of antimicrobial treatment.

In patients with localized abscesses, antibiotics reduce fever and other manifestations of systemic response, but only over an interval of 24 to 36 h. Antibiotics should be administered after fluid resuscitation has been initiated to restore adequate visceral perfusion and provide better drug distribution. Particularly in the case of aminoglycosides, nephrotoxicity is exacerbated by impaired renal perfusion.

Antimicrobial agents are begun when the diagnosis of intraabdominal infection is suspected. This is often before an exact diagnosis is established and before results of appropriate cultures are available. Accordingly, the clinician must anticipate the pathogens most likely to be encountered at the site of infection. Antibiotics used for intraabdominal infections should be active against enteric gram-negative facultative and obligate anaerobic bacilli. The identity and density of microorganisms depend on the site of the gastrointestinal tract perforation. In general, gastric, duodenal, and proximal jejunal perforations release small numbers of gram-positive aerobic and gram-negative anaerobic organisms into the peritoneal cavity. These organisms are generally susceptible to β-lactam antibiotics and are rapidly eradicated by defense mechanisms in intact hosts. *Candida albicans* or other fungi are cultured from about 20 percent of patients with acute perforations of the gastrointestinal tract. Even when fungi are recovered, antifungal agents are unnecessary unless the patient has recently received immunosuppressive therapy for neoplasm, transplantation, or inflammatory disease, or has recurrent intraabdominal infection.

Microbiologic Specimen Collection. Immediately after the abdominal cavity has been opened, a syringe is used to aspirate pus and fluid free of air. Pus is the best transport medium to maintain the viability of bacteria. The syringe containing pus is taken immediately to the laboratory for processing. If the sample cannot be transferred to media expeditiously, 1 to 2 mL of pus is injected into a sealed anaerobic tube (Port-a-cult) and kept at room temperature. Most facultative aerobes survive transportation and holding in an oxygen-free environment together with anaerobes.

The techniques used in selecting and obtaining microbiologic specimens for culture have a marked effect on the organisms recovered. The specimen collected should be representative of the material associated with the clinical infection. There must be sufficient material to permit complete microbiologic analysis. In many cases this is not possible when a specimen is submitted on a swab. When plastic syringes are used they should be transferred to the laboratory for appropriate inoculation into anaerobic medium within 30 to 60 min or oxygen will diffuse through the plastic. In some cases it may be more appropriate to send a sterile tissue sample. Specimen collection on a cotton-tipped swab is the least desirable method because only a small amount of material can be collected and because many organisms will not grow from swabs. If a cotton-tipped swab is used it should be immediately inoculated into a transport medium.

Bacterial Isolates. The organisms recovered from peritonitis and intraabdominal abscess are very similar and include a mixture of aerobic and anaerobic species. Polymicrobial clinical isolates are obtained in more than two-thirds of clinical series. The number of bacteria isolated depends on the meticulousness of laboratory technique as well as on the quality of the clinical specimen. In most clinical settings, two or three aerobic species are identified, and one or two anaerobic species. In the setting of a research-oriented microbiology laboratory, seven to ten aerobic organisms are identified along with 10 to 15 anaerobic species. The clinical utility of such extensive microbiologic efforts is dubious, but they help us to understand the pathogenesis of these infections. One of the most striking findings is that the bacteria populations from peritonitis or abscess are qualitatively and quantitatively different from those found within the gut lumen.

Of the wide spectrum of microorganisms in the intestines, only a few are capable of causing infection in human beings, and even fewer participate in polymicrobial intraabdominal infections. Comparison of the relative occurrence of bacteria in the normal intestine and their relative recovery in intraabdominal infections reveals distinctive selection patterns that reflect the survival capacity of certain bacteria outside the bowel lumen.

Obligate anaerobic bacteria comprise more than 99 percent of the intestinal flora. After bowel perforation most of these anaerobes can be isolated by appropriate culture techniques. They die off quickly, however, in conditions outside their natural environment. Only as contamination of the abdominal cavity progresses to established infection does selection of the most pathogenic organisms take place, resulting in the typical spectrum of bacteria found in an intraabdominal infection.

Cultures from patients with distal small-bowel perforations grow gram-negative facultative organisms with variable density. Perforations of the distal small bowel often evolve to localized abscess formation and present with peritonitis only after rupture of the abscess. Colonic anaerobes such as *B. fragilis* are sometimes present. In patients with colon-derived intraabdominal infections the peritoneal cavity is contaminated with large numbers of facultative and obligate anaerobic gram-negative organisms.

Subsequent decisions regarding antimicrobial therapy should be guided by the results of intraoperative cultures. Although the appropriate role of antienterococcal therapy is controversial, most authorities believe that specific antienterococcal therapy should be given only when enterococci are the only organisms isolated or when they are isolated from blood. Isolation of enterococci as part of a mixed gram-positive and gram-negative flora should not prompt the addition of ampicillin or vancomycin to the antibiotic regimen. The incidence of treatment failure for patients harboring enterococci and not treated for it is the same as for patients treated with imipenem or other agents effective against enterococci. Enterococci are very low-level pathogens, meaning that they incite little host response and do not cause invasive infection in intact hosts. Patients who have had one major episode of sepsis are sufficiently immunosuppressed that

isolation of enterococci from a second infectious site (including recurrent infection within the abdomen) should mandate specific antienterococcal therapy. If the smear reveals gram-negative bacilli, failure to isolate either facultative or obligate anaerobes on culture does not obviate the need to continue providing antimicrobial agents against both. Antimicrobial susceptibility patterns within each hospital should be heeded in selecting initial empiric therapy.

Empiric Therapy. Antimicrobials are often begun if infection is even a remote possibility. The wisdom of this approach depends on the evidence suggesting an infection, taken against the background risk of harm to the patient. Antimicrobial treatment is not without potential adverse effects, but these generally are perceived as temporally remote and often take the form of changes in hospital- or unit-specific susceptibility patterns. For patients with suspected community-acquired infection, recent onset of malaise, symptoms referable to a specific anatomic area, and findings of fever and localizing tenderness, mass, or evidence of organ dysfunction are often sufficient to begin antimicrobial therapy after appropriate cultures are obtained. Except in certain forms of meningitis, initiation of antibiotic therapy is not time-critical. Antibiotics should be administered after fluid resuscitation has begun, so that distribution of the drug(s) is adequate. As noted earlier, the nephrotoxicity of antibiotic agents, especially of the aminoglycosides, is exacerbated by impaired renal perfusion. In the case of suspected community-acquired infection, knowledge of the endogenous flora giving rise to infection is a valuable guide to the selection of antibiotic therapy while awaiting the results of cultures.

Infections in hospitalized patients, particularly in the intensive care unit, require a different set of criteria for beginning antimicrobial therapy. Such patients often have undergone extensive operative procedures and have numerous noninfectious potential causes for fever. Conversely, infection may be masked by immunosuppression associated with the condition (or treatment) that resulted in hospitalization. Such patients become colonized, and cultures of sputum, wounds, and drain tracts are often positive in the absence of infection. Interpretation of culture results is therefore quite difficult unless positive cultures are obtained from a routinely sterile site such as blood or pleural or peritoneal fluid.

Value of Precise Identification of Infecting Organism(s). In vitro data, especially antimicrobial susceptibility tests, are predictive of the in vivo response of infecting bacteria to antibacterial agents; this allows selection of a specific agent or combination regimen and obviates the need for broad-spectrum therapy. Equally important information is gained from stains of infected fluid collections or other direct examinations such as KOH preparations of cerebrospinal fluid for *Cryptococcus neoformans* or bronchoalveolar lavage fluid for other fungi. While a variety of susceptibility testing techniques are available, automated testing is appropriate for bacteria isolated from most infections except in extraordinary circumstances. Certain organisms do not require routine susceptibility testing. Nonenterococcal streptococci are routinely susceptible to penicillin. Because of the technical problems of performing anaerobic susceptibilities, it is best for such isolates to be identified and then batch-tested on a yearly basis for changes in otherwise predictable susceptibilities. This particularly applies to *B. fragilis* group isolates. Local or regional hospital antimicrobial susceptibility patterns determine initial empiric therapy.

Fluid collections, particularly if purulent, should be obtained for smear culture. Specimens of infected fluid are sent to the laboratory in a capped airless syringe with no needle or collected in appropriate separate aerobic and anaerobic transport media. If the stain reveals a predominance of gram-positive cocci, which may indicate that the enterococci or other fecal streptococci are significant copathogens at the site of infection, the clinician should consider alterations in the antibiotic regime to include agents specifically active against *Enterococcus* species.

If the smear reveals gram-negative bacilli, failure to isolate either facultative or obligate anaerobes on culture does not obviate the need to continue to provide antimicrobial agents against both. Conversely, stain in the presence of purulence will not demonstrate a bacterium if organisms are present at a density less than 10^5/mL. A negative stain should not prompt discontinuance of antibiotics until culture results are available and a clinical response has been achieved.

The disk-diffusion method provides qualitative data about the susceptibility of an organism to a given agent. Quantitative data require serial dilutions of the antimicrobial agent in media. The lowest concentration of the agent that prevents visible growth after an incubation period of 18 to 24 h is known as the *minimum inhibitory concentration* (MIC). The *minimal bactericidal concentration* (MBC) can be determined by subculturing on antibiotic-free medium those tubes that show no growth in the determination of the MIC.

There are a number of common errors in the interpretation of sensitivity results from hospital laboratories. Certain agents such as nalidixic acid, nitrofurantoin, and norfloxacin are tested at concentrations achievable only in urine. Susceptibility results for such agents are not meaningful for the management of systemic infections, and using them may result in treatment failure. Conversely, some nontoxic antibiotics for urinary tract infections, such as ampicillin, are not tested at the high concentrations achieved in urine and may be effective even though "resistance" is reported. Intravascular infections such as endocarditis or catheter-related bacteremias may be inadequately treated by *bacteriostatic* agents despite in vitro susceptibility results suggesting efficacy. Concentrations of bacteria employed in susceptibility testing are considerably below those found in clinical situations. Antibiotics effective at the lower bacterial concentrations may not be effective at the higher inoculum. This dependence of antibiotic efficacy on bacterial concentration, termed the *inoculum effect,* is prominent for the β-lactam antibacterials.

Treatment Response. Treatment response is defined as a diminution in the physical signs of infection, including decrease in fever, in tachycardia, and in local findings of tenderness and organ dysfunction, such as ileus. The more localized the initial infection, the more rapidly response will occur. Conversely, extensive infections such as peritonitis or multilobar pneumonia may respond only slowly. As a general rule, infections should show definite evidence of response within 72 h of initiation of treatment. The absence of response is not an automatic indication that the wrong antibiotic was selected. In most cases of apparent treatment failure the same antibiotic should be continued while a diligent search is made for a localized septic anatomic focus requiring drainage, debridement, or excision.

Selection of Antibacterial Agents

The combination of evidence from in vitro data, animal studies, and clinical trials has led to widespread acceptance of the need to provide empiric antimicrobial therapy directed against *E. coli* and other common members of the family Enterobacteriaceae and against *B. fragilis. B. fragilis* and *E. coli* are the most common isolates from intraabdominal infections and are most likely to cause bacteremia in abdominal sepsis, further attesting to their pathogenicity. The evidence in support of broadening therapy to cover organisms other than common facultative and obligate anaerobes such as *E. coli* and *B. fragilis* is more controversial. Initial empiric coverage of *P. aeruginosa* if these organisms are isolated from the site of infection is associated with a decreased likelihood of persistent or recurrent abdominal infection. Other clinical trials, however, do not demonstrate a high incidence of treatment failure associated with this organism, even if it is not treated.

There are a number of agents that are broadly active against the bacteria found in intraabdominal infections. These are best discussed as classes of drugs including the aminoglycosides, carbapenems, cephalosporins, penicillins plus β-lactamase inhibitors, and quinolones. Aztreonam will be considered as a cephalosporin-class agent. An example of what some consider appropriate antibiotics in peritonitis is provided in Table 32-8. Current sensitivities are listed in Table 32-9.

Table 32-8
Appropriate Antibiotic Choices in Peritonitis*

Secondary Peritonitis
  Monotherapy:
    Ampicillin/sulbactam
    Cefotetan
    Cefoxitin
    Piperacillin
    Piperacillin/tazobactam
  Combination therapy:
    Aminoglycoside/metronidazole *or* clindamycin
    Aztreonam/metronidazole *or* clindamycin
Tertiary Peritonitis
  Monotherapy (seldom possible):
    Imipenem/cilastatin
    Piperacillin/tazobactam
  Combination therapy:
    Aminoglycoside/metronidazole *or* clindamycin *or* imipenem/
      cilastatin
    Aztreonam/metronidazole *or* clindamycin
    Cefepime/metronidazole *or* clindamycin
    Ceftazidime/metronidazole *or* clindamycin
    Ciprofloxacin/metronidazole *or* clindamycin
      For *Enterococcus:*
        Ampicillin *or* piperacillin *or* vancomycin (only if ampicillin-resistant or the patient is allergic to penicillin)
      For methicillin-resistant staphylococci:
        Vancomycin
      For *Pseudomonas:*
        Aminoglycoside *plus* aztreonam *or* cefepime *or* ceftazidime *or* piperacillin/tazobactam *or* imipenem/cilastatin
      For *Candida:*
        Fluconazole *or* amphotericin B

*Reflecting the preferences of the authors. Other antibiotics, alone or in combination, may be appropriate in individual circumstances, as long as the spectrum of activity includes activity against both aerobic and anaerobic gram-negative bacilli.

Table 32-9
Antimicrobial Sensitivities of Commonly Encountered Pathogens to Parenteral Antibiotics Used in Abdominal Infection

	Gram-negative Bacilli	Gram-positive Cocci		Gram-negative Bacilli	Gram-positive Bacilli	Gram-positive Cocci
		Enterococci	Other Strepto-coccus species			
Penicillin	0	++	+++	+	+++	+++
Ampicillin	+	+++	+++	+	+++	+++
Piperacillin	+++	+++	+++	++	+++	+++
Ticarcillin[a]	++	++	+++	++	++	++
Cefazolin[b]	++	0	+++	+	+++	+++
Cefamandole[c]	++	0	+++	+	++	+++
Cefoxitin[d]	++	0	++	++	+++	+++
Cefotaxime[e]	+++	0	++	+	++	+++
Imipenem/meropenem	+++	++	+++	+++	+++	+++
Aztreonam	+++	0	0	0	0	0
Aminoglycosides[f]	+++	0	0	0	0	0
Clindamycin	0	0	++	+++	+++	+++
Metronidazole	0	0	0	+++	+++	+++
β-lactamase inhibitor/Beta-lactam combinations:						
Ampicillin/sulbactam	++	+++	+++	+++	+++	+++
Ticarcillin/clavulanic acid	++	++	+++	+++	+++	+++
Piperacillin/tazobactam	+++	+++	+++	+++	+++	+++

0 = little or no activity; + = some activity; ++ = moderate to good activity; +++ = excellent activity.

[a]Azlocillin, mezlocillin, and carbenicillin have similar spectra.

[b]Includes cephalothin, cephapirin, and cephradine.

[c]Includes cefuroxime, cefonicid, cefotiam, and ceforanide.

[d]Includes cefotetan and cefmetazole.

[e]Includes ceftriaxone, ceftazidime, cefoperazone, ceftizoxime, and cefepime.

[f]Includes gentamicin, tobramycin, netilmicin, and amikacin.

SOURCE: From Solomkin JS, Moulton JS: Diagnosis and management of intraabdominal sepsis, in Rippe JM, Irwin RS, Fink MP, Cerra FB (eds): *Intensive Care Medicine*, 3d ed, Boston, Little, Brown, 1996. Used by permission.

Aminoglycosides. The aminoglycosides have been the mainstay of therapy for serious gram-negative infections for the past thirty years. Because of their potential for nephrotoxicity and ototoxicity, aminoglycosides are less likely to be used as first-choice agents for community-acquired intraabdominal infections. The use of β-lactam antibiotics with clindamycin or metronidazole, β-lactam antibiotics combined with β-lactamase inhibitors, or single-agent imipenem/cilastatin in mixed-flora infections has resulted in clinical results equivalent to or better than those seen with aminoglycoside-based combinations. The aminoglycosides no longer represent a "gold standard" of comparison and need not be used for community-acquired intraabdominal infections.

Hypotensive patients with gram-negative bacteremias have higher survival rates if treated at least initially with aminoglycoside-based combination therapy. Approximately one-third of patients with nonappendiceal intraabdominal infections are bacteremic. While gram-negative organisms do not represent the same risk of endocarditis on normal valves or of metastatic abscess formation seen with *Staph. aureus,* combination bactericidal therapy may result in more rapid clearance of organisms and abbreviate host deterioration. Aminoglycosides should specifically be used in the initial treatment of patients with major intraabdominal infection and hypotension in combination with a β-lactam agent, which is effective against the anticipated gram-negative organisms.

Pharmacokinetics. In contrast to the β-lactam antibiotics, the efficacy of the aminoglycosides depends on the maximal concentration achieved. As the ratio of the concentration of aminoglycoside to the minimum inhibitory concentration (ratio of peak concentration to MIC) is increased, the rate and extent of killing is also increased. Moore and colleagues examined the relationship between plasma aminoglycoside concentrations, MICs for the infecting organisms, and therapeutic outcome. Higher and mean ratios of peak aminoglycoside concentration to MIC (6:1) were correlated with a positive clinical response. In addition to concentration-dependent bactericidal activity, aminoglycosides, like other antimicrobials that affect the synthesis of protein, DNA, or RNA, exhibit persistent suppression of bacterial growth after antimicrobial exposure, which is referred to as a post-antibiotic effect (PAE). This phenomenon allows killing to continue despite drug concentrations well below the MIC of the infecting organism. This translates into prolonged dosing intervals. Cell-wall-active agents such as penicillins and cephalosporins exert a PAE against gram-positive bacteria, but none against gram-negative bacteria. Imipenem exerts a modest PAE against gram-negative bacteria. In general, the greater the concentration-to-MIC ratio, the longer the PAE. The PAE allows aminoglycosides to be administered less frequently, and this in turn lowers the risk of aminoglycoside toxicity.

Nephrotoxicity. Aminoglycoside nephrotoxicity is believed to be caused by its accumulation in the proximal renal tubular cell by the process of adsorptive pinocytosis. Once in the cell, the antimicrobial is taken up by cellular lysosomes. This process is diminished when aminoglycoside tubular fluid concentrations fall below a critical value and becomes saturated at higher concentrations. Neither of these limiting values is known precisely, but 2 and 12 mg/dL, respectively, appear to be of the right order of magnitude. Once incorporated into lysosomes, aminoglycosides inhibit lysosomal phospholipase and sphingomyelinase activity, and if drug exposure is prolonged, proximal renal tubular cell phospholipidosis occurs. The overloaded lysosomes swell and then rupture, releasing aminoglycoside, lysosomal enzymes, and phospholipids into the cytosol. The functional integrity of the cell is disturbed, and the result is cell death.

This proposed mechanism may explain why allowing serum aminoglycoside concentrations to decline below 2 mg/dL ("trough level") before administering the next scheduled dose is effective, and why peak serum concentrations have such a minor influence on the nephrotoxic potential of aminoglycosides. In individuals with normal renal function, once-daily dosing of gentamicin and netilmicin routinely results in serum trough concentrations of less than 0.5 mg/dL. Multiple daily doses of aminoglycosides result in more frequent or more severe nephrotoxicity than do less frequent or once-daily doses of these agents.

Pharmacokinetics in Critically Ill Patients. Traditional aminoglycoside dosing methods such as manufacturer's recommendations or nomograms are based on the assumption that pharmacokinetic parameters such as volume of distribution (Vd) and clearance (Cl) are similar from patient to patient, regardless of severity of illness. In fact, however, there is not only a wide variability in these parameters among non-critically ill patients but also significant variability between non-critically ill and critically ill patients. Traditional dosing methods thus can result in inappropriate aminoglycoside regimens.

Septic and postsurgical patients in intensive care units often require large volumes of fluid for resuscitation with major fluid shifts. Alterations in the concentrations of hormones and vasoactive substances may affect blood flow and organ perfusion and function. Cardiac, respiratory, renal, and hepatic failure occur frequently, alone and in combination, and can significantly alter the absorption, distribution, metabolism, and elimination of many drugs. Critically ill patients with sepsis demonstrate altered aminoglycoside pharmacokinetic values as compared with those not critically ill. Critically ill patients typically are significantly older and have higher serum creatinine concentrations and lower elimination rate constants and total body clearances than non-critically ill patients. The major contributing factor, especially in surgical patients, appears to be volume replacement/resuscitation following operation. These differences require significant alterations in the dosing regimens of the aminoglycosides. In critically ill patients, a decrease in clearance and elimination rate constants means that the conventional 8-h dosing intervals may not be sufficient to maintain trough concentrations of less than 2 mg/dL. Additionally, the increase in distribution volume may require a larger dose of aminoglycoside to achieve therapeutic peak concentrations.

Failure to appreciate a decrease in clearance and an increase in distribution volume in critically ill patients can result in suboptimal aminoglycoside therapy. For critically ill patients, gentamicin and tobramycin doses of 3 to 5 mg/kg/day should be replaced with a higher dose of 7 mg/kg/day administered in two divided doses (i.e., every 12 h) or as a single daily dose.

In addition to the difference in pharmacokinetic parameters between critically ill and non-critically ill patients, there also appears to be a wide variation in aminoglycoside pharmacokinetics among critically ill patients. In addition, there is little correlation between changes in serum creatinine concentration and dosing interval. Serum creatinine levels should not be used as a measure of aminoglycoside toxicity or in order to estimate an appropriate dosing interval; rather, it is necessary in critically ill patients to obtain frequent aminoglycoside serum concentrations.

High-dose intermittent therapy with aminoglycosides is preferable. Patients with major infections have expanded volumes of distribution for aminoglycosides and commonly require 2.5 mg/kg gentamicin or tobramycin to achieve therapeutic levels. Regimens involving high-dose (10 mg/kg) gentamicin or tobramycin given every 24 h have been used. This is based on two key antimicrobial properties of aminoglycosides—dose-dependent killing and a post-antibiotic effect. Several trials have examined once-daily dosing, employing netilmicin, amikacin, tobramycin, and gentamicin. Infections treated have included cystic fibrosis, gangrenous and perforated appendicitis, other intraabdominal infections, gram-negative bacteremias, mixed serious infections, pelvic inflammatory disease, and urinary tract infections. Doses have ranged from 4.5 to 9 mg/kg/day for tobramycin, netilmicin, and gentamicin, and 15 mg/kg/day for amikacin. Peak serum concentrations with the once-daily regimen have been obtained with doses ranging from 8 to 52 mg/dL for tobramycin and netilmicin, 33 to 55 mg/dL for amikacin, and 35 mg/dL for gentamicin.

The patient's immunocompetence may affect the utility of this regimen. In an animal study, once-daily tobramycin was found to reduce the mean bacterial titer in the lungs significantly more than the every-4-h regimen in nonneutropenic animals. In neutropenic animals, however, the once-daily regimen proved to be less effective than the every-4-h regimen, as evidenced by a rapid regrowth of bacteria during the latter 12 to 16 h of the 24-h dosing interval.

β-lactam Antibiotics and β-lactam/β-lactamase Inhibitor Combinations. First-generation cephalosporins, including cefazolin, cephapirin, and cephalothin, have excellent gram-positive activity, moderate gram-negative activity, and no anaerobic activity. Cefonicid, cefamandole, and cefuroxime may be grouped with these agents because none has anaerobic activity. The second-generation cephalosporins cefoxitin, cefotetan, and cefmetazole all have some anaerobic activity, improved facultative gram-negative activity, and less gram-positive coverage. The anaerobic activity of these agents against *B. fragilis* is unimpressive, with about one-third to one-half of tested isolates being resistant. Because of the high incidence of *B. fragilis* and relatively large inoculum loads encountered in colon-derived infections, these agents are best used for prophylaxis and for treatment of low-inoculum infections such as appendicitis.

The third-generation cephalosporins, cefotaxime, ceftizoxime, cefoperazone, ceftriaxone, ceftazidime, and cefepime, have considerable facultative gram-negative activity, but no anaerobic and limited gram-positive coverage. Aztreonam, a monobactam, has activity against facultative gram-negative organisms equivalent to third-generation cephalosporins. It has no gram-positive or anaerobic activity. Metronidazole has remained highly effective against *Bacteroides* species, unlike clindamycin, and is now the preferred agent in combination therapy.

The choice of one third-generation cephalosporin or aztreonam versus another is not a major issue. As experience with these agents has widened, it has become apparent that the differences between agents do not affect outcome. Many hospitals have therefore taken the position that cephalosporins can be grouped into classes within each of which the agents are therapeutically interchangeable. Acquisition costs commonly determine which cephalosporin is used in each class. Ceftazidime is *not* recommended because broad usage is associated with decreasing susceptibility of nosocomial *P. aeruginosa,* and this agent is the only cephalosporin usable for this pathogen. Additionally, ceftazidime therapy is associated with an increased incidence of enterococcal superinfections.

Another, more speculative issue fueling interest in antibiotic regimens other than cephalosporins or penicillin derivatives is the possibility that such β-lactam therapy may exacerbate the degree of sepsis seen in the patient. There is clear evidence that agents such as cephalosporins and penicillin derivatives disrupt the outer membrane of gram-negative organisms, exposing the lipid structures ordinarily facing the interior of the cell and ordinarily hidden by long polysaccharides attached to the lipid core. Antibiotic treatment results in the formation of small bacterial fragments with considerable proinflammatory capabilities. Cultures of gram-negative bacteria treated with β-lactam antibiotics release endotoxin, and culture filtrates induce considerably more TNF-α from mononuclear cells than do filtrates from cultures treated with aminoglycosides, carbapenems, or quinolones.

β-lactamases in Bacterial Resistance. β-lactamases are ubiquitous, and therapeutic use of β-lactam antibiotics has been selected against bacterial strains with increased amounts of enzymes and/or selected enzymes with an extended spectrum of activity. The most important chromosomal enzymes are the Class I enzymes that occur in Enterobacteriaceae and *Pseudomonas* species; these enzymes have a high affinity for β-lactams but hydrolyze the drugs slowly. Some bacteria are able to synthesize large amounts of β-lactamases if challenged with a β-lactam. This induced expression is important for *P. aeruginosa, Enterobacter, Citrobacter, Serratia, Morganella,* and *Providencia* species, for *Proteus vulgaris,* and for bacteria in which enzyme activity is stably derepressed. Once selected, derepressed mutants remain sensitive to carbapenems, cefepime, cefpirome, quinolones and aminoglycosides.

TEM-1 is now the commonest plasmid-mediated β-lactamase. This is followed in frequency by SHV-1, PSE-1 and -4, which confer resistance to ampicillin, amoxicillin, ticarcillin, piperacillin, mezlocillin, cefamandole, and cefoperazone. Mutants have been identified in clinical isolates; these mutants have even broader substrate profiles, including most penicillins, cephalosporins, and aztreonam.

A serine in the active site forms a noncovalent complex with the β-lactam, followed by acylation. During this reaction the β-lactam ring is opened, destroying the drug's activity. This reaction also occurs with the drug's true target, the penicillin-binding proteins (PBPs). In this case, drug binding to the PBP inactivates it and prevents cell replication. For β-lactamases, hydrolysis is much more rapid than for PBPs, and it liberates the enzyme and results in drug inactivation. In vivo susceptibility to hydrolysis depends on the pericytoplasmic concentration of the antibiotic, which often is quite low.

Clinically meaningful problems with β-lactamase induction have most commonly involved *Enterobacter* species. *Enterobacter* species have recently emerged as a major cause of nosocomial gram-negative bacteremia in the intensive care unit, ranking third to fifth in frequency. The organism's ability to rapidly develop resistance to third-generation cephalosporins, resulting in higher mortality rates, has been cause for concern.

Chow and associates reported that the administration of a third-generation cephalosporin within 14 days of *Enterobacter* bacteremia was more likely to be associated with a multiresistant *Enterobacter* species in the initial positive blood culture. Patients infected with multiresistant organisms had a higher mortality rate that was independent of other risk factors such as age and underlying disease. This supports the contention by some that highly resistant organisms may emerge more rapidly as a result of the routine use of cephalosporins. Therefore, when *Enterobacter* organisms are isolated from blood, third-generation cephalosporins should be avoided regardless of in vitro susceptibility.

There is variability from one intensive care unit (ICU) to another in the incidence of *Enterobacter* and other organisms that can induce β-lactamases, and there are also unit-specific organisms with mutated β-lactamases. Therefore susceptibility data of ICU organisms should be reported separately from isolates from other hospital units, and this unit-specific data should be employed to make decisions regarding empiric therapy. Many units have deliberately continued the practice of initiating empiric treatment for suspected gram-negative infection with aminoglycoside/β-lactam combinations because of a relatively high incidence of resistant organisms. The aminoglycosides as well as the carbapenems and quinolones have thus far retained their in vitro activity against these organisms, although carbapenem-resistant *Enterobacter* have been reported.

An alternative strategy to the use of β-lactamase–resistant cephalosporins is to use β-lactams in combination with β-lactamase inhibitors that alone are not potent antibiotics. Sulbactam, clavulanic acid, and tazobactam are efficient inhibitors of β-lactamases from gram-positive and anaerobic organisms. They have lesser activity against the chromosomal β-lactamases seen in Enterobacteriaceae and do not completely compensate for the marginal gram-negative activity of the penicillin derivative. The primary concern has to do with organisms that hyperexpress β-lactamases. Organisms that typically do this include *P. aeruginosa,* and *Enterobacter, Citrobacter, Serratia,* and *Acinetobacter* species. These particular organisms are most commonly encountered in nosocomial infections but are also present in about 15 percent of community-acquired infections.

Carbapenems. Imipenem, a carbapenem derivative, has broad activity against facultative and obligate gram-negative anaerobes and excellent gram-positive activity, excepting methicillin-resistant staphylococci. This agent is formulated with cilastatin, a renal dehydropeptidase inhibitor that prevents renal tubular epithelial metabolism of the drug. In situations where plasma accumulation of the drug occurs, as in high-dose levels or renal failure, the drug may cause seizures. With lower-dose levels (500 mg) and appropriate adjustments for renal failure, this is not a problem.

Meropenem is a synthetic agent with a typical broad carbapenem antibacterial spectrum, but with no evidence of an increased risk of seizures compared with cephalosporin control agents. In several clinical trials in which serious intraabdominal infections were treated with meropenem dosed at 1 g every 8 h the drug has shown efficacy.

Fluoroquinolones. The quinolones are chemical modifications of the basic nalidixic acid structure. They have antibacterial potencies 1000 times greater than that of nalidixic acid and are active against gram-negative and gram-positive organisms. The intracellular target of the quinolones is DNA gyrase, an enzyme involved in DNA breakage and repair. It appears that quinolones actually bind to DNA breaks caused by DNA gyrase, with at least four drug molecules binding per site; the binding is stabilized by the enzyme itself. The quinolones are considered bactericidal and are not susceptible to inoculum effects.

Since quinolones are totally synthesized, a vast array of congeners are possible and it is probable that the number of available oral quinolones will eventually exceed the number of cephalosporins. The currently marketed fluoroquinolones are active against facultative and aerobic gram-negative bacteria. *Streptococcus* and *Enterococcus* species show in vitro susceptibility to quinolones, but other, more effective agents are available. *Staph. aureus* and coagulase-negative staphylococci have become progressively more resistant to fluoroquinolones. These drugs should be considered only as a last resort for treatment of infections caused by multiply antibiotic-resistant gram-positive strains, and only in combination with other antistaphylococcal drugs. Fluoroquinolones have excellent activity against gram-negative bacilli. Activity patterns for ciprofloxacin and ofloxacin are very similar. For *P. aeruginosa,* ciprofloxacin has consistently shown greater in vitro activity. Treatment of *P. aeruginosa* with ciprofloxacin risks development of resistance and is not recommended. Resistance to quinolones occurs primarily through spontaneous mutation of either the A or B subunits of the target DNA gyrase. Mutation rates in *Serratia marcescens* and *P. aeruginosa* appear higher than in other gram-negative organisms, and the mutation rate for *Staph. aureus* is also quite high. Resistance also may arise through changes in bacterial permeability. Norfloxacin, because of its poor absorption and low serum concentrations, should not be used to treat systemic infections.

A primary virtue of the quinolones is a very large volume of distribution. Because of their relatively small molecular size and the absence of localized electrical charges, these agents penetrate well into interstitial fluid and achieve high tissue levels, well in excess of those seen with other, larger molecules. Recognition of the wide volume of distribution and broad susceptibility profiles has led to clinical trials examining their efficacy in serious infections. These trials demonstrate an impressive level of activity in nosocomial gram-negative pneumonia and in serious intraabdominal infections. Ciprofloxacin has been found to show better results than imipenem in the treatment of pneumonia. Patients with *P. aeruginosa* did not fare well in either arm of the trial. Almost all quinolones are excreted through the kidneys, and both ciprofloxacin and norfloxacin have an enterohepatic circulation. Hence there is only a modest increase in half-life for these agents in the presence of renal failure.

One major benefit of currently available quinolones, as compared with β-lactam agents, is their continuing activity against *Enterobacter* and other species that have inducible β-lactamases. Another advantage of quinolone therapy is the potential for oral treatment of serious gram-negative infections, as there are a variety of clinical situations in which prolonged therapy is appro-

priate. These include hepatic abscesses and nosocomial pneumonia. Most significant intraabdominal infections are treated for 7 or more days.

The next generation of quinolones is represented by the agents trovafloxacin and clinafloxacin. These drugs have substantially expanded spectra of activity, including against many ciprofloxacin-resistant gram-negative and gram-positive organisms and against many anaerobic organisms, including *B. fragilis.* These agents also appear to have potential side effects of gene damage and photosensitization, and their futures remain unclear.

Quinolone antibiotics, which act by inhibiting DNA replication, appear to be potentially useful for serious systemic infections and have shown similar activity to imipenem in clinical trials for pneumonia and intraabdominal infection. Available quinolones have little anti-*B. fragilis* activity and should be combined with metronidazole if an anaerobic component of the infecting flora is suspected. Quinolones are applicable because serum levels following oral absorption parallel those seen in intravenous infusion. In patients with anatomically extensive infections such as diffuse peritonitis, prolonged therapy with oral quinolones is attractive.

Dosing of cephalosporin, carbapenem, and quinolone antibiotics should be optimized on the basis of their known pharmacodynamics. Cell-wall-active agents are effective at the minimum inhibitory concentration of the drug for the organism(s) being treated. Increasing the drug concentration substantially above about two to four times the MIC does not increase the rate of killing. Once the drug falls below the MIC, the organism begins regrowth immediately. Dosage regimens for cell-wall-active agents in critically ill patients should involve dosing intervals sufficiently short to maintain serum levels above the MIC. With these agents, relatively small doses should be given frequently to maintain the trough level above the MIC and to avoid the costs and toxicities seen with high doses. This is best accomplished by administering these drugs every four half-lives, with adjustments as needed for renal compromise. There has been interest in infrequent drug dosing with β-lactams; this is most likely to succeed in mild to moderate infections in otherwise intact hosts.

Combination Therapy. One result of the availability of multiple classes of effective antibiotics is the possibility of combination therapy with two effective agents. Combination therapy has several theoretical advantages. A broader spectrum of pathogens can be covered, which is of particular importance when treatment is initiated for suspected sepsis without an identified source. Agents with differing mechanisms of action also may delay or prevent the emergence of resistance and superinfection. Combinations of such agents may act synergistically to enhance killing of organisms.

The time-honored tradition of providing an aminoglycoside along with a β-lactam agent has gained support from two studies of gram-negative bacteremia, demonstrating improved survival in patients with severe acute illness treated with combination therapy as opposed to those treated with a single agent. In a similarly constructed study of *Klebsiella* bacteremia, a similar improvement in severely ill patients treated with combination therapy was noted. Survival rates in both studies were around 70 percent for the combination therapy group as compared to 50 percent for the monotherapy group.

Regimens employing two β-lactam agents have been attempted primarily in the setting of febrile neutropenia. No benefit has been found, and there is concern that coverage with such regimens is not as broad as that obtained with an aminoglycoside-based regimen since the β-lactam antibiotics have similar mechanisms of action.

Pharmacokinetics of Antibiotics. Pharmacokinetic parameters can be used to aid in drug selection. Unlike with the aminoglycosides, the maximum effect of the β-lactam-like agents, including cephalosporins, penicillins, aztreonam, imipenem, and quinolones, is not correlated with the peak/MIC ratio seen with a single dose. Rather, the time over a 24-h period above the MIC is most important. Studies have shown that continuous-infusion cephalosporin therapy is maximally effective. Hence the general rule with these agents is to give relatively small doses frequently—every four half-lives, with any necessary adjustments for renal function—to maintain the trough level above the MIC and thus to avoid the costs and toxicities of higher doses.

Another pharmacokinetic variable of considerable significance is the route of elimination. Most agents are excreted by the urine and achieve high levels there. Imipenem is metabolized by renal tubular epithelial cells. To circumvent this, this agent is supplied with the dehydropeptidase inhibitor cilastatin, which provides high urine levels of intact drug and prolongs the circulating half-life. Agents that are excreted primarily by the liver require no dosage adjustment in renal failure but are associated with a high incidence of diarrhea. Such agents may result in acquisition of an enteric flora that is highly resistant to antimicrobial therapy and an increased risk of antibiotic-associated colitis. Since most nosocomial pneumonias are believed to arise from microaspiration of enteric contents, this greatly limits the utility of these agents in severely ill patients with extrabiliary infections.

This property is extremely helpful, however, in managing complex biliary infections such as those seen after enterobiliary anastomoses, biliary stent placement, and biliary stricture. Cefoperazone, piperacillin, and mezlocillin are eliminated at least in part in the bile, and consequently biliary antibiotic levels are high enough to kill bacteria that are resistant to these agents at levels normally achieved in serum. These antibiotics are effective in treating aminoglycoside-unresponsive gram-negative and *Enterococcus* infections in partially obstructed bile ducts.

Bibliography

History

Altemeier WA: The cause of the putrid odor of perforated appendicitis with peritonitis. *Ann Surg* 107:634, 1938.

Altemeier WA: The pathogenicity of the bacteria of appendicitis peritonitis. *Surgery* 11:374, 1942.

Altemeier WA: Surgical infection of the peritoneum. *Surg Clin North Am* 22:437, 1942.

Friedrich PL: Bacteriological ecology and treatment of diffuse peritonitis (German). *Arch Klin Chir* 68:524, 1902.

Fowler GR: Diffuse septic peritonitis, with special reference to a new method of treatment, namely, the elevated head and trunk posture, to facilitate drainage into the pelvis: With a report of nine consecutive cases of recovery. *Med Rec* 57:617, 1900.

Kirschner M: The therapy of acute suppurative diffuse peritonitis (German). *Langenbecks Arch Chir* 142:53, 1926.

Landman MD, Longmire WP Jr: Neural and hormonal influences of peritonitis on paralytic ileus. *Am Surg* 33:756, 1967.

Multiple Organ System Failure

Bohnen J, Boulanger M, et al: Prognosis in generalized peritonitis: Relation to cause and risk factors. *Arch Surg* 118:285, 1983.

Fry DE, Garrison RN, et al: Determinants of death in patients with intra-abdominal abscess. *Surgery* 88:517, 1980.

Fry DE, Pearlstein L, et al: Multiple system organ failure: The role of uncontrolled infection. *Arch Surg* 115:136, 1981.

Glauser MP, Zanetti G, et al: Septic shock: Pathogenesis. *Lancet* 338:732, 1991.

Goris RJA: Mediators of multiple organ failure. *Intensive Care Med* 16:S192, 1990.

Goris RJA, Boekhorst TPA, et al: Multiple organ failure. *Arch Surg* 120:1109, 1985.

Knauss WA, Draper EA, et al: APACHE II: A severity of disease classification system. *Crit Care Med* 13:818, 1985.

Knauss WA, Wagner DP: Multiple systems organ failure epidemiology and prognosis. *Crit Care Clin* 5:233, 1989.

Clinical Trials

Dellinger EP, Wertz MJ, et al: Surgical infection stratification system for intra-abdominal infection. *Arch Surg* 120:21, 1985.

Nystrom PO, Knaus WA, et al: A proposed standard for trials on intra-abdominal infection. *World J Surg* 14:218, 1990.

Solomkin JS, Meakins JL, et al: Antibiotic trials in intra-abdominal infections: A critical evaluation of study design and outcome reporting. *Ann Surg* 201:29, 1984.

Peritoneal Membrane Structure and Function

Autio V: The spread of intraperitoneal infection: Studies with roentgen contrast medium. *Acta Chir Scand* 130:S1, 1964.

Dumont AE: The flow capacity of the thoracic duct venous junction. *Am J Med Sci* 269:292, 1975.

Dumont AK, Mass WK, et al: Increased survival from peritonitis after blockade of trans-diaphragmatic absorption of bacteria. *Surg Gynecol Obstet* 162:248, 1966.

Florey H: Reactions of, and absorption by, lymphatics, with special reference to those of the diaphragm. *Br J Exp Pathol* 8:479, 1927.

Levine S, Saltzman A: Postinflammatory increase of lymphatic absorption from the peritoneal cavity: Role of diaphragmatic stomata. *Microcirc Endothelium Lymphatics* 4:399, 1988.

Li JC, Yu SM: Study on the ultrastructure of the peritoneal stomata in humans. *Acta Anat* 141:26, 1991.

Molmenti EP, Balfe DM, et al: Anatomy of the retroperitoneum: Observations of the distribution of pathologic fluid collections. *Radiology* 200:95, 1996.

Oya M, Shimada T, et al: Functional morphology of the lymphatic system in the monkey diaphragm. *Arch Histol Cytol* 56:37, 1993.

Raftery AT: Regeneration of parietal and visceral peritoneum: A light microscopical study. *Br J Surg* 60:293, 1973.

Raftery AT: Regeneration of parietal and visceral peritoneum: An electron microscopical study. *J Anat* 115:375, 1973.

Tsilibary EC, Wissig SL: Absorption from the peritoneal cavity: SEM study of the mesothelium covering the peritoneal surface of the muscular portion of the diaphragm. *Am J Anat* 149:127, 1977.

Immunology

Aasen AO: Endotoxin: Role in surgical patients, in Aasen AO, Risberg B (eds): *Surgical Pathophysiology*. Chur, Harwood Medical Publisher, 1990, p 3.

Baggiolini M, Dewald B, et al: Interleukin-8 and related chemotactic cytokines: CXC and CC chemokines (Review). *Adv Immunol* 55:97, 1994.

Ben-Baruch A, Michiel DF, Oppenheim JJ: Signals and receptors involved in recruitment of inflammatory cells (Review). *J Biol Chem* 270(20):11703, 1995.

Bevilacqua MP, Nelson RM, et al: Endothelial-leukocyte adhesion molecules in human disease (Review). *Annu Rev Med* 45:361, 1994.

Buetler B (ed): *Tumor Necrosis Factor.* New York, Raven Press, 1992.

Cerra FB: Multiple organ failure syndrome. *Dis Month* 26:816, 1992.

Dinarello CA: The proinflammatory cytokines interleukin-1 and tumor necrosis factor and treatment of the septic shock syndrome. *J Infect Dis* 163:1177, 1991.

Dunn DL, Roderich AB, et al: Role of resident macrophages, peripheral neutrophils, and translymphatic absorption in bacterial clearance from peritoneal cavity. *Infect Immunol* 49:257, 1985.

Ertel W, Morrison MH, et al: The complete pattern of cytokines in sepsis: Association between prostaglandins, cachectin, and interleukins. *Ann Surg* 214:141, 1991.

Gimson AE: Hepatic dysfunction during bacterial sepsis. *Intensive Care Med* 13:162, 1987.

Hinshaw LB: Tumor necrosis factor in septic shock. *Clin Adv Crit Care* 2:6, 1992.

Moore FA, Moore EE, et al: Gut bacterial translocation via the portal vein: A clinical perspective with major torso trauma. *J Trauma* 31:629, 1991.

Nava E, Palmer RMJ, et al: Inhibition of nitric oxide synthesis in septic shock: How much is beneficial? *Lancet* 338:1555, 1991.

Nuytinck HKS, Offermans XJMW, et al: Whole-body inflammation in trauma patients. *Arch Surg* 123:1519, 1988.

Ochoa JB, Udekwu AO, et al: Nitrogen oxide levels in patients after trauma and during sepsis. *Ann Surg* 214:621, 1991.

Rotstein OD, Pruett TL, et al: Fibrin in peritonitis. V. Fibrin inhibits phagocytic killing of *Escherichia coli* by human polymorphonuclear leukocytes. *Ann Surg* 203:413, 1986.

Shenep JL, Flynn PM, et al: Serial quantitation of endotoxemia and bacteremia during therapy for gram-negative bacterial sepsis. *J Infect Dis* 157:565, 1988.

Swerlick RA, Lawley TJ: Role of microvascular endothelial cells in inflammation. *J Invest Dermatol* 100:111S, 1993.

Ulevitch RJ: Recognition of bacterial endotoxins by receptor-dependent mechanisms. *Advances in Immunology* 53:267, 1993.

van Deventer SJ, Knepper A, et al: Endotoxins in portal blood. *Hepatogastroenterology* 35:223, 1988.

Cellular Participants

Solomkin JS, Cotta LA, et al: Complement activation and clearance in acute illness and injury: Evidence for C5a as a cell-directed mediator of the adult respiratory distress syndrome in man. *Surgery* 97:668, 1985.

Thijs LG, Schneider AJ, et al: The haemodynamics of septic shock. *Intensive Care Med* 16:S182, 1990.

Waydhas C, Nast-Kolb D, et al: Inflammatory mediators, infection, sepsis, and multiple organ failure after severe trauma. *Arch Surg* 127:460, 1992.

Wilmore DW, Smith RJ, et al: The gut: A central organ after surgical stress. *Surgery* 104:917, 1988.

Yamada Y, Hefter K, et al: An in vitro model of the wound microenvironment: Local phagocytic cell abnormalities associated with in situ complement activation. *J Infect Dis* 155:998, 1987.

Open Abdomen and Other Alternatives

Anderson ED, Mandelbaum DM, et al: Open packing of the peritoneal cavity in generalized bacterial peritonitis. *Am J Surg* 145:131, 1983.

Aune S, Normann E: Diffuse peritonitis treated with continuous peritoneal lavage. *Acta Chir Scand* 136:401, 1970.

Bose SM, Kala M, et al: Open management of septic abdomen by Marlex mesh zipper. *Aust N Z J Surg* 61:385, 1991.

Broome A, Hansson L, et al: Open treatment of abdominal septic catastrophes. *World J Surg* 7:792, 1983.

Condon RE: Management of the acute complications of diverticular disease. *Dis Colon Rectum* 19:296, 1976.

Cullen DJ, Coyle JP, et al: Cardiovascular, pulmonary, and renal effects of massively increased intra-abdominal pressure in critically ill patients. *Crit Care Med* 17:188, 1989.

Duff JH, Moffat J: Abdominal sepsis managed by leaving the abdomen open. *Surgery* 90:774, 1981.

Garcia-Sabrido JL, Tallado JM, et al: Treatment of severe intraabdominal sepsis and/or necrotic foci by an "open-abdomen" approach. *Arch Surg* 123:152, 1988.

Heddrich GS, Wexler MJ, et al: The septic abdomen: Open management with Marlex mesh with a zipper. *Surgery* 99:399, 1986.

Kinney EV, Polk HC Jr: Open treatment of peritonitis: An argument against. *Adv Surg* 21:19, 1987.

Leiboff AR, Soroff HS: The treatment of generalized peritonitis by closed postoperative peritoneal lavage. *Arch Surg* 122:1005, 1987.

Mastboom WJB, Kuypers HHC, et al: Small-bowel perforation complicating the open treatment of generalized peritonitis. *Arch Surg* 124:689, 1989.

Schein M: Planned reoperations and open management in critical intraabdominal infections: Prospective experience in 52 cases. *World J Surg* 15:537, 1991.

Stone HH, Strom PR, et al: Pancreatic abscess management of subtotal resection and packing. *World J Surg* 8:340, 1984.

Bacteriology and Antimicrobial Therapy

Barie PS, Christou NV, et al: Pathogenicity of the enterococcus in surgical infections. *Ann Surg* 212:155, 1990.

Bartlett KG, Onderdonk AB, et al: A review: Lessons from an animal model of intra-abdominal sepsis. *Arch Surg* 113:853, 1978.

Beckhouse MJ, Whyte IM, et al: Altered aminoglycoside pharmacokinetics in the critically ill. *Anaesth Intens Care* 16:418, 1988.

Berne TV, Yellin AE, et al: Surgically treated gangrenous or perforated appendicitis: A comparison of aztreonam and clindamycin versus gentamicin and clindamycin. *Ann Surg* 205:133, 1987.

Berne TV, Yellin AE, et al: Meropenem versus tobramycin with clindamycin in the antibiotic management of patients with advanced appendicitis. *J Am Coll Surg* 182:403, 1996.

Bieluch VM, Cuchural GJ, et al: Clinical importance of cefoxitin-resistant *Bacteroides fragilis* isolates. *Diagn Microbiol Infect Dis* 7:119, 1987.

Blazer J, Stone BB, Zinner SH: Efficacy of intermittent versus continuous administration of netilmicin in a two-compartment in vitro model. *Antimicrob Agents Chemother* 27:343, 1985.

Bodenham A, Shelly MP, Park GR: The altered pharmacokinetics and pharmacodynamics of drugs commonly used in critically ill patients. *Clin Pharmacokinet* 14:347, 1988.

Bohnen JMA, Solomkin JS, et al: Guidelines for clinical care: Anti-infective agents for intra-abdominal infection: A Surgical Infection Society policy statement. *Arch Surg* 127:83, 1992.

Chow JW, Fine MJ, et al: *Enterobacter* bacteremia: Clinical features and emergence of antibiotic resistance during therapy. *Ann Intern Med* 115:585, 1991.

Collee JG: Factors contributing to loss of anaerobic bacteria in transit from the patient to laboratory. *Infection* 8:145, 1980.

Cornick NA, Cuchural GJJ, et al: The antimicrobial susceptibility patterns of the *Bacteroides fragilis* group in the United States, 1987. *J Antimicrob Chemother* 25:1011, 1990.

Drasar BS, Hill MJ: *Human Intestinal Flora.* London, Academic Press, 1974.

Elek SD, Conen PE: The virulence of *Staphylococcus pyogenes* for man: A study of the problems of wound infection. *Br J Exp Pathol* 38:573, 1957.

Enander L-K, Nilson F, et al: The aerobic and anaerobic microflora of the gastric remnant more than 15 years after Billroth II. *Scand J Gastroenterol* 17:715, 1982.

Fan ST, Lau WY, et al: Once daily administration of netilmicin compared with thrice daily, both in combination with metronidazole, in gangrenous and perforated appendicitis. *J Antimicrob Chemother* 22:69, 1988.

Finegold SM: *Anaerobic Bacteria in Human Disease.* New York–San Francisco–London, Academic Press, 1977.

Gerding DN, Hall WH: The penetration of antibiotics into peritoneal fluid. *Bull NY Acad Med* 51:1016, 1975.

Gilbert DN: Once-daily aminoglycoside therapy. *Antimicrob Agents Chemother* 35:399, 1991.

Gorbach SL: Antibiotic treatment of anaerobic infections (Review). *Clin Infect Dis* 18(suppl 4):S305, 1994.

Gorbach SL, Bartlett JG: Anaerobic infections. *N Engl J Med* 290:1177, 1974.

Greenlee HB, Gelbart SM, et al: The influence of gastric surgery on the intestinal flora. *Am J Clin Nutrit* 30:1286, 1977.

Hau T: Bacteria, toxins, and the peritoneum. *World J Surg* 14:167, 1990.

Hau T, Ohmann C, et al: Planned relaparotomy vs relaparotomy on demand in the treatment of intra-abdominal infections. The Peritonitis Study Group of the Surgical Infection Society–Europe. *Arch Surg* 130:1193, 1995.

Hilf M, Yu VL, et al: Antibiotic therapy for *Pseudomonas aeruginosa* bacteremia: Outcome correlations in a prospective study of 200 patients. *Am J Med* 87:540, 1989.

Huizinga WK, Warren BL, et al: Antibiotic monotherapy with meropenem in the surgical management of intra-abdominal infections. *J Antimicrob Chemother* 36(suppl A):179, 1995.

Itokazu GS, Danziger LH: Ampicillin-sulbactam and ticarcillin-clavulanic acid: A comparison of their in vitro activity and review of their clinical efficacy. *Pharmacotherapy* 11:382, 1991.

Jacobus NV, Cuchural GJ Jr, et al: In-vitro susceptibility of the *Bacteroides fragilis* group and the inoculum effect of newer beta-lactam antibiotics on this group of organisms. *J Antimicrob Chemother* 24:675, 1989.

Jett BD, Huycke MM, Gilmore MS: Virulence of enterococci (Review). *Clinical Microbiology Reviews* 7:462, 1994.

Johnson AP: The pathogenicity of enterococci (Review). *J Antimicrob Chemother* 33:1083, 1994.

Kapusnik JR, Hackbarth CJ, et al: Single large daily dosing versus intermittent dosing of tobramycin for treating experimental *Pseudomonas* pneumonia. *J Infect Dis* 158:7, 1988.

Kollef MH: The role of selective digestive tract decontamination on mortality and respiratory tract infections: A meta-analysis. *Chest* 105:1101, 1994.

Lau WY, Fan ST, et al: Prophylaxis of postappendicectomy sepsis by metronidazole and cefotaxime: A randomized, prospective, and double blind trial. *Br J Surg* 70:670, 1983.

Leggett JE, Fantin B, et al: Comparative antibiotic dose-effect relations at several dosing intervals in murine pneumonitis and thigh-infection models. *J Infect Dis* 159:281, 1989.

Lennard ES, Dellinger EP, et al: Implications of leukocytosis and fever at conclusion of antibiotic therapy for intra-abdominal sepsis. *Ann Surg* 195:19, 1982.

Lorber B, Swenson RM: The bacteriology of intra-abdominal infections. *Surg Clin North Am* 55:1349, 1975.

Malangoni MA, Condon RE, et al: Treatment of intra-abdominal infections is appropriate with single-agent or combination antibiotic therapy. *Surgery* 98:648, 1985.

Meleney FL, Ollp J, et al: Peritonitis: II. Synergism of bacteria commonly found in peritoneal exudates. *Arch Surg* 25:709, 1932.

Mollitt DL, Tepas JJ III, et al: The microbiology of neonatal peritonitis. *Arch Surg* 123:176, 1988.

Montravers P, Andremont A, et al: Investigation of the potential role of *Enterococcus faecalis* in the pathophysiology of experimental peritonitis. *J Infect Dis* 169:821, 1994.

Nichols RL, Smith JW: Intragastric microbial colonisation in common disease states of the stomach and duodenum. *Ann Surg* 182:557, 1975.

Nicolau DP, Freeman CD, et al: Experience with a once-daily aminoglycoside program administered to 2,184 adult patients. *Antimicrob Agents Chemother* 39:650, 1995.

Nystrom P-O, Johansson L, et al: Intraoperative saline irrigation of the peritoneal cavity in experimental post-traumatic peritonitis. *Acta Chir Scand* 149:509, 1983.

Onderdonk AB, Bartlett JG, et al: Microbial synergy in experimental intra-abdominal abscess. *Infect Immun* 13:22, 1976.

O'Sullivan GC, Murphy D, et al: Laparoscopic management of generalized peritonitis due to perforated colonic diverticula. *Am J Surg* 171:432, 1996.

Patel KB, Nicolau DP, et al: Continuous infusion of beta-lactam antibiotics: A rational dosing approach (Review). *Conn Med* 59:471, 1995.

Salacata A, Chow JW: Cephalosporin therapeutics for intensive care infection, in Solomkin JS (ed): *New Horizons.* Baltimore, Williams & Wilkins, 1993, pp 181–186.

Sanders WEJ, Sanders CC: Inducible beta-lactamases: Clinical and epidemiologic implications for use of newer cephalosporins. *Rev Infect Dis* 10:830, 1988.

Schentag JJ, Plat ME, et al: Aminoglycoside nephrotoxicity in critically ill surgical patients. *J Surg Res* 26:270, 1979.

Solomkin JS: Use of new beta-lactam antibiotics for surgical infections. *Surg Clin North Am* 68:1, 1988.

Solomkin JS: Pathogenesis and management of *Candida* infection syndromes in non-neutropenic patients, in Solomkin JS (ed): *New Horizons.* Baltimore, Williams & Wilkins, 1993, pp 202–213.

Solomkin JS, Dellinger EP, et al: Results of a multicenter trial comparing imipenem/cilastatin to tobramycin/clindamycin for intra-abdominal infections. *Ann Surg* 212:581, 1990.

Solomkin JS, Reinhart HH, et al: Results of a randomized trial comparing sequential intravenous/oral treatment with ciprofloxacin plus metronidazole to imipenem/cilastatin for intra-abdominal infections. The Intra-Abdominal Infection Study Group. *Ann Surg* 223:303, 1996.

Swenson RM, Lorber B, et al: The bacteriology of intra-abdominal infections. *Arch Surg* 109:398, 1974.

Thornsberry C: Review of in vitro activity of third-generation cephalosporins and other newer beta-lactam antibiotics against clinically important bacteria. *Am J Med* 79(2A):14, 1985.

Vogelman B, Gudmundsson S, et al: Correlation of antimicrobial pharmacokinetic parameters with therapeutic efficacy in an animal model. *J Infect Dis* 158:831, 1988.

Wells CL, Rotstein OD, et al: Intestinal bacteria translocate into experimental intra-abdominal abscesses. *Arch Surg* 121:102, 1986.

Wittmann DH, Schassan HH: Penetration of eight beta-lactam antibiotics into peritoneal fluid. *Arch Surg* 112:205, 1983.

Wittmann DH, Schein M, Condon RE: Management of secondary peritonitis (Review). *Ann Surg* 224:10, 1996.

Yellin AE, Heseltine PN, et al: The role of *Pseudomonas* species in patients treated with ampicillin and sulbactam for gangrenous and perforated appendicitis. *Surg Gynecol Obstet* 161:303, 1985.

Primary Peritonitis

Akinoglu A, Bilgin I: Tuberculous enteritis and peritonitis. *Can J Surg* 31:55, 1988.

Clark JH, Fitzgerald JF, et al: Spontaneous bacterial peritonitis. *J Pediatr* 104:495, 1984.

Cromartie RS III: Tuberculous peritonitis. *Surg Gynecol Obstet* 144:876, 1977.

Crossley IF, Williams R: Spontaneous bacterial peritonitis. *Gut* 26:325, 1985.

Reynolds TB: Rapid presumptive diagnosis of spontaneous bacteria peritonitis. *Gastroenterology* 90:1294, 1986.

Sanderson MC, Swartzendruber DJ, et al: Surgical complications of continuous ambulatory peritoneal dialysis. *Am J Surg* 160:561, 1990.

Stassen WN, McCullough AJ, et al: Immediate diagnostic criteria for bacterial infection of ascitic fluid: Evaluation of ascitic fluid polymorphonuclear leukocyte count, pH, and lactate concentration, alone and in combination. *Gastroenterology* 90:1247, 1986.

Diagnosis and Therapy of Secondary Peritonitis

Aprahamian C, Wittmann DH: Operative management of intraabdominal infection. *Infection* 19:453, 1991.

Auguste L, Borrero E, et al: Surgical management of perforated colonic diverticulitis. *Arch Surg* 120:450, 1985.

Debas H, Thomson FB: A critical review of colectomy with anastomosis. *Surg Gynecol Obstet* 135:747, 1972.

Graham RR: The treatment of perforated duodenal ulcers. *Surg Gynecol Obstet* 64:235, 1937.

Krukowski ZH, Matheson NA: Emergency surgery for diverticular disease complicated by generalized and faecal peritonitis: A review. *Br J Surg* 71:921, 1984.

Liebert C, Deweese BM: Primary resection without anastomosis for perforation of acute diverticulitis. *Surg Gynecol Obstet* 152:30, 1981.

Wachs ME, Wolfgang HS: Primary intestinal anastomosis is unsafe in the presence of generalized peritonitis, in Simmons RL, Udekwu AO (eds): *Debates in Clinical Surgery.* St Louis, Mosby–Year Book, 1991, pp 228–239.

Tertiary and Other Forms of Peritonitis

Goris RJA, Boekholz WKF, et al: Multiple organ failure and sepsis without bacteria. *Arch Surg* 121:897, 1986.

Kittur DS, Korpe SW, et al: Surgical aspects of sclerosing encapsulating peritonitis. *Arch Surg* 125:1626, 1990.

Monga NK, Sood S, et al: Amebic peritonitis. *Am J Gastroenterol* 66:366, 1976.

Rotstein OD, Meakins JL: Diagnostic and therapeutic challenges of intraabdominal infections. *World J Surg* 14:159, 1990.

Rotstein OD, Pruett TL, et al: Microbiologic features and treatment of persistent peritonitis in patients in the intensive care unit. *Can J Surg* 29:247, 1986.

Solomkin JS, Flohr AB, et al: The role of *Candida* in intraperitoneal infections. *Surgery* 88:524, 1980.

Sturdy JH, Baird RM, et al: Surgical sponges, a cause of granuloma and adhesion formation. *Ann Surg* 165:128, 1967.

Tinker MA, Burdman D, et al: Granulomatous peritonitis due to cellulose fibers disposable surgical fabrics: Laboratory investigation and clinical implications. *Ann Surg* 180:831, 1974.

Operative Treatment of Intraabdominal Abscess

Altemeier WA, Culbertson WR, et al: Intra-abdominal abscesses. *Am J Surg* 125:70, 1973.

Barnard HL: Address on surgical aspects of subphrenic abscess. *Br Med J* 1:371, 1908.

Crepps TJ, Welch JP, et al: Management and outcome of retroperitoneal abscesses. *Ann Surg* 205:276, 1987.

DeCosse JJ, Poulin TL, et al: Subphrenic abscess. *Surg Gynecol Obstet* 138:841, 1974.

Halasz HA: Subphrenic abscess: Myths and facts. *JAMA* 214:724, 1970.

Halliday P: The surgical management of subphrenic abscess: A historical study. *Aust N Z J Surg* 45:235, 1975.

Ochsner A, DeBakey M: Subphrenic abscess: Collective review and analysis of 3,608 collected and personal cases. *Int Abst Surg* 66:726, 1938.

Stone HH, Mullins RJ, et al: Extraperitoneal versus transperitoneal drainage of the intra-abdominal abscess. *Surg Gynecol Obstet* 159:549, 1984.

Percutaneous Drainage of Intraabdominal Abscess

Casola G, van Sonnenberg E, et al: Percutaneous drainage of tuboovarian abscesses. *Radiology* 182:399, 1992.

Gerzof SG, Robbins AH, et al: Percutaneous catheter drainage of abdominal abscesses: A five-year experience. *N Engl J Med* 305:653, 1981.

Gobien RP, Stanley JH, et al: The effect of drainage tube size on adequacy of percutaneous abscess drainage. *Cardiovasc Intervent Radiol* 8:100, 1985.

Haaga JR: Imaging intra-abdominal abscesses and nonoperative drainage procedures. *World J Surg* 14:204, 1990.

Jeffrey RB Jr, Wing VC, Laing FC: Real-time sonographic monitoring of percutaneous abscess drainage. *AJR* 144:469, 1985.

Johnson WC, Gerzof SG, et al: Treatment of abdominal abscesses: Comparative evaluation of operative drainage versus percutaneous catheter drainage guided by computed tomography or ultrasound. *Ann Surg* 194:510, 1981.

Lambiase RE, Cronan JJ, et al: Percutaneous drainage of abscesses in patients with Crohn disease. *AJR* 150:1043, 1988.

Lambiase RE, Deyoe L, et al : Percutaneous drainage of 335 consecutive abscesses: Results of primary drainage with 1-year follow-up. *Radiology* 184:167, 1992.

McGahan JP: Aspiration and drainage procedures in the intensive care unit: Percutaneous sonographic guidance. *Radiology* 154:531, 1985.

Mueller PR, Ferrucci JR Jr, et al: Lesser sac abscesses and fluid collections: Drainage by transhepatic approach. *Radiology* 155:615, 1985.

Mueller PR, Saini S, et al: Sigmoid diverticular abscesses: Percutaneous drainage as an adjunct to surgical resection in 24 cases. *Radiology* 164:321, 1987.

Mueller PR, van Sonnenberg E, et al: Percutaneous drainage of 250 abdominal abscesses and fluid collections. *Radiology* 151:343, 1984.

Neff CC, Mueller PR, et al: Serious complications following transgression of the pleural space in drainage procedures. *Radiology* 152:335, 1984.

Neff CC, van Sonnenberg E, et al: Diverticular abscesses: Percutaneous drainage. *Radiology* 163:15, 1987.

Nosher JL, Needell GS, et al: Transrectal pelvic abscess drainage with sonographic guidance. *AJR* 146:1047, 1986.

van Sonnenberg E, D'Agostino HB, et al: US-guided transvaginal drainage of pelvic abscesses and fluid collections. *Radiology* 181:53, 1991.

van Sonnenberg E, D'Agostino HB, et al: Percutaneous abscess drainage: Current concepts. *Radiology* 181:617, 1991.

van Sonnenberg E, Mueller PR, et al: Sump catheter for percutaneous abscess and fluid drainage by trocar or Seldinger technique. *AJR* 139:613, 1982.

van Sonnenberg E, Wing VW, et al: Temporizing effect of percutaneous drainage of complicated abscesses in critically ill patients. *AJR* 142:821, 1984.

Acute Cholecystitis and Intestinal Ischemia

Alpern MB, Glazer GM, et al: Ischemic or infarcted bowel: CT findings. *Radiology* 166:149, 1988.

Balthazar EJ, Birnbaum BA, et al: Closed-loop and strangulating intestinal obstruction: CT signs. *Radiology* 185:769, 1992.

Boland G, Lee MJ, et al: Acute cholecystitis in the intensive care unit, in Solomkin JS (ed): *New Horizons.* Baltimore, Williams & Wilkins, 1993, pp 246–260.

Boley SJ, Brandt LT, et al: Ischemic disorders of the intestines. *Curr Probl Surg* 15:1, 1978.

Clark RA: Computed tomography of bowel infarction. *J Comput Assist Tomogr* 11:757, 1987.

Clark RA, Gallant TE: Acute mesenteric ischemia: Angiographic spectrum. *AJR* 142:555, 1984.

DuPriest RW, Khaneja SC, Cowley RA: Acute cholecystitis complicating trauma. *Ann Surg* 189:84, 1979.

Frazee RC, Nagorney DM, Mucha P: Acute acalculous cholecystitis. *Mayo Clin Proc* 64:163, 1989.

Lee ML, Saini S, Brink JA: Treatment of critically ill patients with sepsis of unknown cause: Value of percutaneous cholecystostomy. *Am J Surg* 156:1163, 1991.

Lindemann SR, Tung G, et al: Percutaneous cholecystostomy. *Seminars in Interventional Radiology* 5:179, 1988.

Pancreatic Infection

Adams DB, Harvey TS, Anderson MC: Percutaneous catheter drainage of infected pancreatic and peripancreatic fluid collections. *Arch Surg* 125:1554, 1990.

Balthazar EJ, Robinson DL, et al: Acute pancreatitis: Value of CT in establishing prognosis. *Radiology* 174:331, 1990.

Bassi C, Vesentini S, et al: Pancreatic abscess and other pus-harboring collections related to pancreatitis: A review of 108 cases. *World J Surg* 14:505, 1990.

Bittner R, Block S, et al: Pancreatic abscess and infected pancreatic necrosis: Different local septic complications in acute pancreatitis. *Dig Dis Sci* 32:1082, 1987.

Bradley E III, Murphy F, et al: Prediction of pancreatic necrosis by dynamic pancreatography. *Ann Surg* 210:495, 1989.

Bradley E III, Olson RA: Current management of pancreatic abscess. *Adv Surg* 24:361, 1991.

Ekberg O, Weiber S: The clinical importance of a thick-walled, tender gallbladder without stones on ultrasonography. *Clin Radiol* 44:38, 1991.

Freeny PC, Lewis GP, et al: Infected pancreatic fluid collections: Percutaneous catheter drainage. *Radiology* 167:435, 1988.

Hughes CJ, Ramsey Stewart G, Storey DW: Sequential laparotomy and zipper closure in the management of gross peripancreatic sepsis. *Aust N Z J Surg* 60:467, 1990.

Korobkin M, Callen PW, et al: Comparison of computed tomography, ultrasonography, and Ga-67 scanning in the evaluation of suspected abdominal abscesses. *Radiology* 129:59, 1978.

Lee MJ, Rattner DW, et al: Acute complicated pancreatitis: Redefining the role of interventional radiology. *Radiology* 183:171, 1992.

Lumsden A, Bradley E III: Secondary pancreatic infections. *Surg Gynecol Obstet* 170:459, 1990.

Mirvis SE, Vainright JR, et al: The diagnosis of acute acalculous cholecystitis: A comparison of sonography, scintigraphy, and CT. *AJR* 147:1171, 1986.

Rotman N, Mathieu D, et al: Failure of percutaneous drainage of pancreatic abscesses complicating severe acute pancreatitis. *Surg Gynecol Obstet* 174:141, 1992.

Stanten R, Frey CF: Comprehensive management of acute necrotizing pancreatitis and pancreatic abscess. *Arch Surg* 125:1269, 1990.

Steiner E, Mueller PR, et al: Complicated pancreatic abscesses: Problems in interventional management. *Radiology* 167:443, 1988.

van Sonnenberg E, Wittich G, et al: Percutaneous drainage of infected and noninfected pancreatic pseudocysts: Experience in 101 cases. *Radiology* 170:757, 1989.

Fistulas

Kerlan RK, Jeffrey RB Jr, et al: Abdominal abscess with low-output fistula: Successful percutaneous drainage. *Radiology* 155:73, 1985.

Lambiase RE, Cronan JJ, et al: Postoperative abscesses with enteric communication: Percutaneous treatment. *Radiology* 171:497, 1989.

Papanicolaou N, Mueller PR, et al: Abscess-fistula association: Radiologic recognition and percutaneous management. *AJR* 143:811, 1984.

Torres AJ, Landa JI, et al: Somatostatin in the management of gastrointestinal fistulas: A multicenter trial. *Arch Surg* 127:97, 1992.

CHAPTER 33

Abdominal Wall, Omentum, Mesentery, and Retroperitoneum

John M. Daly, James T. Adams, Gary A. Fantini, and Josef E. Fischer

ANTERIOR ABDOMINAL WALL

General Considerations

The abdominal wall functions in many capacities, serving to pad, protect, and surround the abdominal viscera. Physiologically, the muscles can act to assist bending and posture. Along with the intercostal and neck muscles, the abdominal wall muscles provide accessory respiratory function when needed. Urination and defecation can be initiated and prolonged by voluntarily increasing intraabdominal pressures. Topographically, the anterior abdominal wall is bounded by the flare of the costal margins and the xiphoid process of the sternum above and by the iliac crests, inguinal ligaments, and pubis below. The principal structures that comprise the anterior abdominal wall are the rectus, external and internal oblique, and transversus abdominis and lower intercostal muscles together with their enveloping fascial sheaths and aponeuroses. The linea alba, a tendinous raphe formed by a blending of the aponeuroses of the oblique and transversus muscles in the midline, divides the anterior abdominal wall into two parts and restricts the medial extension of pathologic processes that may arise within it. Deep to the muscles is the continuous transversalis fascia, considered to be the strongest layer of the abdominal wall, and peritoneum.

The blood supply of the anterior abdominal wall is furnished by the superior and inferior epigastric, lower intercostal, lumbar, and iliac circumflex arteries. The venous drainage corresponds to the arteries. Lymphatics in the upper half of the abdominal wall drain to the axillary nodes and those in the lower abdomen to the inguinal and then to the iliac nodes. Studies using radionuclides have shown a broad band in the midabdominal region that may drain in either or both directions. Lymph flow around the umbilicus also may ascend around the ligamentum teres (obliterated umbilical vein) to reach the porta hepatis. The nerve supply is via the intercostal and upper lumbar nerves.

Surgical diseases of the anterior abdominal wall include (1) hernia, (2) infection, (3) primary and metastatic tumors of soft tissue and muscle, (4) rectus sheath hematoma, and (5) desmoid tumor. With the exception of rectus sheath hematoma and desmoid tumor, these conditions are covered in other chapters of this book.

Rectus Sheath Hematoma

Bleeding into the rectus sheath may simulate the acute surgical abdomen. The bleeding usually is the result of rupture of the epigastric artery or veins rather than a primary tear of the rectus muscle fibers. It is often a self-limiting condition, but if it is not recognized, it can lead to an unnecessary emergency surgical procedure.

Anatomy (Fig. 33-1). The rectus abdominis muscle is crossed by three transverse tendinous intersections on its anterior aspect. Its contractile force is divided into three parts. The lowermost part is the longest; therefore, its shortening with contraction is the greatest. There may be a difference of as much as 18 cm in length between extreme contraction and relaxation.

A strong fascial sheath, made up of the aponeuroses of the oblique and transversus abdominis muscles and transversalis fascia, contains the muscle. Anteriorly, the sheath is complete throughout; however, midway between the umbilicus and the pubis, the posterior sheath ends, forming an arched border, the linea semicircularis (of Douglas). Cephalad to this level, the internal oblique aponeurosis splits into two leaves, one passing on either side of the rectus, while below it no such division takes place, and together with the aponeurosis of the transversus abdominis, it passes anteriorly. The rectus muscle below the linea semicircularis is therefore separated from the abdominal viscera only by transversalis fascia and peritoneum. The anterior leaf of the sheath is adherent to the transverse tendons and also to the lateral and medial margins of the muscle; posteriorly, the muscle is free. As a consequence of this anatomic arrangement, when there is bleeding within the rectus sheath below the umbilicus, the free blood may lie against the peritoneum, producing irritation and pain and suggesting an acute intraabdominal process.

The blood supply to the rectus muscle is from the superior and inferior epigastric arteries. The superior epigastric artery enters the rectus sheath from above as a terminal branch of the internal mammary artery and passes caudad behind the muscle to anastomose with the larger inferior epigastric artery coming from below. The inferior epigastric artery, a branch of the external iliac artery, enters the rectus sheath just above the inguinal canal and courses upward along the posterior surface of the rectus muscle. Both arteries give off numerous muscular branches. Two veins accompany each artery. As the rectus muscle contracts, the epigastric vessels must glide beneath it to avoid injury.

Etiology. Rectus sheath hematoma may follow direct trauma to the epigastric blood vessels or occur spontaneously in association with several diseases. It also has been noted after a convulsive seizure. Spontaneous bleeding from the smaller muscular arteries has been reported in (1) infectious diseases, notably typhoid fever, (2) debilitating diseases, (3) collagen diseases, (4) blood dyscrasias such as hemophilia and leukemia, and (5) patients on anticoagulation therapy.

Frequently, however, bleeding occurs without obvious trauma or disease. In these patients, the hematoma usually follows minor straining as in coughing or sneezing. Presumably, the underlying factor is an inelasticity of the artery or vein that prevents the

vessel from accommodating itself to the sudden marked variation in length that the rectus muscle undergoes during contraction and relaxation. Spontaneous rectus hematoma also has been described in pregnancy and in the puerperium. It is not known whether the hematoma is from venous or arterial bleeding. Stretching of the epigastric vessels by a distended abdomen during pregnancy and sudden relaxation after delivery are probably factors causing vessel injury. In the elderly, atheroma of an epigastric artery may predispose the vessel to rupture after minor exertion.

Clinical Manifestations. Rectus sheath hematoma is three times more frequent in women than in men. The condition is rare in children and has a peak age incidence in the fifth decade. A history of previous trauma, sudden muscular exertion, generalized vascular disease, or anticoagulation suggests the diagnosis. Hematomas related to anticoagulation therapy usually become apparent 4 to 14 days after treatment is instituted. The first symptom is pain. This is sudden in onset, sharp, and progressively severe. The pain is felt in the side of the abdomen where the bleeding occurs and remains localized, because the hematoma in the rectus muscle is limited by the confines of its sheath. Usually this is manifest in the lower abdomen and more often on the right side. Anorexia, nausea, but rarely vomiting, tachycardia, low-grade fever, and a moderate leukocytosis are frequent findings. With severe bleeding, signs of peripheral vascular collapse may develop. This is more apt to occur with bleeding below the linea semicircularis, where the peritoneum is only loosely adherent to the rectus muscle and cannot tampon the ruptured epigastric vessel. Tenderness and spasm are frequently present over the site of the hemorrhage. The bowel sounds usually are not altered. There may or may not be a palpable mass, depending on the extent of the bleeding. If present, the mass is tender, does not usually cross the midline, and remains palpable when the patient tenses the rectus muscle (Fothergill's sign). A bluish discoloration of the overlying skin is virtually diagnostic; however, this finding usually does not occur until 3 or 4 days after the patient is first seen.

Rectus sheath hematoma has been mistaken for almost every acute disease of the abdomen. Before the advent of ultrasound and computed tomography (CT), a correct preoperative diagnosis was made in less than 30 percent of patients. Using these scanning techniques, the condition can be diagnosed in most patients by the demonstration of a cystic or complex mass lesion within the confines of the rectus sheath (Fig. 33-2). Above the linea semicircularis, the hematoma is limited medially by the linea alba and confined to one side; below this level, the mass may project across the midline.

Treatment. If the diagnosis is made and the rectus hematoma is not causing severe symptoms, the condition may be managed nonoperatively with bed rest and analgesics. Anticoagulants should be discontinued. It is rarely necessary to abruptly reverse a coagulation deficit when operation is not undertaken. Surgical intervention occasionally is necessary to relieve symptoms of the hematoma or, if the diagnosis is in doubt, to rule out other more serious diseases. With a paramedian incision, the diagnosis becomes obvious when the rectus sheath is opened and free blood is found. The hematoma may be diffuse throughout the rectus muscle or may be a localized clot. Bleeding arteries may be present. Ideally, the hematoma is evacuated without entering the peritoneal cavity. Bleeding points are ligated, and the wound is

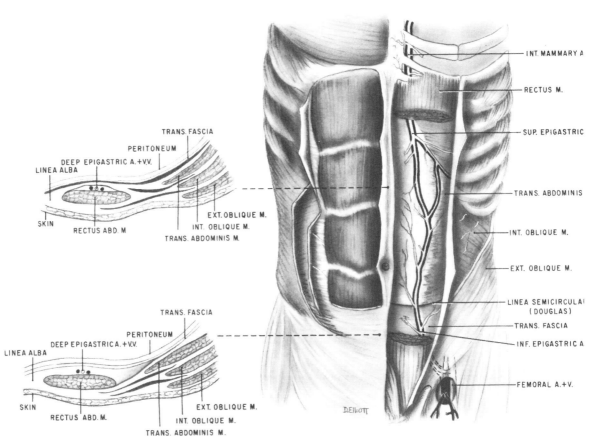

FIG. 33-1. Rectus abdominis muscle and rectus sheath. From the rib margin to a point midway between the umbilicus and the pubis (linea semicircularis of Douglas), the posterior sheath is made up of the posterior leaf of the internal oblique aponeurosis, the aponeurosis of the transversus abdominis muscle, and the transversalis fascia. Below this level, the posterior wall is formed by transversalis fascia alone. The deep epigastric arteries and veins course along the posterior surface of the rectus muscle, so below the linea semicircularis they are separated from the peritoneum by only transversalis fascia.

FIG. 33-2. Rectus sheath hematoma. CT scan of lower abdomen showing an elliptical complex lesion in the left rectus muscle (arrow). The asymmetry of the rectus muscles is an important clue to the diagnosis.

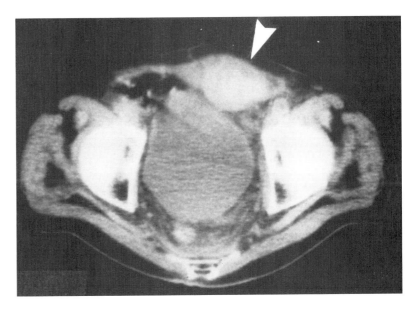

closed without drainage. The prognosis depends on the underlying or concurrent disease but is generally good, and a full recovery can be anticipated.

Desmoid Tumors

The term *desmoid* is derived from the Greek and means "band-like appearance." Desmoid tumors in the past have been characterized as a variant of fibromatosis or fibroma, namely, fibrous tumors of slow growth. More recently, their locally aggressive behavior, their tendency to recur, and the high ultimate mortality rate of patients with fibroma have led them to be reclassified as low-grade malignant lesions, specifically low-grade fibrosarcomas. They are nonencapsulated and rise from the musculoskeletal aponeurotic tissues. Their course is variable, but they proliferate by local invasion and may produce obstruction with invasion of adjacent structures.

Historical Background. The first description of desmoid tumors was in 1832 by John Macfarlane of Glasgow. Muller introduced the term *desmoid* in 1838. Nichols reported the association of desmoids and gastrointestinal polyposis in 1923. The classic paper of Gardner, published in 1953, concerning "kindred 109" (kindred with familial polyposis) suggested the association between desmoid tumors and familial polyposis.

Etiology. Desmoid tumors occur spontaneously in individuals and in patients with familial adenomatous polyposis. The incidence in the general population is thought to be between 2 and 5 cases per 1 million population. Sporadic desmoid tumors occur primarily in the abdominal wall and in extraabdominal sites. They are juvenile or are associated with women of childbearing age, thereby raising the question of estrogen involvement in causation. This hypothesis is supported by in vitro laboratory studies and scattered reports noting the effectiveness of tamoxifen and toremifene in the treatment of desmoids.

Spontaneously occurring desmoid tumors are more common in females, with a ratio of 4.4 to 5:1. There are four major age categories, each demonstrating different biologic properties:

1. *Juvenile desmoid tumors*—predominantly extraabdominal and in females
2. *Fertile*—almost exclusively abdominal and in fertile females
3. *Menopausal*—frequently abdominal with an almost equal sex ratio
4. *Senescent*—occurring in males and females equally and in abdominal and extraabdominal sites.

In patients with familial adenomatous polyposis (FAP), the incidence has been estimated to be between 6 and 31 percent, with an absolute risk of desmoid in the FAP patient at 2.56 per 1000 person-years, a risk 850 times that of the general population. The female-to-male ratio in this group is 1.4:1. The current molecular evidence is consistent with the Knudson antioncogene model. The familial polyposis gene has been mapped to chromosome 5q, and these patients frequently show allele loss on chromosome 5q. It is possible that the polyposis gene behaves as a tumor suppressor gene or antioncogene. For patients with familial polyposis, the first event is the loss of the allele on 5q. The APC gene has been cloned, and approximately 250 mutations have been identified. Studies have revealed a deletion in the (5)(q14q31) region that involves the region q21→22 where the FAP gene is localized in Gardner's syndrome. These abnormalities of the APC gene on the long arm of chromosome 5

frequently result in a truncated protein in which suppression may be lost.

There are numerous extraabdominal abnormalities in patients with FAP. Epidermoid cysts, osteomas, gastric polyps, benign and malignant lesions of the duodenum (specifically around the ampulla of Vater), papillary carcinomas of the thyroid, bilateral fibromatosis of the breast, adrenal adenomas, and pigmented ocular fundus lesions have been reported. Mutations in codons 1445 to 1478 can result in the development of desmoid tumors, but congenital hypertrophy of the retinal pigment epithelium is lacking. Mutations in codons 463 to 1387 regularly manifest congenital hypertrophy of retinal pigment epithelium. The genetic defects in these diseases are being rapidly elucidated.

Pathology. Desmoid tumors usually are solitary and reasonably well defined. They have a hard, rubbery consistency and on the cut surface exhibit a walled grayish white appearance, with white being predominant. The size varies from a few centimeters to a lesion that may weigh several kilograms (Fig. 33-3). There is no true capsule, but a pseudocapsule with multiple projections into the surrounding tissue. This feature (extension into the surrounding tissue) is critical to their surgical management.

Well-differentiated fibroblasts and fibrocytes make up the bulk of the tumor. The degree of cellularity can vary from moderate to almost acellular, but there are few or no mitoses. The cells infiltrate the surrounding muscle, giving rise occasionally to sarcolemmal giant cells.

Local invasion is very common. Symptoms usually are produced by compression or invasion of adjacent muscles, tendons, nerves, periosteum, bones, lymph nodes, and ureters. The tumor does not metastasize to lymph nodes and usually does not invade the skin. Thick-walled hamartoma vascular channels exist within the tumor. Desmoids have been reported to metastasize, but this is extremely rare and has never been observed by us. The differentiation between a desmoid and a low-grade fibrosarcoma is difficult and depends on local behavior and long-term prognosis.

Diagnosis. Because the tumor often interrupts intramuscular and soft tissue planes, there may be some clue to the diagnosis. Invasion of the adjacent muscle and bone may give rise to a periosteal reaction.

On plain abdominal radiographs, visceral displacement or obstruction can occur. When contrast-enhanced studies are performed, thinning, spiculation, and even an occasional extravasation of intraluminal material into the desmoid, occasionally presenting as an abscess, may occur. On excretory urography, displacement of the ureter and compression may be seen.

On ultrasound, the desmoid is a nonspecific, hypoechogenic mass with poor enhancement. It is indistinguishable from rhabdomyosarcoma, hematoma, abscess, or metastatic disease unless there is gas in the abscess. Angiography reveals the expected arterial displacement, occasional neovascularity, and occasional tumor staining. Arterial stretching is the most likely finding. A fibrotic reaction along mesenteric arteries is the most common early manifestation of desmoids.

The most useful radiologic examinations are computed tomography (CT) and magnetic resonance imaging (MRI). These studies usually show a homogeneous soft tissue mass (bright on a T2-weighted image) in which the adjacent viscera are displaced. This can be confused with other soft tissue tumors and lymphoma of the mesentery, which usually has associated retroperitoneal adenopathy.

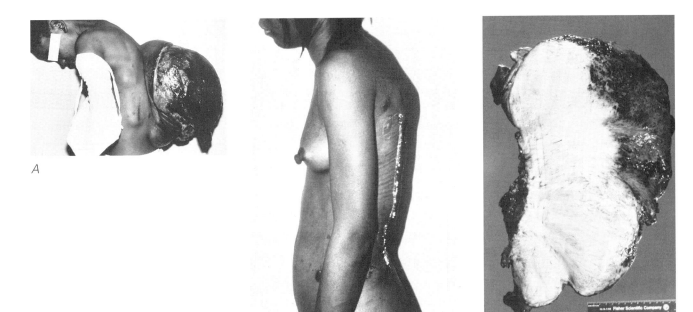

A

B

C

FIG. 33-3. *A.* A young woman with familial adenomatosis polyposis developed a large recurrent soft tissue tumor on her back (note previous scar). *B.* A wide excision and split-thickness skin grafting were performed. *C.* The tumor has a typical gross appearance with dense, white fibrous tissue extending into surrounding tissues.

Management. In a patient with FAP without cancer who develops a soft tissue mass within the first 2 years after colectomy that is adherent to the scar or in the mesentery, biopsy is not indicated. In patients with a spontaneous soft tissue mass in whom there is no reason to suspect a desmoid or in patients with extremity desmoids, adequate tissue biopsy is essential. A longitudinal, incisional biopsy for an extremity mass, which will be excised with the definitive tumor resection, should be performed.

Operative Management. Although ancillary pharmacologic and radiation management has been advocated, complete surgical extirpation of the tumor is the only therapy resulting in long-term remission. The principle is complete excision with a 1- or 2-cm margin of all tissue. Desmoid tumors often invade the surrounding tissue with various pseudopods of microscopic extension; therefore, it is essential to get an adequate tissue margin. Desmoids represent a low-grade fibrosarcoma with a propensity for local recurrence after excision. Every effort must be made at the time of the first operation to eradicate all known disease, which will not always be technically feasible due to the size or location of the tumor.

The following features are contributory to local failure: (1) age between the late teens and 30 years, (2) recurrent disease at presentation, (3) inadequate excision at the time of the first operation, and (4) radiation therapy not administered for gross residual disease.

The extent of the excision must be radical. Thoracoabdominal wall excisions and large abdominal or flank tumor excisions frequently necessitate the use of musculocutaneous flaps to close the defect. Desmoids of the chest wall should be managed with excision of the skin, underlying muscle, and the chest wall, including rib resections. A plastic surgeon should be available to perform the myocutaneous flap and closure. Where possible, artificial mesh should be avoided for reconstruction, especially when there are small bowel anastomoses. If necessary for reconstruction, the underlying viscera should be protected from the foreign mesh material.

Intraabdominal desmoids are difficult to treat because they frequently arise along the superior mesenteric artery and its primary branches, sometimes necessitating massive small bowel resection. An arteriogram can be obtained to track the relation of the vessels to the mass. Radial incisions in the mesentery are performed, identifying the vasculature along the superior mesenteric artery and vein and taking vascular branches in turn. If the situation is favorable, fairly extensive small bowel resection can be undertaken, leaving the blood supply to the proximal and distal small bowel. Desmoids may occur in the mesentery of patients who previously underwent an ileal pouch/anal anastomosis procedure, creating a challenging situation.

For pelvic primary desmoids or recurrences, pelvic exenteration and hemipelvectomy have been performed with discouraging results. Adjunctive therapy with radiation for microscopic or gross disease is essential to prevent local recurrence.

Radiation Therapy. In patients in whom desmoid tumors are unresectable or in patients with gross disease left at the margins, radiation therapy is recommended. At least 55 Gy is necessary, with tumor doses ranging from 4.8 to 61.2 Gy, given in doses of 1.6 to 1.8 Gy per fraction, 5 fractions per week. The port should be designed to cover the tumor bed with a generous overlap margin.

Responses to radiation therapy are varied. Some authors have described the benefits of intraabdominal radiation therapy to the ablation of ovarian function secondary to radiation with the corresponding loss of estrogen being responsible for tumor shrinkage.

Chemotherapy. The behavior of desmoid tumors in response to chemotherapy is erratic. Most authorities claim that it takes up to 27 months for desmoid tumors to respond to chemotherapy. A number of drugs have been used. Current therapy includes a combination regimen of vincristine, actinomycin D, and cyclophosphamide. Most reports are anecdotal, and many patients do not respond. Steroids may or may not be used as an adjunct. Their effect is thought to be secondary to inhibition of prostaglandin synthesis, which is essential to the growth of desmoids.

Pharmacologic Treatment. A number of drugs have been used in the treatment of desmoids, including polynucleotides and theophylline, which are effective in decreasing intradermal growth of tumor cells in mice. Indomethacin with high-dose ascorbic acid also has been used to treat desmoid tumors because of their effect on cyclic AMP and inhibition of ornithine decarboxylase.

Sulindac and other nonsteroidal anti-inflammatory drugs, in conjunction with coumadin, also have been reported to cause regression of desmoid tumors. In our experience, these are ineffective in controlling desmoid tumors. Because estrogens are thought to be involved in causing desmoid tumors, tamoxifen and some of the newer derivatives, such as tomorifene, also are used.

Other combinations of therapy include dicarbazine and doxirubicin, which have been used in the management of unresectable tumors. Iridium-192 implantation for locally advanced and recurrent tumors is advocated.

Some authors advocate no therapy, but this is untenable because of the reclassification of desmoid tumors as low-grade, invasive fibrosarcomas. Patients with FAP should be screened with CT scans after total colectomy because up to 30 percent (depending on the kindred) may manifest desmoid tumors in the surgical scar and in the mesentery.

Prognosis. Approximately 85 to 90 percent of patients will be alive at 5 years after the initial desmoid resection, but many of these patients are less than 30 years of age and may die of their disease over the next 10 years because of inexorable growth of tumor recurrences.

Desmoid tumors of the head and neck pose specific problems. They are found most commonly in the neck area, and radical neck dissection has been advocated at the first appearance. Radical en bloc resection is required with a margin of surrounding normal tissue. Desmoids in the orbit require exenteration, plastic reconstruction, and prosthetic materials. The incidence of recurrence is higher in head and neck lesions.

DISEASES OF THE OMENTUM

General Considerations

The greater omentum consists of a double sheet of flattened endothelium. Between the folds, the epiploic vessels, lymphatics, and nerves pass in areolar tissue enmeshed with a variable amount of fat. The structure hangs in a double fold, or sling, between the greater curvature of the stomach and the transverse colon. At birth, an agglutination of the two layers occurs, creating an apron-like shield overlying the intestinal coils. The right border attaches to the pylorus or first portion of the duodenum, while the left border forms the gastrosplenic ligament. The right

side usually is longer and heavier and may possess tongue-like processes extending into the pelvis. Occasionally, accessory omenta exist attached to the main portion. The size of the greater omentum is related to the amount of fat it contains. It is often huge in obese individuals and very thin and small in emaciated persons. The omentum in infants usually is underdeveloped and may be almost nonexistent. With growth of the individual, there is elongation and thickening of the organ from the deposition of fat within its layers.

As a peritoneal fold, the omentum assumes the mechanical function of a mesentery, i.e., the fixation of viscera and the transmission of a vascular supply. It is not a vital organ and can be removed without disturbance to the individual.

The omentum possesses an inherent motility that allows it to seek out and arrest trouble that may arise within the peritoneal cavity. It has been referred to as the "police officer of the abdomen." The omentum often is found at the site of an intraabdominal pathologic condition, but evidence shows that it has no spontaneous or ameboid activity and that displacement occurs as a result of intestinal peristalsis, diaphragmatic excursions, and postural changes of the individual. The areolar tissue is rich in macrophages that rapidly remove injected bacteria or foreign particles. The usefulness of the omentum in inflammatory processes is related to its bactericidal and absorptive properties and its ability to form adhesions.

Torsion

Torsion of the omentum is a condition in which the organ twists on its long axis, causing vascular compromise. This may vary from mild vascular constriction, producing edema, to complete strangulation, leading to infarction and frank gangrene. For torsion to occur, two situations must exist: (1) a redundant and mobile segment and (2) a fixed point around which the segment can twist.

Etiology. Omental torsion has been classified as primary or secondary. Primary, or idiopathic, omental torsion is relatively rare, and the cause is obscure. Leitner and associates group the causes of primary torsion into predisposing factors and precipitating factors. Among the suggested predisposing factors are a variety of anatomic variations including tongue-like projections from the free edge of the omentum, bifid omentum, accessory omentum, a large and bulky omentum with a narrow pedicle, and obesity associated with irregular distribution of fat within the organ. Venous redundancy relative to the omental arterial blood supply also has been cited as a predisposing factor. The omental veins are larger and more tortuous than the arteries, allowing venous kinking and offering a point of fixation around which twisting can occur. The higher incidence of right-sided omental torsion is related to the greater size and mobility of the right omentum.

Precipitating factors are those which cause displacement of the omentum. These include heavy exertion, sudden change in body position, coughing, straining, and hyperperistalsis with overeating. Primary omental torsion is always unipolar; there is only one locus of fixation.

Secondary omental torsion is associated with adhesions of the free end of the omentum to cysts, tumors, foci of intraabdominal inflammation, postoperative wounds, or scarring, or internal or external hernias. It is more common than the primary type and usually is bipolar; torsion of the central portion occurs between two fixed points. About two-thirds are found in patients with hernias, usually of the inguinal variety. The precipitating factors that cause secondary torsion are the same as those for primary torsion.

Pathology. The omentum in the primary and secondary varieties twists a variable numbers of turns around a pivotal point, usually in a clockwise direction (Fig. 33-4). The whole omentum or, more often, a small portion may undergo torsion. The right side is involved more frequently. Venous return is restricted, and the distal omentum becomes congested and edematous. Hemorrhagic extravasation results in a characteristic serosanguineous effusion into the peritoneal cavity, which, if of sufficient duration, causes acute hemorrhagic infarction and eventual necrosis. If not excised, the mass becomes atrophied and fibrotic and on rare occasions is autoamputated.

Clinical Manifestations. The clinical features of primary and secondary omental torsion are similar. The condition usually occurs in the fourth or fifth decade of life. Males are affected twice as frequently as females. Pain is the initial and predominant symptom. The onset of pain usually is sudden and constant with a gradual increase in severity. Occasionally, the pain is experienced first in the periumbilical region or is generalized. Invariably it becomes localized to the right side of the abdomen, usually the right lower quadrant. This is in keeping with the more frequent involvement of the right side of the omentum. Movement intensifies the pain. Nausea and vomiting occur in

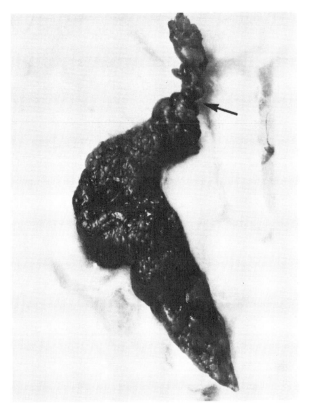

FIG. 33-4. Surgical specimen of primary torsion of the omentum. A small segment of normal-appearing omentum can be seen above the pivotal point (arrow), where it has twisted several times. The omentum below this is congested and hemorrhagic.

less than half the patients. There is moderate leukocytosis and fever that rarely exceeds a rise of 1°C. Tenderness is present, and rebound tenderness and voluntary spasm are frequent findings. A mass may be palpable if the involved omentum is sufficiently large.

The manifestations usually are not sufficient to allow an accurate diagnosis. CT scan has been used in diagnosing omental pathology. This can be a sensitive modality for showing an omental mass but is not usually specific for making a diagnosis of omental torsion. Secondary torsion of the hernial type can be suspected if a tender mass is palpable in the groin. Impressions, in order of frequency, are acute appendicitis, acute cholecystitis, and twisted ovarian cyst. Manifestations usually justify abdominal exploration. The finding of free serosanguineous fluid at the time of laparotomy in the absence of a pathologic condition in the appendix, gallbladder, or pelvic organs should suggest the possibility of omental torsion.

Treatment. Treatment consists of resection of the involved omentum. In patients with secondary torsion, the underlying condition (hernia, cysts, adhesions, etc.) also should be corrected. Postoperative mortality and morbidity are rare.

Idiopathic Segmental Infarction

Idiopathic segmental infarction is an acute vascular disturbance of the omentum. The criteria for diagnosis of this condition are that it is not accompanied by omental torsion, that there is no associated cardiovascular disease or local intraabdominal pathologic condition, and that there is no history of external abdominal trauma, situations that produce secondary omental infarction.

Etiology and Pathology. The condition is precipitated by thrombosis of omental veins secondary to endothelial injury. Halligan and Rabiah summarized the several proposed causes of endothelial damage and thrombosis. These include (1) stretching or primary rupture of the omental veins by a sudden increase in intraabdominal pressure such as that caused by coughing, sneezing, or lifting, especially after ingesting a heavy meal, (2) gravitational pull of an extremely fatty omentum on the omental veins, causing their rupture, and (3) an anatomic peculiarity of the venous drainage of the omentum that predisposes to thrombosis.

The right lower segment of the omentum, which is the most mobile and richest in fat, is the portion usually involved. The area of infarction may vary from 2 to 20 cm at its greatest diameter. Grossly, the involved segment is well demarcated, edematous, and hemorrhagic or gangrenous. It usually is closely adherent to the parietal peritoneum or adjacent abdominal viscera. Microscopically, there is a hemorrhagic infarction with thrombosis of the omental veins and filtration of the omentum with inflammatory cells.

Clinical Manifestations. Most patients are young or middle-aged adults, and there is a 3:1 predilection for males. The manifestations are nonspecific. Patients usually present with a gradual onset of abdominal pain that is steady and virtually always on the right side of the abdomen. Anorexia and nausea are frequent, but vomiting is rare. Diarrhea or constipation is unusual. There is always tenderness and often rebound tenderness over the region of the infarction. Voluntary guarding and, occasionally, spasm also are common. The infarcted segment, if large enough, may be palpable. A slight fever (rarely >38.5°C) and a moderate leukocytosis are usual. The diagnosis can be suspected by finely infiltrated fat giving a "smudged" appearance to the omentum on CT scan.

Treatment. Treatment of this condition is resection of the infarcted area to prevent the possible complications of gangrene and adhesions. A correct preoperative diagnosis is unusual, and most patients are explored for acute appendicitis or acute cholecystitis. The finding of serosanguineous fluid in the abdomen and a normal appendix or gallbladder should indicate disease in the omentum. Postoperative complications are rare.

Cysts

Pathology. Cysts of the omentum are rare. The pathogenesis of these lesions is unclear, but presumably most true cysts are caused by obstruction of lymphatic channels or by growth of congenitally misplaced lymphatic tissue that does not communicate with the vascular system. They contain serous fluid and may be unilocular or multilocular. The cysts have an endothelial lining similar to cystic lymphangiomas. Their size may vary from a few centimeters to over 30 cm in diameter. Dermoid cysts, which are rare, are lined with squamous epithelium and may contain hair, teeth, and sebaceous material.

Pseudocysts of the omentum result from fat necrosis, trauma with hematoma, or foreign-body reaction. These have a fibrous and inflammatory lining and usually contain cloudy or blood-tinged fluid.

Clinical Manifestations. True omental cysts are discovered most frequently in children or young adults but have been reported in the aged. Small cysts generally are asymptomatic and discovered incidentally at laparotomy or at autopsy. Large cysts present as a palpable abdominal mass or produce diffuse abdominal swelling. These may cause symptoms of heaviness or pain or manifestations of possible complications of omental cysts such as torsion, infection, rupture, or intestinal obstruction. Complications are more frequent in children and often produce a clinical picture of an acute surgical condition of the abdomen. The uncomplicated omental cyst usually lies in the lower mid-abdomen and is freely movable, smooth, and nontender.

Plain radiographs sometimes show a circumscribed soft tissue haziness in the abdomen, or after a barium meal, there may be displacement of intestinal loops with pressure on adjacent bowel. The presence of bone or teeth is diagnostic of dermoid cyst. The ultrasound or CT scan shows a fluid-filled mass that often contains internal septations.

Differential diagnosis includes cysts and solid tumors of the mesentery, peritoneum, and retroperitoneal region. An absolute diagnosis can be made only at the time of exploratory surgical procedures. Treatment consists of local excision.

Solid Tumors

The most common solid tumor of the omentum is metastatic carcinoma, which generally involves the omentum by tumor implantation. The primary source is usually the colon, stomach, pancreas, or ovaries. There often is ascites, presumably from "weeping" of serous or blood-tinged fluid from the metastatic implants. Diffuse neoplastic infiltration of the greater omentum produces a distinctive CT scan of a soft tissue mass ("omental cake") separating the colon or small intestine from the anterior abdominal wall (Fig. 33-5).

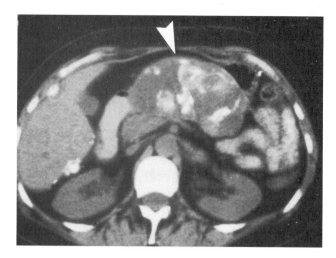

FIG. 33-5. *Omental metastases from ovarian carcinoma. CT scan shows the characteristic soft tissue mass involving the greater omentum ("omental cake") (arrow).*

Primary solid tumors of the omentum are exceedingly rare. They may be benign or malignant. Stout and associates recorded only 24 seen over a 55-year period at a major cancer center. Most are of mesenchymal origin, and about one-half are malignant. Benign tumors consist of lipomas, leiomyomas, fibromas, and neurofibromas. Leiomyosarcoma and hemangiopericytoma are the most common malignant tumors. The malignant tumors spread by direct extension or tumor implants and kill by involvement of vital abdominal organs. The mean age of patients with primary omental tumors is in the fifth decade. Although some patients are symptom-free, about one-half complain of vague abdominal pain. A palpable abdominal mass is present in one-third of patients.

The only treatment is surgical excision. Primary malignant tumors are highly invasive and often require resection of adjacent organs and total omentectomy. The prognosis is poor. Resection of benign tumors is curative, and recurrences have not been reported. Palliative omentectomy for metastatic tumor implants in the omentum has been suggested to control any associated ascites.

MESENTERY AND MESENTERIC CIRCULATION

Mesentery

The mesentery is a reflection of the posterior parietal peritoneum onto the surface of the intestine, where it becomes visceral peritoneum. It connects the intestine to the posterior abdominal wall and transmits blood vessels and nerves. In addition, the mesentery serves as a suspensory ligament of the jejunum and ileum. It is fan-shaped, with the root extending downward and obliquely from the ligament of Treitz (duodenojejunal flexure) at the level of L_2 to the right sacroiliac articulation (ileocecal junction) (Fig. 33-6). The entire root is only about 15 cm in length and allows free motion of the small intestine in any direction, limited only by the length of the mesentery. Within its two fused layers of peritoneum run the intestinal branches of the superior mesenteric artery and accompanying veins, along with

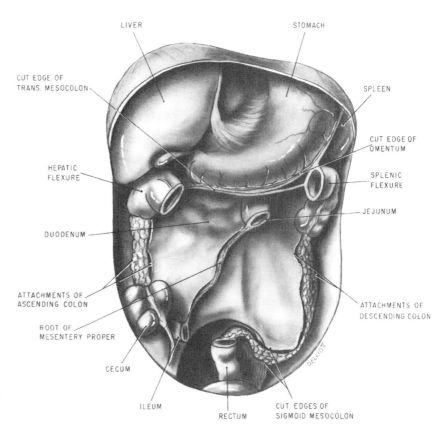

FIG. 33-6. Attachments of the mesenteries. The jejunum, ileum, and ascending, transverse, and descending colons have been removed.

lymphatics, mesenteric lymph nodes, visceral nerve fibers, and a variable amount of adipose tissue.

After the embryonic formation of a distinct intestinal loop, torsion of the loop takes place about the superior mesenteric artery. About the third or fourth fetal month, posterior peritoneal fixation of the colon takes place. The leaves of the mesentery to the ascending colon fuse with the right parietal peritoneum, and those to the descending colon fuse with the left parietal peritoneum. The posterolateral parietal peritoneum then passes directly from the abdominal wall over the ascending and descending colon, respectively, toward the midline and the root of the mesentery proper. For this reason, the mesentery to these portions of the large intestine usually is short or nonexistent. These fusions, however, form surgical cleavage planes allowing bloodless mobilization of the colon with its vascular supply. Within the embryonic mesentery to the ascending colon are the colonic arteries and veins from the superior mesenteric vessels, while those to the descending colon are derived from the inferior mesenteric vessels. On occasion, posterior fusion of the ascending or descending colon is incomplete or does not occur, leaving a well-developed mesentery and allowing free mobility of segments of the large bowel. This anomaly is more frequent with the right colon, predisposing to torsion with resulting intestinal obstruction.

The mesenteries of the transverse colon and sigmoid colon, in contrast to those of the ascending and descending colon, do not fuse with the posterior parietal peritoneum. These remain well developed and are referred to as the *transverse mesocolon* and *sigmoid mesocolon,* respectively. The segment to the transverse colon extends obliquely across the posterior abdominal wall just below the pancreas, remaining fixed at the hepatic and

splenic flexures of the bowel (see Fig. 33-6). The fixation of the splenic flexure is higher than that of the hepatic flexure because of the presence of the liver on the right side. The mesocolon allows the transverse colon to hang over the small intestine. This sagging may be so marked that the transverse colon occasionally reaches the symphysis pubis. Within the transverse mesocolon run branches of the middle colic artery and accompanying veins. Fusion between the mesocolon and the undersurface of the greater omentum from the stomach offers stability that prevents the transverse colon from undergoing torsion.

The sigmoid mesocolon originates at the end of the descending colon in the left iliac fossa and has an inverted V-shape course. It runs diagonally upward along the left iliac artery toward the aortic bifurcation and then bends directly downward into the pelvic fossa, where it is reflected off the rectum. It contains sigmoid vessels and branches of the superior hemorrhoidal vessels from the inferior mesenteric artery and vein. The length of the sigmoid mesocolon determines the location and mobility of the pelvic colon. If the sigmoid mesocolon is long, the bowel may cross the midline. Such a mobile pelvic colon may twist on itself. The sigmoid colon is the most frequent site of torsion producing volvulus of the intestinal tract.

The lateral fixations of the ascending and descending colon and the superior origin of the transverse mesocolon serve to confine the small intestine within the midabdomen. The transverse mesocolon and greater omentum also restrict the small bowel from entering the upper abdomen to become adherent to inflammatory lesions of the stomach, duodenum, gallbladder, or liver.

Defects in the mesenteries are potential sites for internal hernia. Most defects are created inadvertently by the surgeon during the course of intraabdominal operations. On rare occasions, congenital defects occur in areas of the mesentery that are thin and avascular. These usually are found in the mesenteries of the lower ileum, the sigmoid mesocolon, and the transverse mesocolon, the last through a wide avascular space just to the left of the middle colic artery (space of Riolan).

The mesenteries, with the omenta, share bactericidal and absorptive properties and an ability to form adhesions. In this regard, they function to localize and combat intraperitoneal infection and to seal intestinal perforations.

Mesenteric Circulation

The mesenteric vascular bed is of major importance in the maintenance of bodily homeostasis. Under resting conditions, the splanchnic (visceral) vascular bed receives 25 to 30 percent of cardiac output and contains as much as one-third of total blood volume. It has been suggested that this reservoir of blood produces a mechanism for "autotransfusion" during periods of hypovolemia when a relatively large volume of blood can be released rapidly into the circulation by active constriction of the splanchnic vessels. Control of the mesenteric vascular bed is primarily neural via sympathetic autonomic elements carried by the splanchnic nerves. These nerves accompany the celiac, superior mesenteric, and inferior mesenteric arteries and contain α- and β-adrenergic receptors. Stimulation of the splanchnic nerves produces vasoconstriction, with an increase in regional resistance. The mesenteric vasculature also is responsive to a number of pharmacologic agents. Norepinephrine, an α-adrenergic stimulator, produces vasoconstriction, while epinephrine elicits a classic dose-dependent β- or α-adrenergic response, low concentrations producing vasodilatation and higher concentrations producing vasoconstriction. Isoproterenol, a β-adrenergic stimulator, effects a dilator response that can be blocked by propranolol. Nitroglycerine, tolazoline hydrochloride, and papaverine hydrochloride elicit a direct vasodilatory effect; the direct infusion of these agents can be useful in the treatment of nonocclusive mesenteric ischemia. In contrast, the digitalis glycosides produce mesenteric vasoconstriction and may contribute to the pathogenesis of nonocclusive mesenteric ischemia.

Arteries. With the exception of the stomach and duodenum, which are supplied by the celiac artery, and the distal rectum, which is supplied by the inferior hemorrhoidal vessels arising from the internal iliac arteries, the arterial supply to the entire intestinal tract is derived from the superior and inferior mesenteric arteries. The superior mesenteric artery arises from the anterior aspect of the aorta just below the celiac artery at the level of the second lumbar vertebrae. Owing to their anterior origin, lateral aortography is necessary to visualize the origins of the celiac and superior mesenteric arteries. Accurate knowledge of the anatomy of the visceral vessels is of critical importance in the evaluation and treatment of visceral ischemia in the clinical setting. The superior mesenteric artery passes behind the neck of the pancreas but in front of the uncinate process and crosses in front of the third portion of the duodenum to enter the root of the mesentery. The acute angle at which the superior mesenteric artery arises from the aorta may compress the transverse portion of the duodenum between it and the aorta, causing partial intestinal obstruction, a condition referred to as the *superior mesenteric artery compression syndrome*. In addition, this acute angle makes it the most susceptible of the visceral vessels to cardioarterial embolism.

As the superior mesenteric artery continues downward between the two leaves of the mesentery, it gives off 12 or more major branches from its left side to supply the jejunum and ileum (Fig. 33-7). These jejunal and ileal arteries divide and then reunite within the mesentery to form groups, or arcades. Two to five such anastomotic arches are formed and allow collateral pathways for blood to reach the intestinal wall should occlusion of short arterial segments occur. The arcades become more numerous as the terminal ileum is reached. From the terminal arcades, straight branches (vasa recta) alternately pass to opposite sides of the jejunum and ileum. Within the intestinal wall, the vessels run parallel to the circular muscle coat and perpendicular to the direction of the lumen, traversing successively the serous, muscular, and submucosal layers. Each of these terminal arteries supplies only 1 or 2 cm of bowel length. For this reason, they must be preserved as close to the cut margins of the intestine as is technically possible when performing a bowel resection to avoid subsequent necrosis and breakdown of the anastomosis. The terminal straight arteries do not anastomose until reaching the submucous plexuses, where their ramifications anastomose freely. This situation predisposes to serious compromise of the blood supply to the antimesenteric border of the intestine after segmental small bowel resection. To ensure adequate circulation to the antimesenteric portion, it is customary to transect the small intestine obliquely rather than at a right angle (Fig. 33-8).

Arising from the right side of the superior mesenteric artery is the inferior pancreaticoduodenal artery and then, successively, the middle colic, the right colic, and the ileocolic arteries (see Fig. 33-7). Except for the ileocolic artery, these vessels do not form anastomotic arcades until nearly reaching the bowel wall.

The middle colic artery arises below the pancreas, enters the transverse mesocolon, and passing to the right, divides into a right and left branch. The right branch connects with the superior branch of the right colic artery and the left branch with the ascending branch of the left colic artery from the inferior mesenteric artery. It supplies the transverse colon. The location of the main arterial trunk to the right of the midline allows the left side of the transverse mesocolon to be opened through a relatively avascular area (space of Riolan) when performing a retrocolic gastrojejunal anastomosis.

The right colic artery arises just below the middle colic artery and passes to the right just behind the peritoneum. On reaching the midascending colon, it divides into superior and inferior branches, which anastomose, close to the bowel wall, with branches from the middle colic and ileocolic arteries, respectively. The right colic artery supplies the ascending colon.

The ileocolic artery is the terminal branch of the superior mesenteric artery. It supplies several centimeters of ileum, the cecum, the appendix, and the lower portion of the ascending colon. It terminates by dividing into ascending and descending branches. The ascending branch anastomoses with the inferior branch of the right colic artery, while the descending branch forms secondary and tertiary arcades by anastomosing with terminal branches of the superior mesenteric artery within the mesentery proper. From these arcades arise the appendicular artery to the appendix and cecal and ileal branches.

The superior mesenteric artery supplies the intestinal tract (midgut) from the third portion of the duodenum to the midtransverse colon. Collaterals between the inferior pancreaticoduodenal artery and the superior pancreaticoduodenal artery from the gastroduodenal, a secondary branch of the celiac artery,

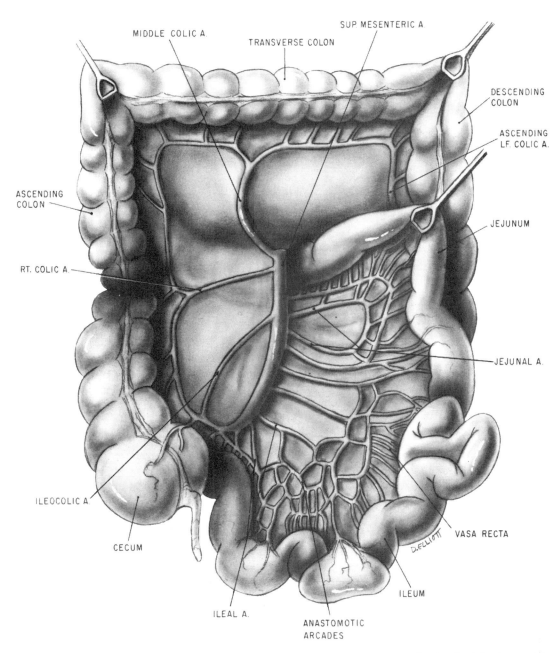

FIG. 33-7. Superior mesenteric artery and its branches. The artery supplies the distal duodenum, jejunum, ileum, ascending colon, and proximal two-thirds of the transverse colon.

enable the third part of the duodenum and proximal 10 to 12 cm of jejunum to survive when the superior mesenteric artery is occluded.

The inferior mesenteric artery supplies the left transverse colon, descending colon, sigmoid colon, and proximal part of the rectum. It arises from the anterior aspect of the aorta at the level of the third lumbar vertebrae and passes downward and to the left, entering the pelvis as the superior hemorrhoidal artery (Fig. 33-9). As it descends, it gives off the left colic and sigmoidal arteries. The left colic artery is the principal branch. It divides into ascending and descending limbs that anastomose with branches from the middle colic and sigmoid arteries, respectively. The sigmoid artery passes into the sigmoid mesocolon

and divides into branches that anastomose with one another, forming several arcades. The lowest sigmoid arcade joins with arcades from the superior hemorrhoidal artery. The superior hemorrhoidal artery continues downward behind the rectum, where it communicates with branches from the middle and inferior hemorrhoidal arteries from the internal iliac artery, giving the rectum a dual source of arterial supply.

The anastomoses between primary branches of the superior and inferior mesenteric arteries form an arcade that passes along the margin of the colon and is referred to as the *marginal artery of Drummond* (see Fig. 33-9). It is situated about 1 cm from the margin of the bowel and extends from the end of the ileum to the end of the sigmoid colon. Through its anastomoses, it gen-

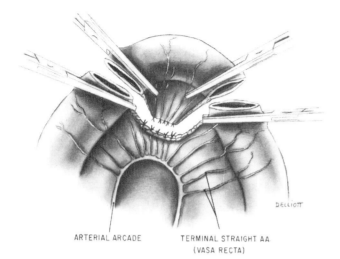

ARTERIAL ARCADE   TERMINAL STRAIGHT AA
                              (VASA RECTA)

FIG. 33-8. *Straight arteries (vasa recta) entering the wall of the small intestine perpendicular to the direction of its lumen. The arteries alternately pass to either side of the intestinal wall. In performing a segmental resection of the small intestine, transecting the bowel obliquely, as indicated, ensures an adequate blood supply to the antimesenteric border.*

erally is capable of supplying the bowel even though one of the major arteries is ligated.

Veins. The venous drainage of the small intestine and colon is through tributaries of the inferior and superior mesenteric veins, which in turn ultimately terminate in the portal vein (Fig. 33-10). The portal circulation begins within the mucosa of the intestine. Small venules coalesce, and the confluent veins pass through the wall of the intestine, emerging alternately in a similar manner to that of the straight arteries entering the bowel wall. These then converge to form a system of venous arcades within the mesentery from which blood enters the main tributaries to the superior and inferior mesenteric veins.

The inferior mesenteric vein is a continuation of the superior hemorrhoidal vein. It passes upward to the left side of the inferior mesenteric artery, receiving tributaries that correspond in name and location to the branches of the artery. The main trunk of the vein does not accompany the artery but rather courses over the duodenojejunal flexure just lateral to the ligament of Treitz and, passing over the body of the pancreas, joins with the splenic vein (see Figs. 33-9 and 33-10). It drains the left side of the large intestine from the upper rectum to the left midtransverse colon. A plexus of anastomoses around the midrectum between the superior hemorrhoidal vein and the middle and inferior hemorrhoidal veins to the internal iliac veins forms a collateral pathway between the portal and systemic circulations. The inferior mesenteric vein generally can be ligated with impunity.

The superior mesenteric vein runs within the mesentery proper lateral to the superior mesenteric artery. It receives tributaries that accompany corresponding branches of the superior mesenteric artery and that drain the entire small intestine and right half of the colon. As it passes over the third portion of the duodenum and behind the neck of the pancreas, it receives the confluence of the inferior mesenteric and splenic veins to become the portal vein.

The venous drainage from the entire gastrointestinal tract passes through the liver via the portal circulation before returning to the heart. Together with the mesenteric lymphatics, it represents the sole means by which ingested food products find their way into the circulation. The normal portal venous pressure is between 12 and 15 cmH_2O; that within the inferior vena cava (systemic pressure) varies between a positive pressure of about 3 cmH_2O during the expiratory phase of respiration to a negative pressure of 1 to 3 cmH_2O during inspiration. Like the vena cava, the portal system does not contain valves, and therefore, the blood flows in the direction of reduced venous pressure.

Lymphatics and Lymph Nodes. The lymph drainage of the small intestine and colon follows the course of the main blood vessels. Those accompanying the inferior mesenteric artery drain to periaortic nodes and then to the superior mesenteric nodes before entering the cisterna chyli of the thoracic duct. Those accompanying branches of the superior mesenteric artery drain into the mesenteric glands within the mesentery, where they are closely related to the vascular arcades. The mesenteric nodes are distributed in three locations: (1) juxtaintestinal, at the last anastomotic branch of the mesenteric arteries before they enter the intestines, (2) intermediate, in the region of the larger anastomosing branches, and (3) central, at the root of the mesentery near the origin of the main mesenteric artery. The nodes are more numerous in the right half of the mesentery, and they increase in size and number as they approach its root. These nodes are the usual site for mesenteric adenitis, tuberculosis, and other inflammatory and neoplastic conditions. From the mesenteric nodes, lymph drains into the superior mesenteric and celiac nodes and then to the thoracic duct.

MESENTERIC VASCULAR DISEASE

Mesenteric vascular disease is not a single entity but rather a syndrome that includes (1) complete occlusion or stenosis of mesenteric arteries by embolism, thrombosis, or obliterative disease, (2) thrombosis of mesenteric (portal) veins, (3) extraluminal obstruction of mesenteric arteries by aortic aneurysm, dissecting aneurysm, fibrous and ligamentous bands, or tumors, (4) aneurysms of the splanchnic arteries, and (5) traumatic injury to visceral vessels. These conditions produce vascular insufficiency or infarction of the affected intestine. Intestinal disease because of impaired circulation is relatively uncommon when compared with the more frequently occurring mechanical obstructions of the mesenteric vessels by adhesive bands, strangulated hernia, and intestinal volvulus.

Occlusions of the mesenteric arteries may be acute and complete (those resulting from emboli or thrombosis), gradual and partial (those resulting from obliterative arterial disease), or acute and complete superimposed on a previously narrowed or stenotic vessel. Collateral vessels permit gradual occlusion of either the celiac or the superior mesenteric artery to be tolerated. Acute occlusion of the celiac or inferior mesenteric artery generally is asymptomatic in an otherwise normal person; acute occlusion of the superior mesenteric artery, if untreated, results in intestinal infarction and death. The superior mesenteric artery at its origin or close to the takeoff of its middle colic branch is the usual site of acute and chronic mesenteric arterial occlusions. Complete occlusion of the inferior mesenteric artery produces symptoms only if there is compromise of collateral blood flow from the superior mesenteric or internal iliac (hypogastric) artery. Clinically apparent venous occlusions are sudden and com-

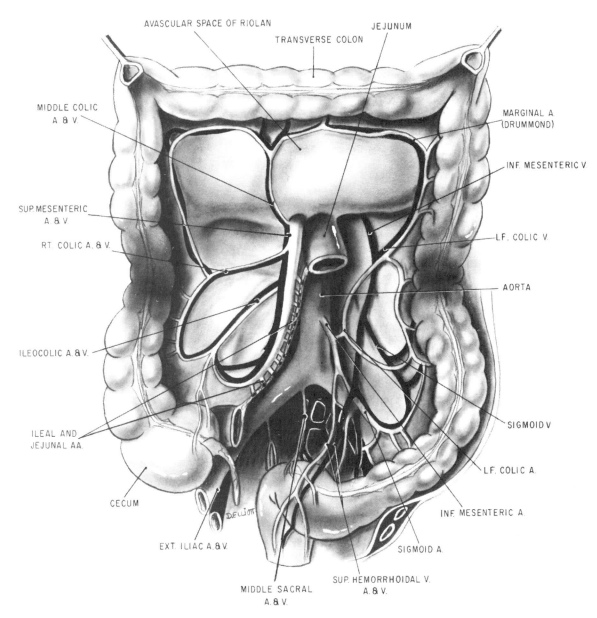

FIG. 33-9. Blood supply to the large bowel. An arterial arcade, formed by anastomoses between branches of the colic arteries, runs along the margin of the large intestine and is referred to as the *marginal artery of Drummond.* This vessel is an important collateral channel between the superior and inferior mesenteric artery distributions and takes on added significance when either of their arteries is stenotic or occluded.

plete and invariably a consequence of thrombosis. Partial mesenteric venous occlusion usually is the result of external compression and is asymptomatic.

The relative incidence of mesenteric arterial as opposed to venous occlusions is not known. When intestinal infarction occurs, it is not unusual to find thrombosis of both sides of the splanchnic circulation at laparotomy or autopsy because initial occlusion of one eventuates in clot formation in the other. The clinical distinction between the two is often difficult. It has been variously estimated that 15 to 20 percent of all significant mesenteric vascular accidents are a result of primary venous thrombosis and that approximately 50 percent are a result of primary arterial occlusion. In the remaining 30 to 35 percent of cases,

intestinal infarction occurs in the absence of major arterial or venous occlusion.

Acute Occlusive Visceral Ischemia

Etiology. Acute occlusion of the superior mesenteric artery may be the result of cardioarterial embolus or in situ thrombosis, with the incidence of each being approximately equal. The steep angle in which the superior mesenteric artery arises from the aorta makes it the most likely target among the visceral vessels to receive embolic material from the heart. Typically, emboli lodge at the origin of the superior mesenteric artery or at the origin of the major distal branch vessels, such as the middle

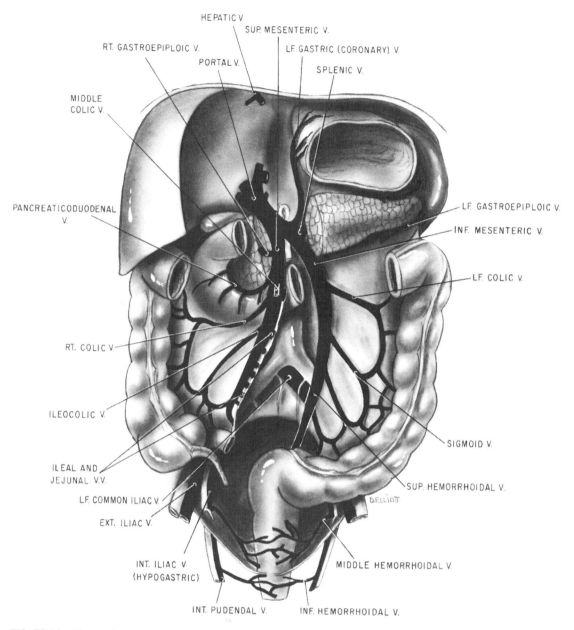

FIG. 33-10. Mesenteric venous circulation, demonstrating communication with the systemic circulation through the middle and inferior hemorrhoidal veins. A similar communication (not shown) exists between the left gastric vein and the azygos system of veins.

colic, right colic and ileocolic arteries (Fig. 33-11). Thrombotic occlusion of the superior mesenteric artery typically occurs at the vessel origin, as a result of progression of a preexisting stenotic atherosclerotic plaque to complete occlusion. The atherosclerotic plaque generally arises in the visceral bearing segment of the aorta and "overhangs" the origin of the visceral vessels. For this reason, atherosclerosis of the visceral arteries is localized to the vessel origin. While this is nearly always true of the celiac artery, it is not uncommon for the atherosclerotic process in the superior mesenteric artery to extend distally over a length of 4 to 5 cm. Less common causes of stenosis and occlusion of the visceral arteries include Takayasu's arteritis, periarteritis nodosa, and thromboangiitis obliterans. Extrinsic compression of

the celiac artery by diaphragmatic fibers (median arcuate ligament syndrome) may produce a chronic visceral pain syndrome.

Whatever the cause, the initial effect of proximal occlusion of the superior mesenteric artery is to cause intense spasm of its distal branches, exacerbating the ischemic insult. Acute occlusion of the origin of the superior mesenteric artery produces ischemia of the small intestine from the level of the ligament of Treitz to the ileocecal valve and of the ascending colon and proximal two-thirds of the transverse colon. Patency of the celiac artery can result in viability of the proximal 10 to 12 cm of jejunum owing to anastomoses between the superior pancreaticoduodenal artery (celiac-based) and the inferior pancreaticoduodenal artery (first branch of the superior mesenteric artery).

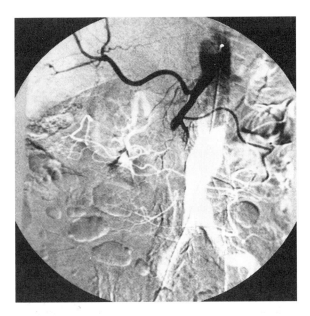

FIG. 33-11. *Selective injection of the superior mesenteric artery, demonstrating embolic occlusion proximal to several jejunal branches. Note the replaced right hepatic artery, taking origin from the proximal superior mesenteric artery.*

Acute occlusion of distal branch vessels, such as the middle colic, right colic, and ileocolic arteries, results in segmental intestinal ischemia that might infarct depending on the status of the collateral circulation.

Pathology. High-grade partial or complete occlusion of the proximal superior mesenteric artery results in intense vasospasm throughout the mesenteric vascular bed, even in areas that would otherwise continue to be directly perfused either by branch vessels originating proximal to the occlusion or by the inferior mesenteric distribution. This observation constitutes the basis for specific catheter-directed pharmacologic therapy.

Because the mucosa is the layer of the intestinal wall most sensitive to ischemia, mucosal sloughing and ulceration, often manifest as gastrointestinal bleeding, are early pathophysiologic events that may be recognized endoscopically. Acutely ischemic intestine will appear pale, and pulsation in the mesentery, which is generally visible and palpable, will be absent. Peristalsis may persist for several hours after the onset of ischemia; the presence of bowel contractility should not dissuade from the diagnosis of acute intestinal ischemia when the findings of pallor and pulselessness are present. As the ischemic process progresses to infarction, over a period of approximately 6 h in the setting of profound complete ischemia, the bowel wall becomes dusky, then cyanotic, and ultimately frankly gangrenous and perforated. Intestinal ischemia and infarction from mesenteric venous occlusion are easily differentiated from those which are purely arterial in origin because the former results in a bowel wall that is intensely hemorrhagic and edematous, along with engorgement of the mesentery. In general, mesenteric venous thrombosis pursues a more virulent course and is less amenable to successful intervention than is mesenteric arterial occlusion.

Clinical Manifestations. Acute intestinal ischemia, regardless of cause, is characterized by pain out of proportion to physical findings. The abdominal pain is acute in onset, intense and diffuse, may be accompanied by vomiting, and is unresponsive to narcotic administration. Occult blood in the stool or frankly bloody diarrhea is a later finding, representing mucosal sloughing. Early abdominal examination is remarkable for a paucity or absence of findings. Localization of abdominal pain and development of peritoneal signs mark the onset of intestinal necrosis.

A history of atrial fibrillation or of a previous cardioarterial embolic event should raise suspicion of embolic occlusion of the superior mesenteric artery. Alternatively, a history of weight loss and food avoidance, along with the stigmata of diffuse atherosclerotic occlusive disease, is suggestive of an acute thrombotic occlusion of a previously stenotic superior mesenteric artery.

Diagnostic Studies. Laboratory investigation is too nonspecific to rule out the diagnosis of acute intestinal ischemia; the diagnosis must be made on clinical grounds and requires a high index of suspicion. Although the leukocyte count may be normal early on, it often increases to greater than 20,000/mm³ as the ischemic process progresses. Hemoconcentration, manifest as a high hematocrit, may be present secondary to fluid accumulation in the extravascular compartment and vomiting. Metabolic acidosis, manifest as a base deficit, may be present, the degree of which is related to the extent and duration of the intestinal ischemic process. Elevation of the serum lactate level similarly reflects the degree and duration of intestinal hypoperfusion. Persistence of a base deficit despite adequate resuscitative measures is indicative of advanced ischemia and most likely intestinal infarction. Elevation of the serum amylase level is a relatively late finding and is often indicative of bowel necrosis.

Plain film findings occur late, if at all, in the course of acute intestinal ischemia and cannot be relied on for diagnosis, although they may be useful in excluding other conditions. A notable exception is that of thumbprinting of the bowel wall because of submucosal edema, which is indicative of intestinal ischemia. More commonly, thumbprinting is seen on double-contrast barium enema examination in the setting of colon ischemia. Plain films of the abdomen in the setting of acute intestinal ischemia reveal only nonspecific air-filled loops of small intestine. Air in the mesenteric or portal venous system is an unusual but ominous diagnostic finding that occurs late in the disease process and signals bowel necrosis.

Ultrasound, computed transaxial tomographic (CTT) scanning, and MRI in the diagnosis of acute mesenteric ischemia are applicable. These modalities may be time-consuming, require radiologic expertise to interpret, offer no possibility of therapeutic intervention, and their diagnostic accuracy at the present time must be considered unproved. Contrast arteriography, including lateral aortography and selective injection of the superior mesenteric artery, remains the single most important diagnostic maneuver in evaluation of the patient with suspected acute mesenteric ischemia.

Prompt arteriography and catheter-based therapies form the basis of an aggressive approach toward the diagnosis and treatment of acute mesenteric ischemia, popularized by Boley and colleagues in the early 1980s, and represent a major advance in the treatment of this highly lethal condition. Arteriography almost always distinguishes between embolic and atherosclerotic occlusive causes of acute mesenteric ischemia. This is a critical determination because the operative approach to mesenteric revascularization is vastly different in each instance. Arteriography demonstrates instances of nonocclusive mesenteric ischemia, which often can be managed successfully nonoperatively with catheter-based pharmacologic therapies.

In the case of cardioarterial embolus, arteriography reveals the level of embolic occlusion, which is typically at the origin of a branch vessel, such as the middle colic or right colic artery, and directs the operative approach to embolectomy. In the case of atherosclerotic occlusion, arteriography reveals the site and length of the occlusion, typically at the origin of the superior mesenteric or celiac artery, and allows planning of operation type, e.g., endarterectomy or bypass. Critical information also is provided regarding suitability of inflow source (usually the supraceliac aorta).

Treatment. Once the diagnosis of acute occlusive mesenteric ischemia has been established at arteriography, continuous infusion of a vasodilator, such as papaverine or nitroglycerine, may be begun directly into the superior mesenteric artery if the origin of this vessel is patent and can be cannulated (Fig. 33-12). This maneuver can be especially useful if an embolus has lodged at the takeoff of the middle colic or right colic artery because it may break the accompanying vasospasm occurring outside the area of ischemia. The catheter may be left in place for ongoing infusion of vasodilator therapy during and after relief of arterial obstruction by surgical embolectomy. When acute mesenteric arterial occlusion has been identified and vasodilator therapy begun, time is of the essence in proceeding to the operating room. Resuscitation of the patient with an intravenous balanced salt solution, nasogastric decompression, establishment of invasive hemodynamic monitoring, optimization of cardiac performance with pharmacologic intervention as needed, and administration of broad-spectrum antibiotics aimed at enteric organisms are supportive aspects of care. These should be instituted on initial assessment of the patient, performed in an ongoing fashion during work-up, and continued in the perioperative period.

At operation, through a long midline incision, initial decision regarding treatment is based on the extent and severity of intes-

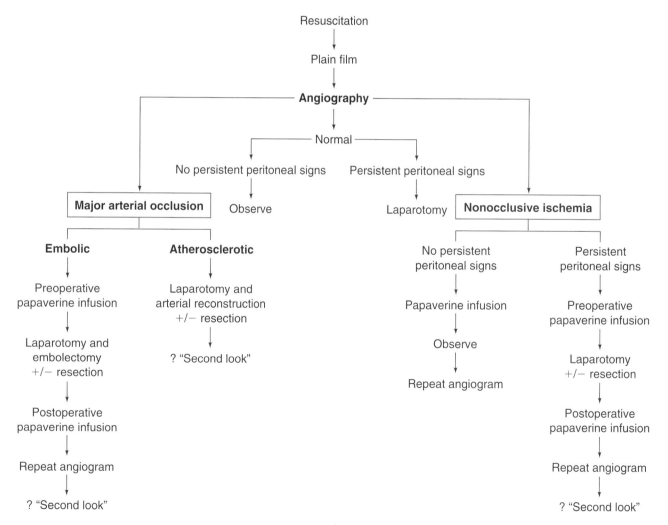

FIG. 33-12. Algorithm for diagnosis and treatment of acute mesenteric ischemia. (Adapted from: *Kaleya RN, Sammartano RJ, Boley SJ: Aggressive approach to acute mesenteric ischemia. Surg Clin North Am 72:157, 1992, with permission.*)

tinal ischemia. Methods of surgical revascularization will be vastly different depending on the cause of the ischemic insult. With embolic or atherosclerotic occlusion, only intestine that is frankly necrotic should be resected initially, followed by an attempt at revascularization. If only a short segment of intestine appears ischemic from an embolus to a distal branch of the ileocolic artery, resection of the affected intestine with primary anastomosis and anticoagulation may be sufficient.

An embolus lodged at the origin of the superior mesenteric artery produces patchy cyanosis of the intestine from the level of the ligament of Treitz to the mid-transverse colon, with many intervening areas of questionable viability. Revascularization of the ischemic intestine by embolectomy of the superior mesenteric artery should be performed. The superior mesenteric artery can be isolated in its midportion as it crosses in front of the fourth part of the duodenum, after the transverse colon has been reflected cephalad and the ligament of Treitz taken down. After anticoagulation with heparin and control of the superior mesenteric artery with atraumatic vascular clamps or doubly looped vessel tapes, a transverse arteriotomy is made, and a small Fogarty balloon embolectomy catheter is passed proximally. The balloon is gently inflated and the embolus extracted. After pulsatile inflow is obtained, an additional pass of the catheter into the aorta is made and any residual thrombus withdrawn. If adequate backbleeding is present and no thrombus is visualized, the Fogarty catheter need not be passed distally, and the arteriotomy can be closed primarily. If thrombus or embolus is encountered at the arteriotomy site, it may be gently teased out, followed by passage of a Fogarty catheter if adequate inflow or backbleeding cannot be readily established. Once embolectomy has been achieved and intestinal circulation reestablished, intestinal viability should be reassessed. Only those areas of intestine which are frankly necrotic should be resected at this time. The routine use of fluorescein injection for intraoperative assessment of intestinal viability cannot be recommended. Intestine that is of questionable viability should be left in situ and reassessed at a planned "second look" laparotomy 24 to 48 h later. The decision to proceed with "second look" laparotomy is made at the time of the initial operation and is not based on the subsequent postoperative course.

At the "second look" laparotomy after successful mesenteric revascularization, it is often found that bowel that appeared to be of questionable viability initially is now clearly viable. This avoids the consequences of massive intestinal resection, such as short-gut syndrome and lifelong parenteral nutrition. All necrotic bowel must be resected at this time, and depending on the extent of intestinal loss, total parenteral nutrition is frequently an important adjunct in the postoperative period.

Necrosis of the midgut from the level of the ligament of Treitz to the mid-transverse colon might be encountered at the time of initial laparotomy. Consequently, there is no point in attempting revascularization because all the end-organ is nonviable. The extent of intestinal resection required is often incompatible with life in the elderly patient, with or without total parenteral nutrition, and the surgeon has a difficult ethical decision. In this circumstance, the most humane course may be to close the abdomen and provide comfort care until death from sepsis inevitably occurs.

In the case of acute mesenteric ischemia resulting from atherosclerotic occlusion of the superior mesenteric artery, with or without associated occlusion or stenosis of the celiac artery, after resection of frankly necrotic bowel, intraoperative efforts are focused on complete visceral revascularization, including revascularization of the celiac artery, if necessary, in addition to the superior mesenteric artery. Techniques of visceral revascularization include transaortic endarterectomy of the origins of the celiac and superior mesenteric arteries via a "trapdoor" aortotomy or bypass. Methods of retrograde bypass from the infrarenal aorta or iliac arteries have been described, but none has proved as durable as antegrade bypass from the supraceliac aorta using prosthetic graft material. Although technically more demanding, transaortic endarterectomy performed via medial visceral rotation is advisable for intestinal necrosis because the need for prosthetic graft material is obviated. Antegrade bypass and transaortic endarterectomy have proved durable, providing symptomatic relief in approximately 95 percent of patients at 1 year and 85 percent at 5 years. After successful revascularization, "second look" laparotomy may be necessary.

The mortality rate after sudden onset of mesenteric ischemia is as high as 85 percent. This can be attributed to delay in diagnosis and the reluctance of many physicians unfamiliar with this entity to proceed with arteriography in a critically ill patient. Using the multimodal approach, Boley and associates reported a decrease in mortality rate to 45 percent. Mortality is higher after acute occlusion by thrombosis compared with embolism.

Reoxygenation of ischemic tissues exacerbates preexisting ischemic injury, especially in an organ with a relatively high cell turnover rate, such as small intestine. This reperfusion injury is mediated by highly reactive free-radical metabolites of oxygen and is characterized by cell membrane injury, phospholipid peroxidation, cell swelling, and in many instances cell death. Bacterial translocation from the intestinal lumen into the circulation has been documented. Injury occurring in organ systems remote from the focus of ischemia-reperfusion, most notably the lung, also has been noted. Mannitol, a tertiary alcohol and scavenger of the deleterious hydroxyl radical, has some efficacy and may be administered in a dose of 25 g before reestablishment of perfusion to ischemic intestine.

Nonocclusive Visceral Ischemia

In up to one-third of patients presenting with the manifestations of acute mesenteric ischemia, lateral aortography demonstrates patency of the main superior mesenteric artery. Selective injection of the superior mesenteric artery reveals multiple segmental areas of narrowing of small and intermediate branch vessels and diminution or absence of a mural intestinal circulation (Fig. 33-13). Nonocclusive mesenteric ischemia occurs in the patient experiencing a prolonged low-flow state, such as that accompanying congestive heart failure complicating acute myocardial infarction or on a chronic basis. The patient usually is hypovolemic from aggressive diuretic therapy aimed at relieving cardiac failure and is receiving cardiac inotropic support and α-adrenergic agents to maintain blood pressure.

Splanchnic vasoconstriction may occur initially on a compensatory basis with profoundly depressed cardiac output. Persistent and intractable splanchnic vasoconstriction results in severe intestinal ischemia. The distribution of ischemia is diffuse from the level of the ligament of Treitz to the mid-transverse colon, and the process often has progressed to bowel necrosis at diagnosis. Nonocclusive mesenteric ischemia can represent the

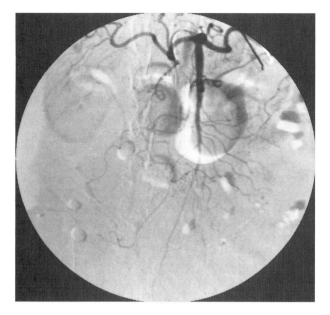

FIG. 33-13. *Selective visceral arteriogram demonstrating diffuse vasoconstriction of the superior mesenteric artery and its branches, characteristic of nonocclusive mesenteric ischemia. Note the common origin of the celiac and superior mesenteric arteries.*

terminal event in a patient with a persistent low-flow state and multiple organ system failure.

Clinical Manifestations. The clinical picture may be identical to that of patients with acute arterial or venous mesenteric occlusions. The patients, however, usually are older, and the infarction develops slowly over a period of several days, during which time there may be prodromal symptoms of malaise and vague abdominal discomfort. Associated congestive heart failure, with or without arrhythmia, is frequent. An unusually large number of patients have been found to be overdigitalized. Infarction of the intestine is preceded by the sudden onset of severe abdominal pain and vomiting. The patient usually becomes acutely hypotensive and develops a rapid pulse. Watery diarrhea is frequent, and the stools may be grossly bloody. The abdomen becomes diffusely tender and rigid. Bowel sounds are diminished and later absent. Fever and leukocytosis are usual, and frequently there is a thrombocytopenia related to intravascular thrombosis. A characteristic early laboratory finding is a markedly elevated hematocrit, which occurs because of the "trapping" of serum in the bowel wall and seepage into the peritoneal cavity. Metabolic acidosis with a significant base deficit is present almost universally.

In disorders in which the splanchnic circulation is thought to be diminished, unexplained abdominal signs and symptoms should be viewed with the possibility of mesenteric vascular insufficiency and intestinal necrosis in mind.

Contrast arteriography, including lateral aortography and selective injection of the superior mesenteric artery, is the most important diagnostic procedure for evaluating patients believed to have acute mesenteric ischemia. In addition, the ability to administer catheter-based pharmacologic interventions is available immediately. Optimization of cardiac function, discontinuation of splanchnic vasoconstricting agents, and infusion of vasodilators such as papaverine or nitroglycerin directly into the

superior mesenteric artery are the recommended therapy. Such infusions can be maintained safely for several days. Serial arteriography over a period of 48 to 72 h might be necessary in order to monitor therapeutic response. Administration of broad-spectrum antibiotics aimed at enteric organisms can diminish bacterial translocation from the gut to the bloodstream. Once peritoneal signs have developed, exploration is necessary.

At initial exploration, only that intestine which is necrotic should be resected, with anticipation of performing a "second look" laparotomy over a period of 24 to 48 h, during which time ongoing vasodilator therapy is administered directly into the superior mesenteric artery. The mortality from nonocclusive mesenteric artery ischemia is in the range of 80 percent in most series, resulting from the presence of bowel necrosis at the time of diagnosis and from the high association of multiorgan dysfunction and preterminal illness in the target population. Improved survivorship has been reported by identifying groups of patients at high risk for this problem, using a policy of aggressive and multiple reoperations, and delaying intestinal anatomosis.

Chronic Visceral Ischemia

Etiology and Pathology. Atherosclerosis of a visceral artery with plaque overhanging or encroaching on the origins of the celiac and superior mesenteric arteries is the cause of chronic visceral ischemia in more than 95 percent of patients. The atheroma may extend into the celiac artery over a length of approximately 1 cm, but it is common for the atherosclerotic process in the superior mesenteric artery to extend distally over a length of 4 to 5 cm. Two of the three main visceral arteries (celiac, superior mesenteric, and inferior mesenteric) must be stenotic or occluded to produce significant gut ischemia because of the rich collateral network.

Other causes of stenosis and occlusion of the visceral arteries include Takayasu's arteritis, periarteritis nodosa, thromboangiitis obliterans, and fibromuscular dysplasia. Obstructing aortic atheroma in the suprarenal segment, termed *"coral reef" atheroma,* can produce visceral ischemia without narrowing the origin of the visceral vessels by restricting aortic flow or embolization. A proposed nonatheromatous cause of chronic visceral ischemic pain is extrinsic compression of the celiac artery by diaphragmatic fibers, known as *median arcuate ligament syndrome.* Extrinsic compression of the celiac artery, however, can be demonstrated by lateral aortography in many patients without symptoms. The existence of this syndrome has been questioned by many and may be insignificant.

Clinical Manifestations. Chronic visceral ischemia is more common in women, with a female-to-male ratio as high as 4:1 in many series. Onset of symptoms usually is in the sixth or seventh decade, and the usual risk factors and stigmata of atherosclerosis frequently are present. The pain of chronic visceral ischemia is dull and persistent, occurring most commonly in the epigastric and periumbilical areas. Often referred to as *intestinal angina,* the pain usually occurs approximately 20 min after eating and may persist for several hours. The pain is exacerbated by ingesting large meals and eating solid foods as opposed to liquids. If the pain is severe, nausea and vomiting occur. Initially the patient complains of constipation and later of diarrhea. There is usually steady progression in the frequency and duration of symptoms. The food-pain relationship leads to a reluctance on

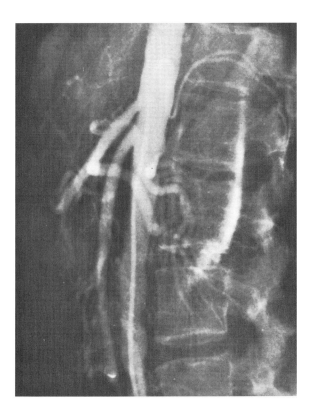

FIG. 33-14. Lateral aortogram demonstrating normal celiac and superior mesenteric arteries.

the part of the patient to eat. The subsequent rapid and severe weight loss characterizes the syndrome. As the intestinal ischemia progresses, a form of malabsorption syndrome occurs that contributes to the weight loss and is manifest by bulky, foamy stools high in fat and protein content. Symptoms of intestinal angina can exist for months or years before the visceral circulation becomes critically curtailed. As the mesenteric occlusive process progresses, patients typically avoid solid foods ("food fear") and drink small amounts of liquid many times per day. This often leads to weight loss and malnutrition, which is contributed to by the decreased nutrient absorptive capacity of the chronically ischemic intestine. Although chronic visceral ischemia produces a well-defined clinical syndrome, it is not always promptly recognized by the clinician, and up to one-third of patients presenting with intestinal infarction have prior symptoms of chronic visceral ischemia that went unrecognized.

Examination usually reveals a thin patient. Auscultation of the abdomen often reveals a bruit in the epigastrium. Stigmata of atherosclerosis are common but not always present. Chronic visceral ischemia may be the initial and only manifestation of atherosclerosis, especially in women under 60 years of age.

Diagnostic Studies. Blood work is not helpful in the diagnosis of chronic visceral ischemia. Duplex ultrasound, combining B-mode ultrasound imaging with spectral analysis of Doppler signals, is useful for identifying high-grade stenoses of the celiac and superior mesenteric arteries. The detection of a stenotic lesion is based on acceleration of the peak systolic velocity of flowing blood across the area of stenosis. In addition to evaluation in the fasting state, repeat evaluation in the post-

prandial state may increase diagnostic accuracy. Because these patients are generally thin, it usually is possible to identify the visceral vessels with B-mode ultrasound.

Contrast arteriography is the definitive method for the diagnosis of chronic visceral ischemia and is the only imaging modality that provides the detailed information necessary to plant treatment. The typical atherosclerotic process is shown in Figs. 33-14 and 33-15. A markedly dilated and elongated inferior mesenteric artery filling the superior mesenteric artery through collaterals is indicative of a superior mesenteric artery stenosis or occlusion (Fig. 33-16). When this finding is noted on a flush aortogram taken in the anteroposterior projection, lateral aortography of the visceral bearing segment of the aorta should be obtained.

When obtaining contrast arteriography, the administration of a dye load to a dehydrated patient with critical stenosis of the visceral arteries can be disastrous because it can precipitate thrombotic occlusion at the site of stenosis with resulting intestinal infarction. Attention to volume status before arteriography is essential, as is hydration before and after arteriography.

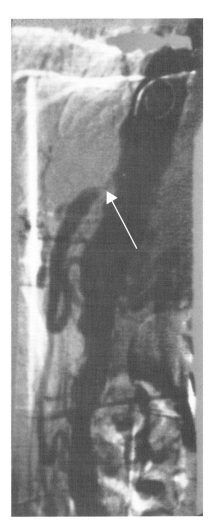

FIG. 33-15. Lateral aortogram demonstrating high-grade stenosis of the celiac artery at its origin and total occlusion of the superior mesenteric artery at its origin. Reconstitution of the superior mesenteric artery distal to the occlusion is noted (arrow).

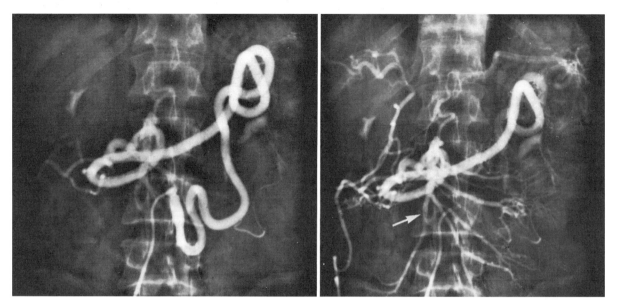

FIG. 33-16. *Left:* Selective injection of the inferior mesenteric artery demonstrating a prominent marginal artery of Drummond filling from a dilated and tortuous inferior mesenteric artery. *Right:* Later film showing filling of the superior mesenteric artery (arrow) through collaterals. The patient had complete occlusion of the celiac and superior mesenteric arteries at their origins.

The arteriographic appearance of median arcuate ligament syndrome is that of extrinsic compression of the celiac artery along its superior border with caudal displacement of the artery. This compression occurs approximately 1 cm beyond the vessel origin, and there is no evidence of atherosclerosis. Poststenotic dilatation of the artery may be present.

Reports of other imaging modalities for the detection of visceral artery stenosis include MRI and MR angiography, conventional CTT scanning and CTT angiography, and various radioisotope techniques.

Treatment. Once the diagnosis of chronic visceral ischemia has been established, hemodynamic status should be optimized. The cardiac function should be closely monitored intraoperatively via flow-directed pulmonary artery catheter or transesophageal echocardiography in anticipation of supraceliac aortic clamping. Afterload reduction to relieve left ventricular wall stress is required during the period of supraceliac aortic occlusion. The goal of the operation is to provide complete revascularization of the ischemic gut. The two principal approaches to mesenteric revascularization are antegrade aortovisceral bypass and transaortic visceral endarterectomy. Both procedures have proved durable, providing symptomatic relief in approximately 95 percent of patients at 1 year and 85 percent at 5 years.

Antegrade bypass from the supraceliac aorta to the celiac or superior mesenteric artery is technically less demanding than transaortic endarterectomy. The supraceliac aorta usually is free from significant atherosclerotic occlusive disease. The gastrohepatic omentum is divided and the stomach and pancreas retracted inferiorly. The left lobe of the liver is mobilized and retracted to the right. The nasogastric tube is palpated easily within the esophagus, which is retracted to the left. The diaphragmatic crura and celiac ganglionic tissue are divided, ex-

posing the supraceliac aorta. Prosthetic graft material, Dacron or expanded polytetrafluoroethylene, is the conduit of choice. The short straight segment of a bifurcated graft will be sewn in end-to-side fashion to the supraceliac aorta, with the limbs of the graft sewn in end-to-end fashion to the celiac and superior mesenteric arteries. The graft limbs should be in the anatomic position, with the limb to the superior mesenteric artery placed in a retropancreatic tunnel (Fig. 33-17). In this way, the prosthesis will resist kinking regardless of the position of the viscera. If only one vessel is to be revascularized, a flanged graft can be used, with attachment of the flanged portion of the graft to the supraceliac aorta.

The anatomic exposure necessary to perform transaortic visceral endarterectomy can be achieved via long midline incision and medial visceral rotation. Medial visceral rotation is accomplished by reflecting the abdominal viscera from left to right, including the stomach, spleen, and pancreas. Only the left kidney is left in anatomic position (Fig. 33-18). After supraceliac aortic clamping, a "trapdoor" aortotomy is created and endarterectomy of the paravisceral aorta and visceral (and, if necessary, renal) artery origins performed (Fig. 33-19). Closure of the aortotomy provides restoration of aortic continuity. Intraoperative duplex scanning provides an excellent method of assessment of technical result.

Mesenteric revascularization using reversed saphenous vein grafts originating from the iliac arteries or infrarenal aorta has been described. Such grafts placed in retrograde fashion are prone to kinking, and long-term durability is not comparable with that of antegrade prosthetic aortovisceral bypass or transaortic visceral endarterectomy.

There have been isolated reports of percutaneous transluminal angioplasty of the visceral arteries in the treatment of chronic visceral ischemia. The number of patients treated has been small, and in almost 20 percent of patients, the planned procedure has

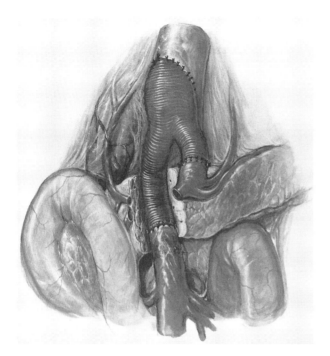

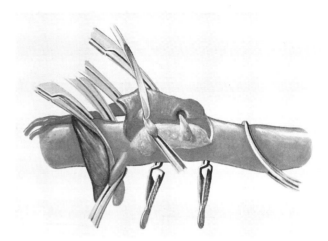

FIG. 33-19. "Trapdoor" aortotomy with endarterectomy of the aorta and origins of the celiac and superior mesenteric arteries, following exposure via medial visceral rotation. (From: *Wylie EJ, Stoney RJ, Ehrenfeld WK: Manual of Vascular Surgery, vol 1. New York, Springer-Verlag, 1980, with permission.*)

FIG. 33-17. Antegrade bifurcation graft from the supraceliac aorta to the celiac and superior mesenteric arteries. The midportion of the pancreas has been cut away to demonstrate the retropancreatic course of the graft limb to the superior mesenteric artery. (From: *Wylie EJ, Stoney RJ, Ehrenfeld WK: Manual of Vascular Surgery, vol 1. New York, Springer-Verlag, 1980, with permission.*)

proved technically impossible because of anatomic considerations peculiar to the visceral arteries. Early follow-up reveals a failure rate of up to 30 percent, necessitating reintervention. Limited applicability and high early failure rate render this a compromise procedure at best, which should be used for patients with prohibitive operative risks.

If operation for median arcuate ligament syndrome is undertaken, narrowing of the celiac artery can be relieved by transecting the constricting fibers of the median arcuate ligament. Concomitant arterial reconstruction may be necessary if the stenosis is persistent or if poststenotic dilatation is present.

Colonic Ischemia

Etiology and Pathology. Colonic ischemia is usually manifest in the elderly population. Causes include atherosclerotic stenosis or occlusion of the inferior mesenteric artery, cholesterol emboli, and the inflammatory arteriopathies. In most instances, no identifiable cause can be found. Iatrogenic causes include operative ligation occurring during extracolonic operative procedures, such as abdominal aortic aneurysm repair. In the setting of chronic occlusion of the inferior mesenteric artery, perfusion of the descending and sigmoid colon is through the collateral circulation emanating from the superior mesenteric artery via the middle colic artery proximally and the internal iliac arteries via the inferior hemorrhoidal vessels distally.

Clinical Manifestations. The presentation is nonspecific, characterized by cramping abdominal pain localized to the left lower quadrant. Compared with the pain of acute ischemia of the small intestine, it is mild in nature. The urge to defecate may be present, followed over a period of 24 h by melena or hematochezia. Physical examination usually reveals tenderness over the area of the involved segment of colon. The descending and sigmoid colon is the most common site of involvement, but any part of the colon can be affected. Colonic ischemia may be reversible, with results ranging from complete healing to stricture formation with obstruction and colonic infarction and perforation. The outcome of colonic ischemia cannot be predicted from

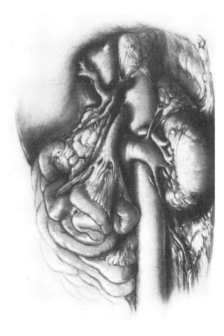

FIG. 33-18. Exposure achieved with left-to-right medial visceral rotation. Note that the viscera, including the spleen and pancreas, have been rotated to the right of the midline. Only the left kidney remains in the anatomic position. (From: *Cunningham CG, Reilly LM, Stoney RJ: Chronic visceral ischemia. Surg Clin North Am 72:231, 1992, with permission.*)

the presenting symptoms unless colonic infarction is obviously present.

Diagnostic Studies. Mild elevation of the white blood cell count is present, but the results of blood work are generally nonspecific. Plain film examination of the abdomen usually is not helpful, although it may demonstrate thumbprinting in up to 20 percent of patients. Thumbprinting consists of multiple round, smooth, soft tissue densities projecting into the air-filled colonic lumen, representative of submucosal edema or hemorrhage. Double-contrast barium enema is the most useful study in detecting colonic ischemia but should not be performed in any patient with signs of peritonitis or when intestinal infarction or perforation is suspected. Findings on barium enema also include transverse ridging and ulceration. CTT imaging may demonstrate thickening of the colonic wall. Flexible sigmoidoscopic or colonoscopic examination often is diagnostic and should be performed with caution in selected patients to avoid converting an ischemic but intact colon to a perforated colon as a result of insufflation and manipulation. Whatever diagnostic modality is used, sequential examination may be required to confirm the diagnosis. Contrast arteriography has little value in the diagnosis of colonic ischemia.

Treatment. When the diagnosis of colonic ischemia is suspected or established, initial treatment consists of parenteral fluid administration with expansion of circulation volume, bowel rest, and administration of broad-spectrum antibiotics aimed at coverage of enteric organisms, including anaerobic bacteria. According to Boley and colleagues, colonic ischemia is reversible in approximately 50 percent of patients, requiring only supportive measures. Approximately 10 percent develop stricture formation, 20 percent persistent colitis, and 20 percent colonic infarction and perforation. Serial abdominal examination and monitoring of urine output and white blood cell count are important in identifying those patients progressing to colonic infarction. Segmental resection of the involved area may be sufficient. Because the bowel is not prepared before operation, resection with end-colostomy and mucous fistula or Hartmann's procedure should be performed. No attempt should be made to prepare the bowel because preparation might precipitate perforation. Late manifestations of colonic ischemia include stricture and symptoms of chronic colitis, either of which can necessitate elective resection.

Mesenteric Venous Occlusion

Etiology. Thrombosis of the mesenteric venous circulation occurs less frequently than that of the mesenteric arterial circulation, accounting for less than 20 percent of all cases of acute mesenteric ischemia. Predisposing conditions include previous deep venous thrombosis, intraabdominal infectious or inflammatory processes, portal hypertension, malignancy, smoking, oral contraception, and the postoperative state. Hypercoagulability because of congenital absence of naturally occurring antithrombotic proteins also has been recognized as a predisposing factor and explains the pathogenesis of cases once thought to be idiopathic. Inherited deficiency or absence of protein S, protein C, and antithrombin III is transmitted in an autosomal dominant pattern and results in recurrent deep venous thrombosis if left untreated. Other hypercoagulable disorders associated with mesenteric venous thrombosis include polycythemia vera, throm-

bocytosis, hyperfibrinogenemia, and myeloproliferative disorders. Up to 50 percent of patients were noted to have previous episodes of mesenteric venous thrombosis.

Pathology. The jejunum and ileum are involved in greater than 80 percent of the commonly affected sites. Colonic and duodenal involvement are unusual, occurring in only 10 percent of patients. A similarly low incidence of duodenal involvement has been noted. Sudden occlusion of the main stem superior mesenteric vein in the dog leads to rapid sequestration of splanchnic venous circulation, stagnation shock, and hemorrhagic infarction of the bowel progressing to necrosis and gangrene. In human beings, ligation of the portal vein or superior mesenteric vein does not produce infarction unless secondary thrombosis extends to the bowel wall and involves the venous arcades and vasa recta. Primary thrombotic occlusion of the visceral veins usually begins in the smaller tributaries. Depending on the extent and location of the propagating clot, the bowel lesion may be represented by small localized areas or extensive segments of infarction. With extensive venous occlusion, thrombosis of the arterial side of the splanchnic circulation often follows, so it becomes impossible to determine accurately whether the occlusion was initially arterial or venous.

Phlebitis secondary to inflammatory disease of the bowel may extend to involve the entire portal system (pyelophlebitis) or give rise to septic emboli that lodge within the liver, causing intrahepatic abscess. This complication of mesenteric venous thrombosis has become less frequent with the advent of antibiotics, and the bowel symptoms usually are overshadowed by those resulting from infection.

Mesenteric venous thrombosis usually results in a segmental and more limited pattern of intestinal ischemia. At operation, the typical appearance is that of a massively edematous bowel wall with bluish discoloration and intramural hemorrhage. The mesentery is edematous, and arterial pulsations are present. Thrombosis of the small-caliber veins adjacent to the bowel wall may be visualized.

Clinical Manifestations. An indication of acute mesenteric venous thrombosis is abdominal pain disproportionate to physical findings. The abdominal pain may be colicky in nature, poorly localized, and accompanied by anorexia and diarrhea, with occult blood or frank blood in the stool. The symptoms accompanying mesenteric venous thrombosis can be insidious and may be present on a subacute basis for a period of 1 to 4 weeks before recognition of the diagnosis or before presentation as an intraabdominal catastrophe. A chronic form of mesenteric venous thrombosis is characterized by persistence of mild symptoms without progression to bowel infarction. The development of persistent, severe abdominal pain with peritoneal signs is indicative of intestinal infarction, which has a mortality rate in excess of 50 percent.

Narcotics usually do not relieve the pain. Bloody diarrhea is more frequent than with arterial occlusions. The bowel sounds are hypoactive or absent. Generalized abdominal tenderness, guarding, and distention are usual; however, true rigidity is not present unless gangrene and perforation of the bowel have occurred. A marked leukocytosis and elevated hematocrit are characteristic findings in venous thrombosis. The latter reflects the trapping of plasma in the occluded bowel segment as arterial blood continues to flow into a splanchnic bed without adequate venous drainage. As with acute mesenteric arterial occlusion, elevations of semen concentrations of phosphate, amylase, and creatinine phosphokinase may be seen. Metabolic acidosis with a base deficit occurs frequently. Abdominal paracentesis yields serosanguineous fluid, which, if foul smelling, makes immediate laparotomy mandatory.

Plain films of the abdomen are generally not helpful. Contrast-enhanced CTT scanning is the most useful diagnostic modality, often demonstrating thrombus in the superior mesenteric vein. Thickening of the bowel wall, as well as air in the bowel wall or portal vein, may be noted as well. Arteriography is not necessary to establish the diagnosis. However, in instances where arteriography is obtained in the acute setting to rule out an arterial etiology, filling defects or nonfilling of the superior mesenteric vein is typically noted and is diagnostic.

Treatment. The cornerstone of therapy rests on early recognition of the disease process and immediate anticoagulation with intravenous heparin. Improved survival correlates with early administration of heparin in several series. In the absence of peritoneal signs, intravenous heparin and supportive therapy may be sufficient. Lifelong anticoagulation with coumadin should be instituted in order to decrease the likelihood of recurrent thrombosis, which is significant even with ongoing anticoagulation. Investigation of the patient and family for hypercoagulability should be carried out.

Those patients in whom peritoneal signs have developed should undergo prompt exploration with resection of infarcted bowel. Intravenous heparin therapy should be started when the diagnosis is established, either preoperatively or intraoperatively. "Second look" celiotomy may be necessary, the need for which should be established at the conclusion of the initial operation. Even with improved methods of diagnosis, reported mortality rates are approximately 30 percent.

The majority of patients with acute mesenteric venous thrombosis have a diffuse thrombotic process with distal extension of clot into the smaller veins, precluding successful venous thrombectomy. Thrombolysis with urokinase as adjunct therapy also has been reported. After successful anticoagulant treatment of mesenteric venous thrombosis, recanalization of the superior mesenteric vein has been demonstrated.

Aneurysms

Visceral artery aneurysms are uncommon. The splenic artery is the most common site, accounting for 60 percent of such aneurysms. The hepatic artery is the second most common site (20 percent), and the remaining 20 percent are aneurysms of the superior mesenteric, celiac, gastroduodenal, left gastric, pancreaticoduodenal, jejunoileal, and inferior mesenteric arteries.

Etiology and Pathology. Visceral artery aneurysms most commonly occur spontaneously; the cause is unknown. Though found in conjunction with atherosclerosis, the atherosclerotic process is not believed to be causative. Recognized causes include fibromuscular dysplasia, connective tissue disorders, infection, pancreatitis, and trauma.

Splenic artery aneurysms are unique, occurring more commonly in women with a ratio of 4:1. Age distribution is nearly equally divided between women of childbearing age in their third decade and women in their sixth or seventh decade of life. Men with hepatic artery aneurysms outnumber women 9:1. Visceral artery aneurysms typically occur in isolation, but they may be associated with other aneurysms of the visceral, aortic, and peripheral arteries.

A relatively large number of aneurysms of the superior mesenteric artery result from mycotic involvement or necrotizing agents. Catheter sepsis, particularly from total parenteral nutrition catheters, may lead to superior mesenteric artery aneurysm when the infecting organism is *Candida* spp.

The size of splanchnic artery aneurysms varies. The majority are less than 2 cm in diameter, but aneurysms of the splenic artery measuring up to 10 cm have been reported. Aneurysms of the superior mesenteric artery and its branches are typically very small, and when rupture occurs, frequently no site of bleeding can be found at laparotomy or at autopsy despite the loss of several liters of blood. In contrast to aneurysms of the abdominal aorta, size does not predict the risk of rupture. It has been estimated that only about 2 to 10 percent of splenic artery aneurysms rupture, whereas the risk of rupture of hepatic, celiac, and superior mesenteric artery aneurysms is high, approximating 30 percent of patients.

Clinical Manifestations and Diagnostic Studies. The majority of visceral artery aneurysms are asymptomatic. Splenic artery aneurysms are most commonly detected on plain film of the abdomen, where concentric calcification of the aneurysm is present in up to 80 percent of patients. Splenic artery aneurysms may present with left upper quadrant pain and pain referred to the region of the left shoulder. Hepatic artery aneurysms may present with right upper quadrant pain, hemobilia, and jaundice. The initial presentation of visceral artery aneurysm in 25 to 40 percent of patients is that of free intraperitoneal rupture with hypotension. The "double rupture" phenomenon has been reported to occur in up to 20 percent of patients with ruptured splenic artery aneurysm. As the initial rupture is contained within the lesser sac, hemodynamic stability is temporarily maintained, only to be followed by free intraperitoneal rupture precipitating hemorrhagic shock.

The incidence of rupture of visceral artery aneurysms is difficult to determine. The rupture rate of hepatic artery aneurysm is estimated at 20 percent and may occur with bleeding into the biliary tract, gastrointestinal tract, or freely into the peritoneal cavity. Mortality rates from rupture also are difficult to determine because many patients bleed to death before diagnosis. Mortality rates from rupture of visceral artery aneurysm are between 35 to 100 percent. Splenic artery aneurysm represents a unique situation because the hormonal and hyperdynamic circulatory changes associated with pregnancy predispose aneurysms of even small diameter to rupture. In the elective setting, selective visceral arteriography should be performed.

Treatment. Resection of the aneurysm, with or without arterial reconstruction, is the accepted treatment. Experience has accumulated with the technique of percutaneous transcatheter embolization, and this has emerged as a viable treatment in selected patients. Indications for intervention in the elective setting are not precise. Since the risk of rupture of splenic artery aneurysm during pregnancy is increased, a splenic artery aneurysm of any size should be repaired before planned pregnancy. The mortality rate associated with rupture for mother and fetus is almost 70 percent. In women of childbearing age, a splenic artery aneurysm measuring 2 cm or greater in diameter or an aneurysm diameter twice that of the caliber of the proximal splenic artery is an indication for intervention. Splenic artery aneurysm occurring in the sixth or seventh decade of life usually should be treated. In the presence of significant comorbidity, splenic artery aneurysms of up to 3 cm can be monitored safely. The rupture rate of hepatic artery aneurysm is approximately 20 percent, with a mortality of at least 35 percent. Therefore, an aggressive approach to intervention is indicated. Indications for repair of hepatic and other visceral artery aneurysms, based on aneurysm diameter, are the same as those for splenic artery aneurysm.

Splenic artery aneurysm is treated by resection of the aneurysm. The spleen can be preserved after resection of an aneurysm of the proximal splenic artery, while aneurysm of the distal splenic artery often necessitates splenectomy. Restoration of splenic artery continuity in order to preserve splenic viability is not necessary because usually the spleen can be perfused adequately by the short gastric circulation. Laparoscopic ligation of the splenic artery for aneurysm also has been described. Percutaneous transcatheter embolization of the aneurysm or occlusion of the main splenic artery on either side of the aneurysm also may be successful. Splenic preservation may be complicated by splenic abscess formation after successful surgical or transcatheter therapy.

Transcatheter embolization is particularly useful for intrahepatic arterial aneurysms and for other visceral artery aneurysms of noncritical vessels that may be difficult to expose at operation. Aneurysm of the proximal hepatic artery (e.g., common hepatic artery) may be treated by simple resection or exclusion because collateral circulation to the liver should be sufficient. Aneurysms of the more distal hepatic artery (e.g., right or left) may necessitate arterial reconstruction with interpositional grafting. Treatment of aneurysms of the celiac and superior mesenteric arteries demands restoration of arterial continuity.

Patients who present with ruptured aneurysms and intraabdominal or gastrointestinal blood loss require immediate resuscitation with fluid and blood and surgical intervention as soon as their condition allows. The bleeding may be so brisk that it will be necessary to take the patient to the operating room while in shock. The chances of finding the open vessel are better if the blood pressure can be elevated. If time allows, preoperative localization by arteriography should be carrier out. When the patient's condition is critical and preoperative studies are not advisable, an operative aortogram may aid in localization of the site of bleeding if it is not obvious at the time of exploration. In the case of a ruptured splenic artery aneurysm, the urgency of the situation usually necessitates a splenectomy to facilitate exposure for ligation of the ruptured artery. Rupture of a celiac artery aneurysm can be treated by ligation, and although most hepatic artery aneurysms also can be treated safely by ligation, an attempt should be made to reconstruct the hepatic artery with a graft. When it is necessary to ligate the hepatic artery, protection should be afforded the liver with large doses of broad-spectrum antibiotics postoperatively. In patients who are not candidates for an operation, catheter embolization of the artery offers a reasonable alternative. Rupture of a main stem superior mesenteric artery aneurysm requires replacement with a graft, preferably of autogenous vein, after excision. Most ruptured aneurysms of the smaller visceral arteries can be treated by ligation. Adequate circulation to the bowel must be ensured and obviously ischemic intestine resected. If there is a question of viability of a long segment of intestine, a "second look" operation in 24 to 36 h may avoid an extensive resection.

The operative mortality for elective treatment of nonruptured splanchnic artery aneurysms is less than 5 percent. The mortality rate is considerably higher once the aneurysm has ruptured and is related to the artery involved. Overall mortality after rupture of a splenic artery aneurysm is about 25 percent, with a 65 percent maternal and 95 percent fetal mortality if rupture occurs during pregnancy. The mortality subsequent to rupture of a celiac or superior mesenteric artery aneurysm is between 40 and 60 percent, whereas rupture of a hepatic artery aneurysm is associated with a 70 percent mortality rate. Death is the result of massive blood loss complicated by the effects of systemic arteriosclerosis, which many patients also have.

Trauma

Etiology. Mesenteric arteries and veins may be injured by penetrating or nonpenetrating abdominal trauma or accidentally during abdominal operations. Often the vessels are lacerated; less frequently, contusion of an artery by blunt trauma results in thrombosis or subsequent aneurysmal formation with rupture.

Most penetrating injuries of the mesenteric vessels are from stab or gunshot wounds, and associated injury to other organs is frequent. Isolated injury to mesenteric vessels after blunt abdominal trauma is rare and usually involves vessels in the mesentery proper or porta hepatis.

Clinical Manifestations. Depending on the size of the vessel lacerated, the rapidity of the bleeding, and associated organ injury, the patient will present with varying degrees of shock, abdominal pain, tenderness, distention, and spasm. Pain referred to the left shoulder is a valuable diagnostic symptom. Plain films of the abdomen are not helpful unless associated visceral rupture has occurred, in which case free air may be seen.

Treatment. Gunshot wounds of the abdomen and most stab wounds should be explored early regardless of physical findings. In nonpenetrating injury, a paracentesis yielding nonclotting blood prompts early operative intervention. Treatment consists of controlling the bleeding vessel. Lacerations of the inferior mesenteric artery or smaller mesenteric arteries and most mesenteric veins usually can be treated successfully by ligation. In the past, few patients with injury to the main trunk of the superior mesenteric artery survived; most died from infarction of the intestine or complications arising from associated organ injury. Currently, if the patient can be resuscitated and reaches the operating room, arterial repair may be possible. This can be accomplished by primary suture or interposition of a vascular graft between the severed ends of the vessel. Every attempt should be made to repair lacerations of the hepatic artery or portal vein. Whether treatment is by ligation or reconstruction, adequate circulation to the intestine should be established and any obviously ischemic bowel resected before closing the abdomen. Long segments of small intestine that are of questionable viability are left in place and reexamined at a second operation 24 h later.

NONSPECIFIC MESENTERIC LYMPHADENITIS

Nonspecific mesenteric lymphadenitis is a common cause of acute abdominal pain in children and young adults. Its existence as a distinct clinicopathologic entity is now well accepted, although the condition received little attention in early medical texts following its initial description by Wilensky and Hahn in 1926. An extensive review of the disease has been reported by McDonald. Because the condition is self-limiting and can be accurately diagnosed only at celiotomy, its true incidence is unknown. It is the most common cause of inflammatory enlargement of abdominal lymph glands, surpassing that resulting from tuberculosis, with which it has been confused in the past. Consideration of the disease is important because of its clinical similarity to several abdominal conditions requiring operative intervention, notably acute appendicitis.

Pathology and Pathogenesis. The lymph nodes primarily involved in nonspecific mesenteric lymphadenitis are those which drain the ileocecal region. The stasis of intestinal contents in the terminal ileum favors absorption of toxic or bacterial products from the bowel lumen, agents that may have a bearing on the pathogenesis of the disease.

The nodes are enlarged, discrete, soft, and pink at first; later they may become firm and white. It is uncertain whether calcification ever occurs in nontuberculous adenitis, and suppuration is rare unless specific bacterial infection is present. Histologically, the involved nodes present a pattern of reactive hyperplasia similar to that found in inflammatory and allergic affections of lymph nodes in other parts of the body. The nodes, with rare exception, prove to be sterile on culture or on animal inoculation. *Yersinia pseudotuberculosis* or *enterocolitica*, two gram-negative coccoid or ovoid organisms, have been insolated from the stool in some cases.

Clinical Manifestations. The disease most commonly occurs in patients under 18 years of age. There is no sex predilection. The signs and symptoms are not particularly characteristic. Very often there has been a recent sore throat or upper respiratory tract infection. Pain usually is the first symptom and varies in intensity from an ache to a severe colic. The mechanism responsible for producing pain is not completely understood. Lymph nodes do not have sensory innervation, and therefore, enlargement of the node by itself should not produce pain. It is probable that the pain is referred from the mesentery, which has an abundance of sensory end organs that are stimulated when the mesentery is stretched during peristalsis. The initial pain usually is in the upper abdomen, but it also may begin in the lower right quadrant or be generalized. Eventually the pain localizes to the right side; an important point in differentiating the disease from acute appendicitis is that the patient is unable to indicate the exact site of the most intense pain. Between spasms of colic, the patient feels well and moves about without difficulty. Nausea and vomiting occur in about one-third of patients, while malaise and anorexia are inconstant symptoms.

The patient often appears flushed, and an associated rhinorrhea or acute pharyngitis is not unusual. Approximately 20 percent of patients have lymphadenopathy elsewhere, most often in the cervical region. The usual finding on examination of the abdomen is tenderness in the lower aspect of the right side, which is somewhat higher and more medial and considerably less severe than in acute appendicitis. The point of maximal tenderness often varies from one examination to the next. An appreciable number of patients also have diffuse or periumbilical tenderness. Rebound tenderness may or may not be demonstrated. Voluntary guarding is sometimes present; however, true muscular rigidity is rare. Early in the attack, the temperature is moderately elevated, 38 to 38.5°C, and at least half the patients have leukocyte counts over 10,000/mm^3.

Differential Diagnosis. The disease is most often confused with acute appendicitis but also must be differentiated from regional enteritis, intussusception, specific bacterial and granulomatous adenitis, and other forms of mesenteric glandular enlargement, such as infectious mononucleosis or lymphoma. The clinical similarity to acute appendicitis is such that in several large series, as many as 20 percent of patients undergoing appendectomy were found to have nonspecific mesenteric adenitis and a normal appendix. Important differentiating factors are the more localized and constant location of the pain and tenderness, the presence of muscle rigidity, and the frequent occurrence of nausea and vomiting in children with appendicitis.

Differentiation from *acute regional ileitis* is at times difficult. Mesenteric adenitis is an almost constant feature of regional ileitis, and indeed, the adenitis is often nonspecific in this disease. An ultrasound that demonstrates mural thickening of the terminal ileum and thickening of the mesentery is characteristic of regional enteritis.

The low incidence of lymphadenopathy in other parts of the body and the brief course of nonspecific mesenteric adenitis are factors in excluding lymphomas and infectious mononucleosis. A peripheral blood smear and a Paul-Bunnell test for sheep red cell agglutinins are also helpful.

Treatment. The prognosis of nonspecific mesenteric adenitis is excellent, and complete recovery from an individual attack can be expected without specific treatment. Death from the disease is extremely rare and occurs only when secondary specific bacterial infection, usually caused by hemolytic streptococci, causes suppuration of the nodes with rupture leading to abscess or peritonitis.

If the condition is mistaken for acute appendicitis, as it frequently is, laparotomy should be undertaken. It is safer to find a normal appendix than to run the risk of allowing acute appendicitis to go on to rupture. The diagnosis is readily established at the time of operation with the finding of enlarged mesenteric nodes in the absence of disease in the appendix or elsewhere in the intestinal tract or abdomen. In view of the tendency for recurrence and the difficulty of differentiating it from appendicitis, appendectomy should be performed.

MESENTERIC PANNICULITIS

Mesenteric panniculitis is a term applied by Ogden and associates in 1965 to describe a process of extensive thickening of the mesentery by a nonspecific inflammatory process. It also has been variously designated *retractile mesenteritis, mesenteric lipodystrophy, lipogranuloma of the mesentery,* and *mesenteric manifestations of Weber-Christian disease.* Many consider it a variant of retroperitoneal fibrosis.

Etiology and Pathology. The cause of the condition is unknown; however, the process apparently results from an insult to the fatty tissue of the mesentery. Trauma, allergy, and subacute infection have all been implicated. The possibility that it is an autoimmune disease also has been suggested. The process usually involves the mesenteric root of the small bowel. Grossly, the normal fat lobulations of the markedly thickened and firm mesentery are lost. Scattered throughout are irregular areas of discoloration, which vary from reddish brown plaques to pale yellow foci resembling fat necrosis. The superior mesenteric vessels, though surrounded by the tumor-like mass of tissue, pass through it unaltered. Histologic sections show inflammatory involvement of the fibroadipose tissue with round cells, foam cells, and giant cells and various degrees of necrosis, fibrosis, and calcification.

Clinical Manifestations. Men are affected more often than women. It is rarely described in children, in whom mesenteric fat usually is scant. The clinical features are nonspecific; they include recurrent episodes of moderate to severe abdominal pain, nausea, vomiting, and malaise, usually in the right side of the abdomen. Radiographs are helpful only if the mass displaces or compresses viscera. CT scan demonstrates mesenteric panniculitis as a localized fat-density mass containing areas of increased density representing fibrosis.

Treatment. Laparotomy is necessary to establish the diagnosis and to rule out other intraabdominal diseases of the abdomen. The widespread involvement of the mesentery precludes doing more than obtaining a biopsy. Because neoplasms of the mesenteric lymph nodes may present a similar gross appearance, several biopsies from different sites should be obtained. Rarely, colostomy of bypass will be necessary to relieve symptoms of obstruction. Treatment of the disease with steroids, immunosuppressive agents, and irradiation has been suggested. The benefits from these are difficult to evaluate because the inflammatory process is self-limiting and seldom causes any serious complications.

TUMORS OF THE MESENTERY

Tumors originating between the leaves of the mesentery are rare. In contrast, malignant implants from intraabdominal or pelvic tumors or metastases to mesenteric lymph nodes are relatively common. Tumors arising from mesenteric lymph nodes occur; however, these are not generally included in a discussion of primary mesenteric tumors.

Pathology. Primary tumors of the mesentery may be cystic or solid. Of these, cystic growths occur more frequently than solid ones in a ratio of 2:1. A number of tissues, including lymphatic, vascular, nervous, and connective tissues, are the source of these tumors. In addition, cystic tumors may arise from embryonic rests (enteroceles or dermoids), from developmental defects (chylous or serous retention cysts), or after trauma (hemorrhagic cysts). A classification of these tumors is shown in Table 33-1.

The majority of cystic mesenteric tumors are benign. Rare exceptions are lymphangiosarcomas, which are true neoplasms arising from lymph channels, and malignant teratomas arising from multipotential embryonic rests. Chylous or lymphatic cysts are the most frequently encountered benign mesenteric masses. These are thought to arise from developmental defects in mesenteric lymphatics creating closed spaces within which fluid accumulates. They may be unilocular or multilocular, have an endothelial lining, contain a grossly cloudy fluid resembling chyle, and often grow to an extremely large size. A similar cause has been ascribed to serous cysts, which are differentiated from chylous cysts in that they contain clear fluid, are invariably unilocular, and may or may not have an endothelial lining. Lymphan-

Table 33-1
Classification of Primary Mesenteric Tumors

Origin	Benign	Malignant
Cystic tumors		
Developmental defects	Chylous cyst	
	Serous cyst	
Lymphatic tissue	Lymphangioma	Lymphangiosarcoma
Trauma	Traumatic cyst	
Embryonic rests	Enteric cyst	
	Dermoid	Malignant teratoma
Solid tumors		
Adipose tissue	Lipoma	Liposarcoma
Fibrous tissue	Fibroma	Fibrosarcoma
Nerve elements	Neurilemoma	Malignant schwannoma
	Neurofibroma	
Smooth muscle	Leiomyoma	Leiomyosarcoma
	Fibromyoma	Fibromyosarcoma
Vascular tissue	Hemangioma	Hemangiopericytoma

gioma of the mesentery is apparently a true neoplasm of lymphatics similar to those found in other parts of the body (cystic hygroma). Grossly and histologically, it is often difficult to differentiate this tumor from a chylous cyst, and in many series the two are grouped in a single category. Traumatic cysts follow external or surgical injury to the mesentery. They are lined with fibrous tissue and usually contain bloody fluid. It is probable that many serous retention cysts are in reality traumatic cysts that have evolved from disruption of mesenteric lymph channels. Enteric cysts are lined with intestinal mucosa and represent duplications of the intestinal tract that do not communicate with the bowel lumen. These and dermoid cysts of the mesentery are exceedingly rare.

Benign solid tumors of the mesentery are more common than malignant ones, and of these, lipomas and fibromas predominate. Recurrence after incomplete excision of histologically benign mesenteric tumors has been reported, and malignant degeneration also has been suggested. Histologically benign tumors can kill by local invasion with mechanical compression of adjacent viscera. The benign tumors of nerve elements and smooth muscles are uncommon. Vascular tumors of the mesentery are rare, and of these, hemangiopericytomas dominate. Ackerman states that liposarcoma is the most frequently encountered malignant tumor of this area, whereas Yannopoulos and Stout report leiomyosarcoma to be the most frequent. Few malignant mesenteric tumors have embolic metastases until very late. They spread by local extension or by peritoneal implants, which occur most often with leiomyosarcomas. As a rule, the malignant solid tumors arise near the foot of the mesentery, whereas solid benign tumors have a greater tendency to develop peripherally near the intestine.

Approximately two-thirds of mesenteric tumors, cystic or solid, are located in the mesentery of the small intestine, usually that of the ileum. Occasionally, they arise in the transverse or sigmoid mesocolon or in the gastrohepatic ligament. In the greater number of cases, the tumor is located peripherally in the mesentery, where it is often adherent to the adjacent intestine. The mobility of the mesentery permits benign and malignant tumors to grow to very large sizes before causing symptoms.

Clinical Manifestations. Early clinical features usually do not differentiate benign tumors from malignant ones. There is an equal sex incidence, although benign cystic tumors are somewhat more common in women and malignant tumors occur more frequently in men. These tumors have been described in children and also the very aged; however, the average age of patients with benign tumors is 45 years, while those with malignant tumors average 55 years old.

The manifestations of mesenteric tumors depend on the size, location, and mobility of the growth. In the majority of patients, symptoms are few or nonexistent, and the tumor is detected during a routine examination. Symptoms appear sooner when the tumor is situated in the periphery of the mesentery near the intestine than when it is located at its root. The patient may experience a sensation of fullness or pressure in the abdomen, particularly after eating. Less frequently, there are frank abdominal complaints. About one-half of patients with malignant tumors complain of abdominal pain, weakness, and weight loss, and one-third have diarrhea, cramps, anorexia, and nausea. Only rarely will the patient present with symptoms of complete intestinal obstruction or symptoms resulting from complications of the tumor per se, such as torsion, hemorrhage, or infarction of the tumor mass. In the absence of intestinal obstruction or these complications, the sole finding will be the presence of a nontender intraabdominal mass, usually in the lower right part of the abdomen. The mass varies in size from a few inches in diameter to one that may fill the entire abdomen. The extremely large masses usually are cystic, in which case they are tense and fluctuant. Cystic and solid tumors of the mesentery are mobile; they can be easily moved from side to side but only slightly in an upward and downward direction.

The differential diagnosis includes a variety of intraabdominal processes. Contrast-enhanced radiographs are helpful only when the mesenteric mass is sufficiently large to cause compression and displacement of the bowel or ureters (Fig. 33-20). They do not differentiate a benign tumor from a malignant one, and in most instances the x-ray studies are not helpful. Calcification in the mass is suggestive of a dermoid or teratoma.

Imaging techniques are the most useful means for diagnosing cystic and solid mesenteric tumors. On ultrasound, a mesenteric cyst appears as a well-outlined, sonolucent transonic abdominal mass. CT demonstrates a simple mesenteric cyst as a nonenhancing near-water-density mass with a thin wall (Fig. 33-21) and a solid tumor as an irregular sheetlike mass of greater density.

Treatment. Surgical excision is the only treatment for benign and malignant lesions. All mesenteric cysts of a size sufficient to be palpated should be removed if at all possible because even benign lesions eventually cause pain and compression of neighboring structures. Benign cystic tumors can be removed by enucleation or local excision, although resection in continuity with the adjacent intestine is often necessary because of possible compromise to the vascularity of the bowel or difficulty in separating the tumor from the intestine. Wide excision together with resection of adjacent intestine is recommended for benign solid tumors, since these have a tendency toward local recurrence and malignant degeneration. Prognosis after adequate excision of cystic and solid benign tumors of the mesentery is excellent.

The outlook for malignant mesenteric tumors depends on whether complete removal is possible and is generally poor. Since malignant growths tend to occur in the root of the mes-

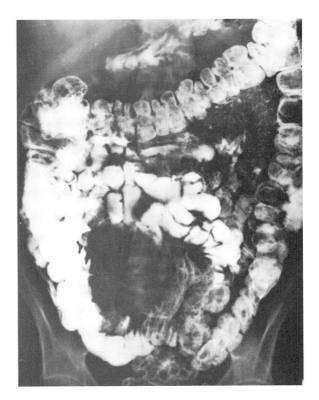

FIG. 33-20. *Small intestinal series showing displacement of bowel loops by a mass lesion in the lower right side of the abdomen. The patient proved to have a large benign fibroma in the mesentery of the terminal ileum. (From: Adams J, Kutner F: Pure fibroma of the mesentery. Am J Surg 111:735, 1966, with permission.)*

entery and often involve the great vessels and vasculature to most of the small intestine and colon, curative resection is often prohibitive. Resectable lesions invariably require removal of a portion of bowel; however, fewer than one-third of the malignant tumors are totally resectable. Since these growths may enlarge

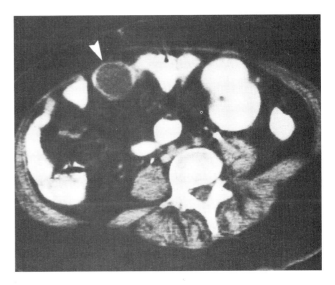

FIG. 33-21. *Mesenteric cyst. CT scan shows a nonenhancing low-density, encapsulated mass in the transverse mesocolon (arrowhead).*

slowly and embolic metastases occur late, it is worthwhile to partially remove them to relieve obstructions, and prolonged survival has been recorded in a few instances. Irradiation therapy offers little, if any, benefit because the tumors are invariably radioresistant. Few patients with malignant primary mesenteric tumors are alive after 5 years. Death results from invasion with obstruction of the gastrointestinal tract leading to perforation and hemorrhage or from metastases to liver and lung.

RETROPERITONEUM

General Considerations

The retroperitoneum consists of that portion of the body which is bounded anteriorly by the peritoneum, posteriorly by the spine and psoas and quadratus lumborum muscles, superiorly by the twelfth ribs and attachments of the diaphragm, and inferiorly by the brim of the pelvis. The lateral margins of the space correspond to the lateral borders of the quadratus lumborum muscles. These limits define both an actual and a potential space, the actual space containing solid organs and major blood vessels and the potential space including soft tissues, nerve elements, and small blood vessels. Since there are no anatomic barriers in this area, pathologic processes may extend easily throughout it and are often bilateral.

Contained within the retroperitoneum are the kidneys, ureters, adrenal glands, portions of the autonomic and peripheral nervous systems, pancreas, abdominal aorta, inferior vena cava, spermatic or ovarian vessels, lymphatics and lymph nodes, and certain portions of the intestinal track, notably the duodenum. The space also contains fatty and areolar tissue and fibrous connective tissue.

The diagnosis of diseases involving the retroperitoneum has been enhanced by the application of such radiographic studies as pyelography, venography, arteriography, ultrasonography, and MRI. Nevertheless, it remains an obscure area of the body, enabling pathologic processes to become advanced before producing symptoms.

The multiplicity of structures within the retroperitoneum gives rise to a variety of pathologic conditions such as (1) idiopathic retroperitoneal fibrosis and (2) primary tumors of the retroperitoneal space.

Idiopathic Retroperitoneal Fibrosis

Idiopathic retroperitoneal fibrosis is a nonspecific, nonsuppurative inflammation of fibroadipose tissue of unknown cause that produces symptoms by the gradual compression of the tubular structures in the retroperitoneal space. It is believed that the disease represents one of the manifestations of a widespread entity termed *systemic idiopathic fibrosis.* Idiopathic mediastinal fibrosis, Riedel's struma, sclerosing cholangitis, mesenteric panniculitis, Peyronie's disease, pseudotumor of the orbit, and perhaps desmoid tumor are other fibromatoses that are considered to be localized forms of systemic idiopathic fibrosis. A factor common to all these diseases is an inflammatory fibrotic process involving areolar and adipose tissue.

Retroperitoneal fibrosis was first described in 1905 by Albarran, a French urologist, who performed ureterolysis for ureteral compression produced by the disease. The first report in English is credited to Ormond in 1948. It has since been referred to as *Ormond's syndrome* but also has been labeled *idiopathic fibrous retroperitonitis, periureteritis plastica,* and *sclerosing retroperitonitis.* Retroperitoneal lipogranulomatosis (xanthogranulomatosis), which can produce a similar clinical picture, may be a granulomatous, prefibrotic stage of retroperitoneal fibrosis.

Etiology. Attesting to the obscure etiology of retroperitoneal fibrosis are the many theories that have been advanced to explain its origin. The possibility that extravasated urine might cause a fibrotic reaction in the retroperitoneum was mentioned by Ormond, and both he and Hackett also suggested that an abortive infection elsewhere might later start an inflammatory reaction in the lymphatic and perivascular tissues of the retroperitoneum. Hache and associates proposed the concept that the fibrosis was the end result of an ascending lymphangitis, adenitis, or periadenitis in the retroperitoneum with the infection arising from chronic or recurrent genitourinary infections or inflammatory diseases of the gastrointestinal tract or pelvic organs. Reports of retroperitoneal fibrosis occurring in patients taking the antiserotonin drug methysergide for headache with reversal of the fibrotic process after discontinuing the medication prompted the theory that the disease may be from a hypersensitivity reaction to the drug. Indirect evidence favoring an immune basis as the cause of the disease is confirmed by the impressive response of some patients to immunosuppressive therapy. It is probable that no single factor is responsible for causing the disease in all patients and that multiple factors may be implicated in any one patient.

Pathology. The gross appearance of retroperitoneal fibrosis usually is that of a plaque of woody, white fibrous tissue that is distributed along the course of the periaortic lymphatics. In about one-third of patients, it is bilateral. The diseased tissue, which may be 2 to 12 cm thick, extends from the sacral promontory to the renal pedicles and laterally to cover the iliopsoas muscle. It is sharply demarcated but not encapsulated. The mass surrounds and constricts but does not invade the regional structures in the retroperitoneum, primarily the blood vessels, nerves, and ureters, to which it becomes adherent.

A localized form has been observed as a circumscribed fibrous reaction surrounding only the ureters, and extensive involvement of the entire retroperitoneum with compression of the duodenum, common bile duct, and pancreas also has been seen. A similar fibrotic process has been described penetrating the diaphragm along the great vessels into the mediastinum, causing superior vena cava obstruction, and also extending into the root of the mesentery, causing intestinal obstruction.

Microscopically, the pattern varies from a subacute cellular process with polymorphonuclear cells, lymphocytes, fibroblasts, and fat cells to a completely hyalinized, relatively acellular sclerosis. Eosinophils, foreign-body giant cells, and small areas of calcification also may be present. Suppuration with abscess formation does not occur. The amount of fat and cellular infiltration and the degree of fibrosis vary between patients and in different biopsy specimens from the same patient. The more cellular picture usually is seen in the early stages of the disease, when there may be systemic signs of inflammation, whereas the dense fibrotic process is found late.

Clinical Manifestations. Retroperitoneal fibrosis is two to three times more common among men. It may occur in children and the aged; however, about two-thirds of the patients are between 40 to 60 years of age.

The protean manifestations of the disease are related to the phase and extent of the process and the structures secondarily involved. Ormond divided the natural history of the disease into three periods: (1) the period of incidence and development, (2) the period of activity, i.e., spread of the cellular and fibrotic process to envelopment of the retroperitoneal structures, and (3) the period of contraction of the fibrotic mass with compression of the involved structures. The disease is self-limiting once the fibrotic stage is reached, a factor of major importance in considering types of therapy.

Early symptoms are vague and nonspecific, but the first complaint is invariably pain. This is dull, noncolicky, and insidious in onset. It usually originates in the flank or low back and often radiates to the lower abdomen, groin, genitalia, or anteromedial aspect of the thigh. The pain is unilateral at first but may become bilateral as the fibrotic process spreads. Anorexia, nausea, diarrhea, generalized malaise, and weight loss variably occur in the early and late phases of the disease. Features of a subacute inflammation such as lower abdominal or costovertebral tenderness, moderate fever, and leukocytosis are often present early. Invariably, the erythrocyte sedimentation rate is elevated. A transabdominal or pelvic mass is palpable in about one-third of patients during some phase of the disease.

Symptoms resulting from compression of the tubular retroperitoneal structures may follow the initial complaints by 1 month to 2 years and reflect the late fibrotic phase of the disease with sclerotic contraction. The major structures involved are the ureters, aorta, and inferior vena cava. These all lie within the same fascial compartment. The aorta is resistant to compression and the inferior vena cava has abundant collaterals, so the symptoms are generally related to ureteral involvement. Partial or complete ureteral obstruction occurs in 75 to 85 percent of patients. The usual site of obstruction is in the lower third of the ureter. The ureteral obstruction usually is functional, rather than organic, as a consequence of cessation of peristalsis in the incarcerated ureteral segment. In the majority of patients, a ureteral catheter can be passed in a retrograde manner.

Dysuria, frequency of urination, and chills and fever occur with secondary infection of a hydronephrotic kidney. These symptoms may be intermittent for years, or a single attack may culminate in sudden anuria from bilateral obstruction. As many as 40 percent of patients have oliguria or anuria with laboratory evidence of azotemia. Clinically, the enlarged kidneys may be palpable, and the urine, if infected, contains white blood cells and bacteria. Hematuria, in the absence of infection, is rare.

Lower extremity edema, presumably from lymphatic and venous obstruction, occasionally occurs and may be unilateral. The level of obstruction in most cases corresponds to that of the ureteral obstruction and can be demonstrated on phlebograms.

Arterial insufficiency resulting from fibrous constriction of the aorta or iliac arteries is uncommon but can occur and may constitute the major problem. The intermittent claudication, rest pain, and limb ischemia are indistinguishable clinically and radiographically from those of atherosclerotic occlusion.

Rarely, the fibrotic process involves the retroperitoneal duodenum and common bile ducts, causing duodenal and biliary obstruction. Mechanical or functional intestinal obstruction resulting from extension into the root of the mesentery or sigmoid mesocolon also is a rare manifestation.

The diagnosis of retroperitoneal fibrosis usually is suggested by the contrast-enhanced radiographs of the urinary tract. Gray-scale ultrasonography and CT scans also have been used for the diagnosis of the entity and for follow-up management. A characteristic CT scan shows a homogeneous soft tissue mass enveloping the ureters, aorta, and inferior vena cava. In contrast to malignant retroperitoneal adenopathy, with which retroperitoneal fibrosis is often confused, there is no anterior displacement of the great vessels. Intravenous pyelography is the most definitive noninvasive diagnostic test. Suggestive of retroperitoneal fibrosis on the pyelogram are (1) hydronephrosis with a dilated, tortuous upper ureter, (2) medial deviation of the ureter, and (3) extrinsic ureteral compression. The medial deviation of the ureter is in contrast to lateral displacement that is characteristically associated with retroperitoneal tumors. Since a variety of conditions can produce a similar picture, final confirmation of the diagnosis can be made only after exploratory operative procedures and biopsy of the fibrotic mass. The differential diagnosis includes the primary retroperitoneal tumors, notably the malignant lymphomas, and metastatic tumor from the kidneys, pancreas, or pelvic organs. Inflammatory conditions to be excluded include tuberculosis, pancreatitis, and intraabdominal inflammation of the intestinal tract.

Treatment. Once the diagnosis is established, the patient should be carefully followed and operative intervention timed properly. Improvement may be anticipated in some patients with supportive measures alone. The onset of urinary tract infection or depression of renal function necessitates operative intervention.

The discontinuance of methysergide is sometimes followed by a reversal of the fibrotic process with an improvement in symptoms. Steroids, antibiotics, and x-ray therapy have been used with inconsistent results. Tamoxifen occasionally produces a beneficial response. The self-limiting nature of the disease and the reports of spontaneous resolution in untreated patients make it difficult to evaluate the results of these therapeutic modalities. Steroids are of theoretical use in the early inflammatory stages to diminish the generation of fibrosis or control a hyperimmune reaction, if one exists. For patients in the prefibrotic stage of the disease with renal insufficiency and prominent constitutional symptoms, steroid-induced regression of the inflammatory edema may reestablish urinary patency and facilitate elective, rather than emergency, surgery. Usually, an advanced stage of fibrosis has been reached before diagnosis.

Surgical treatment is directed toward relief of the tubular obstructions, which are usually urinary, less often vascular, and rarely intestinal. Since the disease is fundamentally a midline process that is often bilateral, a midtransabdominal approach offers the best exposure. Several deep biopsies of the mass should be obtained to eliminate the possibility of an underlying neoplasm, because neoplasms may produce a similar picture, particularly tumors of lymphatic origin. The aorta, inferior vena cava, small bowel mesentery, sigmoid mesocolon, and ureters should be examined for possible involvement.

Ureterolysis with intraperitoneal transplantation is the most effective means of relieving obstruction of the involved ureter. This consists of freeing the ureter from the enveloping mass of fibrous tissue and transferring it into the peritoneal cavity, closing the posterior peritoneum behind it. Lateral reposition of the ureter within the retroperitoneal space has been reported to yield equally good results. A preliminary nephrostomy may be indicated if bilateral ureteral obstruction has resulted in severe renal

Table 33-2
Classification of Retroperitoneal Tumors

Tissue Type	Benign Tumors	Malignant Tumors
Lymphatic tissue	Lymphangioma	Lymphangiosarcoma
Lymph nodes		Lymphosarcoma
		Hodgkin's disease
		Reticulum cell sarcoma
Adipose tissue	Lipoma	Liposarcoma
Fibrous tissue	Fibroma	Fibrosarcoma
Smooth muscle	Leiomyoma	Leiomyosarcoma
Nerve elements	Neurilemoma	Malignant schwannoma
	Neurofibroma	
	Ganglioneuroma	Sympathicoblastoma (neuroblastoma)
		Chordoma
Striated muscle	Rhabdomyoma	Rhabdomyosarcoma
Mucoid tissue	Myxoma	Myxosarcoma
Vascular tissue	Hemangioma	Malignant hemangiopericytoma
Mesothelial tissue		Mesothelioma
Mesenchyme		Mesenchymoma
Extraadrenal chromaffin tissue	Benign pheochromocytoma	Malignant pheochromocytoma
Gland tissue	Adenoma	Carcinoma
Embryonic remnants	Nephrogenic cysts	Urogenital ridge tumor
Cell rests	Dermoid	Teratoma
Miscellaneous	Xanthogranuloma	Synovioma
	Aggressive fibromatosis	Dysgerminoma
		Undifferentiated malignant tumor

impairment with uremia. On rare occasion, it will be necessary to reimplant the mobilized ureter into the bladder or, if this is not technically possible, to perform renal autotransplantation. Aortic or iliac artery obstruction is best treated by arteriolysis or bypass with a synthetic vascular graft.

Symptoms resulting from venous obstruction are best treated with elevation and elastic support to the lower limbs until a sufficient collateral venous system develops. The extent of any permanent venous insufficiency depends on the availability of collateral pathways and the competency of deep vein valves. Release of the obstructed vein from its fibrous encasement may be difficult and hazardous, and bypass procedures for obstruction of the inferior vena cava have been uniformly unsuccessful. The prognosis of the disease is generally good, provided that appropriate treatment has been instituted before the development of irreversible renal damage.

Retroperitoneal Tumors

Primary tumors of the retroperitoneum develop independently from cells distinct from the major retroperitoneal organs such as the pancreas, kidney, adrenal gland, and major blood vessels. The most common malignancies in this area are sarcomas, though lymphomas, extragonadal germ cell tumors, and carcinomas also occur. Approximately 6000 soft tissue sarcomas are noted annually in the United States, and nearly 1000 of these occur in the retroperitoneum. The cause of most soft tissue sarcomas is unclear. Rarely, these tumors are associated with a history of therapeutic radiation usually more than 10 years before onset. The incidence of reported sarcomas after therapeutic radiation is low, ranging from 0.03 to 0.3 percent, with the most common type being malignant fibrous histiocytoma. Exposure to vinyl chloride, thorium dioxide, and other agents is associated with sarcomas. Several familial disorders such as Gardner's syndrome, familial retinoblastoma, neurofibromatosis, and Li-Frau-

mani syndrome are associated with benign and malignant soft tissue tumors. Germ-line mutations of the *p53* tumor suppressor gene on chromosome 17 is present in some of these familial disorders. Retroperitoneal sarcomas are relatively rare mesenchymal and neurogenic tumors often occurring in the fifth or sixth decade of life. Despite their rarity, they should be considered in the differential diagnosis of an unknown abdominal mass.

Pathology. Retroperitoneal tumors generally arise from mesodermal or neuroectodermal tissues or remnants of the embryonal urogenital apparatus. Tumors may arise from fat, aerolar tissue, vascular or nervous tissue, muscle, fascia, lymphatics, and nodal tissues. Tumors of smooth muscle origin, germ cell tumors, teratomas, and other complex lesions also may occur. Table 33-2 provides a classification of benign and malignant characteristics.

Lymphomas and retroperitoneal sarcomas are the most common malignant lesions of the retroperitoneum. Among the later, liposarcomas and leiomyosarcomas are the most frequent, but while it is of pathologic interest to determine the cell of origin of these retroperitoneal sarcomas, it is of greater importance to define their margins, size, and histologic grade to obtain prognosis (Table 33-3). These tumors develop pseudocapsules of collagen, vessels, inflammatory tissues, and tumor cells that extend within the pseudocapsule. Local tumor recurrence is common when these tumors are simply enucleated. Because of their extension within loose retroperitoneal tissue planes and their relationship to vital structures, it is difficult to obtain negative surgical margins during tumor removal. The histologic grade is the most important characteristic to determine prognosis. Grade is defined based on degree of tumor differentiation, nuclear atypia, amount of fibrous/myoid stroma, mitotic activity, cellular pleomorphism, presence of necrosis, and cellularity. The American Joint Commission on Cancer criteria distinguish three grades and tumor sizes 5 cm and less or more than 5 cm to provide prog-

Table 33-3
American Joint Committee Staging Protocol for Soft Tissue Sarcoma

Stage	Grade	Tumor	Nodes	Metastases
IA	1	1	0	0
IB	1	2	0	0
IIA	2	1	0	0
IIB	2	2	0	0
IIIA	3–4	1	0	0
IIIB	3–4	2	0	0
IVA	1–4	1–2	1	0
IVB	1–4	1–2	0–1	1

Characteristics

Histologic grade (G)
  G1 Well differentiated
  G2 Moderately differentiated
  G3 Poorly differentiated
Primary tumor (T)
  T1 ≤5 cm
  T2 >5 cm
Regional lymph nodes (N)
  N0 No regional lymph node metastases
  N1 Regional lymph node metastases
Distant metastases (M)
  M0 No distant metastases
  M1 Distant metastases

SOURCE: From Beahrs OH, et al (eds): *American Joint Committee on Cancer: Manual for Staging of Cancer,* 4th ed. Philadelphia, JB Lippincott, 1992.

nostic criteria, but other systems use only two grades. A low grade is assigned to myxoid and well-differentiated liposarcoma and high grade to rhabdomyosarcoma, synovial sarcoma, and alveolar soft part sarcoma (Table 33-4).

If metastasis occur, it typically spreads hematogenously to liver and lung. Lymph node metastases are rare, occurring in less than 5 percent of patients, except in those with embryonal rhabdomyosarcoma, lymphangiosarcoma, and epitheloid sarcoma, which may be somewhat more frequent. Complete nodal dissections are unnecessary, but gross tumor removal with adequate margins should be attained whenever possible.

The tumors may be solid, cystic, or a combination of both. Their color varies from white (fibroma), to yellow (lipoma), to pink or red (sarcoma) depending on the predominant tissue. They may be single or multiple and vary in size from small outgrowths to tumors weighing as much as 18 kg (40 lb). The predominantly cystic tumors usually are benign, whereas the solid tumors are most often malignant.

Clinical Manifestations and Diagnosis. Because of the great dimension, loose boundaries, and flimsy areolar tissues of the retroperitoneal space, tumors in this location can attain a large size before any symptoms occur. Sarcomas grow along fascial plains and envelop rather than directly invade nearby organs. Symptoms are produced by compression or obstruction of adjacent tissues.

Patients may present initially with a history of an enlarging mass in the abdomen, a vague abdominal discomfort, or a sense of fullness or heaviness. Pain may become severe if compression of adjacent nerves or nerve plexuses occur. Gastrointestinal stromal cell tumors (leiomyosarcomas) may result in nausea, vomiting, intestinal obstruction, and gastrointestinal bleeding. Occasionally, fever, weakness, weight loss, and genitourinary symptoms can occur depending on the size and location of the neoplasm. Pelvic tumors give rise to urinary frequency or rarely anuria. They also may compress pelvic veins resulting in lower extremity swelling and varicosities.

Physical examination reveals the presence of an abdominal mass that is usually nontender, firm, and rubbery. It should be defined as fixed or movable and may involve a flank, the midline, or the entire abdomen. Pelvic tumors can be felt on vaginal and rectal examinations. Examination of the regional nodal areas for metastases should be performed. The scrotum should be examined for the possibility of a testicular neoplasm causing retroperitoneal adenopathy. If there is a question of a testicular mass, ultrasound should be done. The diagnosis of a retroperitoneal tumor often is by exclusion of other abdominal masses such as those involving the kidneys, adrenals, pancreas, aorta, ovaries, or spleen. Laboratory studies such as serum α-fetoprotein and β-human chorionic gonadotropin measurements should be obtained to exclude retroperitoneal germ cell tumors.

The primary roentgenographic diagnostic modality is the CT scan (Fig. 33-22). Use of fast, helical CT scanners allows excellent definition of the extent of the mass, the potential involvement of vital organs or major vascular structures with the primary tumor, and the involvement of the liver, lungs, or peritoneal cavity with metastases. MRI is an excellent diagnostic tool permitting sagittal and coronal views and providing a three-dimensional image to define tumor extent and resectability. Use of contrast enhancement with gallium may be helpful to improve specificity and sensitivity of the examination. These studies can

Table 33-4
Distribution of Adult Retroperitoneal Sarcomas by Histologic Type and Grade

Histology	Low Grade	High Grade	Total (%)
Liposarcoma	34	23	57 (50)
Leiomyosarcoma	6	27	33 (29)
Hemangiosarcoma	3	4	7 (6)
Fibrosarcoma	4	2	6 (5)
Malignant fibrous histiocytoma (MFH)	0	5	5 (4)
Malignant peripheral nerve sheath tumor (MPNT)	1	3	4 (4)
Alveolar soft part sarcoma	1	0	1 (1)
Embryonal rhabdomyosarcoma	0	1	1 (1)

SOURCE: From Jaques D, Coit D, et al: Management of primary and recurrent soft-tissue sarcoma of the retroperitoneum. *Ann Surg* 212:51, 1990.

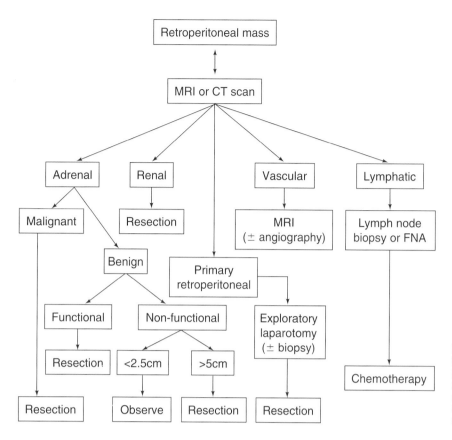

FIG. 33-22. *Management algorithm for patients presenting with a retroperitoneal mass. (Adapted from: Pisters PWT, Brennan MF: Retroperitoneal tumors, in Taylor I, Cooke T, Guillon P (eds): Essential General Surgical Oncology. New York, Churchill-Livingstone, 1996, p 362, with permission.)*

determine tumor size and whether the lesion is solid or cystic. They also are useful for planning the operative approach using abdominal, flank, or thoracoabdominal incisions. Ultrasound, gastrointestinal barium studies, and angiography (aortography) are rarely indicated except when gastrointestinal stromal tumors are suspected.

If lymphoma is suspected as the cause of a retroperitoneal mass, a CT-directed needle biopsy often can be done (Fig. 33-23). Fine-needle aspirates are used, but most pathologists require analysis of cells and stroma for diagnostic accuracy, requiring a percutaneous needle biopsy. The exact location of the retroperitoneal mass, its appearance, and the presence or absence of adenopathy and lymphoma (B) symptoms of fever, weight loss, and night sweats dictate whether a biopsy should be performed. Preoperative tissue diagnosis is useful only if a lesion treated nonsurgically could be determined.

Treatment. Preoperative preparation of the patient should include a mechanical and antibiotic bowel preparation when a bowel resection may be necessary for complete tumor removal. Adjacent involved organs may need to be resected in order to obtain complete gross tumor removal. These organs include the kidney, colon, pancreas, and spleen. Adjacent organ resection may be necessary in 50 to 80 percent of patients in order to obtain complete tumor removal. Tumors of the retroperitoneum should not be enucleated because local tumor recurrence is inevitable. Radical resection of multiple organs is inappropriate when the tumor's margin is the aorta or vena cava. Kidney removal should be contemplated only when the opposite kidney is functioning properly. Knowledge of the exact tumor location,

adjacent structures, and the surgeon's ability to obtain complete tumor removal are critical to operative planning.

Benign retroperitoneal masses can be removed and cured by simple excision. Malignant lesions, such as sarcomas, require

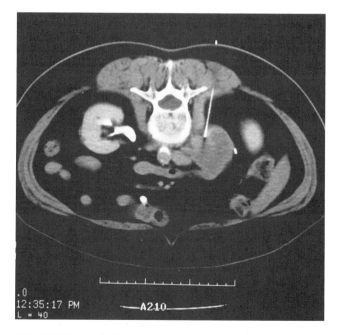

FIG. 33-23. *Needle biopsy of a retroperitoneal mass demonstrated as a ganglioneuroma. Resection was then carried out.*

more extensive resection. Low-grade tumors have a propensity for local recurrence and often become more biologically aggressive with each local recurrence. Distant metastases are less common. High-grade sarcomas have a greater propensity for local and distant metastases. Operative treatment is the most effective form of therapy, with the initial operation providing the greatest opportunity for cure of retroperitoneal sarcomas. Complete surgical resection is the primary determinant of patient outcome, with tumor grade being the next most important factor. Operative mortality should be under 5 percent, with morbidity related to hemorrhage, infection, and delayed intestinal function.

After complete surgical resection of retroperitoneal sarcomas, the 5-year survival ranges from 50 to 70 percent, with the most important determinant being the histologic grade (high grade, 20 to 30 percent and low grade, 70 to 80 percent 5-year survival) of the tumor. Partial tumor resection lowers the 5-year survival outcome to approximately 10 to 30 percent. After resection, the most common pattern of recurrence is at the local tumor resection site. Reoperation and resection of an isolated locally recurrent tumor may be of substantial benefit by improving long-term survival. Strategies to reduce the incidence of locoregional recurrence are important.

Radiotherapy combined with operative resection may be beneficial in reducing the incidence of local tumor recurrence after resection. The dose of radiotherapy must be large, approximately 6000 cGy or greater, to effect substantial benefit. At these doses, the incidence of complications such as intestinal enteritis, fibrosis, and obstruction is prohibitive. A strategy to reduce the radiation dose to normal adjacent organs is to use intraoperative radiotherapy (IORT). One method uses plexiglas cones to move normal tissues aside from the tumor bed, and external-beam treatment is given. Another method uses brachytherapy with radioactive iodine seeds or irridium wires to deliver high doses to the local tumor bed while sparing adjacent tissues. In the former approach, investigators used IORT and external-beam radiotherapy and noted a significant improvement in local control, although painful neuritis was a major side effect. Radiotherapy alone is not curative for treatment of soft tissue sarcomas. Patients with unresectable disease may achieve substantial palliation. Radiation treatment is reserved for patients having pain with unresectable tumors, those who develop tumor recurrence, or those who have positive tumor margins after primary resection.

Chemotherapy does not improve outcome when used in an adjunct setting for adults with retroperitoneal soft tissue sarcomas. For patients with metastatic disease, multidrug chemotherapy uses Adriamycin as the key component. Tumor response can occur in up to 30 percent of patients, but survival outcome benefit has not been demonstrated.

Bibliography

Abdominal Wall

Easter DW, Halasz NA: Recent trends in the management of desmoid tumors. *Ann Surg* 210:765, 1989.

Gocke JE, Maccarthy RL, Foulk WT: Rectus sheath hematoma diagnosed by computerized tomography scanning. *Mayo Clin Proc* 56:757, 1981.

Jones IT, Jagelman DG, et al: Desmoid tumors in familial polyposis coli. *Ann Surg* 204:94, 1986.

Lopez R, Kemalyan N, et al: Problems in diagnosis and management of desmoid tumors. *Am J Surg* 159:450, 1990.

McKinnon JG, Neifeld JP, et al: Management of desmoid tumors. *Surg Gynecol Obstet* 169:104, 1989.

Posner MC, Shiu MH, et al: Desmoid tumor: Not a benign disease. *Arch Surg* 124:191,1989.

Zainea GG, Jordan F: Rectus sheath hematoma: Their pathogenesis, diagnosis and management. *Am Surg* 54:630, 1988.

Omentum

Basson SE, Jones PA: Primary torsion of the omentum. *Ann R Coll Surg Engl* 63:132, 1980.

Baxter NS, Storey DJ, et al: Infarction of greater omentum: Exclusive cause of acute abdominal pain. *Postgrad Med* 79:141, 1986.

Cooper C, Jeffrey RB, et al: Computed tomography of omental pathology. *J Comput Assist Tomogr* 10:62, 1986.

Eitel GG: A rare omental tumor. *Med Rec* 55:715, 1899.

Leitner MJ, Jordan CG, et al: Torsion, infarction and hemorrhage of the omentum as a cause of acute abdominal distress. *Ann Surg* 135:103, 1952.

Rich RH, Filler RM: Segmental infarction of the greater omentum. *Can J Surg* 26:241, 1983.

Schwartz RW, Reames M, et al: Primary solid neoplasms of the greater omentum. *Surgery* 109:543, 1991.

Walker AR, Putnam TC: Omental, mesenteric and retroperitoneal cysts. *Surgery* 178:13, 1973.

Mesentery

Ackerman LV: Peritoneum, retroperitoneum and related structures, in Rosai J (ed): *Surgical Pathology*, 7th ed. St Louis, Mosby, 1989, chap 26.

Ballard JL, Stone WM, et al: A critical analysis of adjuvant techniques used to assess bowel viability in acute mesenteric ischemia. *Am Surg* 59:309, 1993.

Blattner RJ: Acute mesenteric lymphadenitis. *J Pediatr* 74:479, 1969.

Bradbury AW, Brittenden J, et al: Mesenteric ischaemia: A multidisciplinary approach. *Br J Surg* 82:1446, 1995.

Caropreso PR: Mesenteric cysts: A review. *Arch Surg* 108:242, 1974.

Carr SC, Pearce WH, et al: Current management of visceral artery aneurysms. *Surgery* 120:627, 1996.

Christensen MG, Lorentzen JE, Schroeder TV: Revascularisation of atherosclerotic mesenteric arteries: Experience in 90 consecutive patients. *Eur J Vasc Surg* 8:297, 1994.

Cunningham CG, Reilly LM, Stoney RJ: Chronic visceral ischemia. *Surg Clin North Am* 72:231, 1992.

Cunningham CG, Reilly LM, et al: Chronic visceral ischemia. *Ann Surg* 214:276, 1991.

Davis JM, Fantini GA: Remote effects: Lung injury, in Fantini GA (ed): *Ischemia-Reperfusion Injury of Skeletal Muscle*. Austin, RG Landes, 1994, chap 9, pp 143–156.

Durst AL, Freund H, et al: Mesenteric panniculitis: Review of the literature and presentation of cases. *Surgery* 81:203, 1977.

Ellis DJ, Brandt LJ: Mesenteric venous thrombosis. *Gastroenterology* 2:293, 1994.

Fantini GA, Conte MS: Pulmonary failure following lower torso ischemia: Clinical evidence for a remote effect of reperfusion injury. *Am Surg* 61:316, 1995.

Fowler EF: Primary cysts and tumors of the small bowel mesentery. *Am Surg* 27:653, 1961.

Gentile AT, Moneta GL, et al: Usefulness of fasting and postprandial duplex ultrasound examinations for predicting high-grade superior mesenteric artery stenosis. *Am J Surg* 169:476, 1995.

Hallisey MJ, Deschaine J, et al: Angioplasty for the treatment of visceral ischemia. *J Vasc Intervent Radiol* 6:785, 1995.

Harward TR, Brooks DL, et al: Multiple organ dysfunction after mesenteric artery revascularization. *J Vasc Surg* 18:459, 1993.

Harward TR, Smith S, Seeger JM: Detection of celiac axis and superior mesenteric artery occlusive disease with use of abdominal duplex scanning. *J Vasc Surg* 17:738, 1993.

Howard TJ, Plaskon LA, et al: Nonocclusive mesenteric ischemia remains a diagnostic dilemma. *Am J Surg* 171:405, 1996.

Johnston KW, Lindsay TF, et al: Mesenteric arterial bypass grafts: Early and late results and suggested surgical approach for chronic and acute mesenteric ischemia. *Surgery* 118:1, 1995.

Kaleya RN, Boley SJ: Acute mesenteric ischemia. *Crit Care Clin* 11:479, 1995.

Kaleya RN, Sammartano RJ, Boley SJ: Aggressive approach to acute mesenteric ischemia. *Surg Clin North Am* 72:157, 1992.

Katz ME, Heiken JP et al: Intraabdominal panniculitis: clinical, radiographic, and CT features. *AJR Am J Roentgenol* 145:293, 1985.

Kazui M, Andreoni KA, et al: Visceral lipid peroxidation occurs at reperfusion after supraceliac aortic cross-clamping. *J Vasc Surg* 19:473, 1994.

Kitchens CS: Evolution of our understanding of the pathophysiology of primary mesenteric venous thrombosis. *Am J Surg* 163:346, 1992.

Koike K, Moore EE, et al: Gut ischemia/reperfusion produces lung injury independent of endotoxin. *Crit Care Med* 22:1438, 1994.

Kurtz RJ, Heimann TM, et al: Mesenteric and retroperitoneal cysts. *Am Surg* 203:109, 1986.

Matsumoto AH, Tegtmeyer CJ, et al: Percutaneous transluminal angioplasty of visceral arterial stenoses: Results and long-term clinical follow-up. *J Vasc Intervent Radiol* 6:165, 1995.

McAfee MK, Cherry KJ Jr, et al: Influence of complete revascularization on chronic mesenteric ischemia. *Am J Surg* 164:220, 1992.

McMillan WD, McCarthy WJ, et al: Mesenteric artery bypass: Objective patency determination. *J Vasc Surg* 21:729, 1995.

McShane MD, Proctor A, et al: Mesenteric angioplasty for chronic intestinal ischaemia. *Eur J Vasc Surg* 6:333, 1992.

Miani S, Arpesani A, et al: Splanchnic artery aneurysms. *J Cardiovasc Surg* 34:221, 1993.

Nypaver TJ, Shepard AD, et al: Supraceliac aortic cross-clamping: Determinants of outcome in elective abdominal aortic reconstruction. *J Vasc Surg* 17:868, 1993.

Puylaert JB: Mesenteric adenitis and acute terminal ileitis: Ultrasound evaluation using graded compression. *Radiology* 161:691, 1986.

Reilly LM, Ramos TK, et al: Optimal exposure of the proximal abdominal aorta: A critical appraisal of transabdominal medial visceral rotation. *J Vasc Surg* 19:375, 1994.

Rhee RY, Gloviczki P, et al: Mesenteric venous thrombosis: Still a lethal disease in the 1990s. *J Vasc Surg* 20:688, 1994.

Ros PR, Olmstead WW, et al: Mesenteric and omental cysts: Histologic classification with imaging correlation. *Radiology* 164:327, 1987.

Saari TN, Triplett DA: *Yersinia* pseudotuberculosis mesenteric adenitis. *J Pediatr* 85:656, 1974.

Taourel PG, Deneuville M, et al: Acute mesenteric ischemia: Diagnosis with contrast-enhanced CT. *Radiology* 199:632, 1996.

Thorek P: *Anatomy in Surgery,* 2d ed. Philadelphia, JB Lippincott, 1963.

Ward D, Vernava AM, et al: Improved outcome by identification of high-risk nonocclusive mesenteric ischemia, aggressive reexploration, and delayed anastomosis. *Am J Surg* 170:577, 1995.

Weinberger HA, Ahmed MS: Mesenchymal solid tumors of the omentum and mesentery: Report of four cases. *Surgery* 82:754, 1977.

Wilcox MG, Howard TJ, et al: Current theories of pathogenesis and treatment of nonocclusive mesenteric ischemia. *Dig Dis Sci* 40:709, 1995.

Wolf EL, Sprayregen S, Bakal CW: Radiology in intestinal ischemia: Plain film, contrast, and other imaging studies. *Surg Clin North Am* 72:107, 1992.

Yannopoulos K, Stout AP: Primary solid tumors of the mesentery. *Cancer* 16:914, 1963.

Retroperitoneum

Ackerman LV: Peritoneum, retroperitoneum and related structures, in Rosai J (ed): *Surgical Pathology,* 7th ed. St Louis, Mosby, 1989, chap 26.

Adam YG, Oland J, et al: Primary retroperitoneal soft-tissue sarcomas. *J Surg Oncol* 25:8, 1984.

Baker LRI, Mallinson WJW, et al: Idiopathic retroperitoneal fibrosis: A retrospective analysis of 60 cases. *Br J Urol* 60:497, 1988.

Barker CD, Brown JJ: MR imaging of the retroperitoneum. *Top Magn Reson Imaging* 7:102, 1995.

Beahrs OH, Henson DE, et al: Soft tissues, in *American Joint Committee on Cancer Manual for Staging of Cancer,* 4th ed. Philadelphia, JB Lippincott, 1992, pp 131–133.

Boring CC, Squires TS, et al: Cancer statistics. *CA* 43:7, 1993.

Clark CP, Vanderpool D, Preskitt JT: The response of retroperitoneal fibrosis to tamoxifen. *Surgery* 109:502, 1991.

Degesys GE, Dunnick NR, et al: Retroperitoneal fibrosis: Use of CT in distinguishing among possible causes. *AJR* 146:57, 1986.

Hache L, Utz DC, Woolner LB: Idiopathic fibrosing retroperitonitis. *Surg Gynecol Obstet* 115:737, 1962.

Higgins PM, Aber GM: Idiopathic retroperitoneal fibrosis: An update. *Dig Dis* 8:206, 1990.

Jaques DP, Coit DG, et al: Management of primary and recurrent soft tissue sarcoma of the retroperitoneum. *Ann Surg* 212:51, 1990.

Kinsella TJ, Sindelar WF, et al: A 1988 Preliminary results of a randomized study of adjuvant radiation therapy in resectable adult retroperitoneal soft tissue sarcomas. *J Clin Oncol* 6:18, 1988.

Koep L, Zuidema GD: The clinical significance of retroperitoneal fibrosis. *Surgery* 81:250, 1977.

Kottra JJ, Dunnick NR: Retroperitoneal fibrosis. *Radiol Clin North Am* 34:1259, 1996.

Logothetis CJ, Samuels ML, et al: Chemotherapy of extragonadal germ cell tumors. *J Clin Oncol* 3:316, 1985.

Minford JE, Davies P: The urographic appearances in acute and chronic retroperitoneal fibrosis. *Clin Radiol* 35:51, 1984.

Mitchell RJ: Alimentary complications of non-malignant retroperitoneal fibrosis. *Br J Surg* 58:254, 1971.

Osborn DE, Rao PN, et al: Surgical management of idiopathic retroperitoneal fibrosis. *Br J Urol* 53:242, 1981.

Owens LV, Cance WG, Huth JF: Retroperitoneal fibrosis treated with tamoxifen. *Am Surg* 61:842, 1995.

Palleschi J, McAninch JW: Renal autotransplantation for retroperitoneal fibrosis. *J Urol* 125:408, 1981.

Pinson CW, ReMine SG, et al: Long-term results with primary retroperitoneal tumors. *Arch Surg* 124:1168, 1989.

Scavalli AD, Spadaro A, et al: Long-term follow-up of low-dose methotrexate therapy in one case of idiopathic retroperitoneal fibrosis. *Clin Rheumatol* 14:481, 1995.

Sindelar WF, Kinsella TJ, et al: Intraoperative radiotherapy in retroperitoneal sarcomas: Final results of a prospective, randomized, clinical trial. *Arch Surg* 128:402, 1993.

Storm FK, Mahvi DM: Diagnosis and management of retroperitoneal soft-tissue sarcoma. *Ann Surg* 214:2, 1991.

van Doorn RC, Gallee MPW, et al: Resectable retroperitoneal soft tissue sarcomas. *Cancer* 73:637, 1994.

Zornig C, Weh HJ, et al: Retroperitoneal sarcoma in a series of 51 adults. *Eur J Surg Oncol* 18:475, 1992.

Abdominal Wall Hernias

George E. Wantz

Hernias of the abdominal wall are the most common condition requiring major surgery. Despite the frequency of surgical repair, perfect results continue to elude surgeons, and the rate of surgical failure (recurrence) is humbling. The outcome of hernia surgery is highly surgeon-dependent, and Astley P. Cooper's oft-quoted statement of 1804 is still pertinent and an appropriate introduction to this chapter: "No disease of the human body, belonging to the province of surgeons requires in its treatment a greater combination of accurate anatomical knowledge with surgical skill than hernia in all its varieties."

GENERAL CONSIDERATIONS

Definitions. A hernia (Latin, rupture; Greek, bud) is defined as a protrusion of a viscus through an opening in the wall of the cavity in which it is contained. Clinically the important part of the definition is the protrusion, because without the protruding viscus a diagnosis of hernia is essentially impossible. Anatomically the important features of a hernia are the hernial orifice and the hernial sac. The hernial orifice is the defect in the innermost aponeurotic layer of the abdomen, and the hernial sac is an outpouch of peritoneum. The neck of a hernial sac corresponds to the hernial orifice. The size of a hernia is determined by the dimension of the neck and the volume of the distended sac. A hernia is external if the sac protrudes completely through the abdominal wall, interparietal if the sac is contained within the abdominal wall, and internal if the sac is within the visceral cavity. The hernia is reducible when the protruded viscus can be returned to the abdomen and irreducible when it cannot. The manual manipulation required to reduce viscera entrapped in a hernial sac is known as *taxis.*

A strangulated hernia is one in which the vascularity of the protruded viscus is compromised, usually at the neck. Strangulation is most likely to occur in hernias that have small orifices and relatively voluminous sacs. Strangulation is always serious and can be fatal, and the potential for strangulation is the main reason for the repair of hernia. The word "incarceration" is frequently used in connection with a hernia. An incarcerated hernia is nothing more than an irreducible hernia, and the term does not refer, as some surgeons contend, to an irreducible hernia that is on the verge of becoming strangulated. A Richter's hernia is a hernia in which the contents of the sac consist of only one side of the wall of the intestine (always antimesenteric). In a Richter's hernia, strangulation of the bowel wall occurs without concomitant intestinal obstruction.

Sites of Herniation. Hernias of the abdominal wall occur only in areas where aponeurosis and fascia are devoid of the protecting support of striated muscle. Many such sites are normally present, but some may be acquired through muscular atrophy or surgery. Without a counteracting force, the bare aponeurotic areas are subject to the ravages of intraabdominal pressure and give way if they deteriorate or contain anatomic irregularities. Predictably, the common sites of herniation are thus the groin, the umbilicus, the linea alba, the semilunar line of Spieghel, the diaphragm, and surgical incisions. Other similar but rare sites of herniation are the perineum, the superior lumbar triangle of Grynfeltt, the inferior lumbar triangle of Petit, and the obturator and sciatic foramina of the pelvis.

Symptoms and Diagnosis. Some patients have hernias but are unaware of them until the hernia is pointed out to them. The natural history of all hernias of the abdominal wall is slow enlargement to the point of irreducibility and disfigurement, with the risk of strangulation ever present. Symptomatic hernias produce a wide variety of nonspecific discomforts related to the contents of the sac and the pressure by the sac on adjacent tissue. The discomforts produced by hernias are always worse at the end of the day and are relieved at night when the patient reclines and the hernia reduces. Groin hernias are not a cause of testicular pain; groin pain without a demonstrable hernia usually does not indicate or herald the onset of a hernia. Most hernias develop insidiously, but some are precipitated by a single forceful muscular event.

Hernias are easy to diagnose on physical examination. Typically a hernial sac with its contents enlarges and transmits a palpable impulse when the patient strains or coughs. Usually the patient must stand during the examination because it is impossible to palpate a reduced groin hernia with certainty when the patient is supine. Hydroceles may resemble an irreducible groin hernia, but they transilluminate, whereas hernias do not. Hernias undetectable by physical examination can be demonstrated by the radiologist using ultrasonography, computerized tomography, magnetic resonance imaging, and herniography; in the latter a nonirritating contrast agent is injected into the peritoneal cavity. Strangulation produces intense pain in the hernia followed quickly by tenderness, intestinal obstruction, and signs and symptoms of sepsis. A strangulated hernia, in contrast to an irreducible hernia, does not enlarge or transmit an impulse when the patient coughs. Taxis of a strangulated hernia is contraindicated if there is sepsis or if the contents of the sac are thought to be gangrenous.

Indications for Surgery. In general, all hernias should be repaired unless local or systemic conditions in the patient preclude a safe outcome. The possible exception to this generalization is a hernia with a wide neck and shallow sac that is expected to enlarge slowly. Trusses and surgical belts are helpful in the management of small hernias when operation is contraindicated. However, trusses are contraindicated for patients with femoral hernias.

HERNIAS OF THE GROIN

The groin is one of the natural weak areas in the abdominal wall and is the most common site for abdominal herniation. Both sexes of all ages are afflicted, but men are 25 times more likely to have a groin hernia than women.

Hernias arising above the abdominocrural crease are inguinal (Latin, groin), and those arising below the crease are femoral (Latin, thigh) or crural (Latin, leg). Inguinal hernias may be direct or indirect. The sac of an indirect inguinal hernia passes obliquely or indirectly toward and ultimately into the scrotum, in which case it is known as a scrotal hernia. The sac of a direct inguinal hernia protrudes directly outward and forward. Clinically distinguishing an indirect from a direct inguinal hernia is often impossible and is of little importance since the operation to repair them is the same. In men, indirect hernias outnumber

direct hernias at a ratio of 2:1, whereas in women direct hernias are a rarity. Strangulated indirect hernias in men may produce concomitant strangulation of the spermatic cord and testicle.

Femoral hernias are usually considered a separate entity but are actually a form of direct inguinal herniation. Femoral hernias are uncommon, comprising about 2.5 percent of all groin hernias. They occur occasionally in women, especially in multiparous elderly women, but not as frequently as inguinal hernias; in men they are rare. Ten percent of women and 50 percent of men with femoral hernias have or will develop an inguinal hernia. Femoral hernias almost always appear as an irreducible mass about the size of a walnut at the medial base of Scarpa's femoral triangle. A femoral hernia appears irreducible, even though the sac may be empty, because fat and lymph nodes from the femoral canal surround the sac. A solitary enlarged lymph node or a synovial cyst may mimic a femoral hernia exactly. The infrequent reducible femoral hernias may be confused with a saphenous varix.

Strangulated Richter's type femoral hernias occur relatively frequently and carry a significant morbidity and mortality. The diagnosis of such strangulated femoral hernias is invariably delayed because they develop without intestinal obstruction and with minimal local manifestation until the entrapped knuckle of small bowel is gangrenous. A bruit over the femoral vein is an indication that the adjacent femoral hernia is incarcerated or strangulated because the unforgiving hernia compresses the vein.

Both indirect inguinal and femoral hernias are twice as common on the right as on the left. In indirect inguinal hernias this is attributed to a delay in the atrophy of the processus vaginalis that follows the normally slower descent to the scrotum of the right testis. In femoral hernias the right side's predominance is credited to the sigmoid colon's tamponading the left femoral canal.

Epidemiology. Hernias are a common health problem. Exactly how prevalent they are is not known, but the accepted estimated incidence is 3 to 4 percent of the male population. Aging increases the incidence of groin hernias, the likelihood of strangulation, and the need for hospitalization. Strangulation, the most common and serious complication of a groin hernia, increases mortality and morbidity, the need for general or regional anesthesia, and the need for hospitalization. Strangulation occurs in 1.3 to 3.0 percent of groin hernias. Strangulation occurs at the extremes of life and in the elderly is a grave surgical problem. Most strangulated hernias are indirect inguinal hernias, but the femoral hernia has the highest rate of strangulation (5 to 20 percent) of all hernias.

The probability of a groin hernia's strangulating varies with location and duration. For an inguinal hernia the probability of strangulation is 2.8 percent after 3 months from development and increases to 4.5 percent after 2 years; for femoral hernias it is 22 percent at 3 months and 45 percent at 21 months. Femoral hernias require urgent surgery. The probability of strangulation, in both inguinal hernia and femoral hernia, is greatest in the first 3 months, suggesting that patients with a short history of herniation should be referred urgently to a surgeon.

Anatomy of the Groin. Many surgeons have contributed to the study of the anatomy of the groin and groin hernia, and the names of some are eponymically memorialized. The most important contributions were made by Cooper, Anson and McVay, and Fruchaud. Cooper, in a two-volume masterpiece

(1804–1807), was the first to accurately describe and depict the groin. Among other things he named the endopelvic fascia and the transversalis fascia and described the iliopectineal ligament, now called Cooper's ligament. Anson and McVay, in a series of monumental publications beginning in 1937, defined, described, and statistically analyzed the anatomic structures of the groin. Fruchaud, in a spectacularly illustrated two-volume work in 1956 on the anatomy and treatment of groin hernias, unified the hernias of the groin by redefining the weak area of the groin to include the area of occurrence of all the hernias of the groin.

The groin is the area of junction of the lower abdomen and the thigh. The anatomy of the various myoaponeurotic layers and other important structures is illustrated in Fig. 34-1. The only structurally important layer of the groin of concern to hernia surgeons is the innermost aponeuroticofascial layer of the abdomen. It consists of the transverse abdominal muscle, the transverse aponeurosis, and the transversalis fascia. To visualize this layer from the anterior approach, the superficial structures consisting of the external oblique abdominal muscle, the inguinal ligament, and the internal oblique abdominal muscle must be divided, reflected, or partially removed. From the posterior exposure it is necessary to reflect only the peritoneum.

The transverse aponeuroticofascia at the upper border of the femoral sheath is known by North American surgeons as the iliopubic tract, by French surgeons as the bandelette of Thomson, and by English surgeons as the deep crural arch. This portion of the transverse aponeuroticofascia becomes the inferior crus of the deep ring. The superior crus of the deep ring is formed by the portion of the transverse aponeurosis known as the transverse aponeurotic arch. The transverse aponeurosis lies

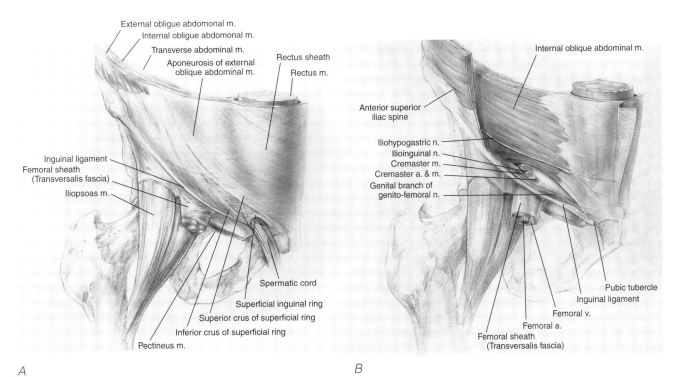

A   *B*

FIG. 34-1. The anatomy of the groin. *A.* The external oblique abdominal muscle and aponeurosis. The inguinal ligament consists of the lowermost fibers of the aponeurosis of the external oblique muscle extending between the anterior superior iliac spine laterally and the pubic tubercle and the superior ramus of the pubis medially. The femoral sheath is derived from the transversalis fascia. The only structure attaching the inguinal ligament to the subjacent femoral sheath and fascia lata is the investing fascia of the external oblique muscle, which is flimsy and is known as the innominate fascia. *B.* The internal oblique abdominal muscle is the middle myoaponeurotic layer of the abdominal wall. The lowermost fibers of the internal oblique abdominal muscle become the cremaster muscle and embrace the mainly inferior aspect of the spermatic cord. The three sensory nerves of the groin are the iliohypogastric and the ilioinguinal nerves and the genital branch of the genitofemoral nerve. The latter nerve is also motor to the cremaster muscle. *C.* The innermost myoaponeurotic layer of the abdominal wall is the transverse abdominal muscle and its aponeurosis. The inguinal ligament has been divided and reflected, revealing its lacunar insertion on the pecten pubis. Aponeurotic fibers of the transverse abdominal muscle along the superior border of the femoral sheath are known as the iliopubic tract. The aponeurosis of the transverse abdominal muscle forms a broad arch superior to the spermatic cord and is known as the transverse aponeurotic arch. The transverse aponeurotic arch is partially hidden by muscle fibers when viewed from the anterior but is clearly apparent from the posterior. *D.* Removal of the three myoaponeurotic layers of the abdominal wall leaves the transversalis fascia that envelopes the entire abdomen and forms the femoral sheath. *E.* The posterior view depicts the deep ring, the transverse aponeurotic arch, the inferior epigastric vessels, and Hesselbach's triangle. *F.* Intraabdominal view of the groin. *G.* Parasagittal section of the groin just lateral to the pubic tubercle illustrates the relationship of the important anatomic structures. (Adapted from: *Fruchaud H: 1956, p 103, Fig. 65, with permission.*)

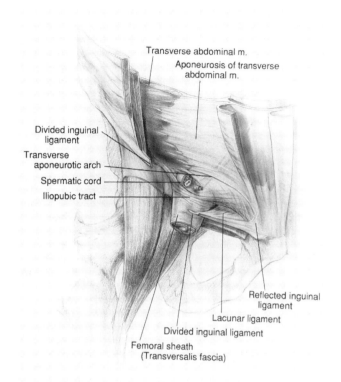

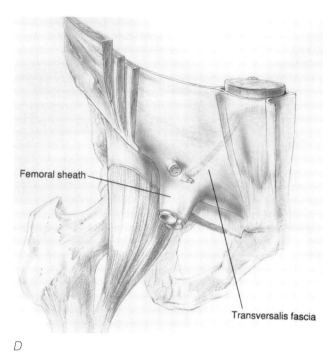

C

D

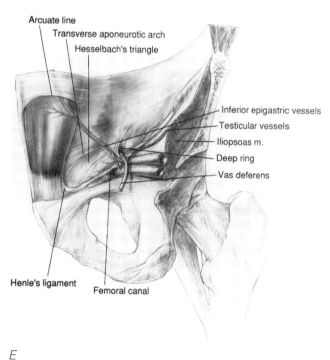

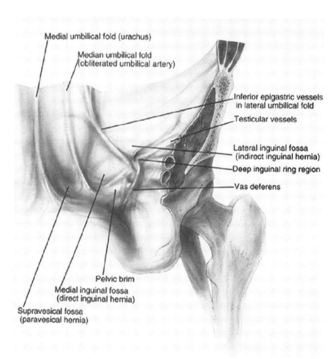

E

F

FIG. 34-1. *C.–F. Continued.*

on the posterior aspect of the transverse abdominal muscle and cannot be seen from the anterior. From the posterior, however, it forms a very obvious broad aponeurotic arch that inserts on

the pectineal line of the pubis (pecten pubis). The portion of the tendon of the rectus abdominis muscle that recurves laterally onto the pecten pubis is known as Henle's ligament.

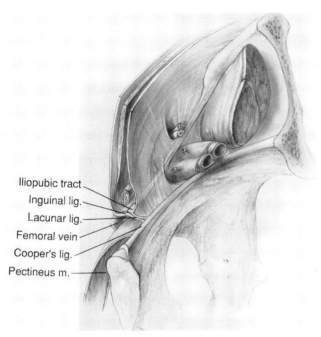

Iliopubic tract
Inguinal lig.
Lacunar lig.
Femoral vein
Cooper's lig.
Pectineus m.

G

FIG. 34-1. *G. Continued.*

The suspended portion of the inguinal ligament is mobile because it is attached to the femoral sheath by the investing fascia of the external oblique abdominal muscle only.

The bulk of the cremaster muscle arising from the lowermost fibers of the internal oblique abdominal muscle embraces the inferior aspect of the spermatic cord in the inguinal canal. The cremaster vessels arise from the inferior epigastric vessels and pass through the posterior wall of the inguinal canal by their own foramen. They are accompanied by the genital nerve and supply the cremaster muscle and the tunica of the testes. They are not part of the spermatic cord and may be divided without damaging the testicle to expose the floor of the inguinal canal during hernioplasty.

A fascial condensation in the region of the inferior epigastric vessels is known as Hesselbach's interfoveolar ligament and is not always obvious. Muscular contraction retracts the ligament and complements the shutter action of the internal oblique abdominal muscle by pulling the cord at the deep ring laterally and superiorly.

The path of the inguinal canal through the abdominal wall is oblique (Figs. 34-1 and 34-2). The anterior wall consists of the aponeurosis of the external oblique abdominal muscle. The posterior wall is the aponeurosis of the transverse abdominal muscle and the transversalis fascia. The angle of entrance of the deep ring is acute medially and obtuse laterally. The transverse aponeurosis and transversalis fascia comprise the medial border of the deep ring. It is fibrous, definable, and palpable and is the margin surgeons repair during hernioplasty. The lateral border of the deep ring is formed by the transverse abdominal muscle.

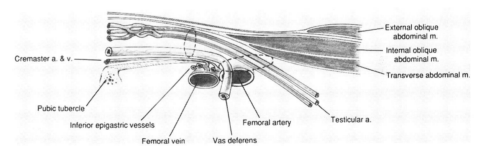

Cremaster a. & v.
External oblique abdominal m.
Internal oblique abdominal m.
Transverse abdominal m.
Pubic tubercle
Inferior epigastric vessels
Femoral vein
Vas deferens
Femoral artery
Testicular a.

FIG. 34-2. Vertical section through the inguinal canal displays the anatomy of the deep ring. The dotted line encircles the spermatic cord in the inguinal canal. The broken line outlines the deep ring. The inferior epigastric artery and vein arise from the iliac vessels directly under the deep ring from the medial border of the deep ring. The cremaster vessels, which are not part of the spermatic cord, arise from the inferior epigastric vessels and penetrate the inguinal floor through their own foramen. They lie on the posterior wall of the inguinal canal (iliopubic tract) and pass to the scrotum near the pubic tubercle.

The path of the inguinal canal through the abdominal wall is oblique. The anterior wall consists of the aponeurosis of the external oblique abdominal muscle. The posterior wall is of the aponeurosis of the transverse abdominal muscle and the transversalis fascia. The angle of entrance of the deep ring is acute medially and obtuse laterally. The transverse aponeurosis and transversalis fascia comprise the medial border of the deep ring. It is fibrous, definable, and palpable and is the margin that surgeons repair during hernioplasty. The lateral border of the deep ring is formed by the transverse abdominal muscle. It is soft, elastic, muscular, and indistinct. The internal oblique abdominal muscle covers the deep ring and forms the shutter mechanism. This muscle obscures the deep ring from view and also prevents palpation of the deep ring from the anterior. Moreover, the lateral border of the deep ring is so blunt that it is indistinguishable and unrecognizable even from the posterior.

The elements of the spermatic cord split proximal to the deep ring; the vas deferens descends with its artery to the seminal vesicles, and the spermatic vessels, lymphatics, and lymph nodes incline superiorly to the region of the kidneys. At the level of the deep ring there is one testicular artery and two or three testicular veins. Distally in the cord and beyond the pubic tubercle are the delicate veins of the pampiniform plexus, from which the testicular veins arise. (From: *Wantz GE: Atlas of Hernia Surgery, 1991, Fig 1-3, p 6, with permission.*)

It is soft, elastic, muscular, and indistinct. The internal oblique abdominal muscle covers the deep ring and forms the shutter mechanism. This muscle obscures the deep ring from view and prevents its palpation from the anterior approach. The lateral border of the deep ring is so blunt as to be indistinguishable and unrecognizable even from the posterior view.

The spermatic cord begins at the deep ring and contains the vas deferens and its accompanying artery, the testicular artery and veins, lymphatics, autonomic nerves, and a variable quantity of fat. Collateral circulation for the testicle is abundant and comes from the vessels supplying nearby structures. Distally in the cord and mainly beyond the pubic tubercle are the delicate veins of the pampiniform plexus from which the testicular veins arise.

The elements of the spermatic cord split proximal to the deep ring, and the vas deferens and its artery descend to the seminiferous tubules, while the spermatic vessels, lymphatics, and lymph nodes incline superiorly to the region of the kidneys. At the level of the deep ring there is one testicular artery and two or three testicular veins.

The iliohypogastric and ilioinguinal nerves and the genital branch of the genitofemoral nerve are the nerves in the groin that are of concern to the surgeon. The iliohypogastric and ilio-inguinal nerves, which intermingle, are sensory to the skin of the groin, the base of the penis, and the medial upper thigh. The position of these nerves, arising from T12 and L1, are variable. The ilioinguinal nerve is found in its typical anatomic position on top of the spermatic cord in only 60 percent of patients. In others its course and position are behind or within the cremaster muscle. Often it cannot be found or it exists in fibers too small to be seen.

The genital nerve is both motor and sensory and innervates the cremaster muscle and the skin of the side of the scrotum and labia. It arises from L1 and L2 and may substitute for the ilio-inguinal nerve when this nerve is deficient. In the inguinal canal, the genital nerve lies on the iliopubic tract, and it accompanies the cremaster vessels to form a neurovascular bundle that is usually divided during anterior inguinal hernioplasty.

Anatomy of Groin Hernia. An indirect hernial sac is actually a dilated persistent processus vaginalis (Fig. 34-3). It passes through the deep ring, lies within the spermatic cord, and follows the indirect course of the cord to the scrotum. At the deep ring the sac occupies the anterior lateral side of the cord. Properitoneal fat is often associated with an indirect hernial sac and is known as a lipoma of the cord, although the fat is not a tumor. Lipomas of the spermatic cord can mimic an indirect hernial sac exactly.

An indirect hernial sac is said to be complete if the sac has descended to the testes and filled the side of the scrotum, and incomplete when it has not. When the processus vaginalis remains completely open, the testicle will be within the sac. This type of hernia is known as a congenital hernia or communicating hydrocele. They are common in infants but rare in adult men.

Retroperitoneal organs such as the sigmoid colon, cecum, and ureters may slide into an indirect sac. They thereby become a part of the wall of the sac and are susceptible to injury during hernioplasty. These sliding hernias often are large and partially irreducible.

Direct inguinal hernial sacs originate through the floor of the inguinal canal, that is, Hesselbach's triangle; they protrude di-

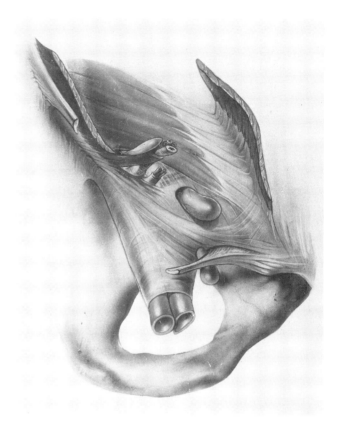

FIG. 34-3. The anatomy of hernial sacs in the groin. Indirect hernial sacs lie within the spermatic cord, pass through the deep ring, and proceed to the scrotum; direct hernial sacs arise through a weakened floor of the inguinal canal; and femoral hernial sacs pass through a parietal defect, which is almost always located in the medial border of the femoral sheath.

rectly; and they are contained by the aponeurosis of the external oblique muscle (see Fig. 34-3). Only rarely do they so enlarge as to force their way through the superficial ring and descend into the scrotum. Direct hernias usually are diffuse and involve the entire floor of the inguinal canal. The less common discrete direct hernias have small orifices and diverticulum-shaped sacs. Direct inguinal hernias also originate lateral to the inferior epigastric vessels and present through the deep ring or interstitially through slips of fatty muscular atrophy in the shutter muscles of the deep ring (see Fig. 34-3). These types of direct inguinal hernia are rare and commonly referred to erroneously as extra-funicular indirect and interstitial indirect hernias, respectively. They do not follow the spermatic cord and enlarge interparie-tally. The inferior epigastric vessels are not a proper anatomic boundary distinguishing a direct hernia from an indirect hernia in all instances, as some surgeons believe. The bladder is a common sliding component of a direct hernial sac.

Femoral hernial sacs originate from the femoral canal through a defect on the medial side of the femoral sheath (see Fig. 34-3). The femoral canal contains one or two lymph nodes, the largest of which is named Cloquet by the French and Rosenmüller by the Germans. These structures are expelled from the femoral canal by a peritoneal protrusion and frequently create a palpable mass. Femoral hernias also occur through the anterior femoral sheath. Prevascular femoral hernias are rare and are most often encountered as a recurrence after inguinal hernioplasty in which the femoral sheath or iliopubic tract has been used in the repair.

Fruchaud's Myopectineal Orifice. Traditionally the hernias of the groin have been defined as separate entities, which creates confusion. Fruchaud's (1956) concept of the anatomy of hernias of the groin is important. Rather than viewing hernias solely by their varied clinical presentation (i.e., indirect, direct, femoral, prevascular, interstitial), Fruchaud emphasized their common origin by noting that all the hernias of the groin begin within a single weak area that he called the myopectineal orifice (Fig. 34-4).

The myopectineal orifice is the area in the groin bounded superiorly by the internal oblique muscle and the transverse abdominal muscle, laterally by the iliopsoas muscle, medially by the rectus muscle and sheath, and inferiorly by the pecten pubis. This bony-muscular framework is bridged and bisected by the inguinal ligament, traversed by the spermatic cord and femoral vessels, and sealed like a drum on its inner surface by the transversalis (endopelvic) fascia only. Therefore the integrity of the myopectineal orifice is dependent on the transversalis fascia. A groin hernia is defined as protrusion of a peritoneal sac through the transversalis fascia spanning the myopectineal orifice. Failure of the transversalis fascia to retain the peritoneum then becomes the fundamental cause of all hernias of the groin.

The inguinal ligament and its broad, recurved, lacunar medial insertion on the pecten pubis are only loosely attached to the adjacent iliopubic tract and transversalis fascia (see Fig. 34-1C and Fig. 34-3). Nevertheless they strongly brace the myopectineal orifice, both separating inguinal herniation from femoral herniation and defining the medial border of the orifice of the femoral canal. The passage of the testicle through the abdominal wall during the embryonic stage weakens and enlarges the myopectineal orifice above the inguinal ligament, predisposing men to indirect and direct inguinal hernias. In women the increased diameter of the true pelvis as compared to men proportionally widens the femoral canal, probably predisposing women to femoral herniation.

Classification. Attempts to classify hernias have been made. These classifications assign numbers and letters to the various types and sizes of hernias of the groin and are intended to pro-

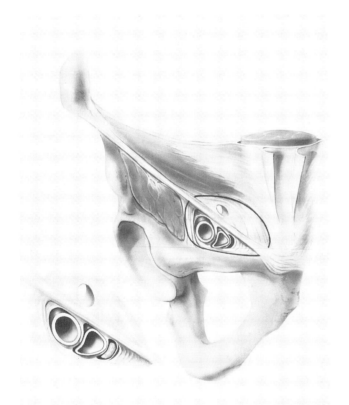

A

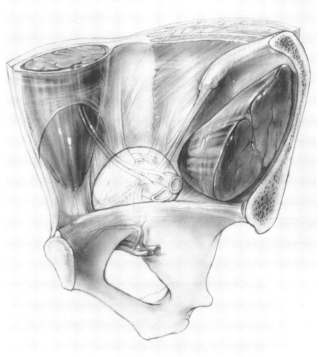

B

FIG. 34-4. Anterior *(A)* and posterior *(B)* views of Fruchaud's myopectineal orifice. The myopectineal orifice is the bony-muscular framework bounded medially by the rectus abdominis muscle and rectus sheath, superiorly by the oblique muscles of the abdomen, laterally by the iliopsoas muscle, and inferiorly by the pecten pubis. It is bridged and bisected by the iliopubic tract, traversed by the spermatic cord and iliac vessels, and spanned and sealed on its inner surface by the transversalis fascia only. All hernias of the groin begin within the myopectineal orifice, be they direct inguinal, indirect inguinal, interstitial inguinal, femoral, or prevascular. The fundamental cause of all hernias of the groin is the failure of the transversalis fascia to maintain the integrity of the myopectineal orifice. In men the superior portion of the myopectineal orifice is weakened by the descent of the testicle; in women the true pelvis is broader than it is in men and may predispose them to femoral herniation by widening the femoral canal. (From: *Wantz GE: Atlas of Hernia Surgery, 1991, Fig 1-2a, b, pp 4–5, with permission.*)

mote a common surgical understanding. Thus far, however, the classifications are incomplete and lack unanimity. Until accord is reached, hernias should be described by their type and location, volume of the sac, and diameter of the neck.

Etiology. Inguinal hernias can be congenital or acquired, and in both a family history of groin hernias is usually strongly positive. Most hernias of the groin therefore may be said to be transmitted genetically. All indirect inguinal hernias are congenital and result from a patent processus vaginalis, with which the patient is born. A patent processus vaginalis is found in 80 percent of newborns and in 50 percent of 1-year-olds. Closure continues until the age of 2 years. The incidence of a patent processus vaginalis in adults is 20 percent. Having the potential for a hernia does not mean that a hernia will develop. Other factors must be present to cause failure of the transversalis fascia to retain the visceral sac in the myopectineal orifice.

The erect stance of human beings, in contrast to that of four-legged animals, promotes herniation by stretching and exposing the groin and, when a hernia is present, permitting the dependent intestines to drop into the hernial sac.

Muscle deficiency contributes to herniation. Congenital or acquired insufficiencies of the internal oblique abdominal muscles in the groin expose the deep ring and the floor of the inguinal canal to the destructive effects of intraabdominal pressure (Fig. 34-5).

Destruction of connective tissue resulting from the physical stress of intraabdominal pressure, smoking, aging, connective tissue disease, and systemic illnesses reduces the strength of the transverse aponeurosis and fascia. Fracture of the elastic fibers and alterations in the structure, quantity, and metabolism of collagen have been demonstrated in the connective tissue structures of the groin in patients with hernias.

Other factors may also have an effect in some cases. Abdominal distention and chronic increase in intraabdominal pressure from ascites and peritoneal dialysis may damage the myopectineal orifice and cause a patent processus vaginalis to dilate.

Fracture deformities of the pelvis and denervation of the shutter mechanism following a low cosmetic appendectomy incision are well-known but uncommon causes of inguinal herniation.

Inguinal hernias of all types occur equally in sedentary and in physically active men. Vigorous physical activity per se is not a cause of inguinal herniation, although strenuous effort may aggravate predisposing factors and precipitate herniation. The notion that carcinoma of the colon is a cause of inguinal hernia is incorrect.

Basics of Groin Hernioplasty. The object of groin hernioplasty is to prevent peritoneal protrusion through the myopectineal orifice. The integrity of the myopectineal orifice is restored in two fundamentally different ways, which are based on Fruchaud's concept of groin hernia, namely, (1) aponeurotic closure of the myopectineal orifice to the extent necessary, and (2) replacement of the defective transversalis fascia with a large synthetic prosthesis. The two methods are sometimes combined.

Hernias are repaired either anteriorly through a groin incision, in which case the structures in and around the inguinal canal must be divided in order to reach the innermost aponeuroticofascial layer, or posteriorly through an abdominal incision, in which case the hernial orifices are exposed directly on entering the properitoneal space. The anterior approach is used in all the classical repairs and for more than a century has been the most popular incision for inguinal hernioplasty. Posterior hernia repairs are called properitoneal hernioplasty. Until recently the distinct advantages of a posterior approach were largely ignored.

Tension is the principal cause of failure of all the hernioplasties that close the myopectineal orifice by aponeurotic approximation. Assiduous efforts to prevent suture-line tension are essential, and sutures must never be drawn up or tied so tightly as to cause necrosis. Permanent monofilament synthetic sutures are preferable.

Synthetic mesh prostheses currently play a major role in the management of all hernias of the groin. Synthetic mesh prostheses are used to patch or plug the myopectineal orifice, to rein-

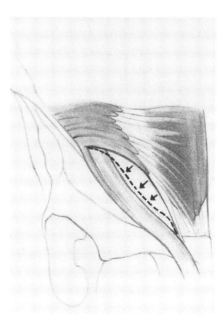

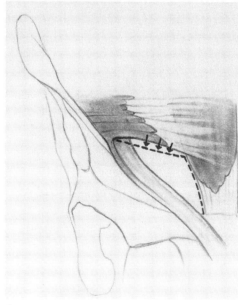

FIG. 34-5. Deficiencies in the lower portion of the internal oblique muscle hinder the shutter mechanism of the deep ring and expose the floor of the inguinal canal to the ravages of intraabdominal pressure. (From: *Wantz GE: Atlas of Hernia Surgery, 1991, Fig 2-3a, b, p 15, with permission.*)

A

B

force a classical repair, and to replace the transversalis fascia. Prosthetic techniques have surfaced in bewildering proliferation, each having enthusiastic proponents.

Anterior Classical Groin Hernioplasty. Only three anterior classical hernioplasties have withstood the test of time and are still used today: the Marcy simple ring closure, the Bassini operation (either in its original form or as performed at the Shouldice Hospital in Toronto), and the McVay-Lotheissen Cooper ligament repair. All produce equally satisfactory results in primary hernias when correctly indicated and are easily performed with local anesthesia in adults. Formerly, recurrent inguinal hernias were fixed by one of the classical repairs, but nowadays prosthetic techniques are preferred, as the results are distinctly better. Classical hernioplasty has three parts: *dissection of the inguinal canal, repair of the myopectineal orifice,* and *closure of the inguinal canal.* The dissection and closure of the inguinal canal are essentially identical in all variants of classical repair, and the repairs vary to the extent to which the myopectineal orifice is repaired.

A complete dissection consists of opening the inguinal canal, preservation (if possible) of the ilioinguinal nerve, division of the cremaster muscle and its neurovascular bundle to expose the deep ring, mobilization of the spermatic cord, division and excision of the posterior wall of the inguinal canal in areas that it is weak, assessment of the transverse aponeurosis, elimination of the peritoneal sac, removal of cord lipomas, and relaxing incisions when necessary (Fig. 34-6). For a successful hernioplasty, the dissection is as important as the repair. Division of the cremaster muscle and of the posterior wall of the inguinal canal are important steps that many surgeons omit, although Bassini routinely used them and surgeons at the forefront of inguinal hernia repair have repeatedly emphasized their importance.

Gentleness and precise, sharp dissection are essential to minimize surgical trauma to the spermatic cord. An important point is never to dissect beyond the pubic tubercle unless absolutely necessary. Hydroceles, cysts of the cord, and other conditions in the scrotum should never be dealt with at the time of inguinal hernia repair because of the risk of damaging the spermatic cord and causing testicular atrophy. Also, the distal portion of indirect hernial sacs should never be dissected from the cord unless absolutely necessary. They should be divided at the neck, with the distal part allowed to remain in situ while the proximal end is dissected beyond the neck and amputated with or without ligation. The retained distal sac will not become a hydrocele, although aspiration of serosanguinous fluid may be necessary in the early postoperative period. Sliding indirect hernial sacs are an exception and must be carefully dissected from the cord because they contain a retroperitoneal organ. Sliding sacs do not require other special treatment and are merely returned to the abdomen. Direct hernial sacs of all sizes are merely inverted and not opened.

Repair of the myopectineal orifice in men includes reconstruction of the deep ring. Contrary to the belief of some surgeons, the anatomy of the deep ring is such that strangulation of the spermatic cord by reconstruction of the posterior wall of the inguinal canal is virtually impossible. Indeed, insufficient repair of the deep ring is the principal cause of indirect recurrence.

The Marcy repair of the myopectineal orifice consists of tightening an enlarged deep ring only. This procedure, com-

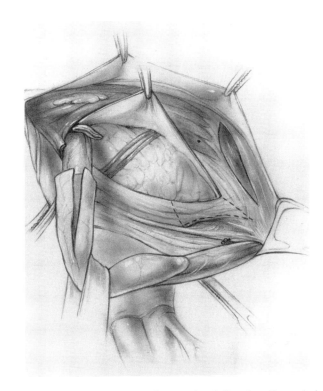

FIG. 34-6. *The appearance of a completed dissection. the groin is ready for a Bassini or Bassini-Shouldice surgical repair. Relaxing incisions are made by reflecting the external oblique aponeurosis medially and incising vertically the exposed aponeurosis of the internal oblique covering the rectus abdominis muscle. Relaxing incisions are beneficial in all hernioplasties except those in women and young men. When performing a McVay hernioplasty, the medial portion of the iliopubic tract, outlined by the dotted line, must be excised to expose the medial edge of the femoral sheath and Cooper's ligament for the placement of sutures.*

monly called simple ring closure, is indicated in men and women who have indirect hernias with only minimal damage to the deep ring (Fig. 34-7). This procedure was clearly illustrated in Marcy's remarkable 1892 book on hernias. Whether or not this is the hernioplasty Marcy claimed he performed in 1871 is uncertain. Marcy persistently claimed that it was, even though his contemporaries never concurred. Students of hernias have conflicting opinions of Marcy's claim to priority for performing the first hernioplasty, although all accredit simple ring closure to him. The operation restores the anatomy of the deep ring by placing one or two sutures in the transverse aponeurotic arch and the iliopubic tract just medial to the spermatic cord.

Simple ring closure is the hernioplasty of choice for women with indirect inguinal hernias. After dividing the round ligament and eliminating the sac, the deep ring is abolished with a few permanent sutures.

The *Bassini-Shouldice hernioplasty* repairs the myopectineal orifice superior to the inguinal ligament—that is, the deep ring and Hesselbach's triangle—and therefore is indicated in all direct and indirect inguinal hernias. Bassini is credited with developing and performing the first modern hernioplasty. Bassini wrote six papers about his surgical technique and experiences between 1887 and 1894, but it was his 1890 paper in German that ignited the enthusiasm of surgeons worldwide. Unfortunately, from the very beginning surgeons misinterpreted Bas-

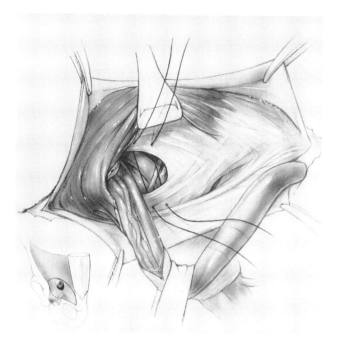

FIG. 34-7. Marcy's simple ring closure consists of a few interrupted stitches approximating the transverse aponeurotic arch and the iliopubic tract which will return the deep ring to its normal size. The blackened area in the inset illustrates the extent of the repair of the myopectineal orifice. *(Main figure is from Wantz GE: Atlas of Hernia Surgery, 1991, Fig. 4-29, p 57, with permission.)*

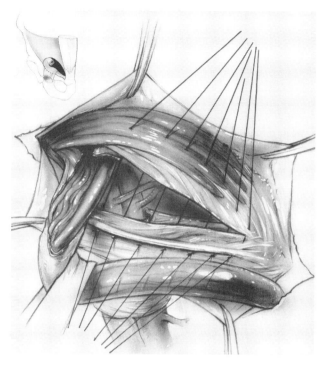

FIG. 34-8. The authentic Bassini hernioplasty consists of approximating the internal oblique abdominal muscle, the transversus abdominis muscle, and the transverse aponeurosis and fascia to the iliopubic tract and the shelving edge of the inguinal ligament with interrupted sutures. The blackened area in the inset illustrates the extent of the repair of the myopectineal orifice. *(Main figure is from Wantz GE: Atlas of Hernia Surgery, 1991, Fig 4-33, p 63 with permission.)*

sini's intent and modified and corrupted the operation. In North America, and to some extent in Europe, the Bassini repair consisted merely of high ligation of the sac and approximation of the conjoined tendon and the internal oblique abdominal muscle to the shelving of the inguinal ligament with interrupted sutures.

The authentic Bassini operation, which is currently performed in Europe and was detailed by Catterina (1932), includes deliberate and complete dissection to expose the anatomy in its entirety and a repair in which the internal oblique abdominal muscle, the transverse abdominal muscle, and the transversalis fascia (Bassini's triple layer) are approximated to both the femoral sheath and the shelving edge of the inguinal ligament with interrupted sutures (Fig. 34-8).

Obney and Ryan, working with Shouldice at his hernia clinic, developed de novo a hernioplasty (1950–1953) that is essentially identical to the original Bassini procedure. The dissection is exactly the same, and the repair approximates the identical myoaponeuroticofascial layers, albeit not with interrupted sutures but by precise imbrication with continuous sutures (Fig. 34-9). The Shouldice hernioplasty is, in fact, the modern equivalent of the original Bassini procedure.

The Bassini-Shouldice hernioplasty produces exceptional results and has become the worldwide standard to which other hernioplasties are compared. Nevertheless, the Bassini-Shouldice procedure has been justifiably criticized because it does not repair the femoral canal and may actually cause some femoral hernias by straining the femoral sheath. In addition, the repair is nonanatomic, because the transversalis aponeurosis is sutured to the inguinal ligament. Consequently some surgeons do not use the inguinal ligament and repair the myopectineal orifice superior to the inguinal ligament by simple edge-to-edge approxi-

mation of the transverse aponeurotic arch and the iliopubic tract. The technique is called the iliopubic tract repair to differentiate it from the Bassini and the Bassini-Shouldice procedures.

The *Cooper ligament hernioplasty* repairs the three most vulnerable areas for herniation in the myopectineal orifice—the deep ring, Hesselbach's triangle, and the femoral canal—and is therefore indicated for the three common types of hernias of the groin (Fig. 34-10). From his anatomic studies, McVay concluded (1942) that the proper structure to which the aponeurosis of the transverse abdominal muscle should be sewn was Cooper's iliopectineal ligament, where it is normally attached, not the inguinal ligament. He was unaware that Lotheissen had reported the procedure (1897) to repair a recurrent hernia in a woman without an inguinal ligament. Lotheissen immediately recognized the importance of the procedure in the treatment of femoral hernia. Lotheissen's Cooper ligament repair is currently known as the McVay hernioplasty in recognition of the man who popularized it.

In the McVay repair the transverse aponeurotic arch is sutured to Cooper's ligament medially and to the femoral sheath laterally. Exposure of Cooper's ligament and the medial border of the femoral sheath is accomplished by excision of the medial portion of the iliopubic tract (see Fig. 34-6). This extra step in the dissection is important for the accurate placement of sutures.

Relaxing incisions are mandatory because there is otherwise too much tension on the suture line. Although many enthusiasts use it routinely, McVay himself used it in only about half of the

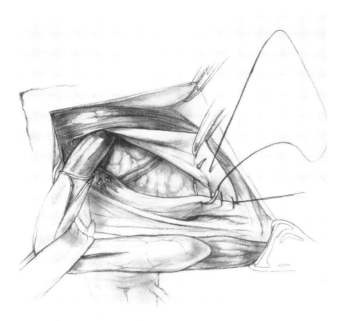

A

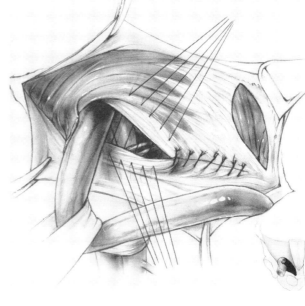

FIG. 34-10. The McVay repair approximates the transverse aponeurotic arch to Cooper's ligament and to the femoral sheath. The suture in the medial side of the femoral sheath is called the transition stitch. Excess tension is always present, and a relaxing incision is mandatory. The blackened area in the inset illustrates the extent of the repair of the myopectineal orifice. *(Main figure is from Wantz GE: Atlas of Hernia Surgery, 1991, Fig 4-44, p 76, with permission.)*

B

FIG. 34-9. The Shouldice-Bassini hernioplasty repairs the innermost aponeuroticofascial layer by imbrication. *A.* A continuous suture approximates the iliopubic tract to the undersurface of the transverse aponeurotic arch. The suture is then returned to its beginning by approximating the free edge of the transverse aponeurotic arch to the shelving edge of the inguinal ligament. *B.* As performed at the Shouldice Hospital, a second continuous suture unites the internal oblique abdominal muscle to the inguinal ligament in two layers. Most surgeons omit the suture and consider it superfluous. (From: *Wantz GE: Atlas of Hernia Surgery, 1991, Fig 4-35, p 65, Fig 4-37, p 67, with permission.)*

hernioplasties he performed; in those with smaller defects he performed what is essentially a Marcy repair.

Closure of the inguinal canal completes the hernioplasty and is the same in all the classical repairs. The aponeurosis of the external oblique abdominal muscle is reapproximated, which thereby incidentally reassembles the superficial ring. The distal stump of a divided cremaster muscle should be attached to the superficial ring to hitch up the testicle.

Special Considerations. *Femoral hernias* with small orifices in women are repaired from below the inguinal ligament with a few sutures (Bassini technique) or corked with a cylindrical plug of polypropylene mesh (see section on Lichtenstein tension-free hernioplasty) because they are rarely associated with hernias above the inguinal ligament (Fig. 34-11). Large femoral hernias in women and all femoral hernias in men, however, are repaired by the McVay Cooper ligament repair or, even better, by a properitoneal permanent prosthesis. Strangulated femoral hernias are preferably approached properitoneally because this provides direct access to the constricting femoral hernia orifice, easy release of the entrapped bowel by incision of the iliopubic tract and lacunar ligament, and ample room for bowel resection. Strangulated inguinal hernias are easily managed through a groin incision.

In indirect hernias in infants, children, and some young men, the myopectineal orifice and its transversalis fascial seal are not damaged and classical repair is unnecessary; merely eliminating the sac cures the hernia. The operation is called *high ligation of the sac* and consists of opening the inguinal canal and, without mobilization of the spermatic cord, identifying, dividing, and tracing the sac to the deep ring, where it is ligated. The operation is similar to the Ferguson and the Halsted II classical hernioplasties that are now largely obsolete.

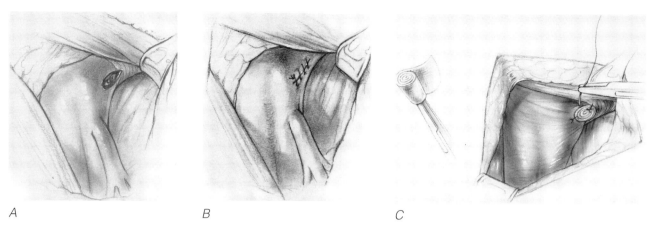

A   *B*   *C*

FIG. 34-11. *Femoral hernia. (A) The defect of small femoral hernias in women are successfully treated by (B) simple aponeurotic closure of the aponeurotic defect or by (C) implanting a cylindrical plug made from a 2-cm-wide strip of Marlex (Lichtenstein technique). Cone-shaped plugs fashioned from swatches of polypropylene mesh may be substituted for cylindrical plugs. Both conical and cylindrical plugs are also used to cork recurrent hernias if the aponeurotic defect is fibrotic and not too large.*

In infant girls the fallopian tube and ovary present commonly in hernial sacs. Testicular feminization is found in 1 percent of females with hernias, especially in cases of bilateral hernias. Therefore female infants with an inguinal hernia should have a buccal smear tested for chromatin. If an infant with normal-appearing external genitalia lacks chromatin, the gonad should be left in the inguinal canal. It will serve as an estrogen generator until after puberty, when it should be removed, because of the risk of malignant degeneration. Consequently, in females, a gonad found in the hernial sac without a fallopian tube should be biopsied for identification.

In boys, exploration of the contralateral groin is commonly performed up to the age of 3 years, especially if unilateral hernia is present on the left. This policy, disputed by some, serves to avoid a second hernioplasty at a later age.

Posterior Hernioplasty. Although the posterior properitoneal approach to repairing hernias was used sporadically in the nineteenth century, credit is generally given to Cheatle (1920) and Henry (1936) for elucidating and popularizing the virtues of the approach. They used a midline incision specifically to repair femoral hernia but recognized the potential of the approach for the repair of inguinal hernias. Nyhus and associates (1959) and later Read were the next to become enthused by the approach to treat both femoral and inguinal hernias, but Nyhus was the surgeon who actually championed the method and ultimately codified it. In this approach the properitoneal space was accessed via a short transverse incision in a lower quadrant rather than through a midline incision. The repair closes the direct space by suturing the iliopubic tract to the transverse aponeurotic arch and narrows the deep ring with a few sutures placed lateral to the spermatic cord.

The results of the properitoneal repair for primary hernioplasty even with a relaxing incision were less than satisfactory, and the procedure never became popular. An exception was the Cheatle-Henry midline approach for strangulated femoral hernias. However, the recent trend of implanting synthetic permanent prostheses for hernia repair has kindled a resurgence in the posterior properitoneal approach, and even Nyhus now buttresses his repairs with polypropylene mesh (Marlex).

Prosthetic Material for Hernioplasty. Nondegradable and biologic-tolerant synthetic mesh prostheses are readily available. Those proven useful are Marlex, Prolene, Trelex, Surgipro, Mersilene, and Gore-Tex. Each has its champions, none is perfect, and in practice the selection of the prosthesis material will be a compromise. They have, for all practical purposes, replaced the inconvenient biologic grafts such as autologous fascia lata.

Marlex, Trelex, and Prolene mesh, which resemble one another, are composed of knitted monofilament fibers of polypropylene. All are porous, slightly elastic, semirigid, and relatively heavy, and they contain plastic memory and buckle when bent in two directions at once.

Surgipro mesh is composed of knitted, braided strands of polypropylene. Its physical characteristics closely resemble those of knitted meshes of monofilament polypropylene.

Mersilene is an open-knitted mesh composed of pure, uncoated, braided fibers of the polyester Dacron. It is porous, soft, light, lacelike, supple, elastic, and without plastic memory; it has a grainy texture that prevents slippage and has only a minimal tendency to buckle when bent in two directions at once.

Gore-Tex is expanded polytetrafluoroethylene (PTFE, or Teflon). It is a nonporous, smooth, supple, fabriclike material containing through-and-through microscopic pores into which fibroblasts grow but through which serosanguineous fluid will not flow.

The prostheses made of polypropylene and polyester desirably incite a prompt fibroblast response and are rapidly integrated in the body with minimal inflammation. Gore-Tex is inert and does not incite fibroplasia or inflammation. It is not integrated in the tissues but rather is segregated by encapsulation. The process of encapsulation is slow, taking as long as 30 to 40 days. Perforated Gore-Tex is available, permitting early fixation and immobilization of the prosthesis during the process of encapsulation. The tendency of intestines to adhere to Gore-Tex is minimal. This feature, which the other permanent prostheses lack, may be advantageous for certain circumstances.

Polyester and polypropylene permanent prostheses should never contact abdominal viscera directly. They provoke binding and intimate adhesions that are difficult to divide and can cause intestinal obstruction and fistulization. Such adhesions can be prevented by interposing the omentum or an absorbable prosthesis between the permanent prosthesis and the bowel. Absorbable prostheses of knitted or woven polyglactin 910 (Vicryl) and polyglycolic acid (Dexon) are available. These prostheses also incite fibroplasia and can cause adhesions. However, they prevent the viscera from touching the permanent prosthesis during mesothelial integration of the permanent prosthesis and prevent grafting of the prosthesis to the viscera. A membranous sheet of Gore-Tex is also available. It is intended to substitute for absorbable meshes for the prevention of adhesions between viscera and polypropylene or polyester prostheses.

Infection and Synthetic Nonabsorbable Prostheses. All the synthetic materials can become sequestered, act like a foreign body and aggravate and prolong infections. Hence the risk of infection is balanced by the risk of recurrence. Theoretically, monofilament mesh ought to tolerate infection better than polyfilament mesh because bacteria can settle into and be hard to dislodge from the interstices of the polyfilament fibers. In practice this is not necessarily true, however, perhaps because the fibers are fine and the braid or twist is loose. The braided, knitted Dacron mesh Mersilene tolerates infection as well as, for example, the nonbraided, solid-fiber polypropylene meshes. If either is infected, integration rather than infection is the rule, provided suitable treatment is instituted and the prosthesis is in contact with healthy tissues and is not sequestered.

Expanded polytetrafluoroethylene (Gore-Tex) is intolerant of early infection because of the slow encapsulation of the material. If an infection develops in the space containing Gore-Tex, the material has to be removed, because there is no chance that it will become incorporated before bacteria have inhabited the microscopic spaces in the material. These spaces are too small to allow entrance of phagocytes and antimicrobial substances.

The management of infections in wounds in which there is a synthetic prosthesis is no different from that of other wounds. All that is needed is the application of sound surgical principles. Superficial infections not directly involving a prosthesis can be expected to heal.

Early infections involving a prosthesis must be treated vigorously and aggressively. The entire prosthesis must be exposed without delay. Failure to expose the entire prosthesis will lead to sinus formation. Local treatment is directed at irrigating purulent material, lysing cellular, fibrous, and fibrinous debris, and destroying the infectious agent. Saline solution, Dakin's solution, granulated sugar, and topical antimicrobial substances are all useful. Complete incorporation can be expected with meshes of both polypropylene and polyester (but not with expanded polytetrafluoroethylene) in 3 to 4 weeks, providing the mesh firmly contacts tissue and is not floating free. Systemic antibiotics, of course, are essential.

Delayed infections involving the prosthesis occur, and the interval between prosthetic implantation and infection may be months or years. In these cases and in all infected prosthetic wounds that have healed with a sinus, it is rarely possible for the prosthesis to become reintegrated, excision of the sequestered mesh is necessary. Only the sequestered mesh must be removed; the integrated mesh can remain.

Prophylaxis of infection is essential. Rigid sterile technique, precise and meticulous surgical technique, and the avoidance of seromas and hematomas with closed suction drains are important. When large pieces of mesh are used, broad-spectrum antibiotics should be administrated intravenously shortly before beginning the operation and continued postoperatively until the closed suction drains, if used, are removed. Intraoperatively, topical antibiotics are also commonly used. Prophylactic antibiotics are not necessary when small prostheses of polyester or polypropylene are used.

Inflammatory granulomas are occasionally encountered during prosthetic incisional hernioplasty. When bacteria are seen in a Gram stain of an inflammatory granuloma, the prudent course is not to implant a synthetic prosthesis. A hernia is a better condition to have than an infected prosthesis. However, Gram stains are not always reliable and may be negative while the culture of the granuloma is positive and grows bacteria. Knowing this possibility, some surgeons have proceeded in the presence of a granuloma to implant prostheses of both polypropylene and polyester successfully. Nevertheless, the correct advice is not to proceed.

Anterior Prosthetic Groin Hernioplasties. *Tension-Free Hernioplasties.* Prosthetic soft-tissue patches have been used for years to reinforce classical repairs but without significantly improving the results. However, when the prosthesis is implanted without a formal repair, thereby obviating tension, results improve dramatically. Lichtenstein credited this idea to R. Newman of Rahway, NJ, but it was Lichtenstein and his group who championed the tension-free hernioplasty and who reported favorable results in a large series of patients (Fig. 34-12). Lichtenstein, aware of the importance of tension as a cause of recurrence, had already developed a tension-free repair for femoral hernias and for recurrent direct and indirect inguinal hernias when the defect is fibrous, circumscribed, and not too large. The technique consists of a prosthetic plug that stoppers the aponeurotic defect (see Fig. 34-11). Lichtenstein got the idea of treating femoral hernias with a plug in the femoral canal from Cheatle, who in 1921 wrote that he "blocked this opening by coiling up into a plug the internal saphena vein."

Marlex, Prolene, Trelex, and Surgipro mesh are interchangeable and are the preferred prosthesis materials for the tension-free hernioplasties because they handle well and become quickly integrated.

The term tension-free was coined by Lichtenstein to describe his prosthetic hernioplasty, in which a formal repair of the parietal defect was not done. However, tension-free hernioplasty has become the generic term for all such hernioplasties performed through an anterior groin incision. Credit for originating the first tension-free and sutureless hernioplasty goes to Stoppa, who in 1969 introduced a properitoneal hernioplasty in which the parietal defects were not closed and peritoneal herniations were prevented by a large piece of unsutured polyester mesh. This hernioplasty is now known by the descriptive term giant prosthetic reinforcement of the visceral sac (GPRVS) and is discussed in the following section.

The Lichtenstein tension-free hernioplasty technique consists of a swatch of polypropylene mesh 8 × 16 cm, partway slit 1 cm from its inferior edge to accommodate the spermatic cord and fashioned for the patient. The mesh is sutured circumferentially to the internal oblique abdominal muscle, the rectus

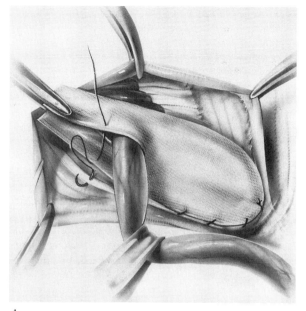

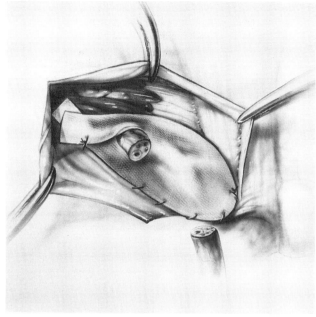

A

B

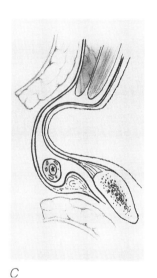

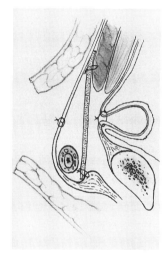

C

FIG. 34-12. Lichtenstein tension-free inguinal hernioplasty. *A.* A patch of polypropylene mesh about 8 × 16 cm is tailored to the patient and sutured to the rectus sheath and shelving edge of the inguinal ligament. Lichtenstein recommends that the superior edge be sutured to the internal oblique abdominal muscle. However, in most instances these sutures are superfluous, as the external oblique aponeurosis will hold the portion of the mesh securely in place. The tails of the mesh must be drawn equally before uniting the lower edge of each tail to the inguinal ligament with a polypropylene suture. *B.* When the procedure is completed, buckling of the central portion of the prosthesis occurs. *C.* No effort is made to repair the hernia, although it is necessary to position a direct inguinal hernia beneath a continuous absorbable suture to make the floor of the inguinal canal smooth. Indirect hernias are dealt with in conventional ways. *(A and B are from Wantz GE: J Am Coll Surg. 183:351, 1996, Fig 1A, B, p 352, with permission; C is from Wantz GE: Atlas of Hernia Surgery, 1991, Fig 6-1, p 98, 1991, with permission.)*

sheath, and the shelving edge of the inguinal ligament. The dissection includes a search for femoral hernias and division of the cremaster muscle, cremaster vessels, and the genital nerve to thin the cord. The tails of the mesh are drawn equally around the cord and the inferior edge of each tail is sutured to the inguinal ligament. For a successful hernioplasty the mesh must be as wide as possible, overlap the rectus sheath by more than 1 cm, extend laterally beyond the shutter mechanism, and snugly embrace the cord.

The Lichtenstein plug is cylindrical and made from a 2- to 2.5-cm strip of polypropylene mesh. For successful use of the plug the defect should be sclerotic and the plug must be wound firmly, fit snugly, and be sutured flush in place with four or more permanent synthetic sutures. The technique is especially useful in the elderly and the infirm with a single parietal defect. It is easily done with unassisted local anesthesia through a small

incision directly over the defect using minimal dissection and without disturbing the spermatic cord.

Gilbert serendipitously discovered that a cone-shaped plug fashioned from a piece of polypropylene mesh approximately 6 × 6 cm, when passed through the deep ring, would retain inverted indirect inguinal hernial sacs and could not be expelled on repeated Valsalva maneuvers (Fig. 34-13). Gilbert placed the cone plug through the deep ring and into the properitoneal space, where, he surmised, it unfolded like an umbrella to occlude the deep ring. The unfixed plug was reinforced with a patch similar in size and shape to that of the Lichtenstein repair but without fixation. He called the procedure the "sutureless hernioplasty" and used it with great success for indirect hernias without defective inguinal floors. Rutkow and Robbins expanded Gilbert's indications and used cone-shaped plugs in both indirect and direct inguinal hernias of all sizes. They used a patented and costly

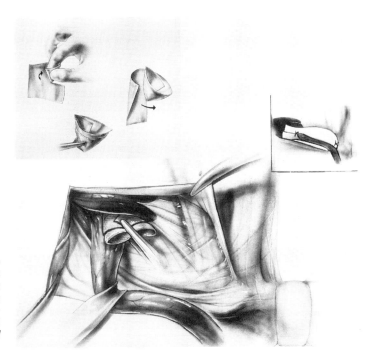

FIG. 34-13. A cone-shaped plug (*upper left inset*) is readily made from a 6- to 8-cm square of polypropylene mesh that has been partially slit and then rolled around the apex of the slit. The plug is inserted apex-first through the deep ring and into the properitoneal space. Gilbert's "sutureless hernioplasty" is completed with a swatch of mesh inlaid to the floor of the inguinal canal *(inset)* usually without sutures. (From: *Wantz GE: J Am Coll Surg, 1996, Figs 3 and 4, p 353, with permission.*)

commercial plug that has no advantages over the handmade cone-shaped plugs. The cone plug is also an effective barrier when merely placed without fixation within the deep ring, and unfolding is not apparent. Indirect hernial sacs are dealt with by conventional techniques, and direct inguinal hernial sacs are merely inverted beneath absorbable sutures. Plugs positioned to invert a diffuse direct inguinal hernial sac as used by Rutkow and Robbins are ineffective because they are expellable without a covering barrier of mesh.

In the tension-free hernioplasties the ilioinguinal nerve and the genital branch of the genitofemoral nerve, when not divided, are allowed to pass with the cord through the newly fashioned deep ring in the prosthesis.

The tension-free hernioplasties are tolerant of technical leeway. For example, the mesh in the Lichtenstein tension-free hernioplasty need not always be sutured to the internal oblique abdominal muscle or even to the inguinal ligament. The tails of the mesh surrounding the cord need not always be overlapped to create a secure newly constructed deep ring, especially when cone plugs are used to retain indirect hernial sacs. In general, tension-free hernioplasties should be tailored to the problem at hand. The tension-free hernioplasty most commonly used in men by the author is Gilbert's sutureless hernioplasty, to which is added a medial point of fixation with a suture on the rectus sheath and a lateral suture to close the tails of the mesh around the cord (Fig. 34-14). The mesh is positioned to allow the inferior edge to roll on the inguinal ligament. In all instances the dissection is minimal and the cremaster muscle and neurovascular bundle are not divided unless the cord is bulky.

The tension-free hernioplasties are contraindicated for hernias resulting from a connective tissue disorder. Also they usually are not needed in women with primary indirect inguinal hernias because simple obliteration of the deep ring always produces excellent results. The tension-free hernioplasties may not be appropriate for repair of most recurrent groin hernias in men

because they necessarily require redissection and remobilization of the spermatic cord, paramount causes of testicular atrophy. Stoppa's GPRVS would be a better choice because it is a posterior hernioplasty providing direct access to the parietal defects, obviating dissection of the spermatic cord and sensory nerves of the groin, and dealing more efficiently with the complex and diverse nature of recurrent hernias.

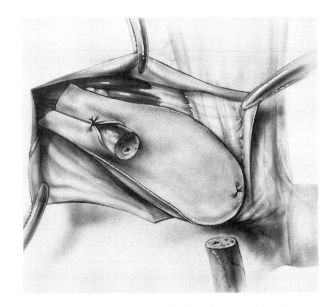

FIG. 34-14. Tension-free hernioplasties tolerate considerable technical leeway. Gilbert's "sutureless hernioplasty," to which is added a polypropylene suture to fix the mesh to the rectus sheath and another to close the tails of the mesh snugly around the cord, suffices for most indirect and direct inguinal hernias. (From: *Wantz GE: J Am Coll Surg. 183:351, 1996, Fig 2, p 352, with permission.*)

The tension-free hernioplasties have been highly touted and aggressively promoted by some of the fabricators of the prostheses and initiators of the procedures. Widespread enthusiasm for them has developed because they are easy to perform even with unassisted local anesthesia, recovery is quick, and results, thus far, are superb. Tension-free hernioplasties are especially suited to the management of simple primary hernias in men but are not the procedures of choice for complex groin hernias or for those with complications.

Posterior (Properitoneal) Prosthetic Groin Hernioplasty. *Stoppa Procedure—Giant Prosthetic Reinforcement of the Visceral Sac.* The properitoneal space is the logical site to implant a prosthesis. The prosthesis is held in place by intraabdominal pressure, and it is remote from the relatively avascular subcutaneous tissues and therefore relatively immune to superficial infection. The myopectineal orifice can be patched or plugged and hernioplasties buttressed with a prosthesis from the posterior approach just as they can be from the anterior (Fig. 34-15). The innovative and revolutionary properitoneal prosthetic technique introduced by Stoppa in 1969 is unique. He proposed eliminating hernias of the groin with a large unresorbable prosthesis that functionally replaces the transversalis fascia. The prosthesis adheres to the visceral sac and renders the peritoneum inextensible so that peritoneum cannot protrude through the myopectineal orifice or adjacent areas of weakness; repair of the defect in the abdominal wall is unnecessary. The operation is technically known by the descriptive phrase giant prosthetic reinforcement of the visceral sac (GPRVS) but is commonly called the Stoppa procedure.

GPRVS is performed bilaterally or unilaterally. In bilateral GPRVS a single large prosthesis is inserted in the properitoneal space of both groins through a midline or a Pfannenstiel incision (Fig. 34-16). The procedure requires general or regional anesthesia and is performed in ambulatory settings. The operation is the procedure of choice for all complex hernias of the groin such as recurrent hernias and hernias associated with connective tissue disorders. It is quick and exceptionally easy to perform, even in the obese, for whom it may be the preferred hernioplasty when they have bilateral hernias. It is the best hernioplasty for patients with primary hernias who prefer or require regional or general anesthesia.

In unilateral GPRVS a large prosthesis is inserted in the properitoneal space of a single groin. Usually it is performed through a transverse abdominal incision, but it also can be performed through an anterior groin incision, both transinguinally

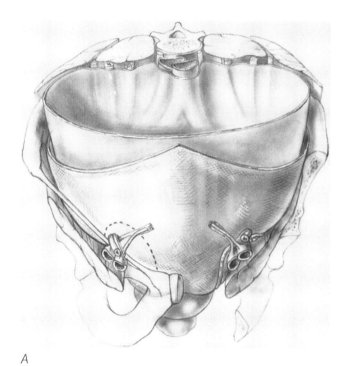

A

FIG. 34-16. Bilateral giant prosthetic reinforcement of the visceral sac. (A) A large prosthesis is implanted via a midline or a Pfannenstiel incision. The mesh extends far beyond the borders of the myopectineal orifice. The properitoneal space is widely cleaved. The pedicle of an indirect hernial sac is encircled (B), the sac divided (C), and the peritoneum is closed. The vas deferens and the testicular vessels are dissected from the parietal peritoneum (D). When freed, they will lie against the parietal wall of the pelvis (parietalization), and the prosthesis will cover the entire myopectineal orifice without a slit for the cord. The prosthesis for bilateral GPRVS is shaped like a chevron and arranged so that the stretch is transverse (E). The width equals the dimension between the anterior superior iliac spine minus 2 cm in a normal patient but can be larger in an obese patient. The vertical dimension equals the distance between the umbilicus and the symphysis pubis. The tails of the chevron are exaggerated to ensure a firm grip of the visceral sac. The prosthesis is implanted by long (30 cm) Wiley or Rochester Péan clamps so that the prosthesis smoothly envelopes the visceral sac. The large dead space may require drainage. The prosthesis is fixed with a single suture to the umbilical fascia only. (From: Wantz, GE: Surg Gynecol Obstet, 169:408, 1989, with permission.)

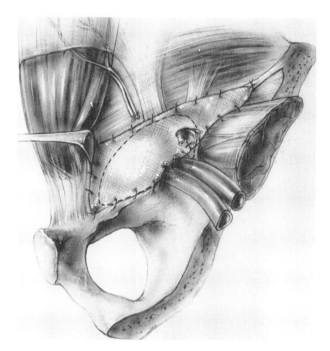

FIG. 34-15. Properitoneal patch prosthetic hernioplasty. The prosthesis is sutured to Cooper's ligament inferiorly and is fixed superiorly by incorporating it in the sutures that close the transverse lower quadrant access incision. A slit in the mesh accommodates the cord; in this case the slit is inferior, but it may be lateral. (From: *Wantz GE: Atlas of Hernia Surgery, 1991, Fig 6-5a, p 105, with permission.*)

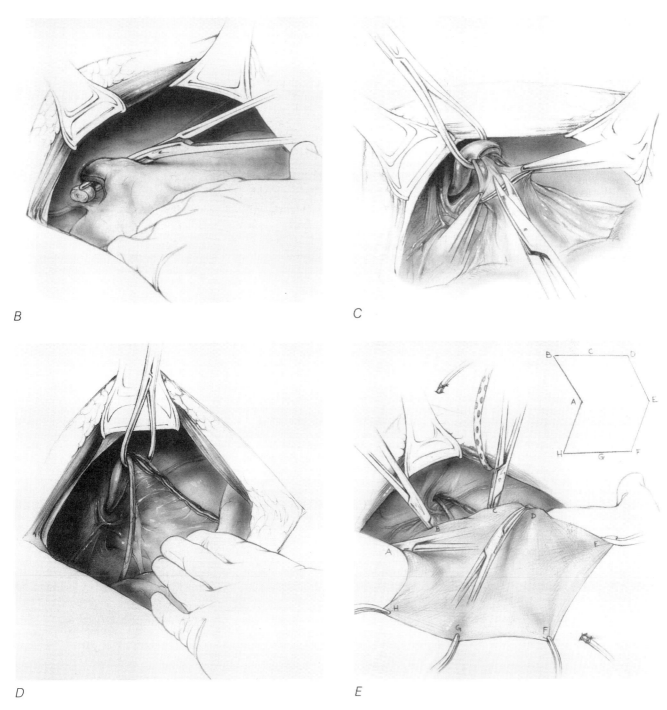

B

C

D

E

FIG. 34-16. *B.–E.* Continued.

or subinguinally (Fig. 34-17). The abdominal incision avoids the dissection of the inguinal canal and is preferred for men with recurrent inguinal hernias after classical repair. Transinguinal GPRVS is indicated when an unanticipated complex groin hernia is encountered, and subinguinal GPRVS is indicated when an unanticipated perivascular femoral hernia is encountered. All forms of unilateral GPRVS can be done in day surgery and with local anesthesia, with the possible exception of transabdominal GPRVS, which more often than not requires general or regional anesthesia.

Ordinarily, a large prosthesis in the properitoneal space would require a slit to accommodate the spermatic cord at the deep ring (see Fig. 34-15). The slit, sutured closed around the elements of the cord, partially holds the prosthesis in place but is also a potential site for peritoneal protrusion. However, a slit in the mesh becomes unnecessary if the elements of the spermatic cord—the vas deferens and the testicular vessels—are dissected from the peritoneum to which they are attached by the transversalis fascia. The elements of the cord can then lie against the wall of the pelvis and the properitoneal prosthesis will cover

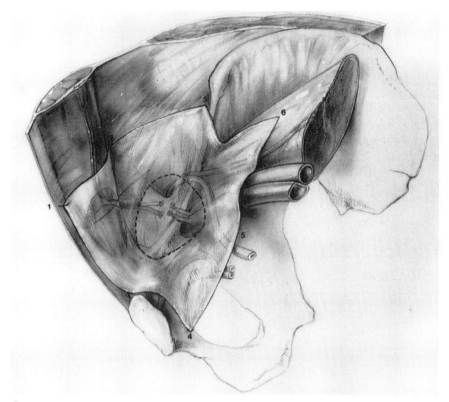

A

FIG. 34-17. *Unilateral GPRVS is the bilateral GPRVS cut in half (A). The prosthesis is shaped somewhat like a diamond (B). It is important that the bottom edge be wider than the top and that the lateral side be longer than the medial side. The width of the prosthesis at the superior edge is equal to the distance from the midline to the anterior superior iliac spine minus 1 cm. The vertical distance is around 14 cm. The length of the inferior-lateral corner increases the measured dimensions by 2 to 4 cm. The exaggerated elongated lateral inferior corner ensures a solid prosthetic grip on the lateral visceral sac. The prosthesis is drawn underneath the superior abdominal wall and fixed with sutures to the midline, to the semilunar line, and to the oblique muscles near the anterior superior iliac spine. The distal prosthesis is implanted with long (30 cm) Wiley or Rochester Péan clamps (C, D). Unilateral GPRVS can be done through an anterior groin incision using the above technique when an unanticipated complex inguinal hernia is encountered. (A is from Wantz GE: Surg Gynecol Obstet, 169:408, 1989, with permission; B, C, and D are from Wantz GE: Atlas of Hernia Surgery, 1991, Fig 6-38, p 141, Fig 6-40, p 146, and Fig 6-42, p 148, with permission.)*

them, the deep ring, and the myopectineal orifice completely. This technique, also devised by Stoppa, facilitates properitoneal prosthetic implantation (see Fig. 34-16).

The prosthetic material of choice for GPRVS is Mersilene because it is supple and elastic, stays in place without sutures, conforms to the complex curvature of the pelvis, and induces prompt fibroblastic integration. Placement of the prosthesis in GPRVS is done with long abdominal clamps. Other prostheses have been used. However, if the semirigid polypropylene meshes are substituted for Mersilene, some fixation will be necessary because they do not conform well. Gore-Tex also requires permanent fixation because encapsulation is very slow.

GPRVS is an efficient, anatomic, and tension-free repair. It is the ultimate hernioplasty. When correctly done, it cures all hernias of the groin, even prevascular femoral hernias, with very rapid recovery and minimal discomfort.

Laparoscopic Repair. Laparoscopic hernioplasty has attracted much attention and deserves comment, even though only

about 5 percent of groin hernias are repaired this way. There is no question that laparoscopic hernioplasty can be done successfully in experienced hands and that in some patients it produces less postoperative pain. The question is whether or not it should be done at all, because it is inherently riskier than open hernioplasty. Prospective randomized studies comparing open repair and laparoscopic repair on a nationwide scale are about to begin. Meanwhile, data from the most experienced laparoscopic hernia surgeons of Western Europe and North America have been published, and their morbidity, mortality, and recurrence rates have been compared with those of surgeons in Western Europe and North America who have specialized in open hernioplasty. The results showed that with the exception of wound infection, the morbidity, mortality, and recurrence rates after laparoscopic hernioplasty are significantly higher than those following open hernioplasty. *The degree of postoperative discomfort should never be the motivating factor in selecting the type of operation.* Rather, the procedure should be selected that will produce the

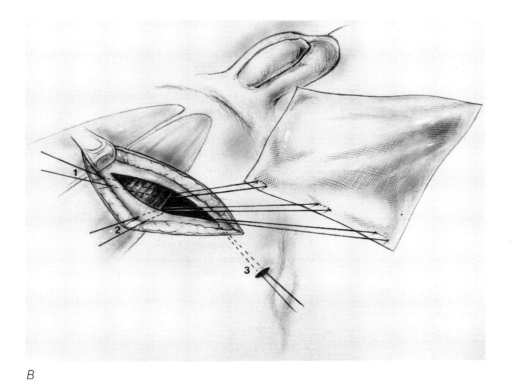

B

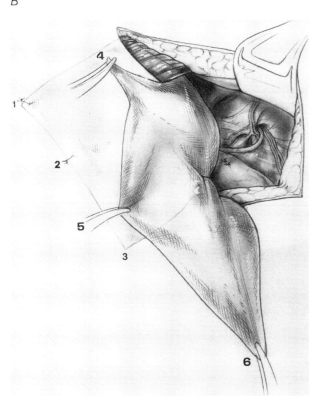

C

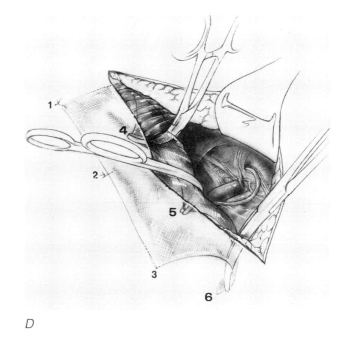

D

FIG. 34-17. *B.–D.* Continued.

best results with the least risks. To date, this is still open hernioplasty. Furthermore, laparoscopic hernioplasty always requires general or regional anesthesia and consumes more of the hospital's resources. Most important, unlike open hernioplasty,

it requires a surgeon who is very experienced and highly skilled with the technique. Open hernioplasty, preferably tension-free hernioplasty, with local anesthesia when possible, remains the procedure of choice for the majority of patients.

Complications. Ischemic orchitis, with its sequela of testicular atrophy, and residual neuralgia are the two important, although uncommon, complications unique to groin hernioplasty. They occur more frequently after anterior groin hernioplasty because the nerves and spermatic cord are necessarily dissected and mobilized. Recurrence also may correctly be considered a complication of groin hernioplasty, though surgeons traditionally have not categorized it as such.

Ischemic Orchitis and Testicular Atrophy. The clinical manifestations of ischemic orchitis develop insidiously, do not become apparent for 2 to 5 days after the hernioplasty, and are frequently misinterpreted initially. The testicle and spermatic cord become swollen, hard, tender, painful, and retracted. The process lasts 6 to 12 weeks and may resolve completely or end in testicular atrophy. Gangrene is unusual and orchiectomy is rarely necessary. The return of the testicle to normal size and shape does not mean that the process is complete, and atrophy of the testicle may not become apparent for as long as a year.

The etiology of ischemic orchitis is thrombosis of the spermatic cord, and the testicular pathology is intense venous congestion. The thrombosis is induced by surgical trauma to the cord, especially that associated with the dissection to completely remove a large indirect hernial sac. Dissection of a scrotal indirect hernial sac damages the delicate veins of the pampiniform plexus, initiates the thrombosis, and coincidentally disrupts collateral circulation (see section on dissection of classical repair).

There is no known successful treatment to prevent atrophy. Antibiotics, anti-inflammatory drugs, and massive doses of steroids are often given. Fortunately the incidence can be minimized by reducing surgical trauma to the cord by never excising the distal part of an indirect sac except when unavoidable; never dissecting beyond the pubic tubercle; and never redissecting an inguinal canal and spermatic cord in a patient who is predisposed to the complication by a previous anterior hernioplasty, vasectomy, hydrocelectomy, or other groin or scrotal surgery. In the latter situations posterior properitoneal prosthetic hernioplasty is the preferred alternative.

Neuralgia. Chronic residual neuralgia may result from surgical handling of the sensory nerves in the groin during hernioplasty or after hernioplasty from constricting scar tissue or adjacent inflammatory granulomas. The intraoperative trauma to the nerve, whether division, stretching, contusion, or suture entrapment, usually is not appreciated at the time. The pain may be localized, diffuse, projected along the course of a nerve, or referred to a nearby site. It may develop early or late, possibly weeks to months after the operation. In most cases the pain is accompanied by changes in mood and behavior. Depression, disturbed interpersonal relationships, and inability to resume work are common and complicate management. A multidisciplinary approach is beneficial.

A well-known cause of residual neuralgia is a neuroma. A neuroma results from a proliferation of nerve fibers outside the neurilemma of a partially or completely divided nerve. The pain from a neuroma varies in intensity, can be induced by changes in position, and is without spontaneous paroxysmal exacerbations. Hyperesthesia is detectable in the area of the lesion, and tapping the site may produce a severe shooting pain. The pain from deafferentation is different from the pain of a neuroma. It is burning and permanent with intermittent paroxysmal exacerbations. The area of involvement is anesthetic at first but becomes hyperesthetic. Typically the onset of deafferentation pain is delayed a week or so, and tapping the site does not produce exquisite pain.

The management of residual neuralgia is difficult. Neurolysis of the involved nerve may afford relief and is more likely to be successful if instituted early. The involved nerve may be identified by local anesthetic nerve blocks. The iliohypogastric and ilioinguinal nerves can be blocked and also divided in the groin. Blocking the genitofemoral nerve with certainty is impossible in the groin. Neuralgia from this nerve is identified by blocking L1 and L2 paravertebrally. Division of the genitofemoral nerve is performed through a flank incision or, preferably, through a laparoscope. Other adjunctive therapy includes analgesics, antidepressants, anticonvulsants, anxiolytics, and transcutaneous electrical stimulation. Injections of steroids in the involved area are sometimes helpful.

The prevention of nerve injury is important since the treatment of neuralgic complications is often unsuccessful. Fortunately they are rare. The sensory nerves should be preserved if possible; this is not always possible, and some small, not readily visible nerves are invariably divided. Occasionally major branches of the sensory nerves or the nerve trunks themselves must be divided in order to accomplish the hernioplasty. Division (usually with ligation) of the genital branch of the genitofemoral nerve is routine in most anterior groin hernioplasties. This virtually never produces genital nerve neuralgia and may suggest that complete division of the nerve is less likely to cause residual neuralgia than other types of nerve trauma. Most nerves require ligature to control bleeding. The ligature may also confine neuroma formation to within the neurilemma.

Recurrences. Very experienced hernia surgeons using classical repairs have been reported to obtain recurrence rates in the range of 1 to 3 percent in a 10-year follow-up. Such results are exceptional, and most surgeons are unable to duplicate them. Recurrences are caused by excessive tension on the repair, deficient tissues, inadequate hernioplasty, and overlooked hernias. Recurrences predictably are more common in patients with direct hernias, especially bilateral direct inguinal hernias, direct hernias presenting on both sides of the inferior epigastric vessels, and in direct hernias combined with an indirect hernia. Indirect recurrences result from insufficient excision of the proximal end of the sac, insufficient repair of the deep ring, and continued atrophy of the shutter mechanism. Most recurrences are direct and are usually in the region of the pubic tubercle, where suture line tension is the greatest. Relaxing incisions are always helpful. Repairing bilateral inguinal hernias simultaneously does not increase suture tension and is not a cause of recurrence, as was formerly believed.

Recurrent hernias require a prosthesis for successful repair. Recurrences after prosthetic patch and plug repairs occur in areas of the myopectineal orifice that are unprotected by the prosthesis, such as the deep ring. Paraprosthetic recurrences result from prostheses that are too small. Recurrences after anterior prosthetic hernioplasty are managed properitoneally with a second prosthesis or anteriorly with a prosthetic plug.

Recurrences after GPRVS occur if the properitoneal space is not cleaved widely enough or if the prosthesis is too small, poorly shaped, or incorrectly implanted. Recurrences after GPRVS usually are approached anteriorly and are managed by adding a prosthetic extension to the existing prosthesis. Alternatively, another permanent prothesis can be implanted transabdominally.

UMBILICAL HERNIA

The umbilicus is one of the weak areas of the abdomen and a common site of herniation. Umbilical hernias occur more frequently in women. Obesity and repeated pregnancies are common precursors, and ascites always exacerbates the problem. Umbilical hernia in adults is acquired and has no relationship to umbilical hernia in children. Strangulation of the colon and omentum is fairly common. Rupture occurs in chronic ascitic cirrhosis, in which case an emergency portal decompression is necessary.

Umbilical hernias are common in infants and close spontaneously if the aponeurotic defect is 1.5 cm or less. Repair is indicated in infants with hernial defects greater than 2 cm in diameter and in all children with umbilical hernia still present by the age of three or four.

The classical repair for umbilical hernias is the Mayo hernioplasty. The operation consists of vest-over-pants imbrication of the superior and inferior aponeurotic segments (Fig. 34-18). Currently, the Mayo repair, although still useful, is infrequently employed. Instead, umbilical hernias with a small parietal defect are merely closed by a to-and-fro, loosely placed polypropylene suture, and those with large parietal defects are managed with a prosthesis in a repair resembling that for incisional hernia.

EPIGASTRIC HERNIA

Epigastric hernia is a protrusion of properitoneal fat and peritoneum through the decussating fibers of the rectus sheath in the midline (linea alba) between the xiphoid process and the umbilicus. Epigastric hernias often are irreducible, invariably have small aponeurotic defects, sometimes are multiple, and often produce discomfort out of proportion to their size. Repair, usually through a vertical skin incision, is easy and similar to that of umbilical hernias.

SPIGELIAN HERNIA

Spigelian hernias are ventral hernias occurring along the subumbilical portion of Spieghel's semilunar line and through Spieghel's fascia. Spigelian hernias are rare and, unless large, are difficult to diagnose because they are interparietal and contained by the aponeurosis of the external oblique muscle. Ultra-

sonography and computerized tomography often reveal symptomatic spigelian hernias too small to detect clinically. Large spigelian hernias may be mistaken for sarcomas of the abdominal wall. Entrapped anterior cutaneous nerves of T10 to T12 produce discomfort resembling spigelian herniation.

Spieghel's fascia is actually aponeurotic and consists of the fused aponeuroses of the internal oblique and the transverse abdominal muscles between the belly of these muscles laterally and the rectus muscle medially (Fig. 34-19). Above the umbilicus the aponeurotic fibers of these muscles crisscross and form a fairly strong barrier. Below the umbilicus the fibers are more or less parallel and may split, permitting the peritoneum and properitoneal fat to protrude through a slitlike defect but to be retained by the overlying aponeurosis of the external oblique abdominal muscle. Although spigelian hernias occur anywhere along the semilunar line, they occur most commonly where Spieghel's fascia is widest and weakest. Spieghel's fascia is widest in the area between the umbilicus and the line connecting it to the anterior superior iliac spine, and it is weakest in the area just beneath the arcuate line and above the inferior epigastric vessels. Spigelian hernias may occur inferior to the epigastric vessels, in which case they are a variant of a direct inguinal hernia.

The neck of a spigelian hernia enlarges laterally by spreading apart the broad muscles of the abdomen. The rectus muscle and sheath inhibit medial enlargement. Small spigelian hernias are simply closed, but large spigelian hernias that are in the muscles require a prosthesis.

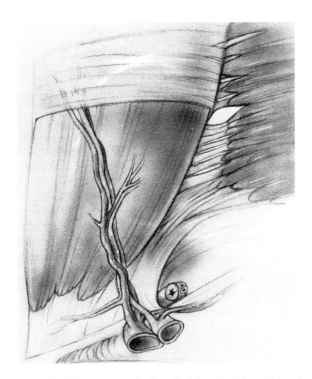

FIG. 34-19. The anatomy of a Spieghel's hernia. Spieghel's hernias occur anywhere along the semilunar line below the umbilicus, but they are most common at the level of the arcuate line that corresponds to the line connecting the anterior superior iliac spines. (From: *Wantz GE: Atlas of Hernia Surgery, 1991, Fig 10-1, p 174, with permission.*)

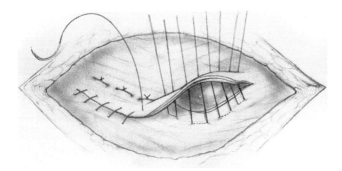

FIG. 34-18. Large umbilical hernias were traditionally repaired by the Mayo technique of vest-over-pants imbrication of the abdominal wall. Today large umbilical hernias usually are managed with a prosthesis, as is done in incisional hernias. (Adapted from: *Wantz GE: Atlas of Hernia Surgery, 1991, Fig 7-4, p 156, with permission.*)

LUMBAR HERNIA

Congenital, spontaneous, and traumatic herniations—all rare—occur through Grynfeltt's superior and Petit's inferior lumbar triangles. They are impossible to repair successfully without a prosthesis or a myoaponeurotic flap. Petit's triangle is an upright triangle bounded by the latissimus dorsi muscle, the external oblique abdominal muscle, and the iliac crest. It is covered by the superficial fascia only. Grynfeltt's triangle is an inverted triangle bounded by the twelfth rib, the internal oblique abdominal muscle, and the sacrospinalis muscle. It is covered by the latissimus dorsi.

The large, diffuse lumbar hernias occurring after kidney excision result in part from muscular paralysis, and aponeurotic defects are usually unidentifiable. They are managed as incisional hernias.

PELVIC HERNIA

Hernias occur in the obturator fossa, in the greater and lesser sciatic foramina, and in the perineum. All are rare and occur mainly in cachectic elderly patients, especially women. Of the hernias in the pelvis, the obturator hernia is most common, and when encountered it is almost always strangulated. Pressure on the obturator nerve causes pain in the region of the hip and of the knee and on the inner aspect of the thigh. This characteristic pain occurs in about half of the patients and is known as the Howship-Romberg sign. A palpable mass on pelvic or rectal examination or in the upper medial part of the thigh is occasionally noted. Prosthetic repair is normally necessary and is preferred unless septic conditions are present.

Perineal hernias occur through the pelvic diaphragm and may be anterior or posterior to the superficial transverse perineal muscle. The anterior perineal hernia is seen only in women and passes into the labia major, while the posterior perineal hernia enters the ischiorectal fossa in men and close to the vagina in women.

PARASTOMAL HERNIA

Parastomal hernias interfere with colostomy irrigations and the adhesion of stomal appliances. Paracolostomy hernias are more common than paraileostomy hernias, and both are more likely to occur when the stoma emerges through the semilunar line rather than the rectus sheath. Parastomal hernias therefore are usually lateral to the ostomy. Moving the stoma to a new location is the traditional method of management and is preferred to local repair. Local repair often fails because the belt muscles lateral to the ostomy lack sufficient aponeurosis. Among the prosthetic repairs, the preferred technique is the Leslie procedure (Fig. 34-20). This method is easy to perform, is nondebilitating, and for the author has essentially replaced transplantation of the stoma. It consists of closing the parietal defect lateral to the stoma in the subcutaneous tissues and then implanting a large piece of Mersilene that has been partially slit to accommodate the stoma and then spread out onto the anterior abdominal wall, to which it is fixed. Broad contact between the mesh and bowel is to be avoided. Mersilene is preferred to polypropylene meshes because it is soft, supple, and conforming. No sutures are placed in the intestinal wall.

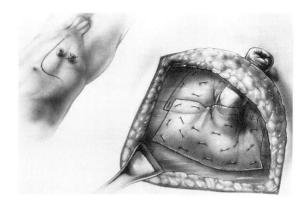

FIG. 34-20. The Leslie parastomal hernioplasty provides simple repair with minimal disability. The skin and subcutaneous tissues are elevated from the abdominal wall and the parietal defect lateral to the stoma is closed with through-and-through permanent sutures. A piece of Mersilene 10 to 15 cm square is slit partway to accommodate the bowel and then spread out onto the abdominal wall, to which it is fixed with staples or sutures. No sutures should be placed in the intestinal wall.

INCISIONAL HERNIA

Incisional hernias are a serious surgical problem. They have a propensity to enlarge, are frequently formidable to repair, and are usually accompanied by serious associated conditions. Patients with incisional hernias are usually obese. Obesity and infection are the two principal causes of this condition. The weight of the panniculus adiposus itself pulls apart the surgical incision, and infection hampers wound healing. Hypertension, cardiac and renal disorders, diabetes, and purulent intertrigo commonly accompany obesity and increase the morbidity of repair.

Eventration Disease. The loss of integrity of the abdominal wall reduces intraabdominal pressure and causes serious disturbances, which Rives appropriately named "eventration disease." The salient feature of the syndrome is respiratory dysfunction. A large incisional hernia produces paradoxical respiratory abdominal motion similar to that of a flail chest. Diaphragmatic function becomes inefficient. The diaphragm no longer contracts against the abdominal viscera and instead forces them into the hernial sac. Appraisal of respiratory function and blood gases is essential.

The detachment of the tendinous insertion of the broad belt muscles of the abdomen aggravates midline incisional hernias. The muscles retract, pull apart the parietal defect, and cause the normally horizontal belly of the rectus muscle to assume a vertical position. Contraction of the rectus muscles then expels rather than retains the abdominal viscera. Ultimately atrophy, fatty degeneration, and fibrosis of the lateral muscles ensue and make tendinous reinsertion of the belt muscle by the midline approximation of the linea alba difficult. In some midline hernias real loss of the abdominal wall may be present as a result of infection, trauma, or repeated laparotomies. In most cases, however, the loss of substance is more apparent than real.

The viscera lose their right of domain in the abdomen in long-standing large incisional hernias. In this instance the reduction of the viscera at operation can cause death by compression of the inferior vena cava and by respiratory failure from forced elevation and immobilization of the diaphragm. The introduction of pneumoperitoneum by Goni-Moreno in 1947 made these formerly inoperable hernias reparable.

Reduced intraabdominal pressure from the hernia also causes edema of the mesentery and stasis in the splanchnic venous system and the inferior vena cava. Distention and atony of the hollow viscera occur, and decreasing the ability to raise intraabdominal pressure and producing difficulties with micturition and bowel movements. Back pain is a common complaint; it is caused by lordosis resulting from retraction of the belt muscles and decreased efficiency of the rectus muscles.

The skin and subcutaneous tissues overlying large incisional hernias are stretched and damaged. The skin becomes atrophic, hypoxic, and devoid of subcutaneous fat. Spontaneous ulcerations develop. Typically they are solitary, occur at the apex of the hernia, and are misconstrued as a pressure sore. They resist healing and require intensive local and systemic antimicrobial therapy to prevent septic complications at the time of hernioplasty.

Obese patients with large incisional hernias are especially at risk for postoperative septic complications, respiratory dysfunction, and pulmonary emboli. Preoperative and postoperative prophylaxis for these problems is essential.

Progressive pneumoperitoneum is a useful technique to prepare patients for incisional hernioplasty because it overcomes some of the disorders of eventration disease. Pneumoperitoneum stretches the abdominal wall and intraabdominal adhesions, facilitates the return of the viscera to the abdomen, and improves diaphragmatic function. The technique of pneumoperitoneum is simple. Air is injected into the peritoneal cavity through a pneumoperitoneum needle that has been inserted with the aid of local anesthesia. The peritoneal cavity is insufflated until the patient experiences shortness of breath or shoulder pain. At first the patient may tolerate only small amounts of air. Sometimes as much as 2 to 4 L may be insufflated initially. Thereafter, air is added as needed at intervals of 1 to 3 days. The pneumoperitoneum is maintained for 10 to 20 days. The patient is ready for operation when palpation reveals flabbiness in the flanks. The inability of the patient to tolerate pneumoperitoneum is a contraindication for incisional hernioplasty.

Incisional Hernioplasty. The object of incisional hernioplasty is anatomic reconstruction of the abdominal wall. This includes closure of the parietal defect, restoration of normal in-

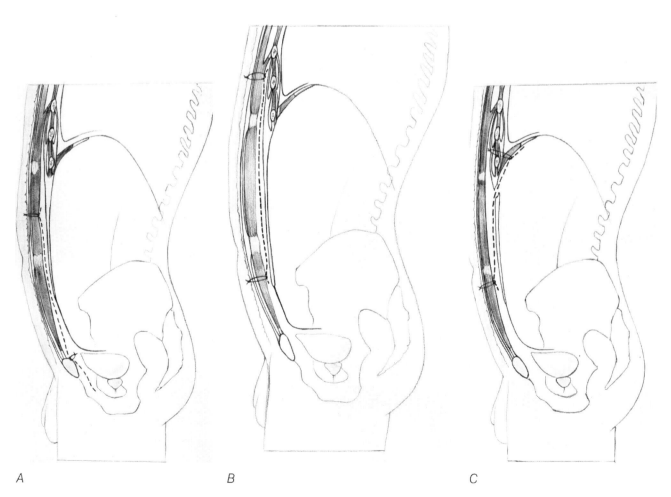

A   *B*   *C*

FIG. 34-21. Parasagittal dissection showing the site of implantation of the prosthesis (broken line) and suture fixation in the Rives-Stoppa incisional hernioplasty in *(A)* subumbilical midline incisional hernias, *(B)* supraumbilical midline incisional hernias, and *(C)* subcostal incisional hernias. (From: *Wantz GE: Atlas of Hernia Surgery, 1991, Fig 11a–c, pp 186–187, with permission.*)

traabdominal pressure, and, in midline hernias, tendinous reinsertion of the lateral abdominal muscles. Most small incisional hernias are managed by simple closure of the aponeurotic defect. However, large incisional hernias with aponeurotic defects greater than 10 cm have a marked tendency to recur. Repairs performed by approximating aponeurosis edge to edge or by the Judd or Mayo technique of imbrication frequently fail and have recurrence rates as high as 50 percent. Consequently most incisional hernias and all recurrent incisional hernias require a prosthesis for a successful repair. Of the many proposed techniques, those developed by Rives and by Stoppa, essentially identical procedures, are preferred. The Rives-Stoppa technique is applicable to all types of abdominal incisional hernias, including postnephrectomy lumbar hernias and parastomal hernias.

In the Rives-Stoppa hernioplasty a very large Mersilene prosthesis is implanted deep to the muscles of the abdominal wall on top of the posterior rectus sheath or peritoneum (Figs. 34-21 and 34-22). The prosthesis extends far beyond the borders of the myoaponeurotic defects and is firmly held in place by intraabdominal pressure (Pascal's principle) and later by fibrous ingrowth. The prosthesis prevents peritoneal eventration in two ways: by rendering the visceral sac indistensible and by solidly uniting and consolidating the abdominal wall. The technique thus uses the same concept and principles as Stoppa's preperitoneal inguinal hernioplasty and, as noted earlier, is known tech-

nically as giant prosthetic reinforcement of the visceral sac (GPRVS).

The knitted elastic Mersilene prosthesis is arranged so that it expands vertically and is inextensible horizontally. The mesh must extend beyond the lateral borders of the aponeurotic defect by 8 to 10 cm. The distance inferiorly and superiorly is less critical, and 4 to 5 cm suffices. Above the umbilicus, the linea alba interferes with the midline placement of the prosthesis, and a slit in the middle of the superior edge of the prosthesis is necessary to allow the prosthesis to protrude upward within the rectus sheath on either side of the linea alba. Traction-fixation sutures proposed by Rives, placed 5 to 6 cm apart, fix the prosthesis circumferentially to the abdominal wall (Fig. 34-23). The lateral traction-fixation sutures also stretch the retracted belt muscles and facilitate midline approximation. Fixation sutures are not needed when the prosthesis extends deep into the space of Retzius or far into the iliac fossa. When the retromuscular space is undissectable, the prosthesis must be implanted intraperitoneally. The intraperitoneal prosthesis must be prevented from touching the viscera either by the omentum or by an absorbable synthetic prosthesis. An absorbable prosthesis is used to substitute for the posterior rectus sheath when it is insufficient.

Aponeurotic closure of the parietal defect is important. The midline closure can withstand greater tension because the pros-

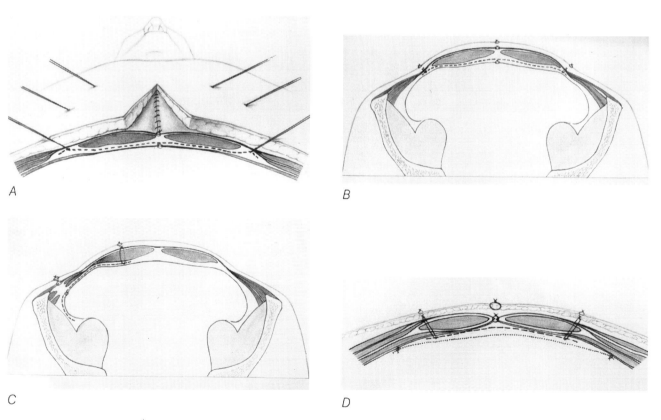

A

B

C

D

FIG. 34-22. Cross-section of the abdominal wall anatomy showing site of implantation of prosthesis (broken line), the lateral extent of the prosthesis, and the suture for traction and fixation of the prosthesis in (A) epigastric region, (B) hypogastric region, and (C) right lower quadrant (appendectomy) incisional hernia. Occasionally the prosthesis must be placed intraperitoneally (D). In these cases the prosthesis must be prevented from touching the bowel, by interposition of omentum or a synthetic absorbable prosthesis. (A, B, and C are from Wantz GE: Atlas of Hernia Surgery, 1991, Fig 11-5a, p 188, Fig 11-5c, p 188, Fig 11-5d, p 189, with permission.)

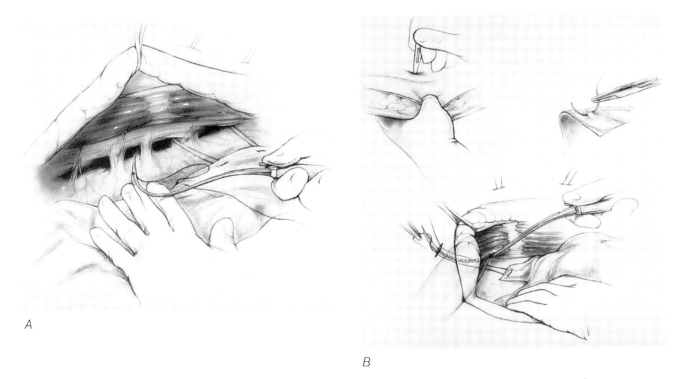

A

B

FIG. 34-23. The retromuscular space has been dissected, exposing the intercostal vessels and nerves. A Reverdin suture needle facilitates the placement of the sutures for prosthetic fixation. (From: *Wantz GE: Atlas of Hernia Surgery, 1991, Fig 11-17a, b, pp 202–203, 1991, with permission.*)

thesis, not the suture line, ultimately unites the abdomen. When necessary, tension can be reduced by 1-cm vertical relaxing incisions arranged quincuncially in the rectus sheath. Each row of overlapping relaxing incisions expands the rectus sheath by 1 cm. Long relaxing incisions are not recommended above the umbilicus and should *never* be made below the umbilicus. Aponeurotic approximation is usually achievable, but when it is not, a second absorbable or nonabsorbable prosthesis inlaid in the aponeurotic defect will ensure stability of the abdominal wall during the healing process. Usually this occurs in the region of the xiphoid process or symphysis pubis. Dead space created by a large prosthesis always requires closed suction drainage to prevent seromas and hematomas and to allow quick fibrous incorporation of the prosthesis in the abdominal wall. The drains on top of the prosthesis are not removed until the drainage is essentially nil.

Infection. Infection is a serious complication and occurs in as many as 10 percent of the cases. For this reason major prosthetic incisional hernioplasties are considered "dirty cases". Management of wound infections involving a synthetic nonabsorbable prosthesis is addressed earlier in the subsection Infection and Synthetic Nonabsorbable Prosthesis.

Bibliography

Abdu RA: Repair of paracolostomy hernia with Marlex mesh. *Dis Colon Rectum* 25:529, 1982.

Anson BJ, McCormick LJ, Cleveland HC: Anatomy of hernial regions: Obturator hernia and general considerations. *Surg Gynecol Obstet* 90:31, 1950.

Anson BJ, McVay CB: Inguinal hernia: the anatomy of the region. *Surg Gynecol Obstet* 66:186, 1938.

Anson BJ, McVay CB: The anatomy of the inguinal and hypogastric regions of the abdomen. *Anat Rec* 70:211, 1938.

Anson BJ, Morgan BH, McVay CB: The anatomy of hernial regions—inguinal hernia. *Surg Gynecol Obstet* 89:417, 1949.

Anson BJ, Morgan BH, McVay CB: Surgical anatomy of the inguinal region, based upon a study of 500 body halves. *Surg Gynecol Obstet* 111:707, 1960.

Anson BJ, Reiman AF, Swigart LL: The anatomy of hernial regions—femoral hernia. *Surg Gynecol Obstet* 89:753, 1949.

Arnbjornsson E: Development of right inguinal hernia after appendectomy. *Am J Surg* 143:174, 1982.

Arnbjornsson E: A neuromuscular basis for the development of right inguinal hernia after appendectomy. *Am J Surg* 143:367, 1982.

Askar OM: Aponeurotic hernias: Recent observations upon paraumbilical and epigastric hernias. *Surg Clin North Am* 64:315, 1984.

Balthazar EJ, Subramanyam BR, et al: Spigelian hernia: CT and ultrasonography diagnosis. *Gastrointest Radiol* 9:81, 1984.

Bassini E: Uber die Behandlung des Leistenbruchs. *Arch Klin Chir* 40:429, 1890.

Bayer I, Kyzer S, et al: A new approach to primary strengthening of colostomy with Marlex mesh to prevent paracolostomy hernia. *Surg Gynecol Obstet* 163:579, 1986.

Berliner SD, Burson LC, et al: The Henry operation for incarcerated and strangulated femoral hernias. *Arch Surg* 127:314, 1992.

Blumberg NA: Infantile umbilical hernia. *Surg Gynecol Obstet* 150:187, 1980.

Brereton RJ: Hernia repair in children. *Lancet* 1:156, 1980.

Cannon DJ, Read RC: Metastatic emphysema, a mechanism for acquiring inguinal herniation. *Ann Surg* 194:270, 1981.

Cheatle GT: An operation for the radical cure of inguinal and femoral hernia. *Br Med J* 2:68, 1920.

Chevrel JP: *Surgery of the Abdominal Wall.* Berlin, Springer-Verlag, 1987.

Chevrel JP, Gatt MT: The treatment of neuralgias following herniorrhaphy: A report of 47 cases. *Postgrad Gen Surg* 4:142, 1992.

Clark JH, Hashimoto EI: Utilization of Henle's ligament, iliopubic tract, aponeurosis transversus abdominis, and Cooper's ligament in inguinal herniorrhaphy. *Surg Gynecol Obstet* 82:480, 1946.

Condon RE: Surgical anatomy of the transversus abdominis and transversalis fascia. *Ann Surg* 173:1, 1971.

Condon RE: Peristomal hernia, in Nyhus LM, Condon RE (eds): *Hernia,* 4th ed. Philadelphia, JB Lippincott, 1995.

Conner WT, Peacock EE: Some studies on the etiology of inguinal hernia. *Am J Surg* 126:735, 1973.

Cooper AP: *The Anatomy and Surgical Treatment of Abdominal Hernia* (2 vols). London, Longmans, 1804, 1807.

Corbitt JD: Laparoscopic herniorrhaphy. *Surg Laparosc Endosc* 1:23, 1991.

Devlin HB: *Management of Abdominal Hernias.* London, Butterworth, 1988.

Fong Y, Wantz GE: Prevention of ischemic orchitis during inguinal hernioplasty with 6454 hernioplasties in male patients. *Surg Gynecol Obstet* 174:399, 1992.

Fruchaud H: *Le Traitement Chirurgical des Hernies de l'Aine chez l'Adulte.* Paris, G. Doin, 1956.

Fruchaud H: *Anatomie Chirurgicale des Hernies de l'Aine.* Paris, G. Doin, 1956.

Gallegos NC, Dawson J, et al: Risk of strangulation in groin hernias. *Br J Surg* 78:1171, 1991.

Ger R, Monroe K, et al: Management of indirect inguinal hernias by laparoscopic closure of the neck of the sac. *Am J Surg* 159:371, 1990.

Gilbert AI: An anatomic and functional classification for the diagnosis and treatment of inguinal hernia. *Am J Surg* 157:331, 1989.

Gilbert AI: Sutureless repair of inguinal hernia. *Am J Surg* 163:331, 1992.

Gilbert AI, Graham MF: Technical and scientific objections to laparoscopic herniorrhaphy. *Problems in General Surgery* 12:205, 1995.

Gilbert M, Clatworthy HW: Bilateral operations for inguinal hernia and hydrocele in infancy and childhood. *Am J Surg* 97:255, 1959.

Glassow F: Femoral hernia: Review of 1143 consecutive repairs. *Ann Surg* 163(pt 1):227, 1966.

Glassow F: The surgical repair of inguinal and femoral hernias. *Can Med Assoc J* 108:308, 1973.

Glassow F: Inguinal hernia repair using local anesthesia. *Ann R Coll Surg Engl* 66:382, 1984.

Gray SW, Skandalakis JE, et al: Strangulated obturator hernia. *Surgery* 75:20, 1974.

Greenberg AG, Saik RP, et al: Expanded indications for preperitoneal hernia repair: The high-risk patient. *Am J Surg* 138:149, 1979.

Griffith CA: Inguinal hernia: An anatomic surgical correlation. *Surg Clin North Am* 39(2):531, 1959.

Griffith CA: The Marcy repair of indirect inguinal hernia. *Surg Clin North Am* 51:1309, 1971.

Griffith CA: The Marcy repair revisited. *Surg Clin North Am* 64:215, 1984.

Gullmo A: Herniography. *World J Surg* 13:560, 1989.

Halverson K, McVay CB: Inguinal and femoral hernioplasty: A 22-year study of the authors' methods. *Arch Surg* 101:127, 1970.

Henry AK: Operation for femoral hernia by a midline, extraperitoneal approach with a preliminary note on the use of this route for reducible inguinal hernia. *Lancet* 1:531, 1936.

Houck JP, Rypins EB, et al: Repair of incisional hernia. *Surg Gynecol Obstet* 169:397, 1989.

Kaplan SA, Snyder WH Jr, et al: Inguinal hernia in females and the testicular feminization syndrome. *Am J Dis Child* 117:243, 1969.

Law NW, Ellis H: Adhesion formation and peritoneal healing on prosthetic materials. *Clinical Materials* 3:95, 1988.

Leslie D: The parastomal hernia. *Surg Clin North Am* 64:407, 1984.

Lichtenstein IL: *Hernia Repair Without Disability,* 2d ed. St Louis, Ishiyaku Euroamerica, 1987.

Lichtenstein IL, Shore JM: Simplified repair of femoral and recurrent inguinal hernias by a "plug" technic. *Am J Surg* 128:439, 1974.

Lichtenstein IL, Shulman AG, et al: The tension-free hernioplasty. *Am J Surg* 157:188, 1989.

Lichtenstein IL: Tension-free techniques held safe and effective for all hernia repairs. *General Surgery News* 9(12):1, 1990.

Light HG: Hernia of the inferior lumbar space. *Arch Surg* 118:1077, 1983.

Lotheissen G: Zur Radikaloperation der Schenkelhernien. *Zbl Chir* 25:548, 1898.

Lytle WJ: Femoral hernia. *Ann R Coll Surg Engl* 21:244, 1957.

Lytle WJ: Deep inguinal ring: Development, function, and repair. *Br J Surg* 57:531, 1970.

Madden JL, Peacock EE: Studies of the biology of collagen during wound healing: I. Rate of collagen synthesis and deposition in cutaneous wounds of the rat. *Surgery* 64:288, 1968.

Madden JL, Peacock EE: Studies of the biology of collagen during wound healing: III. Dynamic metabolism of scar collagen and remodeling of dermal wounds. *Ann Surg* 174:511, 1971.

Madden JL: *Abdominal Wall Hernias: An Atlas of Anatomy and Repair.* Philadelphia, WB Saunders, 1989.

Marcy HO: *The Anatomy and Surgical Treatment of Hernia.* New York, Appleton, 1892.

Mayo WJ: An operation for the radical cure of umbilical hernia. *Ann Surg* 34:276, 1901.

McNaught GHD: Femoral hernia: The rectus sheath operation of McEvedy. *J R Coll Surg Edinb* 1:309, 1956.

McVay CB: The anatomy of the relaxing incision in inguinal hernioplasty. *Quarterly Bulletin of North West University Medical School* 36:245, 1962.

McVay CB: Inguinal hernioplasty: Common mistakes and pitfalls. *Surg Clin North Am* 46:1089, 1966.

McVay CB: The normal and pathologic anatomy of the transversus abdominis muscle in inguinal and femoral hernia. *Surg Clin North Am* 51:1251, 1971.

McVay CB: The anatomic basis for inguinal and femoral hernioplasty. *Surg Gynecol Obstet* 139:931, 1974.

McVay CB, Savage LE: Etiology of femoral hernia. *Ann Surg* 154:25, 1961.

Moosman DA, Oelrich TM: Prevention of accidental trauma to the ilioinguinal nerve during inguinal herniorrhaphy. *Am J Surg* 133:146, 1977.

Moran RM, Blick M, et al: Double layer of transversalis fascia for repair of inguinal hernia: Results in 104 cases. *Surgery* 63:423, 1968.

Munshi IA, Wantz GE: Management of recurrent and perivascular femoral hernias by giant prosthetic reinforcement of the visceral sac. *J Am Coll Surg* 182:417, 1996.

Nehme A: Groin hernias in elderly patients: Management and prognosis. *Am J Surg* 146:257, 1983.

Nyhus LM: An anatomic reappraisal of the posterior inguinal wall, with special consideration of the iliopubic tract and its relation to groin hernias. *Surg Clin North Am* 44:1305, 1960.

Nyhus LM: The recurrent groin hernia: Therapeutic solutions. *World J Surg* 13:541, 1989.

Nyhus LM, Condon RE, et al: Clinical experiences with preperitoneal hernial repair for all types of hernia of the groin, with particular reference to the importance of transversalis fascia analogues. *Am J Surg* 100:234, 1960.

Nyhus LM, Condon RE: *Hernia,* 4th ed. Philadelphia, JB Lippincott, 1995.

Nyhus LM, Klein MS, et al: Inguinal hernia. *Curr Probl Surg* 73:407, 1991.

Nyhus LM, Pollak R, et al: The preperitoneal approach and prosthetic buttress repair for recurrent hernia. *Ann Surg* 208:733, 1988.

Obney N: Shouldice technique for repair of inguinal hernia. *Bull N Y Acad Med* 55:863, 1979.

Orcutt TW: Hernia of the superior lumbar triangle. *Ann Surg* 173:294, 1971.

Peacock EE: Biology of hernia. In: Nyhus LM, Condon RE (eds): *Hernia*, 2d ed. Philadelphia, JB Lippincott, 1978.

Pearl RK: Parastomal hernias. *World J Surg* 13:569, 1989.

Ponka JL: The relaxing incision in hernia repair. *Am J Surg* 115:552, 1968.

Popp LW: Endoscopic patch repair of inguinal hernia in a female patient. *Surg Endosc* 4:10, 1990.

Raynor RW, DelGuercio LRM: The place for pneumoperitoneum in the repair of massive hernia. *World J Surg* 13:581, 1989.

Read RC: Bilaterality and the prosthetic repair of large recurrent inguinal hernias. *Am J Surg* 138:788, 1979.

Read RC: Marcy's priority in the development of inguinal herniorrhaphy. *Surgery* 88:682, 1980.

Read RC: Preperitoneal herniorrhaphy: A historical review. *World J Surg* 13:532, 1989.

Rignault DP: Preperitoneal prosthetic inguinal herniorrhaphy through a Pfannenstiel approach. *Surg Gynecol Obstet* 162:465, 1986.

Rives J with the collaboration of Pire JC, Flament JB, et al: Major incisional hernias. In: Chevrel JP (ed): *Surgery of the Abdominal Wall*. New York, Springer-Verlag, 1987, p 116.

Rutledge RH: Cooper's ligament repairs: A 25-year experience with a single technique for all groin hernias in adults. *Surgery* 103:1, 1988.

Ryan EA: Hernias related to pelvic fractures. *Surg Gynecol Obstet* 133:440, 1971.

Schultz LS, Graber JN, et al: Laser laparoscopic herniorrhaphy: A clinical trial preliminary results. *J Laparoendosc Surg* 1:41, 1990.

Schumpelick V: *Atlas of Hernia Surgery*. Philadelphia, BC Decker, 1990.

Shearburn EW, Myers RN: Shouldice repair for inguinal hernia. *Surgery* 66:450, 1969.

Shulman AG, Amid PK, Lichtenstein IL: The "plug" repair of 1402 recurrent inguinal hernias. *Arch Surg* 125:265, 1990.

Skandalakis JE, Gray SW, et al: *Hernia: Surgical Anatomy and Technique*. New York, McGraw-Hill, 1989.

Smedberg SGG, Broom ARE, et al: Ligation of the hernial sac? *Surg Clin North Am* 64:299, 1984.

Spangen L: Spigelian hernia. *World J Surg* 13:573, 1989.

Spaw AT, Ennis BW, et al: Laparoscopic hernia repair: The anatomic basis. *J Laparoendosc Surg* 1:269, 1991.

Starling JR, Harms BA: Diagnosis and treatment of genitofemoral and ilioinguinal neuralgia. *World J Surg* 13:586, 1989.

Stoppa RE: The preperitoneal approach and prosthetic repair of groin hernias. In: Nyhus LM, Condon RE (eds): *Hernia*, 4th ed. Philadelphia, JB Lippincott, 1995.

Stoppa RE: The treatment of complicated groin and incisional hernias. *World J Surg* 13:545, 1989.

Stoppa RE, Rives JL, et al: The use of Dacron in the repair of hernias of the groin. *Surg Clin North Am* 64:269, 1984.

Stoppa RE, Warlaumont CR: Repair of recurrent groin hernias by the insertion of giant mesh prostheses through the midline preperitoneal approach (GPMPA). In: Madden JL (ed): *Abdominal Wall Hernias: An Atlas of Anatomy and Repair*. Philadelphia, WB Saunders, 1989.

Stulz P, Pfeiffer KM: Peripheral nerve injuries resulting from common surgical procedures in the lower portion of the abdomen. *Arch Surg* 117:324, 1982.

Sugarbaker PH: Prosthetic mesh repair of large hernias at the site of colonic stomas. *Surg Gynecol Obstet* 150:577, 1980.

Thomson A: Cause anatomique de la hernie inguinale externe. *Journal des connaissances médicales pratiques et de pharmacologie* 4:137, 1836.

Thorlakson RH: Technique of repair of herniations associated with colonic stomas. *Surg Gynecol Obstet* 120:347, 1965.

Tingwald GR, Cooperman M: Inguinal and femoral hernia repair in geriatric patients. *Surg Gynecol Obstet* 154:704, 1982.

Wantz GE: Testicular atrophy as a risk of inguinal hernioplasty. *Surg Gynecol Obstet* 154:570, 1982.

Wantz GE: Complications of inguinal hernia repair. *Surg Clin North Am* 64:287, 1984.

Wantz GE: Ambulatory surgical treatment of groin hernia: Prevention and management of complications. *Problems in General Surgery* 3:311, 1986.

Wantz GE: The Canadian repair of inguinal hernia. In: Nyhus LM, Condon RE (eds): *Hernia*, 3d ed. Philadelphia, JB Lippincott, 1989.

Wantz GE: The Canadian repair: Personal observations. *World J Surg* 13:516, 1989.

Wantz GE: The operation of Bassini as described by Attilio Catterina. *Surg Gynecol Obstet* 168:67, 1989.

Wantz GE: Giant prosthetic reinforcement of the visceral sac. *Surg Gynecol Obstet* 169:408, 1989.

Wantz GE: Incisional hernioplasty with Mersilene. *Surg Gynecol Obstet* 172:129, 1991.

Wantz GE: *Atlas of Hernia Surgery*. New York, Raven Press, 1991.

Wantz GE: The technique of giant prosthetic reinforcement of the visceral sac performed through an anterior groin incision. *Surg Gynecol Obstet* 177:497, 1993.

Wantz GE: Special Comment: Personal experience with the Stoppa technique. In: Nyhus LM and Condon RE (eds): *Hernia*, 4th ed. Philadelphia, JB Lippincott, 1995.

Wantz GE: Experience with the tension-free hernioplasty for primary inguinal hernias in men. *J Am Coll Surg* 183:351, 1996.

Williams MH, Frankel SJ, et al: DHA project. *Hernia Repair*, DOH, London, 1993.

Zimmerman LM, Anson BJ: *Anatomy and Surgery of Hernia*, 2d ed. Baltimore, Williams & Wilkins, 1967.

CHAPTER 35

Pituitary and Adrenal

William T. Couldwell, Marie F. Simard, Martin H. Weiss, and Jeffrey A. Norton

Pituitary

William T. Couldwell, Marie F. Simard, and Martin H. Weiss

HISTORICAL BACKGROUND

Although Marie correctly ascribed the clinical syndrome of acromegaly to the presence of a pituitary adenoma as early as 1889, it was not until 1893 that Caton and Paul recorded the first attempt at surgical resection of a pituitary tumor. Their two-stage lateral subtemporal procedure, as suggested by Sir Victor Horsley, was unsuccessful, because the patient died before the operation was completed. Subsequently, Horsley himself, using a lateral middle fossa approach, reported successful surgical resections in eight of ten pituitary tumors operated on between 1904 and 1906. Krause, in 1905, introduced the frontal transcranial approach to the sella turcica; this technique then provided the basis from which the majority of subsequent variations of transcranial approaches were developed.

Kiliani elaborated on Krause's technique with a bifrontal intradural approach to the sella turcica in the hopes that this procedure would offer visualization that would enable a radical intradural resection of all tumor. McArthur, in the first proposal for a predominantly extradural approach to the sella, advocated resection of the supraorbital ridge and the orbital plate to allow dissection to extend posteriorly to the level of the optic chiasm, where subsequent transverse incision of the dura provided access to the intradural compartment.

These basic approaches were modified and improved by a number of the giants of neurosurgical development in the early part of the twentieth century. Modifications described by Frazier, Dandy, Heuer, and Cushing primarily favored the direct intradural approach to the sella turcica and its contents. With the profound influence of these neurosurgeons, by the 1930s most neurosurgical approaches to the pituitary used a transcranial intradural technique, though some neurosurgeons continued to use an extradural approach. Heuer advocated a lateral anterior fossa approach using the landmarks provided by the sphenoid ridge. This approach seemed to be the shortest distance between the inner table of the skull and the sella turcica. Frazier described a frontal transcranial approach beginning at the midpoint between the midline and the lateral sphenoid wing. Cushing preferred a direct midline approach. The dominant neurosurgical teaching during the 1930s and 1940s continued to focus on a transcranial approach to the pituitary. During the 1950s Olivecrona and Ray, major figures in international neurosurgery, promulgated the use of a transfrontal intradural approach to the pituitary while developing extensive experience with hypophyseal ablation, which had become a major adjunct in the management of metastatic breast and prostate carcinoma as well as diabetic retinopathy. Ray, who performed more than 1,000 procedures on the pituitary, emphasized the need for a properly placed low bone flap in order to minimize brain retraction in gaining access to the sella and parasellar areas.

The earliest attempts at transcranial approaches to the pituitary at the turn of the century and shortly thereafter, however, resulted in a mortality rate that was generally considered prohibitive. The 20 percent mortality rate in Horsley's small series of 10 cases referred to above would certainly be unacceptable by modern standards; yet it was significantly better than the experiences of his colleagues, who reported mortality rates ranging from 50 to 80 percent. It should be recognized that this extraordinary incidence of mortality was generally accepted in the efforts at developing intracranial surgery at that time.

As a consequence of these earlier experiences, attempts were made continually to modify surgical techniques as well as adjuvant management protocols in an effort to make the surgical approach to the pituitary a more reasonable option for both surgeon and patient. In this light, Schloffer, a rhinologist from Innsbruck, Austria, recommended the use of a transsphenoidal route as an alternative and presumably safer approach to the sella turcica and its contents. In 1907 he reported the first successful removal of a pituitary tumor using the transsphenoidal approach. The technique of sphenoid sinus exposure subsequently underwent a number of modifications by interested surgeons, the culmination of which was Halsted's description in 1910 of the sublabial gingival incision for the initial stage of sphenoid sinus exposure. After initial disappointments at transcranial efforts, Cushing himself embraced the transsphenoidal approach. He described a technique that combined a number of suggestions that had been made by previous authors and used the sublabial incision described by Halsted (Fig. 35-1). Cushing also adopted the technique of submucous dissection of the nasal septum promulgated by Eiselberg and Kocher and used the headlight described by Kanavel to obtain better visualization into the depths of the operative field during operation. Using the transnasal/transsphenoidal approach during the 15-year period from 1910 to 1925, Cushing operated on some 231 pituitary tumors, with a reported mortality rate of 5.6 percent. This represented the best efforts at surgical exposure and access to the pituitary at the time.

Mortality and morbidity from the use of the transsphenoidal approach were primarily the result of infection, which was frequently associated with postoperative cerebral spinal fluid (CSF) rhinorrhea; hemorrhage and postoperative edema, in contrast, were the causes of the excessive mortality and morbidity asso-

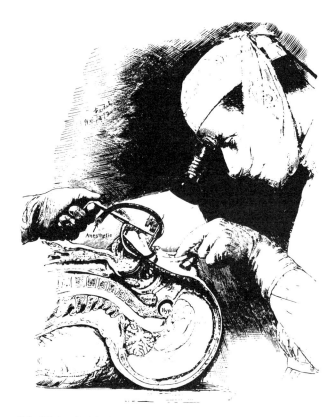

FIG. 35-1. *Cushing's adaptation of the transsphenoidal technique. This 1912 drawing by the renowned medical illustrator Max Brödel shows the technique of the transsphenoidal approach to the hypophysis. Note the sublabial incision adopted by Cushing at the time. (From: Cushing H: The Weir Mitchell lecture: Surgical experiences with pituitary disorders. JAMA 63:1515–1525, 1914, with permission.)*

ciated with transcranial approaches. As Cushing developed expertise and confidence in transcranial surgery, he began again to use the transcranial approach to the pituitary. As he gained experience, he finally reduced his mortality rate with the transcranial approach to 4.5 percent, essentially eliminating any significant difference between the transsphenoidal and transcranial approaches. It was his opinion that visual recovery was more complete after direct decompression of the optic nerves and chiasm, which may well have been the case in those early times. In addition, Cushing recognized that the transfrontal approach allowed more extensive resection of those suprasellar tumors that were complicated by significant lateral extension. Obviously Cushing's intense interest in intracranial surgery must have contributed to his pursuit and development of transcranial approaches to the pituitary. Other distinguished surgeons, however, such as Hirsch and Hamlin, continued to use the transsphenoidal approach, with reports of excellent results. It is reported that Cushing, on the occasion of his seventieth birthday, remarked that the transsphenoidal approach, because of its many advantages, would probably return despite the liabilities that he perceived.

Because of Cushing's dominance in the evolution of neurosurgery in the United States and the outstanding results that he reported, the use of transsphenoidal operations on the pituitary diminished profoundly during this period, until Norman Dott of Edinburgh, a student of Cushing's, refocused attention on this technique. In turn, Dott reportedly introduced Guiot of France to the transsphenoidal approach, and Guiot subsequently influenced the extensive development of this technique by Jules Hardy of Montreal. Having accumulated extensive experience in transsphenoidal microsurgery, these individuals significantly altered and redefined the indications and risks related to the transsphenoidal resection of hypophyseal and parahypophyseal tumors. Hardy propounded the use of intraoperative televised fluoroscopy, the operating microscope that provided both intense focused illumination and magnification, and the design and development of microsurgical instrumentation for work within and about the sella. In addition, refinement of the techniques for closure of the opening between the sphenoid sinus and the intracranial compartment resulted in a profound decrease in the mortality and morbidity associated with the procedure.

In 1908 Horsley, working in conjunction with an engineer, Richard Clark, first proposed a system for stereotactic localization within the brain using a rigid reference frame fixed to the skull. In 1921 Hirsch suggested using this stereotactic technique to approach the sella turcica; unfortunately, this proposal did not receive general acceptance in the neurosurgical community. During the 1950s Talairach and Tournoux, working in France, and Forrest, working in Scotland, reintroduced what they believed was a significant advancement in the stereotactic approach to destruction of the normal pituitary gland. During this time, hypophysectomy for the treatment of the metastatic diseases was a frequently used procedure, and efforts to avoid more extensive surgery were frequently undertaken. Talairach, Tournoux, and Forrest noted that it was possible to advance a straight cannula through the nasal cavity directly to the confines of the sella without encountering any barrier except the floor of the wall of the sphenoid sinus in most patients. Under x-ray visualization, this cannula could subsequently be guided through the anterior wall of the sella, enabling delivery of various destructive agents directly into the gland. Such agents included radioactive materials such as yttrium-90, liquid nitrogen, or even radiofrequency current. These investigators ushered in an active era of stereotaxic pituitary surgery, and some efforts were subsequently made for treatment of pituitary tumors by these techniques. Unfortunately, initial attempts at total hypophysectomy resulted in unacceptable variability in the completeness of hypophysectomy, frequent damage to the oculomotor and optic nerves, and an unacceptably high incidence of CSF rhinorrhea and consequent meningitis. Although these techniques did not find an extensive reception for use in the management of pituitary tumors, refinement in the use of the technique of radiofrequency ablation enabled Zervas to report in 1969 no occurrence of rhinorrhea, meningitis, or local infection in any of 91 consecutive patients who had undergone stereotactic radiofrequency ablation of the normal and abnormal pituitary gland. Subsequent loss of interest in ablation of the normal gland for the treatment of metastatic carcinoma or diabetic retinopathy, however, resulted in a focused effort in transnasal transsphenoidal approach to the pituitary, which today is clearly established as the foremost approach to the sella and selected parasellar lesions.

Radical operative procedures involving the hypophysis carried a prohibitive complication rate before the development of commercially available corticosteroids in the early 1950s. Replacement of these agents in patients who are rendered hypopituitary by the development of a tumor or other mass or as a consequence of surgical extraction of such lesions is essential for successful surgical intercession; commercial availability of the corticosteroids has truly revolutionized postoperative morbidity and mortality in these efforts.

Finally, our understanding of and the diagnosis of pituitary disorders have been revolutionized by two technologies of relatively recent origin—radioimmunoassay techniques, which allow diagnosticians to determine the presence of a number of functional endocrinopathies related to pituitary problems, and high-resolution computed tomography (CT) and magnetic resonance image (MRI) scanning, which allow sophisticated imaging of the pituitary gland itself. These developments have enabled precise definition of functional endocrinopathies, which in turn can be related to visualized structural lesions in and about the pituitary. These technologies, acknowledged by the award of two Nobel Prizes, have contributed immeasurably to the emergence of pituitary surgery as one of the preeminent surgical ventures in sophisticated modern neurosurgery.

ANATOMY

Macroscopic Anatomy

From a surgical standpoint it is crucial to consider the pituitary gland as one component in a complex anatomic region replete with important neural and vascular structures. The pituitary is surrounded by the hypophyseal fossa of the sphenoid bone, known as the *sella turcica,* and is covered superiorly by meningeal tissue forming the *diaphragma sellae.* The pituitary stalk passes through the center of the sellar diaphragm; in some cases the arachnoid also may protrude through this aperture into the sella turcica. The optic chiasm lies superior and anterior to the pituitary stalk and is contiguous anteriorly with the optic nerves and posteriorly with the optic tracts. The hypothalamus, which forms the anterior and lateral walls of the third ventricle, extends from the optic chiasm anteriorly to the mammillary bodies posteriorly over a distance of approximately 10 mm. The cavernous sinuses, which anatomically are more correctly a pair of venous plexuses, border the lateral walls of the sella turcica and extend posteriorly into the petrosal sinuses. Within each cavernous sinus lies the carotid artery, the oculomotor (III), trochlear (IV), and abducens (VI) nerves, and the ophthalmic and maxillary divisions of the trigeminal nerve (V) (Fig. 35-2).

The pituitary gland itself is derived embryonically from the ectoderm. In the normal adult it measures approximately 12 mm transversely, 9 mm anteroposteriorly, and 6 mm in height. In the adult male, the gland weighs about 500 mg, and in the adult female about 600 mg. Through the course of pregnancy and during normal puberty, the gland enlarges.

The pituitary gland is composed of the anterior pituitary or *adenohypophysis,* which accounts for approximately 80 percent of the hypophyseal volume, and of the posterior pituitary or *neurohypophysis.* The adenohypophysis is divided into three regions (Fig. 35-3): (1) the *pars distalis,* which comprises the major portion of the anterior lobe; (2) the *pars intermedia,* which in the human adult is a rudimentary structure composed of colloid-filled cysts located between the anterior and posterior lobes; and (3) the *pars tuberalis,* which is an extension of the pars distalis along the outer aspect of the pituitary stalk. The neurohypophysis is also divided into three regions: (1) the *median eminence,* situated in the hypothalamus, posterior to the optic chiasm, which forms the floor of the third ventricle and is also called

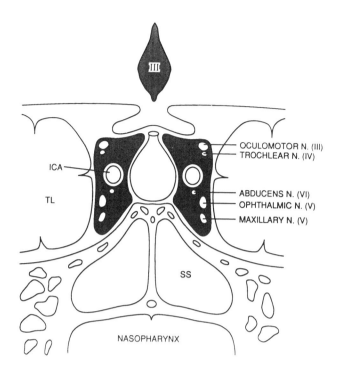

FIG. 35-2. *Anatomy of the sellar and parasellar regions. This coronal diagrammatic representation illustrates the proximity of the pituitary gland to several important neural and vascular structures. The gland is laterally bordered by the cavernous sinuses (shaded in this picture), which contain within their confines or their walls the carotid artery, the oculomotor, trochlear, and abducens nerves, and the first two divisions of the trigeminal nerve. The optic chiasm lies immediately superior to the gland. TL = temporal lobe, ICA = internal carotid artery, SS = sphenoid sinus, and III = third ventricle.*

the infundibulum; (2) the *infundibular stem,* which is the neural portion of the pituitary stalk; and (3) the *neural lobe* or inferior portion of the neurohypophysis, also called the *infundibular process.*

Microscopic Anatomy

Vascular Anatomy. The pituitary gland receives its blood supply from the bilateral superior and inferior hypophyseal arteries, which arise from the intracranial internal carotid arteries. The anterior and posterior branches of the superior hypophyseal arteries irrigate the median eminence and the infundibular stem. Within these structures, they divide to form vascular tufts, which comprise the primary vascular plexus of the hypophyseal portal system. This capillary system drains into the long hypophyseal portal veins, which course down the pituitary stalk anteriorly to supply blood to the anterolateral portion of the adenohypophysis (Fig. 35-4). The posterior adenohypophysis is supplied by the short portal veins originating from the lower infundibular stem. The anterior pituitary has the highest blood flow of any organ in the body (0.8 mL/g/min). The long portal veins supply 70 to 90 percent of its blood flow, and the short portal vessels the remainder. Within the pars distalis, these portal veins join into the secondary capillary plexus of the hypophyseal portal system. This venous plexus drains into the dural sinuses surrounding the pituitary. The hypophysiotropic hormones originating from the hypothalamus flow down the nerve axons and are liberated in proximity to the fenestrated capillaries of the primary hypoph-

yseal portal plexus into which they diffuse. The stimulatory and inhibitory hormones are then transported down the portal veins toward the anterior pituitary. Thus the anterior pituitary gland proper receives blood supply from two portal systems, with no certain direct arterial blood supply; this likely results in less tissue perfusion pressure and an increase in incidence of ischemic loss of function with intrasellar masses. Injury or occlusion of the hypophyseal portal veins can lead to infarction and necrosis of the anterior lobe. The posterior pituitary is supplied by the inferior hypophyseal arteries directly, and hormones are liberated into the surrounding dural sinuses.

Adenohypophysis. The anterior pituitary contains connective tissue, fenestrated capillaries, and epithelial cells organized in a glandular pattern. The distinct epithelial cell types can be characterized by their secretory protein hormones as follows:

1. Growth hormone (GH)-producing cells. Somatotropes comprise approximately 50 percent of the adenohypophyseal cell population and are located in the lateral wings of the anterior lobe. GH is a 191-amino acid polypeptide hormone that opposes the effect of insulin, stimulates the uptake of amino acids, and causes a release of free fatty acids from tissue storage sites. In the liver and other tissues, GH also mediates the synthesis of insulinlike growth factors (IGFs). IGFs induce protein

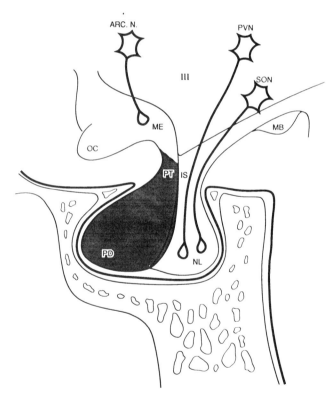

FIG. 35-3. *Anatomy of the pituitary gland. This sagittal diagram of the pituitary gland illustrates the hypothalamus, pituitary stalk, and pituitary gland, located in the sella turcica. The anterior gland or adenohypophysis is composed of the pars distalis (PD), the rudimentary pars intermedia, and the pars tuberalis (PT). The posterior gland or neurohypophysis is composed of the median eminence (ME) (located in the hypothalamus), the infundibular stem (IS), and the neural lobe (NL). The large neurons located in the supraoptic nucleus (SON) and the paraventricular nucleus (PVN) project to the neural lobe, where they store and release oxytocin and vasopressin into the systemic circulation under the appropriate stimulus. OC = optic chiasm, MB = mammillary bodies, Arc. N. = arcuate nucleus*

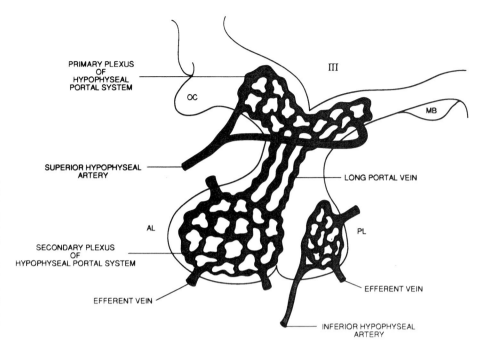

FIG. 35-4. Vascular supply of the pituitary. The pituitary gland receives blood from paired superior and inferior hypophyseal arteries. The long portal venous system originates from the median eminence and infundibular stem to irrigate the anterior lobe (AL) proper. Hypophysiotropic hormones are liberated into this long portal system for transport to the anterior lobe. The posterior gland (PL) receives direct input from the inferior hypophyseal artery. OC = optic chiasm, MB = mammillary body, III = third ventricle.

synthesis in the skeleton and in muscle, and glucose oxidation in adipose tissue; they also stimulate cell replication. The secretion of GH is stimulated by growth hormone-releasing hormone (GHRH) and inhibited by somatostatin. GH and IGF-1 stimulate the release of somatostatin, thereby down-regulating the secretion of GH. GH is secreted in episodic surges occurring every 3 to 4 h. In young people the greatest peaks occur after the onset of deep sleep. Stimuli of GH secretion include insulin-induced hypoglycemia, arginine, exercise, L-dopa, clonidine, propranolol, and GHRH.

2. Prolactin (PRL)-producing cells. The mammotropes, also called lactotropes, represent 15 to 25 percent of the anterior pituitary cells and populate the lateral gland. These cells accumulate during pregnancy and lactation and following estrogen therapy. Prolactin is a 198-amino acid polypeptide known to facilitate the development of breast tissue to ensure the production of milk. Prolactin secretion is stimulated by thyrotropin-releasing hormone (TRH), estrogens, stress, and exercise. Dopamine is acknowledged to be the principal prolactin inhibitory factor (PIF).

3. Adrenocorticotropic hormone (ACTH)-producing cells. Corticotropes constitute approximately 20 percent of the adenohypophyseal cells. They lie within the mediolateral aspects of the pars distalis. ACTH is a 39-amino acid peptide that promotes growth of the adrenal cortex and the synthesis of hormones produced by this gland. ACTH also has melanotropic effects and is responsible for the pigmentation commonly seen in Nelson's syndrome and Addison's disease. ACTH is a fragment of pro-opiocortin. Both the corticotropic and the melanotropic

cells cleave the prohormone into a common precursor containing 130 amino acids (Fig. 35-5). Within the corticotrope there is further cleavage to form ACTH (1-39 amino acids) and β-lipotropin (β-LPH) (1-91 amino acids). β-LPH is cleaved further to form γ-LPH (1-58 amino acids) and β-endorphin (61-91 amino acids). Within the melanotrope ACTH is cleaved into alpha-melanocyte-stimulating hormone (α-MSH) (1-13 amino acids) and corticotropin-like intermediate peptide (CLIP). In human beings the physiologic role of the lipotropins, α-MSH, and β-endorphin is unclear. The synthesis and secretion of ACTH is stimulated by corticotropin-releasing hormone (CRH). Vasopressin, though a weak ACTH stimulant, directly potentiates the effect of CRH. The inhibition of ACTH release is regulated by the negative-feedback effect of cortisol on the corticotrope directly and on the release of CRH at the hypothalamus. ACTH also regulates the release of CRH through a short-loop negative-feedback effect. The secretion of ACTH follows a circadian rhythmicity and occurs in brief episodes during the late sleep period and just before awakening. Rapid release of ACTH also occurs under the stimulation of stress such as pain, fear, noise, extreme cold, fever, hypoglycemia, and hemorrhage.

4. Thyroxin-stimulating hormone (TSH)-producing cells. Thyrotropes constitute approximately 5 percent of the adenohypophysis and are located in the anteromedial region. TSH is a glycoprotein composed of two noncovalently linked moieties, the alpha and the beta subunits. The beta subunit confers biologic activity to the hormone. Thyrotropes secrete not only TSH but also the separate subunits. TSH regulates the synthesis of thyroid hormones, thyroxine (T_4) and triiodothyronine

FIG. 35-5. The processing of pro-opiocortin. Both the corticotropic and melanotropic cells cleave pro-opiocortin into a 130-amino acid precursor (from which ACTH and β-lipoprotein are derived; *right*). ACTH is cleaved from the precursor protein within the corticotrope and is secreted; further processing of ACTH occurs within the melanotrope, producing alpha-melanocyte-stimulating hormone (α-MSH) and corticotropin-like intermediate peptide (CLIP).

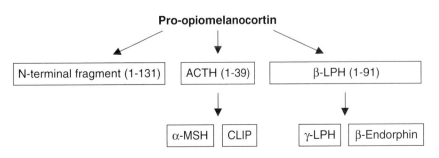

Pro-opiomelanocortin

| N-terminal fragment (1-131) | ACTH (1-39) | β-LPH (1-91) |

| α-MSH | CLIP | | γ-LPH | β-Endorphin |

(T_3), by the thyroid gland. A euthyroid state is maintained through a balance between the stimulatory effect of TRH produced by the hypothalamus and the negative-feedback inhibition of the thyroid hormones on the thyrotrope cells.

5. Gonadotropic-hormone (FSH/LH)-producing cells. Gonadotropes secrete both follicle-stimulating hormone (FSH) and luteinizing hormone (LH) and occupy approximately 10 percent of the anterior gland within its medial region. FSH and LH are glycoproteins formed by two noncovalently linked subunits, the above-mentioned common alpha subunit and the specific beta subunit, which confers the biologic activity to the hormones. Gonadotropin levels are elevated during the first 1 to 2 years of life and rise again with the onset of puberty. FSH stimulates ovarian follicular growth in the female and testicular growth and spermatogenesis in the male. In the female, LH promotes ovulation and luteinization of the ovarian follicle and enhances estrogen and progesterone production by the ovary. In the male, LH supports interstitial (Leydig) cell function and hence the production of testosterone by the testicle. Gonadotropin secretion in the ovulating female is stimulated by gonadotropin-releasing hormone (GnRH) and both positively and negatively regulated by the gonadal steroids. Short-term effects of estrogens are suppressive on basal LH release. With longer duration of exposure to estrogens, particularly at low concentrations, gonadotropin secretion is enhanced. In males, testosterone has a negative-feedback effect on hypothalamic GnRH secretion and on the pituitary gonadotrope cells.

Neurohypophysis. The posterior pituitary lacks a blood-brain barrier and consists of hypothalamus-originating neuronal axons and terminals, specialized glial cells, and blood vessels. As described above, it is divided into three anatomic regions: the median eminence, the infundibular stem, and the neural lobe. The median eminence is composed of three layers: (1) The inner ependymal zone is formed by specialized cells called tanycytes that line the inferior region of the third ventricle. These cells are connected by tight junctions that prevent the passage of CSF into the interstitial fluid of the median eminence. (2) The internal zone contains the supraopticohypophyseal tract, composed of axons of the magnocellular neurons. (3) The external zone contains the parvocellular neuron terminals that form the dopaminergic tuberohypophyseal tract. The supraopticohypophyseal tract and the tuberohypophyseal tract are present also in the infundibular stem and terminate in the neural lobe. Damage to the supraopticohypophyseal and tuberoinfundibular tracts results in atrophy of the posterior lobe as well as of the supraoptic and paraventricular nuclei.

REGULATION OF THE HYPOTHALAMIC-PITUITARY AXIS

Hypothalamic control of the pituitary gland is mediated by two separate neurosecretory systems, known as the *parvocellular* and the *magnocellular* neuronal systems. The parvocellular system consists of small neurons originating in several hypothalamic cell groups that produce the hypothalamic hypophysiotropic hormones, including GHRH, TRH, CRH, GnRH, PIF (probably identical to dopamine), and the growth hormone-inhibiting hormone known as somatostatin (SS). Their axons form the tuberoinfundibular tract, which terminates in the median eminence, where these hormones are released. These various releasing and inhibitory factors regulate adenohypophyseal release of hormones via the portal circulation.

Brain neurotransmitters such as dopamine, norepinephrine, epinephrine, serotonin, acetylcholine, γ-aminobutyric acid, and opioid peptides also can influence anterior pituitary function, primarily by interacting with hypothalamic hypophysiotropic hormone-containing neurons.

The magnocellular system consists of large neural cell bodies located in the supraoptic and paraventricular nuclei. These neurons contain the peptide hormones oxytocin and vasopressin, also known as antidiuretic hormone. Their neural fibers form the supraopticohypophyseal tract, which projects down the infundibular stem and terminates in the posterior lobe, where oxytocin and vasopressin are stored and released into the systemic circulation upon appropriate stimulation. Oxytocin induces smooth-muscle contraction of the uterus, leading to the expulsion of the fetus and the placenta, and contraction of the myoepithelial cells of the breast involved in milk ejection. Vasopressin is released from the posterior lobe of the pituitary into the systemic circulation, where it binds to receptors on renal distal tubules to induce water conservation, and to receptors on precapillary arterioles to elevate mean arterial pressure. The main factor regulating vasopressin release is plasma osmolality through osmoreceptors located in the hypothalamus. As osmolality increases, vasopressin is released to ensure maintenance of serum osmolality and water balance. If a blood loss greater than 10 to 15 percent of the vascular volume is incurred, the low-pressure volume receptors located in the left atrium and in the pulmonary veins and the high-pressure baroreceptors located in the carotid sinus and in the aortic arch will mediate the release of vasopressin. In the advent of hypotension, vasopressin is also carried by the portal venous system to the anterior pituitary, where it regulates the release of ACTH.

DIAGNOSTIC STUDIES

Complete examination of sellar and parasellar regions encompasses both neuroendocrine and anatomic (radiologic) evaluations.

Neuroendocrine Evaluation

Anterior Pituitary. The advent of radioimmunoassay and immunohistochemical methods has greatly enhanced our understanding of the function of the pituitary gland in normal and in pathologic states. The evaluation of the anterior pituitary is indicated in patients who present with signs or symptoms compatible with isolated or multiple hormonal deficits, hyperprolactinemia, hyperthyroidism, diabetes insipidus, a hypothalamic disorder, or with any sellar or suprasellar lesion (Table 35-1). Recognition of any potential hypopituitarism before any surgical endeavor is imperative and may have implications for avoiding complications in the perioperative period.

TSH deficiency can be diagnosed by measuring simultaneously basal serum TSH and thyroid hormone levels. A low serum T_4 in the presence of an inappropriately low TSH level suggests a central cause of hypothyroidism. To assess the TSH reserve within the thyrotropes, thereby distinguishing a hypothalamic from a pituitary defect, a TRH test may be performed. Normally, TSH and both prolactin and GH rise in response to TRH stimulation.

Dynamic tests are required to diagnose a state of ACTH deficiency, because the morning cortisol level is persistently low only when the ACTH deficiency is very severe. The CRH test may be used to distinguish a hypothalamic CRH deficiency from

Table 35-1
Diagnostic Tests to Evaluate Hypothalamic-Pituitary Hypofunction

Thyroid
    Serum TSH, T_4, T_3 resin uptake
    TRH stimulation test (measure serum TSH, prolactin, GH)
Adrenal
    Serum cortisol (8 A.M.)
    Plasma ACTH (if serum cortisol low)
    CRH stimulation test (measure serum ACTH)
Sex hormones
    Serum testosterone (men), estradiol (amenorrheic premenopausal
        women)
    Serum LH, FSH
    GnRH stimulation test (measure serum LH and FSH)
Serum prolactin
Growth hormone
    Serum IGF-1 and growth curve (children and adolescents)
    GH stimulation tests (GHRH, arginine, clonidine, propranolol,
        L-dopa, insulin-hypoglycemia, exercise)

TSH = thyroxin-stimulating hormone; TRH = thyrotropin-releasing hormone; GH = growth hormone; CRH = corticotropin-releasing hormone; LH = luteinizing hormone; FSH = follicle-stimulating hormone; GnRH = gonadotropin-releasing hormone; IGF-1 = insulinlike growth factor-1; GHRH = growth hormone-releasing hormone.

a pituitary ACTH deficiency. The absence of ACTH responsiveness to CRH is diagnostic of a pituitary corticotrope deficiency. The insulin-induced hypoglycemia and the glucagon test will stimulate the entire hypothalamic-pituitary-adrenal axis. The ACTH stimulation test evaluates the capacity of the adrenal glands to secrete cortisol.

Gonadotropin deficiency can be diagnosed by measuring simultaneously basal serum FSH and LH levels and gonadal steroids, estradiol in the premenopausal female and testosterone in the male. In the event of primary gonadal failure, the lack of negative feedback by the gonadal steroids on the hypothalamic GnRH and pituitary LH- and FSH-secreting cells leads to an elevation of LH and FSH. Low circulating gonadal steroid levels associated with inappropriately low gonadotropin levels suggests a hypothalamic or pituitary disturbance. The GnRH stimulation test will evaluate pituitary gonadotrope function. Lack of a secretory response of LH and FSH to GnRH indicates a lesion at the pituitary rather than at the hypothalamic level.

GH levels in the basal state often are low in normal individuals. Measurement of the plasma level of insulinlike growth factor-1 (IGF-1) permits a more accurate diagnosis of a GH-deficient state, because it reflects the integrated 24-h secretion of GH. Stimulatory tests to assess the somatotrope function include sleep and exercise studies, insulin-induced hypoglycemia, and administration of arginine, L-dopa, clonidine, propranolol, or GHRH.

Posterior Pituitary. Central *diabetes insipidus* (DI) refers to a state of relative or absolute insufficient secretion of vasopressin from the posterior pituitary gland. This must be differentiated from renal DI, in which the kidney fails to respond to an appropriate elevation in serum vasopressin level. The diagnosis of central DI may be established by the water deprivation test. This study assesses the patient's ability to concentrate urine in response to an increase in plasma osmolality. Both hypothyroidism and hypocortisolism might cause a decrease in the glomerular filtration rate and thus mask a state of DI. Therefore,

before the test, the patient should be euthyroid and any adrenal insufficiency should be corrected. The diagnosis of DI is based on the development during the test of abnormally concentrated plasma (osmolality > 300 mOsm/kg) and of urine that remains dilute (osmolality < 270 mOsm/kg). Also, the urine volume is not reduced to the expected degree. At the end of the water deprivation period, the administration of exogenous vasopressin will correct these abnormalities (in contrast to renal DI, in which there is resistance to exogenous vasopressin).

Radiologic Evaluation

Radiologic examination of the pituitary should provide information about the bony anatomy of the sella turcica and its surroundings as well as intrasellar contents. Depending on the clinical presentation, the use of more than one imaging modality may be indicated.

The bony anatomy of the sella turcica may be visualized by performing lateral skull x-rays, which may demonstrate enlargement of the sella in cases of intrasellar tumors. Conventional polytomography provides greater resolution. However, if more detailed evaluation of the bone at the base of the skull is necessary, CT using special windows to enhance bony detail is indicated. This study offers the additional advantage of enabling limited soft-tissue resolution of the sella, which is helpful in distinguishing empty sella from a pituitary tumor, as both may result in enlargement of the sella.

For the diagnosis and management of pituitary lesions, the contemporary imaging modalities of CT and MRI have had a revolutionary impact. MRI is superior to CT because of its inherently greater soft-tissue contrast, which allows clear visualization of the optic chiasm, optic nerves, cavernous sinuses, and carotid arteries (Fig. 35-6).

High-field, thin-section MRI appears to be the most sensitive imaging method for preoperative localization of pituitary adenomas. On unenhanced images, focal glandular hypodensity identified on coronal images is the most sensitive predictor of adenoma location. Radiologic evaluation should consist of coronal, sagittal, and axial MRI, with large tumors usually having similar signal intensity to brain on T_1-weighted images. The normal pituitary gland, infundibulum, and cavernous sinuses enhance immediately after administration of gadolinium-DTPA, allowing contrast between the enhancing normal glandular tissue and the low-intensity adenomas. A T_1-weighted image following the infusion of gadolinium-DTPA is the method of choice for the delineation of intrasellar pathology. Shortly after administration, the normal vascular pituitary will increase in signal intensity, and a pituitary tumor will contrast by remaining less intense, being slower to perfuse with the contrast agent (Fig. 35-7). However, after sufficient time for dye uptake into the tumor, it will increase in signal intensity accordingly. After this, the normal pituitary surrounding will "wash out" the contrast before the tumor does; thus the reverse situation will prevail, and the tumor will remain at a higher intensity than the surrounding gland for a period of time. The optimal and most consistent time for visualization is therefore in the early postinfusion period, since the kinetics of dye perfusion and clearance may be variable among patients. Because MRI also offers visualization of the major vessels, the intracavernous carotid artery's proximity to the tumor can be determined; this is especially important in the rare case of severely ectatic carotid arteries that might preclude a transnasal surgical approach because of the risk of vascular injury.

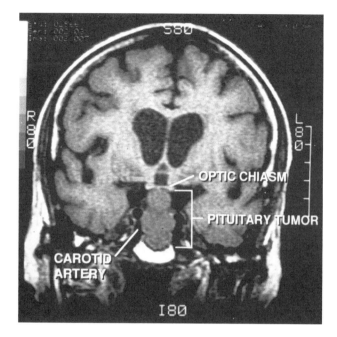

FIG. 35-6. MRI of a patient with a pituitary macroadenoma. A 68-year-old female patient developed progressive visual loss (bitemporal hemianopsia). On the coronal T₁-weighted MRI without contrast enhancement, note the large sellar and suprasellar mass, with compression of the optic chiasm. Also seen are the carotid arteries as signal voids in cross section which contrast to the surrounding soft tissue. The MRI offers soft-tissue resolution superior to that of computed tomography.

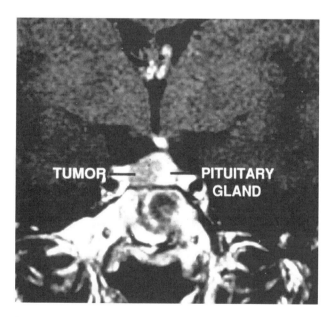

FIG. 35-7. Gadolinium-enhanced MRI of a patient with a pituitary adenoma. This 29-year-old female patient presented with galactorrhea, amenorrhea, and elevation of the serum prolactin level. The administration of the contrast agent gadolinium-DTPA produces an early glandular enhancement, which outlines the low-intensity adenoma.

In summary, MRI should be the primary imaging test used whenever suspected pituitary or parasellar lesion is to be studied noninvasively.

CT may be used if MRI is not available, with direct coronal cuts or with coronal and sagittal reconstruction of axial sections through the sellar region. On unenhanced CT a pituitary tumor usually has a density slightly less than surrounding pituitary or cavernous sinuses. Adenomas may be homogeneous, contain low-density regions of necrosis or cyst formation, or demonstrate intratumoral hemorrhage or calcification. CT also can offer relevant information regarding the bony landmarks by varying the window widths, and it may reveal sellar enlargement or sloping, thinning, or erosion of the sellar floor, all indicative of an intrasellar expansile process. In addition, the presence of calcium in some sellar or parasellar lesions (e.g., craniopharyngioma, meningioma) may be better visualized on CT images, thus providing supplemental information to that obtained by MRI.

ANTERIOR PITUITARY DISORDERS

Postpartum Pituitary Ischemia

Postpartum infarction and necrosis of the pituitary, known as Sheehan's syndrome, leads to hormonal deficiencies. The pathogenesis of this syndrome is still debated, but among the postulated causes of pituitary ischemia at the time of delivery are hemorrhage with hypovolemic shock, and pituitary portal venous thrombosis due to diffuse intravascular coagulation. Panhypopituitarism may develop over an extended period, in some cases being reported 10 to 20 years postpartum. The main clinical features include postpartum failure to lactate, postpartum amenorrhea, and progressive symptoms and signs of adrenal insufficiency and hypothyroidism. Although panhypopituitarism is common, gonadotropic function may be spared or may recover. Diabetes insipidus, although classically considered an anterior gland disease, also occurs in 1 percent of cases.

Pituitary Adenomas

Pituitary adenomas are benign tumors that may originate from any of the pituitary cell types. With today's imaging modalities and radioimmunoassay techniques we are enjoying a new era in the diagnosis and management of pituitary adenomas. Such diagnostic studies have rendered obsolete the earlier morphometric histologic classification of pituitary tumors. Pituitary adenoma is a common incidental sellar abnormality; autopsy and radiologic studies suggest that microadenomas (lesions < 10 mm in diameter) may be present in 22 to 27 percent of older individuals but that macroadenomas (> 10 mm) are quite rare (Fig. 35-8). Hormone secretion by an adenoma may be asymptomatic but is helpful in the differential diagnosis of an incidental mass on MRI.

These tumors are classified according to their secretory product (if any) (Tables 35-2 and 35-3). However, some tumors may secrete multiple hormones (plurihormonal lesions), which may complicate this classification. Another potential confounding factor is in the definition of the term "hormone production." Classically, because cell biologists and pathologists define production as hormone synthesis that is not necessarily associated with hormone release, the endocrinologic status of the patient associated with a particular histological tumor appearance may not be correlated. From a clinical standpoint, however, the true

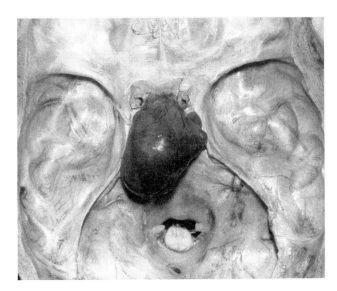

FIG. 35-8. A large null-cell adenoma. This pathology specimen reveals evidence of a large pituitary tumor with marked suprasellar extension. Note the location of the tumor and the proximity of the carotid arteries. (Photo courtesy of Dr. Kalman Kovacs, Department of Pathology, St Michaels Hospital, University of Toronto.)

Table 35-3
Pituitary Adenoma Types and Their Incidence

Type	Incidence	(%)
GH-cell adenoma		
Densely granulated		7.1
Sparsely granulated		8.0
PRL-cell adenoma	28.0	
Densely granulated		0.5
Sparsely granulated		27.5
ACTH-cell adenoma	13.8	
Endocrinologically active		8.1
Silent		5.7
TSH adenoma	0.6	
FSH/LH adenoma	4.4	
Null-cell adenoma	24.7	
Nononcocytotic		17.4
Oncocytotic		7.3
Plurihormonal adenoma	13.4	
GH-cell PRL-cell adenoma		5.2
Acidophil stem-cell adenoma		2.5
Mammosomatotrope-cell adenoma		1.4
Other		4.3
Total	100.0	

GH = growth hormone; PRL = prolactin; TSH = thyroxin-stimulating hormone; FSH = follicle-stimulating hormone; LH = luteinizing hormone.

SOURCE: From Kovacs K, Horvath E: Pathology of pituitary adenomas, in Collu R, Brown GM, Van Loon GR (eds): *Clinical Neuroendocrinology.* Boston, Blackwell Scientific, 1988, with permission.

secretion of the hormone is important, because it determines any hypersecretory endocrinopathy and provides a serum parameter for clinical diagnosis and response to treatment.

Null-Cell Adenomas. *Clinical Manifestations and Diagnosis.* Although tumors that secrete any of the anterior pituitary hormones may grow to sufficient size to become macroadenomas, nonfunctioning adenomas more frequently present, with symptoms of large lesions, such as headache, visual failure, or hypopituitarism. Statistically, null-cell tumors are among the most common types of adenoma found in the pituitary and occur more frequently later in life than secreting tumors. The classic visual triad produced by larger tumors is characterized by optic disc pallor, early loss of central visual acuity, and visual field defects (bitemporal hemianopsia).

In the endocrinologic evaluation of the patient in whom a nonfunctioning pituitary tumor is suspected, an important diagnostic pitfall to be avoided is the misdiagnosis of a prolactin-secreting tumor. Larger adenomas composed of cells other than lactotropes may produce a mild-to-moderate hyperprolactinemia from the so-called stalk-section effect (disconnection hyperpro-

Table 35-2
Classification of Pituitary Adenomas According to Endocrine Function

Adenomas with no apparent hormone function (including alpha-subunit secretors)
Prolactin excess
Growth hormone excess
ACTH excess
TSH excess
FSH/LH excess
Plurihormonal excess

TSH = Thyroxin-stimulating hormone; FSH = follicle-stimulating hormone; LH = luteinizing hormone.

lactinemia-stalk compression causing loss of dopaminergic inhibition to tonic prolactin release), which must be distinguished from a true prolactinoma. Under such circumstances, it is rare to see prolactin levels in excess of 100 ng/mL, at most 250 ng/mL. Consequently, large tumors (> 2 cm) associated with prolactin levels less than 250 ng/mL (and certainly those < 100 ng/mL) should be suspected of being nonfunctional when management strategies are being planned, and one would not expect such lesions to respond to chemical reductions of serum prolactin. Nonsecreting pituitary adenomas can be defined as those that demonstrate no *apparent* clinical or biochemical abnormality indicating hormonal excess, though it must be recognized that the potential exists for the secretion of an as-yet undetectable hormone or its precursor, or an identified hormone may be synthesized in insufficient quantities to be detected by immunoperoxidase methods. Indeed, for this reason, some have considered the term "nonfunctioning" a misnomer. Tumors that secrete the alpha subunit, common to all the glycoprotein hormones, are to be distinguished from the true nonfunctioning tumors; in these cases the alpha subunit may be detected immunohistochemically in tumor specimens and biochemically in the blood and urine, but because it possesses no biologic activity it is of no endocrinologic consequence if secreted. However, the *exclusive* secretion of the alpha subunit may be difficult to determine if each of the glycoprotein hormones has not been independently assayed. For example, TSH-secreting tumors may secrete excessive quantities of the alpha subunit.

With nonfunctioning macroadenomas, varying amounts of hypopituitarism may be present, produced by compression of the gland by tumor or from interference with blood supply leading to infarction of a normally functioning gland.

Therapy. The two objectives of the treatment of *all* pituitary tumors are (1) relief of signs and symptoms attributable to mass effect and (2) correction of endocrine abnormalities—hyposecretion or hypersecretion of adenohypophyseal hormones. When nonsecreting tumors are considered, correction of endocrine abnormalities may be of lesser consequence than is hormonal excess, but it is important to realize that continued growth of the lesion may precipitate hypopituitarism.

The success of medical therapy is predicated on the presence of any associated oversecretion of anterior pituitary hormones. Thus, in the majority of cases of nonfunctioning tumors, no pharmacologic therapy is available. Approximately 10 percent of these tumors will respond to bromocriptine, a dopamine agonist, with a reduction in size. The primary mode of treatment for these tumors should therefore be considered surgical, with other options to be considered (radiotherapy, observation) in patients in whom underlying medical conditions preclude operation.

Prolactin-Secreting Adenomas. *Clinical Manifestations and Diagnosis.* Prolactinomas are the most common functional pituitary tumors. Although they are found pathologically at autopsy with equal frequency in men and women, clinically they present more commonly in women. In a personal series of some 392 PRL-secreting pituitary tumors operated on by one of the authors (MHW), 321 (82 percent) were in female patients. The most common presenting symptom in this group was the development of secondary amenorrhea; approximately 50 percent of those with amenorrhea had associated galactorrhea. Epidemiologically, approximately 5 percent of women with primary amenorrhea and 25 percent of women with secondary amenorrhea (other than those who are pregnant) have a PRL-secreting pituitary tumor as the cause of their clinical symptoms. Because of the readily identifiable symptoms of amenorrhea and galactorrhea, these patients generally present relatively early in the course of evolution of the tumors; this is unfortunately not true in the male population. Since the primary symptom of a PRL-secreting tumor in the male usually is a decrease in libido well before true impotence is observed, this is frequently ascribed to the "aging process" or "functional" causes. Hence males often present at a more advanced age and later in the course of their disease with chiasmal compression and visual compromise.

The diagnosis is secured by radiologic evidence of a pituitary lesion with serial elevations of serum prolactin levels. There exists a rough correlation between the size of the lesion and the serum elevation of prolactin. In addition, local invasion of the tumor into the venous cavernous sinuses is associated with a marked increase in serum PRL level. The PRL level is of great help in determining subsequent management, because the ability to successfully extirpate the tumor is reduced with large and/or invasive lesions.

Therapy. The introduction of an effective medical management potential in the treatment of PRL-secreting tumors came with Food and Drug Administration (FDA) approval of bromocriptine in 1978. The efficacy of bromocriptine (a dopaminergic agonist) in reducing serum prolactin, in addition to reducing tumor size and inhibiting further tumor growth, is well established. The central considerations in treating such patients are the patient's ability to tolerate the medication, and the understanding that in most cases the treatment must continue for the duration of the patient's life. Patients with microadenomas occasionally may be cured with chronic bromocriptine therapy.

With PRL-secreting microadenomas, therapeutic options include medical or surgical management. In our series, 225 of 262 patients (86 percent) undergoing operation for tumors less than 1 cm in size had normal (< 20 ng/mL) postoperative PRL levels (i.e., "chemical cure"). Operative mortality was zero and associated morbidity was low. Strong consideration should be given to surgical intervention in patients who have smaller tumors without significant hyperprolactinemia.

In cases of larger tumors, however, surgical cures are much less frequent (in our personal series, only 63 of 130 [49 percent] of the patients with tumors larger than 1 cm achieved chemical cure). Although no medical therapy will result in cure of a PRL-secreting macroadenoma, only a minority of these patients will remain free of their disease after surgical treatment alone. It is our practice to place *all* patients with large or invasive pituitary tumors with endocrinologically documented prolactin secretion on a trial of bromocriptine initially and to monitor clinical status and radiographic appearance accordingly. All solid primary prolactin-secreting tumors should respond to the medication, both by a reduction in tumor size and by a reduction in prolactin level. The goal of therapy should be absolute normalization of prolactin levels, as a prolonged hyperprolactinemic state may be associated with significant osteoporosis and infertility. Surgical resection of these lesions is indicated only in those patients who are intolerant of the side effects of the medication, unable to afford the cost of the medication for a prolonged period, or in whom sustained tumor reduction is not effected. After operation, if hyperprolactinemia is persistent to some extent, the patient may be able to tolerate markedly reduced doses of bromocriptine to effect long-term control, or else postoperative radiotherapy to bring the residual tumor under control should be considered.

Cushing's Disease. *Clinical Manifestations and Diagnosis.* Cushing's disease is the result of hypersecretion of ACTH by the pituitary. ACTH-secreting tumors are present in over 90 percent of patients with a pituitary source of excess ACTH secretion; in the remaining 10 percent the cause of excess ACTH secretion is diffuse corticotrope hyperplasia from hypersecretion of CRH. The disease affects women approximately eight times more frequently than men. Ectopic ACTH production accounts for 10 percent of ACTH-dependent hypercortisolism and should be ruled out.

Clinical manifestations of the disease include: (1) those due to *glucocorticoid excess* (Fig. 35-9)—central obesity, "moon" facies, dorsocervical and supraclavicular fat pads, proximal muscle wasting, thin skin with ecchymoses and violaceous striae, cataracts, osteoporosis, amenorrhea, diabetes mellitus, growth retardation in children, immunosuppression with fungal infections, and depression; and (2) those due to *peripheral androgen excess*—hirsutism and acne (virilization is unusual), and hypogonadism from increased negative feedback to the hypothalamus and pituitary gland.

The diagnosis of Cushing's disease is confirmed by: (1) increased basal plasma ACTH and cortisol levels in the afternoon and evening with loss of diurnal variation; (2) an elevated 24-h urinary free cortisol excretion (> 100 mg/24 h); (3) a failure of serum cortisol to suppress with the *low-dose dexamethasone suppression test* (1 mg dexamethasone is administered at 11 P.M.; an 8 A.M. plasma cortisol remains higher than 5 mg/dL); and (4) suppression of ACTH after administration of high-dose dexamethasone (overnight 8 mg dexamethasone test or standard two-

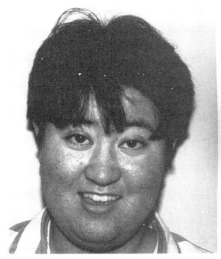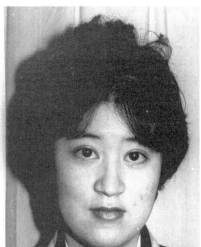

FIG. 35-9. *Cushing's disease. This patient had a microadenoma of the pituitary gland. Note the facial features of glucocorticoid excess, including obesity and acne (left). One year after transsphenoidal resection of the adenoma, the patient shows resolution of these signs (right). (Photo courtesy of Dr. Takanori Fukushima, Department of Neurological Surgery, Allegheny General Hospital, Pittsburgh, PA.)*

day test of 2 mg every 6 h for 2 days). A failure to suppress ACTH secretion with the high-dose dexamethasone suppression test suggests the diagnosis of an autonomous adrenal tumor or ectopic ACTH secretion.

MRI study of the pituitary identifies a microadenoma in around 50 percent of the cases, a macroadenoma less frequently; or the study may appear normal (a small microadenoma below the resolution of the MRI or corticotrope hyperplasia).

Therapy. Fortunately, most patients with Cushing's disease have microadenomas that lend themselves to complete surgical resection. Our experience with these microadenomas has been gratifying; in patients with Cushing's disease who have microadenomas, the series has demonstrated a 91 percent cure rate as defined by laboratory tests. On the other hand, patients with Cushing's disease who have macroadenomas present a serious problem. These tumors are frequently invasive into adjacent dura and bone and consequently defy chemical cure (as defined by laboratory tests) by surgical means alone. For patients with elevated ACTH levels that persist after radical surgical resection, we are currently exploring stereotaxic radiosurgery as a method to eradicate residual sellar and parasellar invasion while sparing adjacent structures (as opposed to standard external beam radiotherapy). If radiotherapy fails, trials of an adrenolytic agent, mitotane, or adrenal enzyme inhibitors, such as aminoglutethimide, metyrapone, and ketoconazole will be required to control the disease. For patients who have failed all modes of nonoperative therapy, bilateral adrenalectomy is recommended.

Acromegaly and Gigantism. *Clinical Manifestations and Diagnosis.* Excess GH secretion produces the clinical syndrome of *acromegaly*. If the excess secretion occurs before the epiphyses of long bones have fused, the result is *gigantism*. GH-secreting pituitary adenomas are the most common cause of excess GH secretion, and the patients present with macroadenomas. Rarely, the disease is a result of the ectopic secretion of GHRH from other tumors.

With gigantism, young individuals may attain great height if the disease progresses unchecked (often greater than 7 feet). After fusion of the epiphyses, GH produces the syndrome of acromegaly, with the soft-tissue and bony enlargement in charac-

teristic locations (Fig. 35-10). Clinical manifestations of these soft-tissue changes include coarsening of facial features, laryngeal enlargement, goiter, thick heel pads, acanthosis nigricans, cardiomegaly, and hepatomegaly. Bony changes are extensive, producing facial prognathism, enlargement of the mandible with increased spacing between the teeth, and bony enlargements of hands and feet. Concomitant with these changes are compressive neuropathies, arthropathies, and osteoporosis secondary to hypogonadism. Metabolic manifestations include associated hypertension, diabetes mellitus, and goiter; hyperhidrosis also is commonly present. Acromegaly affects men and women with approximately equal frequency.

The diagnosis is made by assessing GH secretion. A basal fasting GH level greater than 10 ng/mL is present in 90 percent of those with acromegaly. The diagnosis is confirmed by the *glucose suppression test.* In patients with acromegaly, an oral administration of 100 g glucose fails to suppress the GH level to less than 2 ng/mL at 120 min. As GH is secreted in several peaks throughout the day, a single fasting level may fail to demonstrate GH hypersecretion. The serum IGF-1 level is elevated in those with acromegaly, and this measurement may prove to be more useful because it reflects the integrated pulsatile 24-h secretion of GH and is a more reliable parameter for assessing the disease and to monitor its response to treatment. MRI or CT demonstrates the presence of a pituitary adenoma in more than 90 percent of patients with endocrinologically documented acromegaly.

Therapy. With associated diabetes mellitus, hypertension, and cardiomyopathy in a significant proportion of patients with acromegaly, oversecretion of GH should be considered a "malignant endocrinopathy" that demands complete and expedient treatment. Complete surgical removal of pituitary adenomas that secrete GH usually provides rapid control of elevated GH levels, is capable of producing long-lasting "cure," and is relatively safe. In patients in whom total removal of the lesion is not possible (tumors with large suprasellar extent or cavernous sinus invasion) or in whom surgery is contraindicated, medical therapy should be considered. Patients with elevation of GH and IGF-1 postoperatively should also receive medical therapy. The somatostatin analogue octreotide acetate (Sandostatin) reduces tu-

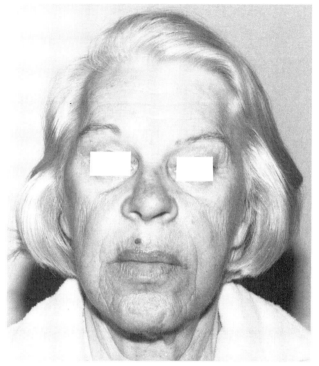

A

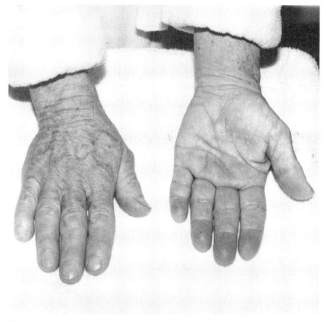

B

FIG. 35-10. A patient with acromegaly. This 70-year-old patient developed coarse facial features and bony changes in her hands and feet over a period of several years. Note the enlargement of the mandible and lips, prognathism (A), and bony enlargement of hands and fingers (B).

mor size in approximately 20 to 50 percent of patients, normalizes GH levels in 50 percent, and normalizes IGF-1 levels in 40 to 80 percent. Present therapy, however, demands parenteral administration or continuous infusion, which dictates careful se-

lection of reliable patients. A long-term parenteral congener, which may be administered every 3 weeks, is currently undergoing clinical trials. Radiotherapy of these lesions, as with other pituitary tumors, is moderately effective but is not without significant adverse effects.

Gonadotroph-Secreting Adenomas. Gonadotroph cell adenomas are uncommon tumors that usually present in middle-aged men with symptoms caused by mass effect: headaches, visual disturbances, and hypopituitarism. Although gonadal function usually is normal, hypogonadism may present in men and women, and some men may present with bilateral testicular enlargement due to FSH hypersecretion. Different hormonal secretory patterns may be encountered: (1) hypersecretion of FSH (the most common anomaly), (2) secretion of biologically inactive LH associated with hypogonadism, (3) hypersecretion of intact LH associated with elevated serum testosterone levels in men and precocious puberty in children, and (4) hypersecretion of alpha subunit. In approximately 50 percent of patients, administration of TRH intravenously induces inappropriate elevations of serum LH and FSH and their subunits. The treatment of these tumors is surgical, with radiotherapy being reserved for patients who are not surgical candidates or in whom total resection is not achieved. Measuring serum LH, FSH, and alpha subunit levels postoperatively can help to determine the extent of tumor removal. For surveillance of tumor recurrence, measurement of basal or TRH-stimulated gonadotrophins or their subunits should be performed.

Thyrotroph Adenomas. TSH-secreting pituitary tumors are rare. Most patients present with invasive macroadenomas. The TSH levels are below 10 mU/L in one third of cases (170), and are usually below 20 mU/L. Most patients present with overt hyperthyroidism and a diffuse goiter. These cases can be differentiated from other causes of hyperthyroidism by a basal alpha subunit-to-TSH molar ratio of less than 1, and exogenous TRH administration may stimulate TSH and alpha-subunit secretion. Many thyrotroph cell adenomas also secrete PRL and GH. Transsphenoidal resection is the treatment of choice. Irradiation is reserved for patients who are not surgical candidates or in whom total resection is not achieved. Irradiation appears to stabilize tumor growth and render the patient euthyroid in approximately one-quarter of cases. Octreotide has been a useful adjunctive therapy while awaiting the ablative effect of radiotherapy. This drug is effective in most patients, rendering them euthyroid and significantly reducing tumor size in many.

Surgery for Pituitary Adenomas. *Preoperative Evaluation.* Any lesion proximal to the pituitary or hypothalamus requires adequate endocrine evaluation preoperatively to minimize the potential for an intraoperative or postoperative catastrophe because of inadequate pituitary reserve. The two most important of these are cortisol and thyroid levels. Because of the universal use of perioperative glucocorticoids in surgery involving this area, the risk of intraoperative hypocortisolemia is generally not a major factor. However, preexisting hypothyroidism can manifest acutely during the early postoperative period, underlining the need for adequate preoperative assessment. In cases with associated hypothyroidism, reestablishment of euthyroidism requires approximately 1 week of treatment before any elective surgical procedure. For this reason complete endocrine evaluation is performed in all patients in whom a pituitary lesion is suspected; normal endocrine function preoperatively, of course, does not guarantee such a state postoperatively, but preoperative function may identify patients in whom a risk of this occurrence should be considered in the perioperative period.

An assessment of electrolyte status is also important in identifying patients with marginal diabetes insipidus who may not comment on the long-standing urinary frequency.

Transsphenoidal Approach. The transnasal transsphenoidal approach is considered the procedure of choice for surgical access to sellar lesions (Fig. 35-11). The increase in popularity of this technique may be attributed also in part to the well-recognized inadequacy of the subfrontal approach for removal of the intrasellar component of the tumor. Moreover, several reports indicate favorable results with the transsphenoidal approach in the management of visual disturbances from macroadenomas, establishing this as the approach of choice for the surgical management of most pituitary tumors, regardless of size. Our assessment of more than 200 patients who presented with visual loss from among our first 1,000 pituitary patients operated on via the transnasal transsphenoidal route yielded evidence of improved vision in 81 percent, unchanged vision in 16 percent, and worsening of vision in 3 percent. These results are similar to those of other large series that have been reported on the efficacy

of the transsphenoidal approach to suprasellar tumors and are equal to or exceed the results of large series of subfrontal explorations for visual loss. In addition, there is clear documentation of the potential for *improvement in pituitary function* after transsphenoidal adenomectomy with careful preservation of normal gland in patients with preexisting hypopituitarism. The efficacy of transsphenoidal surgery in selected patients with microadenomas has been established, with some reports of tumor control in more than 90 percent of the patients. In series including larger tumors, however, a less optimistic rate of 50 to 85 percent tumor control is obtained with surgery alone.

Transsphenoidal microsurgery for both large and small adenomas performed by experienced surgeons has acceptable mortality and morbidity. Of 2,606 patients with microadenomas and 2,677 patients with macroadenomas reported in an international survey, the operative death rates were 0.27 and 0.86 percent, respectively. Direct injury to the hypothalamus seemed to be the major cause of operative death, with delayed mortality attributed to CSF leaks and their attendant septic complications or to vascular injury. Operative morbidity includes persistent or permanent diabetes insipidus, with the incidence ranging from 1.8 percent in one large series to a 17 percent incidence immediately postoperatively with large adenomas. Postoperative CSF fistulas

FIG. 35-11. The transsphenoidal approach. The transnasal transsphenoidal approach is preferred for access to the majority of pituitary adenomas. It offers direct access to the sella turcica and its contents with no brain retraction and minimal morbidity. In contrast, the alternative subfrontal approach may be inadequate for removal of the intrasellar component of the tumor. The current popularity of the transsphenoidal approach was facilitated by the advent of the operating microscope, better microsurgical instruments, and better sources of illumination.

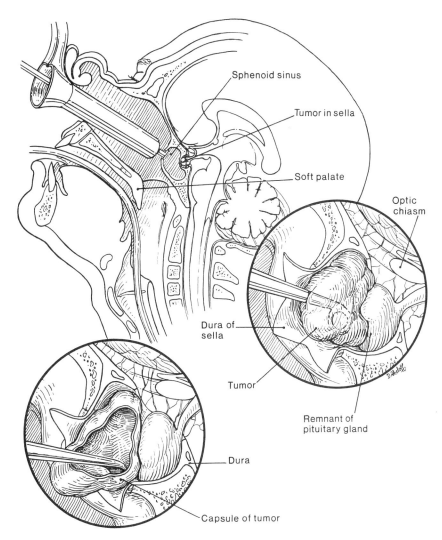

range from 1 to 4.4 percent in different series, depending on the size of the lesion and follow-up time, but they occur most frequently with larger lesions. Other major morbidity (stroke, visual loss, vascular injury, meningitis, cranial nerve palsy) is encountered in 3.5 percent, and minor morbidity (bleeding, nasal or sinus problems, diabetes insipidus, syndrome of inappropriate antidiuretic hormone secretion [SIADH], transient cranial nerve paresis, transient psychosis) occurs in another 3.5 percent of patients. Complications amounted to a small percentage of the overall surgical experience, emphasizing the relative safety of the procedure.

The rare relative contraindications to the transsphenoidal approach include: (1) extensive lateral tumor herniating into the middle fossa with minimal midline mass; these cases may require a primary or secondary transcranial procedure to remove tumor inaccessible by a midline approach; (2) ectatic carotid arteries projecting toward the midline, which are at risk of injury using a transsphenoidal approach; and (3) acute sinusitis, which may delay the procedure for treatment of infection. Previous rhinoplasty or submucous resection may increase the difficulty in developing the dissection planes, but they invariably can be established, and thus this factor should not alone constitute a contraindication to the transnasal approach.

Characteristically these tumors are soft and friable and at surgery may herniate down through the diaphragma sellae after evacuation of the intrasellar component; this may be facilitated if the anesthesiologist performs a Valsalva maneuver intraoperatively. Other techniques to promote herniation include the infusion of air or saline through a previously placed cisternal or lumbar catheter. A pure suprasellar tumor or one that requires suprasellar access may be approached, if necessary, by carrying the bony resection anteriorly over the tuberculum sellae. Such techniques may enable removal of sizable tumors within the suprasellar cistern, subfrontal space, and cavernous sinus; many of these will herniate into the enlarged sella once the intrasellar component has been evacuated.

Once the mass has been resected, attention must be paid to obliteration of the CSF fistula if the arachnoid has been violated. During transsphenoidal procedures in which the arachnoid has been breached, a fascia lata graft of appropriate size is routinely harvested to cover the opening and held in place with a small piece of autologous nasal cartilage or Marlex mesh. The sphenoid sinus behind this graft is then packed with fat obtained at the harvest of the fascia lata graft to further buttress the graft in position. A posterior nasal pack is then placed against the sphenoidal opening to maintain hemostasis and promote sealing of the graft. Using such careful techniques of closure, the incidence of CSF leakage is less than 1 percent, and attendant infectious complications are thus avoided.

Transcranial Approach. There are instances in which the transcranial approach is desirable, as noted earlier, such as when the transsphenoidal approach is hazardous because of the presence of ectatic carotid arteries, or when the tumor spills over into the middle fossa while leaving a small, virtually normal-sized sella turcica. Such lesions generally occur because of an incompetent diaphragma sellae that enables superior and lateral growth of tumor without significant expansion of the sella. Under such circumstances, direct visualization of the tumor by the transcranial approach may be desirable. In addition, there are occasional cases in which the consistency of tumor that is encountered via the transsphenoidal approach is such as to defy an

adequate resection of tumor from this approach. This may require a secondary transcranial procedure if inadequate decompression of the optic mechanism has been established.

The consistency of the tumor is usually that of a soft and friable lesion that is easily debulked with the use of curettes of variable lengths and rotations. The main difficulty encountered with the removal of the lesion is the complicating anatomy related to the vascular supply to the hypothalamus and optic chiasm, in addition to the visual structures themselves. This anatomy may preclude total removal without injury to cranial nerves or the midline neuraxis. In such cases it is certainly more prudent to remove the soft interior and leave a densely adherent capsule than to risk cranial and vascular injury for a lesion that is likely not curable by surgery alone. These patients will invariably need radiotherapy for ultimate tumor control. The goals of the operation should primarily be decompression of the optic apparatus and judicious tumor removal without exposing neural or vascular structures to undue risk of injury.

Perioperative Management. Perioperative glucocorticoids are administered to all patients; this is crucial if preoperative endocrine assessment indicates any hypocortisolemia. Methylprednisolone is given intravenously at sizable dosages of 40 mg (or 10 mg dexamethasone) every 6 h in the immediate perioperative period in those cases with neurologic compromise, usually starting the day before surgery and continuing for 1 or 2 days postoperatively, then in a tapering dosage regimen tailored to the patient's projected glucocorticoid needs as anticipated by the preoperative endocrine assessment and intraoperative findings. In patients without visual compromise, lower dosages of these high-potency glucocorticoids with a more rapid postoperative tapering may be used.

Thyroid function should be assessed preoperatively and normalized before any elective surgical intervention. The stress of surgery can provoke an acute crisis in the patient without sufficient reserve and should be a consideration in patients with an otherwise unexplained alteration in mental status postoperatively.

Serial visual field testing is routinely performed in the recovery room and intensive care unit (ICU) to monitor visual and general neurologic conditions. In the patient with preoperative visual deficit, careful monitoring in the early postoperative period is essential. Both the transfrontal and transsphenoidal routes are successful in improving vision. Immediate postoperative improvement of vision may occur, with a significant improvement usually within the first 2 weeks, but continued improvement may occur for up to 12 months. More important, any *loss* of vision in the postoperative period may indicate an evolving hemorrhagic complication, and emergent CT scanning should be performed. Evidence of hemorrhage on the postoperative scan with a progressive visual deficit would warrant emergent transsphenoidal reexploration.

Blood pressure is carefully monitored; hypotensive events are to be avoided, especially in cases with compressive neurologic deficit in which tissue perfusion is already marginal.

Urine volumes and specific gravities must be followed in concert with sodium levels in order to clearly understand the dynamics of potential postoperative diabetes insipidus. Manipulation of the normal posterior pituitary gland may produce transient fluctuations in serum sodium level.

Before discharge, a morning fasting serum cortisol level is obtained to determine the need for cortisol replacement. Intraoperative evidence of residual normal pituitary gland is also a major guide in such considerations. Thyroid evaluation is usually done at 3 to 4 weeks postoperatively, since autonomous function of the thyroid may persist for some time postoperatively.

Unless clinically indicated, postoperative imaging is not performed for at least 6 weeks postoperatively, and 3 months in most cases. This allows clearance of all operative artifactual changes that might confuse the decision about the implementation of postoperative adjuvant therapy.

Radiotherapy for Pituitary Adenomas. *Primary Radiotherapy.*
Radiotherapy was advocated for the management of pituitary tumors as early as 1907. Radiotherapy per se, however, should not be considered a completely benign therapy or an equivalent alternative to microsurgical resection. Adverse effects from radiation in this region can range from mild to severe. Radiotherapy carries *a significant risk of worsening preexisting hypopituitarism,* with an overt 10 to 15 percent frequency of panhypopituitarism (Fig. 35-12). It also can increase the rate of atherogenesis in the major vessels in the field, and it can cause visual impairment. These complications increase as a function of total treatment dosage. The visual impairment can result from one of several mechanisms, including empty sella syndrome, treatment failure, or direct radiation damage to optic pathways. Other minor complications from radiotherapy include epilation, scalp swelling, and otitis.

In the elderly patient or any patient who has a medical illness in which general anesthesia and surgery pose a significant risk, consideration should be given to primary radiation therapy, following an appropriate clinical diagnosis of a nonfunctioning pituitary tumor. The indications for this nonsurgical approach are strengthened in cases with hypopituitarism. A dose of 4,000 cGy by external beam is considered optimal by most radiotherapists. Reported series of patients treated with radiotherapy alone describe a 50 percent recurrence rate with local control in 75 percent after salvage treatment. Other authors report a local control rate of 50 to 79 percent, with an adequate salvage in cases of recurrence. It has been suggested that late recurrence after radiotherapy, which is not uncommon, may be the result of inadequate dosage. Treatments with 4,500 cGy given in 25 fractions can result in a high (greater than 90 percent) probability of stable long-term control.

The recent development of *stereotactic radiosurgery* (image-directed focal radiotherapy) may provide a safer and more effective method of radiotherapy for pituitary adenomas. Focused radiotherapy may potentially avoid damage to midline neural and vascular structures while delivering high local therapeutic doses to the lesion with great accuracy. Stereotactic radiosurgery offers an alternative for patients who have failed previous microsurgery, and who do not require decompression of the optic apparatus or more rapid normalization of endocrine status. There are few published series with meaningful follow-up for radiosurgery of pituitary adenomas, and optimal dosimetry has not yet been defined. Early reports indicate tumor growth control rates better than 90 percent but a less optimal control rate of endocrinopathy in functional tumors. These results all indicate that stereotactic radiosurgery may be performed for pituitary adenomas with low morbidity. Additionally, these series have demonstrated that the advantage of stereotactic radiosurgery over the use of external fractionated radiation or charged particles is reduction in postoperative hypopituitarism. Present protocols require the tumor to remain a distance of more than 2 mm from the optic nerves or chiasm to avoid visual deficit from radiation.

In the asymptomatic elderly patient with a nonsecreting tumor, intact pituitary function, and no compromise of the visual system, a case can be made for merely monitoring the patient with routine clinical (visual field) and endocrine evaluation, with serial MRI or CT scanning being performed at least yearly; these tumors may exhibit a benign course without reaching symptomatic dimensions within the remaining life expectancy.

Postoperative Radiotherapy. The rationale for the use of postoperative radiation therapy is to reduce the incidence of recurrence, with several studies suggesting improved tumor control with the combination of surgery plus radiotherapy. This is especially true for large and invasive lesions, which manifest an

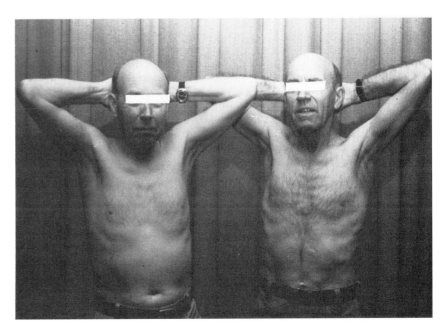

FIG. 35-12. Panhypopituitarism. This striking example of identical twins, in which the brother on the left has long-standing hypogonadism secondary to radiation for a pituitary adenoma. Note the relative loss of masculinizing body hair secondary to the gonadotropic hormonal deficiency. (Photo courtesy of Dr. Peter Singer, Department of Medicine, University of Southern California.)

increased rate of recurrence. This treatment does not ensure recurrence-free survival, but the time to recurrence may be prolonged. Recurrences have been reported up to 18 years after operation; published recurrence rates in series with short follow-up times may therefore be misleading.

With functioning pituitary tumors, evaluation of postoperative endocrine status may give an indication of the effectiveness of the surgical removal; however, in nonfunctioning lesions the judgment of the surgeon supplemented by postoperative imaging are the only parameters to gauge the extent of resection and therefore the risk of recurrence. The surgeon's appreciation of the totality of the resection may not be accurate in the face of an invasive tumor. The lack of a chemical marker in a true nonfunctional tumor makes assessment of cure difficult in the postoperative period. Furthermore, in contrast to prolactin- and GH-secreting tumors, no adjunctive pharmacotherapy is available.

For these reasons, the criteria for selection of patients for postoperative radiotherapy remains controversial. In general, large tumors, which frequently invade the dura and therefore defy surgical excision, should all be considered candidates for postoperative radiotherapy, especially if the patient has hypopituitarism postoperatively. Similarly, with frank cavernous sinus invasion, postoperative radiotherapy would be advocated. In cases in which tumor invasion is not evident and "total" removal has been achieved, observing the patient with routine scanning on a yearly basis can be an appropriate strategy, especially if endocrine function is intact.

OTHER LESIONS

Included in the differential diagnosis of mass lesions that can affect pituitary function are a variety of tumors or cystic lesions in the region of the midline skull base. Many of these can be differentiated from primary pituitary lesions on the basis of the clinical history, physical examination, and radiographic appearance.

Benign Pituitary Cysts

Benign pituitary cysts are a common autopsy finding. They can occasionally become large enough to become symptomatic. These represent a disparate pathologic group of entities that often require histologic evaluation to differentiate. Although pituitary adenomas may contain cystic components and represent the most common cystic lesions of the pituitary, many other cystic lesions are believed to consist of remnants of Rathke's pouch. Rathke's pouch is a transient embryologic structure (third or fourth week of embryonic life) that arises from an outgrowth of stomodeum and elongates to form the craniopharyngeal duct. With further development of the pouch wall to form the anterior lobe of the pituitary, pars tuberalis, and pars intermedia, the residual lumen is reduced to a cleft, which usually regresses. It is hypothesized that persistence and enlargement of the cleft results in a symptomatic Rathke's cleft cyst. The cyst is characteristically lined by a single layer of cuboidal or columnar epithelial cells. Most Rathke's cleft cysts are asymptomatic. Occasionally they enlarge and cause symptoms by local mass effect (hypopituitarism or visual loss). Treatment by transsphenoidal drainage usually is effective.

Less common cystic lesions in this region include arachnoid cysts, pars intermedia cysts, and cysticercal cysts.

Meningiomas

Meningiomas are common tumors that arise from cells of the meninges. Most of these tumors are well-demarcated round or oval tumors that are attached to the dura mater. The vast majority of meningiomas are benign tumors that compress, but do not invade, the parenchyma of the brain. Meningiomas can arise in several locations in and about the sella turcica, the most common of these being the planum sphenoidale, the tuberculum sellae, the anterior or posterior clinoid, or the diaphragma sellae itself. It is distinctly uncommon for such a tumor to present as a completely intrasellar mass. Clinically, patients with meningiomas in these locations present with visual loss or other cranial nerve dysfunction. In contrast to pituitary adenomas, the presentation of visual loss usually is asymmetric; physical examination often yields incongruous and asymmetric visual field defects and optic atrophy. The temporal pattern of visual loss may be acute, gradual, or fluctuating. The pattern of other cranial nerve dysfunction is variable, but involvement of the superior orbital fissure or the cavernous sinus may produce ophthalmoplegia with associated facial sensory deficits (cranial nerve V dysfunction). With larger tumors, variable amounts of pituitary dysfunction can occur from compression of the hypothalamic-pituitary axis.

On unenhanced CT meningiomas are often isodense or hyperdense compared to normal brain. After administration of contrast agent, these tumors enhance markedly on the CT scan and with gadolinium-DTPA on MRI.

The management of meningiomas is primarily surgical, with radiation therapy reserved for lesions that defy removal in younger patients.

Craniopharyngiomas

Though their precise embryologic origin is still debated, these benign squamous epithelium-lined tumors can present at any time of life. Approximately one-half of symptomatic patients present in childhood, making the lesion relatively more common in this age group. Because they are slow-growing, extraaxial tumors, the symptoms produced may be delayed until the tumor has reached considerable size. This is often the case in children, in whom the tumor can reach enormous size, often several centimeters in diameter. However, purely intrasellar tumors in older patients may be only a few millimeters in diameter and might be mistaken for a pituitary microadenoma. Because adults are much more sensitive to impairment in visual function, this is a common presentation in the older age group. Children, in contrast, present more frequently with symptoms of growth retardation secondary to hypothalamic-pituitary dysfunction (Fig. 35-13), or of increased intracranial pressure, often the result of obstruction of midline CSF pathways.

Craniopharyngiomas have a characteristic appearance on skull x-ray or CT scan. The most common location for these tumors is in the suprasellar cistern, but intrasellar lesions are sometimes seen, as are tumors that lie entirely within the third ventricle. In children there is usually erosion of the sella with calcification within or above the sella. This calcification may be missed if only MRI is obtained. Both CT and MRI can demonstrate enhancement of the solid region of the tumor after appropriate contrast agent administration.

Though the primary mode of treatment of craniopharyngiomas is surgical, long-term follow-up results are disappointing, even if the surgeon estimates "total" operative removal. These

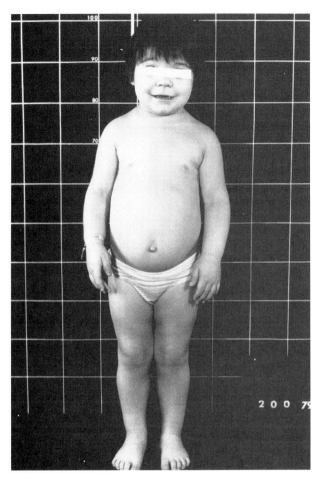

FIG. 35-13. *Hypothyroidism secondary to craniopharyngioma. A 4-year-old female with growth delay, generalized myxedema, obesity, and protuberant abdomen. Endocrinologic evaluation revealed pronounced hypothyroidism, and subsequent radiographic workup revealed a calcified suprasellar tumor.*

tumors are somewhat responsive to radiotherapy, with several studies indicating prolonged interval to recurrence and survival after postoperative radiotherapy.

Optic Chiasm or Hypothalamic Gliomas

Astrocytoma of the optic nerve, the optic chiasm, or the hypothalamus is uncommon in adults but comprises 7 percent of intracranial tumors in children. Chiasmal and hypothalamic lesions are difficult to differentiate clinically or pathologically, and hence are often discussed together. There is an association of these gliomas with neurofibromatosis, but sporadic cases are more frequent. For lesions confined to the chiasm, the presentation is one of monocular or binocular visual impairment with or without optic atrophy. If the optic tract is involved, homonymous hemianopsia may be noted. With larger lesions, hypothalamic involvement is invariable, and children may present with endocrinopathy or lesional obstruction of CSF pathways. Endocrinopathies include precocious puberty or the diencephalic syndrome.

MRI can be helpful in distinguishing this tumor from a craniopharyngioma or a meningioma; coronal views can distinguish whether the chiasm is enlarged with tumor or displaced by another lesion in the suprasellar cistern.

These lesions defy surgical cure. Surgery is used primarily to establish the diagnosis and plan subsequent treatment, which usually is conservative management in young children and radiation in selected older patients.

Suprasellar Germinomas

Germinomas are tumors of germ cell derivation that occur primarily in adolescents and young adults. They occur most commonly within the cranium in the region of the pineal gland, the suprasellar-retrochiasmal region, within the third ventricle, the interpeduncular or quadrigeminal plate regions, or within the pituitary fossa. These tumors are not encapsulated and infiltrate so extensively that complete surgical excision is not possible without producing extensive neurologic deficits. Clinically, patients with suprasellar tumors typically present with diabetes insipidus (present in 95 percent of patients), visual difficulties, or endocrinopathy. Diagnosis usually is made with MRI, in which the tumors are intensely enhanced with administration of intravenous contrast material. Therapy usually consists of surgical biopsy or partial removal followed by radiation or chemotherapy.

Sellar Metastases

Metastases to the region of the sella turcica are uncommon and usually are the result of bony metastases to the region. A variety of tumors have been reported to metastasize to the region of the pituitary gland itself, but these are rare. When metastases do occur to the pituitary gland, the presenting symptoms are those of progressive panhypopituitarism.

Mechanism of spread to the skull base in this area is via venous routes, such as the paravertebral venous plexus, which anastomoses with the venous drainage at the base of the skull. If metastatic cells pass through dural veins, subdural seeding is possible, and contiguous spread through Virchow-Robin spaces allows intracerebral metastases to occur. Direct arterial spread may occur to the region of the posterior pituitary, usually in patients in whom metastatic spread to the lungs has already occurred (the "multistep" metastatic hypothesis).

Lymphocytic Hypophysitis

A rare, presumably autoimmune disorder, lymphocytic hypophysitis is characterized by extensive infiltration of the anterior pituitary with lymphocytes and plasma cells. The pathophysiologic process apparently begins as an acute inflammatory process with diffuse enlargement of the gland. With continued inflammation, the normal pituitary architecture becomes difficult to recognize, and the process might result in diffuse interstitial fibrosis and gland atrophy. The neurohypophysis does not appear to be primarily involved with the process. The rarity of the disorder and the lack of specific radiologic or endocrinologic features have made it difficult to diagnose without a tissue biopsy.

Empty Sella Syndrome

Though not neoplastic, the empty sella syndrome can be mistaken for an intrasellar mass on radiologic imaging. The syndrome results from a herniation of the arachnoid and subarachnoid space of the suprasellar cistern through an incompetent diaphragma sellae. This may be primary, or it may follow pituitary surgery or radiation therapy. CT or MRI will demonstrate an apparently "empty" sella, its contents the same density or signal intensity as CSF. The pituitary stalk and the compressed gland may be visualized and displaced posteriorly. Occasionally, the patient may manifest an associated compressive endocrinopathy.

TRAUMA

Though not common, the pituitary stalk is susceptible to transection in major skull fractures of the base of the skull. In up to 10 percent of fatal head injuries, the stalk is injured. Transection of the pituitary stalk at the skull base results in massive infarction of the anterior lobe, with the subsequent development of panhypopituitarism. It is likely, however, that most pituitary and hypothalamic damage results secondarily from increased intracranial pressure caused by diffuse cerebral swelling.

POSTERIOR PITUITARY DISORDERS

Diabetes Insipidus

Deficient secretion of vasopressin leads to an impairment of water conservation. Excessive volumes of urine are excreted, resulting in increased plasma osmolality and marked thirst. Dehydration can occur if the thirst mechanism is impaired or if the patient does not have access to adequate amounts of water. One-third of the cases of central diabetes insipidus are idiopathic; the other causes include tumors, granulomatous disease, or trauma destroying the hypothalamus, pituitary stalk, or posterior pituitary.

Syndrome of Inappropriate Secretion of Antidiuretic Hormone

Hypersecretion of vasopressin—syndrome of inappropriate secretion of antidiuretic hormone—(SIADH) occurs in 15 percent of hospitalized patients. It leads to impaired water excretion and often manifests few signs other than hypotonicity of body fluids. Evidence of increased total body water, such as edema and hypertension, is absent unless sodium excretion is impaired as a result of some other cause. Renal excretion of sodium is increased (> 20 mEq/L), and urinary osmolality is inappropriately elevated in relation to plasma osmolality. Plasma vasopressin concentrations are inappropriately elevated in relation to plasma hypoosmolality. Reported causes include various central nervous system disorders, neoplastic diseases, pulmonary diseases, and drugs.

Adrenal

Jeffrey A. Norton

HISTORICAL BACKGROUND

In the mid-sixteenth century (1563), Eustachius published the first accurate anatomical drawings of the human adrenal glands and the kidneys with the proper anatomic relationships to the aorta and inferior vena cava. Nearly two and a half centuries later, in 1805, Cuvier described the anatomical division of each adrenal gland into the cortex and the medulla. In 1855 Thomas Addison described the cachexia, weakness, gastrointestinal symptoms, weak pulse, bronze skin color, and fatal prognosis associated with untreated adrenal insufficiency, a condition that still bears his name. Following Addison's treatise, Brown-Séquard demonstrated in experimental animals that the adrenal glands were essential for life.

In 1886 Frankel first described the adrenal tumor that we call a pheochromocytoma. Physiologists Oliver and Sharpey-Schafer noted that there was a substance in the adrenal medulla that dramatically raised the blood pressure of dogs, which they named "adrenalin" in 1895. Two years later Abel, at Johns Hopkins, made a similar observation, and called the substance epinephrine. In 1901 he demonstrated that epinephrine would not maintain life in an adrenalectomized animal. In 1902 Kohn demonstrated that chromaffin-positive cells were present in the adrenal medulla, the carotid body, paraganglia in the abdomen, and the organ of Zuckerkandl. In 1912 the pathologist Pick named an adrenal tumor "pheochromocytoma" for the dark color of the tumor with the characteristic chromaffin reaction. The first successful resections of a pheochromocytoma were performed in 1926 by Roux in Switzerland and Charles Mayo in the United States. Subsequently, Jaffe and others proved that pheochromocytomas were associated with paroxysmal hypertension.

Around 1912 Harvey Cushing had studied and documented the condition that now bears his name. In 1932 he reported 11 patients with moon face, truncal obesity, hypertension, polyphagia, polydipsia, polycythemia, and susceptibility to bruises and infections. Many of the patients were known to have had adenomas of the pituitary. In 1930 Hartman and associates purified adrenocortical extracts that were able to keep adrenalectomized animals alive. In 1934 Kendall, of the Mayo Clinic, obtained crystals from adrenal cortical extracts that retained adrenocortical activity. One of these crystallized extracts, compound E, was named "cortisone." Ten years later, Kendall and coworkers were able to synthesize cortisone.

In 1952 a potent mineralocorticoid was isolated from beef adrenal gland by Grundy and associates. It was purified and called "aldosterone." Three years later, in 1955, Conn described a patient and the clinical syndrome associated with a tumor that secreted excessive amounts of aldosterone (Conn's syndrome). In 1962, Bartter and colleagues described another form of hyperaldosteronism associated with elevated levels of renin secondary to hyperplasia of the renal juxtaglomerular apparatus. The two syndromes can be distinguished from each other by measurement of plasma renin levels, which are undetectable in Conn's syndrome.

In 1865 DeCrecchio first described the condition of congenital adrenal hyperplasia occurring in a female pseudohermaphrodite. Later, in 1887, Phillips reported four similar patients who died from salt wasting. In 1939 Butler hypothesized that the salt-wasting was from adrenal insufficiency, and in 1950 it was established that salt wasting could be treated with cortisone. Bartter and associates demonstrated that patients with salt wasting had elevated circulating levels of adrenocorticotropic hormone (ACTH), further supporting the hypothesis of adrenal insufficiency.

EMBRYOLOGY

The adrenal gland and medulla arise from separate embryologic tissues. In the fourth week of gestation, cells destined to become the adrenal cortex develop from the mesoderm medial to the urogenital ridge. At the sixth week of gestation, these developing cells are penetrated by nerve fibers, through which medullary cells will migrate (Fig. 35-14). By the eighth week of gestation, the cortex has formed two distinct zones: a large and centrally located fetal zone, and a thin rim of cortex that will become the cortex in the adult. Throughout this period, proliferation of cells occurs largely in the outer cortex, suggesting that the same cells give rise to the fetal and the definitive zones. Around the same time, the fetal adrenal circulation is established, with several arteries entering the adrenal gland from the aorta and a central vein that drains the adrenal effluent. During the second and third months of gestation, the weight of the adrenal glands increases from 5 to 80 mg, and the adrenals then are much larger than the

adjacent kidneys. After the twentieth week of gestation, growth of the adrenal cortex is dependent on stimulation from the pituitary gland. Anencephalic fetuses are born with an atrophic adrenal fetal zone. After birth, the fetal zone involutes, and the three zones of the adult adrenal cortex develop.

During the development of the fetus, primitive adrenocortical cells may widely migrate. Accessory adrenocortical tissues have been identified within the broad ligament, near the celiac axis, adjacent to the ovarian or testicular veins, and around the kidney or uterus. Less common locations include other abdominal organs and, rarely, the lungs, spinal nerves, and brain. These ectopic rests of adrenal tissue can be a significant problem because they can cause persistent or recurrent hypercortisolism in a patient with high levels of ACTH production (Fig. 35-15).

The adrenal medulla arises from the primitive sympathetic nervous system, derived from the neuroectoderm. These cells differentiate into neuroblasts that migrate ventrally from the neural crest to form the sympathetic ganglia, and into the pheochromoblasts that form catecholamine-secreting or chromaffin cells. In the fetus, neuroblasts and pheochromoblasts are found in the adrenal medulla and extraadrenal sites. The organ of Zuckerkandl, located near the origin of the inferior mesenteric artery, is the most common site for extraadrenal catecholamine-secreting tissue. The widespread occurrence of extraadrenal chromaffin cells accounts for the location of extraadrenal pheochromocytomas later in life.

ANATOMY

The adrenal glands are paired structures in the retroperitoneal space, lying at the level of the eleventh thoracic vertebra, and anteromedial to the upper pole of the kidney (Fig. 35-16). The normal adrenal gland measures about 5 by 2.5 cm and weighs from 3 to 6 g. Adrenal weight may increase by approximately 50 percent during periods of stress and during pregnancy. The adrenals are supplied by numerous small arteries arising from the aorta and the celiac, superior mesenteric, inferior phrenic, and renal arteries. The arteries are short and are located mainly on the medial side of each adrenal gland, most coming directly off the aorta. Phrenic branches are found along the superior medial margin of the adrenal gland, and renal branches along the inferior medial margin. These arteries join and anastomose over the surface of the gland, and numerous small, unbranched arter-

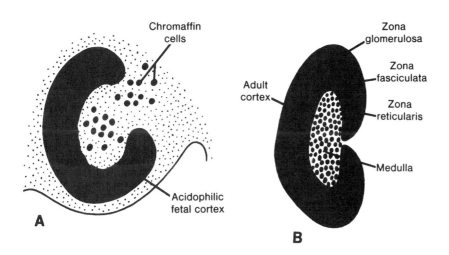

FIG. 35-14. *A. Chromaffin (sympathetic) cells penetrating the fetal cortex of the adrenal gland. B. At a later stage of development, the definitive cortex surrounds the medulla almost completely. (From: Sadler TW: Langman's Medical Embryology, 5th ed. Baltimore, Williams & Wilkins, 1985, with permission.)*

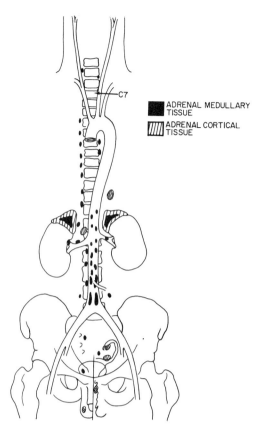

ADRENAL MEDULLARY
TISSUE

ADRENAL CORTICAL
TISSUE

FIG. 35-15. Location of ectopic adrenal tissue. The location of ectopic adrenal medullary tissue is shown in black; cortical tissue is shown in the shaded areas. The incidence of extraadrenal medullary tissue is very high compared to the incidence of extraadrenal cortical tissue, and while functioning extraadrenal medullary tissue occurs in about 1 in 8 cases of medullary hyperfunction, it occurs in fewer than 1 in 1000 cases of adrenocortical hyperfunction.

ies descend through the capsule. Nitric oxide concentration is an important local factor for maintaining high local levels of blood flow to the various zones of the cortex and the medulla. Adrenal blood empties through a single central vein into the inferior vena cava on the right, and the renal vein on the left. The short, wide configuration of the right adrenal vein makes catheterization of the vein for hormone sampling difficult and results in a greater probability of life-threatening hemorrhage during removal of the right adrenal gland.

The adrenal cortex has a characteristic chrome yellow color and is divided into three zones: the zona glomerulosa, the zona reticularis, and the zona fasciculata. The outer cells of the cortex are the aldosterone-secreting cells of the zona glomerulosa. The inner cells of the cortex are the cortisol-secreting cells of the zona fasciculata. The middle cortical cells are the adrenal androgen-secreting cells of the zona reticularis. The center of the adrenal gland, the medulla, contains the catecholamine-secreting cells. Medullary cells are chromaffin positive.

ADRENAL CORTEX

Physiology

The adrenal gland secretes five major steroid hormones: cortisol, aldosterone, progesterone, testosterone, and estradiol. The major

biosynthetic pathways of adrenal steroid synthesis from cholesterol are shown in Fig. 35-17. It is advantageous to think of these pathways as three distinct points of origin: one in the zona glomerulosa, producing aldosterone, a second in the zona fasciculata, producing cortisol, and a third in the zona reticularis, called the adrenal androgen/estrogen pathway that produces testosterone, estradiol, and estrone. Each pathway requires enzyme reactions and approximately five steps from cholesterol to the end product.

Aldosterone. Aldosterone causes the kidney to retain sodium, which increases the extracellular fluid volume. Aldosterone secretion is regulated primarily by the renin-angiotensin system, with potassium, atrial natriuretic hormone (ANH), and dopamine also making important contributions. The factors that stimulate aldosterone secretion have direct effects on the kidney and vasculature and provide maintenance of the extracellular fluid volume, concentration of extracellular potassium, and blood pressure. When intake of salt is restricted and blood volume is contracted, an increase in secretion of renin, and subsequently of angiotensin II, stimulates the secretion of aldosterone (Fig. 35-18). Renin is produced and secreted by the juxtaglomerular cells, which are differentiated smooth muscle cells located in the renal afferent arteriole. An area of the distal tubule near its origin, the macula densa, lies in proximity to the juxtaglomerular cells at the hilus of the glomerulus. The four factors that control renin release by the juxtaglomerular cells are: baroreceptors located within the afferent arteriole, the macula densa, the sympathetic nervous system, and the negative feedback of angiotensin II (see Fig. 35-18). Angiotensin II and aldosterone

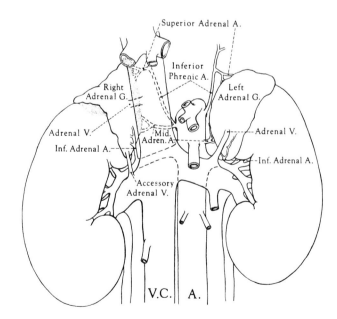

FIG. 35-16. Location and blood supply of the adrenal glands. There is great variation in the arterial blood supply of the glands, but it generally comes from three sources: a branch from the renal artery, a branch from the aorta, and a branch from the inferior phrenic artery. There usually is only one main vein on each side; on the left the adrenal vein opens into the left renal vein, and on the right it opens into the inferior vena cava. Occasionally there are very small accessory adrenal veins such as that illustrated here for the right adrenal gland.

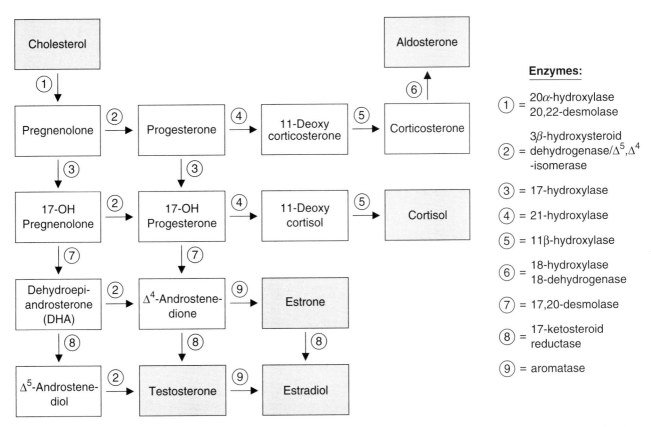

FIG. 35-17. Major pathways of adrenal steroid biosynthesis. Major precursor and end product hormones are shaded. Key enzymes are numbered.

increase the reabsorption of sodium from the renal tubule to restore the extracellular fluid volume. Conversely, when salt intake is increased and extracellular fluid volume is expanded, the formation of angiotensin II from renin is decreased, ANH is secreted by the heart, and the secretion of dopamine by the adrenals also increases. ANH and dopamine inhibit aldosterone secretion and sodium excretion by the kidney. The serum level of potassium also exerts an effect on aldosterone secretion. Hyperkalemia stimulates aldosterone secretion, but hypokalemia inhibits it.

FIG. 35-18. The renin-angiotensin-aldosterone cascade.

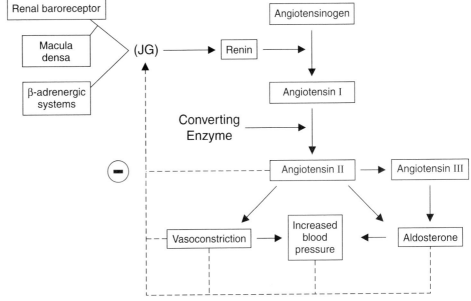

Table 35-4
Effects of Glucocorticoids

System	Effect
Carbohydrate metabolism	↑ Glucose
	↑ Glycogenolysis and gluconeogensis
	↑ Glucose uptake
Protein metabolism	↑ Protein catabolism
Lipid metabolism	↑ Mobilization of free fatty acids
Circulation	↑ Cardiac output
Musculoskeletal	Muscle weakness, osteoporosis
Anti-inflammatory	↓ Permeability
	↓ Leukocyte function
	↓ Antibody formation
	↓ Resistance to infections
Connective tissue	↓ Collagen synthesis
	↓ Healing
CNS	Euphoria; psychosis
Eye	Cataracts

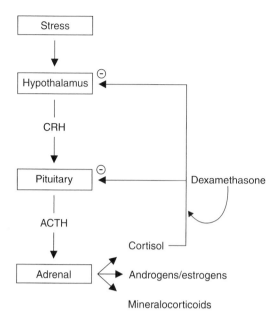

FIG. 35-20. *Model of control and stimulation of cortisol secretion through the hypothalamic-pituitary-adrenal axis.*

Cortisol. Glucocorticoids serve essential functions in human beings without which life cannot be sustained (Table 35-4). Glucocorticoid secretion is pulsatile and assumes a circadian pattern, with peak secretion before awakening in the morning (Fig. 35-19). Glucocorticoid secretion is stimulated by stress and inhibited by the negative-feedback effects of cortisol (Fig. 35-20). All physiologically important effects on cortisol secretion are mediated through adrenocorticotropic hormone (ACTH). ACTH has a short plasma half-life. The rapid metabolism of ACTH combined with the pulsatile pituitary secretion causes rapid changes in plasma ACTH levels. Several hormones can stimulate the release of ACTH from the pituitary gland, including antidiuretic hormone and epinephrine, but the most important is corticotropin-releasing hormone (CRH). CRH is secreted in episodic bursts by the paraventricular nuclei of the hypothalamus, which explains the pulsatile secretion of ACTH. Plasma levels of cortisol exert a negative feedback on secretion of ACTH and CRH at the level of the pituitary and the hypothalamus, respectively.

Sex Steroids. During normal human sexual development, the adrenal gland matures through a specific process called adrenarche. Adrenarche results in adrenal secretion of dehydroepiandrosterone (DHA), DHA sulfate, androstenedione, testosterone, and estrone (see Fig. 35-17). DHA and DHA sulfate are plasma markers of adrenarche, because more than 90 percent of plasma levels come from adrenal secretion. Gonadal secretion only contributes to the plasma levels of the other steroids.

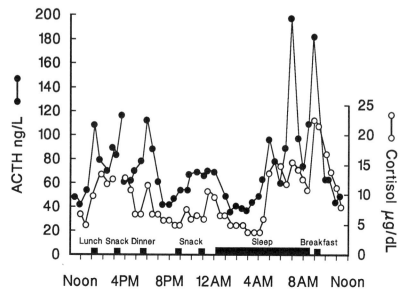

FIG. 35-19. *The pulsatile and circadian pattern of ACTH and cortisol secretion.*

Pathology

Hyperplasia. Hyperplasia is defined as an increased number of cells and is associated with an increased function or compensatory change. In patients with Cushing's disease (excessive production of ACTH by a pituitary tumor), the adrenal gland is approximately twice normal size. The weight of a hyperplastic adrenal gland increases from a normal range of 3 to 6 g, to a range of 6 to 12 g. Microscopically, there is a widened inner zone of the compact zona reticularis and a sharply demarcated outer zone of clear cells. In patients with ectopic ACTH production by a nonpituitary tumor, the microscopic appearance of adrenal glands is similar, but the weight is greater, from 12 to 30 g. Primary pigmented micronodular adrenal hyperplasia (1- to 5-mm nodules with pigmented appearance and normal glandular weight) is a hyperplastic condition of the adrenal gland that is not associated with excessive ACTH secretion. It occurs more commonly in children and can occur in a familial pattern.

Adrenal Cortical Adenoma. Adrenal adenoma is a benign neoplasm of adrenal cortical cells that may produce symptoms secondary to excessive hormone secretion that is not controlled by normal feedback mechanisms. A cortical adenoma does not exceed 5 cm in diameter and weighs less than 100 g. Some cellular pleomorphism and tumor necrosis may be present, but usually the cells are homogeneous and bland with little mitotic activity. It is difficult to distinguish adenoma from carcinoma on the basis of cellular morphology. Adenomas produce syndromes of hypercortisolism and hyperaldosteronism but seldom produce adrenogenital syndromes. Larger tumors (> 6 cm) producing adrenogenital syndromes usually are carcinomas.

Adrenal Cortical Carcinoma. Adrenal cortical carcinoma is a malignant neoplasm of adrenal cortical cells demonstrating partial histologic and functional differentiation. Adrenal cortical carcinomas are rare, comprising 0.05 to 0.2 percent of all cancers. Women develop functional adrenal cortical carcinomas more often. There is a bimodal occurrence by age with a peak incidence of less than 5 years, and a second peak in the fourth and fifth decade of life. Adrenocortical carcinoma is described as part of a complex hereditary syndrome that includes sarcoma, breast, and lung cancer.

Adrenal cortical carcinomas are larger than 6 cm and weigh between 100 and 5000 g. Areas of necrosis and hemorrhage are common. Invasion and metastases can occur. Microscopically, the appearance is variable. Cells with large nuclei, hyperchromatism, and enlarged nucleoli are all consistent with malignancy. Vascular invasion, desmoplastic bands, and mitoses are suggestive of malignancy. Immunostaining profiles of adrenocortical carcinoma and adenoma are similar. The only reliable criterion is the presence of nodal or distant metastasis.

Cushing's Syndrome

Cushing's syndrome (endogenous hypercortisolism) is caused by the secretion of ACTH by a pituitary tumor (Cushing's disease), by the secretion of cortisol by an adrenal tumor, or by the ectopic secretion of ACTH by a nonadrenal tumor. Determining the cause of the hypercortisolism entails performing multiple tests in a logical sequence (Fig. 35-21). Treatment should aim to cure the hypercortisolism and eliminate any tumor that threatens the patient's health while minimizing the chances of endocrine deficiency or long-term dependence on medications.

Clinical Manifestations. The signs and symptoms of Cushing's syndrome are widespread and diverse, and nearly every organ in the body is affected (Table 35-5). Although hypercortisolism is the most common hormonal symptom complex for adrenal cortical tumors, Cushing's syndrome is rare, with an estimated incidence of 10 per million population. It can occur in children. Weight gain is the most common symptom of patients with hypercortisolism. Obesity is usually truncal, and patients have thinning of extremities due to muscle wasting. Increased fat in the dorsal neck region combined with kyphosis secondary to osteoporosis gives the appearance of a "buffalo hump." The face is round and "moon" shaped (Fig. 35-22). Blood pressure is mildly increased secondary to excessive mineralocorticoid secretion. Striae appear as reddish-purple broad skin marks along the flank. Hirsutism consists of excessive fine hair on face, upper back, and arms. Virilization, including clitoromegaly, deep voice, and balding, and is more commonly associated with malignant adrenal cortical tumors. Glucose intolerance with hyperglycemia is mild, and patients seldom require insulin. Muscle weakness is common and can be exacerbated by hypokalemia. Menstrual irregularity or amenorrhea is one of the most common signs of hypercortisolism; men have decreased sexual drive and impotency. Dilatation of superficial blood vessels and thinning of subcutaneous tissue can give the face a ruddy appearance. Mental changes vary from mild depression to severe psychosis. Impaired immune function may cause opportunistic infections, including cryptococcosis, aspergillosis, nocardiosis, and *Pneumocystis carinii* infection. These infections add to morbidity and may be lethal. Children may be diagnosed by an arrest of normal growth and short stature.

Diagnosis. The early diagnosis of Cushing's syndrome depends on an awareness of the different signs and symptoms associated with the disorder and the ability to discriminate these findings. The initial workup is to establish the presence of hypercortisolism. The next step is to determine whether the hypercortisolism is "pituitary-dependent" or "pituitary-independent," and the last step is to determine the exact cause of the hypercortisolism (see Fig. 35-21). Diagnostic laboratory methods yield the correct diagnosis for the presence and the cause of the hypercortisolism in nearly every case. The best screening test for the diagnosis of hypercortisolism is the measurement of 24-h urinary free cortisol. Urinary excretion of free cortisol is directly proportional to the amount of free cortisol in the plasma. As the cortisol-binding globulin becomes saturated (plasma cortisol levels of 20 μg/dL), small increases in cortisol secretion produce exponential increases in urinary free cortisol. Another test for the determination of hypercortisolism is the single-dose dexamethasone suppression test. It works because of the absence of normal feedback that occurs in all forms of hypercortisolism. Normal individuals given 1 mg dexamethasone orally at 11:00 P.M. have plasma cortisol levels below 5 μg/dL at 8:00 A.M. the next day. Patients with hypercortisolism have levels higher than 5 μg/dL. This test has a few false-negative and a few false-positive results. However, a single-dose dexamethasone test with suppression and a normal level of urinary free cortisol (< 100 μg/day) exclude hypercortisolism.

Determination of plasma ACTH levels may be useful to discriminate the cause of hypercortisolism. Patients with primary adrenal tumors or primary pigmented micronodular adrenocortical hyperplasia have undetectable or low plasma ACTH levels.

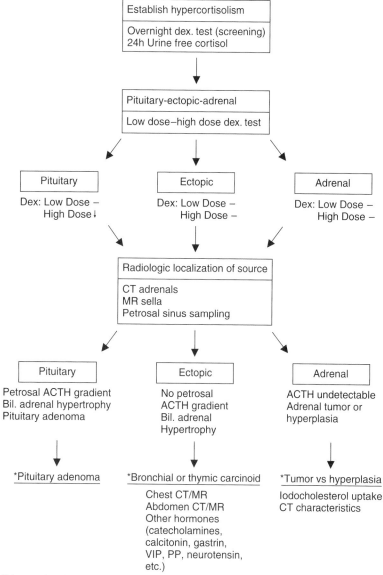

FIG. 35-21. *Flow diagram for the evaluation of a patient with endogenous hypercortisolism.*

Table 35-5
Clinical Manifestations of Cushing's Syndrome

	Percent
Truncal obesity	95
Hypertension	85
Glucosuria and decreased glucose tolerance	80
Menstrual and sexual dysfunction	75
Hirsutism and acne	70
Striae	70
Muscle weakness	65
Osteoporosis	55
Easy bruisability	55
Poor wound healing	55
Psychiatric disturbances	50
Edema, hypokalemic alkalosis	40
Polyuria	15

SOURCE: Harrison TS, Gann DS, et al, 1975.

Pituitary tumors have intermediate plasma levels of ACTH, and ectopic ACTH-producing tumors have very high levels. Radio-immunoassays for ACTH in plasma have been unreliable because of platelet-associated enzymes that degrade ACTH and result in falsely low levels. Samples must be collected in prechilled tubes on ice to improve reliability. Urinary 17-ketosteroid levels can help to distinguish an adrenal adenoma from a carcinoma. Low levels (< 10 mg/day) suggest an adrenal adenoma, and very high levels (> 60 mg/day) suggest adrenal cancer or ectopic ACTH syndrome.

Three diagnostic tests are most useful in determining the cause of hypercortisolism: the CRH test, the dexamethasone suppression test, and the metyrapone test. In patients with an ACTH-secreting pituitary tumor (Cushing's disease), administration of corticotropin-releasing hormone 1 μg/kg body weight increases plasma levels of ACTH and cortisol, but in patients with alcoholism, depression, or other stress diseases the response is blunted. The CRH test also may distinguish a pituitary tumor

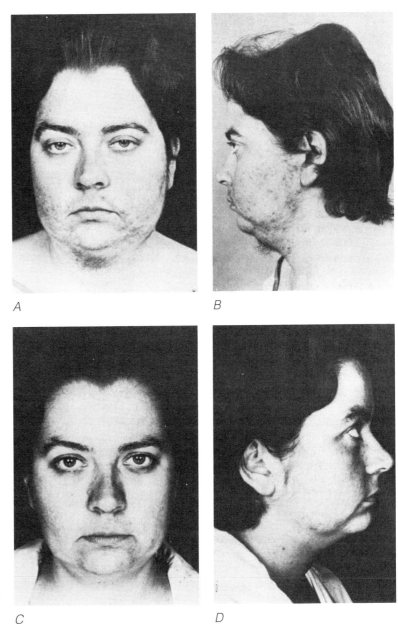

FIG. 35-22. Facial appearance of a patient with Cushing's disease before *(A, B)* and after *(C, D)* remission was achieved with treatment with cyproheptadine. *(From: Hsu TH, Gann DS, et al: Cyproheptadine in the control of Cushing's disease. Johns Hopkins Med J 149:77, 1981, with permission.)*

from ectopic ACTH secretion. In patients with ectopic ACTH secretion, plasma ACTH and cortisol levels after CRH administration do not increase.

The dexamethasone suppression test is the most useful test in establishing the cause of hypercortisolism and in determining whether the cause is pituitary-dependent or pituitary-independent. In normal individuals urinary levels of 17-hydroxysteroid, or free cortisol, will be suppressed by low-dose (2 mg) dexamethasone. In patients with hypercortisolism the urinary level of free cortisol is not suppressed by low-dose dexamethasone. High-dose dexamethasone (8 mg/day) will suppress urinary levels of free cortisol to less than 50 percent of baseline levels in patients with pituitary-dependent hypercortisolism (Cushing's disease), but it will not suppress levels in patients with primary adrenal cases of hypercortisolism or ectopic ACTH syndrome. The dexamethasone suppression test has an accuracy of approximately

95 percent. The metyrapone test, which causes stimulation of ACTH release in patients with pituitary Cushing's disease, can be complementary to the dexamethasone suppression test. Combining the tests results in greater accuracy rates than are obtained with the use of either test alone.

Radiologic Evaluation. Computed tomography (CT) of the sella turcica has been reported in various studies to detect a tumor in only 0 to 15 percent of patients with pituitary-dependent Cushing's disease, and minor abnormalities in 23 to 60 percent. Most ACTH-secreting pituitary tumors are microadenomas (< 5 mm). Pituitary magnetic resonance imaging (MRI) studies, even with gadolinium, have similar resolution. In patients with pituitary-dependent hypercortisolism, CT and MRI may be normal, but bilateral petrosal sinus sampling for ACTH concentrations detects the side with a tumor in most cases. Petrosal sinus sampling is the best method of differentiating a pituitary from an ectopic ACTH-producing tumor. The study requires bilateral sampling of the inferior petrosal sinus and peripheral veins for plasma ACTH levels before and after CRH. A petrosal sinus to peripheral plasma ACTH ratio of more than 3.0 after CRH administration correctly identifies patients with Cushing's disease (sensitivity is 100 percent), with few false positive results (specificity is 100 percent). Petrosal sinus sampling also provides correct localization of the ACTH-producing microadenoma in most patients. This is a relatively new and invasive study. It requires a significant degree of expertise by the radiologist, but it is the study of choice to diagnose and localize pituitary tumors in patients with Cushing's disease.

Adrenal CT can reliably distinguish cortical hyperplasia from tumor (Fig. 35-23). CT has great sensitivity ($>$ 95 percent), but it lacks specificity. In a patient with Cushing's syndrome, early detection of an adrenal neoplasm by CT simplifies the workup. CT can be used to image the primary tumor, plus local and distant metastases in patients with adrenocortical cancer. Approximately 15 percent of patients with Cushing's syndrome have a primary adrenal neoplasm as the source of the hypercortisolism. Diagnosis of a unilateral adrenal tumor requires the detection of a normal adrenal gland on the contralateral side. Adrenal hyperplasia also may be detected if both glands appear enlarged. MRI can add specificity to the sensitivity of CT. MRI may be able to distinguish adrenal adenoma from carcinoma, and a pheochromocytoma may be recognized by the brightness of the lesion on T_2-weighted MRI. Adrenal adenomas appear darker than the liver on T_2-weighted imaging. Carcinomas, whether primary adrenocortical or metastatic, appear as bright as or slightly brighter than the liver on T_2-weighted imaging. Pheochromocytomas appear much brighter (3$\times$) than the liver on T_2-weighted imaging. Different adrenal sequences have been used to better distinguish adrenal masses. Although some of these sequences have been useful, none is unequivocal, and each has been associated with exceptions and false results (Fig. 35-24).

Radioisotope imaging of the adrenals with labeled iodocholesterol, such as ^{131}I-6-beta-iodomethyl norcholesterol, can be useful in distinguishing adrenal adenoma from hyperplasia. It can help in differentiating a benign cortical neoplasm (adenoma), which usually takes up iodocholesterol, from a malignant cortical neoplasm (carcinoma), which usually does not take up the tracer. This is not absolute, because adrenal cortical carcinomas may take up iodocholesterol and be "hot" on scan. Iodocholesterol scan can be the study of choice in patients with primary pigmented micronodular hyperplasia in which CT appears normal, but bilateral adrenal uptake confirms the diagnosis. It can be used to image ectopic rests of adrenal tissue in patients who have had bilateral adrenalectomy but still have evidence of hypercortisolism. The disadvantages of radioiodocholesterol scans include exposure to radiation, limited isotope availability, and poor imaging of malignant adrenal neoplasms.

Interpretation. Once the laboratory tests have confirmed endogenous hypercortisolism, the workup should pinpoint the cause. If an adrenal cortical neoplasm is the source of the hypercortisolism, the workup will show (1) a tumor on CT or MRI (see Figs. 35-23 and 35-24), (2) low plasma ACTH levels, and (3) no suppression of urinary cortisol with high-dose dexamethasone. If there is no tumor but there are low ACTH levels and lack of suppression with dexamethasone, primary micronodular

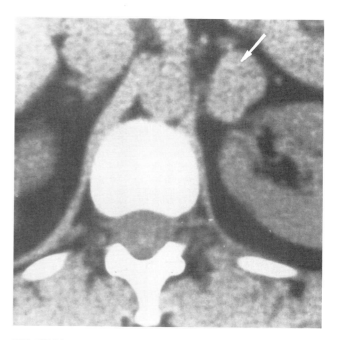

FIG. 35-23. CT image of a left adrenal aldosteronoma *(arrow)*.

adrenal cortical hyperplasia must be excluded by iodocholesterol scan or petrosal sinus sampling for ACTH levels. If there is an adrenal tumor, dexamethasone does not suppress urinary cortisol, and ACTH levels are consistently elevated, as are urinary catecholamines. Vanillylmandelic acid (VMA) and metanephrines must be measured to exclude an ACTH-producing pheochromocytoma.

In patients with ectopic ACTH syndrome, the studies should suggest: (1) bilateral hyperplasia of adrenals on CT, (2) elevated ACTH levels in plasma, (3) no cortisol suppression with high-

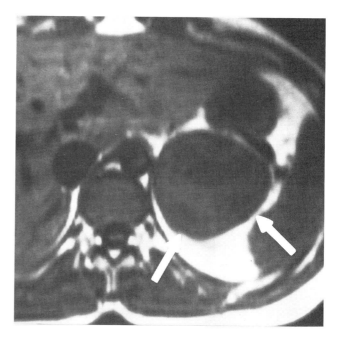

FIG. 35-24. MRI of a left adrenal carcinoma *(arrows)*.

dose dexamethasone, and (4) no evidence of lateralization of ACTH plasma levels on petrosal sinus sampling with CRH. Small-cell lung cancer is the most common ectopic ACTH tumor. Bronchial carcinoid tumors potentially are the most common curable ectopic ACTH tumor. Lobectomy is required because a significant number of patients will have nodal metastases. If the results are inconsistent, a sampling of petrosal sinus should be analyzed for ACTH levels to determine the diagnosis of ectopic ACTH syndrome.

If the patient has a pituitary tumor, the following results are expected: (1) bilateral hyperplasia of the adrenal glands, (2) mildly elevated plasma ACTH levels, (3) suppression with high-dose dexamethasone, and (4) lateralization with petrosal sinus sampling.

Adrenal Insufficiency (Addison's Disease)

Destruction of the adrenal cortex is the most common cause of primary adrenal insufficiency, but the adrenal medulla usually is spared. Adrenal insufficiency may be secondary to an abnormality in the hypothalamus or the pituitary, the so-called secondary adrenal insufficiency. Primary adrenal insufficiency can be caused by an autoimmune adrenalitis, tuberculosis, adrenomyeloneuropathy, fungal infections, AIDS, metastatic carcinoma, familial isolated glucocorticoid deficiency, and adrenal surgery to remove a cortisol-secreting tumor or both adrenal glands. Secondary adrenal insufficiency can be caused by pituitary tumor, craniopharyngioma, pituitary surgery or radiation, sarcoidosis, histiocytosis, empty sella syndrome, hypothalamic tumors; most commonly, it is iatrogenic secondary to long-term glucocorticoid administration. Primary or secondary adrenal insufficiency may lead to adrenal crisis perioperatively if the hypothalamic-pituitary-adrenal axis cannot generate an appropriate stress level of cortisol (see Fig. 35-20). Acute adrenal insufficiency is an uncommon clinical condition, but if it is untreated the consequences may be catastrophic.

Diagnosis. The symptoms and signs of primary and secondary adrenal insufficiency include: tiredness, weakness, mental depression, anorexia, weight loss, dizziness, orthostatic hypotension, nausea, vomiting, diarrhea, hyponatremia, hyperkalemia, anemia, leukocytosis, and eosinophilia. In secondary adrenal insufficiency, hyperpigmentation also may occur. Considering the possible diagnosis of acute adrenal insufficiency can be crucial in some critically ill patients.

Spontaneous adrenal insufficiency secondary to adrenal hemorrhage or adrenal vein thrombosis must be considered in a patient with upper abdominal or flank pain, abdominal rigidity, vomiting, confusion, and hypotension. To exclude the diagnosis of adrenal insufficiency in a patient, the best diagnostic study is the corticotropin (ACTH) stimulation test. In the short ACTH stimulation test 250 μg of cosyntropin is given intravenously or intramuscularly before 10 A.M.; plasma cortisol is measured before cosyntropin is given and 60 min after. The adrenal function is normal if the basal plasma level is at least 20 μg/dL and there is an increment of more than 7 μg/dL over basal levels at 60 min after cosyntropin administration.

Management. If the diagnosis of acute adrenal crisis is suspected, hydrocortisone should be given intravenously (Fig. 35-25). To verify the diagnosis, blood levels of cortisol, glucose, sodium, potassium, blood urea nitrogen, and creatinine should be determined, and a complete blood count should be performed. Treatment begins before results of the studies have returned, with the administration of a 200-mg bolus of hydrocortisone intravenously, followed by a rapid infusion of glucose and saline solution to correct hypoglycemia and dehydration. Patients who have adrenal crisis will have a low plasma cortisol level (< 18 μg/dL), hyponatremia, hyperkalemia, leukocytosis with eosinophilia, azotemia, and hypoglycemia. Another 100 to 200 mg of hydrocortisone should be administered over the next 24 h. If the patient has acute adrenal crisis, there will be a rapid response to the intravenous hydrocortisone and fluid. The high doses of hydrocortisone should be continued for several days and eventually tapered to a maintenance dose (hydrocortisone 12 to 15 mg/m^2 body surface area per day). If the patient has primary adrenal insufficiency (bilateral adrenalectomy), then administration of mineralocorticoid will be required when maintenance doses of hydrocortisone are reached (fludrocortisone 0.1 to 0.2 mg/day). If there is no response to the hydrocortisone bolus, adrenal crisis is unlikely, steroid treatment should be discontinued, and another source for the symptoms should be sought.

Patients with primary or secondary adrenal insufficiency must receive glucocorticoid treatment during surgical procedures (Fig. 35-26). If there is any question about the need for replacement therapy for a patient who has been on therapeutic glucocorticoids previously, a corticotropin stimulation test can be used to determine whether perioperative glucocorticoids are necessary. The amount of perioperative steroid treatment depends on the magnitude of the surgical procedure. Patients undergoing major operations, such as a Whipple procedure, coronary artery grafting, thoracotomy, or esophagectomy, should receive 100 to 150 mg hydrocortisone before operation and 50 mg intravenously every 8 h for 2 days after surgery, then 25 mg intravenously every 8 h for another 3 days. After this time, the usual maintenance daily dose can be initiated. Patients undergoing surgical procedures of moderate magnitude, such as cholecystectomy, appendectomy, joint replacement, colectomy, and hysterectomy, should receive hydrocortisone 50 to 75 mg intravenously before operation and then another 50 to 75 mg intravenously over the remainder of the day of the operation. Another 50 to 75 mg hydrocortisone is administered on postoperative day one, and the usual daily steroid dose may be given on postoperative day two. Patients undergoing procedures that can be done under local anesthesia, such as hernia repair or dental procedures, should receive hydrocortisone 25 mg intravenously preoperatively only, and the usual daily dose should be administered on the first postoperative day.

Patients undergoing surgical treatment of endogenous hypercortisolism require glucocorticoid replacement. Steroids are not given preoperatively because these patients are already hypercortisolemic. Instead, hydrocortisone 100 mg intravenously is given after the removal of the adrenal tumor, the pituitary tumor, or the second hyperplastic adrenal gland. Administration of hydrocortisone is continued at a dose of 50 mg intravenously every 8 h for 2 days, and then at a dose of 25 mg intravenously every 8 h for another 3 days. The final replacement dosage of hydrocortisone is 12 to 15 mg/m^2 body surface area per day. This dosage may be adjusted as necessary to prevent symptoms of adrenal insufficiency. In patients who have undergone unilateral adrenalectomy for a cortisol-producing adenoma, replacement hydrocortisone continues until the hypothalamic-pituitary-adrenal axis has recovered. A corticotropin stimulation test

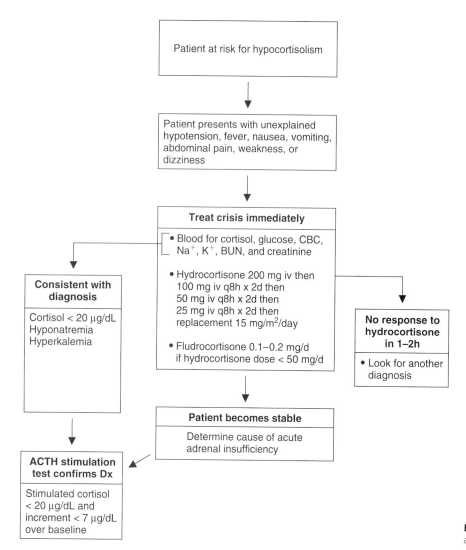

FIG. 35-25. Management of patient with acute adrenal insufficiency.

should be performed every 3 to 6 months to assess recovery of function. When a normal response to cosyntropin is detected, the replacement dose of hydrocortisone can be discontinued. Careful follow-up is necessary, because it takes 18 to 48 months for recovery in most patients.

Primary Hyperaldosteronism (Conn's Syndrome)

Diagnosis. Excessive secretion of aldosterone is the cause of hypertension in patients with primary hyperaldosteronism. The most common cause of primary hyperaldosteronism is an aldosteronoma (aldosterone-secreting tumor); second is idiopathic adrenocortical hyperplasia (IAH) in which excessive aldosterone is secreted; and least common is adrenocortical carcinoma. Primary hyperaldosteronism is diagnosed primarily by an elevated plasma level of aldosterone and a decreased plasma level of renin (see Fig. 35-18). This suggests that the pathologic process is independent of renin. Diagnosis of secondary hyperaldosteronism, which occurs with renal artery stenosis, cirrhosis, and conditions of decreased kidney perfusion, depends on the detection of concomitant elevations in plasma levels of renin and aldosterone (Table 35-6).

High blood pressure measurement, low serum levels of potassium (< 3.9 mEq/L), high plasma levels of aldosterone and low plasma levels of renin are important for the diagnosis of primary hyperaldosteronism. The symptoms of primary hyperaldosteronism may include muscle weakness, muscle cramps, polyuria, and polydipsia. These symptoms probably caused by hypokalemia and can be ameliorated with medications. Systolic hypertension may not be present, but diastolic hypertension is seen commonly.

An important alternative in the differential diagnosis is essential hypertension that is being treated with potassium-wasting diuretics. When a patient is being evaluated for primary hyperaldosteronism, all diuretics and antihypertensive medications should be stopped and a 24-h urinary excretion of potassium measurement obtained. In most patients with primary hyperaldosteronism urinary excretion of potassium will be excessive (> 30 mEq/24 h). Essential for the diagnosis of primary hyperaldosteronism is concomitant measurement of plasma levels of aldosterone and renin. Patients with primary hyperaldosteronism have elevated plasma levels of aldosterone and low levels of renin. The ratio of plasma level of aldosterone to renin activity

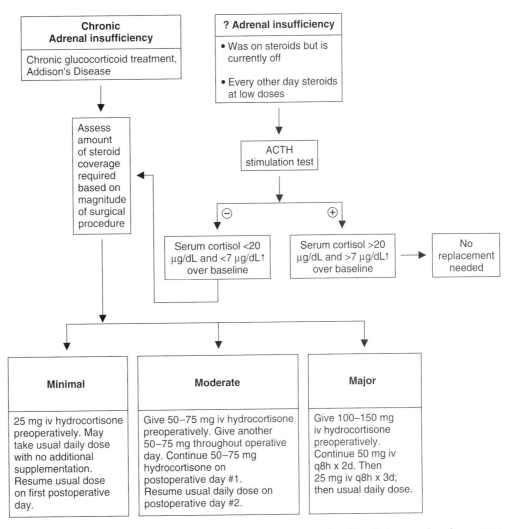

FIG. 35-26. *Management of patient with adrenal insufficiency undergoing surgery.*

usually is greater than 30. Confirmatory evidence for the diagnosis of primary hyperaldosteronism is based on an inability to reduce plasma aldosterone levels and raise plasma renin activity after administration of the antihypertensive medication captopril. In normal individuals and in patients with essential hypertension, captopril decreases plasma levels of aldosterone and increases plasma levels of renin. In patients with primary hyperaldosteronism, administration of captopril does not change plasma levels of aldosterone and renin. A post-captopril plasma aldosterone level above 15 ng/dL and an aldosterone-to-renin ratio higher than 50 are consistent with the diagnosis of primary hyperaldosteronism.

When the diagnosis of primary hyperaldosteronism has been established, the next consideration is the cause—whether the patient has idiopathic adrenocortical hyperplasia or an aldosteronoma (see Table 35-6). The determination of the cause is critical for treatment because drug therapy is indicated for one, and surgery for the other.

CT can accurately image a high proportion of aldosteronomas (75 to 90 percent) and also can image the contralateral adrenal gland (see Fig. 35-23), but it may miss small tumors (1 cm or

less). In patients with an aldosteronoma, the opposite adrenal cortex should appear thin and atrophied on CT. The CT identification of an adenoma in one adrenal gland and a thin-appearing contralateral gland is pathognomonic for aldosteronoma.

Iodocholesterol scans with ^{131}I-beta-iodomethyl-19-norcholesterol also can image a high proportion of aldosteronomas (90 percent). An advantage of this study over CT is that the presence of increased uptake suggests that the imaged glands are functional and responsible for the excessive steroid production. CT is more sensitive and more widely available and uses less radiation per study than iodocholesterol, but in certain patients with equivocal studies, iodocholesterol scans can be helpful. In patients with IAH as a cause of hyperaldosteronism, the iodocholesterol scan shows symmetrical uptake in both adrenal glands, but in patients with aldosteronoma, the study shows uptake only by the tumor.

Some patients with hyperaldosteronism have equivocal results in both CT and iodocholesterol scans. In these patients the study of choice for distinguishing between a tumor and hyperplasia is sampling of the adrenal veins for aldosterone (Fig. 35-27). The procedure is performed by simultaneous selective

Table 35-6
Evaluation of Patient with Hyperaldosteronism

Diagnosis of Primary Aldosteronism	
Measure	Result
Blood pressure	Hypertension
Serum potassium levels	Hypokalemia (serum K$^+$ <3.9 mEq/L)
Urinary potassium levels	Elevated urinary K$^+$ excretion (>25–30 mEq/day)
Plasma aldosterone and plasma renin activity	Ratio >30 (elevated aldosterone and low renin)

Etiology of Primary Aldosteronism: Idiopathic Adrenal Hyperplasia (IAH) Versus Neoplasm		
Measurement	IAH	Neoplasm
Serum 18-hydroxycorticosterone	<90 ng/dL	>100 ng/dL
High-resolution CT scan	Normal adrenals	Tumor (tumors <7–10 mm may be missed)
Iodocholesterol scan	Symmetric uptake bilaterally	Uptake or tracer by benign adenoma (malignant tumor may not take up tracer)
Spironolactone	Fair response	Good response
Adrenal vein sampling with ACTH	Aldosterone levels elevated from both adrenal veins and greater than simultaneous peripheral sample	Aldosterone levels elevated on side with tumor and levels increase with ACTH, contralateral side equal to simultaneous peripheral samples

catheterization of adrenal veins and a peripheral vein. Plasma levels of aldosterone and cortisol are measured at each site before and after administration of ACTH. Aldosteronomas make aldosterone in response to ACTH. A unilateral elevation of aldosterone level or of the aldosterone-to-cortisol ratio indicates the presence of an aldosterone-secreting adenoma. Bilateral high levels of aldosterone that are similar and that are higher than peripheral levels are consistent with IAH. Adrenal venous sampling is more sensitive than CT in prospective studies.

Treatment. The treatment of primary hyperaldosteronism depends on the cause. Idiopathic adrenal hyperplasia is best managed medically with spironolactone, nifedipine, and/or amiloride, in conjunction with other antihypertensive drugs. Because aldosterone-secreting tumors usually are small and benign, the method of choice for surgical resection of these tumors is laparoscopic adrenalectomy. The laparoscopic procedure is associated with less pain, less morbidity, and shorter convalescence than open approaches, including the posterior approach. Prospective randomized studies have not been performed, but early results suggest that the tumor resection is similar and the morbidity markedly less.

It is important to know, however, whether the results of resection of an aldosteronoma have been entirely satisfactory. A high proportion of patients initially become normotensive and normokalemic, but 20 to 30 percent of patients develop recurrent hypertension within 2 to 3 years. It is hypothesized that prolonged preoperative hypertension from an aldosteronoma may alter renal function, which then leads to persistent postoperative hypertension despite complete resection of the tumor. Few cases of recurrent benign aldosteronomas have been described, and aldosterone-producing adrenocortical carcinomas are very rare (2 percent of all carcinomas). Surgical removal of aldosteronoma

clearly is indicated and in most patients is beneficial, if not curative.

Hypoaldosteronism

Hypoaldosteronism is a selective deficiency of aldosterone secretion without alteration in cortisol production. It results in postural hypotension and persistent severe hyperkalemia that may be associated with muscle weakness and cardiac arrhythmias. Hypoaldosteronism can result from inborn errors in aldosterone biosynthesis, failure of the zona glomerulosa secondary to an autoimmune adrenal disease in association with a critical illness, altered function of the renin-angiotensin system with hyporeninemic, hypoaldosteronism, unilateral adrenalectomy for an aldosterone-producing adenoma, and drug inhibition of aldosterone.

Hypoaldosteronism rarely has been reported after surgical excision of an aldosteronoma. After removal of an aldosterone-producing tumor, it is not routine practice to supplement with mineralocorticoids. However, some patients may develop significant hyperkalemia and hypotension lasting several days to several months after adrenalectomy. These patients should be treated with fludrocortisone (0.1 to 0.2 mg/day). This treatment will totally correct the fluid and electrolyte abnormalities and normalize the blood pressure. This treatment should be continued for several months, but it is not permanently necessary.

Adrenogenital Syndrome

Adrenogenital syndrome is commonly associated with congenital adrenal hyperplasia (CAH). CAH is a group of inherited diseases that are caused by defective activity in one of five enzymes that contribute to the synthesis of cortisol from cholesterol in the adrenal cortex (see Fig. 35-17). The term *adrenal hyperplasia* comes from the adrenal enlargement under the influence of

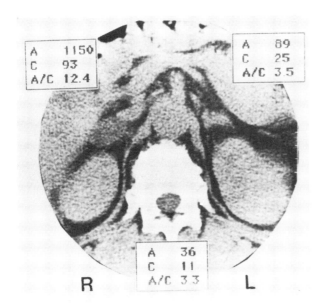

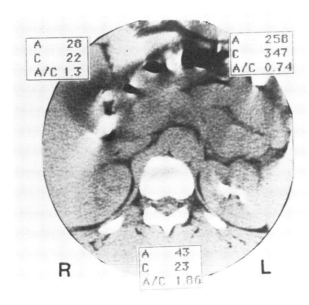

FIG. 35-27. Comparison of CT scan and adrenal vein sampling for localization of aldosterone-producing adrenal adenoma. A. CT scan reveals a right-sided adrenal mass and an increase in the venous plasma ratio of aldosterone (A) to cortisol compared with the peripheral A/C ratio of 3.3, confirming the presence of a right-sided lesion, which was removed at surgery. B. CT scan and adrenal venous sampling in patient with biochemical testing diagnostic of primary hyperaldosteronism both failed to reveal a step up in the A/C ratio. Note that although the A and C concentrations are increased on the left side, the A/C ratio is low. The patient actually had a right-sided aldosterone-producing adenoma. Sampling on the right side was negative because the catheter had been erroneously positioned in a mesenteric branch rather than in the adrenal vein.

ACTH in an effort to compensate for inadequate cortisol synthesis. The term *adrenogenital syndrome* refers to the associated finding of ambiguous external genitalia because of an incidental deficiency or excess production of adrenal androgens. Each en-

zyme deficiency produces a characteristic alteration in the ratio of precursor hormone to hormone that helps with the diagnosis. The different hormonal abnormalities are associated with different clinical features, including abnormal development of the external genitalia, pseudohermaphroditism, abnormal serum levels of sodium and potassium, abnormal values for blood pressure, and abnormal somatic growth.

The most common form of CAH is caused by a deficiency of the cytochrome P-450 enzyme 21-hydroxylase (over 90 percent). The remainder are caused by a deficiency of the following enzymes in order of prevalence: 11-hydroxylase, 17-hydroxylase, 17,20-lyase, and 3β-hydroxysteroid dehydrogenase (see Fig. 35-17). The mode of inheritance is autosomal recessive. The molecular genetics of most of the enzyme deficiencies have been identified, e.g., the CYP21 structural gene encoding 21-hydroxylase is part of the HLA complex on chromosome 6p21.3. The treatment for these conditions is glucocorticoid replacement therapy given in daily doses. Surgical therapy may be indicated for the ambiguous genitalia; this involves clitoroplasty and vaginoplasty in virilized females. Improved surgical techniques have provided superior results in single staged procedures by experienced surgeons.

Patients with adrenocortical carcinoma or adenoma may present with signs and symptoms of excessive sex hormone secretion that may be combined with clinical features of hypercortisolism. In children the signs of increased androgen production include: rapid growth, premature development of pubic and facial hair, acne, genital enlargement, increased muscle mass, and deep voice. The signs of increased estrogen production include gynecomastia in boys and precocious breast enlargement and/or vaginal bleeding in girls. In women the signs of excess androgen production include hirsutism, acne, amenorrhea, infertility, increased muscle mass, deep voice, and temporal balding. In men, hyperestrogenism presents with gynecomastia, decreased sexual drive, impotence, and infertility. In women, hyperestrogenism presents primarily with irregular menses in premenopausal women, and dysfunctional uterine bleeding or vaginal bleeding in postmenopausal women. The workup requires measurement of 24-h urinary 17-ketosteroids, 17-hydroxysteroids, urinary free cortisol, and, depending on virilization or feminization, serum determination of testosterone or estrogen. Virilization secondary to an adrenal neoplasm usually indicates adrenal cortical carcinoma. In the evaluation of a patient with virilization, CT or MRI of both adrenals is indicated to rule out an adrenal neoplasm.

Adrenal Mass

High-resolution CT scans have resulted in a new diagnostic problem: an asymptomatic adrenal mass seen on CT. Unexpected adrenal masses are seen in 0.6 percent of abdominal CT scans. The majority of these are benign, nonfunctional adrenal cortical adenomas, which occur in nearly 10 percent of autopsies.

A flow diagram for a suggested evaluation of an incidental adrenal mass ("incidentaloma") is given in Fig. 35-28. Two questions arise: is it functional or is it cancer?

The surgeon should obtain a careful history and physical examination, including blood pressure, signs of Cushing's syndrome, hypertension, virilization, feminization, change in menstrual history, and evidence of occult malignancy (stool guaiac, Pap smear, anemia). Laboratory evaluation should include a 24-h urine collection for free cortisol, vanillylmandelic acid

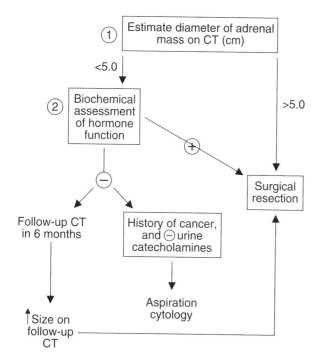

FIG. 35-28. *Flow diagram for the management of an incidentaloma.*

(VMA), metanephrines, and catecholamines. The 24-h urinary level of free cortisol is indicated to rule out Cushing's syndrome, and the urinary catecholamines to rule out a pheochromocytoma. The serum potassium concentration is used to exclude an aldosteronoma. Plasma levels of aldosterone and renin should be measured in any patient with hypertension and hypokalemia. Hormonal screening for an excess of androgens or estrogens is indicated only in patients with clinical signs suggestive of these disorders.

The size of an adrenal mass on CT is an important determinant of a potentially malignant tumor. Adrenal cortical carcinomas generally are larger than 5 cm in diameter, and benign lesions are less than 5 cm, but a smaller lesion should not be totally ignored. Early diagnosis may lead to discovery of a smaller adrenal cortical carcinoma that can lead to better prognosis and survival. CT can only distinguish benign from malignant neoplasms by criteria such as size, direct invasion, and detection of distant metastases. MRI of the adrenal glands has similar resolution to CT (see Fig. 35-24) but may be able to distinguish among adrenal cancer, metastases, pheochromocytoma, and adenoma on the basis of characteristics seen with different sequences.

Fine-needle aspiration for cytology of an adrenal mass has limited ability to differentiate benign from malignant primary adrenal tumors. Fine-needle aspiration might be catastrophic in a patient with an unsuspected pheochromocytoma, and therefore normal levels of urinary catecholamines are necessary to exclude a pheochromocytoma before needle biopsy is performed. In patients with suspected metastatic disease to the adrenal gland or lymphoma, needle aspiration may be helpful. In patients with known primary cancers, the presence of adrenal metastases can be confirmed by aspiration cytology. Because it cannot distinguish between benign and malignant primary adrenal neoplasms,

fine-needle aspiration cytology should not be performed unless adrenal metastases are suspected.

CT and biochemical assessment should be performed on each patient with an incidentaloma. The adrenal mass diameter is carefully measured; a size greater than 5 cm is an indication for surgical resection. If the tumor is hormonally functional, adrenalectomy also is indicated. If the patient has a history of cancer, fine-needle aspiration may be considered to exclude adrenal metastases. If the mass is smaller than 5 cm and nonfunctional, a 6-month follow-up CT examination is indicated to reevaluate the mass's size. If the mass has grown, then surgical excision is necessary. If there is no change, then the mass is likely to be an adenoma, and subsequent CT scans are unnecessary.

Treatment of Adrenal Cortical Neoplasms. *Adenoma.* The indication for resection of an adrenal adenoma is excessive hormone production. The definitive treatment is complete removal of the adrenal gland with the adenoma. The laparoscopic approach is becoming the method of choice to remove benign adrenal tumors because it can achieve complete resection with less pain and morbidity. In patients who are undergoing resection of an adrenal tumor that produces cortisol, steroid replacement during and after surgery is required, but mineralocorticoid replacement is not. Postoperative glucocorticoid replacement (12 to 15 mg hydrocortisone/m^2 body surface area) may be necessary for as long as 2 years. After removal of an aldosteronoma or a virilizing adenoma, hormone replacement therapy usually is not necessary (see section Hypoaldosteronism). Surgical resection of an adenoma is curative. Larger lesions weighing 50 to 100 g that appear benign histologically (no mitoses and no vascular invasion) need careful long-term follow-up to exclude carcinoma. Laparoscopically resected tumors require close long-term follow-up to eliminate the possibility of spillage of tumor cells resulting from handling the gland during the procedure.

Carcinoma. Surgical resection is the only curative treatment for carcinoma of the adrenal cortex. If the carcinoma is intimately associated with the kidney, liver, or diaphragm on the right, or with pancreas on the left, removal of part or all contiguous structures may be necessary at the time of operation. The surgeon needs adequate imaging of the extent of disease, which can be achieved by CT or MRI. CT or MRI should include the chest to rule out metastatic disease above the diaphragm. If the right adrenal gland is involved and the inferior vena cava is compressed, an inferior vena cava contrast study or caval ultrasonography is useful to assess tumor extension into the vena cava. If resection of one kidney is indicated, an intravenous pyelogram or an intravenous contrast CT study is necessary to verify that the contralateral kidney is functioning. A complete bowel preparation is used in case the tumor is found to invade bowel. Though patients with hypercortisolism have impaired healing, adrenal tumor resection can be performed with acceptable morbidity and an operative mortality of 3 percent.

The surgical staging of adrenal carcinoma is: stage I, tumor smaller than 5 cm without local invasion, nodal, or distant metastases; stage II, same as stage I except that tumor is larger than 5 cm; stage III, tumor with local invasion or positive lymph nodes; and stage IV, tumor with local invasion and lymph nodes or distant metastases. Most patients (70 percent) present with stage III or IV disease.

The definitive initial treatment for adrenal carcinoma in all stages of disease, including locally aggressive stage III disease, is en bloc resection. This procedure may require a combined thoracoabdominal approach. Surgical resection of localized disease can be curative. Some recommend adjuvant mitotane therapy after surgical resection to improve survival, but this therapy is not proved. If complete resection of all tumor cannot be achieved, tumor debulking should be attempted to decrease the amount of cortisol-secreting tissue and to minimize complications due to tumor mass. In patients who undergo definitive resection steroid hormone levels should be monitored postoperatively. CT and MRI also are used to detect local recurrences or pulmonary metastases. If a recurrence is detected, it can be removed surgically. Prolonged disease-free intervals have been reported after resection of hepatic, pulmonary, and cerebral metastases from adrenal cortical carcinoma. When complete resection of recurrent tumor or metastases is not possible, tumor debulking may be useful in the case of selected hormonally active, slow-growing tumors. Palliation of bony metastases may be achieved by radiation therapy. Abdominal radiation therapy is not useful in reducing local recurrences.

Patients with recurrent or metastatic adrenal cortical carcinoma usually are treated with mitotane. Mitotane has direct effects on steroid metabolism and usually is associated with a decrease in urinary 17-hydroxysteroids and 17-ketosteroids and improvement in the signs and symptoms of hypercortisolism, but it seldom provides objective antitumor responses. Other chemotherapeutic agents also have been ineffective, though responses have been reported with doxorubicin, alkylating agents, cisplatin, and etoposide.

Treatment of adrenal cancer is ineffective. Surgical cure may be feasible only in stage I or stage II tumors confined to the adrenal gland. In these patients the mean duration of survival is 5 years. In patients with invasion of contiguous structures at presentation, median survival is 2.3 years. For all patients, the 5-year survival rate is 10 to 35 percent, reflecting the fact that most patients present with locally advanced or distant disease. Most clinicians still recommend aggressive surgical re-resection of locally recurrent or metastatic cancer, but even with this aggressive intervention the 5-year survival rate is 10 to 20 percent. Future challenges for better treatment of adrenal cortical carcinoma include earlier diagnosis and better chemotherapy than mitotane.

Ectopic ACTH Syndrome

The diagnosis of ectopic ACTH syndrome requires the presence of Cushing's syndrome and bilateral adrenal hyperplasia, but no evidence of a pituitary tumor. In ectopic ACTH syndrome ACTH is produced by a tumor that is not within the pituitary gland. Early indication of the disorder is hypercortisolism and severe hypokalemia (potassium < 3.3 mEq/L). The laboratory diagnosis depends on the measurement of high plasma levels of ACTH and cortisol that are unaffected by high-dose dexamethasone and do not increase with CRH. Petrosal sinus sampling for ACTH detects low plasma levels of ACTH in the venous blood draining the pituitary gland that do not increase with CRH. After the diagnosis has been made, the primary therapeutic goal is to locate and eradicate the neoplasm that is secreting ACTH. Two difficulties are localizing the tumor in some patients, and treating an aggressive, metastatic malignant tumor in others.

Ectopic ACTH-producing tumors in approximate order of decreasing incidence are: oat-cell or small-cell lung cancer, carcinoid tumor of the bronchus, thymic carcinoid, pancreatic islet cell tumor, medullary carcinoma of the thyroid gland, pheochromocytoma, midgut carcinoid, ovarian adenocarcinoma, pancreatic cystadenoma, and adenocarcinoma of unknown site. Procedures indicated to localize the ACTH producing tumor include chest and abdominal CT, chest and abdominal MRI, urinary catecholamines determination to screen for pheochromocytoma, measurement of plasma calcitonin level to rule out medullary thyroid carcinoma, and inferior petrosal sinus sampling with CRH in patients in whom a pituitary ACTH-secreting tumor cannot be excluded by other tests. Any suspicious finding in the chest or abdomen can be unequivocally confirmed by fine-needle aspiration and radioimmunoassay for ACTH on the aspirate.

The goal of surgery for patients with ectopic ACTH-producing tumors is to locate and resect (unless it is a small-cell lung carcinoma) the neoplasm. A true cancer resection (lobectomy with lymph nodes) is indicated for patients with bronchial carcinoid tumors, because one-half have lymph node metastases. These tumors are treatable, and approximately 75 percent of patients are cured by surgical resection. The proper therapy for ACTH-producing neoplasms depends on the diagnosis (the exact tumor type that is producing ACTH) and the extent of disease. Any of these tumors may be malignant and metastasize. In some patients with ectopic ACTH production, the entire tumor burden cannot be removed, and therapy should be directed toward correcting the life-threatening metabolic and hormonal abnormalities. Hypokalemia and excess mineralocorticoid activity can be managed with potassium supplementation and spironolactone. Hypercortisolism may be managed with metyrapone, amino glutethimide, or mitotane. Bilateral adrenalectomy might be indicated for patients who have tumors that cannot be identified despite numerous radiologic studies and patients who have stable but unresectable metastatic disease whose hypercortisolism cannot be controlled medically. Bilateral adrenalectomy can be performed with the posterior approach via two separate hockey-stick incisions or with the lateral laparoscopic approach through two separate sequential procedures. Patients undergoing bilateral adrenalectomy need glucocorticoid and mineralocorticoid replacement therapy postoperatively.

ADRENAL MEDULLA

Physiology

In responding to severe stress and confrontation (the so-called fight-or-flight response), the autonomic nervous system plays a critical role. The autonomic nervous system consists of the parasympathetic nervous system, which uses acetylcholine as a neurotransmitter, and the sympathoadrenal system, which uses catecholamines. The sympathoadrenal system consists of a sympathetic neuronal component with norepinephrine as the main neurotransmitter at sympathetic neuroeffector junctions, and an adrenomedullary secretory hormone epinephrine, the main hormone secreted into the bloodstream. This system influences cardiovascular, metabolic, and visceral activity in the resting organism and determines the physiologic consequences of every motion and emotion.

The chromaffin tissue of the adrenal medulla and the sympathetic ganglia originate from the neural crest (see Fig. 35-15).

The term *chromaffin* refers to the appearance of intracellular granules, which turn brown when stained with oxidizing agents. The small amounts of epinephrine secreted by the adrenal medulla into the bloodstream is not necessary to maintain blood pressure, but adequate release of norepinephrine at sympathetic nerve endings is critical for maintenance of normal blood pressure, especially during periods of upright posture. The major cellular supply of catecholamines is stored in secretory granules in both nerve endings and the adrenal medulla. A smaller pool of catecholamines is concentrated at the peripheral portion of sympathetic neurons and is released during stimulation. After sympathetic nerve stimulation some of the norepinephrine may spill into the circulation. It is converted in the liver by two enzymes, catechol *O*-methyltransferase and monoamine oxidase to normetanephrine and vanillylmandelic acid (VMA). These metabolites and the small fraction of unmetabolized norepinephrine that escapes into the bloodstream are excreted in the urine. After sympathetic nerve stimulation, most of the norepinephrine is taken up again by the neuron and stored in vesicles for future use. Monoamine oxidase in the cytoplasm of the neuron inactivates any norepinephrine that leaks out. Epinephrine released into the bloodstream from the adrenal medulla is metabolized primarily by the liver into metanephrine and VMA. These metabolites, plus small amounts of unmetabolized epinephrine, are excreted in the urine. Release of norepinephrine from neurons is primarily responsible for controlling blood pressure during upright posture. Release of epinephrine from the adrenal medulla is primarily responsible for the systemic effects of catecholamines observed during episodes of severe stress.

Pheochromocytoma

Pheochromocytomas arise from chromaffin cells that are widespread and associated with sympathetic ganglia throughout the body during fetal life. After birth, most chromaffin cells degenerate. However, most chromaffin cells in the adrenal medulla persist. This may be why 85 to 90 percent of pheochromocytomas are in the adrenal medulla, but pheochromocytomas can arise wherever there is a sympathetic ganglion. Extraadrenal pheochromocytomas may occur in any part of the body, including in the carotid body, in the heart, along the aorta (both thoracic and abdominal), and in the urinary bladder. The most common extraadrenal location is the organ of Zuckerkandl, which is near the origin of the inferior mesenteric artery to the left of the aortic bifurcation (Fig. 35-29). Extraadrenal pheochromocytomas are often malignant. Bilateral adrenal pheochromocytomas usually occur in familial syndromes, including multiple endocrine neoplasia (MEN) type IIA and type IIB. The right adrenal gland is more commonly affected than the left.

Pheochromocytomas from symptomatic hypertensive patients usually measure 3 to 5 cm in diameter and weigh approximately 100 g. They appear tan to gray in color, and are soft and smooth. Larger tumors may be cystic from necrosis, and they may have calcification. Microscopically, pheochromocytomas are arranged in cords or alveolar patterns. Tumors generally are clearly separated from the adrenal cortex by a thin band of fibrous tissue.

The pathologic distinction between benign and malignant pheochromocytomas is not clear. Most reports suggest that only 10 percent of pheochromocytomas are malignant, but some suggest that 23 to 46 percent of pheochromocytomas are malignant. These different results may partly reflect the referral patterns of different institutions, but they may indicate a true higher inci-

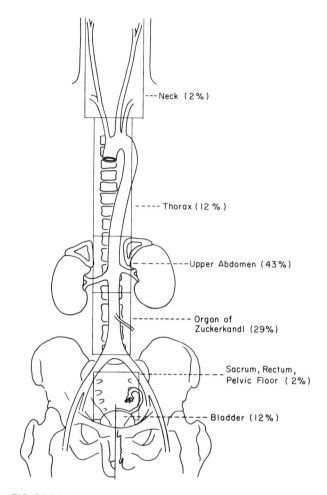

FIG. 35-29. *Location of pheochromocytomas in ectopic sites. About 10 to 15 percent of pheochromocytomas are located in ectopic sites, principally concentrated in the areas shown.*

dence of malignancy. Malignant pheochromocytomas tend to be larger and weigh more, although this is not an absolute pathologic criterion. The only absolute criteria for malignancy are the presence of secondary tumors in sites where chromaffin cells are not usually found, and the identification of visceral metastases.

Associated Syndromes. Approximately 10 percent of pheochromocytomas occur as part of an inherited condition. Pheochromocytomas are associated with endocrine and nonendocrine inherited disorders. Bilateral adrenal medullary pheochromocytomas are components of multiple endocrine neoplasias type IIA and type IIB. Familial pheochromocytoma also has been described. Affected individuals have bilateral adrenal pheochromocytomas and no other manifestation of MEN syndromes. In other families, extraadrenal pheochromocytomas have been reported in the same location in affected individuals. Pheochromocytomas occur in approximately 25 percent of patients with von Hippel-Lindau's disease and in less than 1 percent of patients with neurofibromatosis and von Recklinghausen's disease.

Clinical Manifestations. Pheochromocytomas secrete excessive amounts of unregulated catecholamines, and usually patients have significant hypertension. Pheochromocytomas can cause anxiety attacks, episodic hypertension, or sustained hy-

Table 35-7
Symptoms and Signs of Pheochromocytoma

Symptoms:	Adult	Child
Persistent hypertension	65	92
Paroxysmal hypertension	30	8
Headache	80	81
Sweating	70	68
Palpitation, nervousness	60	34
Pallor of face	40	27
Tremor	40	
Nausea	30	56
Weakness, fatigue	25	27
Weight loss	15	44
Abdominal or chest pain	15	35
Dyspnea	15	16
Visual changes	10	44
Constipation	5	8
Raynaud's phenomenon	5	
Convulsions	3	23
Polydipsia, polyuria		25
Puffy, red, cyanotic hands		11
Signs:		
BMR over +20 percent	50	83
Fasting blood sugar over 120mg/100mL	40	40
Glycosuria	10	3
Eye ground changes	30	70

Approximate Percent

SOURCE: From Hume DM, Astwood EB, Cassidy CE: Grune & Stratton, 1968.

pertension. The patient classically describes "spells" of paroxysmal headaches, pallor, palpitations, hypertension, and diaphoresis (Table 35-7). Some patients with pheochromocytoma have only mild labile hypertension, while others have sudden death secondary to a myocardial infarction, or cerebrovascular accident from uncontrolled episodic hypertension. Patients with pheochromocytoma may have signs of chronic hypovolemia, such as orthostatic hypotension, or lactic acidosis secondary to excessive alpha-adrenergic stimulation and vasoconstriction. The majority of these patients have mild weight loss, but obesity does not exclude the diagnosis. Diabetes mellitus may be induced by

Table 35-8
Differential Diagnosis of Pheochromocytoma

Illness	Associated Conditions
Hypertension	Essential hypertension, renovascular hypertension
Headaches	Migraine, cluster
Tachycardias	Paroxysmal atrial and nodal tachycardia
Endocrine abnormalities	Thyrotoxicosis, menopause, hypoglycemia, diabetes
CNS disorders	Diencephalic seizures, autonomic hyperreflexia, increased intracranial pressure due to tumors, infection, or stroke, lead poisoning
Tumors	Carcinoid, neuroblastoma
Pregnancy	Preeclampsia, eclampsia thyrotoxicosis or simple hypertension of pregnancy

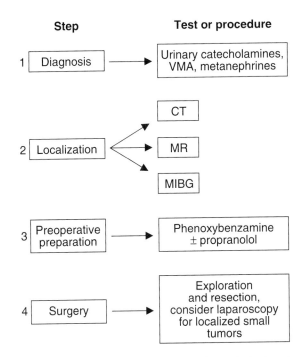

FIG. 35-30. Flow diagram for diagnosis and treatment of pheochromocytoma.

chronic excessive catecholamine secretion. Fever of unknown origin has been caused by an unexpected pheochromocytoma. Pheochromocytomas may produce multiple hormones like catecholamines and ACTH. In these patients symptoms of both pheochromocytoma and hypercortisolism are present. Other conditions may mimic pheochromocytoma and are included in the differential diagnosis (Table 35-8).

Diagnosis. The diagnosis of pheochromocytoma is based on measuring excessive excretion of catecholamines and their metabolites in the urine. The best study is a 24-h urine collection for catecholamines, metanephrine, and vanillylmandelic acid. The 24-h urinary level of VMA has the greatest sensitivity (97 percent) and the best specificity (91 percent) (Fig. 35-30). Because pheochromocytomas secrete catecholamines episodically, 24-h urinary measurements are more sensitive than a plasma level, which reflects only the level at the moment at which blood is sampled. Elevated levels of norepinephrine more commonly occur with extraadrenal pheochromocytomas because of the physiology of catecholamine secretion, and elevated levels of epinephrine commonly occur with adrenal pheochromocytomas.

The clonidine suppression test can be used as an additional study to determine whether a patient has a pheochromocytoma and is recommended in the diagnosis of a pheochromocytoma when plasma catecholamine levels are mildly elevated (500 and 2000 pg/mL). In normal individuals and in patients with idiopathic hypertension, clonidine suppresses plasma levels of catecholamines, and in patients with pheochromocytoma it does not. Few false-positive or false-negative results have been reported. The author recommends relying on urinary levels of catecholamine metabolites.

Localization Studies. CT and MRI have been effective for localization of pheochromocytomas (Fig. 35-31). These studies are noninvasive and sensitive and are able to detect tumors ap-

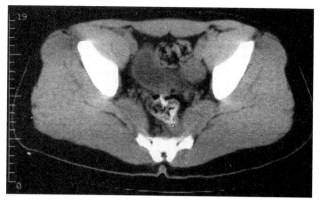

A

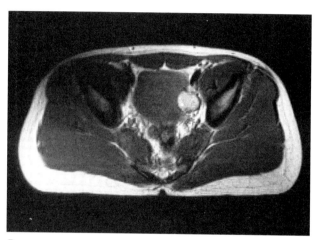

B

FIG. 35-31. *A. A mass is visualized in the left perivesicular region on abdominopelvic CT scan in this hypertensive patient. B. MRI confirmed that the lesion was a pelvic pheochromocytoma, as it enhanced with T$_2$-weighted imaging.*

proximately 1 cm in diameter. MRI may be more specific because of its ability to distinguish various types of adrenal tumors on the basis of imaging characteristics, but CT has several advantages over MRI. CT scans are less expensive and more available than MRI. A major advantage of MRI is that there is no radiation exposure, and it can be used to image pheochromocytomas during pregnancy. MRI has accurately imaged an intrapericardial pheochromocytoma and distinguished it from the cardiac chambers.

A nuclear medicine imaging study for the localization of pheochromocytomas is scanning with ^{131}I labeled metaiodobenzylguanidine (MIBG). MIBG is similar to norepinephrine and is taken up and concentrated in catecholamine-synthesizing tissue. The sensitivity of MIBG scanning is between 78 and 86 percent in sporadic pheochromocytoma, approximately 91 percent in malignant pheochromocytoma, and 94 percent in familial pheochromocytoma. MIBG scanning is safe, noninvasive, and efficacious for the localization of pheochromocytomas, including those arising in extraadrenal sites, and malignant disease. False-positive results with MIBG scintigraphy are rare (tumors such as medullary thyroid carcinoma and neuroblastoma may take up the tracer), which accounts for the high specificity (98 to 100

percent) of the study. False-negative results can occur and have an incidence of 13 to 20 percent, which lowers sensitivity. False-negative results may be more common in patients with multiple tumors and metastatic disease.

Treatment. *Preoperative Preparation.* When the diagnosis of pheochromocytoma has been made and the tumor has been localized, an essential component of preoperative preparation is alpha-adrenergic blockade. Patients receive phenoxybenzamine 10 mg orally two or three times a day (see Fig. 35-30). If tachycardia develops (heart rate > 100 beats/min), beta-adrenergic blocking agents (propranolol) are indicated. Propranolol should never be started before alpha blockade, because unopposed vasoconstriction may worsen hypertension. Phenoxybenzamine increases the total blood and plasma volume in patients with pheochromocytoma. Lactic acidosis can occur in patients with pheochromocytoma, and therefore measurement and correction of arterial blood pH should be performed before the induction of anesthesia.

Alpha-methyltyrosine is another drug that is useful for preoperative preparation of these patients. It is a competitive inhibitor of tyrosine hydroxylase, the rate-limiting step in catecholamine biosynthesis. It reduces catecholamine production by 50 to 80 percent in patients with pheochromocytoma. The usual dose of 250 mg four times a day may be increased to a maximum dose of 3 to 4 g per day. The calcium antagonist nifedipine with phenoxybenzamine or nicardipine alone (60 to 120 mg/24 h) has been used to control hypertension in patients with pheochromocytoma. Both of these newer drug strategies appear to work as well as phenoxybenzamine.

Intraoperative Management. If a patient with pheochromocytoma is elderly or has had cardiac complications, right heart catheter monitoring should be maintained during surgery. On the morning of surgery, an arterial catheter and peripheral intravenous catheters are inserted. Arterial CO_2 is measured to rule out acidosis. Despite preoperative preparation, during manipulation of the tumor marked changes in blood pressure can occur. Hypertensive episodes are controlled with alpha-adrenergic blocking agents, such as phentolamine (Regitine) or smooth muscle relaxers, such as sodium nitroprusside. Nitroprusside usually is chosen because of its rapid onset and short duration. With the use of intravenous nitroprusside, blood pressure can be continuously titrated to acceptable levels. The use of preoperative preparation and intraoperative regulation of blood pressure with nitroprusside greatly reduces operative morbidity and mortality.

The operation is performed via a transabdominal approach, with a bilateral subcostal or a long midline incision. Preoperative localization studies can effectively guide the exploration, but the entire abdomen is nevertheless carefully visualized and palpated. Some have argued that localization procedures are so sensitive and specific that focused direct approaches may be preferred. Small intraadrenal pheochromocytomas have been removed using laparoscopic techniques. Laparoscopic procedures decrease pain and shorten the recovery time, but laparoscopic adrenalectomy is still considered experimental for resection of pheochromocytoma.

Extraadrenal pheochromocytomas can be difficult to find (see Fig. 35-29). The most common locations of intraabdominal extraadrenal pheochromocytomas are in the hilar region of the kidneys, and in the chromaffin tissue along the aorta from the celiac axis to the aortic bifurcation (Fig. 35-32). The organ of Zuck-

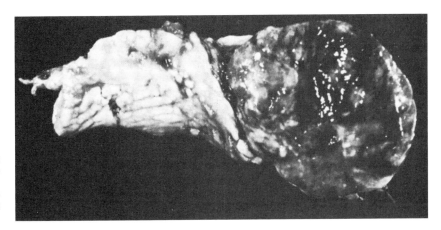

FIG. 35-32. Specimen of a pheochromocytoma from a child. The tumor lay in close proximity to the adrenal gland and was resected en bloc. (From: *Schwartz DL, Gann DS, Haller JA: Endocrine surgery in children. Surg Clin North Am 54:363, 1974, fig 1, p 365, with permission.*)

erkandl near the inferior mesenteric artery is the most common extraadrenal location, and pheochromocytomas have been removed from the urinary bladder. Multiple locations, metastatic potential, and multiple tumors support the need for a complete exploration of the entire abdominal cavity. The "rule of tens" may be of value in the management of pheochromocytomas; 10 percent are malignant, 10 percent are extraadrenal, and 10 percent are bilateral. Bilateral adrenal pheochromocytomas are widely believed to occur primarily as part of a familial syndrome. In patients with MEN type II, some suggest that nearly 100 percent have or will develop bilateral benign adrenal medullary pheochromocytomas, and others suggest that the incidence of bilaterality, although high, may be significantly less (70 percent). The question of whether or not to remove both adrenals is controversial; the author recommends removing only the adrenal gland with an identifiable tumor.

Malignant Pheochromocytoma. Malignant pheochromocytomas are thought not to occur in MEN syndromes and are present in approximately 10 percent of patients with pheochromocytoma. Some reports indicate that substantially more than 10 percent of sporadic pheochromocytomas may be malignant. Pathologic analysis has not been helpful in predicting which tumors are malignant. Patients who develop metastases might not develop them for many years after surgery (Fig. 35-33). After removal of a pheochromocytoma, most recommend lifetime follow-up with measurement of blood pressure and urinary levels of catecholamines. It appears that with careful follow-up the true incidence of malignant pheochromocytoma may be greater than 10 percent.

The basic principles in treatment of malignant pheochromocytoma are to resect recurrences or metastases whenever possible and to treat hypertensive symptoms by catecholamine blockade. Painful bony metastases respond well to radiotherapy. Localized or solitary soft-tissue masses, even when metastatic to the liver or lung, should be resected surgically. Combination chemotherapy with cyclophosphamide, vincristine, and dacarbazine, a regimen that is effective for metastatic neuroblastoma, has also been beneficial for patients with metastatic pheochromocytoma. The regimen has a 60 percent response rate, including some complete responses. Survival data of patients with malignant pheochromocytoma are difficult to obtain because of the rarity of the tumor. In two large series, the 5-year survival rates for patients with malignant pheochromocytoma were 36 and 60 percent.

Neuroblastoma

Neuroblastoma is the fourth most common pediatric malignancy. The median age at diagnosis is 2 years. Half of all malignancies diagnosed within the first year of life are neuroblastomas, and the mortality of children with neuroblastoma diagnosed in the first year of life is lower than that of older children. Neuroblas-

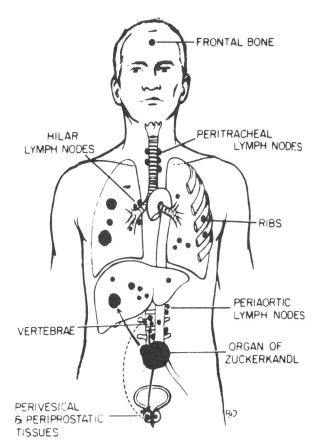

FIG. 35-33. Locations of tumor metastases from a primary malignant pheochromocytoma in the organ of Zuckerkandl. (From: *Mellcow MM, Unson AC, Veenema RJ: Malignant nonfunctioning pheochromocytomas of the organ of Zuckerkandl masquerading as a primary carcinoma of the prostate with metastases. J Urol 110:97, 1973, fig 5, p 100, with permission.*)

toma has been associated with genetic diseases, including neurofibromatosis, Beckwith-Wiedemann syndrome, and trisomy 18. Neuroblastoma has a biologic characteristic unique among human cancers, namely, the capacity to spontaneously differentiate and regress. It is believed that some children with this life-threatening disease are spontaneously cured by their immune system, and these malignant tumors then become benign ganglioneuromas.

Neuroblastoma is believed to arise from the embryonic neural crest. It is called a small round blue cell tumor because it is composed of dense nests of cells separated by fibrovascular bundles. The characteristic electron microscopy finding is dense core secretory granules. Neuroblastoma may be difficult to distinguish from other small round blue cell tumors of childhood, which include Ewing's sarcoma, lymphoma, rhabdomyosarcoma, and other peripheral nerve tumors. An important adjunct to the diagnosis of neuroblastoma is the detection of tumor markers in the serum and urine. The most commonly used marker is urinary excretion of catecholamines. Elevated 24-h urinary levels of homovanillylmandelic acid and VMA are detected in 65 and 90 percent, respectively, of patients with neuroblastoma. Levels of catecholamines in urine are correlated with prognosis, i.e., higher levels are found in patients with more extensive disease.

Neuroblastoma can occur anywhere along the sympathetic nervous system. The most common sites of tumor are in the adrenal gland (40 percent), the paraspinal ganglia (25 percent), the thorax (15 percent), and the pelvis (5 percent). Thoracic primary tumors are more common in children younger than 1 year of age. Metastatic tumor is detected in approximately 50 percent of infants and 67 percent of older children at the time of diagnosis. Metastases usually involve lymph nodes, bone marrow, bone, liver, and subcutaneous tissue. Pulmonary metastases are rare.

Clinical Manifestations. The most common presenting sign and symptom is an abdominal or flank mass, which must be distinguished from Wilms' tumor. Thoracic neuroblastoma commonly presents as a posterior mediastinal mass identified on a routine chest radiograph. Thoracic tumors may cause signs and symptoms of respiratory distress or spinal cord compression.

Neuroblastoma in the neck presents with a cervical mass; the diagnosis can be supported by the signs of Horner's syndrome, suggesting that the mass involves the sympathetic ganglia. Pelvic neuroblastoma commonly involves the organ of Zuckerkandl and may present with urinary symptoms or as a pelvic mass.

There are unusual symptoms and signs associated with neuroblastoma: (1) Some neonates with neuroblastoma have subcutaneous blue-tinged nodules, the so-called "blueberry muffin" sign of neuroblastoma. (2) Some have acute cerebellar and truncal ataxia, which is associated with neurologic involvement but favorable outcome. (3) Some present with severe secretory diarrhea similar to the adult Verner-Morrison syndrome; in these patients the neuroblastoma is producing vasoactive intestinal polypeptide (VIP), which can be measured in the plasma. (4) Neuroblastoma may present with periorbital metastases that cause proptosis and ecchymosis; this is secondary to invasion and involvement of the retro-orbital tissues. (5) Some patients have diffuse bone marrow involvement with neuroblastoma without an obvious primary tumor.

Radiology and Staging. CT is the best imaging study for patients with neuroblastoma and should be performed to determine the extent of disease. CT detects abdominal neuroblastoma with a high degree of accuracy, and calcifications are identified in most tumors. MRI has similar accuracy to CT, and it may be able to image intraspinal extension and vascular invasion more effectively.

Useful nuclear medicine studies include the technetium diphosphonate bone scan and ^{131}I-MIBG because of its preferential uptake by cells with adrenergic secretory granules. Bone scan is the best study to determine bony involvement, and MIBG scan can image some metastatic disease that is not expected.

The goal of the imaging studies is to stage the total extent of tumor. Prognosis and treatment depend on the stage of disease at presentation. The most widely used staging system is the international staging classification for neuroblastoma (Table 35-9).

Treatment. Treatment depends on the stage of disease. For patients with localized disease (stage 1 and 2), surgical resection is the mainstay of treatment. In patients with cervical, mediastinal, and pelvic tumors complete resection usually is feasible.

Table 35-9
Staging System for Neuroblastoma, Recommended Treatment and Survival

Stage	Definition	Recommended Treatment	5-year Survival (%)
1	Tumor confined to primary site	Surgical resection	90
2A	Unilateral localized tumor that cannot be completely excised	Surgical resection with radiation and chemotherapy	85
2B	Unilateral localized tumor that has positive lymph nodes	Surgical resection with radiation and chemotherapy	80
3	Tumor that crosses midline *or* unilateral tumor with contralateral lymph node metastases	Surgical resection with radiation and chemotherapy	60
4	Dissemination of disease to distant sites	Chemotherapy	20
4S	Primary tumor with dissemination only to liver, skin, or bone marrow	Chemotherapy	40

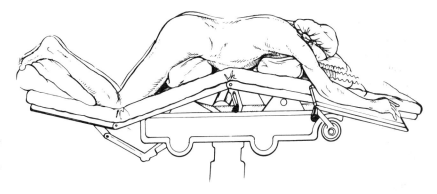

FIG. 35-34. Positioning of the patient on the operating table for the posterior approach to adrenalectomy. (From: Harrison TS, Gann DS, Edis AJ, Egdahl RH (eds): Surgical Disorders of the Adrenal Gland: Physiologic Background and Treatment. Grune & Stratton, 1975, fig 4-1, p 124, with permission.)

Most localized abdominal neuroblastomas involve major vessels, which is stage 2A disease with localized tumor that cannot be completely excised. In unresectable abdominal tumors, biopsy specimens are taken, and then the tumor is treated with radiation or chemotherapy; a subsequent reattempt to remove it might be necessary. If complete resection can be achieved in this fashion, prognosis is the same as with initial resection. In patients with metastatic disease that can be controlled by chemotherapy, resection of the primary tumor may prolong survival. Patients with functional neuroblastomas may need to undergo debulking surgery to alleviate the signs and symptoms of hormonal excess, such as hypertension or diarrhea. If all distant tumor is eliminated by chemotherapy, residual primary tumor mass is excised, although this has not demonstrated improved survival.

Radiation therapy has clearly defined roles in children with lymph node metastases (stage 2B and 3). It also has been useful in infants with spinal cord compression. Neuroblastomas are highly chemoresponsive, and sometimes they are curable with chemotherapy. Response rates for single agents are: cyclophosphamide 59 percent, cisplatin 46 percent, epipodophyllotoxins 30 percent, vincristine 20 percent, dacarbazine 14 percent, melphalan 24 percent, and ifosfamide 20 percent.

The 5-year survival rates for stage 1 and 2 disease are 90 and 85 percent, respectively. For patients with stage 3 disease, the 5-year survival rate is 60 percent, and for patients with stage 4 disease it is 20 to 40 percent. Although surgery is curative for patients with localized, completely resectable neuroblastoma, and there are active chemotherapeutic drugs for patients with distant disease, the overall survival rate of children with neuroblastoma needs to be improved.

ADRENALECTOMY

Posterior Approach. This approach is used for resection of small benign tumors of the adrenal gland, e.g., an aldosteronoma or a cortisol-secreting adenoma. It also can be used for resection of hyperplastic glands in hypercortisolemic patients with primary pigmented micronodular hyperplasia, and for adrenalectomy in patients with Cushing's disease in whom transsphenoidal surgery has failed. The patient is placed supine on the operating table and general anesthesia is induced. The patient is then turned to the prone jackknife position (Fig. 35-34). The chest and the pelvis are padded by rolls so that the abdominal contents fall anteriorly away from the retroperitoneum. A curvilinear hockey-stick incision (bilateral incisions if bilateral adrenalectomy is indicated) is fashioned from the tenth rib to the

posterior superior iliac spine (Fig. 35-35). The superior part of the incision is 3 fingerbreadths from the midline, and the lower part is 4 fingerbreadths, resulting in the curvilinear or hockey-stick shape. The incision is made through the skin, subcutaneous tissue, and the latissimus dorsi muscle to the posterior lamella of the lumbodorsal fascia. This is incised, and the sacrospinalis muscle is retracted medially. The twelfth rib (and occasionally the eleventh rib as well) is removed subperiosteally. The anterior lumbodorsal fascia is incised, and the intercostal neurovascular bundle is clamped and divided. The retroperitoneum is entered. The kidney, which is surrounded by Gerota's fascia, is palpated at the depth of the incision. Care is taken to separate the pleura from the diaphragm without entering the thoracic cavity. The diaphragm is divided with the Bovie electrocautery knife to expose the adrenal gland, which lies within the fat at the superior edge of the incision. Gerota's fascia is incised. The kidney is

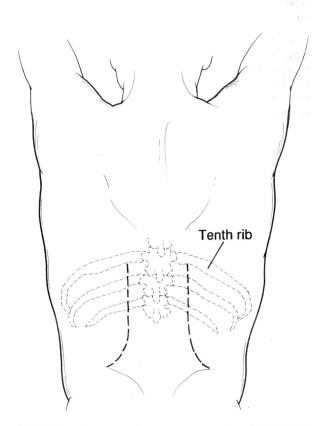

FIG. 35-35. Skin incisions for posterior approach to adrenalectomy.

Tenth rib

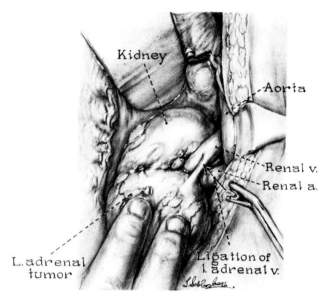

FIG. 35-36. *The left adrenal vein is visualized where it enters the left renal vein. The adrenal vein is ligated twice with 2-0 silk ties, clipped, and divided. The aorta and the left renal artery are located medially.*

identified and retracted inferiorly with the hand. After division of Gerota's fascia at the superior edge of the incision, the chrome yellow adrenal cortex is visualized.

The adrenal gland is freed with blunt dissection. On its medial, inferomedial, and superomedial margins are the arterial feeding vessels, which are small and numerous. These vessels are identified with blunt dissection, hemoclips are applied, and the vessels are divided. The adrenal vein is ligated toward the end of the resection. On the left side, the adrenal vein may be found at the inferomedial border of the adrenal gland, diving

away from the operating surgeon as it empties into the renal vein (Fig. 35-36). On the right side, the adrenal vein may be found on the superomedial border of the adrenal gland, where it empties directly into the inferior vena cava. The right vein is wide and short, and if torn can cause life-threatening hemorrhage. The adrenal vein is ligated with a 2-0 silk tie, and the adrenal gland is removed (Fig. 35-37).

At the time of closure, the diaphragm is not reapproximated. If the thorax has been entered, pleural air is evacuated with a tube while the lungs are hyperinflated by the anesthesiologist, and the pleural opening is closed with a running suture. The anterior and posterior lamella and the lumbodorsal fascia are closed; the skin is closed. In patients with Cushing's syndrome, the closure should be meticulous because wound complications are common.

Laparoscopic Approach. The laparoscopic approach to adrenalectomy has developed as a result of technologically improved equipment and the quest for less invasive and less painful operative procedures. This method of adrenalectomy is suited for small aldosteronomas or cortisol-secreting adenomas. It also is indicated for resection of hyperplastic adrenal glands. Although laparoscopy has been used in a few patients with small pheochromocytomas, it is not recommended because of the need for more tumor manipulation with the instruments and the inability to control the adrenal vein at an early stage of the procedure. Experience in open adrenalectomy is recommended for surgeons who choose to perform laparoscopic adrenalectomy, because difficult laparoscopic dissections can require emergent conversion to open procedures.

The patient is positioned in the lateral decubitus position with the affected adrenal side superficial for laparoscopic adrenalectomy. The operating table is flexed, and the kidney rest is extended. An inflatable bean bag is used to secure the patient in the operating lateral position. Generous padding is used, espe-

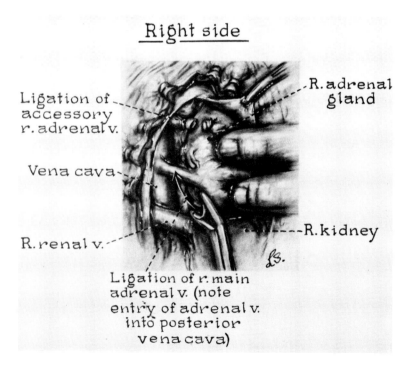

FIG. 35-37. *In the posterior approach to right-sided adrenalectomy, the right adrenal gland has been dissected free from Gerota's fascia. The adrenal vein exits from the medial aspect of the gland and enters the inferior vena cava posterolaterally. The adrenal vein is clipped flush with the inferior vena cava. Care must be taken not to injure the inferior vena cava and to search for an accessory right adrenal vein, which has been divided in this figure.*

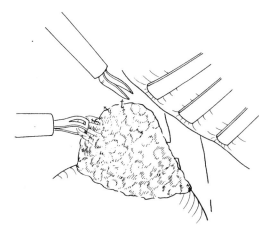

FIG. 35-40. Laparoscopic right adrenalectomy. (From: *Jones DB, Wu JS, Soper NJ: Laparoscopic Surgery: Principles and Procedures. St Louis, Quality Medical Publishing, 1997, with permission.*)

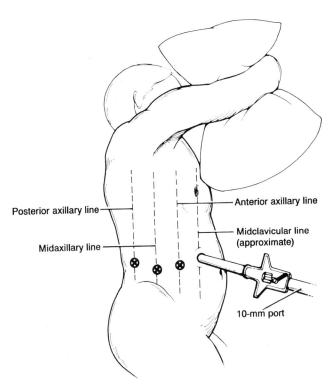

FIG. 35-38. Port placement for laparoscopic adrenalectomy.

cially in patients with hypercortisolism. A transperitoneal approach is used from this lateral position. Four ports are placed transversely across the upper abdomen approximately 2 to 4 fingerbreadths below the costal margin from the midclavicular line to the posterior axillary line (Fig. 35-38). The abdominal cavity is entered through the anterior port site and insufflated with CO_2 gas to a pressure of 12 to 15 mmHg. A videoendoscope is inserted through one port and operating instruments that include retractors, dissecting forceps, grasping forceps, irrigation, electrocautery, laparoscopic ultrasound probe, and harmonic scalpel

are inserted through other ports. On the left side the splenic flexure of the colon must be mobilized, and the spleen and the tail of the pancreas are mobilized anteriorly. The adrenal gland is identified with the use of the ultrasound probe by scanning over the superior and medial border of the kidney (Fig. 35-39). On the right side, the adrenal gland is exposed by dissecting and mobilizing the right lobe of the liver anteriorly. The ultrasound probe can be used to determine the precise location of the adrenal gland. The gland is dissected and removed in a fashion similar to the open procedure, described previously, except that the ultrasonic coagulation-cutting instrument (harmonic scalpel) is used to induce hemostasis in the small arterial branches to the gland. Large hemoclips are applied to the adrenal vein (Fig. 35-40). The resected gland is placed in a bag to avoid spillage while it is manipulated through the small incisions. The small skin and fascial incisions are closed. The laparoscopic approach to adrenalectomy is associated with less pain and a faster return to normal function than the open procedures. In experienced hands, the conversion rate from laparoscopic to open procedures is acceptably low.

Anterior Approach. The anterior approach for adrenalectomy is the recommended approach for potentially malignant adrenal tumors and pheochromocytomas. This approach is chosen because it provides access to the entire abdomen for accurate staging of any lymph node or liver metastases. It also allows better control of the inferior vena cava and other great vessels in the resection of malignant tumors, and it allows the surgeon to visualize and palpate along the sympathetic chain, which is a common extraadrenal site of pheochromocytoma. Some authors have stated that the use of newer localization studies has reduced the importance of this indication.

The abdominal cavity is entered through a midline incision or a bilateral subcostal (chevron) upper abdominal incision (Fig. 35-41). A fixed upper abdominal retractor, e.g., the Thompson or the Omni, aids exposure. The left adrenal gland is approached by dividing the ligaments between the spleen and the diaphragm and mobilizing the spleen and the tail of the pancreas out of the retroperitoneum. Alternatively, the left gland may be approached by opening the lesser sac and mobilizing the splenic flexure.

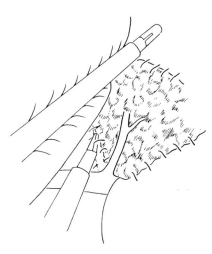

FIG. 35-39. Laparoscopic left adrenalectomy. (From: *Jones DB, Wu JS, Soper NJ: Laparoscopic Surgery: Principles and Procedures. St Louis, Quality Medical Publishing, 1997, with permission.*)

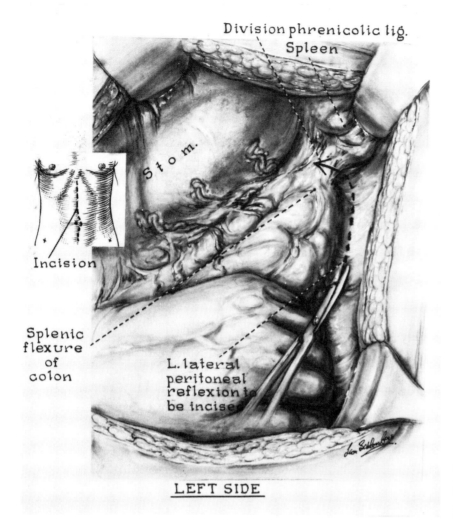

FIG. 35-41. The inset shows a standard long midline incision for anterior adrenalectomy and abdominal exploration. To remove the left adrenal gland, the left colon is mobilized by dividing the left lateral peritoneal reflection, the phrenicocolic ligament, and the gastrocolic ligament.

Once the lesser sac is entered, the pancreas can be elevated by dividing the inferior border and identifying the adrenal gland, which is posterior to the pancreas. The complete mobilization of the spleen and the pancreatic tail is preferred because it avoids the need to work in a deep hole with poor visualization. The left adrenal vein runs along the inferomedial border and empties into the left renal vein. With the anterior approach, the adrenal vein can be easily ligated early in the procedure, and doing so is preferable in resecting pheochromocytomas. After ligation and division of the left adrenal vein, hemoclips are applied to the small arteries that course along the medial border of the adrenal gland, and the arteries are divided (Fig. 35-42).

The right adrenal gland can be exposed by dissecting along the inferior vena cava underneath the liver, or mobilizing the entire right lobe of the liver as is done during a liver resection. The second method is preferred because it allows better exposure of the right adrenal gland, which is nestled underneath and to the right of the inferior vena cava. The right adrenal vein easily can be exposed after mobilization of the right lobe of the liver at the superior medial border of the gland, where it drains into the inferior vena cava (Fig. 35-43). After ligation and division

of the vein, hemoclips are applied to the arteries along the medial border, and the arteries are divided.

The open anterior approach to the adrenal gland is associated with more pain and longer hospitalization than the laparoscopic approach. It is indicated for larger tumors and pheochromocytomas, though some pheochromocytomas are resected laparoscopically.

Thoracoabdominal Approach. The thoracoabdominal approach to adrenalectomy is indicated for large, clearly malignant tumors that may involve adjacent organs, such as the liver, kidney, pancreas, spleen, or the inferior vena cava. The patient is positioned with the side of the tumor upward so the chest and abdomen can be entered. The incision is through the eleventh intercostal space, across the costal margin, and into the abdomen. Each adrenal gland is exposed in the same manner as previously described for the anterior approach. The resection proceeds in a similar fashion. The thoracoabdominal approach is associated with more postoperative pain than the other approaches, but it is indicated for some tumors because of their size and direct invasion of contiguous structures.

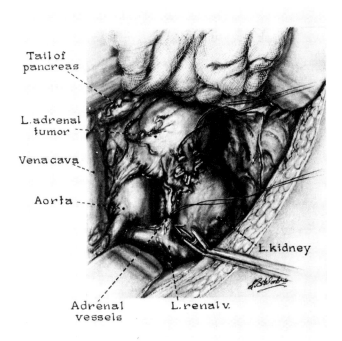

Tail of pancreas

L. adrenal tumor

Vena cava

Aorta

L. kidney

Adrenal vessels   L. renal v.

FIG. 35-42. The spleen and stomach are retracted superiorly and protected with large packs. The peritoneum along the inferior border of the pancreas has been incised, revealing the left adrenal tumor and kidney. The aorta lies medially. The left adrenal vein is ligated above its junction with the left renal vein. Small feeding vessels have been divided.

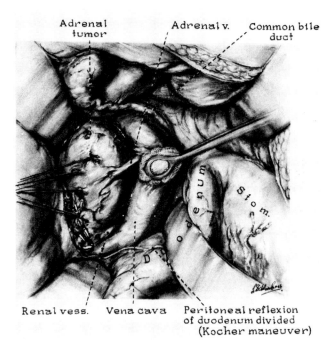

Adrenal tumor   Adrenal v.   Common bile duct

Renal vess.   Vena cava   Peritoneal reflexion of duodenum divided (Kocher maneuver)

RIGHT SIDE

FIG. 35-43. The anterior transabdominal approach to the right adrenal gland requires mobilization of the right colon inferiorly and the stomach and duodenum medially. Retraction of the liver superiorly brings the inferior vena cava, adrenal gland, and kidney into view. Gentle retraction of the inferior vena cava medially reveals the right adrenal vein entering the inferior vena cava posteriorly. The adrenal vein is divided between silk ligatures and clipped at its junction with the vena cava. The rest of the gland is resected as described previously for the left side.

Bibliography

Pituitary

Historical Background

Caton R, Paul FT: Notes of a case of acromegaly treated by operation. *Br Med J* 2:1421, 1893.

Collins WF: Hypophysectomy: Historical and personal perspective. *Clin Neurosurg* 21:68, 1974.

Cope UZ: The pituitary fossa and the methods of surgical approach thereto. *Br J Surg* 4:107, 1916.

Cushing H: Surgical experiences with pituitary disorders. *JAMA* 63:1515, 1914.

Cushing H: *Intracranial Tumors, Notes upon a Series of Two Thousand Verified Cases with Surgical Mortality Percentages Pertaining Thereto.* Springfield, IL, Charles C Thomas, 1932.

Dott NM, Bailery PA: Consideration of the hypophyseal adenomata. *Br J Surg* 13:314, 1925.

Forrest APM, Brown PAP: Pituitary radon implant for breast cancer. *Lancet* 268:1054, 1955.

Frazier CH: An approach to the hypophysis through the anterior cranial fossa. *Ann Surg* 57:145, 1913.

Guiot G, Thebaul B: L'Extirpation des adénomes hypophysaires par voie transsphénoidale. *Neuro-Chirurgie* 1:133, 1959.

Hamlin H: The case for transsphenoidal approach to hypophyseal tumors. *J Neurosurg* 19:1000, 1962.

Hardy J: L'Exerese des adenomes hypophysaires par voie transsphénoidale. *Union Med Can* 91:933, 1962.

Heuer GJ: The surgical approach and the therapy of tumors and other lesions about the optic chiasm. *Surg Gynecol Obstet* 53:489, 1931.

Hirsch O: Endonasal method of removal of hypophyseal tumors with a report of two successful cases. *JAMA* 55:772, 1910.

Horsley V: Address in surgery: On the technique of operation on the central nervous system. *Br Med J* 2:411, 1906.

Horsley V, Clark RH: The structure and function of the cerebellum examined by a new method. *Brain* 31:45, 1908.

Kiliani OGT: Some remarks on tumors of the chiasm, with a proposal how to reach the same by operation. *Ann Surg* 40:35, 1904.

Krause F: Hrinchirurgie (Freilegung Do Hypophyse). *Deutchse Klin* 8:953, 1905.

McArthur LL: An aseptic surgical access to the pituitary body and its neighborhood. *JAMA* 58:2009, 1912.

Olivecrona H, Luft R: Experiences with hypophysectomy in man. *J Neurosurg* 10:301, 1953.

Ray BS, Pearson OH: Hypophysectomy in the treatment of advanced cancer of the breast. *Ann Surg* 144:394, 1956.

Talairach J, Tournoux P: Appareil de stéréotaxic hypophysaire pour voie d'abord nasale. *Neuro-Chirurgie* 1:127, 1955.

Zervas N: Stereotaxic radiofrequency surgery of the normal and abnormal pituitary gland. *N Engl J Med* 280:429, 1969.

Anatomy

Antunes JL, Murasko K, et al: Pituitary portal blood flow in primates: A Doppler study. *Neurosurgery* 12:492, 1983.

Asa SL, Kovacs K: Histological classification of pituitary disease. *J Clin Endocrinol Metab* 12:567, 1983.

Baker BL: Functional cytology of the hypophyseal pars distalis and pars intermedia, in Greep RO, Astwood EB (eds): *Handbook of Physiology,* sec 7, *Endocrinology,* vol 4, *The Pituitary Gland and Its Neuroendocrine Control,* part 1. Washington, DC, American Physiology Society, 1974.

Besser GM (ed): The hypothalamus and pituitary. *J Clin Endocrinol Metab* 6:entire issue, 1977.

Browstein MJ, Russel JT, et al: Synthesis, transport, and release of posterior pituitary hormones. *Science* 207:373, 1980.

Cross BA, Leng G (eds): The neurohypophysis: Structure, function, and control. *Prog Brain Res* 60:entire issue, 1983.

Daughaday WH: The adenohypophysis, in Williams RH (ed): *Textbook of Endocrinology.* Philadelphia, WB Saunders, 1981.

Frentz AG: Prolactin. *N Engl J Med* 298:201, 1978.

Knigge KM, Scott DE: Structure and function of the median eminence. *Am J Anat* 129:223, 1970.

Kovacs K: Pathology of the neurohypophysis, in Reichlin S (ed): *The Neurohypophysis: Physiological and Clinical Aspects.* New York, Plenum, 1984.

Kovacs K, Horvath E, et al: Anatomy and histology of the normal and abnormal pituitary gland, in DeGroot LJ (ed): *Endocrinology,* vol 1. Philadelphia, WB Saunders, 1989.

Page RB: Pituitary blood flow: A review. *Am J Physiol* 243:E427, 1982.

Pardridge WM, Frank HJL, et al: Neuropeptides and the blood-brain barrier, in Martin JB, Reichlin S, Bick KL (eds): *Neurosecretion and Brain Peptides.* New York, Raven, 1981.

Rhoton AL Jr, Hardy DG, et al: Microsurgical anatomy and dissection of the sphenoid bone, cavernous sinus, and sellar region. *Surg Neurol* 12:63, 1979.

Wilhelmi AE: Chemistry of growth hormone, in Knobil E, Sawyer WH (eds): *Handbook of Physiology.* Washington, DC, American Physiological Society, 1974.

Regulation of the Hypothalamic-Pituitary Axis

Bisset GW: Milk ejection, in Knobil E, Sawyer WH (eds): *Handbook of Physiology, Endocrinology,* vol 4, part 1. Washington, DC, American Physiological Society, 1974.

Browstein MJ, Russel JT, et al: Synthesis, transport, and release of posterior pituitary hormones. *Science* 207:373, 1980.

Cocchi D, Muller EE: Control of anterior pituitary function, in Collu R, Brown GM, Van Loon GR (eds): *Clinical Neuroendocrinology.* Cambridge, MA, Blackwell Scientific, 1988.

Daniel PM, Prichard MML: The human hypothalamus and pituitary stalk after hypophysectomy or pituitary stalk section. *Brain* 95:813, 1972.

Fuchs F: Role of maternal and fetal oxytocin in human parturition, in Amico JA, Robinson AG (eds): *Oxytocin: Clinical and Laboratory Studies.* Amsterdam, Elsevier, 1985.

Hayward JN: Functional and morphological aspects of hypothalamic neurons. *Physiol Rev* 57:574, 1977.

Joseph SA, Knigge KM: The endocrine hypothalamus: Recent anatomical studies. *Res Publ Assoc Res Nerv Ment Dis* 56:15, 1978.

Labrie F, Godbout M, et al: Mechanism of action of hypothalamic hormones and interaction with peripheral hormones at the pituitary level, in Motta M (ed): *The Endocrine Function of the Brain (Comprehensive Endocrinology).* New York, Raven, 1980.

Lees PD, Pickard JD: Hyperprolactinemia, intrasellar pituitary tissue pressure, and the pituitary stalk compression syndrome. *J Neurosurg* 67:192, 1987.

MacLeod RM: Regulation of prolactin secretion, in Martini L, Ganong WF (eds): *Frontiers in Neuroendocrinology,* vol 4. New York, Raven, 1976.

Martin JB: Brain regulation of growth hormone secretion, in Martini L, Ganong WF (eds): *Frontiers in Neuroendocrinology.* New York, Raven, 1976.

Morley JE: Neuroendocrine control of thyrotropin secretion. *Endocr Rev* 2:396, 1981.

Oppizzi G, Petroncini MM, et al: Relationship between somatomedin-C and growth hormone levels in acromegaly: Basal and dynamic evaluation. *J Clin Endocrinol Metab* 63:1348, 1986.

Palkovits M: Catecholamines in the hypothalamus: An anatomical review. *Neuroendocrinology* 33:123, 1981.

Porter JC, Reymond MJ, et al: Secretion of hypothalamic dopamine into the hypophysial portal structure, in Tolis G, et al (eds): *Prolactin and Prolactinomas.* New York, Raven, 1983.

Reichlin S: Anatomical and physiological basis of hypothalamic-pituitary regulation, in Post KD, Jackson IMD, Reichlin S (eds): *The Pituitary Adenoma.* New York, Plenum, Medical Book Co, 1980.

Renaud LP: A neurophysiological approach to the identification, connections, and pharmacology of the hypothalamic tuberoinfundibular system. *Neuroendocrinology* 33:186, 1981.

Schally AV, Coy DH, et al: Hypothalamic peptide hormones: Basic and clinical studies, in Li CH (ed): *Hormonal Proteins and Peptides.* New York, Academic Press, 1979.

Scharrer E, Scharrer B: Secretory cells within the hypothalamus. *Res Publ Res Nerv Ment Dis* 20:170, 1939.

Schrier RW, Berl T, et al: Osmotic and nonosmotic control of vasopressin release. *Am J Physiol* 236:F321, 1979.

Silverman AJ, Zimmerman EA: Magnocellular neurosecretory system, in Cowan WM, et al (eds): *Annual Review of Neuroscience,* vol 6. Palo Alto, Annual Reviews, 1983.

Verney EB: Absorption and secretion of water: The antidiuretic hormone. *Lancet* 2:739, 1946.

Neuroendocrine Evaluation

Abboud CF: Laboratory diagnosis of hypopituitarism. *Mayo Clin Proc* 61:35, 1986.

Bayliss PH, Gill GV: The investigation of polyuria. *J Clin Endocrinol Metab* 13:294, 1984.

Kleinberg DL, Frantz AG: Human prolactin: Measurement in plasma by in vitro bioassay. *J Clin Invest* 50:1557, 1971.

Lin T, Tucci JR: Provocative tests of growth hormone release. A comparison of results with seven stimuli. *Ann Intern Med* 80:464, 1974.

Ontjes DA, Ney RL: Tests of anterior pituitary function. *Metabolism* 21:159, 1972.

Radiographic Evaluation

Daniel PM, Prichard MML: Studies of the hypothalamus and the pituitary gland with special reference to the effects of transection of the pituitary stalk. *Acta Endocrinol* 80(suppl 201):1, 1975.

Davis PC, Hoffman JC Jr, et al: MR imaging of pituitary adenoma: CT, clinical, and surgical correlation. *AJR* 148:797, 1987.

Karnaze MG, Sartor K, et al: Suprasellar lesions: Evaluation with MR imaging. *Radiology* 161:77, 1986.

Kaufman B: The "empty" sella turcica: A manifestation of the intrasellar subarachnoid space. *Radiology* 90:931, 1968.

Lundin P, Nyman R, et al: MRI of pituitary macroadenomas with reference to hormonal activity. *Neuroradiology* 34:43, 1992.

Roppolo HMN, Latchaw RE: Normal pituitary gland. 2: Microscopic anatomy-CT correlation. *AJNR* 4:937, 1983.

Molitch ME, Russel EJ: The pituitary "incidentaloma." *Ann Intern Med* 112:925, 1990.

Newton DR, Dillon WP, et al: Gd-DTPA-enhanced MR imaging of pituitary adenomas. *AJNR* 10:949, 1989.

Peck WW, Dillon WP, et al: High resolution MR imaging of pituitary microadenomas at 1.5 T: Experience with Cushing's disease. *AJR* 152:145, 1989.

Smallridge RC, Smith CE: Hyperthyroidism due to thyrotropin-secreting pituitary tumors: Diagnostic and therapeutic considerations. *Arch Intern Med* 143:503, 1983.

Snow RB, Johnson CE, et al: Is magnetic resonance imaging useful in the operative approach to large pituitary lesions? *Neurosurgery* 26:801, 1990.

Stein AL, Levenick MN, et al: Computed tomography versus magnetic resonance imaging for the evaluation of suspected pituitary adenomas. *Obstet Gynecol* 73:996, 1989.

Steiner E, Imhof H, et al: Gd-DTPA enhanced high-resolution MR imaging of pituitary adenomas. *Radiographics* 9:587, 1989.

Weiner SN, Rzeszotarski MS, et al: Measurement of the pituitary gland height with MR imaging. *AJNR* 6:717, 1985.

Wolpert SM, Molitch ME, et al: Size, shape, and appearance of the normal female pituitary gland. *AJNR* 5:263, 1984.

Wray SH: Neuro-ophthalmologic manifestations of pituitary and parasellar lesions. *Clin Neurosurg* 24:86, 1977.

Anterior Pituitary Disorders

Sheehan HL, Stanfield JP: The pathogenesis of post-partum necrosis of the anterior lobe of the pituitary gland. *Acta Endocrinol* 37:479, 1961.

Pituitary Adenomas—Pathology

Bassetti M, Spada A, et al: Morphological studies on mixed growth hormone (GH)- and prolactin (PRL)-secreting human pituitary adenomas: Coexistence of GH and PRL in the same secretory granule. *J Clin Endocrinol Metab* 62:1093, 1986.

Kovacs K, Horvath E: Pathology of pituitary adenomas, in Collu R, Brown G, Van Loon GR (eds): *Clinical Neuroendocrinology*, chap 13. Boston, Blackwell Scientific, 1988.

Thapar K, Kovacs K, et al: Classification of pituitary tumors, in Wilkins RH, Rengachary SS (eds): *Neurosurgery*, 2d ed. New York, McGraw-Hill, 1996, pp 1273-1289.

Pituitary Adenomas—Medical Therapy

Alford FP, Arnott R: Medical management of pituitary tumors. *Med J Austr* 157:57, 1992.

Barkan AL, Kelch RP, et al: Treatment of acromegaly with the long-acting somatostatin analog SMS 201-995. *J Clin Endocrinol Metab* 66:16, 1988.

Barkan A, Lloyd RV, et al: Treatment of acromegaly with SMS 201-995 (Sandostatin): Clinical, biochemical, and morphologic study, in Lamberts SWJ (ed): *Sandostatin in the Treatment of Acromegaly.* New York: Springer, 1988, pp 103-108.

Barnard LB, Grantham WG, et al: Treatment of resistant acromegaly with a long-acting somatostatin analogue (SMS 201-995). *Ann Intern Med* 105:856, 1986.

Baumann G: Acromegaly. *Endocrinol Metab Clin North Am* 16:685, 1987.

Bevan JS, Webster J, et al: Dopamine agonists and pituitary tumor shrinkage. *Endocr Rev* 137:220, 1992.

Couldwell WT, Simard MF, et al: The Management of prolactin and growth hormone secreting pituitary adenomas, in Schmidek HH, Sweet WH (eds): *Operative Neurosurgical Techniques.* Philadelphia, WH Saunders, 1995, pp 305-313.

Ezzat S, Snyder PJ, et al: Octreotide treatment of acromegaly: A randomized, multicenter study. *Ann Inter Med* 117:711, 1992.

Frohman LA: Therapeutic options in acromegaly. *J Clin Endocrinol Metab* 72:1175, 1991.

Harris AG, Prestele H, et al: Long-term efficacy of Sandostatin (SMS 201-995, octreotide) in 178 acromegalic patients: Results from the International Multicenter Acromegaly Study Group, in *Sandostatin in the Treatment of Acromegaly.* New York: Springer, 1988, pp 117-125.

Herman V, Fagin J, et al: Clonal origin of pituitary adenomas. *J Clin Endocrin Metab* 71:1427, 1990.

Klibanski A, Zervas NT: Diagnosis and management of hormone-secreting pituitary adenomas. *N Engl J Med* 324:822, 1991.

Molitch ME: Pregnancy and hyperprolactinemic woman. *N Engl J Med* 312:1364, 1985.

Orth DN: Medical Progress: Cushing's syndrome. *N Engl J Med* 332:791, 1995.

Thorner MO, McNeilly AS, et al: Long-term treatment of galactorrhea and hypogonadism with bromocriptine. *Br Med J* 2:419, 1974.

Thorner MO, Perryman RL, et al: Rapid changes of prolactinoma volume after withdrawal and reinstitution of bromocriptine. *J Clin Endocrinol Metab* 53:480, 1981.

Vance ML, Evans WS, et al: Drugs five years later: Bromocriptine. *Ann Int Med* 100:78, 1984.

Vance ML, Thorner MO: Prolactinomas. *Endocrinol Metab Clin North Am* 16:731, 1987.

Pituitary Adenomas—Surgical Therapy

Adams CBT: The management of pituitary tumors and post-operative visual deterioration. *Acta Neurochir (Wien)* 94:103, 1988.

Arafah B: Reversible hypopituitarism in patients with large adenomas. *J Clin Endocrinol Metab* 62:1173, 1986.

Bevin JS, Adams CBT, et al: Factors in the outcome of transsphenoidal surgery for prolactinoma and non-functioning pituitary tumor, including pre-operative bromocriptine therapy. *Clin Endocrinol* 26:541, 1987.

Black PMcL, Zervas N, et al: Incidence and management of complications of transsphenoidal operation for pituitary adenomas. *Neurosurgery* 20:920, 1987.

Ciric I, Mikhael M, et al: Transsphenoidal microsurgery of pituitary macroadenomas with long-term follow-up results. *J Neurosurg* 59:395, 1984.

Cohen AR, Cooper PR, et al: Visual recovery after transsphenoidal removal of pituitary adenomas. *Neurosurgery* 17:446, 1985.

Collins WF: Pituitary tumor management: An overview, in Tindall GT, Collins WF (eds): *Clinical Management of Pituitary Disorders.* New York, Raven, 1979, pp 179-186.

Couldwell WT, Weiss MH: Strategies for the management of non-secreting pituitary adenomas, in Cooper PR (ed): *Neurosurgical Topics: Contemporary Diagnosis and Management of Pituitary Adenomas.* Park Ridge, IL, AANS Publications Committee, 1991, pp 29-37.

Couldwell WT, Weiss MH: Defining postoperative values for successful resection of prolactinomas. *J Neurosurg* 85:990, 1996.

Faria MA, Tindall GT: Transsphenoidal microsurgery for prolactin-secreting pituitary adenomas. *J Neurosurg* 56:33, 1982.

Grigsby PW, Simpson JR, et al: Prognostic factors and results of surgery and postoperative irradiation in the management of pituitary adenomas. *J Radiat Oncol Biol Phys* 16:1411, 1989.

Guiot G: Considerations on the surgical treatment of pituitary adenomas, in Fahlbusch R, Werder KV (eds): *Treatment of Pituitary Adenomas.* 1st European workshop. Stuttgart, Thieme, 1978, pp 202-218.

Hardy J: Transsphenoidal microsurgery of the normal and pathological pituitary. *Clin Neurosurg* 16:185, 1969.

Hardy J: Transsphenoidal hypophysectomy. *J Neurosurg* 34:582, 1971.

Kayan A, Earl CJ: Compressive lesion of the optic nerves and chiasm: Pattern of recovery of vision following surgical treatment. *Brain* 98:13, 1975.

Laws ER, Fode NC, et al: Transsphenoidal surgery following unsuccessful prior therapy. *J Neurosurg* 63:823, 1985.

Orth DN: Medical Progress: Cushing's syndrome. *N Engl J Med* 332:791, 1995.

Post KD, Biller BJ, et al: Selective transsphenoidal adenectomy in women with galactorrhea-amenorrhea. *JAMA* 242:158, 1979.

Schloffer H: Erfulgreiche operation eiwes hypophysewtunions auf nasallam. *Weg Wien Klin Wochamschr* 20:621, 1907.

Serri O, Rasio E, et al: Recurrence of hyperprolactinemia after selective transphenoidal adenomectomy in women with prolactinoma. *N Engl J Med* 309:280, 1983.

Sheline GF: Treatment of non-functioning chromophobe adenomas of the pituitary. *Am J Roentgenol* 120:553, 1974.

Tyrell JB, Brooks RM, et al: Cushing's disease: Selective transsphenoidal resection of pituitary microadenomas. *N Engl J Med* 298:753, 1978.

Valtonen S, Myllymaki K: Outcome of patients after transcranial operation for pituitary adenoma. *Ann Clin Res* 18(suppl 47):43, 1986.

Warnet A, Timsit J, et al: The effect of somatostatin analogue on chiasmal dysfunction from pituitary macroadenomas. *J Neurosurg* 71:687, 1989.

Weiss MH: Transnasal transsphenoidal approach, in Apuzzo MLJ (ed): *Surgery of the Third Ventricle.* Baltimore, Williams & Wilkins, 1987, pp 476-494.

Weiss MH, Wycoff RR, et al: Bromocriptine therapy of prolactin-secreting tumors: Surgical implications. *Neurosurgery* 12:640, 1983.

Wilson CB, Dempsey LC: Transsphenoidal microsurgical removal of 250 pituitary adenomas. *J Neurosurg* 48:13, 1978.

Wilson CB: A decade of pituitary microsurgery. The Herbert Olivecrona Lecture. *J Neurosurg* 61:814, 1984.

Zervas NT: Surgical results in pituitary adenomas: Results of an international survey, in Black PMcL, et al (eds): *Secretory Tumors of the Pituitary Gland.* New York, Raven, 1984, pp 377–385.

Pituitary Adenomas—Radiation Therapy

Aristzabal S, Caldwell WL, Avila J: The relationship of time dose fractionation factors to complications in the treatment of pituitary tumors by irradiation. *Int J Radiat Oncol Biol Phys* 2:667, 1977.

Baglan R, Marks J: Soft-tissue reactions following irradiation of primary brain and pituitary tumors. *Int J Radiat Oncol Biol Phys* 7:455, 1981.

Chun M, Masko GB, et al: Radiotherapy in the treatment of pituitary adenomas. *Int J Radiat Oncol Biol Phys* 15:305, 1988.

Eastman RC, Gorden P, et al: Radiation therapy of acromegaly. *Endocrinol Metab Clin North Am* 21:693, 1992.

Flickinger JC, Nelson PB, et al: Radiotherapy of nonfunctional adenomas of the pituitary gland. *Cancer* 63:2409, 1989.

Gramegna A: Un cas d'acromégalie traité par la radiothérapie. *Rev Neurol* 17:15, 1909.

Gunz JC, Backlund EO, et al: The effects of gamma knife surgery of pituitary adenomas on tumor growth and endocrinopathies. *Stereotact Funct Neurosurg* 61(suppl 1):30, 1993.

Howlett TA, Plowman PN, et al: Megavoltage pituitary irradiation in the management of Cushing's disease and Nelson's syndrome. *Clin Endocrinol Oxf* 31:309, 1989.

Kramer S: The value of radiation therapy for pituitary and parapituitary tumors. *Can Med Assoc J* 99:1120, 1968.

Littley MD, Shalet SM, et al: Hypopituitarism following external radiotherapy for pituitary tumors in adults. *A J Med* 70:145, 1989.

McCollough WM, Marcus RB, et al: Long-term follow-up of radiotherapy for pituitary adenoma: The absence of late recurrence after greater than or equal to 4500 cGy. *Int J Radiat Oncol Biol Phys* 21:607, 1991.

Noell KT: Prolactin and other hormone producing pituitary tumors: Radiation therapy. *Clin Obstet Gynecol* 23:441, 1980.

Pollock BE, Kondziolka D, et al: Stereotactic radiosurgery for pituitary adenomas: Imaging, visual and endocrine results. *Acta Neurochir* 62(suppl 1):5, 1994.

Rush SC, Newalt J: Pituitary adenomas: The efficacy of radiotherapy as the sole treatment. *Int J Radiat Oncol Biol Phys* 17:165, 1989.

Salinger DJ, Brady LW, et al: Radiation therapy in the treatment of pituitary adenomas. *Am J Clin Oncol* 15:467, 1992.

Stephanian F, Lunsford LD, et al: Gamma knife surgery for sellar and suprasellar tumors. *Neurosurg Clin North Am* 3:207, 1992.

Tran LM, Blount L, et al: Radiation therapy of pituitary tumors: Results in 95 cases. *Am J Clin Oncol* 14:25, 1991.

Urdaneta N, Chessin H, et al: Pituitary adenomas and craniopharyngiomas: Analysis of 99 cases treated with radiation therapy. *Int J Radiat Oncol Biol Phys* 1:895, 1975.

Witt TC, Kondziolka D, et al: Stereotactic radiosurgery for pituitary tumors. *Radiosurgery* 1:1, 1995.

Other Lesions in the Region of the Sella

Carmel PW, Antunes JL, et al: Craniopharyngiomas in children. *Neurosurgery* 11:382, 1982.

Couldwell WT, Weiss MH: Pituitary parenchymal metastasis from adenocarcinoma of the prostate. *J Neurosurg* 71:138, 1989.

Cushing H, Eisenhardt L: *Meningiomas: Their Classification, Regional Behaviour, Life History, and Surgical End Results.* Springfield, IL, Charles C Thomas, 1938.

Gregorius FK, Hepler RS, et al: Loss and recovery of vision with suprasellar meningiomas. *J Neurosurg* 42:69, 1975.

Haughton VM, Rosenbaum AE, et al: Recognizing the empty sella by CT: The infundibulum sign. *AJR* 136:293, 1981.

Hoff JT, Patterson RH Jr: Craniopharyngiomas in children and adults. *J Neurosurg* 36:299, 1972.

Hoyt WF, Baghdassarian SA: Optic glioma of childhood: Natural history and rationale for conservative management. *Br J Ophthalmol* 53:793, 1973.

Iraci G, Gerosa M, et al: Gliomas of the optic nerve and chiasm. *Childs Brain* 8:326, 1981.

Jalalah S, Kovacs K, et al: Rhabdomyosarcoma in the region of the sella turcica. *Acta Neurochir (Wien)* 88:142, 1988.

Matson DD, Crigler JF Jr: Management of craniopharyngioma in childhood. *J Neurosurg* 30:377, 1977.

Pituitary Trauma

Adams JH, Daniel PM, et al: Transection of the pituitary stalk in man: Anatomical changes in the pituitary glands in 21 patients. *J Neurol Neurosurg Psychiatry* 29:544, 1966.

Graham DI, Hume Adams J, et al: Pathology of brain damage in head injury, in Cooper PR (ed): *Head Injury,* 2d ed. Baltimore, Williams & Wilkins, 1987, p 80.

Treip CS: Hypothalamic and pituitary injury, in Sevitt S, Stoner HB (eds): *The Pathology of Trauma. J Clin Pathol (R Coll Pathol)* 4(suppl 23):154, 1970.

Posterior Pituitary Disorders

Bartter FC: Syndrome of inappropriate secretion of antidiuretic hormone. *Dis Mon* (Nov):1–47, 1973.

Bartter FC, Schwartz WB: The syndrome of inappropriate secretion of antidiuretic hormone. *Am J Med* 42:790, 1967.

Cobb WE, Spare S, et al: Neurogenic diabetes insipidus: Management with dDAVP (1-desamino-8-D arginine vasopressin). *Ann Intern Med* 88:183, 1978.

Randall RV, Clark EC, et al: Classification of the causes of diabetes insipidus. *Mayo Clin Proc* 34:299, 1959.

Adrenal

Adrenal Cortex

Avgerinos PC, Yanovski JA, et al: The metyrapone and dexamethasone suppression tests for the differential diagnosis of the adrenocorticotropin-dependent Cushing syndrome: A comparison. *Ann Int Med* 121:318, 1994.

Candel AG, Gattuso P, et al: Fine-needle aspiration biopsy of adrenal masses in patients with extra-adrenal malignancy. *Surgery* 114:1132, 1993.

Chrousos GP, Schuermeyer TH, et al: Clinical applications of corticotropin-releasing factor. *Ann Intern Med* 102:344, 1985.

Corenblum B, Kwan T, et al: Bedside assessment of skin-fold thickness: A useful measurement for distinguishing Cushing's disease from other causes of hirsutism and oligomenorrhea. *Arch Int Med* 154:777, 1994.

Cunningham DS, Cutler GB Jr: Spontaneous vulvar necrotizing fasciitis in Cushing's syndrome. *Southern Med J* 87:837, 1994.

Decker RA, Elson P, et al: ECOG mitotane and adriamycin in patients with ACC. *Surgery* 110:1006, 1991.

Doherty GM, Nieman LK, et al: Time to recovery of the hypothalamic-pituitary-adrenal axis after curative resection of adrenal tumors in patients with Cushing's syndrome. *Surgery* 108:1085, 1990.

Doppman JL, Reinig JW, et al: Differentiation of adrenal masses by magnetic resonance imaging. *Surgery* 102:1018, 1987.

Dunnick NR: Adrenal carcinoma. *Radiol Clin North Am* 32:99, 1994.

Gagner M, LaCroix A, et al: Early experience with laparoscopic approach for adrenalectomy. *Surgery* 114:1120, 1993.

Geisinger MA, Zelch M, et al: Primary hyperaldosteronism: Comparison of CT, adrenal venography, and venous sampling. *AJR* 141:299, 1983.

Go H, Takeda M, et al: Laparoscopic adrenalectomy for Cushing's syndrome: Comparison with primary aldosteronism. *Surgery* 117:11, 1995.

Jensen JC, Pass HI, et al: Recurrent or metastatic disease in select patients with adrenocortical carcinoma. *Arch Surg* 126:457, 1991.

Limper AH, Carpenter PC, et al: The Cushing syndrome induced by bronchial carcinoid tumors. *Ann Intern Med* 117:209, 1992.

Luton JP, Cerdas S, et al: Clinical features of adrenocortical carcinoma: Prognostic factors and the effect of mitotane therapy. *N Engl J Med* 322:1195, 1990.

Magiakou MA, Mastorakos G, et al: Cushing's syndrome in children and adolescents: Presentation, diagnosis, and therapy. *N Engl J Med* 331:629, 1994.

Nieman LK, Chrousos GP, et al: The ovine corticotropin-releasing hormone stimulation test and the dexamethasone suppression test in the differential diagnosis of Cushing's syndrome. *Ann Intern Med* 105:862, 1986.

Oldfield EH, Doppman JL, et al: Petrosal sinus sampling with and without corticotropin-releasing hormone for the differential diagnosis of Cushing's syndrome. *N Engl J Med* 325:897, 1991.

Orth DN: Cushing's syndrome. *N Engl J Med* 332:791, 1995.

Pasieka JL, McLeod MK, et al: Adrenal scintigraphy of well-differentiated (functioning) adrenocortical carcinomas: Potential surgical pitfalls. *Surgery* 112:884, 1992.

Pass HI, Doppman, JL, et al: Management of the ectopic ACTH syndrome due to thoracic carcinoids. *Ann Thorac Surg* 50:52, 1990.

Perry RR, Nieman LK, et al: Primary adrenal causes of Cushing's syndrome: Diagnosis and surgical management. *Ann Surg* 210:59, 1989.

Pommier R, Brennan MF: An 11-year experience with adrenocortical cancer. *Surgery* 112:1963, 1992.

Ross NS, Aron DC: Hormonal evaluation of the patient with an incidentally discovered adrenal mass. *N Engl J Med 323*:1401, 1990.

van Heerden JA, Young WF Jr, et al: Adrenal surgery for hypercortisolism: Surgical aspects. *Surgery* 117:466, 1995.

Adrenal Medulla

Irvin GL, Fishman LM, et al: Pheochromocytoma: Lateral vs anterior operative approach. *Ann Surg* 209:774, 1989.

Krempf M, Lumbroso J, et al: Use of [131]Im iodobenzylguanidine in the treatment of malignant pheochromocytoma. *J Clin Endocrinol Metab* 72:455, 1991.

Lairmore TC, Ball DW, et al: Management of pheochromocytomas in patients with multiple endocrine neoplasia type 2 syndromes. *Ann Surg* 217:595, 1993.

MacDougall IC, Isles CG, et al: Overnight clonidine suppression test in the diagnosis and exclusion of pheochromocytoma. *Am J Med* 84:993, 1988.

Nakabeppu Y, Nakajo M: Radionuclide therapy of malignant pheochromocytoma with ^{131}I-MIBG. *Ann Nucl Med* 8:259, 1994.

Perry RR, Keiser HR, et al: Surgical management of pheochromocytoma with the use of metyrosine. *Ann Surg* 212:621, 1990.

Proye C, Thevenin D, et al: Exclusive use of calcium channel blockers in preoperative and intraoperative control of pheochromocytomas: Hemodynamics and free catecholamine assays in ten consecutive patients. *Surgery* 106:1149, 1989.

Sheps SG, Jiang NS, et al: Recent developments in the diagnosis and management of pheochromocytoma. *Mayo Clin Proc* 65:88, 1990.

Wu LT, Dicpinigaitis P, et al: Hypertensive crises induced by treatment of a malignant pheochromocytoma with a combination of cyclophosphamide, vincristine, and dacarbazine. *Med Pediatr Oncol* 22:389, 1994.

CHAPTER 36

Thyroid and Parathyroid

Gregory P. Sadler, Orlo H. Clark, Jon A. van Heerden, and David R. Farley

Thyroid

Gregory P. Sadler and Orlo H. Clark

HISTORICAL BACKGROUND

Goiters (from the Latin *guttur*, throat) have been known since 2700 B.C., long before the thyroid gland was recognized. The thyroid gland was first documented by the Italians of the Renaissance period. Leonardo da Vinci originally depicted the thyroid in his drawings as two separate glands on either side of the larynx. The term thyroid gland (Greek *thyreoeides*, shield-shaped) is attributed to Thomas Wharton in his *Adenographia* (1656), although Bartholomeus Eustachius had used the description previously; his work, however, was not published until the eighteenth century. In 1619, Hieronymus Fabricius ab Aquapendente recognized that goiters arose from the thyroid gland. It was Albrecht von Haller in 1776 who classified the thyroid as a ductless gland. Many functions were imaginatively ascribed to the thyroid gland, including lubrication of the larynx, providing a reservoir of blood to prevent engorgement of the brain, or beautifying women's necks.

Treatment of goiter was varied; marine preparations, such as burnt seaweed, were among the most effective. In 1811 Bernard Courtois discovered iodine in the ash of burnt seaweed. Surgery of goiters was hazardous, with an exceedingly high complication and mortality rate. The first accounts of thyroid surgery were given by Roger Frugardi in 1170. Failing response to medical treatments, two setons were inserted at right angles into the goiter and tightened twice daily until the goiter separated. The open wound was then treated with caustic powder and left to heal.

Thyroid surgery continued to be hazardous (mortality over 40 percent) until the mid-nineteenth century, when advances in general anesthesia (1840s), antisepsis (1860s), and hemostasis (1870s) enabled surgeons to perform thyroid surgery with significantly reduced mortality. The most notable thyroid surgeons were Emil Theodor Kocher (1841–1917) (Fig. 36-1) and C.A. Theodor Billroth (1829–1894), who performed thousands of operations with increasingly successful results. As patients survived longer, however, problems emerged that had not been previously encountered. After total thyroidectomy, patients became myxedematous with cretinous features; the changes were more noticeable in children. Kocher coined the term "cachexia strumipriva" and wrongly attributed it to operative tracheal trauma giving rise to chronic asphyxia. Felix Semon suggested that myxedema was secondary to the loss of thyroid function, a view originally treated with skepticism. This was later proved true by Victor Horsley's studies on monkeys undergoing total thyroidectomy.

The first successful treatment of myxedema was achieved in 1891 by George Murray when he prepared an extract of sheep's thyroid that he injected subcutaneously into a patient. The following year, Edward Fox demonstrated that oral therapy in the form of "half a sheep's thyroid, lightly fried and taken with currant jelly once a week" was equally effective.

Few of Billroth's patients developed myxedema, but William Halsted suggested that this was because of a difference in operative technique. Kocher was extremely neat and precise, operating slowly in a bloodless field. He removed all the thyroid, and his patients developed myxedema but rarely suffered laryngeal nerve damage or postoperative tetany. Billroth, however, worked rapidly and with less concern for hemorrhage. He often removed the parathyroid glands but left more thyroid tissue and therefore encountered postoperative hypoparathyroidism but rarely myxedema. In 1909 Kocher received the Nobel Prize for medicine in recognition "for his works on the physiology, pathology, and surgery of the thyroid gland."

EMBRYOLOGY

A clear understanding of the developmental embryology and anatomy of the thyroid gland is essential for the clinician performing a thorough physical examination of the gland and aids in evaluating diagnostic images. Knowledge of possible developmental anomalies and the thyroid gland's relationship to the parathyroid glands and other neck structures is vital in performing safe and effective thyroid operations.

The thyroid gland originates from the base of the tongue in the region of the foramen cecum. Embryologically, it is an offshoot of the primitive alimentary tract. The endoderm cells in the midline of the floor of the pharyngeal anlage thicken and form a median thyroid anlage, which migrates caudally into the neck (Fig. 36-2). The anlage descends along a tract that runs anterior to the structures that form the hyoid bone and the larynx; it is composed of epithelial cells that provide the follicular cells of the thyroid. As it descends, it is joined laterally by a pair of components originating from the ultimobranchial bodies of the fourth and fifth branchial pouches. These lateral components supply the C cells of the thyroid, which secrete calcitonin. When the C cells become neoplastic, the result is medullary carcinoma of the thyroid. An understanding of this anatomy explains why medullary carcinoma usually is located in the upper poles of the thyroid and virtually never in the isthmus or pyramidal lobe. The thyroid gland forms follicles by the end of the tenth week of gestation and concentrates iodine and produces colloid by the end of the twelfth week.

ANOMALIES

Rarely, the thyroid gland, whole or in part, descends more caudally. This results in thyroid tissue located in the superior mediastinum behind the sternum, adjacent to the aortic arch or be-

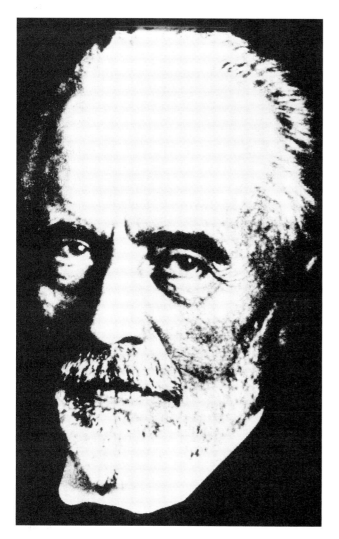

FIG. 36-1. *Emil Theodor Kocher of Berne (1841–1917). Regarded by many as the "father" of thyroid surgery, he received the Nobel Prize for medicine (1909) in recognition of his work on the thyroid gland.*

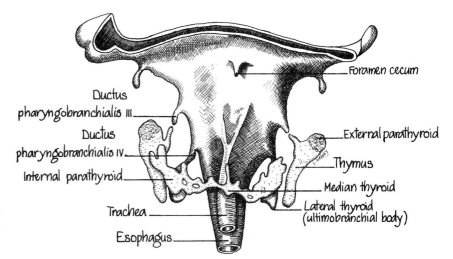

FIG. 36-2. Ventral view of model of pharynx of 14.5 mm embryo (early seventeenth week). (From: *Rogers WM: Normal and anomalous development of the thyroid, in Werner SC, Ingbar SH (eds): The Thyroid, 3d ed. Hagerstown, MD, Harper & Row, 1971, with permission.*)

tween the aorta and the pulmonary trunk, within the upper portion of the pericardium, or in the interventricular septum. The following types of anomaly can be encountered.

Pyramidal Lobe. The migratory tract of the developing thyroid gland is known as the thyroglossal tract or duct. Normally the duct atrophies, although it may remain as a fibrous band. In about 80 percent of people, the distal end that connects to the thyroid persists as a pyramidal lobe projecting up from the isthmus, lying just to the left of the midline (Fig. 36-3). In the normal individual the pyramidal lobe is not palpable, but in disorders resulting in thyroid hypertrophy (e.g., Graves' disease, diffuse nodular goiter, or lymphocytic thyroiditis), the pyramidal lobe usually is enlarged and palpable.

Lingual Thyroid. The median thyroid anlage sometimes fails to develop, resulting in athyreosis, or it may develop but fail to descend, leading to a lingual thyroid (Fig. 36-4). Lingual thyroid is estimated to occur in 1 in 3000 cases of thyroid disease. It occurs more commonly in females, and some develop hypothyroidism. In these patients, the lingual thyroid is the only functioning thyroid tissue, although a normally situated thyroid also may be present.

Presentation usually is dependent upon the size of the lingual thyroid. An asymptomatic posterior lingual mass may be discovered because of physiologic thyroid hyperactivity. If tumor formation occurs the patient presents with symptoms of a posterior oral swelling. If the thyroid tissue continues to enlarge, symptoms such as a choking sensation, dysphagia, dyspnea, and dysphonia may predominate.

Diagnosis is established by scanning with radioiodine (^{123}I) (Fig. 36-5) or technetium (^{99m}Tc). Treatment consists of thyroid suppression with thyroxine; operation for symptoms or an enlarging mass is rarely necessary and may result in hypothyroidism.

Malignancy is rare, occurring in less than 3 percent of patients with symptomatic lingual thyroids. Diagnosis in these cases may be established by fine-needle aspiration cytology (FNAC) or biopsy.

Thyroglossal Duct Cyst. Thyroglossal duct cysts are midline structures containing thyroid epithelium; they may occur anywhere along the course of the thyroglossal duct, though typ-ically they are found between the isthmus of the thyroid gland and the hyoid bone (Fig. 36-6). The cysts usually cause few symptoms but may become infected, prompting the patient to seek medical advice.

Diagnosis may be established by asking the patient to protrude his or her tongue; when the tongue is protruded, the thyroglossal duct cyst moves upward. Treatment is by surgical excision and should include the thyroglossal duct remnant. As the duct may pass anteriorly to, posteriorly to, or through the hyoid bone, the central portion of the hyoid bone is removed to minimize the possibility of recurrence (the Sistrunk procedure).

About 1 percent of thyroglossal duct cysts contain thyroid cancer, and approximately 25 percent of patients with thyroglossal duct cysts that contain papillary cancer have papillary cancer elsewhere within the thyroid gland. Occasionally squamous cell carcinomas develop in thyroglossal duct cysts. Medullary thyroid cancers are not found in thyroglossal duct cysts.

Lateral Aberrant Thyroid. Lateral aberrant thyroid tissue is rare. It is believed that the so-called "lateral aberrant thyroid" is almost always a well-differentiated papillary carcinoma (exhibiting a follicular pattern) that has metastasized to a cervical chain lymph node, replacing the node with tumor. Diagnosis of lateral aberrant thyroid should direct the clinician to search for the primary thyroid tumor, which is almost always present in the ipsilateral lobe of the thyroid. In some patients the primary thyroid cancer is microscopic. Normal ectopic thyroid tissue may be present in the neck; it is always in the central neck (the migratory path of the normal thyroid), it is not situated in lymph nodes, and it is benign.

ANATOMY

The normal adult thyroid gland is light brown in color and firm in consistency, weighing 15 to 20 g. It is formed by two lateral lobes connected centrally by an isthmus. The lobes are approximately 4 cm long, 2 cm wide, and 20 to 40 mm thick, with the isthmus 2 to 6 mm thick. The lateral lobes run alongside the trachea, reaching the level of the middle thyroid cartilage superiorly. Laterally, the lobes are adjacent to the carotid sheath and the sternocleidomastoid muscles; anteriorly, they are adjacent to the strap muscles (sternothyroid and sternohyoid). In ap-

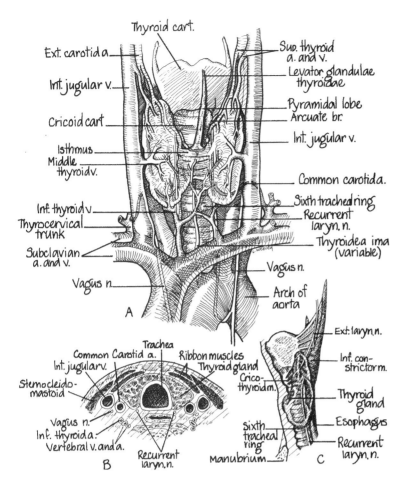

FIG. 36-3. The thyroid gland. A. The gland has been presented as a transparent structure to show the relationship to the vessels and nerves. The path of the inferior thyroid artery can be followed. B. Cross-section through the isthmus of the thyroid gland. C. The thyroid gland viewed from the left side. The gland is in relation to two nerves (recurrent and external laryngeal), two tubes (esophagus and trachea), and two muscles (inferior constrictor and cricothyroid).

proximately 80 percent of individuals, a pyramidal lobe is present, usually just to the left of the midline, extending upward from the isthmus along the anterior surface of the thyroid cartilage. It is a remnant of the thyroglossal duct (see Fig. 36-3).

The four parathyroid glands usually are closely related to the thyroid gland, found on the posterolateral surface of the lobes, within 1 cm of the inferior thyroid artery in 80 percent of individuals. The upper parathyroid glands are more dorsal or pos-

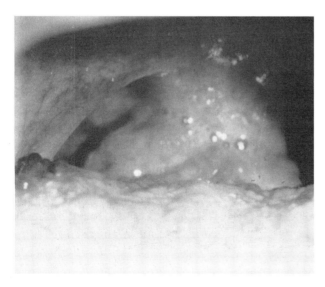

FIG. 36-4. Large lingual thyroid gland located at the posterior of the tongue.

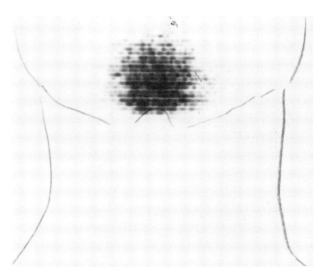

FIG. 36-5. Radioiodine scan of the patient in Fig. 36-4, demonstrating all activity to be above the hyoid bone rather than in the neck.

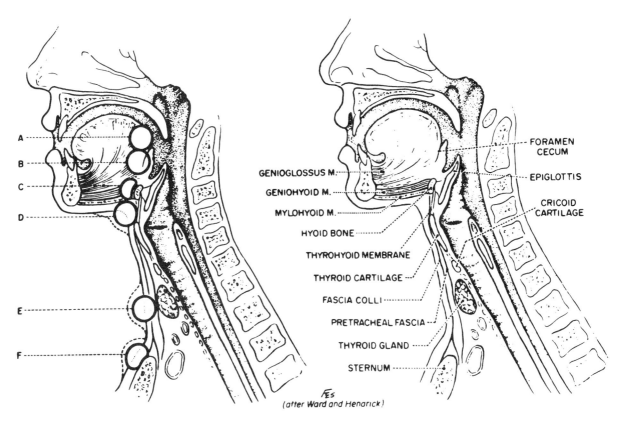

FIG. 36-6. Drawing demonstrating the possible locations of thyroglossal cysts. (A) In front of foramen cecum; (B) at foramen cecum; (C) suprahyoid; (D) infrahyoid; (E) area of thyroid gland; (F) suprasternal. (From: *Sedwick CE, Cady B, 1980, with permission.*)

terior and usually are situated at the level of the cricoid cartilage. The lower parathyroid glands are more variable in position but usually are anterior to the recurrent laryngeal nerves. The thyroid gland is enveloped by a loosely connecting fascia that is formed from the partition of the deep cervical fascia into anterior and posterior divisions. The thyroid is attached to the trachea and suspended from the larynx. It moves upward with elevation of the larynx on swallowing. The true capsule of the thyroid is a thin, fibrous layer, densely adherent, that sends out septa that invaginate the gland, forming pseudolobules. Thyroid nodules are palpable in about 4 percent of adults; smaller, occult nodules can be detected by ultrasound or at postmortem examination in more than 50 percent of older adults.

The thyroid gland has an abundant blood supply provided by four major arteries. The paired superior thyroid arteries arise as the first branch of the external carotid artery, approximately at the level of the carotid bifurcation, and descend several centimeters in the neck to the superior pole of each thyroid lobe. Here the arteries divide into anterior and posterior branches as they reach the gland. The paired inferior thyroid arteries arise from the thyrocervical trunk of the subclavian arteries and enter the gland from a posterolateral position. Occasionally a fifth artery, the thyroidea ima, is present, originating directly from the aortic arch or the innominate artery and ascending in front of the trachea to enter the gland in the midline inferiorly. A rich venous plexus forms under the capsule and drains to the internal jugular vein on both sides via the superior thyroid veins (which run with the superior thyroid artery) and the middle thyroid veins, which can vary in number, passing from the lateral aspect of the lobes. The inferior thyroid veins leave the inferior poles bilaterally, usually forming a plexus that drains into the brachiocephalic vein. Lymphatic drainage of the thyroid gland is primarily to the internal jugular nodes. The superior pole and medial isthmus drain to the superior groups of nodes, and the inferior groups drain the lower gland and empty into pretracheal and paratracheal nodes.

Innervation of the gland is by sympathetic fibers from the superior and middle cervical sympathetic ganglia. The fibers enter with the blood vessels and are vasomotor in action. Parasympathetic fibers are derived from the vagus nerve and reach the gland via branches of the laryngeal nerves.

Microscopically, the thyroid is divided into lobules that contain 20 to 40 follicles. There are roughly 3×10^6 follicles in the adult male thyroid gland. The follicles are spherical and average 30 μm in diameter. Each follicle is lined by cuboidal epithelial cells and contains a central store of colloid secreted from the epithelial cells under the influence of the pituitary hormone, thyroid stimulating hormone (TSH). The second group of thyroid secretory cells are the C cells or parafollicular cells, which contain and secrete the hormone calcitonin. They are found as individual cells or clumped in small groups in the interfollicular stroma, abutting between follicular cells. They are located in the upper poles of the thyroid lobes, reflecting their origin as neuroectodermal cells derived from the ultimobranchial bodies, and are part of the amine containing precursor uptake decarboxylase (APUD) series described by Pearse.

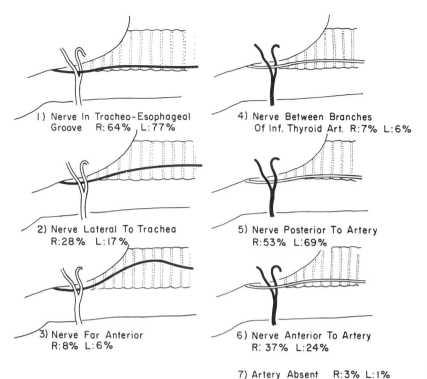

1) Nerve In Tracheo-Esophageal Groove   R:64%   L:77%

2) Nerve Lateral To Trachea   R:28%   L:17%

3) Nerve Far Anterior   R:8%   L:6%

4) Nerve Between Branches Of Inf. Thyroid Art.   R:7%   L:6%

5) Nerve Posterior To Artery   R:53%   L:69%

6) Nerve Anterior To Artery   R:37%   L:24%

7) Artery Absent   R:3%   L:1%

FIG. 36-7. Relationship of the inferior thyroid artery to the recurrent laryngeal nerve.

Laryngeal Nerves. It is important to note the close relationship of the thyroid gland to the recurrent laryngeal nerves and the possible variations in the course of the recurrent nerves. The recurrent laryngeal nerves supply the intrinsic muscles of the larynx, and damage to one of them leads to ipsilateral vocal cord paralysis. Similarly, the external branch of the superior laryngeal nerve, which innervates the cricothyroid muscle, also is at risk during thyroid surgery. Damage of either nerve may result in a disability of phonation.

Identification of the nerves, rather than attempting to avoid them, should be standard practice for the surgeon. The recurrent laryngeal nerves originate from the vagus nerves. On the right side, the recurrent nerve originates where the vagus nerve crosses the first part of the subclavian artery; the nerve loops under the subclavian artery and ascends slightly obliquely to enter the larynx at the level of the cricoid cartilage and posterior to the cricothyroid muscle. The left recurrent nerve branches from the vagus as it crosses the aortic arch and loops posteriorly around the ligamentum arteriosus before it ascends medially in the tracheoesophageal groove to enter the larynx opposite the contralateral nerve. The variable course taken by the recurrent nerves is demonstrated in Fig. 36-7. The right recurrent nerve is in the tracheoesophageal groove in 64 percent of people, compared to 77 percent on the left. The nerve is lateral to the trachea on the right in 28 percent of people and in 17 percent on the left. In a minority of people the nerve is anterolateral to the trachea (right 8 percent, left 6 percent), exposing it to accidental division during subtotal lobectomy. A misconception is that the recurrent laryngeal nerves run behind the inferior thyroid artery, but this is true in only 53 percent of people on the right and 69 percent on the left. In others the nerve's course is anterior to the artery (right 37 percent, left 24 percent), or between branches of

the artery (right 7 percent, left 6 percent). Failure to identify the course of the nerves can lead to accidental damage.

The recurrent laryngeal nerves are not always recurrent; in about 1 percent of people one of the nerves is nonrecurrent. This occurs almost exclusively on the right in association with a vascular anomaly of the right subclavian artery; rarely, it occurs on the left with dextrocardia or situs inversus. In these situations, the nerve arises from the vagus to run directly to the larynx, often in close proximity to the superior thyroid vessels, and may be at risk when these vessels are transected (Fig. 36-8).

The superior laryngeal nerve arises from the vagus near the base of the skull and descends medial to the carotid vessels. At the level of the hyoid bone it divides into two branches, one sensory (internal branch), and the other motor (external branch).

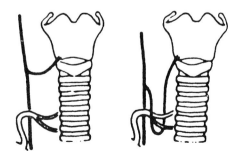

FIG. 36-8. "Nonrecurrent" right laryngeal nerves, coursing near the superior pole vessels *(left)* or around the inferior artery *(right)*. Because of the abnormal location of "nonrecurrent" laryngeal nerves they are more likely to be damaged during surgery. (From: *Skandalakis JE, Droulis C, et al: The recurrent laryngeal nerve. Am Surg 42:629, 1976, with permission.*)

The external branch runs on the lateral surface of the inferior constrictor muscle and descends to innervate the cricothyroid muscle (Fig. 36-9). This muscle alters vocal cord tension and affects the pitch of the voice. In most instances the nerve runs in close proximity to the superior pole vessels, and in 21 percent of people it is closely related to the vessels and is at significant risk if it is not identified at operation. To avoid injury, the superior pole vessels should be individually ligated and divided low on the thyroid gland and dissected laterally to the cricothyroid muscle.

PHYSIOLOGY

Through release of its principal hormones, thyroxine (T_4) and triiodothyronine (T_3), the thyroid gland influences the metabolic rate of all tissues. Increased secretion increases the metabolic rate; conversely, the rate decreases when secretion is decreased. Release of T_4 and T_3 is stimulated by the anterior pituitary hormone thyrotropin or thyroid-stimulating hormone (TSH). Secretion of TSH is directly suppressed by T_4 and T_3 (a negative feedback loop). TSH release also is stimulated by the hypothalamic hormone thyrotropin-releasing hormone (TRH). Thyroid hormone production is influenced by numerous physiologic, pathologic, and pharmacologic factors.

Iodine Metabolism. The formation of thyroid hormones is dependent on the availability of exogenous iodine. The average daily iodine requirement is 0.1 mg. Iodine is found principally in fish, milk, and eggs. In the United States, iodine is

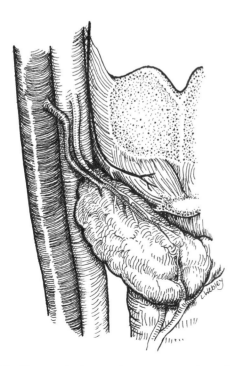

FIG. 36-9. *The superior laryngeal nerve runs on the surface of the cricothyroid muscle (80 percent) or in the muscle (20 percent). In about 20 percent of patients, it runs with the superior pole vessels. The superior pole has been reflected anterolaterally. The superior pole vessels should be ligated on the thyroid gland to avoid injury to this nerve. (From: Clark OH: Endocrine Surgery of the Thyroid and Parathyroid Glands, St Louis, CV Mosby, 1985, with permission.)*

routinely added to bread and salt in order to reduce the frequency of iodine deficiency. Iodine is rapidly converted to iodide in the stomach and jejunum and is absorbed into the bloodstream within 1 h; and from there it is distributed uniformly throughout the extracellular space (Fig. 36-10). Iodide is actively transported into the thyroid follicular cells by an ATP-dependent process. The thyroid-serum iodine ratio under normal conditions is about 50:1, and most of the body's store of iodine is found in the thyroid gland (90 percent). Thyroid-serum ratios can be as high as 500:1 in certain instances, such as iodine deficiency or Graves' disease.

One-third of the loss of iodine from the plasma is accounted for by thyroid concentration, and the other two-thirds through renal excretion. In studies involving radiolabeled iodine, all the iodine is concentrated within the thyroid or excreted in the urine within 48 h, and the plasma and tissues are mostly cleared of iodide. Evidence of labeled iodine in serum is accounted for by secretion from the thyroid gland in the form of thyroid hormone.

Synthesis of Thyroid Hormone. Steps in the synthesis of thyroid hormone are: (1) active trapping and concentration of iodide in the follicular cell; (2) rapid oxidation of iodide to iodine; (3) linkage of iodine with tyrosine residues in thyroglobulin; (4) coupling of these iodotyrosines (monoiodo- and diiodotyrosine) to form the active thyroid hormones T_4 and T_3. Active accumulation of iodide in the thyroid gland is stimulated by TSH, acting via a specific membrane receptor located in the thyrocyte plasma membrane. This mechanism is probably through changes in cyclic adenosine monophosphate (cAMP). Once inside the thyroid cell, the iodide diffuses through the cytoplasm to the apical membrane. It remains in its free state for a short time before being oxidized by peroxidase and hydrogen peroxidase. Iodine rapidly links to tyrosine residues present in abundance in thyroglobulin, a thyroid-specific protein, resulting in the formation of two separate molecules, monoiodotyrosine (MIT) and diiodotyrosine (DIT). Two molecules of DIT combine to form tetraiodothyronine, or thyroxine (T_4); a molecule of MIT and DIT combine to form 3,3',5-triiodothyronine (T_3) or 3,3'5'-triiodothyronine, reverse T_3 (rT_3). The coupling steps are catalyzed by peroxidase in the presence of H_2O_2 and also are rate dependent on TSH.

When iodide transport is defective or when oxidation to iodine is impaired because of disease or pharmacologic agents, goiter or hypothyroidism may result. The antithyroid drugs (propylthiouracil, methimazole, and carbimazole) inhibit the oxidation of iodide to iodine by competitive inhibition of peroxidase and also may interfere with the coupling reaction. In high doses iodide also inhibits iodine trapping. It also has an antithyroid action by inhibiting the proteolysis involved in the release of thyroid hormone. Potassium iodide tablets often are administered to people exposed to radiation leaks involving radioactive forms of iodine, such as nuclear accidents, because it blocks trapping by the thyroid gland.

Storage, Secretion, and Metabolism of Thyroid Hormone. T_4 and T_3 are bound to thyroglobulin and are stored in the colloid of the thyroid follicles. Release of the active hormones is by a process of endocytosis. The colloid is taken up by the follicular cell as discrete packets (endosomes), which then fuse with lysosomes containing hydroxylases. Hydrolysis results in production of all component parts, T_4, T_3, rT_3, MIT, and DIT. Through a process of deiodination most of the iodide is released

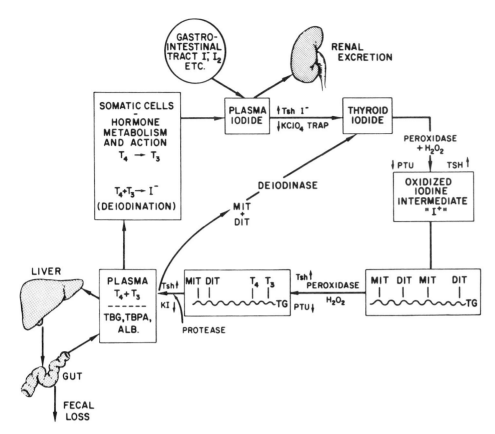

FIG. 36-10. *The iodide cycle. Ingested iodide is trapped in the thyroid gland, oxidized, and bound to tyrosine to form iodotyrosines in thyroglobulin. Coupling of iodotyrosyl residues forms T_4 and T_3. Hormone secreted by the gland is transported in the serum. Some T_4 is deiodinated to T_3. The hormone exerts its metabolic effect on the cell and is ultimately deiodinated. The iodide is reused or excreted by the kidneys. A second cycle goes on inside the thyroid gland with deiodination of iodotyrosines generating iodide, which is reused without leaving the thyroid. (From: DeGroot LJ, Stanbury JB, Larsen PR, Refetoff S, 1984, with permission.)*

from MIT and DIT and reused in the follicle. The iodothyronines are more resistant to this process and are secreted; these steps also are TSH dependent.

The active thyroid hormones circulate in the plasma attached to plasma proteins, principally the carrier proteins, thyroid hormone–binding globulin (TBG), thyroid hormone–binding prealbumin (TBPA), and albumin. About 99.98 percent of thyroid hormone circulates in the plasma bound to protein, and the remaining 0.02 percent is unbound and is the free, *active physiological fraction.* In some conditions TBG may be increased, usually as a result of estrogen effects of pregnancy or the contraceptive pill. This results in a higher circulating amount of T_4 because of increased serum binding capacity. In this situation, *active free T_4* levels remain unaltered.

T_3 is the more potent of the two thyroid hormones (rT_3 is biologically inert), although its circulating plasma level is much lower than that of T_4; the ratio is 10:1 to 20:1. T_3 is less tightly bound to protein in the plasma than T_4, and so it enters tissues more readily. T_3 is three to four times more active than T_4 per unit weight, with a half-life of about 1 day, compared to about 7 days for T_4. Though the thyroid gland produces some T_3 and rT_3, it is known that 75 percent of T_3 is produced by the extrathyroidal conversion of T_4 to T_3 in the peripheral tissues. Almost 85 percent of T_4 is converted peripherally to metabolically inert rT_3 or T_3. Some studies suggest that T_4 is a prohormone and that T_3 is the only hormone acting at the cellular level.

Molecular Basis of Thyroid Hormone Action. Thyroid hormones are transported across the plasma membrane of tissues by an ATP-dependent transport system. Uptake by the tissue is rate-limited by the amount of free hormone available at the tissue level. At the cellular level T_3 is the active hormone, and its activity is mediated through T_3 receptors located in the cell nucleus. The receptors bind to regulatory genes and modify the expression of these genes.

T_3 receptors belong to a group of hormone-responsive nuclear transcription factors. There are two types of T_3 receptor genes, α and β, located on chromosomes 17 and 3. Expression of T_3 receptors is tissue specific. T_3 receptors $\alpha 1$, $\alpha 2$ and $\beta 1$ mRNA are expressed in almost all tissues, but some T_3 receptors are expressed only in certain tissues, e.g., $\beta 2$ is found only in the brain. The brain contains mostly α receptors, the liver β receptors, and cardiac muscle expresses both.

Deiodination and Excretion. Deiodination of thyroid hormones is effected by three different types of deiodination enzymes, which are tissue specific. The released iodine is returned to the blood, where it reenters the metabolic pool. The residual T_3 and T_4 are conjugated with glucuronic acid, which renders the hormones water soluble and facilitates excretion in urine and bile, or sulphate. Some of the excreted iodothyronines are reabsorbed from the small intestine, constituting the enterohepatic circulation. About one-third of total body clearance is effected through the bile, but up to 50 percent of the thyroxine may be reabsorbed. Significant amounts of thyroid hormone and iodine may appear in the milk of lactating mothers.

Regulation of Thyroid Activity. The principal homeostatic control of thyroid hormone secretion is the hypothalamic-pituitary-thyroid axis. The basophil cells of the anterior pituitary produce TSH, which directly regulates thyroid function. TSH acts on the thyroid cell to promote thyroid hormone production at all levels, enhancing iodine uptake, increasing synthesis, and raising secretion of T_4. TSH also has a secondary action on thyroid gland growth, increasing cellularity and vascularization of the gland. Secretion of TSH is regulated at two levels. Thyrotropin-releasing hormone (TRH), is produced by the hypothalamus and reaches the gland via the hypophyseal portal system to stimulate TSH release (Fig. 36-11). TRH binds to high-affinity TRH receptors on the anterior pituitary cells. Originally it was thought that TRH exerted its action of TSH release via adenylate cyclase and cAMP, but now it is believed that postreceptor activation is via the phospholipase-C–based hydrolysis of inositol phospholipids, leading to Ca^{2+} and diacylglycerol activation of protein kinase C. Release of TRH from the hypothalamus is suppressed by T_3, acting in a feedback loop. TRH has been shown to be equipotent in stimulating release of prolactin from the pituitary and TSH.

More important to thyroid hormone regulation is the direct feedback exerted on the pituitary by the level of thyroid hormone in the blood. Raised levels of thyroid hormone suppress TSH and TRH secretion, and lowered levels promote secretion. Iodine deficiency increases the goitrogenic effects of TSH on the thyroid.

ASSESSMENT OF PATIENTS WITH THYROID DISEASE

Thyroid disease may be divided into two types: problems relating to function (hyperthyroidism/hypothyroidism) and thyroid masses. The two types are not mutually exclusive and patients frequently present with both problems.

History. Obtaining an accurate history is essential in assessing thyroid disease. Symptoms such as dysphagia, dyspnea,

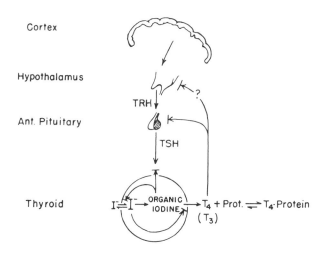

FIG. 36-11. *Schema of the homeostatic regulation of thyroid function. Secretion of TSH is regulated by a negative feedback mechanism acting directly on the pituitary and is normally inversely related to the concentration of unbound hormone in the blood. Release of TSH is induced by TRH secretion, which sets the level of the pituitary feedback mechanism. Factors regulating secretion of TRH are uncertain but may include the free hormone in the blood and stimuli from higher centers. Autoregulatory control of thyroid function also is shown. (From: Ingbar SH, Woeber KA: The thyroid gland, in Williams RH (ed): Textbook of Endocrinology, 4th ed. Philadelphia, WB Saunders, 1968, with permission.)*

and choking are frequently encountered in patients with goiter and may be exaggerated by patients raising their arms above their heads (Pemberton's sign). Pain is uncommon. Localized pain may suggest malignancy, especially medullary thyroid cancer, whereas pain radiating to the ear often is observed in patients with thyroiditis or hemorrhage within the thyroid gland. A change in the character of the voice should also be of concern because it may suggest involvement of the recurrent laryngeal nerves in a malignant process, with vocal cord paralysis. A past history of exposure to radiation, family history of benign or malignant thyroid disease, living in an iodine-deficient area, or ingestion of goitrogenic drugs also are significant.

Physical Examination. Thyroid masses rise on swallowing; most thyroid swellings are accurately discernible by observing the patient swallow. Failure to observe before palpating the thyroid gland may lead to missing a large retrosternal goiter arising from beneath the sternum and clavicles.

Palpation usually is performed from behind while the patient is sitting in a chair with the neck slightly extended and should include palpation of the gland while the patient swallows. A landmark is the cricoid cartilage; the isthmus almost always crosses a fingerbreadth below the cricoid. The normal thyroid gland usually is not palpable unless the patient has a particularly thin neck. The thyroid gland may be diffuse and bilaterally enlarged (goiter), as encountered in conditions such as Graves' disease (hyperthyroidism), Hashimoto's thyroiditis, or multinodular goiter. A unilateral mass may be palpated, as in a colloid nodule, follicular adenoma, or carcinoma.

The cervical chain of lymph nodes should be assessed as well as the nodes in the posterior triangle. The jugular nodes immediately adjacent to a thyroid nodule often are involved in patients with a papillary thyroid cancer. A Delphian node should be palpated for just above the thyroid isthmus and cricoid cartilage.

Fine-Needle Aspiration Cytology (FNAC). Fine-needle aspiration cytology is a simple and low-risk technique that is an integral part of thyroid assessment in the outpatient setting for patients with thyroid nodules. A 23-gauge needle is inserted into the thyroid swelling, and several passes are made while aspirating the syringe. Cells are placed on prelabeled dry glass slides; some are then immediately placed in 70% alcohol while others are air dried. These slides are stained by Papanicolaou or Wright's stains and observed under the microscope. Skilled cytopathologists can accurately diagnose the majority of thyroid diseases using this technique, with a high degree of specificity. This test is less accurate in patients with thyroid nodules and a history of familial nonmedullary thyroid cancer and in patients with a previous history of exposure to low-dose therapeutic radiation. Benign and malignant thyroid tumors are common in such patients, and the tumors usually are multifocal.

Tests of Thyroid Function. *Thyrotropin (TSH, reference range 0.15–4.2 μU/mL).* Thyrotropin secretion from the anterior pituitary is controlled via a negative feedback loop by serum T_3 and T_4 levels. In cases in which high T_3 and T_4 levels are encountered (Graves' disease, toxic nodular goiter), TSH levels will be accordingly low and may be undetectable. When T_4 levels are low (primary thyroid destruction, e.g., end-stage Hashimoto's thyroiditis), TSH levels will be correspondingly high. Many clinicians believe that the circulating level of TSH is the single most sensitive test of thyroid function.

Older radioimmunoassays have been replaced with more sophisticated immunometric assays, using monoclonal antibodies that target two separate sites (increasing specificity) on the TSH molecule. One monoclonal antibody is labeled with a nonradioactive marker, allowing readings with an accuracy down to 0.005 μU/mL. A reference range of normal TSH levels has been established in euthyroid patients, against which levels from the test subject can be compared.

Total Thyroxine (TT$_4$, reference range 55–150 nmol/L) and Free Thyroxine (FT$_4$, 12–28 pmol/L). Total thyroxine concentration reflects the fraction of T$_4$ bound to TBG and other carrier proteins in the serum and also the amount of free T$_4$ in circulation. T$_4$ production from the thyroid is dependent on TSH from the pituitary and an adequate intake of iodine in the diet. When T$_4$ production from the thyroid is increased, the bound and free T$_4$ levels rise (FT$_4$ remains in equilibrium with bound T$_4$), resulting in an increase of TT$_4$. When T$_4$ production from the thyroid decreases, bound and FT$_4$ levels drop, which leads to decreased TT$_4$ levels. Conditions leading to a changes in the level of TBG (e.g., estrogen intake) can alter the level of TT$_4$ (as binding sites increase), but are not reflected by changes in circulating FT$_4$, and so the individual remains euthyroid.

Free T$_4$ estimates are not performed as a routine screening tool in thyroid disease. Use of this test is confined to cases of early hyperthyroidism in which TT$_4$ levels may be normal but FT$_4$ levels are raised. In patients with end-organ resistance to T$_4$ (Refetoff syndrome) T$_4$ levels are increased, but TSH levels usually are normal.

Total Triiodothyronine (TT$_3$, reference range 1.5–3.5 nmol/ L) and Free Triiodothyronine (FT$_3$, 3–9 pmol/L). Levels of total T$_3$ or free T$_3$ are not used as a routine investigation of thyroid function. FT$_3$ is most useful in confirming the diagnosis of early hyperthyroidism, in which levels of FT$_4$ and FT$_3$ rise before TT$_4$ and TT$_3$. Most T$_3$ production comes from the peripheral conversion of T$_4$, and this process may be inhibited by conditions such as starvation illness (low T$_3$ syndrome) or by the effect of certain drugs (e.g., propranolol). There is a rare condition of T$_3$ thyrotoxicosis in which levels of TT$_4$ in the hyperthyroid patient are normal and radioiodine uptake is normal but the TT$_3$ level is raised. This condition is more common in patients from endemic goiter areas and in patients with small solitary thyroid nodules.

HYPERTHYROIDISM/THYROTOXICOSIS

Thyrotoxicosis is the clinical syndrome that results when excessive levels of active thyroid hormone are secreted into the circulation. There are many causes of thyrotoxicosis, but two predominate: Graves' disease (diffuse toxic goiter) and toxic solitary or multinodular goiter (Plummer's disease). The rarer conditions causing thyrotoxicosis are listed in Table 36-1. Conditions resulting in increased thyroid hormone production, such as Graves' and Plummer's disease, or secondary hyperthyroidism because of a TSH-secreting pituitary tumor should be distinguished from conditions in which there is a leak of thyroid hormone, i.e., patients with subacute painless or painful thyroiditis. Hyperthyroidism also can result from taking thyroid hormone (factitious hyperthyroidism), from struma ovarii, from increased secretion of human chorionic gonadotropin with a molar pregnancy, and from rare metastatic thyroid cancers that secrete thyroid hormone.

Table 36-1
Causes of Hyperthyroidism

With increased thyroid hormone secretion
    Graves' disease
    Toxic nodular goiter
    Toxic thyroid adenoma
    Jod-Basedow hyperthyroidism
Without increased thyroid hormone secretion
    Subacute thyroiditis
    Functioning metastatic thyroid cancer
    Struma ovarii

Graves' Disease (Diffuse Toxic Goiter)

Graves' disease is the most common form of thyrotoxicosis. Although originally described by the Welsh physician Caleb Parry in a posthumous article in 1825, the disease is known as Graves' disease after Robert Graves, a physician from Ireland, who described three patients in 1835. Graves' disease is about six times more common in women, and although it may develop at any age, it is most prevalent in young adults (20 to 40 years of age). Associated extrathyroidal manifestations of this autoimmune disease include exophthalmos, pretibial myxedema, dermopathy, acropachy, and vitiligo.

Pathogenesis and Pathology. Graves' disease is an autoimmune disorder in which pathogenic thyroid-stimulating antibodies or immunoglobulins are directed at the TSH receptor on thyroid follicular cells. Binding of the antibodies stimulates the receptors and leads to excess thyroid hormone secretion, which characterizes the condition. Originally the responsible antibody was thought to be long-acting thyroid stimulating antibody (LATS), described by Adams and Purves in 1956. It is apparent now that a whole family of antibodies contribute to the development of the disease. Thyroid-stimulating immunoglobulins (TSI) or antibodies (TSAb) attach to and stimulate the TSH receptor, and TSH-binding inhibiting immunoglobulins (TSII) or antibodies (TBIA) block the TSH receptor. Current practice is to group all these antibodies together under the term thyroid receptor antibodies (TRAb).

What initiates Graves' disease and antibody production is unclear. One theory suggests a defect in the suppressor T lymphocytes allowing helper T cells to stimulate the production of TSI from helper B cell clones. Another theory is that an immune response is launched to altered antigens on the follicular cell surface, an observation supported by the fact that Graves' disease and ophthalmopathy occur more frequently in patients who have been irradiated to the head and neck. Genetic factors also are clearly involved; identical twins have a 50 percent chance of developing the condition if the twin has it, compared to a 30 percent chance in fraternal, nonidentical twins. This is probably through increased frequency of leukocyte antigen expression (HLA-b8 and DR3 in Caucasians and HLA-Bw35 in Japanese).

Macroscopically, the thyroid gland in patients with Graves' disease is diffuse and smoothly enlarged, and the gland's vascularity also is increased. Microscopically, the gland is hyperplastic, and the epithelium is columnar, with minimal colloid present. The nuclei exhibit mitosis, and papillary projections of hyperplastic epithelium are common. There may be aggregates of lymphoid tissue, and vascularity is markedly increased.

Clinical Features Common to All Forms of Thyrotoxicosis. The clinical symptoms and signs of thyrotoxicosis are the same in patients with Graves' disease and toxic nodular goiter, except that patients with Graves' disease usually have more severe hyperthyroidism and have extrathyroidal manifestations of disease. Attention should be paid to a family history of autoimmune thyroid disease, including Graves' disease, Hashimoto's thyroiditis, and other autoimmune disorders.

Manifestation of the increased caloric turnover may be evident. Patients develop heat intolerance, increased thirst, sweating, and weight loss despite adequate caloric intake. Women may develop amenorrhea and decreased fertility and have an increased incidence of miscarriage. Cardiovascular manifestations are tachycardia or atrial fibrillation. In cases in which high-output cardiac failure ensues, signs and symptoms of congestive cardiac failure such as dyspnea and peripheral edema or even anasarca may become evident. Adrenergic stimuli may be particularly distressing, and fatigue, agitation and excitability, disturbed sleep pattern, emotional lability, hyperkinesis, and tremor may be present. In marked cases, psychosis can develop. Diarrhea or increased bowel frequency are the most common gastrointestinal manifestations and run an intermittent course during the disease.

On physical examination, weight loss and facial flushing may be evident. The skin may be warm and moist, and patients often have inappropriate sweating in a cool environment. African-American patients often note darkening of their skin. Examination of the pulse usually reveals tachycardia or atrial fibrillation (the latter is especially apparent in the elderly). Cutaneous vasodilation leads to a widening of the pulse pressure and a rapid falloff in the transmitted pulse wave (collapsing pulse). A fine tremor, muscle wasting, and proximal muscle group weakness with hyperactive tendon reflexes often are present.

Clinical Features Specific to Graves' Disease. Graves' disease is characterized by the classic triad of goiter, thyrotoxicosis, and exophthalmos. These features may occur singularly or in any combination. Additionally, patients present with a goiter that is characteristically diffuse, enlarged, and smooth. Evidence that the whole gland is enlarged is demonstrated by enlargement of the pyramidal lobe, which can be palpated as it crosses the cricoid cartilage (Fig. 36-12). Patients with Graves' disease also may have onycholysis or thyroid acropathy, hair loss, pretibial myxedema (3 to 5 percent) (Fig. 36-13), and gynecomastia (3 to 5 percent). An audible bruit resulting from markedly increased vascularity of the gland can be heard over the gland in up to 50 percent of patients. Splenomegaly also may be present.

Exophthalmos may be present in association with thyrotoxicosis (Graves' ophthalmopathy) or as an isolated condition with no evidence of thyrotoxicosis (euthyroidal or ophthalmic Graves' disease). The condition is characterized by: (1) spasm of the upper eyelid, with retraction revealing the sclera above the corneoscleral limbus (Dalrymple's sign) and lid lag (von Graefe's sign); (2) external ophthalmoplegia; (3) exophthalmos with proptosis; (4) supraorbital and infraorbital swelling; and (5) congestion and edema of the conjunctiva (chemosis) (Fig. 36-14). The exophthalmos is a result of increased retro-orbital tissue and can be assessed objectively with an exophthalmometer (Hertel), which measures the distance from the lateral bony orbital margin to the anterior surface of the cornea. Protrusion may

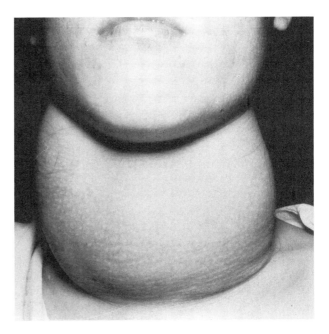

FIG. 36-12. The goiter in Graves' disease is diffusely enlarged and smooth. Evidence that the whole gland is enlarged may be confirmed by palpation of the pyramidal lobe of the thyroid as it crosses the cricoid cartilage. The goiter illustrated here was large enough to be viewed from behind the patient.

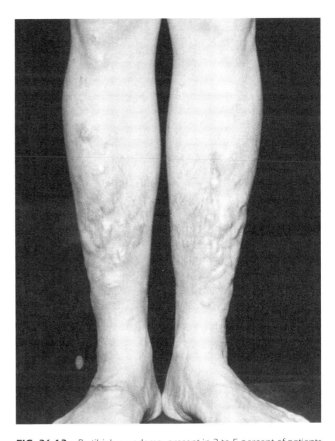

FIG. 36-13. Pretibial myxedema, present in 3 to 5 percent of patients with Graves' disease.

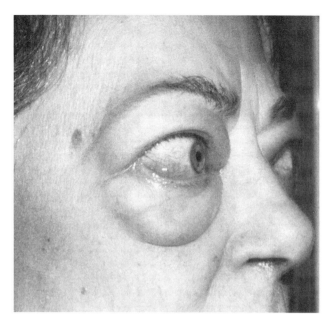

FIG. 36-14. Graves' ophthalmopathy may present in association with thyrotoxicosis or in isolation (euthyroidal or ophthalmic Graves' disease). Eye signs demonstrated in this patient are exophthalmos with proptosis, supraorbital and infraorbital swelling, congestion, and edema of the conjuctiva (chemosis).

lead to ophthalmoplegia, an inability to move the eyeball (upper rotation being most commonly restricted), leading to diplopia. If proptosis is progressive, optic nerve damage and blindness may occur, usually preceded by decreasing visual acuity and increasingly impaired color vision. This condition is commonly referred to as malignant exophthalmos. An urgent ophthalmic opinion should be sought. Marked protrusion can result in chemosis, in which the sclera and conjunctiva become inflamed, with itching, lacrimation, photophobia, and, eventually, ulceration.

The pathogenesis of ophthalmopathy is controversial; the cross-reaction of the thyroid antigen and ocular muscle antibodies is a possible explanation. Continued hyperthyroidism and hypothyroidism aggravate exophthalmos and should be avoided. Histologically, a diffuse lymphocytic infiltration of the retro-orbital tissues occurs, followed by fibroblast activation with glycosaminoglycan (a mucopolysaccharide) production leading to edema and fibrosis.

Diagnostic Findings in Graves' Disease. Thyrotoxicosis is characterized by an autonomous thyroid function and decreased or undetectable level of TSH in association with elevated concentrations of circulating T_3 and/or T_4. Raised levels of circulating thyroid autoantibodies are usually detected in the serum. A radioactive thyroid scan with ^{123}I is characterized by diffuse uptake throughout the gland. An uptake of 45 to 90 percent is usually observed (Fig. 36-15).

Treatment of Graves' Disease. Three treatment modalities are available for patients with Graves' disease: medical management in the form of antithyroid drugs, thyroid ablation with radioactive ^{131}I, and subtotal or total thyroidectomy. The treatment chosen depends on the age of the patient, the severity of the disease, the size of the gland, any coexistent pathology, including associated ophthalmopathy, and other factors such as patient's preferences and pregnancy.

Antithyroid Drugs. The hyperdynamic peripheral adrenergic effects of thyrotoxicosis can be alleviated by administering beta-blocking agents. These drugs have the added effect of decreasing the peripheral conversion of T_4 to T_3. Propranolol is the most commonly prescribed medication. It reduces the heart rate, controls tremor, and to some extent relieves the agitation that these patients have. Beta blockers have no apparent effect on the overall remission rate of thyrotoxicosis.

The main antithyroid drugs are propylthiouracil (PTU) and methimazole (Tapazole) in the United States and carbimazole (in the United Kingdom). These drugs act by inhibiting the organic binding of thyroidal iodine and also inhibit the coupling of iodotyrosines. Propylthiouracil also influences the extrathyroidal conversion of T_4 to T_3. These medications have no effect on the underlying cause of the disease, although there is evidence that propylthiouracil decreases thyroid autoantibody levels.

These drugs also can cross the placenta, inhibiting fetal thyroid function, and they are excreted in breast milk. Side effects of treatment include skin rashes (1 percent), fever, peripheral neuritis, polyarteritis, granulocytopenia (which is reversible on discontinuing treatment), and, rarely, agranulocytosis (1:250). In rare instances, aplastic anemia, which has a poor prognosis, has been documented. Patients should be monitored for these possible complications and warned to stop medication and seek medical advice should they develop a sore throat or fever.

Standard medical treatment is to start the patient on 100 to 300 mg propylthiouracil three times daily, *or* 10 to 30 mg methimazole, initially three times daily and then once daily, *or* 40 mg carbimazole daily. Beta blockers are often used initially, before the diagnosis is made, to treat tachycardia and may be added for symptomatic relief. Patients are observed regularly on an

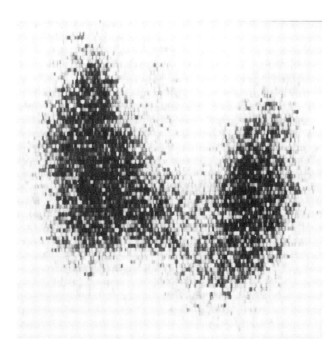

FIG. 36-15. Radioiodine scan (^{123}I) in a patient with thyrotoxic Graves' disease demonstrating uniform uptake throughout the gland.

outpatient basis, and the dose of antithyroid medication is titrated as needed in accordance with TSH and T$_4$ levels. Most patients have improved symptoms in 2 weeks and become euthyroid in about 6 weeks. The regimen described here is in wide use, though some physicians add thyroxine 0.05 to 0.10 mg to prevent hypothyroidism (the blocking/replacement regime). The length of treatment with antithyroid drugs is controversial. For patients with small, diffusely enlarged glands or larger glands that decrease in size in response to treatment with antithyroid medication, the relapse rate after treatment for 12 to 18 months is about 50 percent. Patients with larger diffuse glands or toxic nodular goiter develop recurrent hyperthyroidism when the antithyroid medication is discontinued, and hence definitive treatment with thyroidectomy or radioiodine therapy is indicated.

Radioactive Iodine Therapy (^{131}I). Most patients in the United States undergo treatment with radioiodine. The major advantages of this form of treatment are the avoidance of a surgical procedure and the concomitant risks of recurrent laryngeal nerve damage and hypoparathyroidism, reduced overall treatment costs, and ease of treatment. The major disadvantage is the high incidence of hypothyroidism requiring lifelong thyroxine replacement therapy, the slower correction of the hyperthyroidism, and a higher relapse rate after initial treatment, necessitating further therapy. Radioiodine therapy also has more of an adverse effect on ophthalmopathy than does thyroidectomy.

Patients most suitable for ^{131}I therapy are those with small or moderate-sized goiters, those who have relapsed after medical or surgical therapy, and those in whom antithyroid drugs or surgery are contraindicated. Younger patients (under 35 years of age) usually are treated with thyroidectomy, and older patients are treated with ^{131}I. Radioiodine therapy is contraindicated in women who are pregnant or breast-feeding. Relative contraindications are ophthalmopathy (in which progression of eye signs has been documented), patients with isolated thyroid nodules or toxic nodular goiters, and young age (i.e., especially children and adolescents). Although there is no evidence of long-term problems with infertility or increased incidence of cancer in children who have been treated with ^{131}I, most specialists are reluctant to treat children in this manner and suggest thyroidectomy (usually near-total) for this age group. Children treated with radioiodine for Graves' disease have an increased risk of developing hyperparathyroidism.

Patients should be euthyroid before ^{131}I therapy and should stop all antithyroid drugs for 2 to 3 weeks before treatment in order to allow for adequate uptake into the thyroid. Treatment is provided in the form of a drink of ^{131}I sodium iodide, the dosage of which usually is calculated with a formula based on gland volume and ^{131}I uptake; the typical initial dose is about 10 mCi of ^{131}I (approximately 8500 cGy). Cure rate after initial therapy is dosage dependent; with 5 mCi, cure rate is 70 percent; with 10 mCi, 87 percent; and with 15 mCi, 96 percent. The higher the initial dose, the earlier the onset and the higher the incidence of hypothyroidism.

After standard treatment with radioiodine most patients become euthyroid within 2 months. Approximately 15 percent of patients are hypothyroid at 1 year, with a 3 percent increment each year thereafter. Six months after radioiodine treatment, 50 percent of patients are euthyroid, and the remainder are hyperthyroid or already hypothyroid. Patients need long-term follow-up with TSH levels monitored on a regular basis. Close monitoring is essential, because hypothyroidism and recurrent hyperthyroidism aggravate Graves' ophthalmopathy.

The complications of ^{131}I treatment include: (1) exacerbation of thyrotoxicosis with arrhythmias; this usually becomes apparent within 10 days and may be a particular problem in the elderly, precipitating cardiac failure or death; (2) overt thyroid storm (rare but potentially life threatening); (3) hypothyroidism; (4) risk of fetal damage in patients who are pregnant (women are advised not to become pregnant for 6 months to 1 year after treatment); (5) worsening of eye signs, noted to be more common after ^{131}I treatment than after surgery (33 percent compared to 16 percent); and (6) hyperparathyroidism.

Surgical Treatment. Surgery is advised when radioiodine treatment is contraindicated, such as for young patients, patients with Graves' ophthalmopathy, pregnant patients, patients with suspicious thyroid nodules in Graves' glands, and patients with large toxic nodular goiters with relatively low levels of radioiodine uptake. Thyroidectomy is the treatment of choice in patients with very large goiters and severe thyrotoxicosis at initial presentation. There is a higher failure rate with ^{131}I treatment in these groups, necessitating additional therapy. In the United States radioiodine is the usual treatment for patients over 35 years of age with Graves' disease; in the United Kingdom and many other countries thyroidectomy is more frequently used because it is associated with less hypothyroidism and more rapid correction of hyperthyroidism. The objective of thyroidectomy for Graves' disease should be the complete and permanent control of the disease with minimal risk of morbidity in terms of nerve and parathyroid damage.

Patients should be euthyroid before operation with antithyroid drugs that should be continued up to the day of surgery. Many physicians prefer to treat patients with Lugol's iodine solution (3 drops twice daily) in the 10 days before operation, and some use propranolol. Preoperative treatment with iodine reduces the vascularity of the gland. All these measures decrease the risk of thyroid storm, which can be precipitated by surgery in unprepared patients.

Whether subtotal, near-total, or total thyroidectomy should be performed is controversial. The most commonly undertaken procedure, and perhaps the safest in terms of morbidity, is bilateral subtotal thyroidectomy, in which about 1 to 2 g of thyroid tissue is left on both sides, or a total lobectomy on one side and a subtotal thyroidectomy on the other side (Hartley-Dunhill procedure), leaving about 4 to 5 g of thyroid tissue.

Total thyroidectomy can be performed with minimal risk of morbidity and is the operation of choice in patients with coexisting eye disease. Catz and Perzik reported no progression in 66 of 70 patients with total thyroidectomy. Similarly, Winsa and colleagues reported that ophthalmopathy stabilized or improved in 96 percent of patients 6 months or more postoperatively, which may be the result of removal of the antigenic stimulus. In their series of patients undergoing total thyroidectomy for Graves' disease, 21 of 25 patients not previously treated with ^{131}I had normalization of TSH-receptor antibodies (TRAb) at 2.5 years.

Advantages of thyroidectomy over radioiodine treatment are: immediate cure of disease and decreased long-term incidence of hypothyroidism. Initial series probably overstated the incidence of hypothyroidism because they failed to account for later recovery of thyroid function. Other advantages include a decreased number of outpatient visits and the potential removal of a coexisting thyroid carcinoma. Disadvantages are: possible recurrent laryngeal nerve injury (approximately 1 percent), hypoparathyroidism (usually transient in approximately 13 percent and permanent in 1 percent), hematoma, and hypertrophic scar formation.

Recurrent thyrotoxicosis usually should be managed by radioiodine treatment, because reoperation carries a higher morbidity risk; when tissue has been left on one side, the risk of complications is less. Long-term follow-up should be maintained for all patients, with clinical review and yearly TSH measurement to detect the possible late onset of hypothyroidism or recurrent hyperthyroidism.

Treatment of Exophthalmos. The severity of Graves' ophthalmopathy is independent of thyrotoxicosis; data suggest, however, that recurrent hyperthyroidism and hypothyroidism aggravate the eye problems. Some reports suggest that total thyroidectomy alleviates the eye disease. It is unproved whether total thyroidectomy is preferable to near-total or subtotal thyroidectomy. Total thyroidectomy should be undertaken only in patients with severe exophthalmos when they are well prepared.

Severe or malignant exophthalmos is rare. Treatment is essentially symptomatic; steroid eye drops or systemic steroids (60 mg prednisolone daily) should be used initially to alleviate chemosis. When symptoms are more severe upon awakening, patients should tape their eyes closed at night, and the head of the bed should be elevated. Patients whose eyes are worse during the day should wear glasses to protect the eyes from sun and wind and should use artificial tears to protect against drying.

Lateral tarsorrhaphy to oppose eyelids helps to alleviate drying and subsequent chemosis and corneal ulceration. In extreme situations, retro-orbital radiation or orbital decompression may be necessary to save vision.

Toxic Nodular Goiter

Toxic nodular goiter, also known as Plummer's disease, is a consequence of one or more thyroid nodules trapping and organifying more iodine and secreting more thyroid hormone independently of TSH control. Toxic nodular goiter occurs most often in areas of endemic goiter. It has been documented that most "hot" or "autonomous" thyroid nodules have TSH-receptor (common) or *gsp* (less common) mutations.

Hyperthyroidism in patients with toxic nodular goiter is milder than in patients with Graves' disease, and the condition is not accompanied by the extrathyroidal manifestations of ophthalmopathy, pretibial myxedema, vitiligo, or thyroid acropathy. Ingestion or administration of iodides, e.g., iodine supplements or intravenously administered contrast agents, may precipitate iodine-induced hyperthyroidism (Jod-Basedow phenomenon).

Patients with toxic multinodular goiter (MNG) are older at presentation than those with Graves' disease. The thyroid-gland goiters characteristically have one or more nodules on palpation. Symptoms such as dysphagia and dyspnea may be present. Some goiters are retrosternal. Symptoms are often mild, and atrial fibrillation in the elderly is frequently the only clinical finding apart from the goiter. The diagnosis is suggested by the history and physical examination and confirmed by documenting a suppressed serum TSH level and raised thyroid hormone level. Antithyroid antibodies usually are not present.

Therapy with antithyroid medication or beta blockers alleviates symptoms but usually is less effective than in patients with Graves' disease. Radioiodine therapy is not as effective as in

Graves' disease because of lower uptake, and hence these patients require larger doses of radiation. ^{131}I uptake is localized to one or more autonomous toxic nodules, and the remaining thyroid tissue is suppressed. ^{131}I ablation may be used in patients who are unsuitable for surgery, but because of the high failure rate with this treatment, thyroidectomy is considered the treatment of choice. For solitary nodules, nodulectomy or thyroid lobectomy are the treatments of choice, because cancer is rare. For toxic multinodular goiter, lobectomy on one side and subtotal lobectomy on the other side is recommended for most patients, negating the need for bilateral reoperation in cases of recurrent disease.

Thyroid Storm

Thyroid storm is life-threatening but is rarely encountered during thyroidal—or other—surgery. Most patients with thyroid storm have had known or unknown untreated hyperthyroidism, and thyroid storm is precipitated by an infection (typically pharyngitis or pneumonitis), labor, administration of iodine (such as amiodarone), or after ^{131}I treatment.

Signs and symptoms resemble those of severe thyrotoxicosis, with profound tachycardia, fever, and confusion. Disorientation associated with dehydration from vomiting, diarrhea, and fever may occur and, in extreme cases, adrenergic hyperactivity can lead to overt mania; coma may result as a late event.

The best management is prophylaxis. Patients with hyperthyroidism should be euthyroid before operation. The history and examination of patients admitted for procedures requiring a general anesthetic should identify undiagnosed hyperthyroidism. In cases of thyroid storm, patients can be treated in the acute phase with a combination of fluid replacement, antithyroid drugs, beta blockers, sodium iodate solution or Lugol's iodine solution, hydrocortisone, and a cooling blanket. Sedation may be necessary in cases of agitation with hyperactivity. Aspirin should be avoided because it increases free thyroid hormone levels. In extreme cases peritoneal dialysis or hemofiltration may be effective in lowering serum T_4 and T_3 levels.

HYPOTHYROIDISM

Hypothyroidism is the clinical syndrome that arises when there is a deficiency in the circulating levels of thyroid hormone. In neonates the disease is termed *cretinism* and is characterized by neurological impairment and mental retardation. Early treatment lessens the neurological deficits. Hypothyroidism also may be associated with Pendred's syndrome (deafness and hypothyroidism) and Turner's syndrome. In adults, onset of symptoms is insidious and the patient may be unaware of changes. Causes of hypothyroidism are listed in Table 36-2. The two principal causes of hypothyroidism in the United States are autoimmune thyroiditis and iatrogenic mechanisms such as thyroidectomy, radiation treatment, or medications. Iodine deficiency and dyshormonogenesis are other causes of hypothyroidism and goiter.

Clinical Manifestations. When the thyroid gland fails to develop or function in utero, children are born with cretinism and characteristic facies similar to those of Down syndrome and dwarfism (Fig. 36-16). Failure to thrive is apparent, and mental retardation often is severe. Immediate treatment with thyroid hormone at birth can lessen the neurological and intellectual deficits. Hypothyroidism at birth also can occur because of blocking

Table 36-2
Causes of Hypothyroidism

Primary
    Autoimmune thyroiditis
        Hashimoto's thyroiditis
        Primary myxedema
    Iatrogenic
        Thyroidectomy
        ^{131}I therapy
        Antithyroid drugs
    Congenital (cretinism)
        Thyroid dysgenesis
        Dyshormonogenesis
    Inflammatory
        Subacute thyroiditis
        Riedel's thyroiditis
    Metabolic
        Iodine deficiency
Secondary
    Hypopituitarism
    Hypothalamic hypothyroidism
    Peripheral resistance to thyroid hormones

antibodies from the mother. Hypothyroidism developing in childhood or adolescence is termed *juvenile hypothyroidism;* these children appear younger than their chronologic counterparts and may develop abdominal distention, umbilical hernia, and rectal prolapse. Mental performance may be impaired, but severe retardation is uncommon. Hypothyroidism secondary to autoimmune thyroiditis is far more prevalent in females (80 percent of cases). In adults symptoms in general are nonspecific, including tiredness, weight gain, cold intolerance, constipation, and menorrhagia.

Myxedema is the term given to severe hypothyroidism. In these patients facial features change because of the deposition of glycosaminoglycans in the subcutaneous tissues, leading to facial and periorbital puffiness. The skin becomes rough and dry and can develop a yellowish tinge from reduced conversion of carotene to vitamin A. Hair loss may be marked, with characteristic loss of the outer two-thirds of the eyebrows; remaining hair becomes dry and brittle. Enlargement of the tongue may impair speech, which is already slowed, in keeping with the impairment of mental processes. Untreated dementia may develop *(myxedema madness)*. Abdominal symptoms may predominate. Patients may complain of a nonspecific, dull abdominal pain accompanied by distention and constipation. Libido and fertility are impaired in both sexes.

Cardiovascular changes include bradycardia and cardiomegaly, and a pericardial effusion might be present. Hypotension may be evident with a reduced cardiac output, and some patients develop shortness of breath and pulmonary effusions. Cardiac failure is uncommon. When hypothyroidism occurs as a result of pituitary failure and low TSH levels (secondary hypothyroidism), features of hypopituitarism may be present, such as pale, waxy skin, loss of body hair, and atrophic genitalia.

Laboratory Findings. Hypothyroidism is characterized by low circulating levels of T_4 and T_3. Raised TSH levels are found in primary thyroid failure, whereas in secondary hypothyroidism TSH levels are low. Secondary hyperthyroidism is rare and can be diagnosed by measuring TSH after a TRH challenge. The TSH level is low and does not increase in response to TRH. Autoimmune thyroid disease is characterized by the presence of thyroid autoantibodies (antithyroglobulin, antimitochondrial, or anti–thyroid-peroxidase [anti-TPO]). Other findings in hypothyroidism include anemia, diminished voltage with flattening or inversion of T waves on electrocardiogram, slow alpha waves with loss of amplitude on electroencephalogram, and raised levels of serum cholesterol (>300 mg/dL). In myxedema, comatose patients also have hyponatremia and CO_2 retention.

Treatment. Treatment of hypothyroidism is simple, inexpensive, and effective. Thyroxine is the treatment of choice and is administered in dosages varying from 50 μg to 200 μg per day. Patients are instructed to take tablets in the morning, usually without other medications, or at mealtime to assure good absorption and to avoid any sleep interference.

Young and otherwise healthy individuals tolerate initial starting doses of 100 μg of thyroxine per day, but elderly patients, patients with coexisting heart disease, and patients with profound hypothyroidism are less tolerant of thyroxine and should be started on a lower dose, such as 25 μg to 50 μg, slowly increasing the dose over weeks to months to attain a euthyroid state. An electrocardiogram should be obtained before treatment of patients with severe hypothyroidism for comparison if chest pain develops. Thyroxine dosage is titrated against TSH levels, which should return to normal. Thyroxine supplementation also must be determined by the clinical response of the patient. Whether or not patients with subclinical hypothyroidism (normal T_4, slightly raised TSH) should be treated is controversial. Evidence suggests that patients with subclinical hypothyroidism and increased antithyroid antibody levels should be treated, because

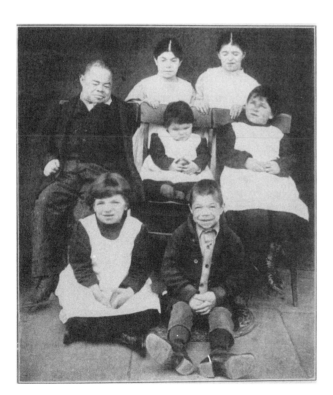

FIG. 36-16. *Children born with cretinism develop facies similar to that of Down syndrome or dwarfism. Immediate treatment of affected children at birth may lessen the neurological and intellectual deficits, which frequently are severe.*

they progress to more severe hypothyroidism. Patients with mild hypothyroidism may benefit from small doses of T_4, as the hypercholesterolemia, which accompanies hypothyroidism in this group of patients, is improved by therapy.

Patients who present with myxedema coma, in contrast to the patients with mild to moderate hypothyroidism, require emergency treatment with large doses of intravenous thyroxine (400 μg) followed by 100 μg/day. These patients usually are hyponatremic and hypocapnic and need careful monitoring in an intensive care unit.

THYROIDITIS

Autoimmune Lymphocytic Thyroiditis (Hashimoto's Thyroiditis)

Chronic lymphocytic thyroiditis, more commonly known as Hashimoto's thyroiditis or disease, after the physician who first described the condition in 1912, is an autoimmune thyroid disease and is the most common cause of hypothyroidism. It is ten times more common in women and more prevalent in the 30- to 60-year-old age group, with a prevalence of about 20 cases per 1000 women and an annual incidence of 1 to 2 new cases per 1000 women in the population. Autoimmune thyroiditis may be familial; up to 50 percent of first-degree relatives of patients with chronic autoimmune thyroiditis have thyroid antibodies inherited as a dominant trait. Chronic autoimmune thyroiditis is encountered in children but is rare in those under 5 years of age. In adolescents 40 percent of goiters are from autoimmune thyroiditis. Other predisposing conditions to autoimmune thyroiditis include Down syndrome, familial Alzheimer's disease, and Turner's syndrome. It is more common in areas of iodine excess. Studies suggest that thyroid cells in Hashimoto's thyroiditis have increased FAS receptors and that interleukin-1 induces abnormal FAS expression and triggers apoptosis or increased programmed thyroid cell death.

Pathology. In Hashimoto's disease the thyroid gland typically is firm and mildly enlarged. The enlargement usually is symmetrical. Frequently the pyramidal lobe also is enlarged. Histologically, there is follicular and Hürthle cell hyperplasia associated with lymphocytic and plasma cell infiltration and formation of lymphoid follicles. The disease is usually focal but gradually extends to involve the whole gland. Epithelial cell degeneration occurs with fragmentation of the basement membrane, and remaining epithelial cells enlarge and demonstrate oxyphilic changes (Hürthle or Askanazy cells). As lymphocytic infiltration progresses, the thyroid tissue degenerates and may be replaced by fibrous tissue.

Clinical Manifestations. Approximately 20 percent of patients with Hashimoto's thyroiditis present with signs and symptoms of hypothyroidism; a few patients present with hyperthyroidism (Hashitoxicosis). Most patients are euthyroid when the diagnosis is made. The most common presenting symptom is a tightness in the throat, often associated with a painless, nontender enlargement of the thyroid gland. Compression of the trachea or a recurrent laryngeal nerve is rare. Rapid enlargement of the thyroid gland should raise suspicion of thyroid lymphoma or carcinoma. Palpation usually demonstrates a diffusely enlarged, firm, often granular thyroid gland; in some cases the gland also is nodular. Usually the pyramidal lobe is enlarged. Evidence of other autoimmune conditions, such as disseminated lupus, rheumatic arthritis, and myasthenia gravis, may be present.

Diagnostic Findings. In early Hashimoto's thyroiditis, patients may present with a transient rise in serum thyroid hormone levels, but as the disease progresses, the serum TSH level rises as serum T_4 and T_3 levels fall. The diagnosis is confirmed by the presence of circulating antithyroid antibodies. These antibodies are directed against the membrane-bound enzyme involved in thyroid hormone synthesis, thyroid peroxidase (TPO), formerly called antimitochondrial antibodies, in almost 100 percent of patients and against thyroglobulin in about 50 percent of patients. FNAC examination of the thyroid gland occasionally is useful in confirming the diagnosis of Hashimoto's thyroiditis and in patients in whom malignancy is suspected.

Treatment. In the absence of compressive symptoms, patients demonstrating goiter, with or without evidence of hypothyroidism, are best treated with thyroid hormone. Reduction in thyroid goiter size with thyroxine treatment is variable but is more commonly seen in younger patients. Surgical intervention is indicated for patients complaining of obstructive symptoms, for cosmetically unacceptable goiters, or when thyroid cancer (other than lymphoma) is found. Thyroxine therapy with long-term follow-up monitoring of TSH levels is recommended.

Subacute Thyroiditis (De Quervain's Thyroiditis)

Subacute thyroiditis, also known as de Quervain's, granulomatous, or giant cell thyroiditis, is an uncommon, acute inflammatory disease of the thyroid. It is thought to be precipitated by a viral infection, although the exact cause is unknown. It is commonly encountered in North America but is relatively rare in the United Kingdom and Europe. The disease may be responsible for up to 10 percent of patients with hyperthyroidism in the United States. It affects women five times more often and usually is seen in patients 20 to 40 years of age.

Clinical Manifestations. Patients usually present with fever, malaise, and unilateral or bilateral thyroid pain and a recent history of an upper respiratory tract or viral infection may be given. Some patients complain of the symptoms of thyrotoxicosis, including palpitations, sweating, and heat intolerance, which are caused by the release of thyroid hormones from disrupted follicles in the inflamed thyroid gland. Palpation of the thyroid gland may reveal a tender, firm gland with mild unilateral or bilateral enlargement.

Pathology and Diagnostic Tests. Histologically, the disease is characterized by an acute inflammatory reaction of the thyroid gland. Degenerative thyroid follicles are surrounded by giant cells forming granulomas, which may be demonstrated on FNAC. Laboratory investigations demonstrate an elevated erythrocyte sedimentation rate (ESR) associated with a neutrophilia. Thyroid function tests usually show elevated levels of thyroid hormones (T_4 and T_3) with suppression of TSH. As the disease resolves, thyroid hormone levels return to normal, although the TSH level can remain low for some time. In contrast to Graves' disease, radioiodine uptake in the acute stage of the disease is low or negligible, because the released thyroid hormone, as result of inflammation, suppresses the serum TSH concentration.

Treatment. Usually treatment with nonsteroidal anti-inflammatory drugs (NSAIDs) for pain relief is all that is necessary. Treatment with NSAIDs should be continued for several weeks after the disease has resolved in an effort to prevent recurrence. Beta blockers (e.g., propranolol) in the initial stages of the disease can be useful for relief of thyrotoxic symptoms. In the more severe cases it might be necessary to prescribe steroids for short periods. Prednisolone 40 mg once daily for 1 to 2 weeks, followed by a gradual reduction of the dose over the ensuing month, is recommended in such cases.

The disease usually lasts 1 to 6 weeks and resolves spontaneously. In some cases the disease lasts from several weeks or months and runs a course alternating between bouts of exacerbation followed by periods of remission. Most patients have complete resolution of the disease, although 10 percent of patients experience permanent hypothyroidism and require thyroxine replacement therapy.

Riedel's Thyroiditis

Riedel's thyroiditis is a rare disease of the thyroid characterized by a marked dense, invasive fibrosis that may extend beyond the thyroid capsule and involve surrounding structures. Fibrosis may involve the strap muscles, blood vessels, trachea, esophagus, and, on occasion, the parathyroid glands, which leads to hypoparathyroidism. Severe cases can result in the patient's becoming hypothyroid. The cause of the condition is unknown, but it may be part of a more generalized condition known as fibrosclerosis that causes fibrosis in other parts of the body, including the retroperitoneum, mediastinum, lacrimal glands, and bile ducts (sclerosing cholangitis).

Patients usually present with symptoms of compression such as hoarseness, stridor, and dyspnea. In more progressive cases involving the esophagus, dysphagia may be present. There often is rapid enlargement of the thyroid gland, which on palpation is "woody," hard, and nontender. Laboratory investigations usually are normal.

Riedel's thyroiditis resembles anaplastic thyroid cancer, except that the goiter is smaller. Diagnosis usually is established by FNAC, although open biopsy occasionally is needed. Treatment with tamoxifen and steroids often is helpful. Isthmectomy to relieve compressive symptoms or to establish the diagnosis is necessary in some patients. Most operations are difficult because of the loss of tissue planes and should only be embarked on by experienced surgeons. Thyroxine replacement therapy is necessary in patients with hypothyroidism.

Acute Suppurative Thyroiditis

Acute suppurative thyroiditis is rare. It is predominantly a disease of childhood or adolescence and is invariably associated with an acute upper respiratory tract infection. The disease is manifested by acute thyroid pain associated with dysphagia, fever, and, occasionally, rigors. The most common bacterial causative agents are streptococci, staphylococci, and pneumococci, but it also can be caused by *Escherichia coli* and *Coccidioides immitis.*

Suppuration usually is unilateral but may extend into the deep spaces in the neck, invading the trachea, esophagus, or mediastinum. FNAC with smear and culture is diagnostic. Treatment consists of intravenous antibiotics and drainage of any abscess. Thyroid lobectomy rarely is required. Most patients recover completely and are euthyroid.

GOITER

Simple or nontoxic goiter is an enlargement of the thyroid gland in a euthyroid patient, not associated with any neoplastic or inflammatory process. It may be diffuse and symmetrical or nodular. Several forms of goiter have been described.

Familial Goiter. Familial goiters usually are regarded as goiters caused by an inherited enzymatic defect (dyshormonogenesis) that may cause impairment of iodine accumulation, organification, or coupling of iodotyrosine in the thyroid gland. The inborn error of metabolism generally is inherited as an autosomal recessive trait, but dominant traits have been described. Familial goiters usually are associated with hypothyroidism, although patients may remain euthyroid. Familial goiter also is associated with deafness (Pendred's syndrome).

Endemic Goiter. Endemic goiter is defined as thyroid enlargement affecting a significant number of inhabitants of a particular locale. The most important factor in the development of this condition is iodine deficiency. It is most commonly encountered in mountainous areas where the iodine content of drinking water is particularly low. Most countries throughout the world have had one or more areas where endemic goiter was encountered; in the United States it was formerly in the Midwestern mountainous regions. Administration of iodine, usually as an additive in table salt, has proved successful as a prophylaxis in reducing the incidence of this condition.

Sporadic Goiter. Sporadic goiter is the term given to a goiter for which no definitive cause can be established. It excludes goiters caused from thyroiditis and neoplasia as well as endemic goiter.

Pathology. The thyroid gland may be diffusely enlarged and smooth, or enlarged and markedly nodular. In the early stages of the disease, the gland may be hyperplastic and diffusely enlarged, a condition that may be reversed by the administration of iodine or thyroid hormone. Nontoxic nodular goiter is a multinodular gland in which the nodules vary considerably in size and number. Nodules are filled with gelatinous, colloid-rich material, and scattered between nodules are areas of normal thyroid tissue. Gross or microscopic cyst formation may be present, with evidence of degeneration, hemorrhage, and calcification.

Clinical Manifestations. Most patients with goiters are asymptomatic. The most common symptom is a sensation of pressure in the neck coupled with a mass. If the goiter enlarges significantly, patients may complain of compressive symptoms such dysphagia or dyspnea. Paralysis of a recurrent laryngeal nerve is rare and should raise the suspicion of malignancy. On occasion a recurrent laryngeal nerve is stretched over a rapidly enlarging thyroid nodular cyst and ceases to function. Goiters may extend into the thorax and become retrosternal (Fig. 36-17), which may be associated with an impedance of venous return in the jugular veins (Fig. 36-18) and consequent facial flushing. Such flushing is accentuated by the patient's raising his or her arms above the head (positive Pemberton's sign). Sudden pain, frequently associated with rapid enlargement of the thyroid gland, usually is related to hemorrhage into a colloid nodule or cyst.

Examination reveals a diffusely enlarged, soft thyroid goiter in patients with simple goiter or an enlarged gland with nodules of varying size and firmness in multinodular goiter (Fig. 36-19). In patients in whom one nodule predominates, or is painful, or

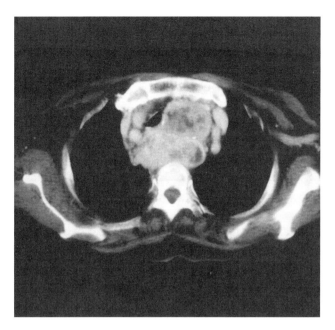

FIG. 36-17. Retrosternal extension of a nodular goiter. Note the displacement and compression of the trachea.

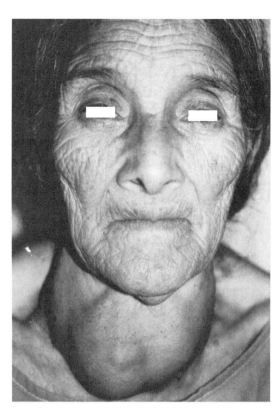

FIG. 36-19. Multinodular goiter in an elderly patient. Nodules vary in size and firmness. When one nodule is prominent, painful, or has recently enlarged, FNAC is recommended.

has recently enlarged, FNAC is recommended because it is sensitive and specific in the diagnosis of colloid nodule.

Results of laboratory investigations usually are normal, although in patients over the age of 60 years with long-standing multinodular goiters (>17 years), a significant number develop thyrotoxicosis (Plummer's disease). Most of these hyperthyroid patients have a suppressed TSH and increased T_3 level but normal T_4 (T_3 toxicosis).

Treatment. Most euthyroid patients with small, diffuse, simple goiters need no treatment. If the goiter is of significant size, treatment with thyroxine may depress TSH stimulation of the thyroid gland and reduce hyperplasia, decreasing goiter size or preventing increases in size. Endemic goiter is managed by the administration of iodine. Surgery should be reserved for patients with cosmetically unacceptable goiters, compressive symptoms, or retrosternal goiters or when malignancy is suspected or demonstrated on FNAC.

SOLITARY OR DOMINANT THYROID NODULE

Solitary thyroid nodules are present in about 4 percent of the population of the United States. Thyroid cancer has an incidence of 40 new cases per 1,000,000 people. The vast majority of thyroid nodules are benign and do not require removal. The physician or surgeon should be able to perform an accurate clinical assessment of any thyroid nodule, appreciate the risk factors of thyroid cancer, and be able to evaluate which patients would benefit from surgery.

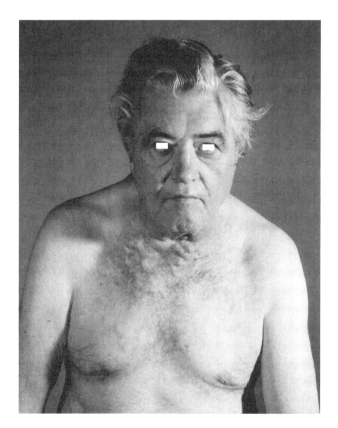

FIG. 36-18. Retrosternal extension of a large goiter has resulted in a marked impedance of the superior vena cava in this patient, as indicated by the dilated veins over the chest wall. Further impedance was evident when the patient raised his arms above his head (Pemberton's sign).

Risk Factors for Cancer. Two groups are at risk for having carcinoma of the thyroid: patients exposed to low-dose radiation to the head and neck regions and patients in whose family another member has developed thyroid cancer. Medullary thyroid cancer, which is the greatest risk factor because it may be inherited as an autosomal dominant trait, can be diagnosed by testing for a RET point mutation. Approximately 6 percent of patients with papillary thyroid cancer have familial disease. Papillary thyroid cancer also occurs more commonly in patients with Cowden's syndrome and familial polyposis.

Irradiation of the Head and Neck. A history of low-dose ionizing radiation (<2000 rad) to the thyroid gland places the patient at increased risk for developing thyroid cancer. The risk increases linearly from 6.5 to 2000 cGy; beyond this the incidence declines as the radiation causes destruction of the thyroid tissue, although patients who receive 4000 cGy for treatment of Hodgkin's disease have been shown to have a higher incidence of thyroid cancer. Low-dose therapeutic radiation was used to treat conditions such as "enlarged thymus" in an effort to prevent "sudden crib death" (150 cGy), tonsils and adenoids to prevent the need for tonsillectomy (750 cGy), acne vulgaris (1500 cGy) and other conditions such as hemangioma, ringworm, and scrofula.

There is a 40 percent chance that patients presenting with a thyroid nodule and a history of radiation have thyroid cancer. Of those patients who have thyroid cancer, the cancer is located in the nodule in 60 percent of patients and in the remaining 40 percent of patients the cancer is in another area of the thyroid gland. In children living near the Chernobyl nuclear power plant, where an accident caused radiation leakage in 1986, there has been a 60-fold increase in thyroid cancer, with most cancers occurring in those who were infants at the time of exposure.

Thyroid cancer in patients with a history of radiation exposure tends to be of the papillary type and frequently is multifocal with a higher incidence of lymph node metastases. To prevent higher doses of radiation exposure to the thyroid, scanning with ^{123}I or ^{99m}Tc has largely replaced scanning with ^{131}I in most hospitals.

Evaluation. Most thyroid nodules are benign and are colloid nodules or adenomas. To distinguish between suspicious thyroid nodules that may be malignant and benign thyroid nodules, certain issues should be considered.

Because 40 percent of patients with a solitary nodule or multiple thyroid nodules with a history of previous head and neck irradiation will have cancer of the thyroid gland, a history of external radiation to the head or neck is important. The age and gender of the patient are also important. Thyroid nodules in children and elderly patients are more likely to be malignant. Solitary nodules also are more common in men over 40 and women over 50 years of age. Signs that should prompt concern are rapid enlargement of an old or new thyroid nodule, symptoms of local invasion (e.g., unilateral vocal cord paralysis), or compressive symptoms (e.g., dysphagia and dyspnea from invasion into the trachea and esophagus).

Approximately 15 percent of solitary thyroid nodules are malignant, and in hard solitary thyroid nodules the risk of malignancy is two or three times higher. When the apparently solitary nodule is found to be a dominant nodule in a multinodular thyroid gland, the incidence of thyroid cancer in this nodule is less than 5 percent. An exception to this is a history of previous head and neck irradiation or a history of familial thyroid cancer. Lesions that are hard, gritty, or fixed to surrounding structures such as the trachea or strap muscles are probably malignant. The presence of palpable cervical lymphadenopathy adjacent to a thyroid nodule should be suspected as a carcinoma. Cervical lymphadenopathy because of metastatic thyroid cancer may be present when no thyroid nodule is palpable. These patients almost always have a thyroid cancer that usually is present in the ipsilateral thyroid lobe. This cancer may be microscopic and demonstrated only after careful sectioning of the thyroid gland.

Investigations. *Fine-Needle Aspiration Cytology.* The procedure of choice in evaluating thyroid nodules is fine-needle aspiration cytology (FNAC). The test is fast, is minimally invasive, has few risks, causes little discomfort to the patient, and has been shown to be specific and sensitive. It has replaced radionuclide and ultrasonographic imaging in the preoperative evaluation of thyroid nodules.

Ninety percent of nodules can be categorized into the following groups: *benign,* 65 percent; *suspicious,* 15 percent; *malignant,* 5 percent; and *nondiagnostic,* 15 percent. The incidence of false-positive results is about 1 percent, and false-negative results, about 5 percent.

FNAC is the investigation of choice in patients with thyroid nodules, but it has limitations. The proportion of patients with suspicious cytology results ranges from 11 to 20 percent. Most have follicular or Hürthle cell neoplasms, and 20 percent of these patients have a thyroid malignancy. There is no accurate method of predicting which of these patients has a thyroid cancer, because the diagnosis depends on demonstrating capsular or vascular invasion, which is not possible on FNAC. The technique also is less reliable in patients who have previous irradiation to the head and neck or have a family history of thyroid cancer, as many of these patients have multifocal lesions.

When a cyst is encountered on FNAC it should be drained completely, which is curative in about 75 percent of simple cysts (Fig. 36-20), although some require a second or third aspiration. If the cyst persists after three attempts at aspiration, unilateral

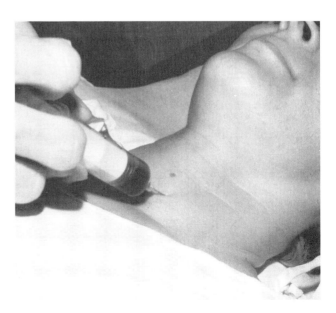

FIG. 36-20. *Aspiration of a simple thyroid cyst.*

thyroid lobectomy is recommended. In cases in which the cyst is larger than 4 cm in diameter or is complex (i.e., has solid and cystic components), thyroid lobectomy is recommended, because these cysts have a higher incidence of malignancy (15 percent).

Thyroid Imaging. Ultrasonographic Imaging. Ultrasound evaluation of the thyroid gland is helpful for detecting nonpalpable nodules and for differentiating solid from cystic nodules. It provides a noninvasive and inexpensive method of following the size of suspected benign nodules diagnosed by FNAC. This is especially useful in determining whether the nodule or the surrounding normal thyroid tissue decreases in size when the patient is treated with thyroid hormone. Ultrasonographic imaging has no role in screening for thyroid nodules in asymptomatic patients.

CT and MRI. Computed tomography and magnetic resonance imaging usually are unnecessary in the evaluation of thyroid tumors except for large or retrosternal lesions and for assessing suspected invasion into surrounding structures. MRI is more accurate than CT in distinguishing recurrent or persistent thyroid tumor from postoperative fibrosis.

Thyroid Isotope Scanning. Scanning the thyroid with ^{123}I or ^{99m}Tc can indicate the functional activity of a nodule and of the thyroid and correlate the location of palpable nodules with the nodules seen with scanning. Scanning with ^{131}I has been largely replaced by ^{123}I or ^{99m}Tc scans to lower the dose of radiation delivered to the thyroid gland during the investigation. Nodules that trap less iodine than the surrounding thyroid tissue are termed "cold," nonfunctional, or hypofunctional (Fig. 36-21). Almost 85 percent of nodules on scanning are cold, and these lesions have a 10 to 25 percent chance of malignancy. Of the 5 percent of nodules shown to be "hot" on scanning, approximately 1 percent are malignant. Thyroid scanning is recommended in the assessment of thyroid nodules only in those patients who have follicular thyroid nodules on FNAC.

Laboratory Findings. Thyroid function tests are not useful in the assessment of patients with thyroid nodules, because most patients with thyroid cancer are euthyroid. In those patients presenting with hyperthyroidism and a solitary nodule, the chances of the nodule's being malignant are very low. Serum thyroglobulin levels cannot differentiate benign from malignant thyroid nodules unless the levels are extremely high, in which case metastatic thyroid cancer should be suspected. Thyroglobulin levels are useful in following patients who have undergone total thyroidectomy for thyroid cancer, excluding medullary thyroid cancer, and also for monitoring patients with nodules being followed nonoperatively. Serum calcitonin levels should be obtained in patients with a family history of medullary thyroid cancer or multiple endocrine neoplasia type II (MEN II) and where FNAC demonstrates medullary thyroid cancer to be present. Patients who are RET oncogene positive should always have a 24-h urine collection with measurements of levels of vanillylmandelic acid (VMA), metanephrine, and catecholamine to rule out a coexisting pheochromocytoma.

Treatment. The algorithm for the diagnosis of a thyroid nodule is shown in Fig. 36-22. When a diagnosis of colloid nodule is made cytologically, thyroidectomy is not necessary except for cosmetic or symptomatic reasons, and these patients can be safely observed. A second FNAC is recommended 6 to 8 months after the initial FNAC if the nodule enlarges. Patients

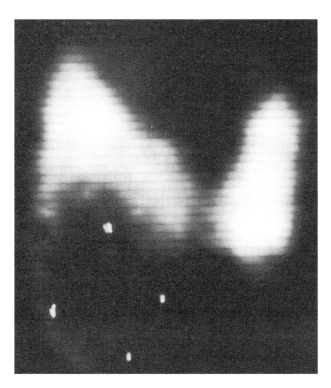

FIG. 36-21. *Radioiodine scan demonstrating a "cold" nodule in the right lower lobe. About 85 percent of nodules are shown on scanning to be "cold." Such lesions have a 10 to 25 percent chance of being malignant.*

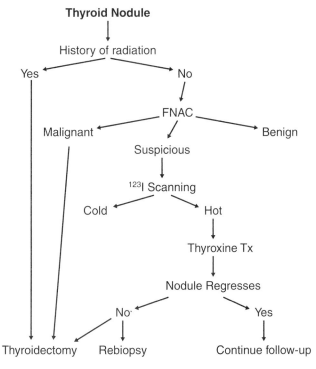

FIG. 36-22. *Algorithm for the diagnosis of thyroid nodule.*

with benign nodules should undergo ultrasound determination of the size of the lesion and a baseline thyroglobulin level should be obtained. Patients may be prescribed thyroxine in doses sufficient to maintain a serum TSH level between 0.1 and 1.0 μU/mL. Approximately 50 percent of these nodules significantly decrease in size in response to the TSH suppression of this regimen. Thyroidectomy should be performed if a nodule enlarges or develops in a patient whose serum thyroglobulin increases despite TSH suppression therapy with thyroxine. An exception to this general rule is the patient who has had previous irradiation of the thyroid gland. In these patients total or near-total thyroidectomy is recommended with FNAC because of the high incidence of thyroid cancer (40 percent).

Thyroid lobectomy is recommended in patients in whom a thyroid cyst has recurred after three aspirations and in patients with a cyst that is larger than 4 cm or is found to be a complex cyst on ultrasound examination. Signs and symptoms such as pressure, hoarseness, dysphagia, vocal cord paralysis, dyspnea, adjacent cervical lymphadenopathy, or recent rapid increase in size of a thyroid nodule (unless FNAC demonstrates hemorrhage) all favor thyroid lobectomy. Patients with a thyroid nodule and a family history of papillary or Hürthle cell cancer probably warrant thyroidectomy. Patients with medullary carcinoma or MEN II with an elevated basal or stimulated calcitonin level or positive RET oncogene also should have a total thyroidectomy, even in the absence of a palpable mass.

MALIGNANT TUMORS

In the United States thyroid cancer occurs in about 40 per 1,000,000 people each year and accounts for less than 1 percent of all malignancies. Thyroid cancer is responsible for six deaths per million persons annually. Most patients present with a palpable swelling in the neck, which initiates assessment through a combination of history, palpation, and FNAC examination. Diagnosed correctly and managed properly, most patients with differentiated thyroid carcinoma of follicular cell origin are curable.

Several different types of primary thyroid carcinoma are recognized, although 90 to 95 percent of thyroid carcinomas are *differentiated* tumors of follicular cell origin (differentiated thyroid cancer) giving rise to papillary, follicular, or Hürthle cell carcinoma. About 6 percent of patients with papillary and Hürthle cell cancer have familial disease; follicular and anaplastic thyroid cancer are more common in patients from iodine-deficient areas. Medullary thyroid cancers account for about 6 percent of thyroid cancers, and approximately 30 percent of these tumors are familial.

Molecular Basis of Thyroid Tumors

Oncogene *(onc)* is the title given to a gene that contributes directly to tumor genesis. Cellular oncogenes *(c-onc)* or proto-oncogenes are cellular genes that can give rise to oncogenes when they are altered or when their expression is modified. The modified genes may encode for a mutated receptor on the cell surface, resulting in an abnormal growth signal being transmitted to the nucleus through overexpression of the receptor or by the receptor's being continually (constitutively) activated. Inappropriate cell division results and may lead to malignant transformation. The fact that these genes have survived in the evolu-

tionary process and play a role in cell transformation suggests that proto-oncogenes are involved in the normal control of cell growth and differentiation.

Several oncogenes are involved in thyroid tumor genesis. Mutations in TSH-receptor and Gs genes are found in hyperfunctioning thyroid nodules, for example, and probably constitutively activate the adenylate cyclase–protein kinase A signal transduction pathway, leading to a well-differentiated tumor. An oncogene that has a significant role in the development of papillary thyroid cancer is the RET oncogene. Rearrangement of this gene occurs in papillary thyroid cancer (PTC) and is more common in childhood thyroid cancers. Point mutations involving RET have been demonstrated in patients with familial medullary thyroid cancer, MEN IIA, and MEN IIB.

The RET proto-oncogene encodes for a tyrosine kinase receptor on the cytoplasmic membrane; the ligand has been identified as glial cell line–derived neurotrophic factor (GDNF). RET is expressed during embryogenesis in the nervous and excretory systems. Disruption of RET results in developmental abnormalities in these systems, including the enteric nervous system (Hirschsprung's disease). Tumors arising from the neural crest cells (medullary thyroid cancer and pheochromocytoma) also contain RET point mutations. The RET gene is located on chromosome 10, and rearrangement of RET by fusion with heterologous genes creates transforming oncogenes, which have been implicated in the pathogenesis of PTC. These oncogenes are RET/PTC1, RET/PTC2, and RET/PTC3.

Not all patients with PTC possess the RET/PTC gene, and expression markedly varies geographically, e.g., being low in Japan (3 percent) and high in Italy (34.6 percent). It also is more common in thyroid cancers in children that develop after radiation exposure. In vitro irradiation induces RET/PTC formation, and 66 percent of the papillary thyroid cancers that were removed from patients living near Chernobyl demonstrated RET/PTC1 and RET/PTC3.

A second oncogene associated with PTC is TRK-A, found on chromosome 1, which encodes for a cell surface receptor for nerve growth factor. Mutated *ras* oncogenes have been demonstrated in a wide variety of human tumors and occur more frequently in human thyroid tumors of follicular origin. Point mutations in *ras* occur in thyroid adenomas and multinodular goiters, as well as follicular carcinoma, and are believed to be an early mutation.

A molecular defect associated with the development of follicular adenoma is allelic loss of genes on the short arm of chromosome 11 (11q). Deletion of 3p accompanies transformation from follicular adenoma to a follicular adenocarcinoma.

The p53 gene is a tumor suppressor gene encoding for a protein (p53) that acts as a transcriptional regulator. Its function is to maintain genomic integrity. Point mutations in the p53 gene result in a protein that lacks this ability, which in turn results in proliferation of malignant cells. A mutated p53 gene is found in most anaplastic thyroid cancers and in thyroid cell lines.

Papillary Carcinoma

Papillary carcinoma is the most common of thyroid malignancies, accounting for 80 percent of all thyroid cancers. It is the predominant thyroid cancer in children (75 percent) and in people who were previously exposed to radiation in the neck (85 to 90 percent). Papillary carcinoma occurs more often in women, with a 2:1 female-to-male ratio, and the mean age at presentation is 30 to 40 years.

Pathology. Papillary thyroid cancers, including mixed papillary follicular carcinoma and the follicular variant of papillary carcinoma, usually are hard and whitish and remain flat on sectioning with a blade, rather than bulging as does normal tissue or benign nodular lesions. Macroscopic calcification, necrosis, or cystic change may be apparent. Smaller tumors occasionally may be present inside thyroid cysts.

Histologically, papillary carcinomas may exhibit papillary projections, a mixed pattern (papillary/follicular structures), or a pure follicular pattern with intranuclear inclusions. The diagnosis is established by characteristic cellular features. Cells are cuboidal with pale, abundant cytoplasm, crowded nuclei, and intranuclear cytoplasmic inclusions, the so-called *Orphan Annie cells* (Fig. 36-23). A characteristic fibrovascular stroma with calcium deposits *(psammoma bodies)* may be present. Tumors that exhibit papillary features such as *mixed tumor* or the *follicular variant* of papillary carcinoma should be classified as papillary carcinomas because they act biologically as papillary carcinomas. Multifocality in papillary carcinoma is common (30 to 87.5 percent) and is a minor risk factor in prognosis. Papillary cancers exhibit a propensity for lymphatic spread within the thyroid and to local lymph nodes (paratracheal and cervical chain). Papillary tumors may invade local structures such as the trachea, esophagus, and recurrent laryngeal nerves and rarely are encapsulated. Blood-borne metastases usually are a late feature.

Macroscopically, there are three recognized forms of papillary thyroid cancer, each based on the size and extent of the primary disease. *Minimal or occult/microcarcinoma* tumors originally included papillary cancers up to 1.5 cm in diameter. They now are defined as tumors of 1 cm or less in size with no evidence of local invasiveness through the thyroid capsule and that are not associated with lymph node metastases. They are nonpalpable and usually are incidental findings at operative, histologic, or autopsy examination. Studies have demonstrated occult papillary thyroid cancer to be present in 2 to 36 percent of thyroid glands removed at autopsy. Recurrence rate in patients with tumors 1.5 cm or smaller after removal is about 7 percent and the mortality about 0.5 percent. *Intrathyroidal* tumors are greater than 1 cm and are confined to the thyroid gland, with no evidence of extrathyroid invasion. *Extrathyroidal* tumors are locally advanced with invasion through the thyroid capsule into adjacent structures. All types of primary thyroid cancers can be associated with lymph node metastases and invasion into intrathyroidal blood vessels or occasionally distant metastases. Long-term prognosis is better for intrathyroidal lesions.

Other types of papillary carcinoma of the thyroid are: tall cell, columnar, diffuse sclerosing, clear cell, trabecular, Hürthle cell, and poorly differentiated variants. Most of these variants behave more aggressively. Angioinvasion also predicts more recurrences and a worse prognosis, but coexisting lymphocytic thyroiditis suggests fewer recurrences and a better prognosis. There usually is no significant difference in management.

Clinical Manifestations. Most patients are euthyroid and present with a slow-growing painless mass in the neck. Accompanying symptoms, which usually are associated with advanced locally invasive disease, may include dysphagia, dyspnea, and hoarseness. Ipsilateral enlarged cervical lymph glands also may be present and most commonly are encountered in younger patients. Nodal involvement may be more apparent than the primary lesion; the so-called *lateral aberrant thyroid* usually is a cervical lymph node that has been invaded by metastatic cancer.

Distant metastases are uncommon at initial presentation (1 to 15 percent), depending on whether detected by physical examination and symptoms or by radioiodine scanning and thyroglobulin determination after thyroidectomy. Distant metastases to the lung are more commonly encountered in children, although up to 20 percent of all patients ultimately develop distant disease (Fig. 36-24).

Thyroid cancer often is suspected by history or physical examination. In most cases the diagnosis is easily established in the outpatient setting by FNAC, which is specific and sensitive in papillary, medullary, and anaplastic thyroid cancer. Radioiodine thyroid scans are not necessary in preoperative evaluation. CT and MRI are used selectively in patients with extensive local or substernal disease or lymph node involvement.

Prognostic Indicators. Ideal treatment objectives for thyroid cancer are detailed in Table 36-3. In order to compare the merits of different surgical therapies, a method of accurately assessing various prognostic factors is necessary.

AGES Scale. This is a postoperative prognostic scale of risk of dying from papillary cancer. Factors taken into account are Age, pathologic tumor Grade, Extent of disease and Size of tumor. Two groups are identified with this system: low-risk patients (young, with well-differentiated tumors, no metastases, and small primary lesions) and high-risk patients (older, with poorly differentiated tumors, local invasion, distant metastases, and large primary lesions). Of 860 patients in one study, 85 percent were in the low-risk group, with a cancer risk mortality of 2 percent at 25 years; the cancer risk mortality in the high-risk group was 46 percent.

MACIS Scale. This more sophisticated postoperative scale is a modification of the AGES system. Factors assessed are distant *M*etastases, *A*ge at presentation (<40 or >40 years), *C*om-

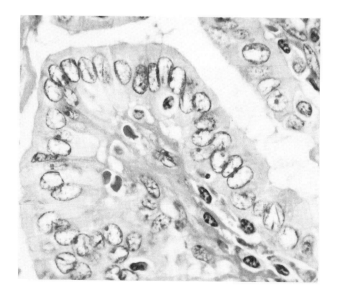

FIG. 36-23. Photomicrograph of papillary carcinoma demonstrating "Orphan Annie nuclei," a characteristic cellular feature of papillary thyroid cancer.

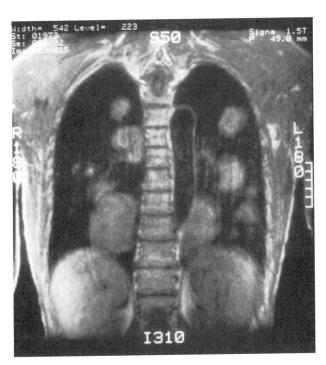

FIG. 36-24. MRI scan of a patient with familial papillary thyroid cancer demonstrating numerous metastatic deposits in both lung fields.

Table 36-3
Treatment Objectives in Differentiated Thyroid Cancer

1. Eradicate primary disease
2. Reduce the incidence of local/distant recurrence
3. Facilitate the treatment of metastases
4. Cure the maximum number of patients
5. Achieve all of the above with minimal morbidity

pleteness of original surgical resection, extrathyroidal *I*nvasion, and *S*ize of original lesion (in cm) (Fig. 36-25).

DNA Ploidy. Measurement of DNA ploidy is of some use in prognosis because aneuploidy is noted in 10 percent of all papillary carcinomas but is present in 25 to 50 percent of patients who die from thyroid cancers. Aneuploid DNA measurements are encountered infrequently in papillary thyroid cancers among survivors.

The most significant single prognostic indicator overall is distant metastases, especially to bone. Local invasion of the primary tumor through the thyroid capsule into the adjacent structures increases the mortality tenfold over matched patients with intrathyroidal tumors.

The other frequently used classification systems are AMES (*A*ge, *M*etastases, *E*xtent, *S*ize) and TNM (*T*umor size, *N*odal involvement, and *M*etastases to distant sites). Patients less than 45 years of age without distant metastases usually are considered to be at low risk.

Surgical Treatment. When patients are found to have a *minimal* papillary thyroid carcinoma in a thyroid specimen removed for other reasons, unilateral thyroid lobectomy and isthmectomy usually is sufficient surgical treatment unless there is angioinvasion or the tumor is at the margins of resection. Similarly, in rare cases of encapsulated papillary thyroid carcinoma, total lobectomy is all that is needed. In all other patients with papillary thyroid cancer, total or near-total thyroidectomy is the procedure of choice.

The Case for Total Thyroidectomy. There are several arguments for the treatment of papillary carcinoma by total thyroidectomy: multifocal disease, decreased incidence of local recurrence, reduced risk of anaplasia in any residual tissue, facilitation of diagnosing unsuspected metastatic disease by ra-

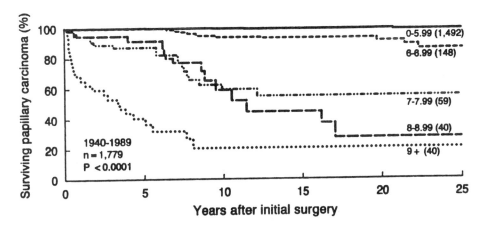

FIG. 36-25. Survival time for patients with papillary thyroid cancer related to MACIS score. A prognostic scale for predicting survival of patients with papillary thyroid cancer, which was devised at the Mayo Clinic. The following patient details and tumor characteristics are assessed and allotted a score: *M*etastases, *A*ge at presentation, *C*ompleteness of original surgical resection, and *I*nvasion and *S*ize of original tumor. Scores are totaled to give a definitive MACIS score. Higher scores are associated with a worse prognosis. MACIS score = 3.1 (if age ≤ 39 years) *or* 0.8 × age (if age ≥ 40 years), + 0.3 × tumor size (in cm) + 1 (if incompletely resected), + 1 (if locally invasive), + 3 (if distant metastases present). (Modified from: Hay ID, et al: Predicting outcome in papillary thyroid carcinoma. *Surgery* 114:1051, 1993, with permission.)

dioiodine scanning or treatment with [131]I (reducing incidence of distant recurrence), and greater sensitivity of blood thyroglobulin levels to predict recurrent or persistent disease.

Multifocal disease in papillary carcinoma is well documented (up to 85 percent). Unilateral lobectomy therefore may leave residual disease in the contralateral lobe. Recurrence rates in the contralateral lobe after thyroid lobectomy range from 4.2 to 26 percent. In one study, the recurrence rate was 19 percent at 10 years after lobectomy versus 11 percent in similar patients treated with total thyroidectomy.

Whether total thyroidectomy has any survival advantage over near-total thyroidectomy (total lobectomy with subtotal resection of the contralateral lobe) is unclear. Studies from the Mayo Clinic demonstrated that in low- and high-risk AGES categories local recurrence was higher after lobectomy than after total or near-total resection. Total thyroidectomy did not have better survival rates than near total thyroidectomy. It is suggested that subtotal resection on the side opposite the tumor decreases the chances of damage to the parathyroid and the recurrent laryngeal nerve. This argument is valid in the case of patients whose parathyroid glands are anteriorly located on the thyroid, so that some thyroid tissue is left to preserve the blood supply to the parathyroid glands. When the parathyroid glands are situated off the thyroid gland, there is little benefit in leaving thyroid tissue. In experienced hands the incidence of permanent hypoparathyroidism or nerve damage after total thyroidectomy is about 1 percent. Differentiation of the residual thyroid cancer to anaplastic carcinoma occurs in about 1 percent of patients and is almost always fatal.

Total thyroidectomy, by removing all residual normal thyroid tissue, facilitates the uptake of radioactive ^{131}I extrinsic to the gland and helps identify and ablate metastatic thyroid cancer. Once all thyroid tissue has been removed, thyroglobulin levels should remain below 3 ng/mL; by monitoring thyroglobulin levels, disease progress can be followed. When thyroglobulin levels increase, recurrent disease must be present and appropriate screening with ^{131}I should be done.

The patient with a thyroid nodule that is suspected to be papillary thyroid cancer should have FNAC performed. When papillary thyroid cancer is diagnosed, the definitive operation can be done without confirming the diagnosis on histologic examination. Patients with a nodule that might be papillary cancer should be treated by thyroid lobectomy, isthmectomy, and removal of any pyramidal lobe or adjacent lymph nodes. When intraoperative frozen-section examination of a lymph node or of the primary tumor confirms carcinoma, completion total or near-total thyroidectomy should be performed. If a definitive diagnosis cannot be made, the operation is terminated. When final histology confirms carcinoma, completion total thyroidectomy usually should be performed. For patients who have minimal papillary thyroid cancers confined to the thyroid gland without angioinvasion, no further operative treatment is recommended. Treatment with thyroid hormone to suppress TSH is recommended. Patients at low risk should have serum TSH levels between 0.1 and 1.0 μU/mL, whereas patients at high risk should have serum TSH levels suppressed to less than 0.1 μU/mL.

Local recurrence is a serious complication, with a disease-related mortality rate of 33 to 50 percent. Patients with nodal recurrence usually do better than those with tumor recurrence in the thyroid bed or with distant metastases. Lymph node metastases in the lateral neck in patients with papillary carcinoma usually should be managed with modified radical neck dissection, and en-bloc dissection of all fibrofatty tissue and lymphatic tissue. The jugular lymph node chain is removed, while preserving the sternocleidomastoid muscle, the internal jugular vein, and the spinal accessory nerve (which are all taken in a radical dissection). Dissection of the posterior triangle and suprahyoid dissection usually are not necessary but should be performed when appropriate. Prophylactic neck node dissection is not necessary in patients with papillary thyroid cancer, because micrometastases appear to be ablated with radioiodine therapy. Survival rates for the different treatment modalities are summarized in Fig. 36-26.

Follicular Carcinoma

Follicular carcinoma, which accounts for about 10 percent of thyroid malignancies, is decreasing in incidence in the United States. This cancer occurs more often in women, with a female-to-male ratio of 3:1, and it presents in an older age group, mean age at presentation of 50 years, compared to a mean age of 35 in patients with papillary carcinoma. Follicular carcinoma occurs more frequently in iodine-deficient areas, and a rare form of familial disease is reported in patients with dyshormonogenesis.

Pathology. Follicular carcinoma usually is solitary and approximately 90 percent are surrounded by a tumor capsule. Follicular carcinoma differs from papillary carcinoma in that vascular invasion and hematogenous spread to bone, lung, and liver is seen more commonly than lymphatic spread, which usually is encountered in late stages. Lymph node metastases occur in less than 10 percent of patients. Histologically, follicles are present, but the lumen may be devoid of colloid. Architectural patterns depend on the degree of differentiation demonstrated by the tumor.

Two types of follicular carcinoma are recognized. In *minimally invasive tumors* there is evidence of invasion into but not through the tumor capsule at one or more spots. Previously, these tumors may have been reported as *atypical adenomas,* although there are reports of metastases occurring, and they should be regarded as low-grade carcinomas. In the second type, *frankly invasive tumors,* there is evidence of vascular invasion or tumor invasion through the tumor capsule. Tumor infiltration and invasion may be apparent at surgery, with tumor thrombus in the middle thyroid or jugular veins.

Clinical Manifestations. Follicular cancers usually present as solitary thyroid nodules, occasionally with a history of rapid size increase, and long-standing goiter. When hemorrhage into the nodule has occurred, pain may be a presenting feature, but usually the tumors are painless. At initial presentation cervical lymphadenopathy is uncommon, although distant metastases are more frequently encountered than papillary carcinoma. Rarely, follicular cancers may be hyperfunctioning (1 percent), and patients may present with signs and symptoms of thyrotoxicosis.

Unless distant metastases have been confirmed as follicular thyroid cancer, definitive preoperative diagnosis usually is not possible in follicular thyroid carcinoma. This is because FNAC is unable to distinguish between follicular cells from a benign follicular adenoma and from a carcinoma. Approximately 20

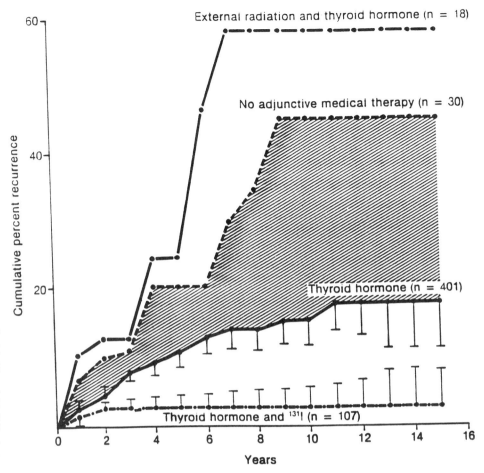

FIG. 36-26. Cumulative recurrence rates of papillary thyroid cancer in patients when follow-up was 1 year or longer, separated by type of medical treatment used postoperatively. Shaded area represents difference resulting from treatment with thyroid hormone. (From: *Mazzaferri EL, Young RL, et al: Papillary thyroid carcinoma: the impact of therapy in 576 patients. Medicine (Baltimore) 56:171, 1977, with permission.*)

percent of all FNAC aspirates showing follicular cells are carcinomas; the remaining 80 percent are adenomas.

Surgical Treatment and Prognosis. Patients diagnosed by FNAC as having a follicular lesion should undergo thyroid lobectomy, including the isthmus and the pyramidal lobe. Intraoperative frozen-section examination usually is not helpful but should be performed when there is evidence of capsular or vascular invasion or when adjacent lymphadenopathy is present. Total thyroidectomy should be performed when thyroid cancer is diagnosed, except in patients with minimally invasive follicular cancers because the prognosis in these patients is so good. In older patients, when follicular neoplasms diagnosed by FNAC are greater than 4 cm and macroscopically suspicious for cancer, some surgeons proceed with total thyroidectomy, because the risk of cancer is about 50 percent. A diagnosis of invasive carcinoma necessitates completion total thyroidectomy primarily so that ^{131}I can be used to detect and ablate metastatic disease. Prophylactic nodal dissection is unwarranted because nodal involvement is infrequent, but therapeutic neck dissection is recommended.

The cumulative percentage of patient mortality from follicular thyroid cancer is about 15 percent at 10 years and 30 percent at 20 years. Factors that significantly worsen long-term prognosis are; age over 50 years at presentation, tumor size greater than 4 cm, higher tumor grade, marked vascular invasion, extra-

thyroidal invasion, and distant metastases at the time of diagnosis.

Hürthle Cell Carcinoma

Hürthle cell tumors are considered by the World Health Organization classification to be a variant of follicular cell neoplasms. Tumors contain sheets of eosinophilic cells packed with mitochondria. They are derived from the oxyphilic cells of the thyroid gland, and although the function of the cells is unknown, Hürthle cell tumors possess TSH receptors and produce thyroglobulin. Only about 10 percent of these tumors trap radioiodine.

Hürthle cell carcinomas account for approximately 3 percent of thyroid malignancies. They differ from follicular carcinoma in that they are more often multifocal and bilateral, are more likely to metastasize to local nodes (25 percent), and usually do not take up [131]I. Hürthle cell neoplasms usually are diagnosed by FNAC, and about 20 percent of these tumors are found to be malignant. There is controversy as to whether all Hürthle cell neoplasms are malignant. Grant and colleagues reported that the mortality rate was less than 1 percent of 642 patients with Hürthle cell adenoma. Adenomas, as in follicular neoplasms, have no vascular or capsular invasion, whereas cancers do have vascular or capsular invasion.

Management is similar to that of follicular neoplasms, with lobectomy, isthmectomy, and pyramidal lobe resection being sufficient surgical treatment for unilateral Hürthle cell adenomas. When Hürthle cell neoplasms are found to be invasive on intraoperative frozen-section or definitive paraffin-section histology, then total thyroidectomy should be performed. These patients should also undergo routine central neck node removal, similar to patients with medullary thyroid cancer, and modified radical neck dissection when lateral neck nodes are palpable. T$_4$ treatment is recommended postoperatively.

Although radioiodine scanning and ablation usually are ineffective, they probably should be considered to ablate any residual normal thyroid tissue and occasionally ablate tumor, since there is no other good therapy. ^{99m}Tc-sestamibi scanning has been reported to be useful for detecting persistent local or metastatic disease. The mortality rate from Hürthle cell cancer is higher than from follicular thyroid cancer.

Medullary Carcinoma

Medullary thyroid cancer (MTC) accounts for about 5 percent of thyroid carcinomas. Although MTC was originally classified as an anaplastic tumor, Hazard and associates recognized that it was a separate entity, because patients survived longer than they did with anaplastic carcinoma. Williams determined that medullary thyroid cancer arose from the parafollicular or C cells of the thyroid. These cells are neuroectodermal and originate from the ultimobranchial bodies of the fourth and fifth branchial pouches. They descend to join the thyroid gland proper and are concentrated mainly in the superior poles laterally. This also is where C-cell hyperplasia is most evident and where medullary thyroid cancers develop. Pearse demonstrated the ability of the C cells or parafollicular cells to secrete calcitonin, a 32-amino-acid polypeptide that has an opposing action to parathyroid hormone (PTH) in that it is an antihypercalcemic hormone and lowers serum calcium levels. In some animals, especially those that lay eggs with shells, calcitonin is a significant regulator of calcium metabolism, but in human beings it has only minimal physiologic effects.

In 1966 Sipple described a postmortem case in which thyroid cancer, hyperplastic parathyroid glands, and pheochromocytoma coexisted; additional review of 500 cases of pheochromocytoma showed thyroid cancer to be six to fourteen times more frequently associated with this condition than expected. Since these initial observations, families have been identified whose members have only MTC; have MTC, hyperparathyroidism, and pheochromocytoma (MEN IIA or Sipple's syndrome), and patients with MTC, pheochromocytoma, ganglioneuromatosis, and Marfan's syndrome (MEN IIB). Patients with MEN IIA also may have Hirschsprung's disease and lichen cutaneous amyloidosis. Patients with von Hippel–Lindau disease also appear to be prone to developing pheochromocytoma and medullary thyroid cancer.

Pathology. Medullary carcinomas are located in the middle to upper thyroid poles (in keeping with the embryological origin of the C cells). Tumors typically are unilateral (75 percent). With familial cases, C-cell hyperplasia and multicentricity are prevalent, and 90 percent of the patients have bilateral tumors.

Microscopically, tumors are composed of sheets of infiltrating neoplastic cells separated by collagen and amyloid. Marked heterogeneity is present; cells may be polygonal or spindle-shaped. The presence of amyloid is a diagnostic finding, but immunohistochemistry for calcitonin has superseded it as a di-

agnostic tumor marker. C-cell hyperplasia is a premalignant precursor of MTC. These tumors also stain positively for carcinoembryonic antigen (CEA), histaminase, and calcitonin gene–related peptide (CGRP).

Tumors spread initially to local lymph nodes in the neck and the superior mediastinum. Distant blood-borne metastases to liver, bone (frequently osteoblastic), and lung usually arise later in the disease. Local invasion into the trachea and esophagus also occurs.

Clinical Manifestations. Patients with MTC usually present with a neck mass that may be associated with palpable cervical lymphadenopathy (15 to 20 percent). Local pain is more common in patients with these tumors, and local invasion may produce symptoms of dysphagia, dyspnea, or dysphonia. The female-to-male ratio is 1.5:1. About 70 percent of the patients have sporadic disease, and age at presentation typically is between 50 and 60 years, though patients with familial disease present at a younger age.

Tumors may secrete a variety of peptides including calcitonin, calcitonin gene–related peptide, CEA, histaminadases, prostaglandins E$_2$ and F$_2$-alpha, and serotonin. Patients with extensive metastatic disease frequently develop diarrhea, which can be debilitating. The reason for this is unclear, although increased intestinal motility, impaired intestinal water and electrolyte flux might be responsible.

Between 2 and 4 percent of patients with MTC develop Cushing's syndrome as a result of ectopic production of ACTH. Kidney stones occur in patients with primary hyperparathyroidism, and hypertension occurs in those with pheochromocytoma.

Diagnosis. Diagnosis of MTC is established by history, physical examination, raised serum calcitonin or CEA levels, and FNAC of the thyroid mass. Attention to family history is important. Since it is not possible to distinguish sporadic from familial disease at initial presentation, all new patients with MTC should be screened for RET point mutations and for pheochromocytoma by measuring 24-h urinary levels of vanillylmandelic acid (VMA), catecholamine, and metanephrine. Serum calcium level also should be observed. A coexisting pheochromocytoma should be ruled out, because operation on a patient with an undiagnosed pheochromocytoma can result in a hypertensive crisis and death.

Familial Disease. MTC is sporadic (70 percent of new cases) or familial (30 percent of new cases). Familial MTC occurs as MEN IIA, as MEN IIB, or as familial MTC without other endocrinopathies. It also may occur in association with papillary thyroid cancer.

MEN IIA. These patients have a syndrome characterized by MTC, pheochromocytoma, or adrenal medullary hyperplasia and hyperparathyroidism. C-cell hyperplasia is present in all of them and normally is detectable by screening before the development of pheochromocytoma. Bilateral pheochromocytomas are detectable in more than 50 percent of the patients with the syndrome and occasionally is the presenting feature. Hyperparathyroidism (25 percent), Hirschsprung's disease, and cutaneous amyloidosis are present in some patients.

MEN IIB. MTC, bilateral pheochromocytomas, and ganglioneuromas affecting mucosal surfaces are found in patients with this condition. Patients have a characteristic facies with a thickened tongue and lips (Fig. 36-27). Marfanoid features, slipped

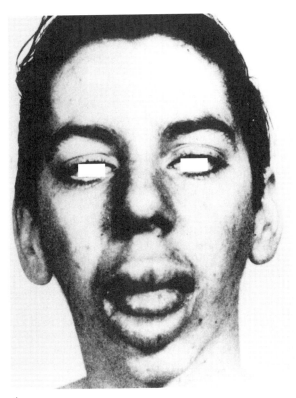

A

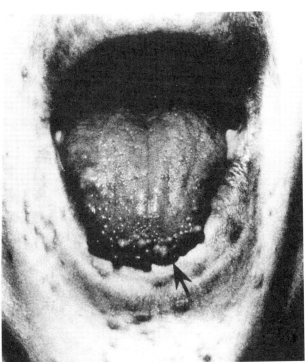

B

FIG. 36-27. Patients with MEN IIB have characteristic facies with *A.* marfanoid features and *B.* thickened lips, scalloping of the tongue, and mucosal ganglioneuromas.

epiphysis, and pectus excavatum also may occur. Patients with MEN IIB have the most aggressive medullary thyroid cancers; patients with familial MTC without other endocrinopathies have the least aggressive thyroid cancers.

Screening of patients with familial MTC for RET point mutations on chromosome 10 has replaced using provocation testing with pentagastrin or calcium-stimulated calcitonin levels to make the diagnosis. Calcitonin and CEA are used to identify patients with persistent or recurrent MTC. The specific phenotypes of MTC are also associated with specific RET mutations (familial MTC, 768 and 804; MEN IIA, 609, 611, 618, 620, and 634; MEN IIB, 918).

Treatment. Most clinicians agree that total thyroidectomy is the treatment of choice for patients with MTC because of the high incidence of multicentricity and the more aggressive course. Because tumors are of C-cell origin, radioiodine therapy and levothyroxine sodium TSH suppression therapy usually are not helpful. The central compartment nodes from carotid sheath to trachea frequently are involved early in the disease process and always should be meticulously cleared along with paratracheal nodes (central neck node dissection). In patients with palpable cervical nodes or involved central neck nodes, ipsilateral or bilateral, bilateral modified radical neck dissection is recommended. Similarly, patients with MTCs larger than 2 cm should undergo ipsilateral prophylactic modified radical neck dissection, because more than 60 percent of these patients have nodal metastases.

If superior mediastinal lymph nodes are noted at operation they also should be removed, although it is rarely necessary to perform a median sternotomy. Surgeons should be prepared to sacrifice the recurrent laryngeal nerve when it is involved in the tumor mass. Though this does not occur frequently, the possibility should be discussed with the patient preoperatively.

Tumor debulking in cases of metastatic disease or local recurrence should be undertaken. This frequently ameliorates symptoms of flushing and diarrhea, and it helps in decreasing the risk of death resulting from recurrent central neck disease.

External-beam radiotherapy for patients with tumors at resection margins or unresectable tumors is controversial. It is recommended for patients with unresectable residual or recurrent tumor, although the results are debatable. There is no effective chemotherapy regimen.

When patients have associated conditions such as pheochromocytoma or hyperparathyroidism, these conditions also require careful evaluation. Pheochromocytomas should be operated on first, before thyroidectomy is performed. In most cases pheochromocytomas can be removed laparoscopically. In patients who have hypercalcemia at the time of thyroidectomy, the parathyroid glands should be identified and, when abnormal, selectively removed. In patients with normocalcemia, efforts should be made to preserve the parathyroid glands, which should be marked with a stitch or clip in patients with MEN IIA. When a normal parathyroid cannot be maintained on a vascular pedicle, it should be removed, biopsied to confirm that it is a parathyroid, and then autotransplanted to the forearm of the nondominant arm.

Postoperative Follow-up and Prognosis. Patients should be assessed at regular postoperative intervals, and serum calcitonin and CEA levels should be monitored regularly. Calcitonin level is more sensitive for detecting persistent or recurrent disease, and CEA for predicting outcome. In a study of 123 patients with MTC, Russell and colleagues reported that 67 percent of the patients whose MTC was confined to the thyroid were clinically and biochemically (calcitonin) free of disease (mean follow-up time 5.5 years), compared to only 8 percent of patients who had extrathyroidal spread. A later paper from the same group reported on 31 patients who, despite having adequate primary operations for MTC, had persistently raised calcitonin levels. The 5- and 10-year survival rates for these patients were 90 percent and 86 percent, respectively, with only two patients dying from MTC. Postoperatively raised calcitonin levels are frequently encountered and are a cause for concern signaling the need for evaluation.

When recurrent or metastatic MTC is suspected and suggested by rising calcitonin levels, localization studies for occult or clinically apparent disease should be used. The investigative tools available include CT, MRI of the neck and mediastinum, ultrasound examination, and selective venous catheterization (with calcitonin assay), including hepatic vein and jugular sampling after pentagastrin stimulation. An increase in the hepatic veins before an increase in the cervical veins indicates hepatic metastases. Nuclear imaging studies with ^{131}I metaiodobenzyl-guanidine (MIBG), dimercaptosuccinic acid (DMSA), and ^{99m}Tc-sestamibi all have been used but are only occasionally helpful. Positron-emission tomography (PET) scanning appears to be useful in selected patients. Some clinicians examine the liver laparoscopically to rule out liver metastases.

Ultimately prognosis is related to disease stage. The 10-year survival rate is approximately 80 percent, and only 45 percent in those patients with lymph node involvement. Survival also is significantly influenced by disease type. It is best in patients with familial non-MEN medullary thyroid cancer, followed by those with MEN IIA, then those with sporadic disease, and it is worst in patients with MEN IIB. Patients with tumors that stain poorly for calcitonin and with a heterogeneous antibody uptake do worse than patients in whom calcitonin staining is increased and homogeneous.

With the identification and localization to chromosome 10 of the gene that causes MTC, it is now possible to screen family members and identify children at risk of developing MTC. Performing thyroidectomy at the C-cell-hyperplasia stage or before, after the age of 5 years, will prevent MTC and improve survival rates. Patients with MEN IIA and MEN IIB are at risk for pheochromocytoma.

Anaplastic Carcinoma

This tumor is one of the most aggressive malignancies, with few patients surviving 6 months beyond diagnosis. The incidence of anaplastic carcinoma has dropped to about 1 percent of thyroid carcinomas in the United States. The decrease in incidence is probably a result of the decrease in iodine-deficient (endemic) goiter, which was a precursor for this condition. Most anaplastic carcinomas arise from differentiated thyroid cancers. There is a female-to-male ratio of 1.5:1, and the majority of tumors present in the seventh and eighth decade of life. Presentation before the age of 50 years is rare.

Pathology.   Tumor growth is extremely rapid, with macroscopic invasion of surrounding tissues. Lymph node involvement frequently is present. Microscopically, sheets of cells are seen, with marked heterogeneity. Cells may be spindle-shaped, polygonal, or large, multinucleated cells. Foci of more differentiated cells may be seen, either follicular or papillary in pattern. Anaplastic tumors originally described as small-cell are recognized to be lymphomas or less commonly medullary carcinomas of the thyroid gland and should be treated as such.

Clinical Manifestations.   Patients typically are elderly females with a history of a lump in the neck that has been present for some time before rapidly enlarging and becoming painful. Associated symptoms such as dysphonia, dysphagia, and dyspnea are common. The tumor is hard and may be fixed to surrounding structures or may be ulcerated (Fig. 36-28). Lymph nodes usually are palpable at presentation. Evidence of metastatic spread also may be present. Diagnosis is confirmed by FNAC revealing characteristic giant and multinucleated cells. Incisional biopsy to confirm the diagnosis rarely is necessary.

Treatment.   All forms of treatment have been disappointing. Tennvall and colleagues reported on 33 patients treated prospectively over an 8-year period with initial hyperfractionated radiotherapy with doxorubicin, then debulking thyroidectomy, followed by completion of radiotherapy and chemotherapy. Using this regimen, only four patients (12 percent) survived more than 2 years, and few patients died of suffocation because of central neck disease. Although the overall survival rate remains very poor, this treatment is recommended until better treatment results are documented.

Lymphoma

Approximately 1 percent of thyroid malignancies are lymphomas, and most of the primary thyroid lesions are of the non-Hodgkin's B-cell type. Although the disease can arise as part of a generalized lymphomatous condition, most thyroid lymphomas develop in patients with chronic lymphocytic thyroiditis (Hashimoto's thyroiditis). Chronic antigenic lymphocyte stimulation has been suggested to result in lymphocyte transformation.

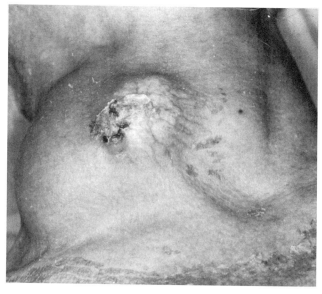

FIG. 36-28.   *Anaplastic thyroid cancer adherent to surrounding structures and ulcerating through the overlying skin.*

Patients usually present with symptoms similar to those of patients with anaplastic carcinoma, although the rapidly enlarging neck mass often is painless. Because there is frequently co-existing Hashimoto's thyroiditis, patients may be clinically hypothyroid or may already be receiving thyroxine treatment. Most patients presenting with thyroid lymphoma are elderly women. The diagnosis usually is suggested by FNAC, although needle-core or open biopsy may be necessary for definitive diagnosis. When nodal dissection is being performed, taking a biopsy sample of lymph node often helps to clarify the diagnosis.

Patients with thyroid lymphoma usually respond rapidly to chemotherapy (CHOP—cyclophosphamide, doxorubicin, vincristine, and prednisone), and combined treatment with radiotherapy and chemotherapy is often recommended. Thyroidectomy and nodal resection are used to alleviate symptoms of airway obstruction in patients who do not respond quickly to chemotherapy or chemotherapy and radiotherapy.

Prognosis depends on the histologic grade of the tumor and whether the lymphoma is confined to the thyroid gland or is disseminated. The overall 5-year survival rate is about 50 percent; patients with extrathyroidal disease have markedly lower survival rate compared to those with intrathyroidal disease—40 percent versus 85 percent. Although there are no prospective studies, similar remission rates have been reported for patients who underwent diagnostic biopsy plus adjuvant therapy alone (85 percent), compared to debulking surgery plus adjuvant therapy. These findings support the argument for chemotherapy and radiotherapy for most patients.

Metastatic Carcinoma

The thyroid gland is a rare site of metastases from other cancers, including kidney, breast, lung, and melanoma; the most common metastatic tumor to the thyroid is hypernephroma. Approximately 3 percent of bronchogenic carcinomas metastasize to the thyroid, and these metastases account for 20 percent of secondary metastases to the thyroid.

Clinical examination and the history often suggest the source of the metastatic disease, and FNAC usually provides definitive diagnosis. Resection of the thyroid, usually lobectomy, may alleviate symptoms in symptomatic cases.

SURGERY OF THE THYROID

Patients who have had any change in voice or any previous neck surgery should have a preoperative vocal cord assessment, by direct or indirect laryngoscopy. Patients should be euthyroid at operation. On the operating table, a sandbag should be placed between the patient's shoulder blades, the head supported by a ring, and the neck extended to provide optimal exposure.

Operative Technique. A Kocher transverse collar incision is sited in a skin crease about 1 cm below the cricoid cartilage and carried through the platysma muscle (Fig. 36-29). The length of the incision varies, typically around 5 cm, and it should be symmetrical. Longer incisions are necessary in patients with larger tumors, in patients with a short, fat neck or whose neck cannot be extended, and in patients with low-lying thyroid glands. The upper flap is dissected in an avascular subplatysmal plane anterior to the anterior jugular veins and deep to the platysma muscle, to the level of the thyroid cartilage. The lower flap is then mobilized in a similar manner, to the suprasternal

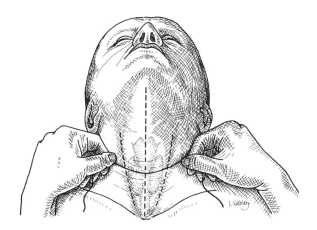

FIG. 36-29. Technique for marking the neck skin incision for thyroidectomy. The center of the incision should be placed 1 cm caudal to the cricoid cartilage and should conform to normal skin lines. (From: *Clark OH, Endocrine Surgery of the Thyroid and Parathyroid Glands. St Louis, CV Mosby, 1985, with permission.*)

notch. Skin towels and a self-retaining retractor are applied. Meticulous hemostasis in thyroidectomy facilitates the identification of the parathyroid glands and the recurrent laryngeal nerves, reducing the possibility of inadvertent damage.

The thyroid gland is exposed via a midline incision through the superficial layer of the deep cervical fascia between the sternohyoid and sternothyroid muscles (Fig. 36-30). Care should be taken not to disrupt the veins on the thyroid surface. On the side to be dissected first, the more superficial sternohyoid muscle is separated from the deeper sternothyroid muscle by blunt dissection. The dissection proceeds laterally until the ansa cervicalis

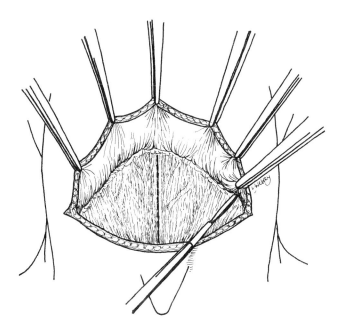

FIG. 36-30. The upper flap is dissected in an avascular subplatysmal plane and the thyroid gland is exposed via a midline incision through the superficial layer of the deep cervical fascia. (From: *Clark OH, Endocrine Surgery of the Thyroid and Parathyroid Glands. St Louis, CV Mosby, 1985, with permission.*)

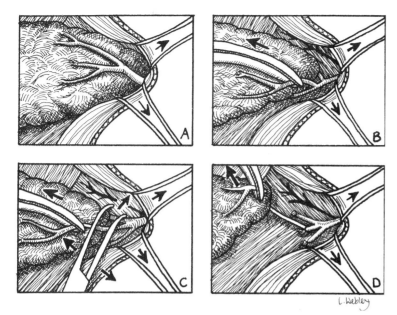

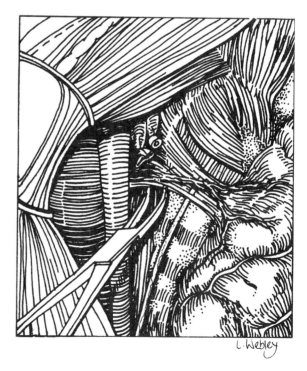

FIG. 36-31. Dissection of the upper thyroid pole should be close to the thyroid to avoid possible injury to the external branch of the superior laryngeal nerve as it runs over the cricothyroid muscle. Superior pole vessels are dissected, ligated, and divided on the thyroid gland to avoid injury to the nerve. (Modified from: *Lennquist S, et al: The superior laryngeal nerve in thyroid surgery. Surgery 102:999, 1987, with permission.*)

is noted on the lateral edge of the sternohyoid muscle and the medial aspect of the internal jugular vein. The deeper sternothyroid muscle is dissected free from the thyroid gland by blunt or sharp dissection, exposing the middle thyroid vein or veins laterally. The thyroid lobe is retracted anteromedially by finger traction and the lateral tissues swept posterolaterally by a pledget. The middle thyroid veins are divided and ligated. In rare cases the strap muscles must be divided in order to gain access to a large thyroid tumor. When this maneuver is necessary, the muscles should be divided high so that innervation from the ansa hypoglossal nerve is preserved. Occasionally a thyroid cancer invades the strap muscles; in this situation the involved muscles should be removed en bloc with the thyroid.

The superior thyroid pole is identified by retracting the thyroid inferiorly and medially. The tissues lateral to the upper pole of the thyroid and medial to the carotid sheath can be mobilized quickly by blunt dissection, because there are no nerves in that region. The upper pole of the thyroid is then mobilized caudally and laterally. The dissection plane should be close to the thyroid to avoid possible injury to the external branch of the superior laryngeal nerve. An effort should be made to identify and preserve the branch of the external laryngeal nerve that supplies the cricothyroid muscle. The branch is visible in about 80 percent of patients on the cricothyroid muscle (Fig. 36-31). The superior pole vessels are then individually identified, skeletonized, and doubly ligated low on the thyroid gland.

When the superior pole vessels have been ligated and divided, the tissues posterolateral to the superior pole can be swept away from the thyroid gland in a posteromedial direction. The direction is important because it reduces the chances of damaging the vessels supplying the upper parathyroid glands. The recurrent laryngeal nerves enter the larynx at the level of the cricoid cartilage, passing under or through Berry's ligament and entering the larynx deep to the cricothyroid muscle (Fig. 36-32).

At this point it should be possible to identify the upper parathyroid gland. The upper gland usually is situated at the level of the cricoid cartilage. The lower parathyroid gland is found most commonly just below where the inferior thyroid artery and re-

current laryngeal nerve cross. In approximately 80 percent of patients the glands are located within 1 cm of the artery. The lower parathyroid gland usually is situated anterior to the recurrent laryngeal nerve, and when it is not, it is usually located in the thymus or in parathymic fat (Fig. 36-33).

The thyroid is completely mobilized by gently sweeping dorsally all tissue along the posterolateral border away from the

FIG. 36-32. The recurrent laryngeal nerve runs through the posterior superior suspensory ligament of the thyroid (Berry's ligament) before entering the cricothyroid muscle. An artery and vein are always present in this area. (From: *Clark OH, Endocrine Surgery of the Thyroid and Parathyroid Glands. St Louis, CV Mosby, 1985, with permission.*)

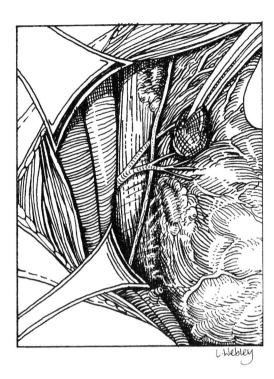

FIG. 36-33. *The parathyroid glands usually are located within 1 cm of the inferior thyroid artery (80 percent), and the inferior parathyroid gland usually is located just below where the artery and the recurrent laryngeal nerve cross. (From:* Clark OH, Endocrine Surgery of the Thyroid and Parathyroid Glands. *St Louis, CV Mosby, 1985, with permission.)*

thyroid. All vessels are ligated and divided on the thyroid capsule to minimize the possibility of devascularizing the parathyroids. No tissue should be clamped or divided that might be or contain a recurrent laryngeal nerve.

Parathyroids that are ischemic, or are situated very anteriorly on the thyroid gland, or have been removed along with the thyroid lobe, should be examined after removal. They should be biopsied and confirmed by frozen-section examination, minced into 1-mm cubed pieces, and implanted into a small pocket in the ipsilateral sternohyoid muscle, with a silk suture or clip marking the site.

The recurrent laryngeal nerves should be identified; the nerve is located more medially on the left and runs more obliquely on the right. The most difficult part of the operation usually is during the dissection where the recurrent nerve passes through Berry's ligament. It is here that the nerve is in close proximity to the thyroid, tethered down by the ligament, through which runs a small artery, and it is here that the nerve is most commonly injured. If bleeding occurs at this site it should be controlled by gentle pressure before identification of the nerve to avoid injury, and then the vessels are all ligated. Use of electrocautery to control bleeding should be strictly avoided.

A pyramidal lobe is present in about 80 percent of patients and should be dissected free superiorly to the level of the thyroid cartilage or higher and removed in continuity with the thyroid lobe and the isthmus. One or more lymph nodes are often present just cephalad to the isthmus of the thyroid gland (Delphian node) and should be removed with the thyroid.

When lobectomy is performed, the isthmus is divided flush with the contralateral gland and oversewn. When total thyroidectomy is performed, the same procedure is followed on the contralateral side. If a subtotal thyroidectomy is being performed (for Graves' disease or multinodular goiter), normal practice is to perform a total lobectomy on one side and a subtotal lobectomy on the other side. Removing all thyroid tissue on one side has the advantage of obviating the need to reoperate on one side in cases in which reoperation may be necessary, and the possibility of damage to the recurrent laryngeal nerve and parathyroid on that side during future procedures is reduced.

Subtotal lobectomy is achieved in a similar fashion to lobectomy, but after division of the superior thyroid pole, arterial clamps are placed along the length of the lobe, anterior to the insertion of the inferior thyroid artery, usually leaving approximately 1 to 2 cm^3 (4 to 8 g) of thyroid tissue. The thyroid is oversewn and secured to the lateral tracheal fascia to encourage hemostasis. Suction drains rarely are necessary. They can be used when there is a large space, e.g., after removing a large substernal goiter. Strap muscles are reapproximated with absorbable sutures, as is the platysma, and the skin is closed with subcuticular sutures or clips.

Surgical Removal of Intrathoracic Goiter

In 99 percent of the patients, intrathoracic goiter can be removed via a collar incision in the neck rather than resorting to a sternotomy. Patients with substernal goiters who have had previous thyroid operations, some with invasive malignant tumors, and patients with no thyroid tissue in the neck may require a median sternotomy.

Vascular connections in the neck are identified, ligated, and divided. The superior pole vessels and the middle thyroid veins are identified and ligated first. Dividing the isthmus may help with subsequent mobilization of the substernal goiter from beneath the sternum.

Several large 1-0 or 00 sutures are placed deeply into the goiter, and through a combination of traction and blunt dissection the thyroid usually can be delivered into the neck from its substernal location. In patients with a very large colloid goiter, the colloid occasionally may be evacuated to permit delivery, but this maneuver usually is unnecessary, and it is contraindicated if cancer is present. Although 1 percent of goiters contain cancer, the frequency of cancer in substernal goiter is as high as 10 percent in some series.

In approximately 1 percent of patients, part or all of the thyroid gland is intrathoracic. This usually is a consequence of extension or migration of the thyroid into the mediastinum rather than aberrant glandular tissue. The blood supply usually originates in the neck rather than the mediastinum. These goiters are more difficult to remove because it is difficult to apply traction.

Substernal goiters occasionally are too large to deliver via a neck incision, and a sternotomy is required. In patients in whom thyroid cancer is suspected or demonstrated in an intrathoracic gland, attempts should be made to avoid rupture of the thyroid capsule.

Because the blood supply to the thyroid gland, thymus gland, and lower parathyroids primarily is derived from the inferior thyroid arteries in the neck, median sternotomy usually is unnecessary. Sternotomy is indicated in patients in whom the intrathoracic gland is cancerous and mediastinal node involvement or metastatic cancer deep in the mediastinum has been demonstrated by scanning. When sternotomy is indicated, the sternum usually should be divided to the level of the third intercostal space and then laterally on one side at the space between the third and fourth ribs (Fig. 36-34). Median sternotomy provides excellent exposure of the upper mediastinum and lower neck.

Neck Dissection for Nodal Metastases

Lymph nodes in the central compartment (medial to the carotid sheath) are frequently involved in metastatic spread in patients with papillary, medullary, and Hürthle cell carcinomas. In these patients all central neck nodes should be removed at the time of the primary procedure, preserving the recurrent laryngeal nerves and, when possible, the parathyroid glands, autotransplanting them when necessary, after histologic confirmation, into the sternocleidomastoid muscle. Removal of all central nodes is important in patients with medullary and Hürthle cell carcinoma because of the high frequency of microscopic tumor spread and because these tumors do not take up radioiodine and cannot be ablated with ^{131}I.

In patients with thyroid cancer with palpable cervical lymph nodes or in cases of medullary carcinoma when the thyroid lesion is larger than 2 cm, a modified radical neck dissection usually should be performed. This operation is possible via extension of the collar incision laterally to the anterior margin of the trapezius muscle (MacFee incision). The internal jugular vein, the spinal accessory nerve, and the sternocleidomastoid muscle are preserved unless they are invaded or adhered to tumor. During dissection all tissue in the anterior triangle of the neck from the hyoid bone to the clavicle is removed. Dissection along the spinal accessory nerve is most important because this is a frequent site of metastatic disease. The deep dissection plane is the anterior scalenus muscle, the brachial plexus, and the medial scalenus muscle. The phrenic nerve is preserved on the scalenus anterior muscle, as are the cervical sensory nerves in most patients.

Complications of Thyroid Surgery

The mortality rate from thyroidectomy is low. In two large series, Gould and colleagues reported no mortality in more than 1000 consecutive patients. Similarly, Colcock reported no deaths in his personal series after 1954. Morbidity is approximately 13 percent. Serious morbidity occurs in fewer than 2 percent of patients. Complications specifically attributable to thyroidectomy include nerve damage or respiratory problems, bleeding with hematoma formation, hypoparathyroidism, wound infection, keloid formation, and, rarely, thyroid storm.

Injury of the Recurrent Laryngeal Nerve. Permanent recurrent laryngeal nerve injury is a relatively uncommon event, with a rate of approximately 1 percent; the rate is probably lower in patients with benign disease and higher in patients with large, invasive, or recurrent thyroid carcinomas. Injuries may be temporary, caused by traction or stretching of the nerve, or permanent, caused by division or ligation of the nerve. Injuries may be unilateral or bilateral. Recurrent laryngeal nerve injury leads to vocal cord paralysis, with the vocal cord assuming a paramedian position. In cases of bilateral nerve damage, the cords may obstruct the airway and lead to acute respiratory distress immediately after extubation. Reintubation and, occasionally, subsequent tracheostomy are needed. Unilateral nerve damage leads to paralysis of the ipsilateral vocal cord, with the cord lying in a paramedian position, usually resulting in a hoarse or husky voice. Because the nerve also is sensory to the larynx and because the vocal cords do not approximate, patients also describe choking and coughing when drinking fluids.

When damage is temporary, vocal cord function usually returns within 6 months, but it may take 1 year. When function has not returned by 6 to 12 months, injection lateral to the cord with Teflon mobilizes the cord to the midline and improves the voice. Occasionally the contralateral cord compensates and vocal cord paralysis may be unnoticed, so all patients should have direct or indirect laryngoscopy to evaluate vocal cord function before reoperation. Speech therapy also helps some patients with vocal cord dysfunction and should be done before Teflon injection.

Identification of the recurrent laryngeal nerves during surgery has been shown to decrease the incidence of permanent damage, although transient paralysis is more common. When nerves are not identified, transient paralysis is reduced, but the incidence of permanent damage is three or four times higher. Disease-specific risk factors for permanent nerve damage, in order of frequency, include recurrent thyroid cancer or recurrent goiter, thyroid cancer, large substernal goiters, chronic lymphocytic thyroiditis, Graves' disease, and euthyroid nodular goiter.

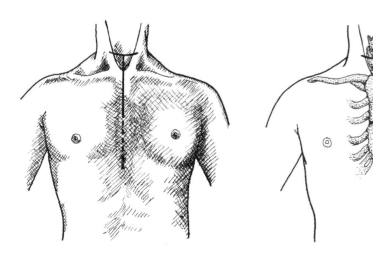

FIG. 36-34. Division of the sternum to the level of the third intercostal space usually is sufficient to provide exposure of the upper mediastinum and lower neck. When indicated, a full median sternotomy may be performed.

A rare cause of injury to a laryngeal nerve is that it is a nonrecurrent laryngeal nerve. This anomaly occurs in about 0.5 percent of patients and is almost always encountered on the right side. Awareness of this possibility reduces the risk of nerve injury when the recurrent nerve cannot be identified at the usual site.

Meticulous hemostasis, precise dissection between the thyroid capsule and sheath, and care dissecting Berry's ligament, where injuries are most likely to occur, all help to reduce the possibility of damage. The right recurrent laryngeal nerve takes a more oblique course in the neck as it loops around the subclavian artery, whereas the left recurrent laryngeal nerve loops around the ligamentum arteriosus and assumes a more midline position in the tracheoesophageal groove. Either nerve may branch before it enters the larynx posterior to the cricothyroid muscle at the level of the cricoid cartilage.

Injury of the External Branch of the Superior Laryngeal Nerve. Injury to the external laryngeal nerve results in difficulty shouting or singing high notes (the nerve is also called the "high note nerve"). The risk of injuring the nerve can be greatly reduced by retracting the strap muscles laterally to provide adequate visualization of the superior thyroid pole. A plane is opened by blunt dissection between the thyroid pole and the cricothyroid muscle bed. In about 80 percent of patients the nerve can be seen on the cricothyroid muscle. The superior thyroid vessels are individually ligated and divided low on the thyroid gland, rather than taken all together in one large bloc to avoid injury to the external laryngeal nerve. If these steps are followed, injury to the nerve is uncommon (2 percent).

Hypoparathyroidism. The chances of permanent hypoparathyroidism after thyroidectomy vary with the size and degree of invasion of the tumor, the type of pathology, the extent of the procedure, and the experience of the surgeon. Total thyroidectomy and central neck compartment clearance in medullary thyroid carcinoma has a higher incidence of subsequent hypoparathyroidism than does subtotal thyroidectomy for multinodular goiter (2 percent versus 0.5 percent), because all of the central neck fibroadipose and lymphatic tissue should be removed in patients with medullary carcinoma. After most operations the serum calcium level falls by about 1 mg/dL. Symptomatic postoperative hypoparathyroidism after thyroidectomy usually is transient and resolves in most cases within a few days without treatment and with calcium supplementation when treatment is necessary. When the serum phosphorus level is low or normal, there is less concern in the hypocalcemic patient than when it is high, because the latter suggests hypoparathyroidism.

In most instances, postoperative hypoparathyroidism is a result of parathyroid ischemia from bruising and partial interruption of parathyroid blood supply. This situation can be avoided by dissection along the thyroid capsule and gently teasing the parathyroid gland on a broad plane of tissue away from the thyroid gland in a posterolateral direction. This decreases the risk of disruption of the parathyroid blood supply, derived from the inferior and superior thyroid arteries. Hypoparathyroid patients usually exhibit early tingling and numbness around the lips, followed by the same sensation in the fingers. A positive Chvostek's sign (twitching of the lips after tapping over the facial nerve) is usually present. When hypocalcemia is not treated, patients may progress to carpopedal spasm. Symptoms occur when the calcium level falls below 8 mg/dL. Hypocalcemia also increases anxiety and respiratory alkalosis. Hyperventilation can cause tetany with or without associated hypocalcemia. Patients with postoperative hypocalcemia are treated initially with approximately 1 g of calcium every 4 h if symptomatic. When the serum calcium level remains low, intravenous calcium (1 to 10 ampoules of calcium gluconate or calcium chloride) can be given over several hours. Extravasation into the subcutaneous tissues can cause tissue necrosis. Treatment with calcitriol (Rocaltrol) 0.25 to 1.0 μg twice daily is occasionally necessary. In patients with persistent symptoms, the serum magnesium level should be evaluated.

Postoperative Management of Differentiated Thyroid Cancer

Thyroid Hormone. After thyroid surgery for carcinoma, patients should be placed on thyroxine. This is necessary as replacement therapy in patients who have undergone total thyroidectomy but has the additional effect of suppressing TSH and reducing the growth stimulus to any possible residual thyroid cancer cells. TSH suppression reduces tumor recurrence rates, particularly in patients with papillary cancer. Thyroxine should be administered to ensure that the patient remains euthyroid, with circulating TSH levels about 0.1 μU/L in low-risk patients or less than 0.1 μU/mL in high-risk patients.

Thyroglobulin Measurement. Thyroglobulin levels in patients who have undergone total thyroidectomy should be below 2 ng/mL when the patient is taking thyroxine, and below 3 ng/ml when the patient is not taking thyroxine. A thyroglobulin level above 3 ng/mL is highly suggestive of metastatic disease or persistent normal thyroid tissue, especially if it increases when TSH levels increase when thyroid hormone treatment is discontinued in preparation for radioiodine scanning. In this situation, radioiodine scan should be performed.

About 95 percent of patients with persistent or recurrent thyroid cancer of follicular cell origin will have thyroglobulin levels higher than 3 ng/mL. High-risk patients should also have a CT or MRI scan of the neck and mediastinum for early detection of any persistent or recurrent disease.

Radioiodine Therapy. Metastatic differentiated thyroid carcinoma can be detected and treated by radioactive iodine in about 75 percent of patients. Screening and treatment are facilitated by the removal of all normal thyroid tissue, which effectively competes for iodine uptake and is the most compelling of arguments in favor of total thyroidectomy for differentiated thyroid carcinoma. Radioiodine is more effective in young patients, even with occult pulmonary metastases, and less effective in older patients with less well differentiated thyroid cancers.

Most follicular carcinomas concentrate iodine. One exception is the Hürthle cell carcinomas, of which only about 10 percent take up iodine. Screening with radioactive iodine is a more sensitive test of metastatic disease than chest x-ray or CT but less sensitive than serum thyroglobulin determination. Micrometastases in the chest are detectable by radioiodine scanning even when chest x-rays show no evidence of disease. Approximately 75 percent of these patients have been successfully treated after receiving ablative doses of ^{131}I for micrometastases, especially when total thyroidectomy has been performed. The success rate of treating macro–pulmonary metastases with ^{131}I is less than 10 percent. TSH suppression with thyroxine after treatment with ^{131}I should be used.

Radioactive iodine scanning and treatment follow a standard protocol after initial or completion total thyroidectomy. Patients should have their levothyroxine therapy discontinued for approximately 8 weeks before the scanning with ^{131}I. During the first 6 weeks of this time they are given a synthetic triiodothyronine (T_3); this decreases the period (and discomfort) of hypothyroidism, because T_3 has a half-life of about 1 day, whereas T_4 has a half-life of about 1 week. The T_3 is then discontinued for remaining 2 weeks, which allows TSH levels to rise. A low-iodine diet also is recommended during these 2 weeks immediately before scanning.

In most centers, a screening dose of about 2 mCi of ^{131}I is administered and the uptake is measured at 24 h. The uptake in most patients should be less than 1 percent, with no "hot" spots in the neck or elsewhere (remnant normal thyroid or metastases). The most frequent cause of a hot spot in the neck after initial screening is residual thyroid tissue in the thyroid bed. If there is significant uptake (>1 percent), then a therapeutic dose of ^{131}I, 30 to 50 mCi in low-risk patients and 100 to 200 mCi in high-risk patients, is recommended. Some physicians omit the scanning dose of ^{131}I for patients who are thyroglobulin positive, especially if the thyroglobulin level increases when the patient is hypothyroid in preparation for scanning or treatment. For these patients a scan should be performed 5 to 7 days after the treatment dose; about one-third will become thyroglobulin and radioiodine-uptake negative, which documents a therapeutic benefit.

After scanning and treatment, patients are placed again on levothyroxine (normal dose is about 125 μg/day) and observed over follow-up with serum thyroglobulin determinations and physical examination at regular intervals. Patients with previously positive scans and patients with serum thyroglobulin levels over 3 ng/mL usually need another ^{131}I treatment after 6 to 12 months. The maximum dose of radioiodine that can be administered at one time is approximately 200 mCi with a cumulative dose of 1000 mCi.

External Beam Radiotherapy and Chemotherapy. External beam radiotherapy is required occasionally to control unresectable locally invasive or recurrent disease. It also is of value for the treatment and control of pain from bony metastases when there is no appreciable radioiodine uptake.

Multidrug chemotherapy and adriamycin have been used with little success in disseminated thyroid cancer; remission sometimes occurs, but cure is rare. Taxol has been reported recently to be of some value in patients with incurable disease.

Parathyroid

Jon A. van Heerden and David R. Farley

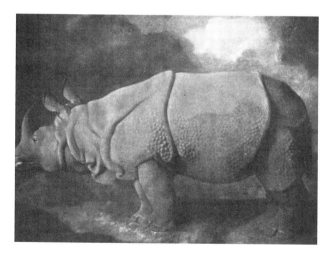

FIG. 36-35. Indian rhinoceros in the London Zoological Gardens, 1849.

HISTORICAL BACKGROUND

In 1849 Sir Richard Owen, curator of the London Zoological Gardens, performed an autopsy on a rhinoceros that had been given to the London Zoo by the government of India (Fig. 36-35). Owen's original description of the mysterious structures he found within the neck of the rhinoceros remains an accurate assessment of the normal parathyroid gland—"a small, yellow, glandular body . . . attached to the thyroid at the point where the veins emerge." In 1879 Anton Wölfer documented the relationship between total thyroidectomy and the ensuing tetany in the first such patient operated on by C.A. Theodor Billroth. The first description of the parathyroid glands in human beings was that by Ivar Sandström, a medical student in Uppsala, Sweden, in 1880 (Fig. 36-36). He suggested that these glands be named the *glandulae parathyroideae*. The function of these structures was unknown at that time.

Friedrich von Recklinghausen, in 1891, described the fibrocystic disease of bone produced by hyperparathyroidism. The first association of hyperparathyroidism with osteitis fibrosa cystica (von Recklinghausen's disease) was made by Askanazy in

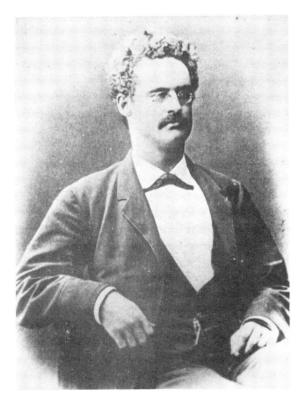

FIG. 36-36. *Ivar Sandström, Uppsala, Sweden, 1877.*

1903. In the same year, Erdheim recorded the coexistence of a parathyroid tumor and a pituitary tumor, foreshadowing the description of multiple endocrine neoplasia almost 50 years later. In 1909 serum calcium level determination became possible, and the association between serum calcium level and the parathyroid glands was established.

The first patient to be operated on for a parathyroid abnormality was a 38-year-old male who underwent a successful parathyroidectomy in 1925 by Felix Mandl. The patient had severe bone pain secondary to advanced osteitis fibrosa cystica. His condition dramatically improved after the operation, and he lived for another 7 years before dying of recurrent hyperparathyroidism or renal failure. In 1926, at the Massachusetts General Hospital, Edward Churchill, assisted by an intern named Oliver Cope, operated for the seventh time on the famous sea captain Charles Martell (Fig. 36-37) for severe primary hyperparathyroidism. No parathyroid abnormalities were identified in any of Captain Martell's previous six cervical explorations. It was only at the time of the seventh operation that an ectopic adenoma was found in the substernal position. Captain Martell died 6 weeks after the successful seventh operation, most likely from laryngeal spasm after a subsequent surgical procedure to relieve ureteral obstruction secondary to stones.

The first successful parathyroidectomy for hyperparathyroidism based on an accurate preoperative biochemical diagnosis was performed in 1928 by Isaac Y. Olch at the Barnes Hospital in St. Louis, Missouri, on a 56-year-old female. At operation, a 3 × 3 cm adenoma was found attached to the left lower lobe of the thyroid gland. Postoperatively the patient developed life-threatening tetany, with her serum calcium dropping as low as 4.5 mg/dL. The patient recovered and lived for many years, although she required lifelong supplemental oral calcium lactate.

ANATOMY

The superior parathyroid glands arise from the fourth branchial pouch in conjunction with the ultimobranchial bodies. Because of this association, the superior parathyroid glands remain in close proximity to the posterior portion of the upper thyroid lobes. This position is fairly constant, and superior parathyroid glands located in ectopic sites are less common in comparison to the inferior glands. When the superior glands enlarge, they tend to "descend by gravity" into or along the tracheoesophageal groove and may be inferior to the inferior parathyroid glands (Fig. 36-38). When true embryologic descent of the superior glands does occur, the descent is in a posterior plane (Fig. 36-39). When such glands descend, they can be located in the posterior or middle mediastinum, with the aortopulmonary window being the most common site. The superior parathyroid glands usually are found in close association with the posterior aspect of the middle and upper thirds of the thyroid gland (Fig. 36-40). In this position, they are in close proximity to the cricothyroid membrane entrance of the recurrent laryngeal nerve and usually cephalad to the superior thyroid artery.

The inferior parathyroid glands arise from the third branchial pouches in conjunction with the thymus. Given this important association, and since the embryologic journey is a longer one, ectopic sites for the inferior glands are more common and more widely distributed than ectopic sites for superior glands (Fig. 36-41). With rare exceptions, thymic tissue is intimately related to inferior glands in ectopic locations. Ectopic sites range from

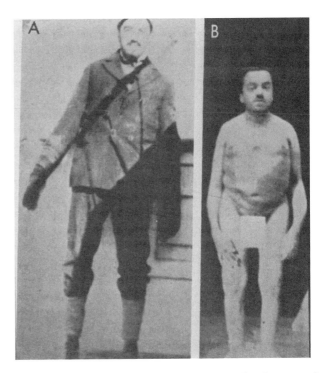

FIG. 36-37. *Captain Charles Martell, before and after the onset of hyperparathyroidism.*

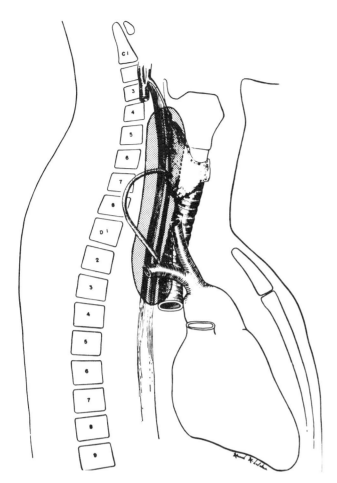

FIG. 36-38. Posterior versus inferior descent of superior and inferior parathyroid glands.

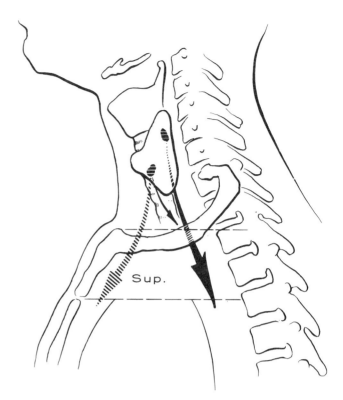

FIG. 36-39. Posterior location of superior parathyroid glands whether undescended, in normal position, or overdescended.

an intrathymic parathyroid gland located in the anterior-superior mediastinum to an undescended inferior parathyroid gland (parathymus) located superior to the superior parathyroid gland. Undescended inferior glands are most often found at the angle of the mandible anterior to the carotid artery but may be seen as high as the base of the skull.

The normal inferior glands are more variable in location than superior glands (see Fig. 36-40B). The most common site (approximately 60 percent) for inferior parathyroids is within a circle 2 cm in diameter centered on a point that is on the posterolateral aspect of the lower pole of the thyroid gland. The majority of the remaining normal inferior parathyroid glands will be found in the thyrothymic tongue of tissue (thyrothymic ligament), which extends inferiorly from the lower pole of each thyroid lobe to the thymus gland, usually located in the anterior mediastinum (Fig. 36-42).

A normal parathyroid gland usually weighs less than 50 mg, measures approximately $3 \times 3 \times 3$ mm, and may be difficult to differentiate from adjacent fatty tissue. Parathyroid glands are more yellow-brown than normal fatty tissue, and close observation will invariably reveal small "grains of salt" on their surface, an observation that aids in differentiation from surrounding fatty tissues. Normal glands have more clearly defined margins, which aids in this differentiation and which has led to their being

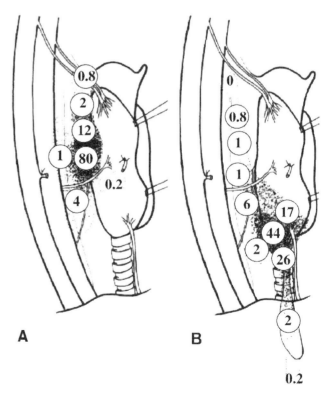

FIG. 36-40. Most common anatomic locations of *(A)* the posterior parathyroid glands, and *(B)* the inferior parathyroid glands. The numbers represent the percentages of glands found at the different locations. (From: *Akerstrom G, Malmaeus J, Bergstrom R: Surgical anatomy of human parathyroid glands. Surgery 95:14, 1984, with permission.*)

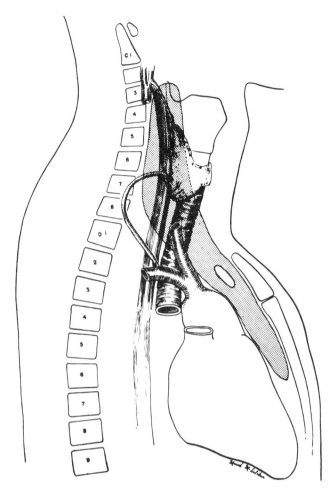

FIG. 36-41. *Possible location of inferior parathyroid glands, whether undescended, in normal position, or overdescended.*

described as looking like "the tongue of a jaundiced humming-bird."

PATHOLOGY

Primary hyperparathyroidism may be due to parathyroid adenoma(s), hyperplasia, or, rarely, carcinoma. Of these causes, a parathyroid adenoma is by far the most common, accounting for 90 percent of cases. In almost 2 percent of patients with adenomatous disease, double adenomas are present. Parathyroid hyperplasia (multiglandular disease) may be found in nearly 8 percent of patients with sporadic hyperparathyroidism. The incidence of hyperplasia increases markedly and may be universal in patients with hyperparathyroidism that occurs in families with multiple endocrine neoplasia (MEN) type I or II, and in patients with non-MEN familial hyperparathyroidism. Parathyroid hyperplasia is seldom equal or even symmetrical. This "unequal hyperplasia," if misinterpreted by the surgeon, may lead to a mistaken diagnosis of single versus multiglandular disease. Parathyroid carcinoma, as a cause for hyperparathyroidism, is exceedingly rare, occurring in less than 1 percent of patients with this disease.

Differentiation between the causes of hyperparathyroidism is of paramount importance, because the selection of appropriate surgical treatment depends on it. This delineation is made primarily by the operating surgeon identifying the pathology encountered at the time of surgical exploration. A structure that looks like a little kidney in the neck or mediastinum is virtually pathognomonic for single-gland disease. Finding multiple enlarged glands somewhat "paler than a normal kidney" suggests multiglandular disease. The pathologist can be of great help to the surgeon, and vice versa. Unequivocal histologic identification of the causes of primary hyperparathyroidism can be difficult without the surgeon's description of the gross characteristics of all glands. With small biopsy specimens alone of parathyroid glands, it can be extremely difficult for the pathologist to accurately differentiate histologically between a truly normal gland, a parathyroid adenoma, or a hyperplastic parathyroid gland. Our own preference is to avoid taking biopsy specimens of normal-appearing glands and to rely on visual inspection of the remaining glands and the histology of the excised abnormality to determine the diagnosis.

Normal parathyroid glands contain primarily chief cells, with occasional oxyphil cells. An adenoma is typically defined as an enlarged parathyroid gland that is made up of solid sheets of chief cells, oxyphil cells, or varying combinations of both with a rim of compressed normal parathyroid tissue (Fig. 36-43). This compressed rim of normal tissue is present in only 20 to 30 percent of parathyroid adenomas. The histology of parathyroid hyperplasia may be difficult to discern unless the nature of the other parathyroid glands is placed in context (Fig. 36-44). His-

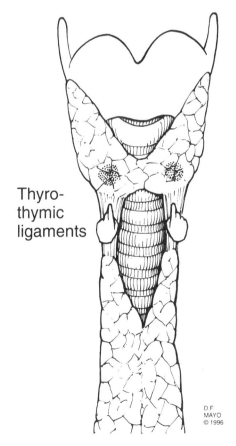

FIG. 36-42. *The thyrothymic ligaments "pointing" to the inferior parathyroid gland.*

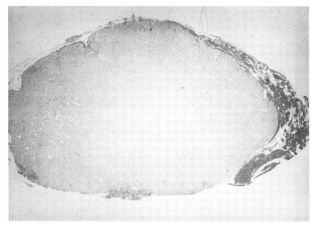

A

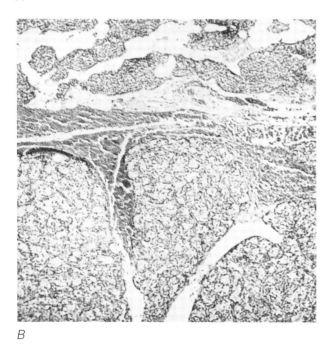

B

FIG. 36-43. *Parathyroid adenoma. A. Solid tumor with compressed normal parathyroid on the right. B. Parathyroid adenoma (below) with normal gland above.*

tologically, the presence or absence of parathyroid fat cells has been believed by some authorities to be of help in the diagnosis of parathyroid hyperplasia; the higher the percentage of fat cells, as demonstrated by fat staining, the lower the chances of hyperplasia, and vice versa.

The macroscopic appearance of the parathyroid glands, as visualized by an experienced parathyroid surgeon, continues to be the most accurate means of identifying the various types of parathyroid pathology.

PHYSIOLOGY OF CALCIUM HOMEOSTASIS

Parathyroid Hormone (PTH). In patients with primary and tertiary hyperparathyroidism, the secretion of parathyroid hormone is abnormal and excessive. In secondary hyperparathyroidism, PTH secretion is increased, but appropriately so. The

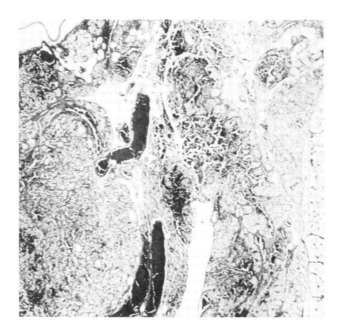

FIG. 36-44. *Parathyroid hyperplasia demonstrating nodular formation.*

effect of PTH in human beings is to increase serum calcium concentration (Fig. 36-45). Hypercalcemia occurs because the principal actions of PTH involve the following:

1. Increase of bone osteoclast and osteoblast activity.
2. Increase in rate of conversion of 25-hydroxycholecalciferol (25-hydroxyvitamin D_3) to 1,25-dihydroxycholecalciferol (1,25-dihydroxyvitamin D_3) in the kidneys by stimulation of 1α-hydroxylase activity.
3. Increase of gastrointestinal absorption of calcium by enhancing vitamin D synthesis.
4. Increased excretion of bicarbonate by the kidney.
5. Decrease in serum phosphate level by increasing the excretion of urinary phosphate.

PTH is a single-chain polypeptide of 84 amino acids. The entire polypeptide is referred to as *intact PTH,* a hormone that has a half-life of 2 to 5 min. The *N*-terminal PTH portion

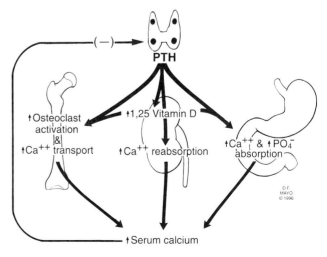

FIG. 36-45. *The physiologic action of parathyroid hormone (PTH).*

(1–34), also called the amino (N) terminal, is biologically active, with a half-life of 2 min. The C-terminal PTH portion (35–84) or carboxyl (C) terminal, is biologically inactive, with a half-life of approximately 30 min. Among other effects, PTH acts to promote bone resorption and to increase calcium absorption from filtered urine in the renal tubule.

Calcium. Calcium is the principal regulator of parathyroid hormone release. This regulation is mediated by calcium receptors or other receptors on the parathyroid cell surface. A membrane protein that has been proposed to constitute such receptors (calcium ion–sensing receptor [CaR]) demonstrates reduced expression in hyperparathyroidism and seems causally related to the relative insensitivity of the secretion to external calcium in pathologic parathyroid cells. This protein consequently may be an important cause for the hypercalcemia of this disorder. Modulating the functions of such proteins comprises interesting means of future therapy in several disorders of mineral metabolism. Increased knowledge of these proteins and parathyroid pathophysiology may clarify the presence of relevant mutations, secretory derangements, and propensity for cell growth, from which accurate classification of parathyroid diseases and improved treatment strategies might evolve.

Calcium is the most abundant cation in human beings, and its distribution within cells is essential for virtually all physiologic functions. Calcium balance in a normal individual is tightly regulated. The body contains approximately 1000 g of calcium, with minimal variations from day to day in serum calcium concentration (Fig. 36-46). Total serum concentrations, as tested by routine laboratory analysis, are accurate as long as serum protein concentrations are normal. Total calcium level must always be considered in its relationship to plasma protein levels, especially serum albumin (for each gram per deciliter of alteration of serum albumin above or below 4.0 mg/dL, there is a 0.8 mg/dL increase or decrease in protein-bound calcium and thus in total serum calcium).

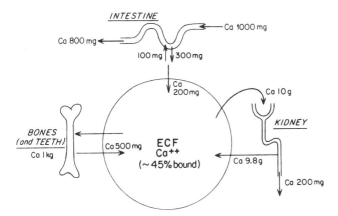

FIG. 36-46. *Overall calcium balance in a normal individual. Of the 1 g of elemental calcium ingested, net absorption is 200 mg (300 mg true absorption, 100 mg endogenous fecal secretion). Balance is achieved by renal excretion of 200 mg calcium, because equivalent amounts of calcium are laid down and removed from the skeleton on a daily basis. (From: Brown EM, LeBaff MS: Pathophysiology of hyperparathyroidism, in Rothmund M, Wells SA Jr (eds): Progress in Surgery. Parathyroid Surgery, vol 18. Basel, Karger, 1986, p 13, with permission.)*

Vitamin D. Vitamin D_3 (cholecalciferol) is vital to calcium homeostasis. It is absorbed through the gastrointestinal tract and synthesized in the skin and is converted by the liver to 25-hydroxycholecalciferol, which is subsequently converted to its active form, 1,25-dihydroxycholecalciferol in the kidneys by the enzyme 1α-hydroxylase. Vitamin D_3 increases the absorption of calcium from the gastrointestinal tract and promotes phosphate retention; it elevates serum calcium and phosphate levels and in turn enhances the mineralization of bone.

A fall in serum calcium concentration stimulates secretion of PTH, which, among other effects, results in a rise in vitamin D_3 synthesis. Vitamin D_3 then acts peripherally to raise the serum calcium concentration toward normal. Vitamin D_3 promotes bone resorption and enhances absorption of calcium and phosphorus from the gut. An elevation of the serum calcium level reduces PTH secretion and the formation of vitamin D_3. Both effects tend to lower serum calcium concentration.

PRIMARY HYPERPARATHYROIDISM

Primary hyperparathyroidism is the hypercalcemic condition generated as a result of overproduction of PTH by one or more parathyroid glands. PTH enhances gastrointestinal absorption of calcium, stimulates the production of vitamin D_3, and inhibits renal calcium excretion. PTH secretion from the parathyroid glands is inversely related to serum calcium levels and is tightly regulated. In primary hyperparathyroidism, the normal negative feedback loop is altered, and inappropriately elevated PTH levels occur in the face of hypercalcemia.

The incidence of primary hyperparathyroidism in the United States is estimated to be 1:700, with a female-to-male ratio of nearly 3:1. Primary hyperparathyroidism is the most common cause of hypercalcemia observed. Only advanced malignancy is a more common cause of hypercalcemia in hospitalized patients in the United States. Of the nearly 100,000 cases diagnosed yearly in the United States, most occur in postmenopausal women, in whom the incidence is nearly 1:200. The incidence of this disease appears to have decreased over the past decade, for unknown reasons.

Etiology. While the exact cause or stimulus that brings about the autonomous production of PTH remains unclear, pathologically the disease is manifested by three separate entities. Most commonly, primary hyperparathyroidism is caused by the benign enlargement of one (90 percent) or, occasionally, two (2 percent) parathyroid glands, a condition referred to as benign parathyroid adenoma(s). Less common is the occurrence of multiple gland enlargement (8 percent), which is referred to as multiglandular hyperplasia. Parathyroid carcinoma is a rare (less than 1 percent), often lethal, cause of hyperparathyroidism.

Clinical Manifestations. Before calcium levels were routinely included in serum chemistry analysis in the late 1960s, and before their routine use in the 1970s as an adjunct for general medical examinations, the diagnosis of primary hyperparathyroidism was rarely considered, typically only in patients with renal stones, bony abnormalities, or severe mental changes. Patients with primary hyperparathyroidism had variable symptoms: renal stones (64 percent), bone disease (20 percent), peptic ulcer disease (12 percent), and hypertension (4 percent). Walter St. Goar, in 1957, first used the mnemonic "Hyperparathyroidism is a disease of stones, bones, and abdominal groans" to remind physicians to consider this diagnosis in patients with varied complaints. With time, the triad of St. Goar has been extended to include other nonspecific regional symptoms of hypercalcemia pertaining to the abdomen, kidney, bone, constitutional, and neurologic manifestations (Fig. 36-47).

Over half of all patients diagnosed with primary hyperparathyroidism are asymptomatic, and the disease is discovered by routine serum chemistry analysis showing hypercalcemia. After successful surgical management of primary hyperparathyroidism, nearly all patients realize that they had in fact been symptomatic.

Evaluation. The diagnosis of primary hyperparathyroidism is most commonly one of exclusion. It is most commonly considered when serum chemistry analysis reveals hypercalcemia. A focused history in symptomatic and asymptomatic patients is important to rule out medicinal use that might cause hypercalcemia and obscure the diagnosis—most commonly thiazide diuretics, but also lithium and excessive ingestion of vitamin A or vitamin D. Consumption of extraordinary amounts of milk or antacids might alert the clinician to the diagnosis of the milk-alkali syndrome. Questions regarding renal failure, dehydration, immobilization, and Paget's disease can lead to identifying the cause of the hypercalcemia. Endocrine abnormalities such as adrenal insufficiency, and either hyperthyroidism or hypothyroid-

ism are similarly rare causes of hypercalcemia. Granulomatous diseases such as sarcoidosis, tuberculosis, coccidiodomycosis, histoplasmosis, and berylliosis can elevate serum calcium levels. It is to critical to evaluate hypercalcemic patients for previous or current malignancy with possible bony metastases. The malignant causes of hypercalcemia include renal cell carcinoma, multiple myeloma, and squamous or small cell lung cancer. Over 90 percent of patients with hypercalcemia have primary hyperparathyroidism or malignancy, most commonly metastatic from the prostate or breast, as the source of their elevated serum calcium levels.

A family history of multiple endocrine neoplasia or benign familial hypocalciuric hypercalcemia (BFHH) is critical. MEN and BFHH usually occur in younger patients with a known genetic predisposition. BFHH involves sufficient retention of calcium to cause hypercalcemia. Unlike patients with primary hyperparathyroidism, BFHH patients have unusually low urinary calcium excretion. Cervical exploration in these patients is of no benefit and is contraindicated.

Physical examination of patients with primary hyperparathyroidism is rarely of diagnostic aid, but it is important to assess for neck masses, voice abnormalities or hoarseness, cervical lymphadenopathy, and mobility of the cervical spine. Neck masses most commonly represent benign thyroid nodules but could be the rare parathyroid cancer. Hypercalcemia coupled with a firm cervical mass with hoarseness or a recent change in voice would indicate involvement of a recurrent laryngeal nerve secondary to this rare malignancy. As a corollary, parathyroid adenomas, regardless of their size, are rarely palpable. While cervical lymphadenopathy can be observed with parathyroid carcinoma, this finding would more likely represent a recent upper respiratory infection or a more common malignant process such as metastatic lung, thyroid, or oropharyngeal cancer. Assessing cervical mobility is important if the patient eventually becomes a surgical candidate with the need for neck extension to facilitate surgical exposure.

While band keratopathy is easily detectable in most patients undergoing ophthalmologic examination with hyperparathyroidism, keratopathy and other ocular changes are not specific; all patients with hypercalcemia show ocular changes. Most patients with primary hyperparathyroidism have no other signs or symptoms; the only likely physical findings of interest would be those to help exclude the diagnosis or to create the suspicion of malignancy as the source of hypercalcemia.

Formerly, a solitary test result showing hypercalcemia was repeated to verify the hypercalcemic state. Today, given the accuracy of serum calcium determination, a single analysis is cost effective and sufficient. After a thorough history and physical examination of an otherwise healthy patient with no risk factors for hypercalcemia, the diagnosis of primary hyperparathyroidism is virtually certain if hypercalcemia exists and the serum PTH level is inappropriately high. "Inappropriately high" does not necessarily mean outside the normal serum range (usually 1 to 5 pmol/L). Given a normally functioning feedback loop, serum PTH levels in an otherwise healthy patient with hypercalcemia should be virtually zero. Nearly 20 percent of patients with primary hyperparathyroidism have an inappropriately normal level of PTH in the presence of hypercalcemia. Serologic testing of patients with primary hyperparathyroidism usually generates consistent results: hypophosphatemia, hypercalcemia, and elevated PTH levels (Fig. 36-48). In any patient in whom the di-

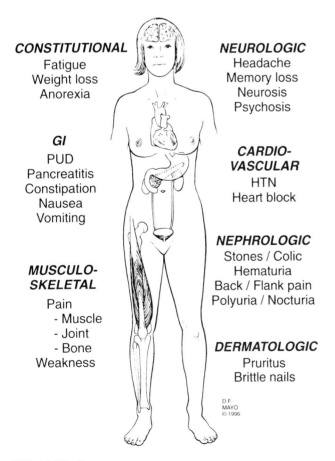

CONSTITUTIONAL
Fatigue
Weight loss
Anorexia

GI
PUD
Pancreatitis
Constipation
Nausea
Vomiting

MUSCULO-SKELETAL
Pain
- Muscle
- Joint
- Bone
Weakness

NEUROLOGIC
Headache
Memory loss
Neurosis
Psychosis

CARDIO-VASCULAR
HTN
Heart block

NEPHROLOGIC
Stones / Colic
Hematuria
Back / Flank pain
Polyuria / Nocturia

DERMATOLOGIC
Pruritus
Brittle nails

D.F.
MAYO
© 1996

FIG. 36-47. *Symptoms and signs of hyperparathyroidism. (PUD = peptic ulcer disease; HTN = hypertension.)*

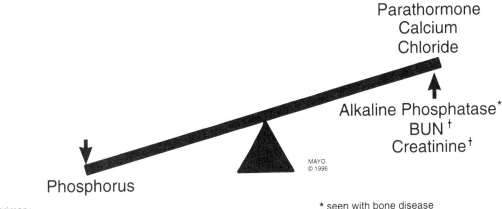

Parathormone
Calcium
Chloride

Alkaline Phosphatase*
BUN†
Creatinine†

MAYO
© 1996

Phosphorus

FIG. 36-48. *Serology of primary hyperparathyroidism.*

* seen with bone disease
† seen with renal disease

agnosis of primary hyperparathyroidism is not secure, additional testing is mandatory. Some examples include:

1. Intravenous pyelography or ultrasonography to rule out renal cell carcinoma (a rare cause of hypercalcemia resulting from the secretion of a parathyroid hormone related protein PTHep)
2. Protein gel electrophoresis to rule out multiple myeloma and sarcoidosis
3. 24-h urine collection for calcium determination to eliminate BFHH
4. Chest x-ray to exclude sarcoid, fungal diseases, or a malignancy of the lungs or mediastinum
5. Mammography in postmenopausal women

Imaging. Radiologic studies are unnecessary unless previous neck operations have been undertaken. Some advocate the use of preoperative ultrasonography in the hopes of avoiding bilateral exploration and minimizing operative time and morbidity, but surgical exploration remains the most accurate localization modality. Use of ultrasonography, computed tomography (CT), magnetic resonance imaging (MRI), venous sampling, and nuclear scintigraphy is not cost effective for initial cervical exploration in patients with primary hyperparathyroidism.

In patients who are undergoing reoperation, in whom dissection is more hazardous, ultrasonography of the neck is helpful to the operating surgeon. Similarly, technetium-99m-sestamibi (Cardiolite) scanning has great sensitivity in identifying missed parathyroid tissue in the neck as well as in the mediastinum. Venous sampling, CT, and MRI are helpful in identifying aberrantly located glands, but they are expensive and less accurate. Our preference when performing a reoperation is to use ultrasonography with fine-needle aspiration of any suspicious cervical masses. If ultrasonography is equivocal, we proceed with technetium-99m-sestamibi scanning.

Treatment. With success rates higher than 98 percent for initial operations, the indication for surgical intervention is the diagnosis of primary hyperparathyroidism. Given the negligible operative mortality and minimal morbidity associated with first-time parathyroidectomy, virtually all patients who have no prior neck operations should be offered exploration. Given the safety and success of primary cervical exploration, concomitant surgical procedures ranging from minor (breast biopsy, dilatation and curettage) to major (cardiopulmonary bypass and cholecystectomy) may be considered. With success rates of roughly 90 percent in reoperative cases, repeat exploration for recurrent or per-

sistent hyperparathyroidism is generally indicated if the offending gland has been localized in imaging studies.

Solitary parathyroidectomy, without biopsy of other glands, is sufficient treatment for solitary adenomas. Instances of double adenomas require both offending glands to be removed. Therapy for four-gland or multiglandular hyperplasia is controversial; our preference is three and one-half gland parathyroidectomy. Total parathyroidectomy with reimplantation of approximately 50 mg in the neck or forearm is another viable option. The use of the rapid (15 min) intact immunoreactive parathyroid hormone (iPTH) assay allows intraoperative assurance of removal of the offending (or sufficient) tissue. The indications for such intraoperative serological testing are rare.

Postoperative laboratory analysis reveals normocalcemia within 24 to 72 h in nearly all cases. Transient hypocalcemia is common with removal of large adenomas, resections involving four-gland hyperplasia, and in patients who have had prolonged hyperparathyroidism. The cause of postoperative hypocalcemia is invariably bone hunger or hypoparathyroidism. Bone hunger and hypoparathyroidism are differentiated by analysis of the serum phosphate and PTH levels. Bone hunger is identified by low phosphate levels associated with transient hypocalcemia after parathyroidectomy. PTH levels are within the normal range. The aparathyroid state is diagnosed by elevated phosphate levels and abnormally low PTH levels.

Hospitalization of patients without complications usually is an overnight stay. Serum calcium levels should be checked to demonstrate the equilibration of calcium before discharge. Obtaining a follow-up serum calcium level is appropriate in 1 or 2 months and yearly thereafter to assess for persistent or recurrent hyperparathyroidism.

The goals of cervical exploration in patients with primary hyperparathyroidism are as follows:

1. *Identification of the pathology.* In practice, this most commonly consists of the identification of a solitary adenoma (90 percent). A less common occurrence is multiglandular disease (8 percent) involving diffuse hyperplasia, which may be unequal. Identification of dual adenomas (2 percent) or parathyroid carcinoma (1 percent) is rare.
2. *Removal of sufficient pathologic tissue to restore normocalcemia.* The ideal postoperative result in these patients is a normocalcemic state with no need for supplemental calcium or vitamin D therapy. Transient hypocalcemia is sometimes unavoidable if severe osteopenia is present preoperatively, with ensuing postoperative bone hunger. Postoperative

hypocalcemia or hypercalcemia may be caused by errors in cervical exploration: not finding the offending pathology (most often in single-gland disease); finding the diseased tissue but excising insufficient amounts of it (multiglandular hyperplasia), with resultant hypercalcemia; overly aggressive exploration with biopsies and possible injury to normal glands in single-gland disease; or excising too much hyperplastic tissue in multiglandular disease, with resulting hypocalcemia.

3. *Minimal postoperative morbidity and mortality.* The operative mortality in most reported series is less than 1 percent, which attests to the safety of cervical exploration. Complications and morbidity involve wound infection, cervical hematoma, injury to the inferior or superior laryngeal nerves, postoperative hypocalcemia, and, perhaps most commonly, poor cosmesis. All such complications should occur in less than 1 percent of patients.

To achieve these goals, cervical exploration should be undertaken with the conviction that parathyroid pathology exists and requires identification and removal. Cervical exploration should not be undertaken to make or confirm the diagnosis of hyperparathyroidism. A gentle technique that delivers a bloodless operative field is imperative. Poor visualization may result in disruption or fracture of parathyroid tissue with subsequent functional regrowth, the so-called parathyromatosis. The surgeon who is unfamiliar with parathyroid embryology should not undertake cervical exploration for hyperparathyroidism. It is important be unhurried when performing this procedure. The surgical adage "The slower one operates, the sooner the operation is over" applies to this operation.

Technique. Although cervical exploration for primary hyperparathyroidism can be performed under regional blockade supplemented by intravenous sedation and local anesthesia, general anesthesia with endotracheal intubation is preferable in most patients. After induction of general anesthesia, both arms are tucked at the patient's sides with careful attention to any interference with the previously placed intravenous lines and with particular attention to possible pressure points on the patient's elbows and wrists. The midline placement of a folded surgical towel beneath the patient's scapulae and a 5- to 10-degree downward tilt of the head of the operating table facilitates exposure of the lower portion of the neck. Cervical extension should be minimized in older patients to avoid undue postoperative neck pain. It is prudent to ask all patients to demonstrate the degree of extension they can achieve voluntarily without discomfort. Sandbags are placed alongside the patient's head to avoid any side-to-side movement during the operation (Fig. 36-49).

It is important for cosmesis that the patient's chin, thyroid cartilage, and suprasternal notch be aligned vertically before an incision is made. Failure to establish this alignment may result in an asymmetric and unsightly incision. A thyroid surgical drape is placed with tie-tapes passing behind each earlobe and anchored at the head of the table with a single hemoclip (see Fig. 36-49).

A collar incision is made approximately two fingerbreadths above the suprasternal notch, which usually means the incision is situated over the cricoid cartilage. The surgeon should look carefully for obvious skin creases slightly above or below this site; if there are any, they should be used for improved cosmesis. The length of the incision is approximately 10 cm. The planned site should be marked in a linear fashion by applying pressure to the imaginary line with a suture. The course of the incision extending laterally above both clavicles should be carefully inspected and equalized, ensuring cosmesis. An incision that is

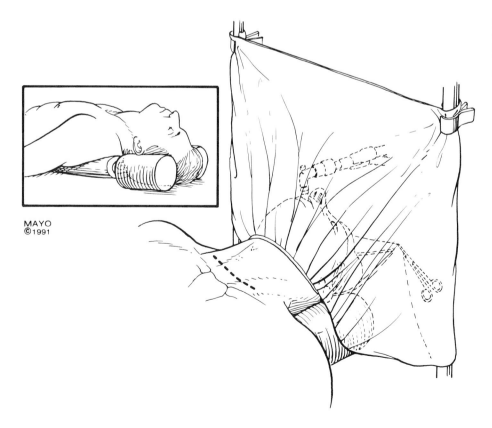

FIG. 36-49. Placement of sandbags on each side of the head to prevent rotation during the procedure *(inset)*. Thyroid drape in position with site of collar incision marked.

MAYO
©1991

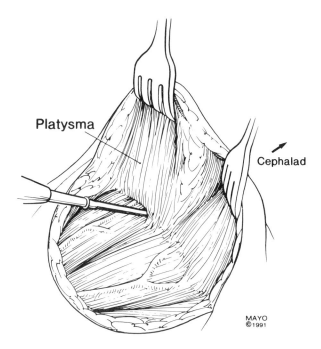

FIG. 36-50. Subplatysmal dissection with electrocautery.

higher on one side than the other is noticeable and troublesome to the patient. The table is positioned with the patient's head and chest elevated approximately 15 to 20 degrees to the horizontal.

The skin incision is made and, with use of electrocautery, the platysma muscle is identified and divided. This muscle is ex-

tremely thin, usually measuring no more than 1 to 2 mm in thickness. The avascular plane, just deep to the platysma, should be searched for. If the dissection at this stage is carried too deep, there will be unnecessary bleeding because of injury to the anterior jugular veins. By placing sharp rake retractors and tensing the platysma anteriorly, the avascular plane immediately beneath the muscle can be easily developed superiorly to the level of the thyroid cartilage. There should be no bleeding during this stage of the operation. Minimal dissection is required inferiorly, usually just enough to allow placement of a self-retaining retractor (Fig. 36-50).

The midline is readily identified by finding the thin, avascular fascial plane connecting right and left strap muscles. This plane is divided with electrocautery. This dissection is carried posteriorly until the thyroid isthmus is clearly identified. Occasionally, small veins cross this midline space; if these are encountered, they should be isolated, ligated, and divided. A meticulous and bloodless operative technique is mandatory. Even minimal bleeding will render identification of parathyroid glands, particularly normal glands, extremely difficult. Once the thyroid isthmus has been identified, traction is applied laterally to the strap muscles with retractors that work against digital medial retraction of the thyroid lobe.

Anterior and medial displacement of the thyroid lobe brings the middle thyroid vein into view. The vein is isolated, ligated, and divided. The carotid sheath should appear in the posterior aspect of the dissection. Clamps are placed on the inferior and superior aspects of the thyroid lobe, and the thyroid gland is elevated anteriorly, superiorly, and eventually medially. This elevation of the thyroid lobe is required for accurate identification of the parathyroid glands (Fig. 36-51).

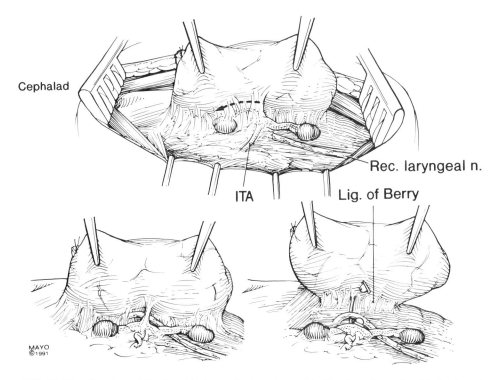

FIG. 36-51. Elevation of the thyroid lobe by Kocher clamps. Identification of parathyroid glands and course of recurrent laryngeal nerve.

The superior parathyroid glands usually are found in close association with the posterolateral aspect of the superior pole of the thyroid lobe. The superior thyroid pole seldom needs to be taken down to visualize the superior parathyroid gland as long as there is anterior and medial displacement of the thyroid lobe. The inferior parathyroid gland, in contrast, is intimately involved with the inferior aspect of the thyroid gland and the thyrothymic tongue of fat (thyrothymic ligament) that extends inferiorly toward the mediastinum. Many inferior parathyroid glands are subcapsular, i.e., attached to the inferior aspect of the thyroid lobe and covered by a thin layer of fibrous tissue. This does not represent an intrathyroid parathyroid gland, as is often erroneously assumed. To be truly intrathyroid, the parathyroid gland should be circumferentially surrounded by thyroid parenchyma.

If the superior parathyroid gland is not visualized, the tracheoesophageal groove should be explored digitally. Enlarging superior parathyroid adenomas often descend into this groove and can be palpated accurately by inserting a finger into the avascular space immediately superior to the inferior thyroid artery (Fig. 36-52). Such glands are often located inferior to the inferior parathyroid glands. The parathyroid glands can be found from as high as the angle of the mandible or the base of the skull (undescended parathymus) to as low as an intrathymic location in the anterior mediastinum or in the aortopulmonary window in the posterior mediastinum.

In the hands of an experienced surgeon, a negative exploration usually is the result of an unusual variation in embryologic descent. The following rule is useful in this situation: If the superior parathyroid gland is not found in its conventional position, the surgeon should search inferior to the inferior parathyroid gland for the superior parathyroid gland (tracheoesophageal groove); conversely, if the inferior parathyroid gland is not found inferior to the superior parathyroid gland, the surgeon should search superior to the superior parathyroid gland for the inferior parathyroid gland (undescended parathymus). If these simple maneuvers are unsuccessful, the surgeon should become suspicious that the offending parathyroid gland might be in one of the following locations:

1. In the thymus. A fairly complete transcervical thymectomy should be performed to search for the missing inferior gland.
2. Within the thyroid. Truly intrathyroid glands are exceedingly rare. Most so-called intrathyroid parathyroid glands are inferior parathyroid glands located beneath the thin veil of the thyroid capsule and can be easily teased off the thyroid.
3. In the carotid sheath. This is extraordinarily rare, but opening the carotid sheath should be considered when all other possibilities have been ruled out.
4. Lateral to the carotid sheath. This location is even more unusual than in the carotid sheath, but the parathyroid gland can hide laterally.

Routine bilateral exploration is recommended in all patients. If a single adenoma is identified, excision of this adenoma, without biopsy of normal glands, is suggested. If hyperplasia is documented, all but approximately 50 mg of clearly viable parathyroid tissue is excised and routine transcervical thymectomy is performed. With the approach outlined, surgical success should approach 99 percent. Permanent laryngeal nerve palsy or hypoparathyroidism occurs in less than 1 percent of patients.

Persistent and Recurrent Hyperparathyroidism

Almost twenty years ago, Wexler stated, "Persistent hypercalcemia in suspected hyperparathyroidism is due to an improperly

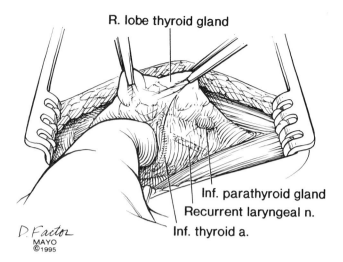

FIG. 36-52. *Digital exploration of the tracheoesophageal groove.*

performed primary operation." This statement is as true today as it was then. A faulty operation is the cause for the vast majority of patients with persistent or recurrent hyperparathyroidism.

Persistent hyperparathyroidism is defined as elevated serum calcium levels that do not return to normal after an operation for biochemically proved hyperparathyroidism; this situation should be differentiated from the less common situation of recurrent hyperparathyroidism in which at least 6 months of well-documented normocalcemia occurs after cervical exploration for hyperparathyroidism before hypercalcemia is documented again.

The results of reoperation for recurrent or persistent hyperparathyroidism do not parallel those achieved for the initial operation. Regardless of the surgical expertise involved, reoperative cure rates are uniformly 10 to 20 percent lower (i.e., 80 to 90 percent success rates) than those obtained in first-time operations (95 to 99 percent). In addition, postoperative morbidity involving recurrent laryngeal nerve palsies, postoperative hematomas, and permanent hypocalcemia are three to five times higher than the rates anticipated after first-time explorations (<1 percent).

The principal factors contributing to persistent or recurrent hyperparathyroidism are varied (Table 36-4). A systematic, logical approach to management is required (Fig. 36-53), with a concerted effort by all members of a multidisciplinary team.

The initial step is to reconfirm the diagnosis of hyperparathyroidism. In particular, the possibility of benign familial hypocalciuria hypocalcemia must be excluded, because cervical exploration is of no benefit to patients with BFHH. This diagnostic

Table 36-4
Factors Contributing to Persistent/Recurrent Hyperparathyroidism

1. Surgical inexperience
2. Lack of knowledge regarding parathyroid embryology
3. Presence of more than one adenoma (2–3 percent)
4. Presence of more than four parathyroid glands (5–10 percent)
5. Benign seeding (parathyromatosis)
6. Parathyroid carcinoma
7. Erroneous diagnosis

MANAGEMENT ALGORITHM

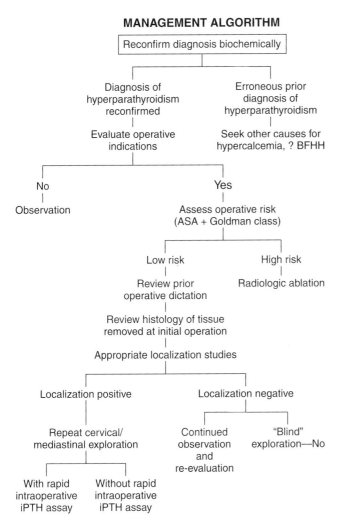

FIG. 36-53. *Algorithm of the approach to the patient with persistent/recurrent hyperparathyroidism.*

Table 36-5

American Society of Anesthesiologists (ASA) Physical Status Classification

Class	Description	Risk of Operative Mortality (%)
Class I	A healthy patient	<0.1
Class II	A patient with mild systemic disease	0.5
Class III	A patient with severe systemic disease that is not incapacitating	4.4
Class IV	A patient with an incapacitating systemic disease that is a constant threat to life	23.5
Class V	A moribund patient who is not expected to survive 24 h with or without operation	50.8

two most commonly used modalities are angiographic embolization and ultrasound-guided alcohol ablation; the latter technique is somewhat safer in the high-risk patient and is gaining worldwide acceptance.

When repeat exploration is warranted, the surgeon should review the prior operative report. It is important to know what tissue was removed and from which site. Additional clues may be obtained regarding the thoroughness of the previous operation. Statements in the report may lead to finding pathologic tissue in more common locations rather than in unusual hiding places.

The pathologist should review previously excised tissue to ascertain whether it was in fact parathyroid tissue and not thyroid or lymphatic tissue and whether any histologic evidence is present to suggest single-gland versus multiglandular disease or parathyroid carcinoma.

The radiologist should be consulted regarding the most appropriate localizing modality for the patient under consideration. In contrast to primary operations for hyperparathyroidism, in

trap may be avoided by obtaining a 24-h urine collection for calcium determination. The clinician must be concerned with the hypercalcemic patient who has 24-h urine calcium levels of less than 100 mg. If diagnostic uncertainty persists, the urine calcium–to–creatinine ratio should be calculated. In BFHH patients, this ratio invariably is less than 0.01. The formula for calculating this ratio, the fractional excretion of calcium, is:

$$FE\ Ca^{2+} = \frac{Urinary\ Ca^{2+}(mg/total\ volume) \times serum\ creatinine\ (mg/dL)}{Serum\ Ca^{2+}(mg/dL) \times urinary\ creatinine\ (mg/total\ volume)}$$

Although the indication for operation for primary hyperparathyroidism is the diagnosis itself, this is not the case in patients who are undergoing reoperation. Risk assessment in this situation is of great importance. Objective data that are helpful in evaluating the anesthetic risks can be obtained. The criteria most often used are those of the American Society of Anesthesiologists physical status classification (Table 36-5) and of the Goldman multivariate index of cardiac risk (Table 36-6).

While cervical exploration invariably is well-tolerated, if the operative risk is unacceptably high, consideration should be given to nonsurgical means of parathyroid tissue ablation. The

Table 36-6

Multivariate Index of Cardiac Risk in Noncardiac Surgical Procedures

Preoperative Factor	Points
S3 gallop, congestive heart failure	11
Myocardial infarction ≤6 months	10
Abnormal ECG rhythm other than PACs	7
≥5 PVCs/min	7
Age ≥70 years	5
Intraperitoneal operations	3
Important valvular stenosis	3
Poor general medical conditions; e.g. renal failure, electrolyte imbalance, bedridden, chronic liver disease	3

Risk of Postoperative Cardiac-Related Death	
Points	Risk (%)
0–5	0.2
6–12	1.6
13–25	2.3
>26	55.6

PACs = premature atrial contractions; PVCs = premature ventricular contractions.

Table 36-7
Comparison of Different Localizing Studies in Patients Undergoing Reoperation

Procedure	Accuracy (%)
Noninvasive	
Ultrasonography (small-part/real-time)	56–76
Thallium-technetium subtraction scan	78
Technetium-99m-sestamibi scanning	58–88
Compute axial tomography	11–79
Magnetic resonance imaging	65
Invasive	
Selective venous catheterization and sampling	44–88
Selective angiography	49–73
Ultrasound-guided fine-needle aspiration	73

which preoperative localization is not indicated, localization in the reoperative setting is crucial. A wide variety of localizing modalities are in use (Table 36-7). The most popular modalities are radionuclide scanning with technetium-99m-sestamibi and ultrasonography (Fig. 36-54). Sestamibi scanning reaches sensitivity rates of over 90 percent and is particularly useful for parathyroid tissue located in the mediastinum (Fig. 36-55). A powerful adjunct to ultrasonography is liberal use of ultrasound-guided fine-needle aspiration (Fig. 36-56), not only for cytologic review but also for the measurement of iPTH. A high level confirms that the image seen is parathyroid tissue.

If all localizing modalities are negative, blind exploration should not be performed. Clinical and biochemical monitoring with interval reevaluation is the more prudent course to follow.

Although a repeat cervical or mediastinal exploration is considerably more difficult than a primary exploration, accurate preoperative localization enables the surgeon to perform a more focused exploration (e.g., unilateral cervical exploration, lateral

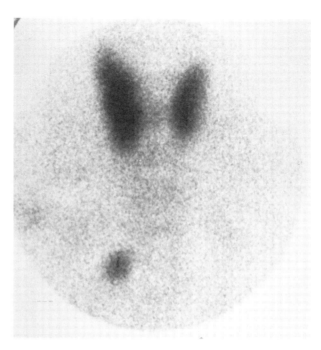

FIG. 36-55. Technetium-99m-sestamibi scan demonstrating right superior mediastinal activity compatible with a parathyroid adenoma.

cervical approach, thoracoscopic mediastinal exploration, mediastinal exploration, or a Chamberlain parasternal approach). Imaging studies of the abnormally located parathyroid gland minimize surgical morbidity and increase success rates. A recent adjunct in these difficult scenarios is the rapid iPTH assay, which can be performed and completed before finishing the operation. The assay is especially helpful for reexplorations in patients with multiglandular disease.

SECONDARY HYPERPARATHYROIDISM

Secondary hyperparathyroidism is an uncommon clinical disorder that develops in patients with chronic renal failure or intestinal malabsorption. PTH secretion appropriately increases be-

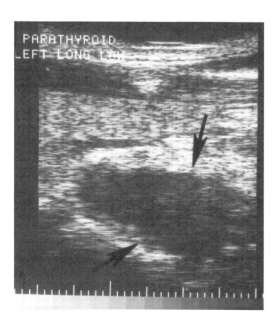

FIG. 36-54. Small-part ultrasound (10 MHz) image demonstrating left anterior sonolucent defect *(arrows)* compatible with a parathyroid adenoma.

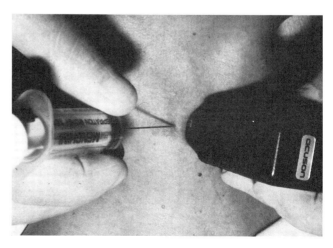

FIG. 36-56. Ultrasound-guided fine-needle aspiration.

cause of hypocalcemia caused by hyperphosphatemia (renal failure) or dysfunctional calcium and vitamin D absorption (malabsorption).

Etiology. Calcium and phosphorus levels are inversely related. As chronic renal failure worsens and hypocalcemia occurs secondary to rising phosphate levels, the parathyroid glands secrete PTH in an attempt to counteract the hypocalcemic effects of renal failure. Compounding the problem is abnormal renal function that causes diminished 1α-hydroxylase activity, which is necessary for proper vitamin D production. Because of the high content of aluminum in renal dialysate and the need to take phosphate-binding medications, patients on hemodialysis or oral phosphate binders can develop aluminum accumulation in bone, (aluminum intoxication), which contributes to osteomalacia and further PTH stimulation.

The cause of PTH stimulation with malabsorption syndromes is that calcium and vitamin D absorption is hindered to the point of hypocalcemia. Although PTH elevation is significant in renal failure and malabsorption, calcium regulation remains tight, and patients with either disease remain normocalcemic.

Clinical Manifestations. The diagnosis of secondary hyperparathyroidism often is made serologically before any symptoms are identified by the patient. When symptomatic, the most problematic feature for patients with secondary hyperparathyroidism usually is severe bone pain related to renal osteodystrophy. Less commonly, patients complain of soft-tissue calcifications (calcium tachyphylaxis) or pruritus. Others may develop bony fractures secondary to bone reabsorption.

Treatment. Initial therapy of secondary hyperparathyroidism is nonsurgical. In renal failure, dietary restriction of phosphate along with consumption of oral phosphate binders counteracts the underlying cause, hyperphosphatemia. In renal failure and malabsorption, oral calcium supplementation along with vitamin D ingestion is helpful. Altering the dialysate to minimize aluminum content and maximize calcium content is beneficial in renal failure patients.

Removing three and one-half parathyroid glands or total parathyroidectomy with reimplantation of a portion of tissue is indicated in secondary hyperparathyroidism for: (1) uncontrollable bone pain, (2) bone fractures, (3) intractable pruritus, (4) symptomatic ectopic calcifications, or (5) intractable disease that cannot be controlled medically. The preference is to excise three and one-half parathyroid glands and leave in situ approximately 50 mg of clearly viable parathyroid tissue.

TERTIARY HYPERPARATHYROIDISM

Tertiary hyperparathyroidism represents the continuation of secondary hyperparathyroidism; parathyroid tissue under the constant stimulation of hyperphosphatemia, and subsequent hypocalcemia, autonomously produces PTH and creates hypercalcemia. This rare situation is seen most commonly in patients with long-standing renal dysfunction who undergo successful renal transplantation.

Surgical removal of parathyroid tissue in tertiary hyperparathyroidism rarely is necessary. Most instances of tertiary hyperparathyroidism are short-lived; PTH levels eventually return to normal under the control of a functioning transplant kidney that corrects or improves hyperphosphatemia. Should persistent, au-

tonomous overproduction of PTH occur with a well-functioning transplanted kidney, operative intervention is indicated.

MULTIPLE ENDOCRINE NEOPLASIA AND HYPERPARATHYROIDISM

Multiple endocrine neoplasia (MEN) is a collection of syndromes with an autosomal dominant pattern of inheritance. Hyperparathyroidism is one factor among many to consider in patients with endocrine abnormalities (Fig. 36-57). The hallmark of the pathology in all MEN syndromes, regardless of the organ involved, are multicentricity and bilaterality.

MEN I. Formerly known as Wermer's syndrome, MEN I includes pituitary, parathyroid, or pancreatic neoplasms. Given enough time, all patients with MEN I develop primary hyperparathyroidism. Tumors of the pituitary (15 to 50 percent) and pancreas (30 to 80 percent) are less common.

MEN IIA & IIB. All patients with Sipple's syndrome (MEN IIA) develop C-cell hyperplasia and, subsequently, medullary thyroid carcinoma if total thyroidectomy is not performed prophylactically. Adrenal medullary hyperplasia/pheochromocytoma (approximately 50 percent) and parathyroid abnormalities (10 to 25 percent) are less common but important to rule out. Patients with MEN IIB also can develop medullary thyroid carcinoma and adrenal neoplasms along with a marfanoid habitus, a typical facies (Fig. 36-58), and mucosal neuromas (Fig. 36-59). Chief-cell hyperplasia of the parathyroid glands is uncommon. MEN IIB is inherently virulent, and malignancy shortens the patient's life span if prophylaxis is not undertaken.

Clinical Manifestations. Over 75 percent of patients with MEN have a long and classic family history of endocrine abnormalities. The genetic abnormalities appear linked to changes in the long arm of chromosome 11 in MEN I and in the centromeric region of chromosome 10 in MEN II. Medical surveillance and genetic testing can identify abnormalities before they become symptomatic, but with time, patients with MEN present with complaints of visual changes, kidney stones, ulcer pain, or diabetes (MEN I); neck masses and hypertension (MEN IIA);

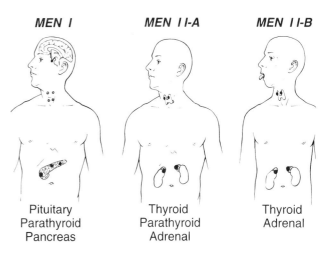

FIG. 36-57. *Endocrine gland involvement in patients with multiple endocrine neoplasia.*

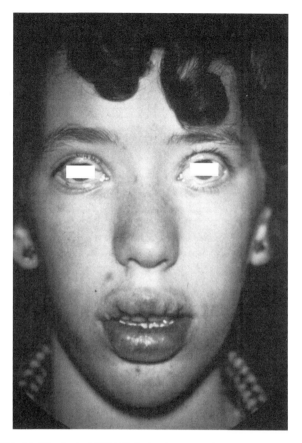

FIG. 36-58. Typical MEN IIB facies demonstrating neuromas of the lips and eyelids.

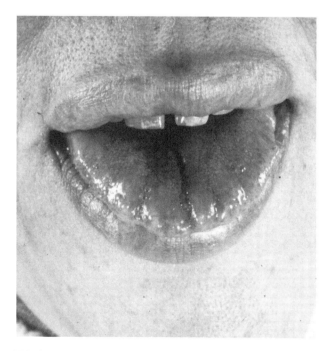

FIG. 36-59. Close-up of MEN IIB patient demonstrating tongue and lip neuromas.

Table 36-8
Serologic Surveillance for MEN

Serologic Marker	Associated Disease
MEN I	
Calcium	Hyperparathyroidism
Prolactin	Pituitary adenoma
Gastrin/insulin/VIP	Pancreas or duodenal neoplasm
MEN II	
Calcitonin	Medullary thyroid hyperplasia/carcinoma
Calcium	Primary hyperparathyroidism
Potassium	Aldosteronoma
Urinary catecholamines	Pheochromocytoma
Urinary cortisol	Adrenal hyperplasia or adenoma

and buccal and lingual nodules, hypertension, neck masses, and a marfanoid habitus (MEN IIB).

Evaluation. Patients with suspected MEN should undergo serologic surveillance of the appropriate markers of disease (Table 36-8). A classic family history for medullary thyroid carcinoma/hyperplasia warrants genetic testing for the ret-proto-oncogene. Such testing is important in children with normal serum calcitonin levels. Prophylactic thyroidectomy in the face of a positive ret-proto-oncogene and normal calcitonin levels is aggressive but appropriate therapy for these children, who otherwise develop a medullary thyroid malignancy.

Treatment. After a thorough work-up, operative intervention is suggested in order to minimize the ravages of primary hyperparathyroidism. Therapy for this syndrome is often less important than for the associated thyroid, pancreas, or adrenal disorders.

Treatment of primary hyperparathyroidism in MEN patients involves removing all but 50 mg of parathyroid tissue. A true solitary adenoma is unusual in these patients because of their propensity for multiple tumors. Given classic chief-cell hyperplasia, surgical options include a three and one-half gland parathyroidectomy or total parathyroidectomy with autotransplantation of heterotopic tissue. The concept of removing all but 50 mg of viable tissue is most important. Given the propensity of MEN patients to have more than four functioning glands, a thorough exploration and a transcervical thymectomy should be a routine part of the operation. It is not uncommon for these patients to have five or six parathyroid glands.

HYPERCALCEMIC CRISIS

Hypercalcemic crisis represents the life-threatening systemic condition brought on by elevated serum calcium levels (generally 13.0 mg/dL or higher).

Clinical Manifestations. Symptoms are varied and range from neuromuscular changes with mild fatigue and irritability to coma. Signs of dehydration are prominent. Gastrointestinal manifestations include anorexia, nausea, vomiting, and weight loss. Cardiac dysrhythmias, most commonly secondary to a shortened Q-T interval, may occur and can be lethal. Cancer cachexia may be evident in patients presenting with skeletal metastases. A palpable neck mass in the face of hypercalcemic crisis is considered a parathyroid carcinoma until proved otherwise. Therapy is initiated before attempting to differentiate the cause of hypercalcemia.

The list for the differential diagnosis is theoretically long, with any cause of hypercalcemia included, but in the vast majority (more than 90 percent) of cases it comes from advanced malignancy or primary hyperparathyroidism.

Treatment. Intravenous saline resuscitation is started and advanced to achieve a diuresis of higher than 100 mL/h. Dehydration is prominent with hypercalcemic crisis, and volume resuscitation (often 4 to 5 L) is the cornerstone of therapy. Once the patient appears adequately hydrated and urine output is more than 1 mL/kg/h, loop diuretics are given to stimulate a natriuresis and subsequent calciuresis. Cardiac dysrhythmias typically resolve with hydration and the subsequent decrease in the serum calcium level. Should dysrhythmias persist or become symptomatic, they are treated with standard agents for dysrhythmia. When hypercalcemia persists in the face of aggressive resuscitation and diuresis, the addition of mithramycin, phosphate binders (e.g., pamidronate), vitamin D, estrogen, calcitonin, or steroids may be useful. Hypercalcemia in patients with advanced malignancy and skeletal metastases can be difficult to normalize.

Patients with hyperparathyroidism usually can be stabilized with simple hydration and diuresis. Identification of a cervical mass on physical examination in the face of hypercalcemic crisis foreshadows a diagnosis of parathyroid carcinoma. Vocal cord function should be checked and the diagnosis of malignancy discussed with the patient. Ultrasonography may be useful while resuscitation is under way, or in the rare patient who is critically ill from persistent hypercalcemia. If a large adenoma is identified, hypercalcemia can be resolved quickly with a focused exploration and parathyroidectomy. With hemodynamic stability, regardless of the results of ultrasonography, operative intervention is undertaken early in patients with primary hyperparathyroidism. If the diagnosis of primary hyperparathyroidism is secure, even in comatose patients or in those with hemodynamic instability despite volume resuscitation, operative intervention should not be delayed. Postoperative transient hypocalcemia is common, and frequent calcium assessment is prudent because of the previous instability of these patients.

PARATHYROID CARCINOMA

Carcinoma of the parathyroid glands accounts for less than 1 percent of reported cases of hyperparathyroidism. In one study, 38 of 5010 patients with hyperparathyroidism were found to have parathyroid carcinoma (0.8 percent). Somewhat higher incidences have been reported in Japan, although the reason for this is unknown. The criteria that should alert the clinician to the possibility of this diagnosis can be divided into preoperative, intraoperative, and histopathologic findings.

Preoperative Findings. *1. Palpable neck mass.* An identifiable mass is present in 40 to 50 percent of patients with parathyroid carcinoma; this is in striking contrast to the incidence of less than 1 percent of this sign in patients with nonmalignant primary hyperparathyroidism. When found on physical examination, a mass secondary to parathyroid carcinoma has the expected characteristics of malignancy—firmness and fixation to surrounding tissue.

2. Markedly abnormal biochemistry. In patients with parathyroid carcinoma, the biochemical parameters used for the diagnosis of hyperparathyroidism are highly abnormal. Mean serum calcium levels usually are greater than 13.0 mg/dL (normal range is 8.9 to 10.1 mg/dL), parathyroid hormone levels are elevated tenfold, and alkaline phosphatase levels are elevated threefold. In our practice, any patient found to have a serum calcium level above 13.0 mg/dL is presumed to have a parathyroid carcinoma until proved otherwise.

3. Complications of hyperparathyroidism. Clear-cut symptoms of hyperparathyroidism should alert clinicians to the possibility of the diagnosis of parathyroid carcinoma. In one study, bone disease, renal insufficiency, and nephrolithiasis occurred in 91 percent, 84 percent, and 56 percent, respectively, of patients with parathyroid carcinoma, which are considerably higher than the rates found in nonmalignant hyperparathyroidism.

Intraoperative Findings. The surgeon should suspect the presence of a parathyroid carcinoma after finding a parathyroid mass that is firmer than the usual soft, friable, nonmalignant parathyroid gland. When a gland has been transformed from the normal bean shape and kidney color to an irregular, pale white and is adherent to any of the surrounding structures, the diagnosis of malignancy is almost certain.

Histopathologic Findings. Most parathyroid carcinomas weigh more than 2000 mg, but weight does not aid in the diagnosis. The hallmark of malignancy histologically are the presence of a thick, fibrous capsule, fibrous septa interdigitating throughout the tumor, and the enlargement, hyperchromasia, and variation of nuclear size. Clear-cut invasion through the capsule to involve adipose tissue, nerves, thyroid gland, or surrounding muscle usually is present (Fig. 36-60).

Treatment. The treatment of choice is en bloc surgical resection of the tumor and the involved surrounding structures. This treatment usually involves a total thyroid lobectomy on the affected side. Regional nodal metastases are uncommon, but lymph nodes should be assessed and, if involved, surgically treated by appropriate resection, which may include a modified radical neck dissection. Adjuvant external beam radiotherapy or multimodality chemotherapy have been used with limited success. Symptomatic hypercalcemia is controlled with mithramycin and biphosphonates. Malignant recurrence after initial operative resection occurs in at least 66 percent of cases. When recurrent disease is seemingly localized, repeat surgical resection—repeated as often as can be safely performed—is optimal. Nonsurgical treatment modalities are inadequate. Most patients with parathyroid cancer will undergo one or more explorations ranging from cervical exploration to thoracotomy or craniotomy. In a study of 43 patients, the 3-year and 5-year survival rates were 84 and 69 percent, respectively. The cause of death often was attributed to the metabolic consequences of hypercalcemia and not to the local effects of malignancy.

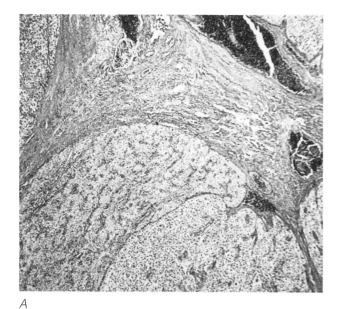

A

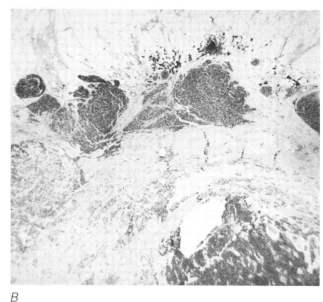

B

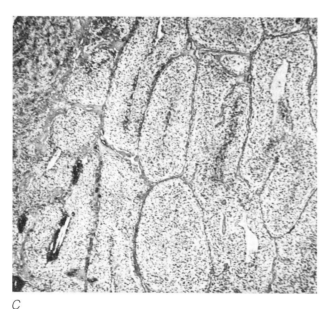

C

FIG. 36-60. Parathyroid carcinoma. *A. Classic fibrous bands. B. Invasion through the capsule. C. Trabecular pattern.*

Bibliography

Thyroid

History

Harrison BJ, Welbourn RB: History of Thyroid Surgery, in Wheeler MH, Lazarus JH (eds): *Diseases of the Thyroid: Pathophysiology and Management.* London, Chapman and Hill, 1994, chap 1, pp 11–18.

Pearse AGE, Polak JM: Cytochemical evidence for the neural crest origin of mammalian ultimobranchial cells. *Histochemie* 27:96, 1971.

Welbourn RB: *The History of Endocrine Surgery.* New York, Praeger, 1907.

Werner SC: Historical resumé, in Braverman LE, Utiger RD (eds): *The Thyroid: A Fundamental and Clinical Text,* 6th ed. Philadelphia, JB Lippincott, 1991, chap 1, pp 3–6.

Anatomy

Hilger AW, Thompson SD, et al: Papillary carcinoma arising in a thyroglossal duct cyst: A case report and literature review. *J Laryngol Otol* 109:1124, 1995.

Livolsi VA: Developmental biology and anatomy of the thyroid, including the aberrant thyroid, in: *Surgical Pathology of the Thyroid.* Philadelphia, WB Saunders, 1990.

Physiology and Tests of Thyroid Function

Björkman U, Ekholm R: Biochemistry of thyroid hormone formation, in Greer MA (ed): *The Thyroid Gland.* New York, Raven, 1990, pp 83–125.

Brent GA: The molecular basis of thyroid hormone action. *N Engl J Med* 331:847, 1994.

Burrow GN: Thyroid hormone biosynthesis, in Burrow GN, Oppenheimer JH, Volpé R (eds): *Thyroid Function and Disease.* Philadelphia, WB Saunders, 1990, pp 11–40.

Franklyn JA: Thyroid hormone action, in Wheeler MH, Lazarus JH (eds): *Diseases of the Thyroid: Pathophysiology and Management.* London, Chapman and Hill, 1994, pp 29–40.

John R, Lazarus JH: Hormone measurements, in Wheeler MH, Lazarus JH (eds): *Diseases of the Thyroid: Pathophysiology and Management.* London, Chapman and Hill, 1994, pp 107–115.

Jones KE, Chin WW: Differential regulation of thyroid hormone receptor mRNAs by thyrotropin-releasing hormone. *Endocrinology* 128:1763, 1991.

Hennemann G, Docter R, et al: Thyroid hormone production, transport, and metabolism, in Wheeler MH, Lazarus JH (eds): *Diseases of the Thyroid: Pathophysiology and Management.* London, Chapman and Hill, 1994, pp 21–27.

Kaye TB: Thyroid function tests: Application of newer methods. *Postgrad Med* 94:81, 87–90, 1993.

O'Leary R, O'Connor B: Thyrotropin-releasing hormone. *J Neurochem* 65:953, 1995.

Hyperthyroidism

Caruso DR, Mazzaferri EL: Intervention in Graves' disease: Choosing among imperfect but effective treatment options. *Postgrad Med* 92:117, 128–129, 133–134, 1992.

Catz B, Perzik SL: Total thyroidectomy in the management of thyrotoxic and euthyroid Graves' disease. *Am J Surg* 118:434, 1969.

Patwardhan NA, Moront M, et al: Surgery still has a role in Graves' hyperthyroidism. *Surgery* 114:1108, 1993.

O'Brien T, Gharib H, et al: Treatment of toxic solitary thyroid nodules: Surgery versus radioactive iodine. *Surgery* 112:1166, 1992.

Roti E, Minelli R, et al: Clinical review 80: Management of hyperthyroidism and hypothyroidism in the pregnant woman. *J Clin Endocrinol Metab* 81:1679, 1996.

Russo D, Arturi F, et al: Thyrotropin receptor gene alterations in thyroid hyperfunctioning adenomas. *J Clin Endocrinol Metab* 81:1548, 1996.

Thyroiditis

Dayan CM, Daniels GH: Chronic autoimmune thyroiditis. *N Engl J Med* 335:99, 1996.

Jordan RM: Myxedema coma: Pathophysiology, therapy, and factors affecting prognosis. *Med Clin North Am* 79:185, 1995.

Edwins DL, McGregor AM: Medical aspects of thyroid disease, in Lynn J, Bloom SR: *Surgical Endocrinology.* London, Butterworth Heinemann, 1993, chap 24, pp 294–311.

Giordano C, Stassi G, et al: Potential involvement of fas and its ligand in the pathogenesis of Hashimoto's thyroiditis. *Science* 14:960, 1997.

Goiter and Thyroid Nodules

Burch HB: Evaluation and management of the solid thyroid nodule. *Endocrinol Metab Clin North Am* 24:663, 1995.

Cooper DS: Clinical review 66: Thyroxine suppression therapy for benign nodular disease. *J Clin Endocrinol Metab* 80:331, 1995.

Gharib H, Goellner JR, et al: Fine-needle aspiration cytology of the thyroid: A 12-year experience with 11,000 biopsies. *Clin Lab Med* 13:699, 1993.

Gharib H, Goellner JR: Fine-needle aspiration biopsy of the thyroid: An appraisal. *Ann Intern Med* 118:282, 1993.

Mazzaferri EL: Management of a solitary thyroid nodule. *N Engl J Med* 328:553, 1993.

Siperstein AE, Clark OH: Surgical therapy, in Braverman LE, Utiger RD (eds): *The Thyroid: A Fundamental and Clinical Text,* 6th ed. Philadelphia, JB Lippincott, 1991, chap 84, pp 1129–1137.

Carcinoma

Ain KB: Papillary thyroid carcinoma: Etiology, assessment, and therapy. *Endocrinol Metab Clin North Am* 24:711, 1995.

Azadian A, Rosen IB, et al: Management considerations in Hürthle cell carcinoma. *Surgery* 118:711, 1995.

Fraker DL: Radiation exposure and other factors that predispose to human thyroid neoplasia. *Surg Clin North Am* 75:365, 1995.

Grant CS, Hay ID, et al: Local occurrence in papillary thyroid carcinoma: Is extent of surgical resection important? *Surgery* 104(6):954, 1988.

Grossman RF, Tu SH, et al: Familial nonmedullary thyroid cancer: An emerging entity that warrants aggressive treatment. *Arch Surg* 130:892, 1995.

Harness JK, Thompson NW, et al: Differentiated thyroid carcinoma in children and adolescents. *World J Surg* 16:547, 1992.

Hay ID, Bergstralh EJ, et al: Predicting outcome in papillary thyroid carcinoma: Development of a reliable prognostic scoring system in a cohort of 1779 patients surgically treated at one institution during 1940 through 1989. *Surgery* 114:1050, 1993.

Hazard SB, Hawk WA, Crile G Jr: Medullary (solid) carcinoma of the thyroid: Clinicopathological entity. *J Clin Endocrinol Metab* 19:52, 1959.

Kaplan ED: Thyroid and parathyroid, in Schwartz SI, Shires GT, Spencer FC: *Principles of Surgery,* 6th ed. New York, McGraw-Hill, 1994, chap 36.

Levin KE, Clark AH, et al: Reoperative thyroid surgery. *Surgery* 111:604, 1992.

Mazzaferri EL, Jhiang SM: Long-term impact of initial surgical and medical therapy on papillary and follicular thyroid cancer. *Am J Med* 97:418, 1994.

Moley JF, Wells SA, et al: Reoperation for recurrent or persistent medullary thyroid cancer. *Surgery* 114:1090, 1993.

Miccoli P, Antonelli A, et al: Prospective, randomized, double-blind study about effectiveness of levothyroxine suppressive therapy in prevention of recurrence after operation: Result at the third year of follow-up. *Surgery* 114:1097, 1993.

Moley JF: Medullary thyroid cancer. *Surg Clin North Am* 75:405, 1995.

Moreno A, Rodriguez JM, et al: Encapsulated papillary neoplasm of the thyroid: Retrospective clinicopathological study with long-term follow up. *Eur J Surg* 162:177, 1996.

Ozata M, Suzuki S, et al: Serum thyroglobulin in the follow-up of patients with treated differentiated thyroid cancer. *J Clin Endocrinol Metab* 79:98, 1994.

Pyke CM, Grant CS, et al: Non-Hodgkin's lymphoma of the thyroid: Is more than biopsy necessary? *World J Surg* 16:604, 1992.

Sadler GP, Wheeler MH: Parathyroid and thyroid cancer, in Taylor I, Cooke TG, Guillou P (eds): *Essential General Surgical Oncology.* London, Churchill Livingstone, 1996, chap 18, pp 189–202.

Samaan NA, Schultz PN, et al: The results of various modalities of treatment of well-differentiated thyroid carcinomas: A retrospective review of 1599 patients. *J Clin Endocrinol Metab* 75:714, 1992.

Sanders LE, Rossi RL: Occult well-differentiated thyroid carcinoma presenting as cervical node disease. *World J Surg* 19:642, 1995.

Scheumann GF, Gimm O, et al: Prognostic significance and surgical management of locoregional lymph node metastases in papillary thyroid cancer. *World J Surg* 18:559, 1994.

Shaha AR, Loree TR, et al: Prognostic factors and risk group analysis in follicular carcinoma of the thyroid. *Surgery* 118:1131, 1995.

Sipple SH: The association of pheochromocytoma with carcinoma of the thyroid gland. *Am J Med* 31:163, 1961.

Soh EY, Clark OH: Surgical considerations and approach to thyroid cancer. *Endocrinol Metab Clin North Am* 25:115, 1996.

Sweeney DC, Johnston GS: Radioiodine therapy for thyroid cancer. *Endocrinol Metab Clin North Am* 24:803, 1995.

Tennvall J, Lundell G, et al: Combined doxorubicin, hyperfractionated radiotherapy, and surgery in anaplastic thyroid carcinoma: Report on two protocols. The Swedish Anaplastic Thyroid Cancer Group. *Cancer* 74:1348, 1994.

Molecular Basis of Thyroid Cancer

Akslen LA, Varhaug JE: Oncoproteins and tumor progression in papillary thyroid carcinoma: Presence of epidermal growth factor receptor, c-erbB-2 protein, estrogen receptor related protein, p21-ras protein, and proliferation indicators in relation to tumor recurrences and patient survival. *Cancer* 76:1643, 1995.

Baker JR Jr, Fosso CK: Immunological aspects of cancers arising from thyroid follicular cells. *Endocr Rev* 14:729, 1993.

Burns JS, Blaydes JP, et al: Stepwise transformation of primary thyroid epithelial cells by a mutant Ha-ras oncogene: An in vitro model of tumor progression. *Mol Carcinog* 6:129, 1992.

Lemoine NR, Wright NA: The molecular pathology of cancer. Introduction. *Cancer Surv* 16:1, 1993.

Nikiforov YE, Nikiforova MN, et al: Prevalence of mutations of ras and p53 in benign and malignant thyroid tumors from children exposed to radiation after the Chernobyl nuclear accident. *Oncogene* 13:687, 1996.

Salvatore D, Celetti A, et al: Low frequency of p53 mutations in human thyroid tumours: p53 and Ras mutation in two out of fifty-six thyroid tumours. *Eur J Endocrinol* 134:177, 1996.

Santoro M, Grieco M, et al: Molecular defects in thyroid carcinomas: Role of the RET oncogene in thyroid neoplastic transformation. *Eur J Endocrinol* 133:513, 1995.

Sozzi G, Bongarzone I, et al: Cytogenetic and molecular genetic characterization of papillary thyroid carcinomas. *Genes Chromosomes Cancer* 5:212, 1992.

Sugg SL, Zheng L, et al: ret/PTC-1, -2, and -3 oncogene rearrangements in human thyroid carcinomas: Implications for metastatic potential? *J Clin Endocrinol Metab* 81:3360, 1996.

Takahashi M: Oncogenic activation of the ret protooncogene in thyroid cancer. *Crit Rev Oncog* 6:35, 1995.

Surgery

Clark OH: Surgical anatomy, in Braverman LE, Utiger RD: *The Thyroid: A Fundamental and Clinical Text,* 6th ed. Philadelphia, JB Lippincott, 1991, chap 25, pp 563–571.

Jatzko GR, Lisborg PH, et al: Recurrent nerve palsy after thyroid operations: Principal nerve identification and a literature review. *Surgery* 115:139, 1994.

Lekacos NL, Tzardis PJ, et al: Course of the recurrent laryngeal nerve relative to the inferior thyroid artery and the suspensory ligament of Berry. *Int Surg* 77:287, 1992.

Mack E: Management of patients with substernal goiters. *Surg Clin North Am* 75:377, 1995.

Wagner HE, Seiler C: Recurrent laryngeal nerve palsy after thyroid gland surgery. *Brit J Surg* 81:226, 1994.

Tietgens ST, Leinung MC: Thyroid storm. *Med Clin North Am* 9:16984, 1995.

Parathyroid

Historical Background

Eknoyan G: A history of the parathyroid glands. *Am J Kidney Dis* 26:801,1995.

Sandström I: On a new gland in man and several mammals (glandulae parathyroideoe). English translation by Carl M. Seipel, *Bull Hist Med* 6:192, 1938.

Taylor S: Hyperparathyroidism retrospect and prospect. *Ann R Coll Surg Engl* 58:255, 1976.

Thompson NW: The history of hyperparathyroidism. *Acta Chir Scand* 156:5, 1990.

Embryology and Anatomy

Mansberger AR Jr, Wei JP: Surgical embryology and anatomy of the thyroid and parathyroid glands. *Surg Clin North Am* 73:727, 1993.

Pearce SHS, Brown EM: The genetic basis of endocrine disease. Disorders of calcium ion sensing. *J Clin Endocrinol Metab* 81(6):2030, 1996.

Pathology

Weiland LH: Practical endocrine surgical pathology, in: van Heerden JA (ed): *Common Problems in Endocrine Surgery.* Chicago, Year Book Medical Publishers, 1989, pp 223–230.

Primary Hyperparathyroidism

Farley DR, van Heerden JA, Grant CS: Are concomitant surgical procedures acceptable in patients undergoing cervical exploration for primary hyperparathyroidism? *Mayo Clin Proc* 66:681, 1991.

Kjellman M, Sandelin K, et al: Primary hyperparathyroidism. Low surgical morbidity supports liberal attitude to operation. *Arch Surg* 129:237, 1994.

Sacks BA, Pallotta JA, et al: Diagnosis of parathyroid adenomas: Efficacy of measuring parathormone levels in needle aspirates of cervical masses. *AJR* 163:1223, 1994.

Shaha AR, Jaffe BM: Cervical exploration for primary hyperparathyroidism. *J Surg Oncol* 52:14, 1993.

Sofferman RA, Nathan MH, et al: Preoperative technetium Tc 99m sestamibi imaging: Paving the way to minimal-access parathyroid surgery. *Arch Otolaryngol* 122:369, 1996.

van Heerden JA, Grant CS: Surgical treatment of primary hyperparathyroidism: An institutional perspective. *World J Surg* 15:688, 1991.

Persistent and Recurrent Hyperparathyroidism

Doherty GM, Weber B, et al: Cost of unsuccessful surgery for primary hyperparathyroidism. *Surgery* 116:954, 1994.

Grant CS, van Heerden JA: Surgical management of persistent and recurrent primary hyperparathyroidism: The problem of hyperplasia. *Acta Chir Austriaca* 112:50, 1994.

Goldman L, Caldera DL, et al: Multifactorial index of cardiac risk in noncardiac surgical procedures. *N Engl J Med* 297:845, 1977.

Hopkins CR, Reading CC: Thyroid and parathyroid imaging. *Semin US, CT, MRI* 16:279, 1995.

Kao PC, van Heerden JA, et al: Intraoperative monitoring of parathyroid procedures by a 15-minute parathyroid hormone immunochemi-luminometric assay. *Mayo Clin Proc* 69:532, 1994.

Lee VS, Wilkinson RH Jr, et al: Hyperparathyroidism in high-risk surgical patients: Evaluation with double-phase technetium-99m-sestamibi imaging. *Radiology* 197:627, 1995.

MacFarlane MP, Fraker DL, et al: Use of preoperative fine-needle aspiration in patients undergoing reoperation for primary hyperparathyroidism. *Surgery* 116:959, 1994.

Marx GF, Maeto CV, et al: Computer analysis of postanesthetic deaths. *Anesthesiology* 39:54, 1973.

McBiles M, Lambert AT, et al: Sestamibi parathyroid imaging. *Semin Nucl Med* 25:221, 1995.

Mitchell BK, Merrell RC, et al: Localization studies in patients with hyperparathyroidism. *Surg Clin North Am* 75:483, 1995.

Rodriguez JM, Tezelman S, et al: Localization procedures in patients with persistent or recurrent hyperparathyroidism. *Arch Surg* 129:870, 1994.

Tezelman S, Shen W, et al: Persistent or recurrent hyperparathyroidism in patients with double adenomas. *Surgery* 118:1115, 1995.

Thompson GB, Mullan BP, et al: Parathyroid imaging with technetium-99m-sestamibi: An initial institutional experience. *Surgery* 116:966, 1994.

Weber CJ, Sewell CW, et al: Persistent and recurrent sporadic primary hyperparathyroidism: Histopathology, complications, and results of reoperation. *Surgery* 116:991, 1994.

Secondary Hyperparathyroidism/Tertiary Hyperparathyroidism

Packman KS, Demeure MJ: Indications for parathyroidectomy and extent of treatment for patients with secondary hyperparathyroidism. *Surg Clin North Am* 75:465, 1995.

Multiple Endocrine Neoplasia and Hyperparathyroidism

O'Riordain DS, O'Brien T, et al: Surgical management of primary hyperparathyroidism in multiple endocrine neoplasia types 1 and 2. *Surgery* 114:1031, 1993.

O'Riordain DS, O'Brien T, et al: Medullary thyroid carcinoma in multiple endocrine neoplasia types 2A and 2B. *Surgery* 116:1017, 1994.

Hypercalcemic Crisis

Allo MD: Hypercalcemic crisis, in: van Heerden JA (ed): *Common Problems in Endocrine Surgery.* Chicago, Year Book Medical Publishers, 1989, pp 151–155.

Parathyroid Carcinoma

Rosen IB, Young JE, et al: Parathyroid cancer: Clinical variations and relationship to autotransplantation. *Can J Surg* 37:465, 1994.

Vetto JT, Brennan MF, et al: Parathyroid carcinoma: Diagnosis and clinical history. *Surgery* 114:882, 1993.

Wynne AG, van Heerden JA, et al: Parathyroid carcinoma: Clinical and pathologic features in 43 patients. *Medicine* 71:197, 1992.

CHAPTER 37

Pediatric Surgery

Philip C. Guzzetta, Kathryn D. Anderson, R. Peter Altman, Kurt D. Newman,
and Jay J. Schnitzer

INTRODUCTION

Pediatric surgery combines the technical challenge of performing complex operations in neonates, the appeal of solving a wide array of problems in many anatomic locations, and the immense satisfaction of caring for children and offering them a long normal life. The approach to surgical problems in children should consider the long-term effects of the therapy as well as its immediate success rate. The resiliency of children to major surgical stress must always be balanced against their intolerance to inaccurate fluid and medication administration. The gratitude of a parent whose child has been saved by surgery is an additional benefit of this unique specialty.

GENERAL CONSIDERATIONS

Fluid and Electrolyte Balance. In an infant or child, the margin between dehydration and fluid overload is small. The infant is born with a surplus of body water, but within a few days this is excreted. At birth and for the first 10 days of life, fluid requirements are 65 to 100 mL/kg (750 to 1000 mL/m^2). Daily maintenance fluids can be calculated by the formula: 100 mL/kg up to 10 kg, add 50 mL/kg for 11 to 20 kg, and add 25 mL/kg for each kilogram of weight thereafter. Because I.V. fluid orders are written as milliliters per hour, this can be conveniently converted to 4 mL/kg/h up to 10 kg, add 2 mL/kg/h for 11 to 20 kg, and add 1 mL/kg/h for each additional kilogram. For example, a 26-kg child has a maintenance fluid requirement of $(10 \times 4) + (10 \times 2) + (6 \times 1) = 66$ mL/h. Fluid for maintenance is generally provided as 5% dextrose in $\frac{1}{4}$ or $\frac{1}{3}$ normal saline. For short-term intravenous therapy, sodium 5 meq/kg/day and potassium 2 meq/kg/day will satisfy the daily need. Fluid and electrolyte losses secondary to protracted vomiting or diarrhea are corrected by modifying this formula according to the measured losses. In the infant the normal serum osmolarity is between 280 and 290 mO/L.

Newborns have the ability to concentrate their urine well by the fifth day of life; thus urine concentration as well as output must be considered when ordering I.V. fluids postoperatively. Daily electrolyte determinations are performed in infants on I.V. alimentation to obviate the serious sequelae of hypoosmolarity or hyperosmolarity. If the child has a significant ongoing fluid loss (e.g., from a nasogastric tube), it is best to properly replace that loss with I.V. fluids at least every 8 h.

Whatever the formula used to calculate fluid replacement for the infant or small child, there is no substitute for collecting and analyzing fluid losses and replacing the depleted constituents precisely.

Acid-Base Equilibrium. Acidosis in children is an ominous sign unless it is the result of a chronic bicarbonate loss from the gastrointestinal tract or an acid accumulation as in chronic renal failure. Acute acidosis usually implies inadequate tissue perfusion, and the cause of acidosis must be sought. Treatment of acute acidosis with a base deficit of greater than 5 is to administer sodium bicarbonate in the following dose: base deficit $\times$ weight in kilograms $\times$ 0.5 (in newborns). In small children, the last factor in the equation should be 0.4, and it should be 0.3 in older children. The dose should be diluted to 0.5 meq/mL because full-strength sodium bicarbonate is hyperosmolar. One-half the corrective dose is given, and the serum pH is measured again. During cardiopulmonary resuscitation (CPR), one-half the corrective dose can be given as an I.V. bolus and the other half given slowly I.V.

Alkalosis is usually caused by hyperventilation or stomach acid loss. In the ventilated child, hyperventilation can be corrected easily by decreasing the respiratory rate or tidal volume. In the child with gastric fluid loss, I.V. fluids of 5% dextrose, 0.5% normal saline, and 20 mEq KCl/L usually correct the alkalosis. This is the preferred replacement fluid in children with pyloric stenosis and alkalosis.

Blood Volume and Blood Replacement. A useful guideline for estimation of blood volume for the infant is 85 mL/kg of body weight. When packed red blood cells are utilized, the transfusion requirement is calculated as 10 mL/kg, which roughly is equivalent to a 500-mL transfusion for a 70-kg adult. In the child, coagulation deficiencies rapidly may assume clinical significance after extensive blood transfusion. It is advisable to have fresh frozen plasma and platelets available if more than 30 mL/kg have been transfused. Plasma is given in a dose of 20 mL/kg and platelets are given in a dose of 1 unit/5 kg. Each unit of platelets consists of 40 to 60 mL of fluid and the platelets can be spun down to a platelet "button" in infants who require restricted fluid administration.

Hyperalimentation and Nutrition. The physiologic nutritional demands imposed on the growing infant are well recognized. When these are compounded by illness and the need to repair tissue and heal surgical wounds, the risks of protein-calorie malnutrition are considerable. Thus parenteral nutritional support has been integrated into the management of infants and children with surgical illnesses. When the gastrointestinal tract is not usable because of mechanical, ischemic, or inflammatory disorders, several options for nutritional support are available. Techniques for delivering calories by a central or a peripheral venous route have been refined to the point where the caloric needs of all patients can be satisfied. Central venous catheters continue to be the most common route for administering I.V. hyperalimentation for an extended period of time. Peripheral I.V. alimentation, utilizing less concentrated but greater volumes of solutions, in combination with I.V. lipid supplements has eliminated the need for central alimentation in some patients. The infusion of all solutions utilized for alimentation, indeed any I.V. solution in an infant or small child, always should be controlled by a properly alarmed constant infusion pump. To prevent the development of trace metal deficiencies, supplementary copper, zinc, and iron are provided to patients receiving long-term parenteral nutritional support.

By using these techniques, positive nitrogen balance can be accomplished for all infants and children. Refinements and advances in the techniques of parenteral nutrition have had an enormous impact on the survival of pediatric surgical patients. Despite the remarkable advances in I.V. alimentation, enteral feeding is always the preferred route, and every effort is made to use the gastrointestinal tract by mouth or by tube feeding as quickly as possible.

Venous Access. Obtaining reliable vascular access in an infant or child is a major responsibility of the pediatric surgeon. The goal always must be to place the catheter in the least invasive, least risky, and least painful manner and in a location that is most likely to allow use of the catheter without complications for as long as needed. Regardless of the size of the patient, most infants requiring short-term I.V. medications and nutrition can be managed by peripheral percutaneous I.V. catheter placement. For long-term I.V. access in small infants, use of Silastic central venous catheters is best. These are usually placed by cutdown in infants and by a percutaneous technique in older children. When a central venous catheter is placed by cutdown, the preferred sites are external jugular vein, facial vein, or proximal saphenous vein. Secondarily, the internal jugular vein may be used with a purse-string suture placed at the venotomy site to prevent venous occlusion. The catheters are tunneled to an exit site separate from the venotomy site. Currently, most central venous catheter placement by cutdown is done in the operating room under general anesthesia.

The percutaneous placement of central venous catheters in infants can be done with success in experienced hands. The risk of doing this procedure blindly in an infant always must be weighed against the benefit of avoiding a venous cutdown. In the infant with multiple central venous lines placed by cutdowns, the percutaneous approach may be the only reasonable option. Regardless of whether the catheter is placed by cutdown or percutaneously, a chest x-ray to confirm central location of the catheter tip and no chest complication from the placement is mandatory. We do this routinely within the operating room before the child is awakened.

Despite the technologic advances in the design of small catheters, the complication rates for central venous lines in infants are high. Sepsis from the catheter approaches a 10 percent incidence in many series, and superior or inferior vena caval occlusion is a significant risk, particularly in the smallest premature patients. We make every effort to feed the infants by the enteral route as soon and as completely as possible to minimize the length of time they depend on I.V. nutrition.

Thermoregulation. Infants or children compromised by disease are extremely thermolabile. Premature infants are particularly susceptible to changes in environmental temperature. Because they are unable to shiver and lack stores of fat, their potential for thermogenesis is impaired. Since these patients lack adaptive mechanisms to cope with the environment, the environment must be regulated. Attention to heat conservation during transport of the infant to and from the operating room is essential. Transport units incorporating heating units are necessary for premature infants. In the operating room, the infant is kept warm by the use of overhead heating lamps, a heating blanket, warming of inspired gases, and coverage of the extremities and head with occlusive materials. During abdominal surgery, it is best to use an adhesive plastic sheet to avoid sheets that are wet and cold. All fluids used to irrigate the chest or abdomen must be warmed to body temperature. Constant monitoring of the child's temperature is critical in a lengthy procedure.

Pain Control. The various physiologic responses of both neonates and fetuses to painful stimuli have been studied, and the results refute a commonly held belief that such patients do not have mature enough nervous systems to sense pain in a manner similar to adults. Despite concern that respiratory depression might result from administration of narcotic analgesics in infants, if the medications are given in the proper dose and with a proper time interval, they have an acceptable safety margin. In our hospital, virtually all parenteral analgesics are given intravenously. For all patients with an adequate understanding of the administration system, patient-controlled analgesia (PCA) is an excellent method of pain control. There is no fixed age below which PCA is not offered; however, patients below the age of 7 years generally are poor candidates for PCA.

Some attempts at parent-controlled analgesia have been made, but the emotional involvement of the parents and their desire to see the child pain-free rather than comfortable have limited the usefulness of that approach. Whenever possible, the use of anesthetic blocks, such as caudal tetracaine for hernias or thoracic epidural blocks for chest surgery, are encouraged. Two to three days of excellent pain relief can be obtained by epidural catheter administration of narcotics and/or local anesthetics, and such patients are monitored closely postoperatively. All pediatric patients having surgery, including circumcision, have pain, and should be given appropriate analgesia by the appropriate route to control that pain.

Minimally Invasive Surgery. New technology has allowed many procedures that traditionally were done as open procedures to be done using video-assisted, minimally invasive techniques in infants and children, regardless of size. Laparoscopic cholecystectomy, splenectomy, Nissen fundoplication, appendectomy, and placement of peritoneal dialysis and ventriculoperitoneal shunts are performed routinely with less morbidity than their open counterparts. Laparoscopic assessment of the asymptomic side in inguinal hernia and localization of the nonpalpable testicle are also becoming commonplace.

Laparoscopic pyloromyotomy is comparable with the open technique, but not demonstrably superior. Thoracoscopy for evacuation of empyema, lung biopsy and thoracic mass excision or biopsy also has gained wide acceptance in pediatric surgery.

LESIONS OF THE NECK

Thyroglossal Duct Remnants

Pathology and Clinical Manifestations. The thyroid gland buds off the foregut diverticulum at the base of the tongue in the region of the future foramen cecum at 3 weeks of embryonic life. As the fetal neck develops, the thyroid tissue becomes more anterior and caudad until it rests in its normal position. The "descent" of the thyroid is intimately connected with the development of the hyoid bone. Residual thyroid tissue left behind in the migration may persist and present in the midline of the neck as a thyroglossal duct cyst. The mass is most commonly appreciated in the 2- to 4-year-old child when the baby fat subsides and irregularities in the neck are more readily apparent. Usually the cyst is encountered in the midline at or below the level of the hyoid bone and moves up and down with swallowing or with protrusion of the tongue. Occasionally it presents as an intrathyroidal mass. Most thyroglossal duct cysts are asymptomatic. If the duct retains its connection with the pharynx, infection may occur, and the resulting abscess will need drainage, occasionally resulting in a salivary fistula. Submental lymphadenopathy and midline dermoid cysts can be confused with a thyroglossal duct cyst. Rarely, midline ectopic thyroid tissue masquerades as a thyroglossal duct cyst and may represent the patient's only thyroid tissue. Therefore, if there is any question regarding the diagnosis or if the thyroid gland cannot be palpated in its normal anatomic position, it is advisable to obtain a nuclear scan to confirm the presence of a normal thyroid gland. Although rarely the case in children, in adults the thyroglossal duct

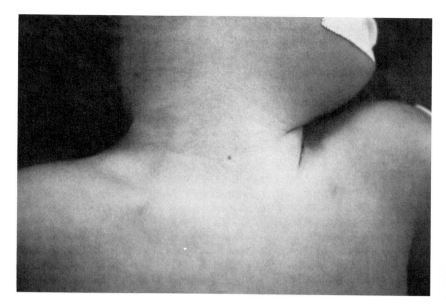

FIG. 37-1. Branchial cleft sinus tract opening at the anterior border of the sternocleidomastoid muscle.

might contain thyroid tissue that undergoes malignant degeneration.

Treatment. If the cyst presents with an abscess, treatment should consist of drainage and antibiotics. Following resolution of the inflammation, resection of the cyst in continuity with the central portion of the hyoid, and the tract into the pharynx, plus ligation at the foramen cecum (the Sistrunk operation), is curative. Lesser operations result in unacceptably high recurrence rates, and recurrence is more frequent following infection.

Branchial Cleft Anomalies

Paired branchial clefts and arches develop early in the fourth gestational week. The first cleft and the first, second, third and fourth pouches give rise to adult organs. The embryologic communication between the pharynx and the external surface may persist as a fistula (Fig. 37-1). A fistula is seen most commonly with the second branchial cleft, which normally disappears, and extends from the anterior border of the sternocleidomastoid muscle superiorly, inward through the bifurcation of the carotid artery, and enters the posterolateral pharynx just below the tonsillar fossa. The branchial cleft remnants may contain small pieces of cartilage and cysts, but internal fistulas are rare. A second branchial cleft sinus is suspected when clear fluid is noted draining from the external opening of the tract at the anterior border of the lower third of the sternomastoid muscle. The treatment is surgical, and complete removal of the cyst and tract is necessary for cure. Dissection of the sinus tract is facilitated by passing a fine lacrimal duct probe through the external opening into the tract and utilizing this as a guide for dissection. Injection of a small amount of methylene blue dye into the tract also may be useful. A series of two or sometimes three small transverse incisions in a "stepladder" fashion is preferred to a long oblique incision in the neck, which is cosmetically undesirable (Fig. 37-2).

Cystic Hygroma

Etiology and Pathology. Cystic hygroma (lymphangioma) occurs as a result of sequestration or obstruction of devel-

oping lymph vessels in approximately 1 in 12,000 births. Although the lesion can occur anywhere, the most common sites are in the posterior triangle of the neck, axilla, groin, and mediastinum. The cysts are lined by endothelium and filled with lymph. Occasionally unilocular cysts occur, but more often there

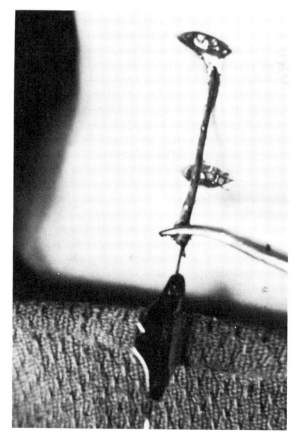

FIG. 37-2. "Stepladder" incisions for removal of branchial cleft sinus tract.

are multiple cysts "infiltrating" the surrounding structures and distorting the local anatomy. A particularly troublesome variant of cystic hygroma is that which involves the tongue, floor of the mouth, and structures deep in the neck (Fig. 37-3). Adjacent connective tissue may show extensive lymphocytic infiltration. The mass may be apparent at birth or may appear and enlarge rapidly in the early weeks or months of life as lymph accumulates; most present by age 2 years. Extension of the lesion into the axilla or mediastinum occurs about 10 percent of the time and can be demonstrated preoperatively by chest x-ray, ultrasound (US) or computed tomographic (CT) scan. Occasionally cystic hygromas contain nests of vascular tissue. These poorly supported vessels may bleed and produce rapid enlargement and discoloration of the hygroma. The diagnosis of cystic hygroma by prenatal US, before 30 weeks' gestation, has detected a "hidden mortality" as well as a high incidence of associated anomalies, including abnormal karyotypes and hydrops fetalis.

Infection within the cysts usually caused by *Streptococcus* or *Staphylococcus* may occur. In the neck this can cause rapid enlargement, which may result in airway compromise. Rarely, it may be necessary to carry out percutaneous aspiration of an infected cyst to relieve respiratory distress.

Treatment. Surgical excision is the treatment of choice. Total removal may not be possible because of the extent of hygroma and its proximity to and intimate relationship with adjacent nerves, muscles, and blood vessels. Radical ablative surgery is not indicated for this benign lesion. Conservative excision and unroofing of remaining cysts is advised, with repeated partial excision of residual hygroma if necessary, preserving all adjacent crucial structures. Postoperative wound drainage is important and is best accomplished by closed-suction technique. Despite this, fluid may accumulate beneath the surgically created flaps in the area from which the hygroma was excised, requiring multiple needle aspirations. Injection of sclerosing agents (OK-432 or bleomycin) with favorable results has been reported, but widespread use of these agents has not been seen in this country.

Cervical Adenitis

Enlarged tender lymph nodes are usually the result of bacterial infection (*Staphylococcus* or *Streptococcus*). Treatment of the primary cause (e.g., otitis media or pharyngitis) with antibiotics often is all that is necessary. However, when the involved nodes become fluctuant, incision and drainage are indicated, followed by appropriate wound care and dressing changes. More chronic forms of lymphadenitis, including infections with tuberculosis and atypical mycobacteria, as well as cat-scratch fever, require further work-up to make the diagnosis. In certain cases, extensive excision of the involved nodes will be necessary.

Torticollis

Fibrosis of the sternocleidomastoid muscle in infancy may produce shortening of the muscle and rotation of the head towards the opposite side. In two-thirds of cases, a mass may be palpated in the affected muscle. Histologically, the lesion is characterized by the deposition of collagen and fibroblasts around atrophied muscle cells. For up to 80 percent of patients, operation may not be needed, and physical therapy may be of some benefit. When necessary, surgical transection of the affected muscle is curative.

RESPIRATORY SYSTEM

Congenital Diaphragmatic Hernia (Bochdalek)

Pathology. During formation of the diaphragm, the pleural and coelomic cavities remain in continuity by means of the pleuroperitoneal canal. The posterolateral communication is the last to be closed by the developing diaphragm. Failure of diaphragmatic development leaves a posterolateral defect known as Bochdalek hernia. This anomaly is encountered more commonly on the left.

Incomplete development of the posterior diaphragm allows the viscera to fill the chest cavity. The abdominal cavity is small and undeveloped and remains scaphoid after birth. Both lungs are hypoplastic, with decreased bronchial and pulmonary artery branching; lung weight, lung volume, and DNA content are decreased, all more severely evident on the ipsilateral side. On rare occasions lung development is less adversely affected, signaling a greater chance of survival of the infant.

Prenatal US is successful in making the diagnosis of congenital diaphragmatic hernia (CDH) in the unborn child as early as 15 weeks' gestation. US findings include herniated abdominal viscera, abnormal anatomy of the upper abdomen, and mediastinal shift away from the herniated viscera. Herniation appears to be a dynamic process in which the viscera move in and out of the chest in some fetuses.

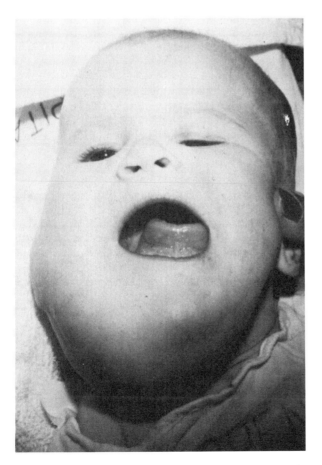

FIG. 37-3. Infant with a large cystic hygroma of the neck and floor of the mouth.

Prenatal criteria for a high-risk fetus include polyhydramnios, early diagnosis, a dilated stomach in the chest, and low lung-thorax ratio. Amniocentesis with karyotypes may show chromosomal defects, especially trisomy 18 and 21. Associated anomalies, once thought to be uncommon, are identified in 40 percent of these infants, most often of the heart, brain, genitourinary system, craniofacial structures, or limbs. Prenatal repair of CDH has had some success, and recent work has suggested that prenatal obstruction of the trachea may exert a salutary effect on lung growth.

Following delivery, the bowel fills with air, and the mobile mediastinum shifts to the opposite side of the chest, compromising air exchange in the contralateral lung. Respiratory failure occurs as a combination of the effect of hypoplasia of the lungs, persistence of fetal circulation as a result of pulmonary hypertension, and the mechanical compression of the lungs from the herniated viscera. Chest x-ray is diagnostic (Fig. 37-4).

Treatment. Many infants are symptomatic at birth due to hypoxia, hypercarbia, and metabolic acidosis, and prompt cardiorespiratory stabilization is mandatory. The goal of preoperative therapy is to reverse the persistent pulmonary hypertension that results in right-to-left shunting across the open foramen ovale and the ductus arteriosus. Improvement in the infant's status is apparent by improved oxygenation and ventilation. Immediate surgical repair is no longer performed. Instead the infant is stabilized by mechanical ventilation with 100% oxygen. Hyperventilation is no longer widely practiced and the infants are

often ventilated by high-frequency oscillation to avoid the pulmonary ravages of high inflating pressures. The goal of preoperative therapy is to prevent or reverse pulmonary hypertension and metabolic acidosis and provide adequate oxygen delivery. Levels of hypercarbia once considered unthinkable are tolerated. Newer techniques, such as intratracheal pulmonary ventilation and liquid ventilation, may offer some improved survival. The use of nitric oxide has been disappointing in correcting the pulmonary hypertension associated with CDH.

Infants with CDH who fail to respond, and remain severely hypoxic despite optimal care are candidates for treatment of their respiratory failure by extracorporeal membrane oxygenation (ECMO). Venovenous or venoarterial bypass is used. Venovenous bypass is established with a single cannula through the internal jugular vein, with blood removed from and infused into the right atrium by separate ports. Venoarterial bypass is used preferentially by some centers because it provides the cardiac support that is often needed. The right atrium is cannulated by means of the internal jugular vein and the aortic arch through the right common carotid artery (Fig. 37-5). As much of the cardiac output is shunted through the membrane oxygenator as needed to provide oxygenated blood to the infant and remove carbon dioxide. The infant is maintained on bypass until the pulmonary hypertension is reversed and lung function, as measured by compliance, is improved. This is usually seen within 7 to 10 days but in some infants may take up to 3 weeks to occur. Newborns who do not demonstrate significant improvement over this time have pulmonary hypoplasia that will not benefit from further extracorporeal life support.

The timing of diaphragm repair is controversial. Some surgeons perform early repair on bypass; others wait until the infant's lungs are fully recovered, repair the diaphragm and discontinue bypass within hours of surgery. Still others repair the diaphragm only after the infant is off bypass.

Operative repair of the diaphragmatic hernia is best accomplished by an abdominal approach. Through a subcostal incision the abdominal viscera are withdrawn from the chest, exposing the defect in the diaphragm. The anterior margin is often apparent, while the posterior muscular rim is attenuated. Most infants who need ECMO support prior to hernia repair have large defects, often lacking the medial and posterior margins. Prior to the availability of ECMO therapy, most of these infants died.

If the infant is heparinized on bypass, minimal dissection of the muscular margins is performed. Electrocautery is used liberally to minimize postoperative bleeding. About three-fourths of infants repaired on bypass require prosthetic material to patch the defect, suturing it to the diaphragm remnant or around ribs or costal cartilages for the large defects. If there is adequate muscle for closure, a single layer of nonabsorbable horizontal mattress suture is used to close the defect. Just before the repair is complete, a chest tube is positioned in the thoracic cavity and connected to 4 to 5 cmH_2O of suction.

Anatomic closure of the abdominal wall may be impossible after reduction of the viscera. Skin flaps are elevated and closed, creating a ventral hernia that may be closed using a Goretex patch. Rarely, a Silastic "silo" must be placed because the skin cannot be approximated.

If the diaphragm has been repaired on ECMO, weaning and decannulation are accomplished as soon as possible. All infants are ventilated postoperatively to maintain postductal arterial oxygenation of 80 to 100 torr. Very slow weaning from the ven-

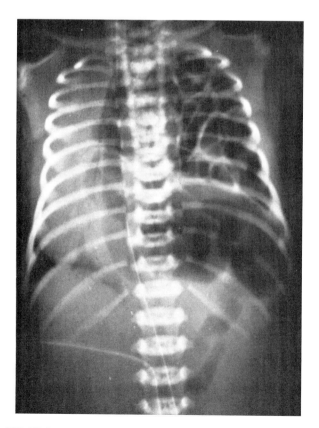

FIG. 37-4. *Chest x-ray of infant with congenital diaphragmatic hernia. Note mediastinum shifted to contralateral chest and absence of normal gas pattern in the abdomen.*

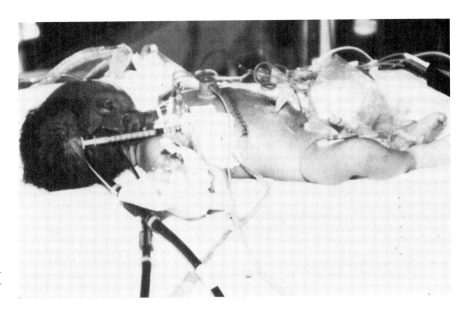

FIG. 37-5. Infant with right-sided congenital diaphragmatic hernia undergoing extracorporeal oxygenation.

tilator is necessary to avoid recurrent pulmonary hypertension. Oscillation ventilation may be switched to conventional ventilation as part of the process of weaning.

Currently there are no absolute criteria that successfully exclude the use of ECMO for these infants. Severe hypoxia or hypercarbia does not select infants who uniformly are nonsurvivors. At present, over 60 percent of infants with congenital diaphragmatic hernia who are supported by ECMO can be expected to survive.

Congenital Lobar Emphysema

Congenital lobar emphysema (CLE) is a rare condition manifested during the first few months of life as a progressive hyperexpansion of one or more lobes of the lung. It can be life-threatening in the newborn period but in the older infant causes less respiratory distress. Air entering during inspiration is trapped in the lobe; on expiration, the lobe cannot deflate and progressively overexpands, causing atelectasis of the adjacent lobe or lobes. This hyperexpansion eventually shifts the mediastinum to the opposite side and compromises the other lung. CLE usually occurs in the upper lobes of the lung (left greater than right), followed next in frequency by the right middle lobe, but it also can occur in the lower lobes. It is caused by intrinsic bronchial obstruction from poor bronchial cartilage development or extrinsic compression. Approximately 14 percent of children with this condition have cardiac defects, with an enlarged left atrium or a major vessel causing compression of the ipsilateral bronchus.

Symptoms range from mild respiratory distress to full-fledged respiratory failure with tachypnea, dyspnea, cough, and late cyanosis. These symptoms may be stationary or they may progress rapidly. Diagnosis is made by chest x-ray which shows a hyperlucent affected lobe with adjacent lobar compression and atelectasis with varying degrees of shift of the mediastinum to the opposite side and compression of the contralateral lung (Fig. 37-6). If definitive diagnosis is unclear by chest x-ray, CT scan may be helpful. Unless foreign body or mucous plugging is suspected as a cause of hyperinflation, bronchoscopy is not advisable because it can produce more air trapping and cause life-

threatening respiratory distress in a stable infant. Treatment is resection of the affected lobe, which may need to be done in urgent circumstances. The prognosis is excellent.

Congenital Cystic Adenomatoid Malformation

The clinical presentation of this lesion can be quite variable and lead to errors in diagnosis. The malformation consists of cystic proliferation of the terminal airway, producing cysts lined by mucus-producing respiratory epithelium, and elastic tissue in the cyst walls without cartilage formation. There may be a single cyst with a wall of connective tissue containing smooth muscle. Cysts may be large and multiple (type I), smaller and more numerous (type II), or resemble fetal lung without macroscopic cysts (type III). Most frequently located in the left lower lobe, this lesion can occur in any lobe and may occur in both lungs simultaneously. In the left lower lobe, type I may be confused at birth with a congenital diaphragmatic hernia. Clinical symp-

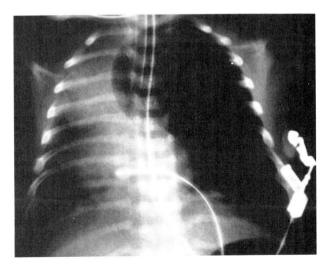

FIG. 37-6. Congenital lobar emphysema of the left upper lobe. Note mediastinal shift from air trapping.

toms may range from none at all to severe respiratory failure. The cyst(s), whether single or multiple, can produce air trapping and thus be confused with congenital lobar emphysema. They also can be involved with repeated infections and produce fever and cough in older infants and children, and be confused with pulmonary sequestration or pneumatoceles.

The diagnosis often can be made by chest x-ray. In certain cases, US or CT scan may be definitive. US evaluation of the fetus may suggest the diagnosis prenatally, and in the newborn US may be useful, especially to distinguish between adenomatous malformation and congenital diaphragmatic hernia. In older children who present with repeated infections, it may be wise to rule out sequestration by Doppler US or aortography. Resection is curative and may need to be performed urgently in the infant with severe respiratory distress. Lobectomy is usually required and the children do well following this procedure.

Pulmonary Sequestration

Pulmonary sequestration is uncommon and consists of a mass of lung tissue, usually in the left lower chest, occurring without the usual connections to the pulmonary artery or tracheobronchial tree. There are two kinds of sequestration. Extralobar sequestration is usually a small area of nonaerated lung separated from the main lung mass, with a systemic blood supply, located immediately above the left diaphragm. It is commonly found in cases of CDH. Intralobar sequestration more commonly occurs within the parenchyma of the left lower lobe but can occur on the right. There is no major connection to the tracheobronchial tree, but a secondary connection may be established, perhaps through infection or via adjacent intrapulmonary shunts. The blood supply is systemic from the aorta, often multiple, and frequently originates below the diaphragm (Fig. 37-7). Venous drainage of both types can be systemic or pulmonary. The cause of sequestration is unknown but most probably involves an abnormal budding of the developing lung that picks up a systemic blood supply and never becomes connected with the bronchus or pulmonary vessels.

Extralobar sequestration is asymptomatic and is usually discovered incidentally on chest x-ray. If the diagnosis can be confirmed, e.g. by CT scan, resection is not necessary. Diagnosis of intralobar sequestration, on the other hand, is usually made after repeated infections manifested by cough, fever, and consolidation in the posterior basal segment of the left lower lobe. Increasingly the diagnosis is being made in the early months of life by US, and color Doppler often can be helpful to delineate the systemic arterial supply. An arteriogram may be helpful in the older child in whom US of the chest is difficult, to help delineate the origin of the systemic blood supply and make surgical excision safer. Removal of the entire left lower lobe is usually necessary since the diagnosis often is made late after multiple infections. Occasionally the sequestered part of the lung can be removed segmentally. Prognosis is excellent.

Bronchogenic Cyst

Bronchogenic cysts can occur anywhere along the respiratory tract from the neck out into the lung parenchyma. They can present at any age. Histologically, they are hamartomatous and usually consist of a single cyst lined with respiratory epithelium and containing cartilage and smooth muscle. They are probably embryonic rests of foregut origin that have been pinched off from the main portion of the developing tracheobronchial tree

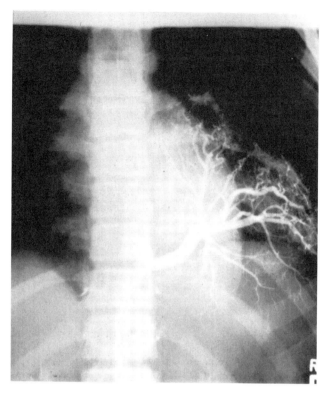

FIG. 37-7. Arteriogram showing large systemic artery supply to intralobar sequestration of left lower lobe.

and are closely associated in causation with other foregut duplication cysts associated with the esophagus. Bronchogenic cysts may be seen on prenatal US but are discovered most often postnatally incidentally on chest x-ray and may be completely asymptomatic. They may, however, produce symptoms, depending on their anatomic location. In the paratracheal region of the neck they can produce airway compression and respiratory distress. In the lung parenchyma, they may become infected and present with fever and cough. In addition they may cause obstruction of the bronchial lumen with distal atelectasis and infection. Chest x-ray usually will show a dense mass, and CT scan (Fig. 37-8) or magnetic resonance imaging (MRI) will delineate the precise anatomic location of the lesion. Treatment is resection of the cyst. Resection may need to be undertaken in emergency circumstances for airway compression. The prognosis is excellent.

Bronchiectasis

Bronchiectasis is an abnormal dilatation of the bronchi and bronchioles associated with chronic suppurative disease of the airways. Usually the children have an underlying congenital pulmonary anomaly, cystic fibrosis, or immunologic deficiency. Bronchiectasis also can result from infection secondary to a neglected bronchial foreign body. The symptoms include a chronic cough, often productive of purulent secretions, recurrent pulmonary infection, and hemoptysis. The diagnosis is suggested by a chest x-ray that shows increased bronchovascular markings in the affected lobe. Historically, a bronchogram was required to demonstrate the saccular or fusiform distortion of the peripheral bronchi. Chest CT delineates these lesions of bronchiectasis

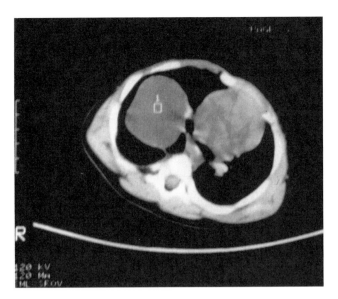

FIG. 37-8. CT scan showing bronchogenic cyst. Patient presented with fever and cough.

with excellent resolution. The preferred treatment for bronchiectasis is medical, consisting of antibiotics, postural drainage, and avoidance of inhaled pollutants. Lobectomy or segmental resection is indicated for localized disease that has not responded appropriately to medical therapy.

Foreign Bodies

Airway. Aspiration of foreign bodies most commonly occurs in the toddler age group. The material aspirated is often the ubiquitous peanut, but there is a plethora of small objects that youngsters put into their mouths that can be aspirated. A solid foreign body often will cause air trapping, with hyperlucency of the affected lobe or lung seen especially on expiration (Fig. 37-9). Oil from the peanut is very irritating and may cause pneumonia. Delay in diagnosis can lead to atelectasis and infection. The most common anatomic location for a foreign body is the right main stem bronchus or the right lower lobe. The child usually will cough or choke during eating but may then become asymptomatic. Total respiratory obstruction with tracheal foreign body may occur, but usually respiratory distress is mild if present at all. A unilateral wheeze is often heard on auscultation. This wheeze often leads to an inappropriate diagnosis of "asthma" and may delay the correct diagnosis for some time. Chest x-ray will show a radiopaque foreign body, but in the case of nuts, seeds, or plastic toy parts, the only clue may be non-deflation of the affected lobe on an expiratory film or fluoroscopy. Bronchoscopy confirms the diagnosis and allows removal of the foreign body. This can be a very simple procedure or it may be extremely difficult, especially with a smooth foreign body that cannot be grasped easily or one that has been retained for some time. Bronchiectasis may be seen as an extremely late phenomenon after repeated infections of the poorly aerated lung and may require partial or total resection of the affected lobe.

Esophagus. The most common foreign body in the esophagus is a coin. Again, toddlers are most commonly affected. The coin is retained in the esophagus at one of three locations: the

cricopharyngeus, the area of the aortic arch, or the gastroesophageal junction, all areas of normal anatomic narrowing. Symptoms are variable depending on the anatomic position of the foreign body and the degree of obstruction, but occasionally include respiratory distress from compression of the trachea or inability to swallow saliva and drooling. Many children are totally asymptomatic. The chest x-ray is diagnostic in the case of a coin. A contrast swallow may be required for nonradiopaque foreign bodies. Coins lodged within the upper esophagus for less than 24 hours usually can be removed safely by an experienced physician in the emergency room. For all other situations, the treatment is by esophagoscopy, rigid or flexible, and removal of the foreign body. In the case of sharp foreign bodies such as open safety pins, extreme care is required on extraction to avoid injury of the esophagus itself. Diligent follow-up is required after removal of foreign bodies such as batteries, which can cause strictures, and occasionally, a foreign body calls attention to a pre-existing stricture.

ESOPHAGUS

Esophageal Atresia and Tracheoesophageal Fistula

Perhaps no pediatric surgical condition has had as gratifying progress as the treatment of esophageal atresia and tracheoesoph-

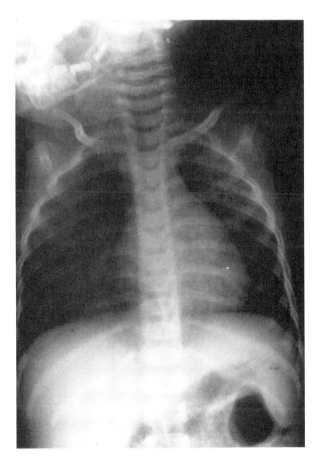

FIG. 37-9. Radiolucent foreign body of the right main stem bronchus. Expiratory film shows air trapping in right lung and mediastinal shift to left.

ageal fistula. In the early decades of the twentieth century, all babies born with this anomaly died. In 1939 Ladd and Leven achieved the first success with a complicated management plan that involved gastrostomy and fistula ligation, followed by esophageal reconstruction with a skin tube. Over 50 years ago, Cameron Haight in Ann Arbor, Michigan, performed the first successful primary anastomosis for esophageal atresia. This landmark achievement has been followed by steady improvement in survival for babies born with this condition. Currently most infants survive unless an associated major anomaly supervenes. This progress has resulted not only from refinements in surgical technique, but also from advances in nutrition, respiratory care, antibiotics, anesthesia, cardiology, genetics, and imaging technology.

Etiology and Pathology.   The cause of this malformation is uncertain; however, it almost certainly relates to the common embryologic origin of the esophagus and trachea. Normally they divide into separate tubes by 34 to 36 days' gestation, at which time the submucosal and muscular layers of both esophagus and trachea are apparent. When this separation is incomplete, a wide spectrum of malformations may result. The most common esophageal malformation (85 percent) occurs as a blind-ending upper esophageal segment. The lower portion of the esophagus connects to the trachea (Gross-Vogt type C) (Fig. 37-10). The lower esophageal fistula usually joins the trachea at or just above the tracheal bifurcation, admitting inspired air into the stomach and, in a retrograde fashion, gastric juice into the lungs.

Associated congenital anomalies are common and are the most significant factor influencing survival. Frequently esophageal atresia occurs as part of a collection of defects known by the acronym VATER or VACTERRL (*v*ertebral, *a*norectal, *c*ardiac, *tr*acheoesophageal, *r*enal, *r*adial, *l*imb). In nearly 20 percent of the infants born with esophageal atresia, some variant of congenital heart disease occurs.

Clinical Manifestations.   The earliest and most obvious clinical sign of esophageal atresia is regurgitation or drooling.

Feedings are followed by choking or coughing, indicating aspiration. Abdominal distention is a prominent feature, occurring when inspired air is transmitted through the fistula into the stomach. This sign differentiates "pure" esophageal atresia, in which no air can pass into the gastrointestinal tract, and the abdomen is therefore scaphoid.

Regurgitated gastric juice passes through the fistula and into the trachea and lungs, leading to chemical pneumonia. The pulmonary problems are compounded by atelectasis, which derives from diaphragmatic elevation secondary to gastric distention. The diagnosis may not be confirmed at the initial newborn examination by a physician, unless an attempt is made to pass a tube into the stomach. Nurses who are feeding the baby and observing behavioral patterns such as the accumulation of mucus or saliva often make the early diagnosis. In recent years, the diagnosis has been made prenatally with US examination. Polyhydramnios arouses suspicion, and failure to visualize a fetal stomach with US is suggestive of the diagnosis of esophageal atresia.

For many surgeons, the demonstration of a tube coiled in an air-filled upper pouch on a plain film is adequate to diagnose esophageal atresia. For others, a contrast x-ray study is required to confirm the diagnosis. Contrast medium instilled into the pouch outlines the blind upper esophagus (Fig. 37-11). It also may document the existence of an upper pouch fistula. Tracheal air enters the stomach via the fistula and establishes the presence of a tracheoesophageal communication on the x-ray. The condition of the lungs and the existence of pneumonia or atelectasis are also essential information. Examination of the heart and great vessels with echocardiography is important to exclude cardiac defects and verify the location of the aortic arch. In a stable infant, bronchoscopy at the time of repair allows localization of the level of the fistula, exclusion of upper pouch fistulas, and identification of a laryngeotracheoesophageal cleft.

Treatment.   With the diagnosis secure, the following measures should be instituted immediately: (1) infant warmer; (2)

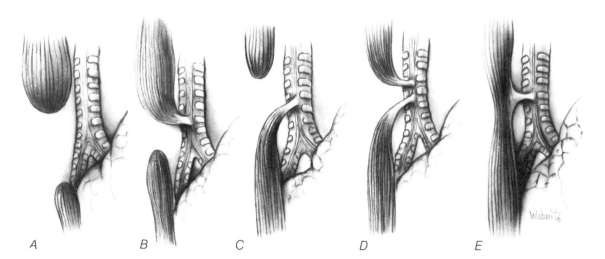

FIG. 37-10.   *Five major varieties of esophageal atresia and tracheoesophageal fistula. A. Esophageal atresia without associated fistula. B. Esophageal atresia with tracheoesophageal fistula between proximal segment of esophagus and trachea. C. Esophageal atresia with tracheoesophageal fistula between distal esophagus and trachea. D. Esophageal atresia with fistula between both proximal and distal ends of esophagus and trachea. E. Tracheoesophageal fistula without esophageal atresia (H-type fistula).*

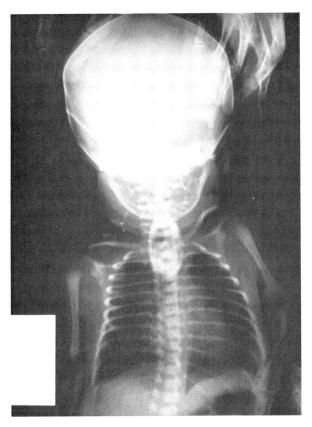

FIG. 37-11. Type C esophageal atresia with tracheoesophageal fistula. Catheter is coiled in upper pouch. Gas below diaphragm confirms the presence of a tracheoesophageal fistula.

30-degree head-up position; (3) route for I.V. therapy; (4) antibiotic treatment (even if pneumonia is not yet clinically manifest); and (5) sump catheter suction in the upper pouch. It has become apparent that the major determinant of poor survival is the presence of other severe anomalies; low birth weight and pneumonia are seldom risk factors for death. The optimal management strategy has evolved and is based on the physiologic status of the infant. If the infant is stable, a primary repair is undertaken. If unstable, the repair is delayed until the problems are resolved and the infant can safely undergo a major operation.

Primary Surgical Correction. The operative technique for primary repair is depicted in Fig. 37-12. The keys are careful division of the fistula with closure of the tracheal opening and adequate mobilization of the upper esophagus to permit an anastomosis without tension. The operation for primary repair of esophageal atresia and tracheoesophageal fistula has changed little since its description by Cameron Haight, although most surgeons now perform a single-layer anastomosis rather than the original two-layer. The transpleural approach may be easier, but the retropleural approach offers advantages. Exposure with this method is perfectly adequate, and protection of the lung by maintaining its pleural envelope has a salutary postoperative effect. More important, an anastomotic leak will not communicate with the pleural cavity. A leak can be drained directly from the mediastinum posteriorly with decreased morbidity. Although once routine, gastrostomy is rarely performed in the stable group of infants having primary repair.

Care must be taken when mobilizing the distal esophagus to avoid devascularization, since the blood supply is segmental from the aorta. Most of the esophageal length is obtained from mobilizing the upper pouch, since the blood supply travels via the submucosa from above. Livaditis showed that incising the muscle of the upper pouch circumferentially produced remarkable lengthening without compromising blood supply. This approach is useful if the distance between the two pouches precludes anastomosis without producing undue tension.

Delayed or Staged Repair. For infants with serious coexisting anomalies or extreme prematurity, survival is limited. For these infants, a gastrostomy is placed and repair delayed. Nutritional support, coupled with suction of the upper pouch and gastrostomy drainage, makes it possible to maintain infants with esophageal atresia and tracheoesophageal fistula indefinitely. Growth and weight gain are achieved, pulmonary status is cleared, and the congenital anomalies are studied and corrected. Some infants, particularly premature ones with noncompliant lungs, will not stabilize and require urgent division of the fistula. Anastomosis of the esophagus is accomplished at a later date.

Surgical correction of esophageal atresia with tracheoesophageal fistula leads to a satisfactory outcome with nearly normal esophageal function in most patients. Overall survival rates of greater than 90 percent have been achieved in patients classified as stable. Unstable infants have an increased mortality (40 to 60 percent survival) because of potentially fatal associated cardiac and chromosomal anomalies. However, the use of the staged procedure also has increased the survival in these high-risk infants.

Postoperative Course and Complications. The infant is maintained on parenteral nutrition for several days after repair. The chest tube is assessed daily for the presence of saliva indicating a leak. Many surgeons obtain a contrast swallow 1 week after repair to assess the caliber of the anastomosis and to look for a leak. If there is no leak, the infant is begun on feedings. A leak at the anastomosis usually heals without intervention, particularly if the pleural envelope has been maintained and drainage accomplished from the mediastinum via the retropleural route. Improved management of infection, nutrition, and respiratory support in infants has contributed to success in handling anastomotic leaks.

Strictures are not infrequent (10 to 20 percent), particularly if a leak has occurred. A stricture may become apparent at any time, from the early postoperative period to months or years later. It may present as choking, gagging, or failure to thrive, but often becomes clinically apparent with the transition to eating solid food. A contrast swallow or esophagoscopy is confirmatory, and simple dilatation is usually corrective. Occasionally, repeated dilatations are required.

"Recurrent" tracheoesophageal fistula may represent a missed upper pouch fistula or a true recurrence. The mediastinal infection seen with an anastomotic disruption may cause recurrence of the tracheoesophageal fistula. This complication may be difficult to identify and requires another operation to divide the tracheoesophageal fistula.

It has become apparent that even after repair, esophageal motility and the anatomy of the gastroesophageal junction are altered, potentially leading to gastroesophageal reflux. The clinical manifestations of this reflux are similar to those seen in other infants with primary gastroesophageal reflux. An antireflux pro-

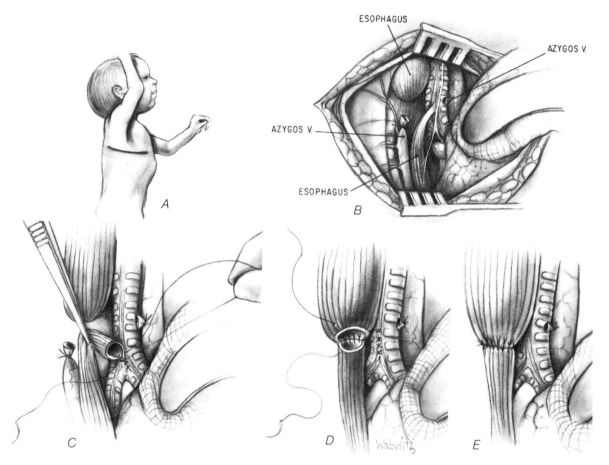

FIG. 37-12. Primary repair of type C tracheoesophageal fistula. *A.* Right thoracotomy incision. *B.* Azygos vein transected, proximal and distal esophagus demonstrated, and fistula identified. *C.* Tracheoesophageal fistula transected and defect in trachea closed. *D.* End-to-end anastomosis between proximal and distal esophagus (posterior row). *E.* Anastomosis completed.

cedure, such as a Nissen fundoplication, is used to prevent further reflux, but the child may have feeding problems after antireflux surgery as a result of the innate dysmotility of the distal esophagus.

Isolated Esophageal Atresia

Among those infants born with esophageal anomalies, 8 percent have isolated esophageal atresia. Characteristically, infants with isolated esophageal atresia present with a scaphoid abdomen, since the gastrointestinal tract is devoid of air. The x-ray finding of a blind upper pouch and the absence of air below the diaphragm is pathognomonic of isolated esophageal atresia without fistula.

The ideal surgical management is based on conservation of the native esophagus. Many surgeons perform a gastrostomy for feeding and wait 6 to 10 weeks for the upper pouch to dilate and elongate. On imaging studies, if it looks as though the two ends can be approximated, primary anastomosis is attempted. If the ends do not reach, however, esophagostomy with the upper esophageal pouch brought to the skin of the left side of the neck allows drainage of saliva and prevents aspiration. Esophageal replacement with a colon segment or reversed gastric tube is then recommended at 1 year of age.

Isolated (H-Type) Tracheoesophageal Fistula

In rare instances (4 percent), an isolated congenital fistula connecting the trachea to the esophagus may exist. In this anomaly, both the trachea and the esophagus are otherwise normal, with no narrowing or obstruction. Infants with this condition seem to swallow normally. The clinical features are subtle; weeks or months may elapse before a correct diagnosis is made. The presence of an H-type tracheoesophageal fistula is suggested by the following triad of symptoms: (1) choking when feeding, (2) gaseous distention of the bowel, and (3) recurrent aspiration pneumonia. Diagnosis usually can be confirmed by cine contrast x-ray studies or by bronchoesophagoscopy. Definitive treatment consists of dividing the fistula. Surgical closure of the esophagus and trachea must be meticulous, and encroachment on the lumen of the trachea must be avoided. The fistula is usually accessible to surgical repair through an incision just above the clavicle.

Laryngotracheoesophageal Cleft

Another variant of the failure of the trachea and esophagus to separate results in a communication that may be confined to the larynx or extend over the entire length of the trachea to the carina. The diagnosis is suggested by recurrent aspiration and is confirmed with bronchoscopy. The cleft is frequently present in association with esophageal atresia. The early management consists of tracheostomy, gastrostomy, and antireflux operation. At a later time the cleft is closed. Although once always fatal, most of these defects can now be repaired successfully.

Corrosive Injury of the Esophagus

The toddler age group is the most vulnerable to injury by ingestion of corrosive substances. Curiosity may lead a child to ingest crystals or an unknown liquid especially if it is placed in a drinking container. Since children gulp rather than taste, a single mouthful can cause severe injury. Both strong alkalis and strong acids produce injury by liquefaction or coagulation necrosis, and since all corrosive agents are extremely hygroscopic, the caustic will cling to the esophageal epithelium. Injury and therefore subsequent strictures occur at the anatomic narrowed areas of the esophagus, cricopharyngeus, midesophagus, and gastroesophageal junction. A child who has swallowed an injurious substance may be symptom-free but usually will be drooling and unable to swallow saliva. Most corrosives are swallowed accidentally by children and the volume ingested is limited to a single swallow because of the noxious taste and pain. Distal injuries to the stomach are therefore less common than in adults. However, the child must be observed carefully for signs of peritoneal irritation.

There is no effective immediate antidote. Diagnosis is by careful physical examination of the mouth and endoscopy with a flexible or a rigid esophagoscope. It is important to endoscope only to the first level of the burn in order to avoid perforation. Early barium swallow may delineate the extent of the mucosal injury, and it is important to realize that the esophagus may be burned without evidence of a mouth injury. Steroids have not been shown to alter the development of stricture or modify the extent of injury and therefore are no longer used, but antibiotics are continued for 3 weeks after injury. Circumferential esophageal injuries with necrosis will almost certainly stricture and therefore will be dealt with most safely by a gastrostomy and a string inserted either through the esophagus immediately or at a repeat esophagoscopy 3 weeks later. Dilatation is attempted after a minimum of 3 weeks to avoid perforation and is restricted to established strictures. For more severe injuries, retrograde dilatations are safest, using graduated dilators brought through the gastrostomy and advanced into the esophagus via the transesophageal string. For less severe injuries, dilatation may be attempted in antegrade fashion by either graded bougies or balloons. Perforation during dilation is extremely rare in experienced hands. Treatment of an iatrogenic perforation is controversial and ranges from nonoperative treatment with closed chest drainage to immediate operative closure. Abandonment of the esophagus is usually not necessary if recognition is prompt and treatment timely. Dilatations are continued as often as necessary, with the goal of keeping the child out of the hospital and eating a normal diet until the stricture is resolved or it is clear that esophageal substitution is required. Strictures have resolved as late as 6 months to a year after injury. Every attempt should be made to preserve the native esophagus.

Esophageal Substitution

Esophageal substitution is required less frequently than heretofore. The incidence of caustic strictures has been markedly diminished by the introduction of child-proof containers, and there have been successes with end-to-end anastomosis after a period of growth in infants with isolated esophageal atresia or wide gap esophageal atresia with fistula. However, these conditions are still the major indications for esophageal substitution in children. The options for esophageal substitution are the colon (right colon or transverse/left colon), reversed gastric tube, gastric pull-up or pedicled or free, grafts of the jejunum. The right colon is based on a pedicle of the midcolic artery, the left colon, on a pedicle of the midcolic or left colic artery (Fig. 37-13). Gastric tubes are made from the greater curvature of the stomach based on the pedicle of the left gastroepiploic artery. When the whole stomach is used, the vascularity is supplied by the right gastric artery. The route of the neoesophagus to the neck is at the surgeon's discretion. The substernal and left transthoracic route are still the most popular. Bringing the substitute through the posterior mediastinum, either following blunt esophagectomy in the case of caustic stricture or by creating a new tunnel in the case of esophageal atresia, avoids a thoracotomy and ensures the straightest path from neck to abdomen. Long-term follow-up has shown that all methods of substitution can support normal growth and development, and the children enjoy reasonably normal eating habits. Because of the potential for late complications such as ulceration and stricture, follow-up into adulthood is mandatory, but complications appear to diminish with time.

Gastroesophageal Reflux

Gastroesophageal reflux (GER) occurs to some degree in all children. GER is considered to be pathologic when it interferes with nutrition, causing failure to thrive; damages the esophagus, causing bleeding or stricture formation; or it leads to pulmonary

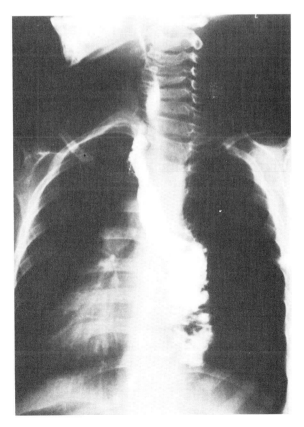

FIG. 37-13. Retrosternal coloesophagoplasty.

problems such as reactive airway disease, aspiration pneumonia or apnea. Failure to thrive and pulmonary problems are particularly common in infants with GER, whereas strictures and esophagitis are more common in older children and adolescents. The majority of children with severe GER that is unresponsive to medical therapy are neurologically impaired.

Clinical Manifestations. A history of repeated episodes of vomiting in an infant is the clearest indication of GER after obvious anatomic obstruction at or beyond the pylorus has been excluded. When the vomiting is associated with failure of normal development or chronic respiratory symptoms, the likelihood of pernicious GER is increased.

A child suspected of having GER is evaluated with a barium swallow to rule out an anatomic obstruction in the stomach or duodenum and a 24-h pH probe study to determine the severity of the reflux. The radioisotope "milk scan" is used to evaluate gastric emptying but is not obtained routinely if the upper gastrointestinal study shows normal gastric emptying. Endoscopy with biopsies to prove esophagitis is utilized only in selected patients.

Treatment. Most patients with GER are treated initially by conservative means. In the infant, propping and thickening the formula with rice cereal are generally recommended, although some authors prefer a prone, head-up position. In the infant unresponsive to position and formula changes and the older child with severe GER, medical therapy is based on gastric acid reduction with an H_2 blocking agent (i.e. ranitidine) and a prokinetic agent (i.e. cisapride). Surgery is indicated if medical therapy has failed to prevent complications of GER or there is an anatomic abnormality such as a large hiatal hernia or esophageal stricture. In children less than 1 year old or those unable to swallow because of neuromotor problems, a gastrostomy is performed routinely with the antireflux procedure.

Antireflux surgery is either by a complete (i.e. Nissen) or partial (i.e. Thal) fundic wrap around the distal esophagus. These procedures can be done safely in children laparoscopically. Postoperative complications of gagging, pulmonary problems and wrap breakdown with recurrent GER are quite high in children with neurologic impairment.

GASTROINTESTINAL TRACT

Pyloric Stenosis

Clinical Manifestations. Hypertrophic pyloric stenosis occurs in approximately 1 in 300 live births and is the most common surgical cause of vomiting in infancy. The typical infant is 4 to 6 weeks of age, male, and the first born child. Nonbilious vomiting, becoming increasingly projectile, occurs over several days to weeks. Eventually the infant will develop a nearly complete obstruction by the second to fourth week of life, and will not be able to hold down even clear liquids. This invariably proceeds to severe dehydration if not treated. These infants develop a metabolic alkalosis with severe depletion of potassium and chloride ions. The serum pH level is high, whereas the urine pH level is high initially but eventually drops as the severe potassium deficit leaves only hydrogen ions to exchange with sodium ions in the distal tubule of the kidney.

The diagnosis of pyloric stenosis usually can be made on physical examination by palpation of the typical "olive" in the right upper quadrant and the presence of visible gastric waves on the abdomen. When the olive cannot be palpated, US in experienced hands will diagnose the condition accurately in 95 percent of patients.

Treatment. Pyloric stenosis is not a surgical emergency. Fluid resuscitation with correction of electrolyte abnormalities and metabolic alkalosis is essential before induction of general anesthesia for operation. For most infants, I.V. fluid containing 5% dextrose and 0.45% saline with added potassium of 2 to 4 meq/kg over 24 h at a rate of approximately 150 to 175 mL/kg for 24 h will correct the underlying deficit. After this resuscitation, a Fredet-Ramstedt pyloromyotomy is performed (Fig. 37-14). Postoperatively, I.V. fluids are continued for several hours after which small frequent feedings of dilute formula or breast milk are offered and are gradually increased to full strength and full volume over the next 24 to 48 h. Most infants can be discharged home within 48 h following surgery.

Intestinal Obstruction in the Newborn

Bilious (green) vomiting is the most common presenting symptom in a newborn with intestinal obstruction. If the abdomen is not distended and the abdominal plain films show complete obstruction with no distal air, then the obstruction is most likely at the level of the duodenum or the pylorus. If there is incomplete obstruction with some gas more distally in the bowel, then an upper gastrointestinal series is mandated to diagnose malrotation with possible midgut volvulus. If, however, the abdomen is distended, the obstruction is most likely more distal. The physical examination will determine whether or not the anus is patent. Calcifications on the abdominal plain film may indicate meconium peritonitis; pneumatosis and/or free abdominal air indicates necrotizing enterocolitis (NEC) with or without intestinal perforation. Otherwise a contrast enema will show whether there is a microcolon indicative of jejunal-ileal atresia or meconium. If a microcolon is not present, then the diagnoses of Hirschsprung's disease, small left colon syndrome, and meconium plug will be entertained.

Duodenal Malformations

Duodenal obstruction may be complete as in duodenal atresia or partial as in duodenal web or stenosis, annular pancreas, and malrotation of the midgut. A prenatal US may show duodenal obstruction by demonstrating fluid filled cystic structures in the upper abdomen. Associated polyhydramnios is common and presents in the third trimester. In 85 percent of infants with duodenal obstruction, the entry of the bile duct is proximal to the level of obstruction, such that vomiting is bilious. Abdominal distention is not present because of the proximal level of obstruction. In those infants with obstruction proximal to the bile duct entry, the vomiting is nonbilious. Approximately one third of newborns with duodenal atresia have associated Down's syndrome (trisomy 21). The "double bubble" seen on the air contrast upper gastrointestinal series is characteristic of duodenal atresia, with small amounts of air seen distally if obstruction is incomplete (Fig. 37-15).

A naso- or orogastric tube is passed to decompress the stomach and duodenum and the infant is given I.V. fluids to maintain adequate urine output. The infant should be evaluated thoroughly for other associated anomalies, especially cardiac, since surgery is non-emergent. However, surgery should not be delayed if mal-

sia. Most surgeons will perform a duodenoduodenostomy to correct the anomaly using either a standard side-to-side or proximal transverse-to-distal longitudinal (diamond shaped) anastomosis with appropriate suture. An annular pancreas is never divided. Webs can be excised through a vertical duodenal incision, the mucosal oversewn, and the duodenotomy closed horizontally. Gastrostomy tubes are not placed routinely. Recently reported survival rates exceed 90 percent. Late complications from repair of duodenal atresia occur in approximately 12 to 15 percent of patients and include megaduodenum, intestinal motility disorders, duodenogastric reflux, gastritis, peptic ulcer, gastroesophageal reflux, choledochal cyst, and cholelithiasis with cholecystitis.

Intestinal Atresia

Fetal mesenteric vascular accidents are likely to be the cause of most cases of intestinal atresia, based on a large amount of experimental and clinical data. The incidence of intestinal atresia has been estimated to be between 1 in 2000 to 1 in 5000 live births, with equal representation of the sexes. Clinically the infants with jejunal or ileal atresia present with bilious vomiting and progressive abdominal distention. The degree to which the

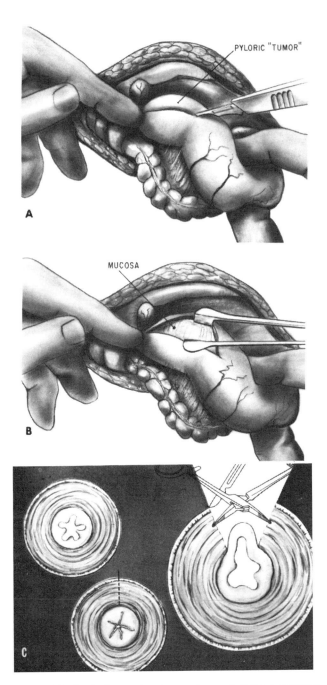

FIG. 37-14. Fredet-Ramstedt pyloromyotomy. *A.* Pylorus delivered into wound and seromuscular layer incised. *B.* Seromuscular layer separated down to submucosal base to permit herniation of mucosa through pyloric incision. *C.* Cross section demonstrating hypertrophied pylorus, depth of incision, and spreading of muscle to permit mucosa to herniate through incision.

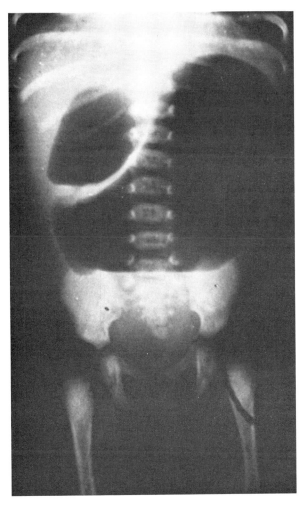

FIG. 37-15. Air-contrast study of an infant with congenital duodenal obstruction. Note size of stomach and distended duodenum, forming the "double bubble."

rotation is the cause of duodenal obstruction or if malrotation is present with intrinsic duodenal obstruction.

Once the work-up is complete and the infant is stable, he or she is taken to the operating room and the abdomen entered through a transverse right upper quadrant supraumbilical incision under general endotracheal anesthesia. Associated anomalies found at the time of the operation include annular pancreas, malrotation, anterior portal vein, second distal web, and biliary atre-

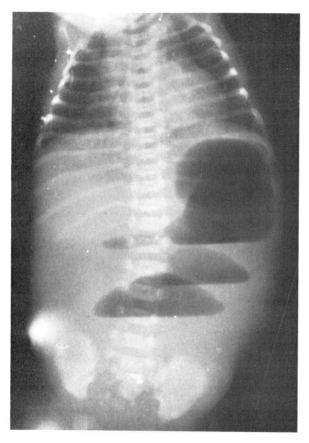

FIG. 37-16. *Newborn intestinal obstruction showing several loops of distended bowel with air-fluid levels characteristic of jejunal atresia.*

abdomen becomes distended and the number of obstructed loops on upright abdominal films correlates roughly with the level of the obstruction (Fig. 37-16).

In 12 percent of patients, calcification can be observed on the plain abdominal films diagnosing prenatal perforation and meconium peritonitis. Work-up of the newborn with suspected jejunal-ileal atresia includes a barium enema. The information from this procedure can distinguish small versus large intestinal distention, whether or not a microcolon is present, the level of obstruction, and the position of the cecum.

Surgical correction of the small intestinal atresia is urgent. At laparotomy, one of several types of atresia will be encountered. In type I there is a mucosal atresia with intact muscularis. In type 2 the atretic ends are connected by a fibrous band. In type 3A the two ends of the atresia are separated by a V-shaped defect in the mesentery. Type 3B is an "apple-peal" deformity or "Christmas tree" deformity in which the bowel distal to atresia receives a retrograde blood supply from the ileal colic or right colic artery. In type 4 atresia, there are multiple atresias with a "string of sausage" or "string of beads" appearance. Disparity in lumen size (Fig. 37-17) between the proximal distended bowel and the small diameter of collapsed bowel distal to the atresia has lead to a number of innovative techniques of anastomosis. These include 1) end-to-back technique, fish-mouthing the antimesenteric border of the distal loop; 2) tapering of the proximal distended loop to correspond to the distal loop with end-to-end anastomosis; 3) Bishop-Koop end-to-side union with exteriorization of the distal lumen, and rarely, 4) Mikulicz exteriorization or 5) end ileostomies with delayed anastomosis (Fig. 37-18).

Malrotation and Midgut Volvulus

During fetal development, the midgut supplied by the superior mesenteric artery grows too rapidly to be accommodated in the abdominal cavity. Prolapse into the umbilical cord occurs around the sixth week. Between the tenth and twelfth week, the midgut returns to the abdominal cavity, undergoing a 270 degree counterclockwise rotation around the superior mesenteric artery. The duodenum rotates caudal to the artery, and its C-loop traces this path. The transverse and ascending colon demonstrate the path of rotation of the cecum cephalad to the artery. The duo-

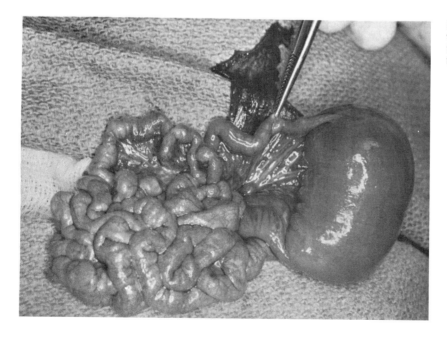

FIG. 37-17. *Operative photograph of newborn with jejunal atresia. Note distended proximal portion; point of obstruction is seen just proximal of forceps.*

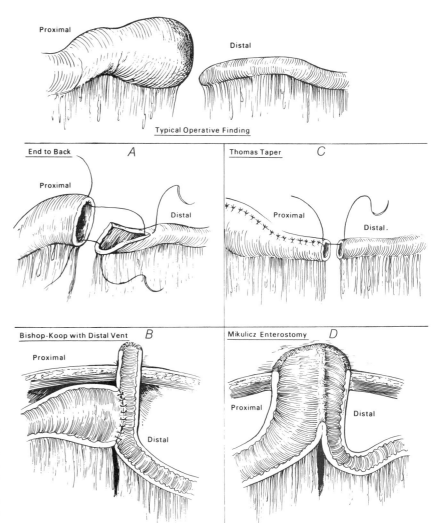

FIG. 37-18. *Techniques of intestinal anastomosis for infants with small bowel obstruction. (Typical operative findings: proximal distention and discrepancy between ends of intestine to be anastomosed.) A. End-to-back distal limb has been incised, creating "fishmouth" to enlarge lumen. B. Bishop-Koop; proximal distended limb joined to side of distal small bowel, which is vented by "chimney" to the abdominal wall. C. Tapering: Portion of antimesenteric wall of proximal bowel excised, with longitudinal closure to minimize disparity in the limbs. D. Mikulicz double-barreled enterostomy is constructed by suturing the two limbs together and then exteriorizing the double stoma. The common wall can be crushed with a special clamp to create one large stoma. The stoma can be closed in an extraperitoneal manner.*

denum becomes fixed retroperitoneally in its third portion, emerging at the ligament of Treitz, and the cecum becomes fixed to the lateral abdominal wall by peritoneal bands. The takeoff of the branches of the superior mesenteric artery elongates and becomes fixed along a line extending from its emergence from the aorta to the cecum in the right lower quadrant. If rotation is incomplete, the cecum remains in the epigastrium, but the bands fixing the duodenum to the retroperitoneum and cecum continue to form. This results in bands (Ladd's bands) extending from the cecum to the lateral abdominal wall and crossing the duodenum with the potential for obstruction. The mesenteric takeoff remains confined to the epigastrium, resulting in a narrow pedicle suspending all the branches of the superior mesenteric artery and the entire midgut. A volvulus may occur around the mesentery, obstructing the jejunum and also cutting off the blood supply to the midgut. Intestinal obstruction and the potential for total vascular compromise of the midgut supervene unless the condition is corrected.

Midgut volvulus can occur at any age, though it is seen most often in the first few weeks of life. Bilious vomiting is usually the first sign of volvulus and all infants with bilious vomiting must be evaluated rapidly to insure that they do not have intestinal malrotation with volvulus. Chronic obstructive symptoms

from Ladd's bands across the duodenum may manifest as intermittent vomiting, but a volvulus presents early with irritability and bile vomitus and later with manifestations of vascular compromise such as bloody stools and eventually circulatory collapse. The index of suspicion for this condition must be high, since abdominal signs are minimal in the early stages. Advanced ischemia of the intestine results in erythema and edema of the abdominal wall, shock and rapidly, death. Abdominal films show a paucity of gas throughout the intestine with a few scattered air-fluid levels. The diagnosis of malrotation is best made by an upper gastrointestinal series that shows incomplete rotation with the duodenojejunal junction displaced to the right. The duodenum may show a corkscrew effect diagnosing volvulus, or complete duodenal obstruction, with the small bowel loops entirely in the right side of the abdomen. Barium enema may show a displaced cecum, but this sign is unreliable, especially in the small infant in whom the cecum is normally in a somewhat higher position than in the older child.

Early surgical intervention is mandatory if the ischemic process is to be avoided or reversed. Volvulus occurs clockwise and it is therefore untwisted counterclockwise. The bands between the cecum and the abdominal wall and between the duodenum and terminal ileum are divided sharply to splay out the superior mesenteric artery and its branches. This brings the straightened duodenum into the right lower quadrant and the cecum into the left lower quadrant. The appendix is removed to avoid diagnostic errors in later life (Fig. 37-19). If the bands have been lysed completely no suturing of the cecum or duodenum is necessary. With advanced ischemia, reduction of the volvulus without the Ladd procedure is accomplished, and a "second look" 24 hours to 36 h later often will show vascular recovery. Frankly necrotic bowel can then be resected conservatively. With early diagnosis and correction the prognosis is excellent. With delays in diagnosis, the infant may succumb or be condemned to the ravages of shortgut syndrome until intestinal transplantation becomes routinely possible.

Meconium Ileus

Meconium ileus produces intestinal obstruction from impaction of meconium in the distal ileum. The ideology of this problem is cystic fibrosis. These infants have deficits of pancreatic enzymes in the intestine producing viscous meconium. Bilious vomiting appears late, following progressive abdominal distention, failure to pass meconium, and impressively dilated loops of small bowel on upright abdominal film without air fluid levels. Small bubbles of gas entrapped in the inspissated meconium in the terminal ileum may produce a characteristic "ground glass" appearance. A contrast enema will demonstrate a microcolon and the terminal ileum filled with pellets of meconium (Fig. 37-20). In patients with prenatal intestinal perforation, intraperitoneal calcifications form, producing an eggshell pattern on plain abdominal x-ray. Patients with uncomplicated meconium-ileus, i.e. patients without intestinal perforation or vascular compromise of the distended ileum, can be treated nonoperatively by a method originally described by Noblett.

Dilute Gastrografin is advanced through the colon under fluoroscopic control into the dilated portion of the ileum. Since Gastrografin acts partially by absorbing fluid from the bowel wall into the intestinal lumen, maintaining adequate hydration of the infant during this maneuver is extremely important. The enema may be repeated at 12-h intervals over several days until all the meconium is evacuated per rectum. If surgical intervention is required because of failure of Gastrografin enemas to relieve obstruction, operative irrigation with dilute Gastrografin or acetylcysteine (Mucomyst) through a purse-string suture may be successful. Alternatively, resection of the distended terminal ileum is performed, the meconium pellets are flushed from the distal small bowel by acetylcysteine, and ileostomies, a Bishop-Koop anastomosis, or an end-to-end anastomosis is performed.

Necrotizing Enterocolitis

Clinical Manifestations. Necrotizing enterocolitis (NEC) is a disease of multifactorial origin that almost exclusively affects stressed premature infants. Common factors found in most infants with NEC include intestinal ischemia, bacterial colonization of the gut, and enteral feedings of synthetic formulas. Hypoalbuminemia may predispose neonates to NEC. Experimental evidence suggests that both ischemia and reperfusion may lead to the intestinal damage seen in NEC. Clinically the first sign of NEC is formula intolerance, evident by vomiting or a large residual volume of a previous feeding in the stomach at the time of the next feeding. Abdominal distention and hematochezia are the next signs of NEC and suggest ileus and mucosal ischemia, respectively. Invasion of the ischemic mucosa

by gas-forming organisms causes pneumatosis intestinalis, which is the pathognomonic radiographic finding in NEC (Fig. 37-21). Development of hepatoportal venous gas suggests a particularly severe form of NEC. Some children, despite appropriate medical therapy, will develop a fulminant course with progressive peritonitis, acidosis, sepsis, disseminated intravascular coagulopathy, and death.

Treatment. In all infants suspected of having NEC, feedings are discontinued, a nasogastric tube is placed, and parenteral antibiotics are given. Free intraperitoneal air and signs of diffuse peritonitis are obvious indications for operation. Children with significant acidosis (pH < 7.20) after volume resuscitation and those with hepatoportal venous gas who do not improve promptly on medical therapy are also considered surgical candidates. In equivocal cases, tapping the peritoneal cavity may aid in the decision to operate if the fluid withdrawn contains bacteria or intestinal contents. Resection of frankly gangrenous bowel should be carried out, and in the vast majority of cases, the intestinal ends are brought out as stomas. When there is massive intestinal involvement, marginally viable bowel is retained and a "second-look" procedure is carried out in 24 h. In the selected neonate weighing less than 1500 grams, drainage of the peritoneal cavity under local anesthesia is an effective method of improving the desperately ill infant, with approximately one-third surviving without additional operations.

Total parenteral nutrition is maintained for at least 2 weeks postoperatively, after which oral feedings of small volumes of dilute formula are gradually introduced. Strictures develop in 20 percent of medically or surgically treated patients, and a contrast enema is mandatory before reestablishing intestinal continuity. If all other factors are favorable, the ileostomy is closed when the child is between 2 and 2.5 kg. Despite the severity of the illness in this premature population, survival rates for NEC approach 80 percent in many series.

Intussusception

Intussusception is a common cause of intestinal obstruction in the infant. It is observed most often in infants between 8 and 12 months of age and is slightly more common in males. The most common cause is hypertrophy of the Peyer's patches in the terminal ileum from an antecedent viral infection. The hypertrophied lymphatic patch becomes drawn into the lumen of the terminal ileum and is moved progressively into the ascending and transverse colon. Polyps, malignant tumors, such as lymphoma, and Meckel's diverticulum may act as lead points for intussusception; such intussusceptions are rarely reduced by air or contrast enema, and thus the lead point is identified when operative reduction of the intussusception is performed.

Clinical Manifestations. Since intussusception is frequently preceded by a gastrointestinal viral illness, the onset may not be determined easily. Typically, the infant develops paroxysms of crampy abdominal pain and intermittent vomiting. Between attacks the infant may act completely well, but as symptoms progress, increasing lethargy develops. Bloody mucus ("currant-jelly" stool) may be passed per rectum. Ultimately, if reduction is not accomplished, gangrene of the intussusceptum occurs.

The pathognomonic physical finding is an elongated mass in the right upper quadrant or epigastrium with an absence of bowel

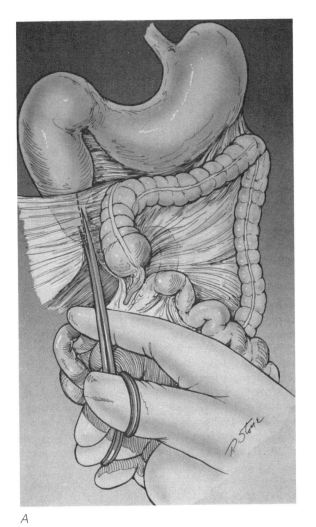

A

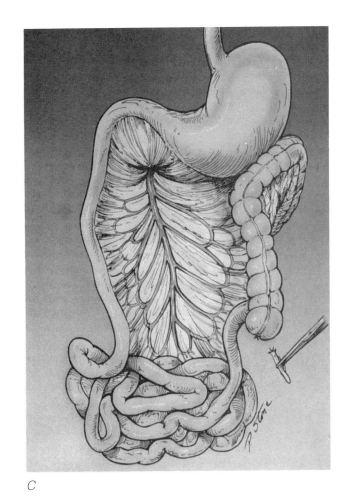

C

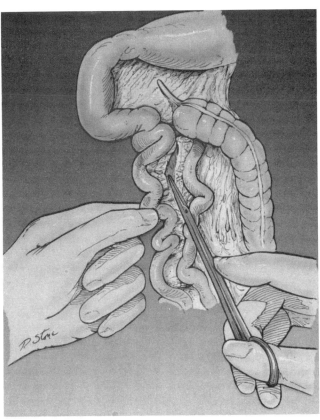

B

FIG. 37-19. Operative correction of malrotation. Lysis of cecal and duodenal bands—Ladd procedure.

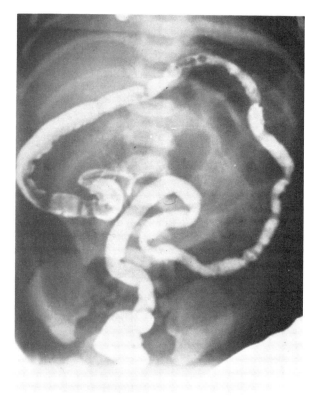

FIG. 37-20. *Barium enema in an infant with meconium ileus. Microcolon is demonstrated. Colonic rotation is normal.*

in the right lower quadrant (Dance's sign). The mass may be seen on plain abdominal x-ray but is more easily demonstrated on air or contrast enema.

Treatment. The air enema is the preferred method of diagnosis and nonoperative treatment of intussusception. Air is introduced with a manometer and pressure should not exceed 120 mmHg. Peritonitis constitutes a contraindication to air enema. The air may push the intussusception before it and accomplish reduction. Free reflux into multiple small bowel loops and an infant who abruptly becomes well are characteristic of successful reduction. Unless both these signs are observed, it cannot be assumed that the intussusception is reduced, and preparations for exploration are made. Despite reports of successful reduction in more than 90 percent of children with intussusception using air enema, most centers are achieving about 60 percent successful reduction with this technique.

If hydrostatic reduction is successful, the infant may be given oral fluids immediately. The incidence of recurrent intussusception is 5 percent whether the intussusception is reduced by operation or by hydrostatic pressure. Failure to reduce the intussusception mandates surgery. Exploration is carried out through a right lower quadrant incision, delivering the intussuscepted mass into the wound. Reduction usually can be accomplished by gentle distal pressure, milking the bowel out of the intussuscipiens, never pulling it out. The blood supply to the appendix is often compromised, and appendectomy is performed. Resection of frankly gangrenous bowel is carried out without attempting reduction of the intussusception. As a rule, primary ileocolic anastomosis can be performed after resection.

I.V. fluids are continued until peristalsis returns. If resection is necessary, prophylactic antibiotics are also administered for 72 h.

Appendicitis

Clinical Manifestations. Appendicitis in children may differ in presentation from the same disease in adults. The incidence of perforation rises dramatically as the age of the patient

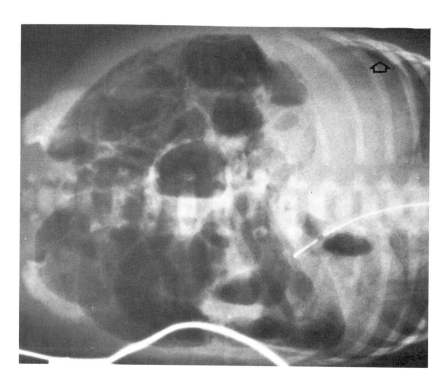

FIG. 37-21. *Left lateral decubitus x-ray study showing characteristic findings of necrotizing enterocolitis. There are distended, separated loops of bowel. Air is seen in the wall of the bowel (pneumatosis). The arrow depicts free air above the liver and below the diaphragm, signifying perforation.*

decreases so that perforated appendicitis occurs in approximately 25 percent of adolescents but 80 percent of children less than 5 years old. The frequency of gastroenteritis and the poor localization of pain in the young child both increase the risk of ascribing the pain to a viral etiology, delaying a visit to the doctor and once seen by the doctor, the low index of suspicion that the problem is appendicitis further delays the correct diagnosis, increasing the risk of perforation.

Once the appendix has perforated, the symptoms may be most consistent with severe gastroenteritis with pain, vomiting and diarrhea, or the child may present with a pattern of intestinal obstruction. An abdominal mass in the lower abdomen, in an ill-appearing child may well be an appendiceal abscess rather than a malignancy.

Sonography has been disappointing in assisting with the diagnosis of appendicitis. Contrast enema and abdominal CT with enteric contrast material are the best radiographic studies to diagnose late appendicitis in the unclear case. In the male, right lower quadrant peritoneal tenderness and leukocytosis should prompt exploration regardless of other signs and symptoms. In the female, ovarian or uterine pathology also must be considered. In girls over 10 years of age, laparoscopy is very helpful in making the correct diagnosis of low abdominal pain and is almost always a successful method of treating that problem. Management of an appendiceal abscess "mass" by drainage percutaneously and I.V. antibiotics has been advocated by some, but most pediatric surgeons prefer early operative drainage of the abscess and appendectomy.

Duplications, Meckel's Diverticulum, and Mesenteric Cysts

Duplications

Duplications can occur at any level in the gastrointestinal tract but are found most commonly in the ileum. They may be long and tubular, but usually are cystic masses lying within the leaves of the mesentery and sharing a common wall with the intestine. Symptoms can include a palpable mass and/or frank intestinal obstruction. Torsion may produce gangrene and perforation, and subtle or massive bleeding may occur. This bleeding comes from ulceration in the duplication or adjacent intestine if the duplication contains ectopic gastric mucosa.

The ability to make a preoperative diagnosis of duplication usually depends on the presentation. Sonography and technetium pertechnetate scanning are the two most helpful diagnostic tests. In the case of short duplications, resection of the cyst and adjacent intestine with end-to-end anastomosis can be performed in a straightforward fashion. If resection of long duplications would compromise intestinal length, multiple enterotomies and mucosal stripping in the duplicated segment will allow the walls to collapse and become adherent. An alternative method is to divide the common wall using the GIA stapler, forming a common lumen. This should not be done in duplications that contain ectopic gastric mucosa. In the patient with a very long duplication or multiple duplications, intraoperative nuclear medicine scanning will ensure complete excision of the ectopic gastric mucosa.

Meckel's Diverticulum

A Meckel's diverticulum is a remnant of a portion of the embryonic omphalomesenteric (vitelline) duct. It is located on the antimesenteric border of the ileum, usually within 2 ft of the ileocecal valve. It may be found incidentally at surgery or may present with inflammation masquerading as appendicitis. Similar to duplications, ectopic gastric mucosa may produce ileal ulcerations that bleed and lead to the passage of maroon-colored stools. Diagnosis may be made by technetium pertechnetate scans when the patient presents with bleeding. Treatment is surgical, and a wedge resection of the diverticulum with transverse closure of the ileum can be performed if the base is narrow. If wedge excision would compromise the ileal lumen, sleeve excision and end-to-end ileoileostomy are performed.

Mesenteric Cysts

Mesenteric cysts are similar to duplications in their location within the mesentery. However, they do not contain any mucosa or muscular wall. Chylous cysts may result from congenital lymphatic obstruction (Fig. 37-22). Mesenteric cysts can cause intestinal obstruction or may present as an abdominal mass. The diagnosis may be made by US or abdominal CT. At operation, surgical excision is preferred sometimes requiring resection of the adjacent intestine. Partial excision or marsupialization should be reserved for cysts involving a large portion of the mesentery.

Hirschsprung's Disease

Hirschsprung's disease results from the absence of ganglion cells in the myenteric plexus of the intestine. Recent findings suggest that mutations in the RET protooncogene may be responsible for many cases of Hirschsprung's disease. The precursors of the ganglion cells are neural crest cells that migrate into the intestine from cephalad to caudad. The process is completed by the twelfth week of embryonic life, but the migration from midtransverse colon to anus takes 4 weeks. This increases the time period of vulnerability for failure of migration and accounts for the fact that most cases of aganglionosis involve the rectum and rectosigmoid. Longer segments of absent ganglion cells also may occur, and total colonic aganglionosis, although rare, is also seen.

Aganglionic colon does not permit normal peristalsis to occur. Functional obstruction therefore supervenes, and the infant may present with complete colon obstruction or with a devastating enterocolitis. The presentation may, however, be much more subtle, with constipation and abdominal distention as the chief findings. Occasionally failure to thrive is the initial sign.

Diagnosis. Infants with Hirschsprung's disease usually will fail to pass meconium in the first 24 h of life, although this history is often difficult to obtain. Barium enema may be unreliable in diagnosing Hirschsprung's disease in the newborn infant because the colon is not dilated enough to show a transition zone. In older infants and children, barium enema will show the size difference between the dilated ganglionic colon and the distal constricted aganglionic rectal segment. The barium enema in total colonic aganglionous usually shows a markedly shortened colon.

Rectal biopsy makes the definitive diagnosis of Hirschsprung's disease. Suction rectal biopsy provides a small piece of mucosa and submucosa without the requirement for anesthesia. Occasionally the suction biopsy is not diagnostic and a full-thickness biopsy is required. The histopathology of Hirschsprung's disease is the absence of ganglion cells in the myenteric plexuses, increased staining of a cholinesterase stain and the presence of hypertrophied nerve bundles. Some surgeons have

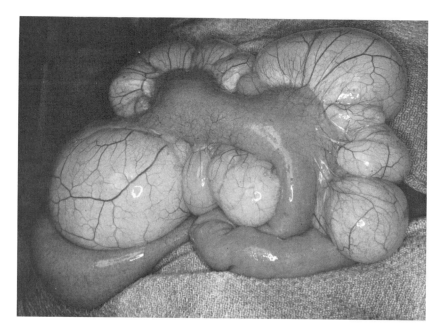

FIG. 37-22. Operative photograph depicting loops of ileum with a large chylous cyst in the mesentery. Note the relationship of the vascular supply to the bowel as it courses over the cyst. In most instances, resection of the involved intestine is necessary.

found the use of rectal manometry helpful, particularly in older children, but it is not as accurate a diagnostic tool as is rectal biopsy.

Treatment. Treatment is surgical in all cases. Some pediatric surgeons prefer to create a colostomy in the newborn period and wait until the child weighs 10 kg before performing a definitive pull-through operation. When a colostomy is done for Hirschsprung's disease, a frozen-section confirmation that ganglion cells are present at the colostomy site is mandatory. Some surgeons advocate primary pull-through operations in newborn infants without colostomy. The intraabdominal dissection can be performed using the laparoscope, even in the newborn. In the older infant and child who have been diagnosed belatedly, it is important to allow the distended hypertrophied colon to return to a normal size before performing a pullthrough. This is usually accomplished by waiting 3 to 6 months after a colostomy is performed.

Three pull-through procedures are currently in use for treating Hirschsprung's disease. The first of these is the original Swenson procedure, in which the aganglionic rectum is carefully dissected in the pelvis and removed down to the anus. The ganglionic colon is then anastomosed to the anus via a perineal approach (Fig. 37-23). In the Duhamel procedure (see Fig. 37-23), dissection outside the rectum is confined to the retrorectal space, and the ganglionic colon is anastomosed posteriorly just above the anus. The anterior wall of the ganglionic colon and the posterior wall of the aganglionic rectum are anastomosed, using a stapling device. In Soave's operation, dissection is entirely within the rectum (Fig. 37-24). The rectal mucosa is stripped from the muscular sleeve, and the ganglionic colon is brought through this sleeve and anastomosed to the anus. Complications with all procedures include enterocolitis, constipation and anastomotic stricture, but long-term results with the three procedures are comparable and generally excellent in experienced hands. These three procedures also can be adapted for total

colonic aganglionosis; the ileum is used for the pull-through or anastomosed to the aganglionic segment of distal colon and rectum to improve absorption.

Imperforate Anus

Imperforate anus occurs in approximately 1 in 5000 live births, affecting males and females almost equally. Failure of descent of the urorectal septum in embryonic life produces a variety of anorectal and cloacal anomalies. The level to which this septum descends determines the separation of the urinary and hindgut systems. Broadly classified, the imperforate anus is characterized as "high" or "low" depending on whether the rectum ends above the levator ani muscle complex or partially descends through this muscle. In high imperforate anus in males the rectum usually ends as a fistula into the membranous urethra. In females, the high imperforate anus often is part of a cloacal anomaly.

The low lesions have a fistula to the perineum. In males this is seen in the median raphe of the scrotum or penis, and in females the most common perineal fistula ends at the posterior fourchette. Since the rectum has descended through the levator complex in low lesions, only a perineal operation is required; this situation occurs in 40 percent of males and 70 percent of females with imperforate anus. Such children will be expected to be continent, since the "muscle of continence," the levator ani muscle, and the rectum are in a normal relationship to each other.

Infants having high imperforate anus require a colostomy in the newborn period, with some kind of pull-through procedure performed at about 2 months of age. Careful assessment of the genital tracts in females and the genitourinary system in all patients with imperforate anus is imperative because of the very high incidence of associated anomalies, particularly in children with a high imperforate anus. Many have associated spinal cord anomalies, particularly tethered cord, and all should be evaluated with spinal US and magnetic resonance imaging MRI. These infants require evaluation for signs of the VACTERRL associ-

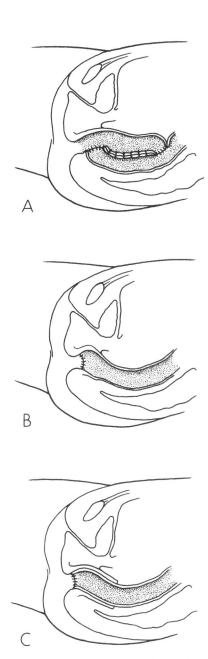

FIG. 37-23. The three basic operations for surgical correction of Hirschsprung's disease. A. The Duhamel procedure leaves the rectum in place and brings ganglionic bowel into the retrorectal space. The common wall, indicated by lines, is crushed to eliminate the septum. B. Classic Swenson operation (1948) is a resection with end-to-end anastomosis performed by exteriorizing bowel ends through the anus. C. The Soave operation is performed by endorectal dissection and removal of mucosa from the aganglionic distal segment and bringing the ganglionic bowel down to the anus within the seromuscular tunnel.

ation (see Esophageal Atresia and Tracheoesophageal Fistula, above), including careful preoperative cardiac assessment.

Diagnosis of imperforate anus is not difficult. The location of the fistula site may sometimes be a problem. Beading of mucus or meconium along the median raphe of the perineum and scrotum denotes a low imperforate anus in the male. Air in the bladder, urinating gas or meconium, and a retrograde urethrogram with contrast material may demonstrate the urinary fistula

of the high imperforate anus in the male. In the female, since most of the lesions are low, careful examination of the perineum, fourchette, and vestibule of the vagina will locate the fistula in most cases. A high fistula in the female may terminate in the vagina and will be harder to demonstrate. If a single perineal opening is seen in the female, a cloacal abnormality is present with urethra, vagina, and rectum opening into a common urogenital sinus. Colostomy is usually delayed for 24 h if no perineal fistula is seen. Cross-table lateral x-ray of the perineum with the buttock elevated may be done to determine the distance between the end of the rectum and the skin. If there is any doubt of the level, it is much safer to perform a colostomy than ruin any chance for continence by an injudicious perineal operation.

Pena and DeVries have devised a posterior sagittal approach for repair of high imperforate anus, dividing the levator ani and external sphincter complex in the midline posteriorly and bringing down the rectum after sufficient length is achieved. The muscles are then reconstructed and sutured to the rectum. Initial reports of results with the posterior sagittal anorectoplasty have been encouraging for both the primary and secondary procedures for high imperforate anus as well as cloacal anomalies. Pena also recommends this approach in the female with a rectovestibular fistula.

JAUNDICE

Biliary Atresia

Pathologic jaundice implies persistent elevation of the direct bilirubin level (> 2 weeks, > 2 mg/dL) and may be consequent to cholestasis or obstruction. The incidence of biliary atresia is approximately 1 in 20,000 births, and the condition affects not only the extrahepatic bile ducts but also the liver, which accounts for the biochemical overlap with many of the cholestatic causes of jaundice. Originally, biliary atresia was thought to be a developmental anomaly. There is recent suggestive evidence, however, that the condition may have an immunologic basis. Infectious etiologies have been proposed but never substantiated.

The obliterative process involves the common duct, cystic duct, one or both hepatic ducts, and the gallbladder, in a variety of combinations. Approximately 25 percent of the patients have coincidental malformations, often associated with polysplenia and may include intestinal malrotation, preduodenal portal vein, and intrahepatic vena cava.

Abdominal exploration in an infant with biliary atresia should commence with inspection of the left upper quadrant to determine the status of the spleen and thereby alert the surgeon to the possibility of coexisting anomalies should polysplenia be encountered.

Clinical Manifestations. Jaundice, a constant finding, is usually present at birth or shortly thereafter but may go undetected or may be regarded as "physiologic" until the child is 2 or 3 weeks old.

Initially, the growth and weight gain are normal, but in later stages retarded growth is apparent. As the liver becomes progressively more fibrotic, the patients develop stigmata of portal hypertension, particularly splenomegaly.

Diagnosis. No single test or combination of studies is absolutely reliable but with properly selected tests, it is usually possible to discriminate between cholestatic and obstructive

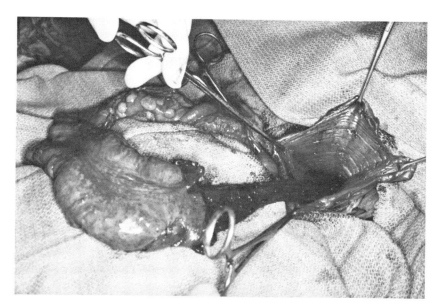

FIG. 37-24. Operative photograph of Soave procedure for Hirschsprung's disease. The seromuscular tunnel has been developed, and the circular muscle of the rectum is clearly seen. The mucosa has been stripped away from this tunnel and can be seen below the normally innervated sigmoid colon. The mucosal sleeve will be pulled through the rectum, and the normal sigmoid colon drawn into the seromuscular tunnel for anastomosis at the anus.

jaundice. Initially, the synthetic functions of the liver are unimpaired. Thus, the serum albumin level and clotting mechanism are normal. In many centers the nuclear scan using technetium 99m IDA (DISIDA), performed after pretreatment of the patient with phenobarbital, has proven to be an accurate and reliable study. If radionuclide appears in the intestine, extrahepatic bile duct patency is ensured. If radiopharmaceutical is normally concentrated by the liver but not excreted despite treatment with phenobarbital, and the metabolic screen, particularly alpha$_1$-antitrypsin determination, is normal, the presumptive diagnosis is biliary atresia. This examination, particularly when complemented by percutaneous needle biopsy of the liver, will establish a diagnosis with a high degree of certainty.

Complementary studies include abdominal US. This examination is reliable only when performed in the fasting patient. It should be emphasized that the presence of a gallbladder does not exclude the diagnosis of biliary atresia; in approximately 15 percent of these patients the distal biliary tract is patent although the proximal ducts are atretic. It is worth noting that the intrahepatic bile ducts are never dilated in the patient with biliary atresia. The sonographer must be alert to the possibility that parallel vascular structures in the porta may be mistakenly interpreted as patent bile ducts. Doppler US will usually resolve confusion.

Neonatal jaundice also may be caused by the *inspissated bile syndrome.* This term is applied to patients with normal biliary tracts who have persistent obstructive jaundice. Increased viscosity of bile and obstruction of the canaliculi are implicated as causes. The condition has been seen in infants receiving parenteral nutrition and is also encountered secondary to hemolysis or cystic fibrosis. In some instances, no etiologic factors can be defined.

Treatment. Historically, a variety of innovative operations have been attempted to promote bile flow from the liver in infants with biliary atresia. Only the hepatoportoenterostomy, developed by Kasai, has stood the test of time and demonstrated promise as a procedure that not only will provide relief of jaun-

dice but also may result in cure. The procedure is based on Kasai's observation that the fibrous tissue at the porta hepatis invests microscopically patent biliary ductules that, in turn, communicate with the intrahepatic ductal system. Transecting this fibrous tissue, invariably encountered cephalad to the bifurcating portal vein, opens these channels and establishes bile flow into a surgically constructed intestinal conduit, usually a Roux en Y limb of jejunum (Fig. 37-25). The likelihood of surgical success is increased if the procedure is accomplished before the infant attains the age of 8 weeks. The outlook is poor for patients after the twelfth week. Bile drainage is anticipated when the operation is carried out early; unfortunately, bile flow does not necessarily imply cure. Prognostic indicators include the rate at which the serum bilirubin level returns toward normal. It has been observed that in patients operated upon before 60 days, jaundice resolves in approximately 2 months, whereas infants having corrective surgery after 60 days rarely become anicteric or do so only after 6 months. Further, in the latter group the transaminases often remain elevated. The outcome is most favorable when the serum bilirubin reaches a level less than 1 mg./dL. Hepatic fibrosis may progress even when bile drainage is achieved. Postoperative cholangitis continues to plague infants having successful portoenterostomy procedures. The incidence and severity of cholangitis may be reduced by external venting of the surgically created biliary conduit and by the long-term administration of antibiotics. Despite these measures, the problem of ascending infection has not been eliminated. Reoperation, with resectional debridement of the portoenterostomy anastomosis, has rescued selected children with intractable cholangitis. Portal hypertension and its sequelae also jeopardize the outcome for some patients even when they have been relieved of jaundice. Gastrointestinal hemorrhage from esophageal varices usually can be managed successfully by endoscopic sclerotherapy or variceal ligation. For some patients portosystemic shunting has been successful in controlling hemorrhage from esophageal varices.

While "cure" may be attained in only 25 to 30 percent of patients after hepatoportoenterostomy, significant palliation and prolongation of life with the native liver has been achieved rou-

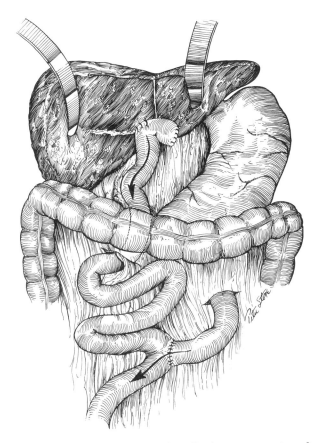

FIG. 37-25. Operative diagram of the Kasai portoenteroectomy for biliary atresia. An isolated limb of jejunum has been brought to the porta hepatis and anastomosed to the transected ducts. The Roux en Y principle has been used to reconstitute intestinal continuity.

Choledochal Cyst

There have been numerous descriptions and classifications based on the location and anatomy of the choledochal cyst. Among the most useful is the classification proposed by Alonso-Lej. The type I cyst characterized by fusiform dilatation of the bile duct into which the cystic duct enters is the most common and clinically relevant. Choledochal cyst is most appropriately considered the predominant feature in a constellation of pathologic abnormalities within the pancreatic-biliary system. Frequently associated with choledochal cyst are anomalous junction of the pancreatic duct and common bile duct, distal bile duct stenosis, intrahepatic ductal dilatation, abnormal histology of the common bile duct, and hepatic histology ranging from normal to cirrhotic. These features are encountered in varying degrees and combinations and constitute the anatomic spectrum of the malformation.

The causation of choledochal cyst is controversial. Babbit proposed an abnormal pancreatic biliary duct junction, with the formation of a "common channel" into which pancreatic enzyme secretions are discharged, with resulting weakening of the bile duct wall by gradual enzymatic destruction, leading to dilatation, inflammation, and finally cyst formation. It should be noted, however, that not all patients with choledochal cyst demonstrate an anatomic common channel.

Choledochal cyst is more common in females than in males (4:1). The so-called classic symptom complex of pain, mass, and jaundice is actually encountered in fewer than half the patients. The more usual presentation is that of episodic abdominal pain, often recurrent over months or years, and generally associated with only minimal jaundice that may escape detection. If the condition persists unrecognized, sequelae including cholangitis, cirrhosis, and portal hypertension are almost inevitable.

Diagnosis. With the increasing use of antenatal US, choledochal cyst is frequently diagnosed in the fetus. For the older child or adolescent, US and CT scanning are the diagnostic mainstays. These studies will demonstrate the dimensions of the cyst and define its relationship to the vascular structures in the porta, as well as the intrahepatic ductal configuration. Endoscopic retrograde cholangiopancreatography (ERCP) is reserved for patients in whom confusion remains after evaluation by less invasive imaging modalities.

Treatment. The surgical options include internal drainage by cystenterostomy and surgical excision. The morbidity from the former is excessive. The cyst wall is composed of fibrous tissue and is devoid of mucosal lining. Anastomotic obstruction from scarring is inevitable. Further, the thick-walled fibrous cyst does not contract after drainage but rather persists as a receptacle for stagnant bile, and complications related to biliary stasis militate against internal drainage procedures. An additional, and perhaps the most serious, consequence of cyst retention is the development of malignancy arising within the cyst wall. The incidence of this aggressive and highly lethal neoplasm further supports the recommendation for cyst resection.

In most circumstances, the caliber of the common hepatic duct cephalad to the choledochal cyst is normal. Successful resection of the cyst requires circumferential dissection, entering the posterior plane between the cyst and portal vein to accomplish removal. The pancreatic duct, which may enter the distal

tinely with the probability of 5 year survival exceeding 60 percent. For the child afflicted with biliary atresia in whom the Kasai operation fails, or succeeds only temporarily, liver transplantation remains the final hope for salvage. It is generally acknowledged that a prior Kasai operation does not adversely affect on the results of subsequent transplantation. In the era of orthotopic and living related transplantation there is little justification for repeated operations attempting to salvage a failed Kasai operation. Biliary atresia has been the most common indication for transplantation in pediatric recipients, and the 1-year survival rate exceeds 80 percent.

Biliary Hypoplasia

In some infants coming to surgery with a presumptive diagnosis of biliary atresia, an operative cholangiogram may demonstrate the gallbladder and extrahepatic biliary system to be patent, albeit diminutive hence, *biliary hypoplasia*. Hypoplasia of the extrahepatic biliary system is associated with hepatic parenchymal disorders that cause severe intrahepatic cholestasis. Included among these are alpha$_1$-antitrypsin deficiency and arteriohepatic dysplasia (Alagille's syndrome). The primary pathology resides within the liver and not the bile ducts; therefore, portal dissection and portoenterostomy are not indicated in these patients. Rather, a generous liver biopsy is obtained and the operation terminated.

cyst, is vulnerable to injury during distal cyst excision but can be avoided by not dissecting into the pancreatic parenchyma.

For the patient in whom the anatomy of the porta is obscured and distorted by pericystic inflammation, an alternative technique is proposed. An arbitrary plane is entered within the posterior wall of the cyst that allows the inner lining of the back wall to be dissected free from the outer layer that directly overlies the portal vascular structures. The lateral and anterior cyst, as well as the internal aspect of the back wall, is removed. The outer posterior wall remains behind. In either circumstance, cyst excision is accomplished, with reconstruction using normal or near-normal proximal bile duct and a mucosal union between the biliary system and intestinal tract. The likelihood of postoperative anastomotic stricture with attendant sequelae is minimized. Further, the risk of malignant tumor is reduced although not completely eliminated.

DEFORMITIES OF THE ABDOMINAL WALL

Embryology

The abdominal wall is formed by four separate embryologic folds—cephalic, caudal, and right and left lateral folds—each of which is composed of somatic and splanchnic layers. Each of the folds develops toward the anterior center portion of the coelomic cavity, joining to form a large umbilical ring that surrounds the two umbilical arteries, the vein, and the yolk sac or omphalomesenteric duct. These structures are covered by an outer layer of amnion, and the entire unit composes the umbilical cord. Between the fifth and tenth weeks of fetal development the intestinal tract undergoes a rapid growth outside the abdominal cavity within the proximal portion of the umbilical cord. As development is completed, the intestine gradually returns to the abdominal cavity. Contraction of the umbilical ring completes the process of abdominal wall formation. Failure of the cephalic fold to close results in sternal defects (such as congenital absence of the sternum or the pentalogy of Cantrell. Failure of the caudal fold to close results in exstrophy of the bladder and, in more extreme cases, exstrophy of the cloaca. Interruption of central migration of the lateral folds results in omphalocele. Gastroschisis, originally thought to be a variant of omphalocele, probably results from a fetal accident in the form of intrauterine rupture of a hernia of the umbilical cord.

Umbilical Hernia

Failure of timely closure of the umbilical ring leaves a central defect in the linea alba. The resulting umbilical hernia is covered by normal umbilical skin and subcutaneous tissue, but the fascial defect allows protrusion of abdominal content (Fig. 37-26). Hernias less than a cm in size at the time of birth usually will close spontaneously by three years of life. Sometimes the hernia is large enough that the protrusion is disfiguring and disturbing to both the child and the family. In such circumstances early repair may be advisable. When the defect is small and spontaneous closure likely, delay of surgical correction until 4 or 5 years of age is appropriate. Incarceration is rarely seen in an umbilical hernia. Unlike treatment for inguinal hernia of infants and young children, attempts at reduction of an incarcerated umbilical hernia are unwise. Repair of uncomplicated umbilical hernia is performed through a small curving infraumbilical incision that fits into the skin crease of the umbilicus. The fascial defect is re-

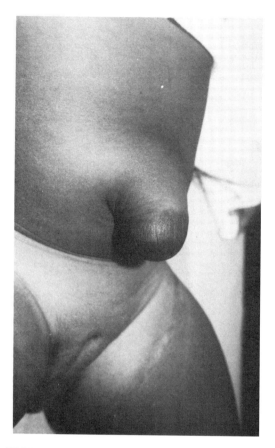

FIG. 37-26. *One-year-old female with large umbilical hernia. Early repair is indicated because of size.*

paired with permanent or long-lasting absorbable, interrupted sutures in a transverse plane. Fascial flaps or other complicated umbilical hernia repairs that have been recommended for adult patients are unnecessary in children. The umbilicus should never be excised in the repair of umbilical hernias in the childhood period.

Patent Urachus

During the development of the coelomic cavity, there is free communication between the urinary bladder and the abdominal wall through the urachus, which exits adjacent the omphalomesenteric duct. Persistence of this tract results in a communication between the bladder and the umbilicus (Fig. 37-27). The first sign of a patent urachus is moisture or urine flow from the umbilicus; consequently, recurrent urinary tract infection can result. The urachus may be partly obliterated, with a remnant remaining beneath the umbilicus in the extraperitoneal position as an isolated cyst, which may be identified by US. Such a cyst usually presents as an inflammatory mass inferior to the umbilicus. Initial treatment is drainage of the abscess with cyst excision as a separate procedure once the inflammation has resolved. Diagnosis of patent urachus is most reliably made by a cystogram in the lateral projection. Surgical correction is carried out via extraperitoneal exposure of the infraumbilical area. After identification, excision of the urachal tract with closure of the bladder is curative.

ratory effort. The omphalocele sac can be treated with desiccating substances such as Mercurochrome, but most infants in the United States are treated surgically. Indications for nonoperative therapy of an omphalocele are (1) a newborn with a giant omphalocele and other life-threatening anomalies whose correction takes precedence over repair of the omphalocele, (2) the neonate with other anomalies that complicate a surgical repair of the omphalocele, and (3) a newborn with severe associated anomalies that may not be consistent with survival.

When the abdomen cannot be closed primarily without undue tension, a temporary measure is placement of a "silo" of Silastic material sutured to the fascia around the circumference of the defect as an exterior cover without skin. This technique also can be used for gastroschisis when necessary. The main principle in the use of the plastic material is steady pressure with gradual reduction of the plastic envelope within 7 days to close the fascia without excessive tension. Today most infants, even those with large omphaloceles, can be salvaged. The persistent mortality rate of 20 to 30 percent from pediatric centers reflects the serious cardiac and chromosomal anomalies associated with this malformation.

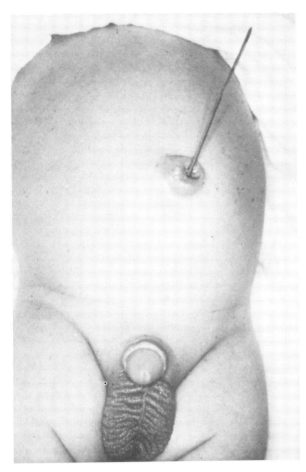

FIG. 37-27. Probe in opening of umbilicus revealing a patent urachus.

Omphalocele

Prenatal US will identify many of these defects permitting genetic evaluation and counselling. Postnatally, an omphalocele (Fig. 37-28) presents as a mass of bowel and solid viscera in the central abdomen, covered by translucent membrane. The size varies from about 1 cm in diameter to huge defects containing much or all of the abdominal viscera. In the latter forms, the bowel has lost its right of domain in the abdominal cavity, and closure is difficult. Frequently the liver occupies much of the defect and does not tolerate compression. The diagnosis is made by inspection. Infants born with omphaloceles are prone to other anomalies. There is a 60 to 70 percent incidence of associated anomalies, especially cardiac and chromosomal abnormalities. Special syndromes such as exstrophy of the cloaca (vesicointestinal fissure) and the Beckwith-Wiedemann constellation of anomalies (macroglossia, macrosomia, hypoglycemia, and visceromegaly) include omphalocele.

Immediate treatment after delivery of an infant with omphalocele consists of covering the lesion with saline-soaked gauze and wrapping the trunk circumferentially. No pressure should be placed on the omphalocele sac in an effort to reduce its contents, because pressure can lead to rupture of the sac or may interfere with abdominal venous return, or impede respi-

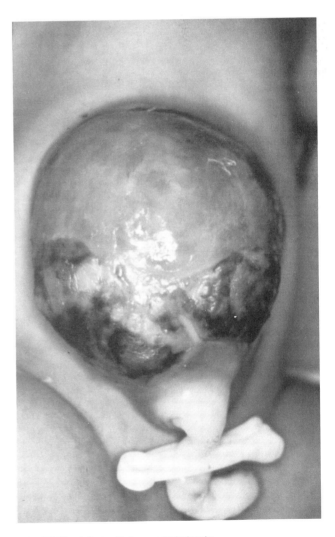

FIG. 37-28. Infant with large omphalocele.

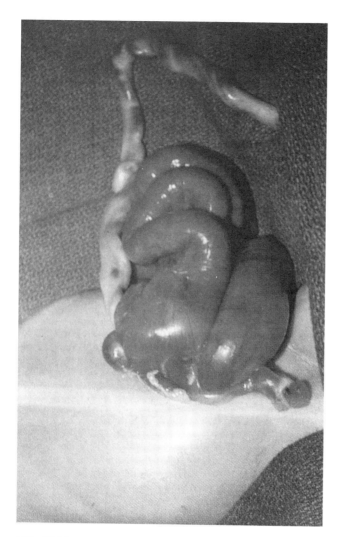

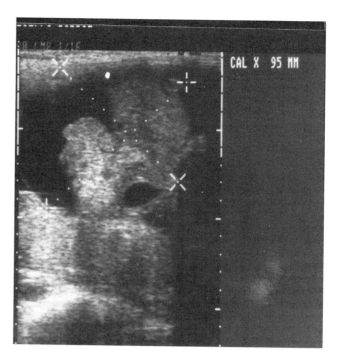

FIG. 37-30. Prenatal US of 32-week gestational age fetus with gastroschisis.

FIG. 37-29. Newborn with gastroschisis. The intestine has escaped through a defect just to the right of the umbilicus. The intestine is edematous and matted, indicating that these loops have been floating freely in the amnion for some time.

Treatment. All infants born with gastroschisis require urgent surgical treatment. The intestine can be returned to the abdominal cavity, and a secure, primary surgical closure of the abdominal wall is possible in many instances. Mechanical stretching of the abdominal wall aids in successful primary closure; however, for those infants whose intestine has become thickened and edematous, the construction of an extraabdominal compartment from Silastic sheeting is beneficial (Fig. 37-31). As in the surgical correction of omphalocele, the prosthetic pouch allows gradual enlargement of the abdominal cavity and accommodation of the intestines. Care must be taken so that increased abdominal pressure does not cause inferior vena cava compression that may impede venous return to the heart or di-

Gastroschisis

Shaw first suggested that gastroschisis is simply a hernia of the umbilical cord that ruptures after the complete development of the abdominal wall. The defect that permits escape of the intestines is located at the junction of the umbilicus and normal skin. The defect is almost always to the right of the umbilicus. Infants with gastroschisis have a large amount of intestine on the surface of the abdominal wall (Fig. 37-29). The umbilicus becomes partly detached, allowing free communication with the abdominal cavity. The intestine lying free outside of the abdominal cavity may be glistening, moist, and normal in appearance, suggesting that the rupture occurred immediately before or during delivery of the infant. More commonly, the intestine is thick, edematous, discolored, and covered with an exudate. Unlike infants born with omphalocele, associated anomalies seen with gastroschisis are confined to bowel atresia, further substantiating the mechanics of this abnormality. Currently, prenatal US may detect gastroschisis, permitting counselling and elective controlled delivery (Fig. 37-30).

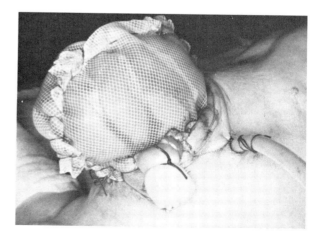

FIG. 37-31. Close-up of Silastic prosthesis for temporary covering of gastroschisis. The remnant of the umbilicus is seen in the center of the photograph. A gastrostomy tube is present.

aphragmatic pressure preventing normal respiratory excursion. Intestinal function may not return for several weeks, and is especially delayed if the bowel is thickened and edematous. In these infants, the advent of I.V. alimentation has been lifesaving. The survival rate for infants with gastroschisis exceeds 90 percent in many series.

Exstrophy of the Cloaca (Vesicointestinal Fissure)

Exstrophy of the cloaca represents one of the severest forms of embryologic derangement. In infants with cloacal exstrophy, the normal ventral closure of the pelvis and the abdominal wall is imperfect. Major components of cloacal exstrophy are (1) omphalocele, (2) exstrophy of the bladder, (3) external intestinal fistula through the bladder (enterovesical fistula), (4) epispadias in males, (5) imperforate anus, and (6) foreshortened colon. In addition, there is often an associated orthopedic deformity of the lower limbs.

Treatment of these complicated anomalies should be done in conjunction with a pediatric urologist and pediatric orthopedist to gain maximal function with a minimal number of procedures. An ileostomy and primary closure of the omphalocele usually are possible. The small piece of distal colon should be preserved for future anal and vaginal reconstruction. Timing of bladder and urinary reconstruction needs to be individualized, depending on the child's anatomy. While most patients suffer a number of physical limitations, many have the potential for functional rehabilitation, which justifies aggressive surgical efforts on their behalf.

Prune-Belly Syndrome (Eagle-Barret Syndrome)

Prune-belly syndrome is characterized by the findings of lax lower abdominal musculature, dilated urinary tract, including the bladder, and undescended testes bilaterally. It occurs almost exclusively in males (Fig. 37-32). Despite the impressive dilatation of the urinary tract, most of the children with prune-belly syndrome have adequate renal parenchyma for growth and development, at least early in life. In the past, aggressive "reconstruction" of the urinary tract was attempted, but currently a conservative approach is favored unless there is a specific area that requires drainage due to obstruction, not just dilation.

The testes are invariably intraabdominal and bilateral orchidopexy can be performed in conjunction with abdominal wall reconstruction at 6 to 12 months of age. Despite orchiopexy, fertility in a boy with prune-belly syndrome is unlikely. Abdominal wall repair is best accomplished with a large curving transverse incision in the lower abdomen extending into the flanks, the so-called "smile" incision. The combination of conservative treatment of the urinary tract and aggressive treatment of the undescended testes and abdominal wall has given many of these children a reasonably normal lifestyle.

Inguinal Hernia

Inguinal hernia results from a failure of closure of the processus vaginalis, a finger-like projection of the peritoneum that accompanies the testicle as it descends into the scrotum. Closure of the processus vaginalis should occur a few months prior to birth, which explains the high incidence of inguinal hernias in premature infants. In children, the male:female incidence of inguinal hernia is 10:1. Infants are at high risk for incarceration of an inguinal hernia because of the narrow inguinal ring. Differentiating between an incarcerated inguinal hernia and a hydrocele can be difficult, even with scrotal transillumination, and the symptomatic infant with a scrotal inguinal bulge must be evaluated by an experienced surgeon. Most often the incarcerated hernia can be reduced. The infant is sedated, and moderate bimanual pressure is applied by compressing the sac from below while a gentle counterforce downward is provided from the examiner's hand above the inguinal ring. Occasionally, these hernias will reduce spontaneously after sedation is given and the continuous struggling and crying are terminated. Following reduction of the incarcerated hernia, the child is admitted for observation, and herniorrhaphy is performed within the next 24 h to prevent recurrent incarceration. If the hernia cannot be reduced, or if intestinal obstruction is obvious, emergency operation, with reduction and repair, is necessary.

When the diagnosis of inguinal hernia is made in an otherwise normal child, operative repair should be planned, since spontaneous resolution does not occur. The frequency of a patent processus vaginalis on the side opposite the obvious hernia remains controversial. Data from laparoscopic evaluation of the normal appearing side revealed an incidence of greater than 30 percent patent processus vaginalis, regardless of the age or gender of the patient.

An inguinal hernia in a female frequently contains an ovary rather than intestine. Although the gonad usually can be reduced into the abdomen by gentle pressure, it often prolapses in and out until surgical repair is carried out. In some patients, the ovary and fallopian tube constitute one wall of the hernial sac (sliding hernia), and in these patients the ovary can be reduced effectively only at the time of operation. If the ovary is irreducible, prompt hernia repair is indicated to prevent ovarian torsion or strangulation.

When fluid fills the processus vaginalis, the patient has a hydrocele. The hydrocele may be associated with a hernia, may have a patent processus vaginalis too small for intestine to pass into (a communicating hydrocele), or may have no communication with the peritoneal cavity. When a hydrocele is diagnosed in infancy and there is no evidence of a hernia, observation is proper therapy until the child is older than 12 months. If the hydrocele has not disappeared by 12 months, invariably there is a patent processus vaginalis, and operative hydrocelectomy with excision of the processus vaginalis is indicated. When the first signs of a hydrocele are seen after 12 months of age, the patient should undergo elective hydrocelectomy, which in a child is always performed through a groin incision. Aspiration of hydroceles is discouraged, since almost all without a patent processus vaginalis will resorb spontaneously, and those with a communication to the peritoneum will recur and require operative repair eventually.

Operative repair of an inguinal hernia or hydrocele is accomplished through a small incision in a skin crease in the groin directly over the internal inguinal ring. The external oblique muscle is opened, and the cord structures and hernia sac are elevated into the wound, taking care not to grasp the vas deferens. The hernia sac is dissected to the internal ring and doubly suture ligated. The distal part of the hernia sac is dissected down to the testicle and widely opened to prevent a postoperative hydrocele. When the hernia is very large and the patient very small, tightening of the internal inguinal ring or even formal repair of the inguinal floor may be necessary, although the vast majority of children do not require any treatment beyond high ligation of

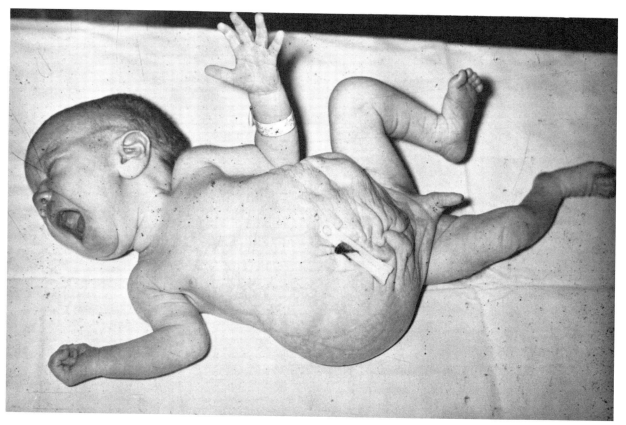

FIG. 37-32. *Eagle-Barrett (prune-belly) syndrome. Baby with congenital absence of the abdominal musculature, showing lax, flaccid abdomen. This syndrome occurs in males and is associated with severe malformation of the urinary collecting system and undescended testicles bilaterally.*

the hernia sac. Inguinal hernias in children recur in less than 1 percent of patients, and recurrences usually result from missed hernia sacs at the first procedure, a direct hernia, or a missed femoral hernia. All children should have local anesthetic administered either by caudal injection or by direct injection into the wound. Spinal anesthesia in preterm infants decreases the risk of postoperative apnea when compared with general anesthesia.

GENITALIA

Cryptorchidism

The term *undescended testicle* describes that testicle that has been interrupted in its normal route of descent into the scrotum. Such a testicle may reside in the posterior abdomen, in the internal inguinal ring, in the inguinal canal, or even at the external ring. The testicle begins as a thickening on the urogenital ridge in the fifth to sixth week of embryologic life. In the seventh and eighth months the testicle descends along the inguinal canal into the upper scrotum, and with its progress the processus vaginalis is formed and pulled along with the migrating testicle. At birth, approximately 95 percent of infants have the testicle normally positioned in the scrotum.

A distinction should be made between the undescended testicle and the ectopic testicle. An ectopic testis, by definition, is one that has passed through the external ring in the normal pathway and then has come to rest in an abnormal location overlying

either the rectus abdominis or external oblique muscle, or the soft tissue of the medial thigh, or behind the scrotum in the perineum. A congenitally absent testicle results from failure of normal development or an intrauterine accident leading to loss of blood supply to the developing testicle.

Clinical Manifestations. Usually a unilateral undescended testicle can be felt in the inguinal canal or in the upper scrotum. Occasionally, the testicle will be difficult or impossible to palpate, indicating either an abdominal testicle or congenital absence of the gonad. Patients with a nonpalpable testicle are routinely laparoscoped before inguinal exploration to identify an abdominal testicle. In patients with bilateral undescended testicles, it is appropriate to study the serum gonadotropin level, since the serum luteinizing hormone level is elevated in patients without gonadal tissue.

Reasons for surgical placement of the testicle in the scrotum are (1) diminished spermatogenesis, (2) malignant degeneration, (3) increased trauma (to a testicle located at the pubic tubercle), (4) increased incidence of torsion, and (5) psychological. The reason for malignant degeneration is not established, but the evidence points to an inherent abnormality of the testicle that predisposes it to incomplete descent and malignancy rather than malignancy as a result of an abnormal environment.

Males with bilateral undescended testicles are infertile. When the testicle is not within the scrotum, it is subjected to a higher temperature, resulting in diminishing spermatogenesis. Mengel and coworkers studied 515 undescended testicles by histology and demonstrated a decreasing presence of spermatogonia after 2 years of age. Consequently it is now recommended that the undescended testicle be surgically repositioned by 2 years of age. Despite orchidopexy, the incidence of infertility is approximately two times higher in men with unilateral orchidopexy compared to men with normal testicular descent.

Treatment. The use of chorionic gonadotropin occasionally has been effective in patients with bilateral undescended testes, suggesting that these patients are more apt to have a hormone insufficiency than children with unilateral undescended testicle. If there is no testicular descent after a month of endocrine therapy, operative correction should be undertaken. A child with unilateral cryptorchidism should have surgical correction of the problem.

Some patients who have an absent testis are greatly bothered by this anatomic deficiency. Prostheses of all sizes are now available and can be simply inserted into the scrotum, achieving normal appearance and a normal structure for palpation. Any patient who has an undescended testicle corrected surgically should be examined yearly by his surgeon until his midteen years. At that time, the individual should undergo thorough explanation about the possibility of malignant degeneration and be instructed in self-examination, which should be carried out at least twice a year for life.

Vaginal Anomalies

Anomalies of development of the vagina constitute a spectrum from simple defects (imperforate hymen) to more complex forms of vaginal atresia, including distal, proximal, and, most severe, complete. These defects are produced by abnormal development of müllerian ducts and/or urogenital sinus. The diagnosis is made most often by physical examination. Secretions into the obstructed vagina produce hydrocolpos, which may present as a large abdominal mass. US may help delineate the anatomy. The type of surgical repair depends on the extent of the defect. Simple imperforate hymen or a low transverse septum may be excised readily by a perineal approach. Other forms of vaginal atresia require complex reconstructive surgery, which may include mobilizing vaginal remnants down to the perineum, creating skin flaps, or using a colon segment as a neovagina.

Ovarian Cysts and Tumors

Ovarian cysts and tumors occur infrequently in childhood. They may be classified broadly as nonneoplastic or neoplastic. Nonneoplastic lesions include cysts (simple, follicular, inclusion, paraovarian, or corpus luteum), endometriosis, and inflammatory lesions. Neoplastic lesions are classified based on the three primordia that contribute to the ovary: mesenchymal components of the urogenital ridge, germinal epithelium overlying the urogenital ridge, and germ cells migrating from the yolk sac.

Most commonly, children with an ovarian mass complain of abdominal pain. Other signs and symptoms include a palpable abdominal mass, evidence of urinary obstruction, symptoms of bowel obstruction, and endocrine imbalance. The surgical approach depends on the appearance of the mass at operation, i.e., whether it is benign-appearing or is suspicious for malignancy. In the case of a simple, benign ovarian cyst, conservative excision is recommended, sparing ovarian tissue. If a lesion appears malignant, (1) ascites and peritoneal washings should be col-

lected for cytologic study, (2) the liver and diaphragm are inspected carefully for metastatic disease, (3) an omentectomy is performed, (4) pelvic and paraaortic lymph nodes are biopsied, (5) the primary tumor is resected completely, and (6) the contralateral ovary is carefully inspected and, if appropriate, bisected and biopsied.

An increasing number of ovarian cysts are being detected by prenatal US. In the past, surgical excision was recommended for all cysts greater than 5 cm in diameter because of the perceived risk of ovarian torsion. More recently, it has become apparent from serial US examinations that many of these lesions will resolve spontaneously. Complex cysts of any size require surgical intervention. Surgeons have four options for managing simple cysts: (1) follow the lesion sonographically and operate if it fails to resolve over several months, (2) drain the cyst percutaneously by ultrasound-guided needle aspiration, (3) drain the cyst by laparoscopically guided needle aspiration, and (4) excise the cyst by conventional operation.

Ambiguous Genitalia (Intersex Syndromes)

Normal sexual differentiation occurs in the sixth fetal week. In every fetus, wolffian (male) and müllerian (female) ducts are present until the onset of sexual differentiation. Normal sexual differentiation is directed by the Y chromosome in a genetic switch initiated by the *s*ex *d*etermining *r*egion of the *Y* chromosome (SRY). SRY is located on the distal 1A1 end of the short arm of the Y chromosome, adjacent to the pseudoautosomal region where small deletions in this area were known to be associated with sex reversal. Thus, SRY provides a genetic switch that initiates gonadal differentiation in the mammalian urogenital ridge. Müllerian inhibiting substance (MIS), a member of the transforming growth factor (TGF-β) family, results in regression of the müllerian duct, the anlagen of the uterus, Fallopian tubes, and the upper vagina. MIS gene transcription is initiated by tissue specific (gonadal ridge) and developmentally appropriate expression of the triple alpha-helical SRY protein that binds to the promoter region of the MIS gene in a sequence specific manner.

Simplistically, in the absence of SRY in the Y chromosome and in the presence of a duplicated X chromosome, the urogenital ridge differentiates as an ovary. In the absence of MIS that is produced by the Sertoli cells of the differentiated testis, the müllerian duct derivatives, i.e., the vagina, uterus, and Fallopian tubes, are preserved or fail to undergo regression. Thus the female phenotype prevails. In order for the male phenotype to develop, the embryo must have a Y chromosome, the SRY must be normal without point mutations or deletions, testosterone and MIS must be produced by the differentiated gonad, and the tissues must respond to these ligands via an appropriate receptor. Testosterone stimulates maturation of wolffian duct structures into epididymis, vas deferens, and seminal vesicles; simultaneously, the MIS produces regression of the female structures. Any disruption of the orderly steps in sexual differentiation may be reflected clinically as variants of the intersex syndromes (Fig. 37-33). These may be classified as (1) true hermaphroditism (with ovarian and testicular gonadal tissue), (2) male pseudohermaphroditism (testicles only), (3) female pseudohermaphroditism (ovarian tissue only), and (4) mixed gonadal dysgenesis (usually underdeveloped or imperfectly formed gonads).

Male pseudohermaphroditism is found in genotypic males with bilateral testes; however, the duct structures of many of

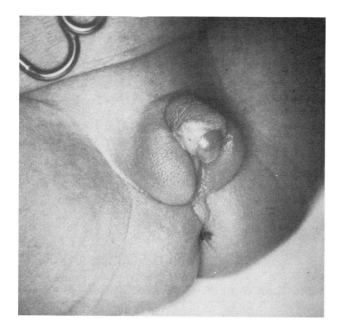

FIG. 37-33. *Ambiguous genitalia, manifest as enlarged clitoris and labioscrotal folds in a baby with the adrenogenital syndrome. This configuration can be confused with a normal penis and undescended testicles.*

these patients differentiate partly as phenotypic females, resulting from defects in androsynthesis or incomplete müllerian regression. Female pseudohermaphroditism is found most commonly in patients with congenital adrenal hyperplasia who are unable to synthesize cortisol due to abnormally low levels of any one of five enzymes. In 90 percent of cases, deficiency of 21-hydroxylase causes adrenocorticotropic hormone (ACTH) to stimulate the secretion of excessive quantities of adrenal androgen, which masculinizes the developing female. These infants are prone to salt loss and can experience collapse at about 1 week of age. The rarest intersex form, that of the true hermaphrodite, is usually found with XX karyotype. These children have ambiguous genitalia and their gonad pattern may show an ovary and a testicle, or an ovotestis.

In the differential diagnosis of patients with intersex anomalies, the following diagnostic steps are necessary: (1) evaluation of the genetic background and family history; (2) assessment of the anatomic structures by physical examination and x-ray studies; (3) chromosome studies; (4) determination of biochemical factors in serum and urine; and (5) when necessary, laparotomy and gonadal biopsy. Genetic females should be assigned the female gender, regardless of the degree of virilization. For genetic males, the gender assignment will depend on anatomic considerations, specifically the size of the phallus, since at this time satisfactory surgical techniques do not exist to reconstruct an inadequate phallus. The physicians presented with a newborn infant with ambiguous genitalia must make the gender assignment rapidly, to minimize the emotional impact on the family, and accurately, since a change later causes irreparable anguish. Assignment to one of four major groups of defects described above can be made readily using two screening criteria: (1) the presence of gonadal symmetry or asymmetry, and (2) the presence of a chromatin mass or Barr body or the absence of fluo-

rescence of the distal long arm of the Y chromosome. After the correct designation to one of the major categories, the specific pathoetiology can be determined at a more deliberate pace.

Gonadal symmetry is determined by the position of one gonad relative to the other, either above or below the external inguinal ring. If the gonadal position is symmetric, both gonads lie either above or below the inguinal ring, suggesting a diffuse etiologic basis for the abnormality. For example, in either male or female pseudohermaphroditism, a biochemical defect affects both gonads equally, such that the gonads are symmetric. In contrast, in mixed gonadal dysgenesis or true hermaphroditism, asymmetry is observed if there is a predominance of testicular tissue on one side and ovarian tissue on the other side, in which case the testicular gonad is descended and the ovarian gonad is undescended.

With more than one X chromosome present in the karyotype, the inactivated X chromosome (Barr body) can be found tangentially in the nucleus, which is the case with female pseudohermaphroditism (adrenogenital syndrome) or in most cases of true hermaphroditism. Conversely, Barr bodies are absent in patients with male pseudohermaphroditism and mixed gonadal dysgenesis. At centers that perform analyses to mark the distal long arm of the Y chromosome, instead of chromatin analysis with Barr bodies, fluorescent Y positive nuclei are seen with male pseudohermaphrodites and mixed gonadal dysgenesis, and fluorescent Y negative nuclei are seen with female pseudohermaphrodites and true hermaphrodites. With this algorithm, a preliminary diagnosis that assigns the patient to one of four major groups can be established with 80 to 90 percent accuracy within the first 24 hours of life.

After complete evaluation, certain plastic surgical procedures are required to harmonize the external genitalia with the sex of rearing. Operations to reduce the size of the enlarged clitoris have been developed that spare the sensation and function of the clitoris. Plastic procedures to exteriorize the vagina or separate it from the urethra are necessary in patients born with a urogenital sinus. When male assignment is appropriate for an infant with ambiguous genitalia, hypospadias repair will be necessary. When contradictory gonads or ovotestes are present, removal of these structures is required to prevent the possibility of hormone secretion or malignant degeneration. For psychological adjustment of some teenage male patients with inadequate or absent gonads, the insertion of testicular prostheses may prove beneficial. Children with endocrine deficiency may require lifetime exogenous supplementation. Prompt recognition of infants with intersex anomalies, followed by appropriate sex assignment and proper treatment, prevents the social and psychological derangements that have occurred in the past because of delayed diagnosis or inappropriate gender assignment.

NEOPLASTIC DISEASE

Cancer is the second leading cause of death in children. Approximately 11 percent of the deaths of children in the United States are due to malignant diseases (Fig. 37-34). In the past 30 years there has been a marked increase in the survival of patients with childhood cancer. This improvement can be attributed to better diagnostic imaging techniques; new chemotherapeutic agents; collaborative approaches to surgery, chemotherapy, and radiation therapy; and multi-institutional studies evaluating new treatments and protocols. This unified approach to diagnosis,

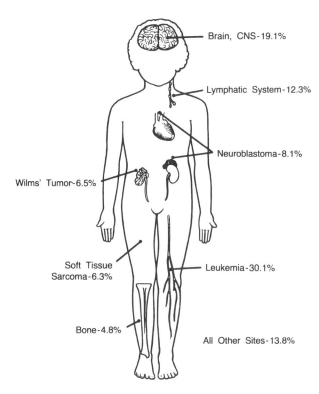

FIG. 37-34. *Most common sites of cancer in children.*

staging, and therapy has proved useful in the management of the more common pediatric solid malignancies, such as Wilms' tumor, hepatic tumors, rhabdomyosarcoma, neuroblastoma, and teratoma. Advances in the understanding of molecular biology, immunology, pharmacology, and tumor biology surely will lead

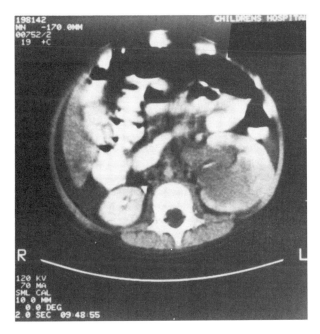

FIG. 37-35. *CT scan from a patient with Wilms' tumor. Note the mass and distortion of the left kidney.*

to improvements in care in the next decade. Best results are achieved in institutions with special skill in the care of children and with access to the latest multimodality and multidisciplinary protocols.

Wilms' Tumor

Wilms' tumor is an embryonal neoplasm of the kidney that usually presents as an asymptomatic mass in the flank or upper abdomen. The peak age of incidence is between 1 and 5 years. This tumor has been associated with congenital anomalies such as aniridia, the Beckwith-Wiedemann syndrome, urinary tract defects, hemihypertrophy, and chromosomal deletion, suggesting a possible hereditary influence. Specific Wilms' tumor suppressor genes have been discovered and cloned (WT1 and WT2), mutations or deletions of which may be responsible for the development of Wilms' tumors.

Before operation, all patients suspected of Wilms' tumor should be evaluated radiographically. Abdominal and chest CT scans and US are the mainstays of the work-up. US confirms the presence of a mass and localizes it to the kidney. It can demonstrate the presence of renal vein or vena caval extension, crucial information before embarking on surgical intervention. The CT scan usually will show a large intrarenal mass (Fig. 37-35). Furthermore, the scan provides important preoperative data such as the tumor status of the contralateral kidney and the presence of local or distant spread. MRI is finding an increasing role in the imaging of these tumors.

The key to staging and treatment is surgical intervention. A generous transabdominal transverse incision is used to ensure adequate exposure for removing the primary tumor, to evaluate the opposite kidney, and to inspect the rest of the abdomen. The tumor and kidney are completely resected with care to avoid tumor spillage. Whenever possible the renal vein should be clamped before the tumor is mobilized, to prevent tumor embolization. If there has been contiguous spread of the tumor into adjacent organs, the operation may be expanded to include part of the liver, spleen, diaphragm, pancreas, or stomach. Lymph nodes are sampled to assist with staging.

Following operative removal of a Wilms' tumor, the need for chemotherapy and/or radiation therapy is determined by the histology of the tumor and the clinical stage of the patient (Table 37-1). Patients with disease confined to one kidney, totally re-

Table 37-1
Wilms' Tumor Staging and Prognosis

			4-yr Survival (%)	
Stage		Incidence (%)	FH*	UH†
I.	Limited to kidney and completely excised	42	97	89
II.	Extends beyond kidney and totally excised	22	94	68
III.	Residual tumor confined to the abdomen	22	88	68
IV.	Distant metastases	9	82	55
V.	Bilateral renal involvement	5	84	16

*FH = favorable histology.

†UH = unfavorable histology.

moved surgically, receive a short course of chemotherapy and can expect a 97 percent 4-year survival, with tumor relapse rare after that time. Patients with Stage II and III disease with favorable histology receive a longer course of combination chemotherapy. Patients with Stage IV disease or unfavorable histology require longer and more intensive chemotherapy. Radiation therapy is used for the advanced stages. Even in Stage IV, cure rates of 80 percent are being achieved. The survival rates are worse in the small percentage of patients considered to have unfavorable histology. Actinomycin D and vincristine are the major chemotherapeutic agents used. Adriamycin and cyclophosphamide are used in advanced stages. Despite the enormous contribution of chemotherapy and radiation to improved survival, surgical excision remains the primary treatment. In selected patients, preoperative chemotherapy is used to shrink massive tumors or to reduce tumor bulk when bilateral disease is present. In the case of massive tumors, this approach may reduce tumor spill and make operations safer. With bilateral disease it allows for conservation of renal tissue at the time of resection.

Current protocols designed by the National Wilms' Tumor Study (NWTS) focus on decreasing therapy for low-risk patients and on intensifying therapy for high-risk patients. Additionally, new strategies are required for children with recurrent disease, since the present outlook with conventional therapy is dismal. Long-term follow-up is required for all children treated for Wilms' tumor because of the increasing recognition of second malignancies.

Neuroblastoma

Neuroblastoma is the third most common pediatric malignancy. Over 60 percent arise in children under the age of 5 years. Neuroblastomas arise from the neural crest cells and show different levels of differentiation. The tumor originates most frequently in the adrenal glands, posterior mediastinum, neck, or pelvis but can arise in any sympathetic ganglion. The clinical presentation depends on the site of the primary and the presence of metastasis.

Two-thirds of these tumors are first noted as an asymptomatic abdominal mass. The tumor may cross the midline, and a majority of patients will already show signs of metastatic disease. The patient should be evaluated by CT scan and US, which usually show displacement and occasionally obstruction of the ureter of an intact kidney. Since these tumors derive from the sympathetic nervous system, catecholamines and their metabolites will be produced at increased levels and may produce symptoms. Measurement of VMA and HVMA in serum and urine aids in the diagnosis and in monitoring adequacy of future treatment and recurrence. Elevations of serum ferritin and neuronspecific enolase levels correlate with poor prognosis. Increased copy number of the N-myc gene is an important indicator of poor prognosis.

Although CT scan, bone marrow biopsy, and radionuclide scans are important adjuncts to preoperative staging, surgical evaluation and excision, when possible, are essential. The main hope of cure is to resect the tumor completely, because chemotherapy and radiation therapy have not altered survival significantly in the past 20 years. Abdominal tumors are approached through a transverse incision, and every attempt is made to resect the tumor completely. Thoracic tumors may be approached through a posterolateral thoracotomy and often have an intraspinal component necessitating laminectomy and intraspinal re-

Table 37-2
Neuroblastoma Staging System

I.	Tumor confined to structure of origin
II.	Tumor extends beyond structure of origin but not across midline
III.	Tumor extends contiguously across midline
IV.	Distant metastatic disease
IVs.	Patients who would otherwise be Stage I or II but have remote disease confined to one or more of these sites: liver, bone marrow, or skin

SOURCE: Adapted from Evans AE, D'Angio GJ, Randolph J: A proposed staging for children with neuroblastoma. Children's cancer study group A. *Cancer* 27:374, 1971, with permission.

moval. Many staging classifications have been developed to predict survival and to stratify patients for treatment protocols (Table 37-2). The most commonly employed are those developed by the Children's Cancer Study Group and the International Neuroblastoma Staging System.

If the tumor is not resectable, a generous biopsy is obtained for histopathologic classification and determination of N-myc gene copy number, both important determinants of prognosis. Under current experimental protocols, the children receive several courses of chemotherapy to shrink the tumor and then undergo a "second-look" attempt at resection. Protocols incorporating bone marrow transplantation have been used for patients with advanced disease. Even with aggressive chemotherapy protocols, the 2-year survival rate for older children with metastatic disease is 20 percent.

Owing to variability in sites and in biologic behavior, the treatment of neuroblastoma must be individualized. In infants favorable survival may be realized even when there is metastatic spread to bone marrow, liver, or skin (Stage IVs). Over 85 percent of these patients, if less than one year old, will be completely and spontaneously cured. The spontaneous regression of tumor seen in many of these patients has led to much investigation of immunotherapy as a possible therapeutic tool. Although cure rates of greater than 80 percent have been achieved in Stages I and II, the poor survival in the higher stages is discouraging and calls for new therapies and further research.

Rhabdomyosarcoma

Rhabdomyosarcoma is a primitive soft tissue tumor that arises from mesenchymal tissues. The head and neck (36 percent), extremities (19 percent), genitourinary tract (21 percent), and trunk (9 percent) are the most common sites of origin, although the tumor can arise virtually anywhere. The clinical presentation of the tumor depends on the site of origin. The diagnosis is confirmed with incisional or excisional biopsy after evaluation by MRI, CT scans of the affected area and the chest, and bone marrow biopsy. The tumor grows locally into surrounding structures and metastasizes widely to lung, regional lymph nodes, liver, brain, and bone marrow. The staging system for rhabdomyosarcoma is shown in Table 37-3.

The overall survival is 60 percent at 5 years. Prognosis relates to the site of origin, clinical grouping, and histopathology. The prognosis in patients with embryonal pathology is much more favorable than that in patients with alveolar histology. Five-year survival rates are 81 percent in clinical group I, 80 percent in clinical group II, 65 percent in clinical group III, and 27 percent in clinical group IV. The Intergroup Rhabdomyosarcoma Study

Table 37-3
Staging System by Clinical Group for Rhabdomyosarcoma*

I. Localized disease, completely resected, no involved lymph nodes (13%)
II. Localized or regional disease with total gross resection, lymph nodes may be involved (20%)
III. Incomplete resection or biopsy with residual unresected disease (48%)
IV. Distant metastatic disease at diagnosis (18%)

* Adapted from Intergroup Rhabdomyosarcoma Study.
SOURCE: Hays DM, et al: *Curr Probl Surg* 23(3), 1986, with permission.

(IRS) has recently developed a staging system based on TNM principles that may serve as the basis for future studies designed to improve survival.

Wide local excision with adequate "clean" margins is the optimal surgical treatment for localized forms of rhabdomyosarcoma. The potential morbidity of radical amputations or exenteration can be avoided because of progress in chemotherapy and radiation therapy in recent years. Often the approach involves initial biopsy, several courses of chemotherapy, and resection at a "second-look" operation. The standard chemotherapy is a combination of actinomycin D, vincristine, and cyclophosphamide. Treatment is individualized based on the site, group, and histology, but all will receive multimodality therapy.

Teratoma

Teratomas are tumors composed of tissue from all three embryonic germ layers. They may be benign or malignant, may arise in any part of the body, and are usually found in midline structures. Thoracic teratomas usually present as an anterior mediastinal mass. Ovarian teratomas present as an abdominal mass often with symptoms of torsion, bleeding, or rupture. Retroperitoneal teratomas may present as a flank or abdominal mass. The location incidence of teratomas in children is seen in Table 37-4. The goal of therapy is complete surgical excision because the success of chemotherapy and/or radiation therapy seen in other pediatric tumors has not been realized in this group of tumors.

Sacrococcygeal Teratoma

Sacrococcygeal teratoma usually presents as a large mass extending from the sacrum in the newborn period. Many tumors have been diagnosed prenatally by US. In fetuses with evidence of hydrops and a large sacrococcygeal teratoma, prognosis is

Table 37-4
Incidence of Teratoma by Location

Head and neck	5.5%
Mediastinal	4%
Retroperitoneal and abdominal	5%
Sacrococcygeal	40%
Ovary	37%
Testicle	3%
Brain/spinal cord	3.5%
Other	2%

SOURCE: Adapted from Tapper D, Lack EE: Teratomas in infancy and childhood. A 54-year experience at the Children's Hospital Medical Center. *Ann Surg* 198:398, 1983, with permission.

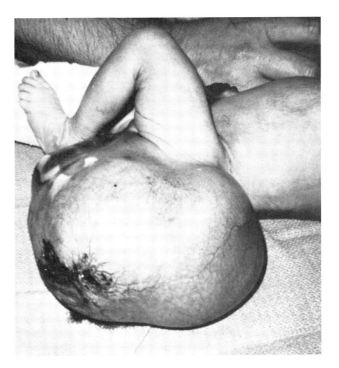

FIG. 37-36. Newborn with huge sacrococcygeal teratoma.

poor, thus prenatal intervention has been advocated in such patients. The mass may be as small as a few centimeters in diameter or as massive as the size of the infant (Fig. 37-36). There is a form of tumor that does not present externally but grows in the presacral space and often presents later in childhood. The differential diagnosis consists of neural tumors, lipoma, and myelomeningoceles.

Most tumors are identified at birth and are benign, but with advancing age the potential for malignant degeneration is high. Complete resection of the tumor as early as possible is essential. The rectum and genital structures are often distorted by the tumor but usually can be preserved in the course of resection. The cure rate is excellent if the tumor is excised completely. Perioperative complications of hypothermia and hemorrhage can occur with massive tumors and may prove lethal in "benign" lesions. With discovery of the tumor in older infants and children, the results are poor because of the high incidence of malignant degeneration. Chemotherapy is indicated in these older children.

Liver Tumors

More than two-thirds of all liver tumors in children are malignant. Hepatoblastoma is the most common malignancy of the liver in children, with most of these tumors diagnosed before 4 years of age. Hepatocellular carcinoma is the next most common, with a peak age incidence between 10 and 15 years. Malignant mesenchymomas and sarcomas are much less common but constitute the remainder of the malignancies. Most children with a liver tumor present with an abdominal mass that is usually painless, which the parents note while changing the child's clothes or while bathing the child.

The patients are rarely jaundiced but may complain of anorexia and weight loss. Most liver function tests are normal. Alpha-fetoprotein levels are elevated in 90 percent of children with hepatoblastomas but are increased much less commonly in other liver malignancies. Radiographic evaluation of these children should include a flat-plate abdominal radiograph, an US study, and a contrast-enhanced abdominal CT scan.

Complete surgical extirpation of the tumor is the primary goal and is essential for cure. For resectable tumors, attempts to reduce the bulk of massive tumors by pretreatment with chemotherapy have met with limited success. The value of radiotherapy is also limited. Previously, hepatic transplantation for unresectable primary lesions had a high incidence of carcinomatosis and death; however, recent results are more encouraging. For hepatoblastoma, about half the patients have completely resectable lesions (Fig. 37-37), and about 80 percent of these can be cured with adjunct chemotherapy. Of all patients with hepatoblastomas, only about 70 percent are long-term survivors. Patients with hepatocellular carcinoma have a worse prognosis because the tumors are frequently multicentric or metastatic. The cure rate for all children with hepatocellular carcinomas is only 25 percent.

TRAUMA

Injuries account for almost half of all pediatric deaths, more than cancer, congenital anomalies, pneumonia, heart disease, homicide, and meningitis combined. Motor vehicle collision involving car occupants or pedestrians is the most common cause of accidental death in children; drowning, burns, and firearms account for a significant segment of the remaining group. Not evident in the mortality statistics is the number of children who sustain injury and recover with a subsequent disability. Improved methods of communication, immediate prehospital care, and rapid transportation to regional centers increase the probability of survival after a major traumatic injury. Because of the complex requirements for resuscitation and treatment of an injured child, it is essential that each regional referral center establish a systematic approach to care.

Management of trauma in children requires immediate recognition and treatment of life-threatening injuries to the head, thorax, and abdomen. Recognition that the child with severe

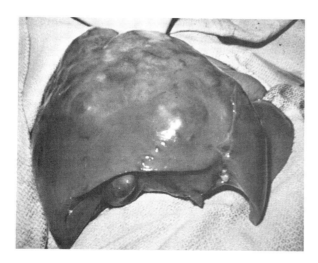

FIG. 37-37. Operative photograph of hepatoblastoma in the right lobe of the liver in an 8-month-old child. Extended right hepatic lobectomy was curative.

head injury manifests a different physiologic response from that of the adult forms the foundation of successful therapy. Aggressive therapy of elevated intracranial pressure results in improved survival; 30 percent of the childhood victims of serious head trauma die, whereas the remainder make a good to excellent recovery. Thoracic trauma occurs in 5 percent of all injured children. Blunt abdominal trauma is common in the pediatric population, the spleen and liver are the most frequent intraabdominal organs sustaining injury. Nonoperative management is a reasonable approach in the child with blunt hepatic or splenic trauma with stable vital signs. Exploratory laparotomy is indicated for a physiologically unstable child despite appropriate fluid resuscitation. These children should undergo laparotomy for hemostasis, and an attempt at splenic salvage by splenorrhaphy is warranted if the child's condition permits. Splenic salvage is important in children to minimize the potential for future overwhelming sepsis. Lap belt injuries are increasingly common in children due to mandatory seat belt laws. Lap-belt injuries may cause serious intestinal trauma and lumbar spine fractures and are poorly diagnosed by the abdominal CT. Peritoneal lavage or laparotomy is indicated in this group of injured children.

Consideration of the unique requirements of the injured child during evaluation and therapy improves outcome and minimizes mortality. Aerophagia proceeding to gastric dilatation can compromise respiration or mimic an abdominal injury; therefore, nasogastric decompression is essential in all children with significant injury. The temperature of injured children might drop precipitously because of the relatively large surface area to body mass ratio. Hypothermia potentiates the deleterious effects of shock and metabolic acidosis. Hypovolemic shock with attendant cellular hypoperfusion requires treatment by infusion of crystalloid solutions at a rate of 20 mL/kg, I.V. push. Urine output (1 mL/kg/h) in children is a useful indicator of adequate fluid resuscitation. Once initial assessment and resuscitation are complete, diagnostic measures with conventional x-rays and CT scan are important. Prompt movement to a pediatric intensive care unit is essential unless a decision for operation is necessary. Complete rehabilitation of the child and the family should be the ultimate goal of every pediatric trauma center. The solution to pediatric trauma is not improved schemes for treatment but rather prevention of injury.

Bibliography

General Considerations

Anand KJS, Hickey RP: Pain and its effects in the human neonate and fetus. *N Engl J Med* 317:1321, 1987.

Mehta S, Connors AF, et al: Incidence of thrombosis during central venous catheterization of newborns: A prospective study. *J Pediatr Surg* 27:18, 1992.

Lesions of the Neck

Guarisco JL: Congenital head and neck masses in infants and children, parts I and II. *Ear Nose Throat J* 70:40, 75, 1991.

Kenealy JF, Torsigliere AJ Jr, Tom LW: Branchial cleft anomalies: A five-year retrospective review. *Trans Pa Acad Ophthalmol Otolaryngol* 42:1022, 1990.

Langer JC, Fitzgerald PG, et al: Cervical cystic hygroma in the fetus: Clinical spectrum and outcome. *J Pediatr Surg* 25:58, 1990.

MacLeod AM, McHugo JM: Prenatal diagnosis of nuchal cystic hygroma. *Br J Radiol* 64:802, 1991.

Ogita S, Tsuto T, et al: Intracystic injection of OK-432: A new sclerosing therapy for cystic hygroma in children. *Br J Surg* 74:690, 1987.

Respiratory System

Atkinson JB, Ford EG, et al: The impact of extracorporeal membrane support in the treatment of congenital diaphragmatic hernia. *J Pediatr Surg* 26:791, 1991.

Bealer JF, Skarsgard ED, et al: The PLUG odyssey: Adventures in experimental fetal tracheal occlusion. *J Pediatr Surg* 30:361, 1995.

Breaux CW, Rouse TM, et al: Improvement in survival of patients with congenital diaphragmatic hernia utilizing a strategy of delayed repair after medical and/or extracorporeal membrane oxygenation stabilization. *J Pediatr Surg* 26:333, 1991.

Harrison MR, Adzick NS, et al: Correction of congenital diaphragmatic hernia in utero: VI. Hard-earned lessons. *J Pediatr Surg* 28:1411, 1993.

Harrison MR, Langer JC, et al: Correction of congenital diaphragmatic hernia in utero: V. Initial clinical experience. *J Pediatr Surg* 25:47, 1990.

Metkus AP, Filly RA, et al: Sonographic predictors of survival in fetal diaphragmatic hernia. *J Pediatr Surg* 31:148, 1996.

Newman KD, Anderson KD, et al: Extracorporeal membrane oxygenation and congenital diaphragmatic hernia: Should any infant be excluded? *J Pediatr Surg* 25:1048, 1990.

Pranikoff T, Gauger PG, Hirschl RB: Partial liquid ventilation in newborn patients with congenital diaphragmatic hernia. *J Pediatr Surg* 31:613, 1996.

Vanamo K, Rintala R, et al: Long-term pulmonary sequelae in survivors of congenital diaphragmatic defects. *J Pediatr Surg* 31:1096, 1996.

Wilson JF, Decker A: The surgical management of childhood bronchiectasis: A review of 96 consecutive pulmonary resections in children with nontuberculous bronchiectasis. *Ann Surg* 195:354, 1982.

Wilson JM, Bower LK, et al: ECMO in evolution: The impact of changing patient demographics and alternative therapies. *J Pediatr Surg* 31:1116, 1996.

Congenital Lobar Emphysema

Gordon I, Dempsey JE: Infantile lobar emphysema in association with congenital heart disease. *Clin Radiol* 41:48, 1990.

Congenital Cystic Adenomatoid Malformation

Harrison MR, Adzick NS, et al: Antenatal intervention for congenital cystic adenomatoid malformation. *Lancet* 336:965, 1990.

Miller JA, Corteville JE, Langer JC: Congenital cystic adenomatoid malformation in the fetus: Natural history and predictors of outcome. *J Pediatr Surg* 31:805, 1996.

Rosado-de-Christenson ML, Stocker JT: Congenital cystic adenomatoid malformation. *Radiographics* 11:865, 1991.

Shackelford GD, Siegel MJ: CT appearance of cystic adenomatoid malformations. *J Comput Assist Tomogr* 13:612, 1989.

Pulmonary Sequestration

Cramer JA, Ford WDA, Furness ME: Pulmonary sequestrations detected by antenatal ultrasound. *Pediatr Surg Int* 11:112, 1996.

Ikezoe J, Murayama S, et al: Bronchopulmonary sequestration: CT assessment. *Radiology* 176:375, 1990.

John PR, Beasley SW, Mayne V: Pulmonary sequestration and related congenital disorders: A clinico-radiological review of 41 cases. *Pediatr Radiol* 20:4, 1989.

Smart LM, Hendry GM: Imaging of neonatal pulmonary sequestration including Doppler ultrasound. *Br J Radiol* 64:324, 1991.

Bronchogenic Cysts

DiLorenzo M, Collin PP, et al: Bronchogenic cysts. *J Pediatr Surg* 24:988, 1989.

Lazar RH, Younis RT, Bassila MN: Bronchogenic cysts: A cause of stridor in the neonate. *Am J Otolaryngol* 12:117, 1991.

Esophageal Atresia and Tracheoesophageal Fistula

Ein SH, Shandling B: Pure esophageal atresia: A 50 year review. *J Pediatr Surg* 29:1208, 1994.

Engum SH, Grosfeld JL, et al: Analysis of morbidity and mortality in 227 cases of esophageal atresia and/or tracheoesophageal fistula over 2 decades. *Arch Surg* 130:502, 1995.

Haight C, Towsley HA: Congenital atresia of the esophagus with tracheo-esophageal fistula: Extrapleural ligation of fistula and end-to-end anastomosis of esophageal segments. *Surg Gynecol Obstet* 76:672, 1943.

Harris J, Kalley B, Robert E: Descriptive epidemiology of alimentary tract atresia. *Teratology* 52:15, 1995.

Poenaru D, Laberge JM, et al: A new prognostic classification for esophageal atresia. *Surgery* 113:426, 1993.

Randolph JG, Newman K, Anderson KD: Current results in repair of esophageal atresia with tracheoesophageal fistula using physiologic status as a guide to therapy. *Ann Surg* 209:525, 1989.

Rokitansky A, Kolankayah A, et al: Analysis of 309 cases of esophageal atresia for associated congenital malformations. *Am J Perinatol* 11:123, 1994.

Spitz L: Esophageal atresia: Past, present and future. *J Pediatr Surg* 31:19, 1996.

Spitz L, Kiely E, et al: Oesophageal atresia: At-risk groups for the 1990s. *J Pediatr Surg* 29:723, 1994.

Corrosive Injury of the Esophagus

Anderson KD, Rouse TM, Randolph JG: A controlled trial of corticosteroids in children with corrosive injury of the esophagus. *N Engl J Med* 323:637, 1990.

Esophageal Substitution

Anderson KD, Noblett H, et al: Long-term follow-up of children with colon and gastric tube interposition for esophageal atresia. *Surgery* 111:131, 1992.

Lindahl H, Louhimo I, Virkola K: Colon interposition or gastric tube? Follow-up study of colon-esophagus and gastric tube-esophagus patients. *J Pediatr Surg* 18:58, 1983.

Gastroesophageal Reflux

Martinez DA, Ginn-Pease ME, Caniano DA: Sequelae of antireflux surgery in profoundly disabled children. *J Pediatr Surg* 27:267, 1992.

Othersen HB, Ocampo RJ, et al: Barrett's esophagus in children: Diagnosis and management. *Ann Surg* 217:676, 1993.

Rode H, Millar AJW, et al: Reflux strictures of the esophagus in children. *J Pediatr Surg* 27:462, 1992.

Smith CD, Othersen HB, et al: Nissen fundoplication in children with profound neurologic disability: High risks and unmet goals. *Ann Surg* 215:654, 1992.

Weber TR: A prospective analysis of factors influencing outcome after fundoplication. *J Pediatr Surg* 30:1061, 1995.

Gastrointestinal Tract

Intestinal Obstruction

Del Pin CA, Czyrko C, et al: Management and survival of meconium ileus: A 30-year review. *Ann Surg* 215:179, 1992.

Grosfeld JL, Rescorla FJ: Duodenal atresia and stenosis: Reassessment of treatment and outcome based on antenatal diagnosis, pathologic variance, and long-term follow-up. *World J Surg* 17:301, 1993.

Kimura K, Mukohara N, et al: Diamond-shaped anastomosis for duodenal atresia: An experience with 44 patients over 15 years. *J Pediatr Surg* 25:977, 1990.

Weber TR, Lewis JE, et al: Duodenal atresia: A comparison of techniques of repair. *J Pediatr Surg* 21:1133, 1986.

Malrotation

Ford EG, Senac MO, et al: Malrotation of the intestine in children. *Ann Surg* 215:172, 1992.

Loyer E, Eggli KD: Sonographic evaluation of superior mesenteric vascular relationship in malrotation. *Pediatr Radiol* 19:173, 1989.

Powell DM, Othersen HB, Smith CD: Malrotation of the intestines in children: The effect of age on presentation and therapy. *J Pediatr Surg* 24:777, 1989.

Necrotizing Enterocolitis

Buras R, Guzzetta P, et al: Acidosis and hepatic portal venous gas: Indications for surgery in necrotizing enterocolitis. *Pediatrics* 78:273, 1986.

Ein SH, Shandling B, et al: A 13-year experience with peritoneal drainage under local anesthesia for necrotizing enterocolitis perforation. *J Pediatr Surg* 25:1034, 1990.

Horowitz JR, Lally KP, et al: Complications after surgical intervention for necrotizing enterocolitis: A multicenter review. *J Pediatr Surg* 30:994, 1995

Weber TR, Lewis JE: The role of second-look laparotomy in necrotizing enterocolitis. *J Pediatr Surg* 21:323, 1986.

Intussusception

Beasley SW, Glover J: Intussusception: Prediction of outcome of gas enemas. *J Pediatr Surg* 27:474, 1992.

Guo J, Ma X, Zhou Q: Results of air pressure enema reduction of intussusception: 6396 cases in 13 years. *J Pediatr Surg* 21:1201, 1986.

Marks RM, Sieber WK, et al: Hydrostatic pressure in the treatment of the ileocolic intussusception in infants and children. *J Pediatr Surg* 1:566, 1966.

Ravitch MM, McCune RM Jr: Reduction of intussusception by barium enema: A clinical and experimental study. *Ann Surg* 128:904, 1948.

Appendicitis

Adolph UR, Falterman KW: Appendicitis in children in the managed care era. *J Pediatr Surg* 31:1035, 1996.

Scholer SJ, Pituch K, et al: Clinical outcomes of children with acute abdominal pain. *Pediatrics* 98:680, 1996.

Hirschsprung's Disease

Carcassone M, Guis J, et al: Management of Hirschsprung's disease: Curative surgery before three months of age. *J Pediatr Surg* 24:1032, 1989.

Cilley RE, Statter MD, et al: Definitive treatment of Hirschsprung's disease in the newborn with a 1 stage procedure. *Surgery* 115:551, 1994.

Edery P, Attie T, et al: Mutation of the endothelin-3 gene in the Waardenburg-Hirschsprung disease. *Nature Genet* 12:442, 1996.

Fortuna RS, Weber TR, et al: Critical analysis of the operative treatment of Hirschsprung's disease. *Arch Surg* 131:520, 1996.

Foster P, Cowin G, et al: Twenty-five years experience with Hirschsprung's disease. *J Pediatr Surg* 25:531, 1990.

Georgeson KE, Fuenfer MM, et al: Primary laparoscopic pullthrough for Hirschsprung's disease in infants and children. *J Pediatr Surg* 30:1017, 1995.

Langer JC, Fitzgerald PG, et al: One-stage vs two-stage Soave pullthrough for Hirschsprung's disease in the first year of life. *J Pediatr Surg* 31:33, 1996.

Levy M, Reynolds M: Morbidity associated with total colon Hirschsprung's disease. *J Pediatr Surg* 27:364, 1992.

Martz TL, Seo T, et al: Gastrointestinal function after surgical correction of Hirschsprung's disease: Long-term follow-up in 135 patients. *J Pediatr Surg* 30:655, 1995.

Swenson O: Early history of the therapy of Hirschsprung's disease: Facts and personal observations over 50 years. *J Pediatr Surg* 31:1003, 1996.

Imperforate Anus

Bliss DP, Tapper D, et al: Does posterior sagittal anorectoplasty in patients with high imperforate anus provide superior fecal continence? *J Pediatr Surg* 31:26, 1996.

deVries PA, Pena A: Posterior sagittal anorectoplasty. *J Pediatr Surg* 17:638, 1982.

Hendren WH: Repair of cloacal anomalies: Current techniques. *J Pediatr Surg* 21:1159, 1986.

Karrer FM, Flannery AM, et al: Anorectal malformations: Evaluation of associated spinal dysraphic syndromes. *J Pediatr Surg* 23:45, 1988.

Pena A: Posterior sagittal anorectoplasty as a secondary operation for the treatment of fecal incontinence. *J Pediatr Surg* 18:762, 1983.

Jaundice

Alagille D, Odievre M, et al: Hepatic ductular hypoplasia associated with characteristic facies, vertebral malformations, retarded physical, mental, and sexual development and cardiac murmur. *J Pediatr* 86:63, 1975.

Alonzo-Lej, Rever WB, Pessagno DJ: Congenital choledochal cyst, with a report of 2 and an analysis of 94 cases. *Int Abstr Surg* 108:1, 1959.

Babbit DP: Congenital choledochal cysts: New etiological concept based on anomalous relationships of the common bile duct and pancreatic bulb. *Ann Radiol* 12:231, 1969.

Broelsch CH, Emond JC, et al: Application of reduced-size liver transplants as split grafts, auxiliary orthotopic grafts, and living related segmental transplants. *Ann Surg* 212:368, 1990.

Chandra RS: Biliary atresia and other structural anomalies in congenital polysplenia syndrome. *J Pediatr* 85:649, 1974.

Davenport M, Kerkar N, et al: Biliary atresia: The King's College Hospital experience (1974–1995). *J Pediatr Surg* 32:479, 1997.

DiNon PW, Balchais PU, et al: Increased expression of intercellular adhesion molecules in biliary atresia. *Am J Pathol* 145:263, 1994.

Endo E, Watanabe K, et al: Outcomes of ileocolic conduit for biliary drainage in infants with biliary atresia: Comparison with Roux-en-Y reconstruction. *J Pediatr Surg* 30:700, 1995.

Kasai M, Kimura S, et al: Surgical treatment of biliary atresia. *J Pediatr Surg* 3:665, 1968.

Laurent J, Gauthier F, et al: Long-term outcome after surgery for biliary atresia: Study of 400 patients surviving more than 10 years. *Gastroenterology* 99:1793, 1990.

Lilly JR: Total excision of choledochal cyst. *Surg Gynecol Obstet* 146:254, 1978.

Lilly JR, Altman RP: Hepatic portoenterostomy (the Kasai operation) for biliary atresia. *Surgery* 78:76, 1975.

Majd M, Reba RC, et al: Hepatobiliary scintigraphy with ^{99m}Tc-PIPIDA in the evaluation of neonatal jaundice. *Pediatrics* 67(1):140, 1981.

Ohi R, Nio M, et al: Long-term follow-up after surgery for patients with biliary atresia. *J Pediatr Surg* 25:442, 1990.

Ohya T, Fujimoto T, et al: Degeneration of intrahepatic bile duct with lymphocyte infiltration into biliary epithelial cells in biliary atresia. *J Pediatr Surg* 30:515, 1995.

Price M, Sartorelli, et al: Management of esophageal varices in children by endoscopic variceal ligation. *J Pediatr Surg* 31:1056, 1996.

Sandler A, Azarow K, Superina R: The morbidity of prior Kasai procedure on liver transplantation for biliary atresia. *J Pediatr Surg* (in press).

Schroeder D, Smith L, et al: Antenatal diagnosis of choledochal cyst at 15 weeks' gestation: Etiologic implications and management. *J Pediatr Surg* 24:936, 1989.

Suita S, Shono K, et al: The prognostic significance of serum bilirubin levels after Kasai's operation in biliary atresia: How normal is the normal range? *J Pediatr Surg* (in press).

Todani T, Watanabe Y, et al: Congenital bile duct cysts: Classification, operative procedures, and review of thirty-seven cases including cancer arising from choledochal cyst. *Am J Surg* 134:263, 1977.

Tsuchida Y, Kawarsaki H, et al: Antenatal diagnosis of biliary atresia (type I cyst) at 19 weeks' gestation: Differential diagnosis and etiologic implications. *J Pediatr Surg* 30: 697, 1995.

Vacanti J, Shamberger R, et al: The therapy of biliary atresia combining the Kasai portoenterostomy with liver transplantation: A single-center experience. *J Pediatr Surg* 25:149, 1990.

Wood RP, Langas AN et al: Optimal therapy for patients with biliary atresia: Portenterostomy ("Kasai" procedure) versus primary transplantation. *J Pediatr Surg* 25:153, 1990.

Deformities of the Abdominal Wall

Caniano DA, Brokaw B, Ginn-Rease ME: An individualized approach to the management of gastroschisis. *J Pediatr Surg* 25:297, 1990.

Fonkalsrud EW, Smith MD, et al: Selective management of gastroschisis according to the degree of visceral abdominal disproportion. *Ann Surg* 218:742, 1993.

Gornall P: Management of intestinal atresia complicating gastroschisis. *J Pediatr Surg* 24:522, 1989.

Gray SW, Skandalakis JE: *Embryology for Surgeons.* Baltimore, Williams & Wilkins, 1994.

Langer JC: Fetal abdominal wall defects. *Semin Pediatr Surg* 2:121, 1993.

Molenaar JC, Tibboel D: Gastroschisis and omphalocele. *World J Surg* 17:337, 1993.

Moretti M, Khaury A, et al: The effect of mode of delivery on the perinatal outcome in fetuses with abdominal wall defects. *Am J Obstet Gynecol* 163:833, 1990.

Nuchtern AG, Baxter R, et al: Nonoperative initial management vs silon chimney for treatment of giant omphalocele. *J Pediatr Surg* 30:771, 1995.

Paidas NJ, Cromblehome TM, et al: Prenatal diagnosis and management of the fetus with an abdominal wall defect. *Semin Perinatol* 18:196, 1994.

Randolph JG, Cavett C, et al: Surgical correction and rehabilitation for children with "prune belly" syndrome. *Ann Surg* 193:757, 1981.

Ricketts RR, Woodward JR, et al: Modern treatment of cloacal exstrophy. *J Pediatr Surg* 26:444, 1991.

Shah R, Woolley MM: Gastroschisis and intestinal atresia. *J Pediatr Surg* 26:788, 1991.

Tunell WP, Puffinbarger NK, et al: Abdominal wall defects in infants: Survival and implications for adult life. *Ann Surg* 221:525, 1995.

Inguinal Hernia

Baguley PE, Fitzgerald PG, et al: Emergency room reduction of incarcerated inguinal hernia in infants: Is routine hospital admission necessary? *Pediatr Surg Int* 7:366, 1992.

Holcomb GW, Morgan WM: Laparoscopic evaluation for contralateral patent processus vaginalis, part II. *J Pediatr Surg* 31:1170, 1996.

Skinner MA, Grosfeld JL: Inguinal hernia and umbilical hernia repair in infants and children. *Surg Clin North Am* 73:439, 1993.

Welborn LG, Rice LJ, et al: Postoperative apnea in former preterm infants: Prospective comparison of spinal and general anesthesia. *Anesthesiology* 72:838, 1990.

Cryptorchidism

Heiss KF, Shandling B: Laparoscopy for the impalpable testes: Experience with 53 testes. *J Pediatr Surg* 27:175, 1992.

Vaginal Anomalies

Tran AT, Arensman RM, Falterman KW: Diagnosis and management of hydrohematometrocolpos syndromes. *Am J Dis Child* 141:632, 1987.

Ovarian Cysts and Tumors

Brandt ML, Luks FI, et al: Surgical indications in antenatally diagnosed ovarian cysts. *J Pediatr Surg* 26:276, 1991.

Croitoru DP, Aaron LE, et al: Management of complex ovarian cysts presenting in the first year of life. *J Pediatr Surg* 26:1366, 1991.

Gribbon M, Ein SH, Mancer K: Pediatric malignant ovarian tumors: A 43-year review. *J Pediatr Surg* 27:480, 1992.

Meizner I, Levy A, et al: Fetal ovarian cysts: prenatal ultrasonographic detection and postnatal evaluation and treatment. *Am J Obstet Gynecol* 164:874, 1991.

Raney RB Jr, Sinclair L, et al: Malignant ovarian tumors in children and adolescents. *Cancer* 59:1214, 1987.

Sakala EP, Leon ZA, Rouse GA: Management of antenatally diagnosed fetal ovarian cysts. *Obstet Gynecol Surg* 46:407, 1991.

Schwobel MG, Stauffer UG: Surgical treatment of ovarian tumors in childhood. *Prog Pediatr Surg* 26:112, 1991.

Ambiguous Genitalia

Donahoe PK, Schnitzer JJ: Evaluation of the infant who has ambiguous genitalia, and principles of operative management. *Semin Pediatr Surg* 5:30, 1996.

Goodfellow PN, Lovell-Badge RA: SRY and sex determination in mammals. *Annu Rev Genet* 27:71, 1993.

Haqq CM, King CY, et al: Molecular basis of mammalian sexual determination: Activation of müllerian inhibiting substance gene expression by SRY. *Science* 266:1495, 1994.

Neoplastic Disease

Ablin AR, Krailo MD: Results of treatment of malignant germ cell tumors in 93 children: A report from the Children's Cancer Study Group. *J Clin Oncol* 9:1782, 1991.

Azizkhan RG, Hause GM: Current biologic and therapeutic implications in the surgery of neuroblastoma. *Semin Surg Oncol* 9:493, 1993.

Bowman LC, Hancock ML, et al: Impact of intensified therapy on clinical outcome in infants and children with neuroblastoma: The St. Judes Children's Research Hospital Experience, 1962-1988. *J Clin Oncol* 9:1599, 1991.

Crist W, Gehan EA, et al: The Third Intergroup Rhabdomyosarcoma Study. *J Clin Oncol* 13:610, 1995.

Douglass EL, Reynolds M, et al: Cisplatin, Vincristine and fluorouracil therapy for hepatoblastoma. Pediatric Oncology Group Study. *J Clin Oncol* 11:96, 1993.

Green DM, Breslow NE, et al: Treatment of children with stage 4 favorable histology Wilms' tumor: A report from the National Wilms' Tumor Study Group. *Med Pediatr Oncol* 26:147, 1996.

Grundy PE, Coppes MJ, et al: Molecular genetics of Wilms' tumor. *Hematol Oncol Clin North Am* 9:1201, 1995.

King DR, Ortega J, et al: The surgical management of children with incompletely resected hepatic cancer is facilitated by intensive chemotherapy. *J Pediatr Surg* 26:1074, 1991.

Koneru B, Flye M, et al: Liver transplantation for hepatoblastoma. *Ann Surg* 213:118, 1991.

Koscielniak E, Jurgens H, et al: Treatment of soft tissue sarcoma in childhood and adolescents. *Cancer* 70:2557, 1991.

Madden SL, Cooke DM, et al: Transcriptional repression mediated by the WT1 Wilms' tumor gene product. *Science* 253:1550, 1991.

Matthay KK, Seeger RC, et al: Allogenic vs autologous purged bone marrow transplantation for neuroblastoma: Report from the Children's Cancer Group. *J Clin Oncol* 12:2382, 1994.

Maurer H, Gehan EA, et al: The Intergroup Rhabdomyosarcoma Study-2. *Cancer* 71:1904, 1993.

Montgomery BT, Kelalis PP, et al: Extended followup of bilateral Wilms' tumor: Results of the National Wilms' Tumor Study. *Gen Urol* 146:514, 1991.

National Wilms' Tumor Study Committee: Wilms' tumor: Status report, 1990. *J Clin Oncol* 9:877, 1991.

Ni YH, Chang MA: Hepatocellular carcinoma in childhood: Clinical manifestations and prognosis. *Cancer* 68:1737, 1991.

Ortega JA, Krailo M, et al: Effective treatment of unresectable or metastatic hepatoblastoma with cisplatin and continuous infusion Adriamycin chemotherapy: A report from the Children's Cancer Study Group. *J Clin Oncol* 9:2167, 1991.

Pappo AS, Shapiro DN, et al: Biology and therapy of pediatric rhabdomyosarcoma. *J Clin Oncol* 13:2123, 1995.

Ritchey ML, Haase GM, et al: Current management of Wilms' tumor. *Semin Surg Oncol* 9:502, 1993.

Shamberger R, Allarde-Segundo A, et al: Surgical management of stage III and IV neuroblastoma: Resection before or after chemotherapy. *J Pediatr Surg* 26:113, 1991.

Tagge EP, Tagge DU, et al: Resection, including transplantation, for hepatoblastoma and hepatocellular carcinoma: Impact on survival. *J Pediatr Surg* 27:292, 1992.

Thompson WR, Newman K, et al: Strategy for resection of Wilms' tumor with vena cava or atrial extension. *J Pediatr Surg* 27:912, 1992.

Trauma

Bond SJ, Gotschall CS, Eichelberger MR: Predictors of abdominal injury in children with pelvic fracture. *J Trauma* 31:1169, 1991.

Cooper A, Barlow B, et al: Epidemiology of pediatric trauma: Importance of population-based statistics. *J Pediatr Surg* 27:149, 1992.

Fallat ME, Hardwick VG: Transport of the injured child. *Semin Pediatr Surg* 4:88, 1995.

Greenwald BM, Ghajar J, et al: Critical care of children with acute brain injury. *Adv Pediatr* 42:47, 1995.

Hall JR, Reyes HM, et al: The outcome for children with blunt trauma is best at a pediatric trauma center. *J Pediatr Surg* 31:72, 1996.

Maksoud JG, Moront ML, et al: Resuscitation of the injured child. *Semin Pediatr Surg* 4:93, 1995.

Moront ML, Eichelberger MR: Advances in the treatment of pediatric trauma. *Curr Opin Gen Surg* 1:41, 1994.

Newman K, Bowman LM, et al: The lap belt complex: Intestinal and lumbar spine injury in children. *J Trauma* 30:1133, 1990.

Peclet MH, Newman KD, et al: Patterns of injury in children. *J Pediatr Surg* 25:85, 1990.

Peclet MH, Newman KD, et al: Thoracic trauma in children: An indicator of increased mortality. *J Pediatr Surg* 25:961, 1990.

Sivit CJ, Taylor GA, et al: Safety belt injuries in children with lap-belt ecchymosis: CT findings in 61 patients. *Am J Radiol* 57:111, 1991.

Taylor GA, Eichelberger MR, et al: Indications for computed tomography in children with blunt abdominal trauma. *Ann Surg* 213:212, 1991.

Wright MF: Update on pediatric trauma care. *Curr Opin Pediatr* 7:212, 1995.

CHAPTER 38

Urology

Margaret S. Pearle, John D. McConnell, and Paul C. Peters

ANATOMY

Kidney. The kidneys are paired retroperitoneal organs that weigh approximately 160 g each in the healthy adult. They are situated within the fascia of Gerota, and a variable amount of perinephric fat is present between the capsule of the kidney and this fascial envelope. Further protection of the kidneys is provided dorsally (posteriorly) by their relationship with the lower ribs, the quadratus lumborum, and the psoas muscles. The ven-

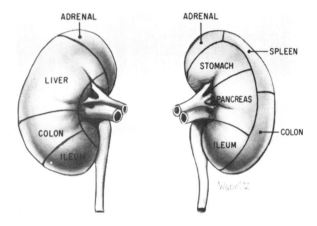

FIG. 38-1. Ventral (anterior) relationships of the kidneys with adjacent organs.

tral (anterior) relationships of the kidney are illustrated in Fig. 38-1. The kidneys lie beneath the diaphragm, with the right kidney usually 1 to 2 cm lower than the left kidney (Fig. 38-2).

The renal arteries originate from the aorta at the upper level of the second lumbar vertebra; the right renal artery is longer than the left because it crosses the midline behind the vena cava. In about two-thirds of the population, each kidney has a single renal artery. Multiple renal arteries occur in normal kidneys but are more prevalent in congenitally malformed or malpositioned kidneys. The main renal artery divides into five major branches, each of which represents an end artery supplying a renal segment. Partial occlusion of any branch produces ischemia, and complete occlusion produces infarction of the involved segment. The ureteral and capsular vessels can provide significant blood flow in the presence of marked renal artery occlusion. The left renal vein crosses the midline ventral to the aorta after it has

received blood from the left adrenal and gonadal veins. The renal lymphatics empty through hilar trunks in the region of the renal artery and vein. Capsular lymphatics travel through the perinephric fat to infradiaphragmatic periaortic nodes. The renal nerves, which receive contributions from T4 to T12, from the vagus nerve via the celiac axis, and from the splanchnic, contain vasomotor and pain fibers. After total renal denervation, such as occurs with transplantation, no persistent abnormalities in renal function occur. The renal pelvis, which usually contains approximately 5 mL of urine, lies dorsal to the renal vessels and has a transitional cell epithelium. The kidney's position, with respect to the vertebral bodies and the axis of a line drawn through the upper and lower calyces, offers a clue to focal diseases of the kidney and adjacent organs. The axis of the kidney often parallels that of the psoas muscle edge, as noted on x-rays of the abdomen (see Fig. 38-2).

Ureter. The ureters are muscular tubes that connect the renal pelvis to the bladder, traversing the retroperitoneal space in a linear course just lateral to the transverse processes of the lumbar vertebrae and crossing the common iliac arteries at their bifurcation. The lower ureter follows the contour of the pelvis and deviates laterally and then medially in a gentle curve to reach the trigone of the bladder above a line drawn between the spinous processes. The normal adult ureter is 28 to 30 cm long and about 5 mm in diameter and has an oblique course through the wall of the bladder. The ureteral orifice is an oblique slit in the trigone.

The function of the ureter is to transmit urine from the renal pelvis to the bladder. Ordinarily, urine is not modified in the ureter. Normally, there are about four peristaltic waves per minute, developing pressures of about 30 mmHg.

The ureteral blood supply originates from the renal, aortic, iliac, mesenteric, gonadal, vasal, and vesical arteries. Free intercommunication between these vessels permits extensive ureteral

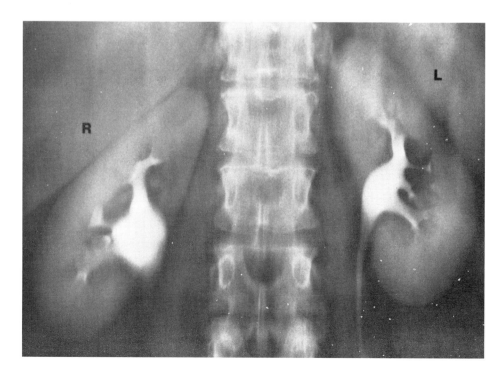

FIG. 38-2. Tomogram from intravenous urogram. Right kidney is lower than left. Axis of left kidney parallels left psoas margin, and right renal axis is slightly deviated because of the more dilated right renal pelvis.

mobilization and transposition. Pain fibers refer stimuli to the T12 through L2 segments, whereas the autonomic innervation is associated with intrinsic parasympathetic motor and sympathetic vasomotor ganglia. The lymphatic drainage is to segmental peri-aortic and caval nodes. The ureter may be drawn medially in retroperitoneal fibrosis and laterally as a result of enlargement of periaortic lymph node involvement with tumor or an aortic aneurysm. It is essential to be aware of the course of the ureter during aortic and pelvic surgery and in difficult dissections of adjacent organs.

Bladder. The urinary bladder is a muscular pelvic organ lined with transitional cell epithelium. It is related to the peritoneum superiorly and posteriorly, the sigmoid colon and rectum in the male, and the uterus, cervix, and vagina in the female. In the male, the bladder is spherical; in the female, the uterus indents the dome. The smooth muscle *(detrusor)* is capable of stretching to a marked degree. The major blood supply originates from the superior, middle, and inferior branches of the hypogastric arteries. The lymphatics drain to the perivesical, hypogastric, and periaortic nodes. The autonomic nerve supply to the bladder is derived from the sacral cord and from the presacral and epigastric plexuses of nerves.

Prostate and Seminal Vesicles. The chestnut-shaped adult prostate surrounds the proximal male urethra. It is firmly attached to the bladder neck and symphysis pubis. Posteriorly, the fascia of Denonvilliers intervenes between the rectum and the prostate and seminal vesicles (Fig. 38-3). Caudad, the prostate rests on the pelvic diaphragm that contains the voluntary external sphincter. The blood supply derives from the inferior vesical, middle hemorrhoidal, and internal pudendal arteries; the venous drainage communicates with an extensive pelvic plexus that empties into the hypogastric veins. This plexus also communicates with Batson's veins, partially explaining the frequently encountered metastatic spread of prostatic carcinoma to the bony pelvis and lumbar vertebral bodies. The prostate receives secretory and motor (parasympathetic) innervation from S3 and S4 and vasomotor (sympathetic) fibers from the hypogastric plexus. The lymphatics drain into the obturator nodes, the external, internal, and common iliac nodes, and then to the periaortic nodes.

The seminal vesicles lie behind the bladder lateral to the ampullae of the vasa deferentia and are closely related to the ureters. Their secretions are rich in fructose, which may be of importance to sperm motility.

Penis and Urethra. The penis is composed of two lateral spongy erectile bodies *(corpora cavernosa)* and a single ventral body *(corpus spongiosum urethrae)* through which the urethra passes. The latter terminates in the glans penis, which is also composed of erectile tissue. As the urethra emerges from the pelvic diaphragm, it enlarges to become the bulbous urethra. The urethra continues as the pendulous urethra, which terminates in the tip of the glans penis (Fig. 38-4). The female urethra corresponds to the prostatic and membranous urethra in the male. It averages 4 cm in length and 32 mm in circumference. The principal blood supply to the penis and urethra originates from the internal pudendal arteries. Somatic sensory innervation of the penis is from S3 and S4 via the ilioinguinal and genitofemoral nerves. Sympathetic vasomotor innervation derives from the hypogastric plexus, whereas the parasympathetic innervation originates from S2, S3, and S4 via the nervi erigentes. The nervi erigentes give rise to the caversonal nerves that course on the posterior surface of the prostate in route to the corpora cavernosa of the penis. Injury to the caversonal nerves during pelvic surgery will lead to impotence. The lymphatic drainage is to the superficial and deep inguinal nodes and then to the external iliac and hypogastric nodes.

Testis and Epididymis. The testis is an ovoid, firm scrotal organ that measures 4 × 2.5 × 2.5 cm. The left testis commonly resides lower in the scrotum than the right. The testis weighs approximately 20 g and is covered by a tough membrane, the tunica albuginea, except at its dorsal aspect, where the epididymis and vascular pedicle are attached. The epididymis is a crescent-shaped body that curves around the dorsal portion of the testis. The vas deferens is a 4-mm-thick walled, firm tubular structure that originates at the inferior pole of the epididymis and follows a cranial course with the spermatic vessels (see Fig. 38-4). The arterial blood supply to the testis and epididymis originates from the aorta just below the renal arteries. The left spermatic vein empties into the left renal vein; the right spermatic vein empties directly into the inferior vena cava. The primary lymphatic drainage from the testis is to the periaortic nodes in the vicinity of the kidney.

DIAGNOSIS

Accuracy of diagnosis is a characteristic feature of the practice of urology. In order to maintain the achievable degree of accuracy, it is essential that a clinical problem be approached in a logical sequence. History, physical examination, laboratory tests, and imaging tests lead to a reasonable estimate of diagnosis. Rarely is a urologic diagnosis made on the basis of surgical exploration.

History

A number of symptoms and signs are characteristic and often diagnostic of pathologic conditions involving the genitourinary system. The patient may spontaneously offer these clues, but in most instances it is necessary to ask proper questions to obtain this information.

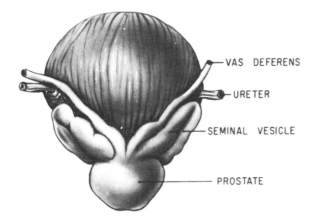

FIG. 38-3. Posterior relationships of the prostate, seminal vesicles, ureters, and bladder.

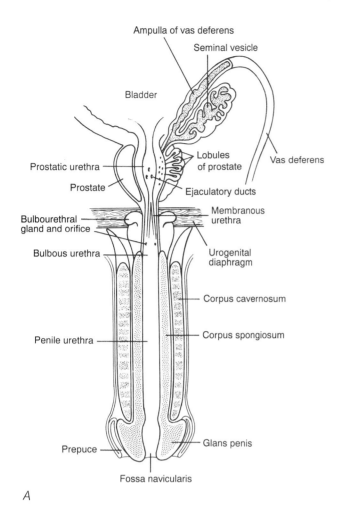

A

Gross Hematuria. The presence of gross blood in the urine is a significant sign that is quite alarming to the patient and warrants further evaluation. The degree of bleeding is not proportionate to the severity of the underlying disease. Even small amounts of blood in the urine occurring on one occasion may be the only indication of a malignant process in the urinary tract. Intermittent bleeding is common; large tumors may manifest with only a small amount of bleeding, whereas small tumors may produce considerable loss of blood. The bleeding originates from lesions that cause erosion or disruption of blood vessels or from inflammatory changes. The common causes are inflammation (including infections), tumors, calculi, and trauma.

In young individuals, gross hematuria is more likely to be the result of infection, and in older patients, it is more likely to be related to tumors and prostatic disease. Any patient with unexplained *asymptomatic* gross hematuria should be evaluated for possible tumor.

It is important to determine whether hematuria appears at the beginning or end of voiding. Initial hematuria suggests lesions distal to the bladder neck, namely, the prostatic and membranous urethra. Predominantly terminal hematuria usually indicates involvement of the proximal urethra, bladder neck, or trigone. Uniform hematuria occurs with lesions of the bladder, ureter, or kidney. The passage of blood clots suggests that the bleeding is quantitatively great because urine inhibits coagulation of blood by the presence of citrate. Long, wormlike clots suggest formation in the ureter. Reddish clots occur with recent bleeding, whereas brownish or grayish white clots indicate a time lapse between the bleeding episode and their passage. These "localizing" signs are not reliable enough to pinpoint the diagnosis. Complete imaging and endoscopic evaluation of the entire urinary tract is usually warranted.

Acute Urinary Retention. *Acute urinary retention* (AUR) is a term that applies to a complete inability to urinate, and this is one of the most distressing symptoms. It should not be referred to as "anuria" because the latter indicates that urine is not being formed. The patient usually complains of lower

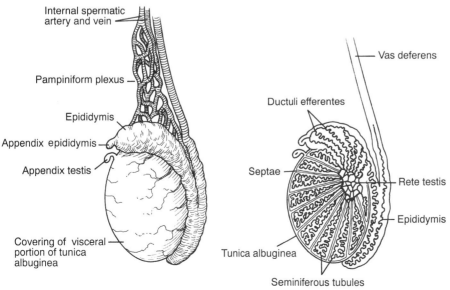

B

FIG. 38-4. Male reproductive and lower urinary tracts noting anatomic features of (*A*) corpora and urethra and (*B*) testis, epididymis, and vas deferens.

abdominal distress, and the bladder is percussible or palpable as a tender suprapubic mass.

Benign prostatic hyperplasia (BPH) is the most common cause of AUR in men. Most have a long-standing history of increasing difficulty in voiding, but occasionally an acute event (e.g., surgery, decongestant medications, etc.) may precipitate AUR in a patient with minimal prior symptoms. By contrast, *carcinoma of the prostate* is accompanied by a much shorter duration of symptoms. The history may be of months rather than years, and the urinary difficulties increase more rapidly. The patient with carcinoma of the prostate seldom presents with urinary retention when the lesion is early and amenable to surgical treatment. The presence of retention in a cancer patient therefore suggests advanced disease, and symptoms of advanced malignancy such as malaise, weight loss, anorexia, and back pain are likely to be encountered. Carcinoma of the prostate can coexist with BPH.

In young males, *prostatic infection* may cause AUR. This results from acute prostate swelling. There is usually an antecedent history of frequent urination and dysuria progressing to acute retention. Fever, chills, and symptoms of systemic infection are common, and abscess formation occurs occasionally. AUR retention may be a manifestation of *urethral stricture.* These patients often have an antecedent history of gonorrhea, transurethral instrumentation, trauma, or radiation therapy. Many will have noted a gradual decrease in the force of the stream.

Neurogenic bladder dysfunction may lead to a progressive increase in residual urine and eventually to complete retention. This may be the first indication of spinal cord disease. In other patients, the retention may be preceded by difficulty in initiating voiding and overflow incontinence related to changes in abdominal pressure exerting force on a markedly distended bladder. Acute retention on a neurogenic basis may follow trauma, pelvic surgery, the administration of general anesthetics, spinal anesthesia, or the administration of certain drugs that influence the innervation of the bladder, bladder neck, proximal urethra, or external sphincter. AUR in women is unusual and may be caused by neurogenic and psychogenic factors or urethral obstructions secondary to carcinoma, stricture, vaginal lesions, or cervical fibroids. A cystocele is seldom the cause of AUR.

Incontinence. *Incontinence* is the involuntary loss of urine that the patient views as socially unacceptable. *Total incontinence* is continuous and not associated with urgency or stress. A vesicovaginal, ureterovaginal, or vesicoperineal fistula may produce total incontinence. Occasionally, an ectopic ureter will open into the vagina, and this also will produce a constant leakage of urine. *Stress incontinence* is the leakage of urine associated with increase in abdominal pressure from coughing, lifting, etc. It is the result of lax pelvic support in women (following childbirth or menopause) and resulting urethral hypermobility or sphincteric dysfunction in men (following prostatectomy). *Urgency incontinence* refers to urinary leakage preceded by the sensation of an urgent need to urinate. This is often the result of a uninhibited contraction of the bladder due to infection, bladder cancer, neurogenic disease, or idiopathic causes. *Overflow, or paradoxical, incontinence* represents a fourth type, in which the bladder retains a large amount of residual urine. With movement, the increased abdominal pressure may cause overflow of a small amount of urine from a distended bladder. This condition may accompany neurogenic diseases of the spinal cord, or it may be the result of long-standing obstructive uropathy with detrusor decompensation. These patients may never really void, intermittently passing small quantities of urine without control. Incontinence of urine is a common manifestation of various neurologic diseases and spinal cord trauma.

Ureteral Colic. Acute obstruction of the kidney or ureter produces very painful distention. Typically, there is sudden unilateral severe crescendo pain in the posterior subcostal region. The localization is frequently so precise that it can be defined by fingertip palpation. Obstruction at the ureteropelvic junction is associated with pain at the costovertebral angle, whereas obstruction lower in the ureter may have the added component of pain in the ipsilateral lower abdomen. With obstruction of the intramural ureter, pain also may be referred to the corresponding side of the scrotum or labia majora. Ureteral colic related to intramural obstruction is often associated with a sudden onset of urgency and frequency.

Lower Urinary Tract Symptoms (LUTS). *Frequency* refers to the patient's voiding an excessive number of times. Frequency of urination should not be confused with *polyuria,* where the patient excretes large volumes of urine at more frequent intervals than normal. Most normal, well-hydrated individuals void four to six times daily and do not arise from sleep to empty the bladder. Frequency may be related to reduction in bladder capacity associated with inflammation, bladder outlet obstruction, effective reduction in functional bladder capacity by increased residual urine, or uninhibited bladder contractions. Frequency is also a symptom of psychological stress.

When patients complain of frequency, it is essential to question them carefully regarding fluid and caffeine intake. It is sometimes of value to have the patient record accurately the time and volume of the amounts of fluid ingested as well as the amount excreted in a 24-h period (frequency-volume chart). It is also essential to note the medications the patient is taking because this may influence urinary frequency considerably. Additional information about the relationship of urinary frequency to work, stress, weekend activity, and vacations is extremely helpful. Many patients seek help from other physicians for this disturbing symptom, which may limit their activities because of the need to be close to a bathroom at all times. A careful history may lead to information that will allow simple modification of habits, intake, and drug therapy to bring relief from this distressing and sometimes incapacitating problem.

Nocturia, awakening at night to void, may be caused by consumption of an excessive amount of fluids before retiring, or it may be an expression of generalized restlessness. With cardiac decompensation, fluids that have accumulated in dependent portions of the body during the day are restored to the circulating blood when the patient maintains a horizontal position, thus causing nocturia. Patients with chronic renal disease who excrete large volumes because of an inability to concentrate the urine and patients on diuretics frequently experience nocturia. Prostatic obstruction and acute or chronic infection of the urinary tract cause nocturia by means of the same mechanisms described for frequency.

Urgency is due to an increase in bladder pressure. Urgency and frequency usually occur together in obstruction and infection. However, urgency can be a normal consequence of voiding postponement for prolonged periods of time. The symptom may be so severe that the patient cannot restrain voiding, resulting in *urgency incontinence.*

Difficult or painful urination is known as *dysuria.* The sensation is commonly described as burning and may be referred to the glans penis or perineum. The symptom may be caused by urinary infection, the passage of clots or calculi, or primary bladder disease. Bladder cancer and other diseases must be excluded when the urine culture is sterile. Severe pain at the termination of or subsequent to voiding is referred to as a *strangury* and may be associated with the presence of a bladder calculus or infection. Difficulty of urination is usually the result of an obstructive uropathy. *Hesitancy,* indicating delayed voiding in response to mental command, is another symptom of chronic obstructive uropathy or sphincter dyssynergia. *Intermittency* refers to the involuntary stopping and starting of the stream during voiding and may be a symptom of obstruction.

Urinary Stream. The stream may lack force and have reduced projection in patients with lower urinary tract obstruction. Prostatic enlargement and urethral stricture are the most common causes. Stenosis of the meatus, which determines the caliber of the urinary stream, may be evidenced by a thin, deviated, or duplicated stream.

Erectile and Ejaculatory Dysfunction. Disorders of sexual function are usually the result of systemic disease processes, such as atherosclerosis. A careful history about medications is essential because certain drugs produce erectile and ejaculatory disturbances. The cause of loss of erection may be endocrinologic, vasculogenic, or neurogenic. In some situations, however, the underlying factor is situational or psychogenic, and this may become apparent during careful history taking. In instances where physical or anatomic abnormality is found to account for impotence, it may be correctable. It can be restored in most patients by medical or surgical therapy.

Physical Examination

Renal Areas. The kidney region can first be examined with the patient in the upright position. Observation may reveal obvious bulging or asymmetry of the costovertebral region. Scoliosis may be present from guarding in the presence of unilateral pain. Herpetic lesions are occasionally encountered on the skin surface of this area and offer a clue to the cause of pain. Gentle palpation of the costovertebral angle areas should be followed by sharp percussion when attempting to disclose an underlying obstructed or infected kidney. If the patient complains of pain in the flank region before examination, it is wise to start the evaluation on the contralateral side.

Thorough examination of the kidney areas should be carried out with the patient supine, knees flexed, and arms at the side. The examiner should stand on the side being examined. The posterior hand is placed parallel to the twelfth rib and below it. The anterior hand is placed 4 cm below the anterior rib cage and parallel to the posterior hand. Renal and retroperitoneal masses can be balloted between the two hands. In slender individuals, the lower pole of the right kidney is often palpable. In others, the kidney may be palpable with deep inspiration. With unusually mobile kidneys, the organ may be more readily palpable in the upright position. Tenderness is usually related to obstruction or infraction and is uncommon with uncomplicated tumors or cysts. The examiner again looks for evidence of asymmetry, rigidity of the costovertebral angle, tenderness, or bulging, which may suggest the presence of an underlying abscess, obstructed kidney, inflammation, or retroperitoneal extravasation of urine or blood.

Ureters. The deep retroperitoneal location of the ureters does not lend itself to palpation. It is unusual to be able to feel them even when they are grossly dilated or to be able to localize a pathologic area within them.

Bladder. Examination takes place with the patient in the supine position. The empty bladder is neither percussible nor palpable. In the markedly distended condition, occurring with chronic obstruction, the bladder may be visible as a large abdominal mass rising out of the pelvis. Under ordinary circumstances, the bladder is not percussible until it contains approximately 150 mL of urine. Persistence of a low abdominal mass following emptying of the bladder by catheterization documents the extra vesical nature of the lesion.

Penis. The penis is examined with the patient in the upright position facing the examiner, who is sitting in a chair, or with the patient in a supine position on the examining table. If the patient is not circumcised, the foreskin should be retracted so that underlying glans, urethral meatus, and inner aspect of the foreskin can be visualized. Additional evaluation of the meatal caliber may be carried out with appropriate instrumentation, if indicated. A recommended means of evaluating the presence of a meatal obstruction is observation of the patient voiding.

Scrotum. Examination of the scrotum is carried out in conjunction with examination of the penis and with the patient in the positions noted above. Some patients are extremely sensitive to examination of this area, and the examiner may elicit a vasovagal response from the patient who is in the standing position. Careful observation and palpation of this region and the use of a small flashlight to transilluminate lesions offer the best means of making an accurate diagnosis.

Scrotal masses have a variety of causes (Fig. 38-5). An indirect *inguinal hernia* may present as a scrotal mass. The enlargement extends up into the inguinal region and often may be reduced with the patient in the supine position.

Epididymitis. Acute *epididymitis* is commonly a result of retrograde extension via the vas deferens from a focus of infection in the prostate, urethra, or bladder. It may follow prostatic massage or instrumentation. The patient is frequently febrile and has a typical straddling gait to minimize contact with the inflamed scrotal contents. The scrotum is exquisitely tender and may contain a mass. The overlying skin is red and edematous. *Chronic epididymitis,* which is a result of incompletely resolved acute epididymitis, presents with an indurated mass that may or may not be tender. *Tuberculous epididymitis* is characteristically nontender, stony hard, and may be associated with irregular indurated beadings of the vas deferens. A *sterile* or *chemical epididymitis* may occur with the retrograde extravasation of fluid into the epididymis secondary to marked increase in intraabdominal pressure associated with heavy lifting while the bladder is distended. The urine is usually sterile in this situation, in contrast to the pyuria often present with acute epididymitis from infection.

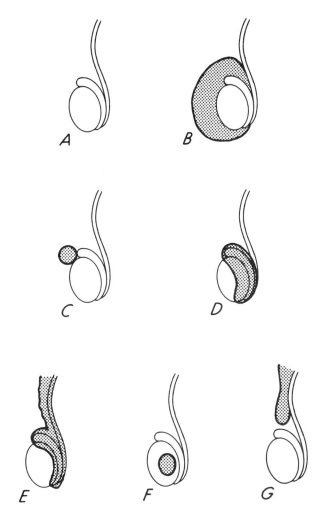

FIG. 38-5. Differential diagnosis of scrotal lesions. A. Normal. B. Hydrocele. C. Spermatocele. D. Epididymitis. E. Epididymovasitis. F. Testicular tumor. G. Hernia.

Varicocele. There is a predilection for the left side, presumably because the left spermatic vein drains into the left renal vein, resulting in higher venous pressures than on the right. Acute onset of a left varicocele after the age of 40 suggests left renal vein occlusion, commonly related to renal tumor. A varicocele on the right side may be secondary to vena caval obstruction or occlusion. This occasionally occurs with tumor thrombus from a renal cancer (hypernephroma) invading and involving the lumen of the vena cava.

The usual type of left varicocele is observed best with the patient in the standing position facing the examiner. The characteristic "bag of worms" appearance and feeling of the scrotum is noted. With the patient in the supine position, the varicocele collapses and usually cannot be palpated. The presence of a varicocele in a patient being examined for infertility can be a significant finding. This is especially true if the patient has a low sperm count with reduced motility of the sperm and changes in sperm morphology.

Hydrocele. *Primary idiopathic hydrocele* can be unilateral or bilateral and represents an increased collection of fluid between the tunica vaginalis and its contents. It is manifested as a nontender mass that is translucent and often obscures palpation of the testis and epididymis. It is ventral, superior, and inferior to the testis and may become very large and symptomatic. *Secondary hydroceles* are the consequence of serous effusion from epididymitis, tuberculosis, trauma, mumps, and occasionally tumors. Aspiration is contraindicated if tumor is suspected. A *communicating hydrocele* is present in a patient with a patent processus vaginalis. In this situation, the scrotal mass fills and empties with varying positions and, in small children, with crying.

Spermatocele. This is a cyst of an efferent ductule of the rete testis. It originates at the head of the epididymis and presents as a transilluminable cystic mass discrete from the testis. Spermatoceles are often bilateral and may be multiple. They are of no consequence except when they reach large proportions or become symptomatic with pain or heaviness. Simple cysts of the epididymis also may occur.

Testicular Tumor. A palpable nodule within the testis represents a malignant tumor until proven otherwise. The lesion is usually firm and nontender and is not transilluminable. It is often first noted by the patient or on a routine examination of this area. Ultrasonography of the scrotum may help in defining the size and location of the lesion. Prompt surgical exploration through an inguinal incision is indicated. One cannot stress enough the importance of being able to detect small lesions of the testis by careful palpation and the significance and urgency of proper management.

Mumps Orchitis. The lesion usually occurs in postpubertal males with acute parotitis. It commonly becomes apparent as the parotitis subsides, 7 to 10 days following the onset of the illness. Patients experience high fever, malaise, and marked testicular swelling. Orchitis can be caused by other viruses as well.

Torsion of the Testis Appendages. *Torsion of the testis* generally refers to torsion of the spermatic cord with a characteristic rotation of the testis (Fig. 38-6) and often an anterior presentation of the epididymis. The patient presents with sudden onset of pain accompanied by scrotal enlargement and edema. The testis, which appears to be elevated because the cord is shortened by twisting, is exquisitely tender. The differential diagnosis between acute epididymitis and torsion of the testis may be difficult. Isotopic scanning of the testes or Doppler ultrasonography may disclose the characteristic ischemia of the involved testis, but false-negative studies are problematic. Because prompt treatment is important to save the testis from infarction, immediate exploration is appropriate, knowing that the intraoperative diagnosis of acute epididymitis may be necessary on occasion to prevent loss of the testis in patients with torsion. Approximately 4 h of torsion appears to be the limit after which the testis is irreversibly damaged. Because of the high incidence of bilateral anatomic predisposition to torsion, bilateral orchidopexy should be performed when surgical treatment for unilateral torsion is undertaken.

Torsion of the testis can occur when there is a long mesorchium connecting it to the epididymis. In such a case, the testis, which is likened to a clapper in a bell, can twist inside the tunica vaginalis and undergo infarction. In this circumstance, the epididymis may lie in its normal position, and the testis, which is enlarged, tender, and hard, is not drawn up high in the scrotum. Another condition of torsion involves the appendix testis. This normally present embryologic remnant lies at the upper pole of

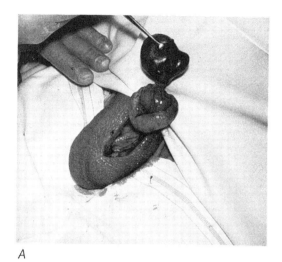

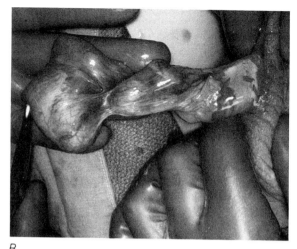

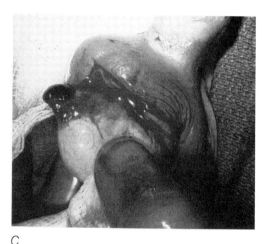

FIG. 38-6. *Types of torsion in infancy and childhood. A. Intravaginal torsion. Note need to open tunica vaginalis to demonstrate torsion. B. Extravaginal torsion. The cord is actually twisted. C. Torsion of the hydatid of Morgagni (appendix testis).*

the testis. When it undergoes torsion, the patient presents with a painful lump on the surface of the upper pole of the testis. Transillumination before major swelling occurs may reveal a characteristic "black dot" sign, which is visualization of the infarcted appendage. Since testicular tumors are rarely tender, they are not likely to be confused with torsion of the appendix testis.

Digital Rectal Examination (DRE). The *prostate gland* can be evaluated best after the patient has emptied his bladder, and it is preferable for the patient to be bending forward over the examining table or bed during the examination. If the patient is unable to stand, he should be examined while lying on his side with knees flexed and facing the standing examiner. If the examiner is right-handed, the patient should lie on his right side. Rectal examination should be carried out carefully, with very little pressure exerted while passing the finger through the anus and while the examining finger is on the prostate gland. Exertion of pressure in this area may produce considerable discomfort and limit the examination. The normal prostate is about 2.5 to 3 cm wide with a 0.5-cm-deep sulcus between the two lobes. It is about 3 to 4 cm from apex to base. Rectal examination is inadequate to define the precise size of the gland; a more accurate estimate by ultrasonography is not routinely warranted.

The consistency of both the normal prostate and the prostate with benign hyperplasia is firm but not hard. Carcinoma of the prostate feels hard, indurated, or nodular. Crepitations are related to multiple prostatic calculi. With benign hyperplasia, the gland can be delineated from surrounding tissues, and the contours are smooth. With advanced carcinoma of the prostate, the surrounding tissues are frequently fixed to the gland, thus eliminating the usual discreteness of the prostatic contour. Extensions of the tumor may proceed into the seminal vesicle area superior and lateral to the prostate. Because 90 percent of carcinomas arise in the posterior portion of the gland, many are readily detectable on rectal examination as induration or a nodular mass. Many men with small prostate cancers have a normal DRE. Acute suppuration of the prostate is accompanied by tenderness or fluctuation and requires an atraumatic examination to avoid dissemination of the infection.

Female Urethra. Pelvic examination of the female patient in the lithotomy position is essential for evaluation of the lower urinary tract. Careful visualization of the urethral meatus can be carried out in this position. The presence of a cystocele or urethrocele can be determined with the patient bearing down and, during examination, with the patient standing. A urethral diverticulum may be detected by gentle pressure against the anterior vaginal wall, milking the urethra from the bladder to the meatus. Pressure in this region against the symphysis may result in release of purulent material or urine from a diverticulum of the urethra.

Urinalysis

A carefully obtained, clean-voided midstream specimen from men and women is usually adequate. A midstream specimen from the circumcised male, without prior cleansing of the penis, is usually satisfactory for culture and microscopic examination. Occasionally, catheterization of the female patient is required to obtain an uncontaminated specimen. The specimen should be examined while fresh, since refrigeration leads to sedimentation of phosphates and storage in a warm environment results in deterioration of formed elements and growth of bacteria.

A clear urine is usually normal. A cloudy urine may be normal if a few drops of dilute acetic acid render it clear, as in phosphaturia. The color may indicate disease, ingestion of certain foods, or administration of medications. Pyridium results in an orange-red color. Methylene blue incorporated in urinary medications leads to varying shades of green and blue. Pink urine may be due to beets or food dyes or to medications such as selenium. Various degrees of bluish gray and brown may be associated with acute porphyria, and bile is readily discernible. The degree and origin of bleeding often can be best estimated by examination of the gross urine specimen.

The odor is often characteristic. A mousy odor that accompanies infection is related to formation of ammonia. A pungent odor is characteristic of necrotic bladder tumors or calculous pyonephrosis. Certain medications, such as ampicillin, have a characteristic and readily identifiable odor in the urine.

Screening examination routinely includes testing for the presence of blood, albumin, glucose, and acetone and determining pH. Because there are no proteins in the secretions of the male genital organs, albuminuria cannot be ascribed to them. The various "dipstick" tests are usually quite reliable and sensitive.

Casts, crystals, and clumps of epithelial cells are identified under low-power microscopic examination, whereas the nature of cells, crystals, and bacteria is determined under higher powers. Following centrifugation, staining with methylene blue facilitates the diagnosis of bacteriuria. Cytologic examination of urine for exfoliated cells may be helpful and may demonstrate clusters of cells with nucleocytoplasmic disparity characteristic of malignancy. Flow cytometry may add additional information regarding possible neoplastic changes. The identification of bacteria in an unspun urine specimen is strongly suggestive of the presence of a urinary tract infection rather than contamination and usually represents more than 100,000 bacteria per milliliter.

Genital Secretions

Urethral Discharge. Collection is accomplished on a glass slide before the patient urinates. Noninfected urethral and prostatic secretions are usually whitish and opalescent; infected secretion is usually yellow and purulent. A heat-fixed and Gram-stained specimen identifies organisms. Gonococcal urethritis is diagnosed by the presence of gram-negative intracellular diplococci. Examination of the wet specimen is helpful in identifying trichomonads. Confirmation of infection is established by adequate culture of the urethral discharge.

Expressed Prostatic Secretions (EPS). The specimen is obtained by gentle massage of the gland and is indicated if symptoms suggest prostatic inflammation. The acutely inflamed prostate should not be massaged. Examination of the normally opalescent fluid reveals a few white blood cells per high-powered field and tiny refractile cephalin bodies. Epithelial cells are present in small numbers. Seminal vesicle secretion presents as a gelatinous and fibrinous tree-shaped cast of the seminal vesicle containing strands and granules. In the presence of prostatic inflammation, the secretions become granular, and many white blood cells (710 per high-powered field) and large clumps are readily seen. A urine culture after prostate examination is required to determine if the inflammation is due to bacterial prostatitis.

Semen Analysis. For purposes of standardization, the specimen should be obtained by masturbation and collected in a dry container after 48 h of sexual abstinence. Examination, performed less than 1 h after ejaculation, normally reveals a volume of 3 to 5 mL with liquefaction complete within 1 h. There should be over 20 million spermatozoa per milliliter with at least 60 percent demonstrating motility and 60 percent appearing morphologically normal. More sophisticated studies of semen may be performed when indicated for the study of infertility.

Endoscopy

Cystourethroscopy. This investigative procedure should be performed in most patients with gross or microscopic hematuria and in selected patients with symptoms of lower urinary tract obstruction or infection. It often can be performed as an office procedure. Flexible and rigid instruments are available. Instillation of a local anesthetic agent into the urethra makes the procedure tolerable. The smallest-caliber instrument that will provide adequate visualization of the bladder and urethra is used. The presence of very small tumors of the bladder can be detected readily, as well as small calculi, the configuration and location of the ureteral orifices, prostate size, urethral strictures or valves, and other pathologic conditions that may be present in the bladder or the urethra.

Ureteropyeloscopy. The ureteral orifice can be dilated, and under direct vision, the full length of the ureter and much of the renal pelvis and calyceal system can be visualized with special instruments. Stones can be manipulated and fragmented with ultrasonic or electrohydraulic probes or with laser, and lesions can be biopsied and treated. This is performed under anesthesia.

Therapeutic Catheterization. An indwelling catheter affords temporary relief of obstruction. Because maintenance for more than 3 days is usually attended by bacteriuria, external collection, such as condom drainage, is more appropriate to improve nursing care of the incontinent patient who has no obstruction. Relative contraindications to urethral instrumentation include acute cystitis, urethritis, prostatitis, and a coagulopathy. In these instances, it is best to pretreat the patient for the infection or bleeding disorder. An exception to the rule is that if obstruction is the predisposing cause of infection, e.g., BPH with retention, immediate drainage by catheterization. Temporary drainage during the acute infection stage may be carried out by suprapubic tap and the insertion of a small polyethylene or plastic tube connected to constant drainage. Therapeutic instrumentation may be applied in the endoscopic removal of calculi or foreign bodies; biopsy or excision of tumors, cysts, or other obstructive lesions; drainage of prostatic abscesses; dilation or incision of urethral strictures or valves; and transurethral removal of prostatic obstruction. Institution of catheter drainage may represent the most important therapeutic measure in obstructions secondary to prostatic hypertrophy or impacted ureteral calculus. Endoscopic insertion of a ureteral stent to bypass an obstructing ureteral stone with concomitant infection can be a lifesaving maneuver.

Catheterization should be performed with aseptic technique and minimal trauma. For routine catheterization in adults, a #16 French or #18 French urethral catheter is the easiest to pass and the least traumatic. Traumatic catheterization may lead to bleeding and urethral strictures. After traumatic catheterization, closed-system drainage should be instituted and efforts made to improve urine output.

Percutaneous Nephrostomy.

This procedure is carried out under local anesthesia as a diagnostic or therapeutic measure. It is used most often to relieve obstruction of the kidney secondary to stone or tumor. In the case of extensive pelvic malignancy (rectal, prostate, etc.), percutaneous nephrostomy may reverse renal failure caused by ureteral obstruction. Stones, pelvocalyceal lesions, and congenital ureteropelvic obstruction can be treated under general anesthesia in an antegrade fashion. An indwelling catheter can be left in place if the obstruction is not relieved.

Imaging Studies

Excretory Urography.

Certain intravenously administered organic substances are filtered and excreted by the kidney. When rendered opaque by iodinization, they opacify the renal parenchyma and collecting system. These agents are potent nephrotoxins and should be used with caution in patients with compromised renal function. It is important to hydrate patients by encouraging fluid intake following examination. Occasionally, the study is followed by anuria and renal failure in elderly, dehydrated, debilitated patients who have evidence of renal dysfunction. The use of other imaging studies is advised for this patient population. Nonionic contrast agents decrease the risk of an allergic reaction, but they are significantly more expensive.

Excretory urography provides excellent visualization of the kidneys (see Fig. 38-2), ureters, and bladder. It is an excellent initial imaging study in patients with hematuria or suspected stone.

The adult male kidney averages 13×6.2 cm on pyelography. The left kidney is usually a few millimeters longer and broader. The kidneys of females are approximately 5 mm smaller in both dimensions. The upper pole of the left kidney lies at mid T12, whereas the right kidney is a half vertebral body lower. In the upright position, the kidney descends one vertebral body. If lines are drawn through the uppermost and lowermost calyces of the two kidneys, they should parallel the lateral margins of the psoas muscles (Fig. 38-7). Any deviation from this axis suggests the presence of a pathologic condition or a variant of normal. The calyces should be adequate in number and delicately cupped. The infundibula are straight and fine. The pelvis points medially and describes a smooth curve without redundancy or tortuosity. There may be several areas of incomplete ureteral visualization due to peristalsis. The diameter of the ureter usually does not exceed 4 to 5 mm. Late upright films should demonstrate emp-

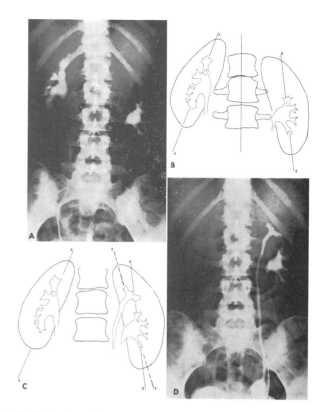

FIG. 38-7. *A and B. Excretory urogram showing complete left ureteral duplicartion and nonvisualizing upper segment. Axis of the left calyceal system (BB) is abnormal. C and D. Left retrograde pyelogram demonstrating the upper segment. Note correct axis of the right kidney (AA) and the corrected axis of the duplicated left pelvocalyceal systems.*

tying of the collecting system and visualization of the urinary bladder. On supine films the contrast material may pool in the fundus of the bladder and lead to the erroneous interpretation of an outlet filling defect. A postvoiding film is helpful in revealing the lower ureter and indicating the amount of residual urine.

Nephrotomography.

More detailed and accurate visualization of the kidney and pelvocalyceal system is available by this excretory urographic technique. Several "slices" of the kidneys are obtained, beginning posteriorly and advancing anteriorly. This eliminates the overlying gas and fecal material in the bowel. Lucent areas such as fat and cysts are more readily identifiable. The poorly prepared patient may be evaluated more satisfactorily than with the standard excretory urography.

Retrograde Pyeloureterography.

This study may be performed during cystoscopy by catheterization of the ureters and is indicated to further evaluate lesions of the pelvocalyceal system and ureter. "Filling defects" of these structures may not be evaluated adequately by excretory urography. Urine may be collected from the kidney for cytologic study and also to determine differential renal function. Instillation of a contrast medium provides a more detailed visualization of these structures and is best done under fluoroscopic control. Improved techniques of excretory urography and nephrotomography have significantly decreased the need for retrograde pyeloureterography. But patients who manifest allergic response to intravenous contrast materials and patients with nonvisualizing or nonfunctioning kidneys can still be evaluated by this method.

Cystourethrography. The bladder and urethra may be evaluated by antegrade or retrograde studies. Fluoroscopic examination of the patient voiding may reveal the dynamics of micturition and evidence of obstruction or reflux of urine. Voiding cystourethrography is a useful diagnostic tool in the evaluation of children with voiding problems or recurrent urinary tract infections to rule out vesicoureteral reflux or urethral obstruction. Isotopic cystograms may be employed for the evaluation of reflux in children and offer decreased radiation exposure.

Antegrade Pyelography. Percutaneous insertion of a small catheter into the pelvocalyceal system may be a valuable diagnostic and therapeutic tool. The procedure is performed under local anesthesia and with fluoroscopic or ultrasonic control. Once the small tube is placed properly within the drainage structures of the kidney, adequate drainage of an obstructed, infected pyohydronephrosis may be instituted, and adequate x-ray visualization of the upper urinary tract may be obtained. Occasionally, a ureter cannot be catheterized from below and may have to be visualized by this technique. It is an extremely valuable technique to use in the seriously ill, toxic patient. Adequate drainage may convert the situation from a surgical emergency to a relatively simple elective procedure in a nontoxic patient. Stone manipulations and ureteral dilations also may be carried out. The percutaneous tract can be dilated, and an instrument can be passed into the kidney, allowing for direct-vision stone fragmentation (nephrostolithotripsy).

Renal Arteriography. Percutaneous transfemoral renal arteriography is useful in the evaluation of possible renal vascular hypertension, and therapeutic dilatation of narrow arteries can be performed (angioplasty). The technique also can demonstrate vascular lesions and thus define the surgical approach. With congenital anomalies of the kidney, arteriography is also helpful, since vascular anomalies frequently coexist and have an important bearing on surgical treatment. Arteriography is also applied to the differential diagnosis of renal masses; a characteristic neovasculature and pooling of opaque material are noted in tumor vessels within the parenchyma, diagnostic for a hypernephroma (Fig. 38-8). Therapeutic infarction of kidneys also may be carried out by this approach.

Digital Subtraction Angiography. This technique provides a means of visualizing the arterial supply of the kidneys on an outpatient basis, with decreased morbidity as compared with standard renal arteriography. A bolus of contrast material is injected intravenously instead of intraarterially, and a computerized subtraction system provides clear visualization of the renal arteries and their branches, as well as of the aorta and other abdominal visceral arteries. Renovascular pathology, such as stenosis or anomalies, can be seen, as well as the presence of multiple renal arteries, which might preclude use of a kidney for donor transplantation.

Vena Cavography. Percutaneous catheterization of the femoral vein with instillation of contrast material provides ade-

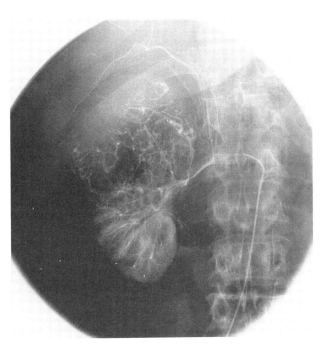

FIG. 38-8. Selective renal arteriography showing large upper pole tumor with pooling ("puddling") of contrast material in the tumor area.

quate visualization of the inferior vena cava. This study is helpful in evaluating patients with carcinoma of the kidney, although it has largely been replaced by magnetic resonance imaging (MRI). Intrinsic involvement and obstruction of the vena cava and renal veins may be present with carcinoma of the kidney. Preoperative evaluation with this study may help determine the most suitable type of surgical procedure.

Renography and Renal Perfusion Scan. A number of isotopes, most of which are gamma emitters, provide an isotopic evaluation of the function and drainage of each kidney. Dehydration, sodium depletion, and tubular blocking agents may alter the curves, and technical factors such as placement of detectors, dose of isotope, and paravenous injection may complicate interpretation. When properly performed, the renogram can be helpful in recognizing nonfunction or reduced function and delayed excretion seen with obstruction. A furosemide (Lasix) challenge may demonstrate delayed "washout" indicative of obstruction. After renal arterial surgical procedures or homotransplantation, renography provides a simple and dependable method of evaluating the vascular status of the organ. Illustrative curves are shown in Fig. 38-9. The use of properly selected isotopes may provide more information about renal perfusion, drainage, morphology, and differential renal function.

Ultrasonography. Improved technology and experience in interpretation have increased the accuracy and applicability of this noninvasive diagnostic modality. The differential diagnosis of renal and scrotal masses has been made easier with ultrasonography. Cystic renal lesions may be readily distinguished from solid tumors. The technique also has provided a means of accurately guiding needles into lesions for biopsy or fluid aspiration. Renal cysts may be punctured and aspirated percutaneously

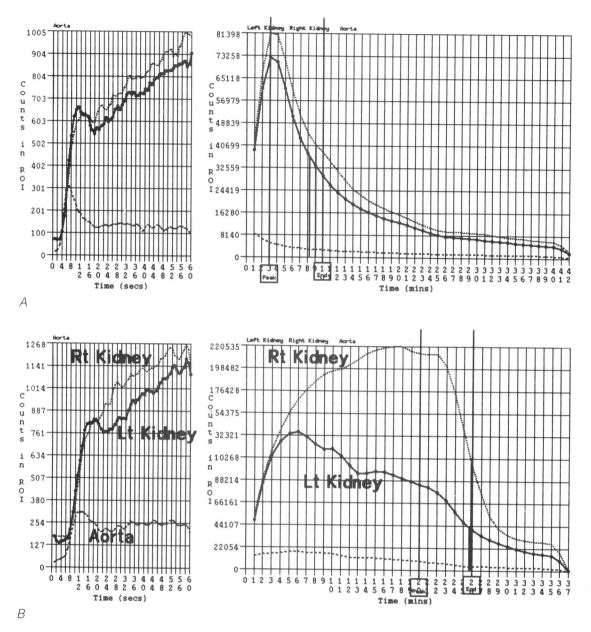

FIG. 38-9. ^{99m}Tc-DTPA Lasix washout renograms. *A. Normal vascular perfusion and normal drainage from both kidneys. B. Left kidney shows continued accumulation of radionuclide until the administration of Lasix, after which the radionuclide washes out normally, indicating absence of obstruction. C. Radionuclide accumulates in left collecting system despite the administration of Lasix, indicating obstruction. D. Right kidney shows reduced perfusion compared with the left kidney and aorta, indicating reduced function.*

and contrast material instilled into the cystic cavity under ultrasonic control for diagnosis and therapy. The noninvasive character of the procedure and the lack of radiation exposure and intravenous injection of contrast material make it a useful outpatient screening test. This is especially important in children, in pregnant women, and in those with compromised renal function. Obstructive uropathy can be ruled out when contrast excretory urography is contraindicated or is not feasible. Transrectal ultrasonography provides a means of early detection and staging of prostatic carcinoma (Fig. 38-10). Biopsies of the pros-

tate can be obtained with ultrasound guidance as an outpatient procedure without an anesthetic.

Computed Tomography (CT). This is one of the most useful and accurate means of evaluating intraabdominal pathology, and it has significantly enhanced evaluation of patients with renal, ureteral, bladder, prostate, and testicular lesions. In some instances it has replaced other modalities such as renal cyst aspirations, angiography, and lymphangiography as a means of diagnosing and staging disease as well as of following patients

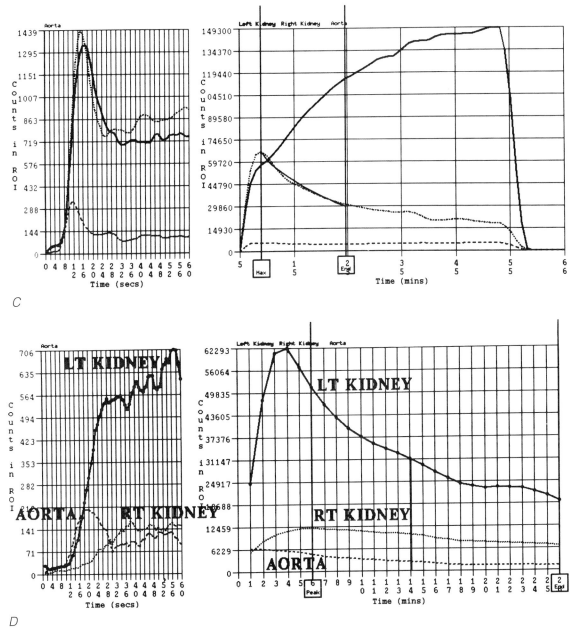

FIG. 38-9. *C, D* Continued.

after a diagnosis has been established and therapy instituted. It is performed with and without contrast material, and lesions of the kidneys can be readily identified as to size, location, extent, and density. Therefore, cystic lesions can be differentiated from solid lesions. Nonopaque filling defects of the urinary tract can be separated readily into stones or soft tissue lesions. Tumor extension, lymph node involvement, and metastases to other organs in the abdomen, chest, and brain can be demonstrated by CT scans.

Magnetic Resonance Imaging (MRI). This imaging study, which requires no ionizing radiation, is applied with increasing frequency for the diagnosis of urologic pathology. The use of contrast agents and MR angiography have increased the diagnostic yield.

Urodynamic Tests: Pressure-Flow, Uroflow, Cystometrics, Urethral Pressure Profiles, and Sphincter Electromyography. These studies are useful diagnostic tools for the evaluation of some patients with micturition dysfunction, including problems from obstruction, neurologic disease, functional disturbances, and dyssynergia. These tests are most commonly indicated to evaluate lower urinary tract symptoms (LUTS) when initial evaluation fails to establish a clear diagnosis.

Biochemical Tests and Radioimmunoassays. Evaluation of renal function, hypertension, electrolyte disturbances, calculous disease, impotence, and neoplasms of the genitourinary tract requires studies involving the use of the biochemistry and radioimmunoassay (RIA) laboratories. Examples include

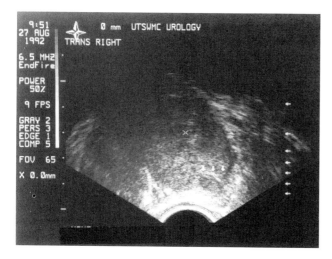

FIG. 38-10. *Transrectal ultrasound. A transverse section of the prostate shows a relatively hypoechoic area that may be indicative of carcinoma and should be biopsied (see arrows).*

blood urea nitrogen, creatinine, creatinine clearance, renin, electrolyte, calcium, phosphorus, serum testosterone, acid and alkaline phosphatase, prostate-specific antigen (PSA), beta subunit of human chorionic gonadotropin, α-fetoprotein, and parathormone determinations.

BLADDER FUNCTION AND DISORDERS

Anatomy and Physiology. Normal micturition requires two simple functions: storage and evacuation of urine. The lower urinary tract includes the bladder, bladder neck, proximal urethra, and external urethral striated sphincter. Smooth muscle in the bladder wall relaxes with filling and accommodates large volumes of urine at low intravesical pressures. The bladder neck and proximal urethra remain closed during urine storage by a combination of mechanisms. First, alpha receptors on bladder neck smooth muscle cells are activated by the sympathetic nervous system, and an increase in muscular tone helps maintain a closed outlet. Second, the proximal urethra shares excursions in intraabdominal pressure exerted on the bladder to avoid an intraluminal pressure difference between the bladder and the urethra. Hypermobility or descent of the bladder neck and base out of a retropubic position can lead to stress urinary incontinence. Third, an increase in external urethral sphincter muscle contraction occurs with transmitted abdominal pressure to the bladder (the guarding reflex) and closes the distal urethra. Normal micturition requires coordination between the bladder and outlet structures whereby a bladder contraction and drop in outlet resistance occur in rapid sequence. The storage and evacuation of urine are regulated by the nervous system.

Smooth muscle cells in the bladder are innervated by short postganglionic axons from ganglia located in the adventitia of the bladder. This short axon system receives afferent input from the pelvic plexus. The pelvic plexus integrates sympathetic and parasympathetic outflow via the hypogastric and pelvic nerves, respectively; these are mixed sensory and motor nerves. The pudendal nerve innervates the external urethral striated sphincter and provides sensory pathways from the penis. Motor pathways to the bladder (pelvic nerve) and external urethral sphincter (pu-

dendal nerve) originate in the S2 to S4 segments of the sacral spinal cord. Sympathetic fibers in the hypogastric nerve arise from T9 to L2 spinal cord segments. The sensations of bladder filling, distention, and pain are mediated by the hypogastric and pelvic nerves. Ascending and descending pathways converge on the dorsal and ventral horns of the spinal cord to regulate the sensory and motor function of the lower urinary tract. Neurons in the pontine reticular formation receive sensory input with bladder filling and coordinate bladder contraction with concomitant lowering of outlet resistance at the bladder neck and external striated urethral sphincter.

Diagnostic Studies. Cystometry and urodynamic testing are used to evaluate abnormalities of urine storage and evacuation. Cystometry is the recording of bladder pressure with filling (gas or water) at a constant infusion rate. Bladder sensation and smooth muscle activity during filling, capacity, and compliance are derived from the cystometrogram (CMG). The CMG is a storage study only and does not provide data on the ability of the bladder to completely evacuate urine. The normal CMG demonstrates an adult bladder capacity of 400 to 600 mL, filling pressure below 15 cmH$_2$O, and the first sensation of bladder filling at one-third bladder capacity. A strong continuous bladder contraction with reflex neurally mediated relaxation of the bladder neck, proximal urethra, and external urethral sphincter characterizes normal micturition. Urodynamic testing with multiple pressure recordings, urinary flow rate, and electromyographic recording from the external urethral sphincter may be needed to diagnose complex voiding dysfunction.

Neurogenic Bladder Dysfunction

The neurologic level of a lesion disrupting the nerve supply to the lower urinary tract can assist in the diagnosis of neurogenic bladder dysfunction.

Sacral and Infrasacral Disorders. Lesions of the conus medullaris, cauda equina, or pelvic nerves related to trauma, congenital lesions, or neoplasia can disrupt sensory and motor innervation of the bladder and external urethral sphincter (Fig. 38-11). Occult or overt myelodysplasia represents the most common congenital lesion. Sacral agenesis, partial or total, and other anomalies in the caudal regression syndrome often are associated with neurogenic bladder dysfunction. Operation for imperforate anus can damage the pelvic plexus. Most patients suffer from recurrent urinary tract infection and overflow incontinence.

Children with spina bifida usually present with an areflexic bladder and open (fixed) bladder neck. If the meningocele or myelomeningocele has damaged the pathways from the pontine reticular formation, one might see detrusor sphincter dyssynergia, with the potential danger of renal compromise from high lower-urinary-tract pressure (Fig. 38-12). No correlation exists between the neurogenic bladder dysfunction and the level of the vertebral defect. Therefore, urodynamic testing in children with myelodysplasia plays a pivotal role in diagnosis and treatment selection.

Voiding dysfunction following radical pelvic surgery (e.g., abdominoperineal resection, proctocolectomy, radical hysterectomy, low anterior resection) is common and usually results from direct injury to the innervation of the lower urinary tract. Most patients recover function within 4 to 6 months, and conservative management is warranted. Urodynamic testing reveals a smooth,

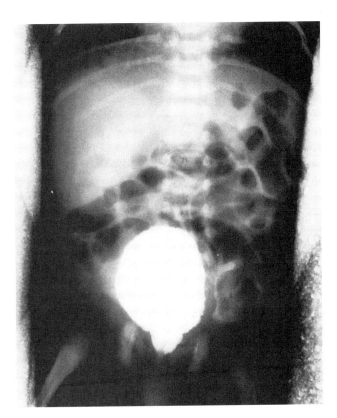

FIG. 38-11. Neurogenic bladder. The normal bladder neck is competent, and the proximal urethra is not normally visualized on a static cystogram. The presence of a trabeculated bladder and a dilated proximal urethra, as seen here, is suggestive of a neurogenic bladder.

large-capacity bladder with no reflex activity. Intermittent self-catheterization at periodic intervals should be instituted early to prevent bladder overdistention, recurrent infection, and overflow incontinence. Long-term antimicrobial therapy is not recommended because of the potential development of resistant organisms. The goals of treatment are preservation of renal function and establishment of urinary continence.

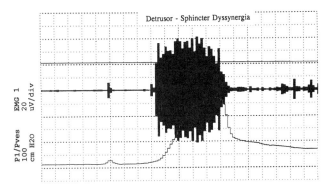

FIG. 38-12. Bladder urethral sphincter dyssynergia. Note hyperactivity of sphincter (large black area) during the time of voiding. In this scenario, the bladder must overcome the increased outlet resistance by raising the pressure in the urinary tract, ultimately resulting in hydroureteronephrosis, reduced renal function, and a small-capacity, high-pressure bladder.

Sensory disorders of bladder innervation may cause the loss of sensation to bladder filling. Tabes dorsalis, posterior spinal cord degeneration, herpetic infection, or diabetes mellitus often leads to chronic overdistention of the bladder and high postvoiding residual urine volumes. Intermittent self-catheterization at periodic intervals is the treatment of choice in these patients.

Suprasacral Spinal Disorders. Spinal cord trauma, vascular compromise, and multiple sclerosis are the most common causes of suprasacral disorders. Spinal cord injury from penetrating trauma or a motor vehicle accident is characterized by an early period of spinal shock and bladder areflexia. A short period of indwelling bladder catheterization is appropriate until the patient is stable. As soon as possible, intermittent catheterization should be started and anticholinergic medication added when bladder function returns. The long-term use of a Foley catheter or suprapubic tube should be avoided because they often lead to chronic resistant infection, urethral erosion, fistula formation, stones, and loss of the bladder as a urinary reservoir.

After the period of spinal shock, most patients develop detrusor-sphincter dyssynergia and are at risk for loss of renal function. Intermittent catheterization, anticholinergic medication, and transurethral sphincterotomy (resection of the external sphincter) with condom catheter drainage have been the mainstays of bladder management in spinal cord injury. With time, the bladder may lose compliance and capacity, thereby placing the kidneys at risk despite frequent catheterization. Augmentation cystoplasty may be used to increase bladder capacity, restore urinary continence, and reduce high intravesical pressures.

Autonomic dysreflexia is a serious medical condition that must be recognized and treated promptly in the spinal cord injury patient. Patients with injuries at T6 or higher are at risk for this autonomic reflex, usually triggered by visceral distention. Elevated blood pressure, sweating, pounding headache, and bradycardia occur with visceral autonomic nervous system activation (bladder distention, fecal impaction, bowel obstruction). Immediate treatment includes relief of the obstruction and the use of alpha-adrenergic blocking agents such as prazosin, terazosin, or nifedipine.

Neurogenic bladder dysfunction is common in patients with multiple sclerosis. This diffuse demyelinating disorder can present with a variety of voiding problems due to the haphazard location of the plaques in the white matter of the spinal cord. Urgency and urgency incontinence are common symptoms. Many patients with multiple sclerosis have detrusor-sphincter dyssynergia with residual urine and must be treated with intermittent catheterization and drugs. Because the disease is characterized by periods of exacerbation and remission, conservative management should be followed along with periodic urodynamic testing.

Supraspinal or Suprapontine Disorders. Coordinated bladder contraction and urethral relaxation are directed by the pontine "micturition center" in the brainstem. Neurologic lesions above the pons usually leave the "micturition reflex" intact. When the lesion affects voiding, it generally results in a loss of voluntary control over urination. Cerebrovascular accident, normal-pressure hydrocephalus, tumor, dementia, and Parkinson's disease represent suprapontine lesions. Urinary incontinence from bladder hyperreflexia presents with complaints of urgency and frequency. Since the lesions are above the pons, detrusor-sphincter dyssynergia does not develop, and renal impairment occurs only when chronic indwelling catheterization is used to manage the urinary incontinence. These patients have lost the ability to inhibit the micturition reflex and are managed best with drugs to inhibit bladder hyperreflexia and timed voiding to keep the bladder empty. Cystometry may show uninhibited bladder contractions at low volumes, which characterize the hyperreflexia seen with suprapontine lesions.

Bladder Rehabilitation. The level and degree (partial versus complete) of a neurologic lesion will determine the pattern of voiding dysfunction and provide prognostic information. Central nervous system structures do not regain function, and complete lesions, after a period of spinal shock, become fixed neurogenic bladder disorders. Maintenance of renal function is the primary goal of management. Intermittent catheterization should be used whenever possible so that the reservoir function of the bladder can remain intact and be augmented if bladder compliance deteriorates. Supravesical urinary diversion is indicated in rare instances, and often a continent pouch or catheter-free diversion can be constructed utilizing segments of bowel. Reconstructive lower urinary tract surgery for neurogenic bladder dysfunction should be done only when a fixed and stable deficit is encountered with the potential loss of renal function or debilitating urinary incontinence.

INFECTIONS

Acute Infections

Pathogenesis. The most common port of entry for urinary tract infection (UTI) is the urethra. Ninety-six percent of pediatric UTIs occur in girls because of the shortness of the urethra. Similarly, in the adult, most UTIs develop in women as a consequence of the short urethra and the superimposed factors of pathogenic organisms, vaginal cell-bacterial adherence, and sexual intercourse. The normal bladder possesses defense mechanisms capable of coping with introduced bacteria. Complete emptying so that no residual urine remains is an additional defense factor. In the obstructed, inflamed, or ulcerated organ, the defense mechanisms are compromised.

Ascending infection is potentiated by any obstructive process, including obstructive uropathy secondary to prostatic hyperplasia, foreign bodies, or bladder tumors. Reflux of infected urine from the bladder can lead to contamination of the ducts of Bellini and to the development of pyelonephritis, predominantly involving the medullary portion of the kidney.

UTIs occasionally are secondary to distant infections such as cutaneous abscesses that undergo hematogenous spread. Hydronephrosis and renal calculi potentiate the risk of hematogenous infection. UTIs rarely are caused by spread from contiguous intestinal infections such as appendicitis, diverticulitis, and regional enteritis.

Bacteriology. The most commonly implicated organism is *Escherichia coli*. Other organisms include enterococci, *Staphylococcus aureus* and *Streptococcus epidermidis*, *Proteus mirabilis*, *Klebsiella*, and *Pseudomonas*. Because most forms of *Proteus* split urea, resulting in an alkaline urine and precipitation of calcium, infections caused by these organisms are often associated with calculi.

Clinical Manifestations. Acute *cystitis* presents with frequency, urgency, and dysuria, with minimal systemic symptoms.

The fever, if present, is usually low grade. By contrast, *pyelonephritis* is usually accompanied by chills, temperatures of 39°C, nausea, and flank pain. The diagnosis of a UTI is established by microscopic analysis of the urine demonstrating bacteria and white blood cells and by culture of the urine to establish the specific pathogens and the sensitivity to antibiotics.

Treatment. The ability to treat UTIs with drugs is enhanced by the unique ability of normally functioning kidneys to concentrate a variety of antibacterial agents in the urine. Drug selection is facilitated by culture and determination of sensitivities, but because these are usually not available in the early stages of treatment, initially the drug is prescribed empirically based on the probable pathogen. Further considerations include the age and general health of the patient, kidney function, history of allergy, previous drug therapy, relative cost of therapy, and possible complications of the drug to be administered.

Drugs that are rapidly excreted by the kidney in high concentrations are ideally suited for the treatment of *uncomplicated lower UTIs*, such as acute cystitis. Most acute UTIs infections are caused by *E. coli* and will respond rapidly to drugs that are usually administered for a period of 7 days or less. Short courses, consisting of single-dose treatment or 1 to 3 days of therapy, also have proved to be efficacious. Some drugs commonly used for the treatment of uncomplicated UTIs are sulfonamides, ampicillin, cephalexin, nitrofurantoin, nalidixic acid, trimethoprim-sulfamethoxazole, and quinolones (e.g., floxacin).

In the patient with manifestations of *acute pyelonephritis* or *sepsis*, drugs that produce high blood and tissue levels are indicated, and drugs that yield only high urinary concentrations are not adequate. Parenteral therapy may be required, and a more prolonged course of other therapy is indicated. When a *Pseudomonas* infection is suspected, the aminoglycosides such as gentamicin, tobramycin, or amikacin may be used. Combination with ampicillin or a cephalosporin provides a broad initial coverage until culture and sensitivity reports are available, at which time specific treatment can be instituted. For less severe "cases," oral quinolones may be sufficient.

The acute infection is sometimes secondary to an anatomic factor (e.g., obstruction or stone) that may require correction to prevent recurrences. Although it is justifiable and essential to treat acutely ill patients before a causative diagnosis is made, a more complete investigation should be carried out as soon as possible. This is especially indicated in patients with complicated UTIs, such as acute pyelonephritis and sepsis. Uncomplicated cystitis in the adult female may require no further evaluation, since the excretory urogram and cystoscopic findings are usually unremarkable in such patients. The male with a single UTI requires evaluation to rule out obstruction, stone disease, or tumor because ascending infection from the urethra is not common except as related to prostatitis in the adult.

The patient who has had a UTI is at increased risk for recurrences, and repeat urinalysis and possibly cultures are indicated in follow-up. Examination of a midstream urine specimen from the male or a clean-catch urine specimen from the female should be performed before or shortly after discontinuing antibiotic therapy. If recurrences occur in the absence of any correctable anatomic abnormality, such as in cystitis in the adult female, long-term, low-dose, suppressive therapy may be required. Drugs suitable for long-term therapy include nitrofurantoin and trimethoprim-sulfamethoxazole. The length of therapy usually is a minimum of 3 months.

Gram-Negative Bacteremia. The urinary tract is a common source of sepsis. Frequently, the bacteremia follows instrumentation in the presence of preexisting UTI that has been ineffectively treated. Parenteral antibiotics should be administered as a prophylactic measure before urethral instrumentation in patients who have had an indwelling catheter for a prolonged period of time.

The patients experience a shaking chill followed by high fever, peripheral vasodilation, and hypotension. The organisms responsible are frequently resistant to the usual drugs and require large doses of parenterally administered antibacterial agents. Bactericidal drugs are preferable to prevent liberation of additional quantities of the endotoxin by the multiplying bacteria. An aminoglycoside, such as gentamicin, tobramycin, or amikacin, and ampicillin, or a similar drug used in combination, has proved to be quite effective for the management of gram-negative bacteremia.

Perinephric Abscess. This usually follows perforation of a renal infection or abscess into the perinephric tissues. In some instances, perinephric abscess may result from direct hematogenous spread or from microabscesses in the kidney that are not apparent. The perinephric infection may be secondary to and is often associated with a struvite renal stone or a staghorn calculus.

The patient presents with an extremely high fever and flank pain. Radiographs reveal nonvisualization of the psoas shadow and concavity of the spine to the side of the lesion. The kidney may be nonfunctioning, and a stone may be seen on the film. Gas can be seen within or outside the kidney shadow if the organism is gas-producing. *Emphysematous pyelonephritis* occurs more frequently in diabetic patients. CT scan provides the most accurate definition of the location and extent of the process.

Papillary Necrosis. Necrosis of renal papillae occurs in patients with diabetes, sickle cell disease, tuberculosis, and excessive ingestion of phenacetin or nonsteroidal anti-inflammatory drugs. In addition to the symptoms related to the associated acute infection of the kidney, renal colic may result from ureteral obstruction by the sloughed papillae. Diagnosis is made radiographically by demonstrating sloughed papillae or by the characteristic appearance of the intravenous pyelogram showing loss of one or more of the papillae (Fig. 38-13). When amputation of the papilla at the cortical-medullary junction is complete and contrast material surrounds the papilla floating free in the calyx, a "ring sign" is present. Loss of renal function may attend papillary necrosis, but recovery usually occurs, and initial measures are directed toward supporting the patient during the acute episode. Specific antibacterial treatment for the involved organism is administered. If the patient remains febrile or septic and there is ureteral obstruction, endoscopic, percutaneous, or open surgical intervention may be required to remove the obstructing soft tissue and to provide drainage.

Urethritis. Acute urethritis is usually a sexually transmitted disease (STD). Included in the acute types of urethritis are those caused by gonorrhea, *Ureaplasma urealyticum, Chlamydia,* and *Trichomonas vaginalis.* Diagnosis is established by microscopy of the gram-stained discharge and confirmed by adequate culture techniques. Reiter's syndrome, consisting of the

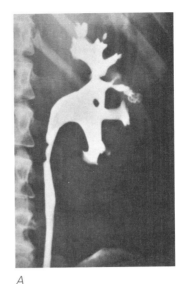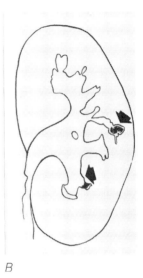

FIG. 38-13. *Renal papillary necrosis. A. Retrograde pyelogram in diabetic renal papillary necrosis. B. Necrotic papillae are indicated by arrows.*

triad of arthritis, nongonococcal urethritis, and conjunctivitis, is considered by many to be of venereal origin and should be included in the differential diagnosis.

Gonorrhea is a common STD. The incubation period is 7 to 9 days, after which the symptoms of acute urethritis are manifested. Urethral stricture is a sequela if the original infection is not adequately treated. Metastatic gonococcal infections include arthritis, tenosynovitis, bursitis, ophthalmitis, perihepatitis, and endocarditis. Gonococcal arthritis, which represents the common manifestation of metastatic involvement, is polyarticular in 80 percent of patients and accompanied by tenosynovitis in 50 percent of the cases. The diagnosis of gonococcal infection is established by demonstration of *Neisseria gonorrhea* (gram-negative diplococci) intracellularly in the urethral discharge and by culture of the organism. Because syphilis and gonorrhea are contracted by the same exposure in some cases, the latter should be excluded by serologic tests. Gonococcal urethral infections are best treated by adequate dosage of penicillin-type drugs. Resistant strains have appeared with increasing frequency; spectinomycin and other antibiotics have been effective in these cases.

Nonspecific urethritis (NSU), or nongonococcal urethritis (NGU), is the most common venereal disease in the male. This is manifest by a translucent, sticky drop on the underwear or liquid that can be milked from the urethra on a daily basis. The organisms most commonly implicated in this infection are *Chlamydia trachomatis* and *U. urealyticum,* which usually can be treated satisfactorily with the tetracyclines. Recurring infections indicate the need to treat the patient and his sexual contacts. *Trichomonas* infections of the urethra and prostate are best treated with metronidazole (Flagyl), including treatment of sexual partner(s).

Bacterial Prostatitis. Acute bacterial prostatitis is usually caused by the same organisms that produce UTIs, and frequently these organisms can be found in the urine. The bacteria may enter the prostate through the urethra and may lie dormant in the many prostatic ducts. Active infection may be precipitated by urethral trauma or instrumentation. Acute prostatitis is particularly common in young, healthy males and is also seen in men in the benign prostatic hyperplasia age range. The organisms associated with urethritis also may be the pathogens of acute prostatitis.

Initial symptoms may be mild and consist of perineal discomfort with increasing frequency, initial hematuria, dysuria, and occasional retention. With progression, the perineal pain becomes continuous and severe and is attended by chills, high fever, malaise, and prostration. The prostate is usually very tender, and examination should be gentle. Leukocytosis is characteristic, and bacteremia is common. In extreme cases, the gram-negative bacteremia may be associated with endotoxic shock. Liquefaction necrosis of the local infection results in the formation of abscesses that may rupture into the urethra spontaneously or as a result of catheterization or transurethral resection.

Culture of the urine should precede administration of antibacterial agents, but these should not be withheld until the culture reports are available. In mild cases, an oral broad-spectrum antibiotic such as a quinolone should be administered for a minimum of 10 to 14 days. Parenteral antibiotics are indicated for patients with chills, high fever, malaise, and/or hypotension. If necessary, the drug may be changed at a later date. The acutely ill patient should be at bed rest, hydrated, and treated with antibiotics until the acute phase of the process subsides. Patients with retention should be catheterized gently with a small indwelling catheter or a percutaneous suprapubic tube. Rectal examination reveals a tender and sometimes warm prostate and should be performed infrequently and gently with great care to avoid dissemination of the infection. Several days of appropriate antibacterial treatment should result in symptomatic improvement and return of temperature to normal. Persistence of symptoms and fever, coupled with a diminished size and force of the urinary stream, suggests the presence of an abscess that may require drainage. CT scan aids in localization.

A significant number of men with the symptoms of chronic prostatitis (pain, frequency, urgency) have sterile prostate fluid and no evidence of inflammation in the expressed prostatic secretions. These men are believed to have chronic pelvic pain syndrome termed *prostatodynia.*

Epididymitis. This condition is characterized by rapid progression of pain and swelling of the epididymis and is usually associated with leukocytosis, fever, malaise, and chills. A UTI often present, with symptoms of frequency, urgency, and dysuria. When this is the case, the offending pathogen can be cultured from the urine. When this is not the case, it is difficult to identify the organism. There can be an underlying prostatic infection. The differential diagnosis includes acute torsion of the spermatic cord or hydatid of Morgagni, spontaneous hemorrhage of a testicular tumor, trauma, or thrombosis of the pampiniform plexus. A radioisotopic scan of the scrotum or ultrasound examination may aid in the diagnosis.

Acute epididymitis can occur after open prostatectomy or might be related to infection secondary to long-term urethral catheterization. Common organisms producing this infection are gonococcus, *E. coli,* and *C. trachomatis.* The latter organism is difficult to culture and is usually surmised to be present.

Treatment consists of symptomatic measures such as elevation of the scrotum, the use of a scrotal suspensory or an ice

bag, and broad-spectrum antibiotic therapy with ampicillin, tetracycline, or aminoglycosides. Epididymoorchitis and abscess formation may occur and require surgical intervention for drainage or excision.

Acute onset of epididymal swelling and tenderness following scrotal trauma or strain in lifting a heavy object provides a problem from a compensation standpoint regarding the entity described as *traumatic epididymitis.* Treatment is usually as noted for infectious epididymitis, but the antibiotic therapy may be withheld. Infection often cannot definitely be ruled out despite the negative urinalysis and cultures.

Chronic Infections

Bacterial Prostatitis. Chronic bacterial prostatitis is characterized by recurring UTIs, low back and perineal discomfort, urinary frequency, urgency, and dysuria. The symptoms are variable, and there may be long periods of remission between symptomatic episodes or signs of UTIs. The prostate usually is not tender, but the expressed prostatic secretion obtained by massage usually shows an increased number of white blood cells with some in clumps. The properly collected specimen may reveal the offending organism on culture.

The commonly prescribed antibacterial agents that are used for the treatment of a UTI or acute bacterial prostatitis may be ineffective in the management of chronic bacterial prostatitis. Failure to achieve adequate levels of these drugs in the nonacutely inflamed prostate may account for this phenomenon and results in a low cure rate for this troublesome condition. The quinolones have largely resolved this problem, although several weeks of therapy may be required. Surgical intervention, such as transurethral resection, does not seem to benefit unless associated obstruction is present because infected prostatic tissue remains after resection.

Nonbacterial prostatitis produces symptoms identical to chronic bacterial prostatitis and may be more common. Inflammatory changes of the prostate are present, with increased white blood cells in the expressed prostatic secretions and negative cultures for bacterial pathogens. *Prostatodynia* is present if both the expressed prostatic secretions and cultures are negative. Symptoms may be similar to those seen with chronic bacterial prostatitis, and therapy is empirical and usually unsuccessful. Management consists of reassurance, as well as muscle relaxants, warm baths, prostatic massage, and other "symptomatic relief" measures.

Cystitis. Chronic cystitis is seldom the end result of recurrent uncomplicated acute bacterial cystitis. The inflammatory process usually extends beneath the mucosa into the submucosal and muscular layers of the bladder and may be associated with white blood cell infiltration and varying degrees of fibrosis, which compromises detrusor function and decreases bladder capacity. Predisposing factors usually contribute to the progressive changes and associated symptoms. These may include urethral stricture, bladder calculi, tumor, diverticula, neurogenic bladder dysfunction, long-standing indwelling catheter drainage, tuberculosis, parasitic infestation, such as schistosomiasis, and vesicoenteric fistula.

Chronic pyuria and often bacilluria are noted, and frequency, urgency, and dysuria are usually present unless catheterization or diversion has been instituted. The diagnostic work-up is directed toward accurate identification of the predisposing factors and the offending pathogen(s). Endoscopic evaluation of the urethra and bladder is usually carried out, as well as biopsy of suspicious lesions, cystourethrography, and cystometrics as indicated. Careful urine collections and appropriate cultures are performed to determine the predominant organisms. Unlike the *E. coli* of acute uncomplicated cystitis, the pathogen is usually one of the more resistant types such as *Pseudomonas, Serratia,* and cocci, and changing organisms are often encountered. When possible, the predisposing factor should be eliminated if symptoms are to be relieved and preservation of the remaining detrusor function is to be accomplished. Chronic antibacterial therapy is often required, and some permanent dysfunction is usually present after treatment.

A form of abacterial chronic cystitis has been identified and termed *interstitial cystitis*. It occurs more commonly in females than in males. The cause remains unknown, and the predominant symptoms are marked urinary frequency, urgency, and suprapubic pain. Cystoscopy may reveal a decreased bladder capacity and increased irritability. Bleeding from the mucosa may occur with bladder distention and production of the so-called Hunner's ulcer.

Biopsies of the bladder mucosa and exfoliative cytology may be indicated to rule out carcinoma in situ or dysplasia of the bladder. Cultures are usually negative, and symptomatic treatment is usually prescribed. As usually is the case in such situations, a number of medical and surgical regimens have been tried. Periodic instillations of dimethyl sulfoxide (DMSO) have proved of little value.

Epididymitis. Persistent induration of the epididymis characterizes this condition. Systemic symptoms and signs are usually absent, and tenderness in the indurated area may be minimal and intermittent. A history of previous acute epididymitis, which may be of the recurrent type, usually can be elicited. A definite cause may be difficult to establish, since culture of a pathogen may be impossible. The differential diagnosis of spermatocele, adenomatoid tumor, tuberculosis, trauma, or underlying testicular tumor has to be considered, especially in the patient in whom there is no previous history of acute infection. Ultrasound evaluation may help rule out a testicular neoplasm or spermatocele. Treatment consists of empirical antibacterial therapy, excisional biopsy, or just periodic observation depending on the size of the lesion, symptoms, and the age of the patient.

Pyelonephritis. The histologic picture of chronic pyelonephritis is characterized by a lack of specificity. Inflammatory changes associated with fibrosis and scarring are noted. Radiologically, there is evidence of loss of parenchyma, calyceal blunting, contracture, cortical scars with an irregular contour, and decreased perfusion and excretion of contrast material. Predisposing factors include vesicoureteral reflux, calculous disease, ureteral stricture, neurogenic bladder dysfunction, urinary diversion, indwelling nephrostomy, or bladder catheter. Treatment is directed toward correction of the predisposing factor and antibacterial therapy. The goal of therapy is preservation of renal function. End-stage renal disease may require dialysis and possibly renal transplantation.

Xanthogranulomatous pyelonephritis is a variant that characteristically presents in middle-aged patients with a poorly functioning kidney. There is often accompanying calculous dis-

ease and *Proteus* infection. Tumefaction can occur with rupture of the process through the renal capsule. It can be confused histologically with renal cell carcinoma because of areas of clear cells that are lipid-laden macrophages. The lesion is occasionally bilateral, does not respond to antibiotics, and progresses to endstage renal disease (Fig. 38-14).

Urinary Tuberculosis. The incidence of urinary tuberculosis is increasing. Renal tuberculosis is the result of hematogenous spread from primary pulmonary or intestinal lesions. Although the involvement is probably bilateral and cortical in most individuals, some lesions progress to healing, whereas others assume clinical significance. Renal tuberculosis is generally undetected and asymptomatic until it ulcerates into the collecting system of the kidney. At that time, the symptoms include gross hematuria, dysuria, frequency, and pyuria with an absence of

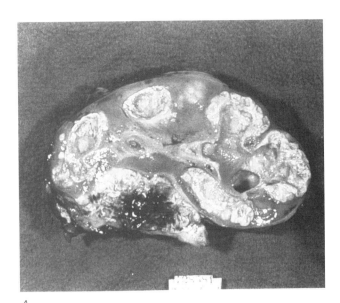

A

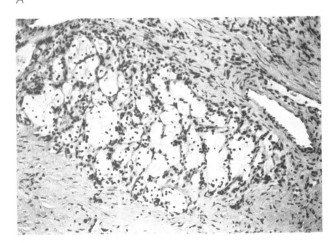

B

FIG. 38-14. Xanthogranulomatous pyelonephritis. *A.* Note excrescences surrounding calyces (grossly yellow). *B.* Micrograph showing clear cells (lipid-laden macrophages) that may lead to confusion with renal cell carcinoma. A stone is often present in the kidney in cases of xanthogranulomatous pyelonephritis.

bacteria on Gram stain. Many of the symptoms are a consequence of cystitis arising from organisms localizing in the bladder secondary to the renal involvement.

Special culture techniques reveal the presence of *Mycobacterium tuberculosis.* Intravenous pyelography demonstrates calcification of caseous abscesses, ulceration of calyces, and failure of visualization of calyces filled with caseous debris (Fig. 38-15). One drug therapy regimen consists of treatment with isoniazid (INH), ethambutol, rifampin, and pyridoxine. The patient is followed by repeated urine cultures and repeated pyelography, which should be performed at 3-month intervals during the first year. Nephrectomy is seldom indicated for renal tuberculosis.

Genital tuberculosis may accompany renal tuberculosis or may exist independently as a result of hematogenous spread. The epididymis is most frequently involved, and spread may take place from this source up the vas deferens to the prostate or through the scrotum in the form of a fistula. The vas deferens may become beaded with involvement. Epididymal tuberculosis may be managed successfully by chemotherapy, and epididymectomy is held in reserve.

NEPHROLITHIASIS

Nephrolithiasis is one of the more common urologic disorders, affecting approximately 5 to 10 percent of the population at some time during their lifetime. Without preventive treatment, the incidence of recurrence is as high as 50 percent within 5 years of the first stone event. Even patients with asymptomatic calculi stand a nearly 50 percent chance of becoming symptomatic within 5 years of diagnosis. Thus the economic and clinical impact of nephrolithiasis is considerable; the total cost of evaluation, hospitalization, inpatient and outpatient treatment, and indirect costs including lost wages has been estimated at $1.83 billion annually.

The surgical management of stone disease has changed dramatically in the past 15 years. Advances in noninvasive and minimally invasive techniques have virtually eliminated the need

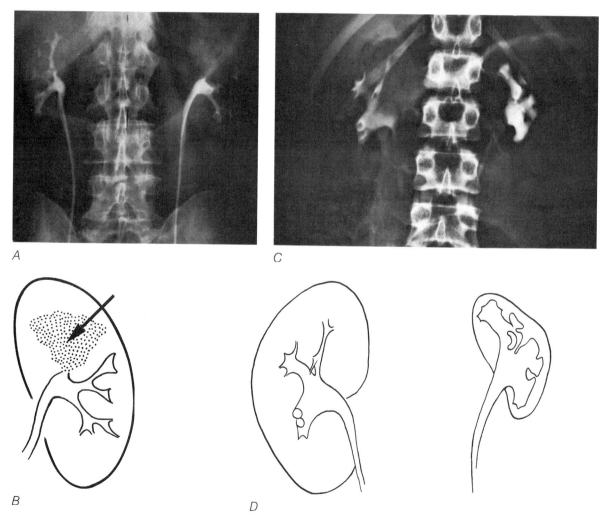

FIG. 38-15. Renal tuberculosis. *A* and *B.* Left upper pole ulcerative tuberculosis. *C* and *D.* Chronic suppurative tuberculous pyelonephritis (left kidney) with atrophy.

for open stone surgery; in 1997, less than 1 percent of patients required open stone procedures. However, the need for a medical prophylactic program has not diminished. Stone recurrences after surgery can be reduced significantly by the initiation of selective medical therapy. With current diagnostic protocols, metabolic abnormalities are identified in more than 95 percent of patients, and in the vast majority of these patients, directed medical and dietary therapy can have a significant impact on the course of the stone disease.

When a patient presents to the emergency room or physician's office with symptoms attributable to a renal or ureteral calculus, the goal is to establish a diagnosis, relieve pain and/or obstruction, identify stone characteristics and anatomic features that affect management, select conservative management versus surgical treatment, and proceed with treatment if indicated. To this end, a careful history, thorough physical examination, selective laboratory tests, and radiographic studies must be obtained (Fig. 38-16).

History. Patients with obstructing renal or ureteral calculi or calculi in transit from the kidney to the bladder typically present with a constellation of symptoms known as *renal colic.* Renal colic is characterized by the abrupt onset, often at night or early morning, of sharp pain originating in the flank and radiating around to the groin or testicle (labia). The sensation of pain in the groin area is attributed to the close proximity of the origins of the blood supply and autonomic nerve fibers supplying the kidney and testicle (ovary). The pain is brief, lasting a few minutes at a time, but recurs in paroxysms. Because the celiac axis innervates the kidneys as well as the stomach and small intestine, renal colic is frequently associated with nausea and vomiting, often confusing the diagnosis with gastrointestinal diseases (acute appendicitis, perforated viscous, colitis, diverticulitis).

The specific location of the pain may reflect the location of the obstructing stone: Stones in the proximal ureter or ureteropelvic junction typically cause flank pain radiating to the groin, stones in the middle ureter (overlying the bony pelvis) are often associated with anterior lower quadrant pain, and stones in the distal ureter may cause bladder irritative symptoms such as urinary frequency and urgency.

Physical Findings. Unlike the patient with an acute abdomen, patients with renal colic characteristically writhe in pain or pace the floor in an attempt to gain relief. Physical examination is remarkable only for abdominal or flank tenderness overlying the site of stone impaction. Palpation of the testes or ovaries fails to reproduce the pain and may rule out the gonads as the underlying source of pathology.

An elevated pulse and blood pressure are common due to pain and are nonspecific. If the obstructing stone is associated with infection, fever or chills may be present; noninfected stones are occasionally associated with a low-grade fever ($\leq 100°F$).

Laboratory Studies. The minimum laboratory evaluation of the patient with suspected renal colic consists of a complete blood count (CBC), serum electrolytes, blood urea nitrogen and creatinine, and a urinalysis. Mild leukocytosis (10,000 to 15,000/mm^3) is common in patients with renal colic due to demargination of white blood cells in response to stress. A white blood

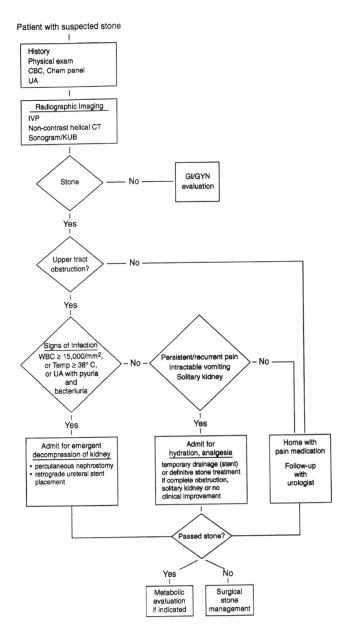

FIG. 38-16. *Algorithm for the management of an acute stone event.*

cell count greater than 15,000/mm^3 should alert the clinician to the possibility of obstructive or nonobstructive pyelonephritis.

An assessment of renal function is indicated to determine the impact of renal obstruction on overall renal function, to determine if intravenous contrast material can be administered safely for radiographic evaluation, and to assess fluid status. Serum electrolytes should be checked to identify any metabolic abnormalities such as acidosis, alkalosis, or hypokalemia.

The urinalysis is an important part of the laboratory assessment because the presence of microscopic hematuria may suggest the diagnosis of renal calculi. The absence of red blood cells in the urine does not preclude the presence of stones; in 10 to 25 percent of patients with an acute stone event, no red blood cells are detected in the urine, particularly in the face of complete obstruction. Mild pyuria may accompany hematuria but often reflects inflammation rather than infection. Significant pyuria, particularly when associated with fever and/or leukocytosis, should raise the suspicion of a UTI, and a urine culture should be obtained.

Additional urine parameters may be helpful in the overall evaluation of the stone patient but contribute less to the acute stone event. Urine pH may suggest the etiology of stone disease. A pH > 7 suggests the presence of urea-splitting organisms and possible struvite stones; in contrast, a pH < 5.5 is associated with uric acid stones. The presence of crystals may reveal the stone composition (hexagonal crystals in cystinuria, pyramidal crystals in calcium oxalate stones).

Radiographic Evaluation. The diagnosis of urinary tract calculi ultimately relies on radiographic confirmation. Radiographic imaging should determine the presence, number, size, location, and occasionally, composition of stones within the urinary tract. For radiopaque calculi, comprising 90 percent of upper tract calculi, a plain abdominal radiograph (kidneys, ureter, and bladder, or KUB) may demonstrate radiodensities highly suspicious for renal or ureteral stones (Fig. 38-17). The addition of oblique views may increase the sensitivity of plain-film radiography by altering which dimension of the stone is penetrated by the x-ray or by projecting the stone away from the spine or bony pelvis, thereby allowing the stone to be visualized. Plain nephrotomograms may prevent overlying bowel gas from obscuring small or faintly opaque renal calculi. Table 38-1 lists various stone compositions in decreasing order of radiodensity.

Extraurinary calcifications may mimic urinary tract calculi and must be distinguished from renal, ureteral, or bladder calculi with the aid of oblique or lateral views that project these calcifications away from the urinary tract. Gallstones, which are characteristically multifaceted, lie in the right upper quadrant and project anterior to the kidney on a right posterior oblique view. Vascular calcifications are often curvilinear and usually identifiable. Renal artery aneurysms are typically circular with a lucent

Table 38-1
Stone Composition in Decreasing Order of Radiopacity

Stone Composition	Radiopacity
Calcium hydrogen phosphate dishydrate (brushite)	Densely opaque
Calcium oxalate monohydrate	Densely opaque
Calcium phosphate (apatite)	Densely opaque
Calcium oxalate dihydrate	Moderately opaque
Magnesium ammonium phosphate (struvite)	Moderately opaque
Cystine	Faint to moderately opaque
Uric acid	Radiolucent

center. Pelvic phleboliths, which are calcified thrombi in pelvic veins, are generally round or oval and contain a lucent center. Phleboliths usually require opacification of the urinary tract to distinguish them from ureteral calculi.

The intravenous urogram (IVU) remains the mainstay of diagnosis of renal and ureteral calculi (Fig. 38-18). The IVU can precisely identify calculi within the urinary tract, assess the degree of obstruction, demonstrate anatomic abnormalities that may predispose to stone formation (medullary sponge kidney, ureteropelvic junction obstruction) or affect treatment decisions (ureteral stricture, calyceal diverticulum), and suggest the presence of sequelae from the obstructing stone (loss of renal parenchyma, forniceal rupture with extravasation of contrast material, mass effect from perinephric abscess). Although radiolucent calculi are not visible on the scout film, opacification of the collecting system may demonstrate a filling defect associated with ureteral obstruction.

Careful monitoring of the IVU as it progresses is critical to the successful diagnosis of the stone and to maximize useful information about the stone and kidney. The study should be modified based on the results of early images (e.g., delayed images or oblique views or the patient in a prone position).

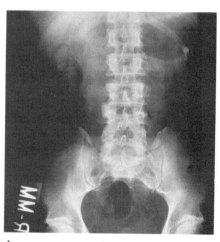
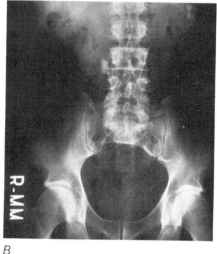
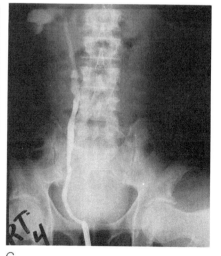

A *B* *C*

FIG. 38-17. *A. KUB view of a large right ureteral stone (between L4–5) somewhat obscured by the spinal column. B. Slightly oblique view of the same patient clearly reveals the large stone in the right proximal ureter. Also noted are two small stones overlying the right kidney and two stones overlying the left kidney. C. A retrograde pyelogram further defined the ureteral and renal anatomy.*

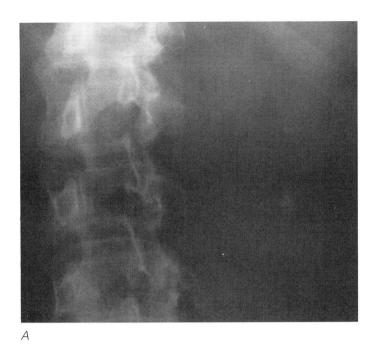

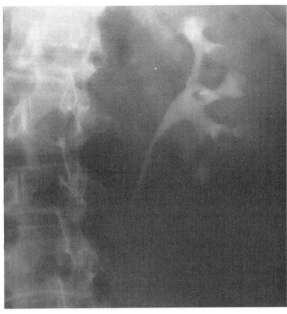

A   B

FIG. 38-18. *A. KUB view shows a calcification overlying the left kidney. B. IVU demonstrates the stone residing in a lower pole calyx without causing obstruction.*

In the acute setting, patients with renal insufficiency or a contrast material allergy can be imaged with a plain abdominal radiograph (KUB) and renal sonography or by retrograde pyelography. Renal sonography is highly sensitive for renal calculi greater than 5 mm in diameter and for detecting hydronephrosis (Fig. 38-19). The quality of the sonogram depends on patient size and imaging technique (i.e., stones in obese patients may easily be missed). Ureteral calculi are poorly imaged, particular in the absence of ureteral dilation, although distal ureteral calculi

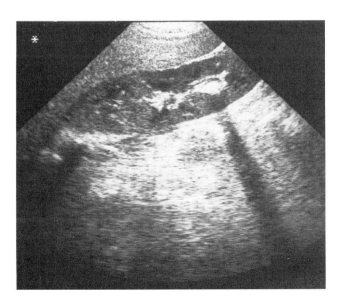

FIG. 38-19. *Longitudinal sonographic image of a kidney in a patient with flank pain and a negative KUB film. A stone in the lower pole of the kidney produces characteristic "acoustic shadowing."*

occasionally may be visualized through the window of a fluid-filled bladder.

Retrograde pyelography is indicated for the patient in whom administration of intravenous contrast material is contraindicated or when the IVU or renal sonogram is inconclusive. Ureteral calculi typically produce a filling defect in the ureter and cause a discrepancy in the caliber of the ureter above and below the defect (dilated above, narrow below).

Non-contrast-enhanced CT scans are very sensitive for detecting calculi of any composition in any location in the urinary tract (Fig. 38-20). However, thin-cut (5-mm) images are necessary to ensure adequate overlap and prevent overlooking small stones. Helical CT, in which images are acquired in a spiral configuration during a single breath hold, eliminates respiratory motion artifact and allows three-dimensional reconstruction of the entire urinary tract. At some institutions, non-contrast-enhanced helical CT has replaced the IVU for the diagnosis of acute flank pain in the emergency room setting. Early results suggest that helical CT is more sensitive than IVU in detecting ureteral stones; even in the absence of a clear-cut stone on CT, secondary signs of obstruction such as perinephric stranding or circumferential soft tissue attenuation can confirm the diagnosis of a ureteral stone with a high degree of accuracy. The advantages of non-contrast-enhanced helical CT are the rapidity of acquisition, the high degree of diagnostic accuracy, and no need for intravenous contrast material; however, the cost of spiral CT currently exceeds that of IVU at most institutions.

Initial Management. The initial effort is directed toward prompt pain relief. Most narcotic analgesics, such as morphine or meperidine, provide adequate analgesia. Intravenous nonsteroidal analgesics, such as Ketorolac, are effective, but caution must be exercised with the administration of these agents because of reported cases of renal failure, particularly in patients

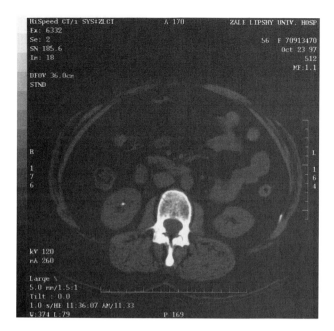

FIG. 38-20. *Thin-cut, non-contrast-enhanced CT scan reveals a small stone in the lower pole of the right kidney in a patient with flank pain and a nondiagnostic IVU.*

with impaired renal function or dehydration. As with other non-steroidal anti-inflammatory medications, Ketorolac causes inhibition of platelet aggregation and may predispose to bleeding, thereby interfering with planned surgical intervention or nephrostomy drainage.

Some investigators have advocated the use of a variety of agents aimed at reducing ureteral peristalsis and renal colic and facilitating stone passage. Intranasal desmopressin, aminophylline, indomethacin, nifedipine, and methylprednisolone have all been used to treat renal colic and facilitate stone passage with variable success. The use of these agents remains sporadic and has not gained widespread acceptance.

Immediate management of patients with renal colic depends on their response to analgesics, their ability to take oral fluids, and the presence of infection. A partially or completely obstructing stone associated with infection, as indicated by a fever, a markedly elevated white blood cell count, or a urinalysis suggestive of infection, mandates immediate decompression of the collecting system. The optimal method of draining the collecting system, whether retrograde placement of a ureteral catheter or placement of a percutaneous nephrostomy tube, is controversial. The advantage of nephrostomy tube placement includes accessibility of the external catheter for irrigation or to monitor urine appearance and output and the option of placing directly into the kidney a larger-caliber tube than is generally accommodated by the nondilated ureter. The advantage of ureteral catheterization is presumed greater patient comfort and less inconvenience with an internalized drainage tube. Regardless of the method of drainage employed, the kidney should be drained promptly and broad-spectrum antibiotics initiated. Urine cultures should be obtained from a voided specimen in the emergency room and a specimen obtained from the kidney at the time of drainage; antimicrobial coverage can be customized based on the identification and sensitivity of the cultured organisms.

The indications for hospitalizing a patient suffering from an acute stone event include failure to gain adequate pain relief with oral analgesics, inability to retain fluids or food because of nausea or vomiting, suspicion of infection, and anuria in patients with a solitary kidney (immediate decompression of the kidney is warranted). The patient may then receive intravenous narcotic analgesics, fluids, antiemetics, and antimicrobial agents if necessary.

Surgical intervention to remove the stone is undertaken if the stone is unlikely to pass spontaneously (≥6 mm in diameter), if the patient experiences persistent or recurrent colic or has persistent high grade obstruction (>1 week), or if occupational requirements mandate prompt treatment (airline pilots).

Despite dramatic advances in the surgical management of stones that has rendered virtually all stones in the urinary tract amenable to a noninvasive or minimally invasive treatment, many ureteral calculi will pass spontaneously without the need for treatment; thus conservative management of selected stones should not be overlooked. The likelihood of spontaneous passage depends on the size and location of the stone at the time of diagnosis. Small stones are likely to pass spontaneously regardless of their location in the ureter; in contrast, stones larger than 6 mm rarely pass spontaneously (<10 percent). Likewise, stones located in the distal ureter at the time of diagnosis stand a better chance of passing than more proximally located stones. A recent review of the literature estimated rates of spontaneous stone passage at 12, 22, and 45 percent for stones in the proximal, middle, and distal ureter, respectively.

The relative indications for treatment of stones in the kidney include large size, pain, location in the renal pelvis with the potential for obstruction, and associated infection or loss of renal function. Asymptomatic calyceal stones have an approximately 50 percent chance of becoming symptomatic within 5 years, and consequently, some authors have advocated prophylactic treatment of these stones as well. Asymptomatic stones that demonstrate continued growth despite preventative medical measures also warrant treatment. Staghorn calculi (large branched stones occupying a substantial portion of the collecting system) always require treatment because of the high incidence of renal failure, sepsis, and loss of renal function (Fig. 38-21).

Surgical Intervention

Appropriate surgical management of renal or ureteral calculi depends on the size, location, and composition of the stone, as well as the anatomy of the collecting system and ureter. Large obstructing renal or ureteral calculi or staghorn calculi may warrant an assessment of renal function before treatment. Substantial loss of renal function from long-standing obstruction or infection may favor nephrectomy over renal-preserving surgery. Radionuclide renal studies assess renal function, perfusion, and drainage with minimal radiation exposure. Unlike radiographic imaging studies, the renogram is unaffected by patient size or body habitus. The finding of 20 percent or less differential function in the stone-bearing kidney suggests an unsalvageable renal unit, and nephrectomy should be considered.

Management of renal and ureteral calculi includes noninvasive, minimally invasive, and open surgical approaches. Open surgery is reserved for complex stones with extensive associated anatomic abnormalities (such as a staghorn calculus in a kidney with numerous stenotic infundibula requiring extensive reconstruction of the collecting system) or stones that have failed min-

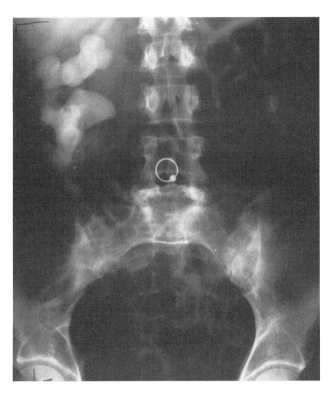

FIG. 38-21. Bilateral complete staghorn calculi in a young woman with recurrent urinary tract infections. The left staghorn calculus is very faintly opaque and was found to be composed primarily of matrix.

imally invasive approaches (e.g., an impacted ureteral calculus in a fixed, scarred ureter that is inaccessible by endoscopic means). The majority of stones, however, are amenable to minimally invasive approaches such as shock-wave lithotripsy, ureterorenoscopy, percutaneous nephrostolithotomy, or laparoscopic uretero- or pyelolithotomy.

Shock-Wave Lithotripsy. The study of shock waves was born from an observation by German scientists that aircraft re-

turning from supersonic flight had pitting on their surfaces, reportedly due to the generation of shock waves that were focused by the contours of the craft onto the surface of the plane. Applying this principle to human study, they observed that shock waves generated under water could be transmitted safely to the body without loss of energy because of the similar acoustic density of water and body tissue. Once the shock wave encountered an object of differing acoustic density, such as a calculus, the energy was released, thereby resulting in stone fragmentation and spontaneous discharge of fragments down the ureter and into the bladder. In 1981, the introduction into clinical practice of this completely noninvasive means of treating stones with shock waves revolutionized the contemporary management of renal and ureteral calculi.

The first lithotripter, designed by Dornier Medical Systems, used an underwater spark plug to generate shock waves that were then focused by means of an ellipsoid reflector (Fig. 38-22). Using biplanar fluoroscopy, the stone was targeted and positioned at the shock-wave focal point. Patients were partially submerged in a large water bath in order to couple the shock waves to the patient. Newer-generation lithotripters differ in the source of shock-wave generation, the means of coupling, the focusing mechanism, the imaging modality, and the anesthesia requirements of the treatment.

With current technology, in excess of 85 percent of stones are amenable to shock-wave lithotripsy (SWL). Most patients are treated on an outpatient basis with the expectation of resuming work within 1 to 2 days. Although SWL has a remarkably low morbidity, it is associated with some complications, either from direct injury to the kidney or from problems associated with passage of stone fragments. Most patients will experience a minimal degree of renal injury, manifested by gross hematuria, but few patients will demonstrate clinically significant hemorrhage (0.1 to 0.7 percent incidence of clinically significant perinephric hematoma).

Incomplete stone fragmentation or fragmentation of a large stone may result in the accumulation of obstructing stone fragments in the ureter (*steinstrasse*) (Fig. 38-23). While some steinstrasses resolve spontaneously, others require intervention such

FIG. 38-22. Dornier HM3 lithotripter. (From: *Steinbock GS, Bezirdjian, L, et al: Extracorporeal shock wave lithotripsy. Surg Rounds 9:45, 1986, with permission.*)

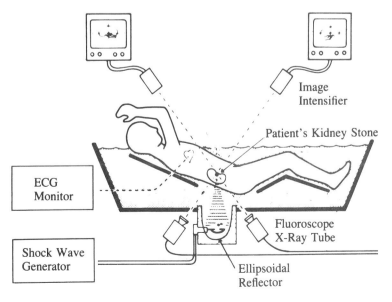

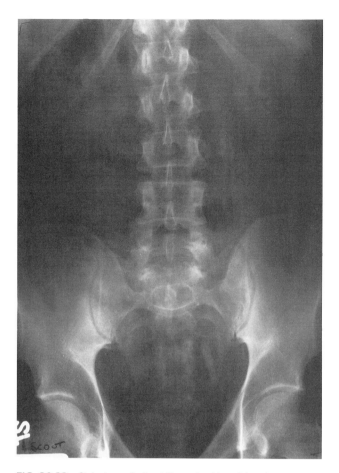

FIG. 38-23. *Steinstrasse in the left proximal (overlying the transverse process of L3) and distal ureter (overlying the sacrum) of a patient who underwent shock-wave lithotripsy for a 15-mm upper-pole renal calculus. Note residual stone fragments in the lower pole of the left kidney as well.*

percutaneous nephrostomy drainage or ureteroscopy with intracorporeal lithotripsy to clear the fragments.

The overall success rate of SWL for renal calculi averages 70 percent using the first-generation Dornier HM3 lithotripter. Success rates vary according to the size, location, and composition of the stone. Stone-free rates vary inversely with stone size; for stones greater than 2 cm in size, stone-free rates drop off substantially. Shock-wave monotherapy for treatment of staghorn calculi is generally discouraged because of the high retreatment rate and the frequent complications attributable to passage of a large volume of stone fragments. SWL monotherapy is reserved exclusively for small-volume staghorn calculi in nondilated collecting systems, a subgroup comprising less than 20 percent of staghorn calculi. The use of a ureteral stent has been shown to decrease the rate of complications and the need for secondary procedures when treating stones greater than 2.5 cm in diameter.

Stone location also influences the outcome of SWL treatment. Higher stone-free rates are achieved with SWL therapy of renal pelvic stones compared with treatment of calyceal stones. In particular, lower-pole stones are associated with the lowest stone-free rates of any renal calculi because of difficulty clearing fragments from the dependent lower-pole calyces. A recent meta-

analysis comparing SWL and percutaneous nephrostolithotomy for the treatment of lower-pole stones favored a percutaneous approach in all size categories.

Stone composition bears directly on the success of SWL, although stone analysis is often unavailable before treatment. Cystine stones are relatively resistant to SWL, and as such, alternative endoscopic treatment is recommended for cystine stones greater than 1 cm in diameter. Calcium oxalate monohydrate stones are hard stones with variable success when treated with SWL. In general, calcium oxalate dihydrate and uric acid stones are easily fragmented with SWL.

Ureteral stones in all locations have been managed successfully with SWL. Modifications of standard patient positioning, such as treatment in the supine or prone position, have enabled treatment of stones in the middle (overlying the bony pelvis) or distal (below the bony pelvis) ureter, which are unable to be targeted with patients on the standard gantry. Early investigators advocated retrograde displacement of ureteral stones into the renal pelvis or bypass of the stone with a ureteral stent prior to SWL therapy because of perceived lower success rates with in situ treatment of ureteral stones. However, several prospective, randomized series have shown that endoscopic manipulation prior to SWL is unnecessary for proximal ureteral stones. No randomized series have evaluated the need for ureteral stents for middle or distal ureteral stones, although several retrospective series suggest that stent placement is unnecessary for stones in these locations as well.

With the introduction of SWL came the sometimes indiscriminate treatment of nearly all renal and ureteral calculi with this noninvasive modality. Now, after nearly 15 years of experience with SWL and extensive analyses of SWL failures, the indications for SWL have been defined more precisely. Staghorn calculi, renal stones greater than 2.5 cm in size, and ureteral stones greater than 1.5 cm in size are best managed endoscopically. Likewise, lower-pole calculi greater than 1 to 2 cm in size may be inappropriate for SWL and will be treated more successfully percutaneously or with ureterorenoscopy. Renal or ureteral calculi associated with distal obstruction, such as ureteropelvic junction obstruction or ureteral stricture, should be managed with an antegrade percutaneous or retrograde ureteroscopic approach in which the stricture can be addressed endoscopically at the time of stone removal. Obese patients pose unique problems for SWL; weight limitations on the gantry or table, difficulty visualizing the stone fluoroscopically or with sonography, and inability to position the stone at the shock-wave focal point because of a skin-stone distance that exceeds the distance to the focal point may all preclude successful treatment.

Percutaneous Nephrostolithotomy. Percutaneous nephrostolithotomy (PCNL) is the endoscopic removal or fragmentation of stones through a tract from the skin into the kidney through the flank. PCNL is generally reserved for large or complex renal or ureteral calculi or for stones associated with anatomic obstruction precluding spontaneous passage of stone fragments after SWL. PCNL fell into disuse after the introduction of SWL, and many urologists lost their percutaneous skills; however, PCNL has experienced a reemergence as the indications for SWL have become more refined.

PCNL requires a general anesthetic and may be performed in conjunction with an interventional radiologist. The procedure is facilitated by placement of a ureteral occlusion balloon catheter into the renal pelvis to opacify the collecting system and to prevent distal migration of stone fragments during intracorporeal lithotripsy. With the patient in the prone position, a small-gauge hollow-bore needle is positioned under fluoroscopic guidance directly into the stone-bearing calyx or into the calyx providing optimal access to the stone. A guidewire is passed through the needle and maneuvered into the collecting system and preferably down the ureter into the bladder. A second guidewire is placed to serve as a safety wire. The nephrostomy tract is then dilated using a high-pressure balloon or sequential graduated dilators, culminating in the placement of a working sheath (usually #30 French in size, or 10-mm inner diameter) through which the endoscope is passed directly into the collecting system.

Stones 1 cm or less in size can be retrieved intact; stones greater than 1 cm in size require some form of power lithotripsy, usually either ultrasonic or pneumatic lithotripsy, to fragment the stone into small pieces that can be extracted or aspirated using suction attached to the end of the hollow lithotripter probe (Fig. 38-24). The use of a flexible nephroscope with fiberoptic imaging allows access to stones in calyces remote from the nephrostomy tract and to stones in the ureter; these stones can be retrieved with flexible graspers or baskets passed through the working channel of the endoscope, or the stone can be fragmented in situ with a flexible laser fiber or electrohydraulic lithotripsy probe.

At the conclusion of the procedure, a ureteral catheter is passed over the working guidewire into the bladder and a large-caliber nephrostomy tube (#22 French) with a central hole in the tip is placed over the ureteral catheter into the renal pelvis to provide urinary drainage and to tamponade the nephrostomy tract. After 24 to 48 h, a nephrostogram is obtained to assess drainage from the kidney and to identify extravasation of contrast from an inadvertent perforation in the collecting system. If residual stone fragments are detected on postoperative imaging studies, "second look" flexible nephroscopy can be performed

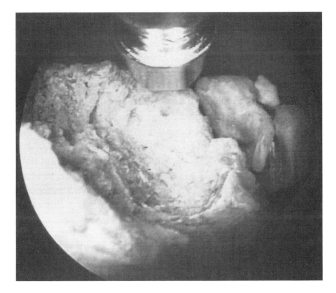

FIG. 38-24. *Endoscopic view through a nephroscope of a large stone in the kidney. At the top of the picture, the hollow metal ultrasonic sonotrode is visible as it fragments the stone and aspirates the fragments.*

under local anesthesia with intravenous sedation to retrieve the remaining stones.

Unlike SWL, stone-free rates for PCNL are independent of stone size and stone location; stone-free rates of 70 to 100 percent have been reported with PCNL. The most common complication associated with PCNL is bleeding; the average decrease in hemoglobin is 1.2 to 2.8 g/dL. In fewer than 1 percent of patients, persistent bleeding from pseudoaneurysm formation necessitates arteriography and transcatheter arterial embolization. The need for renal exploration or nephrectomy is exceedingly rare. Access-related injury to adjacent structures most commonly involves the pleura, which can be traversed in the case of an upper-pole supracostal access. Injury to the spleen, liver, colon, and duodenum have been reported but are rare and generally can be managed conservatively.

PCNL can be performed in association with renal reconstructive surgery; a stricture or narrowing of the infundibulum leading to a stone-bearing calyx (infundibular stenosis) or a short stricture at the ureteropelvic junction (congenital or acquired ureteropelvic obstruction) can be incised endoscopically with a "cold" or "hot" knife, and the stones may be removed simultaneously at the same sitting.

According to the American Urological Association Nephrolithiasis Clinical Guidelines Panel, first-line treatment for staghorn calculi is PCNL, with the addition of SWL and repeat PCNL as needed. Complex stones may require multiple accesses into the kidney in order to render the patient free of stone. In some cases, combination therapy with SWL may be indicated; "sandwich therapy" offers the high success rates of PCNL with the lower morbidity of SWL. Sandwich therapy is a multistage procedure that consists of PCNL followed by SWL and always concludes with flexible nephroscopy for removal of residual fragments remaining after SWL.

Ureterorenoscopy. The introduction of the Hopkins rod lens system and fiberoptic technology paved the way for the development of semirigid and flexible endoscopes that could be passed through the urethra and bladder into the ureter and kidney for inspection and treatment of a variety of pathologic conditions, including stones. Under direct endoscopic vision, the stone can be visualized and extracted intact with a grasper or basket, or it can be fragmented in situ with a variety of intracorporeal lithotripsy modalities: laser (pulsed-dye, alexandrite, neodynium:YAG, or holmium:YAG), electrohydraulic (in situ shockwave generation), or pneumatic (ballistic energy).

Ureteroscopy begins with the successful passage of a guidewire through the ureteral orifice up the ureter and into the kidney via a cystoscope passed into the bladder; for flexible ureteroscopy, a second, safety guidewire is placed. The semirigid ureteroscope is advanced directly into the ureter under endoscopic vision *alongside* the guidewire until the stone is reached. In contrast, the flexible ureteroscope is passed *over* the guidewire and advanced under fluoroscopic guidance to the site of pathology; the guidewire through the ureteroscope is then removed, leaving only the safety guidewire in place (Fig. 38-25). Working instruments are passed through the working channel onto the stone to either retrieve the stone intact or to fragment it into spontaneously passable fragments. A ureteral stent is routinely left in place after ureteroscopy to prevent obstruction and renal colic due to edema at the site of stone manipulation. The stent is

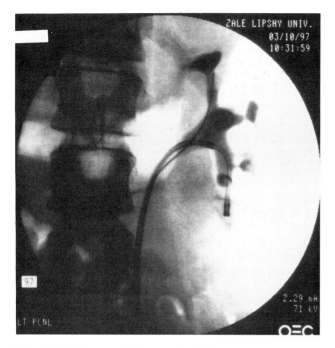

FIG. 38-25. *Fluoroscopic image of a flexible ureteroscope in the lower pole of the left kidney. Contrast material opacifies the collecting system, and a safety guidewire is in place in an upper-pole calyx.*

usually removed in the office with a rigid or flexible cystoscope 3 to 7 days after the procedure.

Recent technology has resulted in miniaturization of ureteroscopes as small as #6.9 French for semirigid and #7.5 French for flexible ureteroscopes; indeed, most small-caliber ureteroscopes can be passed routinely into the undilated ureter. Small-caliber ureteroscopes allow access to virtually any stone in the kidney or ureter. Improvements in ureteroscope design have led to better imaging and larger-caliber working channels, thereby expanding the armamentarium of instruments that can be used in conjunction with the ureteroscope. The introduction of the holmium:YAG laser lithotripsy has raised the upper limit of stone size treatable endoscopically and has made ureteroscopy a reasonable alternative to SWL or PCNL for some moderate to large renal calculi. Ureteroscopy can be performed on an outpatient basis with minimal morbidity. Ureteral perforation and late development of ureteral stricture remain significant, albeit rare, complications of ureteroscopy that render ureteroscopy second-line or salvage therapy for most renal or ureteral calculi after failed SWL.

Laparoscopic Stone Removal. The safety and feasibility of laparoscopic pyelolithotomy and ureterolithotomy have been demonstrated in anecdotal reports in the literature. Laparoscopic stone removal remains a salvage therapy and serves as an alternative to open surgery in the rare case of SWL or endoscopic failure.

Medical Management. Despite dramatic advances in the minimally invasive surgical management of stone disease, the need for a medical prophylactic program remains unchanged. Surgical treatment of renal calculi does not eliminate the risk of stone recurrence; indeed, in one retrospective study, selective

medical therapy reduced the risk of stone recurrence after successful SWL from 0.65 to 0.09 per year.

The selection of patients in need of a metabolic evaluation is controversial. The evaluation of recurrent stone formers or high-risk first-time stone formers (patients with a strong family history of stone disease, associated medical conditions, or nephrocalcinosis) is clearly indicated. The evaluation of first-time stone formers without obvious risk factors is debatable. Nevertheless, first-time stone formers have been shown to have the same incidence and severity of metabolic abnormalities as recurrent stone formers. The decision to pursue a detailed metabolic evaluation must be shared by the patient and the physician.

The first step in evaluation of the stone-forming patient is a careful history. Identification of risk factors such as a family history of stone disease, gastrointestinal disorders, bone disease, nephrocalcinosis, chronic UTIs, or a history of gout should prompt a detailed metabolic evaluation. For first-time stone formers without significant risk factors, a simplified evaluation may suffice.

It is important to identify any medical conditions that may be complicated by renal calculi. Chronic diarrheal syndrome as a result of intestinal disease (Crohn's disease, ulcerative colitis), bowel resection, or pancreatic insufficiency may be associated with uric acid or calcium stones because of dehydration, hypocitraturia, and enteric hyperoxaluria. Gout is frequently associated with uric acid or calcium oxalate stones because of low urine pH and hyperuricosuria. Bone disease may be a result of hyperparathyroidism but in association with brain tumors or peptic ulcer disease may represent multiple endocrine neoplasia syndrome. Recurrent UTIs, particularly with *Proteus, Klebsiella,* or *Pseudomonas,* predisposes to struvite stone formation.

A careful dietary and medication history can elicit environmental factors that predispose to stone formation, such as inadequate fluid intake, salt abuse, a high calcium or oxalate diet, or a purine-rich diet. Stone-provoking medications also may contribute to the risk of stone formation. Acetazolamide, a carbonic anhydrase inhibitor, is associated with metabolic acidosis and may lead to hypocitraturia, hypercalciuria, and an alkaline urine. Calcium supplements or vitamin D, commonly taken for osteoporosis, may cause hypercalciuria. Large doses of vitamin C, which is metabolized to oxalate, may promote calcium oxalate stone formation.

A simplified evaluation includes a careful history, a serum chemistry profile, urinalysis, plain radiograph, and stone composition. The serum chemistry profile may identify systemic risk factors, such as hypercalcemia associated with primary hyperparathyroidism, hyperuricemia associated with gout, hypokalemia, hyperchloremia, and low serum bicarbonate associated with distal renal tubular acidosis or hypophosphatemia associated with renal phosphate leak. Microscopic inspection of the urine may reveal pathognomonic crystals, such as cystine crystals, and dipstick urinalysis may reveal extremes of pH; pH > 7.5 is associated with infection by urea-splitting organisms with subsequent struvite stone formation, whereas pH < 5.5 leads to precipitation of uric acid and subsequent formation of uric acid or calcium stones. In some cases, the stone composition may suggest the underlying metabolic abnormality responsible for stone formation, such as cystine stones and cystinuria, struvite stones and recurrent UTIs, and uric acid stones and low urine pH.

A more extensive evaluation includes 24-h urine collections on a random diet and after 1 week of a low-calcium, low-sodium diet. The urine is assessed for total volume, pH, calcium, oxalate, sodium, uric acid, citrate, magnesium, and phosphorus. A urinary calcium-creatinine ratio measured first while fasting and then after an oral calcium load can distinguish the various causes of hypercalciuria. Bone densities are obtained to assess bone loss prior to consideration of calcium restriction.

With an extensive ambulatory protocol, a diagnosis can be established in more than 95 percent of stone-forming patients. Treatment is then directed at correction of the underlying metabolic derangements and elimination of environmental risk factors. The pathophysiologic categories of stone formation are characterized below (Table 38-2).

Hypercalciuria. Hypercalciuria is a manifestation of a variety of disorders. Absorptive hypercalciuria, the most common form of hypercalciuria, is due to intestinal overabsorption of calcium. The mechanism responsible for calcium overabsorption is unknown; consequently, treatment is aimed at reducing urinary calcium excretion rather than normalizing intestinal calcium absorption. Renal hypercalciuria is less common than absorptive hypercalciuria. The primary defect in renal hypercalciuria is impaired renal tubular reabsorption of calcium. Thiazide diuretics are the mainstay of treatment for both types of hypercalciuria; thiazides directly stimulate calcium reabsorption in the distal tubule and indirectly stimulate reabsorption in the proximal tubule. The hypocalciuric action of thiazides becomes attenuated after 18 to 24 months in absorptive hypercalciuria but is maintained indefinitely in renal hypercalciuria. Consequently, the search for more effective drugs for the treatment of absorptive hypercalciuria has led to the development of a slow-release form of neutral potassium phosphate that has been shown to reduce intestinal calcium absorption and enhance excretion of urinary inhibitors. Preliminary results are encouraging, and clinical trials are currently in progress.

Resorptive hypercalciuria is usually due to primary hyperparathyroidism. Excessive secretion of parathyroid hormone from a parathyroid adenoma leads to bone resorption and increased renal synthesis of 1,25-$(OH)_2D$, which in turn enhances intestinal absorption of calcium; the net effect is elevated serum and urinary calcium levels. Primary hyperparathyroidism is a surgical disease, and parathyroidectomy is the optimal treatment.

Hyperuricosuria. Hyperuricosuria constitutes a risk factor for both uric acid and calcium oxalate stone formation. The most common cause of hyperuricosuria is a purine-rich diet. At low urine pH (<5.5), the undissociated form of uric acid, which has a low solubility, precipitates to form uric acid stones. At pH >5.5, sodium urate formation predominates and promotes calcium oxalate stone formation by serving as a nidus for calcium oxalate crystallization.

Hyperoxaluria. Enteric hyperoxaluria, associated with inflammatory bowel disease or bowel resection, is the most common form of hyperoxaluria. Intestinal malabsorption of fat enhances saponification with divalent cations (magnesium and calcium) in the intestinal lumen, thereby reducing complexation with oxalate and increasing the reservoir of free oxalate available for absorption. Furthermore, poorly absorbed bile salts and fatty acids are thought to increase colonic permeability to oxalate, further increasing serum and urine oxalate levels. Intestinal disease is associated with other metabolic abnormalities as well, such as dehydration, metabolic acidosis, and hypocitraturia. Treatment is aimed at correcting dehydration and reducing the metabolic acidosis. Potassium citrate therapy corrects the acidosis and normalizes urinary citrate. Limitation of dietary oxalate, and in some cases supplementation with calcium citrate, may correct the hyperoxaluria.

Hypocituraturia. Hypocitraturia is associated with a variety of conditions, such as chronic diarrheal syndrome, renal tubular acidosis, or thiazide therapy, or it may be idiopathic and associated with calcium oxalate stones. Potassium citrate supplementation restores urinary citrate, raises urinary pH, and lowers the saturation of calcium-forming salts.

Gouty Diathesis. *Gouty diathesis* describes a stone-forming propensity characterized by a low urinary pH level, which may

Table 38-2
Major Diagnostic Categories of Nephrolithiasis

Condition	Metabolic/Environmental Defect	Prevalence (%)*
Absorptive hypercalciuria		20–40
Type I	Increased gastrointestinal calcium absorption, not correctable with dietary calcium restriction	
Type II	Increased gastrointestinal calcium absorption, correctable with dietary calcium restriction	
Renal hypercalciuria	Impaired renal calcium reabsorption	5–8
Resorptive hypercalciuria	Primary hyperparathyroidism	3–5
Hyperuricosuric calcium nephrolithiasis	Dietary purine excess, uric acid overproduction	10–40
Hypocitraturic calcium nephrolithiasis		10–50
Isolated	Idiopathic	
Chronic diarrheal syndrome	Gastrointestinal alkali loss	
Distal renal tubular acidosis	Impaired renal acid excretion	
Thiazide-induced	Hypokalemia	
Hyperoxaluric calcium nephrolithiasis		2–15
Primary hyperoxaluria	Oxalate overproduction	
Dietary hyperoxaluria	Increased dietary oxalate	
Enteric hyperoxaluria	Increased intestinal oxalate absorption	
Gouty diathesis	Low urinary pH	15–30
Cystinuria	Impaired renal cystine reabsorption	<1
Infection stones	Infection with urease-producing bacteria	1–5

*Represents estimate of relative occurrence based on experience in Dallas. Some patients have more than one abnormality.

or may not be associated with gouty arthritis or hyperuricemia. Gouty diathesis is typically associated with uric acid stone formation but also predisposes to calcium stone formation. In patients with uric acid stones, treatment is directed at raising urinary pH above 5.5 and maintaining a normal urinary uric acid level. Correction of dietary overindulgence in purine-rich foods (meat, fish, poultry) or the administration of allopurinol should normalize the urinary uric acid level. Potassium citrate raises the urinary pH level and results in dissolution of existing uric acid stones and inhibition of new stone formation.

Cystinuria. Cystinuria is an inherited transport disorder that results in excessive urinary excretion of dibasic amino acids (cystine, ornithine, lysine and arginine). In patients with the disorder, the urinary cystine concentration frequently exceeds the solubility of cystine, resulting in stone formation. High fluid intake is critical for maintaining the cystine concentration below the solubility limit. The solubility of cystine varies according to pH and is highest at a pH of more than 7.5. Consequently, alkali therapy may result in dissolution of preexisting stones and prevention of new stone occurrences. When fluid and alkali therapy alone are inadequate to prevent stone formation, the addition of a chelating agent such as D-penicillamine or α-mercaptopropionylglycine reduces cystine concentration by forming a more soluble cysteine-sulfhydryl complex.

Infection Lithiasis. The formation of ammoniomagnesium phosphate, or struvite, stones is due to chronic infection with urea-splitting organisms. The hydrolysis of urea catalyzed by these bacteria leads to ammonium production and an alkaline urine. In this environment, the components of struvite become supersaturated, and crystals form. The mainstay of therapy for struvite stones is surgical removal of the stone and eradication of the offending organism. In some recalcitrant cases, the administration of acetohydoxamic acid, a urease inhibitor, can facilitate stone dissolution and prevention.

BENIGN PROSTATIC HYPERPLASIA

Benign prostatic hyperplasia (BPH) is the most common disorder of the prostate gland. Although seldom life-threatening, BPH can have a significant impact on the aging male's quality of life. In the majority of men affected, the disease produces urinary symptoms that are slightly inconvenient. In others, however, the presence of more bothersome symptoms or the development of more serious sequelae leads to therapeutic intervention. Although surgical removal of the obstructing prostatic tissue offers the highest probability of symptomatic improvement, less effective medical therapies are attractive to some patients because they have less risk.

Natural History. Hyperplastic growth of the prostate begins in many men by the fifth decade of life. By age 80, almost 90 percent of men have histologic evidence of BPH. The normal adult prostate reaches a plateau at a weight of about 20 g at age 30. Then the weight remains stable until approximately age 50, when a process of growth is initiated at an average of 0.5 to 0.8 g/year. In populations, the probability of developing symptoms increases with increasing prostate size. In individual patients, however, the correlation between prostate weight and symptom severity is poor.

The clinical progression of BPH is variable. Approximately one-third of patients being followed by "watchful waiting" will have improvement in symptoms over time, whereas an equal number will have no worsening. The remainder will have symptomatic progression. A small number of men in the latter group will develop more serious sequelae of the disease: urinary retention, recurrent UTIs, bladder stones, bladder failure, or renal dysfunction. The risk of acute urinary retention in men with BPH is approximately 1 percent per year.

Pathogenesis. BPH first develops in the periurethral transition zone of the prostate. The transition zone consists of two separate lobules of tissue immediately external to the preprostatic sphincter (Fig. 38-26). The main ducts of the transition zone arise on the lateral aspects of the urethral wall at the point of urethral angulation near the verumontanum. Proximal to the origin of the transition zone ducts are the glands of the periurethral zone, which also undergo hyperplastic growth. Stromal (smooth muscle and extracellular matrix) and epithelial nodules develop in these zonal compartments, leading to an overall increase in the size of the gland. As the prostate enlarges, the peripheral zone, the most common site for the development of prostatic adenocarcinoma, is compressed between the transition zone and the capsule of the gland.

One of the unique features of the human prostate is the presence of the prostatic capsule, which plays an important role in the development of prostatism. In the dog, the only other species known to develop naturally occurring BPH, symptoms of prostatism rarely develop because the canine prostate lacks a capsule. Presumably the capsule transmits the pressure of tissue expansion to the urethra, leading to an increase in urethral resistance.

Growth of the prostate in aging men is not a uniform process. Some patients develop "global" enlargement of the entire gland, whereas others develop more prominent growth of specific regions of the gland (Fig. 38-27). Extensive growth of the periurethral zone may lead to a "middle lobe" and a resulting ball-valve type of obstruction.

Smooth muscle cells within the prostatic capsule, stroma, and bladder neck have a high density of α_1-adrenergic receptors on their surfaces. Thus tone in the prostatic urethra is influenced by the degree of adrenergic stimulation to the gland, which contributes in a dynamic way to outflow obstruction.

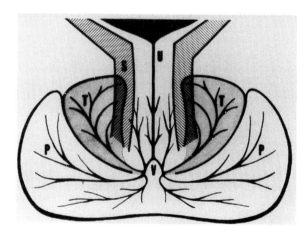

FIG. 38-26. *Diagram of the prostate zonal anatomy. Benign prostatic hyperplasia develops in the transition zone (T) just lateral to the urethra (U) and the preprostatic sphincter (S). The peripheral zone (P) is the most common site of prostate cancer development.*

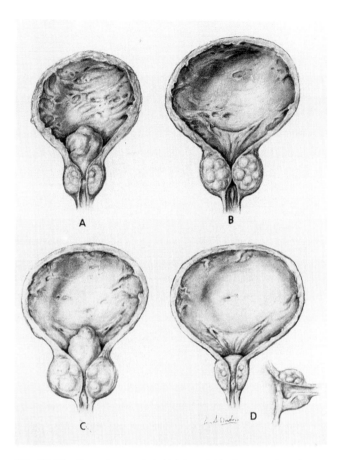

FIG. 38-27. *Prostatic growth is highly variable. Some patients have a predominant middle lobe (A), some have lateral lobe enlargement (B), some have trilobar enlargement (C), whereas others have an obstructing median bar at the bladder neck (D).*

The bladder's initial response to prostatic enlargement is the development of compensatory muscular hyperplasia. Intravesical pressure increases to maintain flow in the face of outflow resistance. Unfortunately, the adaptation is not perfect: Bladder hyperplasia leads to urinary frequency and urgency. In advanced cases, the bladder wall becomes fibrotic, loses compliance, and fails to empty completely. The development of postvoiding residual urine, however, is common and does not invariably lead to urinary retention and hydronephrosis.

The molecular pathogenesis of BPH is uncertain. It is clear that the process requires aging and testicular androgens. BPH does not develop in men castrated before puberty. Testosterone, produced by testicular Leydig cells, is the major androgen in the circulation. After testosterone diffuses into the prostate stromal cell, most of it is converted into a much more potent androgen, dihydrotestosterone (DHT), by the enzyme 5α-reductase (Fig. 38-28). The importance of this amplification step in growth of the prostate is clear from studies of patients with deficiency of the 5α-reductase enzyme who have virtually absent prostates. Both testosterone and DHT bind to the androgen receptor in the epithelial cell to stimulate androgen-dependent cell growth and inhibit the programmed cell death seen on androgen withdrawal. Although androgens do not cause BPH, DHT plays a central role in the pathogenesis of the disease.

Clinical Manifestations. *Symptoms.* Men with clinically significant BPH have a mixture of symptoms that are often termed *LUTS:* lower urinary tract symptoms. Symptoms of urinary frequency and urgency, decreased force of the urinary stream, hesitation in the initiation of flow, intermittency, a sensation of incomplete emptying, and nocturia occur to variable degrees. These symptoms can be quantified by use of a standardized questionnaire developed by the American Urological Association (Table 38-3). Men with AUA symptom scores of 7 or less are seldom bothered by their symptoms and usually can be managed successfully by watchful waiting.

Unfortunately, LUTS is not specific for BPH. UTI, prostatitis, prostate and bladder cancer, urethral stricture disease, and neurogenic bladder disease may all produce identical symptoms. Therefore, further evaluation is necessary (Fig. 38-29).

Baseline Evaluation. A careful history should be taken to exclude causes of urinary tract dysfunction. A history of urethritis, straddle injury, or lower urinary tract instrumentation puts the patient at risk for urethral stricture disease. The presence of dysuria or perineal/suprapubic pain may indicate UTI or prostatitis. Many neurologic diseases, such as stroke, Parkinson's disease, diabetic neuropathy, and disc disease, may alter bladder function. Congestive heart failure, diabetes, and renal insufficiency may lead to polyuria, resulting in urinary frequency and nocturia.

Physical examination must include a careful digital rectal examination (DRE), a limited neurologic assessment to exclude obvious abnormalities, palpation/percussion of the suprapubic area to detect a distended bladder, and an examination of the external genitalia. The DRE is performed to estimate prostate size and to detect asymmetry, induration, or nodularity that may be suspicious for malignancy. Although the size of the prostate does not determine disease severity, the finding of a normal-sized gland on DRE increases the probability that the symptoms are not related to BPH.

Urinalysis must be done to exclude UTI and hematuria. Infection may mimic the symptoms of BPH or be a complication of outflow obstruction. The presence of hematuria should prompt endoscopy and imaging of the kidneys to exclude urothelial and renal malignancy, as well as bladder stones. Bacterial prostatitis may not be associated with pyuria. Therefore, examination of the expressed prostatic secretions and localization cultures should be performed in men with prostatism who also have dysuria or perineal/suprapubic pain.

Measurement of the serum creatinine level is important to evaluate renal function. Even mild degrees of renal insufficiency should be evaluated by renal sonography. Patients with minimal prostatism may develop obstructive uropathy, although rarely.

Although BPH does not appear to be a risk factor for prostatic cancer, *both diseases commonly occur in the same patient.* Digital rectal examination and measurement of the serum PSA level are the best tests to detect prostate cancer. Serum PSA determination is a valuable test in men between the ages of 50 and 75 who have at least a 10-year life expectancy, but PSA is not a specific tumor marker. Approximately 25 to 30 percent of men with BPH will have an elevated PSA level. Since PSA elevation usually prompts the performance of transrectal ultrasonography and biopsy of the gland, this high rate of false-positive results is bothersome. Recently, assays that measure the percentage of

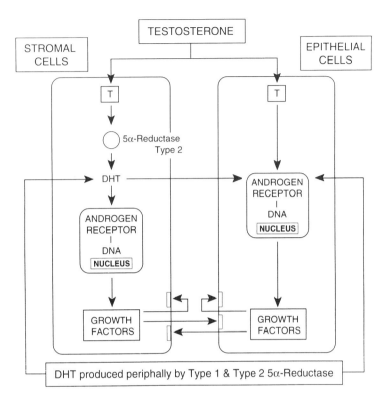

FIG. 38-28. Testosterone (T) diffuses into the prostate epithelial and stromal cell. Testosterone can interact directly with the androgen (steroid) receptors bound to the promoter region of androgen-regulated genes. In the stromal cell a majority of testosterone is converted into dihydrotestosterone (DHT)—a much more potent androgen—that can act in an autocrine fashion in the stromal cell or in a paracrine fashion by diffusing into epithelial cells in close proximity. DHT produced peripherally, primarily in the skin and liver, can diffuse into the prostate from the circulation and act in a true endocrine fashion. In some cases, the basal cell in the prostate may serve as a DHT production site, similar to the stromal cell. Autocrine and paracrine growth factors also may be involved in androgen-dependent processes within the prostate.

PSA in the serum that is unbound to plasma proteins (free PSA) have improved the specificity of PSA testing.

In men with only mild symptoms, and in those who elect medical therapy or observation, more diagnostic testing is not always necessary. If, however, invasive therapy is being considered or the results of the initial evaluation are discordant, further diagnostic testing is indicated (see Fig. 38-29).

Diagnostic Tests. The best noninvasive test to evaluate men with prostatism is the uroflow, measured by an electronic

Table 38-3
The AUA Symptom Scoring Index

	Not at All	Less than 1 Time in 5	Less than Half the Time	About Half the Time	More than Half the Time	Almost Always
1. Over the past month or so, how often have you had a sensation of not emptying your bladder completely after you finished urinating?	0	1	2	3	4	5
2. Over the past month or so, how often have you had to urinate again less than 2 hours after you finished urinating?	0	1	2	3	4	5
3. Over the past month or so, how often have you found you stopped and started again several times when you urinated?	0	1	2	3	4	5
4. Over the past month or so, how often have you found it difficult to postpone urination?	0	1	2	3	4	5
5. Over the past month or so, how often have you had a weak urinary stream?	0	1	2	3	4	5
6. Over the past month or so, how often have you had to push or strain to begin urination?	0	1	2	3	4	5
7. Over the last month, how many times did you most typically get up to urinate from the time you went to bed at night until the time you got up in the morning?						

0 none	1 1 time	2 2 times	3 3 times	4 4 times	5 5 or more times

AUA Symptom Score = sum of questions A1–A7 = ____.

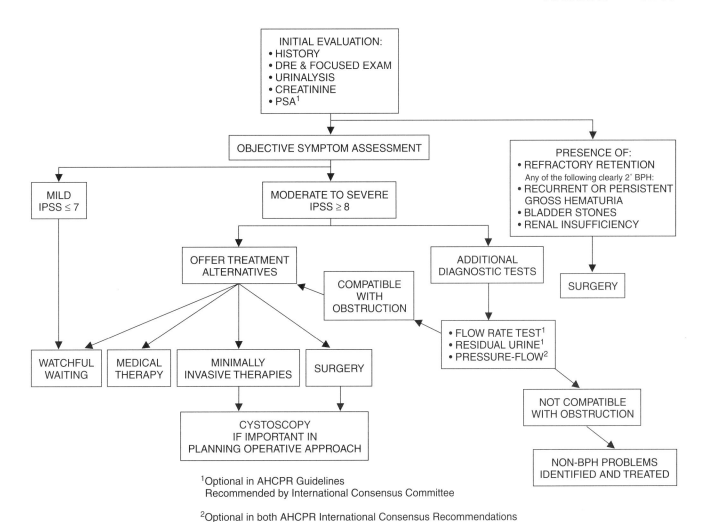

FIG. 38-29. *The decision diagram for the management of BPH recommended by the U.S. government's AHCPR BPH Guideline Panel.*

device that calculates the velocity of urine flow. The maximal urinary flow rate (Q_{max}) is normally greater than 15 mL/s. A reduction in Q_{max} is suggestive of obstruction. Men with normal flow rates and lower urinary tract symptoms are not likely to have BPH as the cause. Unfortunately, uroflow does not distinguish obstruction from poor bladder contractility, nor does it localize the site of obstruction, e.g., BPH versus urethral stricture. Despite these limitations, the test is especially valuable in patient follow-up and in quantifying the response to therapy.

Measurement of the postvoid residual (PVR) by catheterization or ultrasonography is helpful in assessing the bladder's response to obstruction. Large residual urine volumes (>300 mL) may be associated with a higher risk of disease progression. PVR, however, has considerable intraindividual variation, and consensus is lacking about the amount of residual urine that should prompt active therapy.

The most sensitive and specific test to confirm the presence of bladder outlet obstruction is pressure-flow urodynamics. In this evaluation, bladder pressure is measured during urination. High bladder pressures and low flow indicate obstruction. Unfortunately, a significant number of tests are equivocal and are invasive and costly. Urodynamic studies are indicated in patients

at risk for neurogenic bladder disease and in patients in whom the diagnosis of BPH is still uncertain after noninvasive tests.

Endoscopic evaluation of the lower urinary tract by cystourethroscopy can easily distinguish urethral stricture disease from BPH and provide information on prostatic configuration (i.e., the presence of a middle lobe). Endoscopic demonstration of an "obstructing prostate" and bladder trabeculation, however, is of unproved value. Endoscopy should be considered in men before invasive or surgical therapy but is probably not justified in men being treated conservatively.

Renal imaging by excretory urography or by ultrasonography is indicated in the evaluation of BPH in men who have concomitant UTI, hematuria, renal insufficiency, a history of urolithiasis, or previous urinary tract surgery. Renal imaging is not cost-effective in routine cases. Prostatic imaging by ultrasonography can provide much of the same information provided by endoscopy.

Treatment. Men with only mild symptoms or asymptomatic prostatic enlargement should be managed by watchful waiting. By contrast, men who have developed urinary retention, recurrent infections, bladder stones, or renal insufficiency secondary to BPH should be treated surgically. For men with bothersome symptoms, watchful waiting, medical therapy, and surgery should be presented to the patient as treatment options.

Watchful Waiting. Observation is the most appropriate therapy for men with only mild symptomatology (AUA symptoms score <7) (see Fig. 38-29). A significant number of men with moderate to severe symptoms will not progress or will find their symptoms not bothersome enough to warrant therapy. Patients in this group should be seen annually, and the baseline evaluation repeated.

Surgical Therapy. Transurethral resection of the prostate (TURP) is the most common surgical procedure to treat BPH. TURP is clearly the most effective treatment for BPH. Between 80 and 90 percent of patients undergoing TURP experience significant improvement in urinary symptoms and uroflow. The procedure is usually done under regional anesthesia, with tissue removal achieved by an electrocautery-type loop inside a modified cystoscope (resectoscope). The operative mortality for TURP is 1 percent or less, but morbidity rates can be high in elderly patients with underlying cardiovascular disease. Short-term complications include the rare absorption of hypotonic irrigation fluid leading to hyponatremia (TURP syndrome), blood loss requiring transfusion (5 percent), urinary retention, and infection. Long-term complications include urinary incontinence (1 percent), impotence (5 to 10 percent), retrograde ejaculation (78 to 80 percent), and the need for repeat endoscopic surgery for either recurrence, bladder neck contracture, or urethral stricture disease (10 to 15 percent at 8 years). Transurethral laser prostatectomy and electrovaporization techniques have been evaluated, but these have not been shown to be more effective than the standard TURP.

Transurethral incision of the prostate (TUIP) is almost as effective as TURP in glands smaller than 30 g in size. In this endoscopic procedure, one or two incisions are made through the prostatic capsule posteriorly. Without removing tissue, this procedure reduces urethral resistance. The procedure can be done on an outpatient basis and has less risk of retrograde ejaculation, impotence, and blood loss than TURP.

Because of prolonged resection times and the resulting increase in complication rates, very large prostate glands (>60 to 80 g) can be treated by simple retropubic or suprapubic prostatectomy. In these procedures, a lower abdominal incision is made, and the obstructing prostatic tissue is "enucleated" through an incision in the prostatic capsule (retropubic) or in the anterior wall of the bladder (suprapubic). Complication rates for open prostatectomy are probably no higher than for TURP, but incisional morbidity makes TURP the preferred procedure if the size of the prostate does not preclude it.

Medical Therapy. Currently, there are two medical approaches to the treatment of BPH. α-Adrenergic receptor blockers (doxazosin, terazosin, tamsulosin) relax prostatic smooth muscle and partially relieve the "dynamic" component of obstruction. Selective α_1 antagonists achieve significant symptom and flow rate improvement in 30 to 50 percent of men. Side effects of asthenia, headache, dizziness, and orthostatic hypotension occur in 10 to 15 percent of men.

The 5α-reductase inhibitor finasteride reduces intraprostatic dihydrotestosterone levels significantly, without lowering plasma testosterone levels. After 6 months of therapy, the average patient will experience a 20 percent reduction in the size of the prostate. Only one-third of men, however, experience significant improvement in symptoms or uroflow. The major advantage of the drug appears to be a 50 percent reduction in the need for TURP and the risk of AUR. Between 10 and 14 percent of men report sexual dysfunction when treated; otherwise, the drug has no significant side effects. Finasteride lowers the serum PSA level, but this can be corrected simply by multiplying the serum PSA value by 2. Cancer detection does not appear to be compromised.

Minimally invasive treatments for BPH include transurethral needle ablation (TUNA) and transurethral microwave thermal therapy (TUMT). These approaches are safe and effective, but their long-term durability is uncertain.

NEOPLASMS

Renal Parenchymal Tumors

Incidence and Etiology. Renal tumors account for approximately 2 percent of cancer deaths. The frequency in males in twice that in females, and there is a relationship between the incidence and smoking. The histologic origin of most carcinomas in males is from the renal tubular cell, as evidenced by the electron microscopic demonstration of a microvillous brush border on the carcinoma cells.

Pathology. Benign renal tumors (adenomas) frequently are noted on postmortem examinations, but they are rarely clinically significant. There are three major types of malignant tumors of the renal parenchyma. Renal cell carcinoma accounts for 85 percent of these lesions. Grossly, the tumor is yellow, at times pink, and often contains cystic areas of hemorrhage and necrosis. There is a tendency for the tumor to invade its own venous system, extending into the vena cava and even into the right side of the heart. Resection of tumors with this marked intravascular extension is feasible, occasionally using cardiopulmonary bypass, and cures have resulted. Microscopically, the dominant cells appear clear but are often admixed with granular cells.

Wilms' tumor (adenomyosarcoma) characteristically occurs in children and accounts for 14 percent of parenchymal malignancies. Sarcomas arising from interstitial tissue constitute 6 percent of malignancies. Tumors of the collecting system make up 14 percent of renal malignancies but are not considered in the parenchymal category.

Clinical Manifestations. The classic triad of pain, mass, and hematuria occurs late and is seen in its entirety in less than half the patients. Marked variations in the prevalence of these symptoms have been noted in reported series: gross hematuria, 31 to 76 percent; pain, 24 to 75 percent; mass, 6 to 50 percent; fever, 16 percent; metastatic pain, 6 percent. Hematuria is a late manifestation that represents erosion of the tumor into the collecting system. A palpable mass is more frequently present if the tumor involves the lower pole of the right kidney. Pain has been related to stretching of the renal capsule, in which instance it is usually mild but persistent. Sudden severe flank pain may accompany bleeding into the tumor. The passage of blood clots mimics colic from a ureteral stone. Fever is probably caused by necrosis of a tumor. Adult parenchymal tumors are usually not associated with hypertension unless there is a renin-producing tumor. Hypertension is a more frequent accompaniment of

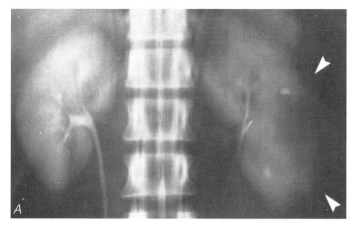

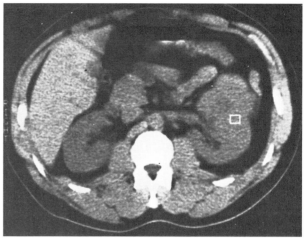

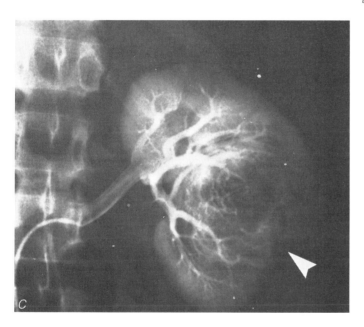

FIG. 38-30. *Renal carcinoma. A. Tomogram shows left renal mass with calyceal distortion (arrows). B. CT scan showing solid left renal mass with irregular contour. Square on mass denotes area selected for density measurement. C. Selective left renal arteriogram reveals characteristic renal carcinoma hypervascularity (arrow).*

Wilms' tumor. Hypertension also has been related to compression of the renal artery with resulting renal ischemia.

Erythrocytemia is present in 2 percent of patients with hypernephroma, which accounts for 7 percent of patients evaluated for polycythemia. Erythropoietin has been extracted from these renal tumors. Hepatic cell dysfunction (Stouffer's syndrome), reversible with removal of the renal carcinoma, has been noted.

Early detection often is the result of abdominal imaging studies, such as CT scans, that have been performed for evaluation of noneurologic conditions. Metastases, which were seen in one-third of patients at the time of diagnosis in the pre-CT scan era (lungs, bones, lymph nodes, and skin), is now seen in fewer than 15 percent of newly diagnosed cases.

Diagnosis. A mass lesion can be seen on an excretory urogram. The uninvolved, functioning portion of the kidney is visualized, whereas the tumor is not. If the renal vein is occluded, the kidney fails to visualize.

Although ultrasonography is helpful in forming the diagnosis, CT usually provides more meaningful information, differentiating between solid and cystic lesions and determining the extent of the tumor and operability (Fig. 38-30). MRI has been used to determine the extent of vascular invasion. The use of arteriography has been reduced because of the more liberal application of CT, but selective renal arteriography provides a "road map" of the arterial pattern that may be helpful if partial nephrectomy is contemplated (Fig. 38-31) and to detect recurrence in the tumor bed. A vena cavagram will identify extension of tumor into that vessel (Fig. 38-32), although MRI is more commonly used for this purpose.

Treatment. Radical nephrectomy with removal of the ipsilateral adrenal and hilar nodes is the standard operation for unilateral renal neoplasms. In this operation, the kidney is removed with the surrounding Gerota's fascia and perinephric fat (Fig. 38-33). Early ligation and division of the pedicle minimize blood loss from the usually present extensive collaterals. Preoperative percutaneous angioinfarction, however, is seldom helpful. For small tumors in the cortex or tumors in a solitary kidney, partial nephrectomy is an appropriate option.

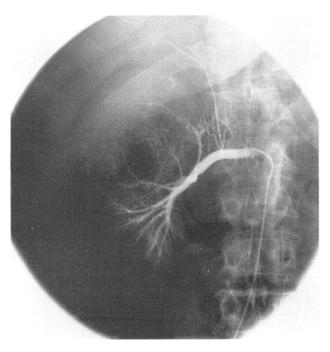

FIG. 38-31. Selective right renal arteriogram showing renal cell carcinoma.

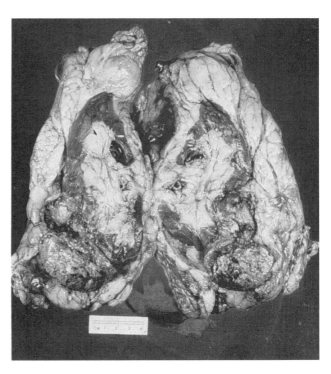

FIG. 38-33. Surgical specimen from a radical nephrectomy. Note that the kidney is within Gerota's fascia and that there is a lower-pole tumor extending from the kidney into the fat beneath Gerota's fascia. Approximately 22 percent of renal cell carcinomas have already extended through the renal capsule into the fat, and thus the tumor might be incompletely resected if the kidney was not removed intact within Gerota's fascia.

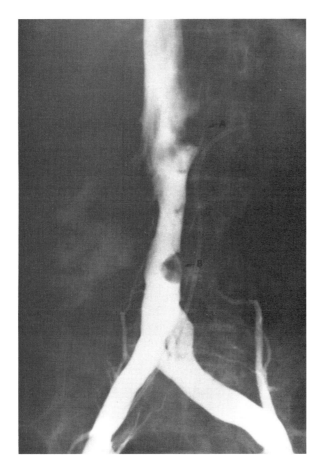

FIG. 38-32. Tumor involvement of vena cava. Renal vein tumor extending into lumen of vena cava (**A**). Direct extension of renal tumor into vena cava (**B**).

Removal of the primary tumor is occasionally followed by regression of metastases. Resection of isolated metastases in the lungs or extremities is associated with prolonged survival. No chemotherapy or immunotherapy has been predictably effective.

Results. Because 80 percent of renal carcinomas are diagnosed by CT in their asymptomatic phase, the 5-year survival now approaches 70 percent. For patients with low-grade local lesions, survival equals actuarial life expectancy. Survival is influenced by histologic type, extension into the perinephric tissues, lymph node, or renal vein involvement, and distant metastases.

Other Parenchymal Tumors

Other solid neoplasms of the renal parenchyma are rarely encountered and are often confused with renal cell carcinoma because of the presence of pain, hematuria, and a solid intrarenal mass.

Oncocytoma. Oncocytoma appears often as a large mahogany-colored, well-demarcated renal neoplasm with a central area of necrosis or a stellate scar, depending on the age of the area of necrosis. The cells have abundant granular eosinophilic cytoplasm (rich in mitochondria) arranged about a space. Most of these oncocytomas have a benign course, but some deaths have occurred from metastatic disease. Some renal cell carcinomas have an oncocytic pattern, making it impossible to distinguish them from oncocytomas.

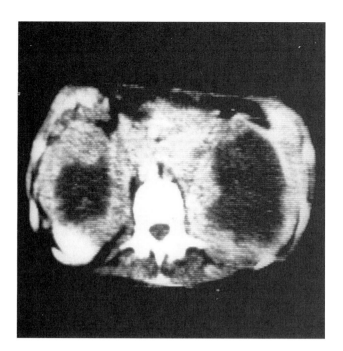

FIG. 38-34. *Hamartoma of the kidney (angiomyolipoma) may present as a unilateral or bilateral renal mass. "Large red kidney." Shown is a CT image of bilateral angiomyolipomas. The large amount of fat in these tumors shows as relatively black areas surrounded by a rim of normal parenchyma. Note the four basic radiographic densities sharply demarcated in this case: air, fat, bone, fluid. Fat is black but not as black as air.*

Angiomyolipoma. Angiomyolipoma (hamartoma) usually occurs as a solitary lesion but sometimes is associated with tuberous sclerosis and should be thought of in patients with adenoma sebaceum, seizures, mental retardation, and renal masses with or without hematuria. The three components vary, but the tumor usually can be differentiated by CT because of its fat content (Fig. 38-34). The lesion is benign and does not of itself usually require surgery but is often operated on because of complications, i.e., hemorrhage or sepsis, or because of confusion with renal cell carcinoma. Bleeding can be controlled by embolization. Rarely the lesion contains an intrarenal neoplasm.

Carcinoma of the Collecting System

Renal Pelvis and Ureter

Tumors of the renal pelvocalyceal system constitute about 14 percent of kidney tumors and are usually transitional cell carcinomas (TCCs); about one-third of patients with TCC of the kidney have TCC of the bladder at the same time. Squamous carcinoma has been associated with calculus in 50 percent of patients. Conversely, only 2 to 3 percent of staghorn calculi have concomitant squamous cell carcinoma.

Transitional cell tumors of the renal pelvis and ureter are histologically similar to their vesical counterparts. They occur more frequently in men and are seldom seen in patients under the age of 50. Gross hematuria and renal colic due to the passage of blood clots are common presenting symptoms. Intravenous pyelography frequently establishes the diagnosis, showing a filling defect in the involved portion of the pelvis or ureter (Fig. 38-35). Differential diagnosis of the filling defects includes blood clot and nonopaque (uric acid) calculi. Calculi can be ruled out by ultrasonography or CT scan.

Urine obtained by ureteral catheter lavage or brushing may demonstrate clusters of abnormal transitional cells. With a flexible nephroscope or ureterscope, direct biopsy can be performed. Transitional cell tumors of the pelvis tend to be multiple, and frequently, there are ureteral implants involving the ureter or the bladder. Treatment consists of removing the kidney, the ureter, and a margin of the bladder around the ureter orifice. The prognosis for survival is markedly reduced when the tumor infiltrates the adjacent parenchyma. Postoperative radiation therapy and chemotherapy have not been demonstrated to be valuable in improving the survival.

Patients with squamous cell carcinoma characteristically have no gross hematuria, flank pain, or mass and frequently present with a resistant urinary infection and markedly reduced function noted on intravenous pyelography. The associated infection or

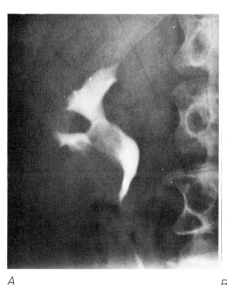

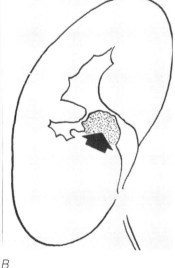

A   *B*

FIG. 38-35. *Carcinoma of the renal pelvis. A. Excretory urogram showing a filling defect in the right renal pelvis due to a transitional cell carcinoma. B. Tumor is indicated by arrow.*

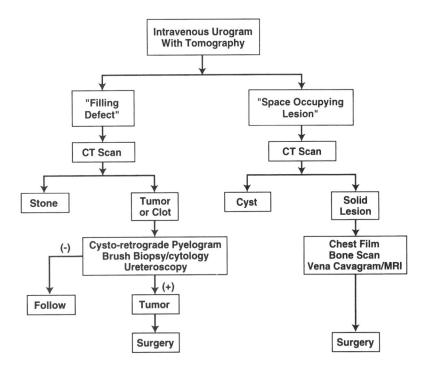

FIG. 38-36. Algorithm for evaluation of a renal lesion. Plan may be altered subject to the age and general health of the patient.

calculus frequently masks the tumor. Ureteral urinary cytology may demonstrate epithelial pearls. The treatment for squamous cell carcinoma is surgical excision, but the prognosis is exceedingly poor because of late diagnosis. Adjuvant radiation therapy and chemotherapy are ineffective.

An algorithm for the diagnosis and treatment of kidney tumors, subject to the age and general health of the patient, is shown in Fig. 38-36.

Urinary Bladder

Incidence and Etiology. The estimated incidence of new cases is approximately 45,000. The peak age incidence is 50 to 70 years of age, and the usual lesion is a transitional cell carcinoma. Approximately 7200 men and 3400 women die from cancer of the bladder annually, accounting for 2 percent of cancer deaths.

Bladder tumors have been related to the prolonged exposure to chemicals that are excreted in the urine as conjugated orthoaminophenols. These include β-naphthylamine and *para*-aminobiphenyl. Certain carcinogenic tryptophan metabolites are present in higher concentrations in the urine of patients with bladder tumors. There appears to be a prevalence of heavy cigarette smokers among the group with bladder tumors. Chronic infection with schistosomiasis and mechanical trauma from calculus also cause metaplasia and neoplasia of the bladder epithelium.

Clinical Manifestations. Gross or microhematuria is the initial sign and is present in 95 percent of patients at the time of diagnosis. Frequency and painful urination are late symptoms that result from sloughing of the tumor, infiltration, and secondary infection. In late cases, the neoplasm can occlude the ureters and lead to hydronephrosis and uremia, manifested by nausea, vomiting, and diarrhea.

The physical findings in early cases are minimal, since the tumor remains within the confines of the bladder. Local exten-

sion of the tumor may result in a nodular induration at the base of the bladder with fixation to the wall of the pelvis. This may be palpated on bimanual examination. Lymphatic spread may involve the pelvic and periaortic nodes. Osseous metastatic lesions are usually osteolytic and may cause nerve root pain.

Malignant cells are demonstrated cytologically by examining a urine specimen or bladder washings. The tumor is demonstrated on an excretory urogram or a cystogram (Fig. 38-37).

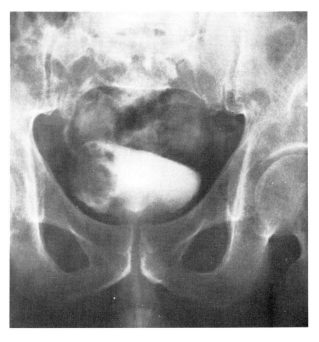

FIG. 38-37. Bladder carcinoma. IVU showing a filling defect on the right side of the bladder due to papillary transitional cell carcinoma.

Cystoscopic examination and cold punch biopsy establish the diagnosis and assess the depth of penetration. Preoperative studies to determine the stage include chest x-ray, CT scan of the abdomen and pelvis, and MRI (especially T2-weighted images).

Treatment. Bladder cancers are categorized as superficial non-muscle-invading lesions and deep tumors with invasion of muscle (Fig. 38-38). Endoscopic resection is suitable for superficial well-differentiated lesions. Intravesicle therapy, such as thiotepa, mitomycin, Adriamycin, or BCG (bacille Calmette-Guérin) can be given to decrease the risk of recurrence. Patients with superficial lesions treated by local therapy require periodic cystoscopic examinations.

For tumors infiltrating the bladder wall, cystectomy with supravesical diversion of urine by means of a cutaneous ureteroileostomy (ileal loop), cutaneous ureterocolostomy (colon loop), continent (catheterizable) supravesical diversion, or orthotopic neobladder is indicated (Fig. 38-39). Continent forms of urinary diversion give patients a significantly improved quality of life.

For patients with advanced nonresectable disease, palliation can be achieved by radiation therapy or transurethral local resection followed by the topical application of chemotherapeutic agents. Diversion of the urine relieves suffering by diminishing bladder stretching and spasm and avoiding the discomfort of voiding. Diversion also will reduce the bleeding and prevent sepsis.

Prognosis. The survival depends on the stage: stage A (T_1), 90 percent 5-year survival; stage B (T_2), 55 percent; stage C (T_3), 13 to 20 percent; stage D, less than 5 percent. Skinner has

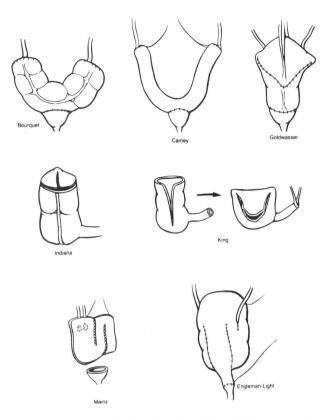

FIG. 38-39. Types of urinary diversion. (*Upper left*) Barquet, using horseshoe-shaped piece of colon to enlarge or replace bladder. Ureters are implanted into the colon. (*Upper middle*) Camey, a horseshoe-shaped piece of small bowel used to enlarge or replace the bladder. Ureters are implanted into the small bowel. (*Upper right*) Goldwasser, using a patch of colon, cecum, or sigmoid folded back on itself (detubularized) with ureters implanted into the bowel. (*Center*) Indiana pouch and King pouch, using ileocecal junction. (*Lower left*) Mainz pouch, using ileocecal junction. (*Lower right*) Endleman-Light, using a pouch made of ileum and sewn to the urethra (a variant of the Hautmann pouch). When the entire bladder is removed, the patient relies only on his external sphincter for continence and may wet the bed at night. (From: *Hinman F (ed): Atlas of Urologic Surgery. Philadelphia, W.B. Saunders, 1989, with permission.*)

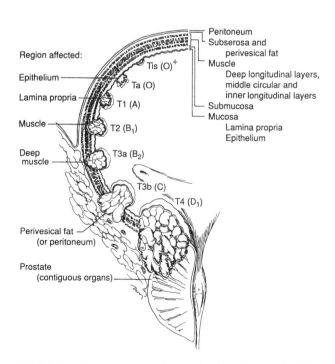

FIG. 38-38. Diagram showing tumors involving the urinary bladder and staging of the tumors according to the depth of penetration of the bladder wall and contiguous organs such as prostate. (From: *Carroll PR: Urothelial carcinoma: Cancers of the bladder, ureter, and renal pelvis, in Tanagho E, McAninch J (eds): Smith's General Urology, 13th ed. Norwalk, CT, Appleton & Lange, 1992, pp 341–358, with permission.*)

reported a 5-year survival of 36 percent for a series of stage D patients who received a combination of *cis*-platinum, cyclophosphamide, and Adriamycin (CISCA). Others have reported equivalent improvement for stage D patients receiving combination chemotherapy.

Prostate

Incidence. In the current era of PSA detection, the incidence of newly diagnosed cases is 400,000 per year, with 45,000 men dying each year. The incidence at autopsy in 65-year-old men is 35 percent; in 90-year-old men it is 70 percent. It is estimated that approximately 5 million men are living with histologic cancer of the prostate. The tumor accounts for 10 percent of male cancer deaths.

Pathology. The causation remains unknown, but an association has been noted to occur when there is atrophy of the gland. Carcinoma can occur in any portion of the gland, and two or three areas are simultaneously involved in about one-third of patients. The apical portion is particularly vulnerable to penetration and spread along the ejaculatory ducts to the base of the gland and the seminal vesicles. The obturator and internal iliac nodes are the first areas of nodal involvement.

The tumor is an adenocarcinoma in more than 90 percent of patients. Criteria of malignancy include small glands in juxtaposition without an intervening stroma, loss of a double layer of nuclei in the acini, capsular invasion, perineural space invasion, and nodal and distant metastases.

Diagnosis. In the past, the diagnosis was suggested by palpating a prostatic nodule on rectal examination. More than 50 percent of prostatic nodules palpated on rectal examination are positive for cancer on biopsy. The liberal use of the PSA screening test has increased the detection rate fourfold in the past decade. PSA levels have been correlated with the clinical extent of disease (Table 38-4). Ultrasonic visualization of hypoechoic areas in the prostate has improved the accuracy of biopsy. An elevated serum acid phosphatase level is characteristic of carcinoma of the prostate, while an elevated alkaline phosphatase level is suggestive of bony metastases.

Early-Stage Carcinoma

This represents disease that is localized to the gland (organ-confined) without extension beyond the capsule or to distant sites. After establishing the diagnosis, the patient should be evaluated for possible radical prostatectomy. The patient's age and general medical condition are important determinants.

The nerve-sparing technique has brought back prostatectomy as the most acceptable treatment for cure. Preservation of the caversonal nerves responsible for erection and maintenance of the external sphincter mechanism have produced a higher incidence of postoperative potency and continence, respectively. Currently, a patient considering radical prostatectomy should anticipate a more than 90 percent incidence of continence. A 50-year-old man will have a 50 to 70 percent chance of remaining potent postoperatively; if the patient is 70, that chance is reduced to 20 percent.

External-beam radiotherapy is an alternative method of treatment. The 5- and 10-year survivals of 75 and 60 percent, respectively, are essentially the same as those achieved with radical prostatectomy. If the patient is not a candidate for either form of therapy, he can be managed with estrogen therapy or other agents to reduce the androgen level or can undergo orchiectomy. In some instances patients have been followed for long periods without specific treatment.

Advanced Carcinoma

The average age of the symptomatic patient who presents with advanced prostatic cancer is 72. Typically, the symptoms are of a few months' duration, with rapid progression of frequency and nocturia leading to acute retention in 28 percent. Weight loss is common; severe back pain occurs in 14 percent and sciatica in 56 percent. Gross hematuria occurs in only 8 percent of patients, and lymphedema secondary to lymphatic obstruction is present in 4 percent.

Rectal examination characteristically demonstrates a fixed, enlarged, nodular, stony hard prostate. The serum PSA level is usually greater than 20 ng/mL; acid and alkaline phosphatase levels are elevated in two-thirds of patients with extension of tumor or metastatic disease. Combined osteoblastic and osteolytic bony metastases are present in 60 percent, whereas isolated osteolytic metastases are rare. Pulmonary metastases occur in some patients and may be miliary in appearance.

Treatment of symptomatic advanced carcinoma consists of androgen blockade therapy and/or orchiectomy. Reduction in serum testosterone to castration levels may be accomplished with surgical castration (bilateral orchiectomy) or with analogues of luteinizing hormone-releasing hormone (LHRH: medical castration). This treatment rapidly improves pain and anorexia and gradually relieves the obstructive urinary symptoms. The addition of oral antiandrogens is of minimal additional benefit in the average patient. If a large residual urine persists, transurethral prostatic resection may be indicated.

X-ray therapy to isolated metastatic bone lesions is also palliative. Corticosteroids in large doses are symptomatically beneficial but have no direct effect on the tumor. Both 5- and 10-year survival rates depend on the stage of disease at the time of institution of therapy. Chemotherapy regimens for advanced cases after endocrine therapy fails have some benefit, especially the combination of alkylating agents with estramustine. Experimental gene therapy and vaccine studies are underway.

Testicular Tumors

Incidence and Etiology. Testicular tumors account for 2 percent of cancers in the male, and the average age at diagnosis is 32 years. Testicular cancer is seen infrequently in blacks. The cause of human testicular tumors is unknown, but they occur 11 times more frequently in undescended testes and 50 times more often in abdominal undescended testes; they may be related to imperfect embryogenesis. Seminomas represent about 40 percent of malignant testicular tumors, embryonal cell carcinomas and teratocarcinomas about 25 percent each, and adult teratomas 8 percent; choriocarcinoma is limited to about 1 to 2 percent. Embryonal carcinomas and teratocarcinomas are the more common lesions in men in their twenties, whereas older men usually have seminomas. Combinations of tumors are common. A nongerminal neoplasm known as the *Leydig cell tumor* makes testosterone and results in precocious puberty in children but is generally asymptomatic in adults. Lymphomas rarely have been reported in men in their sixth and seventh decades. Benign tumors are very rare.

Clinical Manifestations. Patients usually present with a nonpainful "lump" in the testis. On examination, the lesion is firm, nontender, and solid and does not transilluminate. Occasionally tumors are misdiagnosed as simple hydroceles because of the formation of a secondary hydrocele. The diagnosis of epididymitis may be made erroneously in some situations and delay the appropriate diagnostic surgical intervention. In the patient with a testicular tumor, a large scrotal mass also may de-

Table 38-4
Correlation Between Prostrate-Specific Antigen (PSA) and Extent of Disease

PSA	% Capsular Penetration	% Seminal Vesicle	% Lymph Node	N
<15	49	7	2	41
15–40	65	31	21	29
>40	100	87	63	8

velop as a result of rupture of the tumor with formation of a hematocele. Late symptoms of metastatic disease include weight loss, fatigue, hemoptysis, and enlargement of the regional lymph nodes with associated ureteral obstruction.

Diagnosis and Treatment. If a testicular tumor is suspected, surgical exploration is indicated. Ultrasonographic evaluation may be helpful in localization of intrascrotal lesions. Measurement of serum β-chorionic gonadotropin (β-hCG) and α-fetoprotein (AFP) markers should be done prior to surgery, but surgical treatment should not be delayed for the results. If the lesion is confined to the testis on physical examination, an inguinal surgical approach is preferred. The spermatic vessels are occluded before the testis is exteriorized for inspection in order to prevent the spread of tumor. Palpation of induration in the testis is indication for radical orchiectomy, and there is little place for biopsy, because more than 90 percent of solid lesions of the testis in this age group are malignant. In patients with apparent lymphatic or pulmonary spread, the primary tumor should be resected for pathologic evaluation.

Staging has been applied to selection of a therapeutic regimen. Stage A lesions are confined to the testis and cord. Stage B lesions have positive retroperitoneal nodes and are subdivided according to the extent of nodal involvement into B1, B2, and B3. Stage C designates distant metastases above the diaphragm or involvement of visceral organs, including lungs, liver, and brain. Preoperatively, the retroperitoneal nodes are best assessed by CT. In addition to CT-defined nodal involvement, other indications for retroperitoneal node dissection include (1) invasion of lymphatics or blood vessels within the parenchyma by nonseminomatous tumors, (2) invasion of the spermatic cord by nonseminomatous tumors, (3) persistence of a large volume of teratocarcinoma within the testis, and (4) failure of markers to return to normal after removal of testis containing nonseminomatous germ cell elements.

Stage A seminomas usually are treated with 27 to 36 cGy to the abdomen. Stage B seminomas are treated with abdominal radiation therapy and/or chemotherapy with VP-16 and *cis*-platinum. Stage C seminomas receive chemotherapy alone. Stage B and C embryonal cell tumors are treated with chemotherapy alone or followed by retroperitoneal lymph node dissection. Teratocarcinomas are managed with retroperitoneal lymph node dissections. After puberty, teratomas usually are invasive and should be treated in the same fashion as teratocarcinomas. Choriocarcinomas are almost always fatal, but node dissection and chemotherapy are advised.

Prognosis. The 5-year survival depends on the cell type and stage of disease at the time of operation. Currently acceptable 5-year survival figures are listed in Table 38-5.

Table 38-5
Five-Year Survival Rates by Tumor Stage for Patients with Testicular Tumors

Tumor	Stage A	Stage B	Stage C
Seminoma	97	87	80–90
Teratocarcinoma	96	90	<55
Embryonal (choriocarcinoma)	96	93	60–80

Patients who are free of disease for 2 years are usually cured. Chemotherapy for germ cell neoplasms has doubled the survival for patients with advanced disease. Five-year survivals have been in the 90 to 95 percent range for patients with stage A and B nonseminomatous tumors. Ominous signs include high markers at presentation (i.e., beta-chain β-hCG > 8000 mIU/mL, AFP > 1000 IU/mL), failure of markers to normalize, development of intracranial disease, or increasing size of the tumor following node dissection and chemotherapy.

Subsequent therapy depends on the histologic diagnosis. Additional surgical treatment is of little use with choriocarcinoma because this tumor is associated with pulmonary metastases in 81 percent of patients. Pulmonary lesions are present in only 19 percent of patients with seminoma, but bilateral retroperitoneal lymph node resection appears unnecessary for this lesion because it is extremely radiosensitive. Lymph node resection usually is indicated for adult teratomas, embryonal carcinoma, and teratocarcinoma without supradiaphragmatic spread. Lymphadenectomy in such patients increases the 5-year survival and aids in accurate staging of the disease, although observation alone may be considered for select stage A tumors after orchiectomy.

The use of such chemotherapeutic agents as vinblastine, actinomycin, bleomycin, *cis*-platinum, and other drugs in combinations has markedly increased the survival of patients with advanced metastatic testicular tumors. These agents may cause severe hemopoietic changes, especially when combined with x-ray therapy. Adjuvant chemotherapy has been responsible for doubling the number of long-term survivors with advanced disease. Tumor markers (β-hCG and AFP) are valuable aids in diagnosis and follow-up. Figure 38-40 offers an algorithm for the management of the patient with a lesion of the testis.

Carcinoma of the Penis

Carcinoma of the penis develops in the squamous epithelium of the glans and foreskin. The risk of squamous cell carcinoma of the penis is almost eliminated by circumcision in infancy, and the incidence is decreased when the procedure is carried out in adulthood. The lesion is uncommon in the United States, and the average age of onset is over 60. Patients characteristically present with a sore that does not heal or a palpable nodule under the nonretractable foreskin (phimosis). Because of poor hygiene and associated infection, the diagnosis may be difficult. Biopsy provides a definitive diagnosis. Squamous cell carcinoma should be treated by local excision or partial or complete penilectomy and is associated with a 90 percent 5-year cure rate when no distant spread is present. With nodes involved by tumor, the 5-year survival is reduced to 32 percent, and excision of both inguinal and femoral nodes is attended by improved survival.

SEXUAL DISORDERS

Priapism. *Priapism* is defined as prolonged erection without sexual excitement. It results from a variety of vascular disorders. Blood is trapped within dilated arterioles of the erectile tissue by venous occlusion and cannot escape. Priapism differs from true erection in that the glans is not erect and the bulbospongiosus complex is not erect, whereas the corpora cavernosa are.

The most common cause currently is the injection of erection-producing agents by the patient. The antidote is to slowly inject

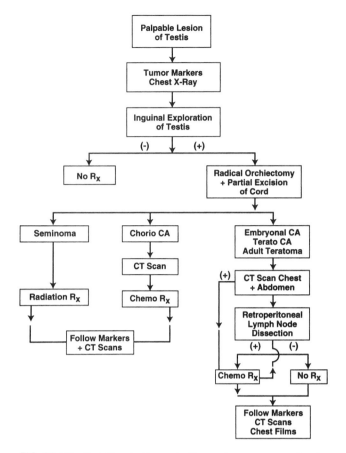

FIG. 38-40. *Algorithm for the evaluation and management of testicular cancers.*

a few milliliters of 1:100,000 epinephrine directly into the corpora to constrict the arterioles and permit spontaneous drainage. If this fails, injection of heparinized saline can be effective, or incision and drainage of the corpora can reverse the process. The Winter procedure, establishing a fistula between the corpora and the glans by incision or with a Tru-Cut biopsy needle, has been successful. Open operations that create shunts between the corpora cavernosa and corpora spongiosa or saphenous vein are seldom used.

Impotence. *Impotence* is defined as the inability to generate or maintain an erection adequate for penetration and sexual intercourse. Orgasm is a separate phenomenon, as is ejaculation. In evaluating the patient, history taking should pay particular attention to the use of antidepressant medications, antihypertensives, and other cardiovascular drugs. A thorough physical examination is essential, and laboratory tests for diabetes and vascular disease should be assessed.

Erection is enhanced by α-adrenergic blockers, e.g., dibenzyline, prostaglandin $E_{1\alpha}$, phentolamine, and papaverine, and is abated by sympathomimetic agents such as epinephrine. Orgasm is mediated through higher cortical centers. A man in whom all major pelvic motor nerves have been severed can experience an orgasm if cutaneous sensitivity persists. This has been noted in men who have undergone pelvic exenteration and insertion of a penile prosthesis. Dry (no ejaculate) orgasm is possible after removal of the entire bladder, prostate, and rectum.

Erection can be effected by use of a vacuum tube device, injection of prostaglandin E_1, or implantation of a solid or inflatable penile prosthesis. Vascular anastomosis for revascularization, i.e., inferior epigastric artery to penile artery or inferior epigastric artery to dorsal vein, is indicated only in younger men with traumatic arterial injury. Nitric Oxide (NO) has been demonstrated to enhance erections during sexual stimulation. The release of NO activates the enzyme guanylate cyclase, which results in increased levels of cyclic guanosine monophosphate (cGMP). This increased level of cGMP produces smooth muscle relaxation in the corpus cavernosum allowing the inflow of blood into the cavernous tissue. Sildenafil (Viagra™) enhances the effect of NO by inhibiting the enzyme which degrades cGMP. This is the first form of oral therapy for erectile dysfunction that has been proved to be effective following sexual stimulation.

Infertility. In evaluating infertility, both partners must be considered. A careful history must be taken from the man and the woman. Does each understand the appropriate timing of sexual activity for conception? Does the woman menstruate regularly? When did her menarche take place? Has she missed periods? Has she noted mucus show midway between her periods? If the patient's menarche occurred between 11 and 15 years of age, if she has not missed any periods, and if she menstruates regularly and has noted midcycle mucus show, there is a 95 percent chance that she is ovulating. A careful pelvic examination and an ultrasonographic examination of the uterus and ovaries determine the presence of any anatomic abnormality.

The man is exclusively at fault in 20 percent of the cases of infertility and a contributing factor in another 30 percent. His history should include questions related to exposures to unusual heat, including the frequent use of hot baths, and hernia repair during infancy. The medications that he has taken should be defined. Specific questions are important to determine if he experiences retrograde or premature ejaculation and if he achieves normal penetration. Physical examination should assess the testis, vas deferens, and epididymis bilaterally and the prostate.

The semen is best taken after 3 days of sexual abstinence. The specimen is allowed to sit at room temperature approximately 30 minutes for liquefaction before microscopic examination. Patients are classified as azoospermic, oligospermic (<20 million sperm/mL), or normospermic. Normally, there are 30 to 100 million sperm/mL, with at least 60 percent showing purposeful motility and less than 40 percent abnormal forms. The ejaculate should be checked for fructose, the absence of which suggests ductal obstruction. Luteinizing hormone (LH), follicle-stimulating hormone (FSH), testosterone, and prolactin levels should be measured. An FSH level over two times normal indicates a germ cell failure that is generally not reversible by treatment.

Failure to ejaculate can be caused by drugs such as α blockers, an incompetent bladder neck following transurethral resection, advanced pelvic atherosclerosis, or diabetes mellitus. The causes of azoospermia include ductal obstruction, germinal aplasia, drug toxicity, and Klinefelter's syndrome. Oligospermia can be a consequence of varicocele, cryptorchidism, or endocrine disorders or the sequela of juvenile mumps orchitis. Infertility associated with normal sperm, sperm counts, and sperm motility can be caused by abnormal sexual habits, prostatitis, gynecologic abnormalities, antisperm antibodies, or a defective acrosomal reaction.

If the man is oligospermic and the couple has tried to conceive for a couple of years under a physician's direction, in vitro fertilization or the use of pooled donor insemination can be tried, with a 15 to 20 percent anticipated success rate.

TRAUMA

Urologic injuries are rarely life-threatening, so the urologic surgeon may not be involved in the early resuscitative efforts of the trauma victim. However, the appropriate management of urologic injuries in the early phase of care may have a significant impact on the long-term outcome and quality of life of these patients. As such, timely urologic consultation is paramount in ensuring a good overall outcome.

Urologic trauma is classified according to the location of injury: upper urinary tract (kidneys and ureters), lower urinary tract (bladder and urethra), and external genitalia (penis, scrotum, and testes).

Kidney

The kidney is the most commonly injured structure in the urinary tract, accounting for 1 percent of all traumatic injuries. Nevertheless, operative intervention is pursued in only approximately 10 percent of renal injuries. The trend toward nonoperative management of renal injuries is the consequence of intense scrutiny of the outcomes of operative and nonoperative management; the end result is an algorithm of care for the trauma victim with upper tract injury that relies heavily on complete radiographic assessment.

The mechanism of renal injury, whether blunt or penetrating trauma, is critical to the decision-making process. The majority of renal injuries (80 to 90 percent) result from blunt trauma, which encompasses direct blows to the flank, falls, and motor vehicle accidents; deceleration injuries are particularly dangerous because they may lead to renal vascular injuries, such as renal artery thrombosis or intimal tearing. Penetrating trauma consists of stab wounds and gunshot wounds.

Initial Evaluation. The first step in the evaluation of the renal trauma victim is to obtain a careful history. The size of the weapon or caliber of the bullet in penetrating trauma, as well as the location of injury (chest, flank, abdomen) in blunt or penetrating trauma, is important in assessing the likelihood and severity of injury. In motor vehicle collisions, the speed of the vehicle and the position of the victim in the car can raise the index of suspicion of renal injury. A history of congenital renal anomalies should be elicited because of an increased likelihood of injury with even seemingly minor trauma. Physical examination includes careful inspection of the chest, abdomen, thorax, and flank for external signs of trauma such as bruising, entry or exit wounds, rib fractures, or abdominal distention.

The urinalysis is the single most important laboratory test in the evaluation of renal injuries. In most patients, a urethral catheter will be placed soon after arrival to the trauma unit, providing early assess to a urine specimen; the exception is the patient with suspected urethral injury, in whom a catheter is not passed routinely. The urine "dipstick" is adequate for the detection of hematuria and precludes the need for microscopic urinalysis, which is time-consuming and inconvenient.

Hematuria will be present in more than 95 percent of patients with renal injury and is the single most important indicator of injury to the kidney. The degree of hematuria, however, does not precisely correlate with the severity of injury. Indeed, hematuria may be absent in a small percentage of renal injuries. In particular, renovascular injuries have no associated hematuria in 24 to 60 percent of patients. As such, a high index of suspicion must be maintained in order to determine which patients need further radiographic assessment.

Radiographic Evaluation. The goal of radiographic assessment is to provide complete and accurate staging of renal injuries in order to determine the need for and to plan operative management. Most blunt renal injuries are minor, however, and can be managed conservatively. Consequently, selective imaging rather than generalized radiographic screening in adult patients with blunt renal trauma avoids low-yield studies in the majority of patients. Adult patients sustaining blunt trauma who have microscopic hematuria but no record of hypotension or shock (systolic blood pressure < 90 mmHg) in the field are exceedingly unlikely to have a major renal injury and may forego radiographic evaluation. Using these criteria, well under 1 percent of major renal injuries will be missed. These criteria do not apply to pediatric trauma patients; in this population, significant renal injury can occur even in the setting of microscopic hematuria without hypotension.

In contradistinction, patients with gross hematuria or those with microhematuria and shock are at significant risk for major renal injury; in one series, 12.5 percent of patients satisfying these criteria sustained major renal lacerations or renal vascular injury. Consequently, all adult patients with gross hematuria or microscopic hematuria and shock and all pediatric patients with hematuria require radiographic imaging (Fig. 38-41).

Patients with penetrating trauma to the kidney require renal exploration unless radiographic imaging clearly delineates injury that can be managed safely nonoperatively in a hemodynamically stable patient. CT scanning is the imaging modality of choice in this setting. For stab wounds, if the site of penetration lies posterior to the anterior axillary line, most injuries can be managed conservatively.

Historically, the IVU has been the initial imaging modality in most cases of renal trauma. This is performed with the rapid intravenous administration of 2 mL/kg of 30% iodinated contrast material after obtaining an initial scout film encompassing the kidneys, ureters, and bladder (KUB). Ideally, the IVU should include nephrotomograms to optimally assess the renal contour. Films are obtained at 1, 5, 15, and 30 minutes after the administration of contrast material if time permits. The IVU should establish the presence of two functioning kidneys, assess renal parenchyma, and delineate the collecting system and ureters. Nonvisualization on IVU implies absence of the kidney or significant renal vascular injury; poor visualization may indicate a major parenchymal injury. Extravasation of contrast material reflects collecting system injury and should prompt further radiographic imaging studies, usually with CT.

In the unstable patient, immediate laparotomy generally precludes a preoperative IVU. In this case, if exploration reveals a retroperitoneal hematoma, an intraoperative IVU should be obtained. An on-table KUB film is obtained, after which 150 mL of iodinated contrast material is administered intravenously. A

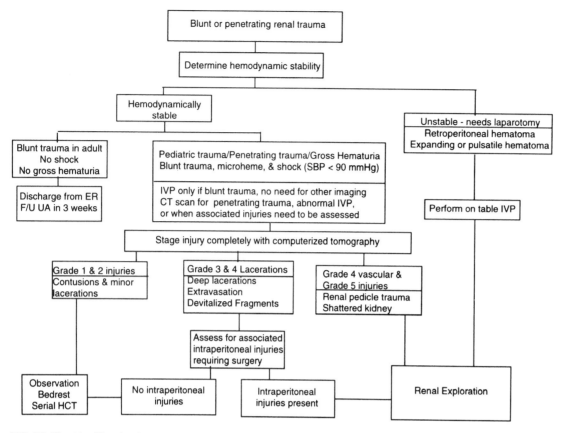

FIG. 38-41. Algorithm for the management of renal trauma. (From: *Wessels H, McAninch JW: Update on upper urinary tract trauma. AUA Update Series. Vol. 15, 1996, with permission.*)

single postcontrast film at 10 or 15 minutes is usually adequate to demonstrate contralateral renal function.

CT scanning is the most informative renal imaging study because it clearly identifies retroperitoneal or intrarenal hematomas, devascularized renal segments, parenchymal lacerations, and urinary extravasation (Fig. 38-42). A completely nonenhancing kidney suggests renal artery injury. In addition, CT demonstrates associated intraabdominal injuries. Consequently,

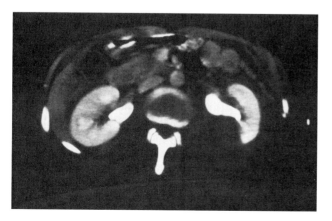

FIG. 38-42. *CT scan in a patient sustaining blunt trauma showing a devitalized (nonperfused) segment in the posterior aspect of the left kidney.*

CT has largely replaced the IVU as the imaging study of choice in the stable trauma patient.

Arteriography demonstrates renovascular injury to the main or segmental renal artery, renal lacerations, and urinary extravasation. However, CT has replaced arteriography in most instances; the advantage of CT over arteriography is its noninvasiveness, the added information provided regarding associated injuries, and clear delineation of a retroperitoneal hematoma (Fig. 38-43). If an arteriogram is performed to evaluate the aortic arch, additional views of the kidney may be helpful. Currently, arteriography is most useful in the delayed setting to evaluate recurrent or persistent bleeding; selective embolization of a bleeding vessel may then be performed concurrently.

Classification. The Committee on Organ Injury Scaling of the American Association for the Surgery of Trauma devised a classification system for renal injuries (Fig. 38-44). Grade I represents renal contusion with or without subcapsular hematoma; these injuries maintain an intact renal capsule and collecting system. Grade II injuries include minor cortical lacerations without injury to the collecting system or extension into the deep medulla. Grade III injuries encompass deep parenchymal lacerations not involving the collecting system. Grade IV injuries involve deep parenchymal lacerations with extension into the medulla and collecting system or contained injury to the main renal artery or vein. Grade V injuries include fractured kidneys or renal artery or vein avulsion.

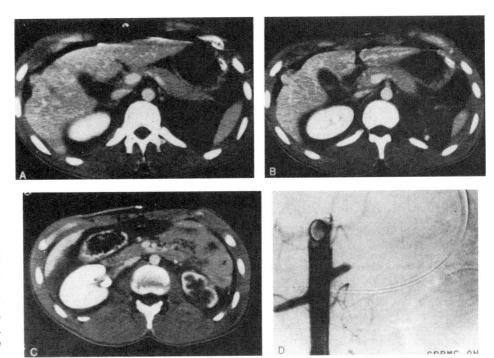

FIG. 38-43. *CT scan. A–C. Visualization of normal, contrast-enhanced right kidney, but in the left kidney, only a cortical rim is enhanced, a classic sign of arterial injury. D. Aortogram demonstrates a complete transverse intimal tear of the main left renal artery. (From: Peters PC, Sagalowsky AI: 1992, with permission.)*

Management of Renal Injury. Absolute preoperative indications for renal exploration include hemodynamic instability due to renal hemorrhage and grade V renal injury. Intraoperatively, the observation of a pulsatile or expanding retroperitoneal hematoma mandates renal exploration. If a preoperative IVU was not obtained, an on-table one-shot IVU should be performed to document contralateral renal function prior to exploration.

A retroperitoneal hematoma encountered at the time of laparotomy should be explored if preoperative radiographic staging was incomplete. If preoperative or intraoperative staging suggests an injury that can be observed safely, the hematoma is left intact.

Relative indications for renal exploration include extensive urinary extravasation, devitalized parenchymal segments, suspicion of renovascular injury, and incomplete staging. By these criteria, grade I and II renal injuries can be managed safely nonoperatively. In contrast, a high incidence of delayed bleeding (23.5 percent) has been noted in grade III and IV injuries that were managed nonoperatively. Grade III or IV renal injuries as-

FIG. 38-44. *Classification of renal injury (see text).*

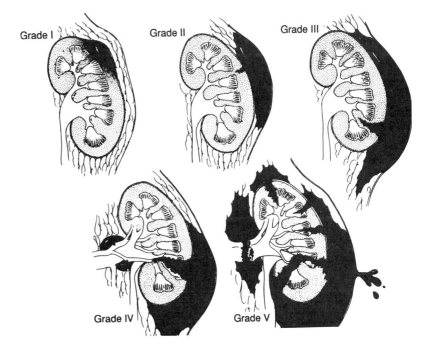

Grade I   Grade II   Grade III

Grade IV   Grade V

sociated with a devitalized renal segment have been shown to have a higher incidence of delayed complications such as urinoma or abscess formation. Consequently, management of grade III and IV injuries is determined by the clinical situation; if laparotomy is performed for associated intraabdominal injuries, repair of grade III and IV injuries is recommended. Urologic complications are more likely to occur when intraabdominal injuries are present. In the absence of associated injuries necessitating laparotomy, grade III and IV injuries can be observed safely with bed rest and serial hematocrit testing. Persistent bleeding or instability mandates surgical exploration or restaging. Arteriography may demonstrate a vascular lesion amenable to selective arterial embolization.

The presence of urinary extravasation does not necessarily mandate renal exploration; in most cases the collecting system will seal spontaneously. However, renal pelvis lacerations are unlikely to seal without intervention, and ureteropelvic junction avulsions require repair. Consequently, visualization of the opacified ureter on CT or IVU is critical in excluding a ureteropelvic junction avulsion. Differentiation between renal pelvic and calyceal extravasation is difficult and may not be possible in the acute setting. As such, persistent urinary extravasation should alert the clinician to a possible renal pelvis injury. In this case, placement of a retrograde ureteral catheter may allow the laceration to seal successfully, obviating the need for exploration and repair.

Major renal vascular injuries require immediate exploration and repair. Small segmental arterial injuries often can be managed nonoperatively with a reasonable expectation of an uncomplicated outcome. In some cases, selective renal arterial embolization may obviate the need for exploration in cases of significant hemorrhage.

Renal artery thrombosis is usually associated with deceleration injury and occurs when stretching of the renal artery leads to intimal tearing and thrombosis. Renal artery thrombosis is difficult to diagnose and treat. Even with prompt diagnosis, successful revascularization occurs in fewer than 30 percent of patients. Furthermore, delayed hypertension occurs commonly even in patients with presumed successful revascularization. Consequently, revascularization is reserved for patients with bilateral renal injury or injury to a solitary kidney. Historically, penetrating injury to the kidney mandated renal exploration. Current teaching, however, suggests that accurate preoperative radiographic staging, usually with CT, can distinguish injuries that require exploration and repair from those which can be managed safely nonoperatively. In the presence of associated injuries requiring laparotomy, renal exploration should be performed. This situation is more likely to occur with gunshot wounds rather than stab wounds.

Operative Management. The preferred approach for laparotomy is a midline transabdominal incision, even in cases of suspected isolated renal trauma. This approach allows inspection of intraabdominal organs and vessels in an expeditious fashion. In most cases, repair of intraabdominal organs or vessels will precede renal exploration unless hemodynamic instability is attributed to renal vascular injury or massive parenchymal bleeding.

The need for early vascular control of the renal vessels is controversial but, in general, is recommended to allow rapid control of bleeding once the hematoma is opened. In most cases,

occlusion of the renal vessels is unnecessary, but in cases of massive bleeding, rapid vascular occlusion may obviate the need for nephrectomy. The renal vessels are identified by incising a "window" in the posterior peritoneum directly over the aorta, just medial to the inferior mesenteric vein. Superior dissection along the anterior surface of the aorta will lead to the left renal vein as it crosses the aorta. The renal arteries are invariably found on either side of the aorta just posterior and superior to the left renal vein. Identification of the right renal vein may require mobilization of the duodenum. Multiple renal arteries are present in 25 percent of patients and occur equally on the right and left sides. Multiple renal veins occur in 15 percent of patients and appear more commonly on the right side.

Once vascular control is attained, the colon is reflected medially, Gerota's fascia is entered laterally, and the hematoma is evacuated. The kidney is then exposed in its entirety. If the kidney is deemed salvageable, devitalized renal parenchyma is debrided sharply, preserving the renal capsule to facilitate later closure. Deep polar lacerations may devascularize a large segment of tissue and are best managed with amputation. Lacerations in the midkidney or small lacerations are debrided, collecting system violations are closed, and bleeding vessels are oversewn. The margins of the laceration are reapproximated with a running absorbable suture through the renal capsule only. If the integrity of the collecting system cannot be ascertained adequately, injection of indigo carmine–stained saline directly into the renal pelvis will facilitate identification of collecting system openings. If a large parenchymal defect is present, the capsule is closed with interrupted mattress sutures over absorbable gelatin bolsters that are wedged into the defect. In the event that no capsule is available for closure, an omental flap is swung over the defect and sutured to the remaining capsular edges. After repair, the kidney is replaced within Gerota's fascia, and a closed suction drain is placed in proximity to the kidney.

Segmental renal vein injuries may be managed with ligation of the vessel. Segmental or main renal artery and main renal vein injuries should be repaired whenever possible. If acute renal artery thrombosis is diagnosed promptly, repair may be attempted with resection of the involved segment and end-to-end anastomosis, bypass grafting with autologous vein or synthetic graft, or autotransplantation.

Complications associated with renal injuries include urinoma or abscess formation, delayed or persistent bleeding, and hypertension. Most of these complications can be managed without the need for reoperation. For urinary extravasation or urinoma formation, retrograde ureteral catheterization or percutaneous antegrade decompression of the collecting system, with or without percutaneous drainage of the urinoma, is adequate in most cases. A perinephric abscess generally also can be drained percutaneously. Delayed bleeding may be managed with selective transcatheter arterial embolization, thereby precluding the need for open exploration. The development of posttraumatic hypertension may be due to renal artery thrombosis, an ischemic renal segment, arteriovenous fistula, or a Page kidney. The hypertension may be managed medically, or partial or total nephrectomy may be necessary. Arteriovenous fistulas are managed with arterial embolization.

Ureter

Because the ureter is mobile and well protected by surrounding retroperitoneal fat and muscle, ureteral injuries are rare. The ureter may be injured, however, as a result of external violence (penetrating or blunt trauma) or by iatrogenic injury during an operation.

Initial Evaluation and Radiographic Imaging. Unfortunately, acute ureteral injuries are associated with few diagnostic hallmarks; consequently, these injuries are frequently missed until the sequelae are apparent. Blunt trauma is rarely associated with ureteral injury except in cases of ureteral avulsion, primarily in children; as such, a high index of suspicion, particularly in cases of deceleration injury, is necessary to identify these injuries. Penetrating trauma requires radiographic imaging of the upper urinary tract and should detect ureteral injury in most cases.

The intravenous urogram detects ureteral injury with a high degree of accuracy. Extravasation of contrast material is pathognomonic, but delayed opacification of the ureter or ureteral dilatation above the site of injury may raise the suspicion of ureteral injury. CT is very sensitive for detecting extravasated contrast material along the ureter and can diagnose ureteropelvic avulsion by the absence of contrast material in the distal ureter.

Retrograde pyelography is generally reserved for delayed diagnosis of missed ureteral injuries. In the multiply injured patient, a retrograde pyelogram is impractical and usually unnecessary; most ureteral injuries are associated with intraabdominal injuries requiring laparotomy, at which time the ureter can be explored.

Operative Management. Acute ureteral injuries diagnosed at initial evaluation should be managed with open surgical repair via a midline transabdominal incision. In the absence of upper tract imaging, an on-table IVU should be obtained to evaluate the function of the contralateral kidney. If the mechanism of injury or path of the projectile placed the ureter at risk, the ipsilateral ureter should be mobilized and inspected in its entirety. Intravenous administration of indigo carmine or direct injection of indigo carmine–stained saline into the renal pelvis can identify subtle ureteral injuries. Alternatively, if the bladder is open, retrograde passage of a ureteral catheter can facilitate identification of a full-thickness ureteral injury.

The principles of ureteral repair include debridement of nonviable tissue, spatulation of ureteral edges, creation of a tension-free, watertight anastomosis over an internal ureteral stent, and drainage of the field with a Penrose or closed-suction drain.

Less than full-thickness ureteral injury or suspicion of blast effect in an apparently intact ureter may be treated with placement of an internal ureteral stent and a retroperitoneal drain. For a partial laceration with viable remaining ureter in continuity, the laceration should be reapproximated over a ureteral stent with interrupted absorbable sutures.

Ureteropelvic junction avulsion is managed with debridement and spatulation of the wound edges and then reapproximation. Placement of a ureteral stent and a closed-suction or Penrose drain is advisable.

Ureteral injury above the iliac vessels usually can be managed with primary ureteroureterostomy (Fig. 38-45). If a large defect precludes primary reanastomosis despite mobilization of the kidney, a transureteroureterostomy may be considered. However, it is always preferable to avoid involvement of the noninjured side if at all possible. Alternative options include autotransplantation or ileal ureter substitution; these maneuvers usually are reserved for elective repair of the injured ureter, and

in the acute setting the ureter may be ligated and a percutaneous nephrostomy performed to establish drainage until the repair can be performed. In rare cases, if a long ureteral defect is present with significant associated vascular or intraabdominal injuries in an unstable patient, nephrectomy may be the best option.

Injury below the level of the iliac vessels is best repaired with a ureteroneocystostomy, in which healthy ureter is anastomosed to the bladder. Mobilization of the kidney and proximal ureter usually provides ample ureter to reach the bladder. If additional distance is needed, a psoas hitch is performed, in which the dome of the bladder is mobilized and then secured to the psoas tendon with several interrupted nonabsorbable sutures. Healthy proximal ureter is then reimplanted into the bladder. For longer defects, a bladder flap is rolled into a tube into which the ureter is reimplanted submucosally (Fig. 38-46).

The same principles of successful repair apply to ureteral injury caused by surgical misadventure. Recognition of these injuries is often delayed until the patient develops a urinoma, abscess, ureterocutaneous fistula, hydronephrosis, or sepsis. In the delayed setting, retrograde pyelography and CT scan can delineate the injury and associated complications. Injury diagnosed within a week of presentation can be repaired surgically at that time if no infection is present. Beyond that period, it is best to manage the injury with percutaneous nephrostomy drainage and an antegrade ureteral stent; a urinoma or abscess should be drained percutaneously. In some cases, 4 to 6 weeks of urinary diversion and stinting may allow resolution of the injury. If a ureteral stricture forms, endoscopic management with endoureterotomy or balloon dilation may be successful.

Bladder

In the adult, the bladder is an extraperitoneal organ relatively well protected from external trauma by the bony pelvis, the symphysis pubis, pelvic floor, and rectum. In contrast, the bladder is an intraperitoneal organ in the child and is susceptible to external injury.

Initial Evaluation. Penetrating trauma to the lower abdomen from gunshot or stab wounds may injure the bladder. Bladder injury may occur from bony spicules generated from a pelvic fracture. Blunt trauma to the bladder may occur from motor vehicle accidents, blows to the abdomen, falls, or crush injuries to the pelvis. A full bladder is particularly susceptible to intraperitoneal rupture from blunt trauma.

Signs and symptoms related to bladder injury are relatively nonspecific and generally consist of vague suprapubic discomfort or inability to urinate. The accumulation of intraperitoneal urine may lead to referred shoulder pain or respiratory distress. In patients at risk for bladder injury, urine should be collected for urinalysis or "dipstick" evaluation. Gross hematuria will be present in over 95 percent of patients with bladder injury.

Radiographic Evaluation. The diagnosis of bladder rupture is established by static cystogram. A Foley catheter is passed into the bladder if there is no suspicion of urethral injury (or after obtaining a retrograde urethrogram if there is), and a scout film is obtained. Approximately 100 mL of water-soluble iodinated contrast material (15 to 30 percent) is instilled into the bladder by gravity drip, and an anteroposterior film is taken. If no gross extravasation of contrast material is seen, further contrast material is instilled until a total of at least 300 mL has been

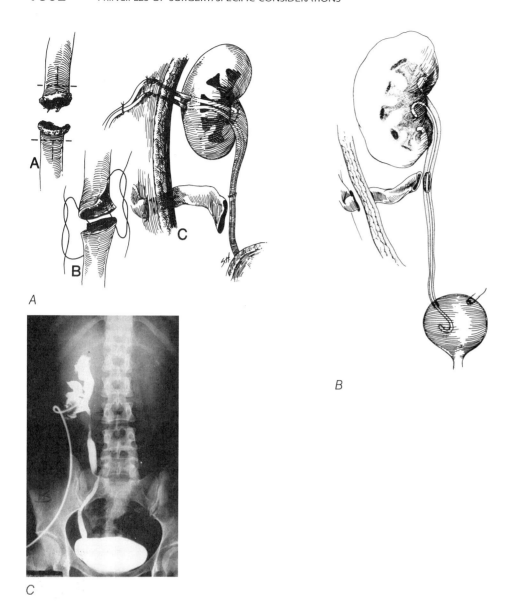

A

B

C

FIG. 38-45. *A. Method of ureteral repair. Note nephrostomy tube and stent and drain near site of repair. B. Recently preferred method shows internal ureteral stent in place with drain near site of repair. The use of a nephrostomy is rarely necessary. C. Antegrade pyelogram in postoperative period shows prompt drainage into the bladder and no urinary extravasation. The nephrostomy tube can be removed safely.*

given. Anteroposterior, both obliques, and postdrain films are obtained. In some cases, subtle extravasation of contrast material is identified only after the bladder has been drained of contrast material. The use of CT cystography has been advocated by some practitioners as a time-saving measure in patients already undergoing CT imaging; the bladder is distended during scanning by clamping the Foley catheter before imaging. The accuracy of this method is controversial; false-negative studies have been reported when the bladder is not actively distended before imaging. However, if retrograde cystography is performed, CT may be used to image the bladder with the expectation of a high degree of accuracy.

Blunt bladder injuries are classified according to the extent and location of injury. Bladder contusion represents a non-full-thickness injury of the mucosa or muscular layer, and no extravasation is identified on cystogram.

Intraperitoneal bladder rupture generally occurs as a result of a sudden blow to the lower abdomen or pelvis, particularly with a full bladder. The dome of the bladder represents the weakest and most vulnerable part of the bladder; as such, the sudden force is transmitted to the dome, which ruptures. On cystography, intraperitoneal extravasation of contrast material outlines loops of bowel and fills the paracolic gutters (Fig. 38-47). Intraperitoneal bladder rupture often occurs in multiply, severely injured patients and, accordingly, is associated with a high mortality rate.

Extraperitoneal bladder rupture occurs with equal frequency compared with intraperitoneal bladder rupture. Extraperitoneal

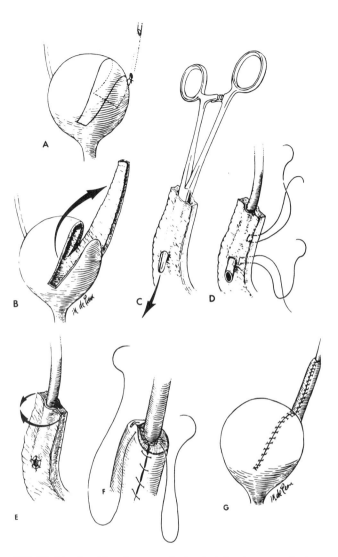

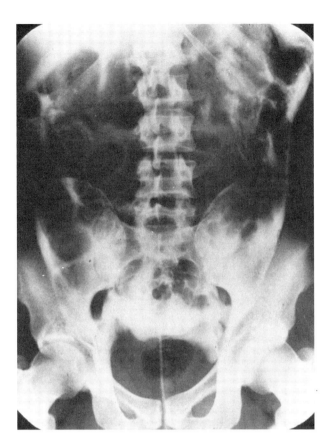

FIG. 38-47. Intraperitoneal rupture of the bladder. Note contrast material outlining loops of bowel and along the paracolic gutter.

FIG. 38-46. Boari flap for ureteral reimplantation in cases of extensive loss of distal ureter. Note creation of the submucosal tunnel to prevent reflux.

rupture is closely associated with pelvic fractures. Indeed, 89 to 100 percent of extraperitoneal bladder ruptures are associated with a pelvic fracture; conversely, only 5 to 10 percent of pelvic fractures are associated with bladder rupture. The typical finding on cystogram is extravasation of contrast material into the pelvis around the base of the bladder. The characteristic "teardrop" deformity represents bladder compression by a large pelvic hematoma (Fig. 38-48). A combination of intraperitoneal and extraperitoneal bladder rupture may occur, usually in conjunction with a pelvic fracture or penetrating injury.

Treatment. Management decisions are based on the location and extent of injury. Bladder contusions require no specific therapy or short-term catheter drainage only.

Intraperitoneal bladder rupture from blunt or penetrating trauma should be explored and repaired via a transabdominal incision so as to allow exploration of the abdomen for associated injuries. If necessary, the bladder opening is extended to facilitate inspection of the bladder neck and trigone. Any extraperitoneal bladder lacerations should be closed from within the

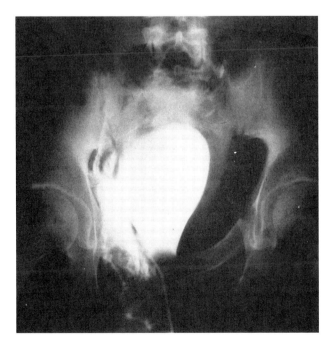

FIG. 38-48. Extraperitoneal rupture of the bladder. Bladder shadow extends to the symphysis. Note flame-shaped extravasation of contrast material. A pelvic fracture is present.

bladder using a single running layer of chromic catgut or polyglycolic suture. The ureteral orifices should be identified and ureteral injury excluded by observing efflux of clear urine from each side; if necessary, intravenous administration of indigo carmine will facilitate identification of the ureteral orifices in an injured, edematous bladder. Passage of ureteral catheters into each ureter helps identification of ureteral or ureteral orifice injury. A large-caliber ($\geq$24 Fr) suprapubic catheter is placed near the dome of the bladder and brought out through a separate stab incision in the bladder and skin.

Most cases of extraperitoneal bladder rupture due to blunt trauma do not require operative intervention and will heal with 7 to 10 days of urethral catheter drainage only. If laparotomy is performed for associated intraperitoneal injuries, however, it is prudent to open the dome of the bladder and repair the bladder injury intravesically. The perivesical hematoma should be left undisturbed to avoid introducing bacteria. No correlation between the degree of extravasation and the size of bladder perforation has been found; accordingly, the decision to formally repair the bladder rather than manage it with catheter drainage should not be based on the degree of extravasation seen on cystography.

Iatrogenic endoscopic intraperitoneal bladder injuries deserve special mention. Provided the patient is hemodynamically stable and shows no signs of respiratory difficulty due to urinary ascites, drainage of the bladder with a large-caliber Foley catheter may be adequate for small perforations typical of endoscopic injury. Bladder injury occurring during laparoscopy may be repaired laparoscopically.

Complications associated with bladder rupture are usually due to failure to diagnose the injury or to adequately drain extravasated urine. Unrecognized extraperitoneal urine collection may result in pelvic abscess formation; intraperitoneal urine accumulation may lead to respiratory compromise and/or peritonitis. Delayed diagnosis of extraperitoneal bladder rupture should be managed with a large-caliber catheter in the bladder and percutaneous drainage of a pelvic abscess. Undiagnosed intraperitoneal bladder rupture requires transperitoneal exploration, drainage of urine or abscess, and closure of the bladder.

Urethra

Although anatomically the male urethra is divided into four regions (penile, bulbous, membranous, and prostatic), for the purpose of trauma, the male urethra is classified as anterior (below the urogenital diaphragm, including the penile and bulbous urethra) or posterior (above the urogenital diaphragm, including the prostatic and membranous urethra). Female urethral injuries are less common than male urethral injuries, and the only anatomic distinction of importance is to recognize bladder neck versus urethral injuries.

Initial Evaluation. Posterior urethral injuries are nearly always associated with pelvic fractures (>90 percent of cases). Crush injuries or penetrating trauma may result in disruption of the attachments of the prostate to the pelvic floor or symphysis pubis.

Anterior urethral trauma is usually associated with blunt straddle injuries in which the bulbous urethra is crushed against the pelvic arch. A direct blow to the perineum also may cause anterior urethral contusion or laceration. Uncommonly, vigorous sexual activity with fracture of the corpus cavernosa additionally

may cause blunt urethral trauma. Penetrating anterior urethral injury may occur with gunshot or stab wounds or as a result of urethral instrumentation.

The patient with a ruptured urethra may be unable to void despite the sensation of feeling full. Most patients with a urethral injury will have blood present at the urethral meatus. In some cases, perineal or penile swelling and ecchymosis will be present. A high index of suspicion of urethral injury must be maintained in any patient with a pelvic fracture.

On physical examination, suprapubic tenderness from a pelvic fracture may be elicited, and perineal or penile contusion may be obvious. On digital rectal examination, the so-called high-riding prostate may be identified, or the prostate may appear to be absent; a large pelvic hematoma causes superior displacement of the prostate when the urethra is disrupted. If blood is seen at the urethral meatus or the prostate is absent or superiorly displaced, urethral catheterization should not be attempted. In the absence of these signs, a careful attempt may be made to pass a urethral catheter.

Injury to the anterior urethra may be associated with disruption of Buck's fascia that surrounds the corporeal bodies and the corpus spongiosum of the urethra. If the urethral injury is contained by an intact Buck's fascia, blood and urine dissect along the penile shaft, producing swelling and ecchymosis of the penis. If Buck's fascia is violated, blood and urine may extravasate diffusely into the perineum, interior thigh, and lower abdominal wall and are limited only by Colles' fascia. Accordingly, a characteristic butterfly hematoma of the perineum and scrotum may be seen (Fig. 38-49).

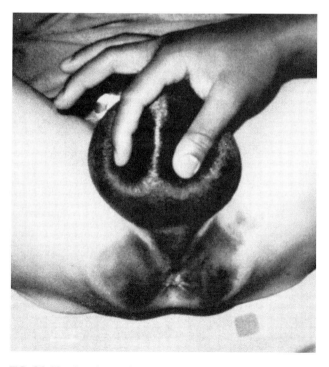

FIG. 38-49. Anterior urethral disruption with violation of Buck's fascia. Note limitation of urine extravasation and hemorrhage by the attachment of Colles' fascia to the fascia of the superficial transverse perinei, resulting in the characteristic butterfly appearance of the hematoma.

Radiographic Evaluation. Retrograde urethrography is the radiographic imaging study of choice for evaluation the patient with suspected urethral injury. In general, this study should precede any attempts to pass a urethral catheter. A scout film is obtained with the patient turned 25 to 30 degrees in the oblique position. A #14 or #16 French Foley catheter is inserted a few centimeters into the urethra, and the balloon is inflated in the fossa navicularis with 1 to 2 mL of water. Water-soluble, iodinated contrast material (15 to 20 mL) is injected into the catheter to distend the urethra, and a film is taken. Alternatively, a catheter-tip syringe can replace the Foley catheter if the meatus is closed tightly around the tip of the syringe; however, this method risks unnecessary radiation exposure to the examiner's hand. If a partial tear is present, contrast material may pass into the prostatic urethra and bladder, and extravasation will be minor. In the case of a complete tear, significant extravasation into the retropubic space is seen, and no contrast material is seen in the prostatic urethra. If no extravasation is identified, the catheter balloon is deflated, and the catheter is advanced into the bladder and the balloon reinflated. A cystogram can then be performed to evaluate the bladder.

Posterior urethral injuries are classified into three types depending on the radiographic appearance of the retrograde urethrogram. In type I injuries, the urethra is stretched from the surrounding pelvic hematoma but remains intact. Type II injuries represent partial or complete rupture of the prostatomembranous urethra at the apex of the prostate just above the urogenital diaphragm. Extravasation is seen superiorly in the pelvis but is limited inferiorly by the urogenital diaphragm. Type III injuries are most common and represent injury to the prostatomembranous urethra as well as the urogenital diaphragm and bulbous urethra. Extravasation occurs both above and below the urogenital diaphragm (Fig. 38-50). With penetrating trauma, extravasation may, in addition, track along the path of penetration.

Anterior urethral injuries are classified only as complete or incomplete, according to whether the urethra remains in continuity as revealed by the flow of contrast material into the bladder on retrograde urethrography. A straddle injury with hematuria but a normal urethrogram is assumed to represent a contusion.

Treatment. *Posterior Urethral Injuries.* No specific therapy is required for type I urethral injuries. However, a large pelvic hematoma may compress the urethra and prevent spontaneous voiding. Therefore, an indwelling urethral catheter may be placed until the patient is able to void spontaneously.

For partial urethral tears, a careful attempt at urethral catheter placement may be performed. The risk of this maneuver is conversion of a partial tear into a complete tear. If a catheter is placed successfully, drainage is continued for 2 to 3 weeks, followed by a voiding cystourethrogram to ensure adequate healing. A safer course of action is placement of a suprapubic tube for a few weeks, followed by a voiding cystourethrogram. After placement of the suprapubic tube, a formal cystogram should be performed to rule out a bladder injury.

The specific treatment for a complete urethral laceration is controversial and ultimately may influence the likelihood of urethral stricture formation, urinary incontinence, or impotence. Options for management include suprapubic cystostomy with delayed surgical repair versus immediate surgical realignment. Immediate attempts at suture repair of the urethral ends is fraught with difficulty and is ill-advised.

In the unstable patient or the patient with complex associated injuries, suprapubic cystostomy and delayed repair constitute the option of choice. Suprapubic diversion is continued for 3 to 9 months or until the pelvic hematoma has resolved. The injury is reassessed at the time with a simultaneous antegrade and retrograde urethrogram to assess the length and location of the injury.

In the hemodynamically stable patient undergoing exploration for associated injuries, immediate surgical realignment is a reasonable option, particularly in the patient with severe prostatic displacement, major bladder neck lacerations, or associated rectal or vascular injuries. Urethral realignment can be accom-

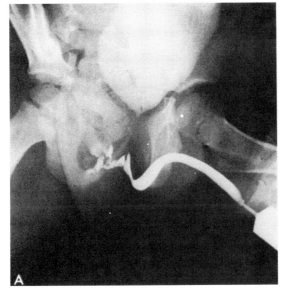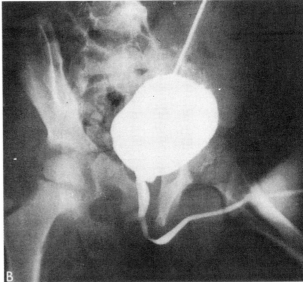

FIG. 38-50. Posterior urethral disruption treated by cystostomy. *A.* Disruption at time of presentation. *B.* VCUG through cystostomy 8 months later showing complete healing.

plished through a variety of techniques. The bladder is opened anteriorly, and a catheter is passed retrograde through the urethra; the catheter can be guided into the bladder by a hand in the wound, or it is passed into the prevesical space, where it is recovered. A second catheter passed antegrade from the bladder into the prevesical space is also retrieved. The two catheters are secured at their tips with a suture passed through their end holes; traction on the bladder catheter guides the urethral catheter into the bladder. The balloon is inflated, and the antegrade catheter is removed. Alternatively, retrograde flexible cystoscopy may reveal the true passageway into the bladder by endoscopic and fluoroscopic guidance. A Councill catheter is passed over the guidewire and positioned in the bladder. If necessary, simultaneous antegrade and retrograde flexible endoscopy may more clearly demonstrate the posterior urethra, thereby facilitating passage of a guidewire into the bladder. A number of investigators have advocated the use of magnetic catheters or sounds to establish continuity between the anterior and posterior urethra (Fig. 38-51).

Advocates of delayed surgical repair versus primary realignment cite conflicting rates of posttraumatic impotence and incontinence. The incidence of impotence and incontinence is likely a function of the severity of the trauma and not the initial treatment method.

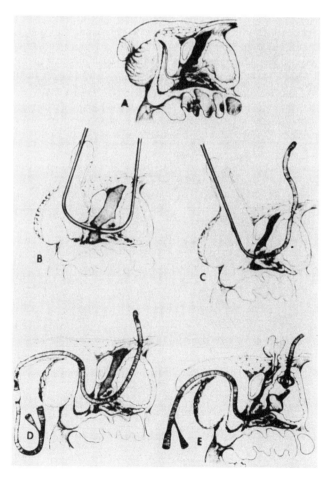

FIG. 38-51. Realignment of posterior urethra using magnetic or interlocking sounds to position a urethral catheter across the injury.

Regardless of the choice of initial management, delayed endoscopic repair has gained popularity for the definitive management of traumatic posterior urethral strictures, which occur in all patients managed with initial suprapubic diversion. A number of endoscopic techniques for reestablishment of urethral continuity have been proposed, including "cut to the light" techniques in which simultaneous antegrade and retrograde endoscopy is used to provide a target (the light from one endoscope) toward which the incision through the other endoscope is directed. Alternatively, a guidewire or needle may be passed through the cystoscope across the urethral scar using three-dimensional fluoroscopic imaging and/or digital rectal guidance to orient instrument passage with subsequent dilation or incision of the obliterated urethra. These techniques usually rely on a period of self-catheterization after removal of the urethral catheter in order to maintain an adequate channel. Advocates of endoscopic techniques cite favorable success rates (61 to 80 percent) and preservation of potency and continence. Detractors of endoscopic means of repair cite the frequent need for repeated procedures to maintain patency.

Despite the enthusiasm for endoscopic repair of posttraumatic posterior urethral strictures, open urethroplasty remains the "gold standard" for establishment of urethral continuity. A recent review of the experience at San Francisco General Hospital revealed a remarkable 97 percent long-term success rate after perineal anastomotic urethroplasty in 82 patients. A successful outcome depends on complete excision of periurethral scar and generous mobilization of the corpus spongiosum to reduce tension on the urethral anastomosis.

Anterior Urethral Injuries. Contusion of the anterior urethra, without urethral laceration, generally requires no specific treatment. Urethral catheterization is indicated only if bladder drainage is required. Partial urethral lacerations with minimal extravasation contained by Buck's fascia can be managed with suprapubic urinary diversion via a punch cystostomy tube for 7 to 10 days. In cases in which urethral continuity is fairly well maintained, careful passage of a urethral catheter is performed, and the catheter is left indwelling for a few days. For more extensive injuries with moderate to severe extravasation and violation of Buck's fascia, formal suprapubic tube placement is recommended.

Complete disruption of the anterior urethra with extensive soft tissue injury requires debridement of devitalized tissue and suprapubic urinary diversion. These injuries may be complicated by hematoma or abscess formation, and close observation with liberal short-term use of parenteral antibiotics is recommended.

Once the soft tissue edema, urinary extravasation, and hematoma have resolved with several months of suprapubic urinary diversion, a voiding cystourethrogram is obtained to determine the length and caliber of the resulting stricture. For short strictures, endoscopic visual internal urethrotomy may be highly successful. For more extensive strictures, primary repair via the perineal route may be accomplished using a free patch graft or a pedicled flap of penile skin to widen the anastomosis.

For penetrating injuries such as stab wounds or low-velocity gunshot wounds, debridement and direct end-to-end anastomosis are advisable. These injuries may be repaired over a catheter by reapproximating spatulated ends; a suprapubic tube is not necessary.

In females, urethral injuries are rare; however, most involve the bladder neck and vagina and require immediate reconstruction in order to maintain continence.

External Genitalia

Penis. Injury to the corpora cavernosa may result in extravasation of blood and urine within or outside of Buck's fascia depending on the extent of injury (Fig. 38-52). These injuries may be caused by penetrating trauma or by blunt trauma sustained during vigorous sexual intercourse when the erect penis encounters the partner's pubic bone. These injuries must be explored, usually through a circumcising incision with degloving of the penis, and the corpora repaired. Rupture of the suspensory ligament of the penis caused by sudden downward flexion of the erect penis requires exploration and repair to maintain penile stability.

Degloving injuries of the penis, usually associated with industrial accidents, mandate surgical debridement and excision of the penile skin distal to the proximal extent of injury; failure to excise distal skin invariably results in severe, permanent penile edema. Skin grafting may be performed when the wound is clean and granulating. Traumatic penile amputation is a rare event, but penile salvage is possible with microsurgical repair of the dorsal penile arteries and vein and selective skin grafting.

Scrotum. Scrotal skin is quite elastic and can be mobilized to cover extensive scrotal defects. Debridement of necrotic tissue

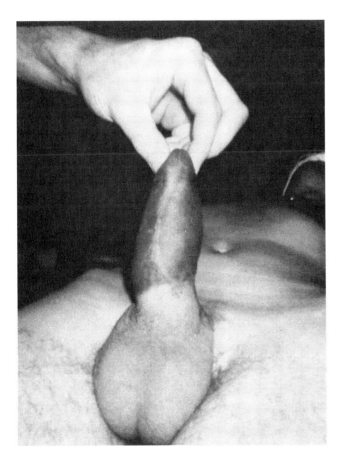

FIG. 38-52. Rupture of corpus cavernosum contained by Buck's fascia.

and foreign bodies is performed. Relatively clean wounds may be closed in layers with absorbable suture; contaminated wounds are managed with dressing changes and subsequently closed primarily or with the use of split-thickness skin grafts. If the remaining scrotal tissue is insufficient to cover the testicles, they may be wrapped daily with warm saline-soaked gauze until granulation tissue is sufficient to allow application of a split-thickness skin graft. Alternatively, the testes may be temporarily placed in thigh pockets.

Testis. Rupture of the testis may occur from either blunt or penetrating trauma. On physical examination, the scrotum is swollen, and the testicle may be indistinct because of surrounding hematoma. Scrotal sonography may help distinguish an intact from a ruptured tunica albuginea, but false-negative studies have been reported. When in doubt, the scrotum should be explored and the testicle examined. Extruded seminiferous tubules are debrided, and the tunica albuginea is closed with absorbable suture. A drain is left in place for 24 hours. A completely shattered testis may require orchiectomy, and patients always should provide informed consent for orchiectomy when undergoing scrotal exploration.

PEDIATRIC UROLOGY

Prepuce. If a boy has not been circumcised, phimosis (constriction of the meatus of the prepuce) can occur, preventing retraction of the foreskin. If smegma accumulates beneath the prepuce, adhesions can develop, preventing retraction. Inflammation of the glans, *balanitis,* can occur; a contraction ring can develop, and the inflammation can extend to the shaft of the penis, *balanoposthitis.* This is reversed by circumcision and prevented by reducing the prepuce and cleansing the glans and coronal area on a regular basis.

Congenital Anomalies

Urethral Meatal Stenosis. This occurs almost exclusively in the male and is believed to be a congenital anomaly. The diagnosis is made by calibration of the meatus using a catheter. The normal neonatal meatus should accept a #10 French sound. Meatotomy is the treatment.

Urethral Valves. These are usually seen in boys and produce variable obstructive changes. There are four anomalies of the male urethra that are not related to intersex problems. These are megalourethra with ballooning of the distal penis, anterior urethral valves, urethral duplication, and posterior urethral valves. Three types of posterior urethral valves were originally described, and a fourth type, a wind-sock valve, was added later. More than 95 percent are type 1 valves, running from the verumontanum to the distal urethra (Fig. 38-53). These are one-way valves; a catheter can be passed easily, but the valves balloon and obstruct the ureter as the child tries to void. There is often a weak or dribbling stream, and the situation can lead to uremia and hypertension. The amount of cystic renal dysplasia is the life-limiting factor (Fig. 38-54). In type 3 valves, the valve acts as a diaphragm or wind sock with a small hole in it.

Diagnosis is made by voiding cystourethrogram and endoscopy, each of which clearly depicts the site of obstruction. Dilatation of the proximal urethra and bladder and marked hydroureteronephrosis are characteristic. Management consists of

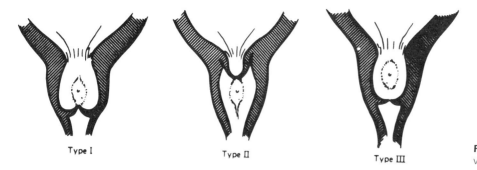

FIG. 38-53. *Types of posterior urethral valves. More than 95 percent are type 1.*

destruction of the valve(s). Preliminary cystostomy or catheter drainage might be required. The prognosis depends on the degree of secondary changes in the proximal collecting system and the renal function at the time of diagnosis.

Neurogenic Bladder. This is usually due to autonomic dysfunction accompanying meningomyelocele. Impaired sensation of filling leads to a large residual urine with overflow incontinence. The patient may present with symptoms of infection, diurnal incontinence, or impaired voiding. Diagnosis is established by excretory urography, voiding cystourethrogram, and cystometry. The latter study reveals a large residual urine with low-pressure, high-volume tracing and lack of sensation of filling until large volumes have been instilled.

Treatment for mild dysfunction can be manual assistance in voiding, coupled with therapy for infection. With moderately

severe involvement, treatment is directed at eliminating the residual urine. This can be accomplished by transurethral resection of the bladder neck. If the children are reminded to void at 2- to 3-h intervals, many become continent. Children can be taught intermittent catheterization when they reach 6 to 8 years of age. For severely compromised urinary tracts with marked loss of renal function, urinary diversion is indicated.

Ectopic Ureteral Orifice. The ectopic ureteral orifice usually drains the upper part of a double kidney, with complete duplication of the ureters. The condition is four times more prevalent in females. In order to be manifest symptomatically, the ectopic ureteral orifice must empty outside the urethral sphincter in the urethra or vagina. The characteristic complaint in the female is urinary incontinence despite normal voiding habits. The ureteral segment drained by the ectopic ureter is frequently not

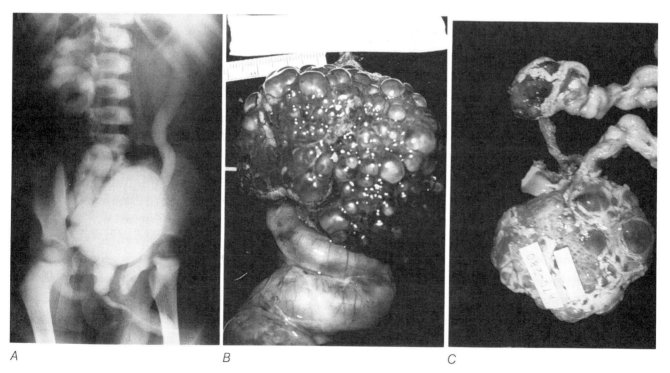

A   *B*   *C*

FIG. 38-54. *A. VCUG. Posterior urethral valves; 95 percent are type 1. Note bulging of urethra proximal to valve and normal urethra distal to valve. Dilated tortuous ureters. B. Cystic renal dysplasia and tortuous ureter. C. Autopsy specimen from child who died early in life from posterior urethral valves and cystic renal dysplasia. Note dilated tortuous ureters.*

visualized on the excretory pyelogram. Treatment is excision of the upper renal segment and ureter in some instances, but at times it is possible to reimplant the ureter into the bladder or into the other pelvis of the duplicated system.

Ureterocele. This is usually associated with a stenotic ureteral orifice. Adult or orthotopic ureterocele is rarely associated with duplication and frequently contains a small stone within its lumen. Infantile or ectopic ureterocele is often associated with duplication of the drainage system. As the intravesical ureter dilates, it forms a cystic mass that can become sufficiently large to obstruct the bladder neck during voiding. Occasionally, the ureterocele prolapses through the urethra (Fig. 38-55). Diagnosis is established by means of delayed films during intravenous pyelography (Fig. 38-56). The opaque-filled intravesical mass has a thin, nonopaque rim (the ureterocele wall) that contrasts with the opacity of the bladder content, giving the appearance of "cobra-head deformity." The pyelogram may show a large filling defect in the bladder and the functioning portion of the duplicated collecting system being pushed laterally and downward (Fig. 38-57), occasionally causing confusion with the pyelographic displacement caused by a neuroblastoma.

Many ureteroceles cause sufficient ureteral obstruction to warrant surgical treatment to preserve renal function. Small lesions can be removed by endoscopic incision or excision. Prolapsing ureteroceles with urethral obstruction require transvesical excision. In children, ureterocele is often associated with ureteral duplication and may be ectopic. Ureteral reimplantation is often required if reflux is present following endoscopic incision of the ureterocele.

Vesicoureteral Reflux. Once urine is transported from the renal pelvis to the bladder, it should not back up into the ureters or kidneys. Vesicoureteral reflux (VUR) is always abnormal. Conditions associated with VUR include posterior urethral valves, prune-belly syndrome (Fig. 38-58), complete duplication of the collecting system, ectopic ureter, ectopic ureterocele, Ask-Upmark kidney (segmental renal hypoplasia), neurogenic bladder, bladder neck obstruction, tuberculosis and other bladder infections, in some instances caused by suprapubic and indwelling urethral catheters, and bladder-urethral dyssynergia.

In adults, often there are no adverse effects of the reflux, particularly when the ureter is not dilated. In children, a number of changes occur secondary to reflux into the ducts of Bellini (reflux nephropathy). VUR runs in families, and asymptomatic reflux is common. Therefore, preadolescent siblings should be screened. A grading system is presented in Fig. 38-59. There is no direct correlation between the severity of renal damage and the grade of VUR. The diagnosis is made by VCUG using radiopaque or, preferably, radioactive material. The appearance of the ureteral orifice on cystoscopy has been correlated with the presence of reflux. The appearance has been described as normal or horseshoe, stadium, or golf-hole shaped. The golf-hole type is the most severe anatomic variety and the most apt to require surgical intervention.

In most cases, VUR can be managed without an operation. Infection occurs secondary to stasis of urine. Residual urine can be minimized by having the patient double-void, i.e., void a second time 10 minutes after completing the initial voiding. Antibiotics are administered until the reflux disappears. Two consecutive VCUGs at least 12 months apart showing no reflux are necessary to conclude that the reflux has disappeared. Recently, submucosal injection of polytetrafluoroethylene or collagen has been shown to eliminate VUR. Reimplantation of the ureter into the bladder is required almost exclusively in young children.

Ureteropelvic Obstruction. Congenital ureteropelvic obstruction is quite common (Fig. 38-60). Trichrome stains have shown that what appears to be a normal ureteropelvic junction actually can have significant replacement of the normal smooth muscle by collagen. Another finding is an anomalous vessel from the aorta to the lower pole of the kidney. During diuresis, the pelvis prolapses over this vessel, tenting and obstructing the ureter. Division of the vessel, however, will not correct the situation because the intrinsic abnormality is in the ureter.

The lesion can present in the newborn as a mass and in the adult with flank pain on hydration, the so-called beer drinker's kidney. There are often associated gastrointestinal symptoms such as nausea and vomiting. Diagnosis is established by excretory urography with delayed films noting impairment of renal excretion of contrast material. When the kidney is forming urine at low volumes, the pyelogram can appear normal.

Because the basic pathologic lesion is a deficiency of longitudinal muscle at the ureteropelvic junction, the treatment is to resect the diseased area and anastomose the renal pelvis to the healthy ureter below. Preliminary nephrostomy is seldom required. If the renal function is markedly reduced and the other kidney is normal, nephrectomy can be the procedure of choice.

Cystic Disease of the Kidney. Although clinically recognizable simple renal cysts are seldom seen in childhood, cystic disease of the kidney occurs more commonly in children. At times, the kidney can be so severely deformed as to be nonfunctioning and present as a lobular flank mass (Fig. 38-61A). In its most advanced form of cystic renal dysplasia, no glomeruli are noted on microscopic examination (see Fig. 38-61B). In *in-*

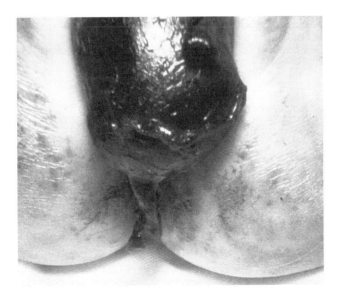

FIG. 38-55. *Prolapse of an ectopic ureterocele through the urethral meatus with complete obstruction of the urethra and impending strangulation gangrene of the ureterocele. The ureterocele can be reduced under anesthesia and then surgically corrected.*

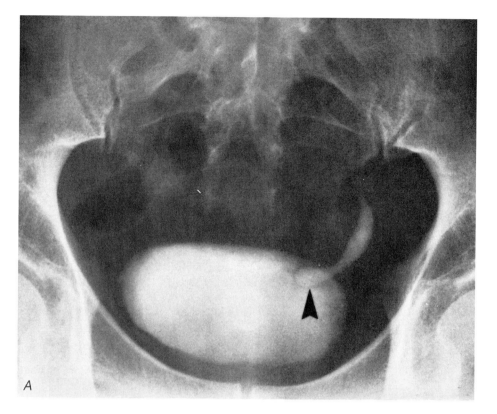

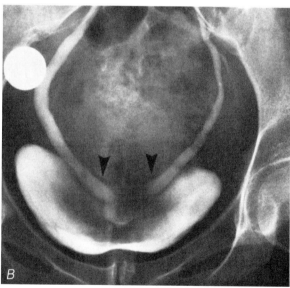

FIG. 38-56. Ureterocele. *A.* Left ureterocele (arrow). *B.* Bilateral ureteroceles (arrows). Note "cobra-head deformity" of the ureteroceles.

fantile polycystic disease there are many cysts throughout the kidney involving all segments of the nephron (Fig. 38-62). Despite the many cysts, the capsule is smooth, and the kidney retains a normal shape. These patients are often diagnosed shortly after birth. The disease is progressive, ultimately requiring dialysis and/or transplantation.

Adult polycystic disease of the kidney is inherited as a mendelian dominant trait and usually becomes manifest when the patient is over 30 years of age. The patients are "4-H Club members"—with headache, hypertension, hematuria, and heredity. The kidneys are large and nodular; many glomeruli are present.

The patients often ultimately progress to renal failure (Fig. 38-63).

Scrotal Contents

Cryptorchidism (see also Chap. 37). Even though it looks full, the scrotum should be palpated to be sure that a testis is present on both sides. About 30 percent of premature males have an undescended testicle; for full-term infants, the incidence is 4 percent. Spontaneous descent occurs in most of these by 1 year of age, when the incidence of undescended testicle is 0.8 percent. The cryptorchid testis must be differentiated from the

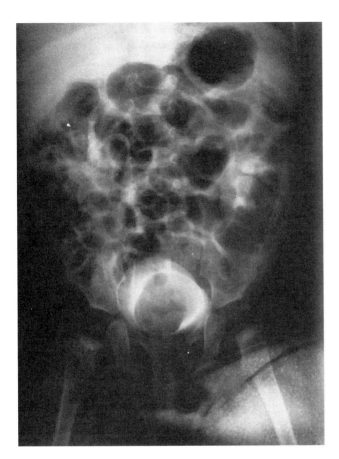

FIG. 38-57. *Ectopic (infantile) type of ureterocele. IVU shows lateral displacement of the left lower moiety of duplicated kidney by the hydronephrotic nonfunctioning upper-pole segment entering the ureterocele.*

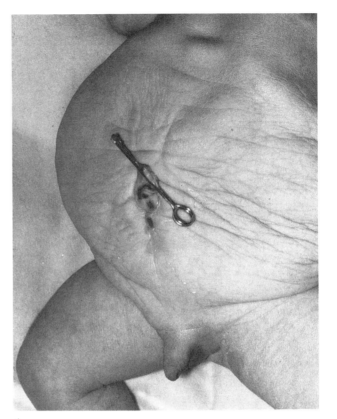

A

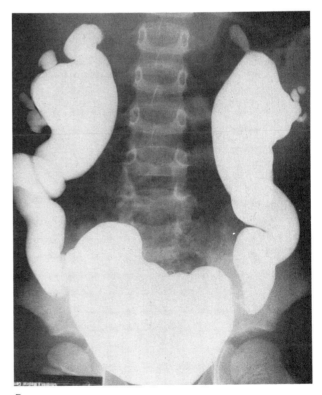

B

FIG. 38-58. *A. Prune-belly syndrome at birth. Note patent urachus, wrinkled abdominal skin, cryptorchidism. B. Cystogram in newborn prune-belly patient showing massively dilated upper tracts.*

retractile testis, which can be brought into the scrotum, and from the ectopic testis, which has already migrated beyond the external ring and can be found in a superficial pouch or in the perineum. The cryptorchid testis often has an associated indirect hernia that should be repaired by high ligation of the sac at the time of orchiopexy.

Nonpalpable testes are frequently found beneath the inguinal ring, but peritoneoscopy or celiotomy may be required to locate them. Bilateral cryptorchidism after 1 year should be treated initially with gonadotropins, resorting to operation in refractory cases. Rudimentary testes (2 to 3 mm) should be removed, and a prosthesis can be substituted. There is an association between cryptorchidism and testicular malignancy, abdominal testes having a higher incidence than inguinal testes. The opposite descended testis also has a higher rate of malignancy.

Testicular Neoplasms.   The most common testicular neoplasm in the adult, seminoma, is rarely seen before puberty. Embryonal carcinoma or its yolk-sac variant is the most common testicular tumor of childhood. Teratoma before puberty can be a benign tumor for which high inguinal orchiectomy is curative. By contrast, teratoma after puberty should be managed as a teratocarcinoma.

The interstitial cell (nongerminal) tumor behaves differently in the child. It has the ability to make testosterone as well as

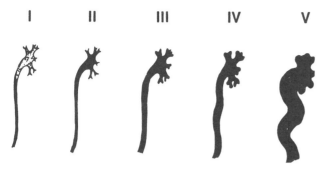

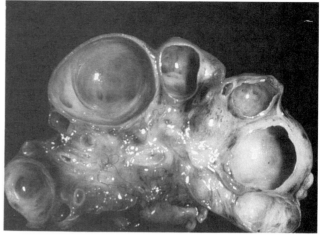

A

FIG. 38-59. The grading system adopted by the International Reflux Study in Children. Contrast material in the collecting system is represented in black. Grade I is assigned if the contrast material enters the ureter but not the renal pelvis. Grade II occurs when contrast material reaches the renal pelvis but does not distend it. Grade III occurs when the collecting system is filled and either the ureter or pelvis is distended but the calyceal demarcations are not distorted. Grade IV is assigned when the dilated ureter is slightly tortuous and the calyces are blunted. Grade V occurs when the entire collecting system is dilated and the calyces have become distorted and indistinct (From: *Arant BS Jr: Vesicoureteral reflux and renal injury. Am J Kidney Dis 10:491, 1991, with permission.*)

possessing 21-hydroxylase activity and has the ability to produce cortisol and 11-beta compounds. In the prepubertal boy it can cause virilization, advanced bone age, male muscular pattern, and evidence of adrenal cortical excess. The tumor is rarely malignant, and high inguinal orchiectomy is curative. Feminizing tumors causing gynecomastia; decreased libido and impotence are uncommon.

Gonadoblastoma occurs more commonly in childhood, usually in patients with gonadal dysgenesis, 80 percent of whom are phenotypic females. It can be bilateral and contain Leydig cells and Sertoli cells, which can exist in the pure form. In childhood, the testis is occasionally the last area cleared in a patient treated for leukemia, and the recurrence of a mass suggests relapse.

Torsion. Torsion of the spermatic cord is classified as extravaginal or intravaginal (see Fig. 38-6). Although torsion can

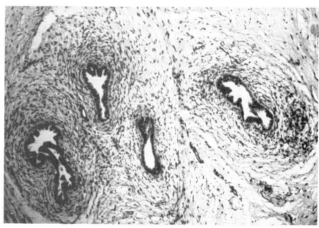

B

FIG. 38-61. Cystic renal disease. A. In its most severe form the kidney appears as a "bunch of grapes." B. Microscopic appearance of A shows no glomeruli.

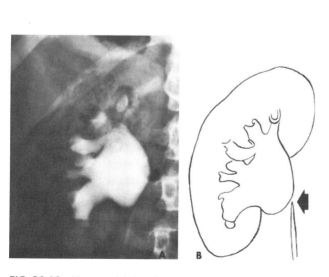

FIG. 38-60. Ureteropelvic junction obstruction (A) due to congenital intrinsic stenosis indicated by arrow in B.

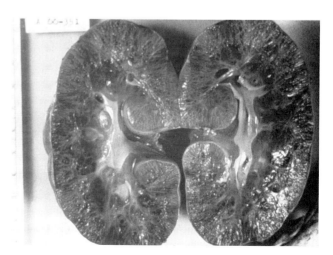

FIG. 38-62. Infantile polycystic kidney disease. Note numerous cysts within the kidney involving all segments of the nephron. Note "tapioca-like" appearance of the cut surface of the kidney.

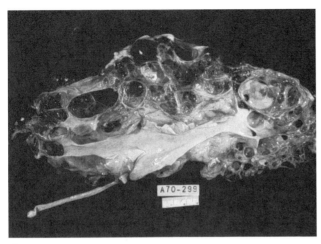

A

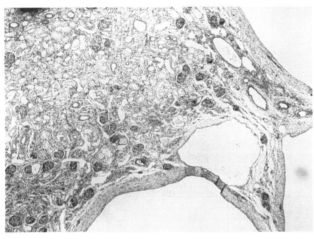

B

FIG. 38-63. *Adult polycystic kidney disease. A. Note numerous cysts causing bumpy outline of kidney. B. Histology shows many glomeruli interspersed between cysts in contrast with cystic renal dysplasia.*

occur at any age, it is more common before puberty, and the extravaginal type is often seen in newborns. Torsion of the appendix testis occurs in one-third of the cases of torsion in infants and small children and is often confused with torsion of the cord and testis. The isotope scan is helpful in making the diagnosis, but getting the scan should not delay surgical repair.

At operation, the tunica vaginalis must be opened to rule out intravaginal torsion. Testicular necrosis is evaluated and a decision made as to whether to remove the testis. After detorting the cord, a bilateral orchiopexy should be performed, suturing the tunica albuginea of the testes, scrotal septum, and tunica vaginalis.

Varicocele. This results from incompetent valves or obstruction of the gonadal vein. It has been noted in 4 percent of college freshmen and occurs more commonly on the left side. The sudden appearance of a varicocele mandates ruling out the presence of a retroperitoneal tumor. After puberty, there is an association between varicocele and subfertility, with the ejaculate demonstrating an increased percentage of abnormally formed sperm. The indications for repair include size, persistent

scrotal pain, rapid growth, and subfertility with abnormal sperm in the ejaculate. An atrophic testis on the side of the varicocele is a late development and not a contraindication to repair. The repair consists of ligating the spermatic vein and its collaterals and removing the varicocele.

Hydrocele and Hematocele (see Fig. 38-5). *Hydrocele* is an accumulation of clear fluid within the tunica vaginalis. As the processus vaginalis descends from the peritoneum into the scrotum, it usually seals off at its upper end, leaving a two-layered sac, the tunica vaginalis, which envelops the testis. If the sac does not fuse, fluid moves back and forth from the peritoneal cavity, and a communicating hydrocele develops. In this case, the child presents with an enlarged scrotal mass that decreases in size overnight. It is repaired as an indirect inguinal hernia. Noncommunicating hydroceles are excised.

A collection of blood within the tunica vaginalis can result from trauma or from rupture of the tunica or testis. This is known as *hematocele* and should be treated by aspiration or open drainage.

Ambiguous Genitalia (see Chap. 37)

Disorders of sexual differentiation are uncommon but challenging cases. The most common cause is the adrenogenital syndrome, which leads to virilization of a genotypic female. The most common form of adrenogenital syndrome is the 46,XX/21-hydroxylase variant that accounts for 90 percent of the cases diagnosed at birth. The anatomic variation ranges from hypospadias in a dysgenetic pseudohermaphrodite to a true hermaphrodite (Fig. 38-64). There can be minimal clitoral enlargement, or the clitoris can mimic a penis. Some of these patients have defects in steroid biogenesis, and adrenal crises have been noted requiring urgent treatment.

Urethral Abnormalities

Hypospadias. This is the most frequent fusion defect of the urethra, occurring in 1 in 300 male births. The abnormality consists of a dorsal hood (absent ventral foreskin), chordee (ventral curvature of the glans penis on the shaft), and proximal location of the urethral meatus. The urethral meatus may be located anywhere from the coronal sulcus to the perineum but is more frequently distal (Fig. 38-65). The more proximal the hypospadias, the more probable is the presence of chordee. Duplication of the urethral orifice may be present, but usually only one communicates with the urethra per se.

Hypospadias results in an abnormal urinary stream. The downward deformity of the glans penis causes the urine issuing from the urethral meatus to be deflected. Infertility is associated with a scrotal or perineal meatus. Hypospadias with the urethral meatus in the scrotal area is often accompanied by bilateral undescended testes and must be differentiated from the adrenogenital syndrome and pseudohermaphroditism. Before performing urethroplasty on such a patient, determination of the genetic sex by karyotyping and adrenal function by determination of 17-hydroxysteroids and 17-ketosteroids is indicated. Visualization of the lower genitourinary tract by means of retrograde opaque contrast studies can disclose the presence of a vagina, and abdominal exploration can reveal that the child's sex organs are female rather than male, in which case excision of the hypertrophied clitoris should be performed.

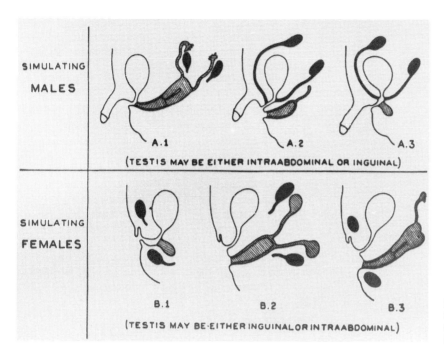

FIG. 38-64. *Anatomic variations in patients presenting with adrenogenital syndrome. The most common variety seen is A-2 caused by 21-hydroxylase.*

Hypospadias should be repaired as soon as adequate phallic tissue is present. The repair is adapted to the anomaly. More than 80 techniques have been described. Some of the popular ones are depicted in Fig. 38-66. Treatment of hypospadias can require staged operations. First the chordee is corrected, and then the urethra is reconstructed. In some cases, stenosis of the original urethral meatus requires meatotomy before the definitive operations are undertaken. One-stage hypospadias repairs are also performed, with simultaneous chordee repair and urethroplasty. Postoperative urethral fistula formation often requires further surgical correction. A minimum period of a few months should be allowed for adequate healing between stages or before a fistula is excised.

Epispadias. This is a dorsally cleft urethra that occurs in 1 in 35,000 births, usually in association with exstrophy of the bladder. It occurs without exstrophy in 1 in 200,000 births (Fig. 38-67). It is the consequence of failure of dorsal fusion. In its most marked form it involves the urethral sphincter and is associated with urinary incontinence. Repair consists of transferring the urethral tube to its normal ventral location, rolling the corpora dorsally into position, and covering the area with skin.

Exstrophy of the Bladder. This is a rare anomaly in which the open bladder is part of the anterior abdominal wall. There is a wide range of deformity. The least complex form is represented by female epispadias with bifid clitoris and a short urethra (Fig. 38-68A). These patients present with urinary incontinence and hematuria at the onset of menstruation. Treatment consists of trigonal tubularization and ureteric reimplantation in the bladder. Another variant is classic exstrophy, with the open bladder serving as the lower abdominal wall, cryptorchidism in males, complete epispadias, and wide separation of the symphysis (see Fig. 38-68B). The most severe form is the cloacal type, in which there is a large omphalocele, the bladder is split, and the bowel protrudes between the split halves, with only a few centimeters of large bowel present (see Fig. 38-68C).

Early reconstruction is indicated, often in the first 24 hours after birth if the bladder capacity is sufficient. Continence-restoring operations are deferred until later in the male. Better

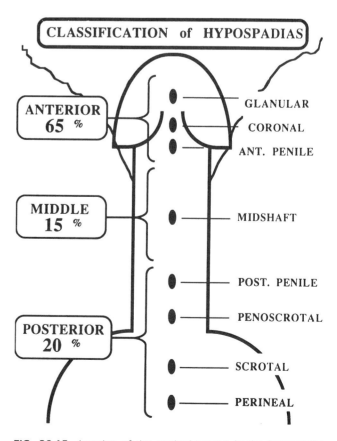

FIG. 38-65. *Location of the urethral meatus in the hypospadias patient.*

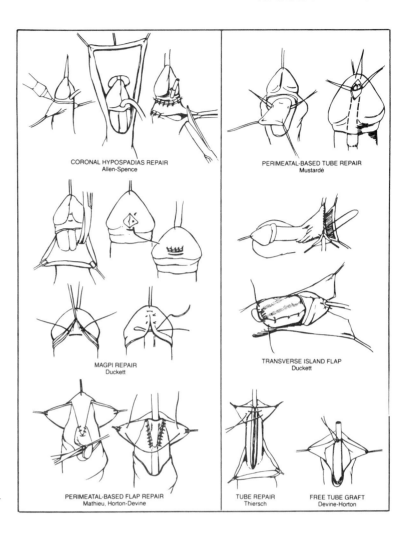

FIG. 38-66. Techniques for repair of hypospadias, depending on the location of the urethral meatus.

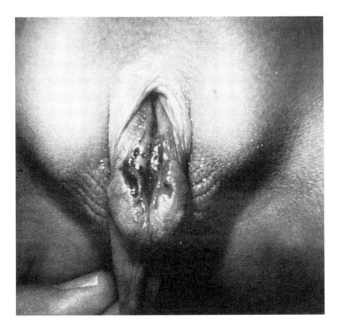

FIG. 38-67. Epispadias without exstrophy. A very rare lesion that usually can be repaired with restoration of continence.

continence results are anticipated in girls. Cloacal exstrophy is converted to classic exstrophy by closing the two halves of the bladder, returning the bowel to the abdomen, and performing a colostomy. Urinary diversion is required in those patients in whom closure is anatomically or functionally unsuccessful.

OPERATIONS ON GENITOURINARY ORGANS

Nephrectomy

The retroperitoneal approach to the kidney was the traditional route, because in the pre-antibiotic era a major proportion of renal operations were performed for pyogenic disease, and the avoidance of contamination of the peritoneum with urine was considered advantageous. Today, the flank or lumbar approach (Fig. 38-69A) remains popular but is supplanted on many occasions by the transabdominal route when early access to the renal vessels is required, as in renal tumor, trauma, or renal vascular disease.

Indications for the lumbar approach include inflammatory renal disease, calculi, perinephric abscess, hydronephrosis, and renal cystic disease. The disadvantages are a limited exposure for abdominal exploration, the fact that the position may be poorly tolerated by the patient, and the fact that it precludes bilateral renal or adrenal exploration. In addition, the lumbar approach

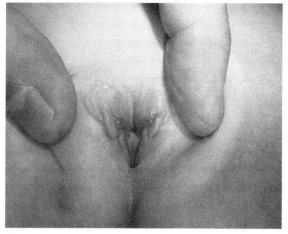

A

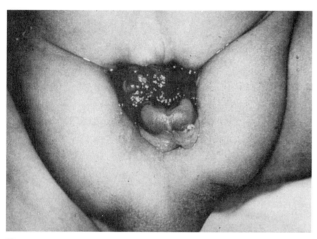

B

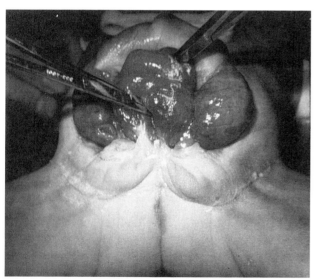

C

FIG. 38-68. *A. Least complex form of exstrophy. Female epispadias. Note bifid clitoris. X-ray of pelvis would show symphysis separated more than 1.7 cm (normal up to 1.2 cm). Other anatomic findings include a very short urethra resulting in incontinence. B. Classic or complete exstrophy. Note complete epispadias and bladder on anterior abdominal wall. C. Cloacal exstrophy, the most severe form of exstrophy. Note bladder split, bowel in between, and short colon.*

makes early control of the renal pedicle without manipulation of the kidney difficult, and therefore, it should not be applied for renal parenchymal tumors.

The lumbar approach may be carried out with the patient in the lateral flexed position, with the involved side on stretch. A modified flank position can be used with a subcostal incision and by remaining retroperitoneal throughout the procedure (see Fig. 38-69*B*). The external and internal oblique muscles are divided in the line of the incision. The transversus muscle is separated, in the line of its fibers, the retroperitoneum is exposed, and the peritoneum is displaced medially. The fascia of Gerota is opened, exposing the kidney and the perinephric fatty tissue.

The important structures within the renal pedicle are located anteriorly (ventrally). During mobilization of the kidney, particular care is necessary in the region of the upper pole because of the adrenal vessels and in the region of the lower pole because of aberrant arteries. Usually the renal artery and vein can be dissected free of fatty areolar tissue so that individual ligation may be performed. The vein is anterior to the artery, and the artery is ligated first if nephrectomy is performed. Under adverse circumstances, a renal pedicle clamp can be used to control bleeding and permit transection of the hilus. Suture ligature of the renal pedicle en masse may fail to control the bleeding and can lead to arteriovenous fistula. Absorbable sutures are often used when infection is present, and drainage is instituted. The incision is closed in layers with chromic catgut or Vicryl, with the exception of the skin, which is closed with nonabsorbable sutures or staples. Nonabsorbable sutures with increased tensile strength, such as Prolene, can be used in the fascia to increase the strength of closure in debilitated patients or in those in whom poor wound healing is expected.

Nephrectomy for a renal carcinoma is carried out through either a transperitoneal, thoracoabdominal, or flank approach with vascular ligation before mobilization and without opening Gerota's fascia, and insertion of a drain is not required.

Partial Nephrectomy (Fig. 38-70)

The exposure for this operation is the same as for nephrectomy and can be done in the flank position or through a subcostal incision with the patient in the supine position. The muscles are incised, and the kidney is exposed. The vasculature is secured first by reflecting the colon and defining the renal pedicle. The ureter can be followed superiorly to a point where it passes beneath the renal vein as a convenient way of locating the pedicle. The artery and vein are then dissected out separately, and a small vascular clamp is placed on the artery. The renal capsule is then incised, and the hub of the knife is used to identify arcuate arteries as the parenchyma is traversed. These arteries are ligated. Calyces that are opened are closed. Absorbable suture must be used for this purpose to avoid stone formation within the kidney. After closure of the calyces, the reflected capsule can be closed over the lower pole of the kidney; a piece of vascularized omentum is sewed to the lower end of the kidney to cover the raw surface. A JP drain is positioned near the site of the kidney repair.

Cutaneous Ureteroileostomy (Ileal Conduit)

Currently, the most popular method of supravesical urinary diversion is cutaneous ureteroileostomy (Fig. 38-71). The major indications for this form of diversion are (1) removal of the

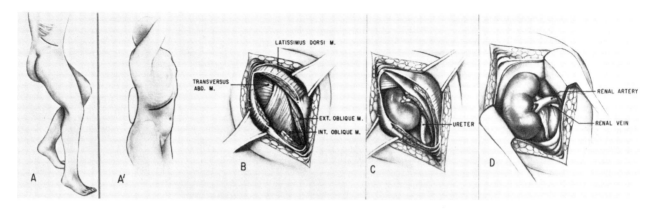

FIG. 38-69. Retroperitoneal nephrectomy. *A.* Standard flank approach. *A'.* Modified flank position and subcostal incision also allow retroperitoneal exposure of the kidney. *B.* Incision through internal and external oblique muscles, transversus abdominis muscle, and latissimus muscle. *C.* Opening the lumbo-dorsal fascia and Gerota's fascia exposes the kidney and ureter. *D.* Mobilization of the kidney reveals the renal vessels medially.

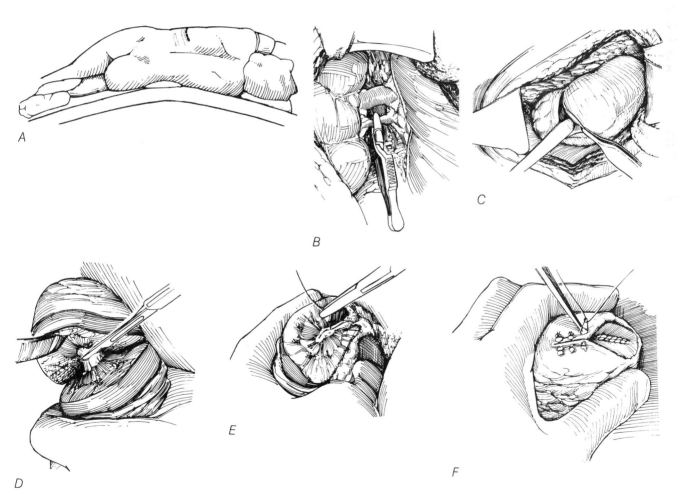

FIG. 38-70. Partial nephrectomy. *A.* Patient in flank position for partial nephrectomy. Incision shown above eleventh rib but may be over or below eleventh or twelfth rib. Note underneath knee is flexed. Flank parallel to ceiling. *B.* Kidney exposed and renal artery clamped. *C.* Incision through kidney capsule, which is reflected. *D.* Division of calyx. *E.* Note that the arcuate vessels have been oversewn with figure-of-eight chromic catgut. Opened calyx is being closed with running 4-0 chromic gut. *F.* Calyx closed. Capsule closure with either running 2-0 chromic gut or, as shown here, interrupted suture tied down over fat.

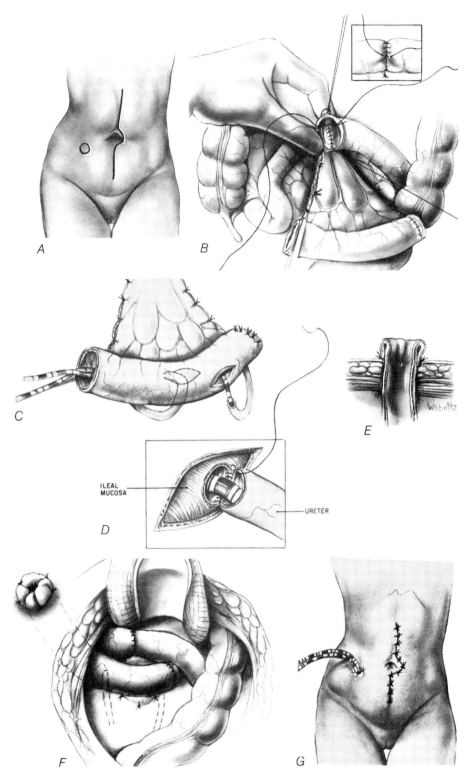

ILEAL
MUCOSA

URETER

Wabnitz

FIG. 38-71. Cutaneous ureteroileostomy (ileal conduit).

bladder and (2) impaired bladder detrusor function. The disadvantages of the procedure are the extent of the operation and the requirement of utilizing a meticulously applied external collection device. These disadvantages are offset by the advantages of the ileal conduit in providing a continuous unobstructed drainage of urine and its versatility in coping with varying anatomic situations. Colon is occasionally used instead of ileum and offers some advantages (colon conduit). Urinary diversion using bowel with modifications to produce continence is also applicable (Koch or Indiana pouch or orthotopic neobladder).

Preoperative preparation is an integral part of the procedure, and the blood volume and cardiac, pulmonary, and renal status should be optimal. Treatment of preexisting infections or metabolic disturbances should be instituted at this time. Mechanical and antibacterial bowel preparation is used preoperatively, but some surgeons use only a mechanical prep for the ileal loop operation. The urinary appliance should be fitted and worn by the patient preoperatively to determine tolerance to adhesive and to identify the optimal location of the stoma.

The ileal loop is best performed through a midline abdominal incision. Before making this incision, it is preferable to create the abdominal wall defect for the ileostomy (see Fig. 38-71A). This results in the creation of a tract through muscles that have not been distorted by the incision and avoids the problem of mechanical obstruction of the ileostomy. The abdomen is then entered. Appendectomy is performed. A well-vascularized segment of the ileum approximately 20 cm in length is selected for the formation of the conduit. The ileum is divided at the selected sites, and the isolated segment is irrigated with saline solution. The continuity of the ileum is restored, and the isolated ileal segment is positioned posterior to the ileoileal anastomosis (see Fig. 38-71B). The proximal end of the ileal segment to be used for the conduit is closed with a continuous inverting chromic catgut suture. The left ureter is brought through the sigmoid mesentery and mobilized to provide length and eliminate the possibility of kinking or obstruction. The full thickness of ureter is sutured to the ileal mucosa. If the left ureter is markedly dilated, an end-to-end ureteroileostomy is performed. Ureteral stents may be used to splint the anastomosis for a few days and to encourage good position of the ureters. The right ureter is anastomosed in a similar fashion over a catheter stent (see Fig. 38-71C, D). The isolated segment of ileum and its mesentery are sutured to the posterior peritoneum to prevent an internal hernia. The distal end of the ileal conduit is brought to the previously prepared abdominal opening. The fascia is secured to the serosa of the ileum to prevent herniation (see Fig. 38-71E). The ileostomy stoma is everted and sutured to the skin and itself (see Fig. 38-71F).

A 1-cm protuberant cuff under no tension is considered optimal. The wound is closed with catgut, Vicryl, or Prolene for the fascial layers and silk or staples for the skin (see Fig. 38-71G). A nasogastric tube is usually necessary postoperatively for 3 to 5 days. Another variation of the procedure involves the joining of both ureters together with one large stoma, which is then anastomosed to the proximal end of the ileal loop as a "cap." This can provide a larger anastomotic opening between the ureters and the segment of ileum and decrease the incidence of the complication of stricture at this vital site. The stoma is usually placed on the right side but can be placed on the left side of the abdomen when indicated.

Cystostomy, Cystolithotomy

Operation on the bladder (Fig. 38-72) is facilitated by filling the organ, because this elevates the peritoneum out of the line of the incision. A low transverse abdominal incision 4 cm above the pubis is carried through the skin (see Fig. 38-72A), subcutaneous tissue, and rectus abdominis fascia (see Fig. 38-72B). The recti are mobilized from their midline attachments and separated (see Fig. 38-72C). The bladder is easily recognized by its characteristic muscular and vascular pattern, and the peritoneum is reflected off the bladder. The bladder is entered longitudinally (see Fig. 38-72D), and if calculi are present, they can be removed digitally or with stone forceps (see Fig. 38-72E). Thorough digital and visual exploration is indicated. Drainage can be provided

by a Malecot cystostomy catheter brought out through a stab wound above the incision (see Fig. 38-72F), or the bladder can be closed primarily. A prevesical tissue drain should be used and brought out through a separate stab wound below the incision (see Fig. 38-72G). The bladder is closed with a one-layer, continuous 0 chromic catgut suture that incorporates the seromuscular wall of the bladder. The rectus fascia is approximated with interrupted 0 chromic catgut or Vicryl sutures. The subcutaneous fat may be approximated with 3-0 interrupted plain catgut sutures and the skin edges with nonabsorbable suture material, such as 4-0 silk, nylon, or staples.

Prostatectomy

Transurethral Prostatectomy. The most commonly performed operation for removal of prostatic obstruction is the endoscopic approach. Following adequate spinal or general anesthesia and dilatation of the urethra, the resectoscope sheath is inserted. Excellent visualization through the resectoscope allows for identification of the ureteral orifices, verumontanum, and external sphincter. With a cutting loop, the prostatic tissue is resected, and hemostasis is secured with electrocoagulation. A catheter is inserted at the end of the procedure, and further hemostasis may be obtained by pulling the catheter bag against the bladder neck and prostatic fossa. This procedure is well tolerated by the patient, with minimal postoperative discomfort and early removal of the catheter. Contraindications to the transurethral resection are inability to place the patient in the lithotomy position, an excessively enlarged prostate gland, and the presence of other intravesical pathologic conditions that warrant open exploration. The skilled operator is able to avoid the complications of excessive bleeding, ureteral orifice injury, perforation, and injury to the external sphincter. The results of this procedure are gratifying, and it can be performed on elderly, debilitated patients with minimal morbidity and mortality.

Suprapubic Prostatectomy (Fig. 38-73). This is performed through the cystostomy approach previously described. The compressed normal prostate represents the pseudocapsule from which adenomatous tissue is mobilized and enucleated by finger dissection. The prostatic urethra and adenomas are removed together. The urethral attachment is transected, and the prostatic fossa is packed while the prostatic arteries that are located on either side of the posterior bladder neck are suture-ligated. Redundant mucosal fragments or small adenomas may be removed by sharp dissection. After the pack is removed, a #22 French, 30-mL urethral retention catheter is inserted. If oozing from the bladder neck or prostatic fossa occurs, gentle traction on the urethral catheter may effect hemostasis. A Malecot catheter and tissue drain are used in similar fashion to that described for suprapubic cystostomy. The suprapubic tube is usually removed in 2 to 3 days and the urethral catheter in 5 to 7 days.

Retropubic Prostatectomy. This is also performed through the incision described for cystotomy. After the bladder wall is identified, the bladder is decompressed, and a 5-cm transverse incision is made 1.5 cm distal to the bladder neck. An alternative approach, known as a *vesicocapsular prostatectomy,* uses a vertical incision in line with the urethra and into the bladder and has the advantages of easier closure and avoidance of the anterior prostatic venous plexus. After the prostatic capsule

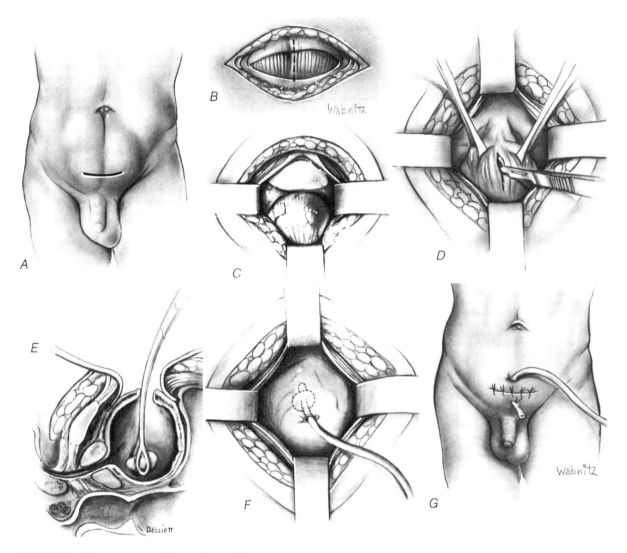

FIG. 38-72. Cystostomy, cystolithotomy (see text).

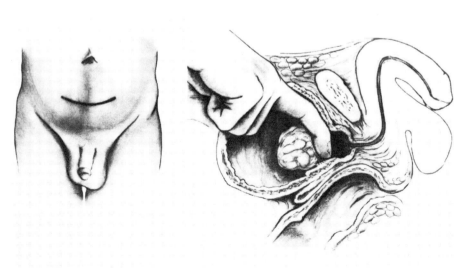

FIG. 38-73. Suprapubic prostatectomy. Through a low transverse abdominal incision, the bladder is entered as described for cystostomy. The bladder mucosa overlying the adenoma is incised, and the prostate is enucleated digitally.

is incised, the adenomas are mobilized by finger dissection. The distal urethra and bladder neck attachments are transected, and hemostasis is effected by suture ligature. The prostatic capsule is closed with interrupted catgut sutures, and a watertight closure is created. The bladder is drained by a urethral retention catheter. Traction on the catheter following retropubic prostatectomy is not as effective for hemostasis as it is following transvesical prostatectomy and may interfere with closure of the capsule. If additional security against catheter obstruction is desired, a suprapubic cystostomy can be performed.

Radical Retropubic Prostatectomy (Fig. 38-74). The modifications of the usual radical retropubic prostatectomy suggested by Walsh enjoy worldwide popularity. A slight Trendelenburg position is used so that the lower abdomen is parallel to the ceiling. The abdomen is opened through a midline incision. The vas deferens is identified on either side and divided between ligatures. The lymph nodes are removed by one of many techniques. Usually the lymphatics surrounding the external iliac vein and those surrounding the obturator nerve as far distally as the exit of the nerve into the obturator foramen and the crossing of the external iliac artery by the superficial iliac vein are removed.

After the nodes are free of tumor, the prostatectomy proceeds. An incision is made through the endopelvic fascia on either side, allowing the prostate to be mobilized and allowing the operator to palpate the apex of the prostate and feel the urethral catheter entering the apex of the prostate. The plexus of Santorini is then dissected off anterior to the urethra and doubly ligated. The prostatic side is suture-ligated. Division between two of these ligatures is then carried out, and one can immediately see the urethra. The neurovascular bundles are then mobilized off the apex of the prostate. The urethra is divided, and at this time sutures are put into the urethra distally. Usually, six 2-0 chromic sutures are placed. After complete division, fragments of rectourethralis muscle are divided, and the prostate is mobilized superiorly. Nutrient vessels to the prostate are ligated between silk ligatures, taking care to preserve the neurovascular bundle back to the base of the prostate.

When the prostate has been elevated to its base, an incision is made over Denonvilliers' fascia, exposing the seminal vesicles and vasa on either side. These are divided between ligatures, taking the nutrient vessel to the seminal vesicle at its tip. Attention is then directed to the prostatovesical junction. The catheter is grasped with a Babcock clamp in the bladder at the prostatovesical junction, helping define its demarcation. Sharp dissection is used to separate the prostate from the vesical neck. The prostate, seminal vesicles, and ampullary portions of the vasa are removed and the area inspected. Hemostasis is achieved by cautery and chromic catgut ligatures. The anastomosis is then completed over a #20 French Silastic catheter by passing the distal sutures (which had been placed previously at the time the urethra was divided). Once these distal sutures have been passed through the vesical neck, the balloon is inflated. When the ligatures are then tied down, one can easily push the bladder against the pelvic outlet. Irrigation is then performed, and the wound is closed in layers. A 10-mm JP drain is placed in the retroperitoneal space near, but not against, the anastomosis to allow for aspiration of any leakage of urine postoperatively.

Hydrocelectomy (Fig. 38-75)

A vertical scrotal incision is usually employed. It is carried through the skin, dartos, and overlying coverings of the hydrocele sac. It is desirable to avoid opening the hydrocele until the sac is totally mobilized. The tunica vaginalis is then opened and the excess tunica excised. Hemostasis is secured with multiple ligatures or electrocoagulation of the small bleeders in the cut edge. The edges of the tunica may be sutured together behind the testis with a continuous 3-0 chromic suture. If hemostasis is satisfactory, this may not be necessary. A drain can be brought out through a stab wound in a dependent portion of the scrotum if the hydrocele is very large, but in most instances a drain is not required. The incision is then closed in layers with absorbable sutures. A scrotal suspensory provides an excellent dressing in the postoperative period, and the use of an ice bag decreases the swelling. Hydrocelectomy in children is carried out through an inguinal incision so that an associated hernia can be repaired at the same time.

Inguinal Orchiectomy (Fig. 38-76)

This approach is used when a testicular tumor is suspected. It provides access to the spermatic vessels before manipulation of the testis. The incision is identical with that performed for repair of a hernia (see Fig. 38-76A), and the spermatic cord is identified at the external inguinal ring. After a rubber-shod or bulldog clamp has been applied to the cord at this level (see Fig. 38-76B), the testis is mobilized from its scrotal attachments and exteriorized through the inguinal incision. The tunica vaginalis is opened to permit examination of the testis, and if the lesion looks or feels neoplastic, the cord is ligated and transected (see Fig. 38-76C). Any solid lesion within the testis is considered potentially malignant, and biopsy is seldom performed. A metal clip is placed in the end of the remaining cord as a marker for future surgery or radiation therapy localization. After the testis has been removed, the inguinal incision is closed. The incision is *not* drained.

Transseptal Orchiopexy

The testis is identified through an inguinal incision that permits mobilization of the spermatic cord and correction of an indirect hernia that usually accompanies the undescended testis. After sufficient length of cord structures is mobilized to permit placement of the testis in the scrotum, a small incision is made in the contralateral scrotum, and a subdartos pouch is prepared to receive the cryptorchid testis. The scrotal septum is incised over a clamp, and traction is applied to the gubernaculum so that the testis is brought down through the scrotal septum into the contralateral scrotum. The septal defect may require a partial closure to prevent the testis from pulling back but should not be closed too tightly because strangulation of the cord could occur. The testis can be brought down on the same side without using the transseptal method if there is absolutely no tension. The scrotal and inguinal incisions are closed, and the patient is usually able to leave the hospital the same day.

Bilateral Vasectomy (Fig. 38-77)

This male sterilization procedure usually is carried out under local anesthesia in an outpatient setting. Previous consultation with the patient and his wife has allowed for careful selection,

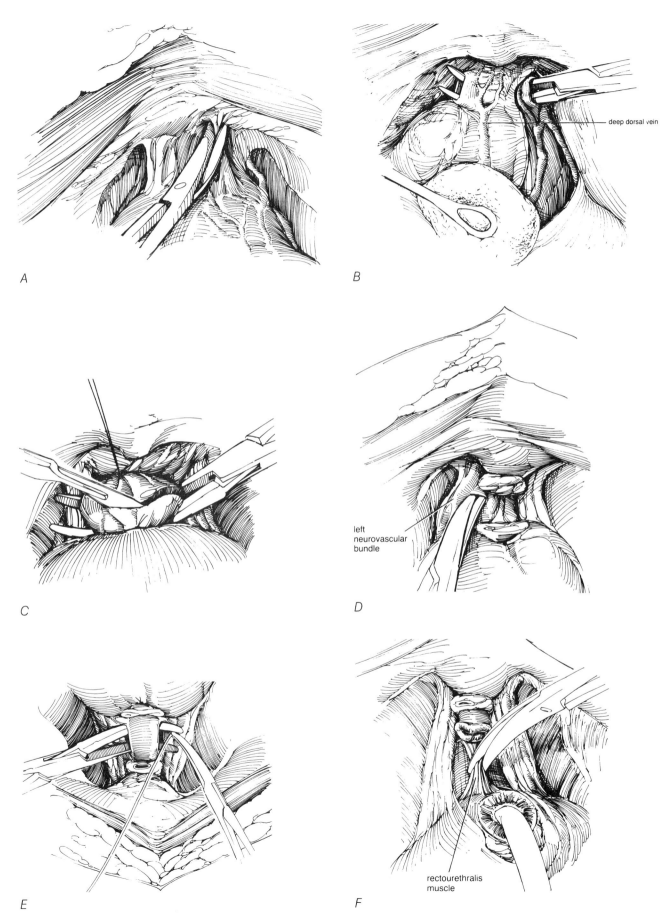

A

B

deep dorsal vein

C

D

left
neurovascular
bundle

E

F

rectourethralis
muscle

FIG. 38-74 *A–F.*

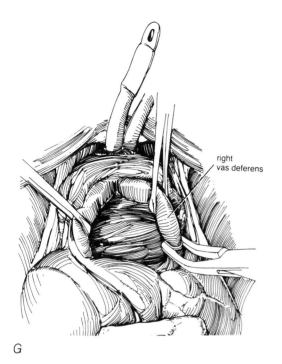

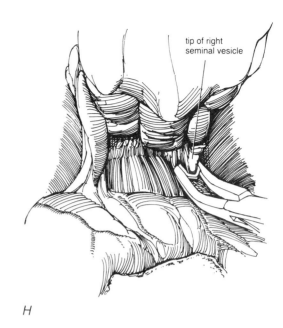

right
vas deferens

tip of right
seminal vesicle

G

H

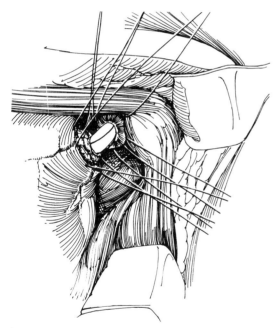

I

FIG. 38-74. Radical retropubic prostatectomy. *A.* Division of puboprostatic ligaments through a midline incision from umbilicus to pubis. *B.* Isolation of dorsal vein
(Santorini's plexus) in preparation for ligation. Endopelvic fascia has been incised. *C.*
Dividing dorsal vein. *D.* Dissecting neurovascular bundle away from adjacent urethra
after dividing dorsal vein. *E.* Dividing the urethra. Urethral sutures may be placed
at this time. *F.* Urethra separated from prostate. Posterior rectourethralis muscle fibers
being divided. *G.* Prostate elevated. Denonvilliers' fascia has been incised, and vasa
and seminal vesicles are being divided. *H.* Left vas and seminal vesical tip have been
divided. Right vas tip has been divided, and now right seminal vesicle tip is being
clipped. *I.* Urethral anastomotic sutures have been placed. A #22 Silastic catheter
has been passed.

instruction to the patient, and the signing of the required papers
for sterilization and informed consent. The scrotum is shaved on
the night before the procedure, and the patient brings a scrotal
suspensory with him to the office. The procedure is carried out
with the patient in the lithotomy or supine position. The vas on
one side is isolated between thumb and index finger of the operator, and the overlying skin is infiltrated with 1% lidocaine or
another local anesthetic agent. The underlying cord is also infiltrated. A towel clip is then used to isolate the vas. A small
incision is made over the vas, and it is delivered into the incision.
An Allis clamp is then used to pick up the vas and separate it

from the surrounding cord structures. The vas is then mobilized
for approximately 3 cm. A segment measuring approximately 1
to 2 cm is excised between clamps. The edges of the vas are
then transfixed with sutures. Another suture is placed approximately 1 cm below the previous suture and tied. The end of that
suture is then passed through the end of the vas and tied, producing a means of bending the vas back on itself so that the
ends are no longer in close proximity. One of the ends also can
be buried in the adjacent tissues to prevent recanalization. An
alternative technique involving electrocoagulation of the lumen
of each end is commonly used. After satisfactory hemostasis has

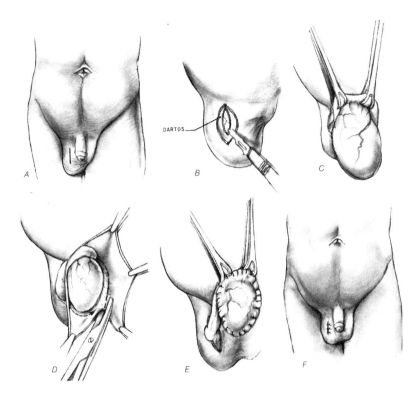

FIG. 38-75. Hydrocelectomy (see text).

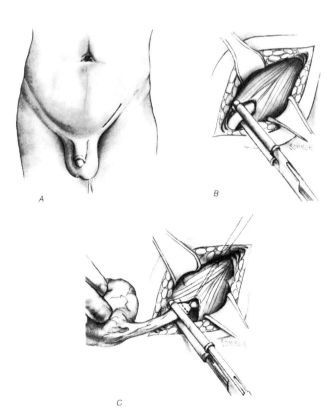

FIG. 38-76. Inguinal orchiectomy. A. An inguinal incision is made. B. The spermatic cord is identified at the level of the external inguinal ring, and the cord is mobilized proximally and then clamped with an atraumatic clamp. C. The testes is mobilized from the scrotum and brought out through the inguinal incision.

been secured, the ends of the vas are dropped back into the incision. The edges of the skin and underlying dartos are then approximated. A similar procedure is then carried out on the other side. Incorporating the underlying dartos in the skin closure provides excellent hemostasis. A collodion dressing is then applied, and the patient uses the scrotal suspensory over a small gauze dressing.

He is instructed to use an ice bag on that area for the remainder of the day and returns to work wearing the scrotal suspensory the following day. He is advised to expect a minimal amount of discomfort, swelling, and ecchymosis. When he resumes intercourse, he continues contraception until an examination of his semen reveals no sperm. This usually requires a period of 6 weeks or at least 10 ejaculations to evacuate the remaining sperm that are distal to the anastomotic sites.

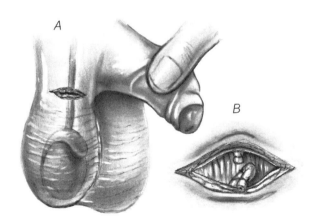

FIG. 38-77. Vasectomy. A. Scrotal incision. B. Double ligation of vasa (see text).

Vasovasostomy (Fig. 38-78)

This procedure is usually carried out in-hospital with the patient under regional, general, or spinal anesthesia. An incision is made in the scrotum, and the underlying cord structures are delivered into view. The previous site of vasectomy is usually palpable unless a large segment of the vas has been excised. Use of the operating microscope facilitates the operation and improves the results. Once the ends of the vas have been isolated, they are excised back to a normal-appearing vas deferens. The ends are then carefully approximated and sutured with 8-0 or 9-0 nylon sutures in a two-layer fashion. Care must be taken to prevent tension on the completed anastomosis. Bleeding is minimal, and the reconstituted vas is then dropped back into the scrotum and the skin and dartos approximated. A similar procedure is then carried out on the other side. The patient is often able to leave the hospital the same day or the following day.

Sperm can begin to appear in the ejaculate as early as 1 month after the procedure, but most often this does not occur until 2 or 3 months following the procedure, at which time the edema may subside enough to allow passage of sperm through the small lumen of the vas deferens. Satisfactory reconstitution with sperm in the ejaculate occurs in approximately 80 percent of cases. A higher percentage of success is reported when microsurgery is used. A satisfactory surgical result does not ensure that a pregnancy will result because other factors such as sperm quality and antisperm antibodies may play a role in persistent infertility.

LAPAROSCOPY IN UROLOGY

Early urologic applications of laparoscopy were confined to diagnostic maneuvers or simple ablative procedures. As the skill and instrumentation of the laparoscopist improved, complex ablative and reconstructive procedures became feasible. Currently, the biggest obstacle to be overcome by the laparoscopic surgeon is the long operative times, and therefore increased cost, that accompany most complex laparoscopic procedures. The recent development of an automated laparoscopic suturing device for tissue approximation has already decreased operative times for a variety of reconstructive procedures, such as laparoscopic pyeloplasty. With further innovations, operative times undoubtedly will decrease, thereby advancing many procedures from the realm of feasible into established clinical practice.

Cryptorchid Testes. One of the earliest urologic application of laparoscopy was in the localization of an intraabdominal cryptorchid testis. With minimal morbidity and an average operative time of about 15 minutes, this diagnostic procedure is highly accurate and remains the procedure of choice for localization of the impalpable testis.

If an intraabdominal testis is identified, a laparoscopic approach can be used to remove the testicle or to translocate it into the ipsilateral hemiscrotum. For the testis located just inside the internal ring or the testis that has easily mobilizable vessels, a single-stage orchiopexy may be performed. If the testicle cannot be sufficiently mobilized to reach the scrotum, a Fowler-Stevens staged orchidopexy may be performed in which the spermatic vessels are laparoscopically clipped or ligated, and the testicle is left in situ to allow formation of collateral blood supply. A staged procedure is performed 6 months later, at which time the testicle is translocated into the scrotum.

Laparoscopic orchiectomy also may be performed via a similar approach. After division of the gubernaculum, the spermatic vessels and vas deferens are mobilized and divided with clips or electrocautery. The testis is delivered to the abdominal wall through a laparoscopic port site.

Varicocelectomy. *Varicocele* refers to a chronic dilatation of the pampiniform plexus that comprises venous drainage of the testicle. Although varicoceles are often implicated in vague testicular pain, the more relevant clinical implication of a vari-

FIG. 38-78. *Vasovasostomy. A. Scrotal incision. B. Excision of ligated (scarred) ends of vas deferens. C. Reanastomosis of ends of vas, restoring continuity.*

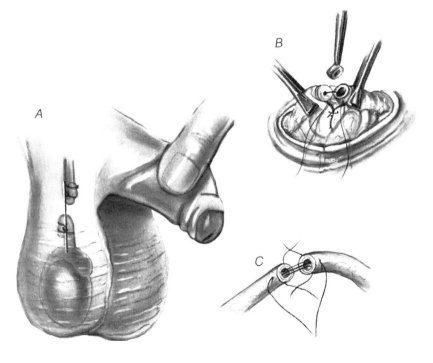

cocele is its potential to cause male subfertility in adults and testicular growth retardation in adolescents.

Repair of a varicocele involves exposure and ligation of the spermatic veins. Laparoscopy is ideally suited to varix ligation because the spermatic cord is one of the more easily recognizable structures laparoscopically. Use of a laparoscopic Doppler probe may facilitate identification of the spermatic artery and help prevent its inadvertent ligation. The success rate, as assessed by physical examination and color Doppler ultrasonography, is more than 98 percent.

The role of laparoscopic varicocelectomy is controversial. Alternative approaches, including an open inguinal or retroperitoneal approach or percutaneous transvenous embolism, are also associated with a high success rate, low complication rate, and rapid convalescence. Indeed, the laparoscopic approach is more time-consuming than the alternative open approaches and is no less invasive than the transvenous approach. As such, the laparoscopic approach may be best suited to bilateral varicocelectomy, in which the time savings and rapid recovery are greatest.

Pelvic Lymphadenectomy.

The use of laparoscopy to sample the obturator lymph nodes in patients with adenocarcinoma of the prostate marked an early application. Previous attempts using radiographic imaging with CT, MRI, or lymphangiography yielded unacceptably high false-negative rates. A minimally invasive means of assessing the pelvic lymph nodes that could preclude a potentially morbid major operation if metastatic disease was identified was an important advance.

The role of pelvic lymph node dissection is to identify patients with clinically localized prostate cancer who are considered for potentially curative treatment (i.e., radical retropubic or perineal prostatectomy, external-beam or interstitial radiation therapy, or possibly cryosurgery) and to exclude patients with metastatic disease (i.e., positive lymph nodes), in whom curative treatment is unlikely and ill-advised. Accordingly, the selection of patients who are suitable candidates for laparoscopic pelvic lymph node dissection (LPLND) is based on identifying patients at high risk for metastatic disease who will benefit from histopathologic staging. The likelihood of positive lymph nodes is based on algorithms that take into account the grade of the tumor, the serum PSA level, and the extent of local tumor as assessed by digital rectal examination and/or transrectal ultrasonography.

LPLND may be performed via a transperitoneal or an extraperitoneal approach. The extraperitoneal approach to laparoscopic pelvic lymphadenectomy offers the advantages of a reduced formation of intraabdominal adhesions, maintaining the integrity of the peritoneal cavity and reducing the risk of tumor spillage into the peritoneal cavity. The confined working area in the retropubic space renders dissection more challenging than in the more spacious peritoneal cavity. Also, the risk of lymphocele formation is greater in the extraperitoneal approach.

The laparoscopic approach yields a lymph node packet that is comparable in content and diagnostic yield with that obtained with open surgery. Compared with open lymph node dissection, however, the laparoscopic approach is associated with less blood loss, reduced pain medication requirements, a briefer hospitalization, and a shorter convalescence. Despite these advantages, the laparoscopic operative time is longer, and the procedure is more costly compared with open surgery.

Bladder Neck Suspension.

Urinary leakage resulting from the loss of normal pelvic support mechanisms is termed *stress urinary incontinence*. The resulting urethral hypermobility allows the bladder neck to assume a dependent position in the pelvis, thereby facilitating transfer of intraabdominal pressure to the bladder; consequently, increases in intraabdominal pressure, such as occurs with coughing or exercise, are associated with urinary leakage.

A number of surgical techniques are available that attempt to replace the bladder neck into a high, fixed retropubic position using a vaginal or abdominal approach. The laparoscopic approach to bladder neck suspension encompasses the high success rates of the abdominal and vaginal approaches and the minimal morbidity of the vaginal approach.

A number of laparoscopic techniques, both intraperitoneal and extraperitoneal, have been described for bladder neck suspension. In most techniques, intracorporeal knot tying is necessary to secure the endopelvic fascia to Cooper's ligament; alternatively, an absorbable clip may be applied to the end of the suture, thereby obviating the need for cumbersome intracorporeal knot tying.

A prospective comparison of laparoscopic bladder neck suspension with an open vaginal bladder neck suspension (Raz procedure) demonstrated comparable 12-month continence rates in the two groups (78 versus 82 percent, respectively). The operative time was significantly longer in the laparoscopic group than in the open group, whereas the hospital stay, pain medication requirement, and length of catheterization were greater in the open group.

Simple Nephrectomy.

The development of means to entrap and morcellate tissue enabled the first laparoscopic simple nephrectomy to be performed in 1990. Since then, the procedure has been performed worldwide for a variety of disorders including end-stage renal disease, renal artery stenosis, and nonfunctioning hydronephrotic kidneys.

The retroperitoneal approach was developed recently to avoid opening the peritoneum with its attendant potential complications. The retroperitoneal approach was hindered by the inability of a pneumoretroperitoneum to create sufficient working space to remove the kidney. The development of a balloon dissector, consisting of a fingerless surgeon's glove mounted on a red rubber catheter, facilitated dissection of the pararenal space and created a working space that could accommodate the pneumoretroperitoneum; the balloon dissector is guided into the retroperitoneal space and inflated with saline to bluntly separate the retroperitoneal tissues along natural cleavage planes.

Compared with traditional open nephrectomy, transperitoneal laparoscopic nephrectomy is associated with a shorter hospital stay, less need for pain medication, and shorter convalescence. However, operative time is significantly longer for the laparoscopic approach. An overall complication rate of 12 percent has been noted in a multi-institutional review, but the complication rate predictably decreased with increasing experience.

The indications for laparoscopic nephrectomy have now been expanded to include live-donor nephrectomy and radical nephrectomy for tumor. Live-donor nephrectomy has been performed using both a transperitoneal and a retroperitoneal approach; in both cases, one port site is extended to accommodate of the intact kidney. When removing a kidney for tumor, a transperitoneal approach is recommended because the limited working space in the retroperitoneal approach is too small to accommodate the large radical nephrectomy specimen.

Adrenalectomy. Laparoscopic adrenalectomy is indicated for aldosteronoma, Cushing's disease due to an adrenal adenoma, or a greater than 6-cm nonfunctioning adrenal mass that has increased in size during a period of observation. Although anecdotal reports of laparoscopic adrenalectomy for pheochromocytoma have appeared, at this time the procedure should be considered investigational for this indication. An appropriate endocrine work-up should be performed preoperatively, and hypertension and electrolyte abnormalities should be corrected.

Both transperitoneal and retroperitoneal laparoscopic adrenalectomies have been described, although experience with the transperitoneal approach is greater. Comparison of laparoscopic adrenalectomy with its open surgical counterpart has revealed a shorter hospital stay, decreased blood loss, and more rapid convalescence in the laparoscopic group. Operative time, however, remains shorter in the open group. Reported complications in several series have been few.

ENDOUROLOGIC MANAGEMENT OF UPPER URINARY TRACT OBSTRUCTION

Upper urinary tract obstruction is the end result of a variety of etiologic factors. Congenital anatomic problems, such as intrinsic narrowing or impingement by a crossing vessel or band of tissue, may contribute to impaired flow of urine from the kidney and are typical of ureteropelvic junction obstruction. Secondary obstruction from previous surgery or radiation or extrinsic compression by a mass is characteristic of ureteral obstruction. Less commonly, secondary causes of ureteropelvic junction obstruction occur, such as previous surgery for congenital ureteropelvic junction obstruction or stricture due to previous stone disease. The distinction is relevant in that the success rates of endourologic procedures differ according to the location of the obstruction and the underlying causes.

In most cases, the diagnosis of ureteropelvic junction obstruction is obvious. Typically, a patient complains of dull flank pain, exacerbated by increased fluid intake or alcohol. An IVU or sonogram demonstrates hydronephrosis with either nonvisualization or delayed visualization of a normal-caliber ureter (Fig. 38-79). However, in some cases, the diagnosis of obstruction is not clear-cut. Accordingly, a quantitative determination of renal drainage is indicated. The diuretic, or Lasix, washout renogram can distinguish between a normal collecting system, a dilated but nonobstructed system, and a dilated, obstructed system (see Fig. 38-9). A radionuclide such as Mag3 or ^{99m}Tc DTPA is administered intravenously. At the point of peak accumulation of radionuclide in the collecting system, Lasix is administered to enhance washout of tracer from the kidney. A gamma scintillation camera quantitates the accumulation and excretion of radiotracer from the collecting system. The time required for half the radionuclide to be excreted from the kidney ($T_{1/2}$) determines the presence or absence of obstruction; a $T_{1/2} < 15$ minutes indicates no obstruction, a $T_{1/2} > 20$ minutes is indicative of obstruction, and anything in between is equivocal. The renogram also determines the differential function of the two kidneys; a functionally significant obstruction may be evident as a loss of differential function from the affected side.

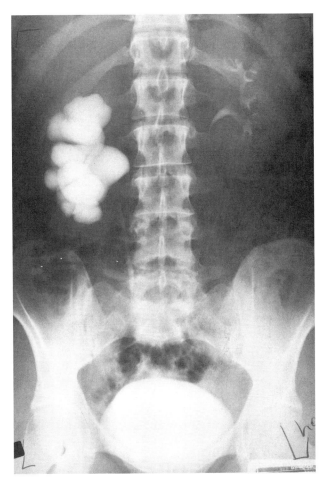

FIG. 38-79. IVU in a young women with right ureteropelvic junction obstruction. Note massively dilated right collecting system and normal-caliber ureter.

If the diuretic renogram is equivocal, a pressure/flow study of the kidney (Whitaker test) may be performed. Dilute contrast material is instilled at a constant rate into the kidney through a percutaneously placed needle, and the differential pressure between the kidney and the bladder is measured. The unobstructed kidney should accommodate an instillation rate of 10 mL/min with a pressure differential of less than 15 cmH$_2$O.

The "gold standard" for surgical repair of the obstructed ureteropelvic junction is the dismembered pyeloplasty, in which the narrowed ureteropelvic junction is excised, along with a segment of markedly redundant renal pelvis if necessary, and the ureter is reanastomosed to the remaining renal pelvis. The procedure is performed through a flank incision, and usually an internal ureteral stent and closed-suction drain are left in place. Success rates approach 95 to 100 percent.

Endopyelotomy. The endourologic management of ureteropelvic junction obstruction is based on the principle of the Davis intubated ureterotomy: A full-thickness incision is made through a narrowed segment, and a tube is placed across the incised segment. After approximately 6 weeks, the epithelial and muscular layers of the ureter regenerate, leaving a normal-caliber ureter. The percutaneous counterpart of the intubated ureterotomy (antegrade endopyelotomy) consists of antegrade passage

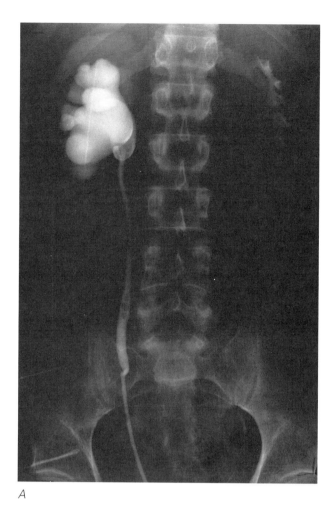
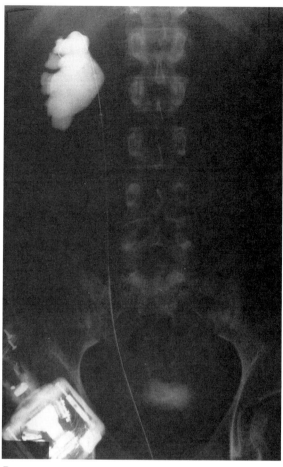

A   *B*

FIG. 38-80. Fluoroscopic retrograde endopyelotomy. *A.* Retrograde pyelogram showing typical right ureteropelvic junction obstruction. *B.* Ureteral cutting balloon catheter, with cutting wire directed laterally, is passed under fluoroscopic guidance until the radiopaque marks straddle the narrowed segment. The balloon is subsequently inflated while activating the cutting wire. *C.* Injection of contrast material after incision reveals extravasation of contrast material, confirming full-thickness incision of the ureteral wall. A ureteral stent has been placed to drain the kidney.

of a nephroscope through a percutaneous tract into the kidney, with endoscopic incision of the narrowed segment using a "cold" or "hot" knife. A nephroureteral stent or an internal ureteral stent and a nephrostomy tube traverse the incised ureter and are left in place for approximately 6 weeks. Alternatively, a retrograde approach through the ureteroscope may be performed, although the procedure is more technically demanding.

In an attempt to simplify the endopyelotomy procedure and avoid placement of a nephrostomy tube, a ureteral cutting balloon catheter was developed that enabled the incision to be performed entirely under fluoroscopic control (Fig. 38-80). The cutting balloon catheter consists of a balloon mounted on a ureteral catheter; a curved cutting wire affixed to either end of the balloon is activated by an electric current when the foot pedal is depressed. The catheter is advanced over a guidewire passed cystoscopically up the ureter into the kidney, and the cutting wire is straddled across the stricture (see Fig. 38-80*B*) Inflation of the balloon with dilute contrast material while simultaneously activating the cutting wire carries the cutting wire into the narrowed ureter and creates a precise full-thickness incision. Ex-

travasation of contrast material on fluoroscopy confirms an adequate incision (see Fig. 38-80*C*). A ureteral stent is left in place for 6 weeks.

The results of endopyelotomy have been good but not quite comparable with open pyeloplasty. In the largest series of antegrade endopyelotomy performed to date (401 procedures), a success rate of 85 percent was achieved. The complication rate from endopyelotomy averages 13 percent; the most feared complication is bleeding, which usually results from transection of a crossing lower-pole vessel.

Areas of current investigation include attempts to identify patients in whom endopyelotomy is most likely to be successful, thereby increasing the success rates of endopyelotomy to those achieved with pyeloplasty. Some investigators have found that the presence of a crossing vessel in the vicinity of the ureteropelvic junction, massive hydronephrosis, and a marked decrease in differential function on the affected side are all negative prognostic factors that are associated with reduced success rates. Current debate has centered on the need for preoperative imaging studies to identify patients with a crossing vessel in the vicinity

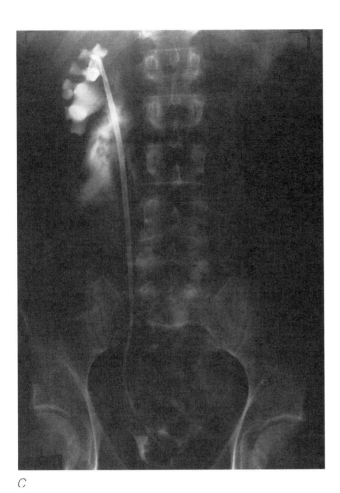

C

FIG. 38-80. *C Continued.*

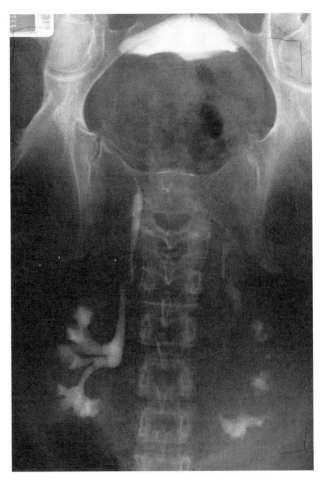

FIG. 38-81. *Middle ureteral stricture (overlying the bony pelvis). IVU demonstrates mild hydroureteronephrosis to the level of the middle ureter. Contrast material is seen passing through a narrow stricture, which on subsequent retrograde pyelogram was shown to be 1 cm in length.*

of the ureteropelvic junction in order to increase the chance of success or decrease the risk of bleeding due to inadvertent incision.

Endoureterotomy. The endourologic management of ureteral strictures is similar to the treatment of ureteropelvic junction obstruction. The cutting balloon catheter may be used to incise strictures in any location in the ureter (Fig. 38-81), although extreme caution must be used when incising a stricture overlying the iliac vessels; in this case, the cutting wire must be directed anteriorly away from the vessels that lie posterior to the ureter in this location. In addition, ureteral strictures may be incised under endoscopic vision (endoureterotomy) using a rigid or flexible ureteroscope and an electrosurgical probe, "cold" knife, or laser. The least invasive means of treating a ureteral stricture is balloon dilation, in which a balloon positioned across the narrowed segment is inflated in order to rupture the fibrotic stricture. All procedures have in common the placement of a ureteral stent for 3 to 6 weeks. The success rate for endoureterotomy is similar to the success rate achieved with endopyelotomy. In one large series, 80 percent of benign ureteral strictures were treated successfully by endoscopic means. Strictures at the ureteroenteric anastomosis after urinary diversion are less successfully treated; although initial success rates approached 75 percent, they continue to drop with successive years after treatment to an average of 32 percent at 3 years.

Bibliography

Abrams P, Blaivas JG, et al: The standardization of terminology of lower urinary tract function recommended by the International Continence Society. *Int Urogynecol J* 1:45, 1990.

Adams JF, Schulam PG, et al: New laparoscopic suturing device: Initial clinical experience. *Urology* 46:242, 1995.

Al-Ali M, Haddad LF: The late treatment of 63 overlooked or complicated ureteral missile injuries: The promise of nephrostomy and role of autotransplantation. *J Urol* 156:1918, 1996.

Allbala DM, Schuessler WW, Vancaille TG: Laparoscopic bladder neck suspension. *J Endourol* 6:137, 1992.

Andersson K-E, Wagner G: Physiology of penile erection. *Physiol Rev* 75:191, 1995.

Appell RA: Retropubic procedures for female stress incontinence, in Webster GD, Kirby R, et al (eds): *Reconstructive Urology*. Oxford, Blackwell Scientific Publishers, 1993, pp 887–894.

Atkinson GO Jr, Patrick LE, et al: The normal and abnormal scrotum in children: Evaluation with color Doppler sonography. *AJR Am J Roentgenol* 158:613, 1992.

Blaivas JG: Treatment of female incontinence secondary to urethral damage or loss. *Urol Clin North Am* 18:355, 1991.

Borghi L, Meschi T, et al: Nifedipine and methylprednisolone in facilitating ureteral stone passage: A randomized, double-blind placebo-controlled study. *J Urol* 152:1095, 1994.

Bowie WR: Approach to men with urethritis and urologic complications of sexually transmitted diseases. *Med Clin North Am* 74:1543, 1990.

Brawer MK, Chetner MP, et al: Screening for prostatic carcinoma with prostate specific antigen. *J Urol* 147:841, 1992.

Brendler CB: Evaluation of the urologic patient: History, physical examination, and urinalysis, in Walsh PC, Retik AB, et al (eds): *Campbell's Urology,* 7th ed. Philadelphia, WB Saunders, 1997, pp 131–157.

Brendler CB, Steinberg GD, et al: Local recurrence and survival following nerve-sparing radical cystoprostatectomy. *J Urol* 144:1137, 1990.

Carroll PR, McAninch JW, et al: Outcome after temporary vascular occlusion for the management of renal trauma. *J Urol* 151:1171, 1994.

Cass AS: Nonstent or noncatheter extracorporeal shock-wave lithotripsy for ureteral stones. *Urology* 43:178, 1993.

Catalona WJ, Hudson MA, et al: Selection of optimal prostate specific antigen cutoffs for early detection of prostate cancer: Receiver operating characteristic curves. *J Urol* 152:2037, 1994.

Catalona WJ, Richie JP, et al: Comparison of digital rectal examination and serum prostate specific antigen in the early detection of prostate cancer: Results of a multicenter clinical trial of 6,630 men. *J Urol* 151:1283, 1994.

Centers for Disease Control and Prevention: 1993 sexually transmitted diseases treatment guidelines. *MMWR* 42(RR-14):1, 1993.

Chandhoke PS, Clayman RV, et al: Endopyelotomy and endoureterotomy with the Acucise ureteral cutting balloon device: Preliminary experience. *J Endourol* 7:45, 1993.

Clark JY, Thompson IM, Optenberg SA: Economic impact of urolithiasis in the United States. *J Urol* 154:2020, 1995.

Cortes D, Thorup JM, et al: Laparoscopy in 100 consecutive patients with 128 impalpable testes. *Br J Urol* 75:281, 1995.

Danuser H, Ackermann DK, et al: Extracorporeal shock wave lithotripsy in situ or after push-up for upper ureteral calculi: A prospective, randomized trial. *J Urol* 150:824, 1993.

Das S, Singer A: Controversies of perinatal torsion of the spermatic cord: A review, survey and recommendations. *J Urol* 143:231, 1990.

de Groat WC: Anatomy and physiology of the lower urinary tract. *Urol Clin North Am* 20:383, 1993.

de Groat WC, Steers WD: Autonomic regulation of the urinary bladder and sexual organs, in Loewy AD, Spyer KM (eds): *Central Regulation of the Autonomic Functions,* 1st ed. Oxford, Oxford University Press, 1990, p 313.

Diamond DA: Intersex disorders, in Stein BS, Caldamone AA, Smith JA Jr (eds): *Clinical Urologic Practice.* New York, Norton, 1995, pp 1547–1565.

Drach GW: Urinary lithiasis: Etiology, diagnosis, and medical management, in Walch PC, Retik AB, et al (eds): *Campbell's Urology,* 6th ed. Philadelphia, WB Saunders, 1992, pp 1065–1077.

Eastham JA, Wilson TG, Ahlering TE: Radiographic evaluation of adult patients with blunt renal trauma. *J Urol* 148: 266, 1992.

El-Abd SA: Endoscopic treatment of posttraumatic urethral obliteration: Experience in 396 patients. *J Urol* 153:67, 1995.

Elliott D, Barrett DM: Long-term follow-up and evaluation of primary realignment of posterior urethral disruptions. *J Urol* 157:814, 1997.

El-Sherif AE, Salem M, et al: Treatment of renal colic by desmopressin intranasal spray and diclofenac sodium. *J Urol* 153:1395, 1995.

Etwaru D, Raboy A, et al: Extraperitoneal endoscopic gasless pelvic lymph node dissection. *J Laparoendosc Surg* 4:113, 1994.

Faerber G, Richardson TD, et al: Retrograde treatment of ureteropelvic junction obstruction using the ureteral cutting balloon catheter. *J Urol* 157:454, 1997.

Fielding JR, Steele G, et al: Spiral computerized tomography in the evaluation of acute flank pain: A replacement for excretory urography. *J Urol* 157:1071, 1997.

Fine JK, Pak CYC, Preminger GM: Effect of medical management and residual fragments on recurrent stone formation following shock wave lithotripsy. *J Urol* 153:27, 1995.

Fried FA, Rutledge R: A statewide, population-based analysis of the frequency and outcome of genitourinary injury in a series of 215,220 trauma patients. *J Urol* 153:314A, 1995.

Gann PH, Hennekens CH, Stampfer MJ: A prospective evaluation of plasma prostate-specific antigen for detection of prostatic cancer. *JAMA* 273:289, 1995.

Gaur DD, Agarwal DK, et al: Laparoscopic condom dissection: New technique of retroperitoneoscopy. *J Endourol* 8:149, 1994.

Gill IS, Clayman RV, McDougall EM: Advances in urological laparoscopy. *J Urol* 154:1275, 1995.

Gill IS, Kavoussi LR, et al: Complications of lapaorscopic nephrectomy in the initial 185 patients: A multi-institutional review. *J Urol* 154:479, 1995.

Glascock JM, Winfield HN: Pelvic lymphadenectomy: Intra- and extraperitoneal access, in Smith AD, Badlani GH, et al (eds): *Smith's Textbook of Endourology.* St. Louis, Quality Medical Publishers, 1996, pp 870–893.

Glassbert KI, Filmer RB: Renal dysplasia, renal hypoplasia and cystic disease of the kidney, in Kelalis PP, King LR, Belman AB (eds): *Clinical Pediatric Urology,* 3d ed. Philadelphia, WB Saunders, 1992.

Glenski WJ, Husmann DA: Nonsurgical management of major renal lacerations associated with urinary extravasation. *J Urol* 153:315a, 1995.

Goel MC, Kumar M, Kapoor R: Endoscopic management of traumatic posterior urethral stricture: Early results and follow-up. *J Urol* 157:95, 1997.

Gonzales ET: Anomalies of the renal pelvis and ureter, in Kelalis PP, King JR, Belman AB (eds): *Clinical Pediatric Urology,* vol 1. Philadelphia, WB Saunders, 1992, p 530.

Guar DD: Retroperitoneal endoscopic ureterolithotomy: Our experience in 12 patients. *J Endourol* 7:501, 1993.

Gupta M, Tuncay OL, Smith AD: Open surgical exploration after failed eneopyelotomy: A 12-year perspective. *J Urol* 157:1613, 1997.

Hershorn S, Thijssen A, Radomski SB: The value of immediate or early catheterization of the traumatized posterior urethra. *J Urol* 148:1428, 1992.

Horenblas S, Van Tinteren H, et al: Squamous cell carcinoma of the penis: III. Treatment of regional lymph nodes. *J Urol* 149:492, 1993.

Howards SS: Treatment of male infertility. *N Engl J Med* 332:312,1995.

Hübner WA, Irby P, Stoller ML: Natural history and current concepts for the treatment of small ureteral calculi. *Eur Urol* 24:172, 1993.

Hussmann DA, Gilling PJ, et al: Major renal lacerations with a devitalized fragment following blunt abdominal trauma: A comparison between nonoperative (expectant) versus surgical management. *J Urol* 150:1772, 1993.

Kerbl K, Clayman RV, et al: Staging pelvic lymphadenectomy for prostate cancer: A comparison of laparoscopic and open techniques. *J Urol* 150:396, 1993.

Koch MO, McDougal WS, et al: Long-term effects of urinary diversion: A comparison of myelomeningocele patients managed by clean, intermittent catheterization and urinary diversion. *J Urol* 147:1343, 1992.

Koraitim MM: Pelvic fracture urethral injuries: Evaluation of various methods of management. *J Urol* 156:1288, 1996.

Kotim L, Koch MO: Impotence and incontinence after immediate realignment of posterior urethral trauma: Result of injury or management? *J Urol* 155:1600, 1996.

Kwon ED, Sandlow JI, Donovan JFJ: Varix ligation, in Smith A, Badlani GH, et al (eds): *Smith's Textbook of Endourology.* St. Louis, Quality Medical Publishers, 1996, pp 894–903.

Labrie F, Dupont A, el al: Serum prostate specific antigen as pre-screening test for prostate cancer. *J Urol* 147:846, 1992.

Leach GE, Yun SK: Post prostatectomy incontinence, parts I and II. *Neurourol Urodynam* 11:91, 1992.

Lepor H: Medical therapy for benign prostatic hyperplasia. *Urology* 42:483, 1993.

Li S, Goldstein M, et al: The no-scalpel vasectomy. *J Urol* 145:341, 1991.

Lingeman JE, Siegel YI, et al: Management of lower pole nephrolithiasis: A critical analysis. *J Urol* 151:663, 1994.

Lingeman JE: Extracorporeal shock wave lithotripsy. *Urol Clin North Am* 24:185, 1997.

Lue TF: Impotence: A patient's goal-directed approach to treatment. *World J Urol* 8:67, 1990.

Lue TF: Erectile dysfunction associated with cavernous and neurological disorders. *J Urol* 151:890, 1994.

Maizels M: Normal and anomalous development of the urinary tract, in Walsh PC, Retik AB, et al (eds): *Campbell's Urology*, 7th ed. Philadelphia, WB Saunders, 1997, pp 1545–1600.

Mandell J, Blyth BR, et al: Structural genitourinary defects detected in utero. *Radiology* 178:193, 1991.

Matthews L, Smith E, Spirnak JP: Non-operative management of major blunt renal trauma: Does urinary extravasation affect outcome? *J Urol* 153:315A, 1995.

McAndrew JD, Corriere JN: Radiographic evaluation of renal trauma: Evaluation of 1103 consecutive patients. *Br J Urol* 73:352, 1994.

McConnell J: Prostatic growth: New insights into hormonal regulation. *Br J Urol* 76(suppl 1):5, 1995.

McConnell J: BPH: Treatment guidelines and patient classification. *Br J Urol* 76(suppl 1):29, 1995.

McConnell JD, Barry MJ, et al: *Benign Prostatic Hyperplasia: Diagnosis and Treatment*. Clinical practice guideline no. 8, AHCPR publication no. 94-0582. Rockville, Maryland, Agency for Health Care Policy and Research, Public Health Service, U.S. Department of Health and Human Services, 1994.

McDougall EM, Clayman RV, Elashry OM: Laparoscopic radical nephrectomy for renal tumor: The Washington University experience. *J Urol* 155:1180, 1996.

McDougall EM, Clayman RV, Fadden PT: Retroperitoneoscopy: The Washington University Medical School experience. *Urology* 43:446, 1994.

McDougall EM, Klutke CG, Cornell T: Comparison of transvaginal versus laparoscopic bladder neck suspension for stress urinary incontinence. *Urology* 45:641, 1995.

McGuire EJ, Fitzpartick CC, et al: Clinical assessment of urethral sphincter function. *J Urol* 150:1452, 1993.

Meretyk I, Meretyk S, Clayman RV: Endopyelotomy: Comparison of ureteroscopic retrograde and antegrade percutaneous techniques. *J Urol* 148:775, 1992.

Micali S, Moore RG, et al: The role of laparoscopy in the treatment of renal and ureteral calculi. *J Urol* 157:463, 1997.

Miller KS, McAninch JW: Radiographic assessment of renal trauma: Our 15 year experience. *J Urol* 154:352, 1995.

Mobley TB, Myers DA, et al: Effects of stents on lithotripsy of ureteral calculi: Treatment results with 18,825 calculi using the Lithostar lithotriptor. *J Urol* 152:53, 1994.

Montie JE: High-stage bladder cancer: Bladder preservation or reconstruction. *Cleve Clin J Med* 57:280, 1990.

Moore RG, Averch TD, et al: Laparoscopic pyeloplastly: Experience with the initial 30 cases. *J Urol* 157:459, 1997.

Moore RG, Peters C, et al: Laparoscopic evaluation of the nonpalpable testis: A prospective assessment of accuracy. *J Urol* 151:728, 1994.

Morey AF, McAninch JW: Reconstruction of posterior urethral disruption injuries: Outcome analysis in 82 patients. *J Urol* 157:506, 1997.

Naber KG: Use of quinolones in urinary tract infections and prostatitis. *Rev Infect Dis* 11(suppl 5):1321, 1989.

Nakada SY, McDougall EM, Clayman RV: Renal surgery, in Smith AD, Badlani GH, et al (eds): *Smith's Textbook of Endourology*. St. Louis, Quality Medical Publishers, 1996, pp 904–954.

Norrby SR: Short-term treatment of uncomplicated lower urinary tract infections in women. *Rev Infect Dis* 12:458, 1990.

Novick AC: Current surgical approaches, nephron-sparing surgery, and the role of surgery in the integrated immunologic approach to renal cell carcinoma. *Semin Oncol* 22:29, 1995.

Novick AC: Renal-sparing surgery for renal cell carcinoma. *Urol Clin North Am* 20:277, 1993.

Ono Y, Katoh N, et al: Laparoscopic radical nephrectomy: The Nagoya experience. *J Urol* 158:719, 1997.

Parra RO: Laparoscopic repair of intraperitoneal bladder perforation. *J Urol* 151:1003, 1994.

Partin AW, Yoo H, et al: The use of prostate specific antigen, clinical stage and Gleason score to predict pathological stage in men with localized prostate cancer. *J Urol* 150:110, 1993.

Pearle MS, Clayman RV: Outcomes and selection of surgical therapies of stones in the kidney and ureter, in Coe FL, Javus MJ, et al (eds): *Kidney Stones: Medical and Surgical Management*. Philadelphia, Lippincott-Raven, 1996, pp 709–755.

Peters PC: Intraperitoneal rupture of the bladder. *Urol Clin North Am* 16:279, 1989.

Podestá ML, Medel R, et al: Immediate management of posterior urethral disruptions due to pelvic fracture: Therapeutic alternatives. *J Urol* 157:1444, 1997.

Porter JR, Takayama TK, DeFalco AJ: Traumatic posterior urethral injury and early realignment using magnetic urethral catheters. *J Urol* 158:425, 1997.

Preminger GM, Clayman RV, et al: A multicenter clinical trial investigating the use of a fluoroscopically controlled cutting balloon catheter for the management of ureteral and ureteropelvic junction obstruction. *J Urol* 157:1625, 1997.

Quillin SP, Brink JA, et al: Helical (spiral) CT angiography for identification of crossing vessels at the ureteopelvic junction. *AJR Am J Roentgenol* 166:1125, 1996.

Ratner LE, Ciseck LJ, et al: Laparoscopic live donor nephrectomy. *Transplantation* 60:1047, 1995.

Ratner LE, Kavoussi LR, et al: Laparoscopic assisted live donor nephrectomy: A comparison with the open approach. *Transplantation* 63:229, 1997.

Resnick NM, Yalla SV, Laurina E: The pathophysiology of urinary incontinence among institutionalized elderly persons. *N Engl J Med* 320:1, 1989.

Richie JP: Neoplasms of the testis, in Walsh PC, Retik AB, et al (eds): *Campbell's Urology*, 7th ed. Philadelphia, WB Saunders, 1997, pp 2411–2452.

Rous SN, Turner WR: Retrospective study of 95 patients with staghorn calculus disease. *J Urol* 118:902, 1977.

Scardino PT, Weaver R, Hudson MA: Early detection of prostate cancer. *Hum Pathol* 23:211, 1992.

Schaeffer AJ: Infections of the urinary tract, in Walsh PC, Retik AB, et al (eds): *Campbell's Urology*, 7th ed. Philadelphia, WB Saunders, 1997, pp 533–614.

Schlegel PN, Goldstein M: Microsurgical vasoepididymostomy: Refinements and results. *J Urol* 150:1165, 1993.

Schulam PG, Kavossi LR, et al: Laparoscopic live donor nephrectomy: The initial 3 cases. *J Urol* 155:1857, 1996.

Scott MH, Porter JR: Extraperitoneal bladder rupture: Pitfall in CT cystography. *AJR Am J Roentgenol* 168:1232, 1997.

Segura JW, Preminger GM, et al: Nephrolithiasis clinical guidelines panel summary report on the management of staghorn calculi. *J Urol* 151:1648, 1994.

Siegel CL, McDougall EM, et al: Preoperative assessment of ureteropelvic junction obstruction with endoluminal sonography and helical CT. *AJR Am J Roentgenol* 168:623, 1997.

Sivit CJ, Cutting JP, Eichelberger MR: CT diagnosis and localization of rupture of the bladder in children with blunt abdominal trauma: Significance of contrast material extravasation in the pelvis. *AJR Am J Roentgenol* 164:1243, 1995.

Skinner DG, Lieskovsky G, Boyd S: Continent urinary diversion. *J Urol* 141:1323, 1989.

Smith EM, Elder JS, Spirnak JP: Major blunt renal trauma in the pediatric population: Is a nonoperative approach indicated? *J Urol* 149:546, 1993.

Smith RC, Rosenfield AT, et al: Acute flank pain: Comparison of non-contrast-enhanced CT and intravenous urography. *Radiology* 194:789, 1995.

Smith RC, Verga M, et al: Diagnosis of acute flank pain: Value on unenhanced helical CT. *AJR Am J Roentgenol* 166:97, 1996.

Smith RC, Verga M, et al: Acute ureteral obstruction: Value of secondary signs of helical unenhanced CT. *AJR Am J Roentgenol* 167: 1109, 1996.

Steers WD, Barrett DM, Wein AJ: Voiding dysfunction: Diagnosis, classification and management, in Lenwater JY, Grayhack JT, et al (eds): *Adult and Pediatric Urology*. Chicago, Year Book Medical Publishers, 1996, pp 1220–1326.

Stein JP, Kaji DM, et al: Blunt renal trauma in the pediatric population: Indications for radiographic evaluation. *Urology* 44:406, 1994.

Steinback E, Stockle M, et al: Conservative surgery of renal tumors in 140 patients: 21 years of experience. *J Urol* 148:24, 1992.

Stoller ML, Wold JSJ, Lezin MA: Estimated blood loss and transfusion rates associated with percutaneous nephrolithotomy. *J Urol* 152:1977, 1994.

Takeda M, Go H, et al: Retroperitoneal laparoscopic adrenalectomy for functioning adrenal tumors: Comparison with conventional transperitoneal laparoscopic adrenalectomy. *J Urol* 157: 19, 1997.

Thomas R, Monga M, Klein EW: Ureteroscopic retrograde endopyelotomy for management of ureteropelvic junction obstruction. *J Endourol* 10:141, 1996.

Thrasher JB, Paulson DF: Prognostic factors in renal cancer. *Urol Clin North Am* 20:247, 1993.

Townsend M, DeFalco AJ: Absence of ureteral opacification below ureteral disruption: A sentinel CT finding. *AJR Am J Roentgenol* 164:253, 1995.

Troxel SA, Winfield HN: Comparative financial analysis of laparoscopic pelvic lymph node dissection performed in 1990–1992 vs 1993–1994. *J Endourol* 10:353, 1996.

VanCangh PJ, Nesa S, et al: Vessels around the ureteropelvic junction: Significance and imaging by conventional radiology. *J Endourol* 10:111, 1996.

Walsh PC: Technique of vesicourethral anastomosis may influence recovery of sexual function following radical prostatectomy. *Atlas Urol Clin North Am* 2:59, 1994.

Walsh PC, Partin AW, Epstein JI: Cancer control and quality of life following anatomical radical retropubic prostatectomy: Results at 10 years. *J Urol* 152:1831, 1994.

Wein AJ, Hanno PM, Gillenwater JY: Interstitial cystitis: An introduction to the problem, in Hanno PM, Staskin DR, et al (eds): *Interstitial Cystitis*. London, Springer-Verlag, 1990, pp 3–15.

Wessells H, McAninch JW, et al: Criteria for noperative treatment of significant penetrating renal lacerations. *J Urol* 157:24, 1997.

Winfield HN, Hamilton BD, Bravo EL: Technique of laparoscopic adrenalectomy. *Urol Clin North Am* 24:459, 1997.

Winfield HN, Donovan JF, et al: Laparoscopic pelvic node dissection for genitourinary malignancies: Indications, techniques and results. *J Endourol* 6:103, 1992.

Wolf JSJ, Elashry OM, Clayman RV: Long-term results of endoureterotomy for benign ureteral and ureteroenteric strictures. *J Urol* 158:759, 1997.

CHAPTER 39

Gynecology

Gregory P. Sutton, Robert E. Rogers, and William W. Hurd

ANATOMY

External Genitalia (Vulva). The vulva is bounded by the symphysis pubis anteriorly, the anal sphincter posteriorly, and the ischial tuberosities laterally (Fig. 39-1). The *labia majora* form the cutaneous boundaries of the lateral vulva and represent the female homologue of the male scrotum. The labia majora are fatty folds covered by hair-bearing skin in the adult. They fuse anteriorly with the anterior prominence of the symphysis pubis, the *mons veneris*. Posteriorly, the labia majora

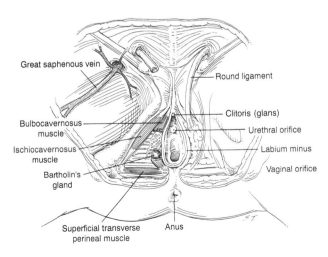

FIG. 39-1. The external anatomy of the vulva.

meet in a structure that blends with the perineal body and is referred to as the *posterior commissure.*

Adjacent and medial to the labia majora are the *labia minora,* smaller folds of connective tissue covered laterally by non-hair-bearing skin and medially by vaginal mucosa. The anterior fusion of the labia minora forms the *prepuce of the clitoris;* posteriorly, the labia minora fuse in the *fossa navicularis,* or posterior fourchette. The term *vestibule* refers to the area medial to the labia minora bounded by the fossa navicularis and the clitoris. Both the urethra and the vagina open into the vestibule. The clitoris lies superior to the urethral meatus; the male homologue is the penis.

Skene's glands lie lateral and inferior to the urethral meatus and occasionally harbor pathogens such as *Neisseria gonorrhoeae.* Cysts, abscesses, and neoplasms may arise in these glands.

Musculature of the Pelvic Floor. The *levator ani* muscles (Fig. 39-2) form the muscular floor of the pelvis. These muscles include, from anterior to posterior, bilaterally, the *pubococcygeus, puborectalis, iliococcygeus,* and *coccygeus* muscles. The first two of these contribute fibers to the fibromuscular perineal body. The *urogenital hiatus* is bounded laterally by the pubococcygeus muscles and anteriorly by the symphysis pubis. It is through this muscular defect that the urethra and vagina pass, and it is the focal point for the study of disorders of pelvic support such as cystocele, rectocele, and uterine prolapse.

Distal or caudad to the levator ani muscles, or *levator sling,* are the superficial muscles that constitute the *urogenital diaphragm.* This structure is bounded by the ischial tuberosities inferolaterally and by the pubic arch superiorly. The lateralmost muscular components of the urogenital diaphragm are the *ischiocavernosus* muscles. These structures parallel and are attached to the inferior rami of the symphysis pubis and, like the *bulbocavernosus* muscles, contain erectile tissue that becomes engorged during sexual arousal. The bulbocavernosus muscles arise in the inferoposterior border of the symphysis pubis and around the distal vagina before inserting into the perineal body.

The *transverse perinei* muscles arise from the inferior rami of the symphysis just anterior to the pubic tuberosities and insert medially into the perineal body, lending muscle fibers to this structure as well.

Internal Genitalia. Figure 39-3 is a view from above of the internal genitalia. The central uterus and cervix are suspended by the lateral fibrous cardinal, or *Mackenrodt's, ligaments,* which insert into the paracervical fascia medially and into the muscular sidewalls of the pelvis laterally. Posteriorly, the uterosacral ligaments provide support for the vagina and cervix as they course from the sacrum lateral to the rectum and insert into the paracervical or *endopelvic fascia.*

The bilateral fallopian tubes arise from the upper lateral *cornua* of the uterus and course posterolaterally and anterior to the ovaries. Each widens in the distal third, or *ampulla.* The ovaries are attached to the uterine cornu by the *proper ovarian ligaments.* These fibrous bands are analogous to the gubernaculum testis in the male and continue laterally from the uterus as the *round ligaments.* These structures exit the pelvis through the internal inguinal ring and course through the inguinal canal and external inguinal ring to the subcutaneous tissue of the mons veneris. They insert into the connective tissue of the labia majora. The ovaries are seemingly suspended from the lateral pelvis

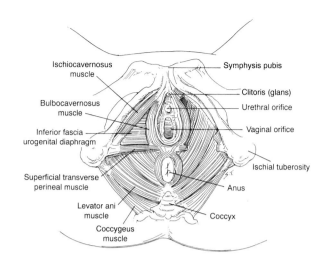

FIG. 39-2. Inferior view of perineal and pelvic muscles.

by their vascular pedicles, the *infundibulopelvic ligaments.* The peritoneum enfolding the *adnexa* (tube, round ligament, and ovary) is referred to as the *broad ligament,* although it is no more ligamentous than the peritoneum overlying the ovarian artery and vein.

The peritoneal recesses in the pelvis anterior and posterior to the uterus are referred to as the *anterior* and *posterior cul de sacs.* The latter is also called the *pouch* or *cul de sac of Douglas.*

On transverse section (Fig. 39-4), several avascular and therefore important surgical planes can be identified. These include the lateral paravesical and pararectal spaces and, from anterior to posterior, the retropubic or prevesical space of Retzius and the vesicovaginal, rectovaginal, and retrorectal, or presacral, spaces. The pelvic brim demarcates the obstetric, or true, from the false pelvis contained within the iliac crests.

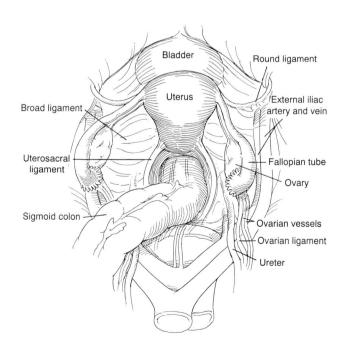

FIG. 39-3. Internal pelvic anatomy, from above.

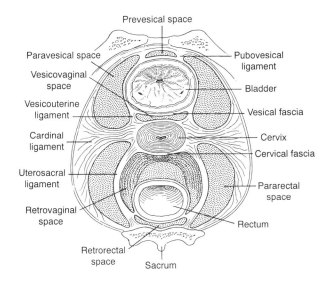

FIG. 39-4. *The avascular spaces of the female pelvis.*

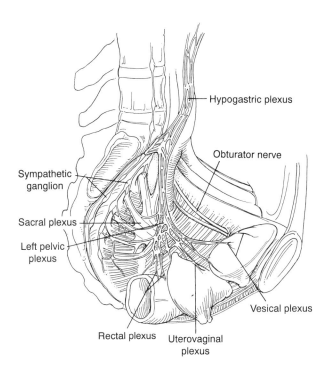

FIG. 39-6. *The nerve supply of the female pelvis.*

The muscles of the pelvic sidewall (Fig. 39-5) include the iliacus, the psoas, and the obturator internus. The blood supply is demonstrated in Fig. 39-5; with the exception of the middle sacral artery, which originates at the aortic bifurcation, the blood supply arises from the internal iliac arteries. The internal iliac, or hypogastric, arteries divide into anterior and posterior branches. The latter supply lumbar and gluteal branches and give rise to the pudendal arteries. From the anterior division of the hypogastric arteries come the obturator, uterine, superior, and middle vesical arteries.

The nerve supply to the pelvis is composed of the sciatic, obturator, and femoral nerves (Fig. 39-6). Sympathetic fibers course along the major arteries and parasympathetics form the superior and inferior pelvic plexi.

The ureters enter the pelvis as they cross the distal common iliac arteries laterally and then course inferior to the ovarian arteries and veins until they cross under the uterine arteries just lateral to the cervix. After travelling around to the cervix, the ureters course downward and medially over the anterior surface of the vagina before entering the base of the bladder.

DIAGNOSIS

Gynecologic History. The gynecologic evaluation includes a general history with special emphasis on the function of the reproductive system. The history should include

Purpose of the visit
Present illness
Menstrual and reproductive history
Past medical, surgical, obstetric, emotional, social, family and sexual history
Medications
Allergies
Family planning
Systems review

The gynecologic history should include the patient's age, date of her last menstrual period (LMP), the number of pregnancies, the number of deliveries, and the number of abortions. Gravidity, parity, and abortions are frequently indicated as G-P-A. The patient's menstrual history should include her age at the onset of menses, menstrual interval (time from the beginning of one period until the beginning of the next), number of days of flow, and some description in regard to the amount of flow (light, moderate, or heavy). The examiner should inquire as to when the patient's last cervical cytology was obtained, and, in patients over 35, the date of the patient's last mammogram should be noted. A description of the patient's current and recent contra-

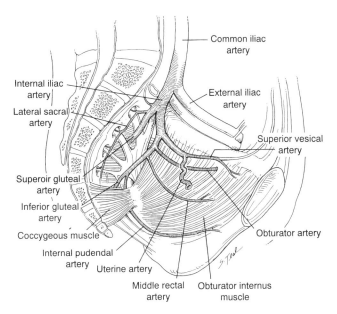

FIG. 39-5. *The muscles and vasculature of the pelvis.*

ceptive methods should be listed. The age of the patient at the time of her last menstrual period is recorded in postmenopausal patients.

Physical Examination. The initial evaluation and the presurgical work-up of a patient should include a general physical examination to include a description of the patient's

Height
Weight
Nutritional status
Blood pressure
Head and neck, including thyroid
Heart
Lungs
Lymph nodes

The gynecologic portion of the examination should document an examination of the breasts, the abdomen, and the pelvis. The pelvic examination is performed on all female patients with a pelvic complaint or on the occasion of their annual gynecologic examination. The patient is examined with her legs comfortably placed in stirrups on an examination table. A good light is essential. Instruments should be warm. Vaginal specula of several sizes must be available.

The external genitalia are inspected, noting the distribution and condition of the pubic hair. The glans clitoris, labia, urethral meatus, and the vaginal introitus are evaluated. The condition of the perineum is noted. The anus and perianal area are inspected.

The speculum is inserted into the vagina, and the vaginal walls and cervix are studied. A cervical cytology is taken at this time. The speculum is removed, and a bimanual examination of the pelvis is performed (Fig. 39-7). The Bartholin, urethral, and suburethral areas are palpated. The vaginal walls are palpated. The cervix is examined, and its consistency, shape, mobility, and tenderness to motion are noted. The uterus and adnexae are evaluated by pressing them between two fingers of the vaginal hand and a hand placed on the lower abdomen. The size, shape, mobility, and tenderness of these organs are noted. After the bimanual examination, a rectovaginal examination should be performed. The middle finger is inserted into the rectum while the index finger is inserted into the vagina. This important maneuver allows the physician to evaluate the posterior surface of the uterus as well as the rectovaginal septum and uterosacral ligaments (Fig. 39-8).

Diagnostic Procedures

Cervical Cytology. Cervical cytology (Pap smear) should be performed beginning at 18 years of age or sooner if the patient is sexually active. Most women should have a cervical cytologic evaluation yearly at the time of their annual pelvic examination. Except in emergency situations, no female in the reproductive age group should undergo a gynecologic surgical procedure in the absence of a recent cervical cytologic evaluation. After total hysterectomy, the Pap smear should be obtained annually in patients treated for cervical neoplasia. After hysterectomy for conditions that did not include cervical neoplasia, the vaginal apex may be screened cytologically every 3 to 5 years, although the cost-effectiveness of continued screening is controversial.

Cervical cytologic specimens are obtained at the time of pelvic examination. The cervix is exposed, and the external cervix

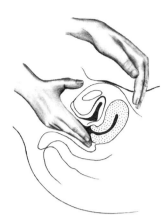

FIG. 39-7. *Bimanual abdominovaginal palpation of the uterus.*

is scraped with a suitable spatula. The material is placed on a slide expeditiously fixed with any of the fixatives favored by the cytology laboratory that serves the practice. A sample of endocervical cells is then collected, either with a cotton-tipped applicator or with one of the specialized cytologic brushes. This specimen is then placed on a slide and fixed in the manner of the previous specimen.

The practitioner should expect a report from the laboratory in the format of the Bethesda classification (Table 39-1) for cervical cytologic reporting. The Bethesda system for reporting cervical cytologic diagnoses was developed in 1988 and improved in 1991; it replaced the original Papanicolaou reporting system and provides a uniform format for cytopathology reports.

All cytologic reports must be studied carefully to determine whether further evaluation or treatment is indicated (Fig. 39-9). Atypical smears or smears with severe inflammation should be repeated generally in 3 months. Persistent (two or more consecutive) atypical smears should be evaluated with colposcopic examination. All smears that indicate dysplasia or neoplasia should be investigated with colposcopy.

Colposcopy is a specialized technique that allows evaluation of the cervix under magnification, enabling the practitioner to do directed biopsies of abnormal areas. In many cases the endocervical canal, which is not directly visible to the colposcopist,

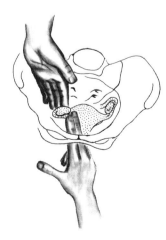

FIG. 39-8. *Bimanual abdominovaginal palpation of the adnexa.*

Table 39-1
The Bethesda Classification for the Classification of Pap Smear Abnormalities

Adequacy of the Specimen
Satisfactory for evaluation
Satisfactory for evaluation but limited by. . .(specify)
Unsatisfactory. . .(specify)

General Categorization
Within normal limits
Benign cellular changes: see Descriptive diagnosis
Epithelial cell abnormality: see Descriptive diagnosis
Descriptive Diagnosis
Benign cellular changes
   Trichomonas vaginalis
   Fungus organisms
   Predominence of coccobacilli
   Consistent with *Actinomyces* sp.
   Consistent with herpes simplex virus
Reactive changes
   Changes associated with inflammation
   Atrophy with inflammation
   Radiation
   Intrauterine contraceptive device

Epithelial Cell Abnormalities
Squamous cell
   Atypical squamous cells of undetermined significance
   Low-grade squamous intraepithelial lesion encompassing human
     papillomavirus
   High-grade squamous intraepithelial lesion encompassing
     moderate dysplasia, severe dysplasia, *carcinoma in situ*
   Squamous cell carcinoma
Glandular cell
   Endometrial cells, cytologically benign in postmenopause
   Atypical glandular cells of undetermined significance
   Endocervical adenocarcinoma
   Endometrial adenocarcinoma
   Extrauterine adenocarcinoma
Adenocarcinoma, NOS
Other Malignant Neoplasms (specify)
Hormonal Evaluation (applies to vaginal smears only)
   Hormonal pattern compatible with age and history
   Hormonal pattern incompatible with age and history
   Hormonal evaluation not possible due to. . .(specify)

is biopsied with a small curette at the time of colposcopic evaluation. Colposcopic examination is important to define the severity and size of a cervical lesion. The colposcopic examination following abnormal cervical cytology will preempt cone biopsy and allow office treatment of cervical dysplasia in most patients. Colposcopy may find a lesion too large for the ablative procedure that was planned and indicate another approach. When an endocervical lesion is found, the biopsy indicates a lesser lesion than cytologic report, or the biopsy is indicative of microinvasion of the cervix, a cone biopsy is indicated.

Office Tissue Biopsy. Biopsy of suspicious lesions of the vulva, vagina, cervix, and uterus should be obtained in the office. Vulvar biopsy is obtained by infiltrating the biopsy site with a small amount of 1% lidocaine using a 27-gauge needle. Ade-

quate biopsies can be obtained using a dermatologic skin punch to the vulvar skin and rotating it slightly. The biopsy then is separated from its base with thumb forceps and a pair of fine scissors. Any bleeding from the biopsy site is controlled with a silver nitrate stick.

Biopsy of vaginal lesions is accomplished under local anesthesia. A 25-gauge needle is helpful to reach lesions in the middle or upper vagina. Most lesions of the vaginal wall can be obtained through the use of specialized cervical biopsy forceps or laryngeal biopsy forceps.

Biopsy of the ectocervix does not require anesthesia. Specialized cervical biopsy punches, such as the Kevorkian or Tischler type, are used. The endocervical canal should be sampled with an endocervical curette such as the Kevorkian or Duncan endocervical curette.

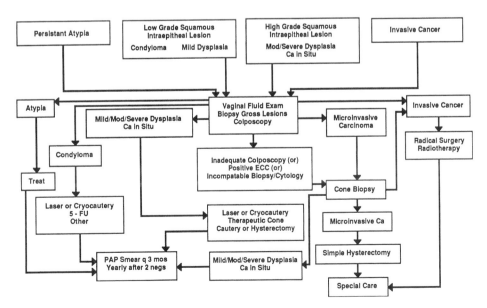

FIG. 39-9. The management of abnormal cytologic findings.

Biopsy of the endometrial cavity is an office procedure. It is essential to be assured that the patient is not pregnant before performing this procedure. A number of instruments are currently available for this biopsy. The Novak endometrial biopsy curette has been replaced largely by sampling devices such as the Pipelle endometrial biopsy instrument or the Vabra suction instrument; these instruments have the advantages of being narrow in caliber, fitting more comfortably into the cervical os, and being entirely disposable.

Vaginal Discharge. The patient's complaint of abnormal vaginal discharge should be investigated. Vaginal secretions that appear abnormal or have a foul odor must be studied. The pH of the vagina, which is normally between 3.8 and 4.4, may be an aid to diagnosis. A vaginal pH of 4.9 or more indicates either a bacterial or protozoal infection. The pH is obtained by dipping a pH tape in the vaginal secretions collected in the vaginal speculum.

Vaginal fluid is collected for study using a cotton-tipped applicator and transferring the sections to a small test tube containing a few drops of saline. The "wet mount" is prepared by placing a small amount of the saline suspension on a microscopic slide with a cover slip and examining it under magnification. The examiner may note motile trichomonads, indicative of *Trichomonas vaginalis;* characteristic "clue cells," indicative of bacterial vaginosis; or pus cells, which may be indicative of a variety of vaginal, cervical, and uterine problems such as gonorrhea, chlamydial or other bacterial infections.

After the initial microscopic examination, a drop of 10% potassium hydroxide is placed on the specimen, and the vaginal material is again evaluated. Potassium hydroxide has the ability to lyse cellular material and enable the practitioner to appreciate the presence of mycelia characteristic of *Candida* vaginitis.

Cultures. Vaginal and cervical cultures are most useful for the detection of sexually transmitted disease. While the diagnosis of gonorrhea might be suspected when gram-negative intracellular diplococci are found on a vaginal smear stained by Gram stain, culture should be obtained to prove the infection. Gonorrhea is cultured on a chocolate agar plate and incubated in a reduced oxygen atmosphere. Cultures are most conveniently collected on a Thayer-Martin medium in a bottle containing a carbon dioxide atmosphere.

Chlamydial infection is suggested by the finding of a characteristic thick yellow mucus (mucopus) in the cervical canal. Mucopus should be collected with a calcium alginate–tipped swab and sent to the laboratory in transport media specifically designated for *Chlamydia.* Some laboratories are now offering urine tests for gonorrhea and *Chlamydia* utilizing the ligase chain reaction (LCR). This test offers improved sensitivity and specificity for gonorrhea and *Chlamydia.*

Pregnancy Tests. A number of pregnancy tests are available for use in the office. These tests measure increased amounts of the beta subunit of human chorionic gonadotropin (hCG) in urine. These urine tests are very sensitive and specific, measuring hCG as low as 50 mIU/mL. Serum tests are even more accurate and sensitive, and they have the advantage that they can be quantitated to give an hCG level. Serial hCG levels are helpful in circumstances where it is important to determine that hCG levels are increasing or decreasing, such as in the management

of threatened abortion, ectopic pregnancy, or trophoblastic disease.

Abnormal Bleeding

After the first menstrual period (menarche), cyclic bleeding is considered the norm but is subject to great variation. Menstrual interval varies from 21 to 45 days (time from the beginning of one menstrual period until the beginning of another). Menstrual duration varies from 1 to 7 days. The menstrual flow is a subjective assessment and varies from light to heavy. Some women experience bleeding at midcycle at the time of ovulation. Abnormal genital bleeding falls into six categories.

Bleeding Associated with Pregnancy. The availability of extremely sensitive pregnancy tests has made it possible to confirm pregnancy in the early days of gestation. Although bleeding can occur in up to 25 percent of all normally pregnant women, this symptom must be considered a threatened abortion until the bleeding is otherwise clarified. In the presence of threatened abortion, the pregnancy test is positive, the cervix is closed, and the uterus is generally consistent with the history of gestation. A threatened abortion is considered inevitable when the cervix is dilated and fetal tissue appears at the cervical os. Abortion is incomplete after a portion of the products of conception has been expelled; it is considered complete after all the products of conception have been expelled. Inevitable and incomplete abortion is generally treated by dilatation and curettage.

Ectopic pregnancy must be considered in any patient with a positive pregnancy test, pelvic pain, and abnormal uterine bleeding. Approximately 20 percent of patients with ectopic pregnancy have no bleeding, but others might complain of bleeding from spotting or hemorrhage.

Gestational trophoblastic disease also causes abnormal bleeding associated with a positive pregnancy test. Most gestational trophoblastic disease is represented by hydatidiform mole. Molar pregnancy is suggested when the uterus is larger than would be expected from the history of gestation, vaginal bleeding, and the passage of grapelike tissue from the vagina. Quantitative gonadotropin levels are almost always greater than expected for the age of gestation. Gestational trophoblastic disease must be differentiated from normal pregnancy. Ultrasound examinations and knowing quantitative gonadotropin levels are helpful in diagnosis.

Dysfunctional Uterine Bleeding. This type of bleeding abnormality is characterized by irregular menses with occasional extended intervals of amenorrhea. When bleeding does occur after one of these periods of amenorrhea, it tends to be extremely heavy. The combination of a period of amenorrhea and extremely heavy bleeding occasionally suggests spontaneous abortion. In the majority of instances, the problem is secondary to failure to ovulate. Evaluation of these patients should include a pregnancy test, which should be negative. Endometrial sampling reveals a nonsecretory or proliferative endometrium. In the presence of extremely heavy bleeding, dilatation and curettage is required on occasion, but in most instances the condition can be managed with cyclic estrogen/progesterone treatment.

Trauma. The bleeding associated with genital trauma may be diagnosed secondary to a history of rape or genital injury. In the premenarchial female, the vaginal canal should be examined carefully for foreign bodies. In the presence of genital bleeding secondary to trauma, the lesion must be evaluated carefully and repaired in the operating room under anesthesia if necessary.

Bleeding Secondary to Neoplasm. Tumors, both benign and malignant, involving the genital tract from the vulva to the ovary, can produce abnormal bleeding. The most important tool in diagnosis is a meticulous pelvic examination that includes visualization of the vulva, vagina, and cervix and careful bimanual examination of the uterus, tubes, and ovaries. Lesions of the vulva, vagina, and cervix that produce bleeding should be biopsied to exclude malignancy.

The most common cause of abnormal bleeding in the reproductive age group is leiomyomas (fibroids). Leiomyomas are almost always benign and are a common cause of menometrorrhagia. Dilatation and curettage is helpful in diagnosing submucous uterine tumor. Pelvic ultrasound and other forms of pelvic imaging are helpful in the diagnosis of uterine fundal tumors.

The bleeding associated with tumors of the fallopian tube and ovary is generally scanty and is almost always associated with a palpable pelvic mass.

Bleeding from Infection. Bleeding is an uncommon symptom of pelvic inflammation. It is associated most often with inflammatory conditions of the vulva, vagina, and cervix. On rare occasions, patients with endometriosis and acute pelvic inflammatory disease have vaginal bleeding.

Bleeding of Nongenital Etiology. Genital bleeding can be associated with coagulopathy secondary to the use of systemic anticoagulants, clotting disorders, or blood dyscrasias.

Pain

Pelvic pain and abdominal pain are common gynecologic complaints. Pain associated with menses is the most common office complaint. Cyclic pain limited to that period just before or with the onset of menses is referred to as *dysmenorrhea*. Pain occurring without a demonstrable pathologic lesion is referred to as *primary dysmenorrhea* and is a common feature of ovulatory menstrual cycles. This condition is usually treated satisfactorily with simple analgesics. In some cases producing periodic disability, the use of ovarian suppression with oral contraceptives may be considered. *Secondary dysmenorrhea* is commonly associated with endometriosis, cervical stenosis, and pelvic inflammation.

Acute pelvic pain must be studied carefully. It may have its origin in abnormal pregnancy, benign or malignant neoplasia, or a variety of nongynecologic diseases.

Pregnancy disorders include threatened abortion, inevitable abortion, incomplete abortion, and ectopic pregnancy.

Neoplasms cause acute pain through degeneration of a myoma or torsion of a myoma or ovarian neoplasm. The spontaneous rupture of an ovarian cyst can produce severe pelvic pain. Pain associated with pelvic malignancy is a late symptom and generally follows other opportunities to diagnose this condition.

Acute pain may be caused by salpingitis or endometriosis. Pain secondary to inflammatory conditions is associated with fever and other evidence of infection in most cases. Pelvic infection secondary to *Chlamydia trachomatis* is the exception to this rule. The possibility of a nongynecologic condition as the cause of pain must be always considered. Appendicitis and other acute gastrointestinal problems are also causes of acute pelvic and abdominal pain. Patients with severe abdominal and pelvic

pain should be evaluated for urinary problems such as renal and ureteral stones as well as inflammatory conditions of the bladder.

In women in the reproductive age group, a differential diagnosis commonly involves appendicitis, ectopic pregnancy, and salpingitis. Readily available, rapidly performed, sensitive, and accurate pregnancy tests have made it possible to quickly exclude the possibility of pregnancy in many situations. Bilateral low abdominal pain increased by movement of the cervix and associated with fever and leukocytosis most often indicates acute pelvic inflammatory disease. Right abdominal pain and tenderness at McBurney's point, associated with a history of gastrointestinal symptoms, on most occasions will indicate appendicitis. In many cases it may not be possible to make a definitive diagnosis in the office, and some form of exploratory operation may be required. Direct visualization of the pelvis can be carried out with a laparoscope. Acute appendicitis, ruptured tuboovarian abscess, torsion of a tube or ovary, or an ectopic gestation may indicate celiotomy. The finding of pelvic inflammation in most cases will dictate medical treatment.

Pelvic Mass

The finding of a pelvic tumor is a common event in reproductive-age women. At one time pelvic examination was the only tool for detection and diagnosis of pelvic tumors, but with increasingly sensitive imaging devices, the surgeon is called to evaluate masses that in the past escaped detection. The clinician must be aware that several physiologic conditions cause enlargement of pelvic organs. Pregnancy should be considered in all cases of uterine enlargement in reproductive-age women. Ovarian enlargement, as a result of ovulation and corpus luteum hematomas, produces masses that are easily palpable and, that may, persist for several weeks. In addition to a carefully performed pelvic examination, abdominal and vaginal ultrasonography is a useful tool. No imaging method will distinguish between benign and malignant disease, however.

Pelvic ultrasonography, computed tomography (CT), and magnetic resonance imaging (MRI) all provide clues to the origin of pelvic tumors. Uterine enlargement may suggest pregnancy, uterine myomata, adenomyosis, or malignancy such as endometrial cancer or sarcoma. Tubal tumors may represent a tubal pregnancy, inflammatory conditions of the tube and hydrosalpinx formation, or a primary fallopian tumor. Ovarian enlargement may suggest endometriosis, ectopic pregnancy, tuboovarian abscess, or benign or malignant tumor of the ovary. The decision to operate is predicated on the patient's age, clinical presentation, and character and clinical course of the mass. If the differential diagnosis points to a strong possibility of ovarian malignancy, the patient should be explored under conditions that will allow for the treatment of a pelvic cancer.

INFECTIONS

Vulvar and Vaginal Infections

Vulvar, perineal, and perianal itching and burning are symptoms that may indicate an inflammatory condition. The area is subject to most of the infections that involve skin on any other part of the body. Vulvar infection may be primary on the vulva or can originate in the vagina.

Mycotic Infection. The most common cause of vulvar pruritus is candidal vulvovaginitis. The infection is most common in patients who are diabetic, pregnant, or on antibiotics. The majority of cases are caused by *Candida albicans,* although other species might be incriminated. The most prominent symptom is itching; burning of the skin, dysuria, and dyspareunia are also common. Diagnosis is confirmed by examination of the vaginal secretions and recognition of the characteristic pseudomycelia. The condition is treated by the topical application of any one of a number of imidazole preparations. Systemic treatment is possible through the oral use of fluconazole.

Parasitic Infections. Pin worms (*Enterobius vermicularis*), which are common in young girls, cause vulvitis. Diagnosis is made by finding the adult worms or recognizing the ova on microscopic examination of perianal material collected on adhesive tape. Mebendazole therapy is indicated.

Trichomonas vaginalis causes primarily a vaginal infection, but the copious vaginal discharge causes secondary vulvitis. The patient complains of heavy, foul-smelling discharge. Diagnosis is made by recognizing the motile flagellates on microscopic examination. Treatment consists of metronidazole 250 mg given three times daily for 7 days.

The vulvar skin is a frequent site for infestation by *Phthirus pubis* (crab lice) and *Sarcoptes scabiei* (scabies, itch mites). The primary symptom of both these infestations is severe pruritus. The adult and immature forms are recognized on close inspection of the skin. Treatment consists of lindane, available for medical use as Kwell.

Bacterial Infections. Many bacteria attack the vulvovaginal region; on occasion, bacteria considered normal inhabitants of the genital tract cause symptoms. The streptococci and staphylococci are the most common offenders.

Gardnerella vaginalis is the most common bacterial pathogen. The vaginal discharge found with this condition is not unlike that found with trichomonal vaginitis. The discharge is thin, gray-green in color. The patient complains of a foul, fishy, or "dead mouse" odor. Diagnosis is made by microscopic study of the vaginal secretions to identify characteristic "clue cells." The condition is treated with metronidazole 500 mg orally every 12 h for 1 week.

Viral Infections. A number of viral infections affect the vulva and vagina, the most common of these being *condyloma acuminatum.* The causative organism is the human papillomavirus. This infection has increased dramatically in the past 20 years. The lesions are characteristic wartlike growths that begin as single lesions but can grow to huge confluent lesions that distort the normal structures. The lesions enlarge rapidly in pregnancy. Diagnosis is suspected on the basis of appearance and confirmed by biopsy. Treatment depends on the destruction of the lesions with caustic agents, cryocautery, laser ablation, or electrocautery. Some large lesions could require surgical removal.

Herpes simplex infection causes painful vesicles followed by ulceration of the vulva, vagina, or cervix. Initial infection is usually widespread, but recurrent infection usually involves a single lesion. Cytologic evaluation of lesions in the vagina is helpful; culture is confirmatory for herpes infection. Once a patient is infected, there is a tendency for the lesions to recur at various intervals for the life of the patient. The attacks may be aborted and the interval between attacks lengthened through the use of acyclovir 200 mg orally five times daily. Active infection in pregnancy carries the risk of newborn infection if the patient delivers vaginally. Cesarean section is recommended in patients in labor with vulvar or vaginal ulceration as a result of herpes simplex infection.

Molluscum contagiosum causes groups of small pruritic nodules with an umbilicated center. The lesions are treated by ablation by cautery, curettage, or corrosive medication.

Pelvic Inflammatory Disease

While pelvic inflammatory disease is basically a medical problem, it has profound surgical implications. It is estimated that there are approximately 1.5 million cases of pelvic inflammatory disease in the United States each year. This condition produced approximately 350,000 hospital admissions and could be responsible for over a hundred thousand surgical procedures annually. The condition might produce infertility in 10 percent of the cases that occur; 3 percent or more of patients will have ectopic pregnancy, and chronic pain is a problem in many others.

Pelvic inflammatory disease is largely limited to sexually active females. Several factors have been recognized as placing the patient at risk: (1) age less than 20, (2) multiple sexual partners, (3) nulliparity, and (4) previous pelvic inflammatory disease.

Pelvic inflammatory disease is classified as *acute* or *chronic.* The most common organisms that produce the condition are *N. gonorrhoeae* and *Chlamydia,* but numerous other organisms have been incriminated. Diagnosis of pelvic inflammatory disease is based on clinical findings. The classic signs include fever, lower abdominal pain with pelvic tenderness, and purulent vaginal discharge. Some patients, however, will have minimal or absent symptomatology, particularly in the presence of a chlamydial infection. The lack of symptoms does not preclude pelvic inflammatory disease and tubal damage. Those patients who present with an acute illness must be studied thoroughly to rule out the possibility of acute appendicitis, ectopic pregnancy, gastrointestinal obstruction or perforation, and urinary stones.

In patients requiring further study, laparoscopy, pelvic ultrasonography, and pelvic CT scanning may be helpful in confirming a diagnosis. When pelvic inflammatory disease is present, laparoscopy will confirm it by finding tubal edema, erythema, and exudate. The presence of a tuboovarian abscess can be confirmed in this manner. Various imaging techniques such as ultrasound and CT scanning may also confirm a pelvic abscess.

Treatment. Women with pelvic inflammatory disease can be treated as inpatients or outpatients, depending on the severity of their disease. Patients with evidence of peritonitis, high fever, or suspected tuboovarian abscess should be admitted to the hospital for observation and intravenous antibiotics. Some specialists believe that all women with pelvic inflammatory disease should be admitted to the hospital for more intensive care, which might preserve their fertility.

The Centers for Disease Control and Prevention recommendations include one of the following outpatient therapy combinations: cefoxitin 2.0 g I.M. with oral probenecid, or ceftriaxone 250 mg I.M. or equivalent cephalosporin, plus doxycycline 100 mg orally two times daily for 10 to 14 days. The first part of the therapy is aimed at *N. gonorrhoeae.* Because cefoxitin is active against the penicillinase-producing gonorrhea, this agent should be used when such strains occur. The doxycycline is added to cover *Chlamydia* either as a single pathogen or as a coexisting agent with *N. gonorrhoeae.*

Follow-up of patients treated on an ambulatory basis should be carried out within 48 to 72 h. If there is no improvement in the patient, she should be admitted for intravenous antibiotics.

Recommendations from the Centers for Disease Control and Prevention for inpatient treatment include cefoxitin 2.0 g I.V. every 6 h plus a loading dose of gentamicin 2.0 mg/kg I.V., followed by a maintenance dose of 1.5 mg/kg I.V. every 8 h. This regimen is continued for at least 48 h after the patient shows clinical improvement. Doxycycline 100 mg orally twice daily is given after the patient is discharged from the hospital, to complete a total of 10 to 14 days of therapy. An alternative regimen is clindamycin 900 mg I.V. every 8 h plus a loading dose of gentamicin 2.0 mg/kg I.V., followed by a maintenance dose of 1.5 mg/kg I.V. every 8 h. This regimen is continued for at least 48 h after the patient improves, following which the patient is discharged on doxycycline 100 mg orally twice daily to complete a total of 10 to 14 days of therapy.

Gentamicin or tobramycin in the doses listed above is given provided the patient has a normal creatinine level. If the creatinine level is elevated, an adjusted dose of gentamicin or one of the other recommended regimens is advised. It is now known that the use of broad-spectrum antibiotics, which must include an antibiotic with anaerobic activity, will result in cures. Some patients may require surgery for persistent abscess or chronic pelvic pain.

Surgical Therapy. Surgery becomes necessary under the following conditions: (1) the intraperitoneal rupture of a tuboovarian abscess, (2) the persistence of a pelvic abscess despite antibiotic therapy, and (3) chronic pelvic pain.

At one time, total abdominal hysterectomy with bilateral salpingo-oophorectomy was considered the procedure of choice when surgery for pelvic inflammatory disease was required. The availability of good antibiotics and a better understanding of the pathophysiology of the disease allow less radical surgery. In young women whose reproductive goals have not been achieved, especially in the presence of unilateral disease, a unilateral salpingo-oophorectomy may be more appropriate than total hysterectomy with removal of both ovaries and fallopian tubes.

The rupture of a tuboovarian abscess is a true surgical emergency. Physical findings are frequently nonspecific. Rupture is most frequently associated with a sudden severe increase in abdominal pain. A shocklike state commonly accompanies rupture. Leukocyte counts are not necessarily increased, and some patients are afebrile. In the days before surgical intervention for this problem was common, mortality approached 100 percent. With prompt surgical intervention and intensive medical management, the mortality rate today is less than 5 percent.

The patient with a ruptured abscess must be explored promptly through a large midline incision. Hysterectomy and oophorectomy are commonly indicated. Operation may be technically difficult because of the distortion and edema secondary to the inflammatory process. Before the extirpation of any pelvic organ, adhesions must be lysed and normal structures, such as ureters and the large and small bowel, identified. At the conclusion of the procedure, the abdomen should be liberally irrigated. If the uterus is removed, the vaginal cuff should be left open for drainage. Patients should be treated with high-dose intravenous antibiotics. Because abdominal wound infection is extremely common in these patients, the rectus fascia should be closed securely with a mass closure of the Smead-Jones type. The skin

and subcutaneous tissue can be closed but frequently are left open for later delayed closure.

ENDOMETRIOSIS

Endometriosis is one of the most common conditions encountered by the pelvic surgeon. It has been estimated that endometriosis will be demonstrated in approximately 20 percent of all laparotomies in women in the reproductive age group. Although the condition occurs in teenage women, it is found most often in the third and fourth decades. Endometriosis persists into the postreproductive years.

The exact cause of endometriosis is unknown, but the most common theory is that it is initiated by retrograde menstruation. The theory is supported by the fact that it is extremely common in women who have congenital anomalies of the lower reproductive tract that would favor menstrual reflux. The most common of these anomalies is an imperforate hymen.

The most common lesions of endometriosis can be recognized as bluish or black lesions, sometimes raised, sometimes puckered, giving them a "gunpowder burn" appearance. Some lesions are white or yellow, but these are less common. The disease is found most commonly on the ovary and in many cases will involve both ovaries. Other involved organs can include the uterosacral ligaments, the peritoneal surfaces of the deep pelvis, the fallopian tubes, rectosigmoid, and a number of distant sites, including the skin or even the lungs, diaphragm, and nasopharynx.

While many patients are asymptomatic even with widespread endometriosis, others have severe pain, particularly dysmenorrhea, and dyspareunia. Other signs and symptoms depend on the location and depth of endometriotic implants. Infertility and abnormal bleeding are common problems.

The complaint of pain is common and in most cases is characteristic of the disease. Pain is associated most often with the menstrual period, characteristically beginning before the flow starts and ending when bleeding is complete. Deep pelvic dyspareunia is commonly associated with this disease, particularly in those individuals with implants involving the uterosacral ligaments or the rectovaginal septum.

The finding of a pelvic mass and tender nodularity of the uterosacral ligament strongly suggests endometriosis. The mass usually represents an ovarian endometrioma, often referred to as a "chocolate cyst" because of its dark-brown fluid contents. Endometriomas are found in approximately a third of women with endometriosis and are often bilateral. Endometriotic involvement of the skin, mucous membranes, or peritoneum is characteristically a bluish discoloration, which will bleed or cause discomfort at the time of menstruation.

Although endometriosis may be suspected on the basis of clinical findings and the patient's history, the definitive diagnosis is made visually, usually with the aid of a laparoscope. Biopsy may be helpful in atypical cases. Medical management of this condition should not be started without a confirmed diagnosis. Laparoscopy offers the best diagnostic opportunity for this disease.

Treatment. Choices of treatment include expectant management only, medical management, and surgery. Patients with minimal endometriosis who are asymptomatic can be cared for through simple observation and management with cyclic oral contraceptives and simple analgesia. The medical management of this condition involves the use of a number of agents in several pharmacologic classes. Progestins have been used for the management of endometriosis for many years. Medroxyprogesterone acetate is given orally. The agent is used in doses of 10 mg two to three times daily and frequently provides symptomatic relief.

Pseudomenopause is currently the most common medical treatment for endometriosis. The most common medications used today for this purpose are the gonadotropin-releasing hormone agonists (GnRH-a). These agents produce a suppression of ovarian function by suppression of both follicle-stimulating hormone and luteinizing hormone as a result of continuous stimulation of pituitary GnRH receptors. These agents have low toxicity, and while they reliably produce the hypoestrogenic effects of hot flashes and vaginal atrophy, these symptoms are generally well tolerated. They can be given by depot injection or daily nasal spray. Because bone loss is also a result of hypoestrogenism, it is recommended that the treatment not be continued for more than 6 months.

In the past, danazol, a weak oral androgen, was used to create pseudomenopause. This agent suppresses pituitary gonadotropins by negative hypothalamic feedback. The resulting ovarian suppression produces endometrial atrophy and regression of ectopic endometrium. Along with vasomotor symptoms and vaginal atrophy, this medication has many other symptoms, including weight gain, muscle cramps, and signs of androgen excess, including oily skin, acne, and hirsutism. For this reason, it has been replaced largely by either GnRH-a or progestin therapy for the medical treatment of endometriosis.

All these medical therapies have been well documented to result in temporary relief in patients with symptomatic endometriosis. In some patients, the effects can be relatively long lasting, but complete, permanent regression of endometriosis is rare with medical therapy. Although these treatments are used widely to enhance fertility, there is little evidence that medical therapy actually increases pregnancy rates compared with expectant therapy.

Conservative surgical therapy for endometriosis has become much more common with the advancement of laparoscopic surgery. At the time of initial diagnosis, superficial endometrial implants can be ablated with electrocautery or laser, and ovarian endometriomas can be removed. This approach appears to result in short-term enhancement of fertility and may give substantial temporary pain relief. In some cases of severe pain, deep retroperitoneal endometriosis implants can be removed either by laparoscopy or laparotomy with good results. However, as with medical therapy, conservative surgical treatment for endometriosis is palliative rather than curative in most patients.

The approach to ovarian endometriomas deserves special consideration. These "chocolate cysts" cannot be treated effectively medically. In general, even large endometriomas can be drained and the cyst lining removed laparoscopically. Although it was recommended in the past to close the ovary with several layers of absorbable sutures, it appears that this approach tends to increase postoperative adhesion formation. For this reason, it is recommended that after hemostasis is achieved, the ovary should be left open to close spontaneously. Other methods to minimize adhesion formation include atraumatic handling of the tissues and the use of a cellulose adhesion barrier (Interceed)

over the surgical site. Several series document pregnancy of about 50 percent rates following conservative operation.

Extirpative surgery is the only permanent treatment for symptomatic endometriosis. Patients with symptomatic endometriosis whose reproductive goals have been achieved may have no interest in preserving their reproductive potential. In these circumstances, extirpation of the endometriosis along with the patient's fallopian tubes, ovaries, and uterus may be the best choice. If extirpative surgery has been chosen, removal of all ovarian tissue has been advocated in the past to prevent the stimulation of residual endometriosis or the development of the residual ovary syndrome. In younger patients, a normal ovary may be spared in some cases. If total hysterectomy with bilateral salpingo-oophorectomy is required, replacement hormone therapy is indicated and recurrence is uncommon. To minimize the risk of recurrent endometriosis, it is recommended that replacement hormones include daily estrogen combined with a progestin such as medroxyprogesterone acetate, 2.5 mg given orally.

ECTOPIC PREGNANCY

Ectopic pregnancy affects a large number of women of reproductive age in this country. The incidence of this condition has increased dramatically in the last two decades. Because of improvements in diagnostic and therapeutic approaches, however, maternal mortality has declined over the same period of time.

Women in the reproductive age group have an increased risk of ectopic pregnancy as they age. Women in the last 10 years of their reproductive life have more than three times the risk of women in the first 10 years of reproductive life. Black and Hispanic women have a higher risk than white women. A history of salpingitis is common in women with ectopic pregnancy. Sterilization protects against ectopic pregnancy, but when sterilization methods fail, the risk of tubal implantation is increased.

The most common complaint of patients with ectopic pregnancy is pain, frequently associated with irregular vaginal bleeding. Approximately 80 percent of affected women will recall a missed menstrual period. Physical findings include abdominal tenderness on cervical motion and adnexal tenderness on bimanual pelvic examination. An adnexal mass may be palpated in approximately 50 percent of patients. As a result of the intraperitoneal bleeding, some patients present in shock.

The most helpful laboratory examination is measurement of the beta subunit of hCG (beta-hCG). Today's test, with a sensitivity of 50 mIU/mL or less, enables the surgeon to confirm the pregnant state in almost all patients at risk for ectopic pregnancy. Once the physician is assured that the patient is pregnant, it must be determined that the pregnancy is in the uterus. Pelvic ultrasonography, particularly when performed with a vaginal transducer, is proving important in differentiating uterine gestations from ectopic gestations.

If the patient's condition is not emergent, the serum level of beta-hCG at 24- to 48-h intervals is followed. In a normally implanted pregnancy, hCG levels will double every 2 days in early pregnancy. The surgeon can separate normally implanted pregnancies from those with impending abortion or those located in an ectopic site.

Ultrasonic evaluation of the pelvis is increasingly important. The vaginal probe enables the clinician to determine whether the developing pregnancy is in the uterus or in the tube at a time when the hCG levels are barely more than 1000 mIU/mL. Significant intraperitoneal hemorrhage also can be visualized by vaginal ultrasound. However, culdocentesis remains an expedient means to determine the presence of hemoperitoneum in an emergency situation. In those patients who do not desire to continue the pregnancy, curettage of the uterus with examination of the tissue can be diagnostic. In the event that fetal tissue is not found, a diagnostic laparoscopy is usually required in the symptomatic patient for definitive diagnosis. In the presence of hemodynamic instability or significant intraperitoneal bleeding that precludes adequate visualization of the pelvis, immediate laparotomy is indicated.

Treatment. Once a diagnosis of ectopic pregnancy has been established, several choices are available for treatment.

Laparoscopic Procedures. The laparoscope has been an important diagnostic tool for the last several decades, but only recently has it become the standard approach for treatment. Linear salpingostomy is the treatment of choice for ectopic pregnancies less than 4 cm in diameter that occur in the distal third (ampullary) segment of the tube. To aid in hemostasis, the mesentery below the involved tubal segment is infiltrated with a dilute vasopressin solution. The tube may then be opened in its long axis along the antimesenteric side with either a laser or a unipolar cutting cautery. The conceptus is then aspirated, and any bleeding is electrocoagulated with bipolar cautery. Closing the tube is not necessary because the tube closes spontaneously in almost every case. If hemostasis cannot be achieved, coagulation of a portion of the mesosalpinx just below the segment may be required. Partial or total salpingectomy is indicated when the pregnancy is located in the isthmic portion of the tube. Bipolar electrocoagulation is used to desiccate a short segment of fallopian tube on either side of the pregnancy, and the pregnancy and tubal segment are removed together. Larger ectopic pregnancies are managed by total salpingectomy because adequate hemostasis is difficult to achieve without extensive tubal damage. For this procedure, the mesosalpinx is serially coagulated with bipolar cautery and transected with scissors. When the uterotubal junction is reached, the tube is desiccated with bipolar cautery, and the entire tube and pregnancy are removed with the aid of a specimen bag and a large port.

Abdominal Operation. In those cases in which the surgeon has elected to perform a laparotomy, the same treatment options exist that were available laparoscopically. In a patient who desires future pregnancy, every attempt should be made to preserve a functional fallopian tube. If linear salpingostomy cannot be performed, consideration should be given to midsegment resection. Midsegment resection invariably shortens the tube but preserves the fimbria, which allows later reanastomosis. Salpingectomy should be reserved for those patients who have completed their reproductive goals, those in whom salpingostomy has failed, or those whose tube has been so completely destroyed by the ectopic gestation that it cannot be salvaged.

Medical Therapy. A relatively new approach to ectopic pregnancy is the use of methotrexate. Conservative criteria for treatment of ectopic pregnancy with methotrexate include serum beta-hCG levels less than 3500 IU/L and vaginal ultrasound that reveals the tubal pregnancy to be less that 3.5 cm in diameter with no visible fetal cardiac motion and no sign of hemoperitoneum. In this situation, studies have shown that administration of intramuscular methotrexate will result in complete resolution of the ectopic pregnancy in 96 percent of the cases. Subsequent tubal patency on the affected side can be documented in approximately 85 percent of the patients so treated. The risk of rupture and intraperitoneal hemorrhage must be made clear to the patient. In these cases, surgical management can be lifesaving. To what degree methotrexate treatment of ectopic pregnancy will replace definitive surgery has yet to be established.

PELVIC SUPPORT DEFECTS

Pelvic support defects include uterine prolapse, cystocele, rectocele, enterocele, urethral detachment, and posthysterectomy vaginal prolapse. The various types of pelvic support defects seldom occur as isolated problems. The forces that produce these defects influence all the organs in the pelvis that are susceptible to injury. Pelvic support defects may be produced by one or more of the following conditions: obstetric injury, conditions that increase abdominal pressure, obesity, decreased estrogen levels, and inherent tissue weakness secondary to genetic or nutritional factors.

Uterine Prolapse. Uterine prolapse is abnormal descent of the uterus relative to the bony pelvis and vagina. If the cervix protrudes through the vaginal introitus, the prolapse is considered partial; if the entire uterus prolapses through the introitus, the condition is considered a total prolapse. To assess this condition, the patient should be examined at rest in a lithotomy position and while straining. The uterus should descend without the use of a tenaculum.

Cystocele and Rectocele. These conditions are due to herniation of the bladder and the rectum into the vaginal canal, generally through a widened vaginal introitus. There are many classifications of these conditions; the simplest is mild, moderate, or severe. A somewhat more useful one is as follows: first degree, a slight bulge in vaginal wall; second degree, a bulge of mucosa that brings the vaginal wall to the introitus; and third degree, the bulge prolapses through the introitus.

Enterocele. An enterocele, herniation of intraperitoneal organs generally at the vaginal apex, most often follows hysterectomy. The hernia sac is lined by peritoneum and can be filled with small bowel, sigmoid colon, and occasionally uterine adnexa. Enteroceles are frequently misdiagnosed as rectoceles. The two conditions can be differentiated by placing one finger in the rectum and another in the vagina, allowing the examiner to palpate small bowel in the hernia sac.

Urethral Detachment. At one time, urethral detachment was called *urethrocele*. When the female urethra loses its normal support, it bulges into the vaginal canal. In the normal state, there is a definite angle produced by the urethra and the posterior wall of the bladder. Urethral detachment results in the angulation approaching 180°. In most cases, the urethrocele coexists with a cystocele.

Stress Urinary Incontinence. Urinary incontinence affects almost 40 percent of all women over 60 years of age and is a common problem for younger women. Some forms of incontinence are surgically correctable. Those conditions improved by operation are frequently associated with loss of the posterior ureterovesical angle, i.e., that angle produced by the posterior wall of the urethra and the posterior wall of the bladder. Mobility in this area, particularly at times of increased abdominal stress such as coughing, laughing, or sneezing, produces involuntary loss of urine.

A patient complaining of the involuntary loss of urine secondary to coughing or sneezing should be evaluated carefully. The surgeon should be certain that the condition is due to distorted anatomy and not to conditions that produce an irritable bladder syndrome.

Incontinent patients are examined initially in the lithotomy position. On straining, the patient generally will exhibit a cystocele or the loss of posterior ureterovesical angle. When asked to cough, there may be a small loss of urine. Movement of the anterior vaginal wall may be observed by placing a Sims speculum or the posterior blade of a medium Graves speculum in the vagina and asking the patient to cough. On occasion, the patient will not demonstrate incontinence in a supine position, and she must be examined in the standing position.

Before considering operation, the patient should be evaluated with a cystometrogram obtained by placing known amounts of water in the bladder and measuring bladder pressure with a manometer. The volume at which the patient feels the first urge to void and the volume at which the patient is unable to tolerate additional fluid are recorded. The amount of fluid in the bladder is reduced by 250 mL, the catheter is removed, and the patient is asked to cough. Most patients with genuine urinary stress incontinence will demonstrate loss of urine. At completion of the study, the patient is asked to void, and residual urine is evaluated by recatheterizing the patient. Normal patients will have the urge to void at 150 to 200 mL. A strong urge to void should be experienced at between 400 and 500 mL. Residual postvoid urine should be less than 50 mL.

Urethral descent may be quantified through the use of a Q-Tip test. The periurethral area is cleansed, and a lubricated Q-Tip is inserted 3 cm into the urethra. The resting angle of the Q-Tip relative to the horizontal is measured. The patient is asked to strain, and the angle that represents the maximum excursion of the Q-Tip is again measured. An excursion of over 20° represents increased urethral mobility, frequently associated with genuine urinary stress incontinence.

Therapeutic Considerations. A decision whether to treat a patient expectantly or surgically depends on the patient's symptomatology. Minor asymptomatic support defects may be treated expectantly or by pubococcygeal exercises. Pubococcygeal exercises involve contracting and relaxing the levator muscle repetitively several times daily. This intervention will not change the anatomic abnormalities of support defects but might give the patient better urinary control. Symptoms that may require surgery include urinary stress incontinence, symptomatic prolapse of the uterus, bladder, or rectum, urinary retention, vaginal ulceration due to prolapse, and constipation secondary to rectal sacculation.

BENIGN TUMORS

Ovarian Tumors

Nonneoplastic Cysts

By definition, a cystic enlargement of the ovary should be at least 2.5 cm in diameter to be termed a *cyst*.

Follicular Cysts. These are unruptured, enlarged graafian follicles. They grossly resemble true cystomas. They can rupture, causing acute peritoneal irritation, undergo torsion and infarction of the ovary or infarction of the tube and ovary, or spontaneously regress.

Corpus Luteum Cysts. These cysts become as large as 10 to 11 cm. They can rupture and lead to severe hemorrhage and occasionally vascular collapse from blood loss. The symptoms and physical findings of these cysts mimic those of ectopic pregnancy, and they are occasionally associated with delayed menses and spotting.

Endometriomas. These account for most "chocolate cysts" and are cystic forms of endometriosis of the ovary.

Wolffian Duct Remnants. These are not ovarian cysts but often cannot be distinguished clinically from tumors of the ovary. They are small unilocular cysts. Occasionally, they enlarge and may twist and infarct. In most instances, they are incidental findings at laparotomy and cause no difficulties or symptoms.

Müllerian Duct Remnants. These can appear as paraovarian cysts or as small cystic swellings at the fimbriated end of the fallopian tube (hydatids of Morgagni).

Nonfunctioning Tumors

Cystadenomas. Serous cystadenomas appear as cysts within translucent walls containing clear fluid and lined by simple ciliated epithelium. They frequently are on a pedicle and may undergo torsion leading to pain and infarction. When encountered surgically, they are adequately treated by simple salpingo-oophorectomy. Many fluid-containing cystic tumors of the ovary are also accompanied by papillary projections and are known as *papillary serous cystadenomas*. Because of epithelial variation in these tumors, it is often difficult to be sure where they fit in the spectrum of benign to malignant disease. A similar problem of malignant potential exists for the *mucinous cystadenoma,* which is a cystic tumor containing sticky, gelatinous material. These mucinous tumors are less likely to be malignant than the serous cystadenomas. About 20 percent of the serous tumors and 5 percent of the mucinous tumors are bilateral.

It is not always possible to be sure by gross inspection whether cystic tumors with solid components are benign or malignant. It is usually necessary to excise the involved ovary completely, even though there is no definite evidence of malignancy. The malignant potential of the cystadenoma is then determined by histologic examination. Some cystadenomas are classified as borderline tumors, or adenocarcinomas of low malignant potential. These (grade 0) carcinomas usually are associated with an excellent prognosis and, if they are unilateral, may be treated by unilateral adnexectomy for women in their reproductive years. Frozen-section examination of the tumor at the time of surgical intervention is necessary to determine the proper course of therapy for patients in the reproductive age group. The opposite ovary should be inspected.

Occasionally, a condition known as *pseudomyxoma peritonei* is encountered; this is a locally infiltrating tumor composed of multiple cysts containing thick mucin. These tumors arise either from ovarian mucinous cystadenomas or from mucoceles of the appendix, both of which commonly coexist. Histologically, they are benign, but by local spread and infiltration they compromise surrounding vital structures. Localized tumors should be excised completely, if possible. Both ovaries and the appendix are removed, even though they grossly appear to be normal.

Mature Teratoma. These germ cell tumors are thought to arise from the totipotential germ cells of the ovary. The tumors often contain calcified masses, and occasionally either teeth or pieces of bone can be seen on abdominal radiographs. Mature teratomas occur at any age but are more frequent in patients between 20 and 40 years. They are benign dermoid cysts. The occasional solid teratoma is usually malignant (immature teratoma).

If a teratoma (dermoid) is encountered in a young woman, it is preferable to shell it out from the ovarian stroma, preserving functioning tissue in the affected ovary. Usually these cysts contain ectodermal, mesodermal, and endodermal tissues, in addition to a thick, greasy, fatty material. If this material is spilled during surgery, a chemical peritonitis may result; therefore, it is important to remove these tumors intact. The opposite ovary should be inspected, but no further operative procedure is performed if the opposite ovary appears normal. In approximately 12 percent of patients, these tumors are bilateral. In patients of childbearing age, some functional ovarian tissue should be preserved. Immature teratomas are treated as a carcinoma of the ovary by hysterectomy and bilateral salpingo-oophorectomy.

Brenner Tumor. These are rare epithelial tumors that usually do not secrete hormones. Histologically, the epithelial elements are similar to Walthard rests and are believed to arise from these. These tumors occur primarily in later life and have a small malignant potential. Simple oophorectomy is usually sufficient therapy, and the prognosis is excellent.

Meig's Syndrome. This pertains to ascites with hydrothorax, seen in association with benign ovarian tumors with fibrous elements, usually fibromas. It is more common to see fluid accumulation with ovarian fibromas that are more than 6 cm in size. The cause of the condition is unknown, but the ascitic fluid may originate from the tumor, as a result of lymphatic obstruction of the ovary. Frequently, this clinical picture is encountered with other ovarian tumors, especially ovarian malignancies, which can produce a cytologically benign pleural effusion; in such cases it is termed a *pseudo-Meig's syndrome*. Meig's syndrome can be cured by excising the fibroma.

Functioning Tumors

Granulosa Cell–Theca Cell Tumor. Pure theca cell tumors (thecomas) are benign, but those with granulosa cell elements may be malignant. It is often impossible to predict their behavior from the histologic features, and prolonged follow-up is necessary in order to judge the nature. Usually, granulosa cell tumors elaborate estrogen, but some of these tumors have no hormone production. In young girls they are characteristically manifested by isosexual precocity, and in elderly women they are sometimes associated with endometrial carcinoma. The tumor can occur at all ages from childhood to the postmenopausal period, but it is most common in later life, with maximal occurrence between the ages of 40 and 60. If the tumor is discovered in the reproductive years and confined to one ovary without signs of surface spread or dissemination, a simple oophorectomy

may be sufficient therapy. If it is discovered in later life, removal of both ovaries with the uterus is indicated.

Sertoli-Leydig Cell Tumors (Arrhenoblastomas). These rare but potentially malignant tumors are associated with androgen output and masculinization. Rarely, they elaborate estrogen. They usually occur in the reproductive age group and appear to contain tubular structures as well as Leydig-type cells. In young patients with a single involved ovary, unilateral oophorectomy is adequate therapy, provided there is no extension of the tumor. For older patients or for those with bilateral involvement, total hysterectomy and bilateral salpingo-oophorectomy are performed.

Struma Ovarii. This term refers to the presence of grossly detectable thyroid tissue in the ovary, usually as the predominant element in dermoid cysts. This tissue occasionally may produce the clinical picture of hyperthyroidism.

Uterine Tumors

Leiomyomas. Uterine leiomyomas are the most common benign tumor in the female pelvis. It is estimated that up to 50 percent of all women at some time in their life have one or more of these uterine tumors. The tumor is never seen before menarche, it grows during reproductive life, and it generally regresses following menopause. The tumors significantly complicate pregnancy by virtue of their rapid growth secondary to the response to pregnancy hormones.

Many leiomyomas are asymptomatic; when they do produce symptoms, they cause pain, abnormal uterine bleeding, infertility, ureteral obstruction, bladder distortion, and pressure symptoms secondary to the enlarged uterus.

Uterine leiomyomata are subject to a number of degenerative changes, including calcification, necrosis (occasionally with liquefaction), fatty degeneration, and occasionally, sarcomatous change. Malignant degeneration occurs in less than 1 percent of all tumors. Uterine myomas may be found in a number of locations within the uterus (Fig. 39-10). The most common location is intramural, but tumors frequently are found just below the peritoneum and occasionally as a pedunculated mass attached

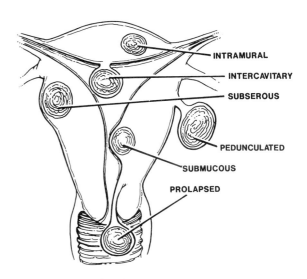

FIG. 39-10. Types of uterine myomas.

to the uterus. Other tumors grow into the endometrial cavity, where they are pedunculated on occasion, prolapsing through the cervix.

Treatment. Most symptomatic tumors can be managed expectantly. When symptoms indicate surgical treatment, consideration must be given to the age of the patient, the number of children she desires, the patient's age, and her reaction to possible loss of reproductive and menstrual function. Surgery should be fitted to the needs and desires of the patient. Therapeutic options might include myomectomy, total abdominal hysterectomy, or transvaginal hysterectomy.

Pedunculated myomas are the easiest to remove because the stalk of the tumor is simply ligated or coagulated and the tumor separated from the uterus. Pedunculated tumors in the endometrial cavity often can be removed with the operative hysteroscope. Similarly, tumors projecting from the external wall of the uterus into the peritoneal cavity can be removed laparoscopically by ligating the tumor pedicle and then morcellating the tumor intraperitoneally for removal or removing the tumor through a cul de sac incision.

Most myomectomies will be performed transabdominally. The most common indication for abdominal myomectomy is the presence of myomas that cause pain, bleeding, or infertility in a patient who continues to desire pregnancy. Before performing myomectomy, the patient must be evaluated completely and counseled about the risk of operation. Blood loss associated with myomectomy frequently exceeds that of hysterectomy. The patient should be advised of the possibility of hysterectomy in the event that myomectomy cannot be effectively performed. It is wise to set aside two or more units of autologous blood for possible operative use. The patient's tubal status should be evaluated with a hysterosalpingogram, and the patient's sexual partner should be evaluated with a semen analysis. In the presence of a very large tumor, chemoreduction of the tumor is currently being performed using a GnRH-a, such as nafarelin, given by nasal inhalation for a period of 3 months, or leuprolide acetate given intramuscularly every month for 2 months. These agents will cause the tumor to regress in size and in most cases provide for less blood loss at the time of operation.

Adenomyosis. *Adenomyosis* is a growth of endometrial tissue in the myometrium of the uterus and is sometimes referred to as *endometriosis of the uterine corpus.* The condition occurs primarily during reproductive years and leads to a thickening of the myometrial wall with subsequent uterine enlargement. Adenomyosis usually occurs in women who have had a number of pregnancies. Occasionally, patients with adenomyosis will complain of dysmenorrhea, and some present with increased uterine bleeding and heavy menstrual flow. However, a number of patients with adenomyosis in hysterectomy specimens have been asymptomatic. Therefore, the association of adenomyosis with heavy menstrual bleeding and dysmenorrhea is questionable.

Polyps. Endometrial polyps can occur at any time after puberty. A *polyp* is a local hyperplastic growth of endometrial tissue that usually causes postmenstrual or postmenopausal bleeding or staining, which is cured by polyp removal or curettage. The polyps are usually benign, but cases of adenocarcinoma of the endometrium arising in a polyp have been reported.

Cervical Lesions. Cervical polyps cause the same symptoms as endometrial polyps. Since they are often quite small and

are visible at the external os, they often can be removed as an outpatient procedure followed by cauterization of the base of the polyp. Nabothian cysts are mucous inclusion cysts of the cervix. They are occasionally associated with chronic inflammation and can be removed easily with a cautery. They are harmless, usually asymptomatic, and generally do not require surgery.

During reproductive years, the portio of the cervix is covered primarily with glycogenated squamous epithelium, and columnar epithelium is normally found centrally near the external os in most women. This exposed columnar epithelium, termed *ectropion* or *eversion,* is usually bright red. Unless accompanied by inflammation and a purulent discharge (cervicitis), it requires no treatment. During adult life, the columnar epithelium is usually replaced by squamous metaplasia, and this physiologic process occurs in the transformation zone at the interface of squamous and columnar epithelium. After menopause, the squamous columnar junction is usually in the endocervical canal.

Vulvar Lesions

The term *leukoplakia* is often used for any white patch of the vulva; it is properly reserved for areas that show histologically atypical epithelial activity. These alterations may precede the development of malignant changes. In many instances, chronically irritated and itchy white areas of the vulva will show sclerosing atrophy of the skin *(lichen sclerosus).* Lichen sclerosus is a pruritic lesion that does not appear to be premalignant. Hyperplastic lesions termed *hypertrophic dystrophies* are found that may be benign (epithelial hyperplasia) or may show atypia, in which case dysplastic changes can be observed. The pruritic symptoms can be helped by topical application of corticosteroids. Testosterone also has been beneficial, especially for the atrophic changes of lichen sclerosus.

Noninvasive malignant change of the surface squamous epithelium of the vulva occurs in the same way as that described for the cervix. Carcinoma in situ of the vulva both histologically and clinically behaves like carcinoma in situ of the cervix. The changes are confined to the squamous elements of the vulva, and the condition is sometimes referred to as *Bowen's disease.* In certain instances, the apocrine glandular elements of the vulva are involved in association with an intensely pruritic area. Histologically, large, foamy Paget's cells are seen, similar to those noted in the breast, although invasive carcinoma occasionally can accompany Paget's cells. Bowen's disease and usually Paget's disease are considered part of the carcinoma in situ complex of the vulva; they are adequately treated by wide local surgical excision (simple vulvectomy). The laser also is used to treat these lesions locally.

MALIGNANT TUMORS

Ovarian Tumors

Ovarian Carcinoma

Ovarian carcinomas are divided histologically into epithelial, germ cell, and stromal malignancies. The majority of the 26,700 or more cases of ovarian cancer diagnosed annually in the United States are of the epithelial type. The median age at diagnosis for epithelial ovarian cancer is 61, and the overall 5-year survival rate for epithelial cancers is 37 percent. Approximately 14,800 women die of this disease in the United States annually.

Although the etiology of ovarian cancer is uncertain, approximately 5 percent of patients with epithelial tumors come from families where one or more first-degree relatives also have the disease. In such families, prophylactic oophorectomy may be considered at the completion of childbearing, especially if specific BRCA1 mutations are identified. Testing for BRCA1 mutations is now available at select centers in the United States. Primary peritoneal carcinomatosis has been reported in women who have undergone prophylactic surgery, however. Life-long screening with CA-125 levels, pelvic examination, and vaginal ultrasonography of women from affected families bears consideration.

The FIGO (International Federation of Gynecology and Obstetrics) staging system for ovarian cancer is outlined in Table 39-2. Early lesions are largely asymptomatic, and advanced tumors may produce only nonspecific symptoms such as early satiety, abdominal distension, and vague gastrointestinal pains. Although an annual pelvic examination is valuable in detecting early ovarian cancer, efforts to establish other cost-effective screening programs using serum markers such as CA-125 and vaginal ultrasound examination are being developed. Vaginal ultrasound is a promising technology that is not presently cost-effective in screening programs. Currently, the majority of women with epithelial cancers have stage III tumors at the time of diagnosis. Widespread peritoneal dissemination, omental involvement, and ascites are the rule rather than the exception in these women.

Table 39-2
FIGO (1986) Staging System for Ovarian Cancer

Stage	Characteristic
I	Growth limited to the ovaries
IA	Growth limited to one ovary; no ascites; no tumor on the external surfaces, capsule intact
IB	Growth limited to both ovaries; no ascites; no tumor on the external surfaces, capsule intact
IC	Tumor either stage IA or stage IB but with tumor on the surface of one or both ovaries, or with capsule ruptured, or with ascites containing malignant cells or with positive peritoneal washings
II	Growth involving one or both ovaries on pelvic extension
IIA	Extension or metastases to the uterus or tubes
IIB	Extension to other pelvic tissues
IIC	Tumor either stage IIA or IIB with tumor on the surface of one or both ovaries, or with capsule(s) ruptured, or with ascites containing malignant cells or with positive peritoneal washings
III	Tumor involving one or both ovaries with peritoneal implants outside the pelvis or positive retroperitoneal or inguinal nodes; superficial liver metastases equals stage III; tumor is limited to the true pelvis but with histologically verified malignant extension to small bowel or omentum
IIIA	Tumor grossly limited to the true pelvis with negative nodes but with histologically confirmed microscopic seeding of abdominal peritoneal surfaces
IIIB	Tumor of one or both ovaries; histologically confirmed implants of abdominal peritoneal surfaces, none exceeding 2 cm in diameter; nodes negative
IIIC	Abdominal implants greater than 2 cm in diameter or positive retroperitoneal or inguinal nodes
IV	Growth involving one or both ovaries with distant metastases; if pleural effusion is present, there must be positive cytologic test results to allot a case to stage IV; parenchymal liver metastases equals stage IV

Treatment. In general, therapy for epithelial ovarian cancer consists of surgical resection and appropriate staging followed by adjuvant radiation or chemotherapy. Women with low-grade early-stage (IA or IB) cancers who have undergone appropriate surgical staging may be treated with surgery without adjuvant therapy. If the lesion is bilateral (stage IB), abdominal hysterectomy and bilateral salpingo-oophorectomy are sufficient. It is in the limited group of patients with unilateral histologic grade 1 or 2 lesions that fertility can be preserved by performing adnexectomy and staging biopsies without removing the uterus or contralateral ovary and fallopian tube. In all other patients (stage IA, grade 3, and stage IB and above), appropriate initial surgery includes bilateral salpingo-oophorectomy, abdominal hysterectomy if the uterus has not been removed on a prior occasion, appropriate staging, and tumor resection.

Staging. Staging indicates surgical resection or biopsy of all potential areas of tumor spread. Thorough staging is imperative in determining appropriate treatment for patients with ovarian cancer. Among patients whose cancer is confined to one or both ovaries at the time of gross inspection, occult metastases can be identified by careful surgical staging in one-third. If staging is improperly performed and adjuvant therapy omitted in patients whose tumors are apparently confined to the ovary, 35 percent will suffer preventable relapse.

Epithelial ovarian cancers disseminate along peritoneal surfaces and by lymphatic channels. The first site of spread is the pelvic peritoneum. Later the abdominal peritoneal surfaces and diaphragms are involved. The omentum is a common site for metastases, as are both the paraaortic and pelvic lymph nodes. Because the abdominal cavity in its entirety is not accessible through a transverse pelvic incision, it is paramount that surgery for ovarian malignancies be performed through a full-length midline abdominal incision. After the peritoneal cavity is entered, the visceral and parietal surfaces are inspected for metastatic disease, and any suspicious areas are biopsied. If ascites is present, it should be aspirated and heparinized. Cytologic evaluation for metastatic cells or clusters is then performed. If no ascites is found, peritoneal washings with balanced salt solution or lactated Ringer's solution are obtained from the pelvis, abdominal gutters, and subdiaphragmatic areas and submitted for cytologic evaluation after centrifugation and fixation.

Patients with histologic grade 1 or grade 2 tumors confined to one or both ovaries (stage IA or IB) require no postoperative therapy if proper staging procedures have been performed. Five-year survival in this group of patients exceeds 90 percent.

Those patients who have stage I, grade 3 lesions, stage IC tumors (malignant peritoneal washings, rupture of tumor, surface excrescences, or ascites), or stage II cancers that are completely resected may be treated equally well with systemic chemotherapy, radiotherapy of the whole abdomen, or a single instillation of intraperitoneal radioactive chromic phosphate. Five-year survival approaches 75 percent in this group of patients.

Women with stage III and IV disease require systemic chemotherapy with cisplatin or carboplatin, generally in combination with paclitaxel or an alkylating agent. Survival at 5 years in such patients may exceed 20 percent, although this rate drops as low as 10 percent at 10 years.

Survival in advanced ovarian cancer is influenced by a number of factors, such as patient age, the histologic type and grade of the lesion, the presence or absence of ascites, and the type of chemotherapy employed. Of prime importance in advanced-stage disease, however, is the volume of tumor remaining after the initial surgical procedure. Many patients with stage III and IV ovarian cancer have diffuse peritoneal, retroperitoneal, diaphragmatic, and mesenteric metastases that resist complete surgical resection. It is often possible, however, to remove large amounts of peritoneal tumor by entering the retroperitoneal spaces and freeing the disease-laden surfaces from the underlying viscera.

It is widely accepted that patients in whom little or no residual disease remains after initial operation, on average, live longer than those in whom a great deal of tumor remains unresected. The terms *debulking* and *cytoreduction* have been introduced to indicate aggressive surgical removal of ovarian cancer. When disease remaining after surgical resection consists of nodules or plaques less than 1 to 2 cm in diameter, the surgical effort is termed *optimal*, and when a larger volume of residual disease remains, the surgical removal is termed *suboptimal*. Because of the survival advantage, every effort should be made to resect as much disease at the time of diagnostic laparotomy as is possible. Since many patients with advanced ovarian cancer are elderly and nutritionally depleted, surgical enthusiasm must be tempered by proper preoperative evaluation and support with appropriate central monitoring and hyperalimentation where indicated. Occasionally it is more prudent to obtain confirmation of the diagnosis, treat with systemic chemotherapy, and then perform definitive surgery when the tumor has diminished in size and the patient has been nutritionally resuscitated.

Resection of nodules involving the small or large bowel is warranted if the exercise results in complete removal of all observed disease. Such procedures are probably not indicated if tumor remains at other sites. After surgical extirpation of the tumor, patients with suboptimal ovarian cancers must be treated with chemotherapy. Approximately 80 percent of these tumors will respond to platinum-based combination therapy; 40 percent of all patients will experience a complete response, or complete resolution of tumor identified on physical examination or radiographic study.

Resection of Advanced Ovarian Cancer. When advanced ovarian carcinoma is discovered at the time of exploratory celiotomy, the first reaction is often one of resignation. There has been a tendency to perform a diagnostic biopsy and close the abdomen without further surgical intervention. In experienced hands, however, successful reduction of tumor volume to nodules 2 cm or less is possible in at least 50 percent of women with advanced ovarian cancer. If the primary surgeon is incapable of obtaining such results, the patient should be referred to one with sufficient expertise in this area. Survival following chemotherapy is inversely related to the volume of residual disease at the time of primary surgery.

Several techniques ensure adequate resection. First, most ovarian cancer is found on peritoneal surfaces and not invading viscera. A retroperitoneal approach thus facilitates mobilization of the involved mesothelium. The lateral aspects of the paracolic gutters may be incised and dissection carried medially to undermine tumor in these locations. The ovarian artery and vein should be identified at this point and securely ligated before division. Once the blood supply to the main body of the ovarian tumor is secured, the adnexa may be mobilized more easily. It is often useful to dissect the ureter from the underlying pelvic peritoneum and retract it laterally with a vessel loop or umbilical

tape. This allows access to the lateral pelvic peritoneum. Tumor nodules on anterior and posterior cul de sac peritoneum may be resected by developing planes in the retroperitoneal spaces and isolating the disease from the underlying bladder, sigmoid colon, and ureters. Opening the pararectal and paravesical spaces facilitates this dissection and also allows access to the uterine vessels, which then may be clamped, ligated, and divided. When the hysterectomy and adnexectomy are complete, the omentum may be resected.

Disease on the right diaphragm may be resected by transecting the falciform ligament and retracting the liver inferiorly. If it serves to remove all remaining tumor, splenectomy may be performed. Resection of small and large bowel may be performed if the operation removes all residual disease. In recent years, use of the ultrasound aspirator has resulted in an increased ability to completely remove tumor, including that which is implanted on the serosal surfaces and mesentery of the bowel. With diligence it is often possible to remove all appreciable disease with this instrument. Another useful addition to the surgical armamentarium is the argon beam coagulator, which carries a stream of electrons into the tissue via an argon jet.

"Second Look" Operations. *"Second Look" Laparotomy.* Ovarian cancer often defies diagnosis because it does not produce symptoms and is detectable neither radiographically nor serologically even in relatively advanced stages. The assessment of ovarian cancer during and after therapy is similarly difficult. Although CT or MRI may identify masses as small as 2 to 3 cm in diameter, neither technique can reliably detect smaller masses, much less the miliary spread so often identified in advanced ovarian cancer.

CA-125 is more sensitive than radiographic or magnetic scanning but is also associated with a number of false-positive results and may not be elevated in patients with mucinous tumors. In addition, approximately half of patients with advanced ovarian cancer whose CA-125 levels normalize during chemotherapy harbor viable and clinically undetectable disease. Radiolabeled monoclonal antibodies raised against epithelial tumor surface antigens may be more sensitive than traditional methods but remain to be proven effective.

The practice of performing exploratory surgery following chemotherapy originated during a time when alkylating agents were used almost exclusively. Because acute nonmyelocytic leukemia is associated with prolonged administration of such agents, a "second look" operation was performed at an interval of 12 to 24 months following primary surgery so that treatment could be stopped in women with no disease. Presently, the duration of postoperative combination chemotherapy is often only 5 to 6 months, and the risk of leukemia is very low. In approximately 20 to 30 percent of patients who receive such treatment, no cancer will be identified at the time of a second operation. These patients have an excellent long-term prognosis. In women who have persistent microscopic disease, the prognosis is also favorable, and in those with persistent gross tumor, the prognosis is relatively poor.

"Second look" surgery is currently used primarily as a research tool. New treatment regimens can be evaluated quickly by performing a "second look" operation, since the findings at such an operation reflect the ultimate clinical outcome and hence the value of the treatment regimen. "Second look" surgery is also valuable in determining when therapy can be discontinued and when further treatment is indicated. If cancer is still present, secondary surgical resection has a beneficial effect on prognosis.

"Second look" laparotomy is performed through a midline abdominal incision. Peritoneal washings are obtained from both abdominal gutters, the diaphragms, and the pelvis. Since persistent cancer is most likely to be identified in sites where there was tumor at the conclusion of the primary operation, these areas are explored first. Any suspicious nodules, thickened peritoneal areas, or adhesions should be biopsied carefully and submitted for histologic evaluation. If no visible tumor is present, a formal staging operation should be performed. Liberal peritoneal biopsies from the above-mentioned sites are obtained, and then pelvic and paraaortic lymph nodes are sampled. Any residual omentum should be excised because it may harbor occult tumor. At the conclusion of "second look" surgery, some consideration should be given to subsequent therapy.

If tumor is identified and can be resected, a Tenckhoff catheter may be placed, through which intraperitoneal chemo- or immunotherapy may be given. If no visible disease is present, a Silastic drain can be inserted for the postoperative administration of radioactive chromic phosphate. Although the morbidity of "second look" surgery is very low, there is no place for this type of operation in patients who wish or who can physiologically tolerate no further treatment at the conclusion of primary combination chemotherapy. Nor is there any reason to reexplore such a patient without the ability or intention to perform a thorough, deliberate staging procedure that can guide subsequent therapy.

Other Secondary Operations. Surgical resection of tumor after chemotherapy or at the time of relapse is termed *secondary cytoreduction.* In the occasional patient who undergoes diagnostic biopsy only before the administration of chemotherapy, early reexploration may be termed *interval cytoreduction.* There is evidence that the surgical removal of extensive tumor is facilitated by the administration of one or two courses of combination chemotherapy. In patients with a massive tumor burden, this approach may not only be safer but also might result in a more successful tumor resection before the completion of chemotherapy. It also promotes the early administration of intraperitoneal chemotherapy.

The importance of secondary cytoreduction is not clearly established. In patients with relapsing ovarian cancer, the prognosis depends in part on the extent of tumor and in part on the type of response to previous therapy. Also important is the interval between primary therapy and relapse. In those who completely responded to platinum combination treatment and who have a disease-free period exceeding 2 years, resumption of platinum-based chemotherapy is very effective. Paclitaxel therapy may be effective in similar situations. It is in such patients that surgical removal of the recurrent tumor is likely to be the most beneficial.

Palliative Surgery. In most cases of advanced ovarian cancer, death is associated with bowel dysfunction or frank obstruction. Although invasion of the small bowel and colon is unusual, growth of the tumor adjacent to the bowel leads to mesenteric compromise and dysfunction usually heralded by distention, nausea, and vomiting. When bowel obstruction occurs early on in the clinical course of ovarian cancer, and particularly if it occurs before the administration of chemotherapy, surgical intervention is warranted and should be aggressive. Resection or bypass of the involved small bowel is indicated; colonic resec-

tion also may be indicated. It is important to perform adequate radiographic studies preoperatively so that obstructed small bowel is not decompressed into a compromised colon.

When bowel obstruction occurs after chemotherapy, the prognosis is unfavorable. Women who develop such difficulties have a limited survival following surgical correction. Surgery is often difficult to perform because of extensive tumor. Laparotomy may be complicated by enteric injury or fistula. Often the best approach in these patients is the use of a percutaneous or endoscopically positioned gastrostomy tube and intravenous fluids or conservative nutritional support. Such a procedure may limit the length of hospitalization and allow the patient to remain in a supportive home environment for a greater period of time.

Laparoscopy in Ovarian Cancer. At present, our ability to resect large ovarian cancers successfully using laparoscopic equipment is limited. In the past, efforts to perform "second look" procedures through the laparoscope were ineffective when compared with laparotomy. However, with the advent of new equipment and techniques, the role of laparoscopy in the staging and treatment of ovarian malignancies is expanding. Several investigators have developed successful methods of performing both pelvic and paraaortic lymphadenectomies using endoscopic equipment. In addition, ultrasonographic and serologic criteria are evolving that will allow the surgeon to more successfully distinguish between benign and malignant neoplasms of the ovary.

Tumors of Low Malignant Potential

These are epithelial tumors of malignant potential intermediate between benign lesions and frank malignancies. Histologically, most are of the serous type. They are distinguished from invasive cancers microscopically by lack of stromal invasion. The median age of diagnosis is approximately 10 years younger than that of patients with epithelial cancers. The vast majority occur in stage I and have a favorable prognosis. Surgery should include abdominal hysterectomy and bilateral salpingo-oophorectomy unless fertility is to be preserved in patients with unilateral lesions. These patients may undergo unilateral salpingo-oophorectomy. Ovarian cystectomy or nonextirpative resections commonly result in recurrences.

Patients with stage III and IV lesions have 5-year survival rates that approach 85 percent after complete surgical resection. There is little evidence that either chemotherapy or radiotherapy administered after surgery improves survival; on the other hand, deaths from chemotherapy-induced leukemia are not uncommon.

Germ Cell Tumors

These tumors occur in women in the first three decades of life and typically grow rapidly, producing symptoms of distention and abdominal fullness. Torsion may occur, producing an acute abdomen. Most are unilateral, and all have a tendency to spread to the paraaortic lymph nodes as well as throughout the peritoneal cavity. Although they are similar in many ways to testicular cancer in the male, there are some differences.

Dysgerminoma, the female equivalent of testicular seminoma, is composed of pure, undifferentiated germ cells. It is bilateral in 10 percent of patients and is occasionally associated with elevated levels of hCG or lactate dehydrogenase (LDH). It is the most common ovarian malignancy diagnosed during pregnancy. Patients bearing dysgerminomas should undergo appropriate staging at the time of the primary resection but need not undergo hysterectomy (if fertility is to be preserved) or removal of the opposite ovary if it is normal in appearance. Secondary operations solely for staging purposes are unwarranted. Adjuvant therapy is unnecessary unless there is evidence of extraovarian spread. Either radiotherapy encompassing the whole abdomen or systemic chemotherapy can be given to patients with metastases. This tumor is exquisitely sensitive to either type of treatment, and the cure rate exceeds 90 percent even in patients with metastases. Chemotherapy has the advantage of preserving ovarian function, whereas radiotherapy results in ovarian failure.

The other germ cell tumors in order of frequency are immature teratoma, endodermal sinus, or "yolk sac," tumor, mixed tumors, embryonal carcinomas, and choriocarcinomas. The first may be associated with elevated levels of alpha-fetoprotein (AFP). Elevated AFP levels are found in all patients with endodermal sinus tumors and mixed tumors that contain this component. Embryonal carcinomas are associated with abnormal levels of both AFP and hCG, and choriocarcinomas secrete hCG.

These tumors are invariably unilateral but may spread by peritoneal, hematogenous, or lymphatic routes. Surgical therapy is much the same as that described for ovarian dysgerminomas. Except for those with completely resected stage I, grade 1 immature teratomas and those with stage I dysgerminoma, all patients with germ cell tumors require systemic chemotherapy. Three courses of a platinum and etoposide-containing combination suffice in those patients whose tumors are completely resected. Cure rates in these patients approach 90 percent. In women with incompletely resected nondysgerminomatous germ cell tumors, cure may still be expected in over 50 percent, but prolonged chemotherapy may be necessary. These tumors are *not* sensitive to radiotherapy.

Carcinoma of the Cervix

Carcinoma of the cervix accounts for about 16,000 cases and 5000 deaths annually in the United States. Risk factors include multiple sexual partners, early age at first intercourse, and early first pregnancy. DNA related to that found in the human papillomavirus has been identified in cervical dysplasia and carcinoma in situ, both precursor lesions, as well as in invasive cancers and lymph node metastases. Other etiologic agents considered in this disease are herpes simplex type II and cigarette smoking.

In no cancer has widespread screening had as profound an impact on mortality as it has in carcinoma of the cervix. Georges Papanicolaou devised the cytologic smear that bears his name in 1943. Since that time, screening programs have dramatically reduced the rate of invasive cervical cancer in countries where this test is widely available. Use of the Pap smear has shifted the frequency of cervical abnormalities toward the premalignant intraepithelial diseases, dysplasia, and carcinoma in situ. Although there are histologic grades of dysplasia leading to carcinoma in situ, all intraepithelial lesions are noninvasive and can be treated successfully using conservative methods.

Eighty percent of all cervical cancers are squamous cell in type and arise from the squamocolumnar junction of the cervix. This epithelial transition zone is found on the face of the cervix or ectocervix in adolescence and, through a process of squamous metaplasia, gradually moves into the endocervical canal as menopause is passed. Dysplasia represents a disordered meta-

plasia and gives rise to epithelial cells that contain increased mitotic rates and nuclear atypia and that lack appropriate maturation within the epithelium. Identification and eradication of intraepithelial lesions before invasion can occur are the goals of cervical cancer screening.

The remainder of cervical malignancies arise in the endocervical canal and are either adenocarcinomas or adenosquamous carcinomas. Although adenocarcinomas are very similar in their clinical behavior to squamous cancers, there is some evidence that adenosquamous cancers are more aggressive. Other rare histologic varieties associated with poor prognosis are neuroendocrine small cell carcinomas and clear cell cancers. The latter are frequently associated with maternal exposure to diethylstilbestrol.

Staging. Cervical cancers spread predominantly by lymphatic channels. The first lymph nodes involved are those in the tissues immediately lateral to the cervix. This region is referred to as the *paracervical* or *parametrial area*. The next lymph nodes to be involved, in order, are those in the obturator fossa, the internal and external iliac chain, the common iliac chain, and the paraaortic lymph nodes. Direct vaginal extension may occur. The lymph nodes in the presacral area may be involved in early stage lesions, and the supraclavicular lymph nodes are the most common site of distant nodal metastases.

FIGO staging for cervical cancer is based on clinical examination, intravenous pyelography, and chest radiography. CT or MRI findings do not affect the clinical stage. The FIGO staging system is illustrated in Table 39-3. Note that the presence of hydronephrosis connotes stage IIIB even if there is no clinical evidence of extracervical spread. Except for selected patients with stage IVA lesions and those with distant metastases, all patients with stage IIB cancer and above are treated primarily with radiotherapy in the United States.

Treatment. *Intraepithelial or Preinvasive Disease.* Abnormal Pap smears must be evaluated by colposcopy and biopsy. Colposcopy is the examination of the cervix with a low-power (10 to 50×) microscope after application of dilute acetic acid to the cervix. The acid solution is mucolytic and serves to desiccate the epithelium, a process that brings out subtle epithelial patterns referred to as white epithelium, punctation, mosaicism, and abnormal vasculature. Abnormal areas must undergo mechanical biopsy or wide excision with a wire loop electrode and are examined histologically. If loop excision is not performed, the endocervical canal should be curetted to exclude epithelial abnormalities in this area, which is difficult to visualize colposcopically.

Once the diagnosis of an intraepithelial process is made and stromal invasion excluded, local therapy can be performed. If there are abnormal cells on the endocervical curettage specimen, a diagnostic cone biopsy is indicated to exclude the possibility of an invasive or microinvasive lesion in the endocervical canal.

Cervical intraepithelial neoplasia is treated in a number of ways. In general, the larger the lesion and the higher the grade of dysplasia, the greater is the failure rate. Similarly, more aggressive therapy yields lower failure rates at increased risk of complications. The most definitive treatment for cervical intraepithelial neoplasia is vaginal or abdominal hysterectomy. This operation is associated with a rate of subsequent dysplasia at the vaginal apex of 1 to 2 percent. This major operation is usually reserved, however, for patients with extensive or high-grade le-

Table 39-3
FIGO Staging System for Cervical Cancer

Stage	Characteristic
0	Carcinoma in situ
I	The carcinoma is strictly confined to the cervix (extension to the corpus should be disregarded)
IA	Preclinical carcinomas of the cervix; that is, those diagnosed only by microscopy
IA$_1$	Minimal microscopically evident stromal invasion
IA$_2$	Lesions detected microscopically that can be measured. The upper limit of the measurement should not show a depth of invasion of more than 5 mm taken from the base of the epithelium, either surface or glandular, from which it originates, and a second dimension, the horizontal spread, must not exceed 7 mm. Larger lesions should be staged as IB
IB	Lesions of greater dimensions than Stage IA$_2$ whether seen clinically or not. Preformed space involvement should not alter the staging but should be specifically recorded so as to determine whether it should affect treatment decisions in the future
IB$_1$	Tumor size no greater than 4 cm
IB$_2$	Tumor size greater than 4 cm
II	Involvement of the vagina but not the lower third, or infiltration of the parametria but not out to the sidewall
IIA	Involvement of the vagina but no evidence of parametrial involvement
IIB	Infiltration of the parametria but not out to the sidewall
III	Involvement of the lower third of the vagina or extension to the pelvic sidewall
IIIA	Involvement of the lower third of the vagina but not out to the pelvic sidewall if the parametria are involved
IIIB	Involvement of one or both parametria out to the sidewall
III (urinary)	Obstruction of one or both ureters on intravenous pyelogram (IVP) without the other criteria for stage III disease
IV	Extension outside the reproductive tract
IVA	Involvement of the mucosa of the bladder or rectum
IVB	Distant metastasis or disease outside the true pelvis

sions, those with recurrent disease after conservative treatment, those in whom adequate follow-up is unlikely, and those with other indications for hysterectomy such as prolapse, abnormal uterine bleeding, pain, or a pelvic mass. Cervical cone biopsy is curative in most cases of cervical intraepithelial neoplasia. In patients in whom the surgical margins of the cone specimen are uninvolved, the risk of recurrence is less than 5 percent. If the surgical margins are involved, half of such patients will develop recurrent disease. This is an outpatient procedure and associated with few serious risks. It may, however, require general anesthesia.

More conservative methods of treating cervical intraepithelial neoplasia include wire loop excision, laser vaporization, and cryosurgery. Loop excision can be done under local anesthesia (paracervical block) in the outpatient setting. The advantage of loop excision is that it removes the diseased area and provides a diagnostic biopsy specimen. The main disadvantage is the relatively large amount of cervical stroma that is taken with the involved epithelium. In cases of cervical intraepithelial neoplasia

confined to the ectocervix, such deep excision is probably unnecessary.

Laser vaporization is usually performed with a carbon dioxide laser, but other laser instruments may be used. The ectocervical transformation zone is ablated to a depth of about 7 mm to ensure the removal of endocervical glandular epithelium. This is a convenient outpatient procedure that results in a clearly visible squamocolumnar junction at the site of treatment. Risks of bleeding and infection are small. Cryotherapy is an inexpensive outpatient procedure that produces a frostbite injury to the ectocervical epithelium. When the cervix reepithelializes, the dysplasia generally does not recur. This is a simple technique that should not be applied to patients with endocervical lesions. The main disadvantage of cryotherapy is obliteration of the squamocolumnar junction, making subsequent colposcopic examination somewhat difficult. In patients with very localized mild dysplasias or low-grade cervical intraepithelial neoplasia, local excision or electrocautery may be sufficient to eradicate the disease.

Microinvasive Cervical Cancer. FIGO (see Table 39-3) subdivides microinvasive cancers into those with "early" invasion (stage IA$_1$) and those in which the tumor measurements are less than 5 mm in thickness and 7 mm in lateral extent (stage IA$_2$). This aspect of the FIGO staging system for cervical cancer fails to distinguish adequately between stages IA$_2$ and IB, however, because both may have occult lymph node metastases requiring regional therapy.

Many prefer the original system of the Society of Gynecologic Oncologists, in which stage IA (microinvasive) tumors may invade to no greater than 3 mm and must lack capability of lymphatic space invasion. Stage IB includes all other cancers clinically confined to the cervix, even if they cannot be visualized on examination. The advantage of this system is that it clearly divides stage I into two treatment groups. Few patients with stage IA cervical cancer have metastases to the lymph nodes. Simple, or extrafascial, hysterectomy without lymphadenectomy is therefore adequate therapy. Five-year survival rates approach 100 percent in these patients. In exceptional patients, cervical cone biopsy or electrosurgical excision may be sufficient treatment, provided close surveillance is possible.

Early Invasive Cervical Cancer (Stage IB and IIA). Stage IB and IIA tumors are associated with a risk of pelvic lymph node metastases of 10 to 15 percent and a risk of spread to the paraaortic nodes of about 5 percent. Treatment must include the regional lymph nodes in these patients. Radical hysterectomy with pelvic lymphadenectomy or definitive radiotherapy is effective treatment in this stage cancer. Prognosis with either modality depends on the size of the primary lesion, the presence or absence of lymph-vascular space involvement, spread to the regional lymph nodes, and status of the surgical margins.

Women with stage IB$_2$ cervical cancers (exceeding 4 cm in diameter), especially those endocervical primaries that distend the cervix circumferentially, may require a combination of radiotherapy and surgery. These large endocervical tumors are referred to as "barrel" lesions and are refractory to surgery or radiotherapy alone. Isodose curves from cesium sources may not encompass the entire tumor (Fig. 39-11). Cure rates with either treatment may be as low as 50 percent.

One current approach to these tumors is the administration of pelvic radiotherapy followed by a cesium implant and subsequent simple hysterectomy. This technique may reduce the number of patients who have persistent invasive cancer in the cervix after radiotherapy and consequently improve survival.

Stage IB_1 lesions and early stage IIA cancers may be treated successfully with radical hysterectomy and pelvic lymphadenectomy. This operation was pioneered by John Clark at Johns Hopkins Hospital in 1895. Radical surgery was transiently eclipsed by the first use of radium in the treatment of cervical cancer by Sjögren and Stenbeck in 1899 and subsequent establishment of the first radium hospital in Stockholm, Sweden, in 1910.

Radical surgery reemerged in the treatment of early carcinoma of the cervix with the advent of the Pap smear and increased diagnosis of early-stage tumors in young women. Because early cervical cancer so rarely spreads to the ovaries, radical hysterectomy need not include oophorectomy. Ovarian preservation is one of the strongest arguments for the use of surgery over radiotherapy, since the latter inevitably results in the premature loss of ovarian function.

Locally Advanced Carcinoma of the Cervix (Stages IIB to IVA). These cancers are treated primarily with radiotherapy. Treatment consists of a combination of external therapy to the pelvis (teletherapy) from a high-energy source such as a linear accelerator and a local dose delivered to the cervix and parametrial tissue (brachytherapy) using a cesium applicator such as a Fletcher-Suite tandem and ovoids (Fig. 39-12). Combination therapy is essential because doses adequate to control cervical tumors exceeding about 1 cm in diameter cannot be given using teletherapy alone. Bladder and rectal tolerances are approximately 6000 rads; higher doses can only be attained by combination therapy.

Cure rates for stage IIB cervical cancers approach 65 percent, and those for stage IIIB, 35 percent. Because the risk of pelvic sidewall lymph node involvement increases with advancing stage, the dose of radiotherapy to this area is advanced with increasing stage. When paraaortic metastases are present in either stage, survival is significantly impaired. Survival for patients with stage IIB carcinoma of the cervix and paraaortic metastases is poorer than that for those with stage IIIB disease and negative paraaortic lymph nodes. Gross paraaortic lymph node metastases may be detected by CT, MRI, or lymphangiography. Microscopic nodal metastases are best detected by retroperitoneal common iliac and paraaortic lymphadenectomy, a relatively simple procedure performed through a "hockey stick" or paramedian incision (Fig. 39-13). The fascial layers are divided, sparing the peritoneum, which is reflected medially to expose the lymph node–bearing areas overlying the major blood vessels.

The finding of metastases in the common iliac or paraaortic chain indicates the need for extended-field radiotherapy encompassing these areas in addition to the pelvis. Even with such therapy, 5-year survival rates are low, seldom exceeding 20 percent. Many consider the presence of paraaortic lymph node metastases to be an indicator of systemic disease, although supraclavicular metastases are present in fewer than 25 percent of such patients.

Recurrent Cervical Cancer. As a rule, patients who develop local recurrences after preliminary surgical therapy are treated most effectively with external- and internal-beam radiotherapy. Although those with lymph node failures may not be curable in this setting, those with vaginal recurrences often can be saved with such an approach. Patients who suffer recurrences at sites distant from the pelvis may be treated with palliative local radiotherapy or chemotherapy with limited success.

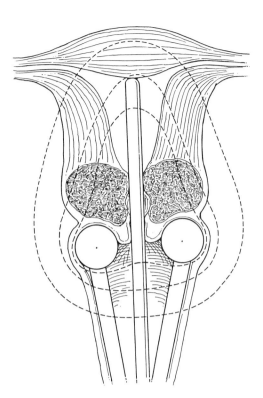

FIG. 39-11. *Radiotherapeutic isodose curves superimposed on a large stage IB "barrel" lesion of the cervix. The upper margins of the tumor may receive an inadequate dose of radiotherapy.*

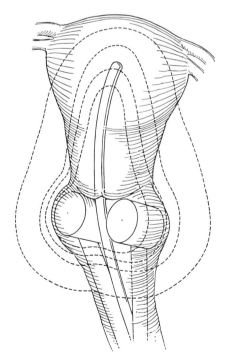

FIG. 39-12. *Fletcher-Suite tandem and paired ovoids. Hollow applicators that can be placed in the uterus and vagina and "afterloaded" once the appropriate position and dosimetry are established.*

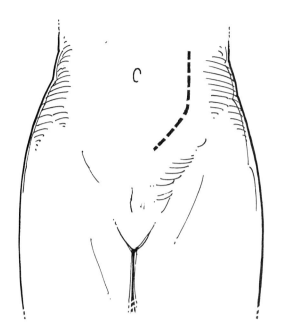

FIG. 39-13. "Hockey stick" incision used for retroperitoneal para-aortic lymph node dissection in cases of locally advanced cervical cancer.

Women who develop recurrent cancer following primary radiotherapy are generally not candidates for curative therapy. If, however, the recurrent lesion is small, the interval to failure is a year or more, and the lesion is unaccompanied by symptoms such as back or leg pain or edema, surgical resection may be possible. Since radiotherapy results in fibrosis of the connective tissues surrounding the cervix, radical hysterectomy is impractical. The risk of vesicovaginal or rectovaginal fistulas is excessive. In addition, surgical margins may be compromised by limited resection in such a situation.

Most gynecologic oncologists prefer to perform pelvic exenteration in such circumstances. Often, an anterior exenteration with en bloc removal of the bladder, cervix, uterus, and upper vagina is feasible. These operations require urinary diversion. Because of radiation exposure, however, an ileal conduit may be associated with urinary leakage from ureteroileal anastomoses. The preferred method of diversion in these patients is the creation of a sigmoid urostomy or transverse colon conduit. Other surgical options include a Koch pouch or the Indiana reservoir (Fig. 39-14), both of which provide a means of urinary continence without an external applicance.

In the case of extensive local recurrences, sigmoid resection may be required in addition to removal of the bladder. A total pelvic exenteration is performed. The sigmoid colon may be brought to the skin as a colostomy or reanastomosed to the rectal stump. Pelvic exenterations may be subclassified as supralevator or infralevator depending on whether this muscular diaphragm is broached (Fig. 39-15). Supralevator exenterations are generally associated with less operative morbidity. An infralevator exenteration is required if tumor involves the middle or lower third of the vagina or the vulva. Vaginal reconstruction in these extensive procedures with gracilis myocutaneous flaps is highly satisfactory (Figs. 39-16 and 39-17).

In general, about half the patients thought to be candidates for pelvic exenteration are found to have intraperitoneal spread or nodal metastases at the time of exploratory laparotomy and, in most centers, do not undergo resection. Of the remaining patients in whom surgery is possible, 30 to 50 percent will develop a second, nearly always fatal, recurrence after surgery. This complex operation should thus be undertaken only in carefully selected patients.

Endometrial Cancer

Endometrial cancer is the most common female genital malignancy, accounting for 34,000 cases annually in the United States. It is a highly treatable cancer, and only 6000 deaths are reported each year. Recently, there has been a disturbing increase in the proportion of fatalities reported in this country.

Risk factors for endometrial cancer include obesity, diabetes mellitus, hypertension, low parity, early menarche, and late menopause. Excessive exposure to estrogens is implicated in the genesis of endometrial cancer and its precursor, endometrial hyperplasia. Women who take estrogens in the menopausal years are known to have a sixfold increase in the risk of endometrial cancer if progestational agents are not taken as well. There is also an increase in the incidence of endometrial lesions in women with a history of chronic anovulation (Stein-Leventhal syndrome) and in those with estrogen-producing ovarian stromal neoplasms such as granulosa-cell tumors.

Endometrial hyperplasia may be divided into simple and complex, depending on the microscopic architecture, and into those with or without atypia. These hyperplasias are thought to be estrogen-dependent. Atypical complex hyperplasias are most likely to give rise to frank adenocarcinomas. They occur in women at an average age that is 5 to 10 years younger than those with frank carcinomas. Simple hysterectomy is the preferred method of treatment for the hyperplasias. In women with underlying health problems that preclude surgical therapy, therapy with progestational agents such as megestrol or medroxyprogesterone acetate may be used with success. Careful monitoring with endometrial biopsy or curettage is required in these patients, however.

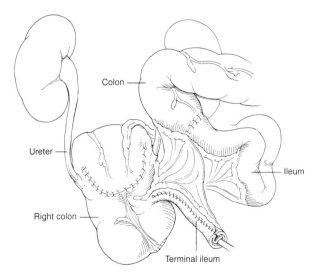

FIG. 39-14. Indiana continent urinary reservoir based on the right colon and terminal ileum. The ileum is plicated to preserve continence.

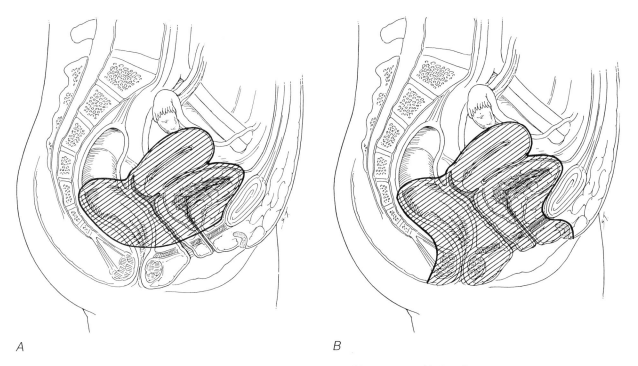

A

B

FIG. 39-15. Pelvic exenteration may be limited to the supralevator space *(A)* or can extend below the levator ani muscle (shaded area) *(B)*.

Both endometrial hyperplasia and carcinoma are often heralded by abnormal perimenopausal or postmenopausal uterine bleeding. This symptom accounts for the early detection and relative curability of these neoplasms.

Treatment. Endometrial cancer is staged according to the FIGO criteria detailed in Table 39-4. Many patients have stage I disease and can be managed successfully with abdominal hysterectomy and bilateral salpingo-oophorectomy. Adjuvant radiotherapy may be required, primarily to reduce the risk of vaginal recurrence. This can be given preoperatively with external therapy or a Fletcher-Suite implant or intrauterine packing (Heyman's or Simon's capsules). Some clinicians prefer to deliver radiotherapy postoperatively after the uterus has been evaluated thoroughly. Either external-beam therapy or vaginal cesium may be used.

Pelvic lymph node metastases occur in about 12 percent of patients with endometrial cancer apparently confined to the uterus. Lymph node metastases have a significant negative impact on survival. Risk factors associated with lymph node spread include high histologic grade (grade 2 or 3), low levels of progesterone receptor, deep myometrial or lymphatic channel invasion, spread to the adnexa, endocervical extension, and unusual histologic variants such as papillary serous or clear cell carcinomas. It is unnecessary to perform lymph node sampling in patients with grade 1 adenocarcinomas confined to the endometrium or inner one-third of myometrium. Other patients should have pelvic lymph nodes sampled at the time of hysterectomy. Therapeutic lymphadenectomy is not advocated; sampling of the external and internal iliac and obturator areas is

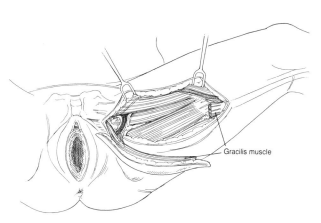

Gracilis muscle

FIG. 39-16. Development of gracilis myocutaneous flaps.

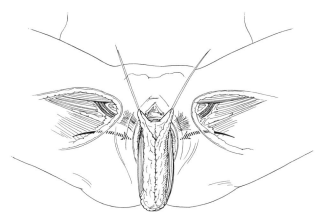

FIG. 39-17. Rotation of the flaps inferomedially and creation of a neovaginal tube that is rotated into the pelvic defect.

Table 39-4
FIGO (1988) Staging System for Endometrial Cancer

Stages	Characteristics
IA G123	Tumor limited to endometrium
IB G123	Invasion to<1/2 myometrium
IC G123	Invasion to>1/2 myometrium
IIA G123	Endocervical glandular involvement only
IIB G123	Cervical stromal invasion
IIIA G123	Tumor invades serosa or adnexae or positive peritoneal cytology
IIIB G123	Vaginal metastases
IIIC G123	Metastases to pelvic or para-aortic lymph nodes
IVA G123	Tumor invasion bladder and/or bowel mucosa
IVB	Distant metastases including intra-abdominal and/or inguinal lymph node

Histopathology—Degree of Differentiation
Cases should be grouped by the degree of differentiation of the adenocarcinoma:

G1	5% or less of a nonsquamous or nonmorular solid growth pattern
G2	6%–50% of a nonsquamous or nonmorular solid growth pattern
G3	More than 50% of a nonsquamous or nonmorular solid growth pattern

Notes on Pathologic Grading
Notable nuclear atypia, inappropriate for the architectural grade, raises the grade of a grade I or grade II tumor by 1.

In serous adenocarcinomas, clear cell adenocarcinomas, and squamous cell carcinomas, nuclear grading takes precedence.

Adenocarcinomas with squamous differentiation are graded according to the nuclear grade of the glandular component.

Rules Related to Staging
Because corpus cancer is now surgically staged, procedures previously used for determination of stages are no longer applicable, such as the finding of fractional D&C to differentiate between stage I and II. It is appreciated that there may be a small number of patients with corpus cancer who will be treated primarily with radiation therapy. If that is the case, the clinical staging adopted by FIGO in 1971 would still apply but designation of that staging system would be noted.

Ideally, width of the myometrium should be measured along with the width of tumor invasion.

sufficient for patients with endometrial cancer. Those with a high likelihood of spread to pelvic lymph nodes (grade 3, outer one-third myometrial or uterine serosal involvement, and those with high-risk histologic subtypes) should undergo sampling of the common iliac and paraaortic lymph nodes, since these areas lie outside the usual fields of pelvic radiotherapy. Patients with papillary serous tumors may develop metastases in the abdominal cavity or omentum much as those with ovarian epithelial tumors.

Another important element of staging endometrial cancer is the evaluation of peritoneal lavage fluid for the presence of malignant cells. About 12 percent of patients are found to have malignant peritoneal cytology. Half have other evidence of extrauterine spread of the disease, but the remainder have no other associated risk factors. Malignant peritoneal cytology increases the risk for intraabdominal failure and treatment for this finding deserves consideration. If external-beam radiotherapy is not used, intraperitoneal radioactive chromic phosphate may be of benefit.

Vaginal hysterectomy is occasionally useful in patients with early endometrial cancer when lymph node metastases are thought to be unlikely. This operation is particularly well suited for massively obese parous patients in whom an abdominal incision would be prohibitively difficult.

It is unnecessary to perform radical surgery in women with endometrial cancer even if there is spread to the cervix (stage II). Although lymphatic spread is important, these cancers also may be disseminated by hematogenous or peritoneal routes. Radical surgery has never been shown to improve survival in comparison with simple hysterectomy and adjuvant radiotherapy. Simple, extrafascial, or complete abdominal hysterectomy is demonstrated in Fig. 39-18 and contrasted with radical hysterectomy. It is critical to remove the ovaries in women undergoing surgery for endometrial cancer because 5 percent harbor occult metastases. Additionally, the source of estrogen secretion in premenopausal women with endometrial cancer should be removed.

In patients with large stage IIB and III lesions, consideration is generally given to preoperative pelvic radiotherapy, since surgery may be otherwise difficult or impossible. These tumors should receive appropriate surgical staging or thorough radiographic evaluation if primary radiotherapy is used.

Pelvic exenteration is rarely necessary in the treatment of patients with endometrial cancer unless it occurs following full irradiation for a preexisting cervical cancer. Such cases are rare, of course.

Radiotherapy alone may be the treatment of choice in patients at excessive risk for operative intervention. Radiotherapy alone produces results inferior to those of surgery or surgery and adjuvant radiotherapy, however, so patients treated without hysterectomy should be selected carefully. Advanced or recurrent endometrial cancer is responsive to progestin or tamoxifen therapy in 30 percent of unselected patients. Lesions that are well differentiated contain higher levels of progesterone receptor and respond more frequently. Only 10 percent of poorly differentiated cancers respond to hormonal treatment. Local radiotherapy or chemotherapy with paclitaxel, doxorubicin, platinum compounds, or combinations may be of benefit in some cases as well.

Vulvar Cancer

Vulvar cancer accounts for about 5 percent of all gynecologic cancers. Although uncommon histologic types such as malignant

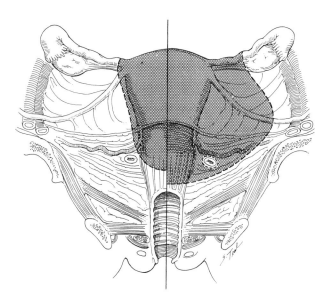

FIG. 39-18. *Extent of simple (extrafascial) hysterectomy depicted on left compared with radical hysterectomy on right.*

melanoma and adenocarcinoma of the Bartholin's gland occur, over 90 percent of vulvar malignancies are squamous carcinomas.

Epidemiologic risk factors include older age, smoking, previous intraepithelial or invasive squamous cancer of the cervix or vagina, chronic vulvar dystrophy (often associated with diabetes mellitus), and immunocompromise (organ transplant recipients, systemic lupus erythematosus). Human papillomavirus-like DNA has been identified in both preinvasive and invasive squamous carcinomas of the vulva. Although the etiology of this cancer is not well understood, it is likely that the human papillomavirus plays an important role.

Spread of squamous carcinoma of the vulva is primarily via the lymphatics of the vulva. Lesions arising in the anterior aspect of the vulva drain preferentially to the inguinal lymph nodes and posterior lesions may drain directly to the lymph nodes of the pelvis.

Stanley Way of Great Britain identified five main groups of lymphatic drainage of carcinoma of the vulva (Fig. 39-19): (1) the superficial inguinal lymph nodes, which lie in the subcutaneous tissue overlying the inguinal ligament, (2) the deep inguinal lymph nodes, which lie along the course of the round ligament in the inguinal canal, (3) the superficial femoral lymph nodes, grouped around the saphenous vein just superficial to the fossa ovalis, with efferents to the deep femoral lymph nodes, (4) the deep femoral lymph nodes, including the most cephalad lymph node of Cloquet or Rosenmuller, and (5) the external iliac lymph nodes.

Since the lymph node of Cloquet receives efferents from the inguinal region and the vulva and drains into the medial portion of the external iliac chain, it is an important sentinel in the route of spread of vulvar lesions. There are also direct lymphatic connections between the clitoris and Cloquet's node.

The 1988 FIGO staging system for vulvar cancer (Table 39-5) is currently accepted. This system requires surgical evaluation of the inguinal lymph nodes and provides a schema in which prognosis and therapy are closely linked with stage.

Treatment. Historically, the single-stage en bloc "extended" radical vulvectomy championed in Great Britain by Way and in the United States by Friedrich Taussig was used to treat all vulvar neoplasms (Fig. 39-20). In this operation, wide margins of skin and subcutaneous tissue around the primary tumor are removed together with underlying lymphatic structures in the groins and the labia majora and minora and clitoris in the vulva. Also removed are the proximal saphenous vein and its tributaries, the superficial circumflex iliac, superficial external pudendal, and superficial inferior epigastric veins.

The deep inguinal lymph nodes are removed by opening the external oblique fascia overlying the inguinal canal; most of the round ligament is removed at the same time.

Pelvic lymphadenectomy is easily performed by opening the transversalis fascia below the inguinal ligament and exposing the external iliac vessels in the retroperitoneal space medial to the psoas muscle. Pelvic lymphadenectomy is probably not indicated in vulvar cancer except in those patients found to have grossly enlarged pelvic lymph nodes on preoperative CT or MRI. Patients with inguinal node metastases are best treated with inguinal and pelvic radiotherapy following resection of the inguinal lymph nodes. In the case of large vulvar primaries or suspicious inguinal lymph nodes, this approach yields better survival rates

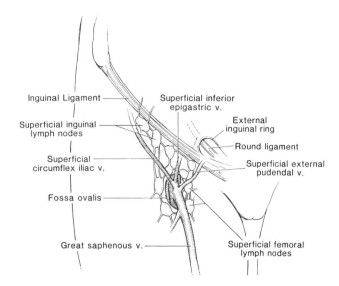

FIG. 39-19. *Lymphatic drainage of the vulva delineated by Stanley Way.*

than those obtained when pelvic lymphadenectomy alone is performed.

Because extended radical vulvectomy is associated with long hospital stays and significant morbidity from wound breakdown and infectious complications, there has been a long-standing interest in more conservative surgery for early vulvar cancer. The first efforts to this end were made in the 1960s. Several investigators introduced the concept of radical vulvectomy and in-

Table 39-5
FIGO Staging of Vulvar Cancer

Stage 0	
Tis	Carcinoma in situ, intraepithelial carcinoma.
Stage I	
T1 N0 M0	Tumor confined to the vulva and/or perineum—2 cm or less in greatest dimension. No nodal metastasis.
Stage II	
T2 N0 M0	Tumor confined to the vulva and/or perineum—more than 2 cm in greatest dimension. No nodal metastasis.
Stage III	
T3 N0 M0	Tumor of any size with
T3 N1 M0	(1) adjacent spread to the lower urethra and/or the vagina, or the anus, and/or
T1 N1 M0	(2) unilateral regional lymph node metastasis.
T2 N1 M0	
Stage IV A	
T1 N2 M0	Tumor invades any of the following:
T2 N2 M0	Upper urethra, bladder mucosa, rectal mucosa, pelvic bone, and/or bilateral regional node metastasis.
T3 N2 M0	
T4 Any N M0	
Stage IV B	
Any T, Any N, M1	Any distant metastasis, including pelvic lymph nodes.

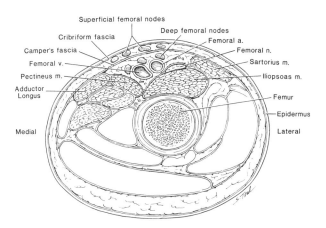

FIG. 39-22. Superficial inguinal lymphadenectomy.

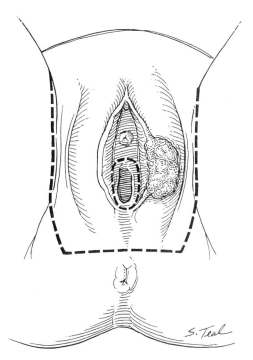

FIG. 39-20. En bloc radical vulvectomy outlined by Way and Taussig.

guinal lymphadenectomy through separate incisions. This approach not only reduces hospital time but also results in fewer major wound complications. This approach, illustrated in Fig. 39-21, has been widely embraced by gynecologic oncologists. Since inguinal node metastases are the result of an embolic process rather than infiltration or direct extension, the approach is

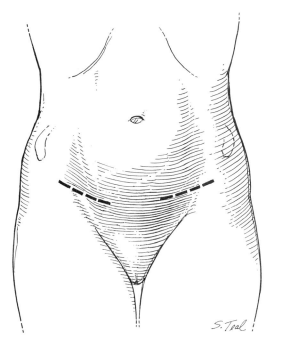

FIG. 39-21. Radical vulvectomy and inguinal lymphadenectomy through separate incisions.

rational. Early concerns regarding recurrence in the skin bridge between the vulvar and groin incisions have been largely allayed by experience with this approach. Recurrence in the skin bridge is usually associated with preexisting large inguinal metastases.

Another area of progress in the surgical management of vulvar carcinoma has been the use of conservative surgery for early lesions of the vulva. Although specific criteria differ slightly, most investigators recognize that squamous cancers of the vulva less than 2 cm in diameter and no more than 1 mm thick, and that are of histologic grade 1 or 2, are associated with a very small risk of inguinal metastases. Such lesions are adequately treated with deep, wide excision, provided skin margins of 1 cm are obtained and the dissection is carried to the level of the superficial transverse perineal muscles. Inguinal lymphadenectomy can be omitted in such patients.

In patients with intermediate lesions located on the labium minus or majus that do not cross the midline or involve midline structures such as the clitoris, perineal body, or perianal area, modified hemivulvectomy and ipsilateral inguinal lymphadenectomy have been used successfully. This approach should be considered if the primary lesion is less than 2 cm in diameter and 5 mm or less in thickness. Lymph node metastases are uncommon in this group of patients and maybe evaluated by frozen section at the time of surgery. The lymph nodes superficial to Camper's fascia (Fig. 39-22) in the groin are removed through a conservative inguinal incision (Fig. 39-23). If these "sentinel" lymph nodes are free of tumor, the risk of involvement of the deep inguinal or femoral lymph nodes is small enough that further dissection may be avoided. The outlines of the modified radical hemivulvectomy are depicted in Fig. 39-24. This excision site may be closed primarily with good results.

Another controversial area in the management of squamous carcinomas of the vulva is that of the patient with locally advanced disease. When extensive vulvar cancer involves more than the distal urethra, the vagina or rectovaginal septum, or the anal musculature, ultraradical surgery may be required. Anterior, posterior, or total pelvic exenteration may be necessary to resect such lesions successfully. The presence of fixed, matted, or ulcerating inguinal lymph nodes presents another problem that may require extensive surgical excision. Following such extirpative procedures, reconstruction of the vulva and groins is accomplished using myocutaneous flaps based on the gracilis, sar-

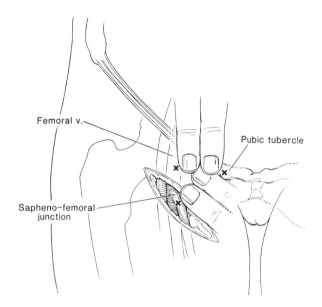

FIG. 39-23. *Incision recommended for superficial inguinal lymphadenectomy.*

torius, or tensor fasciae latae muscles. Approximately 50 percent of patients are cured by such surgical procedures.

In recent years, such locally advanced lesions of the vulva also have been treated successfully with external-beam radiotherapy combined with radiosensitizing drugs such as cisplatin and 5-fluorouracil. At the completion of combination therapy, the areas of involvement are excised widely or biopsied. This approach is associated with results as good as or better than those achieved with ultraradical surgery and generally results in

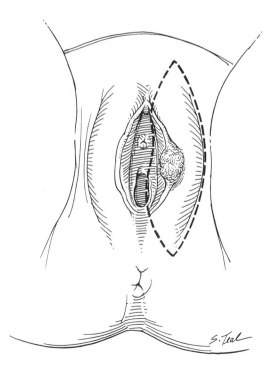

FIG. 39-24. *Extent of modified radical hemivulvectomy for stages I and II squamous cancer of the vulva.*

less morbidity. The need for urinary and fecal diversion is also obviated.

Uncommon Vulvar Tumors

Melanoma. Traditional surgical therapy for malignant melanoma of the vulva has included en bloc radical vulvectomy and inguinofemoral lymphadenectomy. It is now known that lesions less than 1 mm thick or Clark level II lesions may be treated conservatively with wide local excision. The value of inguinofemoral lymphadenectomy is controversial in lesions of greater depth, although primary surgical cure is occasionally achieved in patients with microscopic nodal metastases. Melanomas of the urethra or vagina are usually diagnosed in advanced stages and may require pelvic exenteration for successful management.

Intraepithelial Disease. Intraepithelial disease (Bowen's disease, bowenoid papulosis, vulvar intraepithelial neoplasia, carcinoma in situ) may be treated successfully by removing the involved epithelium. This is characteristically a raised, velvety lesion with sharply demarcated borders that may contain gray, brown, or red pigmentation. Removal is accomplished by simple vulvectomy, where the plane of dissection is limited to the epithelium, or by wide excision. In the case of diffuse intraepithelial disease, a so-called skinning vulvectomy and split-thickness skin graft may be required. This approach is associated with prolonged hospital stays, however, and should be reserved for exceptional cases. Also effective in the treatment of intraepithelial disease are the carbon dioxide laser and the electrosurgical loop.

Paget's disease is an unusual epithelial or invasive process characterized by the presence of distinct "Paget cells" in the involved epithelium. Grossly, the lesion is confluent, raised, red, and waxy in appearance. This lesion also can be excised widely, although the microscopic extent of the disease may exceed the visible margins. Intravenous fluorescein dye and ultraviolet light highlight areas that cannot be detected by the naked eye, and this assists in excision. Frozen-section examination of the surgical margins is also helpful but time-consuming. Paget's disease is occasionally associated with an underlying invasive adenocarcinoma; careful pelvic examination and proctoscopy are indicated in patients with this process.

Bartholin's gland carcinoma represents less than 1 percent of all vulvar malignancies and may be squamous carcinoma, adenocarcinoma, or adenosquamous or adenoid cystic carcinoma. Hemivulvectomy with dissection of the ischiorectal fossa and resection of involved contiguous structures is indicated. Because of the risk of inguinofemoral metastases, groin lymphadenectomy should accompany the vulvar operation.

GYNECOLOGIC OPERATIONS

Dilatation and Curettage (D&C)

At one time dilatation of the cervix and curettage of the endometrial cavity was among the most common surgical procedures performed in this country. Simple office biopsy and medical means of dealing with abnormal bleeding have largely replaced the need for diagnostic dilatation and curettage.

In some cases curettage is necessary for the relief of profuse uterine hemorrhage. It is indicated for removal of endometrial polyp or therapeutic termination of pregnancy and for retained placental tissue following abortion or obstetric delivery.

The patient is placed on the operating table in a lithotomy position, and the vagina and cervix are prepared as for any vaginal operation. The cervix is grasped on the anterior lip with a tenaculum. The cervix is gently pulled toward the outlet of the vagina. Some traction on the cervix is necessary to reduce the angulation between the cervical canal and the uterine cavity. A sound is inserted into the uterine cavity, and the depth of the uterus is noted. The cervical canal is then systematically dilated beginning with a small cervical dilator. Most operations can be performed after the cervix is dilated to accommodate a number 8 or 9 Hegar dilator or its equivalent. Dilatation is accomplished by firm, constant pressure with a dilator directed in the axis of the uterus (Fig. 39-25).

After the cervix is dilated to admit the curette, the endocervical canal should be curetted and the sample submitted separate from the endometrial curettings. The endometrial cavity is then systemically scraped with a uterine curette. The curettings are collected on a small piece of gauze or telfa. The curettings are then placed in the fixative. After the uterus has been thoroughly curetted, a ureteral stone forceps may be used to explore the endometrial cavity, searching for polyps or pedunculated neoplasms within the endometrial cavity. When the procedure is complete, the tenaculum is removed; the tenaculum site is evaluated for bleeding, and, if the puncture sites are bleeding, they are treated with a small amount of silver nitrate.

The major complication of D&C is perforation of the uterus. Perforation is diagnosed when the operator finds no resistance to a dilator or curette at a point where he or she normally would expect it. Perforation generally is treated in an expectant manner. The patient should be watched for several hours for signs of hemorrhage and be warned of the possibility of pelvic infection. A falling hematocrit and other signs of intraperitoneal bleeding indicate the need for laparotomy and control of the bleeding site. Any infection following D&C should be treated with antibiotics.

Uterine curettage is often required for incomplete abortion in the first or second trimester of pregnancy. Dilatation of the cervix in these cases is invariably present. Curettage of the postabortal uterus must be approached carefully because the uterus is extremely soft and perforation can occur with very little warning. Using the largest curette available is a safer choice than a small curette, which tends to cause perforation with less pressure. In the postabortal uterus, the endometrial cavity must be scraped thoroughly until the distinctive gritty feeling of curette against muscle is felt.

In recent years, suction curettage for incomplete abortion, hydatid mole, and therapeutic abortion has become popular. Suction machines fitted with cannulas that vary from 4 to 12 mm in diameter evacuate the uterus in less time and save blood loss. Most of these procedures are accomplished under sedation and paracervical block. Following the curettage, the uterine cavity is explored with a placental forceps or sponge forceps to remove any loose tissue within the cavity. Uterine perforation continues to be a concern when curettage is carried out for incomplete abortion. Perforation of the puerperal uterus is a much more serious problem because the organ is much more vascular than the nonpregnant uterus.

Postoperative bleeding should be modest if the curettage has been complete. Some operators control bleeding with the use of uterotonic agents such as vasopressin and prostaglandin-17-alpha.

Endoscopic Surgery

Endoscopic surgery, including both laparoscopy and hysteroscopy, has assumed a major role in gynecology. Laparoscopy,

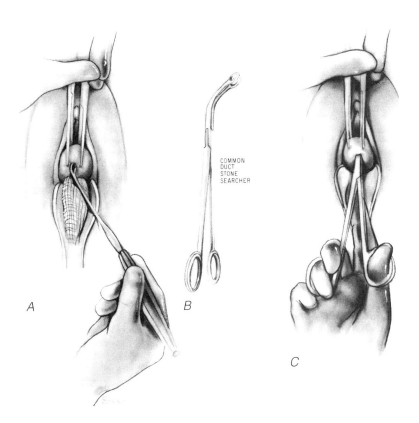

FIG. 39-25. Dilatation and curettage of the uterus.

once used almost exclusively for diagnostic purposes and for tubal ligation, is now being applied to almost every kind of gynecologic procedure. Hysteroscopy has found an expanded role from purely diagnostic to removal of intrauterine pathology and ablation of endometrium for abnormal uterine bleeding. Although the limits of what is possible continue to be defined, the relative safety of some of these techniques in general use remains uncertain.

Laparoscopy

Laparoscopy was developed more than 20 years ago as a diagnostic tool and was soon adapted to perform tubal sterilization techniques. From the beginning, a few intrepid gynecologists used this approach for much more, including lysis of pelvic adhesions, treatment of endometriosis, and removal of ectopic tubal pregnancies. Slowly the role of the laparoscope expanded for conservative surgery and for removal of diseased tissue. More recently, laparoscopic approaches were developed for hysterectomy and gynecologic oncologic procedures. Ongoing research and experience continue to establish which of these approaches represent real advantages to the patients.

General Techniques for Laparoscopy. *Placement of the Veress Needle and Primary Trocar.* The standard method for laparoscopy remains the serial placement through the umbilicus of a retractable-pointed Veress needle for insufflation, followed by a sharp 10-mm primary trocar and sleeve. Although both reusable and disposable instruments are being used, there has been some movement back to sharp reusable instruments because of both cost and safety concerns.

When placing the Veress needle through the anterior abdominal wall, the goal is to minimize the risk of preperitoneal placement while avoiding retroperitoneal vessel injury by the use of proper placement techniques. In patients who are of normal weight or who are overweight but not obese (i.e., less than 200 lb), instruments are placed through the umbilicus toward the pelvis. After the sacral prominence is palpated, the abdominal wall is elevated by grasping the skin and subcutaneous tissue midway between the symphysis pubis and the umbilicus in an effort to maximize the distance between the umbilicus and major vessels. The Veress needle is inserted through the base of the umbilicus at 45° from horizontal.

In the obese patient (>200 lb), the thickness of the abdominal wall requires an alteration of the approach for inserting the Veress needle. If the needle is placed through the base of the umbilicus at 45°, it may not reach the peritoneal cavity (Fig. 39-26). For this reason, it has been suggested that the Veress needle be placed at near 90° from horizontal. To minimize the risk of vascular injury, the umbilicus should be elevated (i.e., supported to avoid depression), and a standard length Veress needle should be used and checked for location as described previously. Following insufflation, a primary 10-mm trocar is also inserted at near 90° from horizontal.

Alternatively, open laparoscopic techniques continue to be refined and more widely applied. For these techniques, the anterior rectus fascia is incised with a scalpel, the peritoneal cavity is entered bluntly, and a blunt-tipped trocar is placed into the peritoneal cavity. Pneumoperitoneum is maintained at the site of entry either by sutures or by mechanisms built into the sleeves such as balloons or fascial threads. Although once reserved for patients with previous surgery, some laparoscopists use these

techniques exclusively to avoid the risk of major retroperitoneal injury and to minimize the risk of bowl injury associated with closed techniques.

Placement of Secondary Trocars. As laparoscopic techniques advanced, the need for secondary trocars increased dramatically. After transillumination to locate the superficial vessels, an attempt is made to laparoscopically locate the inferior epigastric vessels. Secondary trocars are placed under laparoscopic visualization either 3 cm above the symphysis pubis in the midline or 8 cm above the symphysis pubis approximately 8 cm lateral to the midline. At the end of the procedure, the sleeves are removed and the sites observed for signs of hemorrhage. A full-thickness closure of any trocar site more than 5 mm is performed to prevent herniation through the defect.

Power Instruments. Scissors and sutures have long been used for laparoscopic dissections and vessel ligation. However, because of the limitations of laparoscopy, including decreased depth perception and limited field of vision, innovative instruments have been developed for laparoscopic use both for tissue cutting and for vessel occlusion. Initially, unipolar electrosurgery was the only power instrument available, but because of concern about inadvertent damage to adjacent organs, other techniques were developed. Bipolar electrosurgery is excellent for hemostasis but has limited cutting ability. Laser, which can be aimed or placed in the proper location before activation, offers precision and some degree of hemostasis. Recently, an ultrasonic scalpel has been developed that avoids both the smoke and char associated with other power techniques.

Methods for Large-Vessel Occlusion. As techniques to remove tissue with significant blood supplies (e.g., adnexa, uterus) were developed, methods to effectively divide and occlude major vessels also were developed. Laparoscopic suture ligation, using either intra- or extracorporal knot tying, is relatively slow and technically difficult. For this reason, three alternative approaches have been widely applied. Pretied loops, linear stapling devices, and bipolar electrocautery have all been found to be relatively expeditious and effective, although rare cases of delayed bleeding have been reported with all three of these techniques.

Laparoscopic Procedures. *Diagnostic Laparoscopy.* This common procedure involves the placement of a 10-mm lens through an intraumbilical port, often with a 5-mm port placed above the symphysis for manipulation. Pelvic organs are closely inspected in a systematic fashion for signs of disease, and if tubal patency is an issue, a dilute dye solution is injected transcervically (chromopertubation). Biopsies can be obtained if malignancy is suspected.

Tubal Sterilization Procedures. As in diagnostic laparoscopy, a one- or two-port technique can be used. Tubes are occluded in the midisthmic section (approximately 3 cm from the cornua) using clips, elastic bands, or bipolar electrosurgery. With electrosurgery, approximately 2 cm of tube should be desiccated. Pregnancy rates after any of these techniques have been reported in the range of 3 per 1000 women.

Lysis of Adhesions. Pelvic adhesions usually are related to previous infection, either genital (i.e., pelvic inflammatory disease) or extragenital (e.g., ruptured appendix) in origin, or to endometriosis. Adhesions can be associated with decreased fertility or pain and can be lysed mechanically with scissors or any of the power techniques discussed above. Some degree of ad-

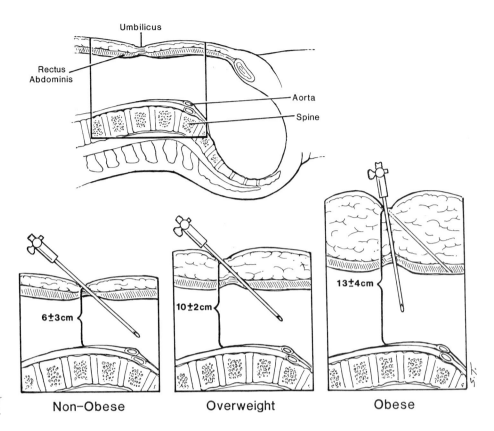

FIG. 39-26. *Changes in the anterior abdominal wall anatomy with weight.*

Non–Obese   Overweight   Obese

hesion re-formation is unavoidable, and residual intrinsic tubal damage continues to interfere with fertility in most patients.

Adhesion re-formation can be minimized by achieving good hemostasis using discrete application of electrosurgery. Postoperatively, intraperitoneal solutions are used commonly to "hydrofloat" the adnexal structures, but controlled studies of their efficacy have been disappointing. Barrier methods have been shown to decrease adhesion formation in both animal and human studies but have not been demonstrated to improve outcome in terms of either subsequent pregnancies or pain relief.

Fulgarization of Endometriosis. Conservative laparoscopic treatment of endometriosis increases fertility and often helps with pelvic pain as well. This condition and the various approaches to treatment were considered earlier in this chapter (see Endometriosis).

Treatment of Ectopic Pregnancy. Laparoscopy has established itself as the primary treatment approach for ectopic pregnancies, a condition considered earlier in this chapter (see Ectopic Pregnancy, Treatment).

Ovarian Cystectomy. The laparoscopic removal of ovarian cysts less than 6 cm in diameter in premenopausal women has become common. Using a multiple-port technique, the peritoneal cavity is inspected for signs of malignancy, including ascites, peritoneal or diaphragmatic implants, and liver involvement. In the absence of signs of malignancy, pelvic washings are obtained, and the ovarian capsule is excised with scissors or a power instrument. The cyst is shelled out carefully and placed in a bag, intact if possible. The bag opening is brought through the lower port incision along with the 10-mm port. The cyst is then drained and the cyst wall removed. Hemostasis of the ovary is achieved with bipolar electrosurgery, but the ovary is usually not closed, since this may increase postoperative adhesion formation. Except in the obvious cases of simple cysts, endometriomas, or dermoid cysts, the cyst wall should be sent for frozen section to verify the absence of the malignancy. If malignancy is detected, immediate definitive surgery, usually by laparotomy, is recommended. All cyst walls are sent for permanent section and pathologic diagnosis.

In many cases the cyst will rupture prior to removal. This is always the case with an endometrioma that contains "chocolate" fluid. On rupture, the cyst contents are thoroughly aspirated, and the cyst wall is removed and sent for pathologic evaluation. The peritoneal cavity is copiously rinsed with Ringer's lactate solution. This is especially important when a dermoid cyst is ruptured, since the sebaceous material can cause a chemical peritonitis unless all the visible oily substance is carefully removed.

Although malignancies are not commonly encountered using these guidelines, there is concern that rupture may worsen the patient's prognosis. Data are accumulating suggesting that cyst rupture may not alter prognosis. Based on conventional wisdom, every effort should be made to remove ovarian cysts without intraperitoneal spillage.

Ovarian cysts larger than 6 cm or those discovered in postmenopausal women also can be removed laparoscopically. Because of the increased risk of malignancy associated with these situations, laparotomy is more commonly used. Laparoscopy may be a reasonable alternative in select patients if standard methods for staging are used in conjunction with appropriate frozen-section evaluation and expedient definitive therapy when indicated.

Removal of Adnexa. Occasionally, all or part of an adnexa must be removed. This may be the case with a large tubal pregnancy, a large hydrosalpinx, or when a small but growing cyst is found in a postmenopausal woman. Using a multiple-port technique, the vascular supply to the tissue is first desiccated with bipolar cautery and then divided with scissors. Alternatively, the ovarian vessels in the infundibulopelvic ligament can first be occluded with one of the techniques described (see Methods for Large Vessel Occlusion). Special care should be taken to identify and avoid the ureter, which lies retroperitoneally as it crosses the ovarian vessels and courses along the ovarian fossa (see Fig. 39-3).

Once the adnexa has been excised and hemostasis is achieved, attention is turned to removing the tissue from the peritoneal cavity. Small specimens can be removed using a retrieval bag via a 12-mm port. The port is removed with the sack, and the fascial incision is enlarged, if required.

For larger specimens, a culpotomy may expedite this procedure. A 12-mm port is placed through the posterior cul de sac under direct visualization. A retrieval sack is placed through the port, and the port and specimen in the sack are removed together. The distensible peritoneum and vaginal wall will allow the removal of a large specimen through a relatively small defect, which can then be closed with a running suture vaginally. Prophylactic antibiotics may decrease the risk of infection.

Myomectomy. Uterine leiomyomas are often approachable via the laparoscope. Hemostasis is assisted by intrauterine injection of dilute vasopressin (10 units in 50 mL) at the site of incision. Pedunculated leiomyomas can be excised at the base using scissors or a power instrument. Intramural leiomyomas require deep dissection into the uterine tissue, which must be closed subsequently with laparoscopic suturing techniques. Because myomectomies are associated with considerable postoperative adhesion formation, barrier techniques are used to decrease adhesion formation.

Removing the specimen can be difficult. In general, morcellation is required, and power morcellators have been developed that significantly expedite this technique. Although leiomyomas of any size or location technically can be removed laparoscopically, it is yet to be proven that either menorrhagia or infertility, the two most common indications for myomectomy, are as effectively treated laparoscopically as they are by laparotomy.

Hysterectomy. Laparoscopy was first used to restore normal anatomy prior to vaginal hysterectomy. More recently, laparoscopy has been used to perform some or all of the actual hysterectomy to avoid laparotomy in patients with known pelvic adhesions, endometriosis, or in whom the uterus is enlarged by leiomyoma. Although multiple variations in technique exist, there are three basic laparoscopic approaches for hysterectomy: laparoscopic-assisted vaginal hysterectomy, laparoscopic hysterectomy, and laparoscopic supracervical hysterectomy. While basic techniques for each of these methods have become somewhat standardized, the indications and relative risk for each remain controversial.

The technically simplest, and probably the most widely applied, is the laparoscopic-assisted vaginal hysterectomy (LAVH). For this procedure, a multiple-port approach is used to survey the peritoneal cavity, and any pelvic adhesions are lysed. The round ligaments are then occluded and divided, and the uterovesicle peritoneum is incised. Next, the proximal uterine blood supply is occluded and divided. When the ovaries are removed, the infundibulopelvic ligaments (containing the ovarian vessels) are divided. If the ovaries are conserved, the uteroovarian liga-

ment and blood vessels are divided and occluded. In some cases, the posterior cul de sac is incised laparoscopically as well. The remainder of the case is performed vaginally, including dissection of the bladder from the anterior uterus, ligation of the uterine vessels, removal of the specimen, and closure of the vaginal cuff.

A laparoscopic hysterectomy (LH) differs from an LAVH in that almost the entire hysterectomy is performed laparoscopically. This procedure is used for the indications listed above and also when lack of uterine descent makes the vaginal approach impossible.

LH is begun in a manner identical to LAVH. But after the proximal uterine blood supply is divided, the bladder is dissected from the anterior uterus. This is followed by a retroperitoneal dissection in which the ureter is identified along it entire pelvic course and the uterine vessels are selectively occluded and divided. The ureterosacral ligaments are likewise divided and the posterior cul de sac incised. The specimen is removed vaginally, and the vaginal cuff is closed.

The third common laparoscopic approach is the laparoscopic supracervical hysterectomy (LSH) This procedure has been advocated for all benign indications for hysterectomy. Technically, it is begun in a manner identical to the first two approaches. But after the proximal vessels are divided and the bladder is dissected from the anterior uterus, the ascending branches of the uterine arteries are occluded and the entire uterine fundus is removed from the cervix. The endocervix is either cauterized or cored out with a special instrument. The fundus is then morcellated and removed through a 12-mm abdominal port or through a special transcervical morcellator. The end result is an intact cervix and cuff, with no surgical dissection performed near the uterine artery and adjacent ureter. This approach avoids both a large abdominal incision and a vaginal incision. According to its advocates, this approach minimizes operating time, recovery time, and risk of both infection and ureteral injury. LH has yet to be widely applied, in part out of concern for the subsequent risk of developing cancer in the residual cervical stump.

Oncologic Procedures. As techniques developed, it became apparent that laparoscopy could be applied to oncologic procedures as well. In addition to the treatment of potentially malignant ovarian cysts, the laparoscopic approach also has been used for "second look" and staging procedures, including peritoneal washes and biopsy, partial omentectomy, and pelvis and periaortic lymphadenectomy. If positive nodes are discovered, treatment options often do not include laparotomy, and thus major surgery can be avoided without compromising patient prognosis. Laparoscopic approaches have been developed for definitive procedures, notably laparoscopically assisted radical vaginal hysterectomy.

A guiding principle is that the same care must be rendered laparoscopically that would be performed by laparotomy with the same or less risk of complications. Until the relative risk of complications and effect on prognosis have been established for these approaches compared with laparotomy, application of the laparoscopic approach in gynecologic oncology will remain highly controversial.

Risks of Laparoscopy. The many unique aspects of laparoscopy contribute to the distinctive complications associated with this approach.

Gas Embolism. Because pressurized CO_2 is used routinely to insufflate the abdomen for laparoscopy, gas embolization continues to be a rare but serious complication. This is related most commonly to misplacement of the Veress needle used for insufflation prior to primary trocar insertion. If the tip of the needle inadvertently enters the aorta or its branches, temporary distal arterial occlusion will result. Since CO_2 is quickly absorbed, no serious sequelae have been reported as a result of embolization, but arterial bleeding from this injury can be serious.

In contrast, inadvertent insufflation of the inferior vena cava or any of its venous branches can be fatal. Massive CO_2 embolism can result in partial or complete pulmonary arterial obstruction. This serious complication can be avoided in most cases by careful determination of Veress needle location prior to insufflation. Techniques for this include (1) ensuring lateral mobility of the needle, since retroperitoneal penetration will prevent this, (2) aspirating through the needle with a syringe, to rule out intravascular placement, and (3) the "hanging drop test," in which a drop of saline placed on the hub of the needle is pulled into the hub of the needle when the abdominal wall is elevated to verify intraperitoneal placement. If any of these tests are not reassuring, the needle should be removed and replaced into the peritoneal cavity.

When CO_2 embolism is encountered, swift recognition and treatment can be lifesaving. Removal of the needle and placement of the patient in left lateral decubitus position are the first steps. In the presence of extreme hypotension, external cardiac massage has been suggested to break up large bubbles. Definitive treatment of this condition is central line placement and aspiration of the gas from the right-sided heart chambers and pulmonary vasculature.

Injury to Abdominal Wall Vessels. Abdominal wall vessel injuries have become more common with the development of more complicated operative laparoscopic procedures that use lateral trocar placement and larger trocars. These vessels include the inferior ("deep") epigastric vessels, the superficial epigastric vessels, and the superficial circumflex iliac vessels (Fig. 39-27).

Injury to the inferior epigastric artery can result in life-threatening hemorrhage. Injury to these or other vessels can result in significant hematoma or postoperative blood loss if unrecognized.

The primary methods to avoid vessel injury are knowledge of the vessels at risk and visualization of them prior to trocar placement when possible. The superficial vessels often can be seen and avoided by transillumination of the abdominal wall with the laparoscope. This is especially true in light-skinned and thin women. In contrast, the larger inferior epigastric vessels cannot be seen by transillumination because of their deeper location. But these vessels often can be seen laparoscopically and avoided as they course along the peritoneum between the lateral umbilical fold of the bladder and the insertion of the round ligament into the inguinal canal.

Because the vessels may not be visible in some patients either by transillumination or laparoscopically, it is important to know their most likely location and place lateral trocars accordingly. Although the traditional location used for lateral trocar placement was approximately 5 cm from the midline, a safer location may be 8 cm or more above the symphysis pubis and 8 cm from the midline, since both the superficial and inferior epigastric arteries are located approximately 5.5 cm from the midline (see Fig. 39-27).

Anatomic variation and anastomoses between vessels make it impossible to know the exact location of all the abdominal wall vessels. For this reason, other strategies also should be used to avoid vessel injury, including the use of trocars with conical tips rather than pyramid tips and the use of the smallest trocars possible lateral to the midline.

Injury to Retroperitoneal Major Vessels. Injury to major retroperitoneal vessels is one of the least common but most serious complications of the closed laparoscopic technique, occurring in approximately 3 per 10,000 laparoscopies. This includes both vessel perforation by the Veress needle with intravascular insufflation and vessel laceration by the 10-mm primary trocar.

Theoretically, the blind placement of sharp instruments through the umbilicus aimed toward the pelvis should rarely, if ever, result in vessel injury because both the aorta and the inferior vena cava bifurcate near level of the umbilicus. Unfortunately, in many patients the aortic bifurcation is at or below the level of the umbilicus, and in most patients the left common iliac vein crosses the midline below the umbilicus. The margin of error may be small, especially in thin patients, where the anteroposterior distance from the umbilicus to the retroperitoneal vessels may be as little as 2 to 3 cm (see Fig. 39-26).

The primary strategy to minimize the risk of vessel injury is to vary the angle of insertion based on the weight of the patient (see Primary Trocar Placement). An alternative strategy to avoid the risk is the exclusive use of an open technique. Although techniques for open laparoscopy have been available for years, the majority of gynecologic laparoscopic procedures are performed using a closed rather than an open technique. Because of the potential advantage of this technique in terms of patient safety, new techniques and instruments continue to be developed and evaluated.

Intestinal Injury. Another potentially serious complication of laparoscopic surgery is injury to either small or large intestines. An unrecognized bowel injury may occur at the time of trocar insertion, especially if the patient has had previous abdominal procedures that often result in bowel adhesions to the

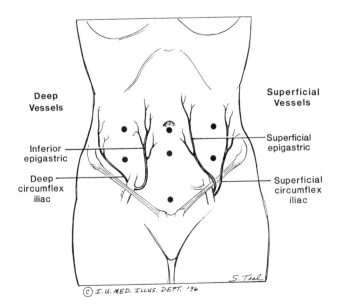

Deep Vessels

Superficial Vessels

Inferior epigastric

Superficial epigastric

Deep circumflex iliac

Superficial circumflex iliac

S. Teal

© I.U. MED. ILLUS. DEPT. '96

FIG. 39-27. Location of anterior abdominal wall blood vessels.

anterior abdominal wall peritoneum. In order to minimize the risk of bowel injury in patients who have undergone previous laparotomy, many gynecologic surgeons recommend the use of an open technique.

Another factor may be the type of primary trocar used. In recent years, disposable laparoscopic trocars have replaced reusable trocars at many hospitals. The extreme sharpness of disposable trocars that make insertion through the anterior abdominal wall easier also may have the potential to increase the risk of bowel injury. In one series, the risk of bowel injury with disposable trocars was approximately three times that previously reported for reusable trocars. Although the majority of these trocars have automatically extending "safety" shields designed to decrease the risk of inadvertent injury to these structures, no study has examined the relative safety of disposable versus reusable trocars.

Another laparoscopic risk to bowel is thermal injuries that may occur when power sources are used, such as electrocautery or laser. Regardless of the cause, major bowel injuries usually become obvious during surgery. Because of the limited field of view, some bowel injuries may not be seen during surgery. These injuries usually manifest 1 to 3 days after surgery, well after the patient has been released following these primarily outpatient procedures.

Urologic Injuries. Bladder injury is an uncommon laparoscopic injury, most commonly occurring as a result of retroperitoneal perforation during lower trocar placement or during sharp dissection of the bladder from the lower uterine segment during hysterectomy. The latter of these two situations is usually recognized intraoperatively; the first sign of the former may be postoperative hematuria or lower-port incisional drainage. Once diagnosed, large defects require layered closure, whereas smaller defects usually close spontaneously within days or weeks with the aid of transurethral catheter drainage.

Ureteral injury may occur as a result of any procedure that requires dissection or ligation of sidewall vessels, such as removal of an adnexa, since the ureter is adjacent to the pelvic peritoneum in the area of the ovarian fossa (see Fig. 39-3). This complication also has been reported after fulgarization of endometriosis on the pelvic sidewall.

Ureteral injuries, including complete ligation, partial resection, or thermal injuries, usually will manifest within hours to days of surgery. Complete obstruction most often manifests as flank pain, whereas the first sign of transection may be symptoms of intraabdominal irritation caused by urine leakage. Transperitoneal thermal injuries resulting from fulgarization of endometriosis may be similar to those after transection, but the appearance of symptoms may be delayed several days until tissue necrosis occurs.

Incisional Herniation. Incisional hernias after laparoscopy were rare prior to the use of large secondary ports (>5 mm) lateral to the midline. In recent times, incisional hernias have become a well-appreciated problem. A small peritoneal defect below the rectus abdominis muscle can allow bowel to become entrapped beneath the anterior rectus abdominis fascia. For this reason, closure of all layers of the incision is recommended whenever trocars greater than 5 mm are used at sites other than the umbilicus, and special needles have been developed for this purpose.

Although umbilical incision hernias also have been reported, fascial closure at the umbilicus is not commonly performed except when a large fascial incision is used for open laparoscopy. This is so both because the risk of herniation at this site is extremely low and because blind closure after removal of the laparoscope may risk bowel injury. Having the patient avoid heavy straining or lifting for 30 days after surgery may minimize the risk of umbilical herniation.

Hysteroscopy

Hysteroscopy, like laparoscopy, has gained widespread support as a very useful technique for both diagnosis and treatment of intrauterine pathology and for ablation of the endometrium as an alternative to hysterectomy for the treatment of abnormal uterine bleeding.

General Hysteroscopic Techniques. *Type of instruments.* Hysteroscopes can be divided into diagnostic, operative, and hysteroresectoscope. The lens for all three is identical. This is usually a fiberoptic lens and light source with an outside diameter of 3 mm and a objective lens that is offset up to 30° from the long axis of the instrument. In contrast, the sleeves for the three types of hysteroscopes vary considerably. The diagnostic sleeve usually has an external diameter of 5 mm and a single direction flow. Because outflow is limited, bleeding may impede a clear intrauterine view.

The operative sleeve, with an external diameter usually less than 10 mm, has a flow-through design with separate channels for input and outflow of distention media. A separate channel is available for placement of fine operating instruments.

The final type of sleeve is the hysteroresectoscope. This is also of a flow-through design and has an integral unipolar resecting loop identical to a urologic resectoscope. The loop can be replaced with a roller bar for endometrial ablation.

Distention Pumps and Media. Because of the small volume of the uterus coupled with its relative nondistensibility and the marked vascularity of the uterine wall, specifically designed pumps are required for hysteroscopy that are relatively high pressure (80–90 mmHg) and low flow. Several companies make CO_2 hysteroinsufflators that have these features and are very useful for diagnostic hysteroscopy. For operative hysteroscopy or for after cervical dilatation, a fluid medium pump is required. Preferably, this should be pressure regulated to approximately 80 mmHg to prevent excess intravasation of distention media. Although gravity alone has been advocated by some, the controllability of this technique is less predictable.

Several distention media have found widespread use. For diagnosis, CO_2 has been found to give excellent clarity. Although it has been found to be extremely safe in general use, fatal gas embolisms have been reported when CO_2 was used after cervical dilatation or intrauterine surgery. This suggests that the use of CO_2 should be avoided after cervical dilatation or any uterine instrumentation.

One of the first operative media used was 32% dextran 70 in dextrose. This syrup-like substance is usually introduced by hand with a large syringe. The advantage is simplicity and low cost. The view is excellent in the absence of bleeding. The disadvantage is the difficulty in completely removing the substance from the instruments. If this solution is allowed to dry in critical movable points, the instrument may "freeze up," and it is very difficult to remove. In addition, intravascular intravasation can result in pulmonary edema.

More recently, aqueous solutions with pressure-controlled pumps have been used. For operative hysteroscopy, where electrosurgery is not being used, it is safest to use a balanced salt solution, such as Ringer's lactate. Moderate fluid intravasation will be of no consequence in a healthy individual. However, intravasation of larger volumes can result in fluid overload, especially in a patient with any cardiac compromise.

When electrosurgery is used for hysteroresectoscope excision of leiomyomas or roller-blade endometrial ablation, a nonconducting solution such as glycine must be used. Significant vascular intravasation can cause hyponatremia, potentially resulting in cerebral edema, coma, or even death. For this reason, protocols must be followed rigorously to detect and treat significant intravasation whenever these solutions are used. Intraoperatively, differences in distention medium input and output should be calculated every 15 min. If the difference is greater than 500 mL, a diuretic should be given. If the difference is greater than 1000 mL, the procedure should be terminated as well. Whenever significant intravasation is suspected, serum sodium level should be checked immediately postoperatively and a few hours later because later hyponatremia, presumably due to transperitoneal absorption, has been reported.

Hysteroscopic Procedures. *Diagnostic Hysteroscopy.*

This common procedure is often performed prior to uterine curettage to identify any focal abnormalities such as an endometrial polyp or a malignancy. This procedure is usually performed in the operating room with either general or regional anesthesia, although it has been performed by some as an office procedure with minimal analgesia.

After determining the position of the uterus, the anterior cervix is grasped with a tenaculum and traction placed to straighten the cervical canal. The lens and diagnostic sleeve are placed into the cervix, and distention medium is introduced with a pressure of 80 to 90 mmHg. The hysteroscope is slowly and carefully advanced toward the fundus, using tactile and visual cues to avoid perforation. The entire uterine cavity is inspected, and any abnormal anatomy is documented. As the hysteroscope is withdrawn, the uterocervical junction and the endocervix are examined.

Directed Endometrial Biopsy. If a focal abnormality of the endometrium is observed, directed biopsy may be more accurate than a simple uterine curettage. The cervix is dilated to allow passage of an 8- to 10-mm flow-through operating hysteroscope, and a balanced salt solution is used for distention. Once the hysteroscope is positioned in the uterine cavity, the area of interest is biopsied under direct visualization.

Polypectomy. If an intrauterine polyp is discovered, the base of the polyp is incised with hysteroscopic scissors, and the polyp is grasped with grasping forceps. The hysteroscope, sleeve, and polyp are removed simultaneously, since most polyps will not fit through the operating channel. Extremely large polyps may have to be removed piecemeal. Any residual base of the polyp may be removed with biopsy forceps.

Uterine Septum Resection. A septum may be resected with scissors, electrosurgery, or laser. Scissors are used most commonly in light of the minimal vascularity of septa and the decreased potential for bowel injury should inadvertent uterine perforation occur. An operating hysteroscope is placed into the uterine cavity, which will appear to be two tubular structures rather than the broad uterine fundus usually encountered. The septum is then evenly divided across the fundus. If scissors are used, rather than a power cutting instrument, the presence of bleeding indicates that the level of resection is shifting from the avascular septum to the vascular myometrium. After surgery, no special device is placed in the uterus because intrauterine synechiae formation is uncommon.

Removal of Intrauterine Synechiae. Intrauterine synechiae are almost always associated with previous uterine curettage, especially when performed in the immediate postpartum period. These synechiae may result in amenorrhea or infertility. The removal of synechiae is performed in a manner similar to that described above for a uterine septum, with some differences. The first is that the anatomy, and thus the visual cues for location of normal uterine wall, is completely unpredictable from patient to patient. Preoperative hysterosalpingography is usually very helpful. Findings can vary from a few small synechiae to complete obliteration of the cavity.

In difficult cases, simultaneous transabdominal ultrasound is extremely helpful in guiding the direction and limits of hysteroscopic resection. Standby laparoscopy should be available in the event of perforation, which is a significant risk in these patients. However, once pneumoperitoneum is achieved, abdominal ultrasound is no longer possible.

Following surgery, some type of intrauterine splint, such as an intrauterine device or a balloon catheter, is often placed to avoid synechia re-formation. Patients are usually placed on estrogen supplementation for a month and prophylactic antibiotics until the intrauterine splint is removed 1 to 2 weeks later.

Intrauterine Myomectomy. Pedunculated or submucosal leiomyoma can be removed safely hysteroscopically with subsequent improvement in both abnormal uterine bleeding and infertility. Because myoma tissue is relatively dense, a power cutting instrument is required. The choices are either laser or, more commonly, electrosurgery. For argon or Nd:YAG laser, a fiber is placed through the operating channel of the operating hysteroscope, and a balanced salt solution is used for distention. When electrosurgery is used via a hysteroresectoscope, an electrolyte-free solution, such as glycine or sorbitol, must be used because a balanced salt solution will dissipate the current and prevent cutting. Use of electrolyte-free solution requires a thorough understanding of the potential risk and prevention of hyponatremia, since fatal complications have been reported with its use (see Fluid Overload and Hyponatremia).

Both pedunculated and submucosal fibroids are shaved into small pieces with either the laser fiber or the hysteroresectoscope. In the case of a pedunculated fibroid, the urge to simply transect the stalk as a first step should be resisted unless the fibroid is 10 mm or less in size. Fibroids that are larger than this are difficult to remove in one piece without excessive cervical dilatation. Morcellation is much easier when the stalk is still attached for stability.

Since the field of view is obscured by multiple pieces of tissue, the hysteroresectoscope is removed and the tissue collected in the urologic pouch. The hysteroscope is replaced in the uterus, and the procedure is repeated until the pedunculated fibroid and its stalk are completely removed, or the submucosal fibroid is shaved flush to the adjacent wall of the uterine cavity. After surgery, some gynecologists will treat the patient with estrogen or place an intrauterine splint as described above (see Removal of Intrauterine Synechiae).

Endometrial Ablation. A recent treatment for abnormal uterine bleeding in the absence of endometrial hyperplasia is ablation of the endometrium using either a laser fiber or, more commonly, an electrosurgical "roller barrel." As described previously for myoma resection, an operative hysteroscope with a balanced salt solution is used for laser resection, and a hysteroresectoscope with an electrolyte-free solution is used for electrosurgery. For both techniques, the endometrium is destroyed down to the myometrium in a systematic fashion starting at the cornua and ending in the lower uterine segment. Electrosurgery has been used for resection of the endometrium with a loop electrode as well as for ablation. Both loop resection and laser ablation may have a somewhat greater chance of subsequent amenorrhea, but both appear to be technically more difficult with a greater risk of perforation than the more widely applied roller-barrel electrosurgical ablation. In general, these techniques result in amenorrhea in half the patients and decreased menstruation in another third over the first year of therapy. However, a large portion of these patients subsequently will require another ablative procedure for bleeding or a hysterectomy for residual bleeding or dysmenorrhea.

A theoretical risk of this approach is the delay of vaginal bleeding if the patient subsequently develops an endometrial malignancy. After several years of using this technique, this has not manifested as a significant risk. Nevertheless, the long-term risk of this problem remains uncertain, and patients undergoing this procedure should be aware of this.

Risks of Hysteroscopy. *Gas Embolism.* Gas embolism

have been reported when using CO_2 for distention after intrauterine surgery. It is recommended that CO_2 not be used for any operative procedure or after significant dilation of the cervix. If symptoms of massive gas embolism occur during diagnostic hysteroscopy, the procedure should be stopped and the patient treated as described above (see Risks of Laparoscopy: Gas Embolism).

Fluid Overload and Hyponatremia. During operative hysteroscopy, significant intravasation of distention medium can occur through venous channels opened during surgery or transperitoneally as a result of any fluid forced through the tubes. Symptomatic fluid overload has been reported with all fluid distention media, including 32% dextran 70 in dextrose. The volume of distention medium introduced through the operating hysteroscope or hysteroresectoscope should always be compared with the volume retrieved using a urologic collection drape. When using a balanced salt solution (e.g., Ringer's lactate), symptomatic fluid overload is treated effectively with diuretics.

When electrolyte-free solutions are used for electrosurgery, the potential exists for serious and even fatal hyponatremia, even without significant fluid overload. Electrolyte-free solutions should not be used for hysteroscopy when electrosurgery is not required. When these solutions are used, careful monitoring of fluid balance should be performed every 15 min to detect intravasation.

Uterine Perforation and Bowel Injury. Uterine perforation is a common risk of uterine dilation prior to hysteroscopy. If it is not possible to distend the uterine cavity when the hysteroscope is placed in the uterus, perforation should be suspected. If no sharp instrument or power source has been placed through the defect, expectant outpatient management is appropriate.

Occasionally, perforation will occur during resection of a septum or leiomyoma or other operative procedures. If any chance of bowel injury exists, laparoscopy to evaluate contiguous bowel for injury is a reasonable precaution.

Intrauterine Synechia. The formation of adhesions between the anterior and posterior uterine walls, referred to as *synechiae*, is an uncommon complication after intrauterine surgery.

Although intrauterine devices, intrauterine catheters, and high-dose estrogen therapy have been advocated to decrease the risk of this complication, the efficacy of these treatments remain uncertain.

Abdominal Procedures

Incisions. The pelvic surgeon must consider a number of factors before beginning a pelvic operation. The most important requirement is that the incision provide adequate exposure for the anticipated procedure. Pelvic surgery is performed through vertical and transverse incisions. The majority of the incisions used in pelvic surgery are shown in Fig. 39-28. The midline incision is the most useful. It is simple and tends to bleed less than incisions made off the midline. The midline incision provides excellent exposure of the pelvis, and, when necessary, the entire abdomen is accessible for operation. This incision is more susceptible to hernia formation and is somewhat more uncomfortable than the transverse incision. The resulting scar occasionally is thicker than incisions made along Langer's lines, resulting in a less desirable cosmetic result.

Transverse incisions are used more often by a pelvic surgeon because the entire incision is centered over the area of operative interest. The incisions are more comfortable postoperatively and

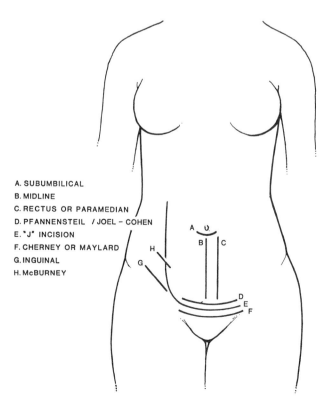

A. SUBUMBILICAL
B. MIDLINE
C. RECTUS OR PARAMEDIAN
D. PFANNENSTEIL / JOEL - COHEN
E. "J" INCISION
F. CHERNEY OR MAYLARD
G. INGUINAL
H. McBURNEY

FIG. 39-28. *Incisions useful for pelvic surgery.*

heal with a lower incidence of dehiscence or hernia formation. The most common transverse incision is the Pfannenstiel incision (Fig. 39-29). The skin is incised transversely approximately 2 cm above the symphysis pubis, and the incision is taken down to the rectus fascia, which is entered transversely. The rectus fascia is dissected bluntly away from the underlying rectus muscles in both a superior and inferior direction. The rectus muscles are separated in the midline, and the peritoneum is opened in the vertical midline.

The Maylard incision carries with it the advantages of a transverse incision but affords more exposure of the pelvis than that provided by the Pfannenstiel. The skin is incised transversely approximately 2 cm above the symphysis pubis, and the rectus fascia is opened transversely but not separated from the underlying rectus muscles. The rectus muscles are cut directly under the fascial incision, and several small bleeders in the body of the rectus muscles are clamped and coagulated. The epigastric artery and vein located just below the lateral edge of the rectus muscles are ligated and cut; the peritoneum is then opened transversely to afford good visualization and access to the entire pelvis.

The Cherney incision provides the advantages of a transverse incision and all the visibility provided by the Maylard incision. The incision is made in the transverse direction in the lower abdomen approximately 2 cm above the symphysis, the rectus fascia is opened transversely, the lower portion of the rectus sheath is dissected free of the rectus muscle, and the insertion of the rectus muscles on the symphysis pubis is visualized. The tendon of the rectus muscle is then cut free of the symphysis pubis, and the muscle is allowed to retract upward. The peritoneum is opened transversely. This incision is repaired by simply sewing the rectus tendon to the lower aspect of the rectus sheath just above the symphysis before closing the rectus sheath at the completion of the operation.

All the incisions used in pelvic surgery have advantages as well as disadvantages. The pelvic surgeon should anticipate the need for surgical exposure in the upper abdomen and in such cases choose a vertical incision. The Pfannenstiel incision is suitable for most operations for benign disease in the pelvis, but if wide pelvic or upper abdominal exposure is needed, the Maylard or Cherney incisions provide better operative exposure.

Hysterectomy for Benign Disease. The abdomen is entered through an appropriate incision. The upper abdomen is examined for evidence of extrapelvic disease, and a suitable retractor is placed in the abdominal wound. The self-retaining bowel is packed out of the pelvis and held in place with a retractor. The uterus is grasped at either cornu with Kocher clamps and pulled up into the wound (Fig. 39-30A). The round ligament is identified and suture ligated and cut (see Fig. 39-30B). If the ovaries are to be removed, the peritoneal incision is extended from the round ligament lateral to the infundibulopelvic ligament

FIG. 39-29. Pfannenstiel incision (see text for description).

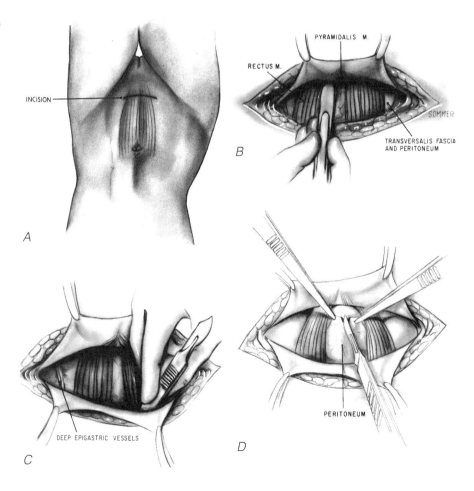

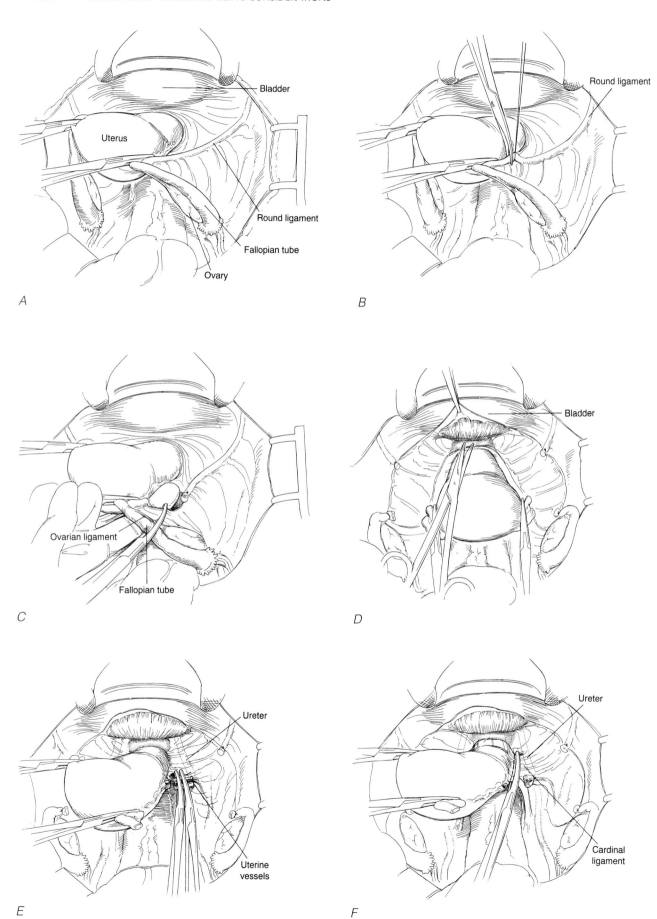

A

B

C

D

E

F

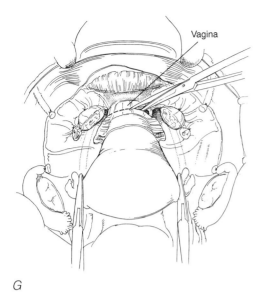

G

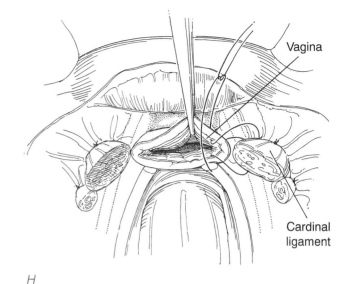

H

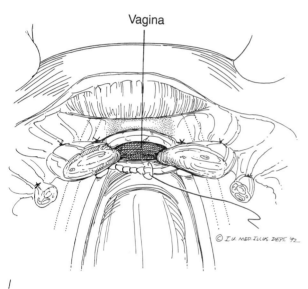

I

FIG. 39-30. Hysterectomy. *A.* The uterus grasped at the cornua. *B.* The round ligament is cut. *C.* The ovarian ligament and fallopian tube are isolated. *D.* The bladder is mobilized. *E.* The uterine vessels are clamped. *F.* The cardinal ligaments are clamped. *G.* The vagina is entered. *H.* The cardinal ligaments are sutured to the vagina. *I.* The vagina is "closed open."

for approximately 2.5 cm. The retroperitoneal space is bluntly opened. The ureter is identified on the medial leaf of the broad ligament. The infundibulopelvic ligament is isolated, clamped, cut, and suture ligated. A similar procedure is carried out on the opposite side.

In the event that the ovaries are not to be removed, after ligating the round ligament, an avascular area in the broad ligament is chosen and the broad ligament bluntly fractured with a finger, producing an opening below the ovarian ligament and fallopian tube (see Fig. 39-30*C*). The fallopian tube and ovarian ligament are clamped, cut, and ligated.

Upward traction is placed on the uterus. The peritoneum in the anterior cul de sac is opened between the ligated round ligaments. The bladder is mobilized by sharply dissecting it free of the anterior surface of the uterus and cervix (see Fig. 39-30*D*). The uterine vessels are skeletonized by transilluminating the fold of the broad ligament and dissecting the avascular tissue off the uterine vessels. The peritoneum on the posterior surface of the uterus is dissected free of the uterus and then cut. Clamps are

placed on the uterine vessels at the cervicouterine junction. The vessels are cut and the clamps replaced with suture ligatures (see Fig. 39-30*E*).

The bladder is again examined to ensure that it has been mobilized sufficiently from the vagina near the cervix. The cardinal ligaments are clamped, cut, and ligated (see Fig. 39-30*F*). Following division of the cardinal ligaments, the uterus is elevated and the vagina entered with scissors or a knife (see Fig. 39-30*G*). The uterus and cervix are cut free of the vagina. Sutures are placed at each lateral angle of the vagina, and the cardinal ligament is sutured to either lateral vaginal angle (see Fig. 39-30*H*). The central portion of the vagina is left open after repairing it with a running absorbable suture (see Fig. 39-30*I*). Pelvic reperitonealization is not necessary. The rectosigmoid colon is allowed to return to the pelvis. The pelvic packs are removed and the small bowel allowed to return to the pelvis. The omentum is placed over the bowel and under the abdominal wound. The abdominal wound is closed in an appropriate manner. In some circumstances, uterine myomata interfere with the operative procedure and myomectomy or supracervical hysterectomy might be accomplished before removing the cervix.

Myomectomy. Myomectomy should be performed through an incision that will allow good visibility of the pelvis. Hemostasis for the procedure is aided by the placement of a Penrose drain (Fig. 39-31A) around the base of the uterus pulled through small perforations in the broad ligament lateral to the uterine blood supply on either side. This "uterine tourniquet" is held in place with a clamp.

Further hemostasis may be obtained by placing bulldog or rubber-shod clamps on the infundibulopelvic ligament in order to control the uteroovarian blood supply. When possible, the uterine incision should be made in the anterior surface of the uterus in order to reduce the incidence of postoperative adhesions. An incision is made through the uterine musculature (see

Fig. 39-31B) into the myoma. The pseudocapsule surrounding the tumor is identified and the tumor is bluntly dissected out with scissors, a knife handle, or a finger. After the tumor is freed of its lateral attachments, it can be twisted to expose a pedicle that frequently contains its major blood supply (see Fig. 39-31C). On occasion, several myomas may be removed through a single incision (see Fig. 39-31D). The uterine wounds are closed with absorbable sutures to obliterate the deadspace and provide hemostasis (see Fig. 39-31E). The uterine serosa is closed with a 000 absorbable suture placed subserosally if possible. A patch of Interceed to cover the uterine incision may prevent adhesion formation (Fig. 39-31F).

Radical Hysterectomy (Modified from Oka-bayashi). The patient is placed in a modified lithotomy position with legs in obstetric stirrups, hips abducted 45° and flexed

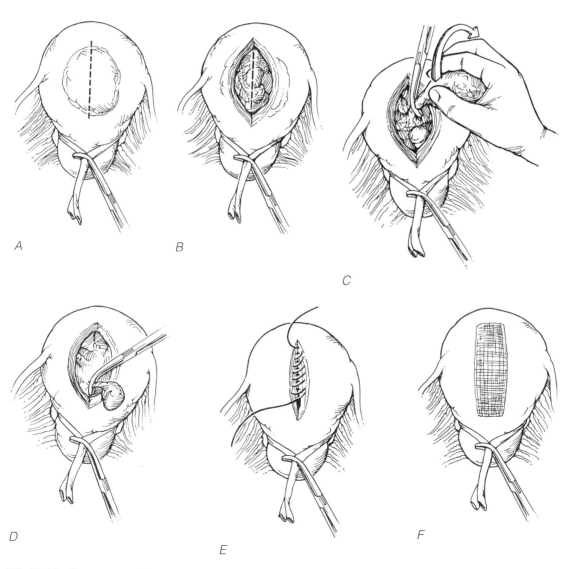

FIG. 39-31. Myomectomy. A. Hemostatic "tourniquet" in place before myomectomy. B. Uterine incision for myomectomy. C. Removal of myoma. D. Several myomas may be removed through a single incision. E. The uterine wound is closed with absorbable suture. F. The uterine wound covered with mesh to retard adhesions.

15°. The peritoneal cavity is entered through a Maylard incision (Fig. 39-32*A*) after ligating and dividing the inferior epigastric vessels. The Maylard incision permits unequaled exposure of structures on the lateral pelvic sidewall. Access to the retroperitoneum is obtained by ligating and dividing the round ligaments (see Fig. 39-32*C*). A U-shaped incision is carried from one lateral abdominal gutter to the other, including the peritoneum of the bladder reflection (see Fig. 39-32*D*). The pararectal and paravesical spaces are opened using blunt digital or instrument dissection, and narrow rigid retractors are placed to maintain exposure (see Fig. 39-32*E*). Pelvic lymphadenectomy is performed by removing lymph nodes from the external, internal, and common iliac vessels (see Fig. 39-32*F*) as well as the obturator fossa (see Fig. 39-32*G*). If there are no pelvic lymph node metastases, paraaortic lymph node sampling is unnecessary. Isolation of the superior vesicle artery by lateral retraction brings the uterine artery into view; this vessel is skeletonized and clipped at its origin from the anterior division of the internal iliac artery (see Fig. 39-32*H*). The branches of the posterior division are generally not visualized at the time of radical hysterectomy. Next, the structures inferior to the uterine artery in the cardinal ligament are clamped and divided, freeing the cervix and upper vagina from the lateral pelvic sidewall.

At this point, the proper ovarian ligaments and the proximal fallopian tubes may be transected between clamps (see Fig. 39-32*J*). After the ovarian vessels are mobilized, the ovaries may be marked with vascular clips and suspended in the lateral abdominal gutters above the pelvic brim. This measure protects the ovaries if postoperative pelvic radiotherapy is to be given. The ureters are carefully detached from the posterior leaves of the broad ligament for a short distance and retracted laterally before the posterior cul de sac is entered and the rectovaginal space developed bluntly (see Fig. 39-32*L*); the uterosacral ligaments are divided. Upward traction on the uterus facilitates dissection of the bladder inferiorly away from the underlying cervix and upper vagina. The ureters are freed from their investment in the paracervical tissue, allowing the bladder and ureters to be displaced inferolaterally, exposing the upper vagina and paravaginal tissues. The tissues are clamped and cut, taking care to remove a 3- to 4-cm "cuff" of vagina with the cervix (see Fig. 39-32*M*).

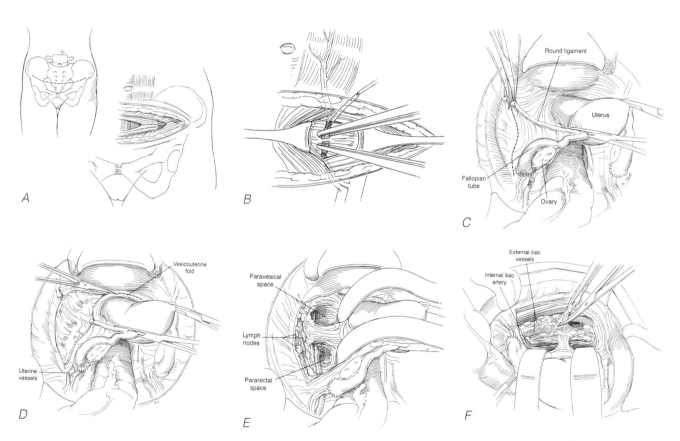

FIG. 39-32. Radical hysterectomy. *A.* Exposure of the inferior epigastric vessels before transection of the rectus muscles. *B.* Ligation of the inferior epigastric vessels before transection of the rectus muscles. *C.* Ligation and division of the round ligaments opens the pelvic retroperitoneum. *D.* First peritoneal incision lateral to the ovarian vessels and across the vesicouterine fold. *E.* Narrow malleable retractors (Indiana Retractors) are placed into the paravesical and pararectal spaces to provide excellent access to the lateral pelvic sidewall and pelvic lymph nodes. *F.* Pelvic lymphadenectomy (external and internal iliac vessels). *G.* Pelvic lymphadenectomy (obturator fossa). *H.* Development of the uterine and superior vesical arteries. *I.* The uterine artery has been clipped and divided near its origin. *J.* The proper ovarian ligament and proximal fallopian tube is clamped and divided if the ovary is to be preserved. *K.* The ureters have been detached from the posterior peritoneum of the broad ligament and are retracted laterally. The rectovaginal space is developed using blunt finger dissection. *L.* Transection of the uterosacral ligaments. *M.* Clamps are placed on the lateral vagina, taking care to remove 3 to 4 cm of the upper vagina.

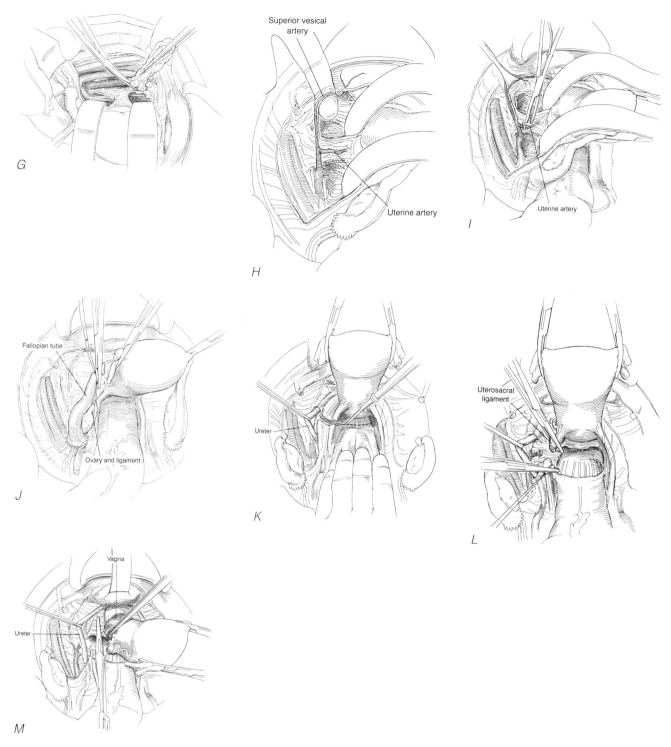

FIG. 39-32. Continued.

The vagina is closed, a suprapubic catheter is inserted, and the abdominal incision is repaired.

Radical hysterectomy is associated with 85 to 90 percent cure rates in patients without lymph node metastases and 65 to 70 percent rates in those with spread to the regional nodes. The primary morbidity is bladder denervation, which occurs to some extent in almost all women undergoing this procedure. Gener-

ally, loss of bladder sensation is the only deficit, although inability to void is not uncommon in the immediate postoperative period. Ureterovaginal fistulas occur in about 1 percent of all patients in recent studies.

Postoperative external-beam radiotherapy may be elected if nodal metastases, positive surgical margins, or parametrial tissue involvement is found. Because bladder and ureteral complications are more common in women undergoing postoperative radiotherapy, surgical candidates must be chosen with care.

Resection of Ovarian Cancer. Radical or modified radical hysterectomy is indicated in the treatment of epithelial ovarian cancer only if peritoneal tumor nodules obliterate the posterior cul de sac or extend to the retroperitoneal spaces. Generally, extrafascial (simple or conservative) hysterectomy (see Fig. 39-18) suffices in the resection of these tumors.

When hysterectomy and salpingo-oophorectomy are completed, the infracolic omentum should be removed by reflecting the fatty organ superiorly, isolating and dividing the right and left gastroepiploic vessels, and dissecting through the avascular posterior leaf before isolating and dividing the vessels in the anterior leaf of the omentum. If the omentum contains a large amount of disease, the gastrocolic omentum should be removed by isolating and dividing the short gastric vessels along the greater curvature of the stomach. In cases of extensive omental involvement, care must be taken not to injure the spleen, stomach, or transverse colon. Generous peritoneal biopsies should be obtained from the right hemidiaphragm, both lateral abdominal gutters, and the anterior and posterior peritoneum of the pelvis.

If gross peritoneal tumor is completely removed, the lymph nodes should be evaluated. The paraaortic lymph nodes may be exposed by reflecting the colon medially. These lymph nodes should be liberally sampled, keeping in mind that the primary venous drainage of the left ovary is the left renal vein and that of the right ovary is the inferior vena cava at the level of the renal vein.

Pelvic lymph node sampling is also an important aspect of surgical staging in ovarian cancer and is completed by removing lymph nodes from the distribution of the external and internal iliac vessels and obturator space above the level of the obturator nerve. This part of the staging procedure is facilitated by first opening the paravesical and pararectal spaces as described for radical hysterectomy above. Lymph node sampling is primarily a diagnostic procedure in the management of early ovarian cancers. There is little evidence that complete lymphadenectomy is therapeutic in patients with advanced and unresected disease.

Vaginal Procedures

Hysterectomy. The removal of the uterus through the vagina is preferred in many cases of myoma, uterine prolapse, intraepithelial neoplasia, and uterine bleeding disorders. Patients are more comfortable, and operative time, hospital stay, and recovery time are shorter than in cases of abdominal operation. Vaginal hysterectomy is an acceptable approach in those patients in whom the uterus descends, the bony pelvis allows vaginal operation, the uterine tumors are small enough to permit vaginal removal, and the patient is amenable to vaginal operation. In the presence of large myomas, pretreatment with a GnRH-a will allow vaginal operation that would have been impossible previously.

The patient is placed in a high lithotomy position, and the pelvis is examined under anesthesia. This examination should confirm previous findings and provide assurance that the operation is possible through the vaginal route. The bladder is not catheterized before operation unless it is greatly distended. A weighted vaginal speculum is placed in the posterior vagina, and the cervix is grasped with a tenaculum and pulled in the axis of the vagina (Fig. 39-33A). The posterior cul de sac is identified

and entered with scissors (see Fig. 39-33B). Mayo scissors are used to circumcise the cervix, and the mucosa is cut down to the pubocervical-vesical fascia (see Fig. 39-33C). The vaginal mucosa and the bladder are sharply and bluntly dissected free of the cervix and the lower portion of the uterus. Care must be taken not to injure the bladder.

When the peritoneum of the anterior cul de sac is identified, it is entered with the scissors, and a retractor is placed in the defect (see Fig. 39-33D). The uterosacral ligaments are identified, doubly clamped, cut, and doubly ligated (see Fig. 39-33E). The second ligature is held long. Serial clamps are placed on the parametrial structures above the uterosacral ligament; these pedicles are cut, and the clamps are replaced with ties (see Fig. 39-33F). At the cornu of the uterus, the tube, round ligament, and suspensory ligament of the ovary are doubly clamped and cut (see Fig. 39-33G). The procedure is carried out on the opposite side, and the uterus is removed. The first clamp is replaced with a free tie; the second clamp is replaced with a suture ligature that is transfixed. The second suture ligature is held long. The pelvis is inspected for hemostasis; all bleeding must be meticulously controlled at this point.

The pelvic peritoneum is closed with a running purse-string suture incorporating those pedicles which were held (see Fig. 39-33H). This exteriorizes those areas which might tend to bleed. The sutures attached to the ovarian pedicles are cut. The vagina may be closed with interrupted mattress stitches, incorporating the uterosacral ligaments into the corner of the vagina with each lateral stitch (see Fig. 39-33I). The vaginal cuff is inspected again for hemostasis. In most cases no vaginal packing is required. A catheter is left in the bladder until the patient has fully awakened and is ambulatory.

On occasion, the uterus, which is initially too large to remove vaginally, may be reduced in size by morcellation (Fig. 39-34). After the uterine vessels have been clamped and ligated, serial wedges are taken from the central portion of the uterus in order to reduce the uterine mass. This procedure will allow the vaginal delivery of even very large uterine leiomyomas.

Pelvic Support Repairs. Most pelvic support defects should be treated by the vaginal route. Vaginal operation allows repair of all support defects and generally allows an opportunity for the use of support structures that will prevent recurrence of prolapse. Uterovaginal prolapse is treated by vaginal hysterectomy. If the ligaments retain their strength, they may be used in a culdoplasty to provide good postoperative vaginal support. In the absence of good uterosacral ligament support, the operator can choose to support the vagina by suturing the vaginal apex to one or the other uterosacral ligament. On rare occasion, a partial colpectomy with colpocleisis may be the surgical method of choice.

Cystocele repair generally follows vaginal hysterectomy. The anterior edges of the vaginal cuff are grasped with Allis clamps, and the vaginal mucosa is opened from the vaginal cuff to the base of the bladder. The bladder is sharply separated from the vaginal mucosa to completely expose the cystocele. A Foley catheter is placed in the bladder, and the bladder neck is identified by palpation. Serial interrupted mattress stitches are used to reduce the bladder by plicating the posterior bladder wall. Cystocele repair is accomplished by placing one or more layers of 2-0 absorbable suture in the bladder wall. After the bladder plication is complete, the vaginal mucosal flaps are trimmed, and

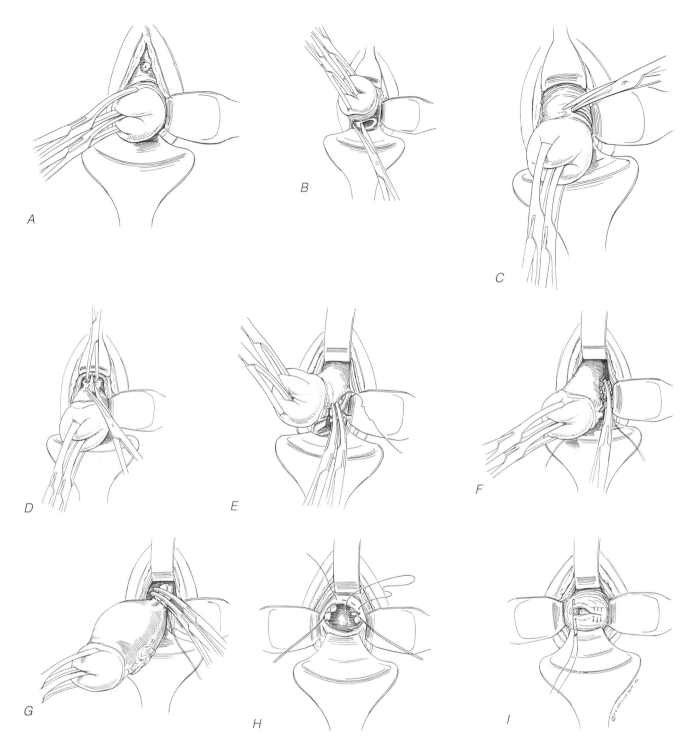

FIG. 39-33. Vaginal hysterectomy. *A.* Traction is placed on the uterus. *B.* The posterior cul de sac is entered. *C.* The vaginal mucosa is circumcised. *D.* The anterior cul de sac is entered. *E.* The uterosacral ligaments are clamped. *F.* The uterosacral ligaments are tied. *G.* The fallopian tube, round ligament, and ovarian ligament are ligated. *H.* The peritoneum is closed. *I.* The vaginal mucosa is closed.

the vaginal mucosa is closed with interrupted 2-0 absorbable sutures. After the cystocele repair is complete the vaginal apex may be closed with interrupted 2-0 absorbable sutures.

If a rectocele repair is required, Allis clamps are placed at the hymenal ring posteriorly, and the posterior vaginal mucosa is opened to a point above the apex of the rectocele. The vaginal

mucosa is separated from the underlying rectum by sharp and blunt dissection. The vaginal mucosa is trimmed to reduce the vaginal luminal diameter, judged to be adequate if two inserted fingers fit the vaginal lumen with ease. The anterior rectal wall is imbricated with either interrupted or running stitches. The imbricating stitches pull the rectum in on itself, eliminating the

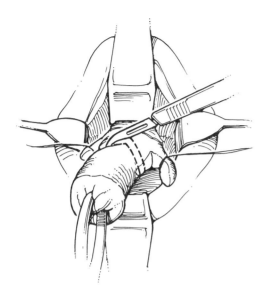

FIG. 39-34. *Uterine morcellation through the vagina.*

rectal hernia when the posterior vaginal mucosa is reapproximated with a running stitch of 2-0 absorbable sutures.

Enterocele. These hernias can exist before hysterectomy, and when they do, they must be recognized and obliterated at the time of uterine removal.

After an enterocele has been diagnosed, it should be repaired in concert with the repair of other pelvic defects. If diagnosis is made at the time of pelvic laparotomy, the defect can be repaired by the abdominal route. The hernia sac can be obliterated using a series of vertical stitches to approximate the anterior rectal wall to the posterior vaginal wall in a technique described by Halban. Moschcowitz described a technique for the treatment of rectal prolapse that serves to obliterate the cul de sac very nicely. The Moschcowitz technique uses concentric purse-string sutures starting at the bottom of the cul de sac to obliterate the hernia.

Enteroceles frequently cause inversion of the vagina. By the time this has progressed far enough to produce symptoms, most of the normal supporting structures have been totally lost. This condition is treated by opening the vaginal mucosa over the enterocele sac, dissecting out the hernia sac, and removing it. The peritoneum is closed at the neck of the hernia with two or more absorbable sutures that approximate the anterior rectal wall to the posterior bladder wall. Anterior and posterior vaginal repairs are performed if appropriate. In most cases, sacrospinous fixation of the vagina will provide a more permanent solution to the vaginal prolapse.

An alternative approach might be an abdominal sacral colpopexy, in which the vagina is supported by a fabric graft placed between the anterior surface of the sacrum and the vaginal apex. If the abdominal route is chosen, either a Moschcowitz or Halban enterocele repair should be performed in association with the surgery.

Surgical Correction of Incontinence. Urethral detachment that causes stress urinary incontinence can be treated with a variety of repairs. A purely vaginal approach to this problem is the Kelly stitch, which involves plication of the periurethral structures at the bladder neck and tends to restore the posterior ureterovesical angle. The failure rate with this procedure is rela-

tively high, and most operators prefer to choose some type of needle procedure such as the Peyrera, Raz, or Stamey procedure when operating vaginally.

The abdominal repair of stress incontinence is accomplished by the Marshall-Marchetti-Krantz procedure or the Birch procedure. The Marshall-Marchetti-Krantz procedure sutures the connective tissue on either side of the bladder neck to the periosteum of the symphysis. The Birch procedure pulls periurethral tissue up to Cooper's ligament if possible. The common denominator of both procedures is the elevation and angulation of the urethra at the bladder neck. Both the Marshall-Marchetti-Krantz and the Birch procedures are most valuable in patients who require repair of only a urethral detachment in the treatment of their urinary stress incontinence.

Pessaries. The vaginal pessary has been used since ancient times. It involves placing a plastic or rubber device into the vagina to support the vaginal apex and the vaginal walls. The device is finding little use in modern gynecology. When pessaries are used, they should be removed at least every 4 weeks. They produce discomfort secondary to pelvic pressure, and vaginal ulceration secondary to pressure necrosis is common.

Injuries Associated with Pelvic Surgery. *Intestinal Injury.* Adhesion formation is the most common antecedent to enterotomy at the time of pelvic operation. When lysis of adhesions is carefully carried out, this complication should occur rarely. Injuries to the small bowel range from serosal tears to through-and-through lacerations. Serosal tears are usually oversewn with a 4-0 nonabsorbable suture. Injuries to the lumen of the bowel are generally repaired using single- or double-layer closure; a single layer of 4-0 absorbable suture followed by an outer layer of interrupted nonabsorbable suture is effective. Lacerations that are extensive or involve multiple areas should be treated by resecting the injured segment.

Injury to the colon may occur during an operation to remove a left adnexal mass. When this injury occurs in a prepared colon, it is primarily repaired in a two-layer closure similar to that used in a small bowel repair. Large injuries may require resection of a segment of the colon.

Injury to the unprepared large bowel is a significant problem. A small wound that is promptly recognized may be treated primarily with a single- or double-layer closure. The patient should be treated with intraoperative and postoperative antibiotics to cover both anaerobic and aerobic organisms. A major injury to unprepared large bowel will require colostomy in most cases.

Ureteral Injury. Ureteral injury at the time of pelvic surgery is uncommon and largely preventable. The ureters are at highest risk when the infundibulopelvic ligament is clamped for removal of an ovary and when the uterine arteries or cardinal ligaments are clamped during the course of hysterectomy. In most cases, visualization or palpation of the ureter before placing a hemostatic clamp will avoid this complication. The ureter is at highest risk in the course of pelvic operation for endometriosis, pelvic inflammatory disease, and pelvic neoplasia. The surgery for most of these conditions allows the dissection of the ureter beginning at the pelvic brim with meticulous exposure down to and through the operative field. Transection of the ureter high in the pelvis may allow primary reanastomosis of the ureter. Ureteral injuries near the bladder generally require ureteral reimplantation into the bladder.

Bladder Injury. The pelvic surgeon must be constantly aware of the proximity of the bladder to the cervix and the anterior portion of the uterine fundus. The bladder must be dissected carefully free of the cervix at the time of hysterectomy. Hemostasis should be meticulous, and large clamps and ligatures should be avoided to prevent devitalization of the bladder wall. Operative entry into the bladder should be recognized immediately. If there is any question about the integrity of the bladder at the time of hysterectomy, a dilute solution of methylene blue will detect the defect and allow for closure.

Bladder injuries must be fully visualized in preparation for repair irrespective of whether they were produced by vaginal or abdominal operation. The surgeon must ascertain that the wound does not involve the ureter and that the resulting repair will not compromise ureteral function. 4-0 polyglycolic acid sutures are placed at either extent of the bladder laceration and held for retraction. The suture does not enter the lumen of the bladder. Once the bladder injury is delineated by the two initial sutures, the wound is closed with 4-0 interrupted polyglycolic acid suture in a running mattress stitch in order to strengthen the first layer and to remove any tension produced by the initial closure. An indwelling catheter should remain in the bladder for 5 to 7 days or until microscopic hematuria has disappeared. Some pelvic surgeons test their repair with a small amount of sterile milk. Milk is preferred to methylene blue or indigo carmine because it will not stain the tissue and therefore allows subsequent testing.

Bibliography

Baggish MS, Sze EH: Endometrial ablation: A series of 568 patients treated over an 11-year period. *Am J Obstet Gynecol* 174:908, 1966.

Copeland LJ: *Textbook for Gynecology*. St. Louis, CV Mosby, 1993.

Herbst AL, Michell D. et al: *Comprehensive Gynecology*, 2d ed. St. Louis, CV Mosby, 1992.

Hoskins WJ, Perez CA, Young RC (eds): *Gynecologic Oncology*. Philadelphia, JB Lippincott, 1992.

Hurd WW, Bude RO, et al: The location of abdominal wall blood vessels in relationship to abdominal landmarks apparent at laparoscopy. *Am J Obstet Gynecol* 171:642, 1994.

Kurman RJ: *Blaustein's Pathology of the Female Genital Tract*, 4th ed. New York, Springer-Verlag, 1994.

Lee RH: *Atlas of Gynecologic Surgery*. Philadelphia, WB Saunders, 1992.

Nichols DH: *Gynecologic and Obstetric Surgery*. St Louis, CV Mosby, 1993.

Rubin SC, Sutton GP (eds): *Ovarian Cancer*. New York, McGraw-Hill, 1993.

Saidi MH, Sadler RK, et al: Diagnosis and management of serious urinary complications after major operative laparoscopy. *Obstet Gynecol* 87:272, 1996.

Shingleton HM, Fowler WC, et al (eds): *Gynecologic Oncology*. Philadelphia, WB Saunders, 1996.

Singer A, Monaghan JM: *Lower Genital Tract Precancer*. Boston, Blackwell Scientific Publications, 1994.

Speroff L, Glass RH, Kase NG: *Clinical Gynecologic Endocrinology and Infertility*, 5th ed. Baltimore, Williams & Wilkins, 1994.

Steege JF: Laparoscopic approach to the adnexal mass. *Clin Obstet Gynecol* 37:392, 1994.

Thompson JD, Rock JA (eds): *TeLinde's Operative Gynecology,* 7th ed. Philadelphia, JB Lippincott, 1992.

CHAPTER 40

Neurosurgery

Julian T. Hoff and Michael F. Boland

GENERAL CONSIDERATIONS

A detailed history and a physical examination are the foundation of neurosurgical diagnosis. Headache, altered consciousness, memory impairment, speech difficulty, visual disturbance, weakness, paresthesia, and incoordination are some symptoms suggestive of central nervous system disease. Historical details suggest a cause (e.g., traumatic, neoplastic, vascular, infectious, degenerative, or metabolic) while neurologic examination permits anatomic localization of the lesion. For patients with nervous system disorders, an accurate history needs to be taken once, but the examination must be repeated and recorded often to gauge the course of the illness and to judge the urgency of other diagnostic steps.

Diagnostic Studies. Once a differential diagnosis is formulated using the information gathered from the history and the examination, diagnostic studies are used to confirm the definitive diagnosis. Common studies include plain film radiography, myelography, arteriography, computed tomography (CT), magnetic resonance imaging (MRI), ultrasonography (USN), electromyography and nerve conduction velocity testing (EMG/NCV), evoked potentials (visual, auditory, and somatosensory), positron emission tomography (PET), electroencephalography (EEG), and cerebrospinal fluid (CSF) analysis.

Plain films, especially of the spine, are useful in trauma and degenerative disorders. Myelography, often combined with CT, is useful for evaluating spinal nerve roots and the spinal cord in trauma, tumor, and degenerative spine disease. CT and MRI provide detailed imaging of both cranial and spinal contents. They are useful in combination for visualization of bone and soft tissues. Arteriography provides detailed information regarding aneurysms, vascular malformations, and atherosclerotic disease. It is an essential tool in the evaluation of cerebral hemorrhage, embolic and thrombotic stroke, and preoperative planning for tumor surgery. USN is an important adjunct in the operating room, providing visualization of tumors, cysts, vascular malformations, and congenital anomalies lying beneath the exposed surface. USN is also used to visualize the brain and spinal cord in newborns.

EMG/NCV helps to assess peripheral nerve and nerve root lesions. It is also used to monitor brachial plexus and peripheral nerve recovery following traumatic injury. Visual and auditory evoked potentials can be employed in comatose patients to monitor the severity of head injury. Auditory potentials are useful in evaluating cranial nerve and brainstem function. Somatosensory potentials continually monitor spinal cord (dorsal column) function and are used often during surgical manipulation of spinal fractures and tumors. PET scans play an important role in epilepsy surgery, preembolization assessment of skull base tumors involving the cavernous sinus, and surgically untreatable vascular anomalies. EEG helps in delineating structural and metabolic disorders and can be employed during cerebrovascular surgery to monitor adequacy of cerebral perfusion. CSF analysis remains essential for many diagnoses, such as bacterial or viral meningitis.

SPECIAL SITUATIONS

Seizures. Seizures are useful clinical signs because the aura, onset, and type of seizure and the postictal state may localize the lesion. Seizures are particularly common in patients with neoplasms. Repetitive seizures should be treated vigorously. Phenytoin (Dilantin) is the drug of choice; 750 to 1000 mg may be given I.V. over 1 h as a loading dose. Supplemental doses usually consist of 100 mg given three or four times a day. Phenobarbital is also useful (32 to 65 mg, three or four times a day), but larger doses may depress consciousness. Diazepam (Valium) given intravenously in divided doses (10 to 50 mg) is highly effective in the control of status epilepticus but is not a good long-term anticonvulsant.

Raised Intracranial Pressure. Almost any space-occupying intracranial lesion can raise intracranial pressure (ICP). Clinical indications of elevated ICP are headache, stupor, diplopia, nausea, vomiting, and neck stiffness. Altered blood pressure and heart rate are late signs; typically the blood pressure is increased and the heart rate is decreased. Apnea may occur if ICP is very high. Raised ICP may be prevented and treated by the following measures.

Hyperventilation. The Pa_{CO_2} should be monitored and maintained at about 35 mmHg. Brain swelling develops when Pa_{CO_2} rises above normal (40 mmHg). A good airway is essential to maintain control of Pa_{CO_2}.

Hypothermia. Because fever causes the brain to swell, the patient's temperature should be controlled by alcohol sponging, antipyretics (aspirin or acetaminophen), and hypothermia blankets. Chlorpromazine (Thorazine, 5 mg I.V. every 3 to 4 h) minimizes shivering during these maneuvers.

Osmotic Diuretics. Mannitol (1.5 g/kg/24 h) causes shrinkage of the brain and reduction of ICP. It should be used only when the clinical situation is desperate; its beneficial effect is transient, and the drug can severely alter serum electrolytes and osmolarity. Urea and glycerol are other osmotic diuretics that may be effective.

Steroids. Dexamethasone (Decadron, 4 to 6 mg every 4 h I.V. or orally) or methylprednisolone (Solu-Medrol, 125 to 250 mg I.M. or I.V. twice daily) lowers ICP by reducing brain edema. The drug probably acts to stabilize the blood-brain barrier.

Infections. CNS infections include meningitis, subdural empyema, brain abscess, and epidural abscess. Antibiotics penetrate the normal blood-brain barrier variably; however, in the presence of meningitis antibiotics are able to penetrate the blood-brain barrier better. Specific antibiotics should be given for specific infections. During the 1 to 2 days required to identify the pathogenic organism, broad-spectrum antibiotics should be given if the infection is life-threatening. Vancomycin (1.0 g I.V. every 12 h) and gentamicin (75 mg I.V. every 8 h) are the drugs of choice while awaiting culture results.

Antibiotics for prevention of CNS infection are rarely indicated. In patients with persistent CSF leakage, a broad-spectrum antibiotic is sometimes used (ampicillin or a cephalosporin).

Fluid Balance. Neurosurgical patients should have low-normal to normal intake and output of fluids (2000 to 2500 mL/24 h for an adult). Free water (5% dextrose in water) should be avoided because it causes brain swelling. The preferred I.V. solution is 5% dextrose in 0.5 normal saline with potassium supplements (40 mEq/day). Fluid balance should be monitored by daily weights and periodic measurements of serum electrolytes. Feedings by gavage may be started early (up to 3 days after injury or operation) provided gastrointestinal function is normal.

Some neurosurgical patients have profound disturbances of fluid balance. Inappropriate antidiuretic hormone (ADH) secretion, which most commonly occurs after head trauma, causes retention of free water, resulting in low serum sodium, high urinary sodium, low serum osmolarity, and high urinary specific gravity. Seizures and coma may be the first clinical signs of inappropriate ADH secretion. The best treatment is fluid restriction.

Diabetes insipidus is also common in patients with neurosurgical illnesses. Urine volume is high and specific gravity is low; serum sodium and osmolarity are high. Seizures and stupor may appear. The condition is treated by administration of I.V. or oral fluids. Sometimes antidiuretic hormone (vasopressin, Pitressin) is required to control urinary loss of water.

Patients who are given steroids, osmotic diuretics, anticonvulsants, and hyperosmolar feedings (typical neurosurgical patients) are prone to developing a hyperosmolar state, sometimes leading to hyperglycemic nonketotic coma. Consequently, careful monitoring of fluid and electrolyte status of the neurosurgical patient is essential.

Coma. *Coma* is a loss of consciousness from which the patient cannot be aroused by any stimulus. *Stupor* implies that the patient can be partially aroused by loud command or painful stimulus but promptly lapses into unconsciousness when the stimulus is withdrawn.

Diagnosis. The diagnosis of coma requires a careful history (generally from friends or relatives of the patient) and a complete physical examination, with specific attention to the neurologic examination. Laboratory and radiologic tests of value include serum electrolytes, blood glucose, and blood urea nitrogen assays, skull x-rays, and CSF examination via lumbar puncture. Medical consultation should be sought promptly.

Coma may be caused by poisoning, such as alcohol, barbiturate, and narcotic overdose; cerebral lesions, such as those caused by trauma, vascular accidents, tumors, infections, and epilepsy; metabolic disorders, such as diabetes mellitus, hypoglycemia, Addison's disease, uremia, hepatic disease, and eclampsia; and other stresses, such as severe infection, shock, asphyxia, heatstroke, and hypoxia. Diagnostic features of common types of coma are as follows.

Acute Alcoholic Intoxication. A history of alcohol abuse, alcoholic breath, flushed face, slow and stertorous respirations, diminished reflexes, and a blood alcohol level above 400 mg/dL establish this diagnosis.

Narcotic Poisoning. Even small doses of narcotics may cause respiratory depression and coma in patients with liver insufficiency, myxedema, emphysema, or head injuries and in debilitated or elderly patients. Findings include cold, clammy, cyanotic skin, pinpoint pupils, respiratory depression, and a feeble and often irregular pulse.

Acute toxicity caused by an overdose of a self-administered narcotic occurs commonly in some localities. The type and purity of the drug are difficult to determine, although a companion or acquaintance may know the patient's drug habits. The examiner should look for needle marks in the arms and legs. Laboratory tests are valuable to determine barbiturate, alcohol, or narcotic levels.

Diabetic Coma. Coma may be precipitated in a diabetic patient by infection or by failure to regulate insulin dosage carefully. Diagnostic features include the following: history of diabetes, gradual onset, with blurred vision and thirst, air hunger or Kussmaul respiration, dehydration (soft eyeballs), acetone breath ("fruity" odor on breath), glycosuria, acetonuria, hyperglycemia, ketonemia, and low plasma bicarbonate level.

Hypoglycemia. Hypoglycemic reactions in diabetics may be precipitated by failure to eat, by vigorous exercise, or by insulin overdose. Mental confusion and bizarre behavior precede coma and convulsions. Tachycardia, sweating, tremors, and vomiting are other manifestations. Low blood glucose level confirms the diagnosis.

Management. *Emergency Measures.* Identify and treat any life-threatening condition immediately. Establish and maintain an airway to provide oxygenation. Insert an endotracheal tube if the respiratory rate is less than 10/min, if the Pa_{O_2} is below 70 mmHg, or if the Pa_{O_2} is greater than 50 mmHg with the patient breathing oxygen through a mask. Monitor arterial blood gases frequently and treat the patient for shock. When no cause for coma is immediately obvious, obtain blood for glucose determination and toxicologic analysis and then administer each of the following: 50 mL of 50% dextrose in water for possible hypoglycemia, 1 mL (0.4 mg) naloxone for possible narcotic overdose, and 100 mg thiamine I.V. for possible Wernicke's (alcoholic) encephalopathy.

General Measures. Observe the patient frequently, record neurologic and vital signs at regular intervals, and change the patient's position often to avoid postural pneumonia and decubitus ulcers. A lateral and slightly head-down position is best for patients who are likely to vomit. A suction machine and an alert attendant near the bedside are essential. Maintain ventilation and monitor urinary output through an indwelling catheter. Maintain fluid, electrolyte, and caloric intake. Nasogastric feeding should be started if the coma lasts more than 2 to 3 days. Avoid administering narcotics, sedatives, and other medications until the diagnosis is established; agitation can then be treated best by administration of parenteral diazepam (2 to 5 mg I.V. every 2 h as needed).

TRAUMA

Trauma is the single most common cause of death in children, adolescents, and young adults. The majority of accidents involving motor vehicles and falls include injury to the brain, spinal cord, and their supporting structures.

Scalp Injury

Scalp injury may cause hemorrhage and subsequent shock if not promptly treated. Bleeding can usually be controlled by a pressure dressing or by clamps applied to the galea aponeurotica. Scalp wounds should be closed as soon as possible. Lacerations that overlie a depressed fracture or a penetrating wound of the skull require debridement and closure in the operating room.

Simple scalp lacerations should be debrided, copiously irrigated, and closed primarily, taking care to approximate both the galea and the skin. A good galeal closure provides excellent hemostasis. Scalp avulsions typically include all layers of the scalp, sparing the underlying periosteum. If the avulsion is small, closure can often be accomplished primarily. Replacement of the avulsed part, employing microsurgical technique, is the preferred method of repair for large scalp avulsions, provided the tissue has been preserved adequately and surgery is not delayed.

If the injured scalp is not viable but the periosteum is intact, split-thickness skin grafts can be used to close the defect. The periosteum must be kept moist before operation. When the periosteum is absent or desiccated, closure is more difficult, since it is through the periosteal layer that the outer skull table receives its blood supply. In this instance, closure can be accomplished using free myocutaneous flaps attached by microsurgical vascular anastomoses.

Skull Fracture

Skull fractures are classified according to whether the skin overlying the fracture is intact (closed) or disrupted (open or compound), whether there is a single fracture line (linear), several fractures radiating from a central point (stellate), or fragmentation of bone (comminuted), and/or whether the edges of the fracture line have been driven inward below the level of the surrounding bone (depressed) or not (nondepressed).

Simple skull fractures (linear, stellate, or comminuted nondepressed) require no specific treatment. They are, however, potentially serious if they cross vascular channels in the skull, such as the middle meningeal artery or the dural venous sinuses. If these structures are torn, an epidural or subdural hematoma may form. A simple skull fracture that extends into the accessory nasal sinuses or the mastoid air cells is considered open, since it is in communication with air.

Depressed skull fractures often require surgical treatment to elevate the depressed bone fragments. If there are no untoward neurologic signs and the fracture is closed, repair may be done electively. Intraoperatively, the dura should be inspected and repaired.

Open skull fractures also require surgical intervention. Linear or stellate, nondepressed open fractures can be treated by simple closure of the scalp after thorough cleansing. Open fractures with severe comminution of underlying bone should be treated in the operating room, where thorough debridement can be carried out. The dura should be inspected to verify that a laceration has not been overlooked. Dural tears should be closed either primarily or with a fascial patch graft to reduce the risk of infection and prevent CSF leakage. Depressed, open skull fractures should be debrided, elevated, and closed in the operating room after preparations have been made for craniotomy, in case broader exposure of the underlying dura and/or brain is necessary.

Basal skull fractures involve the floor of the skull. Bruising may occur about the eye (raccoon sign) or behind the ear (Battle's sign), suggesting a fracture involving either the anterior or middle fossa, respectively. Isolated cranial nerve deficits can be seen in association with this fracture type because the nerves' exit foramina lie at the skull base. The facial nerve is frequently affected, with injury due to laceration or swelling. Most facial nerve deficits resolve spontaneously, so no specific therapy is warranted. On the other hand, complete transections of the facial nerve are usually explored, although the timing of exploration remains a matter of debate.

Any associated CSF rhinorrhea or otorrhea should be treated expectantly. Traumatic CSF leaks typically stop within the first 7 to 10 days. If a leak persists, lumbar CSF drainage can be implemented to seal the leak by lowering CSF volume and ICP. If drainage therapy fails, surgical exploration is indicated and accomplished by oversewing the defect with an intradural fascial patch graft. Fewer than 5 percent of patients require surgical repair. Prophylactic antibiotics are not used routinely because recent prospective studies have failed to demonstrate any benefit from their use.

Brain Injury

Injury to the brain is caused by rapid deceleration, acceleration, rotation, or a combination of these, associated with a blow to the head. The initial impact can produce neuronal and axonal disruption, which constitutes the *primary injury.* Any subsequent complication such as an intracranial hematoma, cerebral edema, hypoxia, hypotension, hydrocephalus, or endocrine disturbance characterizes *secondary injury,* which compounds the initial insult.

Mild head injury is usually not associated with significant primary brain injury, and neurologic deficits are limited to temporary loss of consciousness (concussion). Moderate to severe head injury, on the other hand, is typically associated with deficits that may or may not be reversible. Moreover, this degree of injury is usually accompanied by secondary injury.

Distortional forces causing the primary injury may be great enough to tear intraparenchymal capillaries, superficial subdural bridging veins, or epidural arteries and veins, allowing extravasation of blood and hematoma formation. Cerebral edema occurs in response to vasodilatation and blood-brain barrier disruption. Ischemia from hypotension or hypoxia can produce cell death and consequent cytotoxic edema. Disruption of CSF absorption by contamination of CSF with blood may lead to hydrocephalus. Inappropriate secretion of antidiuretic hormone or the development of diabetes insipidus can aggravate cerebral edema by altering fluid and electrolyte balance. These changes, either separately or in combination, can result in elevation of ICP.

Elevated ICP contributes to secondary brain injury by reducing cerebral perfusion pressure (CPP), which is defined as the difference between mean arterial blood pressure (MABP) and cerebral venous pressure or ICP. Thus when ICP increases and MABP remains stable, CPP decreases. When CPP falls below 70 mmHg, cerebral perfusion is compromised, producing cerebral ischemia and compounding the primary brain injury with a secondary insult.

Intracranial hypertension is one of the most important factors affecting outcome in head injury. For this reason, aggressive management to circumvent cerebral blood flow reduction and secondary injury is imperative. Early resuscitative therapy should be initiated at the scene of the accident if possible with airway control and hyperventilation. In the absence of hypotension, osmotherapy can also be used early to reduce brain bulk.

Rapid clinical assessment is essential. Although extensive neurologic testing is limited in uncooperative or unresponsive patients, certain features of the exam are critical. The Glasgow Coma Scale (Table 40-1), established in 1974, uses a numerical score to evaluate eye opening and verbal and motor behavior, both spontaneously and in response to stimulation. This scale is used to follow the patient's neurologic status and provides information about the ultimate outcome of the patient.

The initial neurologic exam determines whether diagnostic testing is indicated. It is unlikely that patients without headache, lethargy, or a focal neurologic deficit will suffer a secondary complication from their injury. Imaging studies are generally not indicated in the asymptomatic patient. Conversely, symptomatic patients with or without a focal deficit should undergo CT scanning of the head. If CT fails to disclose a lesion despite high clinical suspicion, carotid and/or cerebral angiography may be helpful to identify a vascular abnormality that cannot be appreciated by CT scan.

Treatment. After removal of any traumatic intracranial mass, the goals of management are normalization of CPP and prevention of secondary injury to damaged brain. Intracranial pressure monitoring may be indicated, especially in those patients with marked depression or deterioration in neurologic

Table 40-1
Glasgow Coma Scale

Best motor response	Obeys	M6
	Localizes	5
	Withdraws	4
	Abnormal flexion	3
	Extensor response	2
	Nil	1
Verbal response	Oriented	V5
	Confused conversation	4
	Inappropriate words	3
	Incomprehensible sounds	2
	Nil	1
Eye opening	Spontaneous	E4
	To speech	3
	To pain	2
	Nil	1

NOTE: The coma scale score is the sum of the sectional scores.

function. Comatose patients who require emergency surgery (abdominal, thoracic, orthopaedic, etc.) should also have ICP monitoring, since frequent neurologic examinations are not possible during general anesthesia. Ventriculostomy to measure ICP also allows drainage of CSF, which can lower the pressure significantly. When the ventricular system is collapsed and ventriculostomy not feasible, intraparenchymal monitoring should be established.

Head elevation in the neutral position facilitates venous drainage; sedation reduces posturing and combative activity, both of which elevate ICP; hyperventilation to keep Pa_{CO_2} around 35 mmHg lowers cerebral blood volume and ICP; prophylactic use of anticonvulsants prevents cerebral injury from seizures; mild dehydration with judicious sodium replacement and prompt treatment of SIADH (syndrome of inappropriate antidiuretic hormone secretion) protects the brain from insult secondary to fluid overload; prevention of hypotension reduces the extension of ischemic injury, and aggressive treatment of hypertensive episodes reduces cerebral blood volume and further disruption of the blood-brain barrier; and treatment of hyperthermia avoids an increase in the brain's metabolic demands. All of these management principles may be required simultaneously to achieve optimal homeostasis of the brain.

If ICP remains elevated despite these measures, mannitol (0.5 to 1.0 g/kg I.V.) and furosemide (1.0 mg/kg) can be used to reduce cerebral edema. Deep sedation with narcotics and the use of paralytic agents such as pancuronium may be helpful. Barbiturate coma, once popular in otherwise medically refractory ICP elevation, does not significantly change ultimate outcome and thus is seldom used. Corticosteroids, while occasionally used, have no proved benefit for severe brain injury.

Outcome after head injury depends on many factors. Increasing age and preexisting illness contribute to a poor prognosis. Penetrating injuries, particularly gunshot wounds, are associated with poorer outcome compared with blunt trauma. The presence of an intracranial hemorrhage also implies a suboptimal result. Subdural hematoma has a poorer prognosis than epidural hematoma. Combined subdural and intracerebral hemorrhage has the worst prognosis of all severe head injury subtypes. Other important factors that influence outcome include delay in treatment, multiple trauma, and systemic insults such as acidosis, hypoxia, and hypotension. Predictors of poor prognosis include evidence of brainstem dysfunction on the initial examination and refractory intracranial hypertension within the first few days of injury.

Diffuse Axonal Injury

Diffuse white matter injury is associated with anatomic disruption of axons throughout both cerebral hemispheres. This primary shearing injury is associated with high mortality and substantial neurologic morbidity. It results from rotational forces that are perpendicular to the axis of the white matter, causing axonal transection. Despite severe shearing injury, the brain may appear grossly normal, but numerous axonal transections are seen microscopically in white matter within 2 weeks of injury. Classically, small hemorrhages are present in the corpus callosum and cerebral peduncles on CT scan. Fiber tract demyelinization subsequently develops, extending throughout the cerebral hemispheres and into the brainstem.

Epidural Hematoma

Hemorrhage between the inner table of the skull and the dura mater most commonly arises from a tear of the middle meningeal artery or one of its branches. Arterial bleeding strips the dura from the undersurface of the bone and produces a hematoma, which may increase in size and compress the underlying brain.

An epidural hematoma can also arise from torn venous channels in the bone at a point of fracture or from lacerated major dural venous sinuses. Since venous pressure is low, venous epidural hematomas usually form only when a depressed skull fracture has stripped the dura from the bone and left a space where the hematoma can develop.

Epidural hematoma classically follows a blow to the head that fractures the skull and causes a brief period of unconsciousness. After the patient regains consciousness, there may be a "lucid interval" during which there are minimal symptoms or signs. When the hematoma enlarges, hemispheric compression occurs. With time, the medial portion of the temporal lobe is forced over the edge of the tentorium, causing compression of the oculomotor nerve and dilation of the ipsilateral pupil. Similarly, compression of the ipsilateral cerebral peduncle causes contralateral hemiparesis, which may progress to decerebrate posturing. Coma, fixed and dilated pupil(s), and decerebration are a classic triad indicating *transtentorial herniation.*

Even though epidural hematomas are curable lesions, the mortality rate remains high because the severity of injury is often not recognized early. A patient may be seen during the "lucid interval" and discharged. Later, the patient may become unconscious because of progressive brain compression by the expanding hematoma.

Because of the danger of misdiagnosis, any patient with a history of a blow to the head leading to a period of unconsciousness should have a CT scan (Fig. 40-1). If an epidural hematoma is found, urgent craniotomy is indicated. If the CT scan is normal and the patient's examination shows no neurologic deficit, the patient may be discharged. An accompanying person should be instructed to awaken the patient frequently over the next 24 h to be certain that he or she remains arousable. Any deterioration in consciousness should prompt reevaluation.

Subdural Hematoma

Subdural hematomas may develop when veins bridging the cortex and the dura or venous sinuses are torn or when an intracerebral hematoma extends into the subdural space. They can be large even though the bleeding is of venous (low-pressure) origin.

Acute subdural hematomas are associated with severe head injury and arise from a combination of torn bridging veins, disruption of cortical vessels, and laceration of the cortex. The hematoma is best seen with CT scanning. Evacuation of the clot may lead to significant improvement, but often a major neurologic deficit remains because of the accompanying widespread parenchymal injury.

Subacute subdural hematomas become apparent several days after injury and are associated with progressive lethargy, confusion, hemiparesis, or other hemispheric deficits. Removal of the hematoma usually produces striking improvement.

Chronic subdural hematomas arise from tears in bridging veins, often after a minor head injury. Initially, the hematoma is small. Later, it becomes encased in a fibrous membrane, lique-

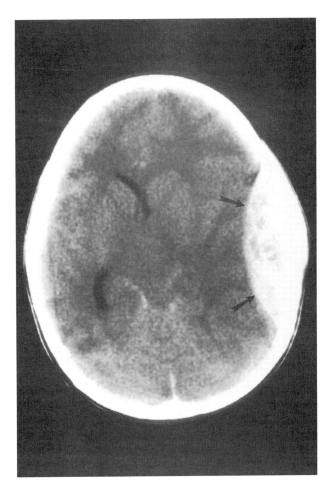

FIG. 40-1. CT brain scan without contrast enhancement. The epidural hematoma (arrows) has compressed the brain, causing a midline shift.

accounts for radiculopathy, characterized by motor and sensory impairment in the corresponding myotome and dermatome (Fig. 40-2). Spinal cord involvement produces myelopathy with variable manifestations.

A complete lesion, clinically defined as total loss of motor and sensory function below the level of injury, is associated with anatomic or physiologic transection of the cord. Acute transections are characterized by areflexia, flaccidity, anesthesia, and autonomic paralysis below the level of the lesion. Arterial hypotension is invariably present when the transection is above T5 because of the loss of sympathetic vascular tone. Common spinal cord syndromes are shown in Fig. 40-3.

Incomplete lesions of the cord may result in the Brown-Séquard syndrome, manifested by ipsilateral loss of motor function and position/vibratory sensation with contralateral loss of pain and temperature sensation below the level of injury. Anatomically, this presentation is explained by hemisection of the cord. The central cord syndrome is characterized by bilateral loss of motor function and pain and temperature sensation in the upper extremities, with relative preservation of these functions in the lower extremities. Typically, the distal upper extremities are more severely affected because the most medial portions of the corticospinal and spinothalamic tracts subserve these areas. The central cord syndrome is often seen following a hyperextension injury of the cervical spine, with or without fracture. The anterior spinal artery syndrome involves bilateral loss of motor function and pain and temperature sensation below the level of the lesion, with sparing of position, vibratory, and light touch sensation. This incomplete lesion develops when the anterior spinal artery is injured, rendering the cord ischemic within the distribution of the anterior spinal artery, affecting the anterior and lateral columns bilaterally. A common cause of anterior spinal artery syndrome is an acutely ruptured cervical disc.

fies, then gradually enlarges. These lesions are more common in infants and the elderly. Typical presentation includes progressive mental status changes, with or without focal signs (hemiparesis, aphasia, etc.). Papilledema may be present. The diagnosis is confirmed by CT scanning. Treatment consists of hematoma drainage by trephination. Craniotomy may be necessary if the fluid reaccumulates.

Spinal Cord Injury

Traumatic injury of the spinal cord may result from vertebral fracture, fracture/subluxation, hyperextension of the cervical spine in the presence of a narrow spinal canal, herniation of intervertebral disc material into the canal, and penetrating injuries such as gunshots or stabbings. Neurologic involvement ranges from mild and transient to severe and permanent. Spinal fracture and cord injury should be suspected in head-injured patients, with or without coma, and in those patients with multiple injuries. It is best to assume that the spine is unstable initially and immobilize the patient on a backboard with a hard cervical collar until careful examination and diagnostic testing are done.

Clinical findings of spinal or spinal cord injury include spinal tenderness, extremity weakness, numbness or paresthesia, respiratory embarrassment, and hypotension. Spinal root involvement

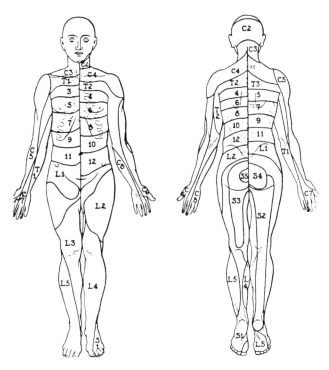

FIG. 40-2. Diagram of sensory nerve root distribution.

SPINAL CORD SYNDROMES

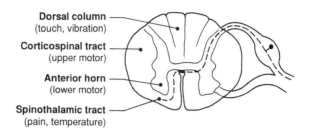

Dorsal column
(touch, vibration)

Corticospinal tract
(upper motor)

Anterior horn
(lower motor)

Spinothalamic tract
(pain, temperature)

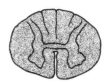

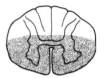

FIG. 40-3. Diagram of spinal cord anatomy and common clinical syndromes that accompany spinal cord lesions.

Trauma to the lumbar spine may produce signs and symptoms of cauda equina compression. Presentation consists of multiple lumbosacral radiculopathies of variable severity. Lower extremity motor, sensory, and reflex functions may be affected, producing variable degrees of weakness, sensory loss (all modalities in the specific distribution of the roots involved), and diminution or absence of reflexes. Bladder distention from detrusor muscle paralysis, flaccidity of the anal sphincter, and loss of perineal sensation are common in severe injuries.

In addition to the neurologic deficit, acute spinal cord injury is accompanied by a variety of systemic responses. If the spinal cord is damaged above C3, respiratory efforts cease, accounting for this injury's high mortality at the scene of the accident. Although spontaneous ventilatory efforts can be initiated with injuries involving C4–C6, tidal volumes are often insufficient, accounting for progressive hypoxia and carbon dioxide retention. Airway obstruction, atelectasis, and pneumonia are common complications. Assisted ventilation is often required early after injury.

Ileus with gastric distention is common, necessitating nasogastric drainage. Similarly, bladder distention occurs because the bladder and pelvic floor muscles are flaccid. Bladder drainage will prevent overdistention, which may be severe enough to cause compression of the inferior vena cava and pelvic veins, impairing venous return to the heart and contributing to systemic hypotension.

Blood pressure is usually low if the cord injury is above the T5 level. This effectively denervates the sympathetic nervous system, which leads to increased venous capacitance and decreased venous return. The resulting hypotension is controlled by the administration of intravenous fluids. Colloid is preferred to reduce the threat of vascular overload and iatrogenic pulmonary edema. Postural changes that will precipitously drop the blood pressure, such as upper body elevation, should also be avoided.

Tachycardia is a common compensatory response to hypotension, but bradycardia is the rule when the cervical cord is damaged and the sympathetic input to the heart is lost. This type of bradycardia does not require treatment unless the patient is

symptomatic or at risk for myocardial infarction or stroke because of age or other debilitating illness. If necessary, treatment with atropine and fluids is effective.

Once the patient is hemodynamically stable, spinal radiographs are essential, but only while the patient remains immobilized on a backboard in a hard cervical collar. Standard views are obtained, ensuring good visualization of the cervicothoracic junction (Fig. 40-4). Comatose and/or severely injured patients with multiple trauma should have good plain-film imaging of the complete spine. Fractured areas can be studied further with CT, using both axial and sagittal views (Fig. 40-5). If no abnormality is found by plain films or CT and a neurologic deficit exists indicating a spinal cord level, MRI or myelography followed by CT should be utilized to identify other causes of cord compromise, such as traumatic intervertebral disc rupture or spinal epidural hematoma.

Treatment. The objectives of treatment are to correct spinal alignment, protect undamaged neural tissue, restore function to reversibly damaged neural tissue, and achieve permanent spinal stability. Reduction and immobilization of any fracture/dislocation must receive top priority to meet these objectives.

Cervical spine malalignment can almost always be reduced by skeletal traction in the neutral position. Traction may be applied using skull tongs or a halo apparatus. Both are seated percutaneously through the outer table of the skull while the patient is kept supine and immobilized. The patient is then transferred to a special bed and traction begun. Frequent lateral view radiographs are obtained to document reduction and prevent overdistraction, which can lead to further cord injury. Once the spinal injury is reduced, traction should be maintained. Frequent follow-up films are then taken to confirm correct alignment.

Sometimes a cervical fracture cannot be reduced by traction alone without jeopardizing spinal cord function. Open reduction, usually through a posterior approach, combined with a fusion procedure may be necessary in those instances. This especially pertains to unilaterally or bilaterally locked facets.

Patients with thoracic and lumbar spine fractures are also treated with immobilization initially. Immobilization is less strict

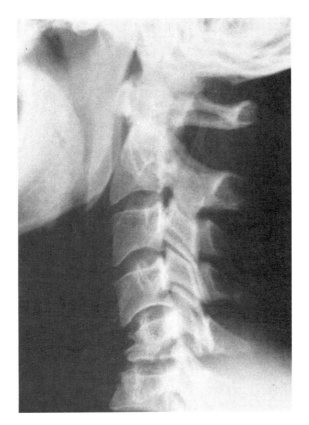

FIG. 40-4. *Cervical spine radiograph, lateral view. The compression fracture at C5 occurred from hyperflexion of the neck.*

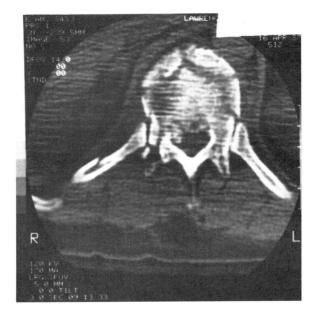

FIG. 40-5. *CT of a compression of the T12 vertebra demonstrating posterior displacement of bone fragments into the right side of the canal resulting in paraplegia. Note the excellent resolution of the fractures in the right pedicle, facet, rib, and multiple fragments of the body.*

compared with that for cervical fractures, but the principles are the same. Patients are kept flat in bed without traction while flexion, extension, lateral bending, and rotational movements are avoided. They typically have fewer systemic complications associated with their neurologic injury but nevertheless require vigilance to prevent neurologic deterioration and provide the best chance for neurologic recovery.

Indications for early operation in patients with spinal cord injury include inability to reduce the fracture/dislocation satisfactorily by closed methods, neurologic deterioration in a patient with an incomplete cord lesion initially, severe compression of the spinal cord by an intraspinal mass shown by myelography or MRI, and a penetrating injury with or without a CSF leak. Open wounds, such as those inflicted by stabbings or gunshots, should be debrided and closed whether the cord injury is complete or incomplete. Early operation to stabilize the spine is warranted because this translates into early mobilization and rehabilitation. Either the anterior or the posterior approach may be used, depending on the nature of the spinal injury and the degree of instability.

If closed reduction is successful and the fracture is stable, external immobilization is necessary for a minimum of 3 months to ensure proper healing. If surgical reduction and/or fixation is necessary, external immobilization is still indicated. For the cervical spine, this involves a halo vest. Certain exceptions include anterior and posterior metal plating procedures in which a hard cervical collar may suffice (Fig. 40-6). The thoracic and lumbar spine usually require a plastic body jacket or plaster cast for a minimum, once again, of 3 months. Plain films are used to follow spinal alignment and the extent of fusion during the recovery period.

If any cord function is preserved immediately after injury, additional function usually returns, provided the cord and spine are protected from secondary injury. Patients with complete injuries rarely recover function below the level of the lesion. Rehabilitation for them is directed toward self-care and vocational readjustment. Most persons with these handicaps can eventually achieve independence. Life expectancy is shortened slightly in paraplegics and significantly in quadriplegics. Long-term problems associated with skin care and recurrent urinary tract infections account for the early mortality rate.

Peripheral Nerve Injury

Peripheral nerve injuries may be categorized functionally. *Neurapraxia* is a temporary loss of function without axonal injury. Structural damage does not occur. The foot that "goes to sleep" after crossing the legs is an example of functional loss without pathologic change. *Axonotmesis* is disruption of the axon with preservation of the axon sheath. Wallerian degeneration of the distal axon fragment occurs. Stretch or prolonged compression causes this functional and structural loss. Regeneration of the proximal axon occurs, but functional recovery depends on associated injuries, the amount of healthy proximal axon remaining after injury, and the age of the patient. *Neurotmesis* is disruption of both the axon and axon sheath with corresponding loss of function. Transection of a nerve causes this phenomenon. Regeneration occurs, but function rarely returns to normal.

Clinically, sensory and motor changes correspond to the peripheral nerve involved. A detailed history and a precise neurologic examination can localize the site of injury with great accuracy. Sensory findings are usually apparent early and remain

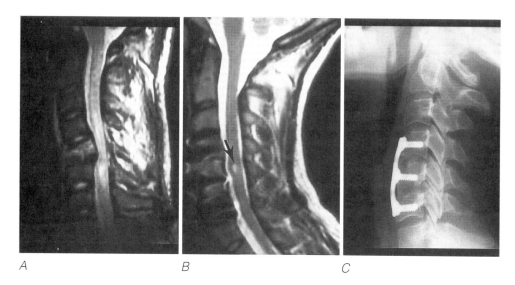

FIG. 40-6. Cervical spine MRI, sagittal view. *A.* Compression fracture of C5 with cord compression. *B.* Decompression of cord by halo traction. *Arrow* shows cord contusion, T_2-weighted image. *C.* Postoperative scan shows C5 body replaced and plate/screw construct for immediate stability.

so until regeneration is nearly complete. Compensatory motor function, often seen in the hand months after injury, is rarely seen acutely. A crude but clinically helpful sign of sensory regeneration is Tinel's sign. Percussion of the skin overlying the length of the injured nerve elicits paresthesias at the site where regeneration is occurring.

Radiographs of the injury site are helpful to look for fracture or foreign body. Electromyography (EMG) is not useful within the first 3 weeks of injury, but this diagnostic aid becomes highly effective to follow the state of the degeneration/regeneration process occurring later. Management decisions are often made depending on EMG findings weeks to months after trauma.

Treatment. Treatment of a lacerated nerve consists of primary repair when the wound is clean and uncomplicated, as in stab wounds, lacerations from glass, and surgical incisions. Secondary or delayed repair is indicated when the wound is dirty or complicated, as in gunshot wounds and avulsions, which disrupt tissue severely, making primary repair less successful. Secondary repair is best accomplished a few weeks after injury, when tissue viability is obvious, the likelihood of infection is reduced, and dissection planes are distinct. If end-to-end anastomosis of nerves is not possible because of tissue loss, nerve grafting using autologous sural nerve may be done. Intraoperative factors such as axial orientation of fascicles, proper coaptation, suture material, hemostasis, and suture line tension determine the outcome.

Nerve injuries in continuity (i.e., resulting from contusion or compression without laceration) are often explored if they do not improve within 6 weeks of injury, whether loss of function is complete or incomplete. Intraneural and extraneural scar tissue at the site of the lesion may prevent axonal regrowth by its constricting effect. Neurolysis releases the regenerating nerve fibers from the impinging scar and may improve functional recovery.

Prompt institution of physical therapy is also indicated for improvement of muscle function and maintenance of joint motion. It is the best means of minimizing the complications of

denervation. The denervated portion of the limb is subject to muscle atrophy and fibrosis, joint stiffness, motor endplate atrophy, and trophic skin changes. The longer the denervation persists, the less likely will good function result.

Regeneration in a peripheral nerve occurs at 1 mm/day (roughly 1 inch per month), so improvement may not be obvious for many months. Factors that adversely affect the return of function include advanced age of the patient, proximal nerve injury, extensive nerve tissue loss, associated soft tissue injury, and presence of mixed sensorimotor function deficits. Unfortunately, incomplete neurologic recovery is often the rule. The use of tendon transfers should be considered to improve functional outcome if neurologic function is inadequate after recovery has ceased.

NEOPLASMS

Nervous system tumors represent almost 10 percent of all neoplasia. Of these, 15 to 20 percent occur in children. Nearly 70 percent of adult tumors are found above the tentorium (supratentorial), whereas 70 percent of childhood tumors are found below (infratentorial). CNS tumors are the most common solid tumors in children. Of all pediatric cancers, they are second in incidence only to leukemia.

The incidence of nervous system neoplasia decreases in the late teen years and begins to peak again by middle age. By then, only 25 percent of intracranial tumors are benign. This percentage, however, rises to 50 percent in the older patient because of the increasing incidence of meningiomas and schwannomas. Overall, there is a slightly greater incidence of tumors in men (55 percent), but schwannomas and meningiomas are more common in women. Of all CNS neoplasms, spinal tumors constitute approximately 15 to 20 percent.

Intracranial Tumors

Intracranial tumors exert both local and generalized effects by their presence within a closed bony structure, arising either from within or on the surface of the brain. Local effects of the tumor are either irritative or destructive. Focal seizures occur because of irritation of adjacent cortex, while a focal neurologic deficit develops because of compressive forces on nearby brain tissue. More generalized effects come from raised intracranial pressure due to the presence of the mass. These may be in the form of obstructive hydrocephalus, hemorrhage, cerebral edema, or simply the bulk of the neoplasm within the closed skull. The symptoms from generalized effects may be headache, occasional nausea and vomiting, decreased level of consciousness, and/or slowed cognitive function. Common tumors are listed in Table 40-2.

Astrocytoma. Astrocytes are glial (stromal or supporting) cells of the brain. Tumors arising from these cells make up over 60 percent of all intracranial tumors.

Low-grade astrocytomas (grades 1 and 2) constitute 5 to 10 percent of all intracranial tumors. When they involve the cerebral hemispheres, they typically arise during the fourth decade. They present with a 1- to 2-year history of illness, producing signs and symptoms such as headache, seizures, vomiting, mental status changes, papilledema, and focal neurologic deficits relevant to the hemisphere involved. On CT scan they appear as low-attenuation lesions with minimal contrast enhancement. These tumors are infiltrative and can rarely be totally excised. Surgery, however, is generally performed for diagnosis and debulking, usually followed by radiation therapy. Five-year survival rate with surgery and subsequent radiation is 35 to 50 percent. Some low-grade astrocytomas may become anaplastic and convert into higher grades of malignancy.

Low-grade astrocytomas of the cerebellum typically develop in children. They are often cystic with hamartomatous features, characteristics that carry a favorable prognosis. These tumors are often totally resectable. Radiation therapy is usually reserved for patients with incomplete resections, and follow-up has demonstrated continued tumor growth. The 10-year survival rate is over 80 percent for this common tumor of childhood.

Brainstem gliomas are also posterior fossa tumors that occur most often in children. The majority are benign astrocytomas. Patients may present with cranial nerve palsies, hemiparesis, and headache, often attributable to hydrocephalus. These tumors usually cannot be removed because of the risk of neurologic injury to the brainstem. They are treated with radiation therapy once a diagnosis is established through either an open or closed biopsy procedure. Prognosis is a function of their location, with 5-year survival rates of 15 to 30 percent.

Optic nerve gliomas are astrocytomas involving the optic pathways anterior to the optic tracts. They occur in the chiasm in 75 percent of cases. Two-thirds of chiasmal tumors also invade the hypothalamus. The peak age for occurrence is 3 to 7 years, but their growth pattern is extremely variable. Some remain stable for years while others are relentlessly progressive. Those occurring strictly within one optic nerve can be excised, but more extensive tumors are generally irradiated. The value of radiation therapy, however, remains controversial.

High-grade astrocytomas (grades 3 and 4) are the most common primary intracranial tumor, constituting 20 to 30 percent of all intracranial tumors and half of all gliomas. Age at discovery ranges from 45 to 65 years. The frontal and temporal regions are most commonly involved. Due to their infiltrative nature, many of these high-grade neoplasms involve both cerebral hemi-

Table 40-2
Brain Tumors

	Percent
Gliomas	40–50
Astrocytoma, grade 1	5–10
Astrocytoma, grade 2	2–5
Astrocytoma, grades 3 and 4 (glioblastoma multiforme)	20–30
Medulloblastoma	3–5
Oligodendroglioma	1–4
Ependymoma, grades 1–4	1–3
Meningioma	12–20
Pituitary tumors	5–15
Neurilemomas (mainly VIIIth nerve)	3–10
Metastatic tumors	5–10
Blood vessel tumors	
Arteriovenous malformations	
Hemangioblastomas	
Endotheliomas	0.5–1
Tumors of developmental defects	2–3
Dermoids, epidermoids, teratomas	
Chordomas, paraphyseal cysts	
Craniopharyngiomas	3–8
Pinealomas	0.5–0.8
Miscellaneous	
Sarcomas, papillomas of the choroid plexus, lipomas, lymphoma, unclassified, etc.	1–3

spheres by invading through the corpus callosum (Fig. 40-7). Histologically these malignant lesions are composed of sheets of anaplastic cells with bizarre nuclei, numerous mitoses, endothelial proliferation, and abundant necrosis.

Patients with malignant gliomas present with a relatively short history of headache, focal neurologic deficit, mental status changes, or seizures. These tumors are readily imaged by CT and MRI, appearing as low-attenuation lesions with marked peritumoral edema and mass effect (Fig. 40-8). Ninety percent show enhancement with intravenous contrast. In spite of aggressive surgery, radiation therapy, and chemotherapy, these tumors are

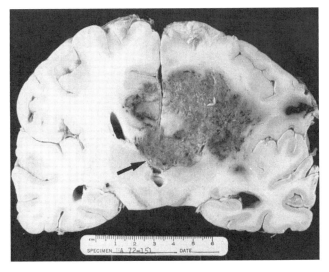

FIG. 40-7. *Postmortem specimen, coronal section. The glioblastoma multiforme is infiltrating, with indistinct margins. It crosses the midline through the corpus callosum (arrow).*

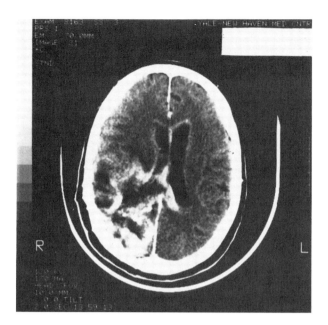

FIG. 40-8. *CT of the brain in a patient with a right hemisphere glioblastoma. Contrast enhancement outlines a central low-density area of necrosis. Tumor extension is clearly demonstrated throughout the parietal and occipital lobes and across the midline to the left occipital lobe.*

subsequent radiation. Still in the early stages of development, immunotoxins toward tumor cells employ antibodies to tumor antigens, thus utilizing the host immune system as a means of destroying the cancerous tissue.

Meningioma. Meningiomas are relatively benign tumors that arise from the arachnoid layer of the meninges, usually occurring in the fourth through sixth decades of life. They affect women more often (65 percent) and arise in a variety of locations. The relative frequency of these locations include parasagittal 29 percent, sphenoid ridge 18 percent, convexity 13 percent, posterior fossa 10 percent, tuberculum sellae 9 percent, olfactory groove 5 percent, middle fossa 4 percent, foramen magnum 2 percent, and 1 percent or less occur in the orbit, gasserian ganglion, tentorium, or ventricular system. Altogether, meningiomas account for about 15 percent of all intracranial tumors.

Parasagittal (falcine) and convexity (hemispheric surface) meningiomas tend to present with seizures, focal neurologic deficits, and signs of intracranial hypertension. Sphenoid wing tumors often present with proptosis, decreased visual acuity, cranial nerve (IIId, IVth, Vth, VIth) palsies, seizures, or the more generalized effects of increased intracranial pressure (Fig. 40-9). Posterior fossa tumors present with cerebellar signs, hydrocephalus, lower cranial nerve palsies, or long tract signs (Fig. 40-10*A, B*). Tuberculum sellae tumors are often accompanied by decreasing vision. Olfactory groove meningiomas may present with the classic Foster Kennedy syndrome of ipsilateral optic nerve atrophy and central scotoma with contralateral papilledema and bilateral loss of smell. Foramen magnum tumors may be difficult to recognize early and are often diagnosed as multiple sclerosis, syringomyelia, or cervical spondylosis. Patients complain of neck pain, clumsiness, and sensory disturbances in the upper extremities as well as gait difficulties.

Either CT or MRI is the principal means of diagnosis. Homogeneous pathologic contrast enhancement is characteristic of these neoplasms. Plain-film skull x-rays show abnormalities in

uniformly fatal. Although younger patients tend to do better, the average survival with surgical plus adjuvant therapy is about 12 months.

Chemotherapy is often used when tumor recurs, when the brain can no longer be irradiated, or when the tumor is not radiosensitive. It can be delivered intravenously, intraarterially, and/or intrathecally. Most drugs are directed at the tumor cells while others indirectly attack the cells by sensitizing them to

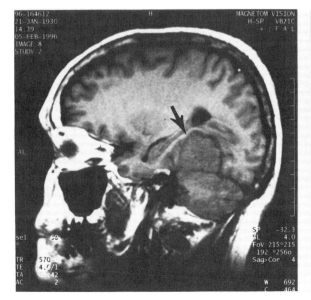
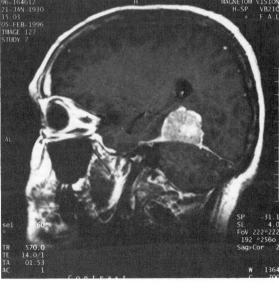

FIG. 40-9. *MRI scan, sagittal view. A. Tentorial meningioma without contrast enhancement (arrow). B. Gadolinium-enhanced lesion.*

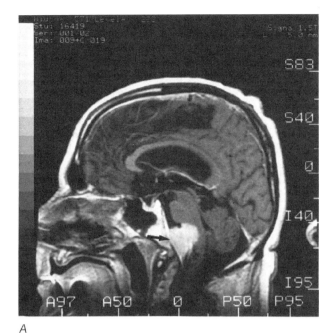

A

B

FIG. 40-10. MRI scan with gadolinium enhancement. *A.* Sagittal view. The posterior fossa meningioma is attached to the skull base (*arrow*). *B.* Coronal view. Note the distortion of the brainstem by the tumor (*arrow*).

50 to 75 percent of patients with meningiomas, showing either tumor calcification, hyperostosis, increased vascular channels, or bone erosion. Angiography classically shows a "blush" in the late arterial phase.

The treatment for meningiomas is surgical. The techniques and goals are individualized for each specific tumor location, taking into account the patient's age and symptoms. In general,

the goal is total excision, including the dura at the site of the tumor's attachment. If the meningeal origin cannot be excised, it is usually cauterized generously. Some meningiomas, such as those along the sphenoid ridge, may be "en plaque" tumors, which are flat and tend to spread along the inner table of the skull. This unique feature often precludes total resection.

The recurrence rate of meningiomas after surgery depends on the completeness of excision initially and the presence of malignant histologic features. If the tumor is totally removed, including its dural attachment, the recurrence rate is about 10 percent. If the dural attachment can only be cauterized, the recurrence rate is 20 percent. With subtotal resection, the recurrence rate is approximately 40 percent. Nonmalignant and malignant meningiomas have 15-year survival rates of 68 and 34 percent, respectively. Radiation therapy is generally reserved for malignant meningiomas, although it has also been used for incompletely removed nonmalignant meningiomas. Highly focused radiation therapy coupled with stereotactic guidance to the tumor site, referred to as radiosurgery, is now available. The single treatment, delivered in a few minutes, is an outpatient procedure. The efficacy of this form of therapy remains debatable, but it is believed to provide prolonged survival.

Medulloblastoma. Medulloblastomas are part of the primitive neuroectodermal class of brain tumors. They are thought to arise from primitive cells of the cerebellum, most likely the external granular layer. They constitute 5 percent of all gliomas and one-third of all fourth ventricular region tumors. Two-thirds of medulloblastomas occur in children, with an average age of onset of fourteen years. In children, these are more likely to occur in the midline, usually within the fourth ventricle, whereas adult tumors are frequently positioned more laterally. They commonly metastasize throughout the subarachnoid space via the CSF and can be found outside the central nervous system.

Children with medulloblastomas commonly present with elevated ICP secondary to hydrocephalus. Cerebellar signs may be prominent, with truncal ataxia and nystagmus. Some patients may present initially with symptoms related to spinal metastases. The diagnosis is generally made by identifying an enhancing mass on CT or MRI. MRI provides better images of this common posterior fossa tumor. Cytologic examination of the CSF is often positive for neoplastic cells.

Treatment involves aggressive surgical removal of tumor, followed by irradiation of the brain. If CSF cytology or spinal myelography or MRI is positive, the spinal axis is included in the radiated field. Chemotherapy is commonly used as well. The 5-year survival rate depends on the extent of tumor resection and the efficacy of radiation therapy. Some centers now report 5-year tumor-free rates of 75 percent in patients who have had gross total tumor resections, radiation therapy, and chemotherapy.

Schwannoma. This benign tumor arises from the Schwann cells that surround axons as they leave the central nervous system via cranial nerves. Schwannomas constitute 8 percent of all intracranial tumors and are almost twice as common in females as males. They occur usually in midlife. If associated with von Recklinghausen's neurofibromatosis, they may be multiple.

Schwannomas usually occur on sensory cranial nerves. The vestibular portion of the acoustic nerve (i.e., acoustic neuroma) is by far the most common site (Fig. 40-11). Depending on their size, these tumors usually produce hearing loss. As they enlarge,

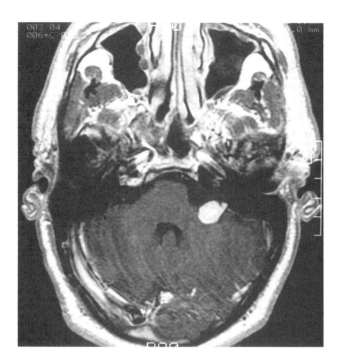

FIG. 40-11. MRI scan with gadolinium enhancement, axial view. The acoustic neuroma is intracranial, with a small portion projecting into the internal auditory canal.

they may create facial numbness by compression of the trigeminal nerve and loss of coordination by compression of the adjacent cerebellar hemisphere. Only very late in their course do they cause facial weakness. Symptoms of increased intracranial pressure due to obstructive hydrocephalus may also present late.

Much less commonly, schwannomas arise from the trigeminal nerve, presenting as a mass in the middle fossa, associated with facial numbness. Some patients complain of lancinating, burning, episodic pain similar to trigeminal neuralgia. Only rarely do other cranial nerves serve as the primary site of origin for schwannomas. These less common sites would be more apt to be involved in cases of neurofibromatosis. Schwannomas occurring in patients with neurofibromatosis are often associated with other intracranial tumors such as meningiomas, astrocytomas, and ependymomas.

The treatment of schwannomas is surgical, with total resection being curative. Microsurgical techniques have reduced the risks of surgery and allowed preservation of cranial nerve function. Acoustic neuromas may be resected via the suboccipital or translabyrinthine approach, with a 95 percent probability of preservation of facial nerve function with small tumors. Even with the largest tumors, preservation is predictable in 50 to 70 percent of cases. The translabyrinthine approach is reserved for those patients who have complete hearing loss due to the presence of the mass. If this loss is incomplete, the suboccipital approach is preferred, allowing for hearing preservation by leaving the middle and inner ear structures intact. Preservation of hearing is directly related to tumor size. Mortality rate for acoustic tumor surgery is a function of tumor size as well, with most deaths occurring in patients with very large tumors.

Ependymoma. These tumors originate from the ependyma, which is formed by cells that line the ventricular system. They constitute 3 percent of all gliomas. Their incidence peaks at the age of 5 years and again at 34 years. They arise below the tentorium, usually within the fourth ventricle, in two-thirds of cases. When they occur above the tentorium, 50 percent are intraventricular. Infratentorial ependymomas are far more common in children.

The presenting symptoms are related to the tumor location. Typically, children harboring fourth ventricular tumors present with headache and vomiting related to associated obstructive hydrocephalus. They also tend to have ataxia secondary to cerebellar compression. Patients with supratentorial tumors present with signs of raised intracranial pressure as well, but this is usually due to brain edema. Focal neurologic deficits are common. These tumors are usually well circumscribed on CT scans as enhancing masses. MRI is the study of choice when the tumor involves the posterior fossa, since it far surpasses the imaging capabilities of CT in this region.

Treatment involves aggressive surgical excision first. Fourth ventricular tumors, however, can rarely be totally removed because they invade the fourth ventricular floor. They are quite radiosensitive, so radiotherapy can prolong survival. The 5-year survival rate with surgery and irradiation for both children and adults is about 50 percent. Chemotherapy is reserved for malignant ependymomas. All ependymomas have a propensity to recur despite aggressive management.

Oligodendroglioma. Tumors arising from oligodendroglial cells (the supporting cells that make myelin in the CNS) make up 4 percent of gliomas and usually occur in the cerebral hemispheres. Half of all hemispheric lesions occur in the frontal lobes. Up to one-third are mixed tumors containing populations of astrocytes in addition to oligodendrocytes. They are considered slow-growing tumors with benign histologic features, but as many as 25 percent may show some degree of anaplasia.

Patients present with a history measured in years; 80 percent have a history of seizures. Patients commonly have focal neurologic deficits and papilledema. These tumors are unique in their tendency to calcify, attesting to their indolent nature. On CT scan, a high percentage show calcification and most have contrast enhancement.

Treatment is maximum surgical resection. Radiation therapy is reserved for those tumors displaying malignant histologic features or for cases of subtotal excision. The 5-year survival rate is 50 to 80 percent. There are well-documented long-term survivors, however, with a reported 20-year survival rate of 10 percent.

Germinoma. These tumors occur most commonly in the region of the pineal gland and have thus been misnamed "pinealomas" in the past. The suprasellar region involving the hypothalamus is the second most common location. They are much more common in males and tend to occur in the second and third decades. They are composed of two cell populations, tumor cells and lymphocytes, and are histologically indistinguishable from testicular seminomas and ovarian dysgerminomas.

Germinomas in the pineal region tend to produce obstructive hydrocephalus and Parinaud's syndrome, characterized by upward gaze paresis, loss of convergence, and small, unreactive pupils. Those in the hypothalamic region may result in diabetes insipidus and emaciation (diencephalic syndrome). Germinomas are extremely radiosensitive and do not require aggressive surgical resection, but biopsy analysis is recommended prior to irradiation. The 5-year survival rate approaches 75 percent after radiation therapy.

Other, related germ cell tumors include teratomas, embryonal cell tumors, endodermal sinus tumors, and choriocarcinomas. These tend to arise in the same locations as germinomas. The germ cell tumors often produce compounds that serve as tumor markers. These markers are identified with immunoassays of the CSF or with immunoperoxidase stains of the tissue under light microscopy. All choriocarcinomas and 10 percent of germinomas secrete beta-human chorionic gonadotropin (beta-HCG). Endodermal sinus tumors produce alpha-fetoprotein (AFP). Embryonal cell tumors typically synthesize both beta-HCG and AFP. Teratomas secrete neither. These markers are useful for confirming the diagnoses and for measuring responses to treatment.

Epidermoid, Dermoid, and Teratoma. Epidermoids and dermoids arise from benign inclusions of epithelial elements within the central nervous system during closure of the embryonic neural groove. Epidermoids contain only stratified squamous epithelium. Dermoids contain skin appendages such as hair follicles, sebaceous glands, and sweat glands in addition to the squamous epithelium. Epidermoids tend to arise off the midline in such locations as the cerebellopontine angle, parasellar region, and in the diploë of the skull. Dermoids, in contrast, usually arise in midline structures such as the cerebellar vermis or the fourth ventricle. They are often accompanied by overlying bone and skin defects. Both tumor types are easily identified on CT and MRI scans. Surgical removal is the preferred treatment. Recurrences are usually managed with further surgery.

Teratomas are more common in children. By definition, they are composed of tumor cells representing all three embryonic germ cell layers. The more differentiated teratomas often contain cartilage and bone. If these elements are primitive, they are considered malignant. Like dermoids, they tend to occur in the midline in such locations as the pineal region, third ventricle, and posterior fossa. Treatment is surgical excision, along with irradiation in certain malignant types.

Hemangioblastoma. These benign tumors are quite vascular and usually occur in the cerebellum. They are uncommon and constitute only 1 percent of intracranial tumors. Typical presentation is in the fourth decade. Fifteen percent of patients have von Hippel-Lindau disease, an autosomal dominant disorder consisting of central nervous system hemangioblastomas, retinal angiomatosis, renal and pancreatic cysts, and renal cell carcinoma. Irrespective of this syndrome, many patients with hemangioblastoma have polycythemia. Sizable neoplastic cysts are present in 60 percent of cases, often with only a small mural nodule of tumor. Total surgical removal is curative. Radiation therapy is used when resection is not possible. Reoperation is recommended for recurrences. The long-term survival is excellent, with up to 80 percent of patients alive at 10 years.

Metastatic Tumor. Twenty-five percent of all intracranial tumors are metastatic. Malignant cells invade the central nervous system hematogenously and tend to lodge at the gray and white matter junction. Metastatic tumors occur singly or multiply and may involve virtually any portion of the brain or, less commonly, spinal cord. Although any malignancy has the potential to metastasize, the most common primary sites are lung, breast, kidney, testis, colon, and skin. The presenting symptoms are determined by the site(s) of the metastases. In general, these commonly include headache, mental status changes, seizures, and hemiparesis.

Metastatic lesions are best imaged with high-resolution MRI, but they may be mimicked by other lesions such as meningiomas, abscesses, primary brain tumors, and even aneurysms. If a metastasis is suspected, a workup to find the primary source is recommended. If the primary site is not identified, an excisional biopsy is indicated to establish the diagnosis.

In general, a symptomatic, solitary lesion that is surgically accessible should be removed. Surgery, however, should not be undertaken for multiple lesions or in patients who are severely afflicted by their primary disease. Treatment should also include preoperative dexamethasone, as in any brain or spinal cord tumor, to reduce adjacent brain edema. Whole brain irradiation is almost always indicated. Prognosis depends on tumor type, with the median survival ranging from 1 to 2 years. Long-term survivors have been reported with surgical removal of solitary brain metastases. Quality of life is almost always improved. There is little evidence that chemotherapy plays a significant treatment role.

Tumor metastasis to the leptomeninges (meningeal carcinomatosis) is also quite common, particularly in the childhood leukemias and in adults with lymphoma, breast and lung cancers, and melanoma. Patients may present with cranial nerve palsies, radiculopathies, or obstructive hydrocephalus. They often have signs and symptoms suggestive of meningitis. Analysis of the CSF is usually critical, often revealing an increased opening pressure, an elevated white cell count and protein level, and a decreased glucose level. There may or may not be identifiable malignant cells, but cytologic examination should always be done.

Treatment of meningeal carcinomatosis usually involves radiation therapy and intraventricular chemotherapy. Methotrexate is a common chemotherapeutic agent. The outlook for patients with leptomeningeal tumor spread is generally poor, but again a few long-term survivors emerge.

Spinal Tumors

Spinal tumors constitute approximately 20 percent of all CNS tumors. They are classified as intradural or extradural. Of the intradural variety, 84 percent are outside the spinal cord (extramedullary) and 16 percent are within it (intramedullary). Intradural tumors are almost always primary CNS tumors, whereas the majority of extradural tumors are either metastatic or primary bone tumors. The majority of intradural spinal neoplasms are benign and can often be excised surgically. Tumors occurring within the cord (intradural, intramedullary) tend to produce weakness, spasticity, and sensory loss. Extramedullary lesions present with radicular pain from nerve root (lower motor neuron) compression as well as with long tract (upper motor neuron) signs from cord compression. Patients with lesions involving the conus medullaris region may have early loss of bladder and bowel function; those with lesions in the cauda equina present primarily with leg pain and only later develop sphincter disturbances.

The definitive study for spinal tumors is MRI, although abnormalities on plain films and myelograms may be diagnostic. Plain films may show widening of the interpeduncular distance, bony erosion, enlargement of neural foramina, or a paraspinous mass. Myelography helps to determine the tumor's relationship to the spinal cord and dura. Postmyelogram CT can further define that relationship.

Neurilemoma and Neurofibroma. Typically benign, these are the most common spinal cord tumors, comprising almost 30 percent of the total. They are usually intradural, extramedullary in location. Of these, 13 percent have extradural extension through an adjacent foramen, producing the classic "dumbbell" shape of the tumor. Fourteen percent are totally extradural. The extradural component tends to enlarge the involved foramen. Treatment is surgical removal. Multiple neurofibromas are associated with von Recklinghausen's neurofibromatosis. In these instances, only symptomatic tumors should be removed.

Meningioma. Meningiomas constitute 26 percent of spinal cord tumors, are benign, and are usually intradural, extramedullary (Fig. 40-12). Fifteen percent occur extradurally. Two-thirds arise in the thoracic spine, affecting women in their fourth through sixth decades in 80 percent of cases. Surgical excision is the treatment of choice.

Ependymoma. Arising from the ependymal cells of the central canal of the cord, these intramedullary tumors constitute 13 percent of all spinal cord tumors. They occur more frequently in males. Nearly 60 percent are found in the conus medullaris region. Ependymomas should be surgically excised. Their distinct borders often allow complete resection; when total removal is not possible, radiation therapy is usually employed.

Astrocytoma. These glial tumors are derived from astrocytes and are often intramedullary. Their incidence is about the same as that of spinal ependymomas. Total excision is rarely possible due to their infiltrative nature. Low-grade astrocytomas, if recurrent, are usually reoperated. Radiation therapy is reserved for the malignant astrocytomas, but this is usually only palliative. While the growth rate of spinal cord astrocytomas is slow, prognosis is generally poor.

Lipoma. Lipomas constitute 10 percent of spinal tumors and are often associated with spina bifida and a subcutaneous lipoma. Although benign, they tend to be intertwined with cord tissue and are usually only partially excised. These do not require radiation, and the mortality is low.

Dermoid. Dermoids are congenital lesions usually found in the lumbosacral area. They often have an associated sinus tract to the skin surface and may present with infection. The treatment is surgical resection, including the sinus tract. The resection of the portion entering the spinal cord is usually incomplete. The long-term prognosis is good.

Metastatic Tumor. Up to 25 percent of all spinal neoplasms are metastatic in origin and most appear in an extradural location (Fig. 40-13). Common primary sites include breast, lung, prostate, and kidney. If the primary site is not known or if the neurologic decline is rapid, treatment is surgical decompression with biopsy. Otherwise, local radiation therapy is the treatment of choice. Other extradural malignant tumors include lymphoma, myeloma, plasmacytoma, chordoma, and osteogenic sarcoma. When significant bone destruction or the surgical decompression renders the spine unstable, surgical stabilization through an anterior or posterior route is often necessary.

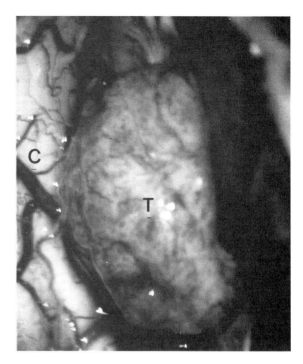

FIG. 40-12. Intraoperative photograph of a meningioma at the C1–C2 level. Note the distinct margin of the tumor (T) and the compressed spinal cord (C).

Peripheral Nerve Tumors

The peripheral nervous system includes the peripheral and cranial nerves, spinal roots, and autonomic nervous system. Tumors can arise from any of these elements. The more common tumors are discussed below. More unusual tumors include gangliog-

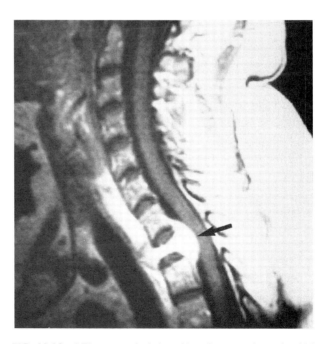

FIG. 40-13. MRI scan, sagittal view. Note the tumor (arrow), which deforms the spinal cord and has replaced the T1 vertebral body.

liomas, neuroblastomas, paragangliomas, chemodectomas, and pheochromocytomas.

Schwannoma. This tumor arises from the peripheral nerve Schwann cells that provide the myelin sheaths for axons. Schwannomas tend to displace the nerve of origin and thus usually present as a painless mass. With continued growth, they can create pain in the distribution of the nerve. As they enlarge, nerve function deteriorates. They tend to arise from sensory nerves but may also be found on motor nerves. The treatment is surgical excision. The nerve of origin can usually be preserved. At times, however, total excision may mean division of the parent nerve. If the nerve serves a significant function, it is preferable to leave a portion of the tumor in order to spare the nerve. This is justified because malignant transformation is rare.

Neurofibroma. Neurofibromas differ from schwannomas in that they actually engulf the nerve of origin, since they arise from the nerve itself. They are often cutaneous, making it difficult to identify one specific nerve of origin. When associated with von Recklinghausen's neurofibromatosis, they are usually multiple. When found singly, treatment is resection. When multiple tumors are present, only the symptomatic ones should be resected. Removal requires sacrifice of the nerve if that nerve is expendable. If the function of the nerve is critical, a portion of tumor should be left attached to the nerve. Unlike in the case of schwannomas, patients with neurofibromas should be followed closely, since these tumors have a higher incidence of malignant transformation.

Malignant Nerve Sheath Tumor. These tumors typically occur after the age of thirty. The treatment of choice is radical wide resection. If there is evidence of muscle or soft tissue invasion, amputation of the involved extremity is recommended. These tumors are generally resistant to radiation therapy.

CEREBROVASCULAR DISEASE

Cerebrovascular disease is the third most common cause of death in the United States and is a significant cause of disability. Death and disability are due either to ischemia causing focal or diffuse infarction or to hemorrhage causing compressive mass lesions. Although discussed separately, cerebrovascular problems producing infarction may become hemorrhagic, and hemorrhagic lesions may lead to infarction.

Ischemic Vascular Disease (Stroke)

Ischemia and subsequent infarction of the brain can occur in the distribution of any of the cerebral vessels; thus any portion of the cerebrum, brainstem, or cerebellum may be affected. Because the carotid circulation provides the greatest blood supply to the brain, ischemia and infarction within its distribution are most common. Ischemia may be the result of diminished flow secondary to stenosis or occlusion of major arteries or due to transient or permanent occlusion of smaller arterioles from intravascular emboli.

The most common cause of stenosis or occlusion of large vessels is atherosclerosis. This disease often develops extracranially at the origin of the internal carotid artery in the neck but may occur in the carotid siphon (that portion of the artery within

the cavernous sinus), the distal internal carotid, or even the proximal middle cerebral artery (Fig. 40-14).

Arterial emboli usually originate either from atherosclerotic ulceration in the region of the carotid bifurcation or from sources within the heart. The heart is a common source of emboli when a mural thrombus forms after a myocardial infarction or as a result of atrial fibrillation. Other risk factors for cerebral ischemia include hypertension, diabetes, hypercholesterolemia, obesity, smoking, and family history of stroke.

Since there is no effective medical or surgical therapy for a completed stroke, the goal of neurosurgical intervention is to identify stroke-prone patients and reduce their risk of cerebral ischemia. These high-risk patients are best identified by a history of transient ischemic attacks (TIAs), which take the form of either transient cerebral ischemia or amaurosis fugax. Transient cerebral ischemia in the carotid circulation usually consists of temporary hemianesthesia, hemiparesis, or aphasia. Amaurosis fugax is transient loss of vision in one eye. Ischemia in the vertebrobasilar system may cause transient diplopia, dizziness, dysarthria, dysphagia, weakness, numbness, loss of vision, or even loss of memory.

Most ischemic episodes last seconds to minutes and rarely longer than 30 min. As long as the neurologic deficit resolves within 24 h, the episode is, by definition, a TIA. A reversible ischemic neurologic deficit (RIND) is one that lasts 24 h to 3 weeks. Ischemic deficits lasting longer are considered completed strokes. Careful questioning of individuals with completed strokes reveals that 60 percent had a prior history of TIAs, 20 percent presented in a slow, stepwise fashion, and only 20 percent were sudden in onset.

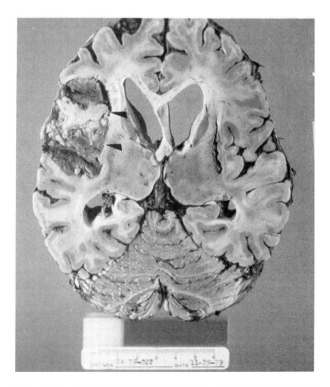

FIG. 40-14. *Postmortem brain specimen, axial plane. Note the sharply demarcated infarct (arrowheads) in the distribution of the middle cerebral artery.*

Patients with TIAs or slow-onset strokes are potential candidates for preventive surgical intervention. Surgical procedures to prevent stroke are directed toward either removal of the source of emboli or augmentation of blood flow to the brain. Operations for these conditions include carotid endarterectomy and microvascular bypass. Potential candidates generally undergo a CT or MRI scan of the brain to evaluate any degree of cerebral infarction and to rule out other diagnoses such as tumor, subdural hematoma, or subarachnoid hemorrhage. Patients then undergo angiography, including the aortic arch and the carotid, vertebral, and cerebral arteries. Noninvasive studies of the carotid circulation are less accurate, although they are useful as screening procedures because of their low risk.

Carotid endarterectomy is indicated when ipsilateral symptoms of cerebral ischemia or amaurosis fugax exist and angiography demonstrates either significant stenosis (usually more than 75 percent) or ulceration in the accessible portion of the common and/or proximal internal carotid arteries (Fig. 40-15). The procedure consists of opening the affected portion of the carotid artery under systemic heparinization and removing the atherosclerotic plaque. The mortality from carotid endarterectomy is about 1 percent and the neurologic morbidity 5 percent in experienced hands.

A number of patients present with cerebral ischemia ipsilateral to an occluded internal carotid artery or with stenosis of the internal carotid or middle cerebral artery that is not surgically accessible. For these patients with inadequate collateral cerebral circulation, a microvascular bypass procedure is sometimes indicated. The most common of these is the superficial temporal artery to middle cerebral artery anastomosis (STA-MCA).

Intracranial Aneurysm

Intracranial aneurysms are diseased dilatations of the cerebral arteries, their walls consisting of ballooned-out tunicae intima, media, and adventitia with a variable degree of intraluminal or mural thrombus. Most are congenital in origin, evolving and developing during life. They may become atherosclerotic. Aneurysms are typically found at the bifurcation of the major vessels of the circle of Willis. Up to 20 percent of patients with aneurysms have multiple aneurysms, and 1 percent demonstrate an associated arteriovenous malformation (AVM). If aneurysms are found more peripherally in the cerebral vasculature, secondary causation such as trauma or infection should be considered.

Over 85 percent of cerebral aneurysms occur in the carotid or "anterior" circulation. Approximately 30 percent arise from the intracranial portion of the internal carotid artery, usually at or near the origin of the posterior communicating artery. Another 30 percent occur in the region of the anterior communicating artery. About 25 percent arise from the middle cerebral artery, usually at its first major branch point, which is commonly a trifurcation. Aneurysms of the vertebrobasilar or "posterior" circulation are most frequently found at the tip of the basilar artery but may occur more proximally along its trunk. The origin of the posterior inferior cerebellar artery is the next most common location.

Patients with intracranial aneurysms most commonly present with signs and symptoms of subarachnoid hemorrhage (SAH). Eighty percent of nontraumatic subarachnoid hemorrhages are caused by aneurysm rupture. The patient notes a sudden severe headache commonly followed by neck stiffness and photophobia due to associated meningeal irritation caused by the subarach-

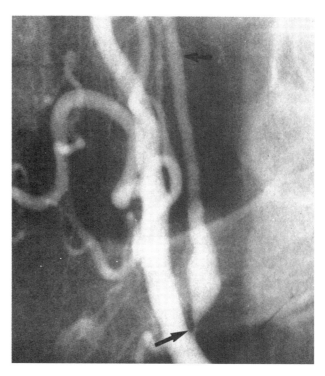

FIG. 40-15. *Arteriogram, common carotid artery, oblique view. Note the stenotic origin of the internal carotid (arrow). The external carotid is relatively unaffected by atherosclerosis.*

noid blood. Transient loss of consciousness may occur. Some patients may develop a focal neurologic deficit or become comatose as a result of the acute rise in intracranial pressure. The severity of the SAH can be graded, as shown in Table 40-3. In general, the lower the grade, the better the outcome.

Not all patients with aneurysms present with symptoms related to rupture. Through mass effect, an internal carotid artery (ICA) aneurysm may compress the optic (IId) nerve (Fig. 40-16*A, B*), causing monocular blindness, or the oculomotor (IIId) nerve, producing a palsy characterized by diplopia, ptosis, and dilated pupil. An ICA aneurysm within the cavernous sinus may compress the abducens (VIth) nerve and create diplopia. A giant aneurysm (larger than 25 mm in diameter) of the basilar tip may block the cerebral aqueduct and create hydrocephalus.

Table 40-3
Subarachnoid Hemorrhage Grading Scale*

Grade I	Asymptomatic or minimal headache and slight nuchal rigidity
Grade II	Moderate to severe headache, nuchal rigidity, but no neurologic deficit other than a cranial nerve palsy
Grade III	Lethargy, confusion, and/or mild focal neurologic deficit
Grade IV	Stupor, moderate to severe hemiparesis, possible early decerebrate posturing, and vegetative disturbances
Grade V	Deep coma, decerebrate posturing, and moribund appearance

*According to the Hunt and Hess criteria.

SOURCE: Adapted from Macdonald RL, Weir B: Pathophysiology and clinical evaluation of subarachnoid hemorrhage, in Youmans JR (ed), *Neurological Surgery*, Philadelphia, WB Saunders, 1996, with permission.

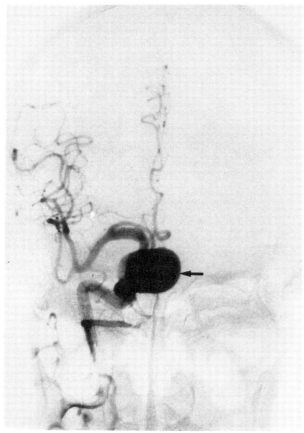

A

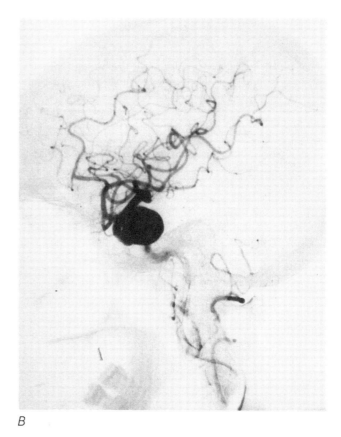

B

FIG. 40-16. Cerebral arteriogram. *A.* AP view. *The large internal carotid aneurysm (arrow) projects medially, where it has compressed the optic nerve. B. Lateral view.*

Rarely, an aneurysm may be large enough to be mistaken for a tumor.

The diagnosis of SAH is usually made clinically and confirmed either by noting blood within the subarachnoid spaces on CT scan or by finding bloody CSF with xanthochromia on a lumbar puncture (LP). The CT scan should be obtained first, since it usually spares the patient an LP and also eliminates the potential risk of brainstem compression from herniation if an unsuspected mass lesion is present. Complete cerebral angiography is then employed to identify and delineate the aneurysm and, at the same time, rule out multiple aneurysms or an associated AVM.

Once the diagnosis of aneurysmal rupture is confirmed, the patient is placed on a medical regimen to reduce the risk of rebleeding. This includes strict bed rest with the head elevated. Stimulation is kept to a minimum. Blood pressure is tightly controlled to keep it below 150 mmHg systolic. Careful observation is necessary to watch for signs of raised intracranial pressure which may be attributable to delayed hydrocephalus. Anticonvulsants are started for seizure prophylaxis. Calcium channel blockers are used to reduce the risk of vasospasm.

The ultimate treatment of aneurysms is microsurgical dissection and obliteration, usually by placing a metallic clip across the aneurysms's neck via a craniotomy. Timing of surgery depends on the clinical grade of the patient (see Table 40-3). Good-grade (I and II) patients should usually undergo operation within 72 hours of rupture. Poor-grade (III and IV) patients should con-

tinue intensive medical management until they improve to a lower grade, if possible, because mortality rises with grade. Surgically accessible unruptured aneurysms should be operated on electively to prevent rupture. Some inaccessible aneurysms can be effectively obliterated by embolization using interventional neuroradiologic techniques.

Complications of aneurysmal rupture include a 30 percent rebleeding rate within the first 8 weeks if the lesion remains unrepaired, hydrocephalus from obstruction of the arachnoid villi by subarachnoid clot, vasospasm, intracerebral hematomas, raised intracranial pressure, and seizures. The most significant and least understood of these is cerebral vasospasm. This phenomenon occurs most frequently within 4 to 7 days after the hemorrhage and results in narrowing of adjacent cerebral arteries. Vasospasm may be noted on angiography without any untoward clinical effects, or it may produce profound and life-threatening cerebral ischemia in the distribution of the involved vessels.

Angioplasty done by interventional neuroradiologic techniques can, in selected cases, increase cerebral blood flow in order to overcome the spasm. Improved perfusion through dilated spastic arterial segments combined with induced hypertension can reverse ischemic neurologic deficits. The use of inotropic support and intravascular volume expansion, usually with colloid and red cell transfusion, is also beneficial. Cardiovascular status is monitored continuously by means of a Swan-Ganz catheter.

Patients who undergo elective clipping of unruptured aneurysms have better outcomes than those with ruptured aneurysms because the brain has not been injured by the subarachnoid hemorrhage. In addition, aneurysms of the internal carotid artery carry less risk than those of the vertebrobasilar system, with the exception of complex anterior communicating artery aneurysms. In general, if the aneurysm can be clipped and vasospasm avoided or effectively overcome, most patients do well.

Arteriovenous Malformation

Arteriovenous malformations (AVMs) occur within the central nervous system as congenital abnormalities that allow blood to be shunted directly from arteries to veins, bypassing the normally interconnecting capillary bed. These malformations may be quite small with only a single feeding artery, or they may encompass several lobes of the brain and arterial feeders from multiple sources. They may occur in virtually any portion of the brain, including the cerebellum and brainstem. In the cerebral parenchyma, where they are most commonly located, the lesion takes on a conical shape, with the apex deep, often reaching the lateral ventricle. Rarely, AVMs occur within the spinal cord, and they may exclusively involve the dura either intracranially or within the spinal canal.

Patients with AVMs tend to develop symptoms before age thirty. The most common initial presentation is hemorrhage (50 percent of cases and 10 percent of all intracerebral hemorrhages, second only to aneurysms). Bleeding usually occurs within the brain substance but may occur within the ventricular system or the subarachnoid space. The patient experiences a sudden headache, often associated with loss of consciousness and/or a neurologic deficit. The next most common presenting symptom is a seizure. In a few cases, seizures may be frequent and refractory to medical therapy. AVMs may also present with the insidious onset of a focal neurologic deficit due to mass effect, increased venous pressure, or vascular steal phenomenon. Occasionally, young patients with severe unrelenting headaches are found to harbor an AVM.

From the time of discovery of an unruptured AVM, the risk of hemorrhage is about 1 percent per year cumulatively. Once an AVM has bled, the risk of rebleeding increases to 5 percent per year. With each hemorrhage, the risk of dying is approximately 10 percent and morbidity at least 15 percent. Smaller AVMs are more likely to bleed than larger ones. Most AVMs remain stable in size, but some enlarge with time. Up to 10 percent have an associated aneurysm on a feeding artery. In these cases, hemorrhage is usually due to rupture of the aneurysm.

An AVM can be identified on contrast-enhanced CT scanning as a hyperdense mass, part of which has a serpentine configuration related to the presence of large draining veins. Its configuration and extent are more easily delineated with MRI. After hemorrhage, an unenhanced CT scan usually demonstrates intracerebral or subarachnoid blood. AVMs may be too small to be seen on CT, so careful angiography may be necessary to identify the source of hemorrhage. Lumbar puncture may be necessary if subarachnoid hemorrhage is suspected clinically but not verified by the CT scan.

In all cases of suspected or proven AVM, complete cerebral angiography must be undertaken to define carefully the extent of the malformation (Fig. 40-17*A, B*). All feeding arteries, including any from the external carotid system as well as the draining veins, must be evaluated. It is only from high-resolution angiography that a treatment decision can be reached. If angiography fails to delineate a lesion despite suspicion, MRI may identify the "angiographically occult" abnormality.

The treatment of AVMs is dependent on the size and location of the lesion, the presenting symptoms, and the age and condition of the patient. Because of the risk of rebleeding, an AVM that has bled should be surgically excised if possible. The treatment decision is more difficult in the patient who presents with seizures. If the patient is young and the malformation is readily accessible, surgical resection is usually recommended, especially when the seizures are medically refractory. Operation involves the microsurgical dissection and resection of the entire malformation, rather than simple ligation of feeding arteries. The results of operation are related to the size and location of the malformation. Overall, the operative mortality is less than 5 percent and the morbidity less than 10 percent.

Alternative or adjunctive methods of treatment include intraarterial embolization and radiation therapy. Using interventional neuroradiologic techniques, particulate matter or glues may be introduced into AVMs via feeding vessels to occlude the vascular shunt nidus. It is rarely possible to obliterate these lesions completely with this method, however. This technique nevertheless can reduce flow through the AVM prior to direct surgical intervention.

Ionizing radiation, on the other hand, has the capability of completely obliterating selected small- to medium-sized AVMs. Focused gamma or proton beam irradiation has demonstrated efficacy, and occasional success with conventional irradiation has been reported. Ionizing radiation causes endothelial proliferation and may take 6 months to 2 years to obliterate the lesion. Focused irradiation is recommended for deep, surgically inaccessible AVMs.

Intracerebral Hemorrhage

Spontaneous hemorrhage is most commonly associated with systemic hypertension and occurs in predictable locations, including the putamen, thalamus, cerebellum, and pons. Hemorrhage can also occur within the various lobes of the brain. Nonhypertensive causes of brain hemorrhage have been discussed above, such as rupture of AVMs and aneurysms and hemorrhage into areas of ischemia. Additional causes include induced or endogenous coagulopathies, primary or metastatic brain tumors, and rare conditions such as amyloid angiopathy.

Chronic hypertension results in lipohyalinosis of the vessel wall, which sets the stage for either vascular occlusion or rupture. Occlusion results in infarction, and rupture produces an intracerebral hemorrhage. The shorter penetrating arteries of the brain appear to be the most vulnerable. The lenticulostriate and thalamoperforating vessels are involved in putaminal and thalamic hemorrhages, and affected basilar branches contribute to pontine hemorrhage.

Although brain hemorrhage is often devastating, it may be surprisingly well tolerated. The hematoma tends to dissect along axonal planes, separating rather than destroying vital structures. If the resultant mass is tolerated by the patient, the blood is slowly resorbed by macrophages along the periphery, leaving only a hemosiderin-stained slit in the brain. Patients may worsen clinically anytime after the initial hemorrhage as a result of associated edema formation.

Hemorrhage into the putamen accounts for the majority of hypertensive hematomas. Presentation is characterized by the

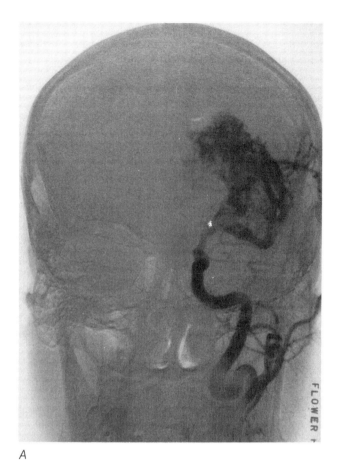

A

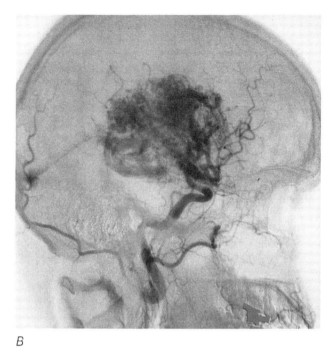

B

FIG. 40-17. *Cerebral arteriogram. A. AP view. The large AVM is supplied mainly by the middle cerebral artery. B. Lateral view.*

lack of headache with gradual development of hemiparesis progressing to hemiplegia. This may be associated with a hemisensory loss, aphasia, hemianopia, and/or ipsilateral deviation of the eyes, depending on the size of the hematoma and its direction of dissection. The patient may, of course, progress into coma if the lesion is large. Similarly, thalamic hemorrhage presents initially with a hemisensory loss and hemiparesis. Localizing features include downward eye deviation with limitation of vertical gaze and small, sluggish pupils due to involvement of the nearby mesencephalon. Headache is uncommon.

Cerebellar hemorrhage is sudden in onset and presents with headache. Vomiting, ataxia, and dizziness are accompanying features. This hemorrhage is extremely dangerous in that it may cause coma and ultimately death due to brainstem compression and acute hydrocephalus. Brainstem hemorrhage (usually pontine) is the most devastating and often presents with quadriparesis, decerebrate posturing, pinpoint pupils, and coma. Most patients do not survive if the hematoma is larger than 1 cm in size. Moreover, those who do survive have a high degree of morbidity.

Lobar hemorrhage is less likely to be associated with hypertension and, in general, is better tolerated by the patient. The symptoms depend on the area of brain involved.

CT scanning has become an invaluable tool in diagnosing and defining brain hemorrhage. CT not only delineates the hemorrhage but also permits assessment of ventricular size, the presence of edema, and often the cause of the hemorrhage (e.g., AVM, tumor, aneurysm). The hematoma appears hyperdense in

the acute phase (Fig. 40-18). With time, as the blood breaks down, the clot progresses to a hypodense lesion. At any time, from days to weeks, the hematoma may demonstrate an enhancing ring. If a vascular lesion is suspected, careful angiography is indicated. In all cases, appropriate coagulation studies should be obtained.

The treatment of brain hemorrhage may be medical or surgical depending on the size of the lesion, its location, and the condition of the patient. Surgical resection is recommended if the patient is deteriorating neurologically, no matter what the size of the hematoma. Cerebellar hematomas are particularly important to remove, since a small change in surrounding reactive edema may result in life-threatening brainstem compression and/or hydrocephalus.

Because hematomas are mass lesions, medical management is directed toward keeping the intracranial pressure under control. If the hemorrhage renders the patient unconscious, hyperventilation and hyperosmolar agents may be required to control ICP. ICP monitoring may be a helpful adjunct to direct treatment. Steroids are useful in controlling brain edema if the patient has bled into a tumor, and coagulopathies should be corrected. Despite medical and/or surgical therapy, mortality and morbidity remain high from all types of brain hemorrhage.

DEGENERATIVE SPINE DISEASE

Anatomy and Pathophysiology. The spinal column is composed of 33 vertebrae making up those divisions labeled

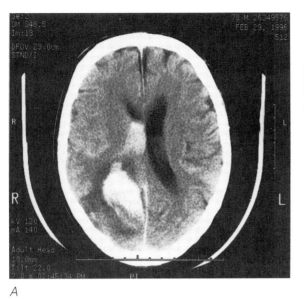
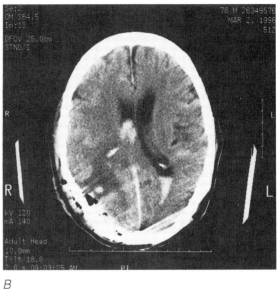

A

B

FIG. 40-18. CT scan, axial view, non-contrast enhanced. *A.* Spontaneous hemorrhage, with rupture into the ventricle. *B.* The hematoma was evacuated urgently.

cervical (7), thoracic (12), lumbar (5), sacral (5 fused), and coccygeal (4 fused). Each vertebra consists of a body, which bears weight, and the posterior elements (pedicles, laminae, spinous and transverse processes), which provide the flexibility and stability to the vertebral column. The spinal canal has an ovoid shape in the transverse plane through the cervical and thoracic regions and assumes a more triangular shape in the lumbar region. Most spine movement occurs in the cervical and lumbar regions. Flexion and extension are greatest in the lower cervical and lumbar segments, and maximum rotation occurs predominantly in the upper cervical and lumbar segments.

The intervertebral disc consists of two parts. The circumferential anulus fibrosus, making up the outer portion, is composed of dense, fibrous tissue. The central nucleus pulposus consists of fibrocartilage, which has little tensile strength but substantial elasticity. The fibrocartilage may fragment acutely or degenerate gradually. It heals poorly because of limited blood supply. The anulus heals well and is buttressed by heavy anterior and posterior longitudinal ligaments. Intervertebral disc disease may occur at any level from C1 to S1. The lower segments of the cervical and lumbar areas are affected most often. Thoracic disc disease is rare.

The spinal cord extends from the cervicomedullary junction at the base of the skull to the conus medullaris at the L1–L2 level. The cord is centrally placed within the spinal canal and moves rostrally and caudally a few millimeters during spinal flexion and extension. Lateral motion of the cord is restricted by intradural dentate ligaments. The blood supply is provided by radicular arteries, which arise from the vertebral arteries and the thyrocervical trunks in the neck, from the intercostal arteries in the thorax, and from the lumbar arteries in the low back. An arterial confluens, the artery of Adamkiewicz, is typically found in the T10–L2 region, usually on the left side. It supplies the lower thoracic cord and conus medullaris.

Three fiber tracts of the spinal cord are important clinically (see Fig. 40-3). The laterally positioned *corticospinal tracts*

carry motor fibers from the cortical upper motor neurons to the spinal lower motor neurons located in the ventral horns of the spinal cord. These tracts cross the midline at the pyramidal decussation in the lower medulla. The *spinothalamic tract,* also positioned laterally, transmits pain and temperature sensation from the contralateral side of the body. Its axons cross through the anterior commissure of the cord within two or three segments of each dorsal root entry zone and ascend to the ipsilateral thalamus. The *dorsal columns* carry sensory fibers conveying position, vibratory, and light touch sensation from the dorsal roots rostrally on the same side, then cross to the opposite cerebral cortex through a decussation in the brainstem.

Dorsal and ventral nerve roots emerge from the spinal cord separately and pass to their respective intervertebral foramina, where they exit from the spinal canal (see Fig. 40-2). The roots join to form a spinal nerve within the neural foramen. In the cervical spine, the roots exit above the corresponding vertebrae; for instance, the C5 root exits above the C5 pedicle. Since there are eight cervical roots, C7 exits above the C7 pedicle and C8 exits below it. Consequently, all roots below C8 exit below the pedicle of their corresponding vertebra.

Lumbar and sacral roots form the cauda equina below the conus medullaris. The sacral roots are more centrally located adjacent to the filum terminale. Because a lumbar root (e.g., L4) passes laterally toward the neural foramen as it descends within the spinal canal, it crosses the adjacent intervertebral disc (e.g., L4–L5) at its extreme lateral edge, hugging the pedicle of the L4 vertebra laterally. The nerve root that descends to the next lowest foramen (e.g., L5) passes across the disc space (e.g., L4–L5) more medially, making that root more vulnerable to disease involving that disc (Fig. 40-19).

Intervertebral Disc Disease

If the nucleus of an intervertebral disc extrudes (herniates) through the anulus, adjacent neural structures may be compressed. In the cervical and thoracic spine, compression of the

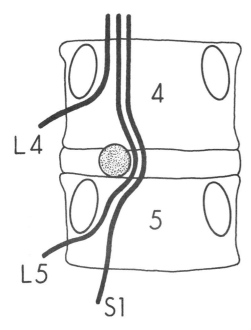

FIG. 40-19. *Diagram of the lumbar spine and nerve roots showing the relationship of the L5 nerve root to the L4–L5 disc space. The common site of disc rupture is stippled.*

spinal cord may result in paraparesis or quadriparesis, depending on the spinal segment involved. At all levels, compression of a spinal root may cause weakness and sensory loss in structures innervated by that root. The severity of the clinical syndrome depends on the site and severity of compression by the displaced disc fragment. In some cases the anulus and adjacent ligament hold, preventing complete extrusion of the fragmented disc. The anulus may only stretch sufficiently to allow the disc to bulge into the spinal canal or foramina, accounting for back and leg pain, but often without neurologic deficit.

Often the nucleus does not extrude, but simply fragments in response to the forces exerted on the spinal column. This is intensified by the concomitant dehydration and loss of elasticity of the disc as it ages. The disc space gradually narrows, the joint becomes loose, and the cartilaginous endplates of the adjacent vertebral bodies abut and wear more quickly. Bony spurs (osteophytes) develop at the joint in reaction to the increased mobility and decreased elasticity.

Formation of osteophytes around the joints of vertebrae, termed spondylosis, is a common disorder that represents the normal process of aging. If an osteophyte forms in a neural foramen, the nerve root passing through may be chronically irritated and compressed. If the osteophyte develops within the cervical or lumbar canal, the cord or cauda equina may be compromised.

The onset of symptoms and signs of an extruded disc fragment may be acute or chronic. Acute symptoms may or may not be related to trauma. In disc disease of the cervical spine, neck and radicular discomfort occur simultaneously. Spinal cord symptoms are rare. There is usually limitation of neck motion, with loss of normal cervical lordosis. With foraminal osteophytes, episodes of cervical discomfort recur over many months or years before radicular symptoms appear. Interscapular aching,

suboccipital headaches, and even chest pain are common complaints.

Nerve root compression produces radiculopathy, often characterized by pain and hypoesthesia in the distribution of the involved root. Associated loss of deep tendon reflex with or without weakness may be seen on examination. Cervical cord compression causes myelopathy characterized by progressive spastic quadriparesis or paraparesis, mild to moderate sensory changes in the lower extremities and trunk with cervical dermatomal sensory loss, weak upper extremities, hyperreflexia, and extensor plantar response.

Cervical Disc Disease

Cervical disc disease must be differentiated from other ailments. These include inflammatory disease of the soft tissues and joints of the arm and shoulder, nerve entrapment syndromes, and neoplasms. The pain must be distinguished from that which accompanies cardiac disease. Spinal infections, congenital lesions, and posttraumatic disorders are other important considerations.

Plain radiographs typically demonstrate loss of the lordotic curve of the cervical spine, with narrowing of one or more disc spaces. Osteophyte formation may be seen. In cervical spondylosis, there is usually radiologic evidence of osteophytes and disc space narrowing at multiple levels. In most cases, the anterior-posterior diameter of the cervical spinal canal is narrowed. Myelography with CT is very useful in the diagnostic workup of nerve root compression. The use of intrathecal contrast medium enhances the power of CT to delineate the lesion. MRI is suitable for investigating myelopathies. In addition to defining the compressive lesion, MRI often shows intrinsic cord abnormalities related to compression. Electromyography may confirm the diagnosis and localize the lesion more specifically, particularly when myelographic defects are multiple.

Treatment. Painful cervical disc disease may be treated medically as long as there is no evidence of a progressive neurologic deficit (motor loss and bowel and bladder dysfunction being most important). Adequate medical therapy includes immobilization of the neck with a soft or hard cervical collar, analgesics, muscle relaxants, and local heat. These methods, in association with a good physical therapy program, provide relief under most circumstances.

Up to 75 percent of patients with cervical disc disease improve following an adequate trial (10 to 14 days) of medical therapy. Some have recurrence of radicular symptoms on return to full activity. In many cases, these patients can be managed for years with intermittent cervical traction and a cervical collar, but some require surgical therapy. For the 25 percent who do not respond to conservative means, operation is often helpful.

There are two approaches for the surgical treatment of cervical disc disease. Anteriorly, nerve roots, spinal cord, or both may be decompressed through discectomy with or without bone graft fusion. The other approach is posteriorly through a laminectomy and/or foraminotomy. The choice of operative direction is based on consideration of the patient's anatomic lesion. Improvement follows operative treatment of symptomatic cervical disc disease by either approach in approximately 80 percent of patients who fail to respond to medical treatment. Surgical treatment of cervical spondylotic myelopathy results in improvement in most cases. Arrest of the progressive myelopathic deficit usually occurs.

Lumbar Disc Disease

Herniated lumbar discs often produce some degree of nerve root compression. The severity of the syndrome depends on the degree of root compression. Occasionally, the entire cauda equina may be involved, resulting in loss of motor and sensory function, including bowel and bladder sphincter control. Sometimes disc rupture may occur in the midline, compressing centrally positioned sacral roots preferentially, without involvement of laterally placed lumbar roots.

Fragmentation of a lumbar disc may occur without extrusion of the nucleus pulposus as described above for cervical disc disease. Because of loss of elasticity within the disc, mobility of the intervertebral joint is increased. The anulus fibrosus may simply bulge without tearing. With time, osteophytes may form around the degenerated disc and encroach on the spinal canal and neural foramina. This degenerative hypertrophy involves the ligamentous structures as well. Stenosis of the lumbar spinal canal is the eventual result, a spondylotic condition common in the elderly.

In the lumbar spine, over 90 percent of clinical problems arise from the L4–L5 and L5–S1 intervertebral discs. Pain is usually chronic, but its onset may be acute when associated with frank herniation. There may be back pain, leg pain, or both. Radiation of low back pain into the buttock, posterior thigh, and calf is usually the same with disease at the L4–L5 and L5–S1 levels. This radiating pain may be exacerbated by coughing, sneezing, or straining. Bending and sitting accentuate the discomfort, while lying down characteristically relieves it. Pain is typically described as aching but frequently has a sharp or shooting element and is limited to one lower extremity. With lumbar stenosis, patients are unable to extend their spine without developing pain, numbness, and/or weakness, usually in both lower extremities. In the upright posture, either standing or walking, the cauda equina becomes relatively ischemic, producing neurogenic claudication. Relief is obtained by sitting or flexing forward (Fig. 40-20).

Palpation usually reveals tenderness over the sciatic notch, the popliteal fossa, or both. Paravertebral muscles may be in spasm. With true nerve root compression, straight-leg raising produces leg pain that is accentuated by dorsiflexion of the foot. Ipsilateral leg pain produced by contralateral straight-leg raising is highly suggestive of lumbar disc herniation. Sensory loss, weakness, and loss of tendon jerks may occur in a variety of combinations and to variable degrees.

Back pain with radiation to the leg has many causes besides lumbar disc disease. The differential diagnosis includes bony abnormalities such as subluxation, degenerative facet fracture, and osteophyte formation; primary and metastatic tumors of the cauda equina, spine, and pelvis; inflammatory disorders, including abscess, arachnoiditis, ankylosing spondylitis, and rheumatoid arthritis; degenerative lesions of the spinal cord; peripheral neuropathies; peripheral vascular occlusive disease including abdominal aortic aneurysm; and gynecologic problems such as endometriosis.

Plain films of the lumbosacral spine can identify congenital or acquired bony changes. Disc space narrowing is an unreliable sign of symptomatic disease, since narrowing of the disc space may occur without clinical symptoms. Flexion and extension lat-

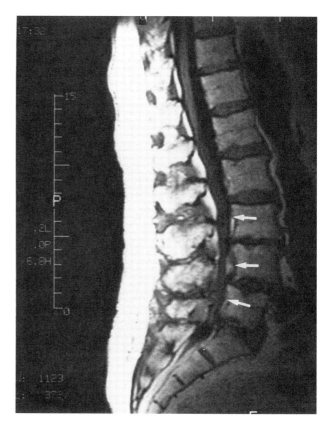

FIG. 40-20. *MRI scan, sagittal view, lumbar spine. Note the progressive narrowing of the spinal canal (arrows) from L2 through S1.*

eral views reveal concomitant instability. Myelography can be diagnostic in symptomatic lumbar disc disease, but CT alone can delineate the lesion in most cases (Fig. 40-21). MRI has replaced myelography and CT at some centers in the workup of lumbar radiculopathy. Electromyography may confirm the diagnosis, especially when physical examination is unable to localize the involved nerve root.

Treatment. Initially medical treatment is indicated in all patients who do not have neurologic deterioration. Bed rest, local heat, analgesics, and skeletal muscle relaxants are usually effective within a few days. Physical therapy and limited exercise often help when the acute episode passes. A back brace partially immobilizes the patient and can minimize muscle spasm. With aggressive conservative management, most patients improve sufficiently to return to full activity. Recurrent symptoms may be treated in a similar fashion, often successfully. Surgical treatment is reserved for the patient with an acute or progressive neurologic deficit, chronic disabling pain, or both. The acute onset of weakness or sphincter disturbance constitutes an emergency, demanding prompt diagnosis and early operation.

Operation usually entails a unilateral laminotomy with removal of the offending disc fragment. Foraminotomy may be necessary in the presence of osteophyte formation. With lumbar stenosis, multilevel laminectomy is curative. Should plain films demonstrate any instability preoperatively, combining the laminectomy with posterior fusion, either with or without instrumentation, is generally indicated. If the imaging studies demonstrate an extruded disc fragment that accounts for the clinical signs

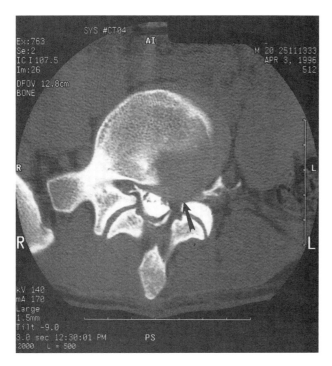

FIG. 40-21. *CT scan following lumbar myelogram, transverse view. The ruptured disc (arrow) has displaced the thecal sac dorsally and laterally.*

and symptoms, 85 to 90 percent of patients recover with surgical treatment. If the syndrome is atypical, the myelogram equivocal, and the patient poorly motivated, operation is less effective. Emotional factors, psychologic disturbances, litigation, and industrial injury play an important role in the eventual outcome, whether the treatment is medical or surgical. Alternatives to the laminotomy approach include percutaneous discectomy done by endoscopic excision of the problematic nucleus pulposus. Clinical results for the alternative approaches are less predictable.

INFECTIONS

The central nervous system may be infected by viruses, bacteria, fungi, and parasites. Development of infection depends on the host's resistance (i.e., immune defenses) and on the infecting agent's virulence. Bone, brain, spinal cord, meninges, and cerebrospinal fluid may be involved separately or in combination. The routes of infection include hematogenous dissemination, local extension from a neighboring source, and direct contamination through an open wound. The infection may be diffuse, as in meningitis, or focal, as in brain abscess.

The clinical spectrum of signs and symptoms of CNS infection varies from nonspecific (such as fever, confusion, and lethargy) to highly specific (such as jacksonian epilepsy and focal neurologic deficits). Consequently, CNS infections present difficult diagnostic and therapeutic problems. Early diagnosis and treatment are critical to achieve a successful outcome.

Bacterial

Subgaleal Abscess. Localized infection between the galea of the scalp and the pericranium constitutes subgaleal abscess. Usually, the process is initiated by contamination of an open

scalp wound by staphylococci, streptococci, or anaerobic cocci. Localized scalp tenderness, warmth, and swelling are signs of abscess formation. Osteomyelitis of the skull may occur secondarily. Subgaleal infections rarely extend intracranially, unless the skull has been penetrated. Treatment includes open drainage, debridement, and systemic antibiotics.

Osteomyelitis. Osteomyelitis may develop from extension of a localized infection, such as sinusitis or mastoiditis, from direct contamination at operation or after trauma, or, rarely, by hematogenous spread from a distant source such as the respiratory or urinary tract. An established skull or spine infection may extend to the epidural space, producing a localized abscess (Fig. 40-22). The usual osteomyelitis pathogens are staphylococci and anaerobic streptococci. Occasionally, gram-negative organisms and fungi are responsible. Treatment consists of drainage, debridement of infected bone, and appropriate antibiotics for a prolonged period, usually 6 weeks.

Epidural Abscess. Spinal epidural abscess is much more common than intracranial epidural abscess. It is characterized by fever, local spinal tenderness, and rapid progression of neurologic deficits, often constituting a medical and surgical emergency. Radicular pain and impairment of cord function, with early motor and sensory deficits including sphincter disturbances, occur within a few days. Most epidural abscesses are caused by local extension of osteomyelitis or by hematogenous spread from a distant suppurative focus. The diagnosis is suggested by the clinical presentation. The CSF often has a markedly elevated protein level with mild pleocytosis. MRI defines the extent of the epidural mass. If the dura is intact, infection rarely extends across it.

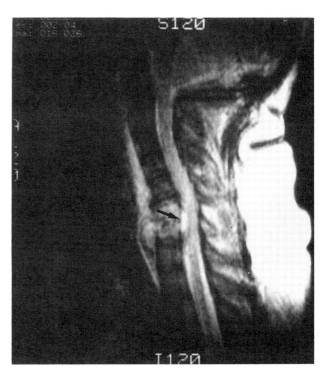

FIG. 40-22. *MRI scan, sagittal view. The disc space and the adjacent vertebral bodies are infected. Epidural pus (arrow) has compressed the ventral surface of the spinal cord.*

The most common causative organisms are *Staphylococcus aureus* and the streptococci. Treatment should be immediate, beginning with broad antibiotic coverage until the offending agent is identified. Specific antibiotic therapy should be continued for a prolonged period, often up to 6 weeks. Surgical drainage is necessary when neurologic deficits progress despite aggressive medical therapy. Corticosteroids in the perioperative period are beneficial in reducing localized edema, although prolonged use can reduce the host immune response to the infection. Recovery of neurologic function is directly related to the duration and severity of impairment before treatment.

Subdural Empyema. Subdural empyema is a purulent infection of the subdural space. It accounts for approximately 25 percent of all intracranial infections and is usually a complication of sinusitis, meningitis, or open contamination of the subdural space at operation or after trauma.

With sinusitis, infection can spread intracranially by transcranial emissary vein thrombophlebitis. Staphylococci, streptococci, and anaerobic cocci are commonly responsible. Once the subdural space is violated, infection can spread over the convexity of the brain. The accumulation of purulent material may be sufficient to produce an intracranial mass, provoking adjacent brain swelling. The clinical result is rapid neurologic deterioration, often with lateralizing signs, coma, and death. Treatment includes craniotomy with debridement, drainage, and intravenous antibiotics. The source of the infection must be treated aggressively. A sinus or mastoid drainage procedure is often required if this is the source. Mortality from acute fulminant subdural empyema from a paranasal source remains about 25 percent.

The diagnosis of intracranial subdural empyema is made readily by CT or MRI scan, but it may be difficult to distinguish from subacute or chronic subdural hematoma. The mass itself may be isodense, necessitating the administration of intravenous contrast. Including the sinuses on the scan may demonstrate the source of infection. Lumbar puncture to obtain CSF for analysis risks transtentorial herniation; thus LP should be avoided if the scan shows significant mass effect.

Spinal subdural empyema is rare. It usually develops from local extension transdurally or through the arachnoid in the presence of meningitis. Spinal cord compression and transverse myelitis may develop. Treatment is emergent, consisting of surgical drainage and prolonged antibiotic administration.

Meningitis. Bacterial meningitis is an acute, purulent infection of the leptomeninges. It is manifested by fever, lethargy, headache, nausea, vomiting, and nuchal rigidity. Seizures occur in approximately 20 percent of patients and cranial nerve palsies in about 5 percent. Coma may develop in up to 10 percent of patients with missed diagnoses, heralding a poor prognosis. Untreated bacterial meningitis is almost always fatal.

A CSF Gram stain may demonstrate the offending organism in 75 percent of cases. Cultures provide a diagnosis 90 percent of the time. When CSF cultures are negative despite high clinical suspicion, as in a mild case or in an incompletely treated case of meningitis, latex agglutination studies are helpful. These immunologic studies are specifically directed at *Streptococcus pneumoniae*, *Haemophilus influenzae*, and *Neisseria meningitidis* and are highly sensitive when an organism is present, even with negative cultures. Blood cultures may be positive and thereby helpful in the diagnosis, particularly with infections caused by *S. pneumoniae* and *N. meningitidis*. CSF pleocytosis with a preponderance of polymorphonuclear cells is typical of untreated bacterial meningitis. CSF glucose level is almost always reduced, and the protein content is typically increased.

Meningitis that develops after a penetrating wound or a neurosurgical procedure is usually caused by staphylococcal, streptococcal, or gram-negative organisms. Meningitis occurring after closed head trauma with either a skull fracture or CSF rhinorrhea is most often caused by *S. pneumoniae*. Ventricular shunt and reservoir infections leading to meningitis are more likely due to *Staphylococcus epidermidis* or *aureus*.

The treatment for acute bacterial meningitis depends on the causative organism, its antibiotic sensitivity, and the primary source of infection from which the meninges were contaminated. The presumed diagnosis is made clinically, a sample of CSF is obtained via lumbar puncture, and broad-spectrum intravenous antibiotics are immediately started. Once culture results are available, the choice of antibiotics is changed to an appropriate single agent. Bacterial endocarditis, pneumonia, sinusitis, concurrent subdural empyema, and brain abscess are sometimes associated with meningitis. Treatment should be directed at both the meningitis and the primary source.

The extent of antibiotic penetration into the CNS varies, depending on the degree of meningeal inflammation. Intrathecal administration of those antibiotics that do not readily cross the blood-CSF barrier may be necessary (the commonly used intrathecal preparations are gentamicin and vancomycin). This is especially true when a foreign body, such as a ventricular shunt, is present. Shunt removal is often necessary despite intravenous and intrathecal antibiotic administration. Rarely, therapy may also include the use of steroids and/or osmotic diuretics if intracranial pressure is elevated as a result of cerebral edema or localized brain abscess.

Complications of bacterial meningitis include communicating hydrocephalus, brain abscess, subdural empyema, and subdural effusions, particularly after *H. influenzae* meningitis in infants. The risk of complications is significantly reduced by prompt, early treatment.

Brain Abscess. Brain abscess is a purulent lesion of brain tissue, beginning as a focal infection, usually in the white matter, surrounded by a typical inflammatory response. The blood-brain barrier becomes disrupted. Necrosis and liquefaction follow the acute inflammatory stage. Eventually, either the process is encapsulated by fibrous granulation tissue or the infection spreads through the parenchyma to the subarachnoid spaces and the ventricular system.

Brain abscess is usually secondary to focal infection elsewhere. Abscesses that develop by direct intracranial extension are usually solitary and are typically found in the frontal and temporal lobes near adjacent nasal sinuses or mastoid processes where the infection began (Table 40-4). Multiple brain abscesses that develop in the septic patient are often related to bacterial endocarditis, pneumonia, and diverticulitis. Cyanotic congenital heart disease with concurrent infection is a frequent source. Direct contamination of the brain through a penetrating wound, especially when accompanied by in-driven bone fragments, is another cause of abscess. Abscess formation is frequent among patients with compromised immunity either from an underlying illness such as HIV infection or during pharmacologic immunosuppression such as in organ transplantation.

Table 40-4
Brain Abscess

Predisposing Condition	Usual Location	Common Organism
Otitis	Temporal lobe	*Streptococcus*
Mastoiditis	Subdural abscess	*Bacteroides*
		H. influenzae
		Gram-negative organisms
Sinusitis	Frontal lobe	*Streptococcus*
	Subdural abscess	*Staphylococcus*
Pneumonia	Multiple brain	Various organisms
Endocarditis	abscesses	(depends on source)
Diverticulitis		
Penetrating wound	Site of trauma	*Staphylococcus*
Neurosurgical postoperative infection	Operative site	*Staphylococcus*

Signs and symptoms of brain abscess are related to its mass effect. Headache, focal, neurologic deficits, and impaired mentation are often noted. There may be little or no evidence of systemic infection, and the patient may be afebrile. Conversely, the patient may be moribund from bacteremia with fever, hypotension, and a markedly elevated white blood cell count. Seizures may occur. Progressive mass effect leads to brain shifts followed by coma.

Contrast CT and MRI are highly accurate in detecting brain abscess and should be done before CSF is sampled (Fig. 40-23). The CSF of patients with brain abscess may be entirely normal, but usually some pleocytosis is noted. The causative organism can be identified and cultured from the abscess itself in 60 to 80 percent of cases, provided cultures are processed carefully for both aerobic and anaerobic organisms. Blood cultures are also helpful, particularly if the abscess is secondary to systemic infection.

In certain cases of early abscess formation or high surgical risk, medical therapy alone with appropriate parenteral antibiotics may be sufficient. The most effective therapy, however, is drainage of purulent material with simultaneous administration of appropriate intravenous antibiotics. Although needle aspiration may be successful, craniotomy with evacuation and removal of the abscess wall may be necessary. Surgical drainage reduces the mass effect, thereby reducing the most critical and dangerous aspect of the infection, and allows accurate bacteriologic analysis.

Results of treatment for brain abscess depend on the patient's neurologic status initially, the efficacy of the antibiotic used, the extent to which the intracranial mass is controlled by surgery, and the effective treatment of the primary source of the abscess. Despite aggressive surgical and medical management, mortality rates associated with brain abscess approach 40 percent, especially in the malnourished, chronically debilitated, or immunosuppressed patient.

Postoperative Infection. Any or all of the pyogenic infections described earlier may develop after operation. Once identified, characterized, and treated with appropriate antibiotics, the infection will almost always subside. Commonly isolated organisms include *Staphylococcus aureus* and *epidermidis*. If a foreign body such as prosthetic material or a ventricular shunt is involved, eradicating the infection becomes more difficult, often requiring a combination of intravenous and intrathecal antibiotics and removal of the foreign material. Occasionally, infections can be treated satisfactorily in the presence of retained foreign bodies, such as a shunt, provided the infection is indolent.

Fungal

Fungi may become pathogenic as a result of depression of the host immune system, prolonged systemic antibiotic therapy, or severe systemic illness. When the CNS becomes infected, it is usually associated with pulmonary fungal infection and depressed host resistance. The CNS involvement may be a diffuse meningitis or a focal abscess. Multiple abscesses may be present. Treatment requires long-term systemic antifungal chemotherapy. Surgical intervention is reserved for drainage of abscesses and resection of symptomatic mass lesions. Hydrocephalus, a potential late complication, is treated with a ventricular shunt.

Parasitic

While relatively uncommon in North America and western Europe, parasitic diseases of the CNS are a major cause of neurologic disability and death worldwide. Control of these diseases remains a public health problem. A major emphasis is placed on their prevention, for once the CNS is infested, therapeutic options are limited. Treatment, both medical and surgical, is usually ineffective or palliative at best.

Cysticercosis. *Taenia solium*, the pork tapeworm, infests the human CNS by transmission of its larvae through the blood

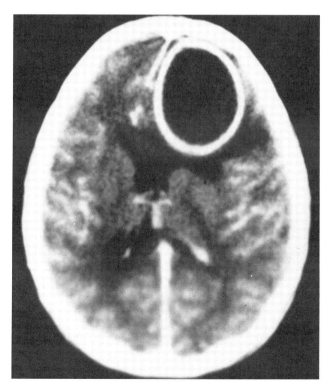

FIG. 40-23. CT scan, axial view, contrast enhanced. The large frontal abscess arose from the adjacent frontal sinus.

following ingestion. It is most prevalent in eastern Europe, Latin America, China, Pakistan, and India. Its presence may take one or all of four forms. Meningeal cysticercosis is characterized by parasitic vesicles throughout the basal cisterns and CSF pathways, usually with resultant hydrocephalus. Parenchymal cysticercosis diffusely involves the brain, sometimes forming large cysts. Seizures and focal deficits are common. The ventricular variety resembles the meningeal form. Obstructive hydrocephalus is commonplace. Spinal cysticercosis may be intramedullary or extramedullary, producing either a transverse myelitis or a compressive myelopathy.

The diagnosis rests on serologic and radiologic testing. The presence of intracranial cysts and calcifications within skeletal muscle is often presumptive of the diagnosis. Praziquantel, an anthelmintic agent, is effective medical therapy for systemic infestation. Anticonvulsants, CSF shunting, and occasional removal of symptomatic cysts are additional treatment options.

Echinococcosis. Hydatid disease is caused by *Echinococcus granulosus*, the dog tapeworm. It is prevalent in southern South America, northern and eastern Europe, Australia, Africa, China, and the Middle East. Humans may serve as intermediate hosts by ingesting the larvae. The liver and lungs are preferentially involved through hematogenous dissemination with subsequent formation of hydatid cysts. When the CNS is involved, cysts are usually solitary, large, and confined to white matter. There is a negligible inflammatory response.

Most cysts produce signs and symptoms related to their mass effect. Diagnosis of the infection is made serologically. CT and MRI of the brain and ultrasonography of the liver and spleen may be definitive. Chest x-ray often shows calcified pulmonary cysts. Treatment consists of patient isolation from the source and surgical removal of symptomatic cysts. Care must be taken to remove the intact cyst to avoid seeding with viable larvae. Hydatid disease of the CNS is disabling, but rarely fatal, provided cysts are removed when they become symptomatic.

CONGENITAL AND DEVELOPMENTAL ABNORMALITIES

Approximately 2 percent of newborns possess some type of congenital abnormality. Sixty percent of these involve the central nervous system, and over half of those are related to defective development or closure of the dorsal midline structures. Many have associated hydrocephalus. The commonly encountered neurologic malformations are listed in Table 40-5.

Table 40-5
Congenital Neurologic Malformations

Arnold-Chiari malformation
Dandy-Walker malformation
Spinal dysraphism
    Meningocele
    Myelomeningocele
    Lipomyelomeningocele
    Diastematomyelia
    Dermal sinus
    Myeloschisis

Spinal Dysraphism

Between 18 and 28 days of embryonic development, the neural groove closes posteriorly in the midline to form the neural tube. This tube is encircled by bone derived from adjacent somites and is covered superficially by skin derived from ectoderm. Abnormal closure of the neural groove, failure of fusion of the adjacent bone, and/or maldevelopment of the overlying ectoderm can lead to a variety of spinal dysraphic states. Thus, dysraphism implies an abnormal fusion of normally united parts.

Failure of the bony structures to close with normal closure of the neural groove is called spina bifida occulta. Patients with this anomaly have a normal spinal cord and normal cord function. The abnormality usually is unnoticed unless seen on plain radiographs. If the meninges fail to close, a meningocele develops, producing a cutaneous abnormality. The underlying neural structures, however, develop normally, so there is no compromise of neurologic function.

Failure of the underlying neural tissue to fuse has been called spina bifida cystica, or more recently, spina bifida aperta. Myelomeningocele, the more common form, involves incomplete closure of the neural groove, usually in the lumbar region, with the abnormal, unfused neural tissue on the dorsal surface, exposed through an associated defect in the spinal column. This may be partially or totally covered with epithelium. The accompanying neurologic deficit usually consists of complete absence of motor and sensory function below the level of spinal cord involvement.

The most severe form of spinal dysraphism is myeloschisis, which is much less common than myelomeningocele. The spinal cord is unfused and presents directly on the surface of the back without overlying meninges or epithelium. It usually occurs at the thoracolumbar region and is virtually always associated with paraplegia and absence of bladder function.

Both myelomeningocele and myeloschisis are associated with hydrocephalus. Hydrocephalus is caused by a developmental abnormality of the hindbrain called Arnold-Chiari malformation, which is associated with the more severe forms of spinal dysraphism. This malformation is composed of caudal displacement of the cerebellar tonsils, vermis, inferior fourth ventricle, and medulla. There is a dorsal kink in the cervicomedullary junction and breaking of the quadrigeminal plate. Associated anomalies include agenesis of the corpus callosum and obstructive hydrocephalus.

The treatment of spinal dysraphism is surgical. Meningoceles are excised and the skin is closed primarily after watertight closure of the posterior meningeal defect. Myelomeningoceles and myeloschises are closed as early as possible to reduce the risk of superficial infection and subsequent meningitis. The goal is to preserve as much neural tissue as possible, untether the spinal cord from surrounding soft tissue, and fashion a dural closure to prevent CSF leakage. Accompanying hydrocephalus is treated by shunting.

Survival of infants with these dysraphic states continues to improve. Those newborns with lower-level lesions have better outcomes than those with higher lesions overall. The more severe the dysraphic state, the higher the morbidity and mortality. Risk of sepsis from bladder infection is reduced with intermittent catheterization when indicated. Timely revision of failed shunts placed for hydrocephalus preserves potential for intellectual development.

Cranial Dysraphism

Cranial dysraphic states are one-tenth as common as their spinal counterparts. Encephaloceles, although rare, are the most common manifestation. They consist of a midline skull defect through which a small portion of brain protrudes. Most encephaloceles are covered with skin, and only some 35 percent have associated hydrocephalus. Once believed to arise from defects in the closure of the primitive neural tube, they probably develop because of an overlying mesodermal abnormality, with subsequent perturbation of underlying cerebral tissue. In North America and Europe, 70 percent of encephaloceles occur in the posterior cranial vault; the remainder are found in the anterior cranial vault. In southeast Asia, this distribution is reversed for unknown reasons.

Surgical repair involves early resection of malformed and devitalized brain and dural closure. The mortality of patients with encephaloceles is extremely variable. Prognostic factors include the size and location of the anomaly, the extent of brain protrusion, and the presence of associated hydrocephalus, seizure disorder, or cerebral dysgenesis. The smaller and more anterior defects generally have a better outcome. Of those who survive, only 35 percent attain normal intelligence.

Hydrocephalus

The term hydrocephalus implies an increase in the amount of CSF within the ventricular system (Fig. 40-24). This is almost always due to a decrease in the absorption of fluid, although there are rare cases of choroid plexus papillomas causing hydrocephalus by an increase in CSF production. Hydrocephalus is traditionally classified as communicating and noncommunicating. In the former, the ventricular system continues to communicate with the subarachnoid spaces outside the brain through the fourth ventricular foramina of Luschka and Magendie. In the noncommunicating variety (often termed obstructive), it does not. The common causes of hydrocephalus vary with age and are listed in Table 40-6.

Infantile Hydrocephalus. Hydrocephalus occurs most frequently between birth and 2 years of age and is most commonly due to congenital abnormalities of the brain. These abnormalities typically produce noncommunicating hydrocephalus. Stenosis of the cerebral aqueduct is one such common congenital anomaly. Another is the Arnold-Chiari malformation, described earlier. The Dandy-Walker malformation produces a markedly enlarged fourth ventricle as a result of congenital obstruction of CSF outflow from the fourth ventricle, with resultant hydrocephalus. Other, less common congenital lesions include arachnoid cysts, vascular anomalies, and congenital tumors.

Acquired hydrocephalus in the infant is often the result of meningitis or intracranial hemorrhage, both potentially causing obstruction of either the CSF absorptive mechanism or the intraventricular pathways. Aqueductal stenosis may develop well after birth because of infection or hemorrhage and thus be considered "acquired." Tumors may also obstruct the outflow of CSF, resulting in noncommunicating hydrocephalus.

Infants with hydrocephalus usually, but not invariably, present with an enlarging head circumference. They often have a tense, bulging anterior fontanelle with distended scalp veins and split cranial sutures. They may appear to have "sun setting" of the eyes, with only the tops of the irises visible (Parinaud's syn-

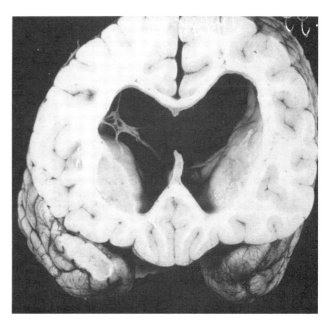

FIG. 40-24. Postmortem brain specimen, coronal section, showing hydrocephalus in a child.

drome). The head may transilluminate because of a lack of cerebral substance. Hydrocephalus usually does not impair the infant initially because the open cranial sutures allow for cranial vault expansion. In the more chronic forms, or in older infants with closed sutures, papilledema, optic atrophy, and VIth nerve palsies may be seen.

Childhood Hydrocephalus. Hydrocephalus in children over 2 years of age may have a more acute presentation because of the decreased ability of the more mature brain and skull to accommodate the increase in CSF. Consequently, raised intracranial pressure may cause headache, nausea, vomiting, lethargy, coma, and even death. Slower onset may result in decreased mentation, behavioral changes, diminished performance in school, VIth nerve palsies, optic atrophy, paralysis of upward gaze, spastic leg weakness, and endocrine (hypothalamic) disorders. Causes of hydrocephalus in this age group include tumors, meningitis, intracranial hemorrhage (both spontaneous and traumatic), and aqueductal stenosis. Ventricular shunt malfunction can cause acute hydrocephalus in the shunt-dependent patient, regardless of the patient's age or the underlying cause of the hydrocephalus.

Adult Hydrocephalus. Hydrocephalus in adults may also result from obstructive tumors, meningitis, and intracranial hem-

Table 40-6
Causes of Hydrocephalus

Congenital	Acquired
Arnold-Chiari malformation	Infectious meningitis
Dandy-Walker malformation	Infectious ventriculitis
Aqueductal atresia/stenosis	Late-onset aqueductal stenosis
Developmental cyst	Intraventricular hemorrhage
Encephalocele	Subarachnoid hemorrhage
Neoplasm	Neoplasm

orrhage, but it may also be more insidious in onset. An entity called normal pressure hydrocephalus occurs in the older population, involving a communicating hydrocephalus with relatively normal intraventricular pressure. The cause remains unknown but is thought to be due to subclinical hemorrhage or infection in the patient's remote past and malabsorption of CSF. The classic symptom triad of ataxia, urinary incontinence, and failing mentation suggests the diagnosis. Treatment is by ventricular fluid shunting.

Regardless of the cause, the treatment of hydrocephalus is essentially the same. Either the cause must be removed (e.g., tumor) or a shunting procedure must be performed to divert accumulated CSF. Sometimes both measures are necessary. The most commonly used procedure is a lateral ventricle to peritoneal cavity shunt with a one-way pressure-regulating valve in the system. If the peritoneal cavity is not suitable for shunting, the distal catheter may be placed in the right atrium of the heart or in the pleural cavity. In selected cases of communicating hydrocephalus, a lumbar subarachnoid to peritoneal shunt may be used. Common complications of indwelling shunts include shunt obstruction and infection.

Craniosynostosis

Craniosynostosis is the premature closure of one or more cranial sutures, typically manifested within the first 6 months of life. Since the brain doubles in size during the first 6 months of life and grows another 50 percent by age two, the cranial sutures must remain open to allow for skull expansion to accommodate this growth. Usually, when one suture fuses prematurely, the brain is not compressed significantly, but the skull will then develop in a distinctly abnormal shape. If more than one suture is fused, brain growth may be restricted.

The sagittal suture fuses prematurely most often. The skull then develops an elongated shape with a narrow biparietal diameter, often referred to as scaphocephaly. The supraorbital ridge may be square-shaped due to overexpansion of the open metopic suture. Associated congenital anomalies are rare.

The next most common suture to be involved is the coronal, which may close prematurely on one or both sides. Unilateral involvement produces an asymmetrically shaped forehead with flattening on the affected side and compensatory enlargement on the opposite side. This is called plagiocephaly and is not usually associated with other abnormalities. Bilateral coronal synostosis produces a more severe foreshortening of the entire anterior fossa and is often manifested by shallow orbits with exophthalmos and hypertelorism. This entity is often associated with inherited congenital disorders such as Crouzon's disease and Apert's and Carpenter's syndromes.

Less common forms of craniosynostosis include premature closure of the lambdoid suture or the metopic suture. With unilateral synostosis of the lambdoid suture, the skull appears flattened in the affected occipital area, which may be confused with birth molding. With premature closure of the metopic suture, the forehead assumes a triangular shape (trigonocephaly). Neither of these forms is associated with other congenital anomalies.

The treatment of craniosynostosis is surgical and generally involves the opening of the affected suture along its entire length. This should be carried out as soon as possible after the diagnosis is made, since early surgical intervention provides the best cosmetic result. In cases of multiple suture involvement, prompt treatment provides early skull expansion to accommodate brain growth.

NEUROSURGICAL MANAGEMENT OF PAIN

The majority of neurosurgical patients have pain, either as their primary complaint or as a secondary manifestation of their disease process. Painful conditions can be categorized as acute processes, such as arm pain from a herniated cervical disc, or chronic processes, such as extremity pain from an invasive neoplasm. For most acute pain states, the cause can be identified and treated, but for chronic pain there is often no ready solution. In this section, the more common neurosurgical procedures available to manage chronic pain will be described.

At one time, the perception of pain was thought to involve a relatively simple system of pathways extending from the peripheral receptors to the brain. It has since been shown that this system is an extremely complex network of pathways, with a considerable amount of modification at multiple synaptic levels. Impulses from pain receptors reach the spinal cord via the dorsal root ganglion and may be significantly modified in the various laminae of the dorsal horn. This information is then relayed to the thalamus, but again may undergo considerable modification in the area of the brainstem reticular formation. This sensory input is subsequently relayed to the cortex for conscious interpretation. Modifiers in this complex system include the endogenous substances endorphins, enkephalins, and substance P. In addition, the psychologic state of the patient influences the perception of painful stimuli.

Traditionally, neurosurgical procedures for chronic pain have been ablative or destructive, but a variety of neuromodulating or stimulating procedures have been developed in recent years. These procedures are generally reserved for those chronic pain conditions that have failed medical therapy.

Cerebrum. In general, few painful states warrant procedures involving the cerebral hemispheres or deep brain nuclei. Bilateral rostral cingulotomies have been performed for treatment of intractable pain. This procedure disrupts the cingulum, a large fasciculus running deep to the cingulate gyrus. It has proved useful for affective disorders involving pain when performed bilaterally.

As the primary relay station for pain impulses, the thalamus has been the target for stereotaxic ablative procedures. Thalamotomies are performed with considerable accuracy and have been used for thalamic pain disorders, phantom limb pain, and pain from invasive tumors. More recently, deep brain electrodes have been placed for stimulation rather than ablation of these structures. In general, thalamic stimulation has proved useful in patients suffering from deafferentation pain, pain that typically does not respond to opiates. Conversely, brainstem stimulation is successful in chronic painful states that are responsive to opiates. Long-term success (control of pain for a minimum of 2 years) is reported to be about 60 and 80 percent for the respective groups.

Cranial Nerves. Trigeminal neuralgia (tic douloureux) is one of the more commonly occurring neuropathic painful conditions. It presents as an intermittent, shocklike pain in one or more divisions of one trigeminal nerve. It most commonly involves the second (maxillary) and/or third (mandibular) division of the nerve and is rarely bilateral. The pain usually lasts for seconds but is extremely severe and may be incapacitating. It is often triggered by touching the face, talking, or chewing. The pain may be present for weeks or months, then spontaneously disappear, only to return with increased severity. For most patients the pain can be controlled initially with phenytoin or carbamazepine, but eventually many will require surgical intervention. A small percentage of patients may have a posterior fossa tumor causing the pain, so evaluation should include a CT or MRI scanning before therapy.

In the past, surgical treatment involved ablation of the involved branch(es) of the trigeminal nerve. This could be accomplished peripherally by surgical section or alcohol ablation of the supraorbital, infraorbital, or inferior alveolar nerves. Pain control through these neurectomies was usually short-lived, however. Experience showed that preganglionic lesions must be made for more permanent relief. Retrogasserian rhizotomy is now carried out by open surgical approaches subtemporally or through the posterior fossa, or percutaneously by placing a radiofrequency electrode through the foramen ovale into the ganglion.

A nonablative approach involves microvascular decompression of the trigeminal nerve in the posterior fossa. The theory behind this approach is that trigeminal neuralgia is caused by external pressure on the nerve by vascular structures (an artery or vein) near its entry into the brainstem. With the use of the operating microscope, the offending artery can be moved or the vein ablated, thus decompressing the nerve. This procedure has a high success rate but carries more risk than the percutaneous method. An advantage is that the nerve's function remains intact.

Spinal Cord. Just like other surgical procedures for chronic pain, those involving the spinal cord have traditionally been ablative. Cordotomy, designed to obliterate the spinothalamic tract (see Fig. 40-3), can be performed by open operation or percutaneously. Anterolateral cordotomy may provide excellent temporary relief of pain for patients with terminal malignancies, but it is rarely effective for chronic benign conditions such as low back, postherpetic, or phantom limb pain.

For selected cases of severe pain of peripheral nerve origin, such as brachial plexus injury, postherpetic neuralgia, traumatic limb amputation, and root avulsion, ablative lesions can be made at the dorsal root entry zones (DREZ) of the spinal cord. These lesions are made with a radiofrequency lesion generator or laser through an open exposure of the cord via a laminectomy. Several levels are usually included. About 50 percent of patients obtain good relief from pain.

Chronic pain that develops in chest, flank, or abdominal incisions may warrant an ablative procedure. Since these regions do not contain critical sensory areas, unilateral dorsal nerve roots may be sectioned to deprive the involved area of sensation. It is necessary to ablate at least three adjacent levels in order to denervate one dermatome adequately because of overlapping sensory distribution. Dorsal rhizotomy may be carried out openly through a laminectomy or percutaneously through radiofrequency thermocoagulation. Pain relief from rhizotomy is good initially, then less so as time passes.

Intrathecal morphine can be given temporarily or permanently by infusion of small but effective doses. This newer method of pain control is particularly effective in debilitated patients with terminal illnesses. The procedure involves the sub-

cutaneous implantation of a constant infusion pump that can be recharged periodically.

In chronic painful states of nonmalignant spinal origin, such as low back and/or leg pain, a nonablative neuromodulation technique may play a role in therapy. This involves transcutaneous excitatory nerve stimulation (TENS), which "blocks" nerve conduction of pain impulses. It is simple, safe, and relatively inexpensive. Electrodes are taped to the skin, usually over the region of the pain or directly over the affected major nerve, and then connected to a small, portable stimulating device. The device has a variable pulse width, frequency, and amplitude, which the patient can adjust in order to achieve maximum pain relief. Use of this device for a brief time often provides long-lasting relief with no untoward side effects. Direct stimulation of the spinal cord by surgically implanted electrodes combined with percutaneous telemetry can also provide relief from chronic pain.

Peripheral Nerve. Pain from a partial or complete nerve injury usually involves the nerve's sensory distribution but may include the whole extremity. Chronic pain developing after an amputation may be present in the remaining portion of the limb at the site of the amputation ("stump pain") or in the nonexistent amputated portion ("phantom pain"). The causation of the pain may be related to the sensory component of the nerve or to its associated sympathetic nerve supply.

With partial or complete peripheral nerve transection, a painful neuroma may form. The usual treatment is excision of the neuroma, with prevention of recurrent formation by burying the nerve end in bone or muscle or wrapping it in tantalum or Silastic. Neuromodulation techniques may also be applied in cases of painful neuromas.

Chronic pain resulting from peripheral nerve injury may be significantly altered by interruption of the sympathetic nerve supply to the affected extremity. The classic example of this dysautonomic state is major causalgia. This term implies a partial injury to a major nerve in an extremity. Minor causalgia is reserved for an injury to a more distal minor sensory nerve, which may also become a source of significant pain. It is also well recognized that a dysautonomic state may be created by major or minor trauma to an extremity that does not involve a peripheral nerve. This has been termed major or minor traumatic dystrophy. The entire collection of causalgias and traumatic dystrophies makes up a syndrome called reflex sympathetic dystrophy.

Major causalgia is most commonly related to partial injury of the sciatic or the median nerve. Typically, symptoms begin in the affected nerve's distribution but may progress to involve the whole extremity. The extremity first becomes swollen, warm, erythematous, and quite sensitive to touch. With time, it becomes cool and pale. Hyperhidrosis (excessive sweating) may follow. Due to lack of joint motion, the normal flexion and extension creases disappear and the skin becomes smooth and flat. Plain radiographs may demonstrate osteoporosis. Eventually the extremity may become completely useless. A constant, burning pain develops and persists throughout these various stages. It may be exacerbated by touching or moving the extremity. Even temperature changes and emotional stress can trigger worsening of pain. Minor causalgia and the traumatic dystrophies may be accompanied by similar, but less severe symptoms.

The treatment of these dysautonomic states is complex. They may be helped by disruption of the sympathetic nerve supply to the extremity. Sympathetic denervation may be extremely rewarding in major causalgia but is less so in minor causalgia and the traumatic dystrophies.

Less severe and more easily treated pain may arise from chronic compression of selected peripheral nerves. The most common are compression of the median nerve at the wrist (carpal tunnel syndrome) and compression of the ulnar nerve at the elbow. Chronic compression may result in pain, paresthesias, numbness, and eventually weakness and atrophy of muscles in the distribution of the affected nerve. These compression syndromes are diagnosed clinically and confirmed by finding denervation and slowed nerve conduction on electromyography and nerve conduction velocity testing. Treatment is surgical decompression of the involved nerve, with prompt and long-lasting relief in most cases.

EPILEPSY AND MOVEMENT DISORDERS

Epilepsy. That removal of specific areas of the brain can cure epilepsy has been known for many years. Inadequate diagnostic tools and poorly defined indications for surgery, however, precluded widespread use of surgery to treat the disease. About 2 million people in the United States have epilepsy, and most undergo treatment for it. Most varieties of epilepsy can be categorized into either generalized (grand mal) seizures characterized by loss of consciousness with tonic/clonic movements, or partial seizures manifested by involuntary movements but no loss of consciousness. Epilepsy can be controlled fairly well by available medications in about 80 percent of patients. Of the remaining 20 percent, nearly 100,000 may benefit from available surgical procedures. Interest in surgical management of epilepsy has increased significantly in recent years because of the availability of accurate physiologic localization of seizure foci and high-quality imaging of the brain by CT, MRI, and PET scanning.

Epilepsy has many etiologies. Congenital anomalies of the brain are relatively common causes in the pediatric age group. Birth injury is also a well-known precursor of seizure disorders in children. Neoplasms and vascular anomalies, including arteriovenous malformations, are common seizure sources in adults. A large number of adults have epilepsy because of mesial temporal sclerosis, a condition that probably results from hypoxia and/or hypermetabolic states during early development of the brain. Some seizures have no known cause.

Patients can be tested effectively in order to select those who can clearly benefit from surgery. Electroencephalography and MRI are initial monitoring tools. More invasive monitoring involves recordings from depth electrodes placed stereotactically and subdural electrodes placed by open craniotomy. Specific foci can be identified with prolonged monitoring using video recording coupled with continuous EEG monitoring. Areas of brain that serve specific functions such as speech and motor/sensory functions can also be identified by specific tests, including PET scanning and functional MRI.

Operation is planned once a focus has been identified that is amenable to surgical resection without undue risk. Often seizure surgery is performed with the patient under local anesthesia. Electrocorticography, which is similar to electroencephalography except that it is performed directly from brain cortex, can further identify the focus of seizures at the time of operation. Stimulation of brain is also used to map the cortex and to identify regions that subserve speech, vision, and sensory/motor functions.

Outcomes of seizure surgery today are often gratifying. Many patients with uncontrolled epilepsy are not able to function in society because of their seizures. About half of those who have uncontrolled seizures can be made seizure-free by surgical techniques. Another one-quarter can have significant reduction in both seizure frequency and seizure intensity by surgical therapy.

Movement disorders. Movement disorders result from a variety of central nervous system diseases and are manifested by abnormal volitional movement. Typical examples are the resting (or "pill-rolling") tremor of Parkinson's disease and the intention tremor that accompanies volitional movement as a consequence of cerebellar disorders. Many treatments have been used since these conditions were first recognized, but most have been ineffective. Because of advances in neurophysiology, neuropharmacology, neuropathology, and anatomic imaging during this century, the balance between excitatory and inhibitory effectors of movement has come to be better understood, and the imbalance responsible for abnormal volitional movements better explained. Improvements in both medical and surgical treatments have resulted.

The symptoms of Parkinson's disease, characterized by resting tremor, cogwheel rigidity, and bradykinesia, were not effectively controlled until it was known that there is a dopamine deficiency in the substantia nigra resulting in inhibition of the voluntary initiation of movement. Dopamine supplements were then developed, and symptoms were often improved.

Surgical treatment began in the 1950s with ablative lesions of the basal ganglia designed to interrupt imbalanced inhibitory/excitatory circuitry and its effect on movement coordination. An ablative lesion in the globus pallidus, called pallidotomy, was not very effective at first, though it did seem to help rigidity and bradykinesia. Similarly, thalamotomy proved to have a modestly beneficial effect on tremor. Neither operation was used extensively because medical treatment, particularly with dopaminergic agents, was generally effective.

Stereotactic methods, particularly pallidotomy, have become popular because medical therapy has not remained effective in many patients over the long term. Escalating doses of medication have often been necessary to control parkinsonism, resulting in widely fluctuating symptoms and signs. Patients who have resting tremor without bradykinesia are considered for thalamotomy, and those with rigidity, bradykinesia, and gaze and balance difficulties are candidates for pallidotomy.

Other movement disorders that respond to ablative lesions in the basal ganglia include essential tremor, intention tremor of multiple sclerosis, and the choreiform movements of Huntington's disease. Hemiballismus and hereditary dystonia can also be treated by stereotactic lesions in the basal ganglia.

RADIOSURGERY

Radiosurgery is a highly focused ionizing radiation derived from an external source delivered to a stereotactically defined intracranial target. Treatment of lesions in the depths of the brain by focused radiosurgery began about 20 years ago. The technique, using the so-called "gamma knife," allows delivery of radiation to a specific target from a variety of sources, ablating the target without significant adverse effects on tissue surrounding it. In some instances, the technique is delivered by fixed cobalt sources delivering photon radiation to the target, aided by a stereotactic frame attached to the patient's head and a computer program coupling the radiation source to the frame on the patient. Identification of the intracranial target is made by CT or MRI scanning, using a computer to relate the target to the stereotactic frame and the patient within it. Other systems involve a similar principle, but the radiation source, delivered by linear accelerator, moves around a fixed target.

Currently radiosurgery is given in a single dose requiring little or no time in the hospital. Fractionated treatments using radiosurgery are being developed, reducing the risk of treatment and increasing its effectiveness. Radiosurgery is used for a variety of conditions, including arteriovenous malformations and neoplasms, and is particularly adaptable to deep intracerebral lesions. It causes sclerosis of vascular structures, resulting in progressive occlusion of arteries, such as those within arteriovenous malformations, and cell necrosis in tumors. Radiosurgery can gradually ablate small to medium-sized arteriovenous malformations with 85 percent efficacy over a 2- to 3-year follow-up period.

Radiosurgery is also used to treat neoplasms, including intracranial schwannomas and meningiomas. In both instances the target is usually well defined and adjacent brain is not involved.

A tumoricidal dose can be delivered in a single shot without significant adverse affects on surrounding tissue. Collimation of the beam allows it to be shaped to fit the anatomic dimensions of the target lesion.

The role of radiosurgery in other tumors, such as metastatic tumors and gliomas, is uncertain at this time. It is probable that metastatic intracerebral lesions will be treated more by this technique in the future because it is relatively noninvasive, and it is probably as effective as surgery for small lesions. Larger lesions are less well suited to radiosurgery because they would require radiation doses larger than can be delivered safely.

Bibliography

Crockard A, Hayward R, Hoff JT (eds): *Neurosurgery: The Scientific Basis of Clinical Practice,* 2d ed. Oxford, Blackwell Scientific Publications, 1992, p 993.

Menezes AH, Sonntag VKH (eds): *Principles of Spinal Surgery,* New York, McGraw-Hill, 1996, p 1525.

Schmidek HH, Sweet WH (eds): *Operative Neurosurgical Techniques: Indications, Methods, and Results,* 3d ed. Philadelphia, WB Saunders, 1995, p 2196.

Wilkins RH, Rengachary SS (eds): *Neurosurgery,* 2d ed. New York, McGraw-Hill, 1996, p 4272.

Youmans JR (ed): *Neurological Surgery,* 4th ed. Philadelphia, Saunders, 1996, p 3729.

CHAPTER 41

Orthopaedics

Randy N. Rosier

GENERAL CONSIDERATIONS

Pain

Anatomy and Physiology. *Definition.* The International Association for the Study of Pain defines pain as "an unpleasant sensory and emotional experience associated with actual or potential tissue damage, or described in terms of such damage." Afferent nociceptive impulses produced by injurious stimulation are transmitted to the central nervous system, where they are given meaning by the perceptual state of the individual. The perceptions of pain are modified by many factors, including past and present experience, state of awareness, concomitant sensory stimuli, and emotional status. Stimulation of peripheral receptors by noxious agents produces a spatiotemporal pattern of nervous impulses that is interpreted as pain within the higher cerebral centers. Teleologically, pain serves the useful function of prevention of tissue damage and is a homeostatic mechanism. It is only in the postoperative setting or when pain becomes chronic that it serves no useful function. Acute pain implies the presence of actual tissue damage or its potential unless the noxious stimulus is removed; it may be associated with autonomic hyperactivity such as hypertension, tachycardia, sweating, and vasoconstriction. Chronic pain implies the absence of a threat of tissue damage yet is described in terms of such damage (discomfort, suffering). Generally pain is considered to be chronic when its duration exceeds 3 to 6 months.

Transduction. Pain is initiated by a stimulus that is detected by nociceptors *(transduction)* and is the most common manifestation of disorders of the musculoskeletal system. Pain can be produced by a wide variety of physical phenomena, including pressure, puncturing, squeezing, tension, and extremes of temperature, and by chemical effects such as change of pH or release of polypeptide mediators, including histamine-like substances, serotonin, bradykinin, and other polypeptides. Prostaglandins may lower the pain threshold for some stimuli, and inflammation accompanied by local acidosis can enhance perception of pain. In addition, a number of local peptide mediators such as substance P are released at sites of injurious stimuli and trigger patterns of nervous activity interpreted as pain.

Transmission. Most cutaneous sensory nerve endings consist of unmyelinated fibers, which produce sensations of pressure, touch, or pain, depending on the impulse pattern invoked. These nerve endings are found also in periosteum, arteries, joint capsules, and synovium, with similar myelinated fibers in muscle. The signal is then transmitted via sensory afferent nerve fibers and dorsal root ganglia to the spinal cord. The smaller-diameter myelinated A-delta and unmyelinated C afferent fibers are those primarily responsible for pain transmission (Table 41-1). Synapses in the dorsal horn interact with other afferents as well as the spinoreticular pathway and transmit information via the spinothalamic tract to the thalamus and somatosensory cortex.

Modulation. Modulation of the nociceptive information occurs in the dorsal horn through a number of neurotransmitters (Fig. 41-1). Descending modulating systems are generally inhibitory and are influenced by multiple factors, including emotional state. Endogenous opioid systems (enkephalins and endorphins) regulate descending modulatory activity, and multiple opioid receptors for these substances have been identified in the central and peripheral nervous system. These same receptors are responsible for the inhibitory effects of opioid analgesics on pain level.

Additional modulation may occur within the dorsal horn, according to the gate theory of pain proposed by Melzack and Wall (Fig. 41-2). This hypothesis involves interactive influences of myelinated and unmyelinated fibers within the dorsal horn, determining the net level of nociceptive output of the transmission cells. Both fiber types are thought to directly excite the transmission cell, while they have opposing effects on the interneurons in the substantia gelatinosa, which also regulate the level of transmission-cell activity. Transcutaneous electrical nerve stimulation as a pain control method is based on this hypothesis, and its efficacy supports the gate theory of pain. Selective stimulation of large-diameter myelinated afferents blocks pain, since

Table 41-1
Peripheral Nerve Fibers

Fiber Type	Diameter	Location	Function
A-alpha	15–25 μm	Myelinated afferents and efferents to muscles and joints	Motor, proprioception
A-beta	15–25 μm	Myelinated afferents and efferents to muscles and joints	Motor, proprioception
A-gamma	15–25 μm	Myelinated efferents to muscle spindles	Muscle tone
A-delta	15–25 μm	Myelinated sensory afferents	Pain, temperature, touch
B	<2 μm	Myelinated preganglionic sympathetic	Autonomic
C (80%)	5–15 μm	Unmyelinated sensory afferents	Pain, temperature, touch
C (20%)	5–15 μm	Unmyelinated postganglionic sympathetic	Autonomic

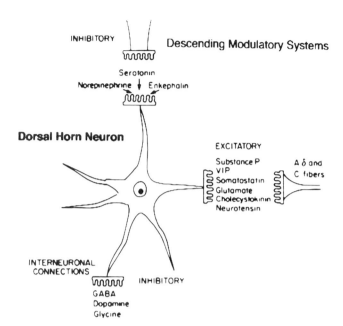

FIG. 41-1. Modulation of pain signals in the dorsal horn of the spinal cord. (Modified from: *Orthopaedic Knowledge Update 3. Park Ridge, IL, American Academy of Orthopaedic Surgeons, 1990, with permission.*)

REFERRED PAIN

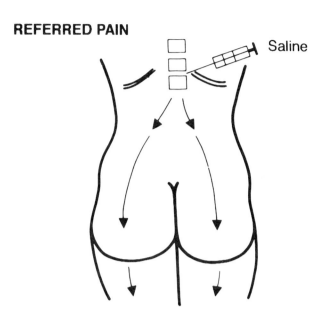

FIG. 41-3. Referred pain radiation after saline injection into the supraspinous ligament. (Modified from: *MacNab I: Backache. Baltimore, Williams & Wilkins, 1979, with permission.*)

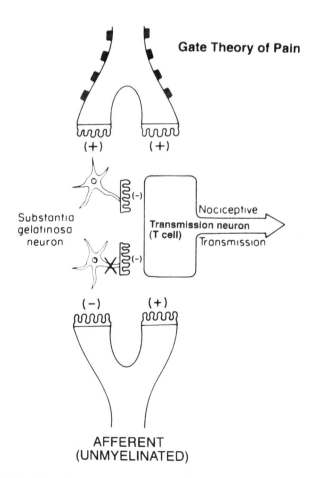

FIG. 41-2. The gate theory of pain. (Adapted from: *Melzack and Wall: Pain mechanisms: A new theory. Science 150:971, 1965.*)

the unmyelinated A-delta and C pain fibers have a high electrical threshold and remain unstimulated. This technique is innocuous, noninvasive, and of great benefit to some patients with postoperative or chronic pain.

Perception. The endpoint in the pain pathway is its *perception* by the patient. Pain occurs with various qualities, such as aching, burning, spasmodic, radiating, lancinating, dull, or sharp. Local pain is felt at the site of injury, while diffuse pain appears to be more characteristic of deep structures, and radicular pain radiates along peripheral nerve pathways, often in association with neurologic deficits such as sensory or motor loss. Referred pain occurs in a location remote from the site of tissue pathology, and represents a misplaced cortical pain perception. Common examples include knee pain as a manifestation of hip joint pathology, and gluteal or posterior thigh and leg pain as a manifestation of spinal pathology. Referred pain tends to follow spinal segmental innervation and must be differentiated from radicular pain. For instance, injection of saline into interspinous ligaments has been demonstrated to cause referred gluteal and lower extremity pain (Fig. 41-3). Radicular pain, however, will follow specific dermatomal distributions.

Tissue Patterns. *Bone.* Bone is not thought to have any sensory endings within it, although the periosteum is richly innervated with both myelinated and unmyelinated nerve endings. Small unmyelinated fibers have been identified in association with blood vessels within bone and probably are sympathetic fibers responsible for bone blood flow regulation. Bony lesions such as tumors or infections cause a deep, boring type of pain that may result from pressure sensation mediated by blood vessel-associated fibers; pain from fractures, in contrast, has a sharper quality and is characteristically relieved by rest.

Muscle/Tendon. Muscle pain may result from direct injury, overuse or chemical irritation from metabolites such as lactic acid resulting from tissue anoxia. Types of local injury causing pain include contusion, partial or complete tendon or muscle rupture, excessive stretch or load under tension (muscle strain), and inflammatory disorders (e.g., myositis). Muscle injury usually is characterized by tenderness of the muscle to palpation and soreness aggravated by movement or voluntary contraction of the muscle. *Muscle spasm* refers to a sustained involuntary muscle contraction, which can cause severe, paroxysmal cramp-like pain and is a common response to muscle injury. Spasm also can result from injury to the innervation of a muscle, as in sciatica, or from metabolic abnormalities such as hypocalcemia, alkalosis, or the presence of toxins such as tetanus. Myalgia, or aching pain in muscle, can occur as a symptom of systemic viral infections, or in association with chronic idiopathic disorders such as fibrositis or fibromyalgia.

Ischemia of muscle causes regional lactic acidosis, which can produce aching pain. More severe degrees of ischemia, usually associated with significant trauma such as fractures, but occasionally seen with excessive exertion, can result in a *compartment syndrome*. Given that muscle is bounded by inelastic fascial compartment coverings, ischemia that causes muscle swelling can result in elevated tissue pressure within muscle compartments, which in turn impedes vascular inflow and starts a vicious cycle of worsening ischemia. The result is severe pain out of proportion to the severity of the initial injury as well as pain with passive stretch of the muscle(s) involved. Emergent surgical release of involved compartments is required to prevent permanent muscle and nerve damage in this condition.

Tendon-related pain is most commonly seen with tendinitis, an inflammation of the tendon and associated sheath (paratenon). Tendinitis usually is a result of overuse, and as such it may reflect the result of mechanical disruption of some of the collagen fibers in a tendon. Common sites include the rotator cuff tendons of the shoulder, the tendons about the wrist, the patellar tendon, and the Achilles tendon. Local tenderness and swelling result, and the pain is generally invoked by contraction of the associated muscle. Tendinitis may presage a rupture of the involved tendon, occasionally seen with the Achilles, patellar, and rotator cuff tendons, and with the tenosynovitis of rheumatoid arthritis in the hand and wrist. Treatment usually involves rest of the affected area and anti-inflammatory medication. Ruptures require surgical repair, and persistent tendinitis may require surgical removal of mechanical causes or tenosynovectomy.

Joint. Joint pain may result from hyperemia or inflammation of synovium, joint effusion producing capsular distention, instability causing traction on capsular or ligamentous structures, or degeneration of articular cartilage. Cartilage is avascular and lacks nerve endings, indicating that pain resulting from cartilage injury or degeneration originates in the underlying bone or adjacent capsule and synovium via secondary mediators.

Neurogenic Pain. Peripheral nerves may cause pain in response to pressure, ischemia, stretching, herpes zoster infection, toxins (lead, arsenic), or metabolic disturbances (vitamin deficiencies, diabetic or alcoholic neuropathies). A characteristic of neurogenic pain is its radicular nature and association with neurologic symptoms such as paresthesias, sensory or motor loss, and secondary muscle atrophy. Hyperesthetic pain may be encountered with herpes zoster infection or Guillain-Barré syndrome, or during axonal recovery from mechanical injury. HIV infection also has been identified as a cause of chronic peripheral neuropathic pain.

Treatment. The mechanism of action of many of the commonly used nonnarcotic analgesics is unknown. Multiple receptors that respond to narcotic medications as well as endogenous analgesics (endorphins) have been identified. For chronic pain from conditions that are not life threatening, efforts are made to avoid the use of narcotics because of the potential for progressive dependence and development of tolerance to the drugs. Nonsteroidal anti-inflammatory and analgesic drugs are useful, and for chronic neurogenic pain antidepressants (amitriptyline) and anticonvulsants (carbamazepine) may be useful.

Postoperatively, patient-controlled analgesia techniques, wherein the patient can self-administer intravenous narcotic medications at low doses as needed, are widely used. This method not only gives better and more even relief of postoperative pain but also has been shown to decrease the total amount of medication needed. The use of epidural anesthesia for surgical procedures also allows the use of the epidural catheter postoperatively for pain control. Local anesthetics or narcotics can be used in conjunction with a pump to deliver minute doses of the agents directly to the epidural space around the spinal cord, usually with total relief of pain.

Implantable subcutaneous or epidural pumps also are useful for continuous delivery of opioids in patients with severe chronic pain such as those with metastatic cancer or AIDS. In selected cases of chronic severe pain involving an extremity, neural ablations with injections of alcohol or phenol have been used successfully to improve pain control.

The topical analgesic capsaicin, which is thought to deplete local tissue stores of substance P, has been used successfully for pain from arthritis and from herpes zoster infection.

Upper Extremity

Wrist and Hand. Radiocarpal, carpometacarpal, metacarpophalangeal, and interphalangeal arthritides frequently cause pain in the region of the wrist and hand, usually with swelling and stiffness of the affected joints. Additional causes include tendinitis, de Quervain's disease, compression of the median nerve at the wrist beneath the transverse carpal ligament (carpal tunnel syndrome), compression of the ulnar nerve beneath the volar carpal ligament (ulnar tunnel syndrome), or radicular pain from compression of these nerves at a more proximal level. Such neurogenic pain can be accompanied by sensory or motor deficits, and when associated with vasomotor trophic changes can indicate the presence of a reflex sympathetic dystrophy (RSD). RSD, which can occur in the upper or the lower extremity after an injury or surgery, is a sustained abnormal reflex caused by efferent activity arising from sympathetic nerves (Fig. 41-4). When the inciting injury is known to involve a major nerve trunk, it is referred to as *causalgia*. The pain typically is described as burning in character, and there is associated hyperesthesia and dysesthesia (painful response to normally nonpainful stimuli), swelling, joint stiffness, vasomotor instability, and marked osteopenia in the region (Sudeck's atrophy). In the upper extremity, adhesive capsulitis of the shoulder may occur with RSD of the hand (shoulder-hand syndrome). Regional sympathetic blockade aids in diagnosis as well as treatment by breaking the reflex arc, and physical therapy and corticosteroids may be helpful.

Afferent Limb

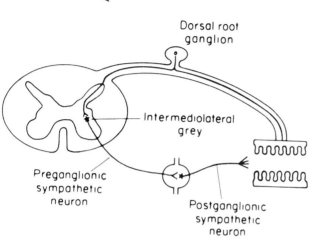

FIG. 41-4. The cycle of reflex sympathetic dystrophy. (Modified from: *Orthopaedic Knowledge Update 3. Park Ridge, IL, American Academy of Orthopaedic Surgeons, 1990, with permission.*)

Elbow. The most common causes of elbow pain are medial or lateral epicondylitis ("golfer's elbow" and "tennis elbow," respectively), arthritis of the elbow joint, and compression neuropathy of the ulnar nerve at the elbow (cubital tunnel syndrome). Treatment is rest, anti-inflammatory medication, and, in refractory cases, surgical release of the affected muscle origin or nerve decompression.

Shoulder. Common causes of shoulder pain include arthritis of the glenohumeral or acromioclavicular joints and impingement syndrome, in which tendinitis and bursitis of the rotator cuff result from impingement of these structures on the coracoacromial ligament. Forward elevation and internal rotation (impingement test) bring the supraspinatus tendon in contact with the coracoacromial ligament, reproducing the pain. Injection of lidocaine and cortisone in the subacromial bursa is helpful diagnostically and therapeutically. In refractory cases, anterior excision of the acromion and coracoacromial ligament (Neer acromioplasty) may be helpful. Impingement chronically can lead to rotator cuff tears, the majority of which can be managed conservatively. Persistent symptoms or complete rupture in a young person are indications for rotator cuff repair. Diagnosis of these lesions is aided by arthrography and magnetic resonance imaging (MRI) scans. Bicipital tendinitis also can present with anterior activity-related shoulder pain, with local tenderness and pain with resisted biceps muscle contraction. Conservative treatment usually suffices. Occasionally rupture of the tendon of the long head of the biceps can occur, particularly in association with impingement syndrome and rotator cuff pathology.

Cervical Origin. Cervical arthritis or nerve root irritation from osteophytes or disc herniations can cause both referred and radicular pain in the shoulder area. In addition, visceral pathology in the heart, lungs, or pleura can be referred to the shoulder or arm. Brachialgia (brachial neuralgia) is characterized by upper extremity pain associated with paresthesias, altered sensation, weakness, and reflex changes in a radicular distribution of the brachial plexus. Occasionally sympathetic plexus disturbances are seen, with vertigo, tinnitus, or visual disturbances. Causes of brachialgia include tumors of the spinal cord or nerve roots, infections, disc herniation, brachial plexus trauma, Pancoast's tumor of the apex of the lung, congenital anomalies of the cord such as syringomyelia, and cervical vertebral subluxations or dislocations. Another possible cause of brachialgia is the thoracic outlet syndrome, in which compression of the brachial plexus and vascular outflow obstruction can result from cervical ribs, anomalous fibrous bands within the scalene muscles, or changes caused by trauma to the clavicle or scalenes. Scalene muscle or rib resection can improve the symptoms if conservative measures fail. Differential diagnosis of the causes of cervical and shoulder pain is aided by radiographs to delineate bony abnormalities, and by computed tomography (CT) or MRI, which can demonstrate both bony and soft-tissue pathology. Cervical strain syndrome (whiplash injury) can result from rapid acceleration or deceleration of the head and is common in motor vehicle accidents. Pain typically is present in the cervical area and often is also referred to the shoulder and arm. Treatment is conservative, with a cervical collar for rest and appropriate medications followed by a cervical isometric exercise program, and, in refractory cases, intermittent cervical traction.

Cervical Disc Disease. Cervical disc herniations most commonly occur at the C4–C6 levels, the region responsible for the majority of flexion/extension motion in the cervical spine. Degenerative changes in the discs or trauma can cause herniation of the gelatinous nucleus pulposus through the annulus fibrosus, allowing impingement on nerve roots or the spinal cord. Neck pain and radicular pain in the distribution of the involved root level(s) can result. Symptoms may be unilateral or bilateral, depending on whether the herniation is central or lateral; in some cases central herniations can cause cord symptoms such as Brown-Séquard syndrome, hyperreflexia below the lesion, incontinence, and gait disturbances. Lateral herniations are the most common, with corresponding local and radicular symptoms. Local paraspinous muscle spasm is common, with rigidity and pain with motion. Vertical compression, particularly with head tilt to the affected side, exacerbates the symptoms, and vertical traction tends to diminish them. Depending on the affected level, the brachioradialis, biceps, or triceps reflexes may be depressed (C5, C6, or C7, respectively), and corresponding muscle weakness or dermatomal sensory changes may be present. Definitive diagnosis can be made by cervical myelography or MRI, along with electromyographic studies to assess the degree and level of neurologic involvement. Treatment consists of cervical traction followed by anti-inflammatory medication and a cervical collar. If neurologic deficit does not respond promptly to traction, surgical discectomy and fusion of the involved vertebrae may be necessary.

Cervical Spondylosis. Degenerative changes in the cervical discs can lead to narrowing of the intervertebral foramina and osteophyte formation in the adjacent facet joints. This can cause impingement on nerve roots, with neck pain and neurologic symptoms as described above for disc herniations. In severe cases the facet joint hypertrophy can lead to stenosis of the cervical spine, resulting in cervical myelopathy as well as radicular symptoms. Sphincter disturbances occur in about one-third of patients, but incontinence is unusual. The causes of the myelopathy are multifactorial but include ischemia to the anterior spinal cord from vascular compression, ligamentous instability that places strain on the cord, and pressure by osteophytes. When conservative measures such as traction, cervical collar, and postural exercises fail to prevent neurologic progression, surgery may be indicated. Anterior interbody fusion (Cloward procedure) and posterior laminectomies or laminaplasty provide relief of symptoms and neurologic improvement in a high proportion of patients. Because of the instability caused by laminectomies, laminaplasty is preferable.

Lower Extremity

Foot and Ankle. The most common causes of foot pain are metatarsalgia and plantar fasciitis, which result from repetitive loading of the metatarsal heads or of the attachment of the plantar ligament to the calcaneus. Appropriate shoe inserts to relieve pressure (heel cups, metatarsal pads or bars, insoles), and anti-inflammatory medication or local cortisone injections generally alleviate the symptoms. In refractory cases surgical release of the plantar fascia or metatarsal osteotomies or head resections are occasionally indicated. Arthritis of any of the joints in the midfoot or forefoot can cause pain, and the first metatarsophalangeal (MTP) joint is particularly susceptible to acute gouty arthritis as well as osteoarthritis. Surgical arthrodesis (fusion) or arthroplasty is occasionally necessary when conservative management is unsuccessful. Additional causes of foot and ankle pain include peroneal tendon subluxation, stress fractures of the navicular or metatarsals, and compression of the posterior tibial nerve at the ankle or distally (tarsal tunnel syndrome). Surgical decompression of the nerve in tarsal tunnel syndrome is not associated with as successful an outcome as it is in treating other compression neuropathies.

Lower Leg. Repetitive loading of the tibia can lead to "shin splints," or activity-related pain and tenderness over the tibia. Several underlying causes have been identified, including an exertionally induced compartment syndrome and a periostitis involving inflammation of the attachments of the posterior tibialis fascia to the tibia. Exercise-induced compartment syndrome can be diagnosed by measuring compartment pressures in the leg before and after strenuous exercise with a slit catheter (see Fig. 41-22*B*). Release of the fascia may be indicated in persistent cases. Stress fractures of the tibia also can occur and present similarly, although radiographs often indicate periosteal reaction, and a nuclear bone scan will be abnormal. Protected weight bearing, alone or with cast immobilization, allows healing. Female runners with amenorrhea have been identified to be at risk for osteopenic tibial stress fractures secondary to decreased estrogen levels.

Pain in the posterior calf can result from partial tears of the medial gastrocnemius muscle; pain was formerly ascribed to rupture of the plantaris muscle. Muscle cramps in the calf, commonly occurring at night, can result from overuse. Deep venous thrombosis in the calf must always be considered in the differential diagnosis of leg pain and usually is associated with diffuse swelling, warmth, tenderness, and pain with passive stretch of the gastrocnemius muscle or toe flexors (Homans' sign). Ultrasonography and venography are important diagnostic aids. Calf pain that progresses with ambulation but is relieved at rest may indicate ischemic claudication. The neurogenic claudication of spinal stenosis continues when the patient stands at rest, which differentiates it from ischemic claudication.

Knee. Traumatic intraarticular derangements of the knee, including tears of the menisci, ligamentous sprains, and osteochondral fractures, are a common cause of knee pain. A history of locking can be found with intraarticular loose bodies, osteochondral defects, or meniscal tears. Arthritis of the knee also can cause pain and local swelling, often with joint space narrowing or osteophyte formation visible radiographically. Because of the common innervation of the medial aspect of the knee and the hip joint by the obturator nerve, knee pain can be a manifestation of hip joint pathology. In these cases local tenderness and swelling of the knee are absent, and forced passive rotation of the hip usually elicits the knee pain.

Anterior knee pain is frequently caused by the patellofemoral pain syndrome, which is often associated with degeneration and fibrillation of the articular cartilage of the patellar facets (chondromalacia). Causes include blunt direct trauma to the patella, malalignment of the extensor mechanism, or recurrent subluxation or dislocation of the patella. Patellar tendinitis (jumper's knee) also can present with anterior knee pain and focal tenderness over the patellar tendon. Diagnosis of chondromalacia is aided by demonstration of patellofemoral crepitus, pain with patellar compression, and tenderness of a patellar facet. Treatment generally is conservative, with isometric quadriceps exercises. If malalignment exists, lateral retinacular release or realignment of the extensor mechanism can be considered, and arthroscopic debridement of chondral fibrillations can be helpful. MRI is often helpful as a noninvasive method for evaluation of intraarticular pathology, including ligament tears, osteochondral fracture, meniscal tears, and chondromalacia and is used increasingly in place of diagnostic arthroscopy.

Hip. An important clinical diagnostic consideration in the evaluation of hip pain is the localization of the site of pathology. Intraarticular hip disorders usually present with anteriorly localized (inguinal) pain, aggravated by weight bearing or by passive rotation of the hip. Referred pain or radicular pain such as sciatica more commonly presents in the gluteal area, as does pain derived from sacroiliac joint pathology. Hip pain can be secondary to osteoarthritis, avascular necrosis of the femoral head, synovitis, septic arthritis, stress fractures of the femoral neck, or avulsion fractures of the anterior inferior iliac spine or the lesser trochanter. Lateral hip pain and tenderness can result from greater trochanteric bursitis, and anteromedial hip pain can be caused by adductor tendinitis, iliopsoas bursitis, or an iliopsoas abscess. With psoas abscess or septic arthritis, the hip tends to be held in flexion and external rotation. Pyriformis syndrome, or entrapment of the sciatic nerve under the pyriformis muscle, causes posterior hip and thigh pain (sciatica) and is aggravated by internal rotation of the hip. Hip flexion contractures frequently result from chronic hip joint pathology.

Low Back

The *low back syndrome* refers to a disease or injury of the lumbosacral spine, of an acute or a chronic nature. There are a wide variety of causes of low back pain; a summary is presented in Table 41-2. Acute low back pain, which is most common in the third to fifth decades, can be activity related, associated with paraspinous muscle spasm, and aggravated by sneezing or coughing. Pain usually is not radicular in nature, but it can be referred to the buttocks or legs. When nerve root irritation is present, paresthesias, neurologic deficits, and radicular radiation of the pain can occur. In the majority of patients with low back pain, no specific pathoanatomic cause can be identified, and treatment is symptomatic. For all idiopathic cases of low back pain, 90 percent of patients recover within 3 months, and 50 to 60 percent of patients with acute back pain recover within 1 week.

In disease processes such as tumors or infections involving the spine, the pain tends to be severe, unremitting, and not relieved by rest. Mechanically caused back pain is activity dependent, while morning pain and stiffness can be associated with ankylosing spondylitis. Examination of the patient should include assessment of the spinal range of motion, straight-leg-raising test for sciatic irritability, and a complete neurologic examination. Low back syndrome is most effectively treated by a short period of bed rest in the semi-Fowler's position (knees and hips flexed), anti-inflammatory medication, local heat, and occasionally muscle relaxants for spasm. Patients mobilized after 2 days of rest have been shown to recover more quickly than those rested 7 days. With subsequent mobilization, isometric back and abdominal exercises are helpful, as is the occasional use of a corset or back brace. Cardiovascular fitness training appears to be important both as a preventive measure against recurrences and for improved functional capacity. Such regimens include regular walking, swimming, or cycling.

Occupational low back pain (OLBP) is one of the most common and costly problems for workers in industry, and it is the second most frequent cause of worker absenteeism. As many as 50 percent of workers in the United States are affected at some time, and low back pain is the most common work-related complaint treated by primary care physicians. This disorder is the leading cause of disability in persons in the 19- to 45-year-old range. Risk factors include repetitive lifting, twisting, whole body vibration, and chronicity, and disability may also be influenced by psychological factors, including work stress and low

job satisfaction. The natural history of OLBP is favorable, with 60 percent of patients improved by 4 weeks and 80 percent by 6 weeks. Initial treatment is conservative, as outlined in the algorithm in Fig. 41-5A. When recovery seems very slow, further evaluation may be indicated as outlined in Fig. 41-5B.

Spondylolisthesis. Spondylolisthesis is a forward subluxation of one vertebral body on another. It can be caused by (1) spondylolysis (a defect in the pars interarticularis), (2) fracture of the posterior elements, (3) congenital facet deficiency, (4) facet deficiency caused by degenerative disc disease, and (5) isthmic elongation of the pars interarticularis. Illustrations of the types of spondylolisthesis are shown in Fig. 41-6. Although back pain may occur along with hamstring tightness, sciatica, and, rarely, neurologic symptoms and signs, spondylolisthesis often is asymptomatic. The L5–S1 articulation is most commonly affected, and the deformity is best visualized on a lateral radiograph, as seen in Fig. 41-7. Pars interarticularis defects (spondylolysis) are best visualized with oblique radiographs and are generally believed to result from incomplete healing of traumatic stress fractures. From 5 to 25 percent of patients presenting in childhood will demonstrate progression of the displacement and can require posterolateral fusion, along with excision of the posterior elements (Gill procedure) if neurologic deficit is present. Otherwise treatment is conservative, with rest and abdominal exercises. There has been renewed interest in reduction of severely displaced vertebral bodies before fusion, as well as in direct repair of pars interarticularis defects.

Sciatica. Sciatica is a symptom rather than a disease, and the term is used to describe radicular-type pain in the lower extremity. Sciatica can be caused by nerve root compression by a herniated disc, tumor, abscess, or osteophyte, or by peripheral nerve compression within the pelvis or gluteal area by tumor, hematoma, or abscess. Disc herniations or degenerative arthritis with facet hypertrophy and foraminal stenosis are by far the most common causes. Inflammatory disorders of nerves and nerve roots also can cause sciatica. Alcoholic or diabetic neuropathy, arsenic or lead poisoning, syphilitic or herpes zoster infections, and vasculitis associated with collagen vascular diseases all have been associated with sciatica.

Disc herniations occur most commonly at the L5–S1 and L4–L5 levels, when a tear or degeneration in the annulus fibrosus allows herniation of the soft, gelatinous nucleus pulposus posteriorly into the spinal canal. Impingement on nerve roots then causes back pain and sciatica, sometimes with radicular neurologic symptoms. Because the posterior longitudinal ligament provides support in the midline, most disc herniations are posterolateral, and hence symptoms often are unilateral. Disc herniations are uncommon in children and in older adults. The low incidence of disc herniations in older individuals probably is related to the age-dependent loss of water content and disc volume. Pain from disc herniations usually is aggravated by sitting, coughing, sneezing, and forward flexion, all of which increase disc pressures. Radicular symptoms also are elicited by straight-leg raising, particularly with additional dorsiflexion of the foot (Lasègue's sign). Depressed reflexes in the affected distribution (knee jerk—L4; posterior tibialis reflex—L5; ankle jerk—S1) as well as associated muscle weakness and dermatomal sensory deficits can be found.

Radiographs may be normal or may show narrowing of the affected disc space. The lesion can be demonstrated radiograph-

Table 41-2
Causes of Back Pain

1. Structural (anomalous or transitional vertebrae, spina bifida, spondylolysis, spondylolisthesis, facet anomalies)
2. Functional (scoliosis, leg length discrepancy, work or postural attitudes, pregnancy, hip or knee flexion contractures)
3. Infections (pyogenic osteomyelitis, tuberculosis, etc.)
4. Inflammatory (arthritis, ankylosing spondylitis, myositis, fibrositis, etc.)
5. Degenerative (osteoarthritis, senile kyphosis, degenerative disc disease, spinal stenosis)
6. Neoplastic (multiple myeloma, giant cell tumor, eosinophilic granuloma, or metastic bone disease from breast, prostate, lung, kidney, or thyroid carcinoma)
7. Traumatic (compression fracture, transverse process or posterior element fracture, ligament sprain or muscle strain, disc herniation)
8. Metabolic (osteoporosis, osteomalacia, hyperparathyroidism, Paget's disease, renal osteodystrophy, pulmonary osteoarthropathy, osteogenesis imperfecta, etc.)

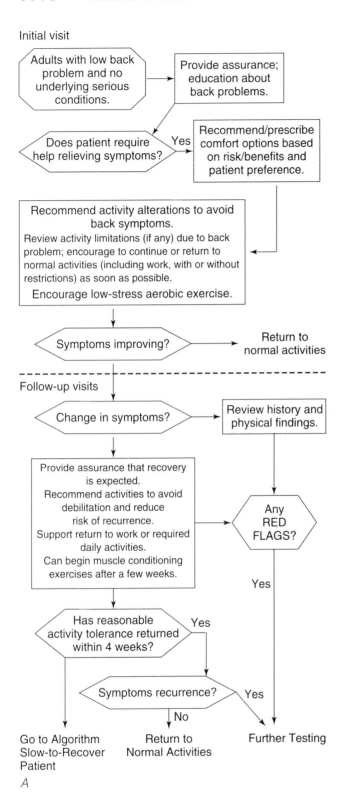

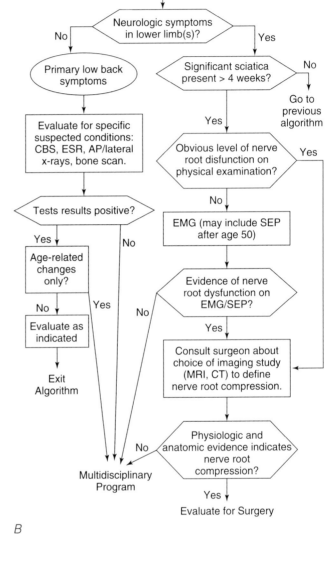

FIG. 41-5. *A.* Medical standards for early care of acute low back pain (LBP); evaluation and treatment algorithm. *B.* Medical standards for slow-to-recover patients (symptoms longer than 4 weeks); evaluation and treatment algorithm. (Adapted with permission from: *The United States Agency for Health Care Policy and Research: Acute low back problems in adults,* in Bigos SJ (ed): *Series: Clinical Practice Guideline No. 14.* Rockville, MD, U.S. Department of Health and Human Services, AHCPR Publication No. 95-0642, 1984.)

ically by CT scan, myelography, or MRI (Figs. 41-8 and 41-9). Treatment usually is conservative initially, with 80 to 90 percent of patients improving spontaneously and not requiring surgery. Helpful therapeutic measures include bed rest, analgesics, abdominal isometric exercises, and sitting in a reclining position, with mobilization as tolerated as the symptoms subside. Avoid-

ance of heavy lifting and bending helps to prevent recrudescence. Surgical excision of the extruded portion of the disc or digestion by percutaneous injection with chymopapain or collagenase into the disc can be effective when symptoms progress despite conservative measures. Fusion at the time of discectomy has not been shown to be of benefit in the absence of spinal

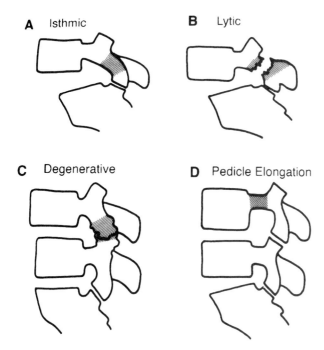

FIG. 41-6. *Types of spondylolisthesis. A. Elongation of the pars interarticularis (isthmic). B. Spondylolytic, from bilateral lysis of the pars interarticularis. C. Degenerative, from arthritic facet subluxation. D. Elongation of the pedicles (seen in osteogenesis imperfecta, osteomalacia, Paget's disease, achondroplasia). (Modified from: MacNab I: Backache. Baltimore, Williams & Wilkins, 1979, with permission.)*

the sacrococcygeal and occipitocervical areas. The most common malignant tumor involving the spine is metastatic carcinoma, usually from a primary tumor in the breast, prostate, lung, kidney, or thyroid gland. Back pain is the usual presenting symptom, but neurologic signs and symptoms, including paralysis, can occur. Lower-extremity hyperreflexia, spasticity, and positive Babinski signs indicate a danger of progression to paralysis and require emergent treatment. Primary benign tumors such as aneurysmal cyst or osteoblastoma are treated by surgical excision, with fusion when necessary. Primary malignant tumors such as chondrosarcoma or chordoma require wide surgical excision, while more radiosensitive lesions such as plasmacytoma or Ewing's sarcoma are treated with radiotherapy and chemotherapy, as are most metastatic lesions. In the presence of spinal instability (defined as a lesion causing a progressive neurologic deficit, or mechanical disruption with the potential to cause such a deficit), surgical decompression through an anterior or a posterior approach, along with fusion and instrumentation, is performed. Decompression without fusion and instrumentation can lead to instability, progressive deformity, and recurrent neurologic deficit. In cases requiring surgical intervention in which the patient has not had prior radiotherapy, postoperative treat-

instability. Microdiscectomy and percutaneous suction discectomy have recently been used as less invasive surgical alternatives but require further validation of efficacy and delineation of indications.

Spinal Stenosis. Spinal stenosis, a narrowing of the spinal canal or neuroforamina, can be acquired, as in the case degenerative disc disease, or congenital, as in achondroplasia. Patients present with back or leg pain, generally exacerbated by standing and walking and, unlike in discogenic back pain, relieved by sitting. Leg pain secondary to spinal stenosis can mimic vascular claudication but is present while standing still, unlike claudication. Neurologic signs, including hyporeflexia and muscle weakness, may be present; sciatic irritability may be evident. Facet arthropathy associated with lumbar spondylosis is readily visualized on lateral and oblique radiographs, but the degree of spinal canal, lateral recess, or foraminal narrowing is better assessed on axial CT or MRI of the lumbar spine (Fig. 41-10). Treatment consists of abdominal isometrics, flexion bracing, and anti-inflammatory medication. Epidural steroid injections can be of some benefit. In refractory cases, wide posterior surgical decompression (laminectomies, facetectomies, foraminotomies) with or without fusion can be undertaken.

Vertebral Tumors. Malignant and benign lesions can occur in the spine as primary tumors. Benign lesions include osteoid osteoma, osteoblastoma, aneurysmal cyst, giant cell tumor, and eosinophilic granuloma. Malignant primary lesions are rare, with the exception of multiple myeloma, and include chondrosarcoma, Ewing's sarcoma, and lymphoma. Chordoma, a rare tumor that evolves from remnants of the notochord, occurs in

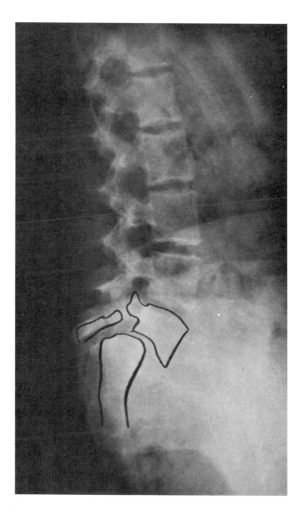

FIG. 41-7. *Radiograph showing a spondylolisthesis of the fifth lumbar vertebra on the first sacral vertebra, with an obvious defect in the pars interarticularis.*

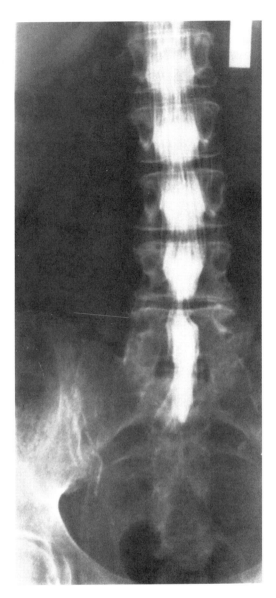

FIG. 41-8. Metrizamide myelogram shows disc prolapse at L4–L5 (left). *(Courtesy of Dr. David W. Stroller.)*

ment after wound healing is indicated to prevent local tumor recurrence.

Vertebral Osteomyelitis. Pyogenic osteomyelitis is usually caused by a *Staphylococcus aureus* infection that starts in the vertebral end plates adjacent to a disc space by hematogenous spread from another infectious focus. Back pain, radiographically visible destruction of the disc space, and sometimes neurologic deficit result. Patients may have systemic symptoms of infection; usually leukocytosis and elevation of the erythrocyte sedimentation rate are present. Marked collapse of the vertebrae with gibbus deformity is unusual with pyogenic infections and is seen more often with tuberculous infection. Acute, fulminating sepsis is more common in children, and chronic osteomyelitis is more common in adults. Radionuclide technetium diphosphonate bone scans and MRI are helpful in diagnosis when radiographic findings are subtle. Figure 41-11 demonstrates the radiographic differentiation between tumor and infection, and

Fig. 41-12 shows the MRI findings in similar lesions. Treatment involves identification of the organism by blood cultures or percutaneous CT or fluoroscopically guided disc space aspiration, followed by immobilization and intravenous antibiotics, usually for 6 weeks. Failure to respond promptly to conservative therapy and the presence of neurologic deficits are indications for surgical debridement with anterior bone grafting to preserve stability.

Chest Wall

Causes of chest wall pain include infections such as herpes zoster (shingles), spinal tumors with intercostal nerve root compression, osteomyelitis, and referred pain from visceral disease of the underlying lung, pleura, mediastinum, or heart. Rib fractures and injuries of the costochondral junctions can cause local pain. Inflammation of the costochondral junctions (costochondritis or Tietze's syndrome) is characterized by painful enlargement and local tenderness, often affecting several ribs simultaneously.

Cumulative Trauma Disorders. Cumulative trauma disorders encompass a spectrum of musculoskeletal problems generally related to repetitive loading or injury to tissues, frequently in a workplace setting (Table 41-3). These disorders may cause pain, swelling, restriction of movement, or neurologic symptoms, depending on the specific condition. Treatment generally involves rest of the affected part, anti-inflammatory medications, and, when possible, workplace modifications based on ergonomic considerations.

DISORDERS OF MUSCLE

Anatomy and Physiology

Muscle fibers consist of multiple bundles of individual muscle cells containing actin and myosin, contractile elements that are

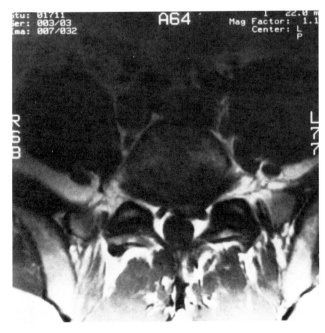

FIG. 41-9. MRI showing disc prolapse at L5–S1. *(Courtesy of Dr. David W. Stroller.)*

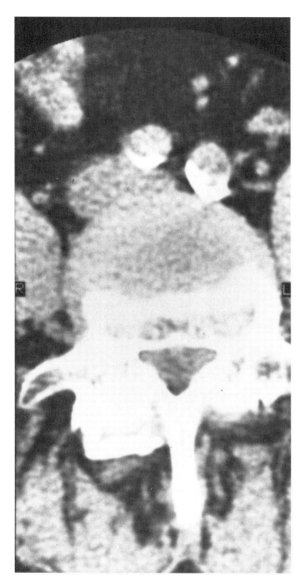

FIG. 41-10. *CT scan of spinal stenosis at L4–L5.*

regulated by neurogenic stimulation of the motor end plates. The macroscopic and microscopic anatomy of muscle is shown in Fig. 41-13. Muscle fibers are divided into two major types having different functional properties. Type I slow-twitch fibers have low glycogen and glycolytic enzyme content, but high mitochondrial oxidative phosphorylation activity and myoglobin content. These fibers function in high-repetition and low-load endurance activities. Type II fast-twitch fibers have higher glycolytic capacity, with subtypes (IIA, IIB, IIC, and IIM) differing in the form of myosin present. Type II muscles are generally involved in activities requiring power and speed. The fiber types can be distinguished histochemically and are genetically determined, with different muscles having differing proportions of fiber types, depending on functional requirements. Type I fibers are fatigue resistant and respond to endurance training, and type II fibers are fatigable, respond to resistance training, and are responsible for muscle hypertrophy. Types of muscular contraction and associated terms are defined in Table 41-4.

Motor paralysis is defined as loss of voluntary control of muscle contraction. Normal muscle has some resting tone, or tension, which is absent with lower motor neuron lesions, causing flaccid paralysis. Tendon reflexes also are abolished with interruption of the lower motor neuron pathway. Spasticity refers to abnormal increases in muscle tone with passive stretch and is caused by loss of normal central inhibitory control resulting from upper motor neuron lesions. Loss of inhibitory control of tendon reflexes with upper motor neuron lesions also causes hyperreflexia and repetitive reflexive muscle contraction in response to stretch, or clonus. Lower motor neuron lesions, disuse, and immobilization result in muscle atrophy. The clinical grading of muscle strength is shown in Table 41-5.

Electrodiagnosis

Stimulation of a peripheral nerve by surface or needle electrodes results in conduction of the stimulus to the motor end plates, with depolarization and resultant muscle contraction. The time for conduction and depolarization, referred to as *latency,* is prolonged in conditions of nerve injury or compression. The nerve conduction velocity, which can be determined by stimulation at two points a known distance apart along the nerve, is useful in localizing peripheral nerve lesions. Electromyography (EMG) is the measurement of electrical potentials within muscles using needle electrodes, both at rest and with voluntary contraction. Spontaneous electrical impulses from individual resting muscle fibers known as fibrillation potentials occur in muscle that has been denervated.

Intrinsic Muscle Diseases

Differentiating myopathies from other causes of muscle weakness or paralysis requires consideration of family history, age of onset, and presence of muscle group involvement without common innervation. Biochemical tests for serum aldolase and creatine kinase and muscle biopsy can be helpful in diagnosis.

Muscular Dystrophies. Muscular dystrophies are hereditary disorders resulting in progressive muscular degeneration. Duchenne's muscular dystrophy is inherited as an X-linked recessive disorder manifesting in male children between the ages of 3 and 6 years. The genetic defect has been identified as a deficiency of a protein called dystrophin, which functions as a calcium transport protein. Duchenne's muscular dystrophy is uniformly fatal, usually by the age of 20 years. Late cardiac and respiratory muscle involvement are the causes of death. The disease presents with difficulty standing and walking, and the child uses the upper extremities to push to an upright posture (Gower's sign). Pseudohypertrophy of the gastrocnemius, deltoids, and quadriceps is common. Equinus contractures of the ankles occur early, as does rapidly progressive scoliosis. Other forms of muscular dystrophy include limb girdle and facioscapulohumeral dystrophies, which have an higher age of onset and are inherited as autosomal recessive and dominant traits, respectively. Facioscapulohumeral dystrophy, with upper-extremity and facial weakness and normal life span, is the most benign.

Pathology. Loss of the integrity of the muscle cell membrane results in progressive degeneration of muscle fibers. Fibers become variable in diameter and rounded rather than polygonal in cross-section and appear hyalinized. Fat and fibrous tissue replace the degenerating muscle fibers, with no evidence of muscle regeneration.

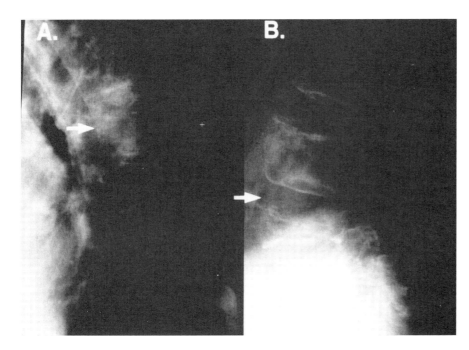

FIG. 41-11. Radiographic appearance of vertebral osteomyelitis *(A)* versus that of metastatic tumor *(B)*. The infection involves the disc space primarily, while tumor involves the bone with preservation of the disc space.

Diagnosis. In addition to the clinical features, serum aldolase and creatine kinase levels are elevated, particularly in the Duchenne form. Urinary creatine and amino acid levels are increased, and creatinine level is decreased. EMG shows lower potentials and a polyphasic pattern during voluntary contraction, and muscle biopsy examination confirms the diagnosis.

Treatment. Given the recent identification of dystrophin deficiency as the cause of muscular dystrophy, the disease is a good candidate for treatment by gene therapy in the future. At present, treatment is symptomatic, with exercise to maintain function as long as possible and bracing or surgery to control deformities. Achilles tendon lengthening is occasionally needed for equinus deformities, and early aggressive treatment of progressive scoliosis with curvature over 25 or 30 degrees is indicated, with posterior rodding and segmental wiring (Luque technique) to maintain sitting balance and prevent restrictive pulmonary compromise.

Myotonias. Myotonic dystrophy is an autosomal dominant inherited disorder of muscle, which usually presents in children or young adults with facial and distal extremity weakness. Stimulation of muscle contraction results in prolonged contraction.

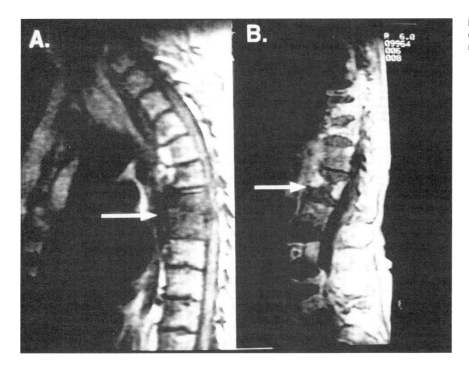

FIG. 41-12. MRI appearance of vertebral osteomyelitis *(A)* versus that of metastatic tumor *(B)*.

Table 41-3
Cumulative Trauma Disorders

Tendon-related disorders	Tendinitis, tenosynovitis
	Epicondylitis (elbow)
	De Quervain's (wrist)
	Dupytren's contracture (hand)
	Trigger finger
	Ganglion cyst (wrist, hand)
Joint-related disorders	Osteoarthritis of most joints
Nerve-related disorders	Carpal tunnel syndrome (median n.)
	Guyon canal syndrome (ulnar n.)
	Pronator teres syndrome (median n.)
	Radial tunnel syndrome (radial n.)
	Thoracic outlet syndrome (brachial plexus)
	Cervical syndrome (radiculopathy)
	Digital neuritis
Muscle-related disorders	Tension neck syndrome
	Muscle sprain and strain
	Myalgia and myositis
Circulatory-related disorders	Hypothenar hammer syndrome
	Raynaud's syndrome
Bursa-related disorders	Bursitis (shoulder, hip, patella, olecranon)

Myotonia congenita (Thomsen's disease) is a hereditary disorder characterized by difficulty initiating voluntary movement. Diagnosis of these disorders is made clinically and by EMG, the presence of elevated serum muscle enzyme levels, and muscle biopsy examination. Contractures do not develop, and surgical treatment is not necessary. Procainamide, prednisone, and quinine can help patients with myotonia congenita.

Myositis. Inflammatory diseases of muscle can cause pain and weakness and can be associated with viral, parasitic, or

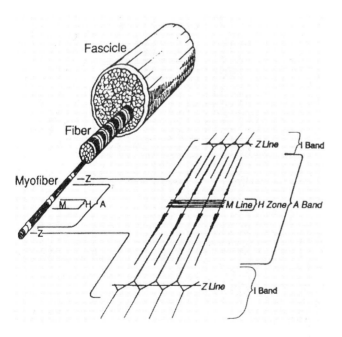

FIG. 41-13. *Organization of skeletal muscle from the microscopic to the macrostructural level. (From: Simon SR (ed): Orthopaedic Basic Science, American Academy of Orthopaedic Surgeons, Rosemont, IL, 1994, with permission.)*

Table 41-4
Definitions Associated with Muscle Contraction

Muscle tone: resting tension in muscles regulated by muscle spindle afferents
Motor unit: muscle fibers innervated by a single motor neuron
Isometric contraction: contraction of a muscle developing tension but without shortening of the muscle (as in quadriceps while doing a leg lift with the knee extended)
Isotonic contraction: generation of constant tension as a muscle shortens (as in lifting a weight)
Eccentric contraction: lengthening of the muscle while under contractile tension (as in lowering a weight)
Isokinetic contraction: generation of maximal tension in a muscle contracting at a constant speed over a full range of motion
Fibrillation: spontaneous resting electrical discharges in individual muscle fibers indicative of denervation
Tetany: sustained maximal involuntary contraction of a muscle

bacterial infections, or with collagen vascular diseases (e.g., dermatomyositis, systemic lupus erythematosus, scleroderma, rheumatoid arthritis). Polymyositis can be treated with corticosteroids, and exercise, physical therapy, and appropriate bracing can be helpful. Muscle biopsy examination reveals inflammatory cells and muscle necrosis, and EMG demonstrates fibrillation potentials, distinguishing polymyositis from muscular dystrophies. In elderly patients, an occult primary malignancy sometimes is associated with polymyositis.

Extrinsic Muscle Diseases (Neurologic Disorders)

Poliomyelitis. Poliomyelitis is an infectious viral disease characterized by central nervous system infection with destruction of anterior horn cells in the spinal cord causing flaccid paralysis. Poliomyelitis, formerly one of the most common diseases causing orthopaedic deformities, is now rarely seen in the United States, because of widespread vaccination. Deformities and leg length discrepancies can result. In about one-third of poliomyelitis patients an initial febrile illness occurs, with headache, malaise, and fever, lasting 48 h. The patient may recover or go on to a second acute phase after 4 or 5 days, which also may resolve without paralysis. Headache, fever, neck stiffness, and muscle spasms may occur during the acute phase, which lasts from several days to a week. Paralysis can develop during the third or fourth day, with loss of deep reflexes and muscle spasm. The lower limbs are more frequently involved than the upper extremities. Death can result from bulbar paralysis with respiratory insufficiency. The convalescent phase follows, and some motor improvement may occur for up to 2 years. Treatment is sup-

Table 41-5
Clinical Grading of Muscle Strength

Grade	Muscle Power
0	Paralysis—no muscle contraction
1	Flicker of contraction without joint excursion
2	Some joint motion, but not against gravity
3	Full joint motion against gravity with no resistance
4	Less than normal strength, but full motion against resistance
5	Normal muscle strength

portive, with physical therapy to maintain joint range of motion and ventilatory support when necessary. Bracing is occasionally needed to assist function of paralyzed extremities. Later, correction of joint contractures, stabilization of flail joints by arthrodesis, and correction of leg length inequalities can be undertaken during the residual phase. Tendon transfers can be useful to improve muscle balance, decrease contractures, or restore functions. Only muscles with a strength grade of 4 or better are suitable for transfer, since one grade of muscle function is lost with transfer (see Table 41-5). A postpolio syndrome has been identified in older adults several decades after disease onset, consisting of increasing weakness in affected muscle groups and fatigue. The cause of this syndrome remains unknown.

Bony Stabilization. For flail joints, when muscles of sufficient strength for transfer are unavailable or bracing is unsuccessful, surgical arthrodesis can be performed. Joint contractures require stretching exercises, splints, or, for severe deformity, surgical release. Epiphysiodesis, the surgical ablation of the growth plate, or bone lengthening/shortening procedures can be used to correct significant limb length inequality.

Treatment of Deformity. Foot deformities are common and can be treated in some cases by orthoses. The most common deformities and functional losses and their corresponding surgical treatments are shown in Table 41-6. Many of the procedures listed are useful also for correction of deformities or functional deficits resulting from neurologic injury from other causes, such as traumatic nerve injuries. Surgical correction of foot deformities may be accomplished by extraarticular subtalar arthrodesis (Grice procedure) in skeletally immature patients, or triple arthrodesis (fusion of the subtalar, calcaneocuboid, and talonavicular joints) in adults (Fig. 41-14). Operations must be individualized according to the deficit. Patients with quadriceps muscle paralysis often are able to stabilize the knee in extension for ambulation with the gluteus maximus and gastrocnemius muscles. Muscle transfers about the hip are variably successful, and if hip subluxation or painful degenerative change occurs, arthrodesis may be needed.

Cerebral Palsy. Cerebral palsy (CP), which occurs in about 3 births per 100,000, can be caused by a number of factors,

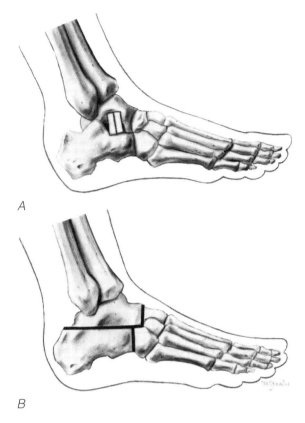

A

B

FIG. 41-14. *A. Grice procedure with a strut of tibial bone graft wedged between talus and calcaneus. B. Triple arthrodesis.*

including birth trauma, childhood head injury, anoxic brain damage, and viral diseases such as encephalitis, measles, and cytomegalovirus. Recent epidemiologic data suggest that a relatively small proportion of CP cases result from perinatal events; the majority are idiopathic and are related to defects in central nervous system development. CP is classified as spastic (50 percent), athetoid (25 percent), ataxic (5 percent), rigid (5 percent),

Table 41-6
Treatment of Deformities Associated with Poliomyelitis

Deformity or Dysfunction	Cause	Treatment
Hindfoot valgus	Anterior and/or posterior tibialis paralysis	Extraarticular subtalar arthrodesis (Grice procedure)
Hindfoot varus	Paralysis of the peronei	Anterior, posterior tibial tendon transfers
Calcaneus deformity	Gastrocsoleus paralysis	Transfer of anterior tibialis or peronei to the calcaneus
Equinus deformity	Paralysis of the anterior tibialis	Transfer of the peronei or posterior tibialis to the dorsum of the midfoot ± triple arthrodesis
Claw hallux	Loss of anterior tibialis	Extensor hallucis recession to the metatarsal and IP joint fusion
Flail knee	Quadriceps paralysis	Anterior transfer of the hamstrings to the patella
Hip	Abductor paralysis	Iliopsoas, tensor fascia lata, or erector spinae transfer to the greater trochanter or hip arthrodesis
Shoulder	Deltoid and/or rotator cuff paralysis	Glenohumeral arthrodesis
Elbow	Paralysis of the biceps and brachialis	Proximal transfer of forearm common flexor origin, or transfer of the pectoralis major or sternocleidomastoid muscle
Paralytic hand	Wrist extensor paralysis	Flexor carpi ulnaris to extensor carpi radialis longus transfer
	Thumb extensor paralysis	Flexor carpi radialis to abductor pollicis longus, extensor pollicis brevis tendons
	Opponens paralysis	Palmaris longus to extensor pollicis longus; 4th flexor digitorum profundus to oppens transfer

or mixed (15 percent). Sixty percent of patients with CP have hemiplegia (ipsilateral upper and lower extremity involvement), with diplegia (both lower extremities) and quadriplegia (all four extremities) being less common. Athetoid types exhibit involuntary repetitive motions that are dysfunctional; ataxia (staggering, broad-based gait) reflects cerebellar dysfunction, and rigidity results from diffuse cerebral involvement usually associated with birth anoxia.

Treatment. Two-thirds of CP patients have an IQ below 70, which compromises treatments that require patient cooperation, such as muscle strengthening, exercise, and gait-training programs. Treatment is directed toward prevention of contractures and surgical correction of deformities that develop from muscle imbalance.

Orthotics. Orthoses are helpful to control varus or valgus deformities of the foot and equinus deformities of the ankle. Long leg braces can help to control knee flexion or valgus deformities and assist in ambulation. Upper-extremity bracing can help to prevent flexion deformities of the wrist and digits and adduction of the thumb. Leg adductor spasticity is common and can cause hip subluxation or dislocation, which becomes painful in about 50 percent of patients who develop it. Abduction bracing can help to prevent this problem.

Surgical Treatment—Lower Extremity. When contractures or deformities progress despite conservative treatment, an operation sometimes is necessary. Surgery also can improve function by improving muscle balance or removing deforming forces. An important adjunct in surgical planning is gait analysis by video recording or dynamic EMG. A major emphasis in the management of the crouched, scissoring gait of patients with CP has been on correction of knee flexion deformities, but evidence suggests that while stance phase of gait is improved, swing phase is not. The rectus femoris muscle has been shown by dynamic EMG to be more active in swing phase, causing inadequate knee flexion and poor toe clearance. Transfer of the rectus femoris to the medial or lateral hamstring muscles has been shown to improve this phenomenon. Excessive length of the patellar tendon also can result from the stretching effect on the rectus femoris when the hamstrings are chronically tight. This can be diagnosed by the presence of patella alta on lateral radiograph or greater passive extension than active extension. Shortening the patellar tendon in conjunction with hamstring lengthening or release can improve gait by correcting these problems.

Equinus deformities of the ankle constitute another common problem that can be corrected by Achilles tendon lengthening. Care must be taken not to overlengthen, as a calcaneus deformity can result, which is difficult to brace. Varus or valgus deformities of the hindfoot can be corrected by a Grice procedure, or by triple arthrodesis at skeletal maturity (see Fig. 41-14). Adduction deformities of the hips are treated by adductor tenotomies along with neurectomy of the anterior branch of the obturator nerve, and if hip subluxation is present varus and derotational osteotomies of the proximal femur with internal fixation may be indicated (Fig. 41-15).

Surgical Treatment—Upper Extremity. An operation on the shoulder is almost never necessary. The most common problems are related to wrist and finger flexor spasticity and thumb adduction deformities. Wrist/finger flexion deformities have been divided into three groups: Type I or mild deformities (digits extend with wrist in less than 20 degrees of flexion) rarely require surgical intervention. Type II or moderate deformities (dig-

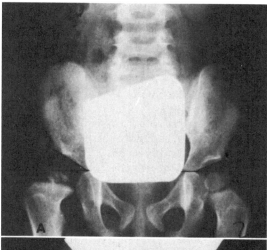
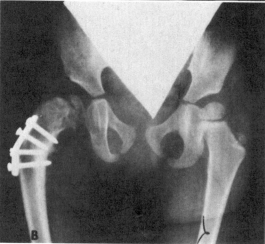

FIG. 41-15. *Hip subluxation in spastic diplegia. A. AP view of the pelvis showing lateral displacement of the right hip. B. AP view of the pelvis showing maintenance of the head in the acetabulum following varus derotation osteotomy.*

its extend with wrist in less than 50 degrees of flexion) benefit from proximal wrist/finger flexor release with dorsal flexor carpi ulnaris transfer. Type III or severe flexion deformities require distal wrist and finger flexor tenotomies, with transfer of the sublimis to the distal profundus tendons. Proximal row carpectomy or wrist arthrodesis occasionally is indicated. Release of the adductor and interphalangeal fusion or tendon transfers can correct thumb-in-palm deformities.

Spinal Deformity. Neuromuscular scoliosis with a C-shaped progressive curve is common in severe cases of CP. Bracing can be of some value for limited or nonprogressive curves. Progression can lead to impaired sitting balance, pelvic obliquity, and ischial decubitus ulcers, and therefore correction of scoliosis with anterior and/or posterior spinal instrumentation and fusion is commonly indicated. Generally, posterior instrumentation with rods and segmental fixation (Luque procedure) from the upper thoracic spine to the sacrum is the preferred approach. With severe rotational deformities in the lumbar spine, anterior instrumentation also may be required.

Myelodysplasia (Spinal Dysraphia). *Myelodysplasia* refers to a developmental defect in the vertebral column associated with a neurologic deficit. *Spinal dysraphia* refers to defects involving failure of fusion of midline structures and may be present without cord involvement (spina bifida occulta), or with a myelomeningocele, a neural tube defect at the level of the lesion. Eighty percent of patients have associated hydrocephalus, and paralysis is generally present below the level of the defect. Antenatal diagnosis of neural tube defects is possible using amniocentesis with assay of alpha-fetoprotein. Supplementation with folate during the first trimester of pregnancy can dramatically reduce the incidence of neural tube defects.

Meningoceles (cystic enlargement of the lower meninges) or myelomeningoceles (cystic enlargement of the meninges and intradural contents) are treated by early closure and shunting for hydrocephalus. Prognosis depends on the degree of neurologic involvement and corresponding level of lower-extremity paralysis and disruption of bowel and bladder function. Patients with lesions below the L4 level will usually be ambulatory, although lower-extremity deformities such as talipes equinovarus and hip subluxation can occur, requiring surgical correction. Additionally, lack of sensory function makes pressure sores a common recurring problem.

Orthopaedic Management. Function is strongly dependent on the level of the neurologic lesion. Patients with lesions below L3 or L4 usually can ambulate but may require orthoses. Maintenance of a plantigrade foot is essential, and 50 percent of patients have foot deformities at birth. Lower-extremity deformities correspond to the level of spinal involvement. Appropriate bracing to minimize progressive contractures and allow ambulation when possible is indicated. Young children with flaccid paralysis of the lower extremities can ambulate and maintain an upright standing position in a parapodium. The energy costs of ambulation with this device are so high, however, that older children and adults are unable to use it and generally are confined to wheelchair. A reciprocating gait orthosis allows ambulation in older patients with meningomyelocele or paralysis secondary to spinal cord injury. Custom-molded orthoses lined with pressure-distributing materials such as Plastizote are important in the prevention of pressure sores from lack of sensation.

Management of paralytic deformities is similar to that with the flaccid paralysis of poliomyelitis. Talipes equinovarus can be quite severe and is treated by posteromedial release or talectomy in severe or recurrent cases. Contractures frequently require release and tendon transfers to remove deforming forces when appropriate muscles are available. The Grice procedure is corrective for valgus hindfoot deformities, and the triple arthrodesis is appropriate for correction of hindfoot deformities in older children (see Fig. 41-14). Maintenance of concentric reduction of the hips can necessitate proximal femoral osteotomies or acetabular osteotomies in severe cases. Spinal deformities include severe kyphosis at the level of the lesion, or scoliosis. Virtually all patients with a functional disturbance of the spinal cord at the level of L3 or higher will develop scoliosis requiring surgical intervention, as compared to approximately 60 percent at the L4 level. Lumbar kyphosis is seen in 8 to 15 percent of patients and is almost always progressive. Kyphectomy with instrumentation and fusion can be helpful, and scoliosis is corrected by posterior rodding with segmental fixation and fusion, occasionally in addition to anterior release and fusion. In addition, tethering of the spinal cord can occur with growth, usually presenting as a worsening of the neurologic deficit. This can necessitate surgical release of the filum terminale.

Degenerative Neurologic Diseases with Skeletal Deformity. *Peroneal Muscle Atrophy (Charcot-Marie-Tooth Disease).* This is an inherited autosomal recessive or dominant trait leading to a degenerative neuropathy, manifested initially in the distribution of the peroneal nerve. Patients develop cavus and varus deformities of the feet and a dropfoot gait. Intrinsic atrophy in the hands also may be apparent. Correction of cavus deformities by midfoot osteotomy and clawtoe deformities by interphalangeal fusions and extensor tendon recession are helpful.

Friedreich's Ataxia. This familial disease begins in childhood, involving the spinocerebellar tracts, corticospinal tracts, and posterior columns. Patients have progressive gait and speech disturbances and scoliosis and foot deformities. Intervention for foot deformities or scoliosis may be indicated early in the course of the disease to maintain ambulation.

Syringomyelia. This degenerative condition of the spinal cord involves destruction of neurons in the central portion of the cord with formation of a cystic cavity, or syrinx. Onset of symptoms usually is in the second or third decade. The intrinsic muscles of the hand are involved initially, followed by progressive loss of motor and sensory function in the upper and lower extremities. Orthopaedic treatment entails bracing for prevention of contractures, or arthrodesis of neuropathic joints. Laminectomy occasionally is indicated to relieve expanding cavities of the spinal cord.

Multiple Sclerosis. This is a progressive demyelinating disease of the central nervous system of unknown pathogenesis. The disease has a variable course, with exacerbations that are sporadic and can be ameliorated by use of ACTH or corticosteroids. Orthopaedic problems include contractures of the ankle, knee, and hip and scoliosis. Treatment involves range-of-motion and stretching exercises, splinting, and occasionally surgical release of contractures. Spinal instrumentation and fusion rarely are indicated. Death can result from progressive muscle weakness causing respiratory failure.

Orthopaedic Management of Stroke. Rehabilitation of stroke patients should begin as early as possible, usually within a few days after the cerebrovascular event. Initially patients exhibit flaccid paralysis, which later can give way to spasticity and the development of contractures. Early physical therapy can maintain mobility and prevent deformity and decubitus ulcers. Persistent spasticity can be temporarily ameliorated by peripheral nerve blocks with phenol or alcohol, but more permanent control generally requires release or tenotomy of the affected muscle groups. The most common deformity is foot and ankle equinus, which can be corrected by Achilles tendon lengthening. Similarly, flexion contractures of the knee and adduction contractures of the hip are corrected by surgical release. Paralysis of the shoulder girdle musculature can lead to a painful "frozen shoulder," which can impede rehabilitation. Active-assisted exercises may help to maintain range of motion, and flexion deformities of the fingers and wrist can be improved by flexor slide, a release of the flexor muscles in the proximal forearm.

POSTURE

Disturbances in Gait

Gait disturbance of mechanical origin must be distinguished from that of neurologic causation. Neurologic gait disturbances include ataxia, hemiplegia, and spasticity. Ataxia, a wide-based, uncoordinated gait, can result from cerebellar lesions, Guillain-Barré syndrome, Friedreich's ataxia, or defects in peripheral sensation and proprioception such as tabes dorsalis or vitamin B_{12} deficiency. Spastic gait, common in cerebral palsy, is characterized by a crouched position with scissoring of the legs. With hemiplegic gait, the patient appears to drag the affected extremity.

Mechanical Disorders. Gait disturbances can be produced by numerous abnormalities of joints, including congenital hip dysplasia or dislocation, slipped capital femoral epiphysis, avascular necrosis of the hip, Legg-Calvé-Perthes disease, and knee joint abnormalities (e.g., arthritis, osteochondritis dissecans, genu valgum, genu varum, meniscal injury). Congenital foot and ankle deformities, such as talipes equinovarus (clubfoot), and limb length discrepancies also can cause a limp. Any condition causing pain on weight bearing in a lower extremity can cause an antalgic gait in which the patient "short steps" on the affected extremity, minimizing the stance phase of gait. Pain in the hip joint can cause an abductor limp, wherein the patient lurches or leans toward the affected side during stance phase to move the center of gravity of the body over the hip, decreasing the abductor force across the joint. With abductor paralysis, a Trendelenburg gait results, in which the pelvis tilts toward the opposite side during stance phase on the affected extremity because of the inability of the abductors to maintain a level pelvis. This also can result from ineffective abductor contraction in congenital hip dislocation or coxa vara. Use of a cane in the opposite hand can reduce the force across the hip joint by a factor of five, the number of times body weight the abductors must contract to maintain the trunk and pelvis level during one-legged stance. In patient with hip problems the use of a cane thus can dramatically improve gait and reduce hip pain when present. Generally, orthopaedic management of a limp requires appropriate diagnostic evaluation and treatment directed toward the cause.

Limb Length Discrepancy. Limb length discrepancies may be secondary to trauma with growth plate injury, shortening of a bone, or growth stimulation from injury. Additionally, congenital aberrations in growth or radiation treatment for tumors can lead to significant and progressive limb length discrepancies in children. Asymmetric growth plate disturbances can produce angular deformities. Orthopaedic treatment includes use of a shoe lift for discrepancies of up to 1 or 2 cm, epiphysiodesis to stop the growth of the longer limb for larger discrepancies, or limb-lengthening or limb-shortening procedures. Growth charts (Moseley chart) are used to plot the growth of the limbs as measured by calibrating radiographs called scanograms versus time. Comparison to normal data allows prediction of the appropriate timing for surgical disruption of the growth plates (usually distal femoral and proximal tibial plates) so that the remaining growth in the short limb will allow leg length equalization at skeletal maturity. Disadvantages include loss of stature, the need to operate on the well leg, and the limitations in the amount of length equalization that can be attained in this manner. For modest discrepancies, however, this is a well-accepted and useful method.

For severe limb length differences a new method of limb lengthening, called *distraction osteogenesis* or *callotasis,* has become popular. This method, first implemented by Ilizarov in the Soviet Union, relies on intramedullary membranous osteogenesis after cortical osteotomy and gradual distraction with an external

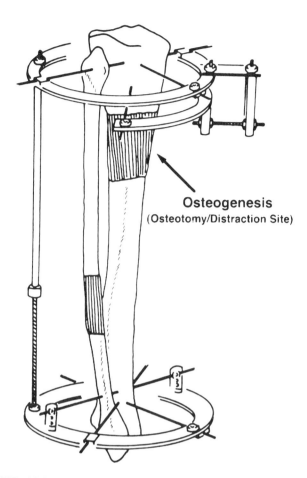

FIG. 41-16. Distraction osteogenesis, or callotasis, or the Ilizarov method of bone lengthening. After corticotomy, the ring fixator is gradually lengthened. Osteoid forms in the gap, and later fully mineralizes when distraction is stopped. (Modified from: *Paley D: Problems, obstacles, and complications of limb lengthening by the Ilizarov technique. Clin Orthop 250:93, 1990, with permission.*)

fixator using small Kirschner wires (K-wires) under tension and circumferential ring supports (Fig. 41-16). The bone can be lengthened by 1 mm daily, and the multiplanar fixation device allows simultaneous correction of angular and rotational deformities. Care is taken at the time of the corticotomy not to disrupt the medullary bone, and the procedure is done through small incisions without any periosteal stripping. Lengthenings of up to 10 cm are obtainable with this method, and more than one bone can be lengthened in an extremity. The method is also useful in the treatment of nonunions.

Spinal Deformities

The spine is characterized by a series of curves that aid its physiologic functions. The cervical and lumbar spine normally exhibit lordosis, while the thoracic spine has a normal kyphosis. The intervertebral discs serve to maintain flexibility of the spine and the function of shock absorption. The discs consist of a tough, fibrous peripheral component, the annulus fibrosus, and a gelatinous central portion, the nucleus pulposus. With age, loss of water content occurs with concomitant loss of disc height.

Kyphosis

Kyphosis is an increase in the normal posterior convexity of the thoracic spine involving a number of vertebral bodies. A *gibbus deformity* is an acute kyphotic angular deformity that may be congenital, posttraumatic, or secondary to tumor or infections such as tuberculosis.

Adolescent Kyphosis. Postural kyphosis, or "round shoulders," occurs in children, occasionally in association with muscular coordination problems. With time, this habitual kyphotic posture can become fixed. Treatment is with extension exercises, and bracing is unnecessary. A discogenic form of adolescent kyphosis that is progressive, known as Scheuermann's disease, also occurs. This disorder is characterized by abnormalities in the growth plates of the vertebral bodies and herniations of disc material into the vertebrae (Schmorl's nodes). Scheuermann's kyphosis tends to be progressive and is generally treated by extension exercises and Milwaukee bracing for more severe deformities. The need for surgical treatment is unusual, but refractory cases with back pain can benefit from staged anterior and posterior fusion with posterior instrumentation.

Osteoporotic Kyphosis. In osteoporotic kyphosis, cumulative effects of compression fractures or anterior wedging of multiple vertebral levels as a result of mechanical failure of osteopenic bone lead to progressive kyphosis in the thoracic spine. Most commonly this is seen in women with postmenopausal osteoporosis. The discs often bulge into the weakened vertebral end plates. Compression fractures can occur as discrete, acute events following minor trauma, or with a more insidious onset and progression, probably the result of multiple microfractures. Back pain is the presenting complaint, and patients may experience loss of height and a roundback deformity (dowager's hump). Neurologic deficit beyond intercostal radicular pain almost never develops despite severe degrees of deformity. Multiple myeloma and metastatic carcinoma also can cause vertebral compression fractures and must be ruled out, as well as osteomalacia, renal osteopathy, and other metabolic derangements. Treatment of acute fractures is with rest, analgesics, and an extension orthosis, followed by extension exercises and therapy for the underlying cause of the osteopenia when possible (see Metabolic Diseases, below).

Scoliosis

Any lateral deviation or curvature of the spine is referred to as *scoliosis*. Because of rotation of the spine, which is almost always a component of the deformity, the abnormality is best demonstrated in physical examination in forward flexion, in which asymmetry of the paraspinous region or rib prominence will be most apparent. Scoliosis has been classified as shown below (modified from Ponseti and Freedman, and R.B. Winter):

I. Nonstructural
  A. Postural scoliosis
  B. Nerve root irritation
    1. Disc herniation
    2. Inflammatory
  C. Muscle spasm secondary to injury
II. Structural scoliosis
  A. Idiopathic
    1. Cervicothoracic
    2. Thoracic
      a. Infantile—age of onset under 3 years
        i. Resolving
        ii. Progressive
      b. Juvenile—age of onset 4–9 years
      c. Adolescent—age of onset 10 years to skeletal maturity
    3. Thoracolumbar
    4. Lumbar
    5. Combined thoracic and lumbar
  B. Osteopathic
    1. Congenital vertebral anomalies
    2. Thoracogenic after thoracoplasty or empyema
    3. Osteochondrodystrophy
      a. Mucopolysaccharidosis
      b. Diastrophic dwarfism
      c. Spondyloepiphyseal dysplasia
      d. Multiple epiphyseal dysplasia
    4. Degenerative disc disease
    5. Postirradiation
  C. Neuropathic
    1. Congenital
    2. Postpoliomyelitis
    3. Neurofibromatosis
    4. Syringomyelia
    5. Charcot-Marie-Tooth disease
    6. Friedreich's ataxia
    7. Cerebral palsy
    8. Spinal muscular atrophy
    9. Meningomyelocele
    10. Dysautonomia (Riley-Day syndrome)
  D. Myopathic
    1. Arthrogryposis multiplex congenita
    2. Muscular dystrophies
    3. Myotonic dystrophy
  E. Metabolic
    1. Osteogenesis imperfecta
    2. Ehlers-Danlos syndrome
    3. Marfan syndrome
    4. Homocystinuria
  F. Tumors
    1. Osteoid osteoma
    2. Eosinophilic granuloma
    3. Spinal cord tumors
  G. Traumatic

Postural Scoliosis. Postural scoliosis occurs in adolescent girls as a characteristically nonprogressive mild left thoracolumbar curve without vertebral rotation that corrects in recumbency. A similar flexible scoliosis can occur with limb length discrepancy and corrects with use of a lift on the short side. Treatment of postural scoliosis is generally with exercises only.

Congenital Scoliosis. Congenital scoliosis occurs as a result of developmental anomalies during embryonic resegmentation of the spine. Unilateral hemivertebrae, fusions of segments, and posterolateral bony bars are the most common abnormalities. When progression of the scoliosis develops, most frequently with unilateral bony bars, fusion of the involved area is necessary. Usually instrumentation is not used, as it increases the risk of paraplegia in these patients. About 20 percent of patients with congenital scoliosis have asymptomatic renal anomalies, and these must be evaluated by intravenous pyelography or abdominal CT or ultrasound studies.

Neuromuscular Scoliosis. Curves with neuromuscular causes such as spinal muscular atrophy, meningomyelocele, cerebral palsy, muscular dystrophies, poliomyelitis, or traumatic paralysis tend to be long, thoracolumbar C-shaped deformities with a high propensity for curve progression. Prognosis depends on the level of the lesion as well as on the age of the patient at the time of onset, with a greater likelihood of progression in younger patients and higher-level lesions. With neurofibromatosis, the curve can be sharp, relatively short, and associated with cutaneous nevi, neurofibromas, or café-au-lait spots. In addition, there may be scalloping of the vertebral bodies and narrowing of the proximal ribs because of neurofibromas of the nerve roots; these curves also have a strong tendency to progress.

Infantile and Juvenile Idiopathic Scoliosis.

Infantile scoliosis presents from birth to age three, while juvenile scoliosis may present up to age ten. The cause is unclear, and the tendency for curve progression is variable. The difference between the rib–vertebral angles on the convex and concave sides of the curve has been correlated predictively with progression, with values greater than 20 degrees indicating a high probability, and less than 10 degrees, a low probability. Early management of the infantile or the early-onset juvenile patients consists of casting in patients up to the age of 4 or 5 years, and bracing thereafter. In patients with progression despite appropriate casting or bracing, surgical intervention is indicated. Generally, anterior and posterior surgery is necessary, with anterior fusion over four or five apical segments only. Subsequent posterior instrumentation can be undertaken without fusion using expandable rods with repeat distractions performed annually until the child is old enough for posterior fusion. In the late-onset juvenile cases about 50 percent will require surgical intervention because of progression with bracing alone. Surgery can be delayed until curves reach a magnitude of 55 to 60 degrees, in an effort to allow maximal spinal growth before fusion. Anterior and posterior fusion is necessary.

Idiopathic Scoliosis. *Pathology.* The underlying cause of idiopathic scoliosis is unknown. There is a familial tendency, particularly in females. Abnormalities of vestibular function have been demonstrated in scoliotic patients as well as defects in posterior column functions of vibratory and proprioceptive sense. Abnormalities in collagen synthesis and proteoglycan content in the intervertebral discs also have been identified in scoliosis but are thought to be secondary changes. Thus a defect in neurologic function has been hypothesized as a possible cause. Progression of the curvature occurs during growth in the majority of cases. The most important factors in determining the risk of progression are age of onset, location of the primary curve, and skeletal or physiologic age. Curves tend to stabilize at skeletal maturity (determined radiographically by fusion of the iliac apophyses), but progression in adulthood of approximately 1 degree per year can be expected.

Clinical Manifestations. Scoliosis is rarely associated with back pain and usually presents as an asymptomatic deformity characterized by asymmetry of the back and chest, accentuated by forward bending. In older adults degenerative changes and pain can occur. Severe scoliosis can result in restrictive pulmonary disease and cor pulmonale. The most common type of idiopathic scoliosis is a right thoracic curve, usually seen in girls (Fig. 41-17). Patients frequently have asymmetrical height of the pelvis when standing, or asymmetrical shoulder height or scapular prominence. Forward bending causes prominence of the paraspinous or rib area on the convex side of the curve. Subtle degrees of asymmetry can be visualized without radiographs by

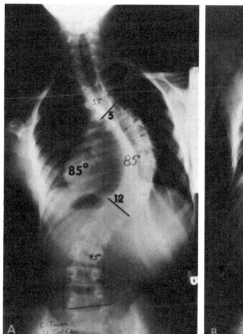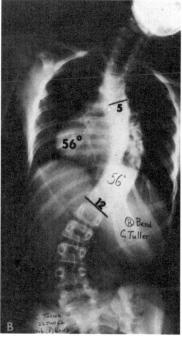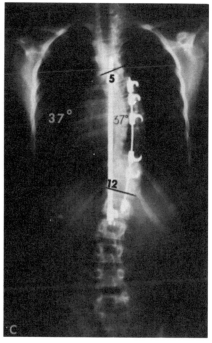

FIG. 41-17. Idiopathic scoliosis treated by Goldstein technique of Harrington rod and massive bone graft. *A.* An 85-degree right thoracic primary curve between T5 and T12. *B.* Lateral bend to the right corrects curve to 56 degrees. *C.* Postoperative correction after Harrington rod instrumentation and bone grafting with massive autogenous cancellous bone. The curve is corrected to 37 degrees and fusion to T1 is performed.

using a Moiré pattern and appropriate illumination to visualize topography of the back; this also has been used as a screening tool.

Radiographic Evaluation. Full-length standing anteroposterior (AP) and lateral radiographs of the thoracic and lumbar spine are necessary, along with supine lateral bending radiographs to assess the flexibility of the curve(s). The primary curve is defined as the longest curve with the greatest degree of angulation and/or the least flexible curve. The degree of angulation (Cobb angle) is measured between perpendicular lines drawn to the end plates of the superior and inferior vertebrae in the curve (see Fig. 41-17).

Treatment. The goal of treatment is to prevent worsening of the deformity. In this regard, careful periodic follow-up is essential to monitor curve progression. For idiopathic scoliosis, nomograms have been developed to predict the risk of progression on the basis of magnitude of curve, skeletal maturity, and age. Observation is the mainstay of conservative treatment, and general spinal exercises to maintain flexibility are advised. For curves greater than 30 degrees with documented progression, bracing with a Milwaukee-type brace or a thoracolumbosacral orthosis is indicated. An alternative but controversial treatment is electrical muscle stimulation on the convexity of the curve, which is used by the patient at night. For curves over 40 degrees with evidence of progression, fusion with instrumentation is indicated. In general, Harrington and Luque rodding posteriorly with sublaminar or transspinous process wiring (segmental stabilization) are the most commonly used techniques. Cotrel-Dubousset posterior instrumentation, which has cross-linkage between the rods, affording greater stability and better preservation of anatomic sagittal contours, also may be used (Fig. 41-18). Spinal cord monitoring (somatosensory evoked potentials) often is used during surgical correction of spinal deformities to decrease the incidence of neurologic deficit. Electrical stimulation of the lower extremities transmits impulses through the spinal cord, causing changes on the electroencephalogram (EEG). Computerized equipment analyzes and monitors the EEG patterns and can give early warning of conduction abnormalities in the cord, allowing preventive modification of the surgical procedure intraoperatively.

Anterior (Dwyer or Zielke) instrumentation occasionally is used in treatment of lumbar or thoracolumbar curves, particularly those of neuromuscular origin, or in adults. Most neuromuscular curves are treated surgically fairly early because of the strong propensity for progression; generally a long fusion from the upper thoracic spine to the sacrum is needed with segmental (Luque) instrumentation. The selection of the extent of the fusion is determined by identifying the vertebra in neutral rotation at the upper and at the lower end of the curve, judged by symmetry of the pedicles and midline position of the spinous process on an anteroposterior radiograph. With Harrington rodding and spinal fusion, postoperative ambulatory immobilization in a body cast or orthosis is necessary, while the more rigid fixation with the Cotrel-Dubousset or Luque technique can obviate the need for this.

Knee Deformities

Genu Valgum

Angular deviations about the knees often are physiologic and rarely require treatment. From birth until about 3 years of age, children have a physiologic varus orientation of the knees (bowleg appearance), which generally corrects spontaneously and converts to a valgus orientation from ages 4 to 8 (Fig. 41-19). The normal adult valgus angle of the knees of 6 degrees is obtained during these years. Physiologic angulations in children of as great as 30 degrees of varus and 20 degrees of valgus can spontaneously correct with growth. Thus the most common treatment approach is parental reassurance and clinical follow-up.

Occasionally progression of the apparent deformity occurs. Causes include vitamin D deficiency (rickets), rheumatoid arthritis, and trauma as well as idiopathic causes. Genu valgum also may be seen in some genetic diseases, such as Morquio's syndrome (mucopolysaccharidosis type IV) and Engelmann's (or Camurati-Engelmann) disease (diaphyseal dysplasia). With progressive deformity, treatment with long leg braces or corrective osteotomy of the proximal tibia or distal femur may be needed.

Genu Varum

Genu varum occasionally fails to resolve spontaneously in infancy, and progression can occur. Physiologic genu varum in an infant is demonstrated in Fig. 41-19. The most common form of genu varum is Blount's disease, a disturbance of the medial proximal tibial growth plate that is seen in infantile and adolescent forms. Persistent excessive medial weight bearing is thought to traumatize the medial growth plate, slowing medial growth and causing the deformity to worsen. Measurement of the metaphyseal-diaphyseal angle provides a means of diagnosis (Fig. 41-20). An angle greater than 11 degrees is consistent with a diagnosis of Blount's disease. In cases with significant deformity or pain, osteotomy of the tibia may be indicated. Stapling of the lateral growth plate is an alternative but less predictable method. Genu varum also may be associated with renal osteodystrophy or achondroplasia, or it may follow trauma to the growth plates about the knee.

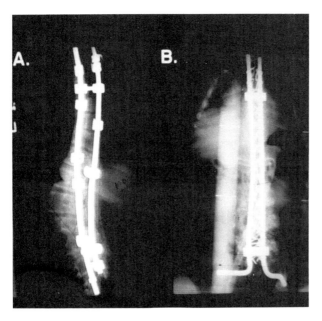

FIG. 41-18. *Spinal instrumentation with Cotrel-Dubousset instrumentation for idiopathic scoliosis (A), and Luque segmental instrumentation for neuromuscular curve (B).*

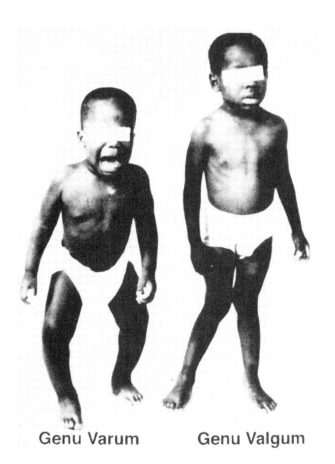

Genu Varum   **Genu Valgum**

FIG. 41-19. Two brothers demonstrating changes in angular growth about the knee. The patient on the left, who is under 2 years of age, exhibits genu varum, while the boy on the right, at 3 years of age, demonstrates genu valgum, illustrating the change from varus to valgus with normal growth. (Modified from: *Orthopaedic Knowledge Update-I, American Academy of Orthopaedic Surgeons, Park Ridge, IL, 1984, p 312, with permission.*)

Foot and Ankle Deformities

Flatfoot (Pes Planus)

Hypermobile or flexible flatfoot is a benign congenital condition that ordinarily is not painful and does not require treatment. Flexibility can be demonstrated by having the child stand on the toes, which usually will reconstitute a normal arch contour, particularly if the flatfoot is in association with Achilles tendon tightness. Treatment with an arch support or orthosis is indicated only for foot pain, excessive shoe wear, or family history of symptomatic flatfoot.

Peroneal Spastic Flatfoot. Although peroneal spastic flatfoot may be caused by inflammatory and traumatic involvement of the tarsal joints, the most common cause is abnormal congenital fusion of tarsal bones, referred to as *tarsal bar* or *tarsal coalition*. The bar may be cartilaginous, particularly in younger children, and may be difficult to visualize on routine radiographs. The most common coalition is the calcaneonavicular bar, followed by talocalcaneal and calcaneocuboid fusions (Fig. 41-21). The oblique radiograph will best demonstrate a calcaneonavicular bar, and an axial radiograph of the hindfoot

is most useful for identifying talocalcaneal coalition. CT scans are also quite helpful when plain-film radiographs are negative. Conservative treatment with anti-inflammatory medications and orthotics can be helpful, but if symptoms persist, resection of the bar with fat or silicone interposition sometimes is necessary. In older adolescents and adults triple arthrodesis may be indicated, especially if degenerative arthritis is present in the adjacent tarsal joints.

Acquired Flatfoot. Flatfoot can be caused by osseous disruption (trauma or infection), ligamentous or tendinous rupture (foot sprain or posterior tibialis tendon rupture), or neuromuscular disorders (poliomyelitis, cerebral palsy, or Charcot neuropathic arthropathy). Acquired flatfoot involves medial and plantar deviation of the head of the talus, frequently accompanied by valgus deformity of the hindfoot (pes planovalgus). Treatment involves supportive measures and orthotics. In cases with severe deformity, pain, or secondary degenerative changes, options for surgical intervention include Grice subtalar or triple arthrodesis, calcaneal or midfoot osteotomy, and posterior tibialis advancement.

Contracture

The term *contracture* implies a permanent shortening and loss of flexibility of muscles, joints, tendons, or fascia. Contractures can be congenital or acquired. Examples of congenital contractures include talipes equinovarus (clubfoot), torticollis, and arthrogryposis multiplex congenita. Acquired contractures of joints can result from periarticular trauma, arthritis, muscle imbalance

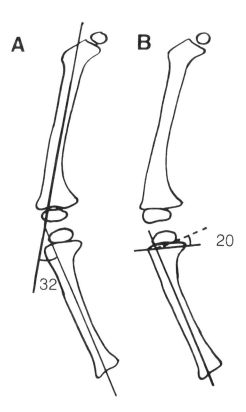

FIG. 41-20. Tibiofemoral angle (A) and tibial metaphyseal-diaphyseal angle (B). A metaphyseal-diaphyseal angle of less than 11 degrees is physiologic.

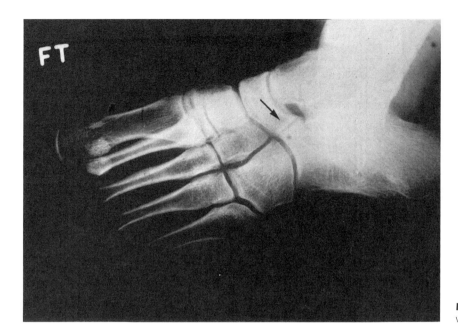

FIG. 41-21. Tarsal coalition with calcaneona-vicular bar *(arrow)*.

(as with cerebral palsy), burns, muscle injury, or idiopathic conditions such as Dupuytren's contracture of the palmar fascia. Contractures of muscles or joints also may occur postoperatively and can be avoided by appropriate strengthening and range-of-motion exercises with the assistance of a physical therapist. The use of continuous-passive-motion machines postoperatively also can help to prevent joint contractures; these have been particularly useful for the knee and also are used occasionally after surgery on the hip or elbow.

Ischemic Contractures (Volkmann's Contracture; Compartment Syndrome). Volkmann first described contractures of the forearm muscles that followed tight bandaging after an elbow fracture in 1875. The contractures result from ischemic muscle necrosis, now recognized as the phenomenon called *compartment syndrome.* All muscle groups in the extremities are bounded by tough, fibrous fascial envelopes called *compartments.* The fascia is relatively unyielding to muscle swelling, which can result from fractures, bleeding, surgery, blunt trauma, or prolonged ischemia (Fig. 41-22A). Elevated pressure within a compartment further compromises arterial inflow, and progressive ischemia ensues. Nerves and muscles within the compartment suffer ischemic injury that can rapidly become irreversible, and severe pain and loss of neuromuscular function occur.

The cardinal signs of compartment syndrome include (1) pain out of proportion to the injury; (2) pain on passive stretch of involved muscles; (3) paresthesias, hypesthesia, or loss of motor function, and (4) diminished or absent pulses, along with coolness or pallor of the extremity consistent with decreased perfusion. Circumferential dressings such as tight bandages or casts can contribute to the development of a compartment syndrome by compromising perfusion, and they must be split or removed at the first signs of a compartment syndrome. If symptoms fail to resolve immediately, compartment pressure measurements must be made. Direct measurement of intracompartmental pressures using a needle or slit catheter with a mercury or electronic manometer is the method of definitive diagnosis of compartment syndrome (Fig. 41-22*B*). Normal compartment pressures are less

than 10 mmHg. Sustained pressures above 30 mmHg indicate impending compartment syndrome, and sustained pressures above 40 mmHg indicate the definite presence of a compartment syndrome.

If untreated, the sustained progressive ischemia causes muscle necrosis and loss of voluntary muscle function. The muscle is replaced by fibrous connective tissue, which leads to severe contractures of the joints powered by the involved muscles. Supracondylar fractures of the humerus and tibial fractures are common causes of compartment syndromes. An exercise-induced compartment syndrome occurs with exercise, causing pain and paresthesias, but is self-limited and resolves after the activity is discontinued. Diagnosis is with postexercise compartment pressure measurements, and treatment is by elective surgical fasciotomy. Contractures and permanent muscle damage generally do not occur in this form of compartment syndrome.

Compartment syndrome is an orthopaedic emergency and requires immediate surgical fasciotomy to prevent irreversible nerve and muscle damage. Severe damage can occur within a few hours. Arteriography often is indicated to rule out arterial damage in cases of posttraumatic compartment syndrome. The compartment pressures that will be tolerated by the extremity without irreversible damage depend on the perfusion pressure; hence with relative hypotension a lower level of compartment pressure will necessitate surgery, and slightly higher levels can be tolerated in a hypertensive patient. Compartment pressures less than 20 mmHg below diastolic blood pressure necessitate surgical intervention in hypotensive patients. The presence of symptoms with compartment pressures above normal is an indication for surgery. The skin and fascia must be left open, and pressures within all compartments in the extremity must be measured and all involved compartments thoroughly released.

EPIPHYSEAL DISORDERS (OSTEOCHONDROSES)

The epiphysis comprises the cartilaginous end of a long bone between the growth plate (physis) and the articular surface.

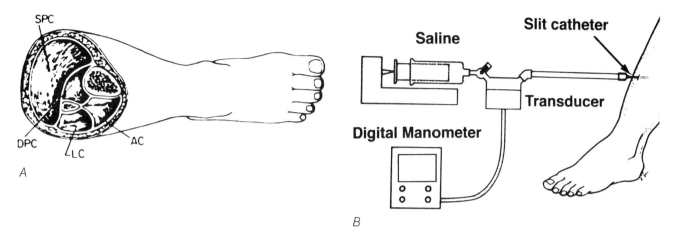

FIG. 41-22. *A. Cross-section demonstrating the compartments of the leg. B. Measurement of compartment pressure with a slit catheter and digital electronic manometer.*

Epiphyses develop secondary centers of ossification, which expand from a central location to replace the cartilaginous epiphysis with trabecular bone through the process of endochondral ossification. At maturity, the only portion of the epiphysis that remains as cartilage is the articular surface. During childhood, a number of disorders of the epiphysis can occur, the etiology of which remains poorly understood. There are several forms of epiphyses, including articular epiphyses, traction epiphyses (apophyses), and atavistic epiphyses. Disorders of the epiphyses were formerly referred to as osteochondritis, but the lack of inflammatory changes histopathologically led to the use of the term *osteochondrosis* as a more accurate description of the various derangements of growth or ossification occurring in epiphyses.

Osteochondroses affect primary and secondary ossification centers. Primary ossification centers (and associated disorders) include:

Scaphoid (Preiser's disease)
Lunate, in adults (Kienböck's disease)
Patella (Köhler's disease)
Talus (Mouchet's disease)
Tarsal navicular (Köhler's disease)

Secondary ossification centers include:

Vertebral epiphysis (Scheuermann's kyphosis)
Humeral head (Hass's disease)
Capitellum (Panner's disease)
Radial head (Brailsford's disease)
Pubic symphysis (Van Neck's disease)
Ischiopubic junction (Oldsberg's disease)
Femoral head (Legg-Calvé-Perthes disease)
Patella (Sinding-Larsen-Johansson syndrome)
Tibial tubercle (Osgood-Schlatter disease)
Calcaneus (Sever's disease)
Metatarsal head (Freiberg's disease)

Cause. The etiology of osteochondrosis remains controversial. In general, vascular disturbance, possibly secondary to trauma, is thought to result in avascular necrosis of the involved epiphysis. In some osteochondroses, such as Osgood-Schlatter disease, there is clear evidence that a traction injury to the epiphysis initiates the pathologic changes. There is some evidence also for an underlying genetic defect in epiphyseal cartilage as a predisposing factor.

Clinical Manifestations. The condition may be unilateral or bilateral, with gradual onset and sometimes a history of antecedent trauma. Pain, joint effusion, limp, limitation of range of motion, and muscle spasm may be present, but the symptoms are often mild.

Radiographic Findings. Osteopenia of the epiphyseal ossification center is present, with areas of increased density. With more severe involvement, fragmentation of the ossification center and deformity and flattening of the epiphysis can occur. The areas of increased density correspond to necrotic bone. The course of the disease usually involves spontaneous revascularization and reconstitution of the ossification center, but there may be residual deformity or growth disturbance.

Legg-Calvé-Perthes Disease

Osteochondrosis involving the hip is primarily seen in boys between the ages of 5 and 9 years and is bilateral in about 10 percent of patients. The pathology is that of osteonecrosis of the ossification center of the femoral epiphysis, but the cause is unknown. The disease has been reported in 1 to 3 percent of patients following transient synovitis of the hip, a disorder clinically mimicking septic arthritis in children but self-limited and resolving spontaneously. In most cases there is no identifiable antecedent event. Epidemiologically, some risk factors have been identified, including delayed bone growth, low socioeconomic status, breech delivery, and being a child of older parents. Coexistence with other osteochondroses such as Scheuermann's disease has been reported and suggests the possibility of an underlying systemic cartilaginous defect. Attention deficit hyperactive disorder has been identified in about one-third of patients with Perthes disease, providing evidence of an underlying genetic predisposing factor. Patients present in the prodromal stage with a limp and hip and/or referred knee pain and loss of motion in the affected hip secondary to muscle spasm initially but later due to deformity of the femoral head. During the active phase, radiographic progression of the disease occurs, but symptoms and muscle spasm resolve or become intermittent. Patients exhibit limitation of abduction and internal rotation, initially due to spasm and later due to flattening and deformity of the femoral head (coxa plana). With the restoration phase the clinical symptoms resolve and the ossific nucleus reconstitutes, although some permanent femoral head deformity and restriction of abduction and hip rotation occasionally remain.

Radiographic Findings. The Caterall classification of the radiographic extent of epiphyseal involvement is the staging system most widely used for prognostication. This staging system has been criticized as insufficiently prospective, since accurate radiographic classification often is not possible until 6 to 8 months after diagnosis. Caterall group I disease exhibits absence of metaphyseal changes or sequestrum formation, with involvement of less than half of the anterior epiphysis. Group II disease shows sequestrum involving the anterior half of the epiphysis, with anterolateral metaphyseal reaction and subchondral fracture line. Group III disease involves more than half of the epiphysis with sequestrum and metaphyseal reaction, and group IV exhibits whole-head involvement with diffuse metaphyseal reaction.

A new classification based on the lateral pillar of the femoral head has been proposed that demonstrates greater predictive value and less interobserver variability (Fig. 41-23). For children with a bone age less than 6 years and lateral pillar involvement of stage A or B, the outcome does not appear to be affected by treatment (i.e., containment). For skeletally older children with stage B involvement, containment by abduction bracing, or femoral or pelvic osteotomy improves outcome.

Waldenström has described four radiographic stages of the disease: (1) failure of ossification center growth and joint space widening; (2) fragmentation with areas of radiolucency; (3) re-ossification with areas of new bone formation; and (4) the healed phase with reconstitution of the epiphysis. The fragmentation stage in a patient with group III involvement is shown in Fig. 41-24.

Studies of the natural history of the disease indicate good, fair, and poor results in about one-third of patients each. Patients with partial (Caterall I and II) involvement have a much better prognosis than those with more extensive involvement (Caterall III and IV). Both clinical and radiologic "at risk" signs that are correlated with a worse prognosis have been identified. Clinical signs include age over 6 years, obesity, progressive loss of hip motion, and adduction contracture. Radiologic signs include defective ossification in the lateral epiphysis, calcification of the epiphysis lateral to the acetabulum, diffuse metaphyseal reaction, lateral subluxation of the hip, and a horizontal growth plate.

Treatment. The differential diagnosis of the disease must include consideration of other disorders that can have similar radiographic changes and clinical presentations, such as hypothyroidism, spondyloepiphyseal dysplasia, multiple epiphyseal dysplasia and sickle cell disease. Treatment is based on containment of the diseased epiphysis within the acetabulum until reossification is complete, which affords the best chance of obtaining a spherical femoral head. The skeletal age and degree of

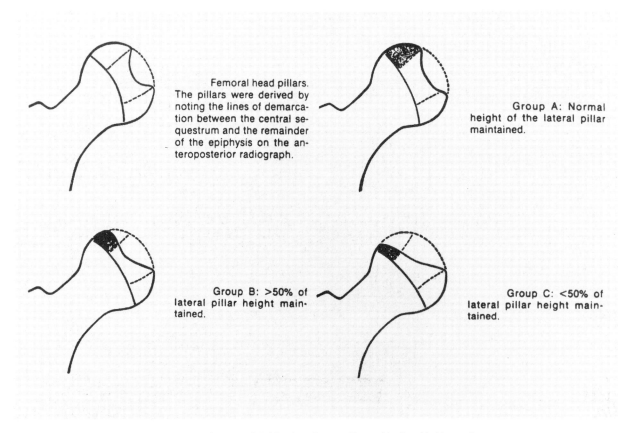

Femoral head pillars. The pillars were derived by noting the lines of demarcation between the central sequestrum and the remainder of the epiphysis on the anteroposterior radiograph.

Group A: Normal height of the lateral pillar maintained.

Group B: >50% of lateral pillar height maintained.

Group C: <50% of lateral pillar height maintained.

FIG. 41-23. The lateral pillar classification for Legg-Calvé-Perthes disease. (From: *Herring JA, Neustadt JB et al: The lateral pillar classification of Legg-Calvé-Perthes disease. J Pediatr Orthop 12:143, 1992, with permission.*)

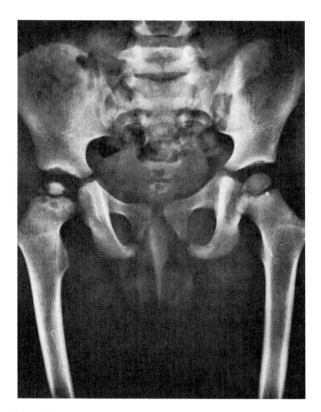

FIG. 41-24. Legg-Calvé-Perthes disease: femoral head osteochondrosis.

Treatment. Treatment is symptomatic and conservative. Immobilization of the knee in an extension or cylinder cast for 4 to 6 weeks may be helpful in particularly symptomatic cases. Symptoms will disappear after fusion of the tibial tubercle apophysis, although enlargement of the tubercle may be permanent. Occasionally a separate ossicle remains within the patellar tendon, and excision can be undertaken for persistent symptoms.

Sinding-Larsen-Johansson syndrome is a similar condition involving the inferior pole of the patella, causing sclerosis and fragmentation. This disorder too is caused by excessive tensile forces on the apophysis and is self-limited and treated symptomatically.

Other Osteochondroses

Köhler's disease of the tarsal navicular occurs in children, with swelling and pain in the area of the navicular. Radiographs show increased density in the navicular ossification center, and treatment is with casting and protected weight bearing until symptoms improve, followed by use of an orthotic arch support (Fig. 41-26). Sever's disease affects the posterior apophysis of the calcaneus in children and can be similar to Osgood-Schlatter disease after a chronic traction injury. Increased radiographic density of the apophysis and pain in the area occur, and treatment is with a heel lift and protected weight bearing when necessary. Freiberg's disease involves the epiphyses of the metatarsal heads, usually the second or third. The cause is unknown, but pathologically, like other osteochondroses, necrosis of bone with repair occurs, and the disease is self-limited and treated

lateral pillar involvement of the epiphysis are important factors in identifying those patients most likely to benefit from containment therapy. For femoral heads in which the diseased portion of the epiphysis is contained within the acetabulum in both neutral and abducted positions, observation alone is needed and the prognosis is excellent. For hips with epiphyseal involvement lateral to the acetabulum, but which are contained with abduction, ambulatory treatment in a walking abduction brace for the duration of the healing (12 to 18 months) is generally recommended. For those few patients with noncontainable epiphyseal involvement with the hip abducted, surgical intervention is necessary to achieve containment. Surgical options include varus osteotomy of the proximal femur or osteotomy of the pelvis to extend acetabular coverage over the femoral head (Salter or Chiari osteotomy) (see Fig. 41-28).

Outcome depends on the staging, final sphericity of the femoral head, and congruity with the acetabulum. Symptoms of degenerative arthritis may present in the fourth to sixth decades in patients with residual femoral head deformity.

Osgood-Schlatter Disease

Osgood-Schlatter disease usually presents in patients 13 to 15 years of age whose history may reveal a precipitating injury. Avulsion or fatigue fracture of the epiphysis is thought to be the underlying cause, with secondary defective ossification and prominence of the tubercle. Pain that is aggravated by quadriceps contraction and tenderness and enlargement of the tibial tubercle are the usual presenting complaints. Radiographs may be normal, or irregularity and fragmentation of the ossification center of the tibial tubercle may be present (Fig. 41-25).

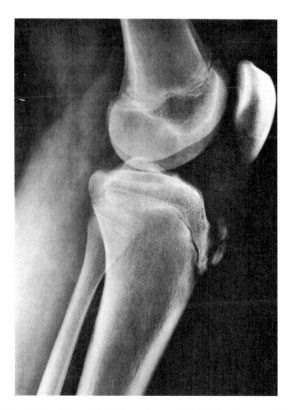

FIG. 41-25. Osgood-Schlatter disease: tibial tubercle osteochondrosis.

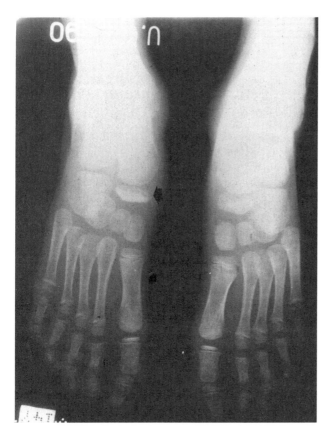

FIG. 41-26. Köhler's disease: osteochondrosis of the tarsal navicular.

with a cast or orthosis with a metatarsal pad to protect the metatarsal head from weight bearing until healing occurs.

CONGENITAL DEFORMITIES

Congenital malformations can be caused by developmental aberrations in utero, environmental influences [radiation exposure, rubella, syphilis, human immunodeficiency virus (HIV), teratogenic drugs, etc.], or hereditary conditions. Overall incidence of congenital malformations diagnosed within 5 years of birth is 23 per 1,000 (Table 41-7). Some of the more common disorders are clubfoot (4.4 per 1,000), spina bifida (3 per 1,000), and hip dislocation (0.7 per 1,000). Metatarsus adductus, valgus hindfoot, unilateral externally rotated leg, internal tibial torsion, or an adducted thigh with external rotation of the leg are conditions thought to result from in utero position, which also may be a contributing factor in the pathogenesis of talipes equinovarus (clubfoot). All of these conditions except talipes equinovarus generally respond to passive stretching exercises, with corrective casts necessary only in refractory cases.

Hip Dislocation. Developmental dysplasia of the hip (DDH) consists of partial or complete displacement of the femoral head from the acetabulum. Epidemiologically, DDH is more common in certain ethnic groups (Navajo Indians, northern Italians, and Japanese), firstborn white females, and in association with other anomalies (torticollis, congenital knee hyperextension or dislocation, and foot deformities). Contributory causative factors include multifactorial inheritance, mechanical factors such as prenatal position, and hormonal influences such as maternal relaxins.

Pathology. In DDH the acetabulum is shallow with a more vertical orientation than normal. It is filled with remnants of ligamentum teres, fat, and fibrocartilage (pulvinar). Overgrowth of the lateral acetabular cartilage occurs in response to pressure of the femoral head (limbus), increasing the obstruction to reduction. A false acetabulum may be present as a depression on the ilium superior to the true acetabulum, lined with periosteum and a fold of the capsule. Ossification of the femoral head is delayed, and the capsule can develop an hourglass-shaped constriction crossed by the iliopsoas tendon. Within a few months of birth, tightness of the shortened adductor muscles develops, causing loss of hip abduction.

Clinical Manifestations. Examination of every newborn's hips in the nursery after birth is essential and effectively detects the majority of dislocated hips. Successful treatment hinges on early diagnosis and intervention. On examination, a hip click can be elicited as the femoral head reduces in the acetabulum with flexion and abduction of the thigh (Ortolani's sign). A similar click occurs with dislocation of the hip by adduction with gentle

Table 41-7
Defects in Embryogenesis and Resulting Deformities

Embryonic Period	Defect	Clinical Deformity
3–3 1/2 weeks	Failure of neural tube closure	Meningomyelocele
4–5 weeks	Defective resegmentation of the spinal somites	Spine anomalies such as unilateral bar or hemivertebrae
5 weeks	Limb bud development	Phocomelia
6 weeks	Long bone formation	Hemimelias, aplasias of long bones
6 weeks	Genetically determined defects in bone and cartilage development	Achondroplasia, osteogenesis imperfecta, mucopolysaccharidoses, osteopetrosis
6 1/2 weeks	Failure of differentiation	Radioulnar synostoses, tarsal coalitions, syndactylies
6 1/2–7 weeks	Faulty regulation of growth by apical ectodermal ridge	Congenital duplications of parts (polydactylies); macrodactyly; limb hemihypertrophy
6–8 weeks	Defective soft tissue development	Amyoplasias, congenital constriction bands, congenital knee dislocation

posterior pressure (Barlow's sign). The gluteal folds will be asymmetrical, and the affected thigh appears shortened when the knees and hips are flexed to 90 degrees (Galeazzi's sign). Limitation of abduction with the hip in flexion may be present at birth but becomes progressively apparent during the first 2 or 3 months. If the dislocation goes undetected the child will have a noticeable limp or waddle when walking begins. Periodic follow-up examinations of the hips in newborns during the first few months are important, and the hip click will disappear, with the limitation of abduction being the most obvious abnormality. Increased lumbar lordosis will be present as the child begins to walk, especially in bilateral dislocations. Milder degrees of dysplasia, with subluxation or shallow acetabulum without frank dislocation, also can occur and are a cause of symptomatic degenerative hip arthritis in adolescents and young adults.

Radiologic Findings. The secondary center of ossification of the femoral head is absent in the newborn and usually appears by 4 to 6 months, although there is a fairly wide range (2 to 10 months). When present, the ossific nucleus should be within vertical lines from the acetabular margin (Perkins' lines) and below a horizontal line drawn through the triradiate growth plate cartilage of the acetabulum (Hilgenreiner's line, Fig. 41-27). The *acetabular index* is the angle of the acetabular roof with Hilgenreiner's line, and normally is 22 degrees. With DDH this angle is greater, and can be as high as 40 degrees. With the hip in abduction, the femoral neck fails to point toward the triradiate cartilage, and Shenton's line (a smooth arc from the lesser trochanter on the femur continuing along the neck and inferior cortex of the pubic bone) is discontinuous. If the ossific nucleus is not present, an arthrogram or MRI will readily demonstrate the dislocated position of the femoral head, although ultrasonography is also an accurate and a less invasive diagnostic modality.

Treatment. In the neonate with DDH, the hip usually can be reduced in flexion and abduction, and treatment is a splint or brace that can maintain this position. The Pavlik harness and Von Rosen splint are two of the more commonly used devices. Flexion of the hip should be 90 to 110 degrees, with slightly less than full abduction. Treatment is for 3 to 6 months, until the acetabular development is normal. In DDH diagnosed in the first few months of life, abduction bracing can also be successful, but radiographic evaluation is needed to be sure that the hip remains reduced. In children under 18 months of age, closed reduction can be attempted under anesthesia. The role of prereduction skin traction, which was advocated in the past, is currently controversial. If concentric reduction can be obtained as judged from radiographs or arthrogram, the patient is placed in a double hip spica cast with the hips flexed to approximately 100 degrees and slightly less than full abduction. Extremes of abduction can impair the blood supply to the femoral head and lead to avascular necrosis. Adductor tenotomy can facilitate the reduction. In children in whom closed reduction cannot be obtained, open reduction is performed using an anterolateral approach, or, in children less than 24 months of age, using a medial approach to the hip. The anterolateral approach in older children facilitates femoral shortening when necessary to achieve reduction. The child is placed in a bilateral hip spica cast with the hips in the position described above to maintain the reduction.

Persistent acetabular dysplasia in children 2 to 5 years old can be corrected by either pericapsular (Pemberton) or innominate (Salter) osteotomy. More extensive procedures such as the Chiari innominate osteotomy are occasionally necessary to obtain superior acetabular coverage of the femoral head in older children (Fig. 41-28).

Dislocation of the Knee. The three types of congenital dislocation of the knee are developmental (thought to be secondary to in utero position), defective embryogenesis (associated with other defects such as DDH), and quadriceps contracture caused by arthrogryposis. The knee is fixed in hyperextension with a variable degree of anterior subluxation or dislocation of the tibia on the distal femur. Treatment depends on the degree of severity and ranges from stretching exercises to surgical quadriceps lengthening followed by cast immobilization.

Pseudarthrosis of the Tibia. Children with this disorder may have a frank pseudarthrosis at birth (usually at the level of the distal and middle thirds of the tibia) or, in milder forms,

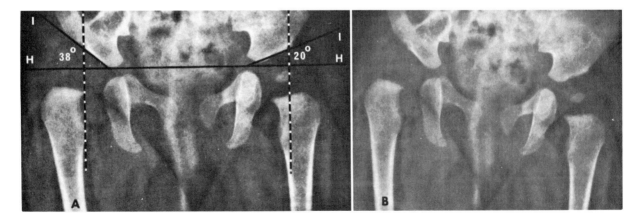

FIG. 41-27. Congenital dislocation of the hip. *A.* The right hip is held in the position of adduction compared with the left. The line parallel with the roof of the acetabulum intersecting Hilgenreiner's line indicates an acetabular index of 38 degrees on the right and acetabular dysplasia. The dotted perpendicular line dropped from the outer margin of the acetabulum shows the proximal capital femoral epiphysis to be laterally displaced, indicating dislocation. The normal left side shows the dotted line at the outer margin of the proximal capital femoral epiphysis. *B.* Right proximal capital femoral epiphysis is much smaller than the left and is laterally displaced.

anterolateral bowing that progresses to pseudarthrosis later. This condition must be differentiated from congenital posteromedial bowing of the tibia, which usually is self-limited. Congenital pseudarthrosis of the tibia is frequently associated with neurofibromatosis. With bowing alone, a total-contact orthosis is used to prevent progression, but once pseudarthrosis develops it can be very difficult to treat. Treatment methods for established pseudarthrosis include intramedullary rod fixation with bone grafting; more recently, free vascularized fibular grafts have been used successfully. Amputation occasionally is necessary in refractory cases.

Metatarsus Adductus. Metatarsus adductus is a common congenital foot deformity also known as metatarsus varus, the cause of which is thought to be related to intrauterine positioning. It occurs in 1 per 1,000 live births, and half of the cases are bilateral. The forefoot is angulated medially, but the deformity is not associated with equinus of the heel. When passively correctable, metatarsus adductus resolves spontaneously. In incompletely correctable deformities, serial manipulation and casting is the accepted treatment. Surgical treatment rarely is necessary and is indicated only in children over the age of 5 years with severe symptomatic residual adductus deformity. Osteotomies of the lateral column (cuboid), medial cuneiform, or metatarsals can accomplish correction.

Talipes Equinovarus (Clubfoot). Talipes equinovarus is a complex deformity consisting of plantar flexion of the ankle, inversion of the foot, adduction of the forefoot, and internal rotation of the tibia (Fig. 41-29). The cause is unknown, and theories include neurologic and vascular defects. Inheritance is variable in pattern, with overall incidence of approximately 1 per 1,000 births, and a 2:1 male preponderance. Siblings have a 1 in 35 probability of the disorder, and identical twins a 1 in 3 chance. The prevailing theory of cause is a single gene predisposing mutation in conjunction with one or more unidentified environmental factors. Talipes equinovarus is associated with other disorders, including myelomeningocele, arthrogryposis, and diastrophic dwarfism.

Pathologic Anatomy. Three-dimensional computer modeling has shown the talus to be externally rotated in the ankle mortise, with 45 degrees of internal rotation of the talar neck (compared to slight internal rotation in the mortise and a 25-degree internal rotation of the neck in normals). The talus is also smaller than normal, and the calcaneus is internally rotated and in varus compared to slight external rotation in normal feet. The tibial tendon sheaths are fibrotic and thickened, and the navicular is subluxated medially on the head of the talus. Radiographically, the calcaneus and talus are more parallel than divergent on a lateral view (Fig. 41-30).

Treatment. Without treatment the condition is permanent and ambulation difficult. Treatment is started immediately in the neonatal period, with stretching exercises and serial plaster casts. Adduction of the forefoot is corrected first, then hindfoot varus, and correction of equinus is not undertaken until these deformities are completely corrected. Conservative treatment is successful in about 50 percent of patients. Surgical correction consists of posteromedial and subtalar release and usually is delayed until the patient reaches 6 to 8 months, but it should not be delayed beyond the age of 1 to 2 years. Complete release of the subtalar joint is best accomplished by a circumferential trans-

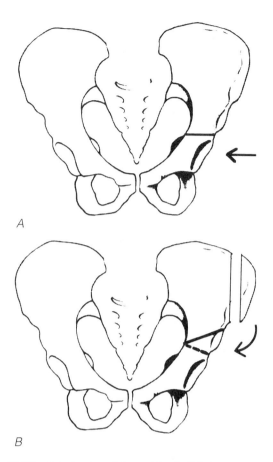

A

B

FIG. 41-28. *Osteotomies of the pelvis. A. Chiari osteotomy, with transverse osteotomy and medial displacement of the acetabulum. B. Salter osteotomy, with oblique cut and graft to inferiorly displace lateral acetabular roof.*

verse incision extending from the lateral side of the hindfoot posteriorly to the medial side, known as the Cincinnati approach.

In recurrent cases, manipulation will not suffice for correction, and posteromedial release is necessary. Lateral transfer of

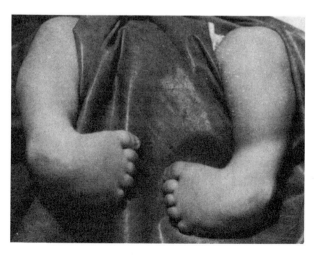

FIG. 41-29. *Characteristic deformities of talipes equinovarus, or clubfoot.*

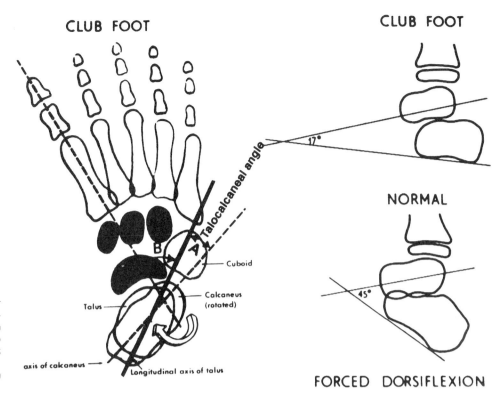

FIG. 41-30. *Talipes equinovarus. The angle between the talus and calcaneus in the anteroposterior projection should be 22 to 45 degrees, and in the lateral projection (with the foot in dorsiflexion), 20 to 45 degrees. In clubfoot, the talus and calcaneus are less divergent, and the angles smaller than normal.*

the tibialis anterior tendon along with Achilles tendon lengthening may also be helpful in patients with mild degrees of recurrence. Incomplete release of the calcaneocuboid joint is believed to be the most common cause of residual adduction or cavovarus deformities. In severe refractory deformities such as those seen with arthrogryposis, talectomy can be necessary to achieve a plantigrade foot.

Convex Pes Valgus (Vertical Talus). Congenital vertical talus (also known as rocker-bottom flatfoot) consists of a dorsal dislocation of the navicular on the head of the talus, with the talus in a more vertical position than normal (Fig. 41-31). The sole of the foot has a rocker-bottom deformity and is not

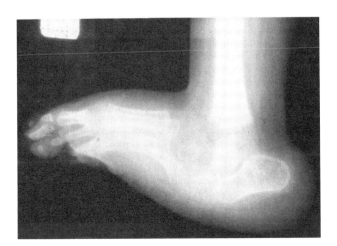

FIG. 41-31. *Congenital vertical talus. Note vertical position of talus and rocker-bottom deformity of foot.*

passively correctable. Vertical talus may be an isolated anomaly, or it may be found in association with meningomyelocele, arthrogryposis, or chromosomal aberrations. Early manipulation and casting can be successful, particularly in milder deformities (referred to as *oblique talus,* in which the first metatarsal aligns with the talus in forced plantar flexion). However, the majority of cases of true vertical talus require surgical correction. Diagnosis is made from the lateral forced-plantar-flexion radiograph, in which the talus and the first metatarsal are not in alignment. Operation is delayed until the patient is 4 to 8 months old and consists of open reduction and pinning of the talonavicular joint, along with lengthening of the Achilles tendon, posterior tibialis, and, when necessary, the toe extensors, peronei, and anterior tibialis tendons. In older children, a Grice subtalar arthrodesis may be necessary. Undiagnosed cases in older children with adaptive bony changes are treated with triple arthrodesis (see Fig. 41-14).

Arthrogryposis Multiplex Congenita (Amyoplasia). Arthrogryposis involves failure of development of muscles and resulting contractures of the extremities. It is not thought to have a genetic basis and is characterized by severe, symmetrical contractures with deformities, including scoliosis, talipes equinovarus, DDH, knee dislocation, internally rotated shoulders, and extended elbows. The individual deformities are treated as described above, but contractures tend to be quite severe, and occasionally osteotomies are needed to improve function and decrease deformity. A genetic variant called distal arthrogryposis has been identified, which affects the digits only.

High Scapula (Sprengel's Deformity). High scapula is caused by embryonic failure of the scapula to migrate to its normal position. The scapula may be attached to the vertebrae by a pathologic band of fibrous tissue and cartilage (omovertebral mass). Other deformities of the spine and ribs are often associated. The scapula is 1 to 4 inches higher than usual, tilted anteriorly, and does not move normally with shoulder motion (Fig. 41-32). Usually it is the cosmetic appearance rather than any functional deficit that brings attention to the disorder. Mild cases need no treatment, but in more severe cases surgical correction can be undertaken, although it is generally delayed until the patient is 3 to 6 years old.

Klippel-Feil Syndrome. Also known as brevicollis and congenital short neck, this syndrome consists of multiple fusions of cervical vertebrae secondary to defective resegmentation of the cervical spine during embryogenesis and is usually not treatable.

Torticollis. Torticollis, also known as congenital wryneck, is caused by unilateral contracture of the sternocleidomastoid muscle, with tilt of the head toward the affected side, rotation to the opposite side, and varying degrees of facial dysplasia. The disorder is thought to be posttraumatic, with a tender swelling in the muscle preceding the deformity. Treatment consists of stretching exercises and, in refractory cases, surgical release of the muscle with cast immobilization or vigorous passive exercises postoperatively.

Cleidocranial Dysostosis. Cleidocranial dysostosis is an autosomal dominant hereditary syndrome exhibiting clavicular aplasia, widened diameter of the cranium, and delayed fontanelle closure. Disability is minimal and treatment usually not needed.

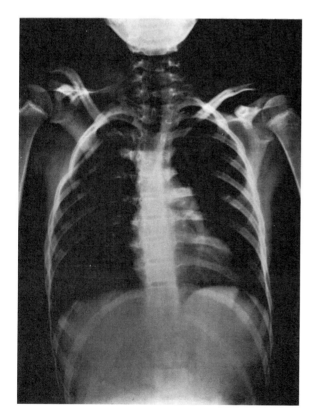

FIG. 41-32. *Radiograph showing the abnormal high situation of the right scapula in Sprengel's deformity.*

Radioulnar Synostosis. This disorder results from defective embryogenesis, with a fusion between the proximal radius and ulna and absence of pronation and supination. Most cases are bilateral, and the degree of deformity or hypoplasia of the proximal radius is variable. Nonfunctional extremes of pronation or supination can be corrected by osteotomy, but resection of the fusion bar has given disappointing results. Resection followed by low-dose irradiation (8 to 10 Gy), a treatment that prevents heterotopic ossification after hip surgery, has been used with some success in prevention of bar reformation.

Madelung's Deformity. This disorder involves progressive volar and ulnar angulation of the distal radius, causing prominence of the distal ulna and abnormality of the shape of the distal radial articular surface. Although wrist pain can occur, most patients are treated conservatively with splinting. Rarely, osteotomy of the distal radius and shortening of the distal ulna is indicated.

Aplasia or Dysplasia of Long Bones. These rare deformities, which do not appear to be hereditary, consist of absence of a bone or part of a bone. The term *congenital skeletal limb deficiencies* is used to describe these disorders collectively. Skeletal deficiencies can be intercalary (an absent segment with bones distal to it intact) or terminal (all bones distal to the lesion absent), and transverse or longitudinal. As an example, absence of the fibula alone would be classified as an intercalary, longitudinal fibular hemimelia. Absence of a hand or foot would be described as a terminal transverse defect (congenital amputation).

Absence of the Radius. The deformity known as radial clubhand is caused by the absence of the radius, which is sometimes bilateral and can be associated with craniofacial anomalies, thrombocytopenia, or Fanconi's anemia (pancytopenia). If the defect is terminal rather than intercalary, the thumb may be absent. Early treatment involves manipulation and splinting and, by the age of 12 months, surgical centralization of the carpus on the ulna. Absence of the ulna is much less common and is associated with digital abnormalities, such as syndactyly, in 90 percent of cases. Treatment is generally nonoperative for the wrist and elbow and focuses on correction of digital abnormalities that impair function.

Fibular Hemimelia. In this disorder, the limb is shortened and the hindfoot usually in equinovalgus position. Involvement is bilateral in 30 percent of cases. For milder cases, limb length equalizations may be possible using the Ilizarov technique; more severe deficiencies may require amputation.

Femoral Hypoplasia. These deformities can range from mild hypoplasia to complete absence of the upper femur. Mild cases are treated by limb length equalization procedures. In more severe cases fusion of the femoral remnant to the ilium or amputation with knee fusion and prosthetic limb fitting has been performed.

GENERALIZED BONE DISORDERS

Composition. Bone is made up of organic and inorganic materials. The organic components include type I collagen (90 percent of the organic matrix), phosphoproteins, bone-specific proteoglycan, sialoprotein, osteonectin, osteocalcin, and growth factors such as transforming growth factor-beta (TGF-β), fibro-

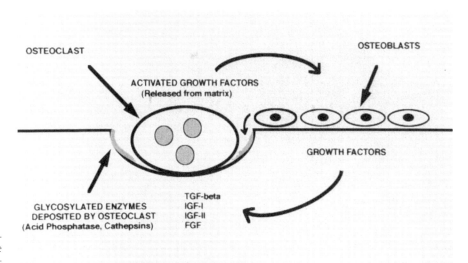

FIG. 41-33. Local coupling of bone formation and resorption. Osteoclasts release and activate growth factors from bone matrix during resorption, and may also deposit glycosylated proteins on the surface. The growth factors stimulate osteoblast progenitor cells to differentiate, and the surface proteins may direct the bone cells to the specific site.

blast growth factors, insulinlike growth factors, and bone morphogenetic proteins. These factors and proteins incorporated into the matrix of bone are responsible for the maintenance of normal bone remodeling processes, and they give bone matrix its osteogenic properties, which make bone grafting possible. Before it is mineralized, the bone matrix secreted by osteoblasts is called *osteoid.*

The inorganic phase of bone consists of hydroxyapatite, a crystalline form of calcium and phosphate, and water, which makes up 8 to 9 percent of bone. Citrate, carbonate, and magnesium also are present. The mineral phase of bone is responsible for its compressive strength, while collagen gives bone its tensile strength. Hydroxyapatite crystals are spontaneously deposited in the "hole zones" formed within the quarter-staggered overlapping array of the type I collagen molecules and later are spread along the fibers by secondary nucleation. Osteonectin, a glycoprotein in bone matrix, may have a role in binding the hydroxyapatite crystals to the collagen. Osteopontin, a phosphoprotein in bone matrix, may be involved in cell attachment to bone, and osteocalcin, a carboxyglutamic acid containing glycoprotein, is thought to be involved in osteoclastic recruitment for the resorption of bone matrix.

Cell Biology. Bone matrix is normally secreted by osteoblasts in discrete layers (lamellae), with the collagen in each successive layer oriented 90 degrees to the adjacent layer. This plywoodlike structure maximizes the mechanical strength of the material. Osteoblasts become entrapped in the secreted matrix and become more quiescent cells known as *osteocytes.* Osteocytes have numerous cell processes called *canaliculi,* which communicate with each other through the bone matrix. In injury and repair processes, bone-forming tumors, and diseases such as Paget's disease, osteoblasts initially secrete woven bone, in which the collagen fibrils have a random orientation. The three-dimensional structure of bone is similar to that of a sponge, with all the bony trabeculae interconnected and the pores containing the bone marrow.

Osteoclasts are multinucleated bone-resorbing cells (also called giant cells) of monocytic lineage that attach to bone surfaces and secrete enzymes that break down organic components of bone matrix. In addition, a proton pump in the plasma membrane of the osteoclast acidifies the region between the cell and the bone surface, dissolving the mineral phase. The cavity excavated by the osteoclast is referred to as a *Howship's lacuna.* Bone is constantly formed and resorbed in the skeleton throughout life. Bone formation and resorption are locally coupled, with osteoblasts always following in the wake of an osteoclast and replacing the resorbed bone with new lamellar bone. Coupling factors such as bone morphogenetic proteins and other members of the TGF-β family are thought to be activated by the acidic environment of the osteoclast and may serve to attract and stimulate osteoblast progenitor cells, accounting for the local coupling phenomenon (Fig. 41-33). When cortical bone undergoes remodeling, osteoclasts tunnel longitudinally within the cortex, forming a cutting cone. Concentric layers of lamellar bone are subsequently deposited, leaving only a narrow central canal that contains vascular channels supplying blood to the bone. This structure is referred to as a *haversian system* or *osteon* (Fig. 41-34).

Enzymes. Osteoblasts contain high levels of alkaline phosphatase, while osteoclasts contain glycolytic enzymes, collagenases, acid hydrolases, and acid phosphatase. Evidence suggests that some of these enzymes, which are glycosylated with mannose-6-phosphate, remain on the resorption surface and can site-direct bone formation through interaction of mannose-6-phosphate moieties with the insulinlike growth factor II receptor of osteoblasts or osteoblast precursor cells. Alkaline phosphatase is thought to be involved in the mineralization process, although its role is not yet understood. Serum levels of alkaline phospha-

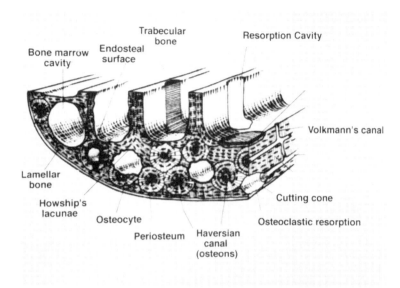

FIG. 41-34. The cellular and structural organization of bone.

tase derived from bone can be elevated in rickets, osteomalacia, Paget's disease, osteosarcoma, and metastatic carcinoma. Decreased levels can be found in achondroplasia, scurvy, hypothyroidism, and a hereditary deficiency of alkaline phosphatase called *hypophosphatasia.*

Ossification. *Endochondral Ossification.* The long bones of the skeleton, with the exception of the clavicle, are formed embryonically from a hyaline cartilage precursor. In the center of the precursor, or anlage, the chondrocytes undergo hypertrophy and begin to calcify the surrounding cartilaginous matrix; this constitutes the primary ossification center. The process extends toward the ends of the long bone, becoming an orderly front of proliferating, hypertrophying, and calcifying cells known as the *growth plate* or *physis.* With ingrowth of the nutrient vessel into the central portion of the forming bone, the calcified cartilage is converted into trabecular bone. Concomitantly, formation of the cortical portion of the bone begins with osteoblastic bone synthesis from the periosteum directly (membranous bone formation), giving rise to the primary bone collar, which also extends from the center toward the ends of the long bone (Fig. 41-35).

During fetal and childhood osteogenesis, endochondral ossification continues in the growth plate, accounting for growth in length of the bone; ossification also occurs within the epiphysis when the secondary centers of ossification appear. Latitudinal growth also occurs at the level of the growth plate by recruitment of cells from the perichondral ring of Lacroix. The diameter of the shaft of the long bones increases through periosteal accretion of new cortical bone with endosteal resorption. The process of endochondral ossification is an integral part of fracture healing by callus formation. Endochondral ossification as it occurs in the growth plate is depicted in Fig. 41-36. The growth plate exhibits a gradient of oxygen and nutrients from the upper proliferating zone to the zone of provisional calcification, and the chondrocytes gradually shift from an aerobic metabolism in the proliferating zone to an anaerobic metabolism in the hypertrophic zone. The hypertrophic chondrocytes acquire high levels

of alkaline phosphatase, accumulate calcium, and secrete calcium-containing matrix vesicles from the plasma membrane that are thought to initially nucleate hydroxyapatite crystals in the matrix.

The proliferation and maturation of the chondrocytes in endochondral calcification are controlled systemically by growth hormone through insulinlike growth factor I, and locally by autocrine growth factors. The most important growth factors known to control chondrocyte proliferation and hypertrophy are TGF-β, basic fibroblast growth factor (bFGF), and parathyroid hormone-related protein (PTHrP). bFGF is produced in the proliferating and resting zones, and defects in FGF receptors are

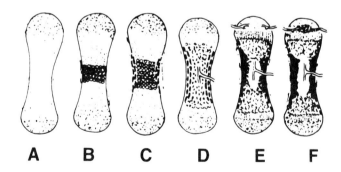

FIG. 41-35. Embryologic development of long bones. *A.* The long bone forms from a mesenchymal precursor (anlage) that differentiates into cartilage. *B.* Hypertrophy of the cells and matrix calcification (primary ossification center) forms in the center of the long bone and progresses toward the ends. *C.* Primary bone collar is formed by osteoblastic activity of the periosteum. *D.* Vascular ingrowth of the nutrient vessel occurs in association with conversion of the calcified cartilage to bone. *E.* The calcification front becomes an orderly plate of cartilage (growth plate, or physis) near the end of the bone, and vascular ingrowth in the epiphysis occurs. *F.* Secondary centers of ossification develop in the epiphyses, expanding centrifugally, with structure and function similar to that of the growth plate, resulting in endochondral ossification of all but the cartilaginous articular surface. (Modified from: *Albright JA, Brand RA (eds): Scientific Basis of Orthopaedics. Norwalk, CT, Appleton: Lange, 1987, with permission.*)

GROWTH PLATE

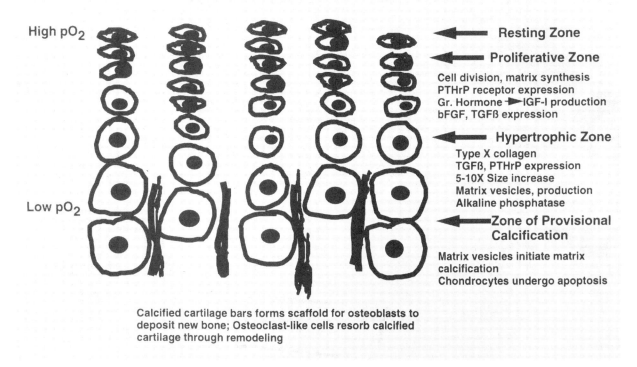

High pO₂

Resting Zone

Proliferative Zone

Cell division, matrix synthesis
PTHrP receptor expression
Gr. Hormone ➤ IGF-I production
bFGF, TGFß expression

Hypertrophic Zone

Type X collagen
TGFß, PTHrP expression
5-10X Size increase
Matrix vesicles, production
Alkaline phosphatase

Low pO₂

Zone of Provisional Calcification

Matrix vesicles initiate matrix calcification
Chondrocytes undergo apoptosis

Calcified cartilage bars forms scaffold for osteoblasts to deposit new bone; Osteoclast-like cells resorb calcified cartilage through remodeling

FIG. 41-36. Structure and function relationships of the growth plate.

responsible for disorders such as achondroplasia and thanato-phoric dysplasia (FGFR3 mutations). PTHrP is produced in the lower proliferating and upper hypertrophic zone and stimulates proliferation while suppressing hypertrophy. PTHrP or PTHrP receptor deletion causes severe lethal disruptions of the growth plate, with loss of the proliferating zone, premature hypertrophy, and defective transformation of calcified cartilage into bone.

The zone of provisional calcification is mechanically the weakest part of the growth plate, accounting for the propensity of children's fractures near the ends of long bones to involve this region. In addition, the hypertrophic chondrocytes produce a unique collagen (type X collagen) that facilitates conversion of the calcified cartilage into bone in the metaphysis. Defects in endochondral ossification may be inherited (achondroplasia) or acquired (vitamin D deficiency rickets).

Intramembranous Ossification. This form of ossification does not involve a cartilage precursor tissue; rather, osteoblasts secrete osteoid and mineralize it directly. Intramembranous or osteoblastic ossification occurs in the calvaria and, as described above, in the periosteum of the long bones. This process is a part of the later phases of fracture healing, in which it gradually supplants endochondral ossification.

Remodeling. As described earlier, bone is continuously forming and resorbing in a locally coupled manner. During growth, remodeling also changes the shape of the long bones, with activity of osteoclasts and osteoblasts particularly in the

cone-shaped metaphyseal area resulting in a narrowing of the diameter of the bone toward the diaphysis. In addition, bone formation and resorption are strongly influenced by mechanical stresses in bone, with net resorption in unloaded bone and increased accretion in loaded bone. Bone is an anisotropic material and develops piezoelectric charges on its surfaces in response to mechanical stresses. Bone cells are thought to respond to these electrical signals, modulating formative and resorptive activities.

Bone Grafting. *Mechanisms.* Bone grafting, the transplantation of bone from one site to another (autologous graft) or from one individual to another (allograft), is an essential part of many orthopaedic surgical procedures. Bone grafts work through one or both of two mechanisms—osteoconduction or osteoinduction. With osteoconduction, the graft may serve to provide a mechanical support and serves as a scaffolding on which host osteoblasts can form new bone and through remodeling eventually replace the graft. This mechanism predominates in cortical bone and large segmental allografts. Osteoinduction is the property of release and activation of bone-inducing matrix proteins from the graft during osteoclastic resorption. Bone morphogenetic protein and other members of the TGF-β family are among the most important factors in this process. When demineralized bone matrix devoid of bone cells is implanted into muscle or subcutaneous tissue, endochondral-sequence bone formation occurs through this osteoinduction phenomenon.

Sites. The iliac crest is generally used as a donor site for cancellous grafting, and the tibia or fibula for cortical bone grafts. A recent development is the use of vascularized bone grafts, wherein an expendable bone such as the midportion of the fibula is removed along with its nutrient vessels. The vessels are then anastomosed to blood vessels in the area of the recipient site using microsurgical technique. This allows bridging of significant bony defects with living bone, which rapidly incorporates. This technique is being used to speed healing of avascular necrosis of the femoral head by inserting a vascularized graft in the femoral neck and head, and for repair of bony defects caused by trauma or tumor resections.

Allografts. Bone allografts are well tolerated immunologically because antigenic cellular proteins make up only a minute fraction of bone. Freezing or freeze-drying further diminishes the antigenicity of bone without impairing its osteoconductive and osteoinductive properties. As a result bone allografts rarely incite rejection reactions and immunosuppression is unnecessary. Osteochondral allografts are used to reconstruct joint surfaces and contain both bone and articular cartilage. They generally are frozen in the presence of a cryoprotectant such as dimethylsulfoxide, which allows preservation of a proportion of the chondrocytes. The collagen and proteoglycan matrix of articular cartilage does not allow penetration of lymphocytes or antibodies; thus cartilage is also an immunologically privileged tissue.

Synthetic Graft Substitutes. Synthetic materials are being used experimentally as bone graft substitutes and show significant promise. Tricalcium phosphate and hydroxyapatite ceramics and corals have been used successfully to fill bony defects and function as osteoconductive substrates. Resorbable synthetic materials such as polyglycolic and polylactic acid are under investigation as vehicles for growth factors. Purified and recombinant bone morphogenetic proteins and demineralized bone matrix have both been used successfully as bone graft substitutes. Table 41-8 lists bone grafting materials with summaries of their properties.

Classifications

I. Developmental disorders
  A. Achondroplasia
  B. Enchondromatosis
  C. Multiple exostoses
  D. Polyostotic fibrous dysplasia
  E. Osteogenesis imperfecta
  F. Osteopetrosis
  G. Osteochondrodystrophies
II. Metabolic disorders
  A. Mineralization defects
    1. Vitamin D deficiency (rickets or osteomalacia)
      a. Nutritional
      b. Malabsorption syndromes
      c. Renal disease
      d. Hepatobiliary disease
    2. Vitamin D-resistant hypophosphatemic rickets
    3. Aluminum-induced osteomalacia
  B. Hormonal disorders
    1. Hyperthyroidism
    2. Hyperparathyroidism
    3. Hypercortisolism (Cushing's disease)
    4. Postmenopausal osteoporosis
    5. Hypogonadism
    6. Pituitary disorders
III. Bone marrow diseases

A. Reticuloendothelial system
  1. Histiocytosis X
    a. Letterer-Siwe disease
    b. Eosinophilic granuloma
    c. Hand-Schuller-Christian disease
  2. Lipoid granulomatosis
    a. Gaucher's disease
    b. Niemann-Pick disease
    c. Xanthomatosis
B. Lymphomas of bone
  1. Hodgkin's disease
  2. Histiocytic lymphoma
C. Hematopoietic system
  1. Leukemia
  2. Multiple myeloma
  3. Hemolytic anemias
    a. Thalassemia (Cooley's anemia)
    b. Sickle cell anemia
    c. Erythroblastosis fetalis
  4. Myelofibrosis
  5. Mastocytosis
IV. Vascular disorders
  A. Paget's disease
  B. Sudeck's atrophy
  C. Massive osteolysis (Gorham's disease, or disappearing bone disease)

Developmental Disorders

Defective cartilage proliferation, calcification, collagen synthesis, and bone remodeling are the most common causes of developmental disorders of bone. Some of these disorders are inherited conditions, and recent advances in molecular biology have allowed identification of specific defects in an increasing number of diseases. Table 41-9 lists musculoskeletal diseases for which the specific genetic defect has been identified.

Achondroplasia. The basic defect in this inherited autosomal dominant disorder is in the proliferation of cartilage due to FGFR3 mutation. Membranous bone development (calvaria, ribs, sternum) is normal, but endochondral ossification is defective. The proliferating zone of the growth plates is shortened and disordered. At birth, the infant has a normal-sized body, large head with a depression of the base of the nose, and short limbs. Shortness of stature because of deficient long-bone growth becomes progressively evident during childhood (Fig. 41-37). Trunk growth remains relatively normal, while the limbs are short, particularly proximally. The hands are short and broad, with digits of equal length. Increased lumbar lordosis may be present, as well as thoracolumbar kyphosis. Intelligence is normal, although life expectancy may be diminished. Genu varum is a common finding, and later in life patients may develop spinal stenosis as a result of decreased spinal canal diameter and interpedicular distance.

Enchondromatosis (Ollier's disease or Dyschondroplasia). This condition, first described by Ollier in 1899, consists of abnormal foci of cartilage within the metaphyses of the long bones. These cartilage rests are referred to as *enchondromas.* The cause is unknown, and the disease is not hereditary. Disturbance of the growth near the ends of the involved bones results in foreshortening, with broadening and cystic changes in the metaphyses. The degree of deformity varies considerably, with some mild cases of enchondromatosis exhibiting no signif-

Table 41-8
Bone Graft Materials

Material	Properties	Disadvantages
Autograft (cancellous)	Optimal biologic behavior; osteoinductive	Limited availability; donor site morbidity
Autograft (cortical)	Structural uses, osteoconductive	Limited availability; and significant donor site morbidity
Autograft (vascularized)	Rapid incorporation, structurally useful; more reliable healing than other types	Prolonged surgical procedure; limited availability and donor site morbidity
Allograft (fresh)	No preservation required articular cartilage viable	Intense inflammatory response; need and availability may not coincide
Allograft (frozen)	Permits cartilage cryopreservation; reduces antigenicity; can be used for cortical or cancellous (can be both osteoinductive and osteoconductive)	Transmissible diseases such as HIV and hepatitis a concern; cannot be sterilized; cartilage viability limited; expensive screening and storage
Allograft (freeze-dried)	Can store indefinitely; cortical or cancellous; decreased antigenicity; can be radiation sterilized	Cannot preserve cartilage; mechanical properties are weakened
Allograft (demineralized)	Osteoinductive, sterile	Expensive; little intrinsic strength; complex processing
Synthetics		
Tricalcium phosphate	Nonantigenic, osteoconductive; restores volume	Unpredictable resorption; no bonding to bone
Hydroxyapatite ceramic	Bonds to bone; osteoconductive; can be shaped to some extent	Brittle; not osteoinductive
Resorbable (polylactic and polyglycolic acid)	Osteoconductive; vehicle for additives; nonantigenic; sterile	Unpredictable resorption; some inflammatory response
Recombinant proteins (BMP2, BMP7, TGF-beta)	Osteoinductive; nonantigenic; sterile	No inherent structural usefulness; expensive; need carrier vehicle
Bioactive silicate	Bonds to bone; osteoconductive	Brittle; not osteoinductive

icant bony distortions. Involvement of the bones of the hand is common. When associated with hemangiomas, the disease is called Maffucci syndrome. The incidence of malignant degeneration of individual lesions into chondrosarcoma occurs in about 25 percent of individuals by age forty and is even more common in Maffucci syndrome. Pathologic fractures caused by weakening of bone by an enchondroma can heal, but the enchondroma will persist, and so curettage and bone grafting is recommended. Malignant degeneration of lesions is managed by local resection and reconstruction when necessary.

Multiple Exostoses (Metaphyseal Aclasis, or Osteochondromatosis). This autosomal dominant hereditary disorder involves outgrowths of cartilaginous lesions from the metaphyses of the long bones as well as occasionally from the pel-

Table 41-9
Genetic Defects in Musculoskeletal Disorders

Disease	Genetic Defect
Osteogenesis imperfecta	Type I collagen
Achondroplasia	FGF receptor 3
Thanatophoric dysplasia	FGF receptor 3
Pseudoachondroplasia	Cartilage oligomeric matrix protein (COMP)
Marfan's syndrome	Fibrillin
Spondyloepiphyseal dysplasia	Type II collagen
Multiple epiphyseal dysplasia	Cartilage oligomeric matrix protein (COMP); type IX collagen
Vitamin D-resistant hypophosphatemic rickets	PEX (endopeptidase with unknown substrate)
Fibrous dysplasia	$G_{s\alpha}$ protein (receptor coupling protein involved in signaling; somatic mutation)
Muscular dystrophy	Dystrophin (calcium transport protein)
Neurofibromatosis type I	Neurofibromin (signal transduction protein)
Neurofibromatosis type II	Schwannomin (links cytoskeleton to plasma membrane)
Schmid metaphyseal chondrodysplasia	Type X collagen
Jansen metaphyseal chondrodysplasia	PTHrP receptor activating mutation
Crouzon syndrome	FGF receptor 2
Diastrophic dysplasia	Sulfate transporter
Apert syndrome	FGF receptor 2
Osteopetrosis	Proton pump; carbonic anhydrase II; MCSF; c-src mutations

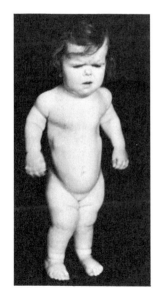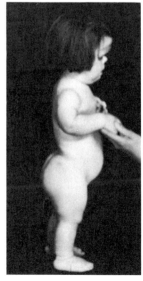

FIG. 41-37. *Achondroplastic girl showing the decreased limb growth, with foreshortening of the stature but normal trunk height.*

vis, ribs, and spine (Fig. 41-38). Extent of the disease is variable, and it is one of the more common skeletal dysplasias. Hereditary multiple exostoses have been mapped to three different chromosomal locations, but the specific genes involved have not been identified. Cartilage-capped exostoses, or osteochondromas, arise from bony surfaces and increase in size during childhood growth. The lesions grow by a process of relatively normal endochondral ossification, forming trabecular bone in the base. They can cause mechanical symptoms as a result of impingement on nerves, joints, tendons, or muscles and, when symptomatic, can be removed surgically. Care must be taken to remove the cartilage cap in its entirety, particularly in children, or local recurrence can result. Genu valgum and progressive ulnar deviation of the hand as well as limb length discrepancies because of asymmetrical limb involvement are other problems that may arise. The most serious complication is malignant degeneration into chondrosarcoma, which has been reported in 1 to 15 percent of affected individuals. This is usually heralded by enlargement of the lesion in adulthood, sometimes in association with pain. Thickness of the cartilaginous cap as assessed by CT or MRI is a good index of malignant transformation, with a thickness of 1 cm suspicious and over 2 cm pathognomonic. Treatment is by wide surgical excision, and metastasis is uncommon.

Polyostotic Fibrous Dysplasia. This disease usually appears in childhood, with development of expansile lytic lesions in the metaphyses and diaphyses of long bones. The pelvis, skull, and bones of the hand also may be involved. Bending deformities from recurrent fractures of the long bones can occur, most commonly in the proximal femur, causing a "shepherd's crook" deformity (varus of the upper femur). Radiographically, the dysplastic bone has a homogeneous "ground glass" appearance as a result of the lack of formed trabeculae (Fig. 41-39). Lesions that are symptomatic or threatening pathologic fracture require curettage and bone grafting as well as internal fixation for stabilization. Cortical bone graft is superior to cancellous graft, which tends to be resorbed by the dysplastic bone. Association with café-au-lait pigmented skin lesions and precocious puberty is termed Albright syndrome. Malignant degeneration has been reported in these lesions but is extremely rare. Fibrous dysplasia occurs also in a monostotic form.

Osteogenesis Imperfecta. Osteogenesis imperfecta is a genetically determined disorder in the structure or processing of type I collagen, with a spectrum of expression. Bone fragility is the unifying clinical manifestation, and four clinical groups have been categorized by Sillence (Table 41-10). While the clinical classification is useful for general treatment and prognosis, recent identification of the specific mutations in the type I collagen gene indicates a wide variety of mutations with differing clinical manifestations. Patients may have blue sclerae, abnormal dentition, deafness, and growth failure. The fetal form (type II) is severe and lethal, the infantile form (type III) less severe but associated with severe deformities, and the adolescent form (tarda, type I) is the most common and least severe form.

Radiographically, the bones may appear normal in type I but tend to be more gracile with decreased trabecular pattern. With more severe involvement, fractures may be evident, and enlargement of the metaphysis and epiphysis may be present, with disorganization of the growth plate into multiple islands of cartilage.

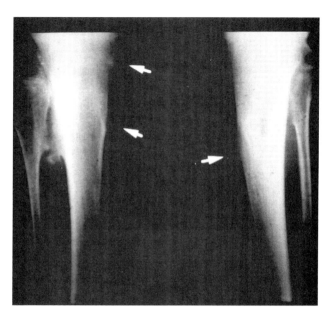

FIG. 41-38. Multiple exostoses, or osteochondromatosis.

Treatment. Osteogenesis imperfecta is treated with orthoses to prevent fractures and correction of deformities by multiple osteotomies with intramedullary stabilization using telescoping rods (Fig. 41-40). Fracture tendency usually decreases at puberty. Correction of scoliosis with posterior instrumentation and

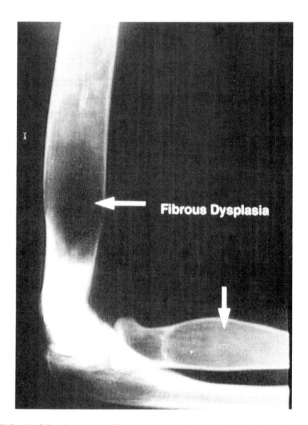

FIG. 41-39. Polyostotic fibrous dysplasia. Note the expansile nature of the lesions, with a homogeneous "ground glass" appearance.

Table 41-10
Classification of Osteogenesis Imperfecta (After Sillence)

Type	Features
I	Bones fragile Blue sclera Growth minimally affected Hearing loss Autosomal dominant inheritance Most common type
II	Crumpled long bones, platyspondylia Beaded ribs Blue sclera Lethal type, with perinatal death Autosomal recessive inheritance
III	Bones twisted, bowed, and fractured Sclera normal at birth, later blue Severe growth failure Autosomal recessive inheritance
IV	Bones fragile Sclera normal Moderate growth failure Dominant inheritance

fusion is helpful in preventing respiratory compromise but can be difficult. A wide variety of systemic therapies, including calcium, phosphorus, vitamin C, vitamin D, fluoride, and calcitonin, have been used without demonstrable beneficial effect.

Osteopetrosis (Albers-Schönberg Disease). This rare skeletal disease is associated with increased density of the bones (Fig. 41-41). It has two forms, an infantile severe form, which is inherited as an autosomal recessive, and an adult (or tarda) milder form, which is an autosomal dominant trait. The central defect is in osteoclastic function, with failure of functional bone resorption and therefore of remodeling. Multiple genetic defects in osteoclast function have been shown to cause osteopetrosis (see Table 41-9). Consequently the medullary cavities are narrowed, with resulting deficiencies of bone marrow activity causing anemia and thrombocytopenia. The bones show persistence of calcified cartilage and woven bone, and absence of osteonal cortical bone. Patients have increased fracture tendency, susceptibility to osteomyelitis, and cranial nerve deficits from skull involvement.

Several patients with infantile osteopetrosis have been cured by bone marrow transplantation, with resumption of bone resorption and remodeling attributable to donor osteoclasts. Bone density in these patients and hematopoietic function returned to normal.

Melorheostosis. This condition, which may involve one or more bones in an extremity, is characterized by endosteal cortical hyperostosis, often described as a "candle dripping" appearance radiographically. The disease is associated with pain

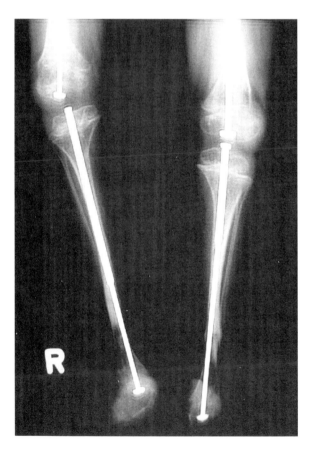

FIG. 41-40. Multiple osteotomies and sliding intramedullary rod fixation in osteogenesis imperfecta.

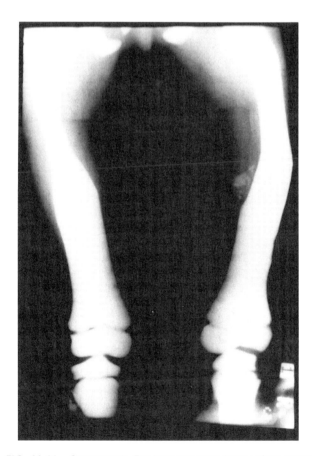

FIG. 41-41. Osteopetrosis. The increased radiodensity of the bones and lack of proper medullary cavity formation result from defective osteoclast function and lack of remodeling. Pathologic fractures, infections, and systemic symptoms from defective myelopoiesis may result.

and contracture of adjacent joints. The cause is unknown, and there is no specific therapy beyond symptomatic treatment.

Metabolic Diseases

Mineralization. Mineralization requires secretion by chondrocytes or osteoblasts of a suitable organic matrix (osteoid or chondroid), within which hydroxyapatite crystals can form. Mineralization defects can result from inadequate availability of calcium and phosphate, interference with crystal formation by drugs or heavy metals, disruption of vitamin D metabolism, or aberrations in the organic matrix.

Scurvy. Scurvy is the clinical condition resulting from a nutritional deficiency of vitamin C, or ascorbic acid. Ascorbate is crucial to the cross-linking process in fibrillar collagen formation, which determines mechanical properties of collagen fibers. Capillary walls are most obviously affected, with microscopic hemorrhage as the hallmark of scurvy. Subperiosteal hemorrhages occur adjacent to the growth plates in the metaphyses of the long bones (Fig. 41-42) and in extreme cases can cause epiphyseal separation. Mineralization in the growth plate is defective, with an irregular and dense mineralization front where transition of the calcified cartilage to bone is impaired. Hemorrhage from the gastrointestinal tract or mucous membranes and subperiosteal hemorrhages present with pain and swelling that can mimic osteomyelitis. Treatment with vitamin C rapidly cures the disease, and within 24 h pain subsides. Protection from weight bearing until reossification occurs is recommended.

Vitamin D Metabolism. Vitamin D (cholecalciferol) is essential for normal bone metabolism and mineralization. Vitamin D is formed from dietary precursor forms, or from ultraviolet irradiation of 7-dehydrocholesterol in the skin. The active form of vitamin D is 1,25-dihydroxyvitamin D_3. 25-Hydroxylation occurs in the liver, and subsequent 1-α-hydroxylation occurs in the kidney. The major function of active vitamin D_3 is to enable absorption of calcium in the gut. Additional effects include a stimulation of renal tubular phosphate reabsorption and bone resorption. The physiologic significance of the bone resorbing effects is unknown, but the mechanism is through stimulation of differentiation of osteoclasts from precursor cells. The 1-α-hydroxylation of vitamin D is up-regulated in the kidney by parathyroid hormone (PTH). Additional effects of PTH include stimulation of bone resorption and decreased renal tubular phosphate reabsorption. The stimulation of bone resorption involves osteoblasts as the target cell, with secondary secretion of an unknown factor that then induces osteoclasts to resorb bone. Calcitonin, on the other hand, activates osteoclast receptors directly to inhibit resorption. While this hormone has therapeutic uses in Paget's disease, hypercalcemia, and some forms of osteoporosis, it is not thought to play a significant role in normal human bone metabolism. Figure 41-43 summarizes the roles of vitamin D and PTH in the regulation of calcium and phosphate metabolism.

Rickets. Rickets is a relative deficiency of the active metabolite of vitamin D (1,25-dihydroxyvitamin D_3) in children, which leads to the inability of chondrocytes to actively mineralize matrix in the zone of provisional calcification of the growth plates. The defect in mineralization has been presumed to be secondary to inadequate calcium absorption in the gut, with inadequate local levels of calcium and phosphate at the mineral-

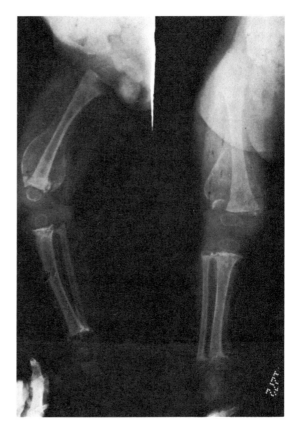

FIG. 41-42. Radiograph of the lower limbs of an infant with scurvy showing the epiphyseal disturbance and calcifying periosteal hematoma formation.

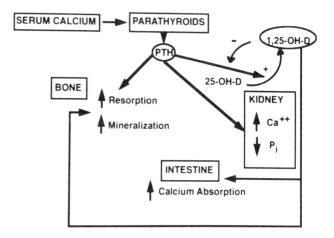

FIG. 41-43. Summary of the regulation of calcium and phosphate metabolism by vitamin D and parathyroid hormone. The major effect of 1,25-dihydroxyvitamin D_3 is stimulation of calcium absorption in the gut. Vitamin D also may stimulate bone mineralization and, at high levels, bone resorption. By negative feedback, 1,25-hydroxyvitamin D_3 inhibits the 1-α-hydroxylase in the kidney, decreasing its own production. PTH secretion from the parathyroid glands is directly regulated by serum calcium levels, with hypercalcemia decreasing secretion and hypocalcemia increasing secretion. PTH causes stimulation of bone remodeling, stimulation of 1-α-hydroxylation of 25-dihydroxyvitamin D_3, increased calcium reabsorption in the distal renal tubule, and decreased phosphate reabsorption in the proximal renal tubule. PTH provides short-term regulation of calcium, while vitamin D provides long-term regulation.

ization front. This can be aggravated by decreased reabsorption of phosphate in the renal tubules, another effect of vitamin D. Some evidence suggests that chondrocytes in the growth plate have vitamin D receptors and can respond to this hormone in a direct fashion as well. Nutritional vitamin D deficiency in children is now rare in the United States, but disruptions of vitamin D metabolism (renal disease, anticonvulsant therapy, malabsorption syndromes) and inherited diseases (vitamin D-resistant hypophosphatemic rickets) can cause rickets.

Pathology. The normal growth plate is a well-defined plate of cartilage approximately 2 mm in thickness that separates the metaphysis from the epiphysis. In rickets, the growth plates are widened and irregular, with patchy decreased mineralization. The proliferative and hypertrophic zones are increased in height and somewhat disordered. The bony trabeculae in the metaphyses are thin, with diminished bone formation. In addition there can be widening and cupping of the metaphyses (Fig. 41-44) and deformities such as coxa vara, tibial bowing, and genu varum or valgus. Other clinical manifestations include gastrointestinal symptoms, irritability, open fontanelles, narrow chest, and prominence of the costochondral junctions (referred to as the "rachitic rosary").

Treatment. Treatment of nutritional rickets is by supplementation with high doses of vitamin D (3,000 U daily; normal daily requirement 400 U). Calcium supplementation enhances the rate of healing. For persistent deformities, correction is delayed until the underlying metabolic defect has resolved, at which time osteotomies can be performed.

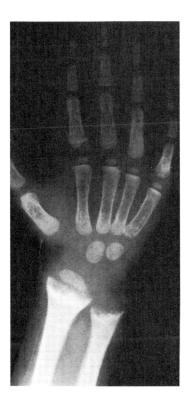

FIG. 41-44. *Radiograph of the hand and wrist of a 3-year-old rachitic child showing the delay in the appearance of the carpal ossification center and the widening of the epiphysis with loss of bone density. (Courtesy of Dr. R. C. Alcheson.)*

Enteropathic Rickets. The most common cause of malabsorptive rickets is celiac, or gluten-sensitive, enteropathy. Chronic diarrhea results in inadequate vitamin D absorption in the gut. The effects of the vitamin D deficiency are exacerbated by periods of rapid growth. The effects on bone and growth plates are similar to those described above, and treatment hinges on the elimination of gluten from the diet and vitamin D supplementation.

Renal Osteodystrophy. Renal disease impairs the 1-α-hydroxylation of vitamin D, causing a functional vitamin D deficiency. Inadequate calcium absorption in the gut causes slight hypocalcemia, which then leads to a secondary hyperparathyroidism. Severe osteopenia results, and in children the clinical picture resembles rickets. In patients on renal dialysis, aluminum contained in phosphate-binding agents (used chronically to decrease phosphate levels) binds to mineralization surfaces and impairs further mineral deposition, a form of osteomalacia. Both glomerular and tubular defects can cause renal osteodystrophy, including Fanconi syndrome (glycosuria, aminoaciduria), Lignac-Fanconi syndrome (impaired tubular phosphate reabsorption), and renal tubular acidosis.

Vitamin D-Resistant Hypophosphatemic Rickets. Vitamin D-resistant hypophosphatemic rickets is a familial disease associated with hypophosphatemia. The syndrome resembles nutritional vitamin D deficiency, except that very high doses of vitamin D in conjunction with phosphate supplementation are required to treat it. The patients are short in stature with disproportionately short limbs, and the disease is inherited as an X-linked dominant trait. The genetic cause of the disease has been identified as a neutral endopeptidase known as PEX, although its substrate is unknown. Oncogenic hypophosphatemia is an unrelated disorder associated with benign soft-tissue tumors that disappears with tumor excision.

Hypophosphatasia. Hypophosphatasia is a rare autosomal recessive hereditary disease characterized by a deficiency of alkaline phosphatase and urinary excretion of phosphoethanolamine. The disease, which is variable in severity, may present in childhood or adulthood, featuring stunting of growth and excessive bone fragility. Hyperphosphatasia is an extremely rare congenital disorder with markedly elevated levels of serum alkaline phosphatase. It is also known as juvenile Paget's disease. The skull and diaphyses of the long bones are thickened, and deformity and fractures can result. There is no effective systemic treatment for either of these disorders.

Osteomalacia. Osteomalacia is defined as a defect in mineralization of adult bone, generally resulting from abnormalities in vitamin D metabolism. As in rickets, causes of osteomalacia include nutritional deficiency, malabsorption, anticonvulsant therapy, and hepatic and renal diseases. In addition, aluminum can induce a mineralization defect, as can chronic use of diphosphonates (a treatment sometimes used for Paget's disease). Anticonvulsants can cause osteomalacia by interfering with vitamin D metabolism in the liver. Histologically, excessive unmineralized surfaces and thickness of the osteoid are observed. The bones become osteopenic, and fractures can result. Nutritional osteomalacia is more common in the elderly than previously recognized, aggravating involutional osteoporosis and the tendency for fractures. A characteristic radiographic finding is

Looser's zones, which are stress fractures extending partly through the bone, usually on the concave side, secondary to mechanical failure in compression. Treatment depends on the underlying cause, but generally involves vitamin D supplementation.

Hyperparathyroid Bone Disease (Osteitis Fibrosa Cystica). Excessive secretion of PTH can cause bone disease as a result of the resorptive effects of PTH on bone. Patients may present with bone pain and tenderness, hypercalcemia, and hypophosphatemia. Common causes are an underlying parathyroid adenoma or adenocarcinoma. Muscle weakness and calcium phosphate renal stones also may be present. Radiographically osteopenia is observed, with subperiosteal resorption in some sites, best seen along the radial borders of the digits and along the distal clavicle. Hemorrhagic cystic lesions (brown tumors) can occur in the long bones but usually resolve with treatment of the underlying hyperparathyroidism. Parathyroidectomy, the treatment of choice, results in spontaneous resolution of the bone disease.

Osteoporosis. In osteoporosis, a common disorder in the elderly, total bone mass and trabecular volume are decreased, but mineralization is normal. Skeletal bone mass reaches its peak at about the age of thirty. Both men and women subsequently lose bone throughout life, though women achieve a lower starting peak mass and have a hormonal acceleration of bone loss due to estrogen loss at menopause. Symptomatic osteoporosis with fractures is therefore much more common in women. Osteoporosis can be primary or secondary to some other process, usually a hormonal abnormality. Table 41-11 lists some of the types of osteoporosis. Type I and type II involutional osteoporosis are the most common. Osteoblasts have been shown to have estrogen receptors and respond to estrogen anabolically, which may explain the accelerated postmenopausal bone loss. Type I osteoporosis generally occurs in women 50 to 75 years of age and is characterized by loss primarily of trabecular bone. PTH levels are decreased in this group. Type II osteoporosis has a 2:1 female preponderance and is found in patients over 70 years of age, with proportionate loss of both trabecular and cortical bone. It is thought to result from depressed renal 1-α-hydroxylase activity associated with aging, leading to inadequate active vitamin D levels and decreased intestinal calcium absorption. Consequently these patients tend to have a mild secondary hyperparathyroidism contributing to their chronic bone loss. Type III patients are similar to type I except that their serum PTH levels are elevated; this group comprises about 10 percent of the postmenopausal form.

Secondary osteoporosis can result from a number of causes, as listed in Table 41-11, which must be ruled out by history, examination, and appropriate laboratory studies. Osteomalacia, with the numerous causes listed previously, must be ruled out as a cause of osteopenia and can be readily evaluated by histomorphometric analysis of a bone biopsy of the iliac crest. Additionally, accurate serum measurements of vitamin D metabolites and PTH levels are now widely available, facilitating evaluation of calcium metabolism. Patients with osteoporosis often present with fractures after minor trauma as the first indication of the disorder. Frequently backache with progressive kyphosis and loss of height are noted. Common locations for fractures are the distal radius, proximal femur, and vertebrae. With acute fracture, patients may have severe back pain, which

Table 41-11
Causes of Osteoporosis

Primary
    Idiopathic
        Juvenile
        Young adult
    Involutional
        Type I—postmenopausal
        Type II—senile
        Type III—increased PTH
Secondary
    Cushing's disease
    Hypogonadism
    Hyperthyroidism
    Diabetes mellitus
    Hyperparathyroidism
    Osteomalacia
        Vitamin D deficiency
        Malabsorption
        Hepatic disease
        Renal osteodystrophy
        Anticonvulsant therapy
    Rheumatoid arthritis
    Malignancy
        Multiple myeloma
        Carcinoma with marrow involvement
        Humeral hypercalcemia secondary to PTH-like peptide

gradually subsides as the fracture heals over 2 to 4 months. Often some residual aching pain persists, but neurologic deficits are extremely rare, even with severe compressions and kyphotic deformity.

Radiology. Radiographically, thinning of the cortices of long bones or vertebral bodies may be noted, with a loss of trabecular pattern and bulging of the discs into the vertebral end plates (Fig. 41-45). Plain radiographs are notoriously inaccurate in the diagnosis of osteoporosis, since the apparent bone density is strongly dependent on radiographic technique. Accurate densitometric measurements have become widely available using

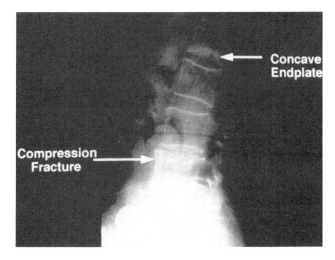

FIG. 41-45. *Osteoporotic spine, with compression fractures, concave vertebral end plates, thin vertebral cortices, and "ground glass" appearance from thinning of trabeculae with loss of normal trabecular pattern.*

quantitative CT scans of the spine, or dual-energy x-ray absorptiometry, which can measure the density of any bone. The accuracy of these techniques is within 1 percent. With dual-energy x-ray absorptiometry, measurements of both the spinal and femoral neck density usually are made to assess the appendicular and the axial skeletal mass. The analysis of spinal mass is demonstrated in Fig. 41-46, which also shows the age-dependent decline in the normal female population, with acceleration during menopause. By comparing the bone density of osteoporotic patients with that of normal control populations, an estimate of the risk of fractures can be made, which is valuable in guiding therapy. Sequential measurements are also helpful in assessing responses to therapeutic interventions.

Treatment. Acute vertebral fractures are treated with a lightweight extension brace, analgesics, and early mobilization. Bed rest aggravates the underlying osteopenia. Other fractures are treated as are those in nonsteoporotic patients (see Fractures and Joint Injuries, below). Endocrine causes, multiple myeloma, and osteomalacia must be ruled out as described above. Calcium supplementation (1,000 to 1,500 mg daily) is generally recommended and can slow the rate of loss. Physiologic doses of vitamin D (400 U daily) help to ensure calcium absorption. In perimenopausal women, estrogen therapy is of proved benefit. Patients who have high-turnover osteoporosis (excessive bone resorption) as judged from histomorphometric or calcium balance studies may benefit from antiresorptive agents such as calcitonin. Bisphosphonates such as etidronate have been used cyclically (a 2-week course every 3 months) to inhibit bone resorption. Since bone is continually forming and resorbing, periodically inhibiting resorption can increase bone mass, since formation continues. Second-generation bisphosphonates, such as alendronate, have been used successfully to increase bone mass in postmenopausal osteoporotic patients by continuous daily oral administration. Fluoride has been used to increase bone formation and bone mass but remains controversial since the new bone formed is woven bone, which is structurally inferior. Prospective, randomized studies have demonstrated no decrease in fracture rates with fluoride therapy. Synthetic androgenic steroids also have been used to increase bone formation rates, as has human growth hormone, but these approaches are still experimental. All osteoporotic patients must be encouraged to begin a regular, progressive program of weight-bearing exercise such as walking, along with general spinal extension and strengthening exercises to help maintain bone mass and prevent fractures.

Pituitary Disturbances. *Pituitary Short Stature.* There are two main types of pituitary dwarfism, Fröhlich's adiposogenital type (short stature associated with obesity, genital hypoplasia, and mental retardation), and the Lorain-Lévi type (short stature without other mental or physical change). The usual cause is a tumor or cyst compressing the pituitary gland, although congenital aplasia also can occur. With the recent availability of recombinant human growth hormone, this form of dwarfism is now treatable.

Hyperpituitary Syndromes. *Gigantism* is caused by excessive growth hormone secretion during childhood and can be accompanied by subnormal mental development. The bones are increased in thickness and length. *Acromegaly* refers to the syndrome associated with excessive growth hormone secretion in the adult. Abnormal bone formation enlarges the alveolar margins of the jaws, leading to elongation of the face and projection of the chin. Prominence of the frontal region of the skull develops as well as increased size of the thorax. The ends of the long bones are enlarged, and the short bones in the hands and feet are elongated and thickened. The usual cause is a pituitary adenoma. Acromegalic patients also may develop arthritis of the spine or other joints that resembles osteoarthritis.

Hypothyroidism (Cretinism). Congenital hypothyroidism leads to short stature, retardation of maturation, and developmental delay. The principal skeletal changes include decreased length of the long bones, thickened cortices, and delayed appearance of the secondary ossification centers in the epiphyses. Irregularity of the ossific nucleus resembles osteochondroses such as Legg-Calvé-Perthes disease in the hips. Closure of the growth plates also is delayed. Thyroid hormone replacement therapy, if started in infancy, cures the disease, and it can produce growth in stature even in adults because of the delayed closure of the growth plates.

Mucopolysaccharidoses. A series of 12 hereditary disorders of mucopolysaccharide metabolism has been described, with identification of the specific enzymatic defect in 10 of them. All affected patients have somewhat thickened, coarse fa-

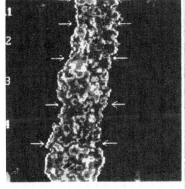

Lumbar Spine

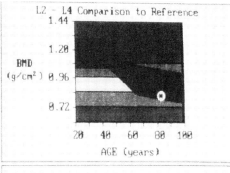

FIG. 41-46. Dual-energy x-ray absorptiometry of the spine in a woman with osteoporosis. The use of two photons of differing energies allows subtraction of all soft-tissue absorption, so the determined densities represent mineral only. The density is compared with normal control population data in the graph on the right, which represents the mean ± 2 SD. Note the age-dependent decrease in bone density, with acceleration in the perimenopausal ages.

cial features, joint stiffness, and short stature. Radiographic findings include oval vertebrae with anterior beaking, coxa valga, and a wide, flat pelvis. Many are associated also with thoracolumbar kyphosis. All forms of mucopolysaccharidosis are inherited as autosomal recessive disorders except type II (Hunter's syndrome), which is X-linked. Mucopolysaccharidosis patients have elevated urinary excretion of dermatan, heparan, or keratan sulfate, depending on the type. The most common forms are type I (Hurler's and Scheie's syndromes—deficiency of α-L-iduronidase) and type IV (Morquio syndrome; type IVA—deficiency of N-acetylgalactosamine-6-sulfatase; type IVB—deficiency of beta-galactosidase). Type I is associated with mental retardation and life expectancy of 10 to 15 years, while type IV patients have normal intelligence and survive well into adulthood.

Paget's Disease (Osteitis Deformans). Osteitis deformans, first described by Sir James Paget in 1876, is a disorder of accelerated regional bone turnover. Ultrastructural studies have demonstrated viral-like inclusion particles in osteoclasts of affected bone, suggesting that the causative agent may be a slow virus. Despite numerous studies, no specific viral etiologic agent has yet been identified. Paget's disease may be monostotic (25 percent) or polyostotic (75 percent). Early in the disease there is excessive osteoclastic resorption and vascularity, followed by abnormal bone formation and sclerosis, with thickening of the trabeculae and cortical bone. In the late phase, dense sclerotic woven bone and marrow fibrosis predominate. The disease begins between the ages of 35 and 50 years and is painful in about 30 percent of patients. Often the diagnosis is made as an incidental finding on a radiograph taken for some other reason. Resorption and formation remain coupled in Paget's disease, so the excessive bone resorption that appears to be the primary defect is accompanied by excessive formation, causing the enlargement of involved bones with cortical and trabecular thickening. Bowing of involved bones such as the tibia and femur may occur, and arthritic changes may develop in adjacent joints. Common locations are the skull, pelvis, lumbar spine, femur, and tibia. Because of the disorganized collagen in the woven pagetic bone, tensile strength is poor. Therefore fractures can occur, more often starting on the tension or convex side of the long bone, and typically transverse in nature.

Skull involvement can lead to enlargement of the cranium and compression of cranial nerves, producing symptoms such as vertigo, deafness, or visual disturbances. Spinal involvement can cause back pain, ankylosis, and spinal cord compression with neurologic deficit. Serum calcium and phosphate levels usually are normal, but the alkaline phosphatase level is markedly elevated and is correlated with the activity of the disease. The urinary hydroxyproline level is elevated as a reflection of collagen breakdown during bone resorption. In a small percentage of patients with Paget's disease, sarcomatous degeneration, usually to an osteosarcoma, develops later in life. Signs of malignant degeneration include radiographic changes with bone lysis or destruction, soft-tissue mass, and progressive pain. The prognosis of pagetic sarcoma is poor.

Radiologic Findings. Early changes consist of lytic resorption of trabecular bone. In the skull this is referred to as *osteoporosis circumscripta,* and in the tibia the phenomenon resembles a flame-shaped area of advancing bone lysis. Later, coarsening of trabecular pattern with thick striations and cortical thickening and enlargement are observed (Fig. 41-47). Vertebral

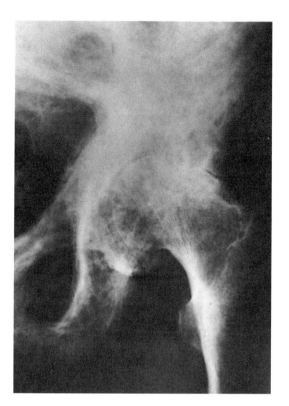

FIG. 41-47. *Radiograph of the pelvis and femur of a patient with Paget's disease.*

involvement is characterized by widening and squaring of the vertebral body and a thickened "picture frame" cortex. Associated joints exhibit degenerative changes with sclerosis and joint space narrowing.

Treatment. There is no cure for Paget's disease, although the symptoms and activity of the disease can be controlled pharmacologically. In asymptomatic patients in whom there is minimal concern about impending fracture, observation alone usually suffices. For symptomatic involvement, treatment is focused on antiresorptive agents (e.g., bisphosphonates such as etidronate or alendronate) or calcitonin. Treatment with calcitonin or diphosphonate is continued until biochemical parameters and symptoms improve, usually about 6 months.

Doses of etidronate higher than 5 mg/kg/day, or continuous treatment for periods longer than 6 to 12 months may be associated with an iatrogenic osteomalacia-like mineralization defect and predispose to fractures. Because bisphosphonates have an antiphosphaturic effect, a slight rise in serum phosphate indicates an effective dose of the medication, which varies depending on the extent of bony involvement. Patients who undergo major surgery should be treated in the perioperative period with calcitonin to prevent postoperative hypercalcemia secondary to immobilization. In cases of spinal involvement with neurologic deficit or impending paraplegia, mithramycin is the drug of choice, producing an immediate and profound inhibition of pagetic activity. It is not suitable for long-term therapy because of hepatic and renal toxicity.

When fractures occur, the incidence of nonunion is greater than normal, and healing more reliably obtains with surgical internal fixation in addition to antipagetic therapy. Sarcomas must be treated by radical resection and prosthetic limb reconstruction or amputation and, if the patient can tolerate the toxicity, chemotherapy.

Bone Marrow Diseases

Diseases of bone marrow constituents can have secondary effects on trabecular bone. The reticuloendothelial tissue of bone is found mainly at the ends of the long bones and in the cancellous bone of the axial skeleton (ribs, spine, skull, pelvis).

Lipoid Granulomatosis. These disorders result from disturbances in lipid metabolism within bone, causing accumulations that displace normal marrow elements. In Gaucher's disease a cerebroside lipoprotein accumulates in histiocytes in the liver, spleen, and bone marrow. Orthopaedic problems include pathologic fractures and avascular necrosis of the femoral head. Symptomatic Gaucher's disease has been treated successfully by exogenous parenteral recombinant alglucerase 3 times per week, with resolution of the bone lesions. Niemann-Pick disease and Tay-Sachs disease involve defective phosphatide lipid and cerebroside proteins, respectively, with primarily neurologic sequelae. All of these disorders can cause formation of tumorlike deposits within the bone marrow, with displacement of normal marrow and trabecular bone. The deposits consist primarily of lipid-laden histiocytes, or "foam cells," and the lesions cause bone destruction without much bony reaction, occasionally resulting in pathologic fractures.

Mastocytosis. Mastocytosis is a systemic disorder that infiltrates bone marrow by mast cells. Release of histamine, serotonin, and other mediators from the mast cells cause characteristic urticaria pigmentosa, a dermatologic condition, as well as pulmonary and a wide range of other symptoms. In the skeleton, mastocytosis can cause lytic or mixed lytic and sclerotic lesions, which may be localized or widespread. The cause of the disorder is unknown, and treatment generally is symptomatic.

Histiocytosis X. This term encompasses a spectrum of clinical disease, with three major forms. Letterer-Siwe disease is the infantile form, which involves hepatosplenomegaly and disseminated bony lesions, and runs a rapidly fatal course in most cases. Hand-Schuller-Christian disease usually occurs in children but occasionally presents in adulthood. The severity varies greatly, and manifestations include the triad of exophthalmos, diabetes insipidus, and skull lesions. In addition, hepatosplenomegaly and hypercholesterolemia can be present, and the disease tends to be progressive.

Eosinophilic granuloma, the least severe form of histiocytosis X, usually presents as a solitary bony lesion that may be painful or cause a pathologic fracture. Two-thirds of patients are under age twenty. Patients who develop multiple lesions usually do so within 2 years of onset, and may go on to develop the Hand-Schuller-Christian variant of the disease. Local tenderness and swelling may be present. Radiographically, eosinophilic granuloma has a highly variable appearance and may cause destructive or permeative bone lysis with periosteal reaction mimicking osteomyelitis or Ewing's sarcoma. In general, however, the radiograph shows well-circumscribed lytic lesions. Involvement of a vertebral body can cause flattening (vertebra plana, or Calvé's disease) and must be differentiated from osteomyelitis.

Treatment. Treatment of systemic forms of histiocytosis is with chemotherapeutic agents such as vinblastine and predni-

sone. Eosinophilic granuloma can be treated with low-dose radiation (2 to 10 Gy), although in long bones at risk of pathologic fracture, curettage with or without bone grafting (depending on the extent of the lesion) may be necessary. Local injection of steroids into symptomatic bony lesions has shown promise in inducing healing.

Chronic Multifocal Recurrent Osteomyelitis. This is a rare disorder of children that presents with swelling, pain, and radiographic findings of lysis, reactive sclerosis, and periosteal reaction resembling osteomyelitis, generally in a metaphyseal location adjacent to a growth plate. Biopsy shows acute and chronic inflammatory cells resembling osteomyelitis, but bacterial cultures are negative, and the disorder is self-limited. Antibiotics have not been proved to have any efficacy in the disorder, and multiple foci may become active at different times during childhood and resolve spontaneously. The disorder has a variable course, but it disappears by skeletal maturity. The disease resembles eosinophilic granuloma in radiographic appearance and clinical behavior, although eosinophils and hepatic or splenic involvement are absent.

Lymphatic and Hematopoietic Systems

Hodgkin's Disease. Hodgkin's disease may involve bone marrow, most commonly in the vertebrae or pelvis. Although bony involvement is frequent, presentation as a primary bone lesion without lymphatic involvement is unusual. The radiographic appearance may be lytic, blastic, or mixed. Generally, dull aching pain is the initial sign of bone involvement. The bony lesions of Hodgkin's disease are responsive to radiation treatment, and the systemic disease responds well to chemotherapy.

Leukemia. Lymphoblastic leukemia is the form that most frequently causes bony changes. The typical radiographic finding is a transverse zone of lucency in the metaphysis adjacent to the growth plate. Diffuse spotty osteopenia and vertebral compression fractures occur, and rarely large focal lytic lesions in long bones are seen. Treatment is aimed at controlling the systemic disease with chemotherapy.

Multiple Myeloma. Multiple myeloma, the most common primary malignancy of bone, is a malignant proliferation of plasma cells within the bone marrow. It usually affects individuals above the age of fifty. There is marrow replacement with tumor cells, and usually secretion of abnormal clonal immunoglobulins. The diffuse marrow involvement leads to anemia and punched out lytic lesions throughout the skeleton (Fig. 41-48). Because there is little reaction to the lesions, bone scans may not demonstrate all lesions, and hence this is one of the few skeletal malignancies in which a skeletal survey using plain radiographs can give a better assessment of the extent of the disease. The massive bone resorption can cause hypercalcemia, and pathologic fractures are common. Abnormal paraproteins produced by the plasma cells can cause renal glomerular damage and amyloidosis. In 50 percent of patients immunoglobulin can be detected in the urine (Bence-Jones protein). Serum electrophoresis may demonstrate the presence of an abnormal globulin, although immunoelectrophoresis is more reliable in establishing the presence of a monoclonal gammopathy.

Clinical Manifestations. Pain in areas of bony involvement is a common initial symptom, as is fatigue. Backache and pathologic vertebral compression fractures are also frequent, and the disease has a male preponderance. The multiple nature of the bony lesions, absence of pulmonary metastases, and osteolytic character of the lesions often suggest the diagnosis prior to bone marrow biopsy or demonstration of a serum or urine paraprotein. Multiple myeloma is a uniformly fatal disease, although it can be controlled for a number of years by systemic therapy.

Treatment. The usual regimen of chemotherapeutic agents includes cyclophosphamide, melphalan, prednisone, and vincristine. The possibility of bone marrow transplantation is under investigation as a potentially curative treatment but remains experimental. Orthopaedic surgical stabilization of pathologic fractures or impending fractures plays an important role in the management and maintenance of ambulatory function. Spinal stabilization and decompression of the cord are often necessary in cases with neurologic deficit that fails to respond promptly to radiation treatment.

Solitary Myeloma (Plasmacytoma). Occasionally solitary plasma cell lesions occur in the long bones, spine, or pelvis. Seventy percent of these patients progress to multiple myeloma, and a circulating monoclonal paraprotein occasionally is found. The usual treatment involves radiation therapy with or without surgical resection, depending on the anticipated morbidity of the surgical procedure. Chemotherapy is usually reserved for those patients who progress to the multiple form.

Hemolytic Anemia. Both thalassemia (Cooley's anemia) and sickle cell anemia produce bone marrow changes in the axial and appendicular skeleton. In the skull, the expansion of the hematopoietic marrow can exhibit a "hair on end" or "sunray" appearance, and bone infarctions can be observed as serpiginous calcified densities in the metaphyses of the long bones. The femoral head may undergo avascular necrosis. Rarely, expansile pseudotumors consisting of hyperplastic bone marrow occur in association with thalassemia.

FRACTURES AND JOINT INJURIES

General Considerations

Definitions. A *fracture* is defined as a linear deformation or discontinuity of bone produced by forces that exceed the ultimate strength of the material. Deformation without fracture can occur with loads that exceed the elastic limit of the bone but not its ultimate strength. This is referred to as *plastic deformation* and is more common in children. *Pathologic fractures* occur when the strength of the bone is below normal, as in infections, tumors, or metabolic bone disease, or after the creation of surgical defects in bone. The direction and magnitude of force applied to a bone and the rate of loading all are important in determining the fracture pattern that will result.

Fractures are described anatomically according to location in the bone (intraarticular, epiphyseal, metaphyseal, diaphyseal), the plane of the fracture (transverse, oblique, spiral), the number and type of fragments, and whether the fracture is open (compound) or closed. Some fracture patterns are illustrated in Fig. 41-49. A spiral fracture is produced by torsional force, and *comminution* refers to presence of multiple fracture fragments.

In an undisplaced fracture a plane of cleavage exists between the fracture fragments without separation. For displaced fractures, the convention is to describe the direction of displacement

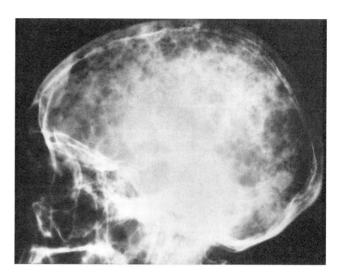

FIG. 41-48. Lytic "punched out" lesions in the skull typical of multiple myeloma.

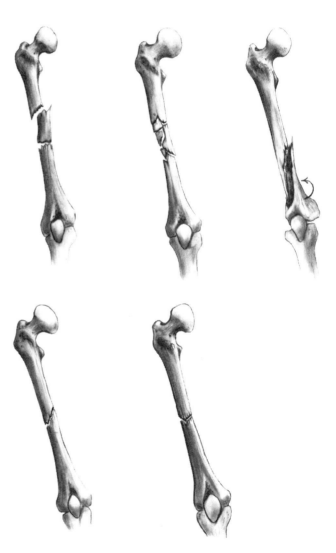

FIG. 41-49. Types of fracture. *Top row,* segmental, comminuted, and spiral; *bottom row,* oblique and transverse.

of the distal fragment with reference to the proximal fragment (medial, lateral, posterior, etc.). Angulation refers to angular deformity between the long axes of the fracture fragments and is also described in terms of the distal fragment's relation to the proximal fragment. Rotational deformity also is expressed in terms of the movement of the distal fragment (internal or external) relative to the proximal fragment.

One of the most important distinctions is whether a fracture is *open* or *closed*. If a fracture communicates with the surface of the skin or mucous membranes, infection is a risk, and this constitutes an orthopaedic surgical emergency. A *stress fracture* occurs when a bone is subjected to repetitive stresses that individually are insufficient to cause fracture but cumulatively lead to fatigue failure. A *compression fracture* results from axial loading of bone with compaction of bony trabeculae; these are seen generally in vertebral bodies. A *greenstick fracture* is an incomplete fracture resulting from failure of a portion of the cortex under tension, with part of the opposing cortex still intact but plastically deformed; these usually are seen in children. A *torus fracture* also retains partial cortical continuity, but with buckling or failure in compression of the opposing cortex (Fig. 41-50).

Diagnosis. The clinical manifestations of a fracture include pain, swelling, deformity, ecchymosis, instability, and crepitus. The diagnosis usually is confirmed radiographically with two radiographs taken at right angles to each other. Joints above and below the fracture site should be included in the radiograph to rule out associated injuries. Occasionally a completely nondisplaced fracture is not apparent on initial films; in this event immobilization with follow-up films 1 to 2 weeks later is indicated.

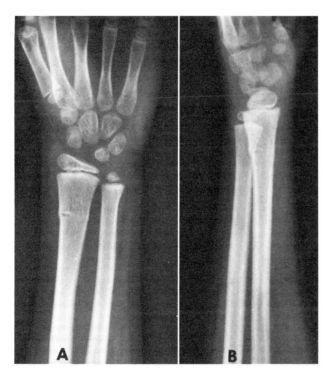

FIG. 41-50. *Torus, or buckle, fracture. A. AP radiograph, on which the radiolucent line is visible proximal to the distal radial epiphysis. B. Lateral radiograph, showing a buckling of the distal cortex of the radius.*

The fracture line can be better visualized after some resorption and early periosteal repair reaction have taken place.

Evaluation of the Injured Patient. Immediate threat to a patient's life from an injured extremity is unusual but can be a consequence of hemorrhage and resulting shock. Associated injuries to the chest, head, and abdominal viscera are potentially more serious and require immediate evaluation and treatment priority. Multiple fractures, even when closed, can cause shock from internal hemorrhage, particularly if major pelvic injuries are present. A closed femoral fracture can readily result in 1 to 2 units of internal blood loss, and shock in adult patients can occur with hypovolemia of 1 to 2 L. Shock is treated by volume replacement emergently with crystalloid such as lactated Ringer's solution to restore blood pressure and perfusion, and as soon as possible with whole blood. Early aggressive treatment of hypovolemic shock greatly reduces the likelihood of morbidity and mortality. Use of pneumatic trousers (MAST—*m*edical *a*nti-*s*hock *t*rousers) during transport may help to maintain blood pressure and decrease blood loss from lower-extremity injuries. Assessment of possible spinal injury is imperative, and transport using a backboard and sandbags or other head supports helps to minimize the chances of causing additional injury. The patient should not be allowed to sit or stand until appropriate spinal radiographs have been taken to evaluate spinal stability.

Evaluation of the Injured Extremity. The injured extremity is evaluated as quickly as possible for neurovascular compromise, soft-tissue and bony injuries, and joint instability. Peripheral pulses and capillary refill are evaluated, and motor and sensory examinations are carried out to the extent of the patient's ability to cooperate. All findings must be carefully documented in the event of later changes.

Emergency Splinting of Fractures. After the neurovascular examination has been performed and soft-tissue trauma or wounds evaluated, fractured extremities are splinted to minimize further injury. Plaster splints, pillow splints, or air splints can be used to stabilize the extremity. Fractures involving the humerus or shoulder can be splinted with a sling. Fractures of the femur are best temporarily stabilized in a traction splint.

Open Fractures. Open fractures constitute an orthopaedic surgical emergency because of the risk of deep infection. Open fractures are generally higher-energy injuries, resulting in more comminution and soft-tissue injury and, consequently, greater impairment of bone blood supply. All these factors contribute to the increased risk of osteomyelitis. Infection in a fracture, once established, can be extremely difficult to eradicate and markedly increases the risk of nonunion. The major aim in treatment of open fractures is the prevention of infection. This is best accomplished by aggressive and immediate debridement of the wound and fracture site in a sterile operative environment, and initiation of empiric intravenous prophylactic antibiotic therapy. Debridement is optimally done within 8 h, and a repeat intraoperative wound inspection and debridement within 24 to 48 h is recommended if significant soft-tissue damage or loss is present. Primary closure of open fractures is rarely, if ever, indicated, and secondary closure after 5 to 7 days or plastic surgical soft-tissue coverage procedures are preferable.

Classification. Open fractures are classified as type I, II, or III, depending on the associated soft-tissue injury. A puncture wound or communication less than 1 cm in length is a type I open fracture. Type II fractures have a wound larger than 1 cm with moderate associated soft-tissue damage. Type III open fractures involve severe soft-tissue injury or loss and are subdivided into subtypes A—soft-tissue injury only; B—severe soft-tissue and bone injury/soft-tissue loss; and C—associated neurovascular injury.

Technique. The following is a general description of the initial management of open fractures.

1. The wound is cultured and covered with a sterile bandage, and the extremity is splinted.
2. Cephalosporin and, with type III or grossly contaminated wounds, penicillin and an aminoglycoside are administered intravenously. Tetanus toxoid or antitoxin is administered, depending on tetanus immunization status.
3. In a sterile operating room environment, the patient is anesthetized, and the extremity is prepared with antiseptic.
4. Skin edges of the wound are excised approximately 1 to 2 mm, and more if clearly avascular or crushed.
5. The wound is thoroughly irrigated with pulsatile lavage using several liters of saline solution.
6. Any devitalized muscle or debris is surgically excised, and the fracture site is exposed. The fracture surface is curetted to remove foreign material, followed again by copious irrigation of the wound with pulsatile jet lavage of saline solution for a total volume of at least 9 L.
7. The fracture is reduced and the skin loosely approximated over a drain, leaving a significant area of the wound open, but covering exposed bone, neurovascular structures, or tendons if possible.
8. The fracture is stabilized with plaster immobilization or, more often, an external fixator to allow wound access. Some type II open fractures can be managed by primary internal fixation with intramedullary devices in the lower extremity or plating in the upper extremity at the time of primary debridement. Additionally, disrupted articular surface fragments can be provisionally stabilized with judicious use of pins or screws.
9. Antibiotics are continued for a minimum of 10 to 14 days postoperatively. Repeat wound inspection and debridement are recommended after 24 to 48 h, especially for type III injuries.
10. If secondary wound closure to achieve bone coverage is not feasible, skin grafts, free tissue transfers, or muscle flaps can be used to obtain adequate soft-tissue coverage for the fracture.

Vascular Injury. Major arterial injury should be suspected in any fracture-dislocation or significant trauma to an extremity. If perfusion to the extremity is disrupted, the maximum time that can elapse before onset of irreversible ischemic damage to muscle and other tissues is 6 to 8 h. Certain injuries are more likely to have associated vascular damage, including supracondylar humeral fractures, knee dislocations, femoral shaft fractures, type III open tibial fractures, and gunshot wounds.

The diagnosis of vascular compromise is not necessarily straightforward, since patients often are unconscious, and peripheral vasoconstriction or arterial spasm may be present. Capillary refill must be assessed, and if pulses are not palpable Doppler examination can be helpful. If there is any doubt about vascular integrity, arteriography as well as appropriate surgical exploration should be carried out.

Compartment Syndrome. One of the most serious complications of extremity trauma or ischemic injury is compartment syndrome, which was discussed earlier (see Contracture). A brief review is appropriate given the extreme importance of early diagnosis and treatment of this complication. The cardinal signs of pain, pallor, pulselessness, and paresthesias are present to variable degrees. Pain with passive stretch of muscles is one of the more reliable indicators of compartment syndrome, and accurate diagnosis is readily made by measurement of intracompartmental pressures using a slit catheter. Pressures in the range of 30 to 40 mmHg constitute an indication for fasciotomy. In patients with prolonged ischemia due to arterial compromise, prophylactic fasciotomies of all compartments distal to the vascular injury should be done concomitantly with reestablishment of perfusion, regardless of whether signs of compartment syndrome are present. In the presence of compartment syndrome, skin closure is contraindicated. The swollen muscle will cause gaping of the fasciotomy incisions, which can be treated with dressing changes and secondary split-thickness skin grafting or with gradual reapproximation of the wound edges using wire sutures or tape strips sequentially tightened daily.

Fat Embolism and the Acute Respiratory Distress Syndrome. Patients who sustain multiple fractures are at high risk for subsequent fat embolism, in which fat droplets from bone marrow enter the systemic circulation and impair pulmonary capillary perfusion via a complex mechanism. The final common pathway of fat embolism and other injuries that result in pulmonary parenchymal dysfunction after multiple-system trauma is severe hypoxemia, or the acute respiratory distress syndrome (ARDS). Fat embolism generally occurs within 24 to 72 h of injury and presents with hypoxemia, tachycardia, tachypnea, fever, restlessness, and confusion. The syndrome is fatal in 10 to 15 percent of cases. Chest radiographic findings are similar to those of other causes of ARDS, with bilateral patchy infiltrates. Petechiae may be present transiently in the axilla, chest, and conjunctiva and thrombocytopenia may occur, with fat droplets visible occasionally in blood specimens and in the urine.

Fat embolism syndrome occurs after total hip and total knee replacement as well as after trauma, but is seen most often following femoral fracture. Treatment of fat embolism syndrome is similar to treatment of ARDS, with administration of oxygen, ventilatory support, and positive end-expiratory pressure as needed to maintain a partial pressure of oxygen of 60 mmHg or better. Moderate-dose corticosteroids (methylprednisolone 9/mg/kg) given prophylactically after trauma has been shown to reduce the incidence of fat embolism from 28.8 to 2.5 percent. The use of corticosteroids in ARDS from causes other than fat embolism remains controversial, however. The other important factor in the management of the multiple-trauma patient that decreases the incidence and severity of fat embolism and ARDS is stabilization of the fractures within the first 24 h of injury. Specific medications such as low-molecular-weight dextran, heparin, and alcohol have not been proved to alter the outcome.

Peripheral Nerve Injuries. Extremity trauma is sometimes accompanied by injuries to peripheral nerves. In the least severe type of injury, neurapraxia, there is interruption of nerve conduction, which will ultimately recover, manifested by a transient complete or partial loss of motor and sensory function. The mechanism of injury is stretch or contusion, and resolution usually occurs within 2 to 3 months. With more severe stretch injuries, axonotmesis, or disruption of the axons with retention of the Schwann cell sheath, can occur. Axonal regeneration may occur with this injury, but only slowly (approximately 1 mm daily), and recovery may be incomplete. In neurotmesis, or complete division of the nerve, regeneration will not occur spontaneously, and surgical repair is necessary.

Assessment of the degree of nerve damage can be difficult unless open reduction of the fracture is needed, in which case the nerve can be explored. Careful documentation of nerve function is essential, as loss of function in a nerve after closed reduction of a fracture is one indication for surgical exploration. In cases of neurotmesis, microsurgical reapproximation of the nerve with fine epineural sutures gives the best chances of recovery. In cases of segmental nerve loss, cable grafting with several lengths of an expendable nerve such as the sural nerve allows some degree of regeneration. Nerve repair can be technically easier after 7 to 10 days, when some thickening of the epineurium due to scarring has developed. Persistent motor deficits in extremities can be managed with orthoses or, later, tendon transfers, depending on the functional loss and remaining available innervated muscles.

Fracture Healing. After fracture, hematoma develops at the fracture site and a clot is formed. Local mediators incite an inflammatory response, and necrosis of bone adjacent to the fracture site occurs as a consequence of disruption of its blood supply. In fractures with severe soft-tissue injury or loss, periosteal stripping, or comminution, the extent of bone necrosis can be significant and the fracture may be delayed in healing or fail to unite.

Stages. Fracture healing occurs in several stages or phases. At the time of fracture (stage of impact), the energy absorbed to failure determines the degree of comminution, soft-tissue injury, and disruption of the bone blood supply. The hematoma, which organizes into a fibrin clot, releases cytokines that attract inflammatory cells from the circulation, initiating the inflammatory stage of fracture healing, which lasts from a few days to 2 weeks. The cytokines released from platelets in the clot, such as platelet-derived growth factor (PDGF) and TGF-β, as well as other factors released from inflammatory cells, are probably involved in stimulating undifferentiated mesenchymal cells (which appear to be derived in large part from the periosteum) to undergo differentiation into fibroblasts, osteoblasts, and chondrocytes. This is accompanied by proliferation of fibrovascular tissue (granulation tissue) in the area of the fracture gap. These events signify the onset of the early reparative stage (or soft callus stage). The osteoblasts form adjacent to the periosteum, while in the more hypoxic area of the fracture gap, differentiation into hyaline cartilage is favored (Fig. 41-51). This fracture callus begins to stabilize the fracture ends and limit motion, leading to progressive vascular ingrowth. The cartilaginous callus, which tolerates hypoxia well and in fact undergoes cellular hypertrophy and matrix mineralization under hypoxic conditions (see Endochondral Ossification, above), begins to go through the endochondral sequence of mineralization. This late reparative stage (or hard callus stage) results in increasing stability of the fracture, and increasing membranous or osteoblastic ossification from the periphery of the callus gradually replaces the endochondral process.

The woven bone is later remodeled into true lamellar bone, a stage that can last from months to years. During this phase the limb is mechanically functional and remodels along lines of stress toward its original shape, with reconstitution of the medullary cavity. Table 41-12 summarizes the events in fracture healing by callus formation. Teleologically it appears that the function of the endochondral calcification is to stabilize the bone, allowing subsequent vascular growth across the fracture

gap to support the more aerobically dependent osteoblastic bone formation. If a fracture is rigidly internally fixed with a metal plate under compression, no callus forms, and the fracture heals by primary remodeling through the activity of osteoclasts and osteoblasts without endochondral ossification.

Factors Influencing Healing. The importance of the periosteum in fracture healing is supported by the observation that fracture healing is accelerated in children, who have much thicker and more cellular periosteal bony coverings. In adults the periosteum is noticeably thinner, and healing is slower. Rates of fracture healing in young and old adults are similar, barring that presence of metabolic bone disease or nutritional deficiencies. Many investigations in animals and human beings have attempted to evaluate substances that stimulate fracture healing, including growth hormone, PTH, various vitamins, and prostaglandins. At this point the evidence is controversial at best. There is no strong evidence that normal fracture healing is accelerated with these types of treatment, although some beneficial effect on delayed union or nonunion remains a possibility. Head-injured patients, who often form abnormal bone and cartilage in muscle or other inappropriate tissues (heterotopic ossification), have accelerated healing of fractures; a factor in the serum of these patients is an anabolic stimulator of osteoblasts in culture, though this factor has not yet been identified.

Articular Cartilage Healing. Unlike bone, articular cartilage has a very limited ability to undergo repair after posttraumatic damage. Articular cartilage has a very orderly structure, with an organic matrix composed of 40 percent proteoglycans, 40 percent type II collagen, and 20 percent glycoproteins, growth factors, and minor collagens such as type IX and type XI (Table 41-13). The collagen fibers in the most superficial layers of cartilage are oriented parallel to the joint surface and gradually change direction to a radial orientation in the deeper layers, with a somewhat random orientation in the transitional zone (Fig. 41-52A). The proteoglycan is a large macromolecular aggregate of subunits consisting of a protein core (aggrecan) with covalently bound branching sulfated carbohydrate groups called glycosaminoglycans (Fig. 41-52B). The predominant glycosaminoglycans are chondroitin and keratan sulfate. These monomer subunits are noncovalently bound to a filament of hyaluronic acid by a small glycoprotein called a link protein. Proteoglycans are responsible for the compressibility, hydration, and mechanical integrity of cartilage.

The earliest responses to an injury such as a laceration of the articular surface are loss of matrix proteoglycans and an attempt, usually unsuccessful, by chondrocytes adjacent to the injury to resynthesize the matrix. Progressive degradation of matrix macromolecules ensues, and the cartilage may fibrillate or split along the radially oriented deeper collagen fibers. If a defect is near the synovial attachment of the joint, cells from this area may migrate into the defect and form fibrocartilage repair tissue. Usually, however, the defect remains and can trigger further areas of progressive degeneration.

If the cartilage defect penetrates the subchondral bony plate, cells from the bone marrow can migrate into the defect and will also allow fibrocartilaginous repair. Fibrocartilage, unlike hyaline cartilage, is mostly composed of type I rather than type II collagen and has inferior wear characteristics, gradually degenerating over a period of years. Fibrocartilaginous repair can be augmented and some type II collagen formation stimulated by

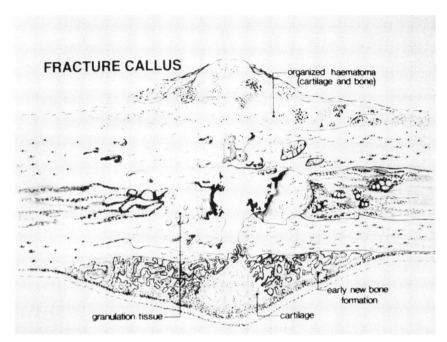

FIG. 41-51. Fracture callus in the reparative stage. Note that cartilage tends to form in the central fracture gap area (endochondral ossification), while periosteally derived osteoblastic bone formation occurs at the periphery of the fracture callus. As the cartilage calcifies it is gradually replaced by bone. (Modified from: *Cruess RL, 1982, with permission.*)

Table 41-12
Stages of Fracture Healing

Stage	Duration	Events
Stage of impact	Seconds	Energy absorbed until failure; comminution, periosteal stripping, and soft tissue injury occur
Stage of inflammation	1–2 weeks	Hematoma attracts inflammatory cells, cytokines released which stimulate mesenchymal cells
Early reparative stage (stage of soft callus)	Weeks to months	Granulation tissue forms in fracture gap; dead bone resorbed; osteoblastic proliferation at periphery; cartilage forms in central area
Late reparative stage (stage of hard callus)	Weeks to months	Cartilage calcifies, gradually replaced by osteoblastic bone formation; clinical union occurs
Remodeling stage	Months to years	Bone tends toward original shape under influence of mechanical stresses; medullary cavity reconstituted

Table 41-13
Articular Cartilage Composition

Component	Proportion	Function
Type II collagen	40%	Structural—shear
Proteoglycan	40%	Structural—compressibility
Glycoproteins	20%	Most unknown; anchorin and chondronectin attach chondrocytes to matrix
Growth factors	Minute	Thought to function in repair and matrix metabolism (TGF-beta FGF, PDGF, IGF)
Type IX collagen	Unknown	Binds proteoglycan to type II collagen
Type XI collagen	Unknown	Regulates fibril diameter

continuous passive motion of the joint. These properties form the basis for current approaches to treatment of chondral defects as well as the rationale for abrasion arthroplasty, or abrading damaged areas of cartilage down to a bleeding bony surface followed by passive motion and protection from weight bearing.

Experimental techniques have evolved to enhance hyaline cartilage repair in animal models as well as in human beings. An approach developed by Caplan and coworkers involves isolation of undifferentiated mesenchymal stem cells from bone marrow aspirates, which are then expanded in tissue culture and implanted in a collagen gel into an articular defect, and results in differentiation into hyaline cartilage. A second approach, developed by O'Driscoll and Salter, uses a periosteal graft attached to the chondral defect by sutures with the cambium layer of the periosteum facing the synovial fluid. This leads to resurfacing of the defect with hyaline cartilage, which can be further enhanced by incubation of the periosteum briefly with TGF-β before reimplantation. Peterson and coworkers have used autologous chondrocyte transplantation to resurface defects in human knee joints. Cartilage is removed arthroscopically from non-weight-bearing regions of the articular surface, and chondrocytes are isolated by enzymatic digestion and expanded in tissue cul-

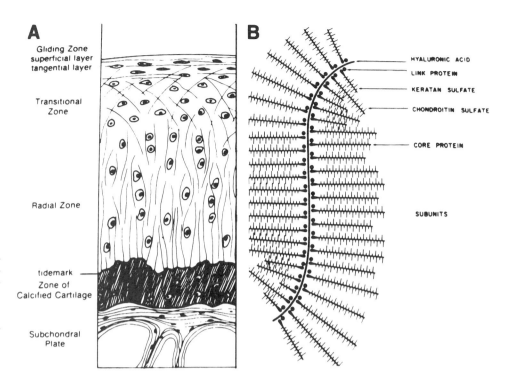

A

Gliding Zone
superficial layer
tangential layer

Transitional
Zone

Radial Zone

tidemark
Zone of
Calcified Cartilage

Subchondral
Plate

B

HYALURONIC ACID
LINK PROTEIN
KERATAN SULFATE
CHONDROITIN SULFATE

CORE PROTEIN

SUBUNITS

FIG. 41-52. *A. Structure of articular cartilage. The change in orientation of the type II collagen fibrils from the superficial to deep layers is shown. B. Structure of the proteoglycan molecule. (Modified from: Albright JA, Brand RA (eds): Scientific Basis of Orthopaedics. Norwalk, CT, Appleton: Lange, 1987, with permission.)*

ture. The chondrocytes are then injected in a collagen gel beneath a periosteal flap sutured to the articular surface over the defect. Early clinical results are encouraging, but these procedures are controversial and the long-term outcome uncertain.

Ligament Healing. Bony injuries to the extremities are frequently accompanied by ligamentous injuries. ligament injuries also can occur independently as a primary injury to a joint; in general these injuries are referred to as sprains. Ligaments heal by progressive scar formation and contracture, and recent studies indicate that repair is improved by early motion in the absence of gross instability. Ligament injuries are graded as type I (stretch but no disruption of fibers), type II (tear of some of ligament fibers), and type III (complete mechanical discontinuity of the ligament). Type I and type II ligament injuries generally are treated by immobilization, or protected motion. Motion and mechanical strain enhance ligament healing. Treatment of type III ligament injuries depends on many factors and can range from nonintervention (as for a type III acromioclavicular separation) to immediate surgical repair or reconstruction (as for a torn anterior cruciate ligament in a competitive athlete).

Delayed Union and Nonunion. *Delayed union* is a somewhat arbitrarily defined term applied to fractures that take longer than average to heal and must be considered in context of the type of fracture and age of the patient. *Nonunion* refers to a condition in which a fracture fails to show progression toward union and in which healing is not expected even with prolonged immobilization. Radiographic examination can show sclerotic bone ends, a persistent fracture gap, and rounding off of the fracture ends. Gross motion can be demonstrable clinically or under fluoroscopic stress testing. The fracture gap usually contains nonmineralized fibrocartilage, although at times a true synovial pseudarthrosis, or false joint, is present. Factors predisposing to nonunion include excessive motion or inadequate im-

mobilization of the fracture, interposed soft tissues, extensive soft-tissue damage, periosteal stripping, devascularization of the bone, and infection. Certain bones have more of a predisposition to nonunion, probably attributable to suboptimal orientation of the local bone vascular supply (such as the tibia, femoral neck, or carpal scaphoid).

Nonunion usually requires surgical intervention such as bone grafting with autogenous or vascularized fibular bone. A growing body of evidence supports the use of electromagnetic stimulation, which can induce a certain proportion of nonunions to heal without surgery. Also, one report suggests that administration of levodopa, which is known to cause a sustained increased level of growth hormone in the serum, can be beneficial in stimulation of healing of ununited fractures. During a 6-month treatment period, over 80 percent of a group of multiply operated patients with nonunion and failed bone grafts healed with this regimen.

Pathologic Fractures. Fractures that occur through bone abnormally weakened by a preexisting condition are termed pathologic. Often these fractures result from significantly less than the usual degree of force needed to cause a fracture. The underlying process may be either systemic (as in osteoporosis) or local (as in a bone tumor or cyst). An example of a pathologic fracture secondary to metastatic carcinoma is shown in Fig. 41-53. Pathologic fractures often require surgical internal fixation to achieve healing, and in patients with carcinomas that commonly metastasize to bone (e.g., breast, prostate, lung, kidney, and thyroid tumors), prophylactic fixation of large lesions in weight-bearing bones decreases morbidity and improves quality of life. Pain on weight bearing is a reliable clinical sign of an impending fracture.

Stress Fractures. Stress fractures are the eventual result of repeated stress to a bone, ultimately causing fatigue failure.

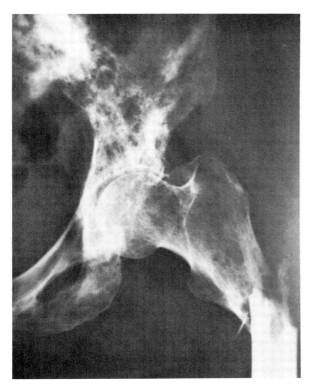

FIG. 41-53. Pathologic fracture. Metastatic carcinoma with pathologic subtrochanteric fracture of the femur. There is diffuse involvement of the adjacent pelvis.

The metatarsals, tibia, fibula, and calcaneus are common sites. Initially radiographs may be negative, but later periosteal reaction will become evident. Nuclear bone scans or MRI can readily demonstrate the lesion in case the radiographs are negative (Fig. 41-54). Treatment usually is conservative, with immobilization and discontinuation of the causative activity.

Growth Plate Injuries. Longitudinal bone growth occurs as previously described in the growth plates, which lie between the epiphyses and metaphyses of the long bones. In children, injuries involving the growth plate are relatively common, and the fractures usually involve the zone of provisional calcification, the mechanically weakest region. Since the germinal cells in the upper growth plate usually are not damaged, fractures that do not cross the plate tend to heal without growth disturbances. The most commonly used classification of growth plate injuries is the Salter-Harris classification, depicted in Fig. 41-55. Type I is a separation of the growth plate and epiphysis from the metaphysis. Type II is similar, with a metaphyseal fragment remaining with the epiphysis. Since the growth plate is intact in these injuries, treatment is with closed reduction, and growth disturbance or premature closure of the growth plate is rare. Fortunately, the majority of epiphyseal fractures are of these two types. Because of the proximity of the fracture to the growth plate, a great degree of remodeling capacity exists, and significant angulations and displacements often heal and remodel uneventfully. Type III injuries are intraarticular, traverse the epiphysis and growth plate, and exit through the zone of provisional calcification. Type IV injuries are similar, but exit through the

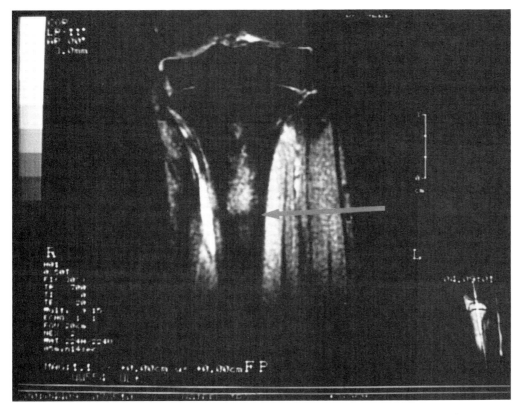

FIG. 41-54. MRI demonstrating transverse stress fracture of the tibia in an adolescent male. The patient had persistent weight-bearing pain, but plain radiographs were normal.

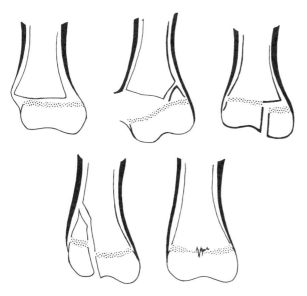

FIG. 41-55. *Salter and Harris classification of epiphyseal injury type I. See text for description.* Top row, *types I, II, and III;* bottom row, *types IV and V.*

metaphysis. Since both these types of fractures cross and disrupt the growth plate, nothing less than anatomic reduction is acceptable, or growth disturbance will result. These fractures are usually treated by accurate open reduction and internal fixation. Type V injuries are difficult to recognize, and result from an axial load or crush injury to the growth plate that later results in premature fusion. Rang has described an additional physeal injury known as type VI, consisting of damage to the perichondral ring on one side of the growth plate. This can lead to a bony bar on one side of the physis acting as a tether and leading to a progressive angular deformity. Careful follow-up and education of the parents is necessary with these injuries to ensure the best clinical outcome, allow planning of any corrective procedures should growth disturbance occur, and minimize the possibility of misunderstanding.

Fractures in Children. Children's fractures present different problems from similar injuries in adults. Nonunion is extremely rare, and fracture healing is more rapid. The challenge is in recognizing and understanding what degree of displacement, angulation, and shortening is acceptable in relation to remaining growth potential. Fracture healing in a young child stimulates the blood flow to the extremity, and this in turn stimulates increased activity of the growth plates, causing the limb to grow at a faster rate than the uninjured extremity. Furthermore, most fractures in children are treated conservatively, whereas a greater degree of surgical intervention is used in fractures in adults.

Closed versus Open Reduction. The optimal method for handling a specific fracture should allow rapid union, reestablish length and alignment of the extremity, restore complete motion in adjacent joints, and return the patient to functional activity with a minimum of morbidity. Furthermore, cost concerns are an increasing pressure on the health care system, and prolonged hospitalization must be at least a distant consideration, obviously with the welfare of the patient taking precedence. For-

tunately technical advances in fracture fixation allow treatment of a wider range of fractures surgically, and prolonged traction in the hospital is much less common than previously. The closed reduction of fractures has the advantages of minimal risk of infection and no further disruption of bone blood supply, and the disadvantages of less precise reduction and prolonged immobilization. Treatment must be individualized to the injury and patient.

Application of Plaster Casts. Circumferential rigid dressings of plaster or fiberglass are an important tool in the treatment of fractures. Plaster is composed of anhydrous calcium sulfate, which solidifies during an exothermic hydration reaction with water. Plaster sets up in a few minutes after addition of water but does not dry completely for 36 to 48 h.

Complications of Cast Treatment. The maximum temperature achieved during setting depends on the water temperature, and use of hot water can result in burns, particularly if the cast is thick or placed on a surface that reflects heat, such as rubber or plastic, during setting. Water used in casting should be lukewarm. After casting for acute injury or surgery, the extremity should be elevated, as swelling within a rigid container can lead to compartment syndrome, as previously described. This is of particular concern in patients who are unconscious or have sensory impairment in the limb. Unrelieved pain, pallor, loss of sensation, development of paresthesias, poor capillary refill, or diminishing motor function are all indications to bivalve the cast. This should be accompanied by cutting the underlying soft padding layer or dressing gauze, which can also become constrictive in the face of swelling. If the symptoms are not promptly relieved, the cast must be removed and the compartment pressures measured as previously described.

Pressure sores, or decubitus ulcers, can occur rapidly in a cast, and tend to occur over bony prominences such as the heel, olecranon, patella, and ischium. Proper molding of the cast, as well as prompt attention to any complaints of pressure or burning pain in an area beneath the cast, are essential to their prevention. The cast also can be windowed and padded to relieve the pressure and prevent skin breakdown; the window is then replaced to prevent window edema.

Types of Cast. When a cast is applied for an acute fracture, it should include the joints above and below the fracture. A long leg cast extends from the upper thigh to the metatarsal bases, and generally the ankle is placed in neutral dorsiflexion and the knee in about 30 degrees of flexion to more easily allow the patient to clear the floor with the immobilized extremity when on crutches. Proper molding above the femoral condyles is important. A cylinder cast extends from the upper thigh to the ankle above the malleoli; it must be well padded above the malleoli and molded above the femoral condyles to prevent it from sliding downward and causing pressure areas around the ankle. A short leg cast extends from the tibial tubercle to the metatarsals; it should be well molded around the malleoli, above the calcaneal tuberosity, in the arch of the foot, and along the shaft of the tibia. A patellar tendon bearing cast is similar to a short leg cast except that it is extended over the knee anteriorly to the midpoint of the patella and is molded over the anterior femoral condyles and patellar tendon to provide partial weight relief of the tibia when weight bearing. Most lower-extremity casts are used with a cast shoe or boot when weight bearing is allowed.

A double hip spica cast, used for immobilization of the hips, is analogous to a plaster pair of pants, usually applied with the hips in some flexion and abduction, and the knees in slight flexion. A single hip spica includes only one leg, and a one and one-half hip spica includes one leg to the toes and the other to just above the knee. Body casts are applied for immobilization of the spine and extend from the groin to the sternum. With improved methods of surgical spinal fixation, molded plastic body jackets often can be used instead of the more cumbersome body cast.

A short arm cast extends from below the elbow to the proximal palmar crease, allowing free flexion and extension of the digits and thumb. If the thumb is included, the cast is referred to as a thumb spica cast. A long arm cast extends from the upper arm to the proximal palmar crease, usually with the elbow flexed 90 degrees. A shoulder spica cast is a body jacket that extends to include the shoulder and elbow, usually with the shoulder abducted and the elbow flexed.

Orthoses. Orthoses and fracture braces are widely used for nonacute treatment of fractures, allowing greater functional use as the fractures heal. These are made of lightweight polypropylene, Orthoplast, or fiberglass and can be custom molded or used in standard sizes. Humeral, tibial, and forearm fracture braces are readily available and can be tightened with Velcro straps as swelling subsides and muscles atrophy. A knee immobilizer with metal staves often can be used in place of a cylinder cast, and adjustable-range-of-motion knee braces that extend from the thigh to the ankle can be helpful in rehabilitating patients after knee, distal femur, or proximal tibial surgery.

External Fixation. External fixation has been used increasingly in trauma treatment in recent years. Threaded pins are inserted into the bone above and below the fracture site and secured to a rigid, adjustable frame to immobilize the fracture (Fig. 41-56). External fixation is particularly helpful in severely comminuted fractures or those with severe soft-tissue damage or loss, since access to wounds is permitted. Pin tract infections are a common complication (incidence 10 percent) but usually respond to local wound care and antibiotics. Occasionally, persistent infection causes loosening of pins and necessitates removal or replacement of one or more pins. An additional advantage of external fixation is in allowing early motion of the joints above and below the fracture, decreasing joint stiffness. External fixation also can be used to help reduce and maintain reduction of comminuted intraarticular fractures by ligamentotaxis (providing traction across the joint, which reduces fracture fragments due to remaining ligamentous and capsular attachments). This is useful in severely comminuted distal radius and tibial plafond fractures.

Another important use of external fixation is in the treatment of acute multiple-trauma patients with severe pelvic fractures and dislocations. Hemorrhage into the pelvis and retroperitoneum can become a life-threatening problem. Application of an anterior external fixator to provisionally stabilize the pelvis and decrease the intrapelvic volume effectively controls intrapelvic hemorrhage. This can be done under local anesthesia in the emergency department, and involves placing two or three pins in each anterior iliac crest and then affixing them to a rigid anterior frame (Fig. 41-57).

One further application of external fixation is in limb reconstruction using the Ilizarov distraction osteogenesis technique, as

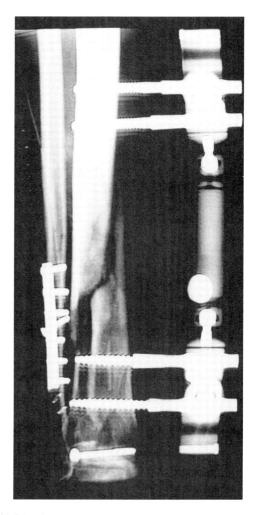

FIG. 41-56. Comminuted open tibial fracture treated by reduction and external fixation, which allows access to wounds and early mobilization of the patient.

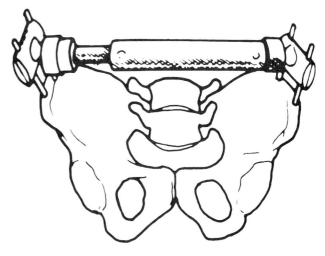

FIG. 41-57. External fixation of the pelvis using an anterior frame, which stabilizes the patient for transport and helps to control hemorrhage.

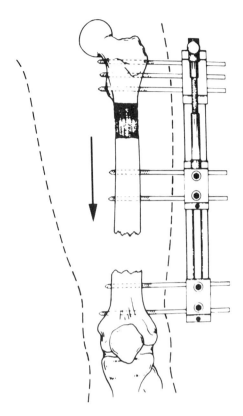

FIG. 41-58. Use of distraction osteogenesis and external fixation to allow bone transport for repair of nonunion with significant traumatic bone loss. After corticotomy, the middle segment of the bone is transported distally toward the nonunion site, with osteogenesis occurring in the proximal gap as it is gradually lengthened.

described earlier for the correction of limb length deficiency. Preliminary results suggest that external fixation may be useful in repairing bony defects caused by traumatic segmental bone loss. A corticotomy is made above the defect, and the segment is gradually transported distally until it abuts the distal fragment. The resulting proximal defect ossifies by the process of distraction osteogenesis (Fig. 41-58).

Traction. Traction is used in orthopaedics to overcome muscle spasm and apply distraction to fracture fragments to re-

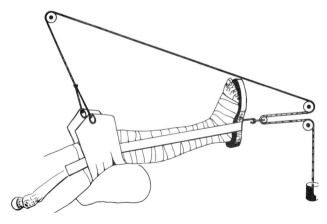

FIG. 41-59. Russell's traction.

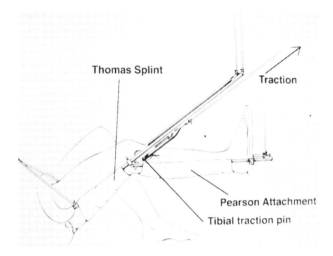

FIG. 41-60. Skeletal traction using balanced suspension with a Thomas splint. The Pearson attachment allows knee motion while in traction, and the arrangement can be used with either a distal femoral or proximal tibial traction pin. (Modified from: *Rockwood CA, Green DP, Bucholz RW, 1991, with permission.*)

duce the fracture. Additional uses include immobilization of long bone fractures until early healing occurs, immobilization and distraction for painful joint conditions, and correction of joint deformities or contractures.

Skin Traction. Skin traction is applied by means of tapes attached to the skin. It is used only when low levels of force are needed, since 10 lbs is the maximum amount of force that the skin will tolerate with this method. Skin traction applied to the foot (Buck's traction) often is used to immobilize hip fractures temporarily before surgery. While skin tapes can be used, a foam boot with Velcro straps is more convenient and more widely used. Russell's traction, used for the treatment of femoral fractures in children, can be used as shown in Fig. 41-59. Alternatively, separate weights can be applied to the femoral sling and the longitudinal foot, a technique known as split Russell's traction. Bryant's traction can be used in infants and small children with femoral fractures. As originally described, the technique consists of skin traction on both lower legs vertically (hips flexed to 90 degrees with knees extended). However, instances of serious vascular compromise of the extremities have been reported with this method; nevertheless, safety can be ensured by limiting its use to children not older than $2\frac{1}{2}$ years of age and applying the traction at a 45-degree inclination rather than directly vertically.

Skeletal Traction. This involves the placement of a Steinmann pin or Kirschner wire percutaneously through the distal femur or proximal tibia in a transverse direction. A traction bow is attached to the pin and a weight applied. The patient is then placed in balanced suspension as shown in Fig. 41-60. Other forms of skeletal traction include halo traction with pins affixed to the skull for cervical spine injuries and olecranon traction overhead for humeral fractures.

Electrical Stimulation. The initial concept that electromagnetic fields or electrical potentials might influence bone formation stemmed from the observed piezoelectric properties of bone, which develops surface charges when mechanically

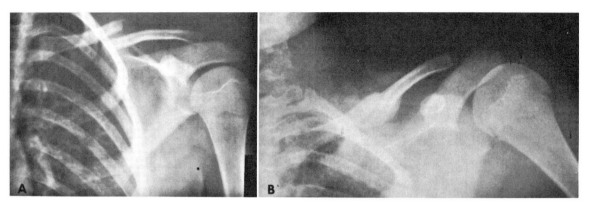

FIG. 41-61. *A. Fracture of the middle third of the clavicle with complete displacement and overriding. B. Healing of a clavicle fracture in 6 weeks with internal callus formation.*

stressed because of its anisotropic nature. Areas of compression develop electronegative potentials, and areas of tension develop electropositive potentials. Increasing clinical and basic research data support the effectiveness of electromagnetic bone stimulation in the healing of nonunions, although the mechanism of action is unknown. The most commonly used form of electrical stimulation involves use of external coils that are attached to a cast and centered over the nonunion site. After 3 to 6 months, union rates of 70 to 80 percent have been reported, but the method remains somewhat controversial, with only a few controlled clinical studies. The biologic events appear to involve stimulation of fibrocartilage at the nonunion site to mineralize. Significant effects of electromagnetic fields on bone formation in various models have been demonstrated by Bassett, Brighton, Rubin, and others. This form of treatment is contraindicated in cases in which the fracture gap is more than 1 cm or half the bone diameter, or in the presence of a synovial pseudarthrosis. Synovial pseudarthrosis can be ruled out by bone scan or aspiration of the site, which will contain synovial-like fluid.

Upper-Extremity Injuries

Shoulder

Full abduction of the shoulder requires motion in the glenohumeral joint, scapulothoracic articulation, acromioclavicular joint, and sternoclavicular joint. Glenohumeral and scapulothoracic motion occur in approximately a 2:1 ratio. For every 10 degrees of forward elevation of the arm, 4 degrees of elevation of the clavicle occurs. Motion at the acromioclavicular joint of 20 degrees occurs during the first 30 degrees of abduction. Because of these complex interactive motions, any disruption of one of these articulations can limit shoulder motion.

Sternoclavicular Joint Injuries. The sternoclavicular joint can be dislocated anteriorly or posteriorly, although anterior dislocations are much more common. These injuries most often occur in motor vehicle accidents or contact sports when force is applied to the shoulder along the axis of the clavicle. While the sternoclavicular joint can be difficult to visualize radiographically, a 40-degree cephalad-angled anteroposterior radiograph, tomogram, or CT scan can aid in evaluation. Differentiation from a Salter type I epiphyseal separation is necessary in young patients, since the medial ossification center often does not appear until age eighteen and fuses by age twenty-five. Posterior

dislocations are dangerous because there may be associated serious damage to retrosternal pulmonary or vascular structures; therefore a very careful examination of the patient should be performed. Closed reduction is accomplished by shoulder retraction with longitudinal traction; for posterior dislocations this must be done under general anesthesia. Subsequently the patient is immobilized in a figure-of-eight harness or plaster to maintain shoulder retraction. Chronic unreduced dislocations that are painful may require excision of the proximal clavicle.

Fractures of the Clavicle. Clavicle fractures are common in both children and adults and usually occur at the junction of the middle and distal thirds. The fracture is caused by either direct downward force on the shoulder or indirect force such as occurs in a fall on the extended arm. Clinically there is swelling and tenderness at the fracture site and pain with movement of the extremity.

Treatment. Although the clavicle is difficult to immobilize, nonunion is unusual (incidence 0.5 percent) with conservative treatment, presumably because of the excellent blood supply in this area (Fig. 41-61). The trapezius and sternocleidomastoid muscles tend to pull the proximal fragment superiorly. Fractures are treated similarly in children and adults, with use of a figure-of-eight device to retract and elevate the shoulders (Fig. 41-62).

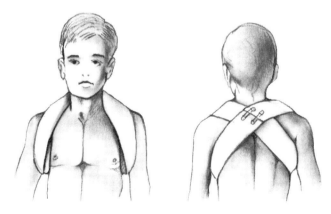

FIG. 41-62. *Figure-of-eight for treatment of a fractured clavicle. The axillae are padded with gauze pads over which a figure-of-eight of felt and stockinet is applied.*

A study comparing figure-of-eight immobilization with a simple sling showed no difference in results. Immobilization is for 4 to 6 weeks, depending on the radiographic evidence of progression toward union. A cosmetic deformity with prominence of the fracture site is the rule, but internal fixation trades the bony prominence for a scar and increases the risk of nonunion. In the rare case in which nonunion does occur, internal fixation with plating and bone grafting usually is successful.

Distal Clavicle Fractures. Fractures of the distal clavicle are less common (incidence 15 percent) and have been classified into three types. Type I fractures, which are lateral to the coracoclavicular ligaments (conoid and trapezoid), are stable and treated with a sling. Type II (interligamentous) fractures exhibit superior displacement of the proximal fragment and detachment of the ligaments. These are unstable, may progress to nonunion, and are best treated surgically by open reduction and stabilization with one or more transacromial pins. Type III fractures involve the articular surface. While stable, they may cause later arthritic symptoms that will require distal clavicular excision.

Acromioclavicular Joint Injuries.

Injuries to the acromioclavicular joint result from downward force on the shoulder and are frequent in contact sports. These injuries are primarily ligamentous sprains of three types. The patient presents with pain, tenderness, and swelling in the area of the joint. Shoulder movement is painful, and there can be palpable or visible prominence of the distal clavicle if there is disruption of the coracoclavicular ligaments, which are the major stabilizers of the joint. Type I sprains involve partial tear of the ligamentous capsule, with no injury to the coracoclavicular ligaments. Type II sprains involve complete tearing of the ligamentous capsule and a grade II sprain of the coracoclavicular ligaments, and hence they can exhibit slight superior subluxation of the distal clavicle radiographically. Type III sprains involve complete tearing of both the capsular and coracoclavicular ligaments, with superior subluxation of the distal clavicle. Radiographic diagnosis is aided by comparison views of the joint bilaterally with and without the patient holding a 10-lb weight, which will accentuate the subluxation. The rare Type IV, V, and VI sprains involve severe posterior or inferior displacements and generally require surgical treatment.

Treatment. Type I injuries are treated with a sling until comfortable and then progressive exercises. Type II injuries can be treated similarly. Type III injuries cannot be reduced nonoperatively and leave a cosmetic deformity if untreated. In less active individuals, conservative symptomatic treatment generally gives good functional results. In patients involved in high-demand activities or with persistent symptoms or major concerns about the deformity, surgical repair or reconstruction usually is indicated. Various approaches include stabilization of the clavicle to the coracoid process with a screw (Bosworth) and reconstruction of the coracoclavicular ligaments using the coracoacromial ligament (Weaver-Dunn procedure). In patients with persistent pain, excision of the distal clavicle usually provides satisfactory results.

Fractures of the Scapula.

Scapular fractures are most commonly seen as a result of violent trauma such as motor vehicle accidents. Consequently associated injuries such as brachial plexus injury and cardiopulmonary trauma are a concern, and these injuries take precedence. Scapular body fractures rarely cause symptoms and usually heal uneventfully. Even with involvement of the glenoid, given the non-weight-bearing status of this joint results of conservative treatment are usually satisfactory, and therefore symptomatic immobilization of the shoulder generally is preferable to more aggressive intervention. In individuals with more than 10 mm of displacement of a glenoid rim fracture comprising more than one-fourth of the joint surface, or with severe separation, or with articular step-off of more than 5 mm, open reduction and internal fixation may be considered.

Acute Anterior Shoulder Dislocations.

Dislocation of the humeral head can be anterior, posterior, or inferior to the glenoid. Anteroinferior dislocations can be subcoracoid or subglenoid. Anterior or anteroinferior dislocations, the most common injuries, are caused by a combination of external rotation and abduction, which tears the anterior capsular structures. Anterior dislocation of the humeral head can tear the anterior glenoid labrum, and a compression fracture of the posterolateral humeral head (Hill-Sachs lesion) can result from impingement on the glenoid.

The patient usually holds the arm in slight abduction and is unable to lower it. A flattening of the deltoid prominence or indentation beneath the tip of the acromion is frequently apparent. Sensation over the lateral deltoid must always be assessed carefully before reduction, as injury to the axillary nerve can occur. Because of spasm, motor function of the deltoid cannot be evaluated until after reduction.

Radiographic Findings. These include inferior and medial displacement of the humeral head on the anteroposterior view (Fig. 41-63). An axillary view may be difficult to obtain, but a

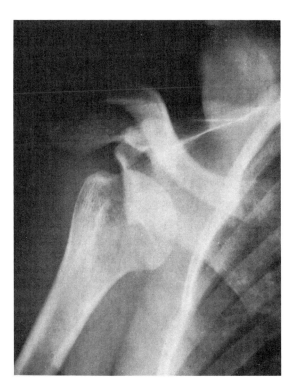

FIG. 41-63. *Anterior subcoracoid dislocation of the shoulder. The articular surface of the humeral head can be seen medial to the glenoid fossa and inferior to the coracoid process.*

transscapular lateral view (Y view) will demonstrate the humeral head lying anterior to the glenoid.

Treatment. The dislocation must be reduced as soon as possible, and unrecognized dislocations may still be reducible within the first 2 weeks. More chronic dislocations and those that cannot be reduced by closed means often require open reduction.

While a number of different reduction maneuvers are acceptable, the basic principle involves longitudinal traction and gentle internal rotation. This can be achieved either by having the patient lie supine while an assistant applies countertraction with a sheet around the chest, or by having the patient lie prone with the arm over the edge of the table with a traction weight attached to the forearm. Adequate sedation and muscle relaxation are essential to counteract muscle spasm. After reduction, the patient is placed in a sling and swathe or shoulder immobilizer with the elbow at 90 degrees and the forearm across the abdomen. Postreduction anteroposterior and transscapular lateral radiographs are essential. Range-of-motion exercises are started after 3 to 4 weeks in younger individuals, and sooner in the elderly because of the predisposition to loss of motion.

Recurrent Anterior Dislocations. A small percentage of patients are subject to recurrent dislocations, sometimes with minor trauma or even with active abduction and external rotation of the shoulder. Occasionally patients complain of recurrent sensation of subluxation without frank dislocation. When spontaneous reduction does not occur, the reduction maneuver is as described above. After a brief period of immobilization until comfortable, appropriate rehabilitation focusing on strengthening the internal rotator muscles is begun. Continued episodes lead to articular damage and are an indication for reconstructive surgery. MRI or arthroscopy can be helpful in surgical planning in that tears of the anterior labrum, which lead to persistent instability, can be identified. Surgical repair focuses on repair of labral tears (Bankhart procedure), anterior capsular and subscapularis repair or tightening (Putti-Platt procedure), or a combination of these techniques. Capsulorrhaphy in conjunction with Bankhart repair has been advocated instead of subscapularis shortening procedures because of restoration of more normal shoulder biomechanics.

Arthroscopic repair of labral tears (Bankhart lesions) associated with pain or instability is increasingly common. Recurrence rates for dislocation are somewhat higher than with open repair, but the surgical procedure is minimally invasive. Shoulder arthroscopy also is useful in diagnosis and in decompression of the rotator cuff by acromioplasty. A superior labral anterior and posterior (SLAP) lesion has been described that typically results from a fall on an outstretched arm and can cause pain and clicking in the shoulder with overhead activities. Depending on the size of the labral tear, arthroscopic debridement or reattachment have been successful forms of treatment.

Chronic Dislocations. Patients with painful chronic dislocations may benefit from arthrodesis of the shoulder in a functional position. Occasionally these injuries are seen in elderly individuals with surprisingly few symptoms and may not warrant surgical intervention.

Posterior Shoulder Dislocations. Posterior dislocations are less common and are seen after seizures or motor vehicle accidents. Physical findings include an inability to externally rotate or abduct the arm, which is held tightly at the side and in internal rotation. The posterior shoulder can exhibit prominence compared to the opposite side, and the coracoid process often is more obvious on the affected side.

Radiographic Findings. On the anteroposterior view findings may be subtle, with loss of the distinct "half moon" overlap shadow seen on in a normal shoulder (Fig. 41-64). Axillary or transscapular lateral views will confirm the posterior displacement. Associated lesser tubercle fractures are common, because of avulsion injury of the subscapularis muscle.

Treatment. Reduction is accomplished by the same methods described for anterior dislocation, except that gentle external rotation is used along with anterior pressure on the posterior humeral head. The shoulder can be immobilized in a shoulder spica cast or brace in 30 degrees of abduction and some external rotation for 3 to 4 weeks. Recurrent posterior dislocations can require posterior capsular reefing or osteotomy of the glenoid with bone block placement.

Fracture-Dislocations of the Shoulder. Dislocation of the shoulder can be associated with fracture of the proximal humerus. Reduction is with maneuvers similar to those for simple dislocations, but usually requires general anesthesia. If reduction cannot be obtained by closed means, open reduction and internal fixation is indicated.

Humerus

Fractures of the Proximal Humerus. Fractures of the surgical neck (proximal metaphysis) of the humerus are common injuries in adults, while in children the anatomic neck (junction of the epiphysis and metaphysis) is involved, usually in a Salter-Harris type II configuration (Fig. 41-65). Treatment is with

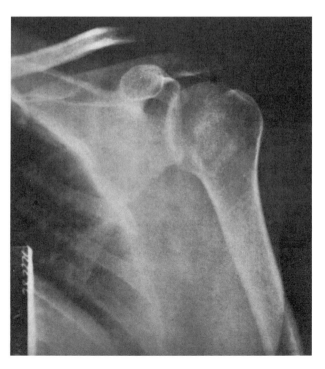

FIG. 41-64. *Posterior dislocation of the shoulder. AP radiograph shows an indistinct border of the humeral head, superimposed on the glenoid rim. There is also a compression fracture in the region of the lesser tubercle.*

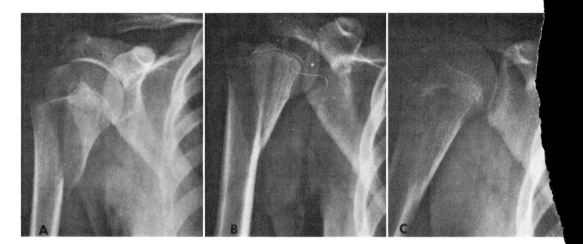

FIG. 41-65. *Fracture of the proximal humerus in a 12-year-old girl. The fracture is an epiphyseal separation with a large metaphyseal fragment attached to the epiphysis. A. Initial fracture position. B. Slight improvement after closed reduction. C. Healed fracture with remodelling changes at 1 year postinjury. The patient has a normal range of shoulder motion.*

closed reduction using longitudinal manual traction, followed by a sling or hanging cast application. A significant degree of angulation can be accepted because of the large range of motion of the shoulder joint. In instances of unacceptable angulation or displacement, percutaneous pinning or open reduction is indicated.

In adults fractures of the proximal humerus may be comminuted, in which case they are classified according to the number of displaced segments (Neer classification). The segments consist of the head, shaft, and greater and lesser tubercles, and displacement is defined as more than 45 degrees of angulation or 1 cm of displacement. Thus fractures are three- or four-part if one or both tubercles are fractured and displaced. Displaced greater tubercle fractures require reduction to maintain function and are repaired using Hawkins's tension band wiring technique. In four-part fractures there is a high incidence of avascular necrosis of the humeral head, and generally replacement of the humeral head with a Neer-type endoprosthesis is advocated, with reattachment of the tubercles to the prosthesis by tension band wiring or heavy nonabsorbable sutures (Fig. 41-66).

In all proximal humerus fractures, early motion is essential to prevent stiffness. Physical therapy is an important part of the treatment, and gentle passive pendulum exercises usually should be started within 1 or 2 weeks.

Fractures of the Humeral Shaft. Humeral shaft fractures may be transverse, comminuted, or spiral, depending on the mechanism of injury (direct versus torsional force). Swelling, pain, crepitus, and instability may be present, and occasionally the fracture is open, particularly with high-energy trauma such as a motor vehicle accident. Careful evaluation and documentation of the neurologic status of the limb is critical, as associated nerve injuries, especially to the radial nerve, are common. Radial nerve injury most commonly occurs with oblique fractures of the distal to middle thirds of the humerus.

Treatment. Generally humeral fractures are reduced by gentle longitudinal traction with adequate sedation or local anesthesia and the patient placed in a coaptation splint (from the axilla medially, around the elbow, and up over the shoulder laterally),

although a long arm splint or plastic humeral fracture brace also may be used. The patient is then placed in a sling and swathe (Fig. 41-67). Neurapraxia occurs in 95 percent of patients with radial nerve injury, but will resolve within a few weeks to 3 months. Therefore the presence of a radial nerve palsy is not an indication for surgical intervention. Loss of the nerve function after closed reduction is indicative of entrapment in the fracture site and warrants exploration. Late exploration is indicated if recovery does not occur within 3 months. If satisfactory reduction cannot be obtained or maintained, surgical treatment with compression plating or intramedullary rodding of the humerus is appropriate. This is also preferred in multiple-trauma patients, who require rapid mobilization to prevent pulmonary and other complications.

Elbow

The elbow functions as a hinge joint, and the proximal and distal radioulnar articulations are important for pronation and supination. Elbow injuries are notorious for causing loss of motion due to capsular fibrosis or ossification (myositis ossificans or, more accurately, heterotopic ossification). In addition to the routine anteroposterior and lateral views, oblique radiographs are helpful in delineating subtle injuries. Because the multiple ossification centers about the elbow appear at differing ages (capitellum—1 to 2 years; medial epicondyle—5 to 6 years; radial head—5 to 6 years; trochlea—9 to 10 years; lateral epicondyle—9 to 12 years), interpretation of radiographs in the context of acute trauma in children can be difficult. Comparison views of the opposite elbow often are helpful.

Fractures of the Radial Head and Neck. These injuries usually result from a fall on the outstretched hand. Patients have limited range of motion of the elbow, localized swelling and tenderness, particularly laterally, and pain with attempted pronation and supination. The greatest problem with these injuries is subsequent loss of motion. Aspiration of the joint and instillation of a small amount of lidocaine will improve range of motion and relieve pain. If the fracture is not severely angulated or displaced, the patient can be treated with a sling and active

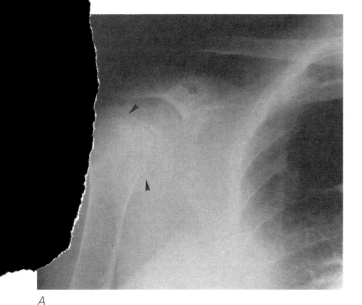

A

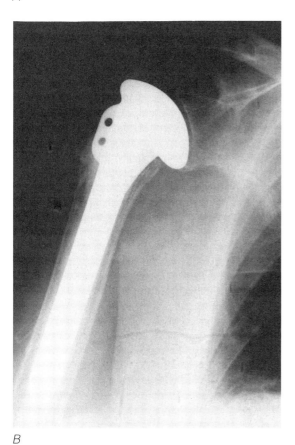

B

FIG. 41-66. *A.* Four-part proximal humeral fracture. Arrows denote major fracture lines. *B.* Neer-type endoprosthetic replacement of the humeral head.

motion begun within 2 weeks to minimize occurrence of flexion contracture. If the radial head is comminuted, excision may be indicated. Long-term follow-up of radial head excision demonstrates proximal subluxation of the radius but minimal symptoms. In cases of associated elbow dislocation with instability, a silicone spacer can be inserted until healing occurs, but it should be removed later to prevent silicone synovitis and fragmentation.

In children a fall on the outstretched hand causes a fracture of the radial neck, as opposed to the radial head fracture that occurs in adults. Closed reduction with varus stress on the elbow and pressure directed laterally on the proximal radius is performed, and the elbow is splinted. Angulation of up to 45 degrees is well tolerated and will remodel, but if greater angulation is present, open reduction may be necessary.

Fractures of the Proximal Ulna. Olecranon fractures occur primarily in adults, either as a result of forced flexion against an actively contracting triceps, or more commonly, from a direct force to the olecranon. In children the usual lack of displacement allows conservative treatment with immobilization in a relatively extended position. In adults, however, the fractures usually are displaced and require open reduction and internal fixation. The most common approach involves the use of tension band wiring, which converts the pull of the triceps into compressive force at the fracture site (Fig. 41-68). More comminuted fractures require excision of fragments and advancement of the triceps aponeurosis to the remaining olecranon, or plating with fixation of the multiple fragments.

Supracondylar Fractures of the Humerus. Supracondylar fractures are the most common fractures about the elbow in children but are rare in adults. The fracture is caused by a fall on the extended elbow, with hyperextension and posterior angulation of the distal condylar fragment. Less than 5 percent of these fractures are of the flexion type. Supracondylar fractures are especially hazardous because of the potential for neurovascular injuries, compartment syndromes, and sequelae such as Volkmann's contracture (discussed earlier under Contracture) and malunion. The brachial artery can be injured or lacerated by the anterior projection of the proximal fragment, as can the median nerve.

Children with displaced supracondylar fractures usually present with marked swelling about the elbow, deformity, and ecchymosis. Circulatory integrity of the forearm and hand as well as neurologic function must be assessed. The distal fragment may be displaced posteromedially (most common) or posterolaterally, and damage to the median or radial nerve can occur. Vigilance regarding development of compartment syndrome is essential.

Treatment. Undisplaced fractures can be treated with a posterior splint with 90 degrees of elbow flexion. Further flexion can be hazardous because of swelling, and all patients should be observed closely after immobilization. Displaced fractures in the past were treated with manipulative reduction and immobilization in as much flexion as tolerated without circulatory embarrassment, or by overhead olecranon skeletal traction. Today, however, the method of fluoroscopically guided percutaneous pinning after closed reduction under general anesthesia is the most widely accepted method. This allows maintenance of more anatomic reduction without the need for excessive flexion of the elbow (Fig. 41-69). Postoperatively the patient is maintained in a posterior splint with not more than 90 degrees of elbow flexion. Circulatory compromise or evidence of compartment syndrome mandates immediate brachial artery exploration and forearm fasciotomies. Pins are removed at 3 to 4 weeks, at which time active range-of-motion exercises are started.

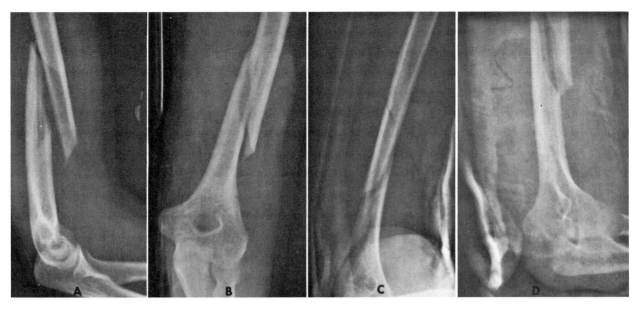

FIG. 41-67. Spiral fracture at the junction of the middle and distal thirds of the humeral shaft. A. Lateral radiograph showing displacement with angulation. B. AP radiograph. C and D. AP and lateral radiographs showing postreduction positions after closed reduction and the application of coaptation splints. The patient had a complete radial nerve palsy (axonotmesis) from which there was complete recovery in 8 months.

Fractures of the Lateral Epicondyle in Children. These injuries result from elbow hyperextension with associated valgus stress. Fractures of the lateral condyle can be difficult to diagnose radiographically, and comparison views are useful (Fig. 41-70). Three stages of displacement have been described: stage I—undisplaced; stage II—minimally displaced; less than 2 mm; and stage III—displaced and rotated. These injuries are not only intraarticular but also cross the growth plate, and therefore any displacement warrants percutaneous pinning, or open reduction

if needed. Complications include nonunion and growth disturbance.

Fractures of the Medial Epicondyle in Children. Valgus injury to the elbow can avulse the medial epicondyle. The treatment of this injury is controversial, and there are pro-

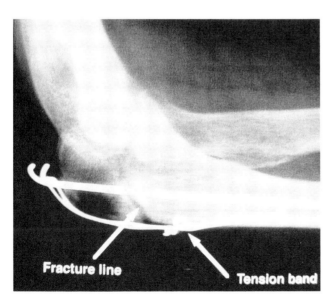

FIG. 41-68. Olecranon fracture internally fixed with tension band wire technique. Tensile force of the triceps mechanism is converted to compressive force at the fracture site.

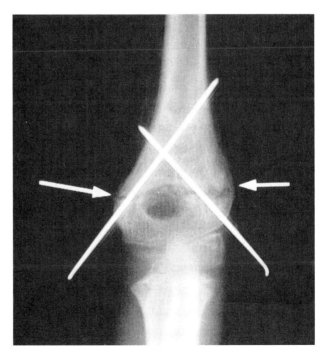

FIG. 41-69. Supracondylar fracture of the humerus, with closed reduction and percutaneous pin fixation.

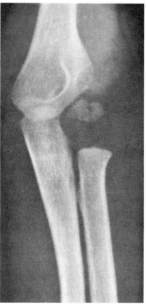

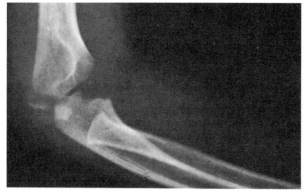

FIG. 41-70. *Lateral and AP radiographs showing Salter-Harris type IV epiphyseal fracture of the lateral epicondyle with displacement and rotation (stage III).*

ponents of accurate reduction and pinning as well as of conservative treatment. However, if the fragment is entrapped in the joint or if ulnar nerve symptoms are present, open reduction and pinning is needed.

Comminuted Fractures of the Distal Humerus.
Comminuted fractures of the distal humerus usually result from a direct blow to the flexed elbow. Discontinuity of the articular surface necessitates open reduction and internal fixation with both interfragmentary screws and medial and lateral buttress plates through a posterior approach. Best visualization of the articular surface is achieved by chevron osteotomy of the olecranon, reflecting the triceps proximally with this fragment, and fixing the olecranon later using an intramedullary screw. The major long-term complication is loss of elbow motion.

Dislocations of the Elbow.
These injuries occur more commonly in children than adults and usually result from a fall on the outstretched forearm with posterior translocation of the radius and ulna. The anterior capsule is torn, as is the medial collateral ligament. These injuries usually are stable after reduction when associated fractures are not present. Immobilization is

with a posterior splint and 90 degrees of elbow flexion, with early institution of motion. Careful neurologic assessment is necessary, since about 10 percent of patients have associated ulnar or median nerve injury.

Fracture-Dislocations of the Elbow. Posterior elbow dislocations in conjunction with fractures of the ulnar coronoid process, radial head, or lateral condyle occur in adults and are much less stable injuries than simple posterior dislocations. Open reduction may be necessary, and if the radial head is fractured, fixation or temporary prosthetic replacement often is necessary to ensure elbow stability in the healing period. Reattachment of an avulsed coronoid fragment also may improve stability by reconstituting the brachialis insertion.

Monteggia Fracture and Galeazzi Fracture-Dislocation. A Monteggia fracture is a fracture of the proximal ulna associated with dislocation of the radial head (Fig. 41-71). A Monteggia-equivalent fracture is fracture of the radial neck in addition and is seen more often in adults. The radial head dislocates posteriorly in 15 percent of patients and anteriorly in 85 percent. This injury illustrates the importance of the principle of obtaining radiographs of the joints above and below the level of a fracture. A single bone fracture in the forearm should always alert one to the possibility of injury to the radioulnar articulation distally or proximally. The Galeazzi fracture-dislocation is an analogous injury with fracture of the radial shaft and dislocation of the distal radioulnar joint.

Closed reduction may be possible, maintaining the elbow flexed and supinated. If the ulna fracture cannot be anatomically reduced, the injury will be unstable and the radial head likely to redislocate. Internal fixation of the ulna, usually by compression plating, may be necessary, but many of these injuries, particularly in children, can be treated closed.

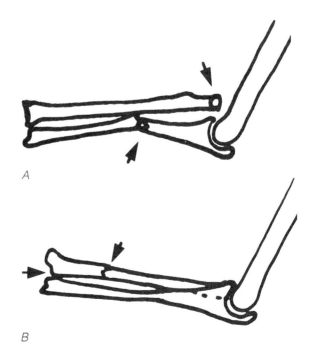

FIG. 41-71. *A. Monteggia injury of the elbow, with dislocation of the radial head and fracture of the proximal ulna. B. Galeazzi injury of the distal forearm, with fracture of the radius and dislocation of the distal radioulnar joint.*

The Galeazzi fracture-dislocation involves a distal-third radius fracture in combination with dorsal dislocation of the distal radioulnar joint. The resultant instability pattern is similar to that of the Monteggia lesion. In adults, plating of the radius and immobilization of the forearm in supination is necessary. This injury is uncommon in children, but closed reduction and immobilization in a long arm cast in full supination usually is successful.

Radial Head Subluxation in Children. Also known as "nursemaid's elbow," this injury results from pulling a child's elbow into sudden extension, and is seen in children under 5 years of age. The elbow can be flexed from 30 to 120 degrees without pain, and the radiographs are normal. The lesion is a tear of the attachment of the annular ligament, allowing escape of the radial head and resulting in entrapment of the annular ligament in the radiohumeral joint. It can be reduced by forceful supination with the elbow flexed 90 degrees, followed by sling immobilization for a week.

Forearm

Fractures. Fractures of the forearm are common in children, but also occur in adults in motor vehicle accidents, falls, and contact sports. Deformity, swelling, and instability may be present. Radiographs must include the elbow and wrist, and careful neurovascular examination of the extremity is critical.

The posterolateral bow of the radius is critical to the maintenance of pronation and supination. In addition, rotational malalignment can occur from the pull of the supinator and biceps on the proximal radius. Anatomic reduction of the fractures with restoration of proper rotation and alignment is essential to a good functional outcome.

Treatment. Closed reduction can be undertaken under axillary nerve block, intravenous sedation, or general anesthesia. Longitudinal traction is applied with the elbow flexed to 90 degrees. After manipulative reduction, the fracture is immobilized in the position of maximum stability. Generally supination for proximal-third fractures, neutral rotation for middle-third fractures, and pronation for distal-third fractures are most appropriate. A long arm cast is applied, with care taken to mold volarly and dorsally along the interosseous membrane to help maintain position. In adults, results of closed treatment are usually inferior to open reduction and internal fixation, and nonunion and malunion rates are significantly higher. Therefore, displaced fractures in adults are ordinarily treated by operative reduction and rigid internal fixation using dynamic compression plates (Fig. 41-72). These plates have eccentrically placed holes that allow significant compression at the fracture site as the screws are seated in the plate. Postoperatively, a plaster long arm splint is applied, but if stable fixation is attained, early motion to restore supination and pronation is a major advantage of internal fixation. In cases of marked comminution or soft-tissue injury, early or primary bone grafting of the fractures is warranted.

Controversy remains over whether the hardware should be removed after fracture healing is achieved (1 to 2 years). In young adults, the stress shielding effect of hardware gradually causes weakening of the cortical bone beneath the plate. In time this results in a stress riser at the edge of the plate, which can lead to a subsequent fracture with less than normal force. On the other hand, incidences of fracture through screw holes (which are also stress risers for a number of months after hardware

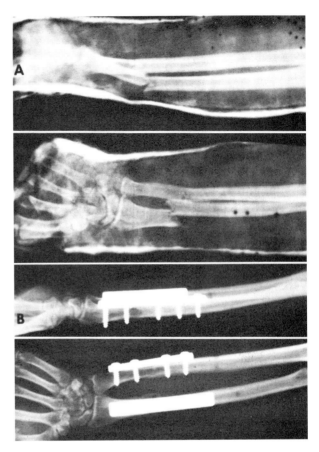

FIG. 41-72. *Fracture of both bones of the forearm with open reduction and internal fixation. A. Lateral and AP radiographs after closed reduction, showing displacement of distal radial fragment. B. Anatomic position after open reduction and fixation with compression plates.*

removal) have been as high as 20 percent after hardware removal. There is no consensus on plate removal at present. Often the plates cause tendinitis or other symptoms, and the patient requests removal despite the risk of refracture. A reasonable approach involves (1) using only the smaller dynamic compression plates in the forearm, which require 3.5-mm rather than 4.5-mm screws; (2) plate removal in symptomatic patients; (3) removal of hardware in young adults; and (4) prolonged protection after plate removal with an orthosis or removable fiberglass cast as well as activity restrictions for 6 months to 1 year.

Forearm Shaft Fractures in Children. Open reduction of these injuries is rarely indicated except when the injury occurs in a teenager without much growth remodeling potential remaining, in which case the fracture is handled as described above for adults.

Greenstick fractures (Fig. 41-73), in which one cortex is fractured but the opposing cortex has undergone plastic deformation and angulation, should be manipulated to complete the fracture; otherwise reduction is hard to achieve. The reduction maneuvers are in other respects similar to those for the adult. Postreduction films are important, as is careful follow-up to ascertain that the reduction is maintained. Greater degrees of angulation can be accepted in fractures in younger children or fractures close to a growth plate, where the potential for remodeling is greater.

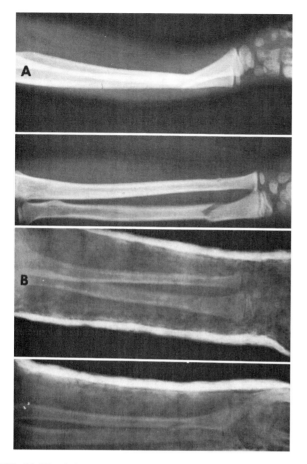

FIG. 41-73. *A. Lateral and AP radiographs of Greenstick fracture of the radius with torus fracture of the ulna. B. Satisfactory position after manipulation and application of plaster.*

Distal Radius

Colles' Fracture. Fracture of the distal radius with dorsal angulation and a "dinner fork" deformity of the wrist was described by Abraham Colles in 1814 (Fig. 41-74). This very common injury occurs as a result of a fall on the outstretched hand. The fracture is most common in patients over 50, often post-menopausal women with some degree of osteopenia. Patients

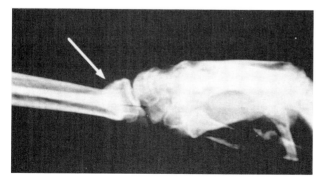

FIG. 41-74. *Colles' fracture. There is dorsal displacement and angulation of the distal radius. After reduction the wrist is immobilized in a position of moderate flexion and ulnar deviation to maintain length and normal volar tilt of the distal radius.*

have deformity, swelling, ecchymosis, and pain in the wrist area. Neurologic injury involving the median nerve occurs, and careful neurologic examination of the hand both before and after reduction is important. Patients occasionally develop an acute carpal tunnel syndrome after reduction, particularly if the wrist is immobilized in a position of extreme flexion. Radiographic evaluation should extend to the elbow to rule out other injuries.

Treatment. Goals of treatment include the minimizing of cosmetic deformity as well as restoration of good wrist and hand function. The usual approach is conservative treatment with closed reduction and plaster immobilization. Generally after regional anesthesia or sedation longitudinal traction is applied using Chinese finger traps with a counterweight to the humerus and the elbow at 90 degrees of flexion. Manipulation then consists of exaggeration of the deformity followed by volar flexion and ulnar deviation along with gentle pressure on the dorsum of the fragment to push it anteriorly. The wrist is then immobilized in a long arm plaster cast in ulnar deviation and flexion—avoiding full flexion because of the potential for median nerve compression. Elevation is continued for a few days to minimize swelling, and early active motion of all digits is encouraged; later shoulder range-of-motion exercises are begun to minimize any stiffness that may occur. In the event of the development of carpal tunnel syndrome, the cast is removed and the wrist placed in the neutral position. If the symptoms fail to resolve, surgical carpal tunnel release is indicated. There is no consensus on whether the wrist should be immobilized in pronation or supination, and hence the neutral position is most commonly used. At 3 to 4 weeks the cast is changed to a short arm cast, which is removed at 6 weeks from the initial injury.

If satisfactory reduction cannot be attained or is lost during the first week of treatment, other methods are used. Manipulation under anesthesia with percutaneous pinning has been used successfully in this situation, preventing recurrent loss of position.

In cases with articular surface disruption, open reduction of the fracture fragments with internal fixation is occasionally indicated to restore a congruous surface of the distal radius. More commonly, however, external fixation is used, allowing ligamentotaxis to achieve reduction of the fracture fragments. One disadvantage of external fixation of distal radius fractures is that marked stiffness of the wrist usually results. Figure 41-75 demonstrates the application of external fixation.

Smith Fracture. A fall on the dorsum of the wrist may cause a reversed Colles' fracture, which is given the eponym Smith fracture. These fractures are characterized by volar angulation and displacement of the distal fragment. Reduction is with longitudinal traction and cast immobilization, but position may be difficult to maintain, and percutaneous pin fixation or open reduction and internal fixation with a volar buttress plate occasionally is necessary.

Wrist

A fall on the outstretched wrist can result in ligamentous injuries, with resultant pain, limitation of motion, and swelling. Ligamentous disruption, particularly when it involves the scapholunate articulation, can result in intercarpal instability patterns and must be carefully evaluated. In addition, these injuries must be differentiated from bony disruptions such as scaphoid fracture, lunate dislocation, or transscaphoid perilunate dislocation.

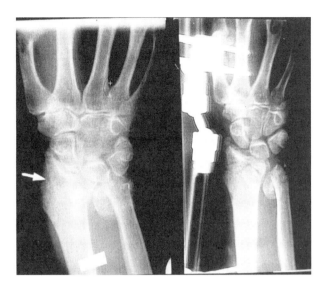

FIG. 41-75. Comminuted intraarticular fracture of the distal radius treated by external fixation.

Fractures of the Scaphoid (Carpal Navicular).

Young adults who fall on the outstretched hand frequently fracture the scaphoid (Fig. 41-76). Signs include tenderness in the "anatomic snuff box," which is formed by the extensor pollicis longus and abductor pollicis longus tendons just over the tuberosity of the scaphoid. In addition to standard anteroposterior and lateral radiographs, an oblique 17-degree view (navicular view) is necessary to adequately visualize the scaphoid. Even with negative films, a nondisplaced fracture may be present when there is reproducible tenderness over the scaphoid. Because the blood supply to the scaphoid enters distally, fractures devascularize the proximal fragment to some extent; consequently healing of this fracture is slow and the nonunion incidence significant. Therefore, in the presence of clinical signs, the patient is placed in a thumb spica cast presumptively and repeat films are obtained out of plaster 3 weeks later (see Fig. 41-76). If radiographs are negative and symptoms resolved, mobilization of the wrist can begin.

Treatment. If the fracture is minimally displaced, thumb spica cast immobilization is initiated; authors differ as to whether a long or short arm cast is necessary, but most prefer a long arm cast at least initially. Average healing time is 12 to 16 weeks, and in some cases can take longer than 6 months.

In cases with displacement or angulation of the scaphoid, open reduction and internal fixation with pins or screws should be performed. In cases of late diagnosis (up to 6 months), union can still occur with prolonged immobilization. When nonunion is not associated with arthritic change in the wrist, autogenous bone grafting is the recommended approach and has a union rate of 92 percent. Electrical stimulation also has been reported to promote union. If degenerative changes are present, radial styloidectomy can provide pain relief and improved function.

Lunate and Perilunate Dislocations.

These injuries are uncommon but can result from traumatic hyperextension of the wrist. Patients complain of pain, swelling, and limitation of motion, and median nerve symptoms may be present. The lunate is displaced anteriorly, best visualized on lateral radiographs. On the anteroposterior view the normal quadrilateral shape of the lunate is more triangular and larger than on the opposite side.

Treatment. Closed reduction can be accomplished by hyperextending the wrist and applying pressure volarly over the dislocated lunate. Afterward the wrist should be immobilized in flexion. If unsuccessful, open reduction through a volar approach is carried out with ligamentous repair and pin fixation. A similar approach is taken with the treatment of transscaphoid perilunate dislocations, in which the lunate remains attached to the distal radius via the radiolunate ligament and the carpus dislocates. Closed reduction of these injuries can be difficult, and open reduction often is necessary to achieve anatomic relationships of the carpal bones. Residual scapholunate dissociation resulting in dorsal or volar intercalated segment instability (depending on the direction of relative flexion/extension of the lunate and scaphoid) can cause late progressive carpal collapse and degenerative arthritis.

Hand

Metacarpal Fractures. Metacarpal fractures can occur from direct trauma, crush injuries, or striking the hand against

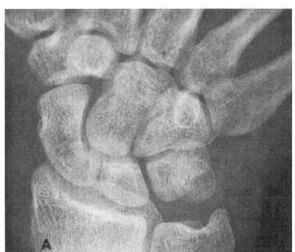
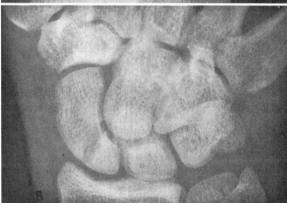

FIG. 41-76. Fracture of the scaphoid. *A.* AP radiograph 1 day after injury is negative for fracture. *B.* Patient had persistent tenderness over the tuberosity. Radiograph at 3 weeks reveals fracture at the junction of the proximal and middle thirds. Fracture subsequently healed without avascular necrosis.

an object. Fractures of the neck of the fourth and fifth metacarpals commonly result from fistfights. Local swelling masks the degree of volar angulation of the metacarpal head. The angular deformity must be assessed on the lateral radiograph, and rotational deformity must be judged clinically by flexing the digit, which should point toward the scaphoid.

Treatment. Metacarpal neck fractures usually are treated by closed manipulation under local anesthesia. For the fourth and fifth metacarpals, an ulnar gutter splint is applied with as much metacarpophalangeal (MCP) joint flexion as possible and the interphalangeal (IP) joints in extension. An important point in immobilization of any injury to the hand is that the collateral ligaments of the MCP joints are lengthened in flexion, and therefore immobilization in extension leads to contracture of the collaterals and difficulty in regaining flexion. Up to 40 degrees of residual angulation can be accepted in the fourth and fifth metacarpals because of the increased mobility of these rays in the anteroposterior direction. If angulation is excessive or involves the more radial rays, percutaneous pinning is necessary to maintain acceptable reduction.

Metacarpal shaft fractures usually can be treated conservatively, but if excessive angulation, displacement, or rotatory malalignment is present, open reduction and Kirschner-wire fixation or plating are occasionally necessary. Comminuted fractures of the metacarpal heads are difficult to treat and should be splinted in a functional position and early motion initiated at 2 to 3 weeks.

Fracture-dislocations of the carpometacarpal (CMC) joint are rare and usually are treated with closed reduction and splinting.

Bennett Fracture. This is an intraarticular fracture of the thumb metacarpal caused by an axial force against the partially flexed bone. The fracture line typically leaves a small volar fragment with the trapezium, while the rest of the metacarpal is pulled dorsally and radially by the abductor pollicis longus muscle. This leads to instability and subluxation or dislocation of the CMC joint. Variants include a rare comminuted type (Rolando fracture) and extraarticular fractures of the proximal metaphysis, which are the most common type and are more stable.

Minimally displaced fractures can be treated by closed reduction and thumb spica casting but must be followed closely because of the propensity for displacement. Because of the inherent instability of the intraarticular fractures, the most common method of treatment involves closed reduction with percutaneous pinning of the metacarpal to the trapezium (Fig. 41-77). If significant incongruity of the joint surface persists despite attempted closed reduction, open reduction and pin or screw fixation are recommended. Rolando fractures are difficult to treat because they can have significant comminution. If the articular surface can be restored by pinning after closed or open reduction, this is the method of choice, but because of the small sizes of the fragments it often is not feasible. In these cases brief immobilization followed by early motion is suggested.

Ulnar Collateral Ligament Injury of the Thumb (Gamekeeper's Thumb). Sudden abduction stress to the thumb can lead to rupture of the ulnar collateral ligament of the MCP joint. The injury was first described in British gamekeepers, who were noted to have a chronic laxity of the ligament caused by chronic repetitive abduction stress when killing game. Falls and ski pole injuries are some of the more common causes today. Stener described a phenomenon that makes conservative

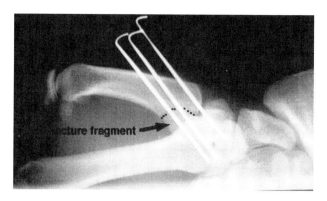

FIG. 41-77. Bennett's intraarticular fracture of the thumb metacarpal, treated by closed reduction and pinning.

treatment of this injury difficult, namely, interposition of the adductor insertion between the ends of the ligament. This occurs in approximately 50 percent of these injuries and precludes healing of the ligament, leading to chronic instability of the joint. The patient usually presents with a painful, swollen thumb MCP joint. The ulnar aspect of the joint is tender, and radiographs usually are normal, although sometimes an avulsion fragment at the base of the proximal phalanx is visible. If standard radiographs are normal, stress radiographs are recommended to demonstrate the instability. This can be appreciated on physical examination as well.

Treatment. For grades I and II ligament sprains, immobilization for 3 to 6 weeks in a thumb spica cast with the thumb in slight adduction is advised. Because of the prevalence of the Stener lesion, for grade III (complete) tears, operative repair is indicated. For ruptures diagnosed later than 2 to 3 weeks after injury, primary repairs are not feasible, and reconstructive surgery is necessary, with tendon grafts or capsular reefing and adductor tendon advancement.

Phalangeal Fractures. Nondisplaced phalangeal shaft fractures are treated by splinting in a position of function (MCP joints flexed approximately 70 degrees and IP joints in only slight flexion). Generally, malleable aluminum splints with foam padding held in place with adhesive tape can be used. For displaced fractures, manipulative reduction may be necessary before splinting.

Small avulsion fractures of the IP joints are treated symptomatically by splinting for 2 weeks followed by range-of-motion exercises. Interphalangeal dislocations are usually dorsal but also may be volar or rotatory. Dorsal dislocations are accompanied by tearing of the volar plate, often with an associated chip avulsion. Rotatory dislocations resulting from twisting injuries are unusual, and they can be irreducible because of soft-tissue interpositions such as buttonhole capture of one condyle through the extensor aponeurosis. Occasionally dorsal IP dislocations are associated with intraarticular fracture of the base of the phalanx.

Interphalangeal Dislocations. Treatment of IP dislocations is with closed reduction followed by buddy taping for 3 to 6 weeks, or by extension block splinting (a dorsal splint that limits full extension but allows active flexion) to allow healing of the volar plate and prevent late hyperextension deformity. Fracture-dislocations involving a portion of the articular surface can be treated by closed reduction with subsequent extension block splinting. If closed reduction is unsatisfactory, open reduction with fixation of the articular fragments can be performed. In cases in which the fragments are small or comminution is present, a volar plate (Eaton) arthroplasty is recommended, with excision of the fragments and advancement of the volar plate into the defect with a pullout wire.

Distal Phalanx Fractures. Crush injuries to the distal phalanx are the most common fractures in the hand. Often there are associated injuries of the nail and nailbed. The most frequent types are comminuted tuft fractures of the distal portion of the phalanx, and transverse fractures of the more proximal base of the phalanx, which may be angulated. The nailbed injuries, which are often neglected, may actually be more of a problem than the fractures themselves.

Initial care is aimed at cleansing any wounds to prevent infection. Drainage of any subungual hematoma by piercing the nail with a hot paper clip or a battery-powered hot wire cautery affords significant pain relief. Late nail deformity is an unavoidable complication of crush injuries, and the patient should be advised of this. Careful repair of any nailbed lacerations with fine absorbable sutures helps considerably in diminishing these problems. If the nail has been avulsed, it is replaced beneath the cuticle after nailbed repair to act as a splint to protect the nailbed and decrease local tenderness. The nail eventually will be pushed off by growth of the new nail. The fracture is then splinted with a protective metal splint for 3 to 4 weeks. Angulated fractures of the distal phalanx should be reduced and, if unstable, pinned with a Kirschner wire before splinting.

Mallet Finger. Forcible flexion of the distal phalanx against active contraction of the extensor mechanism avulses the distal insertion of the extensor tendon from the dorsum of the phalanx, usually with a small fragment of bone (Fig. 41-78). The patient is unable to fully extend the distal phalanx. The injury is generally treated conservatively, with a volar or dorsal splint across the distal interphalangeal (DIP) joint holding it in hyperextension. Most authors believe that immobilization of the proximal interphalangeal (PIP) joint is not necessary. The splinting must be maintained for 6 weeks, and occasionally longer if active extension has not been regained. Some extensor lag may remain after treatment but is usually not problematic. Even if seen late (2 to 3 months after injury), most mallet finger injuries will improve with prolonged (8 weeks) splinting.

If the avulsed fragment of bone comprises more than one-third of the articular surface, operation is indicated, although for small amounts of displacement, conservative treatment as described above is appropriate. With volar subluxation of the distal phalanx, however, repair with a pull-out wire or Kirschner-wire fixation is recommended.

Markedly comminuted intraarticular IP joint fractures are best treated by splinting in a position of function and early arthrodesis if symptoms warrant. Open fractures are treated with irrigation, debridement, and antibiotics, following the general principles of treatment of other open fractures described previously.

Lower-Extremity Injuries

Femur

Before the advent of internal fixation for fractures of the proximal femur, patients were treated with bed rest and traction, and mortality rates were high. Although mortality and morbidity have significantly improved with modern methods of management, hip fractures represent a major challenge to the health care system, with over 275,000 such injuries annually in the United States at an estimated cost of over $3 billion. These fractures generally occur in the 60- to 70-year-old population, and the incidence continues to increase as the number of elderly increases. Femoral neck and intertrochanteric fractures occur with approximately equal frequency and similar epidemiology. The incidence increases with increasing age, with over one-third of women and one-sixth of men over the age of 90 years having sustained a hip fracture. Osteoporosis is a contributing factor to hip fractures, causing decreased mechanical strength of the proximal femur. Mild nutritional osteomalacia also can be a factor but has been found in only about 2 percent of patients with femoral neck fractures. The mortality of hip fractures in the elderly has been reported to be as high as 20 to 50 percent within the first year.

These fractures occur much less commonly in young adults or children, in whom they usually result from high-energy trauma such as motor vehicle accidents. The most serious complications of these fractures are osteonecrosis of the femoral head and nonunion.

Femoral Neck Fractures. Femoral neck fractures are most commonly produced by a fall. The patient usually complains of pain in the groin or thigh and is unable to bear weight on the extremity. The leg usually appears shortened and externally rotated, and any attempt at motion causes severe pain. Trochanteric ecchymosis may be evident. Diagnosis is confirmed by anteroposterior and lateral radiographs of the hip, and careful physical examination is necessary to rule out other injuries to the ribs, upper extremities, or knee. Discontinuity of the trabeculae is seen in both views radiographically, and usually the femoral head is angulated posteriorly on the lateral view.

The most widely used classification of femoral neck fractures is the Garden classification (Fig. 41-79):

Type I—Incomplete fracture (usually impacted in valgus)
Type II—Complete fracture without displacement
Type III—Complete fracture with partial displacement
Type IV—Complete displacement of fracture

Higher incidences of osteonecrosis and nonunion occur with the displaced type III and type IV fractures. The undisplaced type I and type II fractures can be difficult to diagnose, and initial radiographs may be negative. Some patients with undisplaced fractures have surprisingly little pain and are even able to bear weight. Usually internal rotation of the hip will cause pain, and ecchymosis over the trochanter should raise suspicion.

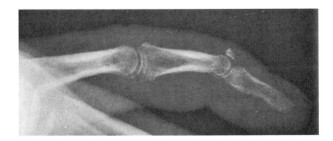

FIG. 41-78. *Mallet finger. Lateral radiograph of a finger with avulsion of the extensor tendon at its bony insertion with minimal subluxation.*

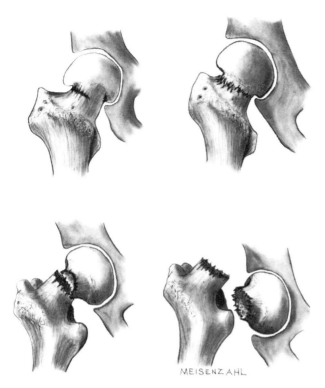

FIG. 41-79. Types of subcapital fracture in Garden classification (see text).

A bone scan or MRI should be performed in any patient with negative radiographs and unexplained hip pain after a fall and will readily demonstrate the fracture in essentially all cases, although the age of the fracture may remain difficult to ascertain.

Treatment. The femoral head has a more precarious blood supply than many bones, given the large surface covered with cartilage, which has no blood vessels. The majority of the blood supply comes in through the neck and through subcapital epiphyseal vessels that run in the inferior capsule, supplied from the medial and lateral circumflex vessels. A small contribution in adults can come from the artery of the ligamentum teres. Disruption of the blood supply occurs with fracture of the neck, accounting for the high incidence of osteonecrosis and nonunion. Mechanical factors such as the high loads across the femoral neck and the fact that little if any external callus formation occurs in these intraarticular fractures further contribute to nonunion. Aspiration of capsular hematoma has been advocated by some to decrease tamponade of capsular vessels, but the effect on development of osteonecrosis remains uncertain.

In elderly patients, surgical treatment allows early mobilization, significantly decreasing morbidity and mortality. Fixation within 24 h has been advocated with hip fractures to minimize osteonecrosis, but more recent data suggest that the most important consideration is achieving medical stability of the patient before surgery. It is generally agreed, however, that fracture fixation and mobilization of the patient as quickly as possible are beneficial. Internal fixation is indicated in nondisplaced fractures and in younger, active individuals even with significant displacement. Displaced fractures in the elderly are treated most commonly by endoprosthetic replacement of the femoral head because of the high incidence of osteonecrosis or nonunion. With

type I and type II fractures, nonunion occurs in less than 5 percent of cases, and osteonecrosis in less than 8 percent, while 10 to 30 percent of patients with type III and type IV fractures develop nonunion and 15 to 33 percent osteonecrosis.

Nondisplaced Femoral Neck Fractures. Type I and type II fractures can be treated conservatively, particularly with fractures impacted in valgus. Because of the frequent inability of the elderly patient to fully cooperate with protected weight bearing and the continued potential for displacement, which would significantly worsen prognosis, internal fixation generally is recommended. In demented, nonambulatory patients with other medical problems, conservative treatment often is indicated. Even medically ill patients, however, usually can tolerate internal fixation, which can be done percutaneously with multiple pins under local anesthesia if necessary. Comparison between sliding compression screw with side plate fixation and multiple parallel threaded-pin fixation has indicated superior union rates with multiple pins or screws, with three pins providing adequate stability (Fig. 41-80). In young adults every effort should be made to preserve the femoral head, even in displaced fractures. Accurate reduction is important in minimizing the incidence of nonunion, and generally varus position or more than 15 degrees of angulation on the lateral should not be accepted. If closed reduction is unsuccessful, open reduction through an anterolateral or posterior approach should be undertaken. Muscle pedicle bone grafting has been advocated to increase union rate and decrease osteonecrosis but remains controversial.

Postoperative Management. Because of the high incidence of thromboembolic disease in elderly patients after hip fracture, many advocate some form of prophylaxis perioperatively. Approaches to this problem include low-dose aspirin, warfarin, antiembolism stockings, and pneumatic compression stockings. Mobilization of the patient is rapid, with sitting in a chair within 24 h of surgery a goal. Weight bearing is protected until the fracture is healed, usually within 4 to 6 months. Follow-up is needed for longer periods, as osteonecrosis may not become radiographically evident for up to 2 years. Viability of the femoral

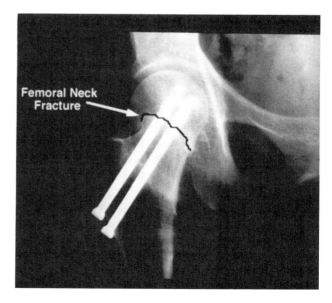

FIG. 41-80. Femoral neck fracture, treated by closed reduction and multiple cannulated screw fixation.

head before or after internal fixation can be assessed by bone scan or MRI. MRI changes of osteonecrosis are present within a few days of blood supply disruption, but after surgery the metal artifact introduced by the pins severely limits usefulness of MRI. In patients who develop osteonecrosis, subsequent collapse necessitates prosthetic replacement. In patients with nonunion and a viable femoral head by conventional or tomographic (single photon emission computed tomography, or SPECT) bone scan, either prosthetic replacement or valgus osteotomy and bone grafting can be undertaken, depending on the age and activity level of the patient.

Endoprosthetic Hip Replacement. In elderly patients the relatively high incidence of nonunion and osteonecrosis with displaced fractures argues for endoprosthetic replacement of the femoral head. If the hip is arthritic, total hip replacement arthroplasty is indicated. Usually cemented arthroplasties are recommended, although in younger or more active patients with complications after attempted femoral head salvage, uncemented porous-coated prosthetic replacement may be considered. Bipolar endoprostheses have a movable articulating surface with a polyethylene liner capturing a smaller spherical ball that is continuous with the intramedullary stem of the device (Fig. 41-81). The motion at both articulating surfaces decreases wear on the acetabulum, and the problem of late acetabular migration (protrusio) is considerably less with bipolar than with earlier fixed-head endoprosthetic designs.

Additional indications for endoprosthetic replacement as opposed to internal fixation include neurologic conditions (parkinsonism, stroke, dementia), metabolic bone disease (renal osteodystrophy, hyperparathyroidism, Paget's disease), and pathologic fractures caused by metastatic carcinoma. With cemented arthroplasty, weight bearing is allowed as tolerated. In patients with preexisting degenerative changes in the joint, total joint replacement rather than bipolar arthroplasty is indicated.

Femoral Neck Fractures in Children. Femoral neck fractures usually occur in children only after high-energy trauma,

such as pedestrian/motor vehicle accidents or falls from a great height. Fractures have been classified as transepiphyseal (with or without dislocation), transcervical, cervicotrochanteric, and intertrochanteric. Transcervical and cervicotrochanteric fractures account for the majority. Pediatric hip fractures are associated with a high incidence of complications, including physeal closure, nonunion, and osteonecrosis of both the femoral head and neck. Displaced fractures are treated by gentle closed reduction and pinning, and nondisplaced fractures by spica cast immobilization with close radiographic follow-up to monitor possible displacement. Intertrochanteric fractures usually can be treated conservatively with a spica cast.

Intertrochanteric and Subtrochanteric Fractures. These fractures occur in the elderly after falls and after significant trauma in younger individuals and generally are mechanically less stable than femoral neck fractures. The instability of the fractures usually results from comminution of the posteromedial cortex in the area of the calcar and lesser trochanter, with a tendency of the fracture to collapse into varus. Patients present with an inability to bear weight, shortening and external rotation of the lower part of the extremity, and often swelling or ecchymosis about the hip.

The considerations for surgical treatment of intertrochanteric and subtrochanteric femur fractures are similar to those described for femoral neck fractures, with internal fixation allowing early mobilization and decreasing significantly morbidity and mortality in the elderly. In younger individuals who can tolerate bed rest or in patients who have medical contraindications to surgical intervention, Russell's or skeletal traction and balanced suspension may be used, but internal fixation is the preferred method of treatment. Union of these fractures may require 4 months or more, however. Surgical intervention consists of open reduction and internal fixation using a sliding compression device with side plate (Fig. 41-82) or an intramedullary fixation device (Zickel nail, gamma nail, or reconstruction nail).

Intertrochanteric fractures have a lower incidence of nonunion than femoral neck fractures, and osteonecrosis of the femoral head is uncommon since its blood supply usually is not disrupted. Treatment of unstable fractures with medial comminution has been controversial, with anatomic reduction, medial displacement, or valgus osteotomies advocated to improve stability. Because a sliding hip screw allows controlled collapse at the fracture site, anatomically reduced fractures often spontaneously impact and medially displace to a more stable configuration. Fixation of a lesser trochanteric fragment, when possible, will also enhance stability. Intramedullary devices have been associated with a high rate of complications in intertrochanteric fractures but are preferred for subtrochanteric fractures. Subtrochanteric fractures have a significant incidence of delayed and nonunion, however, and in the presence of medial comminution primary bone grafting may be indicated.

Postoperative considerations include attention to rapid mobilization, pulmonary hygiene, and thromboembolic prophylaxis, as for femoral neck fractures. Generally, protected weight bearing is indicated until radiographic evidence of healing is present and will depend also on fracture pattern and fixation stability.

Femoral Shaft Fractures. Femoral fractures can occur at any age and generally result from violent trauma. Multiple-trauma patients require evaluation of any associated injuries of the head, abdomen, and chest. Patients exhibit instability of the

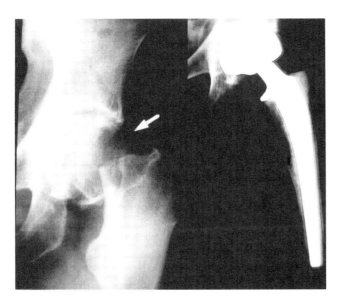

FIG. 41-81. *Displaced femoral neck fracture (Garden type IV). Because of the high risk of osteonecrosis and nonunion, treatment involved replacement of the femoral head with a bipolar endoprosthesis.*

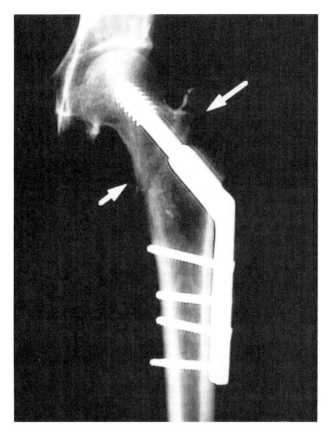

FIG. 41-82. Treatment of an intertrochanteric hip fracture with a compression screw and side plate. The screw can slide within the barrel of the side plate, permitting compression of the fracture site with weight bearing or muscle forces acting across the hip.

extremity, pain with motion, rotational deformity, and shortening of the affected extremity. Neurovascular examination is essential, since there may be injury to the sciatic or femoral nerve or the femoral artery. Associated femoral fracture or knee ligament injuries occur in about 5 percent of patients. In the presence of signs of distal ischemia, arteriography is indicated, followed by immediate vascular exploration for repair or reconstruction and stabilization by internal fixation.

Treatment. Emergency treatment includes stabilization with a splint or traction splint. Open femoral fractures generally result from significant violence and should be handled as described earlier for general treatment of open fractures.

In children femoral shaft fractures are almost always treated conservatively, with modified Bryant's (in infants), Russell's (for ages 2 to 10 years), or distal femoral skeletal traction (for age 10 years and older). If fractures in young children are minimally displaced or shortened less than 1 to 2 cm, immediate spica cast treatment is appropriate. In children 1 cm of overriding is acceptable, since epiphyseal stimulation from the fracture will result in relative overgrowth of the extremity by about that amount. Angular or rotational deformities should be corrected as completely as possible, however (Fig. 41-83). In children treated initially in traction, callus formation will occur within 2 weeks, and the fracture will become nontender. The patient is then placed in a one and one-half hip spica cast for 2 to 4 months, until radiographic evidence of union is present. In children over 12 years of age with multiple trauma, internal fixation of the fracture to facilitate mobilization is often indicated.

The use of two 3- to 4-mm diameter titanium intramedullary nails inserted across the fracture site through the distal femoral metaphysis has been introduced by Rang for use in children as young as 5 years old to allow early mobilization and shorter hospitalization and to obviate the inconvenience of prolonged

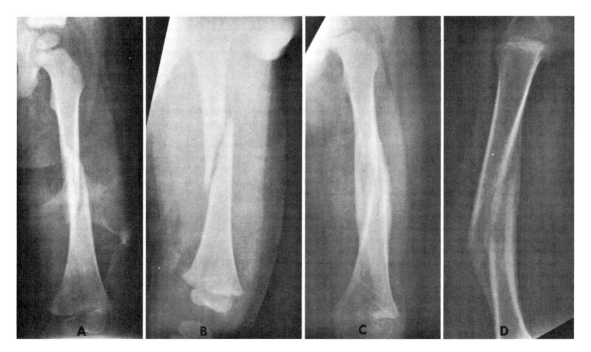

FIG. 41-83. Femoral shaft fracture in a child treated by traction. *A* and *B.* AP and lateral radiographs in satisfactory position in skin traction. *C* and *D.* AP and lateral radiographs of healed fracture showing satisfactory position. The anterior angulation of the fracture site will remodel itself.

spica cast care (Fig. 41-84). One disadvantage of the method is the need for a second surgical procedure for nail removal, but the technique may prove to be a convenient and cost-effective method of treatment.

In adults with medical contraindications to surgery, traction until callus has formed followed by placement in a cast brace or hip spica cast may be appropriate. Conservative treatment of femoral fractures in adults results in a high rate of malunion and knee stiffness, and so the standard method of treatment of most adult femoral fractures is now intramedullary rod fixation. The advent of interlocking nails, which allow multiple screws to be placed through the femur and nail to give rotational and length control proximally and distally, has greatly extended the indications for surgery and is now the method of choice for treatment of comminuted femoral fractures (Fig. 41-85). This form of internal fixation is usually done "closed" under fluoroscopic image intensification, which avoids stripping of the periosteum and promotes more rapid healing. Whether treatment is surgical or conservative, skeletal traction and placement of a Steinmann pin through the distal femur or proximal tibia are needed. The distal femur should be used if knee injury is suspected, but distal locking is technically easier if the traction pin is in the tibia.

Intramedullary nailing facilitates mobilization of the multiple-trauma patient and is recommended within 24 h of injury.

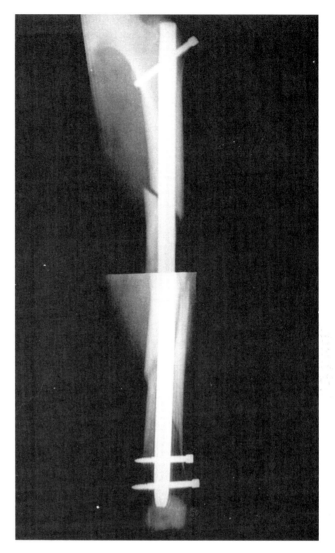

FIG. 41-85. A comminuted femur fracture that has been internally fixed using an interlocking nail, which controls rotation and prevents shortening.

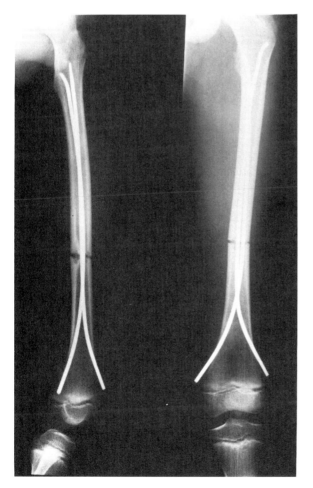

FIG. 41-84. Use of flexible intramedullary nails for fixation of femur fracture in a child. No casting is necessary postoperatively.

Fat embolism and other complications are decreased by early internal fixation. Infection rates with intramedullary fixation are 0.5 to 1 percent, and even with open fractures are in the range of 0 to 4 percent. Infections are treated by rod removal, over-reaming to remove infected bone and granulation tissue, and repeat fixation with a larger rod in conjunction with appropriate antibiotic therapy. Union can be predictably expected in internally fixed femoral fractures in 16 to 20 weeks, and delayed union rates are approximately 1 to 2 percent overall. In the presence of nonunion, fatigue failure will eventually result, and the rod should be removed and replaced with a larger rod, which will result in healing in the majority of cases.

Supracondylar Femoral Fractures. Supracondylar fractures occur in all age groups as a result of motor vehicle accidents, falls, and other accidents. Patients usually present with pain, swelling, and deformity. Supracondylar fractures may be transverse, or T or Y shaped with an intraarticular split of the condyles. Knee stiffness is a major late problem with these fractures. Treatment typically is with skeletal traction through a tibial pin followed by cast-brace mobilization. Patients with multiple trauma should be treated by open reduction and internal fixation with a blade plate, dynamic compression screw and side plate, or intramedullary device. Extensive comminution frequently necessitates primary bone grafting, and emphasis should be on initial accurate fixation of the condyles to ensure a congruous articular surface.

Traumatic Distal Femoral Epiphyseal Separation.
This injury results from hyperextension of the knee in the adolescent. Treatment is with closed reduction and plaster immobilization. Occasionally, percutaneous pin fixation to maintain an unstable reduction is indicated.

Knee

Injuries to the ligaments and menisci of the knee joint are common in athletic activities, including contact sports and skiing. Diagnosis is strongly dependent on clinical examination, since radiographs usually are normal.

Medial Collateral Ligament Injury.
The medial collateral ligament (MCL) consists of both superficial and deep layers, which extend from the medial femoral epicondyle to the medial proximal tibia, blending with the capsule and retinacular structures anteriorly and posteriorly. The anterior portion is tight in flexion, the posterior portion tight in extension, and the middle portion tight throughout the range of motion. With valgus stress to the MCL, the deep capsular portion ruptures first, followed by the tibial collateral (superficial portion) and, with extreme force, the anterior cruciate ligament (ACL).

Clinical findings vary, but with isolated MCL tears they are generally localized to the medial aspect of the knee. Associated hemarthrosis may be noted, and usually there is local swelling and tenderness. With grade I and grade II partial tears, pain with valgus stress with the knee in 20 to 30 degrees of flexion, and slight opening of the medial joint line can occur. Abduction with opening of the joint line of more than 5 mm with valgus stress usually is diagnostic of a grade III rupture of the MCL. Comparison must be made to the other knee, since baseline laxity varies among patients.

Integrity of the other ligaments of the knee also must be established by careful examination to rule out combined injuries. Varus stress testing with the knee in 20 to 30 degrees of flexion, as described above for valgus testing, is used to determine competence of the lateral collateral ligament (LCL) and associated lateral complex. Anteroposterior translation of the tibia on the femur is tested with the knee in 60 to 90 degrees of flexion (anterior drawer test). Rupture of the ACL allows anterior translation and can be evaluated manually or with a device called the KT-1000, which more accurately measures displacements.

The Lachman test is a sensitive maneuver for evaluating anteroposterior motion. The test is performed with the knee in 20 degrees of flexion, with the examiner grasping the distal thigh with one hand and the proximal tibia with the other while applying translatory force. Again, comparison to the uninjured side is essential. Laxity in the Lachman test indicates ACL disruption, as does the pivot shift maneuver, which indicates the presence of anterolateral rotatory instability. This test is conducted by extending the knee with valgus stress applied; a "clunk" in the last 15 degrees of extension indicates anterior subluxation of

the lateral tibia. The reverse test elicits reduction by flexing the knee from full extension, with a "clunk" again indicating reduction of the anterior subluxation. The posterior cruciate ligament (PCL) is examined using the reverse drawer test—forcing the tibia posteriorly with the knee in 60 to 90 degrees of flexion. An alternative method is to have the patient actively extend the knee with the foot fixed and the knee flexed. Anterior translation of the tibia will be observed if the PCL is torn.

Treatment. Isolated MCL tears will heal with conservative management consisting of a hinged cast or brace to prevent valgus stress for 6 weeks, followed by weight bearing as tolerated unless the patient has excessive valgus knee alignment. With combined injuries, surgical repair is warranted.

Anterior Cruciate Ligament Rupture.
Isolated tears of the ACL can result from hyperextension, internal rotation of the tibia on the femur, or a direct blow on a flexed knee. Fifty percent of patients with acute isolated ACL tears have an associated meniscal injury, and MCL or LCL injuries are also common. ACL tears are the most common cause of chronic knee disability among athletes. The chronic rotatory subluxation of an ACL-deficient knee can lead to episodes of giving way and recurrent injury, and in the long term to early degenerative arthritis.

Treatment. Patients with isolated ACL injuries who do not engage in high-demand activity (e.g., older patients and nonathletes) are treated with a period of immobilization to allow healing of secondary restraints followed by an active rehabilitation program stressing hamstring strengthening and graduated quadriceps exercises. If symptomatic instability does not develop, further intervention is unnecessary. In cases of combined instability, surgical repair of the collateral ligament along with primary repair or reconstruction of the ACL is indicated, especially in patients involved in high-demand activities.

Midsubstance ACL ruptures, which are the most common, are difficult to repair primarily and usually require reconstruction with a tendon graft, either from the semitendinosus or the middle third of the patellar tendon. Patellar tendon grafts are also used for late reconstructions and have the advantage that bony blocks removed with each end of the graft can be securely attached within tunnels in the femur and tibia with screw fixation. Synthetic materials (dacron, carbon fiber, etc.) and allografts also have been used, but the autologous patellar tendon remains the most often used substitute. Isometric placement of the graft is essential to prevent tension or laxity throughout the range of motion.

Arthroscopic reconstruction of the ACL using a patellar tendon graft or other material is now a routine approach and allows precise placement of the graft tunnels in the femur and tibia. A small anterior incision is used to harvest the patellar tendon graft without requiring full arthrotomy. This less invasive procedure allows earlier recovery from surgery and earlier mobilization. Meniscal pathology can be treated arthroscopically at the same procedure.

Lateral Collateral Ligament Injury.
The LCL is disrupted by varus stress to the knee, usually in association with injury to the associated lateral complex (posterolateral capsule, arcuate complex, popliteus tendon). The peroneal nerve also may be injured with this mechanism. With complete injuries, surgical repair is generally recommended.

Posterior Cruciate Ligament Injury. The PCL can be injured by a direct blow to the anterior knee, as in hitting a dashboard, or in combination with the ACL in hyperextension injuries. The ratio of PCL to ACL injuries is about 1:10, and isolated injuries do not necessarily cause significant instability. Midsubstance repairs have been associated with poor results, but reattachment of a bony avulsed fragment is recommended when present. Chronic patellofemoral symptoms can result from PCL insufficiency, and if symptoms are significant or if PCL rupture is associated with an LCL disruption, surgical reconstruction, usually with a patellar tendon graft, is advised. The same applies to combined PCL/ACL injuries, in which chronic instability usually follows conservative treatment.

Combined Injuries. Combined multiple-ligament injuries not only increase the likelihood that surgical repair will be necessary but also raise the possibility of knee dislocation. Dislocation can be associated with vascular injury to the popliteal artery with intimal tear or intraluminal thrombus. Vascular injury may be evident immediately or may become evident several days after the injury. Compartment syndrome in the leg also is a serious concern. Arteriography is recommended in all cases of injury to both cruciate ligaments in combination with a collateral ligament injury, in known knee dislocation, and in cases with any suggestion of vascular compromise.

Chronic Ligamentous Instability. Persistent laxity can cause pain and episodic giving way or locking and prevents participation in sports and other activities. Minor degrees of instability are manageable with an exercise program and limitation of high-demand activities. With symptomatic instability, ligamentous reconstruction is indicated. ACL and PCL instabilities are reconstructed as described for acute injuries. Stress radiographs are helpful in defining lax structures causing the instability with MCL and LCL insufficiency, and capsular reefing or other reconstructive procedures are helpful. Rehabilitation and postoperative care are extremely important in optimizing the results of knee ligament surgery, because of the tendency for knee stiffness to develop. For knees with inadequate motion after postoperative rehabilitation, manipulation under anesthesia, or arthroscopic lysis of adhesions followed by manipulation and postoperative continuous passive motion can significantly improve motion. Continuous-passive-motion machines also are useful in improving postoperative knee motion following fracture fixation and other routine knee surgeries.

Meniscal Injuries. The medial and lateral menisci of the knee are composed of fibrocartilage, triangular in cross-section, and serve functions of load transmission, stability, shock absorption, and lubrication. The peripheral 10 to 30 percent of the menisci and the anterior and posterior horn attachments are well vascularized and allow healing of tears. The inner two-thirds of the menisci, however, are avascular, precluding healing. The tibia rotates laterally on the femur with knee extension, and medially with flexion. If this rotation is blocked or forcibly reversed, the meniscus can be injured. Examples include catching a cleated shoe with weight applied to the flexed knee, or twisting the knee while in a squatting position.

The medial meniscus is injured more frequently than the lateral, because of its more constrained by capsular attachments. Several patterns of meniscal injury are illustrated in Fig. 41-86.

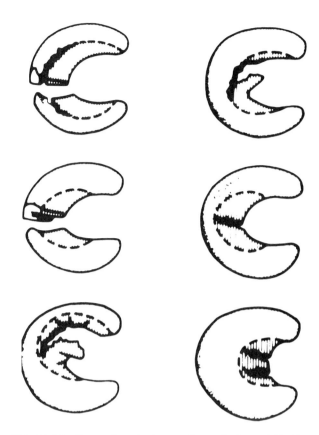

FIG. 41-86. Types of meniscal tears. (From: *Rockwood CA, Green DP, Bucholz RW, 1991, with permission.*)

Meniscal tears are common as sports injuries and can present with effusion, a history of catching or locking, and knee pain. Patients may have joint line tenderness, limited knee motion, and a catching or "click" associated with pain during passive extension of the knee in conjunction with manual rotation of the tibia and varus or valgus stress (MacMurray's test). Clinical diagnosis sometimes is difficult. Arthrography of the knee is fairly reliable in the diagnosis of medial meniscal tears (incidence 95 percent), but substantially less accurate in diagnosis of lateral meniscal tears (incidence 70 percent), owing to the distortion caused by the popliteus tendon. MRI, however, provides extremely accurate diagnosis of internal derangements of the knee of all types, including meniscal tears, osteochondral injuries, and ACL or PCL tears. High signal seen within the menisci also can indicate myxoid degenerative change, which is overinterpreted as a tear.

Treatment. Diagnostic arthroscopy provides another means of diagnosing meniscal injury accurately, and surgical arthroscopy may be performed to repair or excise the torn fragment simultaneously. The menisci are important stabilizers of the knee, and retention of as much well-contoured periphery of the meniscus as possible is desirable. Complete meniscectomy is associated with late degenerative arthritic changes in the affected compartment. For the same reason, peripheral tears in the vascularized portion of the menisci, which will heal, are treated by repair or immobilization. If the joint is unstable, operative repair of the tear with nonabsorbable sutures arthroscopically or by arthrotomy is indicated. If a peripheral tear is of partial thickness or the joint is stable, arthroscopic debridement of the tear followed by immobilization often results in healing. In either case the function of the meniscus can be retained. Meniscal tears in association with instability should not be repaired unless the instability is addressed also, such as by ACL reconstruction for anterolateral rotatory instability.

When intraarticular pathology has been localized by MRI or diagnostic arthroscopy, surgical intervention often can be carried out using arthroscopic technique, and the majority of meniscal lesions, osteochondral lesions, loose bodies, synovial bands, debridement of fibrillated articular cartilage, and abrasion arthroplasty procedures are now done arthroscopically. The advantages of arthroscopic surgery are minimal morbidity, decreased knee stiffness and postoperative pain, and more rapid rehabilitation and return to function. Using a small diagnostic arthroscope in conjunction with a video camera allows documentation of the pathology and viewing of the procedure by others. Small portals are used to introduce the arthroscope and surgical instruments into the joint. Using the technique of triangulation, the surgeon can manipulate objects within the knee, excise torn menisci, and shave or debride cartilage.

Most surgeons use anterolateral and anteromedial portals for diagnosis and most routine procedures. The knee is distended with saline solution injected through a portal in the suprapatellar pouch. Motorized shavers and cutting tools allow rapid resection of synovial, meniscal, or cartilaginous tissue and abrasion of bone to promote fibrocartilage repair. The general technique of surgical knee arthroscopy is illustrated in Fig. 41-87. This technique has more recently been applied to a number of other joints, including the shoulder, hip, ankle, and elbow for diagnosis, and to a limited extent, treatment. For severe meniscal injuries, meniscal transplants (allografts) have been used, but this procedure is experimental and awaits further evaluation of outcome.

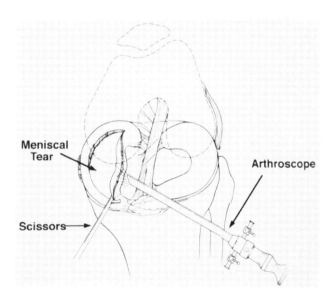

FIG. 41-87. Technique of arthroscopy of the knee. Anteromedial and anterolateral portals just above the level of the joint line are used to introduce the arthroscope, seen here in the lateral compartment, and the surgical instrument, here a scissors in the medial compartment. By triangulation, the instrument and pathology can be visualized while the instrument is manipulated surgically. In this case, resection of a bucket-handle tear of the medial meniscus is demonstrated. (Modified from: *Crenshaw AH, 1992, with permission.*)

Patellar Fractures. Fractures of the patella usually occur as a result of direct trauma to the anterior knee but also can occur with forced flexion of the knee against active contraction of the quadriceps muscle. The patella is an integral part of the extensor mechanism, and disruption of the continuity of the mechanism results in inability to actively extend the knee. Ruptures of the quadriceps tendon or patellar tendon result from the same mechanism of injury and also present with lack of active extension and with tenderness and palpable defect over the ruptured tendon. Fractures may be transverse, comminuted, or stellate.

Treatment. Nondisplaced fractures are treated by immobilization in a cylinder cast in full extension for 6 to 8 weeks. If separation of the fragments is present at the time of presentation or during later treatment, surgical treatment is indicated. If the fracture is comminuted, excision of the smaller fragments, with attachment of the patellar or quadriceps tendon to the larger fragment using wires or heavy nonabsorbable sutures through drill holes, is performed. For transverse fractures, the tension band wiring technique is recommended, with two parallel Kirschner wires placed longitudinally through the fragments and a figure-of-eight wire looped over these anteriorly. This arrangement converts tensile force of quadriceps contraction into compressive force at the fracture site. The retinaculum is repaired and the knee immobilized in a cylinder cast or knee immobilizer in extension. In cases of extreme comminution, primary excision of the patella with retinacular repair is recommended. In all injuries, during extension immobilization active quadriceps exercises are started immediately. Range-of-motion exercises are started at 4 to 6 weeks.

Tendon Ruptures. Ruptures of the quadriceps and patellar tendons are similarly treated, using heavy wire or nonabsorbable sutures through drill holes in the patella, followed by immobilization in extension. After 4 to 6 weeks, immobilization is discontinued and range-of-motion exercises started.

Patellar Dislocation. Lateral dislocation of the patella is relatively common, particularly in young women and girls. Medial dislocation is uncommon but occasionally occurs with severe injury or after poliomyelitis. The higher incidence in females is related to the increased valgus of the knee in women. Hypoplastic development of the lateral femoral condyle also can cause patellar dislocations.

The patient complains of the knee giving way as the patella dislocates laterally and usually then spontaneously reduces. Occasionally the patella becomes entrapped lateral to the femoral condyle and requires manipulative reduction. After reduction the patient may have effusion and mild pain. For an acute first-time dislocation, treatment is with immobilization in a cylinder cast in full extension to allow healing of the torn medial retinaculum, which may decrease the likelihood of recurrence. In some cases a small osteochondral fracture of the patella is present and should be repaired arthroscopically. For recurrent dislocations, initial efforts are directed toward strengthening the quadriceps mechanism with straight-leg-raising exercises. If symptoms of subluxation persist, either a bony or soft-tissue realignment procedure is indicated.

Soft-tissue procedures include lateral retinacular release with or without medial reefing of the retinaculum and Insall's proximal tube realignment procedure (lateral release with imbrication of the lateral retinaculum over the quadriceps tendon to the medial retinaculum). In skeletally mature individuals, the medial advancement of the tibial tubercle of Hauser, or in cases with patellofemoral pain and chondromalacia, the anteromedial elevation of the tibial tubercle of Maquet is applicable. While these procedures all improve the incidence of dislocation and subluxation, pain relief has not been nearly as predictable. The procedure of simple lateral retinacular release has come under greater scrutiny in light of experimental results suggesting that it may be less effective than previously purported. Postoperatively, appropriate quadriceps rehabilitative exercises are important. Progressive chondromalacia necessitates further surgical intervention such as arthroscopic chondral debridement or, in severe cases, patellectomy.

Tibial Plateau Fractures. Fractures of the tibial plateau most commonly occur in the middle-aged or elderly population, although falls from a height or motor vehicle accidents can cause this injury in younger persons. Most often the injury results from a valgus stress to the knee with axial loading. The lateral plateau is more frequently involved (60 percent; medial 15 percent; bicondylar 25 percent). Associated injuries to the medial collateral ligament often occur.

The major types include local compression, split fractures of the lateral plateau, depressed fractures of the lateral plateau, comminuted (split-depression) lateral plateau fractures, and bicondylar fractures. Tomograms or CT scans often are helpful in assessing the extent of the injury, particularly if internal fixation is contemplated.

Treatment. Patients with intact collateral ligaments and less than 10 degrees of instability (less than 10 mm joint line depression) can be treated conservatively, with brace or cast immobilization and protected weight bearing, especially in patients over 50 years of age and those with osteopenia, low-demand activity level, or medical contraindications to operation. Patients with more than 10 degrees of instability in extension or major ligamentous injuries, younger patients, and those with high-demand activity levels are candidates for surgical treatment.

Surgical intervention consists of elevation of depressed articular surfaces, with supportive bone grafting if necessary, and internal fixation ranging from one or more large cancellous screws to medial, lateral, or bilateral buttress plates in more severely comminuted fractures. Ruptured collateral ligaments are repaired primarily. Every effort should be made to avoid varus alignment, which is associated with a worse prognosis. Postoperatively, continuous passive motion aids in recovery of range of motion, and a hinged orthosis or cast brace is used in conjunction with protected weight bearing, which must be continued for 8 to 12 weeks, depending on the quality of the bone, comminution of the fracture, and stability of the internal fixation.

Lower Leg

Tibial Shaft Fractures. Tibial shaft fractures result from direct trauma such as in motor vehicle and motorcycle accidents, sports, skiing, and falls. All age groups are affected, and about 30 percent are open injuries and 70 percent closed. Various fracture patterns occur, depending on the mechanism of injury (Fig. 41-88). The rate of healing is slower in fractures that are open, comminuted, or associated with significant soft-tissue injury.

Undisplaced fractures present with local pain, swelling, and the inability to bear weight, but without obvious deformity. Displaced or angulated fractures exhibit obvious deformity on physical examination. Attention must be given to careful neurovascular examination of the extremity, with especial attention to any signs of compartment syndrome.

Treatment. Closed tibial shaft fractures are best handled by conservative treatment, with closed reduction and long leg casting. Early weight bearing can expedite healing and function. In general, some angulation in the anteroposterior direction is acceptable given the compensatory motion of the knee and ankle in the same plane. Varus or valgus angulation of more than 5 degrees should be corrected if possible by manipulation or wedging of the cast. If adequate alignment cannot be achieved, internal fixation with plating or, preferably, with unreamed intra-

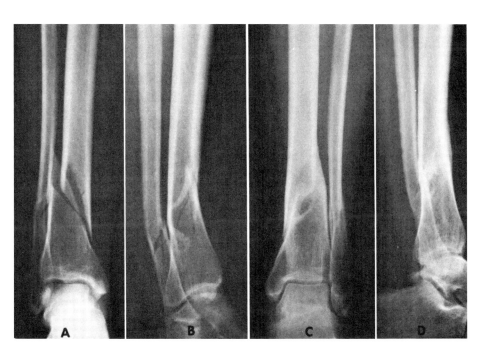

FIG. 41-88. *Fracture of the distal tibia and fibula shafts. A and B. AP and lateral radiographs after injury. C and D. AP and lateral radiographs showing healed fracture in satisfactory position.*

medullary locked or unlocked nailing is advisable. Internal fixation is indicated in the multiple-trauma patient to facilitate immediate mobilization. If significant swelling is present, the patient is admitted to the hospital for elevation and observation of the extremity. Progressive pain or neurovascular symptoms mandate splitting the cast and underlying soft padding, and if the symptoms fail to promptly resolve, measurement of compartment pressures as previously described. The majority of these fractures can readily be treated closed. The cast is changed to a patellar tendon bearing cast or fracture orthosis at 3 to 6 weeks, and weight bearing is permitted as tolerated. Closed tibial fractures generally unite in 12 to 16 weeks, depending on fracture pattern and patient age.

Open fractures of the tibia are treated by primary debridement as previously described. External fixation is the most common approach to fracture stabilization, particularly in grade III injuries (Fig. 41-89). Grade I or grade II fractures can be treated by cast, but if satisfactory alignment cannot be obtained, external or internal fixation is appropriate. The recent development of unreamed locked tibial nails has greatly extended the indications for surgical treatment; several series have shown rates of infection to be no higher than with closed management of grade I and grade II injuries. In cases of significant soft-tissue loss, early coverage with a local gastrocnemius flap (in proximal fractures), a soleus flap (in midshaft fractures), or free vascularized tissue transfers (latissimus dorsi or rectus abdominis) is recommended and decreases the infection rate. Prophylactic fasciotomies at the time of primary debridement decrease the risk of development of compartment syndrome, and neurovascular status should be followed closely postoperatively. Second-look dressing change and debridement is recommended in all grade II and grade III

injuries within 24 to 48 h, and intravenous antibiotics should be continued for 7 to 14 days.

In cases of delayed healing, which is relatively common with open tibial fractures, early posterolateral cancellous bone grafting or fibular osteotomy to improve load transmission across the fracture can be considered. Electrical stimulation is useful in delayed union and nonunion.

Ankle

The tibiotalar articulation functions as a hinge joint, with nearly all rotational motion in inversion and eversion occurring at the subtalar joint. The mortise of the ankle is formed by the downward projecting medial and lateral malleoli, which constrain the motion of the talus. The talus is largely covered with articular cartilage, with the blood supply primarily coming through a ring of vessels surrounding the neck. A normal mortise is required for stability of the ankle and painless motion. Additional stability of the talus in the mortise is provided by the distal tibiofibular ligaments (syndesmosis), interosseus membrane, calcaneofibular ligament laterally, and the deltoid ligament medially.

Ankle injuries are caused by a sudden force that exceeds the strength of either the malleoli or ligaments. Ankle injuries are classified according to the position of the ankle and foot at the time of the injury, based on experimental work by Lauge-Hansen. These positions include supination-adduction, supination-eversion (external rotation), pronation-abduction, and pronation-eversion. Supination-adduction fractures result in transverse fracture of the lateral malleolus with or without adduction fracture of the medial malleolus. Supination-eversion fractures are described in four stages of progressive injury involving tear of anterior tibiofibular ligament, spiral oblique fracture of the lateral malleolus, fracture of the posterior lip of the tibia, and fracture of the medial malleolus or deltoid ligament tear. Pronation-abduction fractures sequentially result in medial malleolar fracture or deltoid ligament rupture, syndesmosis disruption, posterior tibial lip fracture, and supramalleolar fracture of the fibula. Pronation-eversion injuries cause medial malleolar/deltoid disruption, anterior tibiofibular disruption, spiral supramalleolar fibular fracture, and posterior tibial lip fracture.

The injured ankle should be carefully examined for localization of tenderness, swelling, and deformity. Ability to bear weight does not rule out significant injury. The ankle can be splinted with a plaster splint or air splint until radiographs are obtained. Anteroposterior, lateral, and mortise radiographic views are necessary for adequate evaluation of ankle injuries. The mortise view is an AP film taken in 30 degrees of internal rotation, which places the malleoli in the same coronal plane.

Ligamentous Injuries. The most common injury is inversion sprain of the lateral ligaments of the ankle. The anterior talofibular ligament usually is involved, with local tenderness and ecchymosis over it. For grade I and grade II sprains, ambulatory treatment with taping or an air splint is adequate. For more severe grade III sprains, protected weight bearing and cast or splint immobilization are indicated for 2 to 4 weeks, followed by range-of-motion and muscle strengthening exercises. For recurrent inversion sprains, repair of the anterior talofibular and fibular collateral ligaments following the Brostrom-Gould method may provide satisfactory stability without excessive subtalar joint stiffness (Fig. 41-90). Preoperatively, inversion insta-

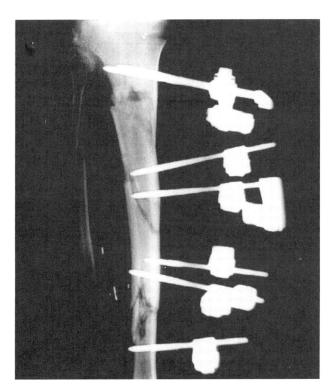

FIG. 41-89. Segmental fracture of the tibia treated with external fixation.

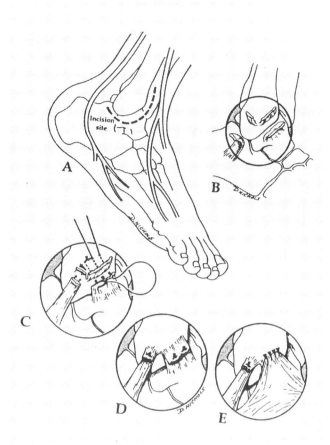

FIG. 41-90. Modified Brostrom (Brostrom-Gould) procedure. *A.* Anterolateral incision. *B.* Arthrotomy leaving a 3-mm cuff of tissue at the fibula. The proximal stump is elevated. *C.* The distal stump of the ligament is sutured into the fibula. *D.* The proximal stump of the ligament is sutured over the distal stump in a pants-over-vest fashion. *E.* The lateral extensor retinaculum is sutured over the repair into the fibula. (From: *Gould JS (ed): Operative Foot Surgery, 1994, with permission.*)

bility is identified by inversion stress radiographs demonstrating more than 10 degrees of difference in the talar tilt as compared to the uninjured side. For patients with generalized ligamentous laxity or failed repairs, reconstruction of the calcaneofibular and anterior talofibular ligaments using a slip of the peroneus brevis tendon can be performed (Evans or Chrisman-Snooks procedures).

Distal Tibiofibular Diastasis. Eversion injuries to the ankle can result in disruption of the anterior and posterior tibiofibular ligaments (syndesmosis), with widening of the ankle mortise. Maintenance of an adequate closed reduction is difficult, since more than 1 to 2 mm of talar shift in a young person causes significant alteration of stresses in the articular cartilage of the ankle joint and is unacceptable. A Maisonneuve fracture is a fracture of the proximal fibula in association with syndesmotic diastasis, resulting from proximal propagation of the external rotation force from the talus along the interosseus membrane.

Surgical treatment of tibiofibular diastasis consists of closed or, rarely, open reduction with placement of a syndesmosis screw through the fibula just above the syndesmosis, affixing it to the tibia. The foot should be in the neutral position and not in plantar flexion, as the narrower width of the posterior talus would allow overreduction and subsequent limitation of dorsiflexion. A short leg cast is applied and weight bearing avoided for 8 weeks to prevent screw breakage, and then the screw is removed and weight bearing permitted as tolerated.

Malleolar Fractures and Dislocations. Undisplaced fractures of the malleoli require immobilization in a cast for approximately 8 weeks. The most common fracture is an isolated, minimally displaced oblique fracture of the lateral malleolus caused by external rotation. Displaced fractures are treated by closed reduction, reversing the direction of applied force that caused the injury. If anatomic restoration of the mortise is not accomplished, open reduction and internal fixation with screws or a small buttress plate is recommended.

Medial Malleolar Fractures. Undisplaced fractures are treated with plaster immobilization. Bimalleolar fractures with disruption of the mortise require accurate reduction, and the majority can be treated conservatively. Closed reduction is performed under local anesthesia or with intravenous sedation, with the leg hanging over the end of the table. Longitudinal manual traction is applied and the foot is inverted and internally rotated as it is brought up to 90 degrees. A well-molded long leg cast is applied and check radiographs obtained. More than 1 to 2 mm of displacement usually requires open reduction and internal fixation. The medial malleolus usually is fixed with one or two screws and the fibula with interfragmentary screws or a small buttress plate (Fig. 41-91).

Posterior Malleolar Fractures. The posterior malleolus usually is fractured in combination with the medial or lateral malleolus. If the fragment comprises less than 30 percent of the articular surface, accurate reduction is not important, but with larger fragments, anteroposterior instability will result from re-

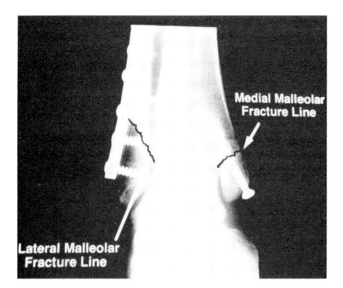

FIG. 41-91. *Bimalleolar ankle fracture. The medial malleolus has been fixed with interfragmentary screws, and the fibula with a small buttress plate.*

sidual displacement. Therefore, with larger fragments, screw fixation after open or indirect closed reduction is indicated.

Pilon Fractures. Pilon fractures are severely comminuted fractures of the ankle and distal tibia, usually resulting from high-energy axial injury, and often involving primarily the anterior lip of the tibial plafond. Vertical compression drives the talus into the tibial plafond, and the entire distal tibia can be comminuted. If excessive comminution is not present, open reduction and internal fixation of the fragments is appropriate. In the face of osteopenia or severe comminution, external fixation, augmented in some cases by limited fixation of one or more larger fragments, is the treatment of choice. Problems with posttraumatic arthritis and ankle stiffness are common with these injuries, and later arthrodesis is often necessary.

Foot

Fractures and Dislocations of the Talus. Talus fractures usually occur through the neck, although the body can be involved. The usual mechanism is forcible dorsiflexion of the foot, impinging the neck on the anterior lip of the distal tibia.

In more severe injuries, subtalar dislocation is associated with the talar fracture. The most severe fracture-dislocations involve dislocation of the talus from both the subtalar and ankle joints, usually with posterior extrusion of the talar body. Isolated subtalar dislocations can also occur without talar neck fractures, either medially or laterally from plantar flexion forces with inversion or eversion.

Hawkins has classified talar fractures as follows:

Type I—nondisplaced fracture of the neck of the talus
Type II—displaced fracture of the talar neck with subtalar dislocation
Type III—displaced talar neck fracture with subtalar and ankle dislocation of the body of the talus
Type IV—displaced talar neck fracture with subtalar, ankle, and talonavicular dislocation

The major complication of these injuries is osteonecrosis of the body of the talus, which is primarily supplied with blood through the neck of the talus. Osteonecrosis has been reported to occur in 0 to 13 percent of type I fractures, 20 to 50 percent of type II fractures, and 83 to 100 percent of type III fractures. The best indication of viability of the talus after treatment of the injury is subchondral lucency in the talus, which should be present 6 to 8 weeks because of disuse resorption.

Treatment. Type I fractures are treated closed, with short leg cast immobilization for 3 months. Type II fractures are treated similarly, but if anatomic reduction of the talar neck is not achieved, open reduction and internal fixation are recommended. All type II injuries require open reduction and internal fixation.

In cases in which osteonecrosis develops, prolonged protected weight bearing in a patellar tendon bearing brace has been advocated. If collapse of the body occurs, secondary arthritis will develop, and ankle arthrodesis is often necessary. The Blair-type fusion, in which a strut of anterior tibial cortex is slid down into the talar neck (with or without screw fixation), is used for this condition.

Isolated subtalar dislocations usually are treated by closed reduction. Occasionally the talar head is buttonholed through the anterior capsule, or interposition of the extensor brevis muscle (medial dislocations) or posterior tibial tendon (lateral dislocations) blocks closed reduction. The dislocations generally are fairly stable after closed or open reduction, and immobilization in a short leg cast for 3 to 4 weeks is followed by range-of-motion exercises.

Calcaneus Fractures. Fractures of the calcaneus usually result from falls from a height, with axial loading of the lower extremity. Ten percent of calcaneal fractures are associated with compression fractures in the thoracic or lumbar spine, and 26 percent with other lower-extremity injuries. The five major types of calcaneus fractures are extraarticular fractures, avulsion fractures, tongue type fractures, joint depression fractures, and comminuted fractures (Fig. 41-92).

Treatment. Treatment is controversial, ranging from brief immobilization with early range-of-motion exercises to internal fixation with bone grafting. Problems caused by fractures of the calcaneus include widening of the heel, loss of height of the hindfoot, and disruption of the subtalar joint, which can result in loss of inversion/eversion and subtalar arthritis. In general all

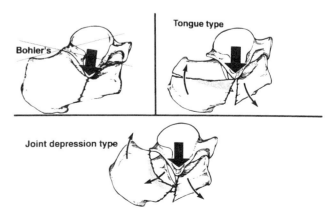

FIG. 41-92. *Types of calcaneus fractures. Böhler's angle is flattened in fractures involving the subtalar joint. (Modified from: Rockwood CA, Green DP, Bucholz RW, 1991, with permission.)*

patients with significant calcaneus fractures should be hospitalized, as severe swelling and skin breakdown can occur. Nondisplaced fractures can be treated with 2 weeks of immobilization followed by active range-of-motion exercises, and protection of weight bearing for 6 to 8 weeks, depending on the fracture type. The most severe fractures involve the subtalar joint, with two major types, tongue and joint depression. In both types, incongruity of the subtalar joint can result, and advocates of no reduction, closed reduction, and open reduction and internal fixation disagree as to which approach to take with these injuries. Böhler's angle (the angle measured between a line across the calcaneal tuberosity and a line across the anterior and posterior subtalar joint; normal range is 25 to 40 degrees) is usually flattened by intraarticular fractures (see Fig. 41-92). CT scans may help to better define the fracture pattern.

There has been renewed interest in internal fixation to anatomically restore the subtalar joint. In young, active patients with intraarticular fractures, current recommendations are for elevation of the subtalar joint with open reduction through a lateral approach, and bone grafting if necessary. The lateral wall is reduced and fixed with a buttress plate, which also stabilizes the medial sustentaculum and sagittal disruption of the calcaneus. Combined medial and lateral approaches can be used. Problems remain, though; lateral wound healing is the most significant early problem, and persistent long-term subtalar stiffness and pain may occur. For severe late subtalar arthritis, subtalar fusion or triple arthrodesis is appropriate. Intraarticular calcaneus fractures require strictly protected weight bearing for a full 3 months.

Metatarsal Fractures. *Fifth Metatarsal Fractures.* Avulsion fractures of the base of the fifth metatarsal are commonly associated with inversion injuries of the foot. The contraction of the peroneus brevis muscle causes the avulsion. The patient often has an associated lateral ankle ligament sprain and presents with pain and swelling laterally, local tenderness, and inability to bear weight.

Treatment ranges from symptomatic (elastic [Ace] bandage wrapping and protected weight bearing on crutches until comfortable) to short leg cast immobilization for 4 to 6 weeks. Fibrous union of the avulsed fragment is common but rarely causes problems. The diaphyseal or metaphyseal fracture of the fifth metatarsal (Jones fracture), usually caused by torsional force on the forefoot, can have markedly delayed healing, and nonunion is common. Some advocate primary internal fixation of the Jones fracture using an intramedullary screw or a small plate, while others endorse conservative treatment with cast immobilization and protected weight bearing for 2 to 3 months, with surgical intervention (internal fixation and local bone grafting) only if nonunion occurs.

Other Metatarsal Fractures. Single metatarsal fractures are readily treated with short leg cast immobilization for 6 weeks. Fracture-dislocations occur at the tarsometatarsal junction, often in association with metatarsal base fractures. Generally, closed reduction is recommended, but open reduction with Kirschner-wire fixation is indicated in some cases. Buckle fractures of the cuboid may be associated with dislocation or subluxation of the tarsometatarsal (Lisfranc) joint. These injuries are unstable and require open or closed reduction with Kirschner-wire fixation of both the medial and lateral columns of the foot.

Phalangeal Fractures. Phalangeal fractures commonly result from direct trauma, such as being struck by a dropped object or striking the toe against an object. Dislocation of the IP or MTP joints also can occur. Treatment is directed at alignment and pain relief. Generally closed reduction can be accomplished, and buddy taping of the affected toe to an adjacent toe is adequate for protection.

Pelvic Injuries

Acetabular Fractures and Hip Dislocations. Dislocation of the hip is caused by force applied to the femur and can be associated with fractures of the acetabulum or femoral head. The most common mechanism of injury is motor vehicle accidents, although falls from a significant height can cause hip dislocations. Position of the limb and direction of applied force determine the direction of the dislocation. Force applied to an abducted hip can result in anterior dislocation, and striking the knee on a car dashboard with the hip flexed and adducted causes posterior dislocations, often with fracture of the posterior wall of the acetabulum (Fig. 41-93). Direct trauma to the greater trochanter can result in medial wall fractures or central acetabular fracture-dislocations.

Thorough evaluation of acetabular fractures requires 45-degree oblique views (Judet view) of the pelvis to assess the integrity of the anterior (iliopubic) and posterior (ilioischial) columns and the anterior and posterior wall (acetabular rim). In addition, CT scans are helpful, particularly with the newer three-dimensional reconstructions, in fully delineating fracture patterns

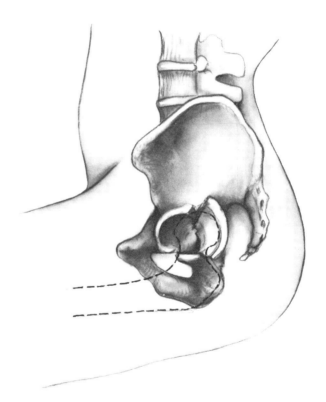

FIG. 41-93. *Posterior dislocation of the hip with fracture of the posterior acetabular rim. Axial force applied to the femur drives the femoral head from the acetabulum and the posterior rim of the acetabulum along with it. Such injuries are common in automobile passengers.*

Table 41-14
Classification of Acetabular Fractures (After Tile)

Type I (posterior types ± posterior dislocation)
   A—posterior column
   B—posterior wall
   C—transverse (intercolumn)
Type II (anterior types ± anterior dislocation)
   A—anterior column
   B—anterior wall
   C—transverse (intercolumn)
Type III (anterior ± central dislocation)
   A—pure transverse
   B—T-shaped fracture
   C—associated transverse and acetabular wall fractures
   D—double column fractures

and demonstrating the presence of any intraarticular bone fragments. Acetabular fractures have been classified by Tile, as shown in Table 41-14, with transverse forms representing a dissociation of the anterior and posterior columns.

Patients with acetabular fractures often have other major injuries, and careful evaluation of the chest, abdomen, spine, and neurologic status is necessary. Prompt reduction of hip dislocations is essential in minimizing the incidence of osteonecrosis of the femoral head.

Anterior Hip Dislocations. These injuries result from forced abduction or anteroposterior force to an abducted thigh; they are much less common than posterior dislocations (10 to 18 percent of hip dislocations). There are two basic types—the superior or pubic type and the inferior or obturator type. The anteriorly displaced femoral head can compromise neurovascular structures. Both types result from abduction and external rotation, but with additional extension for the pubic type and flexion for the obturator type. Femoral head fractures occur in a significant percentage of cases, and late osteonecrosis occurs in about 10 percent. There is a high incidence of late posttraumatic arthritis. The patient presents with the lower extremity abducted and externally rotated. Reduction is accomplished, usually under general anesthesia, by longitudinal traction with subsequent flexion and internal rotation. If the CT scan or radiographs demonstrate intraarticular fragments, arthrotomy and fragment removal is indicated. Postoperatively the patient is maintained in light traction for 1 to 2 weeks, and range-of-motion exercises are initiated. The patient is mobilized on crutches, with protected weight bearing for 6 weeks.

Posterior Hip Dislocations. Posterior hip dislocations can be associated with posterior wall fractures (Fig. 41-94), which significantly impairs stability of the dislocation after reduction if the fragment is large. The patient presents with the thigh adducted, internally rotated, and flexed. Femoral head or neck fractures are sometimes associated, and sciatic nerve injuries are present in 10 percent. Reduction usually is accomplished by longitudinal traction, followed by gentle abduction and external rotation. If the reduction is unstable, fixation of the posterior wall is indicated (see Fig. 41-94). A CT scan to rule out the presence of intraarticular fragments is important, and if any are present, surgical removal is necessary. Promptness of reduction is important to minimize the chances of late osteonecrosis of the femoral head, which has been reported to range from 10 to 50 percent and is often not evident for several years after the injury. After reduction the patient is placed in light traction for 1 to 2 weeks, or until comfortable range of motion is recovered. Protected weight bearing and use of crutches are required for 4 to 6 weeks. Posttraumatic arthritis develops in a high percentage of patients from 5 to 30 years after injury.

Fractures of the Medial and Superior Acetabulum. If the superior dome of the acetabulum is intact, the fracture can be treated with skeletal traction for 8 to 12 weeks, although more aggressive treatment of displaced acetabular fractures is also practiced. In young, active patients, restoration of an anatomic acetabulum presents or decreases the severity of posttraumatic arthritis, and leaves better bone stock for later reconstructive options such as arthrodesis or total hip arthroplasty in the event that arthritic change does occur.

For open reduction and internal fixation of acetabular fractures, anterior (ilioinguinal), posterior (Kocher-Langenbeck), or combined approaches can be used, depending on the fracture

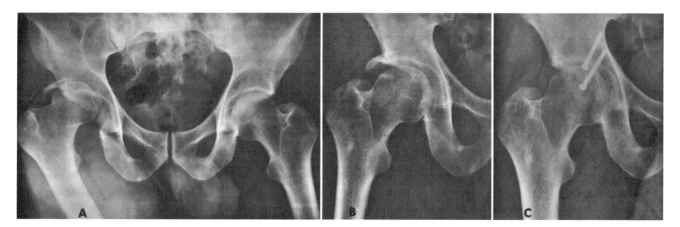

FIG. 41-94. *Posterior dislocation of the hip with fracture of the acetabular rim. A. In this AP radiograph the femoral head on the injured side appears smaller than that of the opposite side and is superiorly displaced. B. AP radiograph showing the relocation of the femoral head with persistent displacement of the acetabular fragment. C. AP radiograph after open reduction and screw fixation of the acetabular fragment.*

pattern. Removal of the greater trochanter by osteotomy makes reduction easier, particularly if there is a transverse intercolumn fracture component, and internal fixation is facilitated by use of newer devices such as pelvic reduction forceps, a femoral distractor, and readily contourable reconstruction plates. Through these approaches, accurate reduction and internal fixation of complex, severely displaced fractures is possible (Fig. 41-95). Generally, the operation is delayed 5 to 7 days until the patient is stabilized, because immediate surgery can be associated with significant blood loss. Postoperative complications include thromboembolic disease, heterotopic bone formation, hip stiff-

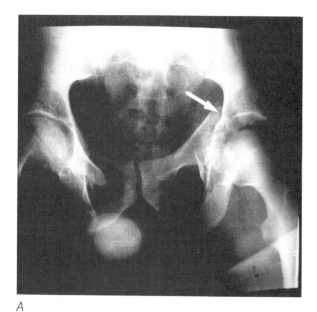

A

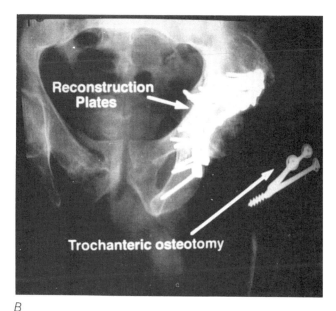

B

FIG. 41-95. *A. Acetabular fracture with transverse component disrupting the anterior and posterior columns. B. Internal fixation involved trochanteric osteotomy and posterior Kocher-Langenbeck approach.*

ness, and late osteonecrosis of either acetabular fragments or the femoral head.

Pelvic Fractures. The pelvis is an intact ring that protects the viscera and transmits mechanical weight-bearing force from the spine and axial skeleton to the lower extremities. Like acetabular fractures, pelvic fractures most commonly result from relatively high-energy trauma such as motor vehicle accidents, although a significant number of pubic ramus fractures occur from simple falls, particularly in the elderly.

Patients present with pain in the pelvic area, inability to bear weight, ecchymosis, and local tenderness. Often these individuals are victims of multiple trauma and are hemodynamically unstable. When the pelvis is fractured or disrupted, a large amount of bleeding into the pelvis and retroperitoneum can occur, aggravated by the fact that the intrapelvic volume is no longer constrained and the tamponade of venous bleeding that would occur with an intact pelvic ring cannot occur. Inlet and outlet views of the pelvis are essential to assess the integrity of the ring, and CT scans are extremely helpful in evaluating the extent of bony and ligamentous disruption.

Treatment. Stabilization of the patient and assessment of associated injuries are essential. If the patient is in shock and does not respond to standard volume replacement therapy, application of an anterior external fixator in the emergency department with two or three pins in each iliac crest can help significantly to contain hemorrhage and stabilize the patient for further diagnostic evaluation. Approximately 10 percent of patients have bladder or urethral injuries, necessitating urologic evaluation. Neurologic function also must be carefully assessed because of possible lumbosacral plexus injuries. Pelvic fractures have been classified by Young into four major types according to the mechanism of injury: lateral compression (LC), anteroposterior compression (APC), vertical shear (VS), and combined mechanism (CM). LC fractures involve pubic rami fractures, with or without sacral compression injury, iliac wing fracture, or disruption of the sacroiliac joint on one side. APC injuries involve symphysis diastasis, with varying degrees of sacroiliac joint disruption. VS injuries involve vertical displacement of one side of the pelvis. A similar classification system has been proposed by Tile, with type A (stable) equivalent to low-grade LC injuries; type B (rotationally unstable but vertically stable) equivalent to higher-grade LC injuries or APC injuries; and type C (rotationally and vertically unstable) equivalent to VS and CM.

The majority of pelvic fractures can be treated without surgical intervention. Type A or LC fractures usually are stable and can be treated conservatively with bed rest and subsequent protected weight bearing. APC injuries are vertically stable but not rotationally stable. Fractures with significant symphysis diastasis (greater than 3 cm) can be treated with placement of an anterior fixator or plating. In multiply injured patients, this approach facilitates rapid mobilization. In APC injuries with significant sacroiliac joint disruption or bilateral disruption, posterior internal fixation with plates or sacral bars often is indicated. VS injuries require skeletal traction, but if there is more than 1 to 2 cm of superior displacement, internal fixation anteriorly and posteriorly should be considered (Fig. 41-96). Sacral and coccygeal fractures generally are treated symptomatically. Neurologic deficits associated with sacral fractures usually occur in traction injuries, and recovery often is poor and not improved by surgical decompression.

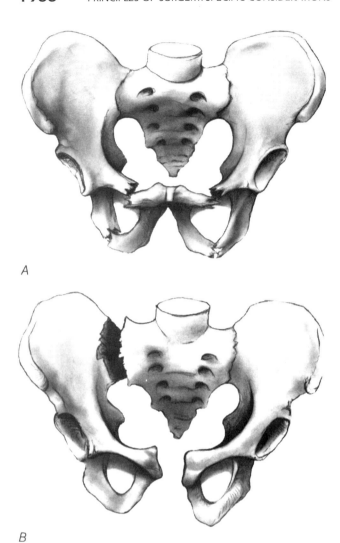

A

B

FIG. 41-96. *A. Displaced fractures of the pubic rami bilaterally resulting from lateral compression type injury. B. Disruption of the hemipelvis by separation of pubic symphysis and sacroiliac joint (unstable vertical shear type injury).*

Spinal Injuries

Fractures and dislocations of the cervical, lumbar, and thoracic spine most commonly follow major trauma such as motor vehicle accidents or falls from a height. Overall prognosis depends on associated spinal cord or nerve root injuries. Any patient who complains of neck or back pain or tenderness after an accident should be assumed to have an unstable spine until adequate radiographic evaluation can be carried out. For neck injuries, sandbags can be used for temporary stabilization and transport, followed by application of a hard cervical collar such as a Philadelphia collar. Patients with thoracolumbar injuries are placed on a rigid backboard for transport. Neurologic examination should be conducted as soon as possible, after attention to chest, abdominal, and other injuries. Anteroposterior and lateral radiographs of the cervical, thoracic, and lumbar spine are obtained before moving the patient from the backboard. Lateral radiographs of the cervical spine must include the C7 level, and generally abnormal findings on the plain radiographs are further delineated by CT scan of the injured area.

Cervical Fractures and Dislocations. Flexion injuries of the cervical spine occur most often at the level of C5 and C7, and can involve anterior compression fracture of the vertebral body, posterior longitudinal ligament tear, and unilateral or bilateral facet subluxation or dislocation. Facet dislocation or fracture presents radiographically with anterior displacement of up to 25 percent with a unilateral facet dislocation (associated also with a rotational difference in the vertebra above as compared to the vertebra below the lesion); bilateral facet dislocation can exhibit anterior displacement of up to 50 percent. Cord injury may be present, depending on the degree of canal compromise.

With an axial load to the cervical spine, burst fractures of the body can occur, with retropulsion of fragments into the spinal canal causing neurologic deficit (Fig. 41-97). Depending on the presence of rotation, flexion, and lateral bending, fractures of the pedicles or lamina occur. CT scans can readily delineate these injuries. Injuries of the spinous processes (clay shoveler's fractures) can occur as an avulsion caused by a sudden stress to the supraspinous ligament.

Axial compressive force can cause fractures of the ring of C1 (Jefferson's fracture). This injury, often subtle on plain radiographs, can be identified by asymmetric widening of the distance between the lateral masses and the odontoid process on the open-mouth anteroposterior view. Fractures of C2 involving the odon-

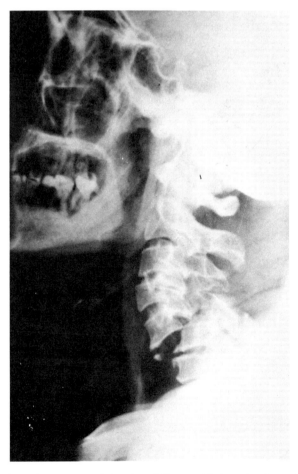

FIG. 41-97. *Fracture-dislocation of C5 upon C6. Lateral radiographs show complete displacement of C5 with fracture of the neural arch. The patient was quadriplegic immediately after his injury.*

toid process or posterior elements (hangman's fracture) result from flexion or extension and rotational forces. In children under the age of 6 years, odontoid injuries can result in an epiphyseal displacement and associated displacement of the atlas upon the axis.

Treatment. Unstable fractures are defined as those with neurologic deficit or potential to cause a neurologic deficit. These injuries must be reduced promptly, usually using tong or halo skeletal traction. The halo consists of four pins inserted under local anesthesia into the outer table of the skull and affixed to a circular ring through which traction can be applied. Additionally, the halo can be attached to a body cast or plastic vest, allowing mobilization of the patient after treatment of the acute injury. Dislocations with fractures are reduced with skeletal traction and confirmed radiographically. Immobilization in a halo vest is maintained for 3 months. Before discontinuation of the vest, flexion/extension lateral radiographs are obtained to be sure that the injury is stable. For bony injuries, healing with immobilization can be anticipated. For severe ligamentous disruptions that do not become stable with immobilization, posterior surgical fusion with spinous process wiring is indicated. This may also be necessary in cases in which satisfactory closed reduction cannot be accomplished.

Patients who present with minimal but progressive neurologic loss may require anterior decompression (for disc herniation) or posterior decompression (for epidural hematoma or depressed laminar fracture). The use of posterior decompression for patients with neurologic deficit is controversial. Late anterior decompression for patients with a complete lesion allows regaining of one root level in about 50 percent of patients. Unsuccessful reduction with persistence of fragments in the spinal canal constitutes another indication for operative exploration. MRI and CT scans can greatly assist in the diagnosis of operable lesions in such situations.

Thoracolumbar Fractures and Dislocations. Fractures and dislocations in the upper thoracic spine are unusual because of the stabilizing effect of the rib cage. Flexion forces can cause compression fractures; this is particularly common in osteopenic fractures, which often are the result of relatively minor trauma. Flexion/rotation injuries result in fracture-dislocations, most commonly in the vicinity of the thoracolumbar junction. Axial loading also can cause burst fractures of the thoracic or lumbar vertebrae, and retropulsion of fragments into the canal with neurologic deficit can result. Flexion/distraction injuries occur in seatbelted passengers in motor vehicle accidents and can cause transverse fractures through the posterior elements and body (Chance fracture).

Treatment. After the patient is stabilized and other acute injuries assessed, appropriate radiographs are obtained with the patient on a backboard as described above, and a careful neurologic examination is carried out. Treatment of the fracture depends on the degree of stability. Compression fractures are treated symptomatically, with a brace and early ambulation. Burst fractures without neurologic deficit are treated with recumbency and a body cast, and spontaneous fusion across the involved discs will often result. Indication of stability of thoracolumbar spine fractures is based in part on the three-column assessment as well as on the neurologic status. Stability is conferred by the vertebral bodies, anterior longitudinal ligament, and discs (anterior column); the posterior longitudinal ligament, pos-terior annulus, and posterior vertebral body (middle column); and the posterior elements (posterior column). The middle column is thought to be the key to stability, and disruption of this column increases the likelihood that surgical stabilization will be necessary. Which columns are involved plays a role in determining whether an anterior or posterior surgical approach will be used.

In unstable fractures or those with neurologic deficit and canal compromise, open reduction with Harrington distraction rodding and indirect reduction or direct anterior decompression and stabilization should be carried out. Patients with paraplegia persisting beyond the period of spinal shock (assessed by return of reflexes such as the bulbocavernosus, usually about 24 h after injury) require posterior stabilization with rodding and fusion, most often with Harrington rods (Fig. 41-98). Metal sleeves (Edwards sleeves) over the rods have been used to improve kyphotic correction, and recently the more rigid fixation of segmental instrumentation (Luque or segmentally wired Harrington rods) has been advocated, particularly in complete neurologic lesions. This allows rapid mobilization of the patient and minimal external support. The cross-linked Cotrel-Dubousset instrumentation also has been used increasingly in trauma, and pedicle screw-fixed rods have been used for lower lumbar fractures.

DISEASES OF JOINTS

Afflictions involving joints are widespread. Degenerative joint disease affects most individuals over the age of 50 with decreased range of motion, although only a small proportion are symptomatic. Injuries that cause fractures also frequently involve joints, and the immobilization associated with prolonged casting for fractures invariably causes some temporary joint dysfunction.

Anatomy. Joints can be diarthrodial (involving articulating cartilage surfaces), or synarthrodial (involving the fibrous junction). Most major joints—the shoulder, knee, and hip—are diarthrodial. Synarthroses include the intervertebral discs, symphysis pubis, and ankle syndesmosis.

Diarthrodial joints are surrounded by a fibrous capsule that is lined with synovium. The synovium secretes the joint fluid, which lubricates the joint and provides nutrition to the articular cartilage.

Articular Cartilage. Normal articular cartilage is blue-white, smooth, glistening, and slightly compressible. The matrix of articular cartilage consists mainly of type II collagen and proteoglycan, with a smaller amount of glycoproteins and minor collagens such as type IX (which coats the type II collagen fibrils and binds them to the proteoglycan in the matrix) and type XI, which regulates fibril diameter. One of the glycoprotein components, chondronectin, binds chondrocytes to the matrix type II collagen. Normal articular chondrocytes do not replicate, although they do synthesize and turn over matrix components. After injury or in degenerative disease, chondrocytes have a limited ability to attempt repair, and they replicate to a limited degree (cloning). Under such conditions they also increase production of proteoglycan. Articular cartilage has no blood vessels and must derive its nutrition from the synovial fluid. The collagen and proteoglycan are maintained in a constrained molecular configuration in cartilage, providing its viscoelastic compressibility and load transmission characteristics. The collagen

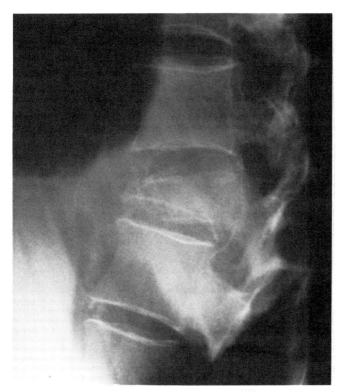

A

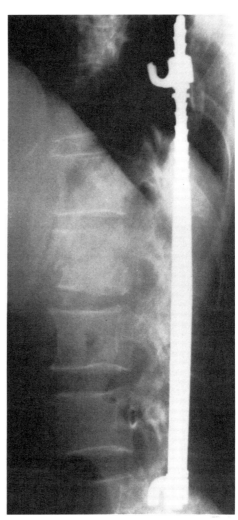

B

FIG. 41-98. *A. Burst compression fracture of L1. B. Harrington rod reduction and fixation shows correction.*

has a specific orientation in articular cartilage, as has been previously discussed.

Synovium. The synovium in a normal joint is only a few cell layers thick. Over ligaments the synovium is quite thin, but in areas of fat pads and loose capsule there is considerable areolar tissue beneath the synovial layer. The synovium is well vascularized from a plexus of vessels beneath the synovial layer. The cells are of three types: type A (macrophage-like, secretory cells); type B (fibroblast-like cells), and type C (dendritic cells of uncertain function).

The secretory cells produce the hyaluronic acid of the synovial fluid, which contributes to its lubricative viscosity. Synovial fluid also contains some plasma proteins, water, and electrolytes. Normal synovial fluid is clear, yellowish, and viscous and contains about 200 nucleated cells (polymorphonuclear leukocytes, lymphocytes, and monocytes).

The synovium is innervated, as is the joint capsule, which in addition to unmyelinated sensory fibers contains proprioceptive fibers. Generally the nerve supply to a joint is from the nerves innervating muscles that act across the joint. Nerve fibers ac-

company arteries into the subchondral bone and provide the basis for bone pain in some inflammatory conditions of joints. The proprioceptive fibers in the capsule and associated ligaments are important in providing information regarding joint position. There are no nerves in articular cartilage.

Articular Cartilage Degeneration. As already noted, articular cartilage has a limited repair capacity. Loss of proteoglycans occurs early after any insult (trauma, chemical, inflammatory, infectious, autoimmune) to a joint. This causes loss of elasticity of the cartilage and swelling with pathologic hydration. Load transmission becomes defective, causing progressive damage to the articular chondrocytes, which respond by replicating and synthesizing matrix molecules. The cells also paradoxically synthesize matrix metalloproteinases (collagenase, stromelysin, and gelatinase), which mediate further matrix breakdown. The mechanical forces on the joint in the context of now abnormal mechanical properties result in fibrillation of the cartilage, and debris from the fragments of matrix induces an inflammatory response. The synovium responds to this with inflammatory infiltration and hypertrophy. Secretion of metalloproteinases from the synovial cells also occurs, further contributing to the matrix breakdown. The vicious cycle of cartilage degradation continues in a self-propagating manner. The final common pathway for all inflammatory, degenerative, and traumatic afflictions of joints is thus progressive cartilage degradation. New therapeutic approaches to the treatment of arthritis involves inhibitors of metalloproteinases or pharmacologic stimulation of the production of the endogenous tissue inhibitor of matrix metalloproteinases.

In response to the activation of latent endochondral calcification in the deep layer of the articular cartilage, the subchondral plate begins to thicken (subchondral sclerosis). This contributes to acceleration of the breakdown of matrix because of stiffening of the subchondral bone with increased loading of the cartilage. The sequence of events in cartilage degeneration is shown schematically in Fig. 41-99.

Examination. The diagnosis of joint disease depends on the following:

1. Clinical history
2. Physical examination of all joints
3. Radiographs
4. Synovial fluid analysis
5. Serologic tests
6. Other imaging modalities, such as MRI and bone scans

Localization of pain, identification of aggravating factors and traumatic incidents, and the presence of swelling, stiffness, and mechanical symptoms of locking are important aspects of the history. Other considerations include the presence of systemic diseases or symptoms.

Clinical Examination. Involved joints should be inspected for swelling, effusion, warmth, and erythema, and unilateral cases should be compared with the opposite side. Range of motion, actively and passively, is assessed and ligamentous stability tested. Presence of muscle atrophy is noted and measured, and regional adenopathy, neurologic examination, and vascular examination of the extremity are carried out. Other joints in both the upper and lower extremities also should be examined, and the range of motion of the cervical and thoracolumbar spine should be assessed.

Radiographic Examination. Standard anteroposterior and lateral radiographs of any involved joint(s) are obtained. If ligamentous instability is present, stress radiographs can be helpful. Joint space narrowing; presence of effusion, intraarticular calcified loose bodies, osteophytes, subluxation, subchondral sclerosis, articular cartilage or meniscal calcification (chondrocalcinosis); and subchondral cyst formation are some of the more important findings that can be detected radiographically. Arthrography and MRI are used to evaluate the possibility of meniscal or rotator cuff lesions. MRI is increasingly useful in the diagnosis of nonosseous lesions in joints, and it can allow assessment of chondral lesions and degenerative changes that are not apparent on plain radiographs.

Synovial Fluid Analysis. The abnormalities in the synovial fluid are specific or nonspecific, depending on the cause of the joint problem. A specific diagnosis can be obtained for infection, gout, and pseudogout (calcium pyrophosphate deposition disease). The technique of aspiration depends on the involved joint and local anatomy. Aspiration through any cellulitic or fluctuant areas suggestive of infection must be strictly avoided to prevent the introduction of bacteria into a joint. The knee is aspirated either medial or lateral to the patella, the ankle anterolaterally at the corner of the mortise, the shoulder anteriorly, the elbow laterally at the radiohumeral joint, the hip anterolaterally or anteriorly, and the wrist dorsally. Sterile preparation and draping and meticulous sterile technique are necessary to prevent infection or contamination of cultures if infection is already present. Fluid is collected in (1) a culture tube, (2) a tube with EDTA to prevent clotting, and (3) an empty tube for chemistry or immunologic analyses.

Normal synovial fluid is slightly straw colored and clear. In inflammatory conditions or infection the fluid ranges from turbid to frankly purulent. In inflammatory conditions, the hyaluronate in the fluid is depolymerized and has decreased viscosity. Adding synovial fluid to 5% acetic acid should form a firm mucin clot that does not separate or fragment with agitation. In inflammatory conditions, a clot might not form or might fragment as a result of breakdown of glycoproteins and mucopolysaccharides in the fluid. The synovial fluid analysis in various disorders is shown in Table 41-15.

Fluid should be cultured for aerobic and anaerobic organisms as well as mycobacteria, fungi, and gonococci, with primary plates, chocolate agar (for gonococcal infection), and broth cultures to detect fastidious organisms.

A total cell count and differential count is performed on fluid in an anticoagulated tube. Joint fluid is examined also for the presence of urate or calcium pyrophosphate crystals after collection in a tube without EDTA or oxalate. After centrifugation of the fluid to concentrate the cells, the sediment is examined using polarized light microscopy. Urate crystals are negatively birefringent and rod-shaped. Calcium pyrophosphate crystals are rhomboidal and weakly positively birefringent. Glucose in joint fluid will also be significantly lower than serum values if large numbers of inflammatory cells are present.

Pyogenic Arthritis

With early diagnosis of septic arthritis and appropriate treatment, the prognosis for maintenance of normal joint function is excellent. The lysosomal enzymes released from white cells in the joint, however, can permanently destroy the articular cartilage and lead to progressive degenerative change if inadequately treated. Joint infections can result from hematogenous spread from septicemia, direct infection from adjacent traumatic

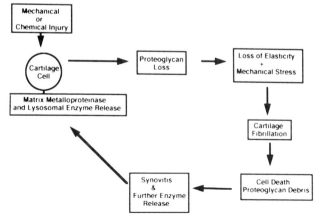

FIG. 41-99. The cycle of cartilage breakdown and degeneration.

Table 41-15
Synovial Fluid Analysis

Clinical Example	Normal	Noninflammatory (Osteoarthrosis)	Inflammatory (Rheumatoid)	Septic (Bacterial)
Color	Clear	Clear yellow	Opalescent yellow	Turbid yellow to green
Viscosity	High	High	Low	Low
WBC/mm³	200	200–2000	200–100,000	>100,000
% PMM leukocytes	<25%	<25%	>50%	>75%
Culture	Negative	Negative	Negative	Positive
Mucin clot	Firm	Firm	Friable	Friable
Glucose (% of serum glucose)	100%	100%	50–75%	<50%
Total protein	Normal	Normal	Elevated	Elevated

wounds or surgery, or extension of an adjacent metaphyseal osteomyelitis.

Staphylococcus aureus and hemolytic streptococci are the two most common organisms that cause pyogenic arthritis. Gonococcal and coliform organisms, *Hemophilus influenzae* (in infants), pneumococci, meningococci, and *Brucella* are other causative agents. With the advent of widespread *H. influenzae* vaccination in children, the incidence of infections because of this organism has dramatically declined.

Septic arthritis occurs in children and adults and is more common in debilitated patients or those undergoing steroid therapy or immunologic suppression.

In patients with hematogenous spread from bacteremia several joints may be involved. Complaints include fever, pain and swelling in the affected joint, chills, and malaise. Elevation of the white blood count and erythrocyte sedimentation rate are common. The affected joint(s) are swollen, tender, erythematous, warm to touch, and painful during range-of-motion maneuvers. The physical findings vary greatly and often depend on the virulence of the organism; indolent infections present with a nearly normal examination.

Radiographs reveal effusion. In more advanced infections, erosions and joint space narrowing occur as consequences of the destruction of the articular cartilage (Fig. 41-100). With chronic infection or a large abscess, subluxation of the joint also may be evident. Diagnosis is made by aspiration of the joint with culture, Gram stain, and analysis of the synovial fluid. The presence of organisms and an elevated white cell count in the fluid are diagnostic. The white cell count in the fluid may range from 25,000/mm³ to more than 200,000/mm³, usually with a high percentage (greater than 90 percent) of leukocytes.

Treatment. In the presence of an elevated synovial white cell count and other signs and symptoms of septic arthritis, antibiotic therapy is started empirically, usually with coverage for *S. aureus* (cephalosporin), streptococci (cephalosporin or a penicillin), and, in children, *H. influenzae* (ampicillin).

Controversy exists as to whether surgical drainage, arthroscopic drainage, or repeated daily aspiration represents the best treatment option. Generally it is agreed that for hip infections, which can result in rapid destruction and secondary osteonecrosis and can be difficult to aspirate, emergent surgical drainage is indicated. Chronic infections with loculation or thick purulence also require surgical drainage. In chronic infections removal of hypertrophic infected synovium can be advantageous. For the knee, arthroscopic drainage may be appropriate. Shoul-

der and ankle infections can be managed either by sequential aspiration or surgical drainage. In general, patients who undergo surgical drainage undergo defervescence and improve clinically more rapidly. Depending on the organism, intravenous antibiotic therapy is indicated for 2 to 4 weeks. If the septic arthritis results from extension from an adjacent osteomyelitis, intravenous antibiotic therapy for 6 weeks or longer is needed. Early joint motion is encouraged to restore nutrition to the articular cartilage and prevent stiffness.

For cases in which articular cartilage destruction progresses despite treatment, late secondary degenerative arthritis can result. Options for treatment when symptoms are severe include arthrodesis, resection arthroplasty, and, in rare cases, joint replacement arthroplasty.

Bone and Joint Tuberculosis

Tuberculous Arthritis. Although skeletal tuberculosis has been rare in the United States since the advent of appropriate antibiotic therapy, the incidence is increasing among immigrants, patients with HIV infection (AIDS), and patients on chronic immunosuppressive therapy. In addition, drug-resistant strains of tuberculosis are now emerging.

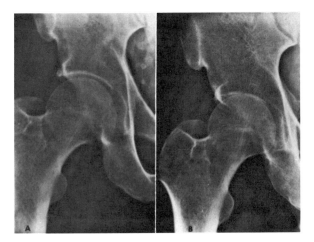

FIG. 41-100. Pyogenic hip joint. A. AP radiograph of hip joint taken 48 h after onset of acute hip pain associated with minor hip injury. Joint space is normal, and no bone changes are seen. B. Three and one-half weeks later there is complete loss of joint space with no bone changes. Cartilage destruction was a result of *Haemophilus influenzae* septic arthritis.

The most common site of skeletal involvement is the spine. The infection starts adjacent to the disc space and spreads across the disc to involve contiguous vertebrae. In the lumbar spine the infection can dissect into the psoas muscles, with subsequent abscess formation. Peripheral joint involvement affects the synovium, bone, and cartilage. Hypertrophic infected synovium (pannus) gradually covers the cartilage surface and erodes the subchondral bone, eventually destroying the cartilage as well. The articular cartilage (radiographically, the joint space) is well preserved until late in the course, unlike in pyogenic arthritis, in the course of which articular cartilage destruction occurs early. The result is complete destruction of the joint with fibrous ankylosis.

Tuberculosis can affect any large joint, and any chronic monarthritis should be suspected of being tuberculous. Pulmonary disease is not necessarily present. The clinical onset is insidious, and symptoms are often present for weeks or months. Limitation of motion and swelling can occur, but marked signs of inflammation generally are absent.

Radiographs usually show soft-tissue swelling and, later, marginal erosions, but the joint space is maintained initially (Fig. 41-101). In children enlargement of the adjacent epiphysis occurs, and in adults with long-standing disease complete destruction of the joint results.

The diagnosis depends on recovery of the organisms from the joint. Demonstration of pulmonary lesions or a positive purified protein derivative test is helpful but not pathognomonic. Joint aspiration and/or synovial biopsy is essential, with demonstration of acid-fast bacilli on smears or positive cultures. Synovial fluid analysis usually demonstrates a leukocytosis of less than 20,000/mm³. If aspiration is not diagnostic, open synovial biopsy is necessary.

Treatment. Therapeutic measures include antibiotic therapy, symptomatic treatment of the involved joint, and surgical debridement. General supportive measures include hydration, rest, and proper caloric and protein intake. Antituberculous chemotherapy is begun, and the treatment is highly successful if initiated before significant necrosis and abscess formation have occurred.

Usually triple-drug therapy with rifampin, isoniazid, and ethambutol is used. In resistant infections, a fourth drug such as streptomycin or para-aminosalicylic acid (PAS) is added. Treatment is for 6 to 12 months. Involved joints should be immobilized by traction or splinting. If there is subchondral bone involvement or if the joint fails to respond to drug treatment, surgical debridement often is indicated. In joints with severe destruction, arthrodesis is the treatment of choice. Patients with disease that has been inactive for 10 years can be considered for total joint arthroplasty, although reactivation rates of infection may run as high as 25 percent.

Tuberculosis of the Spine. Tuberculous spondylitis (Pott's disease) is the most common form of skeletal involvement (Fig. 41-102). The infection can involve the thoracic or lumbar spine. Vertebral destruction results, and multiple levels can be involved, often with kyphotic deformity. Neurologic deficit or paralysis results in severe cases. Treatment involves appropriate chemotherapy and anterior surgical debridement, with abscess drainage and stabilization of the spine with anterior rib strut bone grafts. Antibiotic therapy is continued for 6 to 12 months after operation, and patients are immobilized in plaster body casts until fusion has occurred.

Tuberculosis of the Hip. Initial treatment of tuberculous involvement of the hip joint consists of appropriate antibiotic therapy and light traction. If symptoms continue, open debridement and synovectomy, or in cases of severe destruction, arthrodesis, are applicable.

Gonococcal Arthritis

Gonococcal arthritis is more common in females and results from spread from cervicitis or vaginitis. Symptoms often begin with migratory polyarthralgias, followed by localization in one or two joints. The knee is commonly affected, and systemic

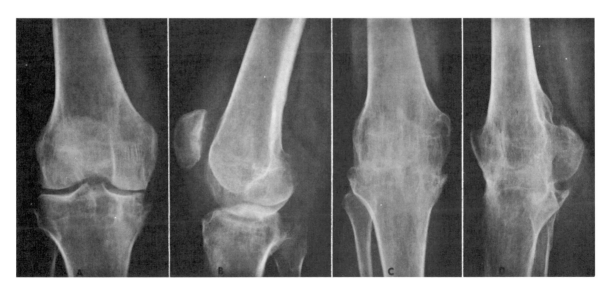

FIG. 41-101. Tuberculosis of the knee joint. *A* and *B.* AP and lateral radiographs of the knee showing erosion of the margins of the medial tibial plateau and medial femoral condyle. There is only minimal joint space narrowing. *C* and *D.* Postsurgical arthrodesis of the knee.

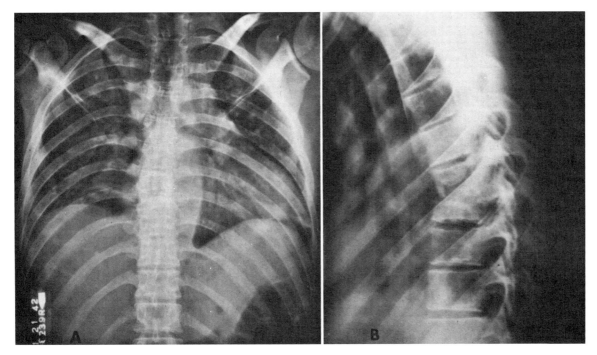

FIG. 41-102. *Spinal tuberculosis (Pott's disease). A. AP radiograph of thoracic spine showing large paravertebral abscess. B. Lateral radiograph of thoracic spine showing disruption of the T7–T8 interspace with kyphotic deformity.*

symptoms are variable, as is the severity of the local findings. Diagnosis depends on identification of gonococcal organisms by joint aspiration and culture. Synovial fluid analysis is compatible with a moderate inflammatory process. Radiographs often reveal no abnormality.

Intramuscular penicillin G 1 to 2 million U/day for 2 weeks is sufficient to eradicate the infection. If persistent purulent effusions are present, serial aspiration may be helpful, but usually this is not needed. If the patient fails to respond to antibiotic treatment, then other diagnoses such as Reiter's syndrome or early rheumatoid arthritis, should be considered. With proper treatment, normal recovery of joint function usually results.

Lyme Arthritis

Lyme disease is a tick-borne (deer tick, *Ixodes dammini*) illness caused by the spirochete *Borrelia burgdorferi.* Affected patients may have intermittent attacks of swelling in one or more large joints, accompanied by a characteristic skin rash (erythema chronicum migrans) that often precedes the arthritis. The intermittent attacks and rash comprise stage I Lyme disease and have an onset 3 to 30 days after a tick bite. Stage II can involve cardiac manifestations and neurologic symptoms such as Bell's palsy. In stage III a chronic low-grade septic arthritis develops. The knee joint is most often involved. Treatment includes tetracycline, penicillin, or erythromycin for 4 weeks.

Rheumatoid Arthritis

Rheumatoid arthritis is a systemic disease that affects not only the joints but the cardiovascular, nervous, and respiratory systems as well. Rheumatoid arthritis affects diarthrodial joints and all the supporting structures, including synovium, tendons, tendon sheaths, and bursal tissues. The synovium characteristically

undergoes inflammatory infiltration and hypertrophy. The hypertrophic synovium (pannus) creeps over the articular surface, destroying the cartilage. At the joint margins the inflamed synovium induces osteoclastic bone resorption and creates periarticular erosions. The cartilage undergoes symmetrical thinning, and the ligamentous structures and capsule of the joints also erode and become lax, allowing joint subluxation. The adjacent bone becomes osteopenic from a combination of increased blood flow, immobility due to pain, and accelerated osteoclastic activity possibly related to inflammatory cytokines. Ultimately the process in a given joint can become "burned out," with subsidence of the inflammation and ankylosis of the joint.

In about 25 percent of patients subcutaneous nodules develop along the ulna, the olecranon, or the dorsal aspect of the fingers or feet. Tendon ruptures from attrition of involved tenosynovium are common, especially in the shoulder and hand. Pericarditis and valvular involvement can occur, and granulomatous lesions can occur in the lungs. Uveitis also is common in rheumatoid patients.

The diagnosis of rheumatoid arthritis in a patient with long-standing disease and deformity is not difficult, but in early stages it may not be straightforward. Arthritis associated with collagen vascular diseases, systemic lupus erythematosus, psoriasis, or dermatomyositis can have a similar presentation. Measurement of rheumatoid factor may be helpful. Rheumatoid arthritis may present with morning stiffness, one or more swollen, tender, or painful joints that persist continuously for weeks to months, subcutaneous nodules, iritis, and symmetrical joint swelling.

The differential diagnosis includes lupus, polyarteritis, erythema nodosum, rheumatic fever, gout, tuberculous arthritis, Reiter's syndrome, hypertrophic pulmonary osteoarthropathy, ochronosis, multiple myeloma, and lymphoma.

Ninety percent of rheumatoid patients have an immunoglobulin in the serum called rheumatoid factor, although in juvenile rheumatoid arthritis only 20 percent are positive. The erythrocyte sedimentation rate is a good index of the disease activity. Synovial fluid analysis reveals leukocytosis of greater than 50,000/mm³. Radiographic findings include joint space narrowing, periarticular erosions, soft-tissue swelling, osteopenia, and joint subluxations (Fig. 41-103). The joint space narrowing tends to be symmetrical or concentric, as opposed to the eccentric narrowing seen with degenerative arthritis.

Treatment involves a team effort on the part of the rheumatologist, orthopaedist, physical therapist, occupational therapist, and social worker. The aim of orthopaedic treatment is to halt disease progression, restore or maintain function, and relieve pain.

Medical Management. Numerous anti-inflammatory medications are available for treatment of the rheumatoid patient. Drugs include analgesics (codeine, aspirin), mild anti-inflammatory/analgesics (ibuprofen, naproxen), high-potency anti-inflammatory/analgesics (phenylbutazone, indomethacin), corticosteroids, and drugs that appear to modify the immune response (gold salts, penicillamine, antimalarials, azathioprine, cyclophosphamide, methotrexate). Corticosteroids are widely used in the management of rheumatoid patients, but usually are reserved for acute exacerbations or life-threatening situations such as vasculitis.

Orthopaedic Management. Efforts should focus on maintenance of muscle strength and range of motion of joints and avoidance of deforming forces. Protection of symptomatic joints with walking aids or splints is helpful. Varus and valgus deformities of the lower extremities can be treated with orthoses. The initial approach should focus on optimization of medical management of the disease. For persistent symptomatic synovitis, surgical synovectomy is helpful in slowing progression of the disease. In the knee, arthroscopic synovectomy can be undertaken and provides similar results to those obtained by arthrotomy. Radiation synovectomy by intraarticular injection of short-half-life isotopes such as dysprosium-165 ferric hydroxide has provided results comparable to those of surgical synovectomy. External beam radiation synovectomy too has been reported to have some success in early rheumatoid arthritis.

Knee. With joint space narrowing and collateral ligament laxity in the knee, instability results. Synovectomy at this stage is ineffective, and generally total knee replacement arthroplasty is indicated. Total knee arthroplasty has evolved to a degree of success comparable to that of total hip arthroplasty (86 to 95 percent good and excellent results at 5 years in total knee and total hip arthroplasty, respectively). Total knee replacement relieves pain and improves ambulatory function (Fig. 41-104). Complications include infection, deep venous thrombosis, and late loosening. Infection requires removal of the prosthesis and all cement and the institution of appropriate intravenous antibiotic therapy, after which exchange arthroplasty can be undertaken, although the success rate is substantially lower than for primary arthroplasty.

Hip. Synovectomy generally is not performed for hip involvement in rheumatoid arthritis. For the patient with disabling pain and stiffness, total hip replacement arthroplasty has been quite successful (see Total Hip Replacement Arthroplasty under Osteoarthritis, below). Complications include infection and loosening of the implants. Although most rheumatoid patients undergoing total joint replacement are treated using cemented components, in younger patients the use of uncemented components, which have porous coatings allowing bony ingrowth, may prove to be acceptable, especially on the acetabular side.

Ankle and Foot. Most rheumatoid deformities about the ankle can be controlled by appropriate bracing. Patients with severe

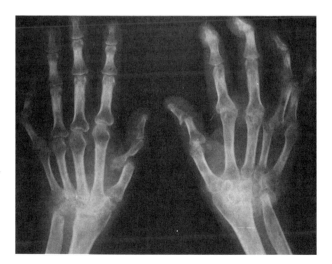

FIG. 41-103. *Radiographic changes in rheumatoid arthritis: severe destruction of radiocarpal articulation with subluxation and ulna deviation at the wrist; loss of ulnar styloid bilaterally; dislocation of the PIP joint of the left thumb and dislocation of the right fourth and fifth finger MCP joints and left MCP joint; diffuse joint space narrowing of many IP joints.*

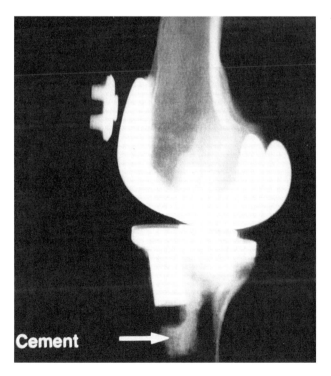

FIG. 41-104. *Rheumatoid arthritis of the knee treated with cemented total knee arthroplasty.*

pain or deformity can benefit from arthrodesis. Total ankle joint replacements have had a high rate of loosening and unsuccessful outcomes and are not currently recommended.

Involvement of the feet with rheumatoid arthritis is quite common. Clawtoe occurs, with dislocation of the MTP joints and flexion of the IP joints, and the resulting painful plantar prominence of the metatarsal heads interferes significantly with ambulation. The Hoffman procedure is used for this problem and has an excellent success rate. It consists of resection of all of the metatarsophalangeal joints, with realignment and temporary Kirschner-wire fixation. Correction of hallux valgus by arthrodesis of the first MTP joint also can be helpful, and in conjunction with the Hoffman procedure on the other toes helps to prevent recurrent lateral drift (Fig. 41-105).

Hand. The hand is one of the most common areas of problematic rheumatoid involvement. The MCP, PIP, and carpal joints and the tenosynovium of both the flexor and extensor tendons can be affected. Laxity of capsules allows ulnar drift of the digits. Ruptures of involved tendons can occur, but can be prevented by early tenosynovectomy. Common tendon ruptures include the extensor digiti minimi, common extensors to the ring and little fingers, extensor pollicis longus, flexor pollicis longus, and finger flexors. Associated carpal tunnel syndrome can occur with flexor tenosynovitis in the carpal tunnel and frequently requires carpal tunnel release with tenosynovectomy. Severe involvement of the MCP joints necessitates silicone replacement arthroplasties. Thumb deformities also are common and require stabilization of the MCP or IP joint by arthrodesis. Similarly, painful involvement of the thumb CMC joint often requires excisional arthroplasty, with tendon or silicone interposition arthroplasty.

Other Upper Extremity Deformities. Elbow involvement can occur in rheumatoid arthritis, with pain, restriction of motion, and instability. Splinting is helpful along with appropriate medical management. In selected cases, arthroplasty is necessary. Fascial interposition arthroplasties have been somewhat successful, but recent advances with unconstrained total elbow replacement suggest improved results over prior devices.

Shoulder involvement also is common, as is involvement of the rotator cuff with the synovitis, often leading to attrition or rupture of the rotator cuff. Results of total shoulder arthroplasty are not as successful as with osteoarthritis, in which the cuff

involvement tends to be less severe, but may nevertheless afford pain relief and improved function.

Spine. Back pain is common in rheumatoid patients, and compression fractures and kyphosis develop as a result of osteopenia, often aggravated by chronic steroid use. More serious potential problems result from involvement of the cervical spine, with instability and the potential for neurologic deficit. Destruction of joints and ligaments can result in basilar invagination or cranial settling, subaxial subluxation, and atlantoaxial subluxation. Cranial settling and atlantoaxial subluxation can result in neurologic deficit, and posterior fusion, decompression, and wiring may be necessary to prevent quadriplegia. Evaluation of the cervical spine in rheumatoid patients is particularly important when considering surgical intervention requiring general anesthesia and intubation, which can be dangerous with instability of the upper spine. Neurologic evaluation of the rheumatoid patient as a part of routine follow-up is also important for this reason.

Osteoarthritis

Osteoarthritis is a term used to describe degenerative changes in diarthrodial joints. The primary change is in the articular cartilage, which becomes soft, loses elasticity, and fibrillates, ultimately resulting in eburnated bone devoid of cartilage. It is the final common pathway of degeneration of joints from nearly all insults, and occurs secondarily in joints previously damaged by trauma, inflammation, or sepsis.

The early changes in articular cartilage degeneration include loss of metachromatic staining, which is a result of the loss of proteoglycans in the territorial matrix of the chondrocytes. Swelling of the cartilage and fibrillation occur subsequently, as previously described. The cartilage grossly appears more yellow and is softer than normal cartilage. Mechanical attrition then causes flaking of debris from the damaged cartilage, which induces mild inflammatory changes in the synovium, contributing to the progressive breakdown by secretion of cytokines and proteases.

With loss of cartilage and eburnation of the underlying subchondral bone, marginal osteophytes develop, often at sites of ligamentous attachments. Reactivation of endochondral ossification in the deep layer of the cartilage as well as the increased abnormal mechanical stresses in the subchondral bone contribute to subchondral thickening and sclerosis. This also supports the vicious cycle of degeneration by increasing mechanical stresses in the cartilage. Subchondral degenerative cysts develop where the subchondral bone marrow has undergone mucoid degeneration, but the mechanism of cyst formation is unknown.

Scarring and fibrosis of the capsule occur, with loss of range of motion. Mild villous synovitis may be present, but synovial fluid cell counts are only mildly elevated (less than 2,000/mm^3). Because of the relatively noninflammatory nature of osteoarthritis, many prefer the term osteoarthrosis.

Osteoarthritis can result from derangement of a joint by any of a wide variety of mechanisms, including congenital hip dysplasia, Legg-Calvé-Perthes disease, slipped capital femoral epiphysis, aseptic necrosis, septic arthritis, hemophilia, gout, pseudogout, and trauma. If no predisposing factor exists, the degenerative process is considered primary. Structural mutations have been identified in the type II collagen gene in patients with osteoarthritis, which may explain at least some forms with familial tendencies. Primary osteoarthritis affects mainly the large

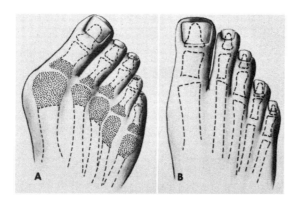

FIG. 41-105. *Hoffman operation used in rheumatoid deformities of the forefoot to relieve metatarsal head pressure and improve toe function and alignment. Metatarsal head and proximal portions of phalanges are excised through transverse dorsal incision.*

weight-bearing joints such as the hips and knees (Fig. 41-106), but generalized forms exist, most often in postmenopausal females, involving multiple joints, including the DIP joints. Osteophytes along the DIP joints are called *Heberden's nodes*. In generalized primary osteoarthritis the course often is more rapidly progressive, with more pronounced clinical signs of inflammation.

Clinical Manifestations. Radiographically, the evidence of degenerative changes in joints increases with age, but only a small proportion of these changes are associated with symptoms. Only 5 percent of patients over the age of 50 years and 20 to 30 percent of patients over the age of 60 years are estimated to have clinical symptoms. The onset of osteoarthritis usually is insidious, with radiographic changes often preceding symptoms. Stiffness is noted after rest and resolves with mild exercise of the joint. Swelling and effusion are often absent. There is no specific diagnostic test for osteoarthritis, although the disease usually is diagnosed radiographically on the basis of eccentric joint space narrowing, osteophyte formation, subchondral sclerosis, and subchondral cyst formation (Fig. 41-107). The radiographic findings and clinical symptoms frequently are poorly correlated.

Treatment. Therapeutic measures include (1) modification of activities to avoid high-impact forces on the joint; (2) anti-inflammatory analgesic medications; (3) weight loss; (4) range-of-motion exercises to minimize contractures; (5) walking aids such as a cane (because of the moment arm of the hip abductors, use of a cane in the contralateral hand results in a fivefold reduction in the forces acting across the joint; (6) orthoses to control instability if present; and (7) avoidance of aggravating activities.

Osteoarthritis tends to be only very slowly progressive, and symptoms can be satisfactorily managed conservatively for many years. When symptoms become intolerable, surgical intervention might be indicated. Procedures include osteotomy, arthrodesis, joint replacement arthroplasty, and resection arthro-

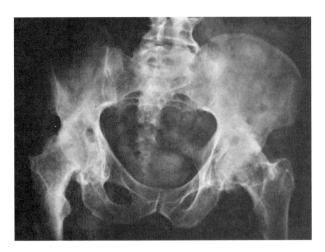

FIG. 41-107. Bilateral osteoarthritis of the hips showing marked osteophyte formation, sclerosis, acetabular cysts, obliteration of joint space, and partial subluxation.

plasty. Arthroplasties provide pain relief and improved range of motion, and osteotomy alters weight-bearing forces to decrease pressure on damaged cartilage and slows progression.

Thumb Carpometacarpal Joint

Osteoarthritis of the thumb CMC joint is much more common in women, particularly after menopause. Patients have pain with motion of the thumb and interference with grasp because of pain. Conservative measures include the use of an orthosis to restrict CMC joint motion in addition to the approaches mentioned above. Rarely, surgical intervention (such as arthrodesis) is necessary. Implant arthroplasty also is useful, but loosening and silicone synovitis can occur. If both the CMC and the intercarpal joints are involved, resection of the trapezium with interposition of a folded segment of flexor carpi radialis tendon has been successful.

Wrist, Elbow, and Shoulder

The need for surgical treatment of osteoarthritis in these joints is relatively uncommon. Wrist pain can be treated by arthrodesis, and for localized intercarpal osteoarthritis limited intercarpal arthrodeses are frequently used. Total replacement arthroplasty is rarely used. Development of unconstrained elbow prosthetic replacements has improved the results of total elbow replacement arthroplasty, and fascial interposition arthroplasty too has been successful in younger patients. Manual laborers can be treated by arthrodesis of the elbow, but this is less commonly done than previously. Posttraumatic degenerative change in the acromioclavicular or sternoclavicular joints can be treated by resection of the joint. Unconstrained total shoulder replacement arthroplasty has provided acceptable results in osteoarthritic patients, and arthrodesis is also quite successful for shoulder arthritis.

Hip

Osteoarthritis of the hip can be primary or secondary to causes mentioned above, including developmental abnormalities of the femoral head or acetabulum. Patients may present with stiffness and pain in the inguinal area or referred pain in the

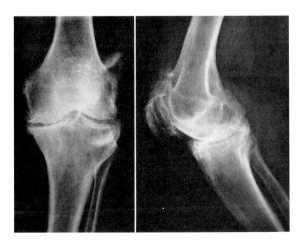

FIG. 41-106. Primary osteoarthritis of the knee. AP and lateral radiographs showing varus deformity of the knee with joint space narrowing and osteophyte production on medial, lateral, and posterior aspects of the tibia, on anterior aspects of the femoral condyles, and on upper and lower poles of the patella. There is minimal cyst formation and sclerosis of subchondral bone of the medial joint space.

knee, usually aggravated by weight bearing. Patients often have an abductor limp (leaning toward the affected side on weight bearing to decrease hip abduction force), and the affected extremity can exhibit shortening from both loss of joint space and hip flexion contracture. Internal and external rotation are limited and provoke pain, particularly with the hip in flexion.

Conservative treatment involves the measures described previously, and use of a cane on the contralateral side may decrease pain and limp dramatically. If conservative measures fail, surgical intervention often is appropriate. Surgical options include osteotomy, arthrodesis, and total hip replacement arthroplasty.

Arthrodesis. For young patients with severe osteoarthritis, the increased risk of long-term failure of total hip replacement militates against this approach. Arthrodesis of the hip provides excellent pain relief and function. Patients require spica cast immobilization for 3 to 6 months. Possible long-term problems include development of low back pain and knee pain from increased stresses on these joints. Preexisting degenerative change or symptoms in these joints contraindicate hip arthrodesis. Bilateral hip involvement also is a contraindication to fusion. Arthrodesis is useful in cases of pyogenic or tuberculous infection of the hip, in which the risk of reactivation after total hip replacement is significant.

Femoral Osteotomy. A number of osteotomies about the hip have been used for osteoarthritis, including medial displacement osteotomy, and varus or valgus osteotomies. These procedures have been more popular in Europe than in the United States, and significant pain relief has been reported in approximately 80 percent of patients. One disadvantage of osteotomies is that subsequent total hip replacement is made technically much more difficult if disease progresses despite osteotomy.

Total Hip Replacement Arthroplasty. Reconstructive procedures about the hip must be compared with the excellent results obtained by total hip replacement. Total hip replacement has been used for primary or secondary osteoarthritis, as well as rheumatoid arthritis. Long-term studies have indicated up to 91 percent implant survival at 15 years for conventional cemented arthroplasties. The major problem with total joint arthroplasty is related to loosening of the prosthetic components, usually at the bone-cement interface (Fig. 41-108). Failure and revision rates as high as 20 to 25 percent at 5 years have been reported in some series. Failure rates are significantly higher in active patients under 40 years of age. A significant factor contributing to late loosening is wear debris of polyethylene and methyl methacrylate cement particles, which incite an inflammatory and macrophage response. Secondary release of local cytokines is thought to lead to bone resorption and consequent loosening. The predominant bone-resorptive cytokines identified in reactive membranes and fluid surrounding loose arthroplasties are IL-1, IL-6, and tumor necrosis factor–alpha. Perioperative or late infection poses the most serious complication of hip arthroplasty, often necessitating removal of the prosthetic components and cement in order to treat the problem definitively.

Uncemented Prosthetic Joint Replacement. Because of the problems associated with prosthetic loosening, efforts have been focused on the development of uncemented, porous-coated prosthetic designs that allow bony ingrowth to provide permanent stability. Designs include sintered metal beads (cobalt-chrome or titanium), sintered titanium wire mesh, and plasma-sprayed ti-

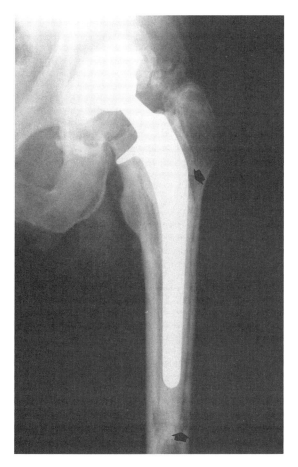

FIG. 41-108. *Radiolucency surrounding femoral component of total hip arthroplasty, indicating periprosthetic bone resorption and loosening.*

tanium bead coatings. Pore sizes of 50 to 400 μm have demonstrated optimum bony ingrowth experimentally, but in retrieval studies, significant areas of porous prostheses have been found to have only fibrous ingrowth. Micromotion greater than 150 μm appears to be associated with fibrous rather than bony ingrowth.

Another problem is dissociation of beads from the device, which may be a result of loosening. In an effort to enhance fixation, hydroxyapatite coatings have been introduced, allowing direct bony bonding. The use of recombinant growth factors also has been explored. Several clinical studies of uncemented hip replacements have been published, and while overall results are acceptable, mild persistent thigh pain and limp appear to be more common than with cemented arthroplasty (Fig. 41-109). Radiolucent lines are frequent around these prostheses, but revision rates have been low. Uncemented knee arthroplasty has been fairly successful on the femoral side, but problems with loosening have occurred with tibial and patellar components.

Infections. The most serious complication of total hip replacement is infection, which may occur immediately after operation or after several months or years. In addition, hematogenous seeding by bacteremia from other causes can result in infection of any total joint arthroplasty. Prophylactic antibiotics in patients who undergo invasive procedures such as dental work, colonoscopy, or cystoscopy is recommended. The use of

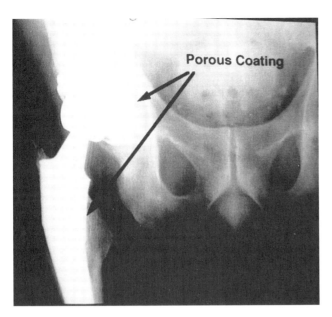

FIG. 41-109. Total hip replacement arthroplasty using a porous-coated prosthesis to allow bony ingrowth for fixation.

clean air laminar flow operating rooms, prophylactic perioperative antibiotics (cephalosporin), and ultraviolet lights during surgery all have been associated with a drop in infection rates to less than 1 percent. Acute infection is treated by immediate debridement, suction/irrigation drainage for 24 to 72 h, and a full 6-week course of intravenous antibiotics. If infection recurs or is chronic, single-stage or two-stage exchange arthroplasty is undertaken. This involves removal of hardware and cement, debridement, and intravenous antibiotic therapy. With primary exchange the arthroplasty is revised using antibiotic-impregnated cement at the time of the debridement. More commonly, secondary exchange is carried out with revision after antibiotic treatment for 6 weeks (for staphylococcal or streptococcal infections) to a year (for gram-negative organisms).

In infected total knees or hips, the placement of antibiotic-impregnated cement beads in the joint at the time of primary debridement can enhance eradication of the infection. A cement spacer has been used in knee arthroplasties also to maintain the joint space until secondary revision is carried out. In some cases, loss of bone stock or presence of virulent organisms precludes revision surgery. In these instances resection arthroplasty (Girdlestone procedure), leaving a pseudarthrosis, provides satisfactory function and pain relief, although walking aids usually are needed permanently.

Heterotopic Ossification. Heterotopic ossification (myositis ossificans) is a frequent complication of total hip arthroplasty (reported incidence varies from 8 to 90 percent) and consists of abnormal bone and cartilage formation in the soft tissues adjacent to the joint. This can limit joint motion and progress to ankylosis in a small proportion of patients. Histologically, endochondral ossification and membranous bone formation are both present and resemble fracture callus. Risk factors include male gender, past history of having formed heterotopic bone, hypertrophic osteoarthritis, ankylosing spondylitis, and diffuse idiopathic skeletal hyperostosis. Heterotopic bone formation often is seen in head-injured and spinal cord–injured patients as

well. Posttraumatic heterotopic ossification can follow muscle contusion and can be mistakenly diagnosed as an osteosarcoma.

Patients at risk for heterotopic ossification can be treated prophylactically with low-dose radiation (8 to 10 Gy) administered within the first 3 or 4 days after operation. This is thought to obliterate the cellular proliferative response. Indomethacin treatment for 6 weeks postoperatively also has been shown to significantly decrease the incidence of heterotopic bone formation. Ankylosis of joints secondary to heterotopic ossification can be treated by surgical excision after the ossification has matured, if postoperative radiation is used to prevent recurrence.

Osteonecrosis of the Femoral Head (Avascular Necrosis). Certain periarticular bony areas are prone to development of osteonecrosis because of their relatively precarious blood supply. The humeral head, femoral condyles, tibial plateau, talus, lunate, scaphoid, and femoral head are the most frequent areas of involvement. Osteonecrosis of the femoral head is the most common and serious of these.

Disruption of the blood supply can result from trauma (femoral neck fracture or hip dislocation), sickle cell anemia, abnormalities of fat metabolism (associated with alcoholism, lipid storage diseases, and corticosteroids), and decompression sickness ("the bends," secondary to nitrogen bubbles causing intraosseous vascular occlusion) and can also be idiopathic. The superior lateral quadrant of the femoral head is most often initially involved, and infarction causes marrow edema and venous outflow obstruction, progressively increasing local intramedullary pressure and widening the area of the infarction. The dead bone is gradually revascularized and replaced by creeping substitution, but during revascularization bone resorption can lead to mechanical failure, with subchondral fractures (crescent sign) indicative of impending joint surface collapse. The net result is flattening of the femoral head, with incongruity of the joint and, usually, rapid progression of secondary osteoarthritis.

Patients complain of hip pain, particularly with weight bearing or rotation of the hip; the infarction also may be clinically silent. When collapse occurs, however, patients almost always have pain and limitation of weight bearing and motion. A high proportion of cases with systemic causes (such as steroid use) have bilateral involvement. The progression may be rapid, over 1 to 2 months, or it may take years for flattening and collapse to cause symptoms. Steroid-induced osteonecrosis has been shown to progress to collapse in essentially all patients.

In patients at risk, the diagnosis should be suspected with a presentation of unexplained hip pain. Radiographs may be normal initially, but sclerotic changes soon develop in the femoral head, followed by subchondral lucency, flattening of the joint surface, and, later, secondary degenerative changes. Although bone scans can demonstrate decreased perfusion early in the evolution of osteonecrosis, MRI is the most sensitive method for detection of early necrosis when radiographs are normal.

Treatment. Treatment of osteonecrosis has been controversial and disappointing overall. Earlier literature supported the use of cortical strut bone grafting (Phemister, Enneking procedures) using tibial or fibular segments placed through the femoral neck to the subchondral bone to support the necrotic segment and prevent collapse. In steroid-induced avascular necrosis, however, a high proportion of patients progress despite this intervention. Ficat and Hungerford have popularized the procedure of core decompression, in which a channel is drilled through the femoral neck into the femoral head to decrease the elevated bone marrow pressure and facilitate healing. Prevention of progression in 90 percent of patients has been reported, but subsequent series have had failure rates as high as 80 percent, making this procedure very controversial. The procedure does provide good relief of rest pain, and, if done early, before there is any evidence of collapse or subchondral lucency, it appears to prevent progression in the majority of patients. Patients are kept on crutches with no weight bearing for 3 months after surgery. Urbaniak has proposed the use of a vascularized fibular graft with microvascular anastomosis to the femoral circumflex vessels to allow more rapid and reliable healing of the strut while mechanically supporting the necrotic segment. This procedure has given satisfactory results even in patients with subchondral lucency or slight collapse, although it is still too early to fully evaluate efficacy. Diagnosis and treatment of osteonecrosis are summarized in Fig. 41-110.

When secondary degenerative arthritis occurs, total hip replacement often is necessary. Arthrodesis has not proved very successful, with a high pseudarthrosis rate, presumably secondary to the bone necrosis. If collapse has occurred but no secondary degenerative changes are evident, bipolar endoprosthetic arthroplasty may be considered, although this is controversial. In general, results of total hip arthroplasty for osteonecrosis are not as good as those for primary osteoarthritis, with a higher loosening rate. In part this is a result of comorbidity caused by steroid use or underlying medical disease.

Knee

Chondromalacia of the Patella. Patellar pain and mild degenerative changes are very common, particularly in young females. Chondromalacia refers to the early changes of degenerative arthritis, with softening and fibrillation of the articular cartilage. The medial facet is most often involved. Chondromalacia may be related to patellar subluxation, dislocation, or chondral contusion from a direct trauma. Patients complain of pain, especially with stair climbing and kneeling, which increase patellofemoral joint contact forces. Physical examination may reveal patellofemoral crepitus, pain with patellar compression, effusion, and tenderness of the patellar facets. Radiographs show patellar tilt or narrowing of the joint space, and articular cartilage degeneration and thinning is readily discernible on MRI. The evolution of chondromalacia to frank osteoarthritis is uncommon.

Treatment. Isometric quadriceps (straight-leg-raising) exercises and use of anti-inflammatory medications, along with avoidance of aggravating activities, often suffice to permit resolution of symptoms. A patellar sleeve-type brace also helps. In refractory cases with quadriceps malalignment, procedures to correct the alignment (as discussed earlier under Patellar Dislocation) can be helpful. Arthroscopic debridement of fibrillated cartilage is helpful in some cases, although the resultant degree of cartilage healing remains a subject of controversy. Arthroscopic debridement of either the patellofemoral or tibiofemoral joint does decrease inflammatory debris in the knee and usually improves symptoms, at least temporarily. In cases in which severe cartilage degeneration is present with exposed subchondral bone, abrasion arthroplasty of the bone surface to bleeding bone is recommended. As discussed previously (see Articular Cartilage Healing), growth of fibrocartilage in the defect then occurs, which allows resolution of symptoms for a number of years. Treatment of end-stage patellofemoral arthritis is with patellectomy.

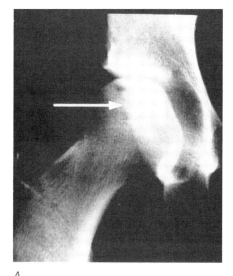
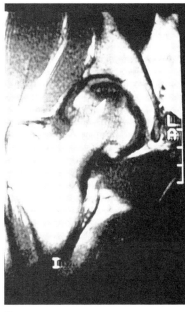
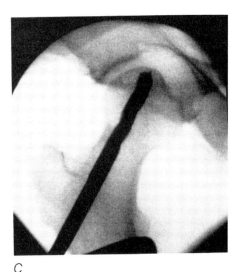

A

B

C

FIG. 41-110. *Diagnosis and treatment of osteonecrosis of the hip. A. Radiograph showing changes of osteonecrosis with sclerosis in the superior lateral aspect of the femoral head. B. T₁-weighted MRI of the hip showing early osteonecrosis, where plain radiographs were normal. C. Treatment by core decompression. A similar channel is used for bone grafting with the earlier Phemister technique or the more recent vascularized fibular transplant grafting.*

Osteoarthritis of the Knee. Osteoarthritis of the knee is common in the aging population and can be associated with varus or valgus deformity, which accelerates the articular cartilage degeneration. Conservative therapy includes nonsteroidal anti-inflammatory medications; an elastic knee brace, which can decrease swelling and pain; and exercises to maintain range of motion and prevent contracture. Patients with varus and medial compartment degeneration (the more common pattern) may benefit from a lateral wedge in the shoe. In cases of unicompartmental (medial or lateral) involvement in the younger patient, osteotomy of the femur or tibia to effect realignment and decrease mechanical stress in the degenerated portion of the joint often is helpful. For varus deformities, valgus osteotomy of the proximal tibia is appropriate, although a significant number of patients progress later. With varus deformities, osteotomy of the distal femur is preferred, because osteotomy of the tibia can result in the joint line's not being parallel to the floor because of the normal valgus of the femur.

Total knee replacement arthroplasty is the treatment of choice for severely symptomatic older patients, with over 90 percent successful results at 5 to 10 years. The considerations are similar to those for total hip replacement arthroplasty, with the major problems being prosthetic loosening and infection. In patients with unicompartmental involvement, unicompartmental knee arthroplasty has been advocated because more bone stock is preserved compared to total knee replacement. Although results of unicompartmental replacement series vary, and loosening remains a significant problem, this is an option for the younger patient. Osteochondral allograft replacement for posttraumatic defects and arthritis about the knee also has been recommended by some, but these techniques remain controversial.

Ankle and Foot

Osteoarthritis in the ankle and foot most often results from trauma. Immobilization of the joint with an ankle lacer or brace and use of a rocker-bottom shoe sole is helpful in controlling pain. In severe cases, arthrodesis of the ankle may be successful. Similarly, subtalar arthritis can be handled by subtalar or triple arthrodesis if bracing is ineffective.

Hallux Valgus (Bunion). Lateral deviation of the great toe (hallux valgus) is a disease of shoe-wearing populations. The incidence is higher in females. With progressive deviation of the toe caused by ill-fitting shoes, the lateral displacement of the flexor and extensor tendons contributes to progression of the deformity. Capsular traction on the MTP joint from the deformity and pressure medially from shoe wear cause exostosis, or osteophyte formation, on the medial metatarsal head, accentuating the deformity and causing pain. The articular cartilage responds to the mechanical incongruity of the joint by progressive degenerative change, and the stiffening of the joint aggravates pain on push-off. Initial treatment efforts are directed at more appropriate shoe wear with wide toe box shoes and insoles or metatarsal pads to alleviate metatarsalgia. In refractory cases, surgical intervention often is indicated.

Over 100 surgical procedures have been devised, suggesting the inadequacy of many of these operations in resolving the deformity and symptoms. One of the most frequent procedures is the Keller bunionectomy, which is a resection of the joint and osteophyte, resulting in a shortened but painless toe (Fig. 41-111A,B). Chevron osteotomy of the distal first metatarsal has

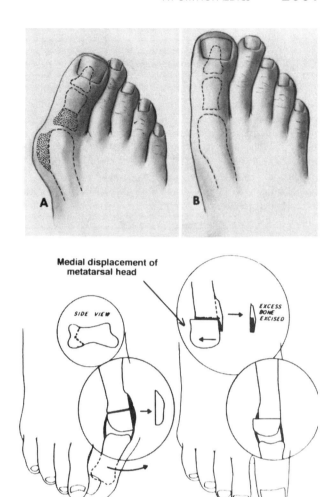

FIG. 41-111. Keller arthroplasty. A. Exostosis and proximal phalangectomy carried out through dorsal medial incision. B. Postoperative position. C. Chevron osteotomy of the distal first metatarsal to allow lateral displacement of the metatarsal head in conjunction with removal of the medial exostosis and tightening the medial capsule. (Modified from: Evarts CM, Surgery of the Musculoskeletal System, 2d ed. New York, Churchill Livingstone, 1990, with permission.)

been used in mild to moderate deformities in the absence of significant arthritic change, with satisfactory results (Fig. 41-111C). If metatarsus primus varus exists, proximal osteotomy of the metatarsal base with or without a distal procedure may be helpful. In adolescents, soft-tissue procedures to release adduction contracture and tighten the medial capsule (Mitchell procedure) are favored.

Gout

Gout is a disease resulting from abnormalities in the metabolism of urate that cause deposition of urate crystals in joints, kidneys, and musculoskeletal soft tissues. Joint deposition is episodic and is associated with acute inflammation and pain. Deposits of urate crystals, called tophi, can occur in bone, cartilage, and synovium. The most common locations are the external ear, olecranon bursa, and around tendons of the distal extremities. Renal excretion can cause stones, and deposition in renal parenchyma can lead to renal damage. Secondary degenerative changes in joints can follow repeated inflammatory episodes.

Clinical Manifestations. The classic presentation is a middle-aged man with an acute, severe monarticular arthritis, usually involving the MTP joint of the great toe (podagra). Swelling, erythema, and severe pain with movement of the joint are typical. The diagnosis is confirmed by demonstration of urate crystals in the synovial fluid. The serum urate level also may be elevated. In chronic gouty arthritis, punched-out periarticular erosions due to tophi may be present radiographically, and later secondary degeneration, with joint space narrowing and subchondral sclerosis, is observed.

Treatment. Colchicine has been used for acute gout episodes since the days of Hippocrates. A dose of 0.65 mg is given every 1 to 2 h until acute symptoms subside; the effect is usually rapid and dramatic. For less acute symptoms, nonsteroidal antiinflammatory medications such as indomethacin or naproxen are effective. Allopurinol, a xanthine oxidase inhibitor widely used prophylactically to lower the serum urate level, is helpful in preventing recurrent attacks and reducing tophaceous deposits. In severe chronic secondary degenerative arthritis, treatment as for osteoarthritis, including joint replacement arthroplasties, is appropriate.

Calcium Pyrophosphate Deposition Disease (Chondrocalcinosis)

Like gout, calcium pyrophosphate deposition disease occurs more commonly in males than in females, and usually in middle-aged patients. Acute inflammatory episodes, termed pseudogout because of their resemblance to gout, are associated with this disease. The knee joint is most commonly involved, and radiographs will demonstrate the calcification of articular or meniscal cartilage. The diagnosis is confirmed by synovial fluid analysis under polarized light, which will demonstrate the weakly positively birefringent rhomboidal crystals of calcium pyrophosphate. The distal radioulnar joint, pubic symphysis, and acetabular or glenoid labrum can also be involved. Treatment is with aspiration and cortisone injection, or with systemic anti-inflammatory therapy in milder cases.

Hemophilic Arthritis

In patients with hemophilia acute hemorrhage in joints exposed to minor trauma leads to joint stiffness and articular cartilage degeneration, particularly with repeated episodes. Spontaneous bleeding occurs only when factor VIII levels are 0, and bleeding with minor injury occurs with levels of 1 to 5 percent. The synovium exhibits villous proliferation with marked brownish staining from hemosiderin. The most commonly involved joint is the knee, followed by the elbow, ankle, and shoulder. The joint assumes a position of maximal volume (knee—flexion of 20 degrees; hip—flexion, adduction, external rotation), and the patient will not move the joint because of pain and muscle spasm. With progressive episodes, joint contractures and eventual destruction of the articular cartilage occur. The characteristic radiographic findings include enlargement of epiphyses in children, and a squared-off appearance of the inferior patella and femoral condyles (Fig. 41-112). An additional concern in hemophiliac patients is HIV infection, which has become the lead-

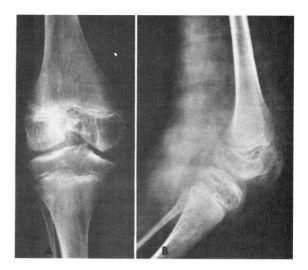

FIG. 41-112. Hemophilic arthritis. *A* and *B*. AP and lateral radiographs of the knee joint showing enlargement of epiphyses of the knee and joint space narrowing, with irregularity and squaring of the lower end of the patella. Note also the soft-tissue swelling about the knee.

ing cause of death in this group. Consequently, infectious processes such as tuberculosis or pyogenic arthritis may have to be considered in the differential diagnosis.

Treatment. Minimizing joint hemorrhage decreases the likelihood of chronic arthritis. Patients should be treated with factor VIII, splinting, and compression wrapping of the joint. Weight-bearing joints are protected on crutches until pain and effusion resolve and motion returns. Bracing may be needed to prevent deformity, and dynamic splints may help to improve contractures. In severe cases of joint destruction, total joint replacement arthroplasty is now feasible, with appropriate coagulation factor replacement to 100 percent levels in the perioperative period.

Synovial Lesions

Pigmented Villonodular Synovitis. Pigmented villonodular synovitis is an inflammatory synovial process of unknown cause that causes monarticular arthritis in children and young adults. Patients present with pain and intermittent, often chronic, swelling. Examination shows swelling and synovial thickening, and aspiration of the joint reveals bloody or brownish hemosiderin-stained fluid. Cytologic examination of the fluid may reveal the presence of hemosiderin-containing macrophages. Early in the course of the disease the radiographs are normal except for soft-tissue swelling or effusion. Later, periarticular erosions and cyst formation occur, and ultimately degenerative change of the articular surfaces with the radiographic features of osteoarthritis supervene.

Histopathologic inspection of the synovium reveals nodules and villous projections, brownish in color, containing fibrous tissue, giant cells, and monocytic cells with hemosiderin granules and hyperplasia of the synovial layer. Both nodular and diffuse forms have been described, with the diffuse form having a higher recurrence rate (approximately 50 percent) than the nodular form (25 percent) after synovectomy.

Treatment of the lesion involves synovectomy. Radiation synovectomy using dysprosium-165 has been reported to give satisfactory results, as has arthroscopic synovectomy of the knee. In joints such as the hip, or in the presence of large masses of the synovial tissue, open surgical synovectomy usually is preferable.

Synovial Chondromatosis. Synovial chondromatosis is a neoplastic-like condition of synovium in which the synovial tissue undergoes chondroid metaplasia, forming nodules of cartilage and bone that can detach and become loose bodies in the joint. The most commonly involved joints are the hip, knee, and shoulder. Three phases have been described, with an initial proliferative phase, a secondary phase of loose body formation, and an inactive phase in which mechanical damage to the joint leads to progressive secondary degenerative arthritis. Patients present with mild pain, effusion, and episodes of locking. Radiographs usually demonstrate the loose bodies, which often are calcified. MRI also is diagnostic and can demonstrate the lesions before calcification of the cartilage. Surgical synovectomy is the treatment of choice.

Ankylosing Spondylitis. Ankylosing spondylitis is one of the group of seronegative spondyloarthropathies with unknown causes. Other members of this group include psoriatic arthritis, Reiter's syndrome, and enteropathic arthritis. Characteristics include sacroiliac and spinal involvement and a higher than normal incidence of human leukocyte antigen (HLA) B27 positively. The incidence of ankylosing spondylitis is 1:1,000, and there is a male predominance. Progressive back pain, stiffness of the spine progressing to ankylosis (bamboo spine), morning stiffness, associated hip arthritis, and age of onset under 40 are common features.

Treatment consists of nonsteroidal anti-inflammatory agents and physical therapy to maintain range of motion. If severe spinal deformity (most commonly severe flexion deformity of the cervical spine) develops, corrective osteotomy occasionally is necessary. Total hip arthroplasty is helpful in cases with severe arthritis of the hips, and care must be taken to consider prophylactic treatment for heterotopic ossification in these patients using indomethacin or postoperative low-dose radiation treatment.

Transient Synovitis of the Hip in Children. Children 3 to 10 years of age may present with sudden onset of hip pain and an inability to walk that can mimic symptoms of septic arthritis. A limp may be noted for several days, and often there is a history of an antecedent viral illness. Radiographs usually are normal, and ultrasonographic examination will demonstrate effusion in the joint. Aspiration is mandatory for cultures and Gram stain to rule out septic arthritis. The white cell count in the aspirate is elevated, in some cases over 50,000/mm^3. The erythrocyte sedimentation rate and peripheral white cell count also may be slightly elevated. If cultures are negative, a brief period of bed rest with light traction will allow spontaneous resolution. A small proportion of these children (2 percent) later develop Legg-Calvé-Perthes disease, and some develop recurrences of transient synovitis, but long-term problems generally do not occur.

Slipped Capital Femoral Epiphysis

Slipped capital femoral epiphysis, which occurs in children (girls aged 10 to 13 years; boys aged 12 to 15 years), consists of a displacement of the capital femoral epiphysis posteriorly and medially with respect to the femoral neck. Boys are affected more frequently (ratio 5:1). The slippage can occur acutely or gradually, and the incidence of bilaterality is 15 to 25 percent. Patients with endomorphic body habitus tend to be affected.

Pathology. Unlike in Salter type I and type II fractures, in which the epiphysis separates through the zone of provisional calcification of the growth plate, in this disorder the separation occurs through the hypertrophic zone above the calcified cartilage. The cause is unknown, and mechanical, endocrine, immunologic, and genetic causes have been proposed. Histologically, the hypertrophic zone of the growth plate is disorganized, and similar disorganization has been identified in preslipped growth plates. Much of the evidence suggests an abnormality in the collagen of the growth plate as the underlying problem.

Clinical Manifestations. The most common presentation is pain in the inguinal area or referred pain in the knee. The patient may have an antalgic gait, and physical examination reveals pain on motion of the joint with loss of internal rotation. With flexion of the hip the thigh externally rotates.

Diagnosis. Diagnosis is made radiographically with biplanar films. Both hips should be included because of the incidence of bilaterality. Preslip radiographic findings include widening of the growth plate. A minimal slip presents with only subtle radiographic findings, but a line projected along the superior femoral neck on the anteroposterior film usually will not intersect the epiphysis. With an acute slip, a tube lateral view is safer than a frog-leg view, which will displace the epiphysis further. Chronic slips exhibit some metaphyseal remodeling, with new bone formation inferior and posterior to the junction of the head and neck.

Treatment. Treatment is aimed at preventing further displacement of the epiphysis. Mild to moderate acute slips are treated by in situ pinning with threaded pins or screws across the physis and into the femoral head (Fig. 41-113). Great care must be taken to ensure that penetration into the joint does not occur, as this can lead to chondrolysis and a poor outcome. It has been demonstrated that a single screw is effective if placed centrally in the epiphysis. Weight bearing is protected until fusion of the growth plate occurs, usually within several months. Severely displaced acute slips (less than 1 to 2 weeks old) can be reduced by gentle traction and then pinned. Manipulative reduction is controversial, because it is associated with an increased incidence of chondrolysis and avascular necrosis. For severe chronic slips, osteotomy of the proximal femur and cuneiform osteotomy of the femoral neck have been recommended.

The complication of chondrolysis occurs more frequently in blacks and females with a slipped epiphysis and leads to rapidly degenerative arthritis. Patients with higher grades of displacement are prone to development of secondary osteoarthritis in the fifth to sixth decades.

Hypertrophic Pulmonary Osteoarthropathy

Hypertrophic pulmonary osteoarthropathy is associated with pulmonary diseases and consists of excessive bone formation adjacent to joints, clubbing of the distal digits, and periosteal new bone formation along shafts of the long bones. Arthritic changes resembling osteoarthritis can develop, and treatment is sympto-

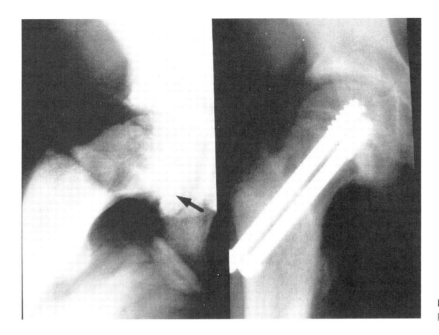

FIG. 41-113. Slipped capital femoral epiphysis, pinned in situ with cannulated screws.

matic. Occasionally resolution of the pulmonary pathology (as occurs after excision of a neoplasm) results in regression of the symptoms.

Neuropathic (Charcot) Arthropathy

A neuropathic, or Charcot, joint is a consequence of diseases that result in denervation or loss of proprioceptive sense in joints. Etiologic conditions include diabetes mellitus, syphilis (tabes dorsalis), lepromatous neuropathy, paraplegia, and syringomyelia.

Affected joints are characterized by progressive, severe, and total destruction, often following minor trauma. Fragmentation of joint surfaces and marked deformity can occur (Fig. 41-114).

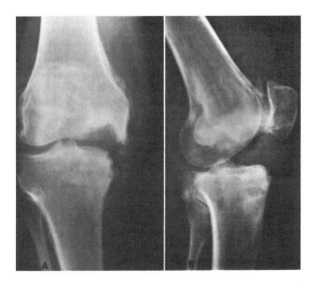

FIG. 41-114. Neuropathic knee due to tabes dorsalis showing marked destruction of medial femoral condyle. Clinically there was marked synovial swelling and effusion with marked instability as a result of the loss of bone substances.

Massive swelling is present, and joint volumes are large, which is a helpful point in differentiating these conditions from chronic septic processes, in which the capsule is scarred and fibrotic and joint fluid volume small. These changes may be attended by gross ligamentous instability. The foot and ankle commonly are involved, although the knee, shoulder, and, rarely, the hip may be affected. Pathologically, synovial biopsy analysis shows moderate hypertrophy, minimal inflammatory infiltration, and fragments of articular cartilage or subchondral bone embedded in the synovial membrane, which are pathognomonic for Charcot arthropathy.

Bracing for control of instability and pain is the mainstay of treatment, and total joint arthroplasty is relatively contraindicated. Arthrodesis is helpful in symptomatic joints when conservative therapy fails, but it is difficult to achieve. With foot and ankle arthropathy in diabetics, below-knee amputation is a common long-term outcome.

TUMORS OF THE MUSCULOSKELETAL SYSTEM

General Considerations

Primary tumors of the musculoskeletal system are rare. The histogenetic type of the tumor is dependent on the tissue of origin. In addition, specific types of lesions tend to occur in particular bones or areas of bones, usually in areas of maximal growth or remodeling. Giant cell tumors (osteoclastomas) occur near the growth plate, where a high level of resorption takes place as part of remodeling; osteosarcomas occur in the metaphysis, where new bone formation is maximal; cartilage tumors involve the metaphysis near the growth plate, and round cell tumors occur in the metaphyseal/diaphyseal bone marrow (Fig. 41-115). These neoplastic processes are thought to represent a derangement of normal growth and bone remodeling functions, which become uncontrolled.

Etiology. The cause of most bone and soft-tissue neoplasms is unknown, but recent molecular biology studies prom-

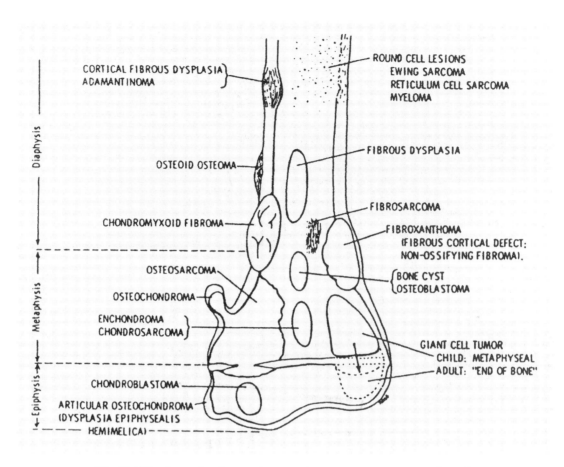

FIG. 41-115. Composite diagram demonstrating the most common sites of specific primary bone tumors. (From: *Madewell et al, Radiol Clin North Am, 1991, with permission.*)

ise to elucidate these mechanisms, with identification of specific genetic mutations and chromosomal aberrations in some tumors, derangements of tumor suppressor gene function, and expression of oncogenes. Most histogenetic tumor types have variable levels of aggressiveness and occur in benign and malignant forms. Table 41-16 illustrates the range of incidence and histogenesis of musculoskeletal neoplasms. The biologic behavior of tumors can vary, as reflected by the pathologic grade of the tumor. While various grading systems exist for different tumors, in general the simplified system adopted by the Musculoskeletal Tumor Society reflects overall gross behavior differences, with benign, low-grade malignant, and high-grade malignant forms.

Characteristics. Musculoskeletal neoplasms are characterized by initial centrifugal growth from a single focus, pseudo-encapsulation (formation of a zone of reactive tissue around the expanding lesion, which in malignant lesions can be focally invaded by the tumor), and a tendency to respect anatomic boundaries early in the evolution of the lesion. These tumors thus tend to spread along fascial planes and tend to remain contained in anatomic compartments, a crucial characteristic in strategies for staging and surgical treatment of these lesions. Anatomic compartments include bones, muscle compartments, joints, skin and subcutaneous tissue, and in some cases, major neurovascular sheaths.

Metastasis. Metastasis of malignant musculoskeletal neoplasms is associated with a poor prognosis. Metastases are most often pulmonary, although some tumors tend also to involve regional lymph nodes, and bony metastases also occur. Brain and visceral metastases are unusual, generally occurring only in terminal end-stage disseminated disease.

Staging. The most widely used staging system for musculoskeletal neoplasms, shown in Table 41-17, has been applied to both soft-tissue and bone lesions. Benign lesions are graded as latent, active, or aggressive. Malignant lesions are staged on the basis of whether they are high grade (stage II) or low grade (stage I), and intracompartmental (A) or extracompartmental (B). Metastatic tumors are all stage III regardless of local extent and have a dismal prognosis. This staging system has shown great value in predicting survival (Fig. 41-116).

Clinical Manifestations. Patients typically present with a history of pain that is often worse at night and usually is not activity related. A mass or swelling may be present, but constitutional symptoms (weight loss, fevers, night sweats, malaise) usually are absent, except in cases with disseminated disease. Lesions adjacent to joints can cause effusion, contractures, and pain with motion. Soft-tissue tumors often are painless unless there is involvement of neurovascular structures. Compression of veins or lymphatics in a limb can cause distal edema, and

Table 41-16
Incidence of Bone Tumors (After Dahlin)

Histology	Benign	% Cases	Malignant	% Cases
Hemopoietic (28%)			Myeloma	24.7
			Lymphoma	3.1
Chondrogenic (27%)	Osteochondroma	12.0	Primary chondrosarcoma	8.7
	Enchondroma	4.3		
	Chondroblastoma	0.7	Secondary chondrosarcoma	0.8
	Chondromyxoid fibroma	0.6		
Osteogenic (25%)	Osteoid osteoma	2.5	Osteosarcoma	9.9
	Osteoblastoma	0.7	Chondroblastic osteosarcoma	6.0
			Fibroblastic osteosarcoma	4.6
			Parosteal osteosarcoma	0.9
Unknown origin (12%)	Giant cell tumor	4.8	Ewing's sarcoma	6.2
			Giant cell tumor	0.5
			Adamantinoma	0.2
Fibrogenic (4%)	Fibroma	1.5	Fibrosarcoma	2.5
Notochordal (3.5%)			Chordoma	3.5
Vascular (0.8%)	Hemangioma	0.6	Hemangioendothelioma	0.1
	Hemangiopericytoma	0.1		
Lipogenic (0.1%)	Lipoma	0.1		
Neurogenic (<1%)	Neurilemmoma	<0.1		

larger masses exhibit a pattern of overlying venous distention. Malignant soft-tissue masses can be firm and fixed to subcutaneous tissue, muscle, or bone, and usually are nontender. Local warmth is evident because malignant lesions induce local angiogenesis. Patients may also present with a pathologic fracture as a manifestation of benign or malignant intraosseous lesions, with bone destruction and subsequent mechanical failure. Pain on weight bearing is an ominous clinical symptom that often indicates an impending fracture.

Evaluation should include a thorough history and physical examination of the affected region, with attention to joint, muscle, neurologic, and vascular structures. Examination of regional and distant lymph nodes is essential, as are pulmonary and abdominal examinations to assess the possibility of metastatic disease.

Radiographic Findings. The plain radiograph is the single most useful study in differential diagnosis of bone lesions. Considerations include the following:

1. Evidence of matrix production (bone formation, calcification)
2. Pattern of growth (permeative, geographic, moth-eaten, loculated, expansile, exophytic)
3. Presence of bony reaction to the lesion (periosteal reaction, sclerotic margination)
4. Zone of transition between the host bone and lesion (narrow or well-marginated versus wide or poorly defined)

Table 41-17
Surgical Staging System for Musculoskeletal Tumors (After Enneking)

Stage	Characteristics	Metastases
Benign		
1	Latent	No
2	Active	No
3	Aggressive	No
Malignant		
IA	Low grade; intracompartmental	No
IB	Low grade; extracompartmental	No
IIA	High grade; intracompartmental	No
IIB	High grade; extracompartmental	No
III	Low or high grade; intra or extracompartmental	Yes

SOURCE: Modified from Enneking WF, Gearen PF, 1986, with permission.

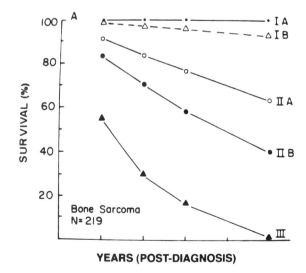

FIG. 41-116. Survival of patients with bone sarcomas according to surgical stage. (Modified from: *Enneking WF, Gearen PF: Fibrous dysplasia of the femoral neck: Treatment by cortical bone grafting. J Bone Joint Surg (Am), 1986, with permission.*)

5. Age of the patient
6. Bone involved (flat bone, long bone, skull, vertebrae, acral bone)
7. Location within the bone (epiphyseal, metaphyseal, diaphyseal)
8. Associated soft-tissue mass, clinical symptoms
9. Presence of solitary versus multiple lesions

Using these criteria, an accurate differential diagnosis can be formulated in most cases. Infection (osteomyelitis) must always be considered given its highly variable radiographic appearance. Metabolic, inflammatory, dysplastic, traumatic, congenital, and degenerative conditions also are always considered. Soft-tissue lesions are better evaluated by MRI than any other type of radiographic study.

Diagnostic Evaluation. Routine laboratory studies include complete blood count and differential; erythrocyte sedimentation rate; serum alkaline phosphatase, calcium, and phosphate levels, renal and liver function studies, and urinalysis. If multiple myeloma is within the differential diagnostic possibilities, determination of serum protein level or immunoelectrophoresis should also be performed. In most instances of primary tumors the majority of these studies are normal. The alkaline phosphatase level may be elevated in osteosarcoma, and the blood count and erythrocyte sedimentation rate are helpful in excluding infection. Further staging studies vary according to the location of the lesion, diagnostic possibilities, age of the patient, and likelihood of malignancy. A bone scan almost always is indicated to assess the activity and extent of the primary lesion as well as to exclude the presence of other lesions. With soft-tissue tumors bone scan is reserved for lesions close to bone or suspected of malignancy. For suspected malignant lesions, other recommended studies include chest radiograph (or preferably CT scan) and abdominal CT scan to exclude metastatic disease. A diagnostic staging algorithm is shown in Fig. 41-117.

Biopsy. For lesions with a radiographically benign appearance, imaging studies of the lesion usually are unnecessary, and the appropriate next step is tissue diagnosis by biopsy. For any potentially malignant lesion, three-dimensional imaging studies (CT or, preferably, MRI) before biopsy are recommended to fully assess the extent of the lesion and to plan the biopsy procedure, minimizing potential contamination of compartments, which could compromise subsequent definitive surgery. Depending on the experience of the surgeon and pathologist, needle or trocar biopsy is appropriate for the majority of soft-tissue and bone tumors. General principles of the biopsy procedure include the following:

1. Biopsy incisions should always be longitudinal on extremities.
2. Needle biopsy tracts and incisional biopsy should be placed so that they can be excised en bloc at the time of resection.
3. Radiographic localization should be done to ensure accuracy.
4. Frozen-section examination should be done to be sure that adequate tissue has been obtained.
5. Cultures and appropriate microbiologic studies should be performed.
6. The bone biopsy cortical window should be as small as possible and oval in shape to minimize the risk of pathologic fracture.
7. Central or necrotic areas should be avoided; biopsy at the periphery of the lesion is most helpful.
8. Exposure of any major neurovascular structures should be avoided.
9. Hemostasis must be obtained to prevent hematoma, which could seed other compartments; for bone lesions suspected of malignancy, the biopsy site should be plugged with methacrylate cement to prevent hematoma.
10. Tourniquet use is helpful for intraoperative accuracy of dissection.

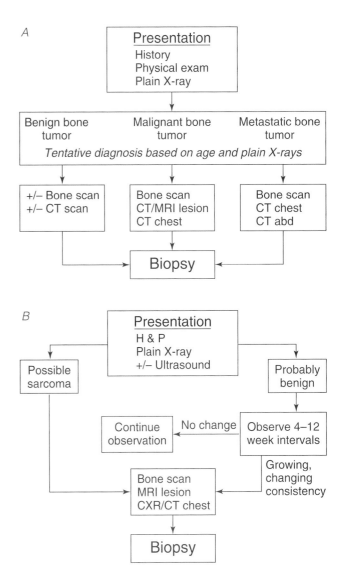

FIG. 41-117. *Staging algorithms for (A) bone tumors and (B) soft-tissue tumors. (Modified from: Kasser JR (ed): Orthopaedic Knowledge Update 5, American Academy of Orthopaedic Surgeons, Rosemont, IL, 1996, with permission.)*

11. Use of a drain with its tract in line with the biopsy incision and near it will facilitate later en bloc resection.
12. Contamination of any uninvolved compartment must be avoided.
13. In general, the surgeon providing definitive treatment should also perform the biopsy whenever possible; this would usually involve a tertiary care referral center.

Treatment. In the treatment of benign and nonmetastatic malignant musculoskeletal tumors the primary goal is eradication of the disease; preservation of limb function is an important but secondary consideration. Long-term results have improved dramatically in the past two decades, and the treatment approach for malignant lesions has changed, with a shift away from amputations and toward limb salvage procedures. The specific treatment varies with the lesion but usually includes a combination of several modalities: surgery, chemotherapy, and radiotherapy. Benign lesions usually are treated surgically. For malignant tumors the primary treatment usually is surgery, with chemotherapy or radiotherapy as a secondary (adjuvant) treatment. Commonly used chemotherapeutic agents include doxorubicin, methotrexate, cyclophosphamide, ifosfamide, vincristine, and actinomycin D. Radiation treatment may be given preoperatively, postoperatively, or by implantation of catheters at operation followed by postoperative loading with short-range isotopes (brachytherapy). Effective doses for control of microscopic disease are generally in the range of 50 to 65 Gy.

Surgical Procedures. Surgical procedures used in treatment of tumors are defined as follows:

1. Intralesional: leaves microscopic and macroscopic residual, as in curettage of a benign lesion.
2. Marginal: removal through the reactive zone of the tumor; may leave microscopic residual in malignant tumors.
3. Wide: removal with some normal tissue beyond reactive zone in all directions.
4. Radical: complete removal of all compartments (bone, muscle, joint) involved with the tumor or its reactive zone.

These surgical procedure definitions are summarized in Fig. 41-118. For benign stage I or stage II lesions, intralesional or marginal excision is adequate, while stage III aggressive lesions require marginal to wide resection for cure. Low-grade (stage I) malignant tumors can be treated with wide surgical resection, with a high probability of local control. High-grade (stage II) malignant lesions can be treated by radical surgical excision, or wide excision plus adjuvant treatment, with comparable low recurrence rates (5 to 10 percent). In the treatment of tumors with similar margins the results of amputation versus resection are

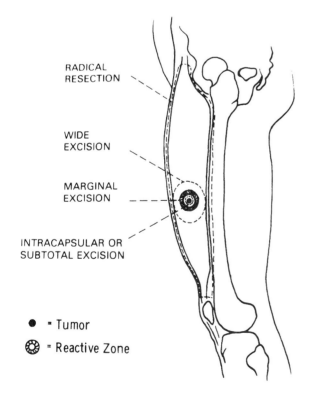

RADICAL
RESECTION

WIDE
EXCISION

MARGINAL
EXCISION

INTRACAPSULAR OR
SUBTOTAL EXCISION

● = Tumor

⊛ = Reactive Zone

FIG. 41-118. *Definitions of surgical margins for bone and soft-tissue sarcomas. (Modified from: Enneking WF, Gearen PF: Fibrous dysplasia of the femoral neck: Treatment by cortical bone grafting. J Bone Joint Surg (Am), 1986, with permission.)*

also comparable, forming the basis for the predominance of limb salvage surgery in recent years.

Technological advances also have contributed to this change in treatment approach, given the availability of custom computer-designed prosthetic implants, which can replace all or part of a bone or joint; osteochondral allografts; new limb lengthening techniques; and microvascular techniques for free tissue transfers of bone and soft tissue. Amputation may still be necessary for tumors in which involvement of major neurovascular structures or multiple compartments precludes resection with preservation of useful limb function. Specific treatment and adjuvant therapies vary according to the histogenetic tumor type and grade, and are summarized in Table 41-18.

Prognosis. Malignant musculoskeletal tumors remain serious and life-threatening diseases, although the prognosis has improved significantly over the past two decades. For stage II lesions 5-year survival rates range from 40 to 80 percent, while for stage I lesions 5-year survival rates are in the 70 to 90 percent range. Local control rates of 90 percent or better can be anticipated in the majority of tumor types. Local recurrence of benign lesions varies with stage and tumor type.

Given that the major problem in the treatment of skeletal malignancies remains late metastatic disease, further scientific advantages in this area are needed. Recent research has identified multiple drug resistance gene expression in patients treated with chemotherapy whose tumors become resistant to the drugs. These genes lead to the production of an ATPase (P-glycoprotein) that pumps a wide variety of drugs out of the tumor cells, maintaining sublethal intracellular levels. Other mechanisms of drug and radiation resistance also exist. Experimental pharmacologic approaches to the enhancement of chemotherapeutic effectiveness by inhibiting these resistance mechanisms are currently under study and show promise for improving outcomes of sarcoma treatment. Other experimental methods of metastatic sarcoma treatment under investigation include the use of immunotherapy, in which the patient's immune system is sensitized to tumor antigens, and bone marrow transplantation, in which high-intensity chemotherapy is followed by the reintroduction of autologous marrow obtained in advance.

Specific Musculoskeletal Tumors

Bone-Forming Tumors

Osteoma. This small, sessile benign body tumor occurs most often in the skull and neither causes symptoms nor requires treatment. It consists of an abnormal excrescence of surface bone. Similar lesions occur posttraumatically on the femur in the area of the adductor magnus insertion (rider's bone), or in relation to the medial collateral ligament of the knee (Pellegrini-Stieda lesion).

Osteoid Osteoma. This benign bone-forming lesion primarily affects patients under 30 years of age and has a male preponderance. Patients present with local pain, which can be quite severe and is often relieved by aspirin. Radiographically, a small (less than 1 cm) lucent lesion (nidus) is seen, typically surrounded by marked reactive sclerosis (Fig. 41-119). Sometimes areas of radiodensity are seen within the lucent lesion, corresponding histologically to disorganized woven bone formation. The lesion gradually regresses over a period of 5 to 10 years, but most patients are unable to tolerate the symptoms and

Table 41-18
Treatments for Musculoskeletal Tumors

Tumor	Chemotherapy	Radiation	Surgery
Osteoid osteoma	No	No	Excision
Osteoblastoma	No	No	Curettage or resection and bone graft
Osteosarcoma	Neoadjuvant and postoperative	No	Wide to radical resection with limb salvage or amputation
Secondary osteosarcoma	If patient can tolerate	Palliative only	Radical resection or amputation
Parosteal osteosarcoma	No	No	Wide surgical resection and reconstruction or wide amputation
Osteochondroma	No	No	Simple excision; all cartilage cap must be removed
Enchondroma	No	No	Curettage and bone graft
Parosteal chondroma	No	No	Marginal to wide resection and bone grafting
Chondroblastoma	No	No	Curettage and bone graft
Chondromyxoid fibroma	No	No	Aggressive curettage or marginal to wide excision and grafting
Chondrosarcoma	No	May be useful as adjuvant for high grade lesions	Wide or radical surgical resection and reconstruction or amputation
Fibroma	No	No	Curettage/grafting
Fibrosarcoma	Adjuvant systemic may improve survival	Yes	Wide to radical resection
Ewing's sarcoma	Yes	Yes	Adjuvant surgery (wide to marginal resection) improves outcome
Unicameral cyst	Steroid injection	No	Curettage and bone graft for latent cysts or with steroid failure
Aneurysmal cyst	No	In unresectable cases	Curettage or marginal excision and grafting
Giant cell tumor	No	Only unresectable cases	Curettage, followed by cementation or cryotherapy
Soft tissue sarcoma	Controversial as adjuvant; does benefit in metastatic disease	Yes—preoperative, postoperative or brachytherapy	Wide resection or amputation and radiation
Metastatic carcinoma	Yes	Yes	Internal fixation of fractures or impending fractures or joint replacement

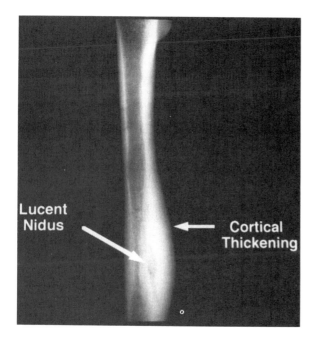

FIG. 41-119. Osteoid osteoma of the femoral shaft, with reactive cortical thickening and radiolucent nidus representing the tumor.

opt for surgical resection of the lesion, which usually is curative if the entire nidus is removed.

Osteoblastoma. Osteoblastoma is a benign bone-forming tumor affecting primarily children and young adults. Any bone may be involved, but the spine, particularly its posterior elements, is most often affected. The lesions are expansile and have a mixed lytic and blastic radiographic appearance. Patients usually present with pain, and treatment involves marginal resection or curettage and bone grafting if resection is not feasible without excessive morbidity. Histologically, vascular stroma, woven bone formation, giant cells, and osteoid may be present, and differentiation from osteoid osteoma is based on clinical and radiographic criteria (i.e., a lesion greater than 1 cm in diameter, without reactive cortical sclerosis) rather than histology. Cellular lesions can easily be confused with osteosarcoma, and careful evaluation by a qualified pathologist is essential to avoid misdiagnosis.

Osteosarcoma (Osteogenic Sarcoma). Osteosarcoma is the most common primary bone malignancy apart from multiple myeloma, although it is nonetheless a rare disease (incidence 2.8/1,000,000). Patients 10 to 25 years of age are most often affected, and the most common sites are areas of maximal bone growth (distal femur—52 percent; proximal tibia—20 percent; proximal humerus—9 percent). Usually the lesions are metaphyseal. Although any bone can be involved, the disease seldom occurs in the small bones of the distal extremities and in the spine. This disease has a number of variants:, (1) "classic" central or medullary high-grade osteosarcoma; (2) periosteal osteosarcoma; (3) parosteal osteosarcoma; (4) osteosarcoma secondary to malignant degeneration of Paget's disease, fibrous dysplasia, or radiation; and (5) telangiectatic osteosarcoma.

Osteosarcoma exhibits a blastic radiographic appearance in most cases because of the neoplastic woven bone formation. The periosteum may be raised off the bone by the tumor mass, causing a fusiform swelling with reactive periosteal bone at the periosteal margins (Codman's triangle). The malignant bone formation may have a sunburst appearance (Fig. 41-120), with invasion into adjacent compartments. Pathologic fractures can occur but are unusual.

Histologically, the tumor consists of small pleomorphic spindle cells, with osteoid and woven bone formation, and there is often cartilage formation as well. Cartilage formation is a prominent feature of periosteal and parosteal variants of osteosarcoma. Telangiectatic variants are lytic and expansile, resembling an aneurysmal bone cyst, and have prominent vascular spaces and relatively sparse bone formation.

Patients present with pain that often is nocturnal and a mass or swelling. Metastatic spread usually is pulmonary, and evaluation of the chest by CT is necessary. Serum alkaline phosphatase levels may be markedly elevated, but laboratory studies are otherwise usually negative. Evaluation also should include bone scan to rule out bone metastases, and CT or, preferably, MRI of the region for surgical planning. Most osteosarcomas present as stage IIB lesions.

Osteosarcoma is not particularly sensitive to radiation, but it does typically respond well to combination chemotherapy. Depending on the extent and location of the lesion, treatment typically involves wide surgical resection or amputation, usually

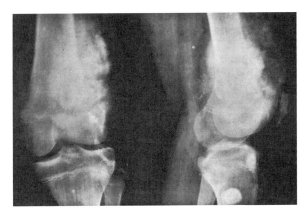

FIG. 41-120. *Osteogenic sarcoma of the femur. The films show characteristic bone destruction, soft-tissue mass, new bone formation, and sclerosis limited to the metaphysis of the lower femur.*

after preoperative (neoadjuvant) chemotherapy. Bone resected in limb salvage operations can be reconstructed by custom prosthetic replacement, arthrodesis, or allografting (Fig. 41-121). Results of combination chemotherapy with resection are better than even radical surgical amputation without adjuvant therapy, with 50 to 70 percent 5-year survival rates and usually better than 90 percent local control (compared with 20 percent 5-year survival rates with radical surgery alone). Pathologic fracture, with contamination of all compartments, can preclude limb salvage surgery. Chemotherapy is continued after surgery for 1 year. Prosthetic designs that can be periodically lengthened by a minor surgical procedure allow limb salvage even in relatively young

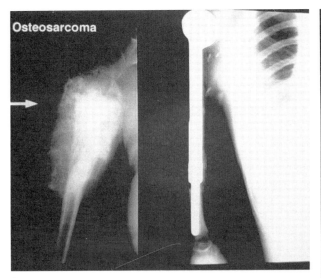

A

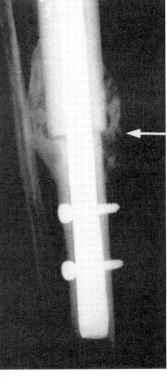

B

FIG. 41-121. *A. Osteosarcoma of the proximal humerus treated by custom prosthetic replacement. B. Osteosarcoma of the proximal tibia treated by resection and an intercalary allograft arthrodesis. Note the incorporation of the allograft at the junction with the host bone. The allograft arthrodesis was internally fixed using an interlocking intramedullary nail.*

children with osteosarcoma, in whom progressive limb length discrepancy might otherwise be a severe problem. Preoperative intraarterial chemotherapy and radiotherapy have been used instead of neoadjuvant systemic chemotherapy, and results appear to be comparable.

Parosteal Osteosarcoma. These tumors occur in a slightly older age group and start adjacent to the periosteum rather than in the bone. The posterior aspect of the femur and proximal humerus and tibia are the most frequent sites. The tumor tends to be well circumscribed and slow-growing and metastasizes only late, usually to the lungs. Histologically, bland spindle cells with woven bone formation, fibrous stroma, and focal cartilage formation are the typical characteristics. These lesions are not sensitive to adjuvant treatments and are treated by wide surgical resection and appropriate reconstruction, or by amputation. Prognosis is significantly better than for conventional high-grade osteosarcoma.

Secondary Osteosarcoma. In older patients, osteosarcoma can arise secondary to a chronic predisposing condition. The most common of these is Paget's disease (malignant degeneration reported in 1 to 10 percent of cases), but osteosarcoma has also been reported in fibrous dysplasia, and rarely with chronic osteomyelitis. As many as 5 to 10 percent of patients subjected to high-intensity radiation therapy for other cancers (sarcoma, lymphoma, etc.) may develop secondary sarcomas 10 to 20 years later, of which one type is osteosarcoma. Secondary osteosarcomas invariably are high-grade aggressive tumors, and prognosis is poor, with a tendency for early metastasis. Most patients in this age group are unable to tolerate the toxicity of intensive chemotherapy, and the usual treatment consists of surgical resection or amputation.

Cartilaginous Tumors

Osteochondroma (Exostosis). This lesion is a common exophytic benign lesion that occurs during childhood, usually in the metaphyses of the long bones (Fig. 41-122). It is thought to result from an aberrant fragment of the growth plate that is left behind and undergoes spontaneous growth. The lesions have a bony base with a cartilaginous cap, from which the growth occurs as it does in normal growth plates during childhood. A multiple hereditary form occurs and was discussed earlier (see Multiple Exostoses under Developmental Disorders). The lesions may cause pain from impingement on tendons, nerves, or muscle and frequently require surgical excision. Growth of the lesion, while not of concern in children, may indicate malignant transformation in adults. A cartilaginous cap thickness of more than 1 cm (assessed by CT or MRI) should arouse suspicion of malignancy. In solitary lesions the risk of malignant degeneration is less than 1 percent, while in multiple lesions it may be as high as 15 percent. Marginal to wide excision of benign or malignant lesions usually is curative if all the cartilage is removed.

Enchondroma. Enchondromas are intramedullary cartilage lesions, often exhibiting calcification and expansion of the bone. The small bones of the hands and feet are commonly involved, but long bone involvement also occurs (Fig. 41-123). The disease occurs in solitary and multiple forms. Patients may present with pain or pathologic fracture. The usual treatment is intralesional resection (curettage) and bone grafting. The most serious concern is the possibility of malignant degeneration, and careful sampling at the time of biopsy is necessary to exclude the possibility of chondrosarcoma.

Parosteal Chondroma. This is a rare benign cartilage lesion arising subperiosteally, often in the humerus or small bones of the hand or foot. The lesions are somewhat more aggressive than enchondromas and are prone to local recurrence. Accordingly, marginal or wide resection and bone grafting is indicated and is curative in the majority of cases.

Chondroblastoma. This is one of the few epiphyseal tumors and occurs most often in the first and second decades of life, when the growth plate is still open. Patients present with pain, joint effusions, or contractures, and radiographs show a lytic lesion with calcifications in the epiphysis (Fig. 41-124). The lesion is composed of chondroblasts, cartilage, giant cells, and vascular stroma. Treatment is by curettage and bone grafting

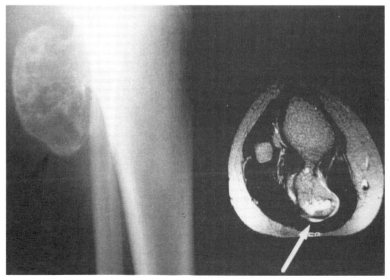

FIG. 41-122. Osteochondroma of the tibia. *A.* Plain film demonstrates a benign appearance, with trabecular bone within the base and calcification in the cartilaginous cap. *B.* CT scan shows a thin cartilage cap, which rules out malignant transformation.

A   *B*

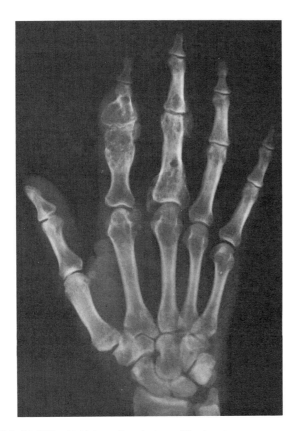

FIG. 41-123. Multiple enchondromas of the hand.

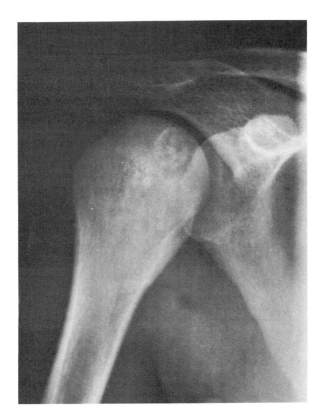

FIG. 41-124. Benign chondroblastoma (Codman's tumor) of the humerus.

and is often challenging because of the intraarticular location of the lesions. A rare malignant epiphyseal cartilage tumor in older adults, clear cell chondrosarcoma, probably represents the malignant degenerative counterpart of chondroblastoma.

Chondromyxoid Fibroma. This rare metaphyseal tumor affects children and young adults, typically arising in the femur or tibia. The lesion is benign, but it exhibits aggressive local behavior, with a high propensity for local recurrence and spread. The radiographic appearance is primarily geographic and lytic with occasional calcifications; an expansile or multilocular appearance with a relatively well-defined zone of transition between the tumor and host bone also is found. Histologic examination reveals a lobular configuration with three components: cellular fibroblastic areas, chondroid areas, and myxoid areas with typical stellate tumor cells. Treatment is by wide or marginal resection and bone graft reconstruction, although aggressive curettage with grafting also has been associated with satisfactory results.

Chondrosarcoma. Chondrosarcoma can be primary or secondary (as discussed above) and affects a broad age range (age 20 to 60 years). The pelvis, femur, tibia, and other long bones can be involved, and lesions closer to the axial skeleton are more likely to be malignant. Intramedullary calcifications are usually evident. Differential diagnosis includes bone infarction and enchondroma. Features of cortical destruction and pain are important indicators of possible malignancy (Fig. 41-125). The tumors are graded as low, intermediate, or high grade of malignancy on the basis of cytologic features and presence of matrix production. Lower-grade lesions can be treated by wide resection, but with high-grade lesions metastatic disease is frequent and the prognosis is poor. Limb salvage surgery often is feasible, but adjuvant treatments are not particularly helpful since these lesions tend to be resistant to chemotherapy and radiotherapy.

Fibrous Lesions

Fibroma. Small intracortical fibrous lesions, referred to as fibrous cortical defects, are common incidental radiographic findings in the long bone metaphyses of children and tend to disappear spontaneously at skeletal maturity. Larger variants, which can progressively enlarge into the medullary cavity and occasionally cause pathologic fractures, are referred to as *nonossifying fibromas.* The tumor consists of bland fibroblastic and histiocytic cells, with osteoclasts and cholesterol clefts from lipid-laden macrophages. A variant of this tumor that ossifies occurs in the mandible (ossifying fibroma). In larger or symptomatic lesions, curettage and bone grafting is indicated, and recurrences after this treatment are uncommon.

Desmoid. This is a rare aggressive fibrous tumor of bone that is analogous to its soft-tissue counterpart, aggressive fibromatosis. Marginal to wide resection is indicated rather than curettage because of the tendency for local recurrence. With aggressive fibromatosis of soft tissues, local invasiveness causes frequent and progressively problematic recurrences after surgical treatment. The lesions do not metastasize and have been treated with wide surgical resection or radiation treatment, with local control rates of approximately 50 percent. Significantly better results have been obtained by marginal to wide local resection in conjunction with moderate-dose (45 to 55 Gy) radiation ther-

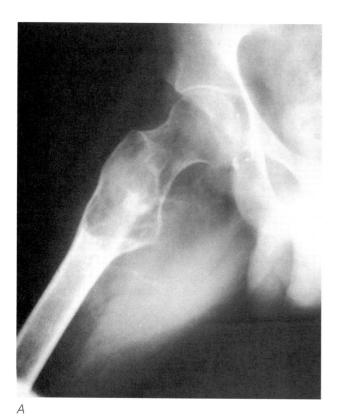

A

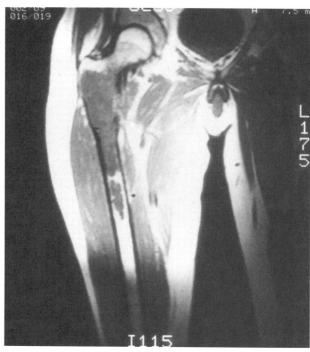

B

FIG. 41-125. *A.* Plain radiograph of proximal femur with primary chondrosarcoma demonstrating lucency and calcification in lesion. *B.* MRI shows marrow destruction and extension of lesion through cortex into soft tissues medially.

apy. Systemic therapy with methotrexate also has been reported to control or cause regression of aggressive fibromatosis.

Fibrosarcoma. Primary fibrosarcoma of bone is rare and is characterized by a geographic lytic radiographic appearance with cortical destruction and associated soft-tissue mass (Fig. 41-126). Some of these lesions are better classified as malignant fibrous histiocytomas, with a mixed cell population. The tumors are moderately radiosensitive, and adjuvant chemotherapy can be effective in improving survival rates. Surgery consists of wide or radical resection and reconstruction rather than amputation, often in conjunction with adjuvant radiation treatment. These tumors also arise as secondary lesions in fibrous dysplasia and Paget's disease and after radiation treatment for other cancers.

Cystic Lesions

Unicameral (Solitary) Bone Cyst. This lesion occurs in children in the metaphysis of the long bones adjacent to the growth plate, most often the humerus or femur, although the radius, calcaneus, and tibia also can be affected. Usually the lesions are painless and may present with a pathologic fracture as the initial manifestation of the disease. The lesions are lytic, expansile, and well marginated (Fig. 41-127), and may be found in the diaphysis in older children as a result of continued growth of the growth plate away from the lesion. In young children fractures heal, but the lesions usually recur, causing recurrent fractures during childhood. The cyst fluid contains high levels of bone resorptive cytokines, presumably produced by the living

tissue and accounting for the aggressive bone resorption in these lesions. At skeletal maturity the cysts tend gradually to disappear. In older children and young adults, the lesions become latent (stage I) and do not progress. Recurrence rates in active (stage II) lesions in younger children after surgical treatment (curettage and bone grafting) average 50 percent. Partial or complete healing of the majority of these lesions has been obtained after intraosseous injection of methylprednisolone, currently the preferred treatment (70 to 90 percent effective with up to three sequential injections). In older children or adults with latent cysts, curettage and bone grafting is effective, and steroid injections appear to have little effect.

Aneurysmal Bone Cyst. This tumor, found most often in children or young adults, consists of a cystic lesion with large vascular spaces, characterized by aggressive, expansile lysis of bone. The tumor is composed of fibrous tissue, vascular spaces with a lining resembling endothelium, giant cells, and reactive bone formation at the periphery. Aneurysmal cysts can arise as a secondary degenerative vascular lesion within another primary benign or malignant bone tumor, such as giant cell tumor or chondroblastoma; however, about half are thought to represent primary lesions. Because recurrence is relatively frequent with simple curettage, local resection with bone grafting is preferable. Embolization has been used successfully in unresectable spinal or pelvic lesions, as has intermediate-dose radiation treatment. Preoperative embolization of large lesions is helpful in decreasing the risk of hemorrhage.

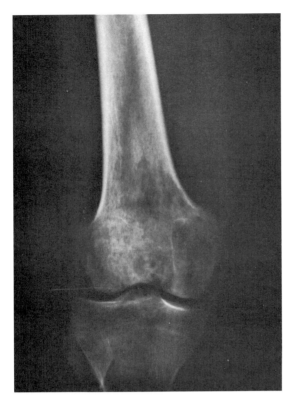

FIG. 41-126. Fibrosarcoma of the lower femur. The films show a lytic lesion, apparently of medullary origin, on the distal end of the femur. The lesion is destroying cortex. There is no evidence of sclerosis and new bone formation or any definite soft-tissue mass.

Round Cell Tumors

Ewing's Sarcoma. Ewing's sarcoma is a highly malignant primary bone tumor of children (age range 5 to 15 years) that tends to arise in the diaphyses of long bones. The spine and pelvis also may be primary sites. The radiographic appearance usually is that of an aggressive lesion, with a permeative pattern of bone lysis and periosteal reaction (Fig. 41-128). Often there is an associated large soft-tissue mass, and patients have systemic symptoms (fever, weight loss) in addition to local pain, which tends to be worse at night. A soft-tissue variant of Ewing's sarcoma, primitive neuroectodermal tumor (PNET), occurs as well, usually exhibiting evidence of neural differentiation immunohistochemically. Differential diagnosis includes osteomyelitis, lymphoma, and eosinophilic granuloma.

Diagnostic evaluation includes chest and abdominal CT scans and bone scan to rule out metastases. Treatment consists of a combination of local radiation therapy and systemic chemotherapy. Five-year survival rates with this approach are around 50 percent. A multimodality treatment that uses adjuvant surgery (wide or marginal resection) has resulted in 5-year survival rates of 75 percent. In young children amputation may be necessary because of the severe compromise of bone growth that can result from the effect of the required levels of radiation on the growth plates.

Histiocytic Lymphoma (Reticulum Cell Sarcoma). This tumor occurs in patients 20 to 40 years of age, usually affecting the diaphyses of long bones. Its radiographic appear-

ance is similar to that of Ewing's sarcoma, with permeation, periosteal reaction, and frequently a large associated soft-issue mass. Pathologic fracture may occur. A significant proportion of patients present with or develop regional or distant lymph node involvement. Treatment consists of radiation to the local lesion in conjunction with systemic chemotherapy. If feasible, resection of the primary tumor improves survival and decreases the risk of local recurrence.

Other Tumors

Giant Cell Tumor (Osteoclastoma). These tumors arise in the epiphyses of young adults, most commonly in the proximal tibia, distal femur, proximal femur, and distal radius. Characteristically the lesion is radiographically purely lytic, well circumscribed, and occasionally expansile with cortical destruction. The lesion often extends to the subchondral surface and can even invade the joint (Fig. 41-129). Although usually benign, a malignant variant occurs in a small proportion of cases, and even the benign lesions are stage III tumors, with local aggressive behavior and a high tendency to recur after surgical treatment. Patients usually present with pain, and pathologic fracture may occur. The tumor consists of monocytic stromal cells, vascular tissue, and sheets of large, multinucleated osteoclast-like cells. The key feature in differentiating these tumors from other tumors that can contain large numbers of giant cells (eosinophilic gran-

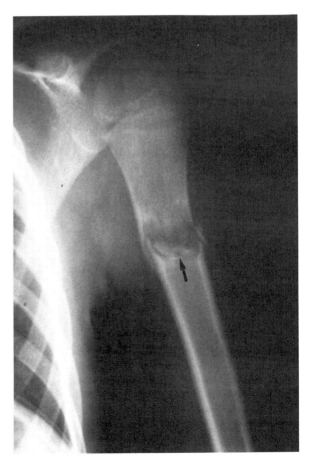

FIG. 41-127. Unicameral bone cyst presenting with pathologic fracture. Note "fallen fragment sign" from a fracture fragment that has fallen through the fluid-filled cyst to the bottom of the cavity (arrow).

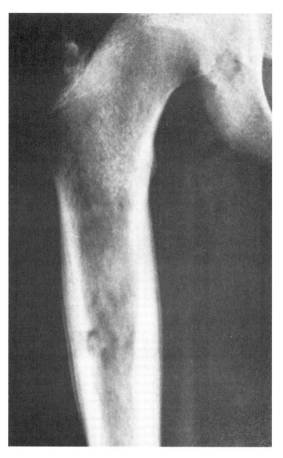

FIG. 41-128. Ewing's sarcoma involving the proximal femur. Note permeative nature of lesion and periosteal reaction.

uloma, brown tumor of hyperparathyroidism, aneurysmal bone cyst, chondroblastoma, osteoblastoma, nonossifying fibroma) is that the oval nuclei of the monocytic stroma resemble those of the giant cells, suggesting a common origin. The most common cause of malignant giant cell tumors is prior radiation therapy

for a benign giant cell tumor, which was a former mode of treatment and can be associated with malignant recurrence in up to 10 percent of cases. Because of this radiation is no longer used in the treatment of giant cell tumor except in dire circumstances (such as unresectable lesions in the spine with threat of neurologic deficit).

The most common treatment of giant cell tumor, curettage of the lesion, is associated with recurrences in 25 to 50 percent of cases. Alternative treatments therefore have included wide resection (usually reserved for recurrent cases) and adjuvant local treatments such as cryotherapy with liquid nitrogen or phenol and, most recently, filling the defect with methyl methacrylate. The lowest recurrence rates have been with cryotherapy and methyl methacrylate cementation. Cementation causes a thermal kill of tissue within several millimeters of the margin in bone as a result of the exothermic reaction that occurs during polymerization of the cement. If local recurrence occurs after cementation, it is readily detectable radiographically as a lucency next to the cement. With bone grafting, remodeling changes in the graft can obscure signs of recurrence. Because these are epiphyseal lesions, the presence of cement next to the articular cartilage may predispose to cartilage degeneration, and in young patients, some advise removal of the cement and bone grafting after 2 years if the patient remains free of recurrence. Given an incidence of joint degeneration of only 15 to 20 percent in longterm follow-up studies, the indications for cement removal are controversial. Control of the lesion with this treatment approach has been successful in 90 percent of cases.

Vascular Tumors

Hemangioma. Hemangiomas of bone often are noted in the spine as an incidental finding. These benign lesions are characterized by endothelial vascular spaces, and because they typically do not cause symptoms management usually is simply observation. A more aggressive lesion is the hemangioendothelioma, which can occur in bone or in the soft tissues and generally is characterized as a low-grade malignancy. In bone the lesions appear cystic and well marginated, with increased local perfusion on bone scan or angiography. Occasionally lesions oc-

FIG. 41-129. Giant cell tumor of the tibia. A. Note the epiphyseal location and well-delineated margins. B. The lesion was treated by curettage and methyl methacrylate cementation. C. To prevent degeneration of the articular cartilage of the ankle joint from the abnormal stress transfer, 2 years later the cement was removed and the defect bonegrafted.

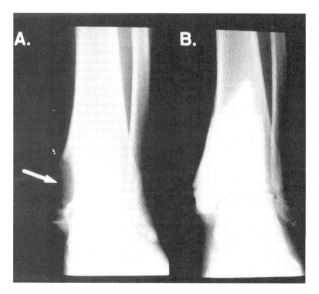
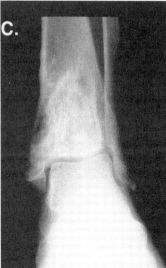

cur in several bones. Treatment is with wide local resection, although curettage with radiotherapy has been successful in some cases.

Angiosarcoma. Angiosarcoma is a highly malignant sarcoma of the bone or soft tissues. The prognosis of this lesion is poor, with early hematogenous spread to the lungs the rule. Amputation or radical resection in nonmetastatic cases is appropriate.

Tumors Arising from Included Tissues

Adamantinoma. Adamantinoma is a rare epithelial tumor occurring in the jaw and occasionally in the tibia or fibula of young adults. The tumor, although malignant, is slow growing and presents with pain and a lytic, multiloculated or bubbly radiographic appearance. The diaphyseal portion of the bone tends to be involved. Treatment is with wide resection or amputation, and adjuvant therapies have not been shown to be effective. Metastasis to the lungs occurs in about 50 percent of cases.

Chordoma. This rare, low-grade malignant neoplasm arises in the sacrococcygeal or occipitocervical area and is thought to develop from embryonic remnants of the notochord. Sixty percent of cases occur in the sacrum or coccyx (Fig. 41-130). Patients present with a mass, neurologic symptoms, or pain. The lesions are slow growing and occur usually in older adults. Differential diagnosis includes plasmacytoma, giant cell tumor, and metastatic carcinoma. The tumor is composed of cords and nests of cells resembling chondrocytes, with typical highly vacuolated "basket" or physaliferous cells. The stroma consists of a basophilic, mucoid, or myxoid ground substance. The location makes wide resection difficult and causes signifi-

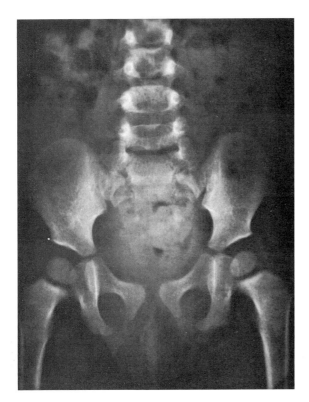

FIG. 41-130. *Chordoma destroying the coccyx of a child.*

cant morbidity, but without treatment the lesion is uniformly fatal, with late pulmonary metastases. The lesions are not responsive to radiotherapy or chemotherapy, and surgical resection is the treatment of choice. Some recent evidence suggests that this tumor may be somewhat responsive to proton beam irradiation.

Soft-Tissue Sarcoma

Soft-tissue sarcomas are more than twice as common as malignant primary bone tumors. Malignant fibrous histiocytoma is the most common type, but a wide variety of other histogenetic types exist, including fibrosarcoma, liposarcoma, malignant nerve sheath tumors (neurofibrosarcoma or malignant schwannoma), rhabdomyosarcoma, synovial sarcoma, lymphoma, primitive neuroectodermal tumor (PNET), and extraskeletal chondrosarcoma. In general these lesions occur in patients over 50 years of age, and the treatment is similar for all tumors despite the differences in histogenesis. Soft-tissue sarcomas are as a rule somewhat sensitive to radiation. While chemotherapy has proved benefit in controlling disease in patients with metastasis and prolonging their survival, its role as an adjuvant therapy is controversial, with the majority of recent data indicating only minimal efficacy in improving outcome. Exceptions to this include rhabdomyosarcoma, PNET, and lymphoma.

Treatment usually involves appropriate staging followed by a combination of surgery and radiation therapy. Achieving wide to radical surgical margins is necessary, and in most cases can be accomplished by a limb salvage operation. MRI is essential in treatment planning and in assessment of local compartment involvement (Fig. 41-131). Radiation therapy may be administered preoperatively or postoperatively by brachytherapy or external beam irradiation. With this approach 90 to 95 percent local control can be anticipated, but a significant proportion of patients (about one-third) succumb to later metastatic disease. In selected cases of soft-tissue and other sarcomas, resection of pulmonary metastases has led to cures in approximately 30 percent of those treated.

Metastatic Bone Tumors

Carcinomas often metastasize to the skeleton, and metastatic lesions are much more common than primary bone lesions in general orthopaedic practice. The five primary cancers with a strong propensity to metastasize to bone are those originating in the breast, prostate, lung, kidney, and thyroid. Multiple myeloma, although technically a primary bone tumor, also must be considered in this group because of its similar age distribution (patients over age 50 years), radiographic presentation, and orthopaedic problems and treatment (pathologic fractures). Over 90 percent of patients with metastatic breast or prostate carcinoma have at least microscopic bone involvement.

The axial skeleton, including the skull, thoracic spine, ribs, lumbar spine, and pelvis, is most commonly involved. The proximal long bones, particularly the humerus and femur, also are affected frequently. Acral (distal) metastases are uncommon and are almost always secondary to lung carcinoma when they do occur. The predilection of particular tumors for bone, and for particular regions of specific bones, is thought to be caused by cytokines, local growth factors, or matrix components that attract and support growth of these lesions in specific areas. Lesions can be blastic (breast, prostate), lytic (breast, lung, myeloma, kidney, thyroid), or mixed (breast, lung) in radiographic appear-

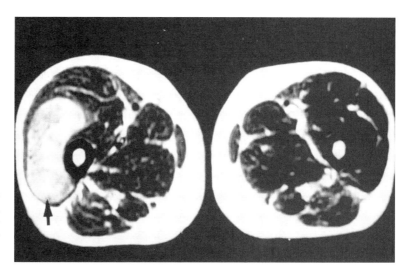

FIG. 41-131. MRI demonstrating soft-tissue sarcoma of the thigh (malignant fibrous histiocytoma), with involvement of the vastus lateralis muscle. Note the tendency to spread along rather than to traverse anatomic boundaries such as the anterior compartment fascia and periosteum.

ance. Blastic or sclerotic lesions are less prone to pathologic fractures.

Patients with multiple lesions may have elevated alkaline phosphatase levels and occasionally are hypercalcemic, a result of secretion of PTH-like protein by some tumors, or more frequently, secondary to massive osteolysis by the tumor cells. The presenting complaint usually is pain in the affected area. Patients with spinal lesions may present with neurologic deficit or back pain. The major orthopaedic problem is that of fracture or impending fracture, with resulting functional disability and pain.

The mainstay of treatment of metastatic disease is radiation therapy, which often controls symptomatic lesions with relatively moderate doses (35 Gy). Larger lesions (larger than 3 cm in a weight-bearing bone), lesions that progress despite radiation, lesions that involve more than one-third of the cortex, and lesions that present with pain on weight bearing (impending fractures) should be internally fixed prophylactically. Fractures are treated surgically if the patient is able to tolerate the procedure medically, since aggressive mobilization significantly improves quality of life. Newer prosthetic implants for joint reconstruction and fracture fixation allow stabilization in the majority of cases (Figs. 41-132 and 41-133). Bracing or casting is rarely successful for pathologic fractures, since pain control remains a persistent problem, and fractures usually will not heal by closed means if irradiated because of the suppression of callus formation by radiation therapy. Exceptions include spinal fractures, which re-

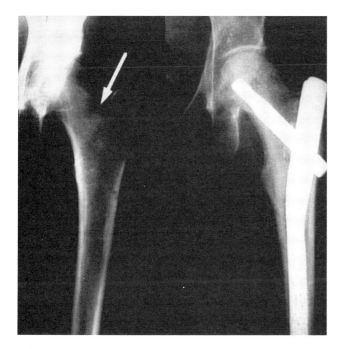

FIG. 41-132. Impending fracture of the proximal femur from metastatic breast carcinoma. Internal fixation using an intramedullary device (Zickel nail) with subsequent radiation therapy allows local control of the tumor and healing of the fracture.

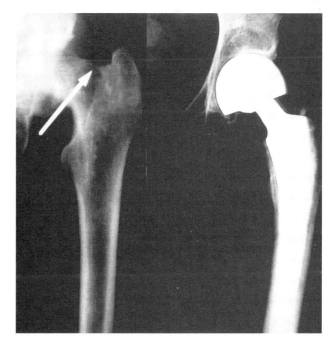

FIG. 41-133. Pathologic fracture of the femoral neck, treated by femoral head excision and endoprosthetic hip replacement. In cases with acetabular involvement, the acetabulum must be replaced as well.

spond to bracing and radiation treatment, but if neurologic deficit occurs they require surgical decompression and internal fixation either anteriorly or posteriorly. If large areas of bone are destroyed, stabilization often necessitates filling the defect with methyl methacrylate cement to supplement hardware fixation. The goals of treatment are maintenance or restoration of function and pain relief, since carcinoma metastatic to the bones is essentially always incurable. Rarely, a solitary metastasis is amenable to curative resection if the primary tumor has been removed; this situation can occur with renal cell carcinoma. Resection or amputation is also considered for pain relief or control of bulky, fungating lesions. Experimental treatments under investigation for metastatic disease, including immunotherapy and bone marrow transplantation, may offer future alternatives to current palliative treatment approaches.

Bibliography

General References

Canale ST, Beaty JH: *Operative Pediatric Orthopaedics.* St Louis, CV Mosby, 1991.

Chapman MW: *Operative Orthopaedics,* 2d ed. Philadelphia, JB Lippincott, 1993.

Crenshaw AH: *Campbell's Operative Orthopaedics,* 9th ed. St Louis, CV Mosby, 1996.

Evarts CM: *Surgery of the Musculoskeletal System,* 2d ed. New York, Churchill Livingstone, 1990.

Kasser JR: *Orthopaedic Knowledge Update 5.* American Academy of Orthopaedic Surgeons, Rosemont, IL, 1996.

Ogden JA: *Skeletal Injury in the Child,* 2d ed. Philadelphia, WB Saunders, 1990.

Rockwood CA, Green DP, et al: *Rockwood and Green's Fractures,* 4th ed. Philadelphia, JB Lippincott, 1996.

Simon SR: *Orthopaedic Basic Science.* American Academy of Orthopaedic Surgeons, Rosemont, IL, 1994.

Tachdjian MO: *Atlas of Pediatric Orthopaedic Surgery.* Philadelphia, WB Saunders, 1994.

Pain

Abram SE: Advances in chronic pain management since gate control. *Regional Anesthesia* 18:66, 1993.

Detmer DE: Chronic shin splints: Classification and management of medial tibial stress syndrome. *Sports Med* 3:436, 1986.

Frieman BG, Albert TJ, Fenlin JM Jr: Rotator cuff disease: A review of diagnosis, pathophysiology, and current trends in treatment. *Arch Phys Med Rehabil* 75:604, 1994.

Frymoyer JW: Back pain and sciatica. *N Engl J Med* 318:291, 1988.

Ginsburg GM, Bassett GS: Back pain in children and adolescents: Evaluation and differential diagnosis. *J Amer Acad Orthop Surg* 5:67, 1997.

Harris IE, Weinstein SD: Long-term follow-up of patients with grade III and IV spondylolisthesis: Treatment with and without posterior fusion. *J Bone Joint Surg* 69A:960, 1987.

Herkowitz HN: A comparison of anterior cervical fusion, cervical laminectomy, and cervical laminoplasty for the surgical management of multiple level spondylotic radiculopathy. *Spine* 13:774, 1988.

Inhofe PD, Garcia-Moral CA: Reflex sympathetic dystrophy: A review of the literature and a long-term outcome study. *Orthop Rev* 23:655, 1994.

Lazarus MD, Chansky HA, et al: Comparison of open and arthroscopic subacromial decompression. *J Shoulder Elbow Surg* 3:1, 1994.

Melzack R, Wall PD: Pain mechanisms: A new theory. *Science* 150:971, 1965.

Montgomery TJ, Yerger B, et al: Management of rotator cuff tears: A comparison of arthroscopic debridement and surgical repair. *J Shoulder Elbow Surg* 3:70, 1994.

Nasca RJ: Surgical management of lumbar spinal stenosis. *Spine* 12:809, 1987.

Neer CS II: Impingement lesions. *Clin Orthop* 173:70, 1983.

Osterman K, Schlenzka D, et al: Isthmic spondylolisthesis in symptomatic and asymptomatic subjects, epidemiology, and natural history with special reference to disk abnormality and mode of treatment. *Clin Orthop* 297:65, 1993.

Pedersen AK, Hagen R: Spondylolysis and spondylolisthesis: Treatment by internal fixation and bone grafting of the defect. *J Bone Joint Surg* 70A:15, 1988.

Ribbers G, Geurts AC, et al: The reflex sympathetic dystrophy syndrome: A review with special reference to chronic pain and motor impairments. *Int J Rehab Res* 18:277, 1995.

Riegler FX: Update on perioperative pain management. *Clin Orthop* 305:283, 1994.

Satomi K, Nishu Y, et al: Long-term follow-up studies of open-door expansive laminoplasty for cervical stenotic myelopathy. *Spine* 19:507, 1994.

Shorter E.: Somatization and chronic pain in historic perspective. *Clin Orthop* 336:52, 1997.

Siddall PJ, Cousins MJ: Pain mechanisms and management: An update. *Clin Exp Pharmacol Physiol* 22:679, 1995.

Sluka KA: Pain mechanisms involved in musculoskeletal disorders. *J Orthop Sports Phys Therapy* 24:240, 1996.

Stewart G, Sachs BL: Patient outcomes after reoperation on the lumbar spine. *J Bone Joint Surg* 78A:706, 1996.

Twycross RG: Management of pain in skeletal metastases. *Clin Orthop* 312:187, 1995.

Willis WD, Westlund KN: Neuroanatomy of the pain system and of the pathways that modulate pain. *J Clin Neurophysiol* 14:2, 1997.

Disorders of Muscle

Boachie-Adjei O, Lonstein JE, et al: Management of neuromuscular spinal deformities with Luque segmental instrumentation. *J Bone Joint Surg* 71A:548, 1989.

Broughton NS, Menelaus MB, et al: The natural history of hip deformity in myelomeningocele. *J Bone Joint Surg* 75B:760, 1993.

Carroll NC: Assessment and management of the lower extremity in myelodysplasia. *Orthop Clin North Am* 18:709, 1987.

Dabney KW, Lipton GE, et al: Cerebral palsy. *Curr Opin Pediatr* 9:81, 1997.

Funasaki H, Winter RB, et al: Pathophysiology of spinal deformities in neurofibromatosis: An analysis of seventy-one patients who had curves associated with dystrophic changes. *J Bone Joint Surg* 76:692, 1994.

Hsu JD, Furumasu J: Gait and posture changes in the Duchenne muscular dystrophy child. *Clin Orthop* 288:122, 1993.

Koman LA, Gelberman RH, et al: Cerebral palsy: Management of the upper extremity. *Clin Orthop* 253:62, 1990.

Roberts A, Evans GA: Orthopedic aspects of neuromuscular disorders in children. *Curr Opin Pediatr* 5:379, 1993.

Shapiro F, Specht L: The diagnosis and orthopaedic treatment of inherited muscular diseases of childhood. *J Bone Joint Surg* 75A:439, 1993.

Smith AD, Koreska J, et al: Progression in Duchenne muscular dystrophy. *J Bone Joint Surg* 71A:1066, 1989.

Sussman MD, Little D, et al: Posterior instrumentation and fusion of the thoracolumbar spine for treatment of neuromuscular scoliosis. *J Pediatr Orthop* 16:304, 1996.

Posture

Aronson J: Current concepts review: Limb-lengthening, skeletal reconstruction, and bone transport with the Ilizarov method. *J Bone Joint Surg* 79A:1243, 1997.

Bridwell KH: Spinal instrumentation in the management of adolescent scoliosis. *Clin Orthop* 335:64, 1997.

Calvert PT, Edgar MA, et al: Scoliosis in neurofibromatosis: Natural history with and without operation. *J Bone Joint Surg* 71B:246, 1989.

Connolly PJ, Von Schroeder HP, et al: Adolescent idiopathic scoliosis. Long-term effect of instrumentation extending to the lumbar spine. *J Bone Joint Surg* 77A:1210, 1995.

Denis F: Anterior surgery in scoliosis. *Clin Orthop* 300:38, 1994.

Gelberman RH, Garfin ST, et al: Compartment syndromes of the forearm: Diagnosis and treatment. *Clin Orthop* 161:252, 1981.

Guidera KJ, Hooten J, et al: Cotrel-Dubousset instrumentation: Results in 52 patients. *Spine* 18:427, 1993.

Gutkowski W, Renshaw T: Orthotic results in adolescent kyphosis. *Spine* 13:485, 1988.

Heckman MM, Whitesides TE Jr, et al: Compartment pressure in association with closed tibial fractures: The relationship between tissue pressure, compartment, and the distance from the site of the fracture. *J Bone Joint Surg* 76A:1285, 1994.

Loder RT, Johnston CE II: Infantile tibia vara. *J Pediatr Orthop* 7:639, 1987.

Marsh DR, Shah S, et al: The Ilizarov method in nonunion, malunion, and infection of fractures. *J Bone Joint Surg* 79A:273, 1997.

McCarthy DM, Sotereanos DG, et al: A cadaveric and radiologic assessment of catheter placement for the measurement of forearm compartment pressures. *Clin Orthop* 312:266, 1995.

McMaster MJ, Ohtsuka K: The natural history of congenital scoliosis: A study of 251 patients. *J Bone Joint Surg* 64A:1128, 1982.

Noonan KJ, Weinstein SL et al: Use of the Milwaukee brace for progressive idiopathic scoliosis. *J Bone Joint Surg* 78A:1996.

Robinson CM, McMaster MJ: Juvenile idiopathic scoliosis. Curve patterns and prognosis in one hundred and nine patients. *J Bone Joint Surg* 78A:1140, 1997.

Rorabeck CH, Fowler PJ, et al: The results of fasciotomy in the management of chronic exertional compartment syndrome. *Am J Sports Med* 16:224, 1988.

Rowe DE, Bernstein SM, et al: A meta-analysis of the efficacy of nonoperative treatments for idiopathic scoliosis. *J Bone Joint Surg* 79A:664, 1997.

Sachs B, Bradford D, et al: Scheuermann kyphosis: Follow-up of Milwaukee-brace treatment. *J Bone Joint Surg* 69A:50, 1987.

Schlenzka D, Poussa M, et al: Operative treatment of adolescent idiopathic thoracic scoliosis: Harrington-DTT versus Cotrel-Dubousset instrumentation. *Clin Orthop* 297:155, 1993.

Epiphyseal Disorders

Carney BT, Weinstein SL: Natural history of untreated chronic slipped capital femoral epiphysis. *Clin Orthop* 322:43, 1996.

Farsetti P, Tudisco C, et al: The Herring lateral pillar classification for prognosis in Perthes disease: Late results in 49 patients treated conservatively. *J Bone Joint Surg* 77B:739, 1995.

Grasemann H, Nicolai RD, et al: The treatment of Legg-Calvé-Perthes disease: To contain or not to contain. *Arch Orthop Trauma Surg* 116:50, 1997.

Hubbard AM, Dormans JP: Evaluation of developmental dysplasia, Perthes disease, and neuromuscular dysplasia of the hip in children before and after surgery: An imaging update. *Am J Roentgenol* 164:1067, 1995.

Martinez AG, Weinstein AL, et al: The weight-bearing abduction brace for the treatment of Legg-Perthes disease. *J Bone Joint Surg* 74A:12, 1992.

Ritterbusch JF, Shantharam SS, et al: Comparison of lateral pillar classification and Catterall classification of Legg-Calvé-Perthes disease. *J Pediatr Orthop* 13:200, 1993.

Sponseller PD, Desai SS, et al: Comparison of femoral and innominate osteotomies for the treatment of Legg-Calvé-Perthes disease. *J Bone Joint Surg* 79A:1131, 1988.

Wang L, Bowen JR, et al: An evaluation of various methods of treatment for Legg-Calvé-Perthes disease. *Clin Orthop* 314:225, 1995.

Wenger DR, Ward WT, et al: Legg-Calvé-Perthes disease. *J Bone Joint Surg* 73A:778, 1991.

Congenital Deformities

Aronson J, Puskarich CL: Deformity and disability from treated clubfoot. *J Pediatr Orthop* 10:109, 1990.

Askins G, Ger E: Congenital constriction band syndrome. *J Pediatr Orthop* 8:461, 1988.

Bassett GS: Orthopaedic aspects of skeletal dysplasias, in Greene WB (ed): *Instructional Course Lectures 39.* Park Ridge, IL, American Academy of Orthopaedic Surgeons, 1990, p 381.

Cheng JW, Au AW: Infantile torticollis: A review of 644 cases. *J Pediatr Orthop* 14:602, 1994.

Choi IH, Kumar SJ, et al: Amputation or limb-lengthening for partial or total absence of the fibula. *J Bone Joint Surg* 72A:1391, 1990.

Cooper DM, Dietz FR: Treatment of idiopathic clubfoot: A thirty-year follow-up note. *J Bone Joint Surg* 77A:1477, 1995.

Crossett LS, Beaty JH, et al: Congenital pseudarthrosis of the tibia: Long-term follow-up study. *Clin Orthop* 245:16, 1989.

Forlin E, Choi IH, et al: Prognostic factors in congenital dislocation of the hip treated with closed reduction. *J Bone Joint Surg* 74A:1140, 1992.

Galpin RD, Roach JW, et al: One-stage treatment of congenital dislocation of the hip in older children, including femoral shortening. *J Bone Joint Surg* 71A:734, 1989.

Ganel A, Horoszowski H: Limb lengthening in children with achondroplasia: Differences based on gender. *Clin Orthop* 332:179, 1996.

Gilbert A, Brockman R: Congenital pseudarthrosis of the tibia: Long-term follow-up of 29 cases treated by microvascular bone transfer. *Clin Orthop* 314:37, 1995.

Haasbeek JF, Wright JG: A comparison of the long-term results of posterior and comprehensive release in the treatment of clubfoot. *J Pediatr Orthop* 17:29, 1997.

Leibovic SJ, Ehrlich MG, et al: Sprengel deformity. *J Bone Joint Surg* 72A:192, 1990.

Mankey MG, Arntz GT, et al: Open reduction through a medial approach for congenital dislocation of the hip: A critical review of the Ludloff approach in sixty-six hips. *J Bone Joint Surg* 75A:1334, 1993.

Schrader LF, Gilbert RJ, et al: Congenital vertical talus surgical correction by a one-stage medial approach. *Orthopaedics* 13:1233, 1990.

Södergård J, Ryöppy S: The knee in arthrogryposis multiplex congenita. *J Pediatr Orthop* 10:177, 1990.

Swanson AB, Swanson GD, et al: A classification for congenital limb malformation. *J Hand Surg* 8:693, 1983.

Viere RG, Birch JG, et al: Use of the Pavlik harness in congenital dislocation of the hip: An analysis of failure of treatment. *J Bone Joint Surg* 72A:238, 1990.

Weiland AJ, Weiss AP, et al: Vascularized fibular grafts in the treatment of congenital pseudarthrosis of the tibia. *J Bone Joint Surg* 72A:654, 1990.

Wilde PH, Torode IP, et al: Resection for symptomatic talocalcaneal coalition. *J Bone Joint Surg* 76B:797, 1994.

Wirth T, Schuler P, et al: Early surgical treatment for congenital vertical talus. *Arch Orthop Trauma Surg* 113:248, 1994.

Generalized Bone Disorders

Barth RW, Lane JM: Osteoporosis. *Orthop Clin North Am* 19:845, 1988.

Borrie MJ, Campbell AG, et al: Osteomalacia in the elderly. *N Engl J Med* 98:989, 1985.

Bulger EM, Smith DG, et al: Fat embolism syndrome: A 10-year review. *Arch Surg* 132:435, 1997.

Cauley JA, Seeley DG, et al: Estrogen replacement therapy and fractures in older women. *Ann Intern Med* 122:9, 1995.

Enneking WF, Gearen PF: Fibrous dysplasia of the femoral neck: Treatment by cortical bone grafting. *J Bone Joint Surg* 68A:1415, 1986.

Friedlaender GE: Current concepts review. Bone grafts: The basic science rationale for clinical applications. *J Bone Joint Surg* 69A:786, 1987.

Liberman UA, Weiss SR, et al: Effect of oral alendronate on bone mineral density and the incidence of fractures in postmenopausal osteoporosis. *N Engl J Med* 333:1437, 1995.

Lindsay R: Managing osteoporosis: Current trends, future possibilities. *Geriatrics* 42:35, 1987.

Mankin HJ: Metabolic bone disease, in Jackson DW (ed): *Instructional Course Lectures 44.* Rosemont, IL, American Academy of Orthopaedic Surgeons, 1994, p 3.

Mirra JM, Brien EW, et al: Paget's disease of bone: Review with emphasis on radiologic features, Part II. *Skel Radiol* 24:173, 1995.

Raisz LG: Local and systemic factors in the pathogenesis of osteoporosis. *N Engl J Med* 318:818, 1988.

Riggs BL, Melton LJ III: *Osteoporosis: Etiology, Diagnosis, and Management,* 2d ed. New York, Raven, 1996.

Selby P: Alendronate treatment for osteoporosis: A review of the clinical evidence. *Osteoporosis Int* 6:419, 1996.

Shapiro F: Osteopetrosis: Current clinical considerations. *Clin Orthop* 294:34, 1993.

Tsuchiya H, Tomita K, et al: Shepherd's crook deformity with an intracapsular femoral neck fracture in fibrous dysplasia. *Clin Orthop* 310:160, 1995.

Fractures and Joint Injuries

Alho A, Ekeland A, et al: Locked intramedullary nailing for displaced tibial shaft fractures. *J Bone Joint Surg* 72B:805, 1990.

Andersen K, Jensen PO, et al: Treatment of clavicular fractures: Figure-of-eight bandage versus a simple sling. *Acta Orthop Scand* 58:71,1987.

Antich-Adrover P, Marti-Garin D: External fixation and secondary intramedullary nailing of open tibial fractures: A randomized, prospective trial. *J Bone Joint Surg* 79B:433, 1997.

Arntz CT, Veith RG, et al: Fractures and fracture-dislocations of the tarsometatarsal joint. *J Bone Joint Surg* 70A:173, 1988.

Bach BR Jr, Jones GT, et al: Arthroscopy-assisted anterior cruciate ligament reconstruction using patellar tendon substitution: Two- to four-year follow-up results. *Am J Sports Med* 22:758, 1994.

Baumhauer JF, Alvarez RG: Controversies in treating talus fractures. *Orthop Clin North Am* 262:335, 1995.

Benson DR: Unstable thoracolumbar fractures, with emphasis on the burst fracture. *Clin Orthop* 280:14, 1988.

Bergman GD, Winquist RA, et al: Subtrochanteric fracture of the femur: Fixation using the Zickel nail. *J Bone Joint Surg* 69A:1032, 1987.

Bezes H, Massart P, et al: The operative treatment of intraarticular calcaneal fractures: Indications, technique, and results in 257 cases. *Clin Orthop* 290:55, 1993.

Biyani A, Ebraheim NA, et al: Thoracic spine fractures in patients older than 50 years. *Clin Orthop* 328:190, 1996.

Blick SS, Brumback RJ, et al: Compartment syndrome in open tibial fractures. *J Bone Joint Surg* 68A:1348, 1986.

Bohlman HH, Anderson PA: Anterior decompression and arthrodesis of the cervical spine: Long-term motor improvement: Part I. Improvement in incomplete traumatic quadriparesis. *J Bone Joint Surg* 74A:671, 1992.

Bolano LE, Grana WA: Isolated arthroscopic partial meniscectomy: Functional and radiographic evaluation at five years. *Am J Sports Med* 21:432, 1993.

Bone L, Bucholz R: The management of fractures in the patient with multiple trauma. *J Bone Joint Surg* 68A:945, 1986.

Bradford DS, McBride GG: Surgical management of thoracolumbar spine fractures with incomplete neurologic deficits. *Clin Orthop* 218:201, 1987.

Bray TJ, Smith-Hoefer E, et al: The displaced femoral neck fracture: Internal fixation versus bipolar endoprosthesis: Results of a prospective randomized comparison. *Clin Orthop* 230:127, 1988.

Bridle SH, Patel AD, et al: Fixation of intertrochanteric fractures of the femur: A randomized prospective comparison of the gamma nail and the dynamic hip screw. *J Bone Joint Surg* 73B:330, 1991.

Brittberg M, Lundahl A, et al: Treatment of deep cartilage defects in the knee with autologous chondrocyte transplantation. *N Engl J Med* 331:889, 1994.

Brumback RJ: The rationales of interlocking nailing of the femur, tibia, and humerus. *Clin Orthop* 324:292, 1996.

Buchko GM, Johnson DH: Arthroscopy-assisted operative management of tibial plateau fractures. *Clin Orthop* 332:29, 1996.

Caplan A, Carlson B, et al: Skeletal muscle, in Woo SL-Y, Buckwalter JA (eds): *Injury and Repair of the Musculoskeletal Soft Tissues.* Park Ridge, IL, American Academy of Orthopaedic Surgeons, 1988, p 213.

Cash JD, Hughston JC: Treatment of acute patellar dislocation. *Am J Sports Med* 16:244, 1988.

Caudle RJ, Stern PJ: Severe open fractures of the tibia. *J Bone Joint Surg* 69A:801, 1987.

Choi KY, Chan WS, et al: Percutaneous Kirschner-wire pinning for severely displaced distal radial fractures in children: A report of 157 cases. *J Bone Joint Surg* 77B:797, 1995.

Cooper RA, Brems JJ: The inferior capsular-shift procedure for multidirectional instability of the shoulder. *J Bone Joint Surg* 74A:1516, 1992.

Covey CD, Sapega AA: Injuries of the posterior cruciate ligament. *J Bone Joint Surg* 75A:1376, 1993.

Cruess RL, Kan K, Bassett CA: The effect of pulsing electromagnetic fields on bone metabolism in experimental disuse osteoporosis. *Clin Orthop* 173:245, 1983.

Cuomo F, Flatow EL, et al: Open reduction and internal fixation of two- and three-part displaced surgical neck fractures of the proximal humerus. *J Shoulder Elbow Surg* 1:287, 1992.

Dalal SA, Burgess AR, et al: Pelvic fracture in multiple trauma: Classification by mechanism is key to pattern of organ injury, resuscitative requirements and outcome. *J Trauma* 29:981, 1989.

Daniel DM, Stone ML, et al: Fate of the ACL-injured patient: A prospective outcome study. *Am J Sports Med* 22:632, 1994.

DeHaven KE, Arnoczky SP: Meniscus repair: Basic science, indications for repair, and open repair, in Schafer M (ed): *Instructional Course Lectures, 43.* Rosemont, IL, American Academy of Orthopaedic Surgeons, 1994, p 65.

Delamarter R, Hohl M: Ligament injuries associated with tibial plateau fractures. *Clin Orthop* 250:226, 1990.

Eaton RG, Malench MM: Volar plate arthroplasty of the proximal interphalangeal joint: A review of ten years' experience. *J Hand Surg (Am)* 5:260, 1980.

Georgiadis GM, Behrens FF, et al: Open tibial fractures with severe soft-tissue loss: Limb salvage compared with below-the-knee amputation. *J Bone Joint Surg* 75A:1431, 1993.

Gomez GA, Kreis DJ Jr, et al: Suspected vascular trauma of the extremities: The role of arteriography in extremity injuries. *J Trauma* 26:1005, 1986.

Grana WA, Buckley PD, et al: Arthroscopic Bankart suture repair. *Am J Sports Med* 21:348, 1993.

Heaps RJ, Degnan GG: A modification for the insertion of the Herbert screw in the fractured or nonunited scaphoid. *J Hand Surg* 21A:922, 1996.

Helfet DL, Koval K, et al: Intraarticular "pilon" fracture of the tibia. *Clin Orthop* 298:221, 1994.

Hooper GJ, Keddell RG, et al: Conservative management or closed nailing for tibial shaft fractures: A randomised prospective trial. *J Bone Joint Surg* 73B:83, 1991.

Hughes LO, Beaty JH: Fractures of the head and neck of the femur in children. *J Bone Joint Surg* 76A:283, 1994.

Jakob RP, Staubli HU, et al: The arthroscopic meniscal repair: Techniques and clinical experience. *Am J Sports Med* 16:137, 1988.

Johnson KD, Cadambi A, et al: Incidence of adult respiratory distress syndrome in patients with multiple musculoskeletal injuries: Effect of early operative stabilization of fractures. *J Trauma* 24:375, 1985.

Johnson RJ, Beynnon BD, et al: Current concepts review: The treatment of injuries of the anterior cruciate ligament. *J Bone Joint Surg* 74A:140, 1992.

Kifune M, Panjabi MM, et al: Fracture pattern and instability of thoracolumbar injuries. *Eur Spine J* 42:98, 1995.

Lansinger O, Bergman B, et al: Tibial condylar fractures: A twenty-year follow-up. *J Bone Joint Surg* 68A:13, 1986.

Letournel E: The treatment of acetabular fractures through the ilioinguinal approach. *Clin Orthop* 292:62, 1993.

Leung KS, Shen WY, et al: Interlocking intramedullary nailing for supracondylar and intercondylar fractures of the distal part of the femur. *J Bone Joint Surg* 73A:332, 1991.

Levine A, Edwards CC: Lumbar spine trauma, in Camins M, O'Leary P (eds): *The Lumbar Spine.* New York, Raven, 1987, p 183.

Lhowe DW, Hansen ST: Immediate nailing of open fractures of the femoral shaft. *J Bone Joint Surg* 70A:812, 1988.

Lipton HA, Wollstein R: Operative treatment of intraarticular distal radial fractures. *Clin Orthop* 327:110, 1996.

Lucas SE, Seligson D, et al: Intramedullary supracondylar nailing of femoral fractures: A preliminary report of the GSH supracondylar nail. *Clin Orthop* 296:200, 1993.

Mack GR, Bosse MJ, et al: The natural history of scaphoid non-union. *J Bone Joint Surg* 66A:504, 1984.

Mammi GI, Rocchi R, et al: The electrical stimulation of tibial osteotomies: Double-blind study. *Clin Orthop* 288:246, 1993.

Matheson GO, Clement DB, et al: Stress fractures in athletes: A study of 320 cases. *Am J Sports Med* 15:46, 1987.

Matta J, Merritt P: Displaced acetabular fractures. *Clin Orthop* 230:83, 1988.

Matta JM, Tornetta P III: Internal fixation of unstable pelvic ring injuries. *Clin Orthop* 329:129, 1996.

Mayo KA: Fractures of the talus: Principles of management and techniques of treatment. *Techn Orthop* 2:42, 1987.

McDonald MG, Burgess RC, et al: Ilizarov treatment of pilon fractures. *Clin Orthop* 325:232, 1996.

Michelson JD: Fractures about the ankle. *J Bone Joint Surg* 77A:142, 1995.

Mindrebo N, Shelbourne KD, et al: Outpatient percutaneous screw fixation of the acute Jones fracture. *Am J Sports Med* 21:720, 1993.

Muller ME, Allgower M, et al: *Manual of Internal Fixation,* 3d ed. Berlin, Springer-Verlag, 1991, p 28.

Nordqvist A, Petersson C: The incidence of fractures of the clavicle. *Clin Orthop* 300:127, 1994.

O'Driscoll SW, Keeley FW, Salter RB: Durability of regenerated articular cartilage produced by free autologous periosteal grafts in major full thickness defects in joint surfaces under the influence of continuous passive motion. A follow-up report at one year. *J Bone Joint Surg (Am)* 70:595, 1988.

Post M: Current concepts in the diagnosis of management of acromioclavicular dislocations. *Clin Orthop* 200:234, 1985.

Prokuski LJ, Saltzman C: Challenging fractures of the foot and ankle. *Radiol Clin North Am* 35:655, 1997.

Reckling FW: Unstable fracture-dislocations of the forearm (Monteggia and Galeazzi lesions). *J Bone Joint Surg* 64A:857, 1982.

Rieger H, Brug E: Fractures of the pelvis in children. *Clin Orthop* 336:226, 1997.

Robinson CM, Court-Brown CM, et al: Hip fractures in adults younger than 50 years of age: Epidemiology and results. *Clin Orthop* 312:238, 1995.

Rubin CT, McLeod KJ, Lanyon LE: Prevention of osteoporosis by pulsed electromagnetic fields. *J Bone Joint Surg (Am)* 71:411, 1989.

Sarmiento A, Gersten LM, et al: Tibial shaft fractures treated with functional braces: Experience with 780 fractures. *J Bone Joint Surg* 71B:602, 1989.

Sidor ML, Zuckerman JD, et al: Classification of proximal humerus fractures: The contribution of the scapular lateral and axillary radiographs. *J Shoulder Elbow Surg* 5:24, 1994.

Silva I Jr, Silver DM: Tears of the meniscus as revealed by magnetic resonance imaging. *J Bone Joint Surg* 70A:199, 1988.

Simonet WT, Cofield RH: Prognosis in anterior shoulder dislocation. *Am J Sports Med* 12:19, 1984.

Simpson NS, Jupiter JB: Complex fracture patterns of the upper extremity. *Clin Orthop* 318:43, 1995.

Stephenson JR: Treatment of displaced intra-articular fractures of the calcaneus using medial and lateral approaches, internal fixation, and early motion. *J Bone Joint Surg* 69A:115, 1987.

Tile M: Pelvic ring fractures: Should they be fixed? *J Bone Joint Surg* 70B:1, 1988.

Tornetta P III, Bergman M, et al: Treatment of grade IIIB open tibial fractures: A prospective randomised comparison of external fixation and non-reamed locked nailing. *J Bone Joint Surg* 76B:13, 1994.

Tscherne H, Lobenhoffer P: Tibial plateau fractures: Management and expected results. *Clin Orthop* 292:87, 1993.

Villar RN, Marsh D, et al: Three years after Colles' fracture: A prospective review. *J Bone Joint Surg* 69B:635, 1987.

Wehbe MA, Schneider LH: Mallet fractures. *J Bone Joint Surg* 66A:658, 1984.

Wheeler DL, Croy TJ, et al: Comparison of reconstruction nails for high subtrochanteric femur fracture fixation. *Clin Orthop* 338:231, 1997.

Whittle P, Russell TA, et al: Treatment of open fractures of the tibial shaft with the use of interlocking nailing without reaming. *J Bone Joint Surg* 74A:1162, 1992.

Zook EG, Guy RJ, et al: A study of nail bed injuries: Causes, treatment, and prognosis. *J Hand Surg* 9:247, 1984.

Zuckerman JD, Skovron ML, et al: Postoperative complications and mortality associated with operative delay in older patients who have a fracture of the hip. *J Bone Joint Surg* 77A:1551, 1995.

Diseases of Joints

Barrett WP, Franklin JL, et al: Total shoulder arthroplasty. *J Bone Joint Surg* 69A:865, 1987.

Boden SD, Dodge LD, et al: Rheumatoid arthritis of the cervical spine: A long-term analysis with predictors of paralysis and recovery. *J Bone Joint Surg* 75A:1282, 1993.

Boyd AD Jr, Ewald FC, et al: Long-term complications after total knee arthroplasty with or without resurfacing of the patella. *J Bone Joint Surg* 75A:674, 1993.

Brittberg M, Lindahl A, et al: Treatment of deep cartilage defects in the knee with autologous chondrocyte transplantation. *N Engl J Med* 331:889, 1994.

Callaghan JJ: Current concepts review: The clinical results and basic science of total hip arthroplasty with porous-coated prostheses. *J Bone Joint Surg* 75A:299, 1993.

Clark CR, Goetz DD, et al: Arthrodesis of the cervical spine in rheumatoid arthritis. *J Bone Joint Surg* 71A:381, 1989.

Culp RW, Eichenfield AH, et al: Lyme arthritis in children: An orthopaedic perspective. *J Bone Joint Surg* 69A:96, 1987.

Donnelly RE, Saltzman CL, et al: Modified chevron osteotomy for hallux valgus. *Foot Ankle Int* 15:642, 1994.

Ghazavi MT, Stockley I, et al: Reconstruction of massive bone defects with allograft in revision total knee arthroplasty. *J Bone Joint Surg* 791:17, 1997.

Goldberg VM, Figgie MP, et al: Use of a total condylar knee prosthesis for treatment of osteoarthritis and rheumatoid arthritis: Long-term results. *J Bone Joint Surg* 70A:802, 1988.

Guerra JJ, Steinberg ME: Distinguishing transient osteoporosis from avascular necrosis of the hip. *J Bone Joint Surg* 77A:616, 1995.

Harris ED Jr: Rheumatoid arthritis: Pathophysiology and implications for therapy. *N Engl J Med* 322:1277, 1990.

Heekin RD, Callaghan JJ, et al: The porous-coated anatomic total hip prosthesis, inserted without cement: Results after five to seven years in a prospective study. *J Bone Joint Surg* 75A:77, 1993.

Herndon WA, Knauer S, et al: Management of septic arthritis in children. *J Pediatr Orthop* 6:576, 1986.

Kavanagh BF, Wallrichs S, et al: Charnley low-friction arthroplasty of the hip: Twenty-year results with cement. *J Arthroplasty* 9:229, 1994.

Kuettner KE: Biochemistry of articular cartilage in health and disease. *Clin Biochem* 25:155, 1992.

Maderazo EG, Judson S, et al: Late infections of total joint prostheses: A review and recommendations for prevention. *Clin Orthop* 229:131, 1988.

Nelson CL, Evans RP, et al: A comparison of gentamycin-impregnated polymethylmethacrylate bead implantation to conventional parenteral antibiotic therapy in infected total hip and knee arthroplasty. *Clin Orthop* 295:96, 1993.

Paliard X, West SG, et al: Evidence for the effects of a superantigen in rheumatoid arthritis. *Science* 253:325, 1991.

Rorabeck CH, Bourne RB, et al: A double-blind study of 250 cases comparing cemented with cementless total hip arthroplasty: Cost-effectiveness and its impact on health-related quality of life. *Clin Orthop* 298:156, 1994.

Samuelson T, Olney B: Percutaneous pin fixation of chronic slipped capital femoral epiphysis. *Clin Orthop* 326:225, 1996.

Shaw BA, Kasser JR: Acute septic arthritis in infancy and childhood. *Clin Orthop* 257:212, 1990.

Skyhar MJ, Mubarak SJ: Arthroscopic treatment of septic knees in children. *J Pediatr Orthop* 7:647, 1987.

Sullivan PM, MacKenzie JR, et al: Total hip arthroplasty with cement in patients who are less than fifty years old: A sixteen to twenty-two-year follow-up study. *J Bone Joint Surg* 76A:863, 1994.

Tumors of the Musculoskeletal System

American Joint Commission on Cancer: Bone and soft tissues, in Beahrs OH, Myers MH (eds): *Manual for Staging of Cancer,* 3d ed. Philadelphia, JB Lippincott, 1988, p 123.

Bell GR: Surgical treatment of spinal tumors. *Clin Orthop* 335:54, 1997.

Bini SA, Gill K, et al: Giant cell tumor of bone: Curettage and cement reconstruction. *Clin Orthop* 321:245, 1995.

Campanacci M: *Bone and Soft Tissue Tumors.* Vienna, Springer-Verlag, 1986.

Capanna R, Dal Monte A, et al: The natural history of unicameral bone cyst after steroid injection. *Clin Orthop* 166:204, 1982.

Elias AD, Antman KH: Adjuvant chemotherapy for soft-tissue sarcoma: A critical appraisal. *Semin Surg Oncol* 4:59, 1988.

Enneking WF, Spanier SS, et al: A system for the surgical staging of musculoskeletal sarcoma. *Clin Orthop* 153:106, 1980.

Frassica FJ, Frassica DA, et al: Ewing sarcoma of the pelvis: Clinicopathological features and treatment. *J Bone Joint Surg* 75A:1457, 1993.

Goodlad JR, Fletcher CD, et al: Surgical resection of primary soft-tissue sarcoma: Incidence of residual tumor in 95 patients needing re-excision after local resection. *J Bone Joint Surg* 78B:658, 1996.

Harrington KD: Metastatic tumors of the spine: Diagnosis and treatment. *J Am Acad Orthop Surg* 1:76, 1993.

Hipp JA, Springfield DS, et al: Predicting pathologic fracture risk in the management of metastatic bone defects. *Clin Orthop* 312:120, 1995.

Huvos AG: *Bone Tumors: Diagnosis, Treatment, and Prognosis.* Philadelphia, WB Saunders, 1991.

Kaiser TE, Pritchard DJ, et al: Clinicopathologic study of sacrococcygeal chordoma. *Cancer* 53:2574, 1984.

Lokiec F, Ezra E, et al: Simple bone cysts treated by percutaneous autologous marrow grafting: A preliminary report. *J Bone Joint Surg* 78B:934, 1996.

Mankin HJ, Gebhardt MC, et al: Long-term results of allograft replacement in the management of bone tumors. *Clin Orthop* 324:86, 1996.

Mankin HJ, Mankin CJ, et al: The hazards of the biopsy, revisited. Members of the Musculoskeletal Tumor Society. *J Bone Joint Surg* 78A:656, 1996.

Marcove RC, Sheth DS, et al: The treatment of aneurysmal bone cyst. *Clin Orthop* 311:157, 1995.

McCollough WM, Parsons JT, et al: Radiation therapy for aggressive fibromatosis, *J Bone Joint Surg* 73A:717, 1991.

Mirra JM, Picci P, et al: *Bone Tumors: Clinical, Radiologic, and Pathologic Correlations.* Philadelphia, Lea & Febiger, 1989.

Mundy GR, Yoneda T: Facilitation and suppression of bone metastasis. *Clin Orthop* 312:34, 1995.

National Institutes of Health, Consensus Development Panel: Limb-sparing treatment of adult soft-tissue sarcomas and osteosarcomas. *JAMA* 254:1791, 1985.

O'Connor MI, Sim FH, et al: Limb salvage for neoplasms of the shoulder girdle: Intermediate reconstructive and functional results. *J Bone Joint Surg* 78A:1872, 1996.

O'Donnell RJ, Springfield DS, et al: Recurrence of giant-cell tumors of the long bones after curettage and packing with cement. *J Bone Joint Surg* 76A:1827, 1994.

Ortiz-Cruz E, Gebhardt MC, et al: The results of transplantation of intercalary allografts after resection of tumors: A long-term follow-up study. *J Bone Joint Surg* 79A:97, 1997.

Rougraff BT, Simon MA, et al: Limb salvage compared with amputation for osteosarcoma of the distal end of the femur: A long-term oncological, functional, and quality-of-life study. *J Bone Joint Surg* 76A:649, 1994.

Ruggieri P, De Cristofaro R, et al: Complications and surgical indications in 144 cases of nonmetastatic osteosarcoma of the extremities treated with neoadjuvant chemotherapy. *Clin Orthop* 295:226, 1993.

Sailer S, Harmon DC, et al: Ewing's sarcoma: Surgical resection as a prognostic factor. *Int J Radiat Oncol Biol Phys* 15:43, 1988.

Schreuder HW, Veth RP, et al: Aneurysmal bone cysts treated by curettage, cryotherapy and bone grafting. *J Bone Joint Surg* 79A:20, 1997.

Scully SP, Temple HT, et al: The surgical treatment of patients with osteosarcoma who sustain a pathologic fracture. *Clin Orthop* 324:227, 1996.

Simon MA: Current concepts review: Limb salvage for osteosarcoma. *J Bone Joint Surg* 70A:307, 1988.

Simon MA, Finn HA: Diagnostic strategy for bone and soft-tissue tumors. *J Bone Joint Surg* 75A:622, 1993.

Skrzynski MC, Biermann JS, et al: Diagnostic accuracy and charge-savings of outpatient core needle biopsy compared with open biopsy of musculoskeletal tumors. *J Bone Joint Surg* 78A:644, 1996.

Toni A, Neff JR, et al: The role of surgical therapy in patients with nonmetastatic Ewing's sarcoma of the limbs. *Clin Orthop* 286:225, 1993.

Weinstein JN: Spinal neoplasms, in Weinstein SL (ed): *The Pediatric Spine: Principles and Practice.* New York, Raven, 1994, p 887.

Wormer RB: The cellular biology of bone tumors. *Clin Orthop* 262:12, 1991.

Yasko AW, Lane JM: Current concepts review: Chemotherapy for bone and soft-tissue sarcomas of the extremities. *J Bone Joint Surg* 73A:1263, 1991.

Surgery of the Hand

Clayton A. Peimer

Philosophically and anatomically, the hand and brain uniquely identify *Homo sapiens.* Throughout history humankind's progress is measured through the evolution of a strong and mobile upper limb with an independently opposable thumb and the cognitive powers to use them. The balance, precision, and specialization of the hand give it a central role. The goal of surgical treatment of the hand is to retain maximum useful part length, independent, stable motion, and unimpaired mobility of sensate parts.

GENERAL CONSIDERATIONS

Examination

Prior records and diagnostic images may precisely define the extent, limitations, and duration of the patient's disorder, and the clinical course. The history should include information of relevant systemic disease such as diabetes, atherosclerosis, neurologic and psychiatric disorders, and other serious diseases or chronic diseases.

The examiner should use the patient's normal anatomy—the contralateral, uninvolved limb—to observe for differences in alignment, contour, and symmetry. Observing the hand and forearm at rest in pronation and in supination, should reveal any swelling, masses, erythema, ulceration, atrophy, anhidrosis, or excoriation (Fig. 42-1). The reproducibility of the patient's active participation in the examination process is important. Responses should be consistent; repeated efforts, such as in grip testing, should produce similar values. Accurate recording of information by the examiner is important (Fig. 42-2).

Light palpation provides information concerning excessive or absent sweating associated with anxiety or insensibility in particular zones, nerve distributions, dermatomes, or body parts. Variations in skin contour, texture, color, temperature, capillary refill, and hair characteristics offer information regarding circulation, nerve supply, masses, and joint swelling. Abnormal, injured, and scarred soft tissues can restrain joint motion, produce skin blanching with attempted active function, or cause visible

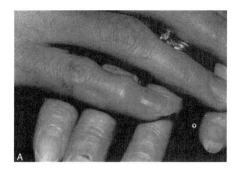
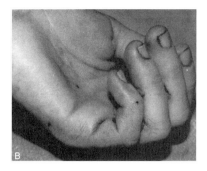
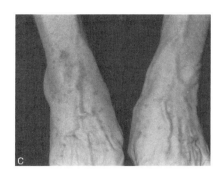

FIG. 42-1. Interruption of normal symmetry and comparison with a known normal render abnormal physical findings more apparent. *A.* Heberden's nodes are strikingly apparent in monarticular degenerative arthritis of the distal interphalangeal joint in the small finger of this woman with youthful, symmetrical, and aesthetically attractive hands. *B.* Interruption of the normal, progressive flexion cascade by absent DIP joint flexion in the middle and ring fingers strongly suggested the diagnosis in this woman, who had lacerated the flexor digitorum profundus tendon in both fingers. *C.* Ulnar wrist synovitis due to rheumatoid arthritis is more evident in the wrist on the left when compared side-by-side with the uninvolved wrist.

Name:
Hospital Number:

Date:
Major Hand: Right/Left
Symptomatic Hand: Right/Left

		ACTIVE MOTION									SENSIBILITY			
		MP		PIP		DIP		Distance From PULP to MPL (cm)		Pinprick		2-Point (mm) static/moving		
		Right	Left	Right	Left	Right	Left	Right	Left	Right	Left	Right	Left	
THUMB	Extension													
	Flexion													
INDEX	Extension													
	Flexion													
MIDDLE	Extension													
	Flexion													
RING	Extension													
	Flexion													
LITTLE	Extension													
	Flexion													

		Right	Left
WRIST	D.F.		
	P.F.		
	R.D.		
	U.D.		
THUMB	ABD		
	ADD		
	PRO		
	SUP		
PINCH (KG/LBS/PSI)			
GRIP (KG/LBS/PSI)			

		Right	Left
FOREARM	Pronation		
	Supination		
ELBOW	Extension		
	Flexion		
CIRCUMFERENCE (CM) 10 CM FROM EPICONDYLE OR AT MPL	Biceps		
	Forearm		
	Palm		

NOTE:

1. 0° = STRAIGHT LINE (FULL EXTENSION). Other figures refer to angles from full extension. Thus 30/70 = locks 30° of extension and flexes to 70°; 40/40 =ankylosed in 40° of flexion.

2. Passive motion, when different from active, is noted in parenthesis.

3. Motions not recorded are considered normal.

A

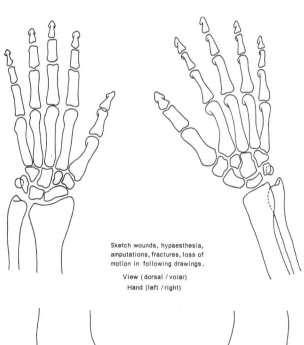

Sketch wounds, hypaesthesia, amputations, fractures, loss of motion in following drawings.

View (dorsal / volar)
Hand (left / right)

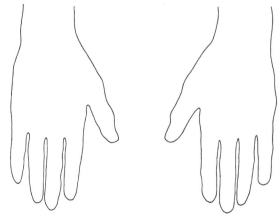

FIG. 42-2. *A* and *B.* Preprinted sheets for recording data from the history and physical examination can be tailored to the individual surgeon's practice to facilitate documentation.

B

"dimpling" of adherent deep structures, such as injured, repaired, or adherent tendons.

The nails and eponychial and paronychial cuticular tissues often mirror systemic disease as well as acute and chronic injury. Nails have a limited range of biologic responses. Splitting and fissuring, onycholysis, and onychorrhexis may reflect loss of nail adherence to the bed matrix after trauma, aging, or malnutrition. The transverse posttraumatic nail crease that parallels the proximal nail fold and advances with growth (Beau's line) represents a single alteration of nail metabolism at the time of trauma. It is common after injury but does not offer a poor prognosis. Multiple transverse grooves (Mee's lines) can occur with diseases such as Hodgkin's disease, malaria, and psoriasis and are normal in the latter part of pregnancy. Pigmented longitudinal bands may occur in melanoma, glomus tumor, and carpal tunnel syndrome. Nail bed pigmentation can be found with systemic sepsis, subungual infection, and benign and malignant tumors (Fig. 42-3).

Motion should be recorded with a small goniometer and strength with a dynamometer. Simple line sketches record sites of injury, swelling, part loss, or dysfunction and can precisely record and communicate findings (Fig. 42-4).

Imaging Studies. Diagnostic imaging includes traditional roentgenography, single- and multiple-phase technetium bone scans, computed tomography (CT), and magnetic resonance imaging (MRI). Most patients should receive plain radiographs in posteroanterior lateral and one or both oblique projections. Radiographs provide information with relatively intermediate sensitivity, high specificity, and reasonable cost. Diagnoses can be missed if only specialized and expensive evaluations such as trispiral or CT, MRI, or bone scans are used.

The x-ray beam must be centered on the part in question. Requesting an x-ray of the hand may be too general for diagnosing a problem in a specific finger. The physician evaluating the imaging studies should receive the history, physical findings, and a working differential diagnosis (Fig. 42-5).

TRAUMA

It is estimated that one-third of musculoskeletal trauma occurs to the upper limb. The annual economic impact from diminished

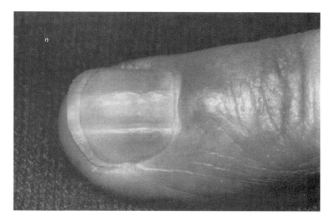

FIG. 42-3. The combination of a firm, translucent swelling of the proximal nail fold with a furrow of the nail distally is characteristic of a pedunculated ganglion (mucous cyst) from the distal interphalangeal joint that has produced chronic pressure on the nail matrix.

and lost hand and upper extremity function runs into the billions of dollars in the United States. The best care is delivered initially, when tissues are fresh and potentially can be salvaged, revascularized, and directly repaired, without the burdens of secondary scar tissue after delayed healing, osteoarticular degeneration, or infection. It is in the acute situation that success is greatest in achieving a potentially functional and aesthetically satisfactory result.

Skeletal Trauma

Forearm and Wrist. The forearm is a two-bone musculotendinous unit with complex biomechanical interactions. The osteoarticular and ligamentous connections of radius, ulna, interosseous membrane, and proximal and distal radioulnar joints allow the variety of hand placement and force transfers. The disruption of any one part of this anatomic and mechanical construct should cause the physician to search also for less obvious injuries elsewhere. Most suboptimal outcomes after forearm fractures can be related to failure to recognize injury to a proximal or distal region, often at the radioulnar joint, or failure to appreciate progressive loss of initial reduction after treatment. Severe neurovascular problems are uncommon, but, when present, they may be related to acute vascular compromise from trauma, immobilization, or compartment syndrome.

The distal radius forms a biconcave articular surface to seat the proximal row of carpal bones, scaphoid, lunate, and triquetrum. The radius articulates distally not only with the carpals but also with the ulna. The length and relationships of these several bones must be considered after trauma. The traumatized limb usually can be compared to a preinjury state by radiographs of the opposite side (Figs. 42-6 and 42-7).

Distal radius fractures have been variously classified, but a guide that integrates assessment of fracture patterns and treatment is useful (Table 42-1). Because there are many variations of fracture patterns in the distal radius, this system simplifies common characteristics and suggests treatment for each generic type of fracture. The treatment for a specific patient should be based not only on the pattern but also on age, hand dominance, occupation, social needs, cognitive and psychosocial factors, and living arrangements.

Radiographically, radius fractures are stable or unstable, displaced or nondisplaced, and with or without involvement of the radiocarpal or radioulnar articular surfaces. The condition of surrounding soft tissues and the presence of associated injury in other regions of the hand, forearm, and elbow are part of the decision-making process. Because these fractures most commonly occur from a fall on an outstretched hand, they result in a bending moment with the axial load through the radial metaphysis, and transient or complete associated neurovascular injuries, particularly to the median nerve at the carpal canal, are common. There may be an associated avulsion fracture of the ulnar styloid process.

The radius is more commonly displaced dorsally, as in Colles' fracture, with impaction, proximal displacement, and dorsal angulation of its distal articular surface. In such cases, the dorsal cortex of the distal fragment is comminuted and has significant prognostic implications for postreduction bone stability when managed entirely by external manipulation and cast or splint fixation (Fig. 42-8). Less frequently, a flexion or bending occurs in a fall, creating palmar displacement (Smith's fracture). When

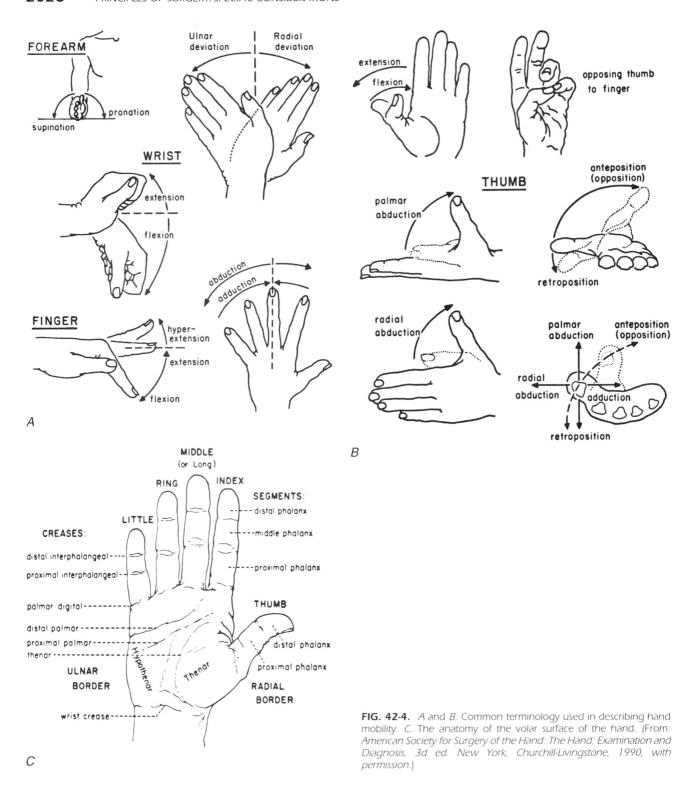

FIG. 42-4. *A* and *B.* Common terminology used in describing hand mobility. *C.* The anatomy of the volar surface of the hand. (From: *American Society for Surgery of the Hand: The Hand: Examination and Diagnosis, 3d ed. New York, Churchill-Livingstone, 1990, with permission.*)

intraarticular, either of these fracture patterns may have associated radiocarpal subluxation, but this problem is more often associated with the volar lip variant, Smith Type 3 or Barton's fracture pattern.

Even nondisplaced fractures can potentially displace during the healing process as resorption and bone remodeling occur at the fracture site. Maintaining a satisfactory degree of length and alignment during healing is important, and patients should be observed every 10 to 15 days with examination and x-rays. This injury may be associated with significant swelling, and circular cast immobilization should not be used initially; cast immobilization should be delayed until initial swelling has subsided. A sugar-tongs forearm and wrist splint may be applied that maintains bone length and alignment while simultaneously controlling forearm rotation without a rigid circumferential shell (Fig. 42-9).

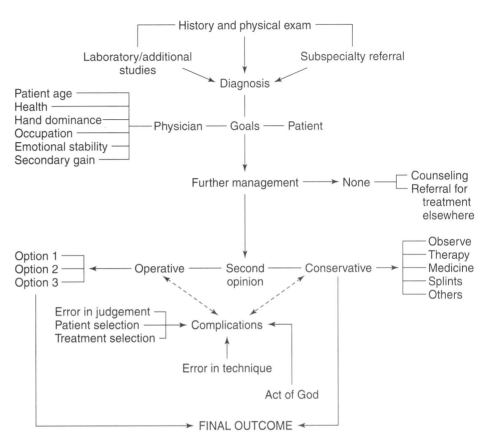

FIG. 42-5. Flow chart providing a graphic summary of the decision-making process. Note that both patient and physician play a necessary role in this process. Also note that a similarity in the goals and expectations of both patient and physician is central to this process.

The displaced dorsal fragment can be reduced comfortably under fracture block anesthesia, with or without addition of intravenous or intramuscular sedation. After sterile skin prepara-

tion a 22-gauge needle is introduced obliquely into the fracture site via overlying skin. Aspiration will reveal when the needle is within the fracture hematoma; 6 to 8 mL 1% mepivacaine hydrochloride (Carbocaine) or lidocaine hydrochloride (Xylocaine) without epinephrine can be injected to produce anesthesia in 10 to 15 min. The typical fracture, with dorsal displacement and angulation from an extension vector, can be reduced by distraction applied by allowing the arm to hang from finger traps placed on the index and middle fingers, with the arm itself serving as a counterweight. A dorsal-to-palmar force is applied over the area of displacement after the fragments have been disimpacted. The wrist is immobilized in neutral forearm rotation with only slight wrist flexion or ulnar deviation to avoid causing sec-

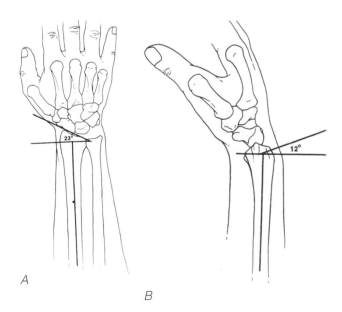

A

B

FIG. 42-6. *A.* This drawing of an anteroposterior view of the distal radius demonstrates its normal angle of inclination of 23 degrees in relationship to the long axis of the radius. *B.* A lateral view demonstrates the normal palmar tilt of 12 degrees of the lunate fossa in its orientation with the long axis of the radius.

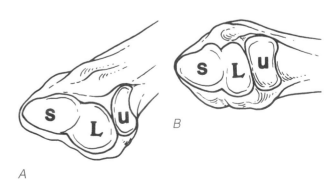

A

B

FIG. 42-7. *A and B.* The articular surface of the distal radius demonstrates articular facets for the scaphoid (S), the lunate (L), and the ulnar head in the sigmoid notch (U).

Table 42-1
Classification and Treatment of Distal Radius Fractures

Classification of Radius Fracture	Treatment Preference
I. Nonarticular, nondisplaced	Cast immobilization
II. Nonarticular, displaced	
A. Reducible, stable	Cast immobilization
B. Reducible, unstable	Percutaneous pins
C. Irreducible	Open reduction/external fixation
III. Articular, nondisplaced	Cast immobilization with or without percutaneous pins
IV. Articular, displaced	Closed reduction
A. Reducible, stable	Percutaneous pins (Kirschner wires) with or without external fixation
B. Reducible, unstable	Closed reduction/external fixation, with or without percutaneous pins, with or without bone graft
C. Irreducible	Open reduction/external fixation with percutaneous pins
D. Complex	Open reduction/external fixation plate fixation with bone graft (with or without percutaneous pins)

ondary compression of the median nerve. The sugar-tongs splint is applied. The width of the plaster should allow adequate space for tissue swelling. The dorsal and palmar edges of the splint should not touch each other. For most adults, a 3-inch plaster width is adequate, but in large individuals 4-inch plaster may be needed, which is applied over generous soft-tissue padding. After reduction and splint application, x-rays are obtained to record the reduction. If fracture realignment is incomplete, or if significant intraarticular displacement (1 mm or more) osteoarticular incongruity remains, repeated manipulative reduction or an alternate method of treatment should be considered.

Patients should have a neurovascular examination before manipulative reduction, and their median nerve sensory status should be assessed again after the application of the plaster splint. Fracture position and neurovascular status must be followed carefully.

After 7 to 10 days, the patient has repeat x-rays. Elevation and digital motion will have diminished swelling significantly in many cases, and the splint may be replaced with a circular cast. Some circumstances may dictate snugging the splint with a replacement circular gauze overwrap and delaying cast application an additional week or two. In young patients, a long arm cast may be preferable; in the older individual, the risk of elbow stiffness is significant, and prolonged immobilization of that joint is not advisable. Elevation of the hand plus finger mobilization and a therapy program that is directed to the entire upper limb, including the shoulder, is started at this time. When the splint is changed into a cast, x-rays are obtained after cast application. Radiographs are repeated every 2 weeks to monitor healing and observe for collapse, angulation, and displacement (Fig. 42-10). Most casts can be removed 6 weeks after trauma, when radiographs demonstrate obvious new bone formation and the fracture region is relatively nontender. If no motion or significant pain is elicited at the fracture site, cast immobilization may be discontinued. Therapists can fabricate a custom thermoplastic resting/protective splint and active motion exercises can begin (Fig. 42-11). The custom splint can generally be discontinued after another 2 to 4 weeks, depending on patient comfort and progress in rehabilitation. Motion exercises for the hand and wrist are followed by progressive strengthening, increasing activities of daily living, and return to function.

Unstable fractures of the distal radius are treated with percutaneous or open fracture pinning under fluoroscopic monitoring. Many of these fractures require an external fixation device to prevent progressive collapse and loss of alignment at the comminuted fracture line. When fractures are significantly impacted, areas of obvious bone loss within the submetaphyseal region after reduction may require bone graft or bone substitute to prevent delayed union or nonunion. Management by open reduction, with the combination of external and internal fixation with plates and screws, is appropriate for the more severe subgroup,

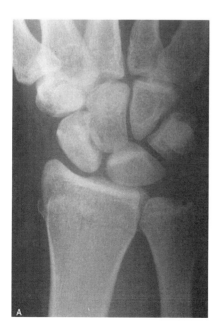

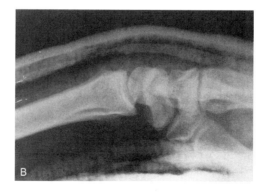

FIG. 42-8. *A and B.* This radiograph demonstrates a nonarticular, nondisplaced (type I) inherently stable fracture of the distal radius.

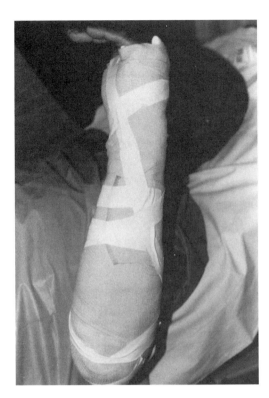

FIG. 42-9. *Application of sugar-tongs splint. The splint can be wrapped with a gently applied Ace bandage, following which full flexion of the metacarpophalangeal joints must be demonstrated.*

most often those of younger age whose injuries are the result of high-impact trauma, such as those sustained in vehicular accidents and mishaps with heavy machinery (Figs. 42-12, 42-13, and 42-14).

Carpal Bone Fractures. The eight carpal bones have a large proportion of their surfaces covered with articular cartilage, a fact that has two clinical implications. First, the limited periosteal attachment offers a tenuous blood supply; after fracture one of the fragments is potentially at risk for avascular necrosis. Second, most carpal fractures are intraarticular injuries. The displaced fracture often needs surgical repair to avoid secondary arthritis from joint surface incongruity. The pattern of carpal fracture or fracture dissociation may not be clearly discernible on standard posteroanterior and lateral radiographs, and oblique views, carpal tunnel projection, and other views may be necessary. If results are still equivocal, trispiral tomography or CT should demonstrate the fracture patterns and fragment positions. When the question of whether or not a fracture is present, a frequent problem with injuries about the radial side of the carpus, especially the scaphoid, the use of technetium bone scan 72 h after trauma is diagnostic.

Scaphoid Fracture. Nearly two-thirds of all carpal fractures are of the scaphoid. This injury occurs most often in males aged 15 to 30 years. Scaphoid fractures occur most commonly through the middle third of the waist or at the juncture of the middle and proximal poles. Diagnosis requires clinical and imaging information. After a fall on the outstretched hand, the patient's wrist is tender at the anatomic snuff box, the hollow between the thumb extensor tendons on the radial aspect of the

wrist, just dorsal and distal to the styloid process of the radius. Pain is elicited and symptoms reproduced with direct pressure over the tuberosity of the scaphoid at the base of the thenar eminence and with passive wrist motion. Routine radiographs in posteroanterior, lateral, and oblique views along with a posteroanterior projection in ulnar deviation to elongate the scaphoid helps to visualize the fracture. If initial radiographs are normal but the history and physical examination suggest the possibility of scaphoid fracture, continuous immobilization in a thumb spica splint or cast is advised. Repeat radiographs in 2 to 3 weeks or technetium bone scan after 72 h will make the diagnosis.

Fracture configuration (Fig. 42-15) and location affect stability and lability of the blood supply. The proximal pole of the scaphoid is supplied from vessels entering the distal two-thirds. Fracture of the proximal third or a smaller fragment risks avascularity in the small proximal fragment, resulting in nonunion and secondary arthrosis. Nondisplaced scaphoid fractures treated with adequate immobilization have a union rate of 90 to 95 percent. Displaced fractures, defined as displacement of 1.0 mm or more, are associated with avascular necrosis in one-half and nonunion in one-half of patients if not reduced and stabilized operatively. Scaphoid fracture fragment displacement of 2.0 mm or more should raise suspicion of an associated intercarpal ligament injury, such as transscaphoid perilunate instability or subluxation.

In the treatment of the nondisplaced, stable scaphoid fracture, one study demonstrated decreased time to union and decreased incidence of delayed and nonunion when long arm, above-elbow thumb spica casts were used for 6 weeks, followed by short arm spica cast for approximately 6 weeks. Immobilization of the wrist in slight flexion and radial deviation relaxes the volar radioscaphoid ligament. The thumb metaphalangeal joint should be included in the cast, at least during the initial 6 weeks. Open reduction and internal fixation can be done effectively with an interfragmentary lag compression screw or with Kirschner wires for all displaced fractures. The screw technique is more stable and allows earlier mobilization.

The use of percutaneous compression screws for immediate internal stabilization of the acute but nondisplaced fracture is increasingly popular outside the United States. Limited experience suggests a more rapid course with decreased acute and long-term disability without significant increase in complications. Interfragmentary screw technique for this bone is technically demanding.

When immediate postinjury imaging does not clearly demonstrate the presence of fracture, immobilization and additional imaging information by standard radiographs in 2 weeks or bone scan after 3 days are necessary to make the diagnosis. Fracture displacement is unacceptable, and 1 to 2 mm of malposition, angulation, or any intercarpal collapse should prompt open repair. Less than 5 percent of nondisplaced fractures result in nonunion, which is defined as absent x-ray evidence of healing 4 to 6 months after injury, while a 50 percent nonunion rate for displaced fractures occurs.

Other Carpal Fractures. The *lunate* most commonly fractures secondary to idiopathic avascular necrosis or lunatomalacia (Kienböck's disease) without a history of acute trauma. The lunate is more radiodense on posteroanterior projection radiographs. Mild radiodensity is not uncommon after carpal injuries and should not be confused with Kienböck's disease. Simple, acute lunate fractures are not common. They should be treated

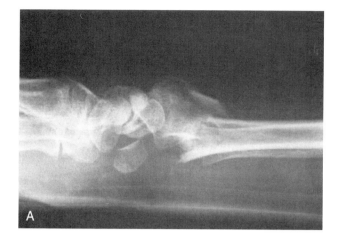

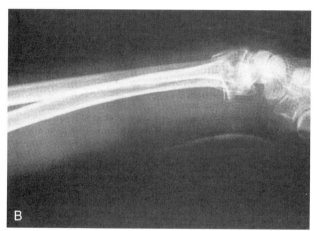

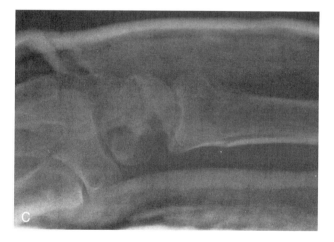

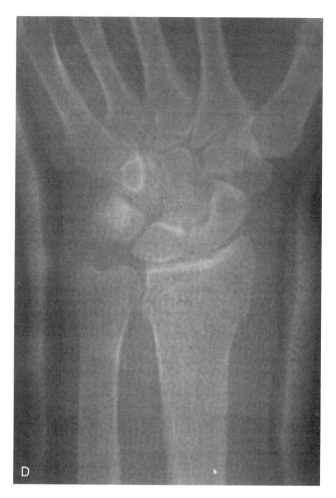

FIG. 42-10. *A and B. A type II, displaced but stable, extraarticular fracture of the distal radius has been treated with closed reduction and application of a sugar-tongs splint. C and D. Ten days later a conversion has been made to a long arm cast, and x-rays demonstrate maintenance of length and alignment.*

with immobilization when nondisplaced; open treatment rarely is required.

Fractures of the *capitate* are uncommon. The proximal pole, like that of the scaphoid, receives its blood supply from vessels that enter distally. Capitate neck fractures are at potential risk for avascular necrosis. When avascular necrosis occurs, usually it is incomplete, that is, temporary. Capitate head collapse is uncommon.

Isolated fractures of the *trapezium* and *trapezoid* are uncommon. Injuries to these bones are often associated with intraarticular fractures of the base of the first metacarpal. Open reduction

is often necessary, with internal fixation by Kirschner wires or compression screws.

Fractures of the *pisiform* usually are secondary to a direct blow to the hypothenar eminence. The fractured pisiform is best seen in carpal tunnel projection radiographs or CT imaging. Excision may be required for displaced fractures, nonunion, malunion, and secondary arthritis. There are two types of fracture of the *hamate:* those involving the body and those of the hamulus (hook). Fractures of the body of the hamate are difficult to diagnose on plain radiographs; imaging may require several oblique projections or CT scan. The patient may have pain re-

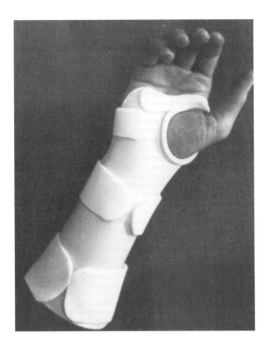

FIG. 42-11. A removable thermoplastic splint with Velcro fasteners is molded to the palmar aspect of the patient's hand and wrist. This provides support between periods of active range-of-motion exercise in the initial mobilization period.

ferred to the dorsal wrist with fractures of the body or hook. Fractures of the body of the hamate heal with immobilization for 4 to 6 weeks. Fractures of the hamulus are more common and usually are the result of a direct force transmitted into the base of the palm from a grasped object. The palm is tender to direct pressure over the hamate; sometimes the discomfort is reported as dorsal. Secondary ulnar neuropathy at Guyon's canal also may be present. Late flexor tendon ruptures have been reported, especially in those whose undiagnosed palmar pain syndrome is treated with repeated steroid injections. Routine radiographs and carpal tunnel views may be negative; CT scan can make the diagnosis. The acute hook fracture should heal in a short arm cast; displaced fractures and symptomatic nonunions are most efficiently treated with excision of the hamulus and smoothing of the fracture base.

Carpal Dislocations and Instabilities. The radiocarpal and intercarpal articulations are not inherently stable on the basis of their osseous anatomy; it is the integration of osteoligamentous anatomy that secures the complex kinematics of wrist function (Fig. 42-16). Most carpal dislocations are caused by an acute axial load with wrist hyperextension. The primary dislocation occurs at the midcarpal joint with dorsal displacement of the capitate. When the capitate displaces, the scaphoid must fracture or its ligaments will tear, allowing it to rotate from a relatively horizontal position to one of vertical malalignment with the proximal pole rotating dorsally. This configuration is called *dorsal perilunate dislocation* (Figs. 42-17, 42-18, and 42-19). These serious and unstable intraarticular injuries, with or without scaphoid fracture or triquetral break, require careful reduction and internal fixation. The majority require open reduction. Direct trauma to the median nerve from impact, by secondary stretching resulting from dorsal displacement of the carpus, or from acute bleeding and swelling within the carpal tunnel, should be elucidated by neurovascular examination. Carpal instabilities of all types should be treated aggressively to prevent chronic instability and dysfunction (Fig. 42-20).

Metacarpal Fractures. Because of their subcutaneous location and relatively rigid proximal articulations, the metacarpals represent one-third of hand and wrist fractures. Failure to recon-

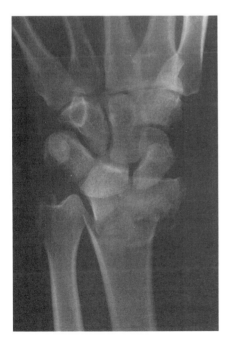
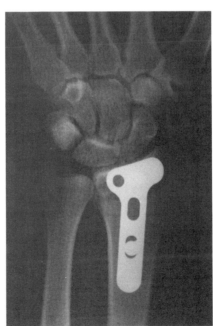
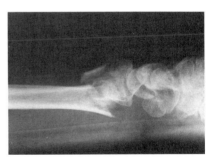
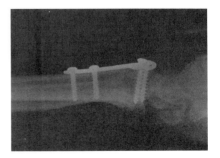

FIG. 42-12. Radiographs of this unstable displaced fracture demonstrate return of length, angle or inclination, and palmar tilt using this dorsal buttress plate.

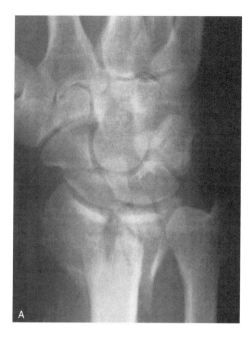

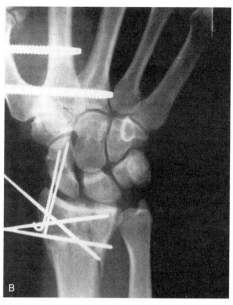

FIG. 42-13. *A. A comminuted unstable intraarticular fracture of the distal radius is seen combined with a transverse fracture of the scaphoid waist. B. The scaphoid fracture has been anatomically fixed with two Kirschner wires, and the distal radius fracture has been managed with a combination of external fixation, internal fixation, and bone grafting.*

stitute the metacarpals may lead to permanent functional deficit. Complication rates after extensive exposure for plate fixation can be high, and the risk of additional injury must be weighed against outcomes expected with conservative measures.

The goal is early restoration of hand function to prevent stiffness. Whether internal or external immobilization is used is immaterial, as long as bone length and articular relationships are preserved and soft-tissue management and therapy techniques can be instituted rapidly.

The metacarpals form a rigid longitudinal arch because of their convexity dorsally. There also is a dynamic transverse arch based on the stable and mobile carpometacarpal articulations of the thumb and those of the ring and little fingers. The thenar and hypothenar muscles mobilize these arches, allowing precision and strength in hand use. Because of stable proximal and distal ligamentous support, isolated fractures of the central third and fourth metacarpals—the middle and ring fingers—are less

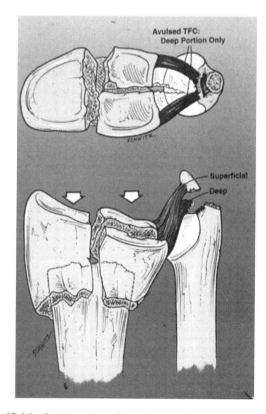

FIG. 42-14. *Both insertions of the triangular fibrocartilage (the styloid and foveal insertions) may be severely damaged when plain x-rays reveal a displaced ulnar styloid fracture through its base. The clinician must thoroughly appreciate the magnitude of soft-tissue injury when assessing x-rays after wrist trauma.*

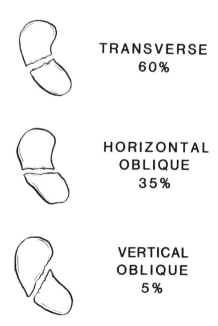

**TRANSVERSE
60%**

**HORIZONTAL
OBLIQUE
35%**

**VERTICAL
OBLIQUE
5%**

FIG. 42-15. *Russe's classification of scaphoid fractures.*

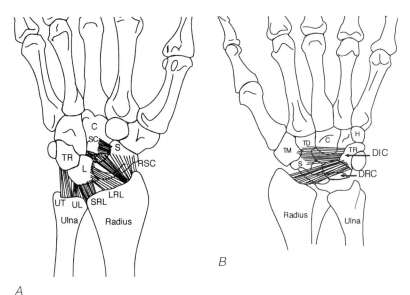

FIG. 42-16. Ligamentous anatomy of the wrist. *A.* Palmar wrist ligaments. RSC = radioscaphocapitate; LRL = long radiolunate; SRL = short radiolunate; UL = ulnolunate; UT = ulnotriquetral; SC = scaphocapitate. The space between the LRL and SRL is where the radioscapholunate ligament (ligament of Testut), now known to be a neurovascular pedicle, enters the radiocarpal joint. Carpals: S = scaphoid; L = lunate; TR = triquetrum; C = capitate. *B.* Dorsal wrist ligaments. DRC = dorsal radiocarpal; DIC = dorsal intercarpal. Carpals: S = scaphoid, TM = trapezium; TD = trapezoid; C = capitate; H = hamate; TR = triquetrum.

likely to shorten, rotate, and angulate. Spiral and oblique fractures that displace do so with shortening and rotation. Metacarpal shortening also may occur by direct bone loss or angular deformity. Midshaft angulation produces a more serious deformity (Fig. 42-21).

Pain and swelling are the hallmarks of metacarpal fractures, as the loose dorsal tissues allow large amounts of edema fluid and fracture hematoma to accumulate. The bony prominence of an angulated fracture apex is always located dorsally because of the pull of the interosseous intrinsic muscles. A skin laceration often connotes an open fracture and mandates surgical treatment. This is important in metacarpal fractures caused by a tooth impact, as in a fight; this results in a contaminated puncture wound at the fracture site or at the metacarpophalangeal joint. Patients with human or animal bites require surgical irrigation of the fracture site or joint plus high-dose antibiotics.

Rotational alignment of a metacarpal fracture is best assessed with the fingers flexed at the metacarpophalangeal joint. With an uncooperative juvenile patient or an unconscious patient, the

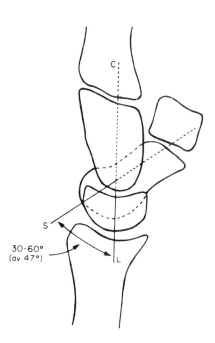

FIG. 42-17. Lateral wrist view demonstrates a normal scapholunate angle of 30 to 60 degrees. The capitolunate angle should be less than 30 degrees. Here both lunate and capitate axes are coaxial.

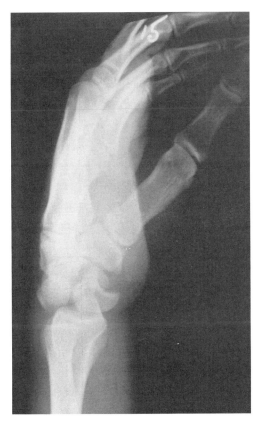

FIG. 42-18. Lateral radiograph of a dorsal perilunate dislocation.

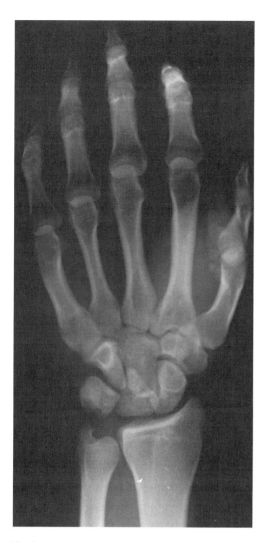

FIG. 42-19. *Anteroposterior radiograph of a dorsal perilunate dislocation.*

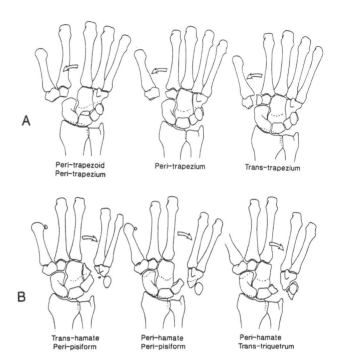

FIG. 42-20. The most common types of axial disruption of the carpus. *A.* Axial-radial disruption. *B.* Axial-ulnar disruption. *(Modified from: Garcia-Elias M, Dobyns JH, Cooney WP, Linscheid RL: Traumatic axial dislocations of the carpus. J Hand Surg 14A:449, 1989, with permission.)*

fifth metacarpals. Closed reduction may be achieved through the combination of direct and counterpressure applied with the finger flexed (Fig. 42-22). The hand should not be immobilized in the position depicted for manipulation. Open reduction usually is not necessary, but when the fracture is unstable and residual or recurring angulation is not acceptable, then internal fixation is required. Metacarpal shaft fractures should be protected when position and angulation are acceptable, but repaired when they

wrist can be passively flexed and extended, with the resulting extrinsic flexor and extensor effect on digital alignment observed. Malrotation or active flexion produces a degree of visible digital overlap. Malrotation and radial-ulnar angulation interferes with hand function and should be corrected.

Fractures of the metacarpal heads are less common, usually the result of direct trauma. The second and fifth metacarpals are most commonly traumatized, with a 3:1 male predominance. As these are intraarticular injuries, a step-off of 1.0 mm or more is significant. Unstable fractures are fixed with pins, screws, or plates.

The metacarpal neck is the most common fracture site. As with displaced and angulated fractures, the cortex on the angulated side usually is comminuted. The normal pull of the intrinsic muscles further flexes the head fragment, making it difficult to maintain reduction. The degree of angulation and the metacarpal involved determines the best treatment for the specific fracture. Because the second and third carpometacarpal joints are rigid, no more than 10 to 15 degrees of palmar angulation of the distal fragment is acceptable. Considerably more angulation (30 to 50 degrees) may be acceptable in the neck region of the fourth and

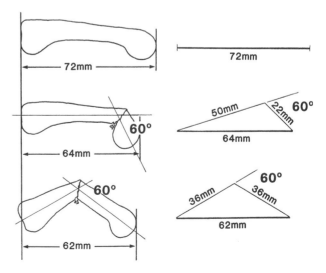

FIG. 42-21. The effect of location of a metacarpal fracture on shortening. 60-degree angulation of a midshaft fracture will produce more shortening than an equivalent angulation at the metacarpal neck.

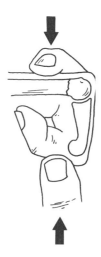

FIG. 42-22. The Jahss "90–90" maneuver for reduction of metacarpal neck fractures. Dorsally directed force along the proximal phalanx (arrows) serves to reduce neck angulation, while rotational control is gained via tightening of collateral ligaments in metacarpophalangeal flexion.

are not. Spiral and oblique fractures undergo malrotation and displacement because of the normal forces of the flexor and extensor tendons and hand intrinsics. Those that are not initially displaced or rotated must be carefully observed. Internal fixation allows more rapid soft-tissue mobilization and often can be treated with percutaneous intermetacarpal pin technique, local block anesthesia, and fluoroscopic monitoring. Some of these fractures require open reduction for fixation (Figs. 42-23, 42-24, and 42-25).

Intraarticular carpometacarpal fracture-dislocations are of functional significance in the mobile fourth and fifth metacarpal-

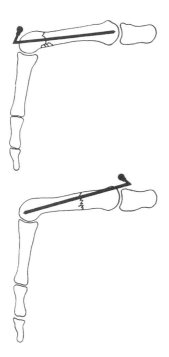

FIG. 42-23. Two methods for percutaneous or open intramedullary fixation of metacarpal fractures.

hamate saddle joints. These mobile joints have tendon insertions around the bases of the metacarpal and periarticular tissue that allow displacement (Figs. 42-26 and 42-27). Reduction is best maintained with internal fixation. Some require open reduction and fixation to restore accurate osteoarticular alignment.

Delayed union and nonunion of closed metacarpal injuries are uncommon. Bone consolidation should be discernible by radiograph within 12 to 16 weeks. Immobilization of the hand for several months seriously risks compromising function. Nonunion may be associated with inadequate immobilization, loss of bone substance, infection, or disruption of blood supply. Digital impairment may result from tendon adhesions directly over a fracture site, secondary small-joint contracture from prolonged immobilization, or scarring of traumatized intrinsic muscles. Simultaneous skeletal stabilization and small-joint mobilization should be achieved.

Phalangeal Fractures. The goal of phalangeal fracture treatment is restoration of anatomy, bone healing, and full functional recovery. Dysfunctional angulation and rotation are not acceptable. Stabilized fracture anatomy must allow rapid mobilization. Each method of fracture care has relative advantages and risks. Less invasive methods may offer less stability, but they inflict less soft-tissue damage. An algorithm for care is outlined in Fig. 42-28. When operation is required, the least traumatic method should be used to avoid violation of gliding structures when possible. The patient's active participation in a rehabilitation program encompassing supervised therapy, custom splinting, and home exercises is critical for recovery of function. Proximal interphalangeal joint motion, particularly extension, can be difficult to regain if an injured, swollen finger is immobilized in flexion. Scar can tether the extensor tendons or prevent the flexors from gliding, impairing grasp and manipulation and preventing return to preinjury employment.

When Kirschner wires are used, they may be buried, and they may then be retrieved in the outpatient setting under local anesthesia after 4 weeks. Sufficient fracture healing usually has occurred by then despite the delayed appearance of significant interfragmentary callus on radiographs. When Kirschner wires are left external to the skin, as in juveniles, pins must be capped and cared for meticulously. Screws and plates usually are not removed until at least 6 to 12 months after fracture healing. Small bone plates and screws need not be removed except to treat symptoms from the hardware.

Finger Ligament Injuries. *Metacarpophalangeal (MP) Joint.* MP joint dislocations can be managed by closed means through gentle reduction and splinting under local anesthesia. If significant residual collateral ligament instability in a particular finger is present, surgical repair is necessary. The small subgroup of irreducible fractures requires operative repair. Patients with acute collateral injuries may have a malrotated finger (Fig. 42-29) because of rotation about the intact ligament. The ruptured ligament region is swollen and tender. Evaluation by gentle passive stress should be done with the MP joint in flexion, a position in which the collateral ligaments are normally tight. Some perform simultaneous radiographic evaluation during this passive stress. Patients with particular discomfort who cannot tolerate soft-tissue stress in order to evaluate joint stability can be examined after 1.0 mL of local anesthetic agent is injected into the joint. Dorsal dislocations that are irreducible are characterized by dimpling of the palmar skin over a prominent met-

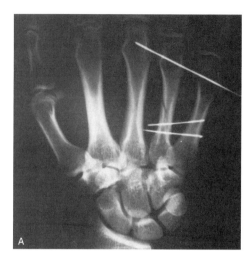

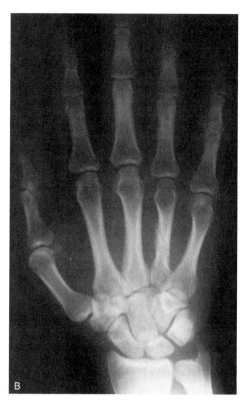

FIG. 42-24. *A.* Percutaneous fixation of short oblique metacarpal shaft fracture. Fixation of both the proximal and distal shaft fragments is recommended for stability in fractures of the fourth and fifth metacarpal shafts. *B.* Uneventful healing at 6 weeks.

acarpal head. Interposed soft tissues can prevent joint reduction. In these cases surgical treatment is required (Fig. 42-30).

Thumb MP joint injuries result from axial load and angular displacement. These injuries often occur when the patient jams the thumb into an object while falling. Disruption of the ulnar collateral ligament of the thumb is called *gamekeeper's thumb,* although the term was originally applied only to chronic ulnar collateral instability. A larger percentage of the injuries are caused by jamming the thumb into snow in a fall while skiing. Collateral laxity at the thumb MP joint is dysfunctional and painful and may lead to late arthritis. After plain radiographs fail to detect the presence of intraarticular fractures, the thumb is carefully examined in about 30 degrees of MP flexion, gently and progressively stressing the suspect collateral ligament (Fig. 42-31). Radiographs may be obtained simultaneously (Fig. 42-32); the stress radiograph is best performed by the examining physician. Treatment of incomplete collateral ligament injuries without associated instability is best done closed, with cast immobilization for approximately 4 weeks, followed by custom-splint immobilization. Soreness may persist for several months.

Complete disruption of the ulnar or radial collateral ligament of the thumb MP joint should be repaired and protected by temporary pin fixation of the joint, which is most likely to give a

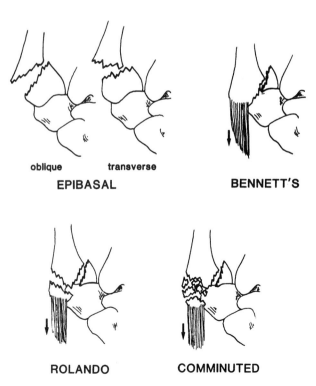

oblique transverse
EPIBASAL **BENNETT'S**

ROLANDO **COMMINUTED**

FIG. 42-26. Four different types of metacarpal base fractures.

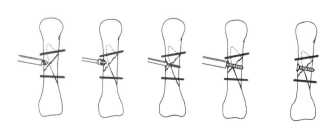

FIG. 42-25. Steps for placement of provisional Kirschner wires and interfragmentary screws.

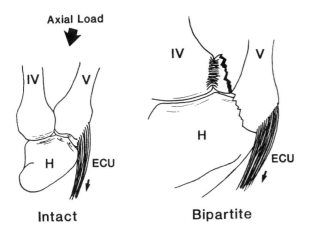

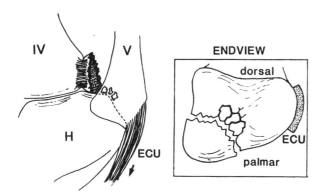

Comminuted

FIG. 42-27. Types of fifth carpometacarpal fracture-dislocations. A bipartite fracture-dislocation, which results from a dorsally directed load on the fifth metacarpal shaft, leaves a minor fragment attached to the fourth metacarpal by the intermetacarpal ligaments. The comminuted fracture-dislocation is a result of axial loading, and the radial facet of the hamate causes a variable degree of central impaction of the fifth metacarpal base.

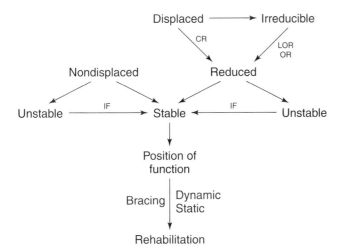

FIG. 42-28. Phalangeal fracture management algorithm. CR = closed reduction; LOR = limited open reduction; OR = open reduction; IF = internal fixation.

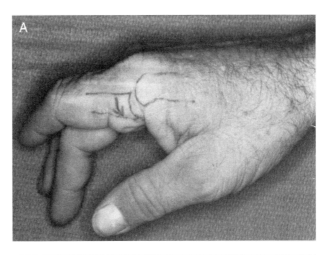

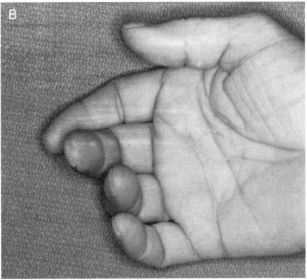

FIG. 42-29. Rupture of the radial collateral ligament of the index MP joint. A. Rupture of the radial collateral ligament allows the radial base of the proximal phalanx to subluxate palmarward and to rotate around the remaining ulnar collateral ligament. B. The rotation at the base of the proximal phalanx becomes magnified over the length of the digit, causing the index finger to overlap the long finger.

better result and shorter period of disability than secondary reconstruction.

Proximal Interphalangeal (PIP) Joint. The tightly congruent osteoarticular contours of the proximal interphalangeal joint make restoration of stable alignment of disrupted or displaced structures essential, allowing safe institution of early mobilization. Stiffness, rather than instability, is the outcome that must be avoided after trauma in the region of the PIP joint. Most dorsal and lateral PIP dislocations can be treated by closed reduction and should be stable. Immobilization for 10 to 15 days allows the patient to recover from the acute posttraumatic effects before a protected mobilization program is started, with buddy tapes to an adjacent finger. Joints without an actual history of displacement, deformity, or reduction by patient, coach, trainer, or physician may have considerable swelling and stiffness if not mobilized early. Dislocations with fractures are more likely unstable (Figs. 42-33 and 42-34). Postoperative immobilization that

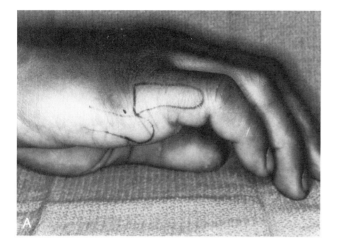
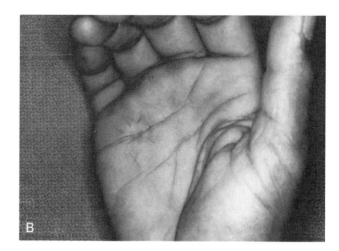
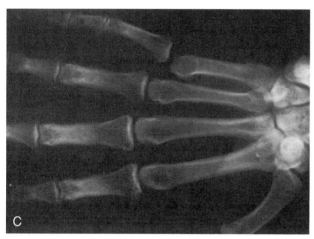
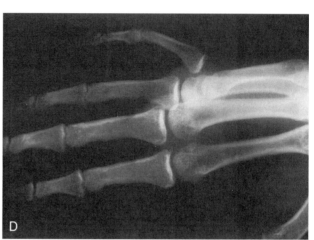

FIG. 42-30. *Dorsal complex (irreducible) dislocation of the MP joint. A. The proximal phalanx rests in bayonet apposition on the dorsal aspect of the metacarpal head. The resulting digital deformity is subtle. B. A palmar skin dimple (outlined here with small radiating marks) is a pathognomonic sign of a complex dislocation. C. The anteroposterior x-ray demonstrates joint-space widening and subtle subluxation. D. An oblique film clearly demonstrates the dorsal dislocation.*

inadvertently stresses an osteoarticular fragment results in post-traumatic instability (Fig. 42-35). The combination of joint surface impaction and ligament disruption have the worst prognosis (Fig. 42-36). These fracture-dislocations have an ultimate outcome that is often unsatisfactory.

Palmar (Volar) PIP Dislocations. In volar PIP dislocations the middle phalanx is displaced palmarward, sometimes resulting in serious instability. This PIP dislocation results from the combination of axial load and palmar vector force, most often during sports activities (Fig. 42-37). Often unrecognized is that this trauma has an associated disruption of the central slip of the extensor tendon and one collateral ligament. Closed reduction and pinning, or open reduction for the irreducible variant, with prolonged postoperative therapy is the rule.

Distal Interphalangeal (DIP) Joint. The DIP joint must be comfortable and stable for precision pinch and power grip. Ideally, rehabilitation after DIP joint trauma restores a pain-free and stable arc of motion, but this is not always possible. Some compromise between stability, motion, and symptoms may be necessary; functional position, near extension, and DIP joint stability are the most critical to regaining a useful hand. Collateral

ligament injuries and dorsal or palmar dislocations may occur at this level. Stable joints for which closed reduction is possible need not be pinned. Percutaneous fixation under fluoroscopic guidance, with maintenance of pin fixation for 4 to 5 weeks, is a useful adjunct, because it allows the rest of the hand to be rapidly mobilized. It is preferable to bury pins in adults and to remove them in an outpatient setting using local anesthesia.

Swelling and discomfort persist after DIP and PIP injury for 3 to 6 months in most patients. Functional recovery of mobility and power occurs slowly. Protection during sports and similar activities may be needed for 6 months or more. It should be explained early to patients that the joint is likely to be sore or swollen for some time; the sooner patients understand this, the more likely they are to accept their role in recovery.

Fingertip Injuries. Conservative treatment, such as healing by secondary intention of fingertip amputations, often results in painful scarring and deformity. There are several requirements for a satisfactory outcome after fingertip amputation: (1) Optimum functional finger length must be maintained, and additional shortening during or as a complication of treatment must be

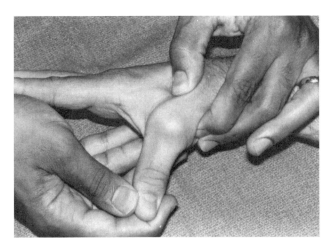

FIG. 42-31. Laxity of 30 degrees more than the uninjured thumb measured in neutral and 30 degrees of flexion are strongly suggestive of a complete ulnar collateral ligament tear. There is no "end point" to the radial deviation of the phalanx.

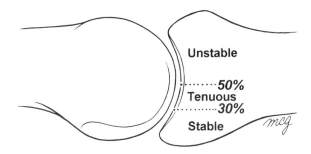

FIG. 42-33. Classification of PIP fracture-dislocations. Stable (type I) injuries involve less than 30 percent of the articular surface and demonstrate no instability on stress testing. Tenuous (type II) injuries involve 30 to 50 percent of the articular surface, but reduction can be maintained with 30 degrees or less of joint flexion. All fracture-dislocations that involve 50 percent or more of the articular surface are unstable. Fractures with 30 to 50 percent joint surface involvement that will only stay reduced with more than 30 degrees of flexion are also classified as unstable.

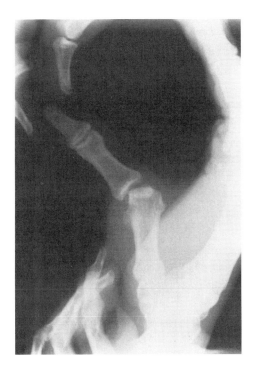

FIG. 42-32. Stress x-ray of a thumb with a complete ulnar collateral ligament tear demonstrates marked instability of the ulnar side of MP joint and radial deviation of the proximal phalanx.

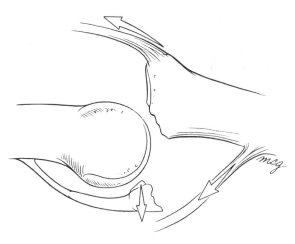

FIG. 42-34. Unstable fracture-dislocation of the PIP joint. The slope of the remaining dorsal articular surface, the pull of the central tendon, and the angulatory moment created by the distal insertion of the flexor digitorum superficialis tendon combine to cause dorsal subluxation of the middle phalanx. The mechanical buttress provided by the volar lip of the middle phalanx is the only support that counteracts these forces. Restoring this buttress is the primary treatment goal for unstable PIP fracture-dislocations.

avoided. (2) The residual tip/pulp requires a resistant and resilient character like normal skin. (3) Excellent fingertip sensibility should be maintained to avoid "blinding" the finger. (4) Finally, bone support for the nail is needed to minimize beaking deformity. Achieving all of these targets simultaneously may be impossible, and choices may be necessary. Anatomy and function in conjunction with the type and level of injury in each patient should be considered (Figs. 42-38 and 42-39).

Which finger is injured and how it was injured influence treatment. For the thumb, every reasonable effort must be made

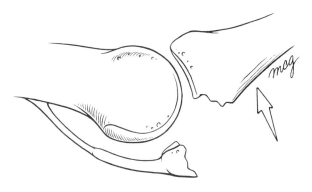

FIG. 42-35. Palmar plate avulsion fracture. Noncomminuted volar lip fractures are caused by forceful hyperextension of the PIP joint.

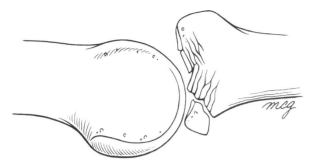

FIG. 42-36. Impaction shear PIP joint fracture-dislocation. Longitudinal loading with the PIP joint slightly flexed or extended causes extensive comminution of the articular surface and impaction of osteochondral fragments into the metaphyseal bone. By definition, the dorsal cortex and some portion of the dorsal articular surface remain intact.

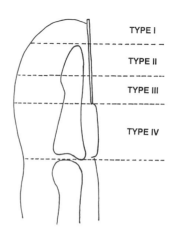

FIG. 42-38. Transverse amputations; classification into four types.

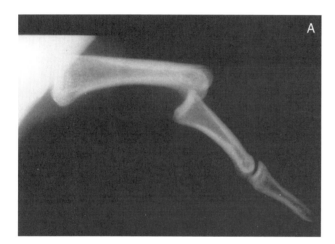

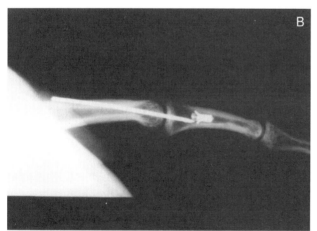

FIG. 42-37. Volar dislocation of the PIP joint. *A.* Lateral radiograph demonstrates the palmar subluxation of the middle phalanx. The rotational component of the injury is recognized by observing a true lateral view of one bone (in this case the middle phalanx) and an oblique view of the opposite joint member (here the proximal phalanx). *B.* Reducible volar dislocations can be managed with closed reduction and percutaneous pin fixation. If surgical repair of the central tendon is elected, suture repair usually is not feasible, because the tendon typically avulses directly off of the bone. The tendon can be secured with a pullout wire or, as in this case, a Mitek suture.

to restore a sensate and durable pulp. Requirements for sensibility are more critical in the index and middle fingers, but they are also significant in the ulnar pulp of the small finger. Amputations can be clean and sharp, but the common avulsion may have a component of avulsion, crush, blast, and burn, as in explosions. Explosions cause extensive trauma to surrounding skin, soft tissue, and neurovascular tissue that requires debridement and, in some cases, staging of the closure. Treatment of partial amputations, crush injuries, and partial devascularizing injuries should be directed toward preserving soft tissues.

Distal phalangeal fractures, including bursting or tuft fractures, are frequently associated with crush trauma and nail bed disruption or lacerations. Nail bed injuries are not always obvious, and subungual hematoma may be the only sign of nail bed injury. Nail bed injuries should be repaired to prevent permanent late nail deformity. Nail bed repairs usually are done with fine 6-0 absorbable suture. After repair, the nail that was removed is replaced beneath the cuticle to splint the bed (Figs. 42-40 and 42-41).

Surgical treatments used to treat fingertip amputations include the following:

Bone Shortening and Primary Closure. This is performed under local or regional anesthesia and consists of debriding

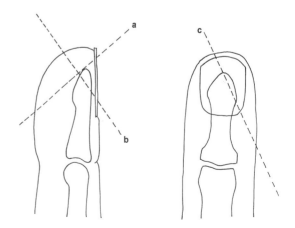

FIG. 42-39. Oblique defects. *A.* Volar oblique. *B.* Dorsal oblique. *C.* Lateral oblique.

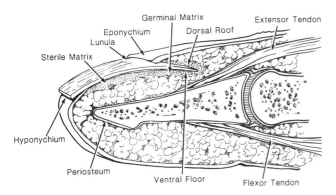

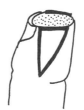

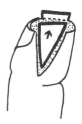

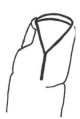

FIG. 42-40. *The pertinent anatomy of the nail bed includes the distal phalanx, nail bed, nail plate, and surrounding soft tissue.*

FIG. 42-42. *Kutler's flap.*

enough bone so that the skin can be closed with a few 5-0 sutures, without tension. Thorough debridement of contaminated or devitalized hard and soft tissues is required. This method affords coverage with soft tissues of normal sensibility, and this well-padded fingertip is not painful, but the cost is some length and at least a portion of the fingernail. Inadequate bone resection produces a fingertip with unpadded bone, resulting in pain during grasping.

Composite Pulp Reattachment. Reapplication of the "composite" of skin and pulp, or skin, pulp, and bone, can be done when the mass of the amputated part is very small. This choice should be reserved for young children. It is best to debride any residual bone. Superficial necrosis of the reapplied part should be expected. In most situations, this is a temporary biologic dressing.

Skin Grafting. Grafts are a means of coverage for skin defects; they are not time consuming and theoretically could be applied to a wide range of fingertip amputations. The major drawbacks are sensory loss in the graft area and the inadequate padding if graft is applied over unpadded bone and periosteum on prehensile surfaces.

The aesthetics of the graft are affected by the donor site. The best cosmetic result for the pulp surface is achieved in all races with split-thickness or full-thickness skin graft taken from the glabrous skin at the hypothenar eminence under local anesthesia. The defect covered with skin graft should be a skin defect, and the recipient bed must have adequate native padding. Skin graft will not satisfactorily protect bone, no matter what the skin donor source. Skin graft to the palm from any area other than glabrous skin produces a result that is relatively hyperpigmented. Split grafts usually are inadequate for pressure and friction surfaces. Toe-to-finger and foot instep-to-hand pulp skin grafting can be performed, but the short-term disadvantages are obvious as compared to full-thickness hypothenar skin as the donor.

Local Flaps. Local tissue transfer from more proximally on the injured finger affords vascularized, padded, and most often sensate tissue. Advancement is by transposition or rotation (Figs. 42-42 and 42-43).

Regional and Distant Flaps. Cross-finger, thenar, and other heterodigital flaps have been used since the early part of the twentieth century, generally for more extensive pulp loss and otherwise uncoverable bone and tendon (Fig. 42-44). These flaps have the advantage of retaining finger length but carry the risk of posttraumatic deformity or dysfunction in an adjacent donor finger. Care must be taken to avoid dysfunction from immobilization of the injured or the donor part because of nonphysiologic positioning during flap healing and before pedicle detachment. Such flaps usually are not sensate.

Replantation and Microvascular Neurosensory Flaps. Microsurgical advances have made finger- and hand-part reattachment possible and allowed reconstruction by composite neurovascular pulp tissue from toes, with or without joints and tendons. The isolated single digit amputation in the adult usually is not suitable for replantation, especially if proximal to the PIP joint, because the functional and aesthetic recovery usually does not justify the morbidity and costs of the replantation procedure. Multiple digit amputations, subtotal hand amputations, amputa-

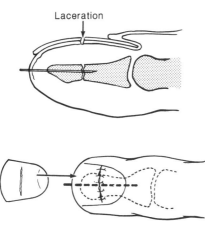

FIG. 42-41. *Unstable fractures of the distal phalanx require reduction and Kirschner-wire fixation. Care is taken to properly align the dorsal cortex of the bone. The nail bed laceration is repaired, and the nail is replaced as a stent for the injury as well as to provide a conforming surface for the healing nail bed.*

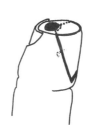

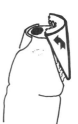

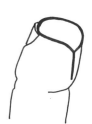

FIG. 42-43. *V-Y advancement flap (Tranquilli-Leali).*

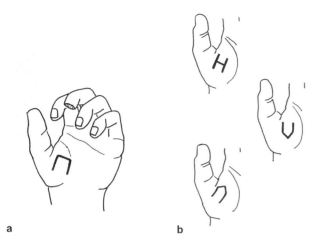

FIG. 42-44. *Thenar flap. A. Classic outline with a proximal pedicle. B. Modification by Smith (top), Dellon (middle), and Melone (bottom).*

tions throughout the upper limb proximal to the hand, and most pediatric amputations should be evaluated for replantation or primary composite microvascular reconstruction (Fig. 42-45).

Soft-Tissue Trauma

Tendon Injuries. *Flexor Tendons.* Flexor mechanism injuries in the hand and fingers are no longer treated by late reconstruction in most patients, because direct primary and delayed primary repairs offer good to excellent results, even when done in the middle of the digits. Satisfactory results are reported in 75 to 98 percent of patients in various series. Flexor tendon repair and functional rehabilitation is a challenge.

Flexor tendons are not difficult to repair, but achieving good function of repaired tendons is difficult, particularly in zones in which multiple tendons of different excursion are in juxtaposition. Tendons must glide, and simultaneously they are restrained by ligaments, such as within the digital sheath and within the carpal canal. Getting flexor tendons to glide after repair remains the problem. The critical operative principle in tendon repair is to achieve near-perfect anatomic alignment of the tendon ends. There should be no gaps at the repair site, and "bunching" of the repair zone should be avoided to permit the repaired tendon(s) to glide within a sheath or pulley system. The zones of flexor tendons are defined by the number of tendons, restraints, and pulleys and the presence or absence of synovial membrane at that specific anatomic level (Figs. 42-46 and 42-47).

In the diagnosis of tendon disruption, the patient often presents with an open wound and loss of active motion. Observing the part at rest (Fig. 42-48) along with active, separate evaluation of the flexor digitorum profundus and flexor digitorum superficialis tendons (Fig. 42-49) makes the diagnosis. A high level of suspicion should be maintained with injuries that have loss of active flexion or extension when x-rays do not show skeletal disruption. Tendon avulsions may occur without attached bone and can be diagnosed only if the examiner is suspicious. Closed, isolated flexor profundus avulsion is most common in the ring finger; the DIP joint will not flex, but the PIP joint does, however painful. For primary or delayed primary repair to be effective, early diagnosis is essential (Figs. 42-50 and 42-51).

Partial tendon lacerations, approximately up to one-third of the tendon's cross-sectional area, do not present serious risk of rupture, but the lacerated edge may catch on a nearby pulley, producing posttraumatic triggering. Lacerations involving 30 to 50 percent of the tendon's cross-sectional area may be treated by epitendinous suture alone. Division of 50 percent or more of cross-sectional area should be treated surgically as though division were complete. Flexor mechanism salvage by graft and staged reconstruction, or by posttraumatic tenolysis or grafting, is beyond the scope of this text. Secondary tenolysis should be reserved for those patients whose fingers have achieved a stable biologic state more than 4 months after trauma. Soft tissues are no longer edematous, maximum active and passive joint mobi-

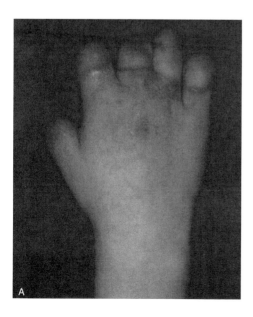

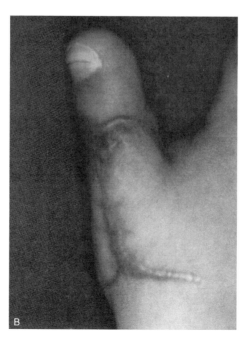

FIG. 42-45. *A. Traumatic amputation of all fingers in a 3-year-old child. B. Reconstruction with a free partial transfer from the great toe.*

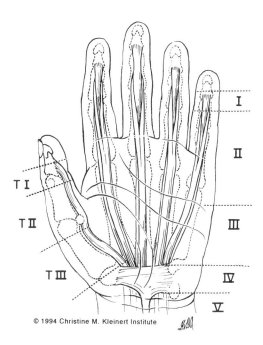

FIG. 42-46. The five flexor tendon zones in the hand and the three zones in the thumb.

© 1994 Christine M. Kleinert Institute

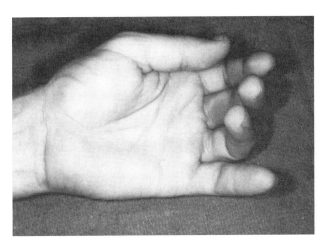

FIG. 42-48. The normal cascade of flexion is disrupted in the injured hand.

lization has been achieved before secondary operation, and the patient must be willing to undergo a second operation for additional recovery.

Extensor Tendons. The superficial location of the extensor tendons on the dorsum of the fingers and hand make them vulnerable to injury, especially when the fingers are flexed. Trauma comes from lacerations, crush impacts, abrasions, and bites. Extensor tendon injuries are more common than those of flexor injuries and are often treated casually in the emergency department.

Extensor dysfunction may result in loss of active flexion from scar tattering and in diminished active extension. The extensor system is more intricate and complex than the flexor system. The interconnections of the *extrinsic* digital extensor tendons

from the muscles in the forearm and tendons in the hand, and the *intrinsic* tendons in which muscles and tendons are in the hand, are complex. The two sets of tendons collaborate to flex the metacarpophalangeal joints and extend the interphalangeal joints. Because excursion of the extensor mechanism is limited over the finger joints, preservation of tendon length is more critical to maintain and restore tendon balance than with flexor tendon injury.

The flexor tendons are thick, round, cordlike structures with spiraling fibers. The extensor tendons are thin and flat, and the longitudinal fibers of the extensors do not hold sutures well. The limited amount of soft tissues about these tendons also makes repairs prone to adherence and scarring.

The extrinsic extensors of the forearm, i.e., brachioradialis and extensor carpi radialis longus, are innervated by the radial nerve, and the extensor carpi radialis brevis muscle by the deep

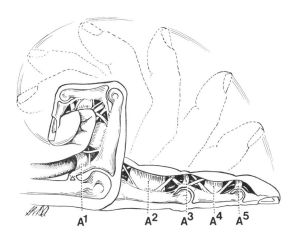

© 1992 Kleinert, Kutz and Associates Hand Care Center

FIG. 42-47. The annular pulley system.

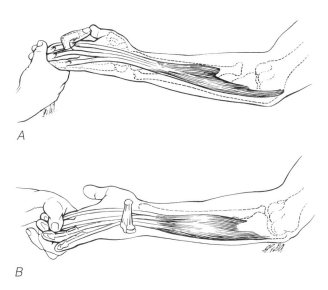

FIG. 42-49. *A.* Examination of the flexor digitorum superficialis tendons. *B.* Examination of the flexor digitorum profundus tendons. *(Modified from Lister G: The Hand: Diagnosis and Indications, 3d ed. London: Churchill-Livingstone, 1993, reprinted with permission.)*

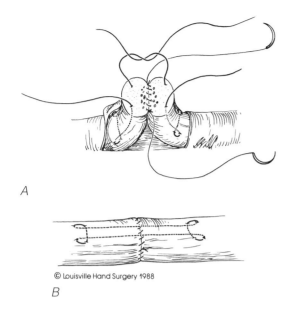

© Louisville Hand Surgery 1988

FIG. 42-50. *A. Debrided tendon ends are aligned and sutured. A permanent core suture is placed so as not to disturb tendon vessels in the volar aspect. B. The completed repair.*

branch of the radial nerve. The posterior interosseous branch of the radial nerve innervates the extensor carpi ulnaris muscle and all proper and common thumb and digital extensors. The tendons cross the wrist through six pulley compartments, serving to extend the wrist and the MP and interphalangeal (IP) joints. These six tendon tunnels are defined by reflections of the extensor retinaculum into the dorsal cortex of the radius and wrist capsule and serve to limit the tendon vector effect of the digital extensors at the wrist joint by maintaining their proximity to the center of axis of wrist motion. Extrinsic digital extensor tendons elevate the proximal phalanx. That is, they extend the MP joint via the aponeurotic sagittal fibers that reach around the lateral sides of the phalanx to insert on the palmar margin of the bone and volar plate, thereby lifting the metacarpal from a broad palmar attachment rather than a single point dorsally. The extrinsic extensor tendon is the only MP joint extensor. Distally, the function of the intrinsic and extrinsic tendons together form the dorsal tendon apparatus in the fingers (Fig. 42-52). The intrinsic tendons arise from the four dorsal and three palmar interosseous muscles. There also are three thenar, three hypothenar, and four lumbrical muscles. The group serves as the primary independent metacarpophalangeal joint flexors and as interphalangeal joint extensors. The MP joint flexor fibers course distally from a palmar position, sending up the transverse aponeurosis dorsally to insert on the lateral edges of the extrinsic extensor tendon in the proximal third of the proximal phalanx (see Fig. 42-52). The direct distal continuation of the intrinsic tendon is the lateral band that continues distally to reach a position dorsal to the center of axis of PIP motion before crossing over the distal third of the proximal phalanx, thereby making it an extensor tendon for both interphalangeal joints. At the metaphysis of the proximal phalanx and the base of the middle phalanx, the extrinsic and intrinsic tendons converge to become conjoined extensors. The central slip inserts into the dorsal lip of the middle phalanx as its direct extensor, but the conjoined lateral bands run along the dorsal

lateral edge of the PIP joint and converge distally over the middle phalanx to become the terminal tendon that inserts into the dorsal lip of the distal phalanx, functioning as this last joint's only extensor.

Because of the normal dorsolateral position of the lateral bands, in certain direct injuries to the dorsum of the finger at the PIP joint the lateral bands may subluxate volarly, hyperextending the terminal joint. This is called the *boutonnière deformity*. When the terminal tendon insertion at the distal interphalangeal joint is avulsed or transected, the distal joint droops and the secondary proximal and dorsal retraction of the lateral bands produces gradual hyperextension at proximal interphalangeal level. This deformity is known as *mallet* or *baseball finger*; it progresses to the *swan-neck deformity* when the PIP hyperextension is added.

The type of injury and the results of surgery vary because of the structural and functional differences in the extensor system from fingertip to forearm. Extensor tendon characteristics have been categorized by eight anatomical zones; the four with odd numbers overlie the joints, and the four with even numbers are the tendon segments between the joints (Fig. 42-53). Generic recommendations for repair methods are illustrated in Fig. 42-54.

Zone 1 (Mallet Finger and Secondary Swan-Neck). Terminal tendon injury may occur by avulsion with or without attached bone fragment, and by transection from laceration or crush (Figs. 42-55 and 42-56). Closed injuries can be successfully treated by closed means; open injuries also may be treated by extension splinting. Open or closed injuries that include fracture of the joint surface with secondary palmar subluxation of the distal phalanx require reduction and internal fixation in neutral extension to restore DIP joint congruence and proper tendon relationships. This permits almost immediate joint plus hand rehabilitation while protecting the repaired tendon and joint and making wound care easier. Otherwise, the terminal joint is rarely pinned. Splints that immobilize the DIP articulation in extension (6 to 8 weeks) but leave the PIP joint unrestrained usually are preferred (Fig. 42-57).

Zone 2. Zone 2 is the area over the middle phalanx where the lateral bands fuse to form the terminal tendon. The lateral bands are connected proximally by the thin triangular ligament. Injuries in this area usually are from laceration with resultant mallet deformity. Direct repair and terminal joint pinning for 6 to 8 weeks is appropriate for open cases; closed splinting for closed injuries without significant fracture is effective.

Zone 3 (Boutonnière). Zone 3 is the area over the PIP joint where the central slip and lateral bands interconnect. Injury may be closed or open and may include avulsion of the central slip, with or without a dorsal bone fragment. The latter injuries require accurate reduction of the joint, bone, and contiguous tendon mechanism. Pinning the PIP joint in extension allows early rehabilitation of the other joints. Untreated, this boutonnière deformity progresses to a fixed PIP joint flexion contracture with secondary hyperextension of the terminal joint. Closed splint or percutaneous pin management may be equally effective for the pure tendon injuries (Fig. 42-58).

Zone 4. The dorsum of the proximal phalanx is covered entirely by the confluent extrinsic extensor tendon and by the two lateral bands arising from tendons of intrinsic muscles. Because of this local anatomy, most tendon injuries in zone 4 are partial and the cut tendon ends do not retract significantly. Only direct inspection can confirm this diagnosis. If interphalangeal joint

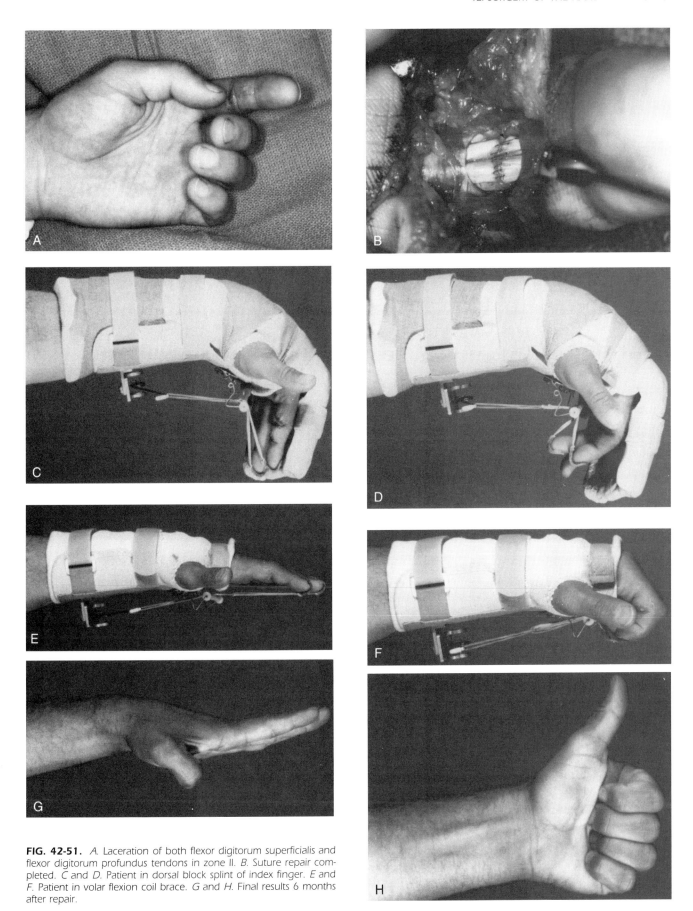

FIG. 42-51. *A.* Laceration of both flexor digitorum superficialis and flexor digitorum profundus tendons in zone II. *B.* Suture repair completed. *C* and *D.* Patient in dorsal block splint of index finger. *E* and *F.* Patient in volar flexion coil brace. *G* and *H.* Final results 6 months after repair.

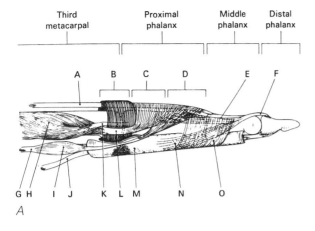

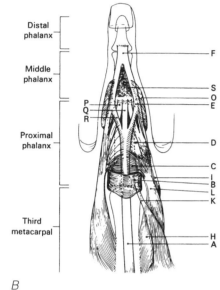

FIG. 42-52. *Diagrammatic representation of the dorsal apparatus of the finger. A. Lateral side, middle finger. B. Dorsum, middle finger. A = extensor digitorum communis tendon; B = sagittal bands; C = transverse fibers of intrinsic muscle apparatus; D = oblique fibers of intrinsic apparatus; E = conjoined lateral band; F = terminal tendon; G = flexor digitorum profundus tendon; H = second dorsal interosseous muscle; I = lumbrical muscle; J = flexor digitorum superficialis tendon; K = medial tendon of superficial belly of interosseous muscle; L = lateral tendon of deep belly of interosseous muscle; M = flexor pulley mechanism; N = oblique retinacular expansion; O = transverse retinacular ligament; P = medial band of oblique fibers of intrinsic expansion; Q = central slip; R = lateral slips; S = triangular ligament. (Adapted from: Smith RJ: Balance and kinetics of the fingers under normal and pathologic conditions. Clin Orthop 104:92, 1974, figs 5 and 6, p 95.)*

mechanism of injury. The incidence of complications is directly related to the delay in treatment. Radiographs are taken to rule out the presence of a foreign body such as a piece of tooth, an intraarticular fracture, or air in the joint, proving contamination. When caused by a bite, the wound is left open and tendon repair is performed secondarily after healing by secondary intention. In a simple laceration, the tendon can be repaired directly. The more dorsal extrinsic extensor tendon and the sagittal band mechanism should be repaired to prevent subluxation of the extensor into the intermetacarpal valley. Closed extensor tendon dislocation is almost always to the ulnar side of the joint and requires tendon and sagittal fiber reconstruction.

Where direct repair is possible, primary and delayed primary repairs are preferable, using suture techniques described in Fig. 42-54. The wrist is immobilized in 30 degrees or less of extension, and the MP joint is splinted at 60 to 70 degrees or treated with a custom dynamic MP extension splint for early passive motion. The PIP and DIP joints are left free.

Zone 6. Zone 6 covers the dorsum of the hand, which includes the metacarpals and distal carpals, where there are four common extensor tendons to the fingers and two proper tendons, one to the index and one to the little finger. The three wrist extensors insert in this region: extensor carpi radialis longus into the dorsoradial base of the second metacarpal, extensor carpi radialis brevis into the dorsoradial base of the third metacarpal, and extensor carpi ulnaris into the ulnar dorsal edge of the fifth metacarpal. The extensor pollicis longus tendon crosses from proximal to distal in a radial to ulnar line. Single or partial tendon laceration may not produce metacarpophalangeal extension loss, because forces are transmitted through the tendinous interconnections extending from adjacent extensors, such as the juncturae tendinum. In most cases, however, the involved finger lies slightly more flexed or is less able to extend than the others. Paradoxically, the affected finger may flex at the MP and extend at the IP joints when the patient attempts active extension be-

extension is normal, a partial tendon injury need not be repaired. Splinting the PIP joint for 3 to 4 weeks usually is adequate.

Zone 5. Lacerations and bite wounds are common at the metacarpophalangeal joint. With open injuries in this region, a human or animal bite should be suspected until otherwise disproved. Bite wounds are serious contaminated injuries requiring primary surgical debridement, irrigation of the wound and joint, and aggressive intravenous antibiotics for 24 to 48 h. Patients may be reluctant to seek treatment early, and many deny the

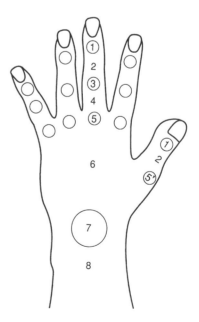

FIG. 42-53. *Diagram of the surgical/topographic zones of the extensor apparatus.*

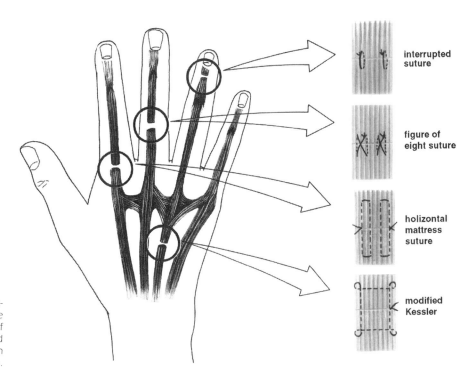

interrupted suture

figure of eight suture

holizontal mattress suture

modified Kessler

FIG. 42-54. *Suture techniques for the extensor tendons. Different techniques are chosen according to the size and quality of the tendon. The interrupted suture is used in zone 1, whereas core-type sutures can be used in thicker tendon tissue in zone 6.*

cause of loss of the extrinsic extensor tendon without disruption of the intrinsics. The tendons are oval in cross-section and thicker here than distally. Core sutures of the type used in flexor repairs are recommended (see Fig. 42-54). Conventional postrepair treatment was immobilization with the wrist in 45 degrees or more of extension and the fingers in mild MP flexion for about 4 to 6 weeks. This is discouraged, however, because patients can become significantly stiff with this protocol. Instead, the wrist should be kept in about 30 degrees of extension and the metacarpophalangeal joints fitted with proximal phalangeal extensor cuffs with the interphalangeal joints free, allowing active flexion and passive extension. Motivated patients may begin this program on the seventh to tenth postoperative day; others are immobilized for double that time. At least one adjacent finger must be included in the splint. Multiple tendon injuries may necessitate including all fingers in splints throughout the rehabilitation protocol.

Zone 7. Zone 7 is the proximal wrist region under the extensor retinaculum in which the extensors traverse the fibro-osseous tunnel in six synovial compartments. Unlike for the flexor pulleys, repair of the extensor retinaculum is relatively easy to perform, but retinacular release should be avoided when possible. To prevent extensor tendon bowstringing, preservation or reconstruction of some portion (40 percent or more) of the proximal or distal retinaculum is critical. Step-cut retinaculum release more easily allows closure without producing a space too tight to allow gliding of repaired tendon(s). Tendon lacerations in this area often are associated with injuries to the nearby radial or ulnar sensory nerve branches, which should be considered at examination and surgery.

Closed rupture of extensor tendons, usually the extensor pollicis longus tendon, is not rare, especially after Colles' fracture and other injuries to the distal radius. Many extensor pollicis longus ruptures occur several weeks or months after nondis-

placed Colles' fractures. It is postulated that fracture hematoma reduces the limited blood supply in the extensor pollicis longus tendon, leading to the attrition rupture. Systemic connective tissue diseases, such as rheumatoid arthritis, and pathologic conditions that produce a sharp bone edge, chronic tenosynovitis, or both, also may contribute to this problem. Attrition ruptures should be repaired by tendon transfer or grafting. Direct repair is almost never possible because of the wide zone of tendon trauma that occurs before breakage.

Zone 8. Trauma to the radial sensory or posterior interosseous nerve branches may occur concomitantly with extensor injuries in the forearm in zone 8. Multiple adjacent muscles or tendons make it difficult to identify individual tendons. The priority of repair is to restore independent wrist and thumb extension and group extension of the fingers. With lacerations at the musculotendinous junctions, the tendons may be seen distally, but proximally their fibrous septa retract into the muscle bellies. For repair at this level, the suture line must include fascia or the intramuscular tendinous septa to prevent pullout and failure of operation. With injuries in the proximal forearm, division of the posterior interosseous nerve alone may produce loss of extensor function by denervation, or it may occur in combination with injury to some or all of the muscles and tendons. After repair, elbow flexion and wrist extension may be needed to reduce tension at the suture line. Thumb extensor injuries are dealt with in manner similar to injuries to the finger.

Tendon Transfers. Tendon transfer is a reconstructive procedure that antedates the twentieth century. Transfers in the upper limb are designed to restore motion in a nonfunctioning part. Tendon transfers are used in isolated peripheral nerve paralysis, for irreparable tendon damage after extensive segmental loss from devastating trauma or in destructive connective tissue diseases such as rheumatoid arthritis, and to rebalance the hand

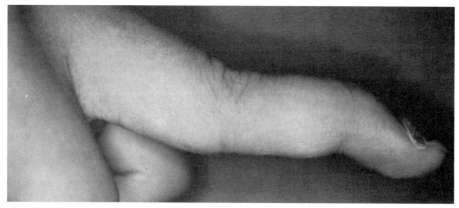

A

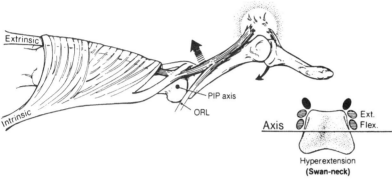

B

FIG. 42-55. *A.* Swan-neck deformity secondary to mallet finger. *B.* Appearance and mechanism. Because of the extensor apparatus lesion, the distal phalanx flexes by the effect of the flexor digitorum profundus tendon *(curved arrow).* The proximal stump of the distal conjoined extensor tendon retracts proximally, and consequently the lateral band and oblique retinacular ligament *(ORL)* are slack at the beginning and later contract and displace dorsally. Because of the concentration of the extensor forces over the middle phalanx, the PIP joint is progressively set in hyperextension *(wide arrow).* Inset: Transaxial representation at the condyle of the proximal phalanx, showing the normal positions of the conjoined lateral bands in extension and flexion of the PIP joint. Dorsally displaced position of the conjoined lateral bands is represented in black.

or provide movement to a spastic or paralyzed limb after central nervous system injury or disease. Upper extremity reconstruction by tendon transfer requires careful patient selection and extended therapy supervision, often with preoperative and postoperative rehabilitation protocols.

Nerve Injury

The upper extremity is innervated by the brachial plexus and several sensory branches arising from the plexus and intercostal nerves (Fig. 42-59). Innervation patterns vary, with intercommunications and fiber exchanges within and between nerves. Nerves are composed of axons and associated Schwann cells enclosed in a basement membrane. Thin collagen fibers called endoneurium are immediately outside this basement membrane; the term *endoneurial tube* refers to the axon and Schwann cell composite. Endoneurial tubes are grouped together to form a variable number of fascicles. Perineurium surrounds each fascicle, composed of concentric layers of flattened cells and collagen fibers. The perineurium creates a diffusion barrier against the surrounding environment, providing the peripheral nerve the equivalent of a blood-brain barrier (Fig. 42-60). Surrounding the layers of perineurium is epineurium. Epineurium that fills the space between fascicles is called *internal* and that surrounding the nerve itself is termed *external* or *outer.* The outer layer is composed of collagen and some elastin fibers. The fascicular organization and internal anatomy of the nerve is not constant over its length. The topographic fascicular organization of the nerve rearranges as branches come off these fascicles. The fascicles move to the perimeter within the nerve as the nerve courses toward the periphery. The internal organization of the nerve reflects the location and position of those final branches.

For normal nerve function to be maintained, the peripheral nerve must glide. Focused tension or compression induces local injury, nerve dysfunction, and symptoms. Compression and traction neuropathies result when a nerve is tethered, especially at or near a joint. The ulnar nerve, for example, has a longitudinal excursion of 10 mm or more proximal to the elbow; the median and ulnar nerves glide nearly 15 mm at the wrist. After injury

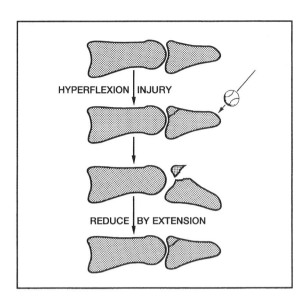

FIG. 42-56. *Mechanism of mallet finger. Hyperflexion injury. (From: Lange RH, Engber WD: Orthopedics 6:1426, 1983, with permission.)*

to a nerve, the nerve is at risk for local scar formation adhesions and secondary traction neuritis from tension focused at the site of adherence.

Classification of nerve injuries, as described by Seddon, is as follows:

Neurapraxia describes paralysis/dysfunction in the absence of nerve degeneration. This dysfunction is often of some duration, though recovery is always achieved in a shorter time than would be required after complete transection and nerve degen-

eration and regeneration. Recovery by definition is invariably complete.

Axonotmesis includes damage to the nerve fibers of a severity that causes complete nerve degeneration. The epineurium and other supporting structures of the nerve are not disrupted, so the internal architecture is relatively well preserved. Spontaneous recovery is the rule, and generally it is of very good quality because the regenerating fascicles are guided into their paths via the intact sheaths. Recovery takes longer than for neurapraxia.

Neurotmesis is when all nerve structures have been divided. Laceration produces neurotmesis, but physical gaps in the nerve may occur even though the epineurial sheath appears in continuity, such as after traction or crush. At the site of damage the nerve will be completely replaced by fibrous tissue, and there is complete loss of anatomic continuity.

Recovery after nerve injury depends on successful reinnervation of sensory or motor end-organs. After denervation, muscles begin to lose their bulk; a loss of cross-sectional area without any loss in muscle fiber count begins within 1 week of denervation. Connective tissue surrounding the muscle undergoes degeneration and thickening. Interstitial fibrosis predominates over time, but passive exercises may delay or prevent this phenomenon. For function to be resumed, motor end-plates must be reinnervated within 18 months of trauma. Sensory end-organs may be usefully reinnervated long after initial injury, but the quality of recovery diminishes with the passage of time.

The result after repair depends on numerous factors: injury level and mechanism, associated bone and soft-tissue loss, residual function, patient compliance and motivation, timing of repair, and supervised rehabilitation. Quantitative postoperative assessment of motor and sensory function should be documented.

Repair should be done with microsutures with the aid of magnification to produce a spatially correct, tension-free suture line.

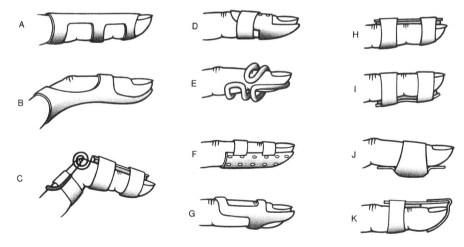

FIG. 42-57. *Various splints: fixation for both DIP and PIP joint (A–C); molded plastic or rubber-coated splints (D–G); aluminum splints (H–K). A. Metal tubed splint by Lewin. B. Frog splint from Richards. C. Combined dorsal DIP aluminum splint and coil splint for PIP flexion. The PIP joint is allowed to extend passively during 3 to 4 weeks of splinting followed by distal component only for an additional 2 weeks. D. Stack splint. E. Rubber-coated wire splint by Abouna and Brown. F. Perforated splint by Kinninmonth, individually made with thermoplastic material to reduce skin irritation. G. Modified Stack splint, with added spaces for extra ventilation in the pulp and on the dorsal surface of the middle phalanx. H. Dorsal padded aluminum splint. I. Volar padded aluminum splint. J. Concave aluminum splint. K. Dorsal padded aluminum splint allows adjustable flexion of the DIP joint.*

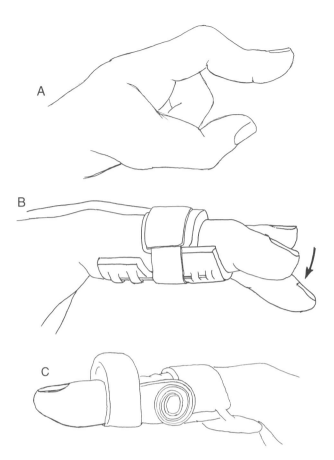

FIG. 42-58. *A. Boutonnière injury. B. The Bunnell-type safety-pin splint. The splint is worn constantly, and the strap on the splint is tightened on a daily basis until full extension of the PIP joint is achieved. The terminal crossbar does not go beyond the distal joint flexion crease, and the patient is instructed to flex the distal joint actively and passively while the proximal joint is held in maximum extension. The splint is used on a continuous basis for several weeks until there is full passive extension of the DIP joint. When this occurs, the length relationships and balance between the central slip and the lateral bands have been achieved and the splint can be discontinued. C. Capener splint.*

Nerve grafts are used when direct repair after segmental loss or fibrosis would require tension at the repair site. Joint posturing into extreme flexion or extension to decrease tension at the nerve repair site should be avoided; nerve graft is substituted for such destructive splinting maneuvers. Primary or delayed primary repair should be done whenever appropriate conditions allow. The combination of group fascicular and epineurial nonreactive microsutures after identification of the internal topography should produce the best anatomic result. Repairs are protected by relaxed joint posturing for about 3 weeks, and the results of repair are maximized by beginning sensory and motor reeducation after reinnervation (Figs. 42-61 and 42-62).

Vascular Trauma and Replantation

The majority of upper extremity replantation surgery is based on microsurgical technique. Ocular loupes are useful for lower magnification and wide-field dissections and are particularly helpful in preparing the ends of nerves and vessels for repair. However,

the operating microscope offers a steady field magnification range of 25× or more. Miniaturized needle holders and instruments, bipolar coagulation, and other modifications are necessary for proper microvessel handling. The typical repair in vessels of 0.5 to 3.0 mm diameter is performed with nonreactive monofilament interrupted sutures to prevent luminal impingement collapse, although microvessel grafts and end-to-side connections also are used (Figs. 42-63 and 42-64). A contaminated soft and bony tissue injury is healed by primary debridement and stabilization of open fractures, repair of extensor and flexor mechanisms, and repair of nerves and vessels (Fig. 42-65).

Each patient should be considered individually on the basis of the location and extent of the injury and the patient's age and condition. Relevant questions include: (1) Can function be obtained from the replanted part? (2) Will that function exceed what can be achieved through amputation closure and possible prosthetic fitting? (3) Will long-term function be improved or compromised by part replantation? (4) Does the potential benefit to the patient outweigh the surgical risks, costs, and loss of productivity?

Segmental, extensive, or multiple-level injuries require repair and reconstruction over an extended area. Neither complete nor near-complete part amputation makes any patient an automatic candidate for revascularization or reattachment. Single finger amputation in the adult, especially at a level proximal to the PIP joint, including both superficialis and profundus tendons and digital nerves is not suitable for replantation in the vast majority of cases. Consideration should be given to replantation for thumb amputations at and proximal to the interphalangeal joint, for single-finger amputations in children, and for partial hand and more proximal wrist, forearm, or arm amputations. In adults over the age of 40 years, repair of the ulnar nerve proximal to the elbow rarely produces a functional result. Crush and avulsion injuries often make it impossible to achieve successful reattachment and revascularization. Reperfusion before tissues are nonviable is essential. Muscle is the most oxygen-sensitive upper-extremity tissue and must be revascularized within 6 h of amputation.

Handling of Amputated Parts. The amputated part should be cleansed under saline solution, wrapped in a saline-moistened gauze, and placed in a plastic bag. The plastic bag containing the part should then be placed on, not packed in, a bed of ice in a suitable container. The part should not be immersed in nonphysiologic solution such as antiseptics or alcohols. The amputated part is never put in dry ice, it is not perfused, and it should not be allowed to freeze.

Preparing the Patient. The patient is stabilized, and a compression dressing is applied to the stump before transport to the replantation center. Intravenous access lines should be started and blood samples drawn while awaiting transportation. If time permits, x-rays of the stump and also of the amputated part can be obtained.

Most replantation centers request that the patient be given intravenous antibiotics, an aspirin suppository (325 mg), and 25 to 50 mL per hour intravenous supplement of low-molecular-weight dextran in dextrose, the latter for antiaggregation platelet effects. Before the patient is transported to the replantation center, someone responsible at the receiving institution must know-

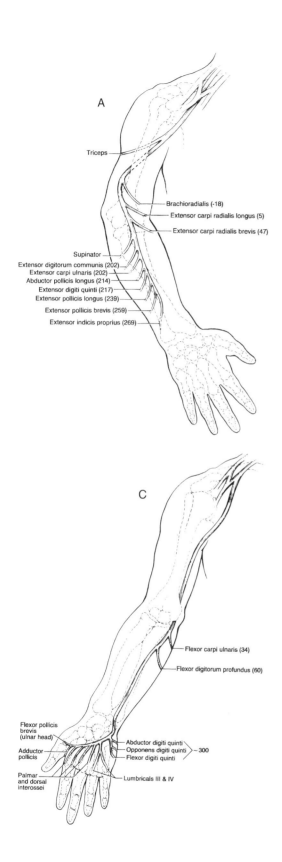

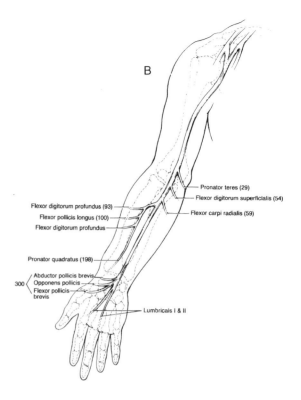

FIG. 42-59. Motor innervation of the arm. *A.* Radial nerve. *B.* Median nerve. *C.* Ulnar nerve. Numbers in parentheses indicate shortest average distances from medial epicondyle to muscle, in millimeters, as determined by Sunderland.

ingly accept the patient as a candidate for part reattachment. Even if the center has an active replant team, its members may be occupied with another case. Accurate communication by telephone, physician-to-physician, is an essential part of replantation triage. Even if the referring physician is unsure of the patient's status, preparations can still be made for possible transport. When the patient is transported, the patient should be told that referral is for evaluation for possible replantation.

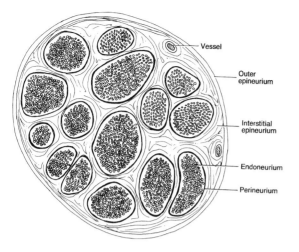

FIG. 42-60. Nerve cross-section. Axons are surrounded by endoneurium and bundled into discrete fascicles. Note the internal epineurium between fascicles supporting longitudinal running vessels.

Amputations (See Chap. 20)

The value of traditional methods to manage amputations is worth emphasis. Digital amputation affects precision pinch and power grip, the latter more significantly if the hand is painful. The treatment principles for fingertip amputation were discussed earlier. It is important that stable soft-tissue and skin coverage over an amputation stump at any level be obtained (Fig. 42-66). If a residual stump is stiff or painful, amputation or amputation revision through the metacarpal can be a functional enhancement. Where a central ray is excised, second-ray transfer or third–fifth intermetacarpal ligament closure preserves and restores metacarpal alignment and the functional contour of the hand (Figs. 42-67 and 42-68).

Complications of Trauma

Compartment Syndrome/Volkmann's Contracture.

In acute compartment syndrome, increased fluid pressure in the tissues contained within a fascial space or subcompartment increases to a level that reduces capillary blood flow below that necessary for continued tissue viability. When untreated, continued pressure elevation produces irreversible muscle and nerve damage because of ischemia, with secondary necrosis, fibrosis,

FIG. 42-61. Algorithm for the evaluation of nerve injuries.

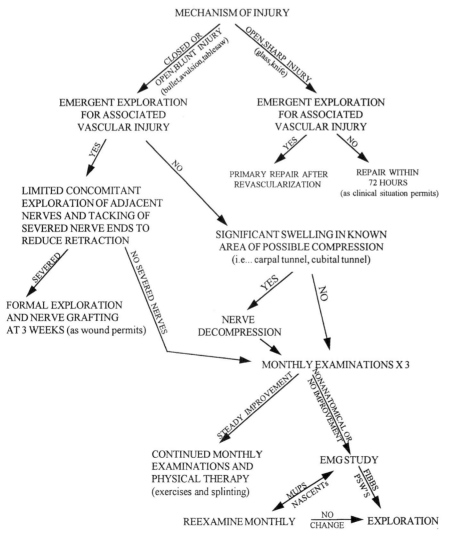

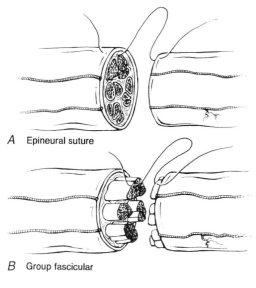

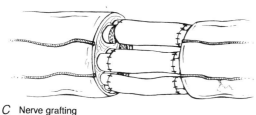

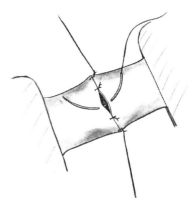

FIG. 42-64. Placement of central suture in anterior wall.

A Epineural suture

B Group fascicular

C Nerve grafting

FIG. 42-62. Techniques of nerve repair. A. Direct epineurial suture using surface vessels for alignment. B. Group fascicular repair. C. Nerve grafting using multiple strands of donor nerve to bridge defect.

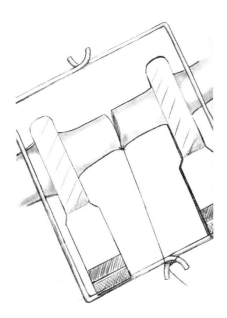

FIG. 42-63. Vessel with first stay suture in place and pulled to proper tension.

contractures, and sensibility deficits or chronic pain. Acute compartment syndrome results from an increase in the volume of fluid within a compartment or limitations on the dimensions of an anatomic compartment. Posttraumatic edema or hemorrhage, hematoma, swelling from infection, or burns increase compartment fluid, as does revascularization. Other causes include venous obstruction and transiently strenuous exercise. Constrictive dressings and casts, excessively tight surgical closure, and prolonged direct limb pressure during unconsciousness with alcohol and drug stupor or during extended surgical procedures add to the limited dimensions of the anatomic compartment.

Acute compartment syndrome is diagnosed clinically but can be confirmed by measurement of intracompartmental tissue pressure. Clinical findings include a swollen, tense, and tender compartment with pain out of proportion to that expected from the originating injury, peripheral sensibility deficits and, finally, motor weakness or paralysis. Pain is accentuated by passive stretch of the affected muscle. Peripheral pulses usually remain intact because systolic arterial pressure usually is well in excess of the dangerously elevated intracompartmental pressure. While blood flow through the major arteries is not impeded, capillary perfusion is compromised by the elevated pressure (30 to 60 mmHg) within the compartment. Pressure measurement devices are confirmatory but not infallible, and in treatment decisions clinical concerns should outweigh specific pressure measurements. Threshold pressure measurements of 30 mmHg or more are consistent with compartment syndrome, and surgical decompression should be prompt. Because tissue perfusion is affected by systemic blood pressure, a lower threshold pressure for fasciotomy should be used in hypotensive patients. While MRI, CT, or ultrasonography may delineate areas of muscle edema or necrosis, these studies do not help with the diagnosis of acute compartment syndrome. Treatment should not be delayed to order and obtain imaging beyond plain radiographs.

Treatment includes removal of all occlusive dressings, wraps, layers, and splints and splitting tight casts and cast padding down to the skin. If symptoms are not rapidly relieved, fasciotomy of the affected areas is required (Figs. 42-69 and 42-70). After surgical decompression, the wounds are left open but dressed to prevent desiccation. Skin closure by direct means or with skin grafting is delayed for 48 to 96 h at a minimum, but may be performed after 5 to 10 days as swelling permits. Hand therapy is started at 48 h.

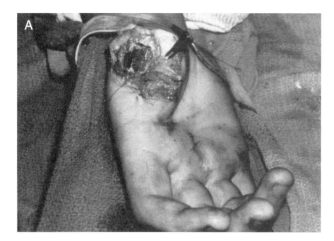

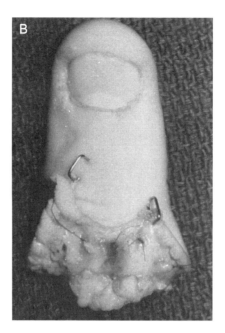

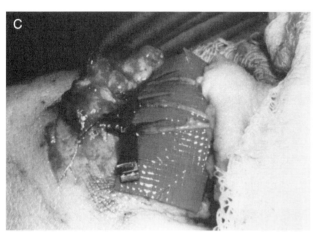

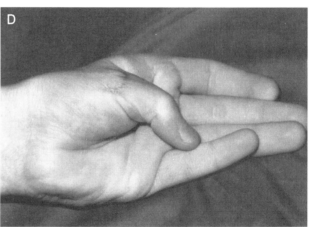

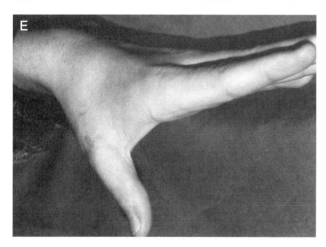

FIG. 42-65. *A. Amputation of thumb at proximal phalangeal level. B and C. Identification and tagging of dorsal veins and subsequent anastomosis. D and E. Palmar abduction and opposition 18 months after replantation.*

Neuromas. Neuromas represent a normal physiologic response after nerve injury. All badly injured and severed nerves form neuromas, but only those neuromas that are exposed, superficial, and likely to be impacted become symptomatic. Only sensory fibers develop painful neuromas (Figs. 42-71, 42-72, 42-73, and 42-74). Medical and surgical management of symptomatic neuromas may be difficult, but prevention is more important. Inadvertent injuries to nerves can be avoided during resection, but with amputation end-nerve divisions are at risk for neuroma formation. Divided nerve stumps should be transposed to deep locations, preferably between or within muscle, or into

bone when padded tissue is scant. In the fingers, where there is often limited soft-tissue padding, the practice of dividing the nerve under traction and allowing it to retract proximally is not as certain a method as leaving the nerve end long and transposing it to a site where it is less likely to be struck but more likely to be protected.

A symptomatic neuroma is a therapeutic challenge. More than a hundred methods of surgical treatment have been described, but no method is universally successful. The symptomatic neuroma should be identified, isolated, and dissected intact. The scar bulb is kept in continuity with the nerve. The

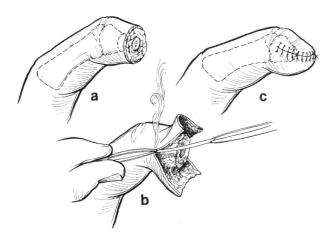

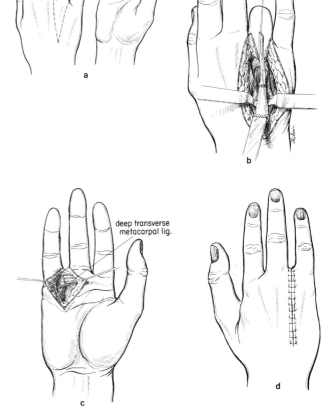

FIG. 42-66. *Schematic of the technique of digital amputation.*

symptomatic nerve and its continuous neuroma are transposed to a deeper, more padded, and often more proximal location, beneath muscle if possible, but within bone when needed. The neuroma bulb is not excised from the nerve because its excision stimulates germination of another neuroma whose contents may not be contained with this secondary procedure.

Reflex Sympathetic Dystrophy. The first clinical description of abnormally exaggerated and prolonged pain after injury is attributed to the Civil War surgeon S. W. Mitchell, who coined the term *causalgia* from the Greek meaning burning pain. Synonyms include inflammatory bone atrophy and Sudeck's atrophy. Reflex sympathetic dystrophy emphasizes the importance of the sympathetic nervous system in posttraumatic pain pathophysiology. Prompt diagnosis and early therapeutic intervention are the most important factors in optimizing clinical and functional outcome. Reflex sympathetic dystrophy is not a disease. It is a complex interaction of physiologic responses initiated by trauma and exacerbated by posttraumatic events. This process is staged by time and inflammatory phase with characteristic changes (Table 42-2) and by descriptive terminology (Table 42-3). The presumptive diagnosis is based on pain, which is often diffuse, burning, and *hyperpathic,* including *allodynia*

FIG. 42-68. *Schematic of the technique of central ray deletion with simple web space closure.*

(pain to light touch), *hyperalgesia* (painful response to nonpainful stimuli), *dysesthesia* (pins and needles following minor stimulus), and *hyperesthesia* (increased sensitivity or pain with nonpainful stimuli). In addition, the clinical diagnosis of reflex

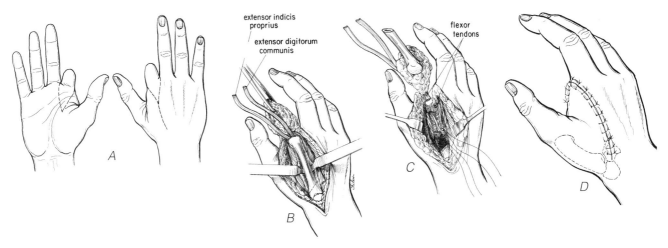

FIG. 42-67. *Schematic of the technique of index ray deletion.*

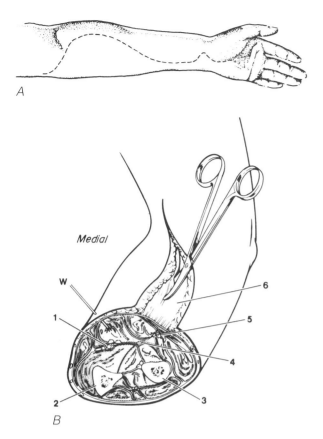

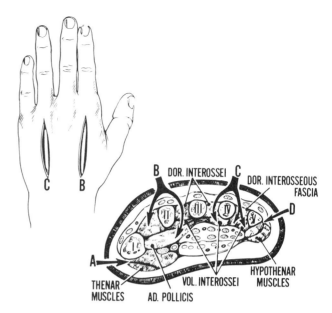

FIG. 42-69. *A.* Incision used for flexor compartment release and median nerve decompression. Incision is extended distally for carpal tunnel release. *B.* Cross-section of left forearm with wick catheter placed and fasciotomy incision illustrated. W = wick catheter; 1 = ulnar nerve; 2 = ulna; 3 = radius; 4 = median nerve; 5 = radial artery; 6 = forearm fascia. (From: *Gelberman RH, Garfin SR, Hergenroeder PT, Mubarak SJ, Menon J: Compartment syndromes of the forearm: Diagnosis and treatment. Clin Orthop Rel Res 161:252–261, 1981.*)

FIG. 42-70. Incisions for intrinsic muscle decompression. Incision *A* allows decompression of the thenar muscles; incision *D* allows decompression of the hypothenar muscles. The two dorsal incisions, *B* and *C*, are placed over the index and ring metacarpal, respectively, each allowing decompression of the adjacent interosseous muscle compartments. The adductor compartment (containing the adductor pollicis muscle) may be decompressed through incision *B.* (From: *Rowland SA: Fasciotomy: The treatment of compartment syndrome,* in *Green DP and Hotchkiss RN (eds): Operative Hand Surgery, 3d ed. New York, Churchill-Livingstone 1993, pp 661–694.*)

BURNS

Approximately 2 million people sustain burns that require medical attention annually in the United States, resulting in almost 500,000 emergency department visits. Isolated hand burns can result in severe functional and aesthetic impairment. The direct

sympathetic dystrophy requires at least three of the following: (1) diminished hand function, (2) joint stiffness, (3) atrophic changes (edema, atrophy, or fibrosis), and (4) vasomotor instability or vasomotor disturbance.

Reflex sympathetic dystrophy presents acutely as a hot, swollen, painful, or dysesthetic extremity. A specific precipitating injury, such as a neuroma-in-continuity or an entrapped peripheral nerve, may not become apparent until the acute manifestations are treated and resolve. In the case of nerve entrapment, careful consideration should be given to surgical decompression. Prolonged discomfort or pain-limited motion does *not* automatically mean that reflex sympathetic dystrophy or a reflex sympathetic dystrophy–like syndrome is present. Patients may have secondary soft-tissue and periarticular fibrosis after trauma or surgery and a focally tender scar, but with pain isolated only to that area, not generalized. Disuse from any cause can result in osteopenia.

Patients with reflex sympathetic dystrophy often require chronic treatments, psychologic support, including counseling and medication, and an extended, intensive, and closely monitored therapy program (Table 42-4). Early recognition and treatment prevents secondary stiffness from joint and tendon adhesions.

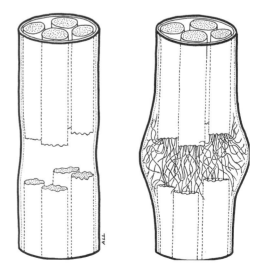

FIG. 42-71. Pseudoneuroma-in-continuity formed after a traction injury. These are seen after traction injuries in which the perineurium remains intact. The axoplasmic flow will accumulate proximal to the point of axonal disruption, forming a fusiform neuroma confined inside the perineurial sheath.

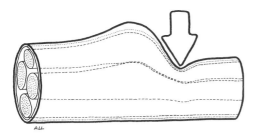

FIG. 42-72. *Pseudoneuroma-in-continuity secondary to severe and chronic nerve compression. The axoplasm accumulates just proximal to the area of compression, mainly in the fascicles closest to the external deforming structure.*

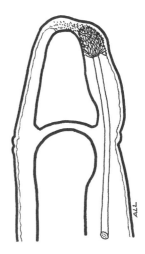

FIG. 42-74. *Terminal neuroma following an amputation (amputation neuroma). The neuroma is quite superficial and gloved by the fibrous tissue formed during the healing of the amputation wound.*

effect of thermal injury to the skin and the consequences of this trauma to hand function include: (1) heat, (2) edema, (3) decreased circulation, and (4) infection. Systemic problems include burn shock, the requirement for fluid resuscitation, secondary immunologic deficits, proteolysis, and the accumulation of secondary toxins.

Management of the burned hand depends on the depth of burn, its surface area, patient age and reliability, and coexisting systemic conditions. Treatment must be individualized. Patients who are reliable and have an adequate support system may be appropriately treated outside of the hospital. Patients with burns that prevent self-care and individuals who have no personal assistance require a more controlled setting.

Primary treatment should focus on preserving viability of soft tissues by preventing secondary wound dehydration via application of a moist or biologic dressing. Blisters can be aspirated to preserve overlying epithelium as a biologic dressing, but if they are leaking and require debridement, the wound should be covered with an occlusive and nondesiccating composite dressing.

Circulation maintenance requires prevention of hypovolemia and avoidance of mechanical obstruction to circulation from en-

veloping eschar. Along with clinical examination, the use of Doppler ultrasonography or a wick catheter for compartment pressure measurement is helpful in assessing vascular sufficiency.

Escharotomy or fasciotomy in a burned extremity may be required to prevent secondary ischemic necrosis. Midlateral incisions are used, whether in the forearm or the fingers. The incision must be deep enough to release all burn eschar and to identify normal tissues at the wound depth. If a single midaxis release does not restore circulation to the periphery, both midaxes must be incised. The neurovascular bundles themselves should be avoided to prevent iatrogenic injury or desiccation after unneeded exposure. The edematous hand may develop an acute carpal or ulnar tunnel syndrome.

Infection is prevented by prophylactic systemic antibiotics in the first 2 days to avoid selection of resistant organisms, but the mainstay of antimicrobial prophylaxis treatment is topical. The most frequently used antimicrobial is silver sulfadiazine (Silvadene), which does not penetrate eschar, is not painful, has broad coverage, prevents desiccation, and can be removed with water, saline solution, or hydrotherapy cleansing. Temporary reversible bone marrow suppression and neutropenia may result from extensive, extended use of silver sulfadiazine. In burn wound sepsis, full-thickness wound biopsy cultures allow diagnosis of sepsis and adjustment of appropriate antibiotics. Surgical debridement of infected burns is necessary, but in widespread burn wound sepsis, mortality may result.

Functional restoration is the most important goal. Most hand burns are on the dorsum because of its exposed position. Deep burns to the palm are more rare except with electrical, chemical, and occasional direct contact thermal burns. Bilateral palmar burns or glovelike burns in children should be considered as evidence of possible child abuse and carefully investigated.

Nonoperative treatment allowing spontaneous healing, and early excision with grafting yield the best functional results in appropriately selected patients. Prolonged inflammation diminishes the chances of recovering hand motion. If initial assessments indicate that the burned hand requires more than 2 weeks before skin healing, early tangential excision and skin grafting

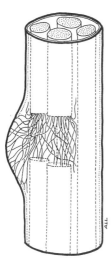

FIG. 42-73. *Lateral neuroma. When a peripheral nerve is partially severed, the regenerating axons that fail to regenerate the distal segment will escape through the epineurial gap, forming a lateral neuroma.*

Table 42-2
Staging of Reflex Sympathetic Dystrophy

	Stage I Acute	Stage II Dystrophic	Stage III Atrophic
Time Frame	0–3 months	3–6 months	6–>12 months
Symptoms	Allodynia	Constant pain	Constant pain
	Hypersensitive	Cold intolerance	Cold intolerance
Signs	Swelling (edema)	Tissue indurated	Thin, atrophic skin
	Redness	Joint stiffness	Dry skin
	↑ Sweating	Dry skin	Cool
Microvascular	↑ Total flow	N1 to ↓ total flow	↓ Total flow
Assessment	↓ Nutritional flow	↓ Nutritional flow	↓ Nutritional flow
X-ray Findings	Mild to moderate osteopenia	Moderate to severe osteopenia	Severe osteopenia

should be undertaken promptly. If spontaneous epithelialization and wound closure are anticipated within 2 weeks, nonoperative treatment with continuous exercises and splinting is appropriate.

Splinting should be given high priority in an antideformity position. Splinting may be done in positions other than the traditional position of function, that is, wrist extension, MP flexion, and IP extension. In dorsal hand burns, the splint position is wrist extension of 30 degrees or less with maximum MP flexion and full IP extension (Fig. 42-75). To preserve the first web, the thumb should be widely abducted palmarward and flexed slightly at the carpometacarpal joint to a position where the radial border of the hand is flat, i.e., the first metacarpal is positioned almost palmar to the second metacarpal. The goal of splinting is to stretch the healing wound and prevent anatomic distortion by scar tissue that can prevent restoration of hand function. Neglected dorsal burns develop metacarpophalangeal hyperextension and interphalangeal flexion deformities, thumb adduction, and wrist flexion contractures (Fig. 42-76). Hand rehabilitation requires a coordinated approach between surgeon and therapist to assure a maximal and timely recovery. At first, hand therapy is directed toward minimizing edema and prevent-

Table 42-3
Definitions of Reflex Sympathetic Dystrophy

From the International Association for the Study of Pain, Taxonomy, Adelaide Consensus Statement 1990

- RSD is a descriptive term for a complex disorder or group of disorders that may develop as a consequence of trauma affecting the limbs with or without obvious nerve lesions.
- RSD consists of pain and related sensory abnormalities, abnormal blood flow and sweating, abnormalities of the motor system, and changes in structure of both the superficial and the deep tissues (tropic changes).
- It is agreed that the term RSD is used in a descriptive sense and not to imply a specific underlying mechanism; not all components will exist at once.

From the Ad Hoc Committee on to the American Association for Hand Surgery

- RSD is a pain syndrome in which the pain is accompanied by loss of function and evidence of autonomic dysfunction.
- Neither pain without autonomic dysfunction nor autonomic dysfunction without pain is sufficient to define the syndrome.
- A more appropriate name for this syndrome may be *sympathetically maintained pain syndrome.*
- Diagnostic criteria include diffused pain, loss of function, and sympathetic dysfunction.

ing deformity. The exercise program starts between the first and fifth posttrauma day to encourage gliding of flexor and extensor tendons and movement of small joints. Therapy eventually progresses to activities of daily living and reintegration into normal life.

Referral of patients requiring postburn reconstruction is made to a specialized center where coverage and therapy techniques are available for hypertrophic scars and contiguous tendon and joint injuries for selected cases.

INFECTION

Bacterial Infection

Skin infections most commonly derive from direct bacterial inoculation. Secondary spread from contiguous sites and hematogenous seeding are less likely. The most common infecting organisms are staphylococcus and streptococcus species; gram-negative, anaerobic, and mixed infections are seen, depending on the inoculation method, e.g., a tooth. Serious, deep infections require hospital admission and extended use of high-dosage intravenous antibiotics. Wound and blood cultures are obtained before antibiotic therapy is started, and adjustments are made as indicated.

Paronychial infections are common. These involve the nail and nail bed, and constitute about 15 percent of hand infections. Occurrence is associated with hangnails, nail biting, finger sucking, and occupations requiring the hands to be damp frequently. Acute infection is always bacterial, creating a localized abscess, but chronic inflammation is most often yeast or fungal, requiring different therapeutic approach (Fig. 42-77).

Herpetic whitlow is an infection of the soft tissues of the distal phalanx or paronychial area by the herpes simplex virus. It is characterized by intense pain and cutaneous vesicles or blisters. The vesicle fluid is clear at first but may become cloudy over a few days. It is important to distinguish this from bacterial infection. Surgical intervention may spread the herpes virus systemically or dispose to local secondary bacterial infection. Only a bacterial abscess needs surgical drainage. Herpetic whitlow is self-limited, generally resolving within 3 to 4 weeks.

Felon is an expanding abscess within the finger pulp, and represents up to one-quarter of hand infections. Felons can also be extremely painful, often reported as throbbing pulp pain. The expanding abscess produces a localized compartment syndrome as a result of the presence of the fibrous septa that normally anchor the pulp skin and subcutaneous tissues to the distal pha-

Table 42-4
Oral and Topical Medications for Reflex Sympathetic Dystrophy

Drug	Usual Dosage	Mechanism	Major Short-term Disadvantage or Side Effects	Contraindications
Amitriptyline (Elavil)	25 mg tid or 50 mg qhs	Inhibits amine pump (decreases norepinephrine uptake)	Drowsiness: antimuscarinic side effects; orthostatic hypotension	With guanethidine sulfate or bretylium
Phenytoin (Dilantin)	100 mg tid	Decreases resting membrane potential; inhibits amine pump; stabilizes synaptic membrane	Minimal drowsiness; serum levels suggested	Long-term use
Phenoxybenzamine hydrochloride (Dibezyline)	40–120 mg/day	Alpha-receptor blocking agent	Orthostatic hypotension	With late-stage RSD
Nifedipine (Procardia)	10 mg tid; may be increased slowly to 30 mg tid (30 mg XL for qd administration available)	Calcium-channel blocking agent; diminishes A–V shunting; increases nutritional flow	Headache; constipation	Concurrent use of beta-adrenergic blocking agents
Corticosteroids	20–80 mg qd prednisone equivalents × 5–40 days	Stabilizes membrane, increases nutritional flow	Adrenal suppression; avascular necrosis; pain (related to dose decreases)	
Carbamazepine (Tegretol)	400–1200 mg in 2 to 3 divided doses	Blocks neural discharges; sodium-channel blocker	Neurological; bone marrow suppression; hepatoxicity; supresion; ataxia	History of bone marrow suppression; hypersensitivity suppression; to tricyclic compounds; concurrent monamine oxidase inhibitors
Clonidine (Catapres-TTS −2, −3)	0.2–0.3 mg patch	Affects adrenergic transmission with marked selectivity for presynaptic sites of vasomotor fibers; alpha-2 adrenergic agonist	Skin irritation; rash surrounding patch; passive absorption of drug varies	Renal disease; heart block; beta-blockers

SOURCE: From Koman LA, Ruch DS, Smith BP, Pollock FE, Poehling GG: Reflex sympathetic dystrophy after wrist surgery. In: Levin LS (ed): *Problems in Plastic and Reconstructive Surgery*. Philadelphia, JB Lippincott, 1992, pp 300–322.

lanx. Felons usually are caused by penetrating direct trauma producing bacterial inoculation. Untreated felons, like other compartment syndromes, compromise local circulation and produce secondary tissue ischemia and necrosis in addition to septic destruction. In surgical drainage additional injury to the finger pulp should be avoided, but an abscess may already point to a superficial location (Fig. 42-78).

Deep-space palmar infections may occur more often in the immunocompromised, drug abusers, elderly, and neglected populations. These are extremely serious infections with secondary systemic symptoms requiring the combination of extended medical and staged surgical therapy (Fig. 42-79).

Tenosynovitis. Acute pyogenic digital tenosynovitis is most frequently a result of direct penetrating trauma. Kanavel's cardinal signs of tenosynovitis include: (1) fusiform digital swelling, (2) semiflexed digital posture, (3) significant pain from passive extension of the finger, and (4) tenderness along the entire flexor sheath. Proper management for this closed-space tenosynovial abscess is surgical drainage and intravenous antibiotics. A high index of clinical suspicion is required for diag-

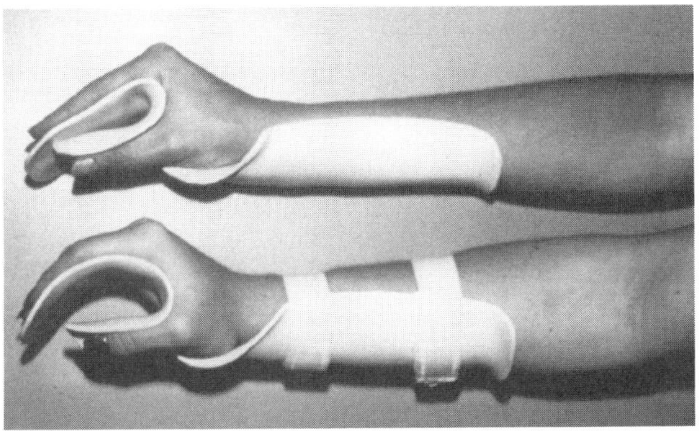

FIG. 42-75. Upper picture demonstrates the antideformity position as advocated by Salisburg. The lower picture shows the traditional functional position of the hand.

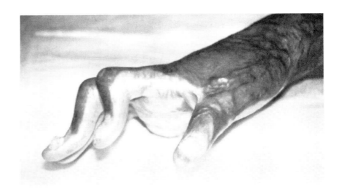

FIG. 42-76. Poor hand splinting resulted in this intrinsic minus hand.

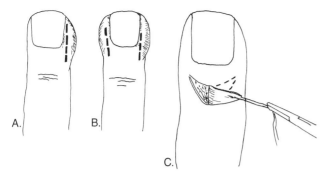

FIG. 42-77. Drainage of a paronychial infection involves opening the involved lateral sulcus with a probe or scalpel blade. Occasionally the incision must be extended proximally (A) or involve both sulci (B). C. A crescent-shaped incision is used to marsupialize chronic paronychia.

nosis. Aspiration of the sheath will confirm the diagnosis. In early cases, systemic antibiotics alone may be considered, but there must be profound resolution within 12 to 24 h; otherwise, prompt operative drainage is necessary (Fig. 42-80).

Arthritis and Osteomyelitis. Septic arthritis and osteomyelitis result from neglected soft-tissue infection and may occur in the undertreated or unhealthy population. These problems require extended surgical and medical therapies and often multiple, staged salvage or reconstructive procedures.

High-Pressure Injection Injuries. These injuries occur from paint and grease guns, hydraulic lines, and diesel injectors that propel material under pressures of up to 7,000 pounds per square inch. Penetration through skin and along extended tissue planes is the rule rather than the exception. These injuries almost always involve the hands. The severity of injury is related most directly to the nature of the injected material. Paint and solvents that are cytotoxic produce intense inflammation in addition to the trauma from the high-force injury. This prolonged inflammatory phase is sometimes mistaken for infection. Such injuries require immediate mechanical and pulse-lavage debridement in order to prevent extended tissue loss (Figs. 42-81 and 42-82).

Nonbacterial Infection

Nonbacterial infections include tuberculous, mycotic, and similar diseases. Granuloma, a collection of macrophages and histiocytes characteristic of the systemic response to these agents, is diagnostic. A high index of suspicion and a careful history are necessary for accurate diagnosis. Patients present with relatively painless, chronic, indolent soft-tissue problems. The patient may recall a local traumatic event. The correct diagnosis often is appreciated only after months or years. For example, the history of a penetrating fish hook injury weeks or months before a nodular or boggy tenosynovitis in a fisherman could suggest an atypical mycobacterial infection to the suspicious clinician. Tissue biopsy and cultures confirm the diagnosis of specific granulomatous disease. The distinction between superficial and deep tissue involvement is important in tubercular and fungal infections, because superficial infections are treated medically and deep infections require surgical debridement. Mycobacterial infection, including tuberculosis and the atypical mycobacteria originally thought to be just saprophytes, occurs primarily as soft-tissue infection with secondary bone and joint penetration. The pathologic atypical mycobacteria include *Mycobacterium marinum, kansasii, avium-intracellulare, fortuitum,* and *chelonei.* Outside of the United States, the organism most frequently producing deformity and destruction of upper extremity function is *Mycobacterium leprae,* Hansen's bacillus. Hansen's disease should be considered in patients from other nations.

CHRONIC SYNDROMES

Tendinitis

De Quervain's Tenosynovitis. Inflammation of the tendons in the first dorsal compartment and the abductor pollicis longus and extensor pollicis brevis became associated with de Quervain after his 1895 report of five cases. This tendon inflammation is one of the most common causes of pain along the radial side of the wrist and the proximal dorsoradial thumb. The problem is more common in women, and particularly in new mothers because of frequent positioning of the wrist into flexion and thumb in extension while carrying or manipulating their infant. As both tendons pass across the radial styloid process in their tendon sheath, they are subjected to angulation and shear.

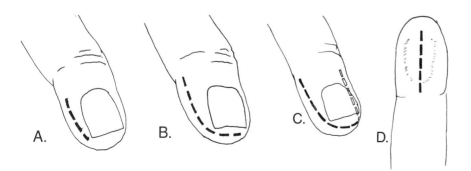

FIG. 42-78. Incision and drainage is the proper management of a felon. A. The proper incision is dorsal to the apex of the distal interphalangeal flexion crease at the junction of the dorsal and glabrous sulci. Usually the incision is lateral. B and C. The incision may be extended to varying degrees around the fingertip as necessary, but it must be carried just volar to the edge of the nail matrix. D. An alternative incision, advocated by some authors, extends longitudinally on the midline of the volar pulp distal to the flexion crease.

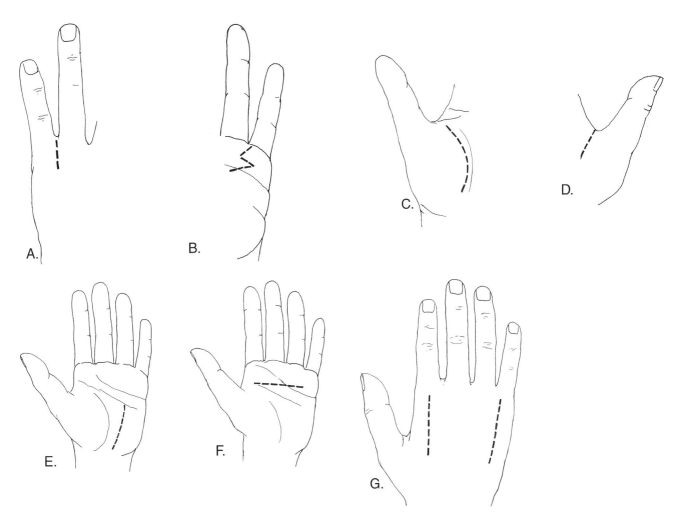

FIG. 42-79. Surgical approaches to deep-space infections. *A* and *B.* Interdigital web space. *C* and *D.* Thenar space. *E.* Hypothenar space. *F.* Midpalmar space. *G.* Dorsal subaponeurotic space.

Patients present with tenderness over the midaxis of the radial styloid process. Active thumb and wrist motion, particularly active thumb extension and passive flexion with wrist deviation, are painful. There may be crepitus over the tendon sheath, occasional locking, or a secondary ganglionic mass. There also may be secondary irritation of the overlying superficial branches of the radial nerve with paresthesias along the thumb and first web (Fig. 42-83). The tendon inflammation causes restriction of activities and motion. In Finkelstein's test, designed to reproduce symptoms by passive traction on these tendons, the patient grasps the flexed thumb under the fingers of the same hand, and then the examiner actively deviates the wrist ulnarly. The test is positive when symptoms are reproduced by this maneuver.

The initial treatment for de Quervain's tenosynovitis includes rest and custom splint support of the wrist and thumb. Oral nonsteroidal anti-inflammatory agents may sometimes be helpful, but injection with a steroid and local anesthetic combination is best. The injection should not be made into subcutaneous tissues, because it can produce fat atrophy or depigmentation in darker-skinned individuals. Once acute symptoms resolve, splinting may be continued for symptom-inducing activities, such as when mothers care for their infants. As with other tendon inflamma-

tions, injection should relieve symptoms adequately and for a minimum of 4 to 6 months to merit repeating.

When symptoms persist or recur, surgery is carried out through a transverse 2-cm incision centered over the thickened radial styloid process. All deeper dissection is done by gentle longitudinal spreading. The branches of the radial sensory nerve are retracted gently and the thickened sheath incised longitudinally. Multiple tendon slips are evident when the abductor pollicis longus is exposed; this tendon is commonly multistranded. The extensor pollicis brevis tendon is in another subcompartment that also must be released separately in up to 90 percent of cases. Many surgeons excise a portion of the sheath; others close it deep to the tendons. Postoperatively, the thumb and wrist are immobilized for 1 week before active motion with decreasing splint protection is started. Resistive exercises begin when they can be tolerated.

Other Wrist Tendinitis. Flexor and extensor sheath tendinitis may occur in any of the dorsal and volar subgroups, including the second through sixth extensor compartments, the flexor carpi radialis tendon tunnel, and at the flexor carpi ul-

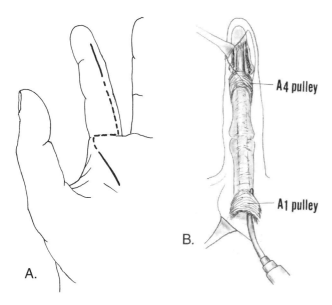

FIG. 42-80. *A.* Generic midaxial digital skin incision may be carried proximally (if necessary) to connect to the proximal portion of the sheath. The incision is kept dorsal to preserve both neurovascular bundles in the palmar flap and to allow the wound to remain open without jeopardizing flap coverage of the affected tendon. *B.* Irrigation catheter placement beneath the A1 pulley is all that is needed to achieve unimpeded irrigation once the sheath distal to the A4 pulley has been excised (the distal pulley is preserved, of course); the distal wound is left *open.*

naris–pisiform and pisotriquetral joint. Chronic inflammation of any tendon compartment is associated with local and radiating symptoms. Passive stretch and resisted active function of the affected tendons reproduces symptoms and confirms the diagnosis in the absence of other clinical or x-ray findings. Flexor tenosynovitis is not rare after prolonged gripping activities, such as in stringed-instrument players and typists. Extensor compartment inflammation may be found with intense repetitive wrist and finger motion from any cause.

More proximally, intersection syndromes can occur where the extensor carpi radialis longus and extensor carpi radialis brevis tendons cross the first compartment tendons at their musculotendinous junctions. These crossover tendon inflammations may sometimes be accompanied by audible and palpable crepitus. Similar presentations may occur with the extensor pollicis longus and extensor indicis proprius tendons.

Trigger Finger. Chronic flexor tenosynovitis or tenovaginitis occurs most commonly in the middle and ring fingers and in the thumb, and most often in postmenopausal females. Patients may not recall an injury that predates symptoms, but many can describe an episode of prolonged use or forceful trauma with impact or hyperextension that immediately preceded the symptom onset. The snapping phenomenon occurs as the flexor digitorum superficialis and profundus tendons, or the flexor pollicis longus in the case of the thumb, pull through a tight A1 flexor pulley at the proximal edge of the sheath. There is debate as to whether tenosynovial inflammation or pulley thickening is the cause. There is a relative lack of volume in the sheath for the tendon, inducing the crepitus, catching or locking, and pain. Many patients have other associated systemic diseases, such as diabetes, connective tissue disease, or additional sites of teno-

synovitis or carpal tunnel syndrome, but the process may be isolated.

Patients presenting with complaints of finger pain, distal palmar pain on grasping, finger catching and locking should be evaluated for systemic and local problems. Thickening of the flexor tendon at the base of the finger, in the distal palm, and palpation of tendon nodule that glides with active finger motion will make the diagnosis. In the locking finger, an audible and palpable snap is noted (Fig. 42-84). Any condition that causes finger stiffness, diminished flexion, or a flexion contracture especially at the PIP joint, snapping or locking can be potentially *mis*diagnosed as trigger finger. Diagnosis is made by careful clinical examination and findings of a localized nodularity and tenderness about the flexor sheath in the distal palm.

Nonsurgical treatment should be offered except for patients with a fixed PIP joint flexion contracture that will not unlock after local anesthetic and steroid injection. Approximately 1 to 2 mL of the mix is injected into the flexor sheath and pulley. At introduction, the needle pierces the skin and tendons at the base of the proximal phalanx/metacarpal head and is then withdrawn slightly. The sheath is aspirated and injection proceeds with gentle pressure. Firm resistance indicates that the needle is in a tendon and needs to be withdrawn or inserted further. Palpable and visible introduction of fluid into the flexor sheath is a successful injection. Most patients improve, but those with continuing and recurring symptoms are candidates for surgery.

Surgery routinely cures the problem, providing long-term relief unless incomplete A1 pulley release, digital nerve injury, or division of the next more distal A2 pulley occurs. With the patient under local anesthesia and with a forearm or elbow tourniquet, a longitudinal incision is made directly over the flexor tendon between the proximal metacarpophalangeal joint flexion crease and the distal palmar crease (Fig. 42-85). The thickened pulley lies directly beneath this skin incision, just dorsal to the fascia and subcutaneous fat layers. The neurovascular bundles are both lateral to the sheath. Longitudinal incision in the sheath is made under direct vision, carefully releasing the proximal and distal extent of the pulley. To assure restoration of unimpeded tendon gliding via active flexion and passive traction, a blunt hook is used. In the thumb, special care is taken to avoid inadvertent division of the radial proper digital nerve, which usually crosses over and is palmar to the flexor tendon proximal to the pulley. Tendon release under direct vision protects this structure. For tendon release in the thumb, an oblique longitudinal or Bruner-style incision is performed (Fig. 42-86).

Direct trauma producing a partial tendon laceration distally may cause a triggering phenomenon in the distal flexor sheath. Systemic diseases that produce tendon nodularity, such as rheumatoid arthritis and gout, may cause similar, but more distal, locking or catching of the tendon. These less common causes require more extended flexor sheath exploration, excision of tendon nodules, and rehabilitation.

Neuropathies

Median Nerve. The median nerve may be compressed anywhere along its course from the cervical roots to the fingertips, but the most common site is within the carpal tunnel, where it is dorsal to the transverse carpal ligament. All anatomic sites of compression must be considered and evaluated in the differential diagnosis of this increasingly common peripheral neuropathy.

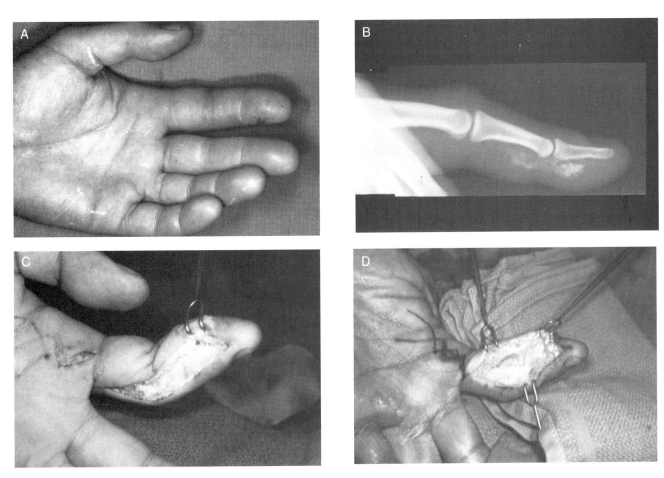

FIG. 42-81. *A.* This 23-year-old autobody worker presented with increasing index finger pain and swelling 4 h after an injury at work when the paint gun he was cleaning accidentally discharged into the ulnar pulp of this finger. *B.* X-ray shows the paint in the flexor sheath and volar soft tissues. *C* and *D.* Sharp debridement and pulse irrigation were performed through an ulnar midaxial incision. Paint products were removed from around the flexor tendon, sheath, and throughout the digital subcutaneous tissues. Meticulous care was required to save the neurovascular bundles during debridement.

Carpal tunnel syndrome results from increased pressure within the rigid carpal canal, producing median nerve ischemia and physiologic dysfunction. Symptoms include paresthesias and numbness in the radial $3\frac{1}{2}$ fingers, burning digital dysesthesias,

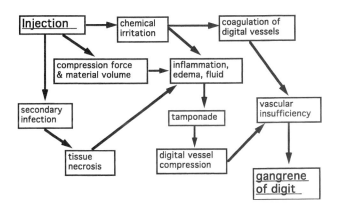

FIG. 42-82. Pathophysiology of high-pressure injection injuries. Multiple mechanisms contribute to tissue damage and gangrene.

and, later in the course, hand weakness or awkwardness. Focal wrist and hand pain are not a part of the syndrome, while nocturnal presence of symptoms is a hallmark of this diagnosis. All treatments are designed to reduce pressure within the canal and relieve nerve compression.

The carpal canal serves as a mechanical conduit for the digital flexor tendons. The carpal bones form the walls and floor or dorsal surface of the canal, and the palmar aspect is roofed by the transverse carpal ligament. Tunnel cross-sectional area is dynamic, with the smallest area probably obtaining at the extremes of wrist flexion and extension. There is debate as to the cause of the increased pressure. Some have postulated tenosynovitis, while other studies have shown collagen, amyloid deposits, and edema as causes.

Eighty percent of carpal tunnel patients are over the age of 40 years. The female/male ratio varies from 4:1 for idiopathic cases, but be as low as 1.5:1 with occupational presentation. A direct connection between carpal tunnel syndrome and forceful or repetitive use of the hands has not been conclusively demonstrated. There are reports of low and high instances among workers in manual industries. Such studies have used clinical criteria alone for the diagnosis and have not eliminated avoca-

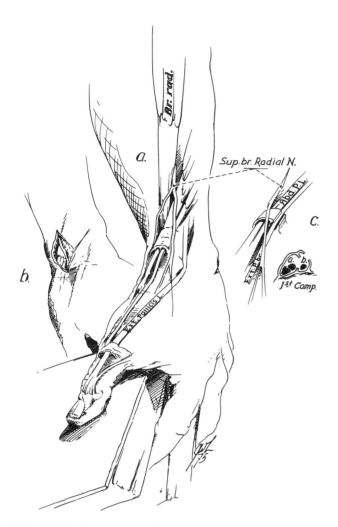

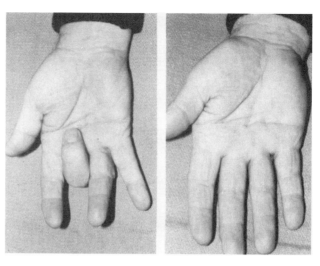

FIG. 42-84. Trigger finger coexisting with Dupuytren's contracture in the same digit. This patient had locking of the middle finger in flexion, which was unrelated to the mild static flexion deformity of the metacarpophalangeal joint caused by the Dupuytren's cord and was relieved by a steroid injection into the flexor sheath.

FIG. 42-83. Anatomy of de Quervain's tenosynovitis. Note the relationship of the radial sensory nerve to the tendons. Note the relationships of the extensor pollicis brevis and abductor pollicis longus tendons within the first extensor compartment. (From: *Burton RI, Littler JW: Entrapment syndromes of the retinacular or restraining systems of the hand, in: Nontraumatic Soft Tissue Afflictions of the Hand. Current Problems in Surgery, Chicago, Year Book Medical Publishers, 1975, with permission.*)

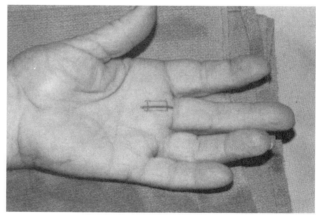

A

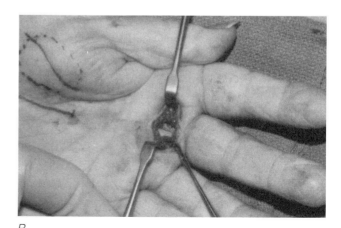

B

tional or systemic disease–induced causes. The causation is probably multifactorial in most patients. Carpal tunnel syndrome has been associated with endocrine disorders, including diabetes, myxedema, hyperthyroidism, acromegaly, pregnancy, and the postpartum state. Chronic infections and hematologic and autoimmune disorders also are associated with carpal tunnel syndrome. Space-occupying lesions such as lipomas, bone abnormalities of the radius or carpals, posttraumatic edema, and hematomas may induce increased pressure within the canal and compromise median nerve function.

The diagnosis of carpal tunnel syndrome is clinical. Classic symptoms include paresthesias, with a predominance of nocturnal or early morning onset, burning or numbness in the median sensory distribution, and awkwardness in use of the hand. On physical examination, direct digital pressure over the median nerve at the carpal tunnel reproduces symptoms within 30 seconds. In Phalen's maneuver, gravity-induced wrist flexion repro-

FIG. 42-85. Longitudinal incision for trigger finger release. *A.* The incision is made in a natural skin crease, over the A1 pulley, between the base of the finger flexion crease and the distal transverse crease of the palm. *B.* The surgical view shows the released A1 pulley and the flexor digitorum superficialis tendon.

duces symptoms within a minute. When direct percussion of the nerve elicits and reproduces paresthesias in the median distribution, it is a positive Tinel's sign. The application of a pneumatic tourniquet to the upper limb to reproduce digital symptoms is of no value in making this diagnosis. Examination should include objective documentation of sensory and motor loss, the former by threshold testing, including vibration and Semms-Weinstein monofilaments rather than innervation density or two-point discrimination. Examination of motor function includes observation for thenar loss and assessing abductor muscle resistance against force (Fig. 42-87).

Electrophysiologic studies provide important confirmatory and differential diagnostic information. Electrophysiologic studies alone do not form the basis for this diagnosis, but surgery should not be done without electrophysiologic evaluation. Electrophysiologic tests are useful when the diagnosis is difficult or when surgical release is contemplated. Underlying peripheral neuropathies and multifocal compressions that are otherwise unsuspected may be uncovered. Electrical studies provide a baseline for later comparison if the response to surgery is disappointing. Evaluation should include studies of the median nerve as well as of a second nerve in the more symptomatic extremity. Comparison of median and ulnar or of median and radial sensory stimulation values at the wrist is useful in confirming the diagnosis. Studies are not necessarily of prognostic value for the response to surgery.

Routine radiographs including the carpal tunnel view are recommended by the American Academy of Orthopaedic Surgery for evaluation and treatment of carpal tunnel syndrome. Radiographs are evaluated for carpal fractures, arthritis, Kienböck's disease, or other problems that could alter treatment. CT and MRI scans are seldom needed, but basic laboratory studies to screen for endocrine and hematologic disorders are helpful. Predisposing medical diseases, such as thyroid dysfunction or rheumatoid arthritis, should be treated and may frequently improve or resolve the neuropathy without surgery. In pregnancy, carpal tunnel syndrome is treated by salt restriction, wrist splinting, analgesics, and, occasionally, diuretics. Local injection may be needed in the third trimester. Most patients recover within about 6 months of delivery.

For acute posttraumatic carpal tunnel syndrome associated with swelling or hemorrhage, loosening of constrictive bandages and moving the wrist from a position at the extreme of flexion or extension may suffice to reverse or significantly improve symptoms. Pressure studies and early surgery may be appropriate for those who do not respond.

Splints and nonsteroidal anti-inflammatory medications are widely used. Splints should fit comfortably and position the wrist in neutral to minimal extension. Splints are worn at night if nocturnal symptoms are a major complaint. Night splinting may be all that is required. With activity-induced symptoms, daytime splint use during provoking tasks may be needed. Oral nonsteroidal anti-inflammatory agents are helpful, with monitoring for possible gastrointestinal and systemic side effects. Although subclinical vitamin B_6 deficiency is a possible cause of carpal tunnel syndrome, no prospective study has demonstrated the efficacy of pyridoxine, but it is nontoxic. Local steroid injection results in improvement in 80 to 90 percent of patients, but there is gradual deterioration over the next 12 to 24 months. As with other sites, injections should not be repeated more than

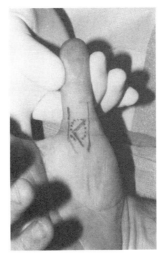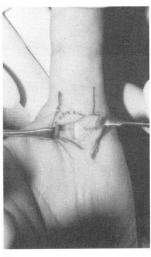

A   *B*

FIG. 42-86. *V-shaped incision for release of trigger thumb. A. A V-shaped flap is raised full thickness, based radially, and centered over the A1 pulley, with its apex at the metacarpophalangeal joint flexion crease. This protects the radial digital nerve of the thumb. B. The surgical view shows the released A1 pulley and the flexor pollicis longus tendon.*

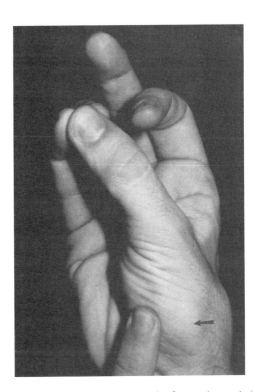

FIG. 42-87. *Palpation of thenar muscles for weakness during opposition. The bulging muscle of the abductor pollicis brevis (arrow), which is consistently innervated by the median nerve, is seen and can be palpated adjacent to the metacarpal while asking the patient to oppose the thumb forcefully to the little finger. Softness in the muscle contraction suggests weakness in this muscle.*

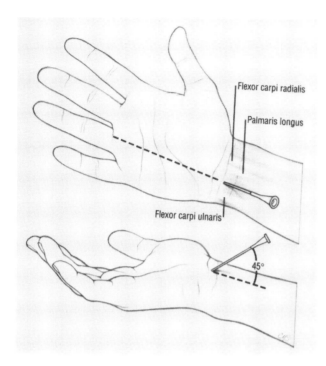

FIG. 42-88. Needle placement for injection of the carpal canal. The needle tip is placed through the skin at the volar wrist crease midway between the flexor carpi ulnaris and palmaris longus tendons at a 45-degree angle. A fine needle is used. If paresthesias are encountered in this location, the needle should be redirected to avoid intraneural injection with corticosteroid. Inadvertent median nerve injection can occur even in this location if the nerve lies ulnarly.

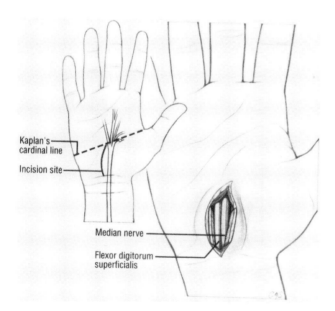

FIG. 42-89. The cardinal line and the incision for open carpal tunnel release. Kaplan has described a line drawn to help localize the motor branch of the median nerve. At the site of intersection of a line dropped from the radial side of the ring finger is the entrance of the recurrent motor branch of the median nerve into the thenar muscles. The gently curved incision for surgical decompression begins at the volar wrist crease in line with the ring metacarpal and parallels the thenar crease to end at the cardinal line.

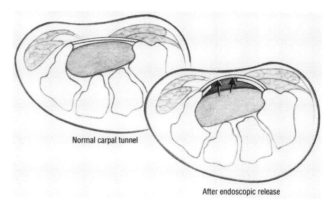

FIG. 42-90. The dual layers of the transverse carpal ligament. The transverse carpal ligament has a deep, rigid layer and a more superficial flexible layer composed of palmar, thenar, and hypothenar fascia. With endoscopic carpal tunnel release, the rigid deep layer separates, but the more flexible superficial layer remains intact. The increased volume within the carpal canal is a result of volar migration of the contents of the canal.

2 or 3 times annually. Inadvertent injection directly into the median nerve will worsen symptoms (Fig. 42-88).

Surgical treatment requires complete division of the transverse carpal ligament for the entire length of the carpal tunnel under direct vision. Surgical failure is most often associated with incorrect diagnosis or incomplete ligament division. Internal neurolysis, flexor tenosynovectomy, concomitant ulnar nerve decompression in Guyon's canal, or carpal ligament reconstruction are not indicated with primary release and may be harmful. Open and endoscopic release can effectively divide the transverse carpal ligament and increase canal volume (Figs. 42-89, 42-90, and 42-91). Open release is performed with the patient supine and under tourniquet control. After limb exsanguination and tourniquet inflation, the field is infiltrated with local anesthetic. Intravenous sedation may be used as a supplement. Incision for open release parallels the thenar crease from the distal end of the transverse carpal ligament to almost the distal wrist crease and is made in line with the third web. The skin should be marked before incision. Small twigs of palmar cutaneous nerve branches are identified during subcutaneous dissection and preserved where found crossing the incision. The palmar fascia is split longitudinally, using a small curved hemostat, from the proximal end of the carpal canal moving distally in the most palmar and ulnar quadrant of the canal. The nerve and flexor tendons beneath and radial to the clamp are continuously identified and protected. The motor nerve to the thenar muscles is identified and protected. The ligament incision roughly parallels the ulnar border of the median nerve and leaves a small tissue flap attached to the hook of the hamate, more ulnarly. The wound is inspected to assure complete division of the ligament, release of the contents, and the absence of soft-tissue and bone anomalies. The median nerve is found in the palmoradial portion of the canal, generally adherent to the underside of the ligament. The nerve may have a central-narrowing, hourglass constriction at the site of maximum compression. The surgeon should avoid manipulating the nerve because this induces more intraneural scarring and interferes both with postoperative nerve gliding and ultimate recovery. After tourniquet release and hemostasis, palmar fascia may be closed, but most surgeons close only the skin,

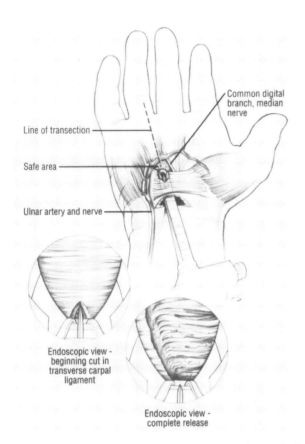

FIG. 42-91. *Endoscopic carpal tunnel release. The safe area for ligament division is in line with the ring finger between the median nerve and the ulnar neurovascular bundle, proximal to the superficial vascular arch. With the resection nosepiece aligned with the ring finger, the transverse fibers of the transverse carpal ligament as seen through the endoscope assures the surgeon that no critical structures intervene between the blade and the ligament. When resection is complete, the rigid portion of the transverse carpal ligament slides apart, creating a trapezoidal defect, decompressing the carpal canal. After this occurs, the nosepiece of the system fits between the cut edges of the ligament; if the endoscope is rolled from one side to the other, only one side of the divided ligament can be seen through the window.*

using a fine monofilament nonabsorbable suture. The wrist is splinted in slight extension for about 2 weeks before therapy is started.

Endoscopic release was introduced to avoid the morbidity of a palmar scar. Studies suggest a more rapid recovery with equivalent increase in canal volume by this approach. The single-portal endoscopic decompression is associated with less perioperative discomfort and shorter immobilization and recovery. After endoscopic release, a canvas wrist splint is offered but not required. Therapy usually can be started within the first postoperative week.

The incidence of inadvertent tissue trauma from open and endoscopic methods has not been determined. The best method for avoiding complications is to operate carefully, in a bloodless field, cutting only what can be seen clearly and identified precisely before it is incised. If the patient continues to have symptoms after surgery, appropriate clinical and adjunctive diagnostic investigation should be undertaken. Incomplete ligament division or inaccurate preoperative diagnosis are the most frequent problems, but patients with hidden agendas of a nonanatomic

nature may experience prolonged wound discomfort and limited recovery. In such situations, the real value of preoperative electrodiagnostics becomes evident.

Ulnar Nerve. Ulnar nerve compression at the elbow, the cubital tunnel syndrome, has been known for more than a century. It has been called posttraumatic ulnar neuritis and tardy ulnar nerve palsy to emphasize the traumatic causation. Distal compression in the canal of Guyon (the ulnar tunnel) at the wrist is a less common problem and more often caused by a space-occupying lesion or direct trauma. The possible sites of ulnar nerve compression in the fibromuscular groove posterior to the medial epicondyle are summarized in Fig. 42-92. All sites of nerve compression must be considered. The differential diagnosis must include medial epicondylitis and its coexistence with ulnar nerve irritation. Some patients have the mechanical problem of a hypermobile or subluxating ulnar nerve. Ulnar traction neuritis with elbow flexion and anterior nerve subluxation reproduce radiating paresthesias in the ulnar two fingers. Patients who have actual motor weakness, and especially the subgroup with intrinsic muscle atrophy and electrophysiologic changes, have a guarded prognosis after delayed decompression.

Patients presenting with medial epicondylitis should be treated for that problem, but the presence of secondary coexistent nerve irritation must be addressed. Those who do not respond to conservative measures as outlined for the carpal tunnel should be treated surgically. At operation, after nerve decompression, the resultant problem of iatrogenic subluxation must be dealt with. Some prefer simultaneous subperiosteal medial epicondylectomy, excising enough of the bony prominence to flatten the skeletal contour of the medial side of the elbow so that flexion/extension does not produce snapping of the nerve over a tissue prominence. Alternatively, submuscular transposition can be performed. There is no clear advantage of one technique over the other in most patients (Fig. 42-93).

Ulnar tunnel decompression at the wrist must include the management of space-occupying lesions which complicate this diagnosis. Ulnar tunnel syndrome is far less frequent than compromise of the median nerve in the carpal tunnel syndrome (Fig. 42-94). Pathologic conditions predisposing to ulnar nerve and

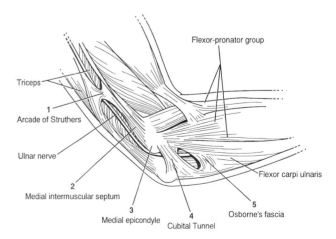

FIG. 42-92. *The five potential areas of ulnar nerve compression around the elbow: (1) the arcade of Struthers, (2) the medial intermuscular septum, (3) the medial epicondyle, (4) the cubital tunnel, (5) Osborne's fascia.*

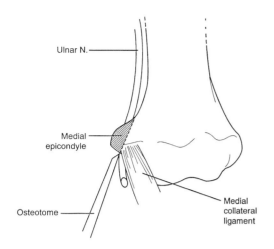

FIG. 42-93. *Medial epicondylectomy. The key here is to excise the midportion of the medial epicondyle without disrupting the origin of the medial collateral ligament. When there is doubt, radiographs can be useful.*

artery compression in the ulnar tunnel should be attended to simultaneously, including excision of a hamulus nonunion, ulnar artery revascularization, or removal of ganglia.

Radial Nerve. Radial nerve entrapment may cause sensory symptoms of paresthesias and dysesthesias in the nerve's afferent muscular and cutaneous distributions in the dorsal forearm, wrist, and hand. Symptoms depend on the primary site of nerve irritation or compression, which is most frequently in the proximal forearm. The term *radial tunnel syndrome* describes a compression neuropathy involving the posterior interosseous nerve branch of the radial nerve. The common presentation is aching discomfort in the dorsal and dorsal-lateral forearm. Patients with

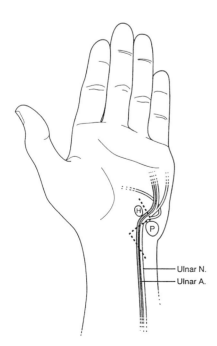

FIG. 42-94. *Incision for exposure of Guyon's canal.*

this problem may have preceding or coexistent lateral epicondylitis, and the distinction between epicondylitis and posterior interosseous nerve compression must be included in the differential workup of all cases of resistant tennis elbow. Unlike epicondylitis, the site of focal tenderness is distal to the epicondyle, over the extensor muscles, at the site where the posterior interosseous nerve passes into the fibromuscular tunnel bounded by the fibrous proximal edge of the superficial heads of the supinator, approximately at the neck of the radius (Fig. 42-95).

Nonsurgical treatment includes rest, activity modification, splint protection, and nonsteroidal anti-inflammatory agents. Injectable steroids do not have a useful role. Electrodiagnostic studies are not helpful because of the deep and variable location of the nerve. Only patients with denervation of the forearm muscles will dependably have electrical changes—and this group should be easy to diagnose clinically before operative decompression.

The radial and posterior interosseous nerves can be decompressed in the proximal forearm and anterolateral elbow region in patients with resistant symptoms. The brachioradialis splitting incision is most efficient (Fig. 42-96).

Radial sensory entrapment distally, Wartenberg's disease or cheiralgia paresthetica, may occur, but usually only after direct trauma to the radial wrist, e.g., after application of handcuffs. Operation is rarely required for this typically transient problem. Radial sensory symptoms of local paresthesias more often coexist with or are secondary to the more common problem of de Quervain's tenosynovitis in the first dorsal compartment. This tendinitis should be excluded in the differential diagnosis and is a more probable reason for nerve irritation than primary entrapment (Fig. 42-97).

ACQUIRED DYSFUNCTION

Dupuytren's Contracture

Although this disorder is associated with the nineteenth-century French surgeon Baron Guillaume Dupuytren, he was not the first to describe it. John Hunter, in 1777, and Sir Astley Cooper, in 1822, described the disease, and Cooper recommended subcutaneous fasciotomy. The pathologic proliferation is primarily of the longitudinal portion of the palmar fascia and its digital expansions palmar and dorsal to the neurovascular bundles (Fig. 42-98). The diagnosis in advanced cases is not difficult, but in early stages the disorder may be confusing. Knuckle pads consisting of fasciotendinous proliferations over the dorsum of the PIP joints, of palmar fascial nodules, or dimpling or pitting of the palmar skin are characteristic findings. While palmar fascial nodules are believed pathognomonic, other masses including, retinacular cysts, tendon nodules, foreign bodies, and trigger finger, occasionally cause confusion. The Dupuytren's fascial nodule does not move with active flexor tendon excursion and is located just deep to the skin and subcutaneous fat. Fascial skin tethering may result in fat bulging on either side of the diseased pretendinous band and cause the skin pits that are characteristic of this pathologic process. Proliferating nodules precede cords, but patients may not present until cords and contractures are present. Joint deformity and contracture is the eventual result of coalescence of nodules with the development of a shortened, pathologic fascial mass. There is no proven relationship to

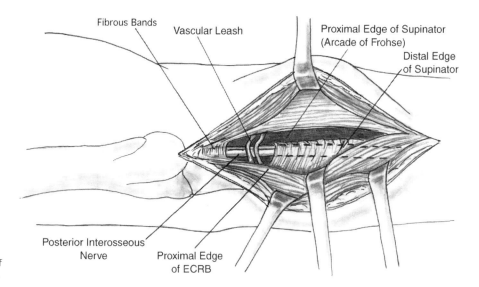

FIG. 42-95. The five potential sites of posterior interosseous nerve compression.

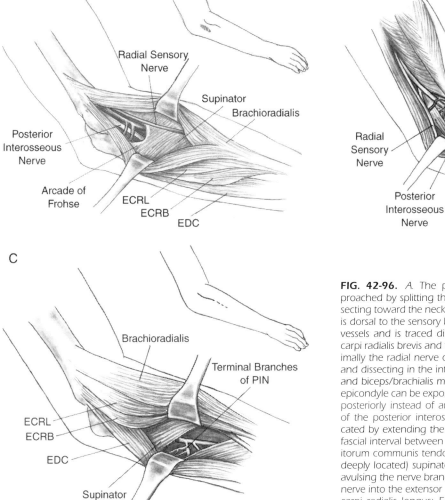

FIG. 42-96. *A.* The posterior interosseous nerve is efficiently approached by splitting the brachioradialis muscle fibers bluntly and dissecting toward the neck of the radius. The posterior interosseous nerve is dorsal to the sensory branch; it is located deep to the leash of radial vessels and is traced distally under the fibrous edge of the extensor carpi radialis brevis and the supinator (arcade of Frohse). *B.* More proximally the radial nerve can be exposed by extending the skin incision and dissecting in the intermuscular space between the brachioradialis and biceps/brachialis muscles more medially. As necessary, the lateral epicondyle can be exposed by turning this extended skin incision more posteriorly instead of anteriorly and proximally. *C.* The distal portion of the posterior interosseous nerve and the lower supinator are located by extending the original skin incision distally and opening the fascial interval between extensor carpi radialis brevis and extensor digitorum communis tendons, continuing proximally to locate the (more deeply located) supinator muscle edge. Care must be taken to avoid avulsing the nerve branches traversing from the posterior interosseous nerve into the extensor digitorum communis muscle. ECRL = extensor carpi radialis longus; ECRB = extensor carpi radialis brevis; EDC = extensor digitorum communis; PIN = posterior interosseous nerve.

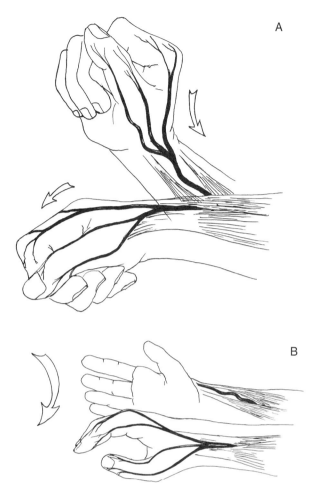

FIG. 42-97. *Radial sensory nerve irritation may occur in response to repetitive physiologic stress. A. The superficial branch of the radial nerve is relatively lax with wrist extension but stretches during flexion and ulnar deviation, such as during hammering. The nerve is tethered proximally, where it exits from deep to superficial through the fascia just dorsal to the brachioradialis muscle. This mechanism generates the neuritic pain during Finkelstein's maneuver, but as paresthesias rather than localized discomfort. B. As the forearm rotates into pronation, the superficial radial nerve stretches and may be compressed between the tendons of the brachioradialis and extensor carpi radialis longus muscles.*

trauma, occupation, handedness, or repetitive use in work or sports.

Dupuytren's contracture is most commonly seen in Caucasian males of Northern European descent who are in their sixth decade or older (Figs. 42-99, 42-100, and 42-101). Hand dominance or trauma are not causes; the male-to-female ratio varies from 2:1 to 10:1. Dupuytren's contracture is familial and is inherited as an autosomal dominant but with variable penetrance. There are significant associations with a number of diseases and conditions, the most prominent of which are diabetes and alcoholism. HIV may be a risk factor.

There is no effective nonsurgical treatment for Dupuytren's contracture. Operation should be reserved for those whose disease is complicated by contracture. Tender palmar nodules are a transient phenomenon, caused by the coexistence of active cellular proliferation and repetitive daily contact, impact, or load. In patients with such complaints, often truck drivers and others

who must grip or lift continuously, padded gloves such as those worn by bicyclists and weight lifters may help. Symptoms resolve within a few weeks or months. Splinting does not prevent later contracture. When the patient can no longer place the hand flat on the table, the Huston tabletop test, operation is indicated. Contracture correction at the MP joint is easier than at the PIP joint, where surgery should proceed when the fixed PIP contracture approaches 45 degrees.

Operating on a patient with Dupuytren's contracture requires a detailed knowledge of normal hand anatomy, palmar fascial structure, and location of the pathology as it applies to the deformity, including pathologic displacement of the neurovascular bundles, which puts them at risk of injury during even the most careful of surgical release procedures (Fig. 42-102). Most patients have the ulnar palm affected first and most significantly. In decreasing order, the fourth, fifth, third, second, and first rays are most frequently involved. The most effective technique is digital fasciectomy as opposed to fasciotomy. The results deteriorate with time, however; surgery does not cure the disease but treats joint deformities, contracture, and dysfunction. Fasciectomy is performed under loupe magnification and exsanguinated pneumatic tourniquet control. Skin flaps are dissected at the level of palmar fascia, preserving the maximum thickness of contiguous skin and subcutaneous tissues to avoid devascularized, over-thinned flaps (Fig. 42-103). Closed fasciotomy is not performed because of the risk of neurovascular injury in this blind release technique.

Postoperative management varies only to a minor degree whether Bruner-style, Z-plasty, or the McCash open-palm incision technique is used. With the open technique, transverse areas at the skin creases minimally affect the recovery protocol. A drain is not necessary. The lessened risk of hematoma and diminished short-term pain afforded by leaving some incisions

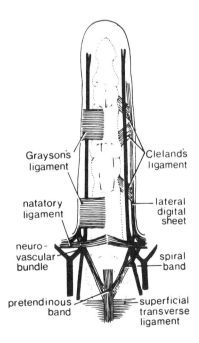

FIG. 42-98. *Normal fascial structures that can become involved with the pathological cords of Dupuytren's contracture. Figure shows the pretendinous band, the spiral bands, the natatory ligaments, the lateral sheet, Grayson's ligaments, and Cleland's ligaments.*

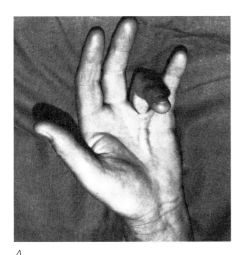

A

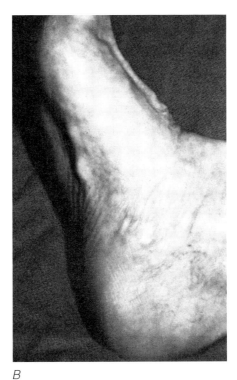

B

FIG. 42-99. *A.* Typical clinical appearance of the hand of a patient with Dupuytren's contracture. *B.* Dupuytren's contracture may involve the foot and present as nodules on the sole. Note that microscopically this material has the exact appearance of low-grade fibrosarcoma. Should the material from the sole be excised, the pathologist must be alerted to the presence of Dupuytren's contracture to avoid a potentially disastrous misreading of the microscopic slide with the obvious tragic consequences.

open and connecting the transverse crease incision via oblique longitudinal incisions avoids the need to dissect under an awning of palmar skin (see Fig. 42-103*D*). A voluminous and moderately compressive dressing is applied, supplemented by a palmar, or palmar and dorsal, plaster splint(s) that maintains the wrist in 35 degrees or more of extension and the MP and IP joints in full corrected extension. Therapy is started under close supervision by the end of the first postoperative week. Rehabilitation

includes active and passive motion and custom extension splinting of released joints at night. Sutures are removed after 2 weeks, depending on wound healing. Soaking and washing, especially when the McCash technique is used, is more an individual choice than required. In addition to wound infection and skin slough, secondary swelling is a serious but uncommon complication. Prolonged pain leading to reflex sympathetic dystrophy is a difficult problem for patient, therapist, and physician. Digital nerves can be injured during operation no matter how expertly the procedure is performed, but such injury must be recognized and repaired.

Arthritis

Inflammatory Arthropathies. The hand is a mirror of many inflammatory arthropathies, not just gout or rheumatoid arthritis (Figs. 42-104, 42-105, and 42-106 and Table 42-5).

Adult and Juvenile Rheumatoid Arthritis. Primary consideration should be given to arthritis because of worldwide prevalence and the severe disability if untreated or, occasionally, when treated aggressively. Rheumatoid arthritis is a chronic systemic disorder of unknown cause whose major manifestation is inflammatory synovitis with secondary bone and tendon invasion and destruction. There may be late tendon dysfunction through nodularity and locking or scarring, joint subluxation, and pain. In most cases, synovitis deformities are symmetrical. Rheumatoid arthritis affects the elbows, wrists, and metacarpophalangeal joints. Proximal interphalangeal involvement is less common but may be significant in a given patient. On radiographs, the hands and feet show some of the earliest signs of periarticular osteopenia, demineralization. The earliest erosions occur along the radial-palmar aspects of the metacarpal heads, at the proximal phalanges, and in the prestyloid recess of the ulna.

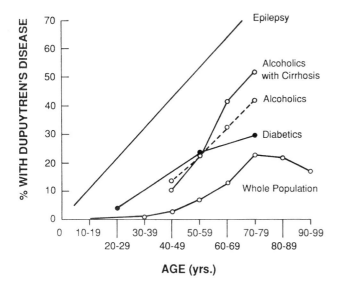

FIG. 42-100. The relationship of age to the percentage of the population with Dupuytren's contracture. Other superimposed lines showing disease incidence by age with epilepsy, alcoholism, and diabetes were constructed from data from multiple sources.

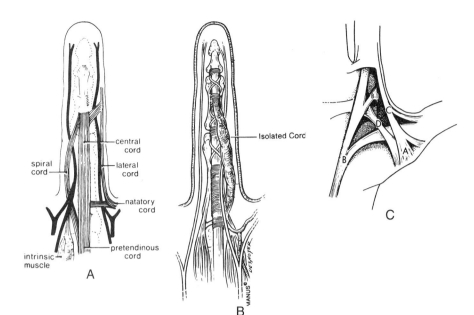

FIG. 42-101. The seven frequently recognized cords of Dupuytren's contracture. *A.* Five of these cords. The four cords in the digit are the central cord, the spiral cord, the lateral cord, and the natatory cord. The palmar cord is the pretendinous cord. *B.* The isolated digital cord of Basset and Strickland. *C.* The intercommissural cord.

Operative intervention is best limited to patients who, despite medical management, have persistent dysfunction because of pain, stiffness, or instability, or those who have progressively worsened function and increased deformities.

Scleroderma or Systemic Sclerosis. This is a generalized vasculitis affecting the skin, gastrointestinal tract, kidneys, and hands, resulting in thickened, dense, and inelastic skin and connective tissues. Pathologic joint involvement occurs in up to 80 percent of the patients. Vasculitis and secondary small-joint de-

formity may combine to produce unstable skin, chronic ulcerations that cannot heal, and secondary infections and painful loss of use (Fig. 42-107).

Psoriasis. This should always be a consideration in the patient with inflammatory arthritis of the hands, particularly with nail deformities and oligoarticular arthritis. Psoriatic arthritis usually affects the distal interphalangeal joints.

Crystal Arthropathies. Crystal arthropathies include gout and pseudogout, which are diagnosed definitively after exami-

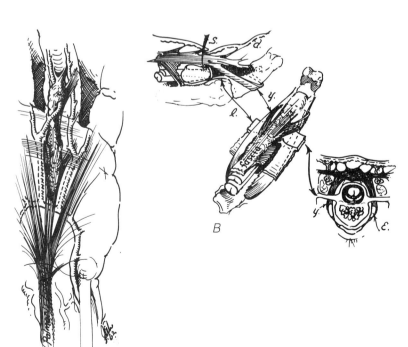

FIG. 42-102. *A.* The anatomy of the palmar fascia is complex when it has been altered by a hypertrophic (Dupuytren's) process; the prime involvement is in the longitudinal fibers and septa. Passing into the digit at the level of the distal palm, the digital nerves may spiral through or around the fascial process itself, making dissection precarious. *B.* As it passes into the finger, the fascia may expand laterally and extend into the fibers of the fibro-osseous sheath or extend into the lateral bands of the extensor mechanism. The vertical septa are second and pass to the deep fascia to form an integral part of the metacarpophalangeal restraint. (From: *Littler JW, The Hand, in Cooper P (ed): Craft of Surgery, 2d ed. Boston, Little, Brown, 1971, pp 1385–1410, with permission.*)

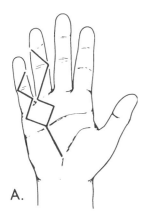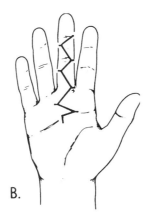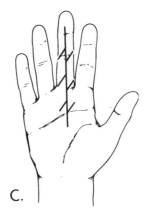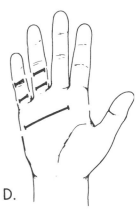

FIG. 42-103. Four skin incisions for the surgical treatment of Dupuytren's contracture. *A.* The zigzag incision with its linear extension proximal to the palmar flexion crease. *B.* The Littler-Bruner incision with small transverse extension. Watson uses these for V-Y-plasty closures; Bedeschi leaves them open in the honeycomb technique. *C.* The longitudinal incision, which is closed by Z-plasty incisions (oblique incision lines). *D.* The transverse incisions of McCash's open-palm technique.

nation of joint aspiration fluid or biopsy specimen. The serum uric acid levels may be normal even in an acute attack. Most patients with hyperuricemia never have acute gouty arthropathy. Calcium pyrophosphate crystalline inflammation, or pseudogout, often affects the wrist, with chondrocalcinosis classically seen on the posteroanterior wrist radiograph at the prestyloid recess (Fig. 42-108).

Noninflammatory Arthropathies. Noninflammatory arthropathies include osteoarthritis, heritable abnormalities of cartilage production, primary and secondary osteonecrosis or osteomalacia, endocrine-associated articular changes from thyroid, parathyroid, pituitary glands and pancreas, hematologic diseases such as hemophilia and hemoglobinopathies, the collagen storage diseases, and miscellaneous bone, nerve, and other connective tissue pathologies, including amyloid. Sarcoidosis is inflammatory.

Osteoarthritis. Osteoarthritis is the most common upper extremity arthropathy. Although classically defined as noninflam-

matory, osteoarthritis is a cartilage disease with at least intermittent low-to-moderate levels of inflammation. Its incidence increases with age. There is a significant hereditary component, especially for women. Patients may demonstrate progressive loss of articular cartilage, seen on radiographs first as diminished joint space, with secondary subchondral sclerosis and marginal bone spurs or lipping. Joint enlargement as a result of lipping usually occurs. The prevalence of distal interphalangeal joint nodularity, Heberden's nodes (Fig. 42-109), is up to ten times greater in women, especially for those with a family history. Secondary, posttraumatic, mechanical osteoarthritis is more common in individuals whose occupations expose them to in-

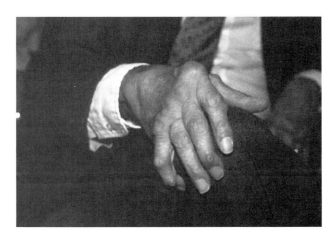

FIG. 42-104. Deformities of rheumatoid arthritis, with marked ulnar deviation, swan-neck deformity, active synovitis, and nodules.

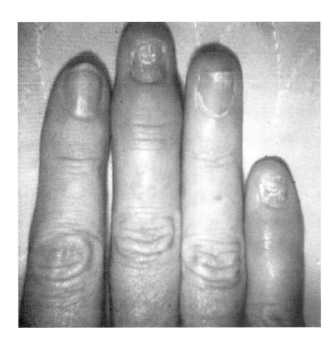

FIG. 42-105. Nail changes typical for psoriasis with distal interphalangeal joint involvement.

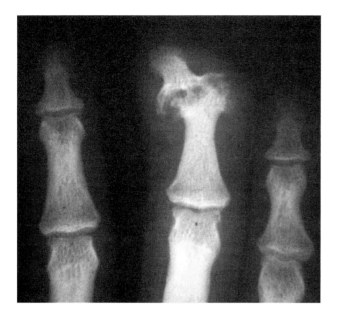

FIG. 42-106. *Radiographic changes in gout.*

juries or repetitive load, motion, and impact. The inflammatory variant often affects the hands, particularly the interphalangeal joints, and can be clinically and radiographically aggressive. The interphalangeal joints (particularly the terminal interphalangeal joints of index and thumb), the trapeziometacarpal, thumb basilar joint, the pantrapezial and radioscaphoid articulations are most frequently affected. With inflammatory problems due to chronic or progressive synovitis, tendon involvement, secondary joint locking and tendon rupture may contribute to symptoms.

Table 42-5
Inflammatory Arthropathies Affecting the Hands

Systemic autoimmune diseases
Rheumatoid arthritis (RA)
Polymyalgia rheumatica
Systemic lupus erythematosus (SLE)
Systemic sclerosis (scleroderma)
Vasculitis
Polymyositis and dermatomyositis
Adult-onset Still's disease
Remitting, seronegative, symmetrical synovitis with pitting edema
   (RS$_3$PE)

Spondyloarthropathies
Ankylosing spondylitis (AS)
Reiter's syndrome
Psoriatic arthritis
Inflammatory bowel disease-associated
Reactive arthritis

Rheumatic fever

Crystal arthropathies
Gout
Calcium pyrophosphate dihydrate (CPPD) deposition disease
Apatite crystal deposition disease

Miscellaneous
Infectious arthritis
Sarcoidosis
Leukemia and lymphoma

Extensor or flexor tenosynovectomies in the lower forearm, wrist, palm, or digits may be necessary and should be combined with a supervised postoperative therapy program to recover motion (Fig. 42-110). When tendon ruptures occur, the attritional defect in tendon substance and segmental tendon loss prevents direct repair and requires tendon graft or transfer (Fig. 42-111). Tendon subluxation may occur as a result of tendon disease or secondarily from joint involvement deep to that tendon.

Focal small-joint deformities are best treated with arthroplasty, especially in MP joints and for the less active, older patient, or with arthrodesis at selected limited intercarpal and interphalangeal joints (Figs. 42-112, 42-113, and 42-114). For successful arthrodesis, selection of operative method is not as important as meticulous, precise technique. Stabilized continuous bone contact over the entire surface to be fused, in the presence of good bone stock with durable soft-tissue coverage, produces a positive outcome. Living bone provides the most durable arthrodesis. With removal of all the unsightly, painful, prominent osteophytes about the dorsal, palmar, radial, and ulnar joint margins, the results are excellent.

Thumb stiffness, pain, and malalignment produce marked hand impairment; the problems are far out of proportion to the lesion because of the critical importance of comfortable thumb mobility and stability in precision and power hand use (Figs. 42-115 and 42-116). Thumb basilar arthroplasty yields functional, aesthetic results.

CONGENITAL DEFORMITIES

Failures of development, separation, and segmentation and intrauterine injury such as amniotic bands or congenital constriction ring syndrome affect mobility, facility, and self-image. Abnormalities of the shoulder and humerus, elbow, forearm, wrist, and hand produce important but different impairments, and all diminish hand facility to different degrees (Fig. 42-117). Among the most common congenital afflictions in the hand are syndactyly and polydactyly (Fig. 42-118). Consideration of repair should begin when the patient is 3 to 6 months of age.

Congenital trigger thumb may present to the primary pediatric caregiver as a snapping that may or may not be painful, but it often presents as a fixed flexion of the terminal thumb joint. Trigger thumbs are rarely locked in extension. Pathologic findings are localized to the flexor pollicis longus tendon and the proximal annular pulley of the thumb. It is not clear whether the tendon enlargement, known as Notta's node, or thickening of the pulley with relative lessening of the internal diameter of the sheath is the primary pathology. Only 10 to 20 percent are bilateral, at times sequential rather than simultaneous. Other trigger fingers may occur in the infant or young child, but only rarely.

Surgery is conservative management. There is no justification for steroid injection in treating congenital trigger thumb. Children who are diagnosed at 12 months of age may be observed for 6 to 12 months for possible spontaneous correction, because waiting does not compromise outcome. At any age, when fixed flexion deformity of the thumb interphalangeal joint produces secondary metacarpophalangeal joint hyperextension, or when a child over the age of 2 years initially presents with symptomatic locking, surgery to release the proximal flexor pulley is in order. The thickened tendon nodule is not debulked or debrided. None

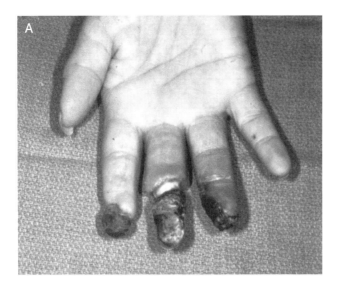

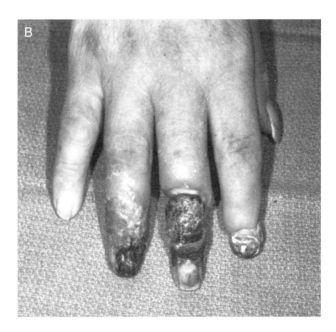

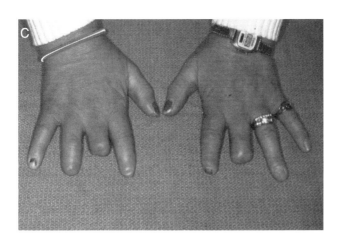

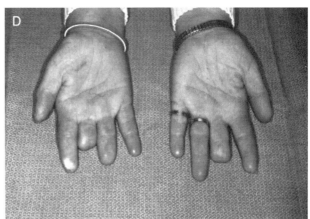

FIG. 42-107. *A and B.* Painful gangrene of the distal phalanx of the right index finger and the middle and distal phalanges of the right long and ring fingers in a patient with scleroderma. *C and D.* After treatment by amputation, with satisfactory relief of pain and excellent return of hand function.

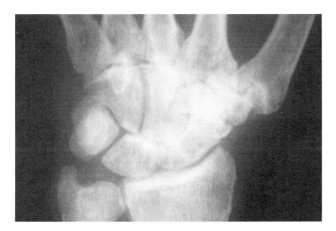

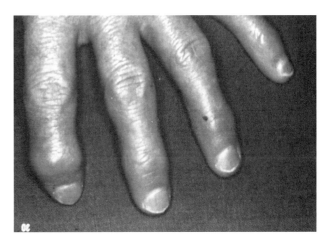

FIG. 42-108. Chondrocalcinosis seen in one of the typical locations for this crystal deposition, at the triangular cartilage of the wrist.

FIG. 42-109. The characteristic appearance of Heberden's nodes in the hand of a patient with osteoarthritis.

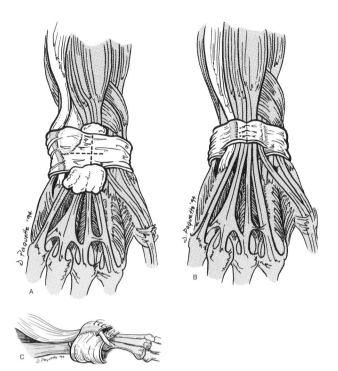

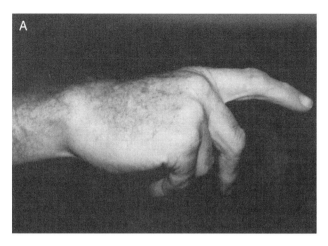

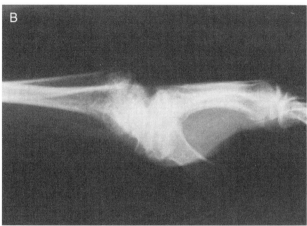

FIG. 42-110. *A.* Dorsal tenosynovectomy is performed through a longitudinal incision centered over Lister's tubercle. The extensor retinaculum over the fourth compartment is incised longitudinally, unroofing adjacent compartments as necessary. *B.* If wrist joint coverage or relocation of extensor carpi ulnaris tendons is necessary after tenosynovectomy, the retinaculum is incised transversely to the level of the fifth compartment. The distal half is placed deep to the extensor tendons, providing a gliding surface. The remainder of the retinaculum is sutured dorsally to prevent tendon bowstringing. *C.* The intact edge of the retinaculum acts as a pulley, restricting volar translation of the extensor carpi ulnaris tendons.

FIG. 42-111. *A.* Rupture of multiple extensor tendons. Lack of active extension of the middle, ring, and small fingers is secondary to rupture of extensor digitorum communis III–V and extensor digiti minimi. Note the prominent ulnar head. *B.* Lateral radiograph demonstrates the arthritic, prominent ulnar head.

of these children has permanent loss of interphalangeal extension. If an interphalangeal joint cannot be fully extended at surgery, it means that the pulley has not been released completely until proven otherwise.

TUMORS

Principles. Localized masses are common in the hand and upper limb, but most are benign. Most have characteristics that assist in making the diagnosis. The relative rarity of malignant tumors of the musculoskeletal system distal to the elbow can lead to misdiagnosis and undermanagement.

Every mass, particularly those that are atypical in appearance or location, should be diagnosed with staging and imaging procedures leading to careful incisional biopsy. Hand masses tend to present earlier, when smaller, because of their superficial location. Enlarging, symptomatic masses are evaluated with history, laboratory studies, imaging by plain films, ultrasonography, scintigraphy, CT scans, or MRI. Biopsy is the last step in diagnosis, and only very small lesions or lesions that are typical should be excised initially.

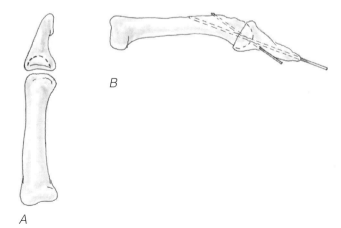

FIG. 42-112. *A.* Bone surface preparation for distal interphalangeal arthrodesis. *B.* Lateral view with Kirschner wires in place.

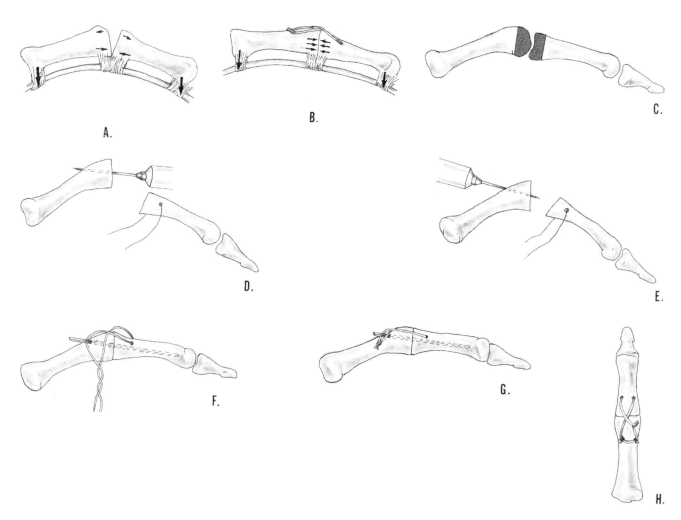

FIG. 42-113. *A.* Flexion of interphalangeal joint creates tension forces on the dorsal aspect and compression forces on the volar aspect of the joint. *B.* Placement of a tension band dorsal to the joint axis neutralizes the tension forces and uses the flexor moment force to apply compression loads across the arthrodesis site. *C–H.* Tension-band technique for proximal interphalangeal joint arthrodesis.

Benign Neoplasms

Benign tumors can be subdivided into three categories:

1. *Latent Benign.* Tumors arising during childhood may heal spontaneously. Most are well encapsulated, with a clearly defined plane between the tumor capsule and normal surrounding tissue. In bone, the growth process is slow, allowing a margin of mature cortical bone to develop and contain the lesion.
2. *Active Benign.* Lesions continue to grow, albeit slowly, and are not self-limited in size or by patient age. The tumor is well encapsulated, but the reactive zone is thicker and less mature than in the preceding category. Within bone, the tumor has an irregular shape that alters the internal or external bone architecture. Surgical management is dictated by determining the grade of the lesion and adequacy of local resection. Operative method is determined by the anatomical setting and the implications for altered musculoskeletal part function.
3. *Aggressive Benign.* Lesions do not metastasize but are more difficult to control locally. These lesions do not have clear zones of capsular containment. Nodules or extensions of the tumor may grow out into nearby normal tissue, such as in Dupuytren's contracture. Excision

through the reactive zone exposes these tumor projections at the surgical margins, allowing microscopic contamination into unaffected tissue. Failure to fully remove the tumor ensures local recurrence.

Malignant Neoplasms

Surgical staging and treatment for true malignant tumors is outlined in Tables 42-6 and 42-7.

Specific Tumors

Ganglion. Joint and tendon ganglions are among the most common benign soft-tissue tumor masses in the upper extremity, representing up to 50 to 75 percent of reported tumors. Although potentially located anywhere, the majority of ganglions are in specific sites: the middorsal wrist; the volar radial wrist; the flexor sheath at the metacarpal flexion crease as a seed or pea ganglion that is extremely small but hard and tender; and at the dorsum of the distal interphalangeal joint and nail base. The latter is associated with secondary nail deformity, such as in mucous cyst, particularly in the older population (see Fig. 42-3).

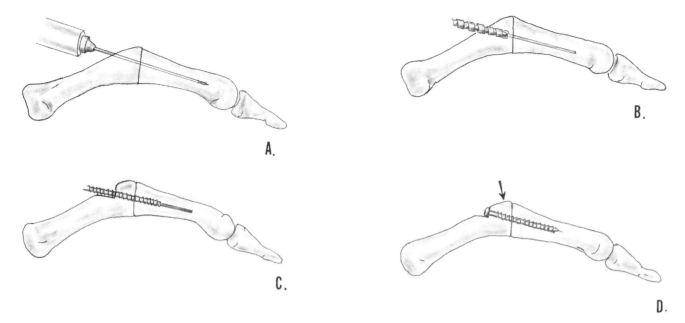

FIG. 42-114. *Compression-screw fixation for proximal interphalangeal joint arthrodesis. A. Smaller-diameter drill bit through proximal and middle phalangeal segments. B. Overdrilling the proximal phalanx with larger-diameter drill bit. C. Screw tap used to tap smaller hole in middle phalangeal segment. D. Compression screw placed. The dorsal bridge (arrow) in the proximal phalanx is subject to fracture when this technique is used.*

Treatment options include closed rupture impact, hypodermic needle aspiration, and operative excision. Rupture by digital pressure or with a swift blow is unnecessarily traumatic and has little chance of succeeding. Aspiration and steroid instillation may be of value, particularly when the expanding lesion has not been diagnosed or is associated with discomfort. At the dorsal

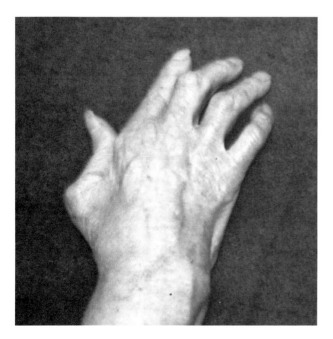

FIG. 42-115. *Thumb with metacarpophalangeal flexion, interphalangeal extension, and carpometacarpal abduction—the boutonnière deformity.*

wrist, the most common site of origin is from the scapholunate interosseous ligament, and the occult ganglion may account for a significant amount of dorsal wrist pain, particularly in the female teenage population. Volar ganglions are most commonly situated between the flexor carpi radialis tendon and the radial artery, at or just proximal to the wrist at the radioscaphoid joint. Most arise from a radiocarpal or intercarpal capsule. Aspiration is helpful and may be entirely curative for the flexor sheath ganglion that appears as a 3- to 10-mm hard mass at or just distal to the metacarpophalangeal joint flexion crease. Aspiration and injection of the mucous cyst distal interphalangeal joint ganglion is less likely to be curative. Repeated drainage increases the risk of joint contamination.

Surgical excision must include the capsular base origin, sometimes referred to as the stalk or root. Deflating the ganglion during operation by incising it before dissecting is much easier than trying to protect nearby cutaneous nerves or vessels while still avoiding an excessively large skin incision around an inflated cyst.

Giant Cell Tumor of Tendon Sheath. Also known as nodular tenosynovitis, fibroxanthoma, giant cell tumor of synovium, and pigmented villonodular synovitis, it is the most common solid soft-tissue tumor in the hand. It is more frequent in females, and patients are generally between the ages of 30 and 60 years. It presents as a firm, lobular, nontender, slowly enlarging mass in the palm, finger, or thumb. It is more frequently seen on the palmar surface, given that synovium is present in the fingers only about the flexor tendons and in the joints. Secondary tendon, joint, and skeletal invasion is well known (Fig. 42-119). Effective treatment requires meticulously complete excision, with care being taken not to injure the neurovascular bundles or the critical flexor sheath pulleys. Recurrences occur

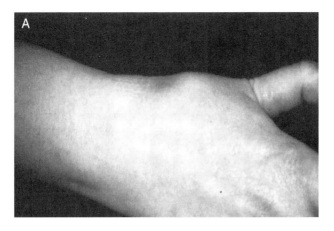
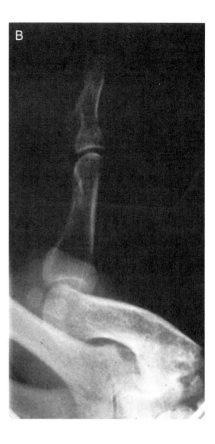
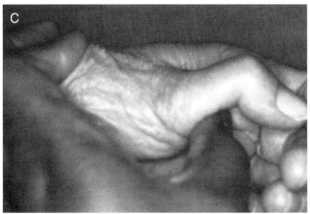

FIG. 42-116. *A, B, and C. Thumb carpometacarpal joint adduction and subluxation with secondary metacarpophalangeal extension and interphalangeal flexion, commonly known as a swan-neck deformity, are seen in these two patients. The patient shown in B and C has primary carpometacarpal degeneration and first metacarpal adduction with secondary, compensatory instability and collapse of the two more distal joints.*

in up to 10 percent of patients within 2 years and may occur up to 10 years later, though late recurrences may be new lesions entirely.

Lipoma. Lipomas are benign tumors that contain mature fat cells. They are rare in people under the age of 20 years. Some are multifocal. Tumors usually are asymptomatic but gradually enlarging soft to moderately firm masses. When they arise near a nerve or in a nerve tunnel, they may cause secondary symptoms. Lipomas can be superficial, subcutaneous, or intramuscular, and in the hand they also may be large and deep. Surgical treatment is for diagnosis of the unknown enlarging mass or for improving functional impairment. Recurrences are rare (Fig. 42-120).

Enchondroma. Enchondromas, the most common cartilage lesion of bone, are most frequently found at the small tubular bones in the hand. They can present at any age, but most are found in young adults. Virtually all enchondromas present as pathologic fractures, although a small number may be found as an asymptomatic enlargement of a bone. Radiographs usually are diagnostic (Fig. 42-121). Surgical treatment may be for diagnosis or therapy. Pathologic fractures may heal, but the tumor

is unlikely to regress spontaneously with fracture union. It is best to treat the fracture and the tumor together, but some patients prefer to allow the fracture to heal while waiting for the tumor to resolve spontaneously. Treating the lesion and the fracture simultaneously limits the disability to just one interval. Thorough lesional curettage is required, and autogenous bone grafting is appropriate; some bones heal without added graft. Incidental discovery of small asymptomatic enchondromas does not mandate treatment. Aggressive and malignant tumors distal to the elbow are uncommon but are more likely to be of soft-tissue origin.

SURGICAL PRINCIPLES

Skin Preparation. Detergents and solutions assist in mechanically debriding skin and also mechanically decrease the microflora population; however, all can irritate skin, and each has limitations.

Alcohols work primarily through the denaturation of proteins and produce the most rapid reduction in microbial counts. They work against most gram-positive and gram-negative organisms. Alcohols are not sporicidal but are active against many fungi and tuberculosis; they also act against some viruses, including

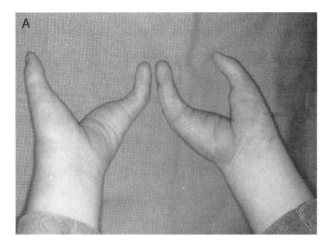

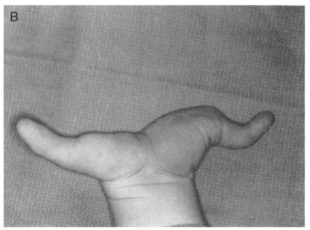

FIG. 42-117. *Two-digit cleft hand, untreated surgically, demonstrates considerable mobility and dexterity.*

Table 42-6
Surgical Staging for Sarcoma

Stage	Grade	Site
IA	Low (G_1)	Intracompartmental (T_1)
IB	Low (G_1)	Extracompartmental (T_2)
IIA	High (G_2)	Extracompartmental (T_1)
IIB	High (G_2)	Extracompartmental (T_2)
III	Regional or distant metastasis (M); any (G); any (T)	

Table 42-7
Musculoskeletal Oncologic Surgical Procedures

Margin	Local	Amputation
Intracapsular	Currettage/debulking	Debulking amputation
Marginal	Marginal excision	Marginal amputation
Wide	Wide local excision	Through bone amputation
Radical	Radical local excision	Disarticulation of extremity

HIV and cytomegalovirus. Alcohols do not have persistent effects.

Hexachlorophene is bactericidal through cell wall destruction and is especially active against gram-positive cocci. It is minimally effective against gram-negative, viral, and fungal organisms. This agent is potentially toxic systemically when absorbed and is not recommended for open wounds.

Iodophors, iodine complexes that irritate the skin less than the iodine/alcohol tincture solutions, are effective against a broad spectrum of gram-positive and gram-negative bacteria, fungi, viruses, and mycobacteria by cell wall penetration and oxidation. Iodophors have almost immediate onset of action, and residual activity declines quickly. Because the iodophors can cause skin irritation, tissue damage, and allergic reactions in some patients,

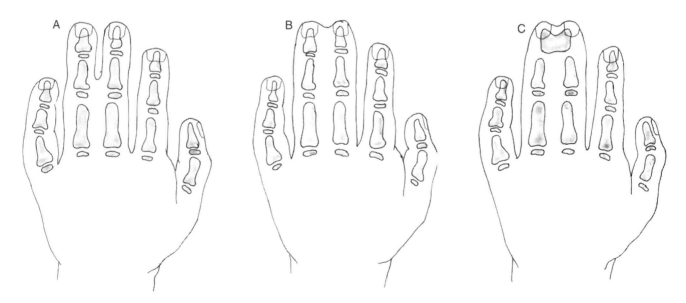

FIG. 42-118. *Syndactyly classification. A. Incomplete simple syndactyly. B. Complete simple syndactyly.*
C. Complete complex syndactyly.

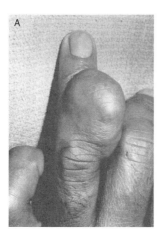
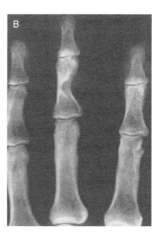

FIG. 42-119. *Giant cell tumor of soft tissue. A. Slowly enlarging soft-tissue mass surrounding middle phalanx. B. Radiograph demonstrating extrinsic pressure from mass causing saucerization and sclerotic reaction of middle phalangeal diaphysis.*

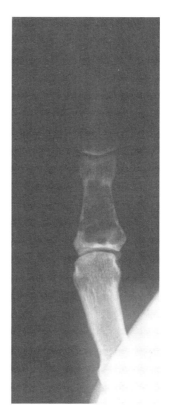

these solutions are not recommended for chronic use on open wounds, because the additional tissue irritation may make the wound more susceptible to late infection.

Chlorhexidine gluconate is a broad-spectrum antibacterial that is effective against many viruses, with limited activity against fungi and the tubercle bacillus. The time of onset of action is intermediate, and residual bactericidal action continues for several hours. Chlorhexidine gluconate alcohol-based solution may provide the added benefit of rapid onset and residual activity with minimal toxicity.

Chloroxylenol or parachlorometaxylenol (PCMX) is active through destruction of microbial cell walls. It has intermediate onset and good activity against gram-positive organisms but only fair activity against gram-negatives, fungi, mycobacterial species, and viruses. It is not toxic and rarely causes skin irritation. It may be a good choice in many situations.

FIG. 42-121. *Enchondroma on the proximal phalanx of the thumb. Radiograph demonstrating lobulated epiphyseal-metaphyseal lucency with endosteal scalloping and thinning. No calcifications are visible.*

Hair Removal. While the conventional wisdom is that routine hair removal eliminates a potential wound contaminant, most studies reveal that hair removal is not a benign procedure and that close skin shaving increases the risk of postoperative wound infection, with risk rising as the time between the shave

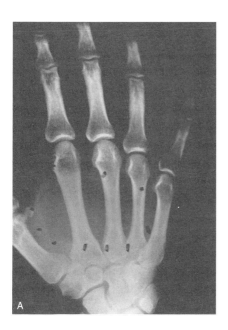
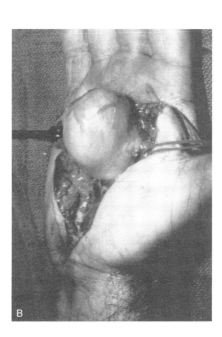

FIG. 42-120. *Large palmar lipoma. A. Radiograph with the water density mass outlined. B. Intraoperative photograph demonstrating large lipoma, which compromised the motor branch of the median nerve.*

and the surgical procedure increases. In a case in which the presence of hair would interfere with wound closure or tissue and skin manipulations, the use of electric clippers or depilatories is preferable, and hair removal should be done at the start of the procedure rather than the day before.

Anesthesia. Regional anesthesia for upper limb surgery offers effective pain control and the avoidance of mental confusion or other side effects from sedatives and general anesthesia (Fig. 42-122). Regional anesthesia is not risk-free or always fully satisfactory; systemic and local reactions may be serious. Appropriate monitoring is mandatory. Forearm or axillary tourniquet is used for most hand surgery, but patients often are not able to tolerate continuous pneumatic tourniquet applications for more than 30 min. Isolated peripheral blocks have more limited usefulness.

Distal peripheral blocks in the upper extremity should always be done without epinephrine added to the anesthetic solution. The injection technique is based on infiltration of anesthetic around the nerve and not directly into nerve substance. Although inadvertent needle entry into nerves is common, without epinephrine in the injection solution and with the use of a fine gauge needle it should present no problem. Should a patient complain of paresthesias, the needle is withdrawn and redirected. Intraneural injection with epinephrine-containing solutions may result in extended intraneural ischemia and secondary fibrosis as well as peripheral vascular compromise, particularly in the digital end-arterial circulation.

Ulnar Nerve Block. Proximal block is among the more useful peripheral techniques (Fig. 42-123). The ulnar nerve is palpated just posterior to the medial epicondyle and injected with 5 to 8 mL 1% mepivacaine hydrochloride without epinephrine via a 23- to 26-gauge needle. The nerve should not be pinned to the epicondyle with the needle; intense paresthesias elicited from neural perforation warrant immediate withdrawal and redirection.

The ulnar nerve at the wrist is in the volar flexor compartment located dorsal to the flexor carpi ulnaris tendon, and just ulnar to the ulnar artery; both nerve and artery are dorsal to the tendon. The dorsal cutaneous branch of the ulnar nerve has already branched 4 to 8 cm proximal to the ulnar styloid process. Initially deep to the flexor carpi ulnaris tendon, it courses dorsally to exit on its dorsal edge distal to the ulnar styloid process, where it can be blocked separately (Fig. 42-124). A fine-gauge needle is inserted into the skin just dorsal and ulnar to the flexor carpi ulnaris tendon; the needle is aimed palmarward and distally, toward the ring finger into Guyon's canal. The skin concavity for needle entry is dorsal to the flexor carpi ulnaris tendon, and easily palpated and visualized during active wrist flexion and ulnar deviation. After needle entry, paresthesias may be elicited, and 5 mL of anesthetic is injected. Aspiration before injection avoids intraarterial injection. The dorsal branch of the ulnar nerve is blocked with an additional subcutaneous infiltration of 2 to 3 mL after first pulling the needle proximally and then redirecting it dorsal and distal to the ulnar styloid.

Radial Nerve Block. The radial nerve is located between the lateral edge of the biceps and the anterior border of the triceps muscles; motor and sensory components can be anesthetized with injection approximately 4 cm proximal to the lateral epicondyle, where the nerve lies on the humerus in this intermuscular space (Fig. 42-125). The needle is aimed distally and in-

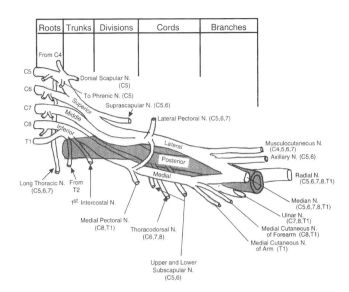

FIG. 42-122. The brachial plexus. Organization of the roots, trunks, divisions, and cords, as well as root origins of peripheral nerves.

serted; paresthesias confirm needle and nerve location. The needle is then withdrawn slightly and 7 to 10 mL of anesthetic is injected, with another 2 to 3 mL of anesthetic infiltrated in the subcutaneous plane, which also blocks the lateral antebrachial cutaneous nerve.

The purely sensory superficial radial nerve emerges at the dorsal edge of brachioradialis tendon 4 to 6 cm proximal to the radial styloid process. As it courses distally, the nerve divides into multiple terminal branches. Subcutaneous anesthetic infiltration at the styloid process of the radius with a total of 6 to 8 mL of anesthetic effectively blocks the superficial radial nerve in this region (Fig. 42-126).

Median Nerve Block. Blocking the median nerve is more difficult in the region of the elbow than in the region of the wrist. At the elbow the median nerve is posterior and ulnar to the brachial artery. A fine hypodermic needle is introduced from a location medial to the palpated brachial artery, aiming distally.

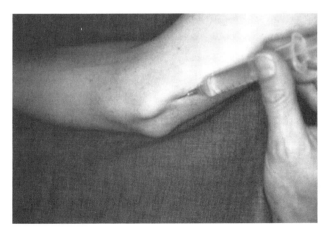

FIG. 42-123. The ulnar nerve is blocked at the elbow with 5 to 8 mL of local anesthetic without epinephrine. A fine-gauge needle is used, aiming distally with care being taken to avoid impaling the nerve.

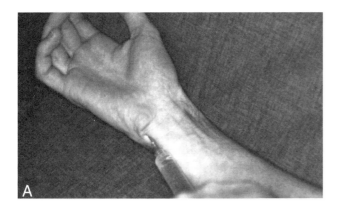

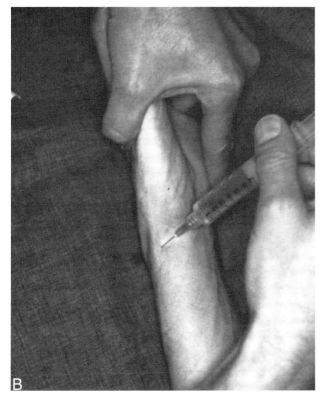

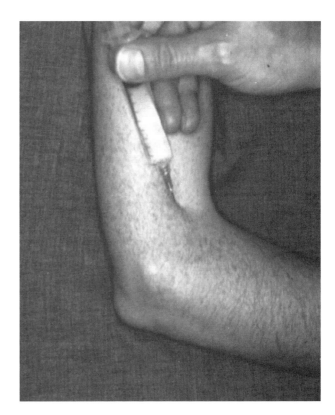

FIG. 42-125. Radial nerve block is done 4 cm proximal to the lateral epicondyle by eliciting paresthesias in the intermuscular groove between the lateral border of the biceps brachialis and brachioradialis muscles.

space (Fig. 42-128). Injecting 6 to 8 mL of anesthetic consistently blocks the median nerve. The palmar cutaneous branch of the median and lateral antebrachial cutaneous nerves can be blocked with another 2 to 3 mL of anesthetic injected subcutaneously, aiming more superficially and 45 degrees radially from the same entry point.

FIG. 42-124. *A.* The ulnar nerve is blocked at the wrist with needle entry *dorsal* to the flexor carpi ulnaris tendon, aiming toward the ring finger in the plane of the palm. Aspiration serves to prevent needle placement in the more radially located ulnar artery during injection. *B.* Subcutaneous block of the dorsal branch is done at the ulnar styloid process.

After aspiration, 8 to 10 mL of anesthetic is injected. If intense paresthesias are elicited, the needle is withdrawn slightly before injection (Fig. 42-127).

The median nerve becomes progressively more superficial as it approaches the wrist, where it lies in the most palmar and radial quadrant of the carpal canal. Proximal to the canal, the nerve is located dorsal and slightly radial to the palmaris longus tendon, and ulnar to the flexor carpi radialis tendon—i.e., between the two tendons. Proper technique avoids the canal contents and the nerve. The most consistent and comfortable skin portal is about 3 cm proximal to the wrist crease. The needle is aimed 30 to 45 degrees dorsal and distal, toward the third web

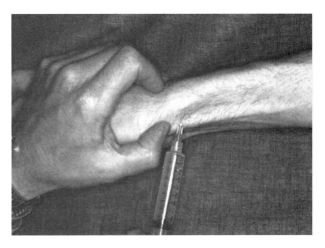

FIG. 42-126. Superficial (sensory) radial nerve block at the wrist is done by subcutaneous infiltration at the styloid process of the radius and along the dorsum of the wrist.

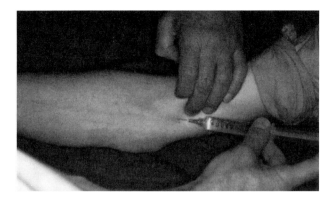

FIG. 42-127. Proximal median nerve block is performed just above the intercondylar line, ulnar and posterior to the palpable brachial artery (index finger).

Digital Nerve Block. The fingers receive their sensory supply from the common digital nerve branches of the median and ulnar nerves. Digital anesthesia can be achieved by injecting the anesthetic into the looser web tissues about the common digital nerves, which is preferable to a ring block in the base of the finger. The so-called ring block technique risks vascular compromise from volume compression when a solution is injected circumferentially about the base of the finger. Digital anesthetic solution should not include epinephrine, because any resulting digital vessel spasm may compromise finger circulation.

Anesthetic is injected retrograde from the web, advancing about 1 cm proximally into the palm, where 2 mL of anesthetic is injected after aspiration. The needle can be withdrawn and turned into the dorsal subcutaneous tissues of the web to ensure anesthesia of the dorsal branch of the digital nerve with another 1 to 2 mL of anesthesia. The technique is repeated on the opposite side of the finger or sequentially in several digits as needed. No more than 5 to 7 mL total of anesthetic solution should be injected for any one finger with this technique (Fig. 42-129).

Flexor Sheath Block. Single-digit anesthesia can also be achieved with injection of 2 mL of anesthetic directly into the flexor sheath. A fine hypodermic needle is introduced into the

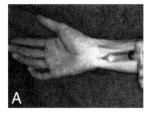
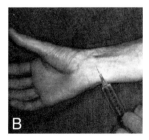

FIG. 42-128. *A.* Median nerve injection at the carpal tunnel is accomplished from a point 3 cm proximal to the transverse carpal ligament, aiming toward the third ray and slightly dorsal in order to stay within the carpal canal and avoid impaling the nerve. *B.* Additional subcutaneous infiltration is done to block the palmar cutaneous and lateral antebrachial cutaneous nerve branches.

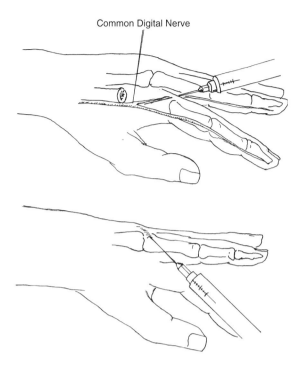

FIG. 42-129. For intermetacarpal digital block, the needle is introduced into the web space, aimed in a proximal and palmar direction, and advanced for a distance of 1 cm. After aspiration, 1 to 2 mL of anesthetic is injected around the common digital nerve. The needle is withdrawn, and an additional 1 to 2 mL is infiltrated in the web and about the dorsum of the metacarpal metaphysis.

flexor tendon from the palmar side at the level of the distal palm or MP flexion crease. Rapid onset of anesthesia can be achieved. This method has the advantage of a single injection but the disadvantage of sometimes failing to completely anesthetize the dorsal divisions of the proper digital nerves.

Tourniquet. The use of tourniquets dates to Roman times, but the device acquired its name from surgical application in eighteenth-century France, from *tourner,* meaning to turn. Hand surgery is performed using an axillary or forearm pneumatic tourniquet. Fingertip procedures can be done using a digital tourniquet made from a $\frac{1}{4}$-inch rubber drain hose or with the finger sleeve cut from a sterile surgical glove; the tip of the finger sleeve is pierced, and the sleeve is placed over the patient's finger and rolled proximally, simultaneously exsanguinating and achieving a tourniquet effect. In the absence of proximal anesthetic blockade, the maximum tourniquet time a patient will tolerate is 30 to 60 min.

Exception in the presence of infections and suspected aggressive and malignant tumors, the arm should be exsanguinated before tourniquet inflation; limb elevation may be used for partial exsanguination. Covering the arm with a fabric stockinette before elastic bandage exsanguination reduces skin shear; this is important in patients with delicate skin, those with connective tissue diseases, and those who are on steroids. Axillary and forearm tourniquet cuffs are best applied over cast padding. Nonsterile pneumatic tourniquets should be draped away from the operative field with an occlusive plastic tape or drape distal to the cuff to prevent wicking of antiseptic solution during extremity preparation and risking chemical burn (Fig. 42-130).

Pneumatic tourniquet pressures of 225 to 250 mmHg for adults and 200 mmHg in children are adequate. Patients with very large or obese arms require higher pressures and larger cuffs, as do hypertensive patients, in whom tourniquet pressure should be at least 100 mmHg over systolic blood pressure. Tourniquet time is limited by the most oxygen-sensitive tissue—muscle—and the most oxygen-sensitive organelle—mitochondria. Continuous tourniquet application should not exceed 3 h. In cases in which longer tourniquet times are required, the tourniquet should be deflated after the wound has been dressed temporarily and left deflated for at least 10 min per hour of prior inflation. Tourniquet complications involve not only ischemia in labile distal tissues but also ischemia and direct injury to skin, nerves, and muscles located immediately beneath the tourniquet. Assuming operative tourniquet time of 30 min or more, at tourniquet deflation tissues show relative, reactive hyperemia driven by the tourniquet-induced hypoxia and directly proportional to the time of tourniquet use. This hyperemia may complicate hemostasis.

The tourniquet is deflated before wound closure; deflation should be immediately followed by 7 to 10 min of direct, moderate wound pressure before electrocautery is used. To avoid hematomas, the wound is closed when an acceptably dry field has been achieved. If oozing persists, a suction drain is used to keep dead spaces empty.

Incisions and Exposures. Skin incisions can be linear, curved, or angled. They may be oriented in longitudinal or transverse directions relative to the limb. Ideally, elective wounds are placed to lie in and about the soft-tissue skin creases. Hand incisions are not made perpendicular to joint creases, so that iatrogenic contracture and unsightly scars are prevented (Fig. 42-131).

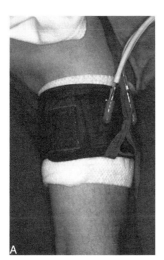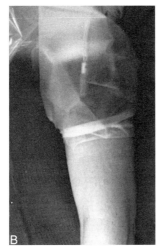

FIG. 42-130. *A. Padding beneath an axillary tourniquet. B. Occlusive drape distal to both tourniquet and padding to prevent wicking of antiseptic solution beneath cuff.*

A sterile skin-marking pen is used to draw out the incisions. Cross-hatching the incision at regular intervals assists in realigning the skin edges for closure (Fig. 42-132). Angles, pedicles, and turns in incisions should not be so narrow as to risk vascular compromise by creating a narrow skin peninsula.

Dressings and Splints. The hand dressing is an intrinsic part of the surgical procedure. The dressing and splint are as important to the outcome as the operation. Application of dressings and splints cannot be delegated without supervision by the responsible surgeon. A poorly applied dressing may destroy or disrupt the intended effect of the operation.

The bottom layer of the dressing should be conforming, nonocclusive, and preferably nonadherent, such as Xeroform or Adaptic. Applied dressing sponges may be dry or moistened for contour. When interdigital dressings are appropriate, a single gauze pad is folded, not twisted, between fingers. The involved fingers or the entire hand is then overwrapped loosely with a Kerlix type of bulky rolled gauze. Padded dorsal or volar splints are applied to maintain the desired position of the operated part.

The generic position for hand immobilization includes splinting the wrist at about 30 degrees of extension, the metacarpophalangeal joints at 70 degrees of flexion, and the interphalangeal joints at 0 to 5 degrees of flexion. The splint is extended to the fingertips, and care is taken to avoid compressing the dressing and splint too tightly and risking circulatory compromise. Fingertips should be exposed for circulation checks in hospital and at home. Hand and arm elevation is encouraged for comfort and for minimizing edema during the first several postinjury and postoperative days. With or without a sling, when the patient is supine, sitting, or walking, the hand is kept at or above the level of the heart.

Postoperative Hand Therapy. Hand therapy is begun early and depends on the specific diagnosis, procedure, and patient. Operative goals include minimizing the time of immobilization, enhancing internal stabilization, preferably with minimal invasion, and allowing early mobilization of skin, joints, and tendons.

Exercises appropriate for the condition and surgery performed are prescribed, and a therapist instructs the patient in these exercises. Exercises should be gentle, not painful, and should take the patient to the limit of potential motion at that time. The therapy program should emphasize soft-tissue mobilization and a decrease of edema. When doing therapy for the hand, mobility in the forearm, elbow, and shoulder should be included, especially in older patients. The use of whirlpools is limited to patients with special needs, such as those with burns and those whose wounds require periodic debridement. Heating the tissues is rarely, if ever, done acutely; ice is often more appropriate for posttraumatic conditions. Use of warm-water or paraffin baths is reserved for chronic conditions of systemic inflammation and periarticular stiffness. After injury, tissue swelling often increases proportionally to heat, worsening the prospects of rehabilitation in those swollen parts.

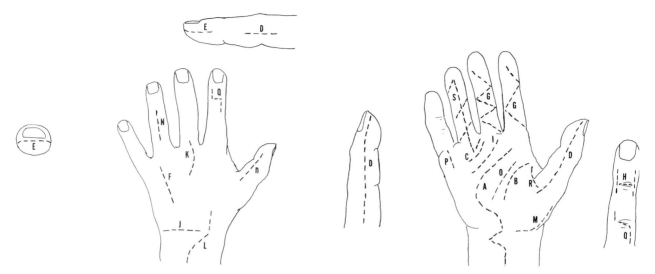

FIG. 42-131. *Common palmar and dorsal incisions in the hand. A. Incision opening the palm or draining the midpalmar space parallels flexion creases, exposes by triangular flap, enters between median and ulnar nerve supplies, and may be extended through the ulnar side of the carpal ligament up the forearm. Curve-crossing creases in wrist avoid contracture. B. Drainage for thenar space parallels thenar crease; must not sever the thenar motor nerve. Pedicles between it and the palmar incision must be wide enough to nourish intermediate skin. C. Drainage of collar button abscess. Avoid the digital nerve. D. Midaxial incisions in digit spare nerves and vessels and do not cause flexion contractures. E. Drainage for pulp abscess, posterior to tactile surface. Should sever the vertical fat columns and not cause tenosynovitis by opening the flexor sheath. F. Dorsal incisions over second and fourth web spaces for decompressing dorsal and volar interosseous compartments. G. Both modifications of Bruner's zigzag volar digital incisions for flexor tendon surgery. H. "H" incision for distal interphalangeal joint debridement or fusion. Terminal extensor tendon may be transected and repaired. I. Incision along the distal palmar crease to expose palmar fascia. J. Transverse incisions parallel wrinkles, thus avoiding conspicuous keloid formation. K. Curvilinear incision on radial side of metacarpophalangeal joints for isolated interphalangeal joint synovectomy or extensor centralization. L. Approach to dorsal wrist. The central axis of the incision is moved radialward or ulnarward for approach to the various dorsal wrist compartments. M. A Wagner incision to approach the carpometacarpal joint of the thumb. Care is taken to avoid crossing branches of the dorsoradial sensory nerve. Abductor pollicis brevis is reflected palmarward/ulnarward. N. Straight dorsal incision for approach to the proximal interphalangeal joint. The elasticity and redundancy of skin over the dorsal PIP joints coupled with the great power of the flexor mechanism eliminates concerns regarding contracture across a joint crease. O. Approach to the midpalm. P. Longitudinal incision over the A1 pulley for trigger finger release. Care is taken to avoid crossing the flexion creases. Incision is made midline on the tendon, avoiding the neurovascular bundles on either side. Q. Incision exposing extensor tendon central slip. R. Short transverse incision for release of trigger thumb. S. McGregor incision, sometimes used in Dupuytren's contracture surgery. After contracture release, flaps are interposed to gain length and avoid linear incisions across flexion creases.*

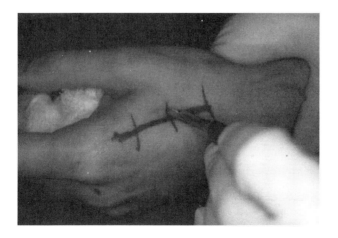

FIG. 42-132. *Preincision scoring the skin for easier, more accurate alignment of wound edges at closure.*

Bibliography

General Considerations

Arateri E, Regesta G, et al: Carpal tunnel syndrome appearing with prominent skin symptoms. *Arch Dermatol* 120:517, 1984.

Mees RA: Eed verschijnsel by polyneuritis arsenicosa. *Ned Tijdschr Geneeskd* 1:391, 1919.

Murphy WA, Totty WG, et al: Musculoskeletal system, in Lee JKT, Sagel SS, Stanley RJ (eds): *Computed Body Tomography with MRI Correlation*, 2d ed. New York, Raven, 1989, pp 899–989.

Scher RK, Daniel CR III: *Nails: Therapy, Diagnosis, Surgery*. Philadelphia, WB Saunders, 1990, pp 130–133, 167–187.

Trauma

Ahlo A, Kankaapaa V: Management of fractured scaphoid bone. *Acta Orthop Scand* 46:737, 1975.

Arzimanoglou A, Skiadaresis SM: Study of internal fixation by screws of oblique fractures in long bones. *J Bone Joint Surg Am* 34:219, 1952.

Ashkenaze DM, Ruby LK: Metacarpal fractures and dislocations. *Orthop Clin North Am* 23:19, 1992.

Atasoy A, Loakimidis E, et al: Reconstruction of the amputated fingertip with a triangular volar flap. *J Bone Joint Surg* 52A:921, 1970.

Beasley RW: Reconstruction of amputated fingertips. *Plast Reconstr Surg* 44:349, 1969.

Belsky MR, Eaton RG, et al: Closed reduction and internal fixation of proximal phalangeal fracture. *J Hand Surg* 9A:725, 1984.

Bennett JE: Upper arm tourniquet tolerance in hand surgery (letter). *Plast Reconstr Surg* 52:660, 1973.

Blair WF, Steyers CM: Extensor tendon injuries. *Orthop Clin North Am* 23:141, 1992.

Bunker TD, Potter B, et al: Continuous passive motion following flexor tendon repair. *J Hand Surg* 14B(4):406, 1989.

Bunnell S: *Surgery of the Hand.* Philadelphia, JB Lippincott, 1944, p 90.

Chow JA, Thomes LJ, et al: Controlled motion rehabilitation after flexor tendon repair and grafting. *J Bone Joint Surg* 70B(4):590, 1988.

Cooney WP: Fractures of the distal radius: A modern treatment-based classification. *Orthop Clin North Am* 24:211, 1993.

Cooney WP, Agee JM, et al: Symposium: Management of intra-articular fractures of the distal radius. *Contemp Orthop* 21:71, 1990.

Cooney WP, Dobyns JH, et al: Fractures of the scaphoid: A rational approach to management. *Clin Orthop* 149:90, 1980.

Cooney WP, Dobyns JH, et al: Nonunion of the scaphoid: Analysis of the results from bone grafting. *J Hand Surg* 5A:343, 1980.

Coonrad RW, Knight WE: Use of the tourniquet in the lower and upper extremities without general anesthesia. *J Bone Joint Surg* 39A:463, 1957.

Cushing H: Pneumatic tourniquet, with especial reference to their use in craniotomies. *Med News* 84:577, 1904.

Dabezies EJ, Mathews R, et al: Injuries to the carpus: Fractures of the scaphoid. *Orthopaedics* 5:1510, 1982.

Drefuss UY, Singer M: Human bites of the hand: A study of one hundred six patients. *J Hand Surg* 10A:884, 1985.

Dushoff IM: Hand surgery under wrist block and local infiltration anesthesia, using an upper arm tourniquet (letter). *Plast Reconstr Surg* 51:685, 1973.

Engkvist O, Lundborg G: Rupture of the extensor pollicis longus tendon after fracture of the lower end of radius: A clinical and microangiographic study. *Hand* 11:76, 1979.

Estersohn H, Sourifman H: The minimum effective midthigh tourniquet pressure. *J Foot Surg* 21:281, 1982.

Flatt AE: Minor hand injuries. *J Bone Joint Surg* 37B:117, 1955.

Gatewood: Plastic repair of finger defects without hospitalization. *JAMA* 87:1479, 1926.

Gellman H, Caputo RJ, et al: Comparison of short and long thumb-spica casts for nondisplaced fractures of the carpal scaphoid. *J Bone Joint Surg* 71A:354, 1989.

Guirguis EM, Bell MSG: The wrist tourniquet: An alternative technique in hand surgery. *J Hand Surg* 15A:516, 1990.

Gutmann E: Effect of delay of innervation on recovery of muscle after nerve lesions. *J Neurophysiol* 11:277, 1948.

Hart RG, Uehara DT, et al: Extensor tendon injuries of the hand. *Emerg Med Clin North Am* 11:637, 1993.

Harvey FJ, Harvey PM: Three rare causes of extensor tendon rupture. *J Hand Surg* 14A:957, 1989.

Heim U, Pheiffer KM: General techniques for the internal fixation of small fracture, and The hand, in *Small Fragment Set Manual: Internal Fixation of Small Fractures,* 3d ed. New York, Springer-Verlag, 1987, pp 31–40, 179–211.

Herbert TJ, Fisher WE: Management of the fractured scaphoid using a new bone screw. *J Bone Joint Surg* 66B:114, 1984.

Hove LM: Fractures of the hand: Distribution and relative incidence. *Scand J Plast Recon Surg* 27:317, 1993.

Howard FM: Ulnar nerve palsy in wrist fractures. *J Bone Joint Surg* 43A:1197, 1961.

Hueston JT: Local flap repair of fingertip injuries. *Plast Reconstr Surg* 37:349, 1966.

Itoh Y, Horiuti Y, et al: Extensor tendon involvement in Smith's and Galeazzi's fracture. *J Hand Surg* 12A:535, 1987.

Jupiter JB, Koniuch MP, et al: The management of delayed union and nonunion of the metacarpals and phalanges. *J Hand Surg* 10A:457, 1985.

Kaempfe F, Peimer CA: Quick fixation of skin grafts. *J Hand Surg* 16A:761, 1991.

Kaplan EB: Anatomy, injuries, and treatment of the extensor apparatus of the hand and fingers. *Clin Orthop* 13:24, 1959.

Klenerman L: The tourniquet in surgery. *J Bone Joint Surg* 44B:937, 1962.

Kutler W: A new method for fingertip amputation. *JAMA* 133:29, 1947.

Lie KK, Magargle RK, et al: Free full-thickness skin grafts from the palm to cover defects of the fingers. *J Bone Joint Surg* 52A:559, 1970.

Mann RJ, Hoffeld TA, et al: Human bites of the hand: Twenty years of experience. *J Hand Surg* 2:97, 1977.

McElfresh E, Dobyns J: Intra-articular metacarpal head fractures. *J Hand Surg* 8:383, 1983.

Neimkin RJ, Smith RJ: Double tourniquet with linked mercury manometers for hand surgery. *J Hand Surg* 8:938, 1983.

Newport ML, Blair WF, et al: Long-term results of extensor tendon repair. *J Hand Surg* 15A:961, 1990.

Nisenfield FG, Neviaser RJ: Fracture of the hook of the hamate: A diagnosis easily missed. *J Trauma* 14:612, 1974.

Novak CB, Kelly L, et al: Sensory recovery after median nerve grafting. *J Hand Surg* 17A:59, 1992.

Patton HS: Split-skin grafts from hypothenar area for fingertip avulsions. *Plast Reconstr Surg* 43:426, 1969.

Pedowitz RA, Gershuni DH, et al: Effects of reperfusion intervals on skeletal muscle injury beneath and distal to a pneumatic tourniquet. *J Hand Surg* 17:345, 1992.

Pedowitz RA, Gershuni DH, et al: Muscle injury induced beneath and distal to a pneumatic tourniquet: A quantitative animal study of effects of tourniquet pressure and duration. *J Hand Surg* 16:610, 1991.

Polivy KD, Millender LH, et al: Fractures of the hook of the hamate: A failure of clinical diagnosis. *J Hand Surg* 10A:101, 1985.

Reyes FA, Latta LL: Conservative management of difficult phalangeal fractures. *Clin Orthop* 214:23, 1987.

Rüedi TP, Burri C, et al: Stable internal fixation of fractures of the hand. *J Trauma* 11:381, 1971.

Russe O: Fracture of the carpal navicular: Diagnosis, nonoperative treatment, and operative treatment. *J Bone Joint Surg* 42A:759, 1960.

Schenck RR, Cheema TA: Hypothenar skin grafts for fingertip reconstruction. *J Hand Surg* 9A:750, 1984.

Seddon HJ: Three types of nerve injury. *Brain* 66:238, 1943.

Steel WM: The AO small fragment set in hand fractures. *Hand* 10:246, 1978.

Stern PJ: Fractures of the metacarpals and phalanges, in Green DP (ed): *Operative Hand Surgery,* 3d ed. New York, Churchill-Livingstone, 1993, pp 695–758.

Stern PJ, Wieser MJ, et al: Complications of plate fixation in the hand skeleton. *Clin Orthop* 214:59, 1987.

Strickland JW: Flexor tenolysis. *Hand Clin* 1:121, 1985.

Sunderland S, Ray LJ: Denervation changes in mammalian striated muscle. *J Neurol Neurosurg Psychiatry* 13:159, 1950.

Szabo RM, Manske D: Displaced fractures of the scaphoid. *Clin Orthop* 230:30, 1988.

Taleisnik J, Gelberman RH, et al: The extensor retinaculum at the wrist. *J Hand Surg* 9A:495, 1984.

Thompson JS, Peimer CA: Extensor tendon injuries: Acute repair and late reconstruction. In Chapman MW (ed): *Operative Orthopaedics.* Philadelphia, JP Lippincott, 1988, pp 1169–1184.

Tsuchida H: Experimental study of the tendon repair: 2nd report. *J Jpn Soc Surg Hand* 9(2):87.

Vaughan-Jackson OJ: Rupture of extensor tendons by attrition of the interior radioulnar joint: Report of two cases. *J Bone Joint Surg* 30:528, 1948.

Verdan CE: Primary and secondary repair of flexor and extensor tendon injuries. In Flynn JE (ed): *Hand Surgery,* 2d ed. Baltimore, Williams & Wilkins, 1975, p 149.

Werntz JR, Chesher SP, et al: A new dynamic splint for postoperative treatment of flexor tendon injury. *J Hand Surg* 14A(3):559, 1989.

Willson RL: Management of acute extensor tendon injuries. In Hunter JM, Schneider LH, Mackin EJ (eds): *Tendon Surgery in the Hand.* St Louis, CV Mosby, 1987, pp 336–348.

Complications of Trauma

Bonica JJ: *The Management of Pain.* Philadelphia, Lea & Febiger, 1953.

Gelberman RH, Szabo RM, et al: Tissue pressure threshold for peripheral nerve viability. *Clin Orthop* 178:285, 1983.

Hargens AR, Akeson WH, et al: Tissue fluid pressures: From basic research tools to clinical applications. The Kappa Delta Award Paper. *J Orthop Res* 7:902, 1989.

Hargens AR, Gershuni DH, et al: Tissue necrosis associated with tourniquet ischemia. Eleventh European Conference for Microcirculation. Garmisch-Partenkirchen, Germany. *Bibliotheca Anatomica* 20:599, 601, 1981.

Matsen FA III, Mayo KA, et al: A model compartmental syndrome in man with particular reference to the quantification of nerve function. *J Bone Joint Surg Am* 59:648, 1977.

Matsen FA III, Rorabeck CH: Compartment syndromes. *AAOS Instr Course Lect* 38:463, 1989.

Mitchell SW: *Injuries of Nerves and Their Consequences.* Philadelphia, JB Lippincott, 1972.

Mitchell SW, Morehouse GR, : *Gunshot Wounds and Other Injuries of Nerves.* Philadelphia, JB Lippincott, 1964.

Mubarak SJ, Hargens AR (eds): *Compartment Syndromes and Volkmann's Ischemic Contracture.* Monographs in Clinical Orthopaedics, vol 3. Philadelphia, WB Saunders, 1981.

Burns

American Burn Association: Guidelines for service standards and severity classifications in the treatment of burn injury. *ACS Bull* 69:24, 1984.

Demling RH: Burns, in Greenfield LJ, et al (eds): *Surgery: Scientific Principles and Practice.* Philadelphia, JB Lippincott, 1993, pp 368–388.

Helm PA: Burn rehabilitation: Dimensions of the problem. *Clin Plast Surg* 19:551, 1992.

Robson MC, Smith DJ Jr: Burned hand. In Jurkiewicz MJ, et al (eds): *Plastic Surgery: Principles and Practice.* St Louis, CV Mosby, 1990, pp 781–802.

Salisbury RE, Nieves SU, et al: Acute care and rehabilitation of the burned hand, In Hunter JM, et al (eds): *Rehabilitation of the Hand: Surgery and Therapy,* 3d ed. St Louis, CV Mosby, 1990, pp 831–840.

Infection

Brown DM, Young VL: Hand Infections. *South Med J* 86:56, 1993.

Cheatum DE, Hudman M, et al: Chronic arthritis due to *Mycobacterium intracellulare:* Sacroiliac, knee, and carpal tunnel involvement in a young man and response to chemotherapy. *Arthritis Rheum* 19:777, 1976.

Dickson-Wright A: Tendon sheath infections. *Proc R Soc Med* 37:504, 1943–1944.

Glass KD: Factors related to the resolution of treated hand infections. *J Hand Surg* 7:388, 1982.

Gunther SF, Levy CS: Mycobacterial infections. *Hand Clin* 5:591, 1989.

Neviaser RJ: Closed tendon sheath irrigation for pyogenic flexor tenosynovitis. *J Hand Surg* 3:462, 1978.

Strombert BV: Changing bacterial flora of hand infections. *J Trauma* 25:530, 1985.

Chronic Syndromes

Belsole RJ: De Quervain's tenosynovitis: Diagnostic and operative complications. *Orthopaedics* 4:899, 1981.

Borg K, Lindblom U: Diagnostic value of quantitative sensory testing (WST) in carpal tunnel syndrome. *Acta Neurol Scand* 78:537, 1988.

Boyes JH: *Bunnel's Surgery of the Hand,* 4th ed. Philadelphia, JB Lippincott, 1964.

Boyle J, Smith N, et al: Vibration white finger. *J Hand Surg Br* 13:171, 1988.

De Quervain F: Ueber eine form von chronischer tendovaginits. *Corresp Blatt Schweitzer Arzte* 25:389, 1895.

Dobyns JH, Sim FH, et al: Sports stress syndrome of the hand and wrist. *Am J Sports Med* 6:236, 1978.

Farkkila M, Pyykko I, et al: Forestry workers exposed to vibration: A neurological study. *Br J Ind Med* 45:188, 1988.

Finkelstein H: Stenosing tenosynovitis at the radial styloid process. *J Bone Joint Surg* 28:509, 1930.

Garcia-Elias M, Sanchez-Freijo J, et al: Dynamic changes of the transverse carpal arch during flexion-extension of the wrist: Effects of sectioning the transverse carpal ligament. *J Hand Surg Am* 17:1017, 1992.

Gellman H, Gelberman R, et al: Carpal tunnel syndrome: An evaluation of the provocative tests. *J Bone Joint Surg Am* 68:735, 1986.

Harter B, McKiernan J, et al: Carpal tunnel syndrome: Surgical and nonsurgical treatment. *J Hand Surg Am* 18:734, 1993.

Harvey FJ, Harvey PM, et al: De Quervain's disease: Surgical or nonsurgical treatment. *J Hand Surg* 15A:83, 1990.

Hymovich L, Lindholm M: Hand, wrist, and forearm injuries: The result of repetitive motion. *J Occup Med* 8:573, 1966.

Kuorinka I, Koskinen P: Occupational rheumatic diseases and upper limb strain in manual jobs in a light mechanical industry. *Scand J Work Environ Health* 5(suppl 3):39, 1979.

Kaplan S, Glickel S, et al: Predictive factors in the nonsurgical treatment of carpal tunnel syndrome. *J Hand Surg Br* 15:106, 1990.

Kruger V, Kraft G, et al: Carpal tunnel syndrome: Objective measures and splint use. *Arch Phys Med Rehabil* 72:517, 1991.

Luchetti R, Schoenhuber R, et al: Assessment of sensory nerve conduction in carpal tunnel syndrome before, during, and after operation. *J Hand Surg Br* 13:386, 1988.

Luopajarvi T, Kuorinka I, et al: Prevalence of tenosynovitis and other injuries of the upper extremities in repetitive work. *Scand J Work Environ Health* 5(suppl 3):48, 1979.

Miller R, Lohman W, et al: An epidemiologic study of carpal tunnel syndrome and hand-arm vibration syndrome in relation to vibration exposure. *J Hand Surg Am* 19:99, 1994.

Moore J: Carpal tunnel syndrome. *Occup Med* 7:741, 1992.

Nau H, Lange B, et al: Prediction of outcome of decompression for carpal tunnel syndrome. *J Hand Surg Br* 13:391, 1988.

Ordeberg E, Sälgeback S, et al: Carpal tunnel syndrome in pregnancy. *Acta Obstet Gynecol Scan* 66:233, 1987.

Stock S: Work place ergonomic factors and the development of musculoskeletal disorders of the neck and upper limbs: A meta-analysis. *Am J Ind Med* 21:895, 1992.

Subcommittee on Clinical Policies, American Academy of Orthopaedic Surgeons: Carpal tunnel syndrome. *Clinical Policies,* 11–13, 1991.

Wand J: Carpal tunnel syndrome in pregnancy and lactation. *J Hand Surg Br* 15:93, 1990.

Wieslander G, Norback D, et al: Carpal tunnel syndrome (CTS) and exposure to vibration, repetitive wrist movements, and heavy manual work: A case-referent study. *Br J Ind Med* 46:43, 1989.

Yoshioka S, Okuda Y, et al: Changes in carpal tunnel shape during wrist joint motion: MRI evaluation of normal volunteers. *J Hand Surg Br* 18:620, 1993.

Zeiss J, Skie M, et al: Anatomic relations between the median nerve and flexor tendons in the carpal tunnel: MR evaluation in normal volunteers. *Am J Roentgenol* 153:533, 1989.

Acquired Dysfunction

Ketchum L: The use of the full thickness skin graft in Dupuytren's contracture. *Hand Clin* 7:731, 1991.

Congenital Deformities

Abouna JM, Brown H: The treatment of mallet finger, the results in a series of 148 consecutive cases and review of the literature. *Br J Surg* 55:653, 1968.

Angelides AC: Ganglions of the hand and wrist, in Green DP (ed): *Operative Hand Surgery,* 3d ed. New York, Churchill-Livingstone, 1993, pp 2157–2171.

Bruner JM: Optimum skin incisions for the surgical relief of stenosing tenosynovitis in the hand. *Plast Reconstr Surg* 38:197, 1966.

Hooper G: Cystic swellings, in Bogumill GP, Gleegler EJ (eds): *Tumors of the Hand and Upper Limb.* Edinburgh, Churchill-Livingstone, 1993, pp 172–182.

Kaplan E: *Functional and Surgical Anatomy of the Hand,* 2d ed. Philadelphia, JB Lippincott, 1965.

Lange RH, Engber WD: Hyperextension mallet finger. *Orthopaedics* 6:1426, 1983.

Lewin P: A simple splint for baseball finger. *JAMA* 85:1059, 1925.

Lowdon IMR: Fractures of the metacarpal neck of the little finger. *Injury* 17:189, 1986.

McCarroll HR Jr: Congenital flexion deformities of the thumb. *Hand Clin* 1:567, 1985.

Segmüller G: *Surgical Stabilization of the Skeleton of the Hand.* Baltimore, Williams & Wilkins, 1977, pp 45–47.

Stack HH, Boyes JH, et al: Mallet finger. *J Bone Joint Surg* 44A:1061, 1962.

Stefanich RJ, Peimer CA: Longitudinal incision for trigger release. *J Hand Surg* 14A:316, 1988.

Watchmaker GP, Mackinnon SE: Nerve injury and repair, in Peimer CA (ed): *Surgery of the Hand and Upper Extremity,* New York, McGraw-Hill, 1996, 1251–1270.

Tumors

Angelides AC: Ganglions of the hand and wrist, in Green DP (ed): *Operative Hand Surgery,* 3d ed. New York, Churchill-Livingstone, 1993, pp 2157–2171.

Greendyke SA, Wilson M, et al: Anterior wrist ganglia from the scaphotrapezial joint. *J Hand Surg Am* 17:487, 1992.

Ragsdale DB, Dupree WB: Neoplasms of the fatty tissues, in Bogumill GP, Fleegler EJ (eds): *Tumors of the Hand and Upper Limb.* Edinburgh, Churchill-Livingstone, 1993 pp 254–278.

Oster LH, Blair WF, et al: Large lipomas in the deep palmar space. *J Hand Surg Am* 14:700, 1989.

Tordai P, Hoglund M, et al: Is the treatment of enchondroma in the hand by simple curettage a rewarding method? *J Hand Surg Br* 15:331, 1990.

Hasselgren G, Forssblad P, et al: Bone grafting unnecessary in the treatment of enchondromas in the hand. *J Hand Surg Am* 16:139, 1991.

Johnson JO: Differential diagnosis and treatment of giant cell lesions, in Boguill GP, Fleegler EJ (eds): *Tumors of the Hand and Upper Limb.* Edinburgh, Churchill-Livingstone, 1993, pp 360–391.

Vander Griend RA, Funderburk CH: The treatment of giant cell tumors of the distal part of the radius. *J Bone Joint Surg Am* 75:899, 1993.

Szabo RM, Thorson EP, et al: Allograft replacement with distal radioulnar joint fusion and ulnar osteotomy for treatment of giant cell tumors of the distal radius. *J Hand Surg Am* 15:929, 1990.

Surgical Principles

Adler VG, Burmon D, et al: Absorption of hexachlorophene from infants' skin. *Lancet* 2:384, 1972.

Alexander JW, Fischer JE, et al: The influence of hair removal methods on wound infections. *Arch Surg* 118:347, 1983.

Ayliffe GAJ: Surgical scrub and skin disinfection. *Infect Control* 4:23, 1984.

Branemark PI, et al: Local tissue effects of wound disinfectants. *Acta Chir Scand* 357(suppl): 166, 1966.

Bridenbaugh LD: Patient management for neural blockage: Selection, management, premedication and supplementation, in Cousins MJ, Bridenbaugh LD (eds): *Neural Blockade in Clinical Anesthesia and Management of Pain.* 2d ed. Philadelphia, JB Lippincott, 1988, pp 191–210.

Butcher HR, Ballinger WF, et al: Hexachlorophene concentrations in the blood of operating room personnel. *Arch Surg* 107:70, 1973.

Chiu, DTW: Transthecal digital block: Flexor tendon sheath used for anesthetic infusion. *J Hand Surg Am* 15:471, 1990.

Cruse PJE, Foord R: The epidemiology of wound infection: A 10-year prospective study of 62,939 wounds. *Surg Clin North Am* 60:27, 1980.

Expert Panel of the Cosmetic Ingredient Review. Final report of the safety assessment for chloroxylenol. Washington, DC, 1984.

Garibaldi RA, et al: The impact of preoperative skin disinfection on preventing intraoperative wound contamination. *Infect Control Hosp Epidemiol* 9:109, 1988.

Hochberg J, Murray GF: Principles of operative surgery: Antisepsis, technique, sutures, and drains, in Sabiston D (ed): *Textbook of Surgery: The Biological Basis of Modern Surgical Practice.* Philadelphia, WB Saunders, 1991, pp 210–220.

Jepsen OB, Bruttomesso KA: The effectiveness of preoperative skin preparations: An integrative review of the literature. *AORN J* 58:447, 1993.

Kaul AF, Jewett JF: Agents and techniques for disinfection of the skin. *Surg Gynecol Obstet* 152:677, 1981.

Kulekampff D, Persky MA: Brachial plexus anaesthesia: Its indications, technique, and dangers. *Ann Surg* 87:883, 1923.

Larson E: Guideline for use of topical antimicrobial agents. *Am J Infect Control* 16:253, 1988.

Larson EL, Eke PI, et al: Quantity of soap as a variable in handwashing. *Infect Control* 8:371, 1987.

Larson EL, Leyden J, et al: Physiologic and microbiologic changes in skin related to frequent handwashings. *Infect Control* 7:59, 1986.

Lily HA, Lowbury EJL: Transient skin flora. *J Clin Pathol* 31:919, 1978.

Lowburg EJL, Lily HA: Disinfection of the skin of operation sites. *Br Med J* 2:1039, 1960.

Lowbury EJL, Lily HA: Use of 4 percent chlorhexidine detergent solution (Hibiscrub) and other methods of skin disinfection. *Br Med J* 1:510, 1973.

MacKenzie I: Preoperative skin preparation and surgical outcome. *J Hosp Infect II* (suppl B):27, 1988.

Maki DJ, Zilz MA, et al: Evaluation of antibacterial efficacy of four agents for hand washing. *Curr Chemother Infect Dis* 11:1089, 1977.

Miller JM, Jackson DA, et al: The microbicidal property of pHisoHex. *Mil Med* 127:576, 1962.

MMWR Update: Research reinforced doubts about need for prep shaves. *Hosp Infect Control* 82, Monograph, 1989.

Reybouck G: Handwashing and hand disinfection. *J Hosp Infect* 8:5, 1986.

Seropian R, Reynolds BM: Wound infections after preoperative depilatory versus razor preparations. *Am J Surg* 121:251, 1971.

Smylie HG, Logie JRC, et al: From PHisoHex to Hibiscrub. *Br Med J* 4:586, 1973.

Winnie AP: *Plexus Anesthesia,* vol 1: *Perivascular Techniques of Brachial Plexus Block.* Philadelphia, WB Saunders, 1983.

CHAPTER 43

Plastic and Reconstructive Surgery

Robert J. Wood and M.J. Jurkiewicz

INTRODUCTION

Plastic surgery is that aspect of the discipline of surgery in which concentration and interest are focused on the restoration of form as well as function. The disorders that the plastic surgeon encounters might be the result of trauma, aging, congenital defects, cancer, or prior surgical procedures. Deformity and its consequences are protean, and hence a plastic surgeon must have versatility, a sure spatial sense, and an appreciation of the profound effects that deformity can have on the human spirit. The foundation for the study of plastic surgery is a thorough education in surgical principles and a detailed knowledge of anatomy, surgical technique, and the biology of wound repair.

The word *plastic* derives from the Greek *plastikos*, meaning to mold. The term *plastic surgery* appeared sporadically in a number of surgical texts through the eighteenth and nineteenth centuries. It was firmly established with the publication of *Plastic Surgery—Its Principles and Practice* in 1919 by John Staige Davis.

Many modern plastic surgical procedures have their roots in ancient times with early practitioners. In the *Sushruta Samhita*, an early text written in the sixth or seventh century B.C. by the practitioner Sushruta, reconstruction of an amputated nose with a pedicled forehead flap and reconstruction of auricular defects with cheek flaps are described. Amputation of the nose remained a common form of punishment in India through the eighteenth century. When this technique was noted by English physicians of the seventeenth and eighteenth centuries it became known as the Indian method of nasal reconstruction. The Roman physician Celsus described operations for the repair of traumatic injuries to the nose, eyelids, ears, and lips in the first century A.D. Another Roman physician, Paulus Aegineta, also described operations for the treatment of facial injuries in the first century A.D.

The Middle Ages produced few known practitioners of reconstructive procedures. The period of the Renaissance marked a resurgence in attempts at reconstructive surgery. During the fifteenth century members of the Branca family in Italy practiced techniques of nasal reconstruction probably derived from Sushruta. Gaspara Tagliacozzi (1545–1599) published *De Curtorum Chirurgia per Insitionem* in 1597. This is believed by many to

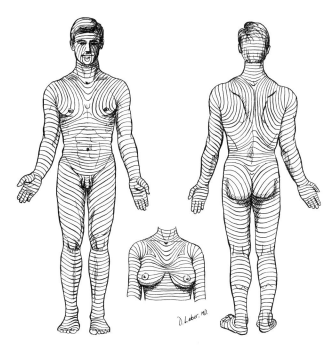

FIG. 43-1. *The lines of minimum tension generally lie perpendicular to the direction of pull of the underlying muscles. Correct incision lines for the sternal, deltoid, and interscapular regions are difficult to determine. Incisions should be made parallel to the lines of minimum tension.*

be the first modern plastic surgery text; it describes the technique of nasal reconstruction using an arm flap.

Baronio described the successful grafting of skin in sheep in 1804. Techniques for human skin grafting were described by Revendin in France, as well as by Ollier and Thiersh in a series of publications during the latter part of the nineteenth century. As with other surgical specialties, great advances in plastic surgery took place during the First and Second World Wars. During the period of the First World War the discipline of plastic surgery became well established by melding techniques of dental surgery, otolaryngology, ophthalmology, and general surgery. In England Sir Harold Gillies, an otolaryngologist, established a center for maxillofacial reconstruction of the many allied military casualties. V. H. Kazanjian is well known for his application of dental techniques to these injuries. In particular, he pioneered the use of prosthetic devices to maintain soft tissue as delayed bony reconstructions were performed. Upon entry of the United States in World War I, Vilray P. Blair of St. Louis became consultant to the surgeon general of the army and organized units to care for soft tissue wounds and maxillofacial reconstruction.

In the period between World Wars I and II academic societies of plastic surgeons were established and the training of plastic surgeons both in the United States and Europe became more formalized. As in World War I, centers for plastic surgery were established during World War II, including centers for reconstructive surgery of the hand. Ever since World War II a unifying theme in the clinical and research work of plastic surgeons has been the transfer of tissue, both autologous and allogeneic. The biology of the transplantation and rejection of skin allografts was studied by Gibson and Medawar, who set the stage for the first successful renal transplantation in monozygotic twins by Joseph

Murray and coworkers in 1954 at the Peter Bent Brigham Hospital in Boston.

The techniques of moving tissues regionally within a patient were advanced by the development of axial pattern flaps, including the deltopectoral flap by Bakamjian in 1965 and the groin flap by McGregor and Jackson in 1972. Transferring muscle and muscle-skin units had been described in the nineteenth century by Tanzini. Lost and forgotten, the work was rediscovered by McCraw, Orticochea, Ger, Vasconez, Bostwick, and others. Since 1974 a great number of muscle and muscle-skin flaps have been developed.

Also during this time the development of microsurgical techniques by Buncke in the United States, Ackland in the United Kingdom, Harii and Ohmori in Japan, and Taylor in Australia made possible the transfer of tissues from distant donor sites. Among the earliest "free flaps" described were transfer of the omentum and groin flap. By 1990 microsurgical transfer of a great number of muscle as well as skin flaps was commonplace, and replantation of traumatically amputated extremities and digits became a standard of care.

In France, Paul Tessier and coworkers in the 1960s pioneered new techniques for reconstruction of deformities of the craniofacial skeleton. This new discipline of craniofacial surgery was rapidly adopted in the United States, and multidisciplinary centers for the treatment of craniofacial disorders were established.

GENERAL PRINCIPLES

Skin Incisions

Perhaps more than in any other surgical specialty the operative results in plastic surgery are readily apparent, to both the trained and the untrained eye. Although a patient may not have an opinion about the adequacy of resection after colectomy for colon carcinoma, the same patient would almost certainly have a strong opinion about the results of rhinoplasty or the repair of a child's cleft lip. Hence in any plastic surgery procedure skin incisions are planned to optimize the resultant scar. Langer has described the skin lines of minimal tension that generally run perpendicular to the long axis of underlying muscles (Fig. 43-1). Gravitational forces also work to produce these lines. The lines of minimal tension, or *Langer's lines*, are very obvious in the face of an older person, in whom they can be seen as the lines of facial expression (Fig. 43-2). An incision planned within or parallel to these lines will result in a narrower and less conspicuous scar than one that runs perpendicular to the lines of minimal tension. Elective incisions may also be placed in areas less obvious to the observer, such as the hairline or eyebrow, or within the eyelids, nares, or mouth.

As the scar matures there is an attendant contraction of the wound. If an incision must cross a joint surface, the direction of the incision should be altered so a linear contracture does not develop that may restrict joint motion. An incision placed across a joint in an oblique or transverse fashion will lengthen the overall scar and change the direction of wound contracture to optimize range of motion.

Excisions of lesions small enough to be closed primarily are frequently performed by an elliptical excision. The long and short axes should be in a ratio of approximately 4:1. Excisions by an ellipse with a long axis that is too short will often result in excess tissue at either end of the closure, or a *dog ear*. Reskin edge, and by transposing additional skin into the wound in the form of a flap.

Skin and subcutaneous tissues may by coapted with suture material, staples, or surgical tape. A great variety of suture material, absorbable and nonabsorbable, is available to the surgeon. Common absorbable sutures include surgical gut, chromic gut,

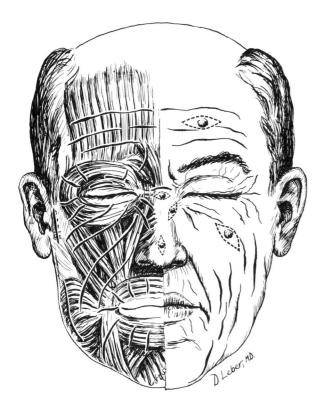

FIG. 43-2. The relation of the lines of minimum tension to the underlying facial muscles. The right side of the drawing shows the direction of elective excisions.

moval of this excess tissue can be performed with a number of techniques, all of which result in a longer but much more acceptable scar. A common technique involves extending the incision in longitudinal fashion and then excising the redundant tissue on one side of the incision (Fig. 43-3).

Wound Closure

Wound healing is a complex process dependent on local and systemic factors as well as surgical technique. Before closing any wound, basic preparation includes debridement of devitalized tissue and removal of foreign bodies and gross wound contaminants. Debridement of devitalized tissue is considered by many to be the single most important factor in the management of a contaminated wound. Nonviable tissue within a wound acts as a culture medium for bacterial growth and also affects leukocyte function by promoting an anaerobic environment within the wound. Tissue viability and the extent of debridement required are best judged by thorough inspection of the wound. In fresh traumatic or surgical wounds skin viability can often be difficult to assess accurately. In these instances the injection of fluorescein dye can be helpful in demarcating devitalized skin. In general, however, viable skin edges and muscle tissue bleed when debrided, and viable muscles contract when stimulated.

Ideally skin should be coapted with minimal or no tension (Fig. 43-4). Excessive tension across a wound can lead to delayed wound healing and a wide scar. The tension across a wound closure can be modulated by undermining the surrounding skin, closing the wound in a layered fashion such that sutures in a deep dermal or subcutaneous plane reduce the tension at the

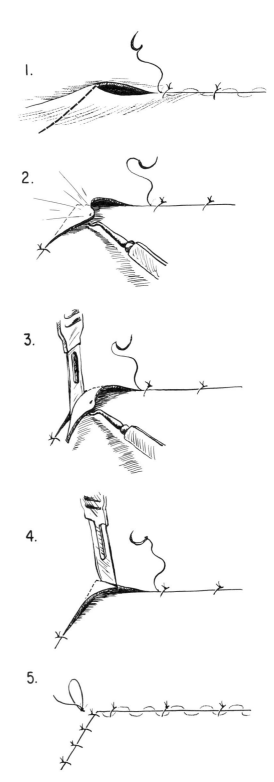

FIG. 43-3. Excision of "dog ears."

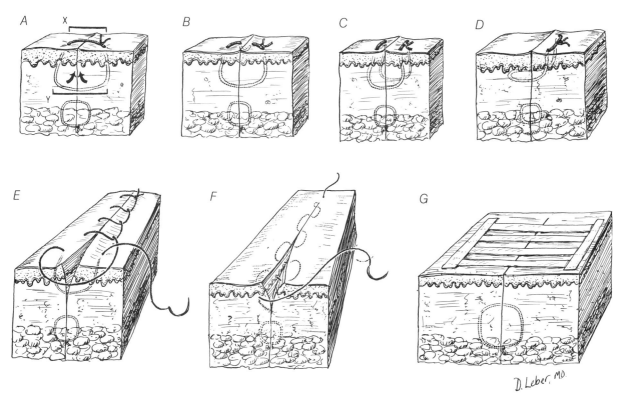

FIG. 43-4. Examples of wound closure. The transcutaneous suture is best placed by ensuring that the deeper portion of the suture (y) is wider than the superficial portion (x). This causes the wound pressures to encourage slight skin edge eversion *(curved arrows)*, an excellent way of preventing edge inversion. *A.* Simple suture. *B.* Vertical mattress suture. *C.* Horizontal mattress suture. *D.* Half-buried mattress suture. This suture is useful for flaps, as it causes minimum interference with blood supply. *E.* Locked simple running suture. *F.* Intracuticular running suture. *G.* Wound closure with porous tape.

polyglactin-910 (Vicryl), polydioxanone (PDS), and polyglycolic acid (Dexon). Plain gut, derived from sheep or beef intestine, loses most of its strength within 7 days. This is commonly used in areas where wound healing is expected to be rapid and suture removal may be difficult. Fine gut suture (6-0) is commonly used for skin closure in the periorbital regions and in facial wounds in children. Chromic gut is treated to resist breakdown by tissue and maintains its tensile strength longer that plain gut. We frequently use this suture within the mouth and nose, where suture removal can be difficult. Tissue reaction to chromic gut can be significant. It is rarely used on the skin of the face. Polyglactin and polydioxanone sutures can be used in subcutaneous tissues. Polyglactin will have lost approximately 70 percent of its tensile strength at 3 weeks, and polydioxanone will maintain approximately 50 percent of its tensile strength at 4 weeks and 25 percent at 6 weeks.

Nonabsorbable sutures include surgical silk, surgical cotton, surgical steel, nylon, polypropylene, and polyethylene terephthalate. Nylon and polypropylene are relatively inert within tissue. These sutures are appropriate for skin closure in both interrupted and running subcuticular "pull-out" fashion, tendon repairs, and microsurgery. A continuous running polypropylene suture in a subcuticular fashion allows the accurate coaption of skin edges and can be left in place without creating suture marks in the skin. A subcuticular polypropylene pull-out suture is our standard for general skin closure. The point where a suture pierces the epidermis will begin to epithelialize at 3 days. This

process is responsible for the permanent suture marks sometimes seen after wound repair. To prevent these permanent suture marks, skin sutures on the face should be removed at 3 to 5 days and the wound stabilized with sterile tape.

Skin Grafts

Skin grafting is one of the most powerful techniques in plastic surgery. By transplanting a sheet of epidermis and a variable thickness of dermis a surgeon is able to close wounds that would otherwise require a more complex flap or free tissue transfer. The technique of skin grafting also allows large areas to be resurfaced, as in the treatment of burns. A skin graft is a sheet of skin including epidermis and a variable thickness of dermis that is completely freed from its native blood supply and transplanted to a recipient site to be closed. Skin grafts may be either full thickness, including all epidermis and dermis, or partial (split) thickness, in which the skin is harvested at some level within the dermis (Fig. 43-5). Partial-thickness grafts are frequently harvested at a thickness of 1/1200 to 1/2000 of an inch. Harvesting skin at this level will leave some dermis as well as epidermal appendages such as hair follicles and sweat glands in the donor site. These epidermal appendages then allow regeneration of new epidermis to close the donor site.

A full-thickness graft, because it includes the entire epidermis and dermis at the donor site, requires that the donor site be closed primarily or left open to granulate and contract. In a full-thickness graft there are no epidermal or dermal remnants to

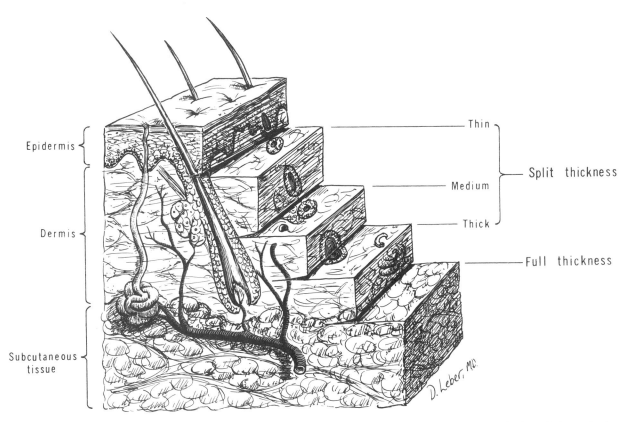

Epidermis

Dermis

Subcutaneous tissue

Thin ⎫
          ⎬ Split thickness
Medium ⎪
Thick ⎭

Full thickness

D. Leber, MD.

FIG. 43-5. *Representation of skin graft donor depths.*

allow epithelialization as in a partial-thickness graft (Fig. 43-6). As a general rule, split-thickness grafts have a greater chance of surviving but will contract up to 40 percent on average. In practice, the type of skin graft is matched to the given clinical situation. Partial-thickness grafts are usually used to resurface burns, as the donor areas will rapidly close and can be reharvested. A full-thickness graft is usually selected to resurface relatively small and critical areas such as an eyelid so that contraction of the grafted tissue is minimal.

There are a number of commonly used donor sites for full-thickness grafts. In selecting a donor site, the surgeon must consider which anatomic location provides the best skin color and texture match to the anatomic area being grafted and the consequences of a scar in the region of the donor site. In general, donor sites that are closest anatomically to the site to be grafted will have a closer match in skin color and texture. Postauricular skin is suitable for grafting the skin of the face. Smaller grafts in this area may be taken and the donor site closed primarily. If necessary the entire non-hair-bearing skin of the postauricular and mastoid region can be harvested and grafted with split-thickness skin, as this area is relatively concealed from a frontal view. The supraclavicular region is another appropriate donor site for a full-thickness graft for the face. This skin will often maintain a pinkish tone to match the face. The antecubital crease and inner aspect of the arm are appropriate donor sites for full-thickness grafts for the hand or finger. These donor sites are usually already prepared in the field during hand cases but have the disadvantage of a frequently prominent scar. Transverse incisions in the area of the wrist flexion crease can be especially troublesome to patients if mistaken by others as self-inflicted or an apparent suicide attempt. The hip flexion crease in the inguinal area is an excellent donor site for full-thickness grafting to the upper extremities and hands. The linear scar usually remains well hidden in a natural skin fold. A limited split-thickness graft may be harvested from the hypothenar region, which gives the best match and texture for the hand. Redundant upper eyelid skin may be harvested with or without underlying orbicularis muscle for full-thickness grafting of the contralateral lid. This is also a well-concealed donor site when the donor incision is oriented within the tarsal fold.

When larger areas are to be grafted, split-thickness skin is frequently harvested from the buttocks, thighs, and abdominal wall. It is desirable whenever possible to keep this donor site in an area that will eventually be hidden by undergarments and bathing suits. The scalp and suprapubic areas provide possible donor sites for split-thickness skin. With the regrowth of hair in the donor site any resultant scar remains well concealed. Thick grafts should be avoided in these areas to prevent alopecia. Scalp donor sites reepithelialize rapidly and permit frequent reharvesting. This technique is useful in treating extensive burns.

Cultured autologous keratinocytes can provide sheets of epithelium that will cover patients who have massive burns. Promising techniques are being developed to provide collagen or dermis matrix to enhance the stability of cultured keratinocytes.

For a skin graft to survive it must be revascularized by the recipient bed. Radiation-damaged tissue and relatively avascular tissue such as tendon or bone are therefore poor recipient sites for skin grafts. For the first 48 h that a skin graft is in contact

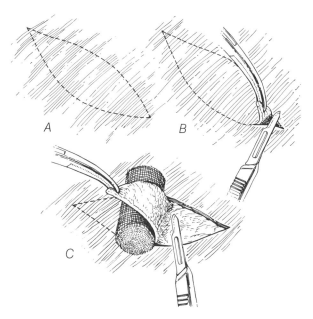

FIG. 43-6. *Full-thickness skin graft. A minimum of subcutaneous fat is raised with the graft.*

with the recipient bed the graft survives by a process known as *plasmatic imbibition*. During this time nutrients diffuse from the underlying bed through the surrounding extracellular fluid and directly into the capillaries and cells of the skin graft. During this period fibrin bonds fix the graft to the recipient bed. At 48 h, vascular buds in the bed have made contact with capillaries within the graft, and circulation is established by a process known as *inosculation*. In this process vessels in the graft bed randomly attach to capillaries in the skin graft or recipient site blood vessels grow into the graft itself and within some of the preexisting capillaries. It remains controversial whether neovascular ingrowth or random inosculation of existing vessels is the primary method of revascularization.

For a graft to be successfully revascularized and survive, a number of conditions must be satisfied. As discussed above, as a rule the recipient bed must be well vascularized. An exception to this is the occurrence of the "bridging" phenomenon, in which a small area of skin graft over avascular tissue is perfused via collateral vessels from adjacent vascularized skin graft. In this event only several millimeters of vascularity are bridged and even then may eventually break down.

Wounds containing more than 1×10^5 bacteria per gram of tissue will not support a skin graft. Heavily colonized wounds are also chronic and poorly vascularized. In these instances simple examination of the wound is often not adequate and quantitative bacteriology may be helpful. A rapid slide technique to predict the number of bacteria per gram of tissue homogenate is examined microscopically and the bacteria per gram of tissue reliably determined.

Contact of the skin graft and the recipient bed must be maintained for the skin graft to survive. Any shear force between the graft and its bed will disrupt revascularization. When a skin graft is applied to the extremities, splinting of proximal and distal joints should be considered to limit motion at the site of the skin graft. Compressive dressings also serve to firmly fix the skin

graft to its bed. Any collection of fluid, such as serum, blood, or purulent material, between the skin graft and its bed will also prevent revascularization. Here again a compressive dressing such as a tie-over dressing can be helpful. Meshing or "pie crusting" the skin graft with a number of small slits in the graft will permit the egress of fluid beneath the graft into the adjacent dressing. Unless a tie-over dressing is applied, examination of the graft on the second postoperative day is recommended. At this point if any fluid collection is noted beneath the graft, that area can be incised and the fluid evacuated.

Split-thickness skin grafts can be harvested by hand or by using a number of power instruments. A drum dermatome such as the Reese dermatome employs an adhesive-coated cylinder that is applied to the skin. As this cylinder is rotated away from the surface of the skin a blade harvests a sheet of skin in a very controlled manner.

Humby knives and Weck knives use a guarded, disposable blade that harvests skin as the knife is advanced tangentially across the body surface with a back-and-forth movement. Power-driven instruments permit the rapid harvesting of large surface areas. These include the Brown or Zimmer air-driven dermatome (Fig. 43-7) and the Padgett electric dermatome. Full-thickness grafts are usually harvested with a No. 10 or a No. 15 blade by elliptical excision. Any fat is then trimmed from the dermal surface to permit dermal contact with the recipient bed. This can be facilitated by rolling the graft around the surgeon's finger with the dermal side exposed and then using a Metzenbaum-type scissors to excise subcutaneous fat.

A number of mechanical devices are available to mesh skin grafts. All these devices produce multiple uniform slits in the graft. When tension is applied perpendicular to these slits, openings appear in the graft and the effective surface of the area is increased. These openings will eventually epithelialize. Meshed skin grafts allow large surface areas to be resurfaced and are particularly useful in large burns. They contour well and allow the egress of any fluid collection beneath the graft during the first 24 h. Meshed skin grafts contract more than sheet grafts,

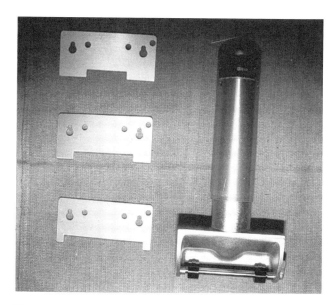

FIG. 43-7. *Power-driven dermatome (Zimmer).*

however, and the aesthetic result is often inferior to that with sheet grafts.

Skin grafts can be secured to the recipient bed by staples, sutures, skin tapes, or the dressing alone. For large burns skin stapling is rapidly done and decreases operating time. We favor fine chromic sutures in the younger child, in whom staple or suture removal can be problematic. Skin grafts are usually dressed with a layer of nonadherent material such as Xeroform or Adaptic next to the graft's surface followed by a layer of sterile absorbent gauze. The dressing is then secured by an occlusive circumferential wrapping of an extremity and tape. A tie-over dressing is helpful for providing compression in areas such as the face where the circumferential wrapping is not possible (Fig. 43-8). Sutures placed circumferentially at the edge of the skin graft are left long and then tied over a standard skin graft dressing beneath a layer of cotton or Dacron fiber. This technique is also used to secure intraoral skin grafts. We substitute a soft dental compound for the fiber bolus in oral tie-over dressings.

The split-thickness graft donor site heals by reepithelialization from epidermal appendages in the dermis. Epithelial cells from sweat glands, hair follicles, and sebaceous glands in the dermis migrate across the surface of the donor area. The donor site is not unlike a partial-thickness burn wound; a donor site from which a thick skin graft has been taken will heal more slowly than one from which a thin graft has been harvested.

The healing process may take from 7 to 21 days, depending on the thickness of the graft. This process is facilitated by a clean, moist environment. Donor sites may be dressed with a layer of Xeroform and Adaptic followed by absorbent gauze or pads. After 24 h the dressing is taken down to the level of nonadherent dressing material. As healing occurs at the donor site the edges of the nonadherent material separate from the underlying skin and may be trimmed. The donor site usually dries after it is left open for 1 or 2 days. We do not favor the use of heat lamps or hair dryers to dry a donor site because it is painful and impedes reepithelialization. The transparent semipermeable dressings, such as Op-Site, are also excellent dressings for donor sites. These have been shown to reduce pain remarkably at the donor site postoperatively. They can be left in place for 1 to 2 weeks as epithelialization proceeds. If an excessive amount of fluid collects under a transparent dressing it may be drawn off

with a syringe and the dressing "patched" with another, smaller piece of transparent dressing using sterile technique.

We prefer to take down the skin graft dressing on the second postoperative day and examine the graft for any fluid collection or signs of infection. If the likelihood of these complications is thought to be small the dressing may be left undisturbed for 5 days for a split-thickness graft and 7 to 10 days for a full-thickness graft. Any unexplained fever, local pain, erythema, or purulent drainage necessitates the immediate removal of all dressings.

Infection can convert a donor site from a partial-thickness to full-thickness skin wound. We treat any signs of infection at the donor site or skin graft site aggressively with frequent dressing changes and topical and appropriate systemic antibiotic therapy. Patients who are debilitated, immunosuppressed, or elderly are also at risk for having the donor site convert to a full-thickness injury. When this risk is judged to be high, the donor site can be grafted with a small amount of widely meshed split-thickness skin.

When the skin grafts and donor sites are epithelialized, any commercially available skin lotion containing lanolin or cocoa butter may be used. Compressive garments can control edema and scar hypertrophy at both the skin graft and the donor site.

Lower-extremity skin grafts are maintained in a nondependent position for 7 days postoperatively. Subsequently, activity is slowly increased from leg dangling to non-weight-bearing to full-weight-bearing ambulation over the next 1 to 2 weeks. During this time frequent examination of the graft is essential and compressive garments or wraps are used for the first week. Activity is then increased as tolerated, with frequent monitoring of the graft for any sign of breakdown. Elastic (Ace) bandages are essential for 4 weeks.

A skin graft undergoes contraction in two phases. Primary contraction occurs as the skin graft is lifted from its donor site. In this phase contraction is caused by elastic fibers within the dermis of the skin graft. Thin grafts with less dermis contract less than thick grafts. The secondary phase of contraction is largely a result of contraction of the recipient bed. This phase begins after 7 to 10 days and continues for as long as 6 months. A number of factors alter the extent of the secondary contraction. Thin grafts contract more than thick grafts, and full-thickness grafts undergo little contraction. Meshed grafts or grafts in which only partial take has occurred contract more as the open areas heal by contraction and epithelialization. Soft, mobile recipient beds tend to contract more than fixed, rigid beds. For instance, skin grafts placed on flexor surfaces often yield troublesome contractures.

Skin grafts, especially those taken below the clavicle, often become darker as they mature. This is often more pronounced with thinner grafts. To minimize hyperpigmentation skin grafts should be protected from ultraviolet light by clothing or sunscreen for a full year postoperatively.

The return of sensation to a skin graft is dependent on the recipient bed and its anatomic location. Heavily scarred beds or beds with poor native sensibility, such as granulation tissue over bone or periosteum, allow minimal regeneration of peripheral nerves into the graft. Two-point discrimination in a skin graft, however, will approach that of surrounding skin if regenerating nerves are not impeded at the level of the recipient bed. The return of sensation can be considered maximal at 2 years.

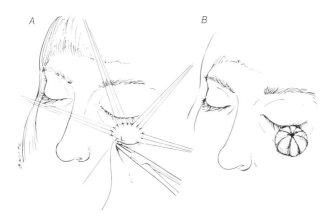

FIG. 43-8. Tie-over dressing.

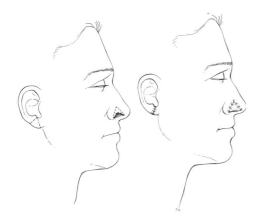

FIG. 43-9. Composite graft. The composite graft from the ear provides both lining and alar skin to the nasal defect.

Skin grafts may be effectively banked by immediately replacing them on their donor site. Grafts stored in this manner may be reharvested easily up to 48 h later. Skin grafts may also be banked by placing them in saline-soaked gauze sponges and storing them at 4°C. If sterility is maintained, grafts stored in this manner remain viable for up to 21 days.

A composite graft is a free graft containing at least two different tissue elements. The most common composite graft is skin and cartilage transferred to a small wedge taken from the ear. This composite graft is commonly used to reconstruct alar defects of the nose (Fig. 43-9). Common composite grafts include skin and cartilage from the auricular concha, skin and fat from the earlobe, and skin and muscle from the eyelid. Revascularization of a composite graft is similar to that in a split-thickness skin graft except that the large ratio of volume to absorptive surface area precludes nourishment from plasmatic imbibition. The general principles involved in skin graft survival also apply to composite grafts. A well-vascularized recipient bed and meticulous technique, including graft immobilization and hemostasis, are imperative for graft survival. As a general rule, all points within the composite graft should be less than 1 cm from the recipient bed, and grafts with a diameter of less than 1.5 cm are safest.

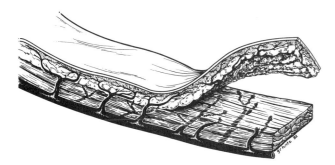

FIG. 43-10. Random skin flap. The segment of skin and subcutaneous tissue elevated from the underlying muscle is no longer nourished by musculocutaneous perforating vessels. The random flap is supplied by a subdermal plexus of vessels.

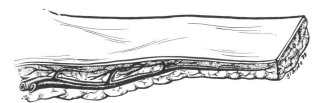

FIG. 43-11. Axial pattern flap. This flap is supplied by a defined cutaneous artery and vein. Examples of the axial pattern flap include the groin flap, deltopectoral flap, and forehead flap.

Flaps

A flap is a tongue of tissue transferred from one anatomic site to another. Vascularity of the transferred tissue is maintained by nutrient vessels within the flap pedicle. The pedicle may either remain attached at its origin or be divided during transfer and reanastomosed to recipient vessels using microsurgical techniques. Microsurgical transfer of tissue is also known as a *free flap.* Flaps are useful for closing defects too large for primary closure and where skin grafting is inadequate. Examples include exposed structures such as brain, blood vessels, bone and joint surfaces, and wounds with poor vascularity, where skin grafting would likely fail. Full-thickness defects in the head and neck are often unacceptable in appearance and function when reconstructed with skin grafts. In these instances flaps may provide better form and function. The reconstructive surgeon may transfer functional units of bone, muscle, and neural tissue for reconstruction of complex defects. Flaps, especially those containing muscle, have proved useful in clearing infection at the recipient site. Muscle flaps have proved to be very immunologically active and are a mainstay in the treatment of problem infections such as osteomyelitis, sternal wound infections, and infected prosthetic materials.

Flaps are classified according to their blood supply. A *random flap* receives blood through the dermal and subdermal plexus (Fig. 43-10). The subdermal plexus receives its blood supply from vessels extending from underlying muscles to the skin. These vessels are sometimes referred to as *musculocutaneous perforators.* Skin flaps that receive their blood supply from cutaneous arteries and veins longitudinally oriented within the substance of the flap are known as *axial pattern flaps* (Fig. 43-11). A *fasciocutaneous flap* contains skin and underlying fascia and is supplied by the vascular plexus within the fascia. A *musculocutaneous flap* contains skin, fascia, and muscle and is supplied by perforating vessels from the muscle to the subdermal plexus (Fig. 43-12). Arterialized flaps have a richer vascular supply and allow for reliable transfer of a greater amount of tissue.

Random Flaps. Random flaps receive their blood supply from the subdermal plexus via musculocutaneous perforators at the base of the flap. These flaps are usually categorized by their type of movement. The *advancement flap* is moved into a defect without lateral or rotational movement. To close a rectangular defect, three sides of an adjoining rectangle of tissue can be incised and undermined with a layer of subcutaneous fat. The rectangle of skin is then advanced into the defect. Small rectangles of tissue at the base of the flap, known as Burow's triangles, may be excised to facilitate advancement. A triangle of tissue may also be advanced as a V-Y advancement flap (Fig. 43-13).

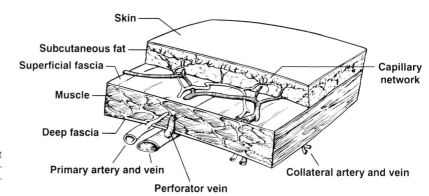

FIG. 43-12. Musculocutaneous flap. Note that branches from the primary vessels nourish and traverse muscle and fascia to ramify throughout subcutaneous fat and the overlying skin.

With this technique a rectangular defect is closed by incising an adjacent triangle of tissue, which is advanced into the defect, closing the secondary defect as a linear incision behind the flap. Advancement flaps generally allow limited movement of tissue. This movement is facilitated in anatomic areas where a relative excess of skin exists or in the elderly patient with loose, mobile skin.

A *rotation flap* is a semicircular flap rotating about a pivot point to close a triangular defect (Fig. 43-14). The secondary defect may then be closed primarily or skin grafted. A small backcut into the base of the flap can facilitate movement of a rotation flap. A *transposition flap* is typically a rectangular flap that rotates about its base to fill an adjacent defect (Fig. 43-15). This allows closure of the defect without undue tension. Here again, a small backcut into the base of the flap may facilitate movement. Any backcut into the base carries some risk of compromising the vascular supply of the flap.

The *Z-plasty* is a particularly useful type of transposition flap (Fig. 43-16). The Z-plasty consists of two triangular flaps, each of which is rotated into the defect left by the other flap. This is frequently used to transfer tissue into a scar or contracture and lengthen it or to reposition a scar within lines of minimal tension. The sides of the two triangles must be equal in length, and the angles may vary between 30 and 90 degrees. For any given

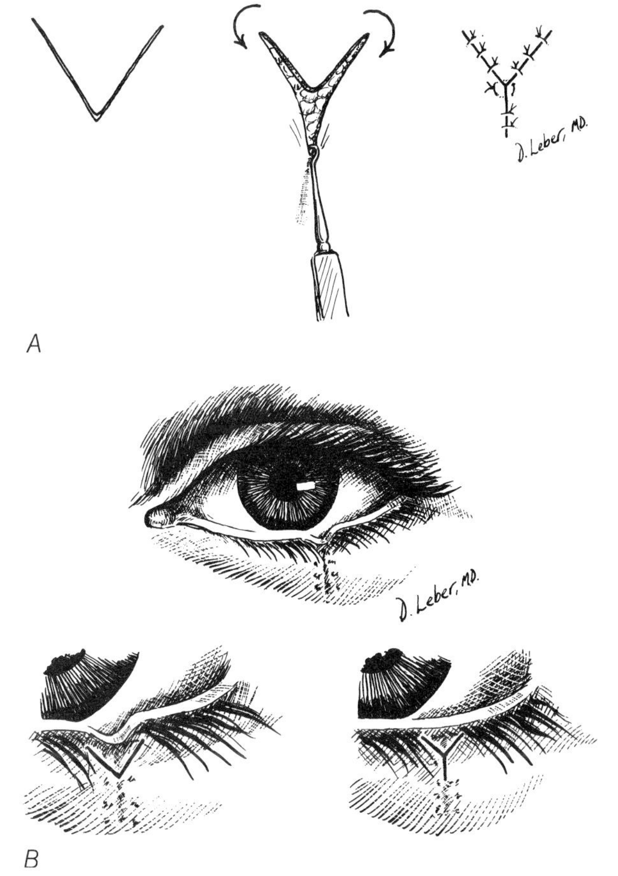

A

B

FIG. 43-13. *A.* The V-Y advancement principle. The apex of the V is advanced along the scar axis, thus lengthening the scar. *B.* Clinical application of a V-Y advancement.

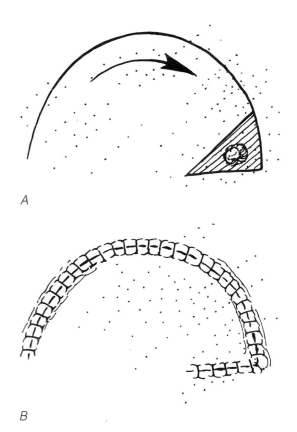

A

B

FIG. 43-14. Rotation flap.

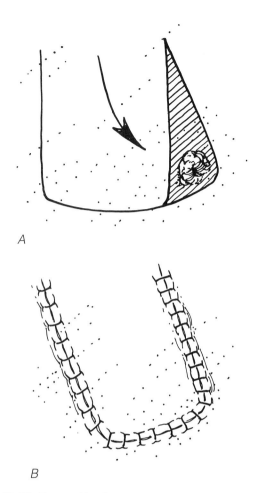

A

B

FIG. 43-15. Transposition flap.

cutaneous artery and an additional distal area of skin that is randomly supplied by the subdermal plexus. The midline forehead flap is based on supratrochlear vessels and is commonly used for nasal reconstruction. The deltopectoral flap receives blood supply from perforating branches of the internal mammary artery through the second, third, and fourth intercostal spaces (Fig. 43-19). Historically, this flap has been a mainstay in the reconstruction of head and neck defects. The groin flap is based on the superficial circumflex iliac artery and has been used to resurface wounds of the hand and upper extremity (Fig. 43-20). An axial pattern flap can be designed around the radial artery to involve skin and subcutaneous tissues of skin and bone. The radial forearm flap can then be transferred to defects of the upper

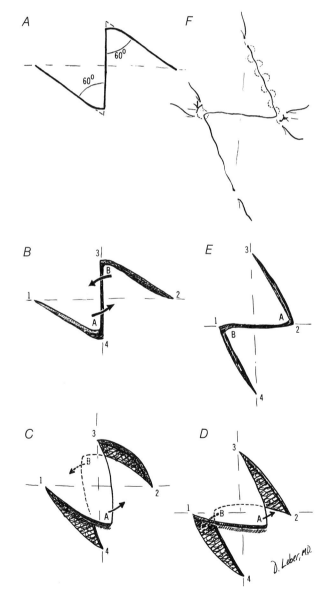

FIG. 43-16. The Z-plasty. Construction of two identical equilateral triangles based on any scar line creates two triangular flaps that together constitute a parallelogram. Interchanging these two flaps will lengthen the original scar line, exchanging the short diagonal of the parallelogram for the long diagonal.

angle, longer triangles will transfer more tissue and provide greater lengthening. Larger angles will also transfer more tissue; however, clinical experience has shown that 60 degrees provides optimal lengthening.

The *rhomboid flap*, or Limberg flap, is another common transposition flap design (Fig. 43-17). To close a rhomboid-shaped defect with internal angles of 60 and 120 degrees, a rhomboid-shaped flap of identical dimensions is designed on the side of the defect judged to have the most available tissue. A *bilobed flap* is a series of two transposition flaps (Fig. 43-18). A properly designed bilobed flap is rotated into the defect as a primary flap, and a secondary flap, whose diameter is half that of the primary flap, is rotated into the defect left by the primary flap. The defect left by the secondary flap is closed primarily. For a bilobed flap to be successful the secondary flap should come from an area of relative skin laxity. An *interpolation flap* is similar to a transposition flap in that a tongue of skin and subcutaneous tissue is rotated about an axis. An interpolation flap, however, is transposed across an intervening bridge of tissue. The deltopectoral flap, discussed below, is an example of an interpolation flap.

Axial Flaps. Axial pattern flaps contain cutaneous vessels running in the longitudinal axis of the flap. They are better vascularized and more reliable than random flaps. The possible length of an axial pattern flap is determined by the length of the

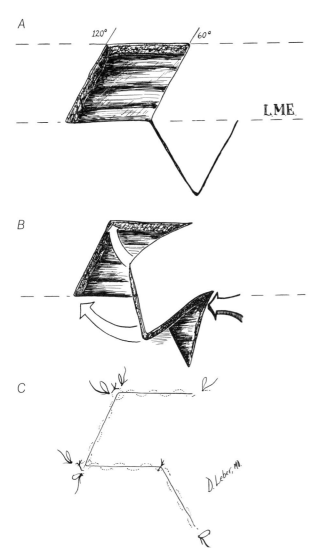

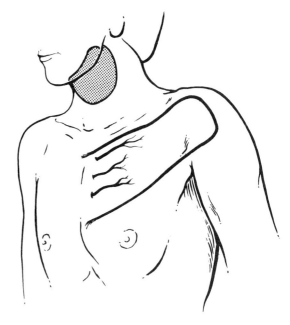

FIG. 43-19. Deltopectoral flap. This axial pattern flap, as illustrated, is being used to close a defect in the neck. Blood supply comes from perforating branches of the internal thoracic artery.

FIG. 43-17. Limberg flap. This is designed by excision of a 60-degree rhomboid, oriented in relation to the lines of minimum tension, also termed line of maximum extensibility (LME). *A.* Excision of the 60-degree rhomboid, correctly oriented. The flap is constructed by extending the short diagonal by its own length and constructing a third side arranged at a 60-degree angle to the extended short diagonal and equal in length to any side. *B.* Elevation and transposition of the Limberg flap. *C.* Closure completed.

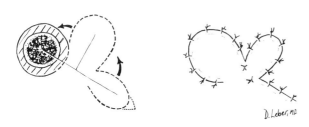

FIG. 43-18. Bilobed flap.

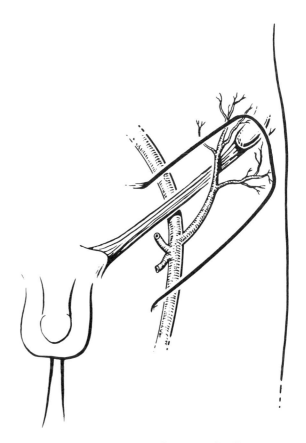

FIG. 43-20. Groin flap. The superficial circumflex iliac artery nourishes this flap in an axial pattern; the diameter of the artery is exaggerated for purposes of illustration.

extremity or transferred with microsurgical techniques to distant sites. The entire greater omentum may be taken as an axial flap based on either the right or left gastroepiploic arteries. The omentum is then available for closing defects of the chest wall and mediastinum (Fig. 43-21). Because of its large surface area, the omentum is particularly useful for extensive wounds such as radiation injuries and sternal wound infections. The omentum readily accepts split-thickness grafts to complete closure.

Fasciocutaneous Flaps. A fasciocutaneous flap consists of skin, subcutaneous tissues, and underlying fascia. Blood supply is derived at the base of the flap from musculocutaneous perforators or direct branches of major arteries. Because this flap includes the vascular plexus immediately superficial to the fascia, it is more reliable than random flaps. Fasciocutaneous flaps are frequently used in the lower extremity. A fasciocutaneous flap can be designed to include perforators from the medial head of the gastrocnemius muscle to close difficult wounds of the middle and proximal thirds of the lower leg. The posterior thigh fasciocutaneous flap is frequently used for closure of ischial pressure sores. This flap includes fascia lata, subcutaneous skin, and tissue of the posterior thigh and includes the descending branch of the inferior gluteal artery. This vessel runs parallel to the posterior cutaneous nerve of the thigh and accounts for the reliability of this flap.

Muscle and Musculocutaneous Flaps. Muscles can be transferred into adjacent defects if their native vascular supply is preserved. The utility of any given muscle flap is limited by the size of the muscle and the length of its vascular pedicle and hence the distance it can be transferred. The defect, both functional and cosmetic, created by the muscle transfer must also be considered. Muscle flaps transfer richly vascularized and very immunologically active tissue into wounds that are ischemic or infected. The bulk of muscle flaps allows contour defects to be resurfaced.

Skin can be transferred with the underlying muscle. Vessels extending directly from the muscle to the overlying skin, known as *musculocutaneous perforators*, account for a significant portion of cutaneous circulation. These perforating vessels define independent vascular territories within the skin that can be transferred as units with muscle. This principle has been rediscovered several times in the past century. Manchot, in 1889, noted that the skin received much of its blood supply from the underlying muscle. Tanzini, in 1906, described the latissimus dorsi myocutaneous unit for breast reconstruction. The concept was again lost until McCraw and colleagues described a number of musculocutaneous flaps and their vascular territories in 1974.

Delay

Partial disruption of the vascular supply to a flap in a preliminary procedure is known as a *delay procedure*. The purpose of a delay procedure is to increase the length of the random portion of the flap that will survive after transfer. In a delay procedure skin incisions defining the flap partially disrupt the subdermal plexus but maintain the primary pedicle. The flap is then replaced in its bed. One week later the flap is lifted out of its native bed and transferred to the recipient site. Clinical experience suggests that delay procedures can increase the amount of tissue a given pedicle can carry. The mechanism of the delay phenomenon remains incompletely understood. There are two general schools of thought. One theory suggests that delay acclimatizes the flap

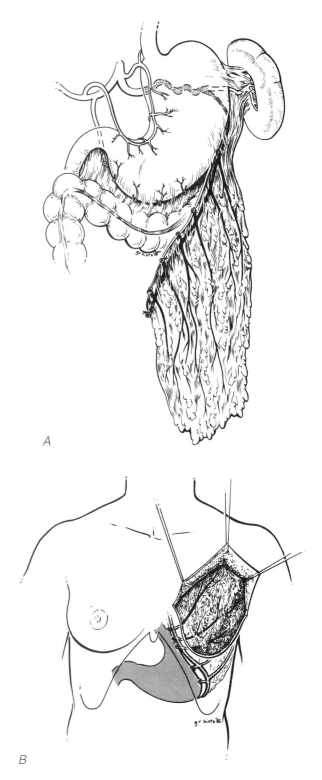

FIG. 43-21. Omental flap. *A.* The greater omentum is dissected free of the stomach and transverse colon. The blood supply is provided via the left gastroepiploic vessels. *B.* A left chest wall defect is filled with the omentum and a split-thickness skin graft applied.

to ischemia, permitting it to survive with less blood flow than would normally be required. Another theory suggests that delay improves vascularity by increasing flow through preexisting vessels, reorganizing the pattern of blood flow to more ischemic areas. In reality, probably both mechanisms contribute to the delay phenomenon.

Free-Tissue Transfer

The development of microsurgery was one of the great advances in plastic surgery of this century. Reconstructive surgeons previously were constrained by the arc of rotation of any given vascular pedicle. Microvascular surgery allows the complete division of a known vascular pedicle and reanastomosis to recipient vessels at a distant site.

Replantation of severed upper extremities was reported by Malt and McKhan in 1964. The first clinical example of free-tissue transfer was reported in 1972, when McLean and Buncke transferred greater omentum to resurface a large scalp defect. Since that time microsurgery has become standard in most large medical centers, and successful reimplantations of severed parts occur on a daily basis. Many series of elective free-tissue transfers report success rates higher than 95 percent. Free-tissue transfer has applications in all areas of reconstruction and is the standard for reconstructing large defects of the head and neck.

In its simplest form microvascular surgery involves the anastomosis of vessels 0.5 to 3.0 mm in diameter in a manner that maintains patency of the anastomosis. This involves not only surgical technique but also controlling the dynamics of the blood flow, the coagulation system, and inflammatory mediators.

Flow through a blood vessel can be described by Poiseuille's law, whereby the volume flow rate through a capillary tube varies directly with the pressure drop and the fourth power of the radius of the tube, and inversely with the length of the tube and the coefficient of viscosity. Clinically blood pressure must be adequately maintained throughout a microvascular procedure. Hypotension or the use of systemic vasoconstrictors to support blood pressure can be disastrous. Blood viscosity is another factor that can be manipulated by the microvascular surgeon by altering hematocrit levels. A hematocrit level between 30 and 35 percent maximizes flow and oxygen-carrying capacity. Poiseuille's law suggests that vessel radius is the single most important factor in determining flow rate. For this reason the largest possible vessels should be selected for anastomosis. When dealing with very small vessels any problem with technique or vasospasm will likely result in failure of the anastomosis.

The coagulation system is best controlled by avoiding traumatized vessels and by performing an anastomosis that coapts intact intima to intact intima. Microanastomoses that expose subendothelial collagen invite platelet aggregation and activate the coagulation cascade. A traumatized artery responds to mediators of inflammation by contraction of the smooth muscle within the vessel wall. Some vasospasm occurs even with careful dissection of vessels. If vasospasm is persistent, it can be controlled by irrigation of the vessel with a solution of papaverine and lidocaine. The spasm of severely traumatized vessels is often refractory. For this reason microsurgeons prefer to operate out of the "zone of injury," the region near the defect that, although grossly intact, is undergoing the metabolic changes of injury at a cellular level. The mediators of inflammation within the zone of injury can lead to vasoconstriction and platelet aggregation. If a surgeon is unable to perform the anastomosis out of the zone of injury, a pharmacologic agent to modulate the coagulation system can be administered. The most commonly used

agents are aspirin, heparin, and dextran. These medications can be given prophylactically before operation or used selectively intraoperatively.

Aspirin blocks prostaglandin synthesis at the level of cyclooxygenase. At lower doses this effect appears to be selective for thromboxane synthesis and platelet aggregation. Aspirin is used in some microsurgical centers as a single preoperative or intraoperative prophylactic dose. Heparin inhibits thrombin production, the production of fibrin from fibrinogen, and the second phase of platelet aggregation. Heparin is usually used selectively in circumstances judged to be unfavorable such as reoperation for thrombosis of a microvascular anastomosis, anastomoses performed with an extensive zone of injury, and replantation. Dextran decreases platelet adhesiveness, alters the structure of fibrin clot to make it more unstable, and enhances blood flow by reducing viscosity and increasing vascular volume. Dextran is frequently given routinely by microsurgeons as an intraoperative bolus at the time of anastomosis, followed by several days of continuous infusion. The role of any agents used to manipulate the coagulation system nevertheless remains poorly defined in microsurgery. Although dextran is still widely used, the trend in elective free flap transfers has been toward less frequent use of anticoagulation therapy. In situations in which mechanical or metabolic factors are not optimal for microvascular anastomosis, such as replantation surgery, extensive zones of injury proximal to the area to be reconstructed, and long periods of ischemia, anticoagulant therapy is commonly used.

Response to Ischemia. Any operation involving free-tissue transfer requires the donor tissue to undergo a variable period of ischemia. Skin and subcutaneous tissue are relatively tolerant of ischemia. Skin can tolerate 24 h of anoxia. Muscle, however, is relatively sensitive to ischemia. Irreversible changes are apparent in muscle tissue after 6 h of warm ischemia. Peripheral nerves are intermediate in their tolerance to ischemia, with irreversible changes appearing at 8 h of warm ischemia. In general those tissues with a low metabolic rate, such as connective tissue, are more resistant to ischemia. Cooling of tissue prolongs viability during ischemia. Traumatically amputated parts should be wrapped in saline-moistened gauze and placed in a plastic bag. The bag should then be packed in ice. When handled in this manner successful digital replantation has been reported after 36 h.

Vascular endothelium appears to be the tissue most sensitive to hypoxia. Changes can be seen in the endothelium after only several minutes of warm ischemia. Hypoxic damage to endothelial cells is thought to be responsible for the "no-reflow phenomenon," in which damage to the sodium pump of endothelial cells leads to cellular swelling of the vascular endothelium and leakage of intravascular fluid to the interstitium. Adenosine triphosphate-depleted red blood cells are less deformable and not able to pass through microcirculation. A combination of endothelial swelling, interstitial edema, and aggregation of rigid red blood cells leads to obstruction of the microcirculation. There is additional evidence that arachidonic acid release by injured endothelial cells and aggregation of granulocytes are also part of the mechanism of the no-reflow phenomenon.

Clinically, the no-reflow phenomenon might be seen in a free muscle flap with an extended ischemic period. Upon microvascular anastomosis, the flap would show progressive decrease in arterial inflow because of increasing arterial resistance within the flap. Finally, despite widely patent anastomoses there would be no arterial inflow or venous outflow. There is no specific treatment for the no-reflow phenomenon at this time. Current research revolves around the use of nonsteroidal anti-inflammatory agents and control of oxygen free radicals.

Microsurgical Technique. Microsurgery involves the use of an operating microscope. This instrument usually includes foot pedals to control focus, a beam splitter with independent objectives to allow the surgeon and assistant to assume positions 180 degrees from each other, a fiberoptic light source, and a solid base to minimize unwanted motion of the microscope during the procedure. Microsurgical instruments perform the same basic functions as macrosurgical instruments, but are particularly small and delicate. They must be handled carefully; simply dropping a microsurgical instrument can damage it beyond repair. A jeweler's forceps is used almost constantly in the surgeon's nondominant hand. This instrument is useful for handling perivascular tissue and sutures. The tips must be precisely aligned, kept free of dried blood and tissue, and meet evenly or suture cannot be reliably handled by the instrument. There are a variety of needle holders available. Most have tips that are angled in relation to the handles. A curved-tip microscissors is useful for dissection. A straight microscissors is use for trimming adventitia of vessels. A vessel dilator is a modified jeweler's forceps with a smooth, tapered, blunt tip. This instrument is helpful for dilating vessel ends for irrigation. Vessel clamps may be either single- or double-approximating clamps. Double-approximating clamps may have a suture holding frame that permits stay sutures to be used during the anastomosis. Closing pressures of microvascular clamps must be below 30 g/mm^2 to prevent extensive damage to the endothelium. Suture material is usually polypropylene or monofilament nylon. The size of the suture used is dependent on the vessel size and ranges from 8-0 to 11-0. Microneedles are usually tapered needles ranging from 30 to 100 μm in diameter.

Vascular Anastomosis. The end-to-end anastomosis is the most common anastomosis performed by the microsurgeon. The vessels to be anastomosed are placed in microclamps and approximated without tension (Fig. 43-22). Adventitia is removed from the vessel ends using the microscissors. The adventitia may be removed as a sleeve by pulling the adventitia off the end of the vessel in the long axis of the vessel and trimming it with straight microscissors. The vessel dilator is then used to dilate the end of the vessel, and the lumen is irrigated with heparinized saline. Frequently a piece of blue or green plastic sheeting is placed behind the microclamps and vessel ends. This prevents adjacent tissue from obstructing the operative field and permits easy visualization of the suture material.

The needle holder is then used to grasp the needle, which is most stable when held perpendicularly to the jaws of the needle holder. The needle should be passed perpendicularly through the vessel wall, released, and regrasped in the vessel lumen. The needle should be passed through the tissue along the curve of the needle. With time, it may be difficult to refrain from passing the needle through both vessel ends in one stroke. This is discouraged, however, as needle placement in the second vessel wall is less precise. The suture is then drawn through the vessels until approximately 10 mm is apparent from the vessel end. To tie a knot, the longer end of the suture is grasped with the nondominant-hand forceps approximately 10 mm from the ves-

sel end. A loop is made by winding the dominant-hand forceps around the suture or creating a loop with the opposite-hand forceps or a combination of these movements. The dominant-hand forceps is then passed through the loop, and the free, short end of the suture is grasped. The free end is pulled back through the loop and the knot secured. A second throw of the square knot can be completed by making a loop in the opposite direction. The loop should be formed near the short end so that the distance traveled by the instruments is small. As the second half knot is made, the nondominant-hand forceps never releases the suture. For most purposes, three half knots will be sufficient. The suture is then cut short end first followed by the long end between forceps and knot. In this manner the suture is always controlled and the needle can be retrieved easily by pulling the needle into the field with the nondominant hand.

A second suture may be placed 180 degrees from the first and the anterior wall completed by placing sutures bisecting the space between each suture. Alternatively the triangulation technique may be used with the first three sutures.

On completion of the anterior wall the microclamps are rotated 180 degrees and the anastomosis is inspected. This is an opportunity to note any suture placed in the back wall and again to irrigate any blood or clot within the lumen. The posterior wall of the anastomosis is then completed in an identical manner.

If the discrepancy of lumen size in the vessels to be anastomosed is greater than 2:1, an end-to-side anastomosis should be performed. The same microsurgical techniques also apply to an end-to-side anastomosis. The adventitia is removed from the area of the anastomosis using a curved microscissors. The media of the vessel is grasped with a jeweler's forceps and the arteriotomy or venotomy made with a straight microscissors. It may be necessary to change the microscissors from the one hand to the other to create two clean scissors cuts. If placed properly, the two scissors cuts will make a neat elliptical hole in the vessel wall. The donor vessel should be trimmed at an angle to reduce turbulence. The end of the donor vessel is often trimmed in a convex form to increase the lumen size at the area of anastomosis (Fig. 43-23). The posterior wall is normally completed first. If the anterior wall is completed first it is often difficult to fully visualize the sutures in the posterior wall. Suturing of anastomosis can be facilitated if the donor vessel can be moved across the field as each side of the anastomosis is completed.

Although not universally accepted, continuous-suture techniques can be used in microsurgery. The principal advantage of a continuous-suture technique is that anastomosis can be completed in less time; in addition, it may be the preferred technique in the anastomosis of vessels with different-sized lumens. The usual disadvantages of continuous-suture techniques include purse-stringing, narrowing of the anastomosis, and suture breakage requiring repeat anastomosis.

When the distance between recipient and donor vessels is too large to allow direct coaptation of vessel ends, vein grafts are required. Vein grafts may be used in head and neck reconstruction, where therapeutic neck dissection or irradiation preclude the use of vessels adjacent to the defect. Lower-extremity trauma with extensive zones of injury also may require vein grafts. The vein graft selected should be as close in size to the recipient vessel as possible. Donor sites for vein grafts include the saphenous vein in the leg and the superficial veins in the dorsum of the hand and ventral forearm.

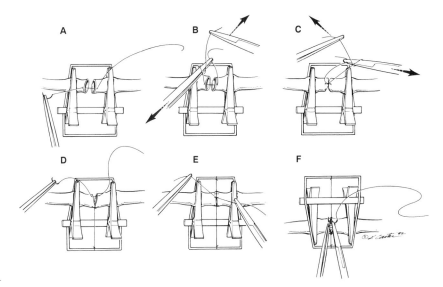

FIG. 43-22. Microvascular anastomosis.

Monitoring Free-Tissue Transfers. The success rate for free-tissue transfer, in most series, is greater than 90 percent. Given the large number of free-tissue transfers performed yearly, this success rate still yields a sizable number of failed grafts. The purpose of any postoperative monitoring system is to identify failing grafts early enough that an appropriate intervention might salvage the graft.

Examination by an experienced physician is the single most reliable test of graft viability. The flap should be examined for temperature, color, capillary refill, and if any doubt remains, response to pinprick. A pale, cool flap with delayed or absent capillary refill indicates arterial obstruction. Flaps that are purplish with rapid capillary refill and prolonged bleeding of dark blood upon needle stick likely have a venous obstruction. Although the clinical examination is usually an accurate assessment of flap viability, it is often not practical to have an experienced

physician observe the flap continuously for the first several days postoperatively. Remote monitoring systems include percutaneous Doppler flow monitoring, laser Doppler, temperature probes, transcutaneous measurements of tissue oxygen tension, and intravenous fluorescein. Clinical experience has not indicated any single monitoring system to be superior. The inexpensive, reliable, and simple free-flap monitoring system has yet to be described.

Tissue Expansion

Human tissue has a well-known ability to expand. This is observed during growth and pregnancy as well as in response to pathologic processes such as tumor growth and morbid obesity. Neumann in 1957 described the first attempt at controlled clinical expansion of soft tissue. He successfully resurfaced an ear reconstruction by placing a subcutaneous balloon in the post-auricular area and inflating it over 2 months. Radovan, in a series of reports beginning in 1976, described tissue expansion with silicone devices. Tissue expansion has become an increasingly important part of reconstructive surgery. The technique provides sensate tissue of similar color and texture to tissue adjacent to the defect.

A wide variety of expansion devices are available to the reconstructive surgeon. In its simplest form the device consists of a silicone reservoir attached to a self-sealing injection port via a variable length of silicone tubing. Using a 23-gauge or smaller needle, saline is injected into the injection port and the reservoir is expanded beneath skin and subcutaneous tissue. Ports may be placed external to the skin or in a subcutaneous position. They should be placed in an accessible location and, if subcutaneous, should be easily palpable. Tissue expanders are also currently available with the injection port integrated into the wall of the expander. These devices require accurate localization of the injection port by palpation or a magnetic locator to prevent inadvertent puncture and deflation of the expander.

The biology of tissue expansion has been extensively studied. When expansion forces are applied to skin, collagen fibers are noted to orient parallel to the expansion force and lose their native orientation. In the first week after placement of the tissue expander epidermal thickening can be noted. This rapidly returns

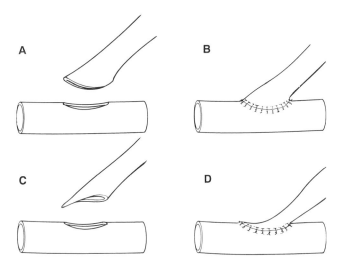

FIG. 43-23. End-to-side microvascular anastomosis. Note the correct manner of fashioning a concave end of the vessel, as in A and B. When cut on a straight-line diagonal, there is a tendency for the vessel actually to be convex, thereby narrowing the anastomosis, as in C and D.

to baseline and probably represents postoperative edema. An increase in melanocyte activity is noted during active expansion and may account for the hyperpigmentation sometimes seen during tissue expansion. A decrease in dermal thickness is noted during and after expansion. The population of myofibroblast cells increases, and elastic tissues become more prominent. Elastin fibers serve to align collagen. With excessive expansion forces elastin fibers are disrupted, leaving collagen in an unnatural orientation. Disruption of elastin fibers might account for stria formation and the permanence of expansion when the expander is removed. Skin with a great deal of intact elastin fibers tends to contract more after expansion.

Tissue expansion increases the vascularity of skin. New vessels are seen in the area adjacent to the capsule. Skin flaps raised in expanded tissue behave similarly to delayed flaps. Compared to unexpanded skin, increased survival length of skin flaps can be expected.

A number of mechanisms account for the new skin formed with tissue expansion. When serial stress loads are applied to skin, collagen and elastin fibers align themselves parallel to the stress, as noted above. As this alignment takes place, the skin stretches. This phenomenon is known as *creep*. As an expander is inflated, adjacent skin is recruited into the area of the expander. It is probable that new tissue is also formed during the expansion process. Increased epidermal mitoses are noted during expansion, and collagen synthesis increases in the dermis.

Suction Lipectomy

Suction lipectomy is said to be the most frequently performed aesthetic procedure in the United States. The procedure involves removal of subcutaneous fat via a blunt-tipped cannula attached to a vacuum pump. The cannula is introduced through small stab incisions, and radial passes are made across the anatomic region where fat removal is desired. The ideal patient for suction lipectomy is young, with localized fat deposits that are unresponsive to diet and exercise.

Suction cannulas range from 1.5 to 10 mm in diameter, and the most popular models have three openings set back from the tip at 120 degrees around the axis of the cannula. A vacuum pump able to generate a negative pressure of 1 atm is then connected to the cannula by flexible tubing. The area to be suctioned is usually injected with a solution of 0.25% lidocaine and 1:400,000 epinephrine. Hyaluronidase (Wydase) is sometimes added to improve the diffusion of the injection fluid. A small stab incision is made along Langer's lines, typically in the groin or suprapubic area for abdominal suction and within the gluteal fold for hip and buttock suction. With the vacuum pump on, the cannula is passed in the subcutaneous plane, creating tunnels radiating from the skin incision. This process is repeated through a second incision such that the radiating subcutaneous tunnels intersect one another. As the procedure progresses the area being contoured is constantly palpated. As a general rule the procedure is terminated when less than 2 cm of skin and subcutaneous tissue can be pinched between the index finger and thumb in the extremities and trunk. The wounds are closed with fine absorbable sutures and a compressive garment is worn for 10 days postoperatively.

Suction lipectomy requires close monitoring of the patient's hemodynamic status. For every 150 mL of fat removed, a 1 percent drop in the patient's hematocrit level can be expected. Fluid shifts dictate that crystalloid must replace fat removed in a 3:1 fluid-to-fat ratio. If more than 1500 mL of fat is removed, autologous blood replacement must be considered. Tumescent technique involves the injection of large volumes of dilute lidocaine and epinephrine solution into the subcutaneous tissue before liposuction. This technique decreases transfusion requirements in cases in which large volumes of fat are removed.

The procedure is generally safe and well tolerated. In 1987 the American Society of Plastic and Reconstructive Surgeons ad hoc committee on new procedures reported a 5-year experience with more than 100,000 suction lipectomies. Eleven deaths and nine major complications were reported within this group. Most cases of death or major morbidity result from hypovolemia, overwhelming sepsis, or embolism, including fat emboli. Although rare, these complications underscore the need for appropriate patient selection and intravenous fluid therapy. Most surgeons give prophylactic antibiotics, but available clinical and laboratory data do not favor any specific prophylactic agent for the fat emboli syndrome.

HEAD AND NECK

Cleft Lip

Two theories are generally held concerning the embryogenesis of cleft lip. The classic theory holds that a cleft lip results from failure of the nasomedial and nasolateral process of the embryo to fuse. The mesodermal penetration theory notes that the embryo is an epithelial bilayer in the region of the face until mesoderm migrates between the bilayers, forming the facial processes. Failure of this mesodermal migration results in clefting. Available evidence favors the mesodermal penetration theory in the etiology of cleft lip.

The primary palate is considered to include the lip, the alveolus, and the hard palate to the incisor foramen. The secondary palate includes the hard palate posterior to the incisor foramen and the soft palate. A cleft lip, then, would also be considered a cleft of the primary palate.

The incidence of cleft lip varies across races (approximately 1/1000 for whites and 0.41/1000 for blacks in the United States). The etiology of cleft lip is thought to be multifactorial. Factors that may increase the incidence of cleft lip include increased parental age, drug use and infections during pregnancy, and smoking during pregnancy. Parents with a cleft lip have an increased risk of producing a child with a cleft lip. The chance of producing a cleft-lipped child with one affected parent is approximately 4 percent. If both parents are unaffected but have a single child with a cleft lip, the risk of the second child's being affected is also approximately 4 percent.

A cleft lip may be unilateral or bilateral and may or may not be associated with a cleft palate (Figs. 43-24 and 43-25). Cleft lips are termed *complete* if the cleft extends into the nostril floor and *incomplete* if a bridge of tissue connects the central and lateral lip. This tissue bridge is sometimes referred to as *Simonart's band*.

Cleft lips are associated with characteristic nasal deformities. For a unilateral cleft lip this consists of inferior and posterior displacement of the alar cartilage on the cleft side. The maxilla and alar base on the cleft side is also deficient, resulting in posterior displacement of the alar base. In a bilateral cleft lip these nasal deformities are bilateral and the columella is usually short. The nose tends to be broad and vertically short.

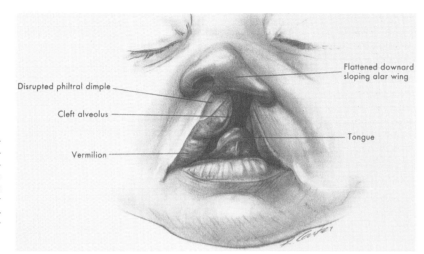

FIG. 43-24. Unilateral cleft lip topography. The upper lip is twisted and shortened in the vertical dimension. The Cupid's bow is incomplete. The vermilion tapers cephalad, and the white line extends into the vestibule. In this instance an alveolar cleft is present, creating a defect in the nasal floor. The alar rim is significantly distorted. (From: Sando WC, Jurkiewicz MJ: Cleft lip, in Jurkiewicz MC, Krizek TJ (eds): Plastic Surgery: Principles and Practice, Vol 1, Ch 5, St. Louis, CV Mosby, 1990, with permission).

Before definitive lip repair is carried out the patient may undergo a course of presurgical oral orthopaedic procedures. In conjunction with an orthodontist, acrylic splints may be fabricated to better align the alveolar segments and effectively narrow the cleft. By adding acrylic or removing it in certain areas of the splint, the orthodontist is able to move the alveolar arches and soft tissues of the lip to facilitate repair. As an alternative to these passive appliances, pin-retained appliances may be used. The appliance is fixed to the palate with metal pins and moves the alveolar segments with a connecting screw that is rotated daily.

Definitive lip repair is carried out when the child's general health and weight permit the safe induction of general anesthesia. The time-honored "rule of tens" is a useful guide to the timing of surgery. According to this rule, lip repair is carried out when the child has attained a weight of 10 lbs, is 10 weeks old, and has a hemoglobin concentration higher than 10 mg/dL. Cleft lip repair is being considered at even earlier ages in otherwise healthy babies.

The cleft lip repair is usually performed under general anesthesia. After marking the proposed flaps, the lip is injected with dilute epinephrine (1:400,000) to facilitate hemostasis. Many different types of cleft lip repair have been proposed. An effective repair must realign the vermilion and cupid's bow of the lip, reconstruct the upper lip and philtrum, and reapproximate the orbicularis oris muscle within the repair. The rotation-advancement repair as described by Millard is the most popular technique for unilateral cleft lip repair (Fig. 43-26). This technique uses a medial rotation flap to realign the vermilion of the lip. The triangular C flap is inset into the defect created by the rotation flap and is used to lengthen the columella. An advancement flap of the lateral side closes the upper lip and nostril sill. At the time of primary lip repair some surgeons will attempt to raise mucoperiosteal flaps within the alveolar cleft. When these flaps are reapproximated across the cleft, a tunnel of periosteum is formed that may support bone growth across the cleft. This technique, known as *gingivoperiosteoplasty*, is facilitated by the use of presurgical oral orthopaedics.

Bilateral clefts of the lip present a great challenge. No technique yet described provides consistently satisfying results. The central portion of the upper lip (prolabium) and maxilla (premaxilla) often project anteriorly away from the lateral lip ele-

FIG. 43-25. Bilateral cleft lip topography. Severely shortened columella, wide, flattened alae, and jutting, often rotated premaxilla are hallmarks of this deformity. (From: Sando WC, Jurkiewicz MJ: Cleft lip, in Jurkiewicz MC, Krizek TJ (eds): Plastic Surgery: Principles and Practice, Vol 1, Ch 5, St. Louis, CV Mosby, 1990, with permission).

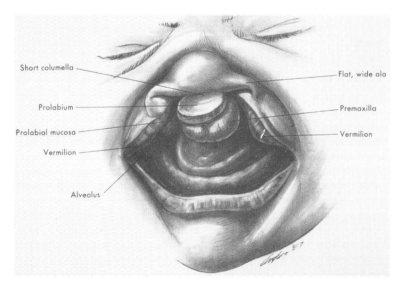

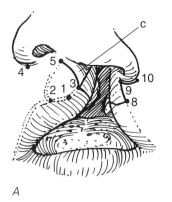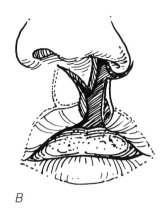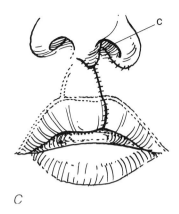

FIG. 43-26. *A.* Millard rotation-advancement cheiloplasty (stippled areas are excised). Landmarks include midline nadir (1) and peaks (2,3) of Cupid's bow, alar bases (4–10), extent of rotation curve (5), commissures (6,7), new Cupid's bow peak on cleft side (8), and tip of advancement flap (9). *B.* Philtrum and Cupid's bow are rotated down to allow advancement into apical defect of tissue from lateral cleft side. Central flap c elongates columella. *C.* In wide clefts horizontal tightness may be created.

ments. Repositioning of the premaxilla is carried out preoperatively with an intraoral appliance or with external traction from tapes or head gear. Current techniques for closure of the bilateral cleft lip use the prolabium to form the upper central lip, closing the cleft with either a straight-line closure or some application of the Z-plasty principle. The prolabium contains no mature muscle, and orbicularis oris muscle continuity must be restored.

Attempts have traditionally been made to protect the cleft lip repair postoperatively. Some surgeons advocate the use of stiff plastic arm cuffs that prevent the child from touching the lip. Feeding by cups and catheter also avoids possible trauma by nippling. This view, however, is not universally accepted. Breast feeding has not been shown to be deleterious to lip repair.

Correction of the cleft lip nasal deformity may accompany primary lip repair. Proponents of this approach typically mobilize the lower lateral cartilage from the overlying nasal skin and reapproximate the cartilage medially with a suture. Timing of the nasal correction remains controversial. Some authors believe that dissecting the nasal cartilages at the time of lip repair carries the risk of injury to these fragile structures and possible disturbances in nasal growth. Another approach to the cleft lip nasal deformity is to perform a rhinoplasty at the age of five or six, before the child enters school. At this time further revisions in the cleft lip repair are also often completed.

Cleft Palate

The hard palate develops from the fusion of the two lateral palatine processes that meet initially in the region of the incisive foramen and then continue to fuse posteriorly until, by the twelfth week of gestation, the uvula is formed. These processes are initially on either side of the tongue but swing upward into a more horizontal position as the tongue migrates down. Clefting results when the fusion of the two palatal processes is incomplete. Clefts of the lip and palate are more common on the left side, probably because this palatal process is the last to assume a horizontal position. The most common cleft is a cleft uvula. This occurs in approximately 2 percent of the population. The second most common type of cleft palate is a left unilateral cleft palate and left unilateral cleft lip or cleft of both the primary

and secondary palates (Fig. 43-27). The incidence of cleft palate alone in the general population is approximately 1/2000.

A unilateral cleft of the primary palate extends from the incisive foramen anteriorly between a canine and an adjacent incisor to the lip. Clefts of the primary palate may be unilateral or bilateral. A cleft of the secondary palate extends from the incisive foramen to the uvula. An incomplete cleft palate does not extend entirely to the incisive foramen, involving mainly the soft palate.

As with cleft lip, the etiology of cleft palate is multifactorial. Animal models have demonstrated that vitamin A, corticosteroids, and phenytoin produce cleft palate when given during pregnancy. Cleft palates commonly are associated with other anomalies at birth.

During speech and swallowing the palate moves both superiorly and posteriorly against the posterior pharyngeal wall to separate the oral pharynx and nasal pharynx. This is known as *velopharyngeal closure*. Effective velopharyngeal closure allows intraoral pressure to be increased for release with certain sounds during speech. A cleft palate allows air to escape through the nose during speech; this is known as hypernasal speech. Because the oral and nasal cavities cannot be effectively partitioned in the presence of a cleft palate, it is also difficult for the patient to create a negative intraoral pressure. This results in an ineffective suck and feeding problems in the infant with cleft palate. Children with cleft palate have an increased incidence of otitis media. This may be related to abnormal insertions of palate musculature and ineffective opening of the eustachian tube. The recurrent otitis media in cleft palate patients can result in hearing loss.

Timing of cleft palate repair remains somewhat controversial. The cleft palate is usually closed when the patient is between 6 and 18 months of age. The dissection involved in cleft palate closure may have a negative effect on facial growth. For this reason many surgeons prefer late closure of the cleft palate. Children who have undergone early closure of their cleft palate, however, tend to develop more normal speech.

Cleft palate closure is performed under general anesthesia using endotracheal intubation. The head is hyperextended, and a

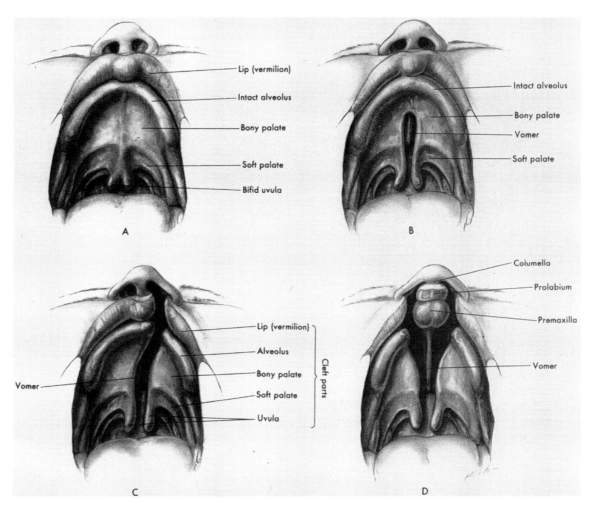

FIG. 43-27. Variations in cleft palate anatomy. *A.* Bifid uvula, the most common cleft palate presentation. In this instance one should search for occult submucous cleft with its physical findings of notched posterior bony plate, or diastasis of levator musculature with midline palatal translucency suggesting underlying fissure. If anteroposterior shortening were severe, resulting in symptomatic velopharyngeal insufficiency, surgical repair might be considered. *B.* Incomplete cleft of secondary palate (posterior to incisive foramen) with intact premaxillary structures. Nasal deformity is usually absent. *C.* Unilateral complete cleft lip and palate. Gap extends entire palatal length, through alveolus and lip and into nostril. Uvula is bifid. Cleft palate is usually shortened in anteroposterior dimension. *D.* Bilateral complete cleft lip and palate. Premaxilla is adrift from adjacent palatine shelves and may be displaced or rotated out of its "keystone" berth. Occasionally it may become locked out anteriorly from a collapsed palatal arch, creating a difficult reconstructive problem. (From: *Sando WC, Jurkiewicz MJ: Cleft lip, in Jurkiewicz MC, Krizek TJ (eds): Plastic Surgery: Principles and Practice, Vol 1, Ch 5, St. Louis, CV Mosby, 1990, with permission*).

retractor such as the Dingman mouthgag is placed to hold the mouth open and retract the tongue and endotracheal tube. The palate is injected with 0.25% lidocaine with 1:400,000 epinephrine solution. Prophylactic intravenous antibiotics are usually administered. A number of techniques are currently used for cleft palate closure. The von Langenbeck palatoplasty is the oldest technique for cleft palate closure still in use today. In this procedure, relaxing incisions are made bilaterally medial to the alveolar ridges, and incisions are made along the margin of the cleft (Fig. 43-28). Bipedicle mucoperiosteal flaps are then raised based on the greater palatine vessels. These flaps are then closed in the midline in two layers. Mucosal flaps may be also raised from the vomer to aid in closure of the nasal layer. Most surgeons believe that it is also important to reconstitute the sling

of the levator veli palatini muscle during cleft palate closure. In patients with cleft palate this muscle abnormally inserts along the margins of the cleft. In the normal palate the levator veli palatini muscle extends from the base of the skull to the middle of the palate, where it decussates with the opposite paired muscle to form a continuous sling. This sling moves the palate posteriorly and superiorly during speech and swallowing (Fig. 43-29). Reconstitution of the levator muscle sling is known as an *intravelar veloplasty*. The bare areas of the hard palate are then left for closure by secondary intention or may be closed primarily in some cases. Critics of the von Langenbeck technique note that it does nothing to lengthen the palate to aid in velopharyngeal closure and that fistulas tend to develop anteriorly where a number of suture lines meet.

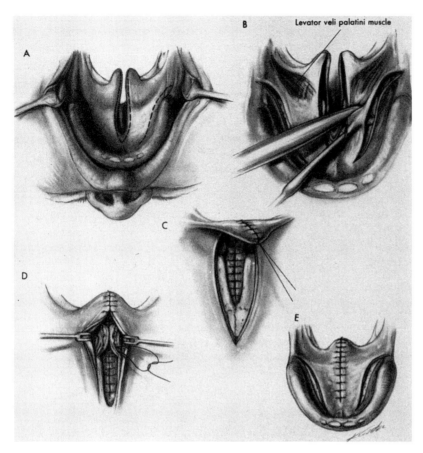

FIG. 43-28. *A.* Von Langenbeck palatoplasty. *B.* Bipedicled mucoperiosteal flaps are elevated. Lateral relaxing incisions allow closure of midline cleft of secondary palate. Veau flap is required on occasion for anterior closure. *C.* Layered closure of nasal mucosa. *D.* Reconstitution of levator muscular sling (optional) and *E.* oral mucoperiosteum complete repair. A drawback of the procedure is that it does not provide anteroposterior lengthening. (From: *Sando WC, Jurkiewicz MJ:* Cleft lip, *in Jurkiewicz MC, Krizek TJ (eds): Plastic Surgery: Principles and Practice, Vol 1, Ch 5, St. Louis, CV Mosby, 1990, with permission).*

The Veau-Wardill-Kilner palatoplasty uses a W-shaped relaxing incision to create mucoperiosteal flaps that are then advanced in a V-Y fashion to close and lengthen the palate. This technique also involves a confluence of incisions anteriorly, and many question whether any permanent lengthening of the palate is achieved.

We prefer Furlow's double-opposing Z-plasty technique for most cleft palates in our practice (Fig. 43-30). This operation uses a Z-plasty on both the nasal and the oral side of the palate to lengthen the palate and to realign the levator musculature. With this technique, relaxing incisions may still be required for closure of the hard palate.

Breakdown of the cleft palate closure will result in a palatal fistula. This allows food and fluid to escape into the nose. Air may also pass through the palatal fistula, resulting in speech disturbances. Small fistulas may be closed by raising adjacent flaps of mucoperiosteum. Large palatal fistulas often require flaps of gingiva or tongue tissue.

After cleft palate closure the palate may still not be able to achieve velopharyngeal closure. The incidence of velopharyngeal incompetence varies among studies, depending on the surgical technique and methods of speech evaluation involved. Historically, 20 percent of patients exhibit velopharyngeal insufficiency after a cleft palate closure. The majority of these patients can achieve satisfactory speech with speech therapy. The remainder require a second procedure to lengthen the palate. The most popular surgical technique for correction of velopharyngeal insufficiency is a superiorly based posterior pharyngeal flap inserted into the free edge of the soft palate. Orticochea has

described a pharyngoplasty designed to create a dynamic velopharyngeal sphincter. In this technique the palatopharyngeus muscles are raised from the lateral pharynx and joined in the posterior midline with an inferiorly based flap of mucosa and the superior constrictor muscle.

A well-trained speech pathologist is best able to evaluate velopharyngeal incompetence and success after corrective surgery. Other useful adjuncts in diagnosis include radiography and nasal endoscopy.

Craniofacial Surgery

Craniofacial surgery principally involves movements of the craniofacial skeleton for reconstruction of acquired or congenital defects. Many of the procedures commonly performed by craniofacial surgeons today were considered too dangerous or the bony movements too unstable until the pioneering work of Dr. Paul Tessier of Paris. These advances were in part made possible by parallel advances in the fields of anesthesia and critical care. In a series of publications during the late 1960s and 1970s Tessier not only clarified the classification of craniofacial anomalies but also described access to the entire cranium and facial skeleton through less conspicuous incisions, and the bony movements necessary to reconstruct craniofacial anomalies.

Craniosynostosis. *Craniosynostosis* is the premature closure of one or more cranial sutures. This occurs in approximately 1/1000 births. The etiology of craniosynostosis remains incompletely defined and is probably multifactorial. Some cases of craniosynostosis, particularly craniosynostosis as part of a cra-

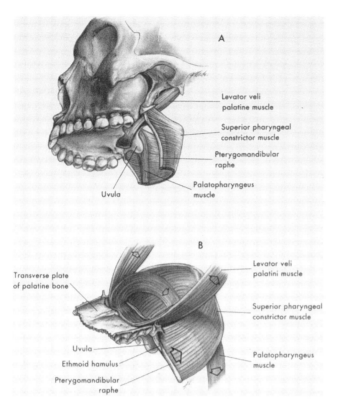

FIG. 43-29. *A. Pharyngeal muscular slings, including levator veli palatini, superior pharyngeal constrictor, palatopharyngeal, and palatoglossus muscles. B. Sphincteric closure of velopharyngeal space is accomplished by the palatopharyngeal sphincter of Willis (superior pharyngeal constrictor and levator), which brings, respectively, the posterior pharyngeal wall forward and the soft palate upward and backward and is assisted by uvular thickening. Palatopharyngeal and palatoglossal arches form with the tongue and the oropharyngeal sphincter. Dually innervated, muscular slings are crucial in the dynamics of phonation and swallowing. (From: Sando WC, Jurkiewicz MJ: Cleft lip, in Jurkiewicz MC, Krizek TJ (eds): Plastic Surgery: Principles and Practice, Vol 1, Ch 5, St. Louis, CV Mosby, 1990, with permission).*

niofacial syndrome, may be secondary to an abnormal cranial base. In these cases abnormal forces from the cranial base could be transmitted to the involved suture through ligamentous structures. Isolated cases of craniosynostosis may also be secondary to abnormal extrinsic forces in utero, such as abnormal fetal position, or weak intrinsic growth forces, such as microcephaly.

Premature closure of a cranial suture results in limitation of growth perpendicular to the line of the suture and compensatory growth parallel to the direction of the suture. Complications of craniosynostosis follow from the brain growing within a restricted bony vault. These problems include intracranial hypertension, optic atrophy, and mental retardation. Hydrocephalus may be secondary to a generalized stenosis of the cranial base.

Craniosynostosis is often classified according to the shape of the skull (Fig. 43-31). It is important to remember that these terms refer not to a disease entity but simply to the morphology of the skull. For instance, a child with plagiocephaly does not necessarily have premature fusion of the coronal suture. *Scaphocephaly* refers to increased length of the skull in the sagittal plane with bitemporal narrowing. This skull morphology is seen with isolated synostosis of the sagittal suture. *Trigonocephaly* describes a midline, keel-like prominence of the forehead that is

seen with premature closure of the metopic suture. *Plagiocephaly* is an asymmetric obliquity or flattening of one side of the skull. This may be either anterior or posterior. Plagiocephaly is seen with synostosis of the coronal or lambdoid sutures. *Brachycephaly* is shortening of the skull in the anteroposterior direction. This is seen with premature fusion of both coronal sutures. *Turricephaly* presents an excessive skull height and can be seen in pansynostosis.

Craniofacial Dysostosis. *Craniofacial dysostosis* refers to a variety of syndromes, most involving some degree of midface (maxilla, orbits) deficiency and craniosynostosis. These syndromes involve complex deformities that are a supreme challenge for the craniofacial surgeon. Reconstruction of these craniofacial syndromes is usually staged, with several procedures during childhood and early adolescence.

Crouzon's Syndrome. Crouzon's syndrome is characterized by hypoplasia of the orbits, zygomas, and maxillae and variable craniosynostosis. The coronal suture is more frequently involved. The syndrome is inherited in an autosomal dominant pattern with variable penetrance. The incidence in the general population is 1/25,000. Patients with Crouzon's syndrome can suffer all the complication of craniosynostosis as well as problems related to exorbitism such as corneal exposure. Midface hypoplasia can lead to malocclusion, airway disturbances, and significant facial deformity (Fig. 43-32).

Apert's Syndrome. Apert's syndrome involves a morphology similar to Crouzon's syndrome with syndactyly of the hands. Most cases of Apert's syndrome are sporadic, although autosomal dominant transmission has been reported. Advanced paternal age is thought to be a factor in some cases. The deformities of the midface are generally more severe than in Crouzon's syndrome. There is also a significant incidence of cleft palate.

Treacher Collins Syndrome. Treacher Collins syndrome, also known as *mandibulofacial dysostosis*, is characterized by hypoplasia of structures derived from the first and second branchial arches. Typically this involves hypoplasia or clefting of the zygomas, external ear deformities, and hypoplasia of the mandible. The syndrome has an autosomal dominant inheritance pattern with incomplete penetrance.

Facial Clefts. A number of rare craniofacial clefts have been described. As with cleft lip and palate, these probably represent failure of mesenchymal migration or incomplete fusion of facial processes. A number of confusing classification schemes have been proposed. In 1976 Tessier proposed a classification system that remains in wide use. In Tessier's system clefts are assigned a number based on their position relative to the sagittal midline (Fig. 43-33). Within this classification system, the standard cleft lip is part of clefts 1, 2, and 3, and Treacher Collins syndrome exhibits some expression of clefts 6, 7, and 8.

Craniofacial Techniques. The majority of craniofacial surgery can be performed through a combination of three well-concealed incisions. A buccal sulcus incision can be made within the mouth to provide wide subperiosteal exposure of the anterior maxilla, the piriform aperture, and the anterior zygoma. A subciliary incision placed just beneath the lower eyelashes is also well concealed and provides access to the orbital floor, the medial and lateral orbital walls, and the anterior maxilla (Fig. 43-34). A bicoronal incision extended from ear to ear trans-

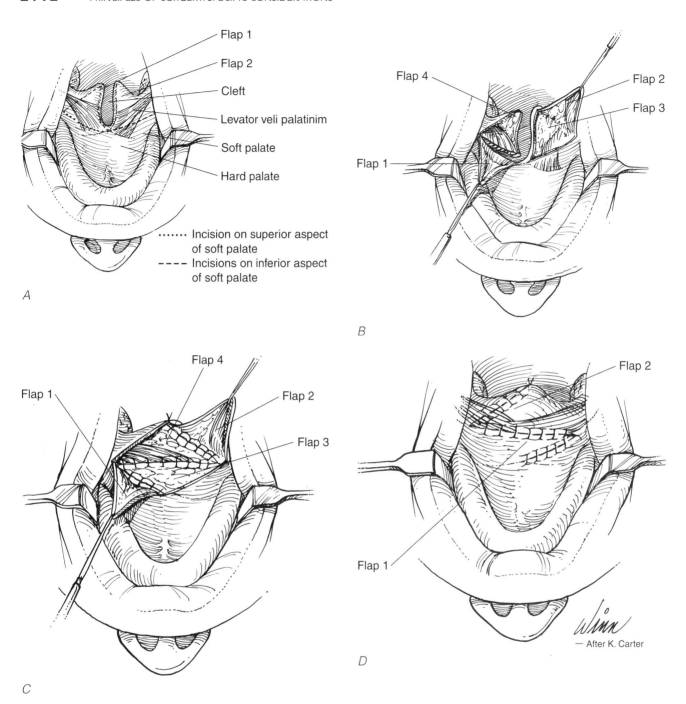

FIG. 43-30. *A. Furlow Z-plasty palate repair. A Z-plasty is constructed straddling the cleft margins with the major axis in the anteroposterior direction. B. Oral mucosa is elevated on side chosen to have anterior base along posterior hard palate margin (flap 1). Contralateral flap (2) is based posteriorly and contains the levator, which has been dissected off the palatine shelf. A second Z-plasty is created at a deeper level with flaps 3 and 4 based in a direction opposite to those of the first-layer Z-plasty so that the nasal mucosal triangular flap (3) is based anteriorly and its contralateral counterpart (4) is based posteriorly and contains not only nasal mucosa but also levator muscle. C. The two layers of Z-plasties are closed separately. Interdigitated flaps bring the levator sling into normal anatomic alignment. D. Anteroposterior lengthening is achieved.*

versely across the scalp allows the surgeon to expose the entire cranial vault, and by reflecting the bicoronal flap anteriorly and dissecting in a subperiosteal plane, the entire bony orbit can be exposed (Fig. 43-35).

Historically, craniosynostosis was treated by strip craniectomy in an attempt to create a patent cranial suture. Simple craniectomy fails to address other abnormalities in the cranial vault and has a high rate of reoperation, as the craniectomy site rapidly

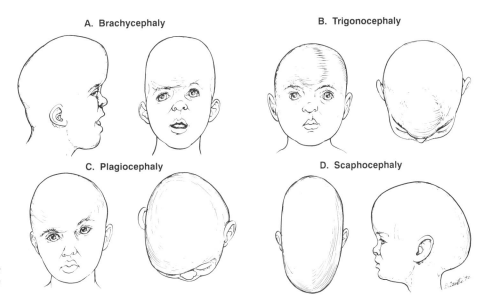

A. Brachycephaly

B. Trigonocephaly

C. Plagiocephaly

D. Scaphocephaly

FIG. 43-31. *The morphology of the cranium and the face associated with craniosynostosis.*

reossifies. Tessier pioneered the advancement of the superior orbit and frontal bone in one piece. This increases intracranial volume to alleviate increased intracranial pressure and also corrects the brachycephaly commonly seen in craniofacial syndromes or coronal synostosis. At the time of frontal bone ad-

vancement, the anterior cranial vault might also be remodeled by shaping and repositioning the bone of the anterior cranium. In a typical patient with coronal synostosis frontal orbital advancement and cranial vault remodeling would be performed as a single procedure before the child is 1 year old (Fig. 43-36).

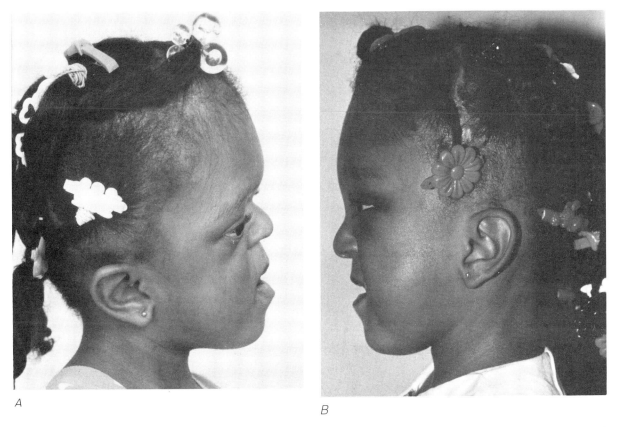

A

B

FIG. 43-32. *A. Crouzon's disease in a 4-year-old girl. The disorder is characterized by malformation of the skull (scaphocephaly), midface retrusion and stenosis, and bilateral exorbitism. B. After LeFort III midfacial advancement.*

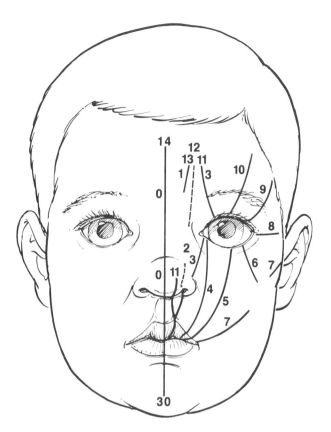

FIG. 43-33. Tessier classification of craniofacial clefts. The clefts numbered below the orbit are facial; those above are cranial. The clefts that involve both regions are designated by two numbers that sum to 14 typically. These clefts can involve both soft tissue and bone.

Children with more complex cranial deformities and severe craniosynostosis syndromes may require repeat frontal bone advancement or further cranial vault remodeling in early childhood. In those patients with midface hypoplasia such as in Apert's and Crouzon's syndromes, a second phase of treatment involves advancement of the midface. By performing osteotomies at the nasofrontal junction, the floor of the orbit, the lateral maxilla, and the pterygomaxillary fissure, the entire midface may be advanced in an anterior direction. This is known as a LeFort III midfacial advancement after the facial fracture of the same

name. Advancement of the midface in this manner serves to correct exophthalmos and improve airway difficulties, and it has a powerful effect on facial appearance. The timing of the LeFort III midfacial advancement is also controversial and varies from early childhood to adolescence. Treatment of the patient with a craniofacial syndrome would typically then be completed by a course of orthodontic treatment and jaw surgery, if necessary, in adolescence.

Hypertelorism. *Orbital hypertelorism* refers to increased distance between the bony orbits. This is seen with midline craniofacial clefts and certain craniofacial syndromes, including Crouzon's and Apert's syndromes. Significant hypertelorism is best managed by an intracranial approach as described by Tessier. In this procedure a bicoronal incision provides exposure for an anterior craniotomy. Osteotomies are then made around the entire orbit and paramedian bone is removed. The orbits are then mobilized and fixed in a more medial position (Fig. 43-37).

Distraction Osteogenesis. Distraction osteogenesis has become a standard part of the craniofacial surgeons' armamentarium. This technique is adapted from the original work of Ilizarov in orthopaedic reconstruction. For some time the healing callus of a surgically created cut in the long bones of extremities are stretched slowly by an extended frame to lengthen the bone. This typically yields 1 mm of lengthening per day of distraction.

After the pioneering work of McCarthy and colleagues, this technique is now widely applied to the mandible of children with hemifacial microsomia and micrognathia. This has proved to be a powerful technique for augmenting the facial bones and even soft tissue of children with severe microsomia.

Orthognathic Surgery. Disproportion of the maxillae and mandible is commonly seen with craniofacial problems. Maxillary hypoplasia is particularly common with cleft lip and palate and may in part be related to the dissection and subsequent scarring of repair. Acquired maxillomandibular disproportion is usually the result of trauma. Maxillomandibular disproportion can result in malocclusion and ineffective chewing. These patients may also have a significant aesthetic deformity.

The patient with maxillomandibular disproportion is best evaluated by team approach. Essential members of this team include a plastic surgeon, an orthodontist, and a prosthodontist. Evaluation includes dental impressions from which plaster models can be made. If surgery is planned, these models can then

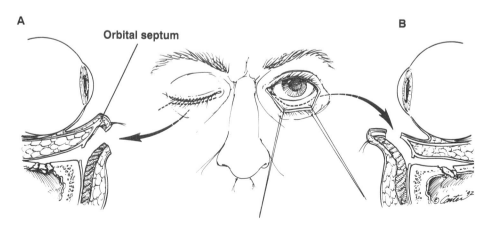

A Orbital septum **B**

FIG. 43-34. *A.* Subciliary incision that traverses skin, muscle, and septum orbitale. *B.* Transconjunctival incision. Typically the incision is extended through the lateral canthus.

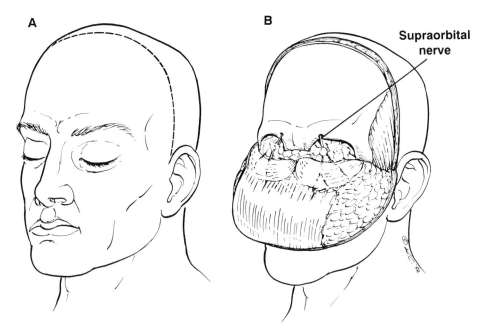

Supraorbital nerve

FIG. 43-35. *A.* The bicoronal incision. *B.* Wide exposure is provided to the orbit and upper facial skeleton.

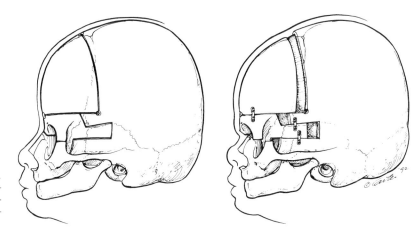

FIG. 43-36. Operative treatment of plagiocephaly. The upper orbital segment and frontal bar are advanced and plated to provide rigid fixation. The segment of frontal bone is cut and contoured to the desired shape and plated to the frontal bone.

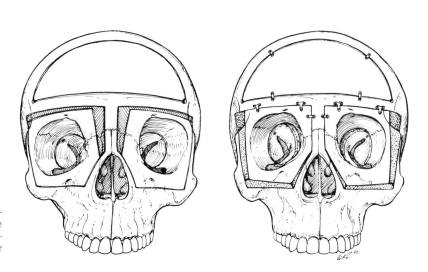

FIG. 43-37. Operative treatment of orbital hypertelorism. The approach is transcranial. Blocks of bone are resected on both sides of the midline; the osteotomies then allow medial translocation of the entire anterior orbits.

be cut and segments repositioned during model surgery. This allows the plastic surgeon and the orthodontist to plan accurately what bony movements are necessary to achieve proper occlusion. Cephalograms or standardized frontal and lateral radiographs of the face and skull provide an outline of the skeletal and soft tissue profile. Measurements between standardized points on the radiograph can then be compared to a database of normal values for age and sex. Minor problems of maxillomandibular disproportion and malocclusion can often be handled by orthodontia alone. Significant skeletal disproportion requires both surgical and orthodontic treatment.

Deformities of the jaws may be classified according to their dental and skeletal relationships. Dental occlusal relationships are normally described by Angle's classification. In this classification *mesial* means close to the dental midline, *distal* means away from the dental midline, *buccal* means toward the outer aspect of the dental arch, and *lingual* means toward the inner aspect of the dental arch. In normal occlusion the mesial buccal cusp of the maxillary first molar lies within the buccal groove of the mandibular first molar. This is known as *class I occlusion.* In *class II occlusion* the mesial buccal cusp of the maxillary first molar is found mesial to the buccal groove of the mandibular fist molar, as might be seen with an abnormally small mandible. In *class III occlusion* the mesial buccal cusp of the maxillary first molar is found distal or posterior to its normal position. This relationship may be seen with an abnormally large mandible or small maxillae.

Micrognathia refers to an abnormally small mandible. *Retrognathia* refers to a mandible of normal size located in an abnormally posterior position. Both retrognathia and micrognathia would typically present with class II occlusion and the appearance of a weak or recessed chin. Mandibular advancement is normally performed by creating osteotomies in the sagittal plane through both mandibular rami. The distal mandible is then advanced into a more favorable position and plates or screws used to hold the advancement rigidly. This technique carries some risk of injury to the inferior alveolar nerve. Nerve transection has been reported in approximately 2 percent of cases, and up to 15 percent of patients may have some evidence of long-term dysfunction (Fig. 43-38).

Prognathia denotes an abnormally large mandible. These patients will often have class II occlusion. Surgical treatment of mandibular prognathism may also be by a sagittal split of the mandibular rami, with posterior repositioning of the distal mandibular segments. Alternatively a vertical osteotomy can be made from the sigmoid notch to just anterior to the angle of the mandible. The distal mandibular segment can then be positioned posteriorly and lingual to the proximal segment of the mandible. This technique has a lower risk of inferior alveolar nerve injury, but fixation is more difficult. Most patients will be placed in intermaxillary fixation for 4 to 6 weeks after vertical osteotomy of the mandible.

The soft-tissue contour of the mandible can be further altered by bony movement of the symphysis. A genioplasty or horizontal osteotomy of the mandible allows the anterior projection of the chin to be augmented or reduced. By advancing or recessing the mentum, the soft-tissue contour of the chin can be significantly altered without changing dental occlusion. Plates or lag screws are used to rigidly fix the bony movement. Chin augmentation can also be achieved with the use of a small silicone prosthesis.

Maxillary deformities of hyperplasia and hypoplasia are also commonly seen by the craniofacial surgeon. Maxillary hypoplasia commonly presents as maxillary retrognathia and class II or class III occlusion. This is commonly seen in cleft lip and palate patients. Maxillary hyperplasia often presents as vertical maxillary excess, also known as the *long face syndrome.* These patients have excessive gingival exposure when smiling and poor lip competence.

Most maxillary deformities can be approached by the LeFort I osteotomy. An incision is made in the upper buccal sulcus and dissection is carried out in the subperiosteal plane. The surgeon then performs a horizontal osteotomy just above the level of the piriform aperture bilaterally. When additional cuts are completed through the base of the nasal septum, the medial wall of the maxillary sinus, and the pterygomaxillary fissure, the maxilla is then free to be repositioned in three dimensions. This technique is usually performed in patients with permanent dentition. Horizontal osteotomy of the maxilla risks damage of tooth buds in patients with deciduous dentition.

In treating maxillary hypoplasia the surgeon would reposition the maxillae anteriorly and rigidly fix the segments with plates and screws according to the preoperative plan. Treating vertical maxillary access will require maxillary bone to be removed and the segments repositioned superiorly.

Facial Fractures

Facial fractures are most frequently caused by motor vehicle accidents and physical assaults. Although the specifics of facial fracture treatment have evolved since the advent of craniofacial

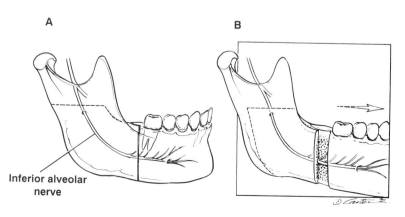

A **B**

Inferior alveolar nerve

FIG. 43-38. Sagittal split osteotomy of the mandible permits advancement of the body of the mandible. Broad apposition of bone and rigid fixation by screws enhances early bone healing.

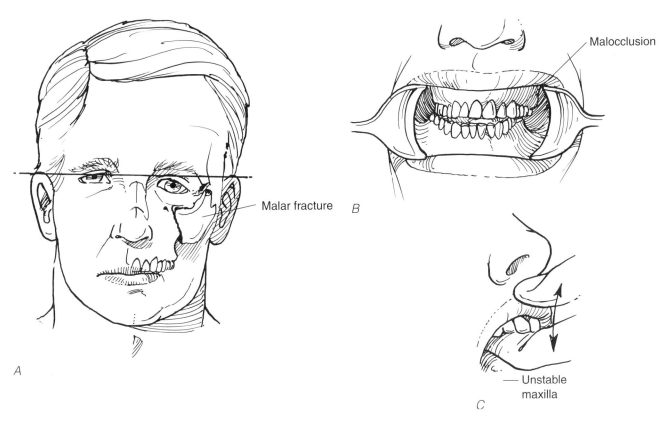

FIG. 43-39. Common physical findings in facial fractures.

techniques in the 1980s, the principles remain the same. The patient with facial fracture is often a multiple trauma patient and requires thorough evaluation. Although the facial fracture is rarely a surgical emergency, other associated injuries frequently require emergency care. For instance, the patient with a gunshot wound to the angle of the mandible is first and foremost a patient with a penetrating neck wound, and the patient with a depressed supraorbital fracture is first and foremost a patient with closed head trauma.

Physical Examination. Examination for facial trauma must be systematic and complete (Fig. 43-39). Proceeding from superior to inferior, the forehead and supraorbital ridge is palpated for any fracture. The orbital rims are also evaluated for any stepoff or irregularity. The ophthalmologic examination must include pupillary responses, extraocular muscle function, and visual acuity. Any enophthalmos, inferior displacement of the globe, or limitation in extraocular muscle function is a sign of orbital fracture. Any patient with signs of direct injury to the ocular globe or an orbital fracture should have a formal ophthalmologic examination. The nose is examined for any gross deformity, the septum is examined for hematoma, and patency of the airway is ascertained. The zygomatic arches are palpated for fractures. Depressed fractures of the zygomatic arch can impinge on the temporalis muscle. It is important to note whether there is pain associated with movement of the mandible or any limitation in mandibular excursion. Fractures of the maxilla frequently run through the infraorbital foramen, and these patients frequently have paresthesia of the upper lip and teeth. Midface stability is assessed by grasping the upper incisors and alveolar ridge with one hand and palpating the nasofrontal junction and

anterior maxilla with the other. An attempt is then made to gently rock the alveolar ridge anteriorly and posteriorly. Occlusion is noted and the patient is asked if his teeth "fit together" as usual. The mandible is palpated for any tenderness or fracture.

Radiologic Examination. The radiologic examination is guided by the history and physical examination (Table 43-1).

Table 43-1
Facial Fracture Radiography

Bone	Radiographic Projection
Mandile	
Condylar and coronoid processes	Right and left lateral obliques of mandible
Ascending ramus and body	
Symphysis, parasymphyseal area	
Body and ascending rami	Posteroanterior of mandible
Condyle and condylar neck	Towne (modified)
	Anteroposterior of base of skull
Anterior arch	Occlusal of anterior mandible
Maxilla and zygoma	Waters (posteranterior oblique)
	Anteroposterior of face
	Lateral of face
Zygomatic arch	Submental-vertex
Orbital floor	Waters
	Stereo Waters
	Laminography
Nasal bone	Superoinferior of nose
	Lateral of nose

Most patients will need clear views of the cervical spine, including odontoid, posteroanterior, and lateral to include the first thoracic vertebrae. The standard facial bone series includes posteroanterior, lateral, and Waters views. Standard views of the mandible include oblique, lateral, and Towne views. A Panorex radiograph will provide an image of the entire mandible, including the temporomandibular joints. This film is necessary in most cases of suspected mandible fracture. Submental vertex films free the zygomatic arches of other bony silhouettes and are useful in diagnosing zygomatic arch fractures (Fig. 43-40).

Computed tomography is the mainstay in diagnosing and planning treatment for orbital fractures. Standard axial slices should be reformatted to provide coronal views of the orbit. These coronal images are extremely helpful in diagnosing orbital floor fractures.

Treatment. *Mandibular Fractures.* Specific mandibular fractures are treated according to the characteristics of the fracture and its anatomic location. The goal in treating any mandibular fracture is restoration of function occlusion with firm healing at the fracture site. Any open mandible fracture requires operative irrigation, debridement, and intravenous antibiotics.

A number of techniques may be employed in the management of mandibular fractures. *Intermaxillary fixation* is the ligation of the maxilla to the mandible with the teeth in occlusion, serving to immobilize the mandible. This may be accomplished by ligating metal arch bars to the upper and lower dental arch and then fixing these bars to each other by means of heavy elastics or wire. Alternatively, when the teeth are in occlusion, mandibular and maxillary teeth may be directly wired together. Intermaxillary fixation requires a patent nasal airway and must

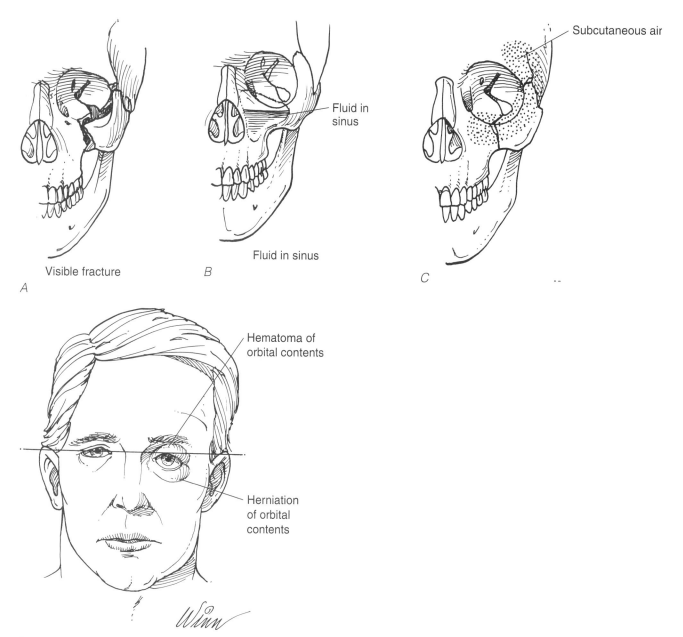

FIG. 43-40. Common radiographic findings in facial fractures.

be used with caution in alcoholics and other patients prone to loss of consciousness or vomiting. Use of intermaxillary fixation is contraindicated in patients with a seizure disorder. *Open reduction and internal fixation* has become the treatment of choice for most unstable fractures of the mandible. Most fractures can be exposed intraorally through a buccal sulcus incision and rigidly fixed with plates and screws. This precludes the need for intermaxillary fixation and allows the patient to resume oral intake on the first postoperative day. It also reduces the possibility of limited mandibular excursion secondary to prolonged intermaxillary fixation. External fixation devices are employed only rarely, for large bony defects and recurrent infections.

Mandibular fractures may be classified as *favorable* or *unfavorable*, according to the manner in which the muscles of mastication serve to distract the fracture. Fractures of the body of the mandible that course obliquely and anteriorly when followed from interior to superior are termed unfavorable. In these fractures the masseter muscle, by pulling on the posterior segment, will displace the fracture (Fig. 43-41). Fractures of the body that course posteriorly in the inferior to superior direction are termed favorable. In these fractures the masseter muscle, by pulling superiorly on the posterior segment, serves to appose the mandibular segments.

Fractures of the rami and mandibular condyles are frequently not greatly displaced by the muscles of mastication. These may be treated with intermaxillary fixation or a soft diet alone if not widely displaced and occlusion is adequate. Widely displaced fractures of the condyle may require open reduction and internal fixation. Fractures of the coronoid process usually do not interfere with occlusion unless the fracture fragments interfere with mandibular excursion. Coronoid process fractures usually may be treated with a soft diet. Fractures of the angle and body of the mandible are subjected to significant stress and motion by the muscles of mastication. These fractures usually require open reduction and internal fixation. Minimally displaced fractures may be treated by internal maxillary fixation. Nondisplaced fractures can be treated with a soft diet alone in selected patients. Fractures of the symphysis and parasymphyseal area also are usually displaced by the muscles of mastication and normally require open reduction and internal fixation. Fractures of the alveolar process may be seen alone or in combination with other fractures of the mandible. These are usually treated by ligating the teeth of the fractured segment to adjacent stable teeth by the application of arch bars.

Nasal Fractures. A nasal fracture is usually diagnosed on the basis of gross deformity and nasal airway obstruction. In patients with craniofacial trauma any deformity should be noted and the nasal airway should be examined with a speculum for patency and the presence of a septal hematoma. Septal hematomas require prompt incision, drainage, and nasal packing to prevent subsequent infection and septal perforation. With early treatment nasal fractures usually can be reduced with closed techniques under local or general anesthesia. Late treatment of nasal fractures usually requires osteotomies to mobilize and adequately reposition the nasal bones.

More severe nasal fractures often occur when the nasofrontal area strikes the steering wheel during a motor vehicle accident. These fractures involve not only the nasal bones but also the nasofrontal junction, the ethmoid sinuses bilaterally, and the medial orbits. These fractures are also known as nasoorbital-ethmoid fractures. Typically the patient with a nasoorbital-ethmoid fracture has a depressed and deformed nasal contour, and *telecanthus*, an increased distance between the medial canthi. The medial canthus inserts into the frontal process of the maxilla and the lacrimal bone in the medial orbit. In a nasoorbital-ethmoid fracture these bones are comminuted and displaced laterally, increasing the distance between the medial canthi (Fig. 43-42). Nasoorbital-ethmoid fractures are best treated by extensive exposure through a bicoronal incision. The multiple small fracture fragments are accurately reduced and wired or plated in place. If the medial canthi remain attached to a large fracture fragment, accurate reduction and rigid fixation of this fragment will reposition the medial canthi. A transnasal wire placed posterior and superior to the native insertion of the medial canthus can also be used to reduce the traumatic telecanthus. This wire is placed as a loop through each medial canthus and then tightened, repositioning the canthi in a more favorable and medial position.

Zygoma Fractures. Fractures of the zygoma commonly occur as isolated fractures of the zygomatic arch or as zygomaticomaxillary complex fractures (Fig. 43-43). Fractures of the zygomatic arch, when depressed, may impinge on the temporalis muscle, causing pain with mandibular excursion. The depression in the lateral face may also be a significant distortion in appearance. Noncomminuted zygomatic arch fractures sometimes may be elevated by sliding an instrument beneath the arch via an incision in the temporal scalp. Comminuted zygomatic arch fractures usually require plating via a bicoronal incision. Zygomaticomaxillary complex fractures result in a depressed malar eminence and infraorbital rim. The fracture lines are typically along the zygomatic frontal suture, zygomatic arch, and infraorbital rim and floor of the orbit, through the infraorbital foramen (Fig. 43-44). These patients typically present with an in-

FIG. 43-41. *A.* Favorable mandibular fracture. *B.* Unfavorable.

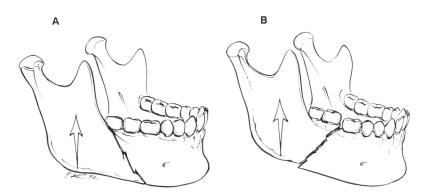

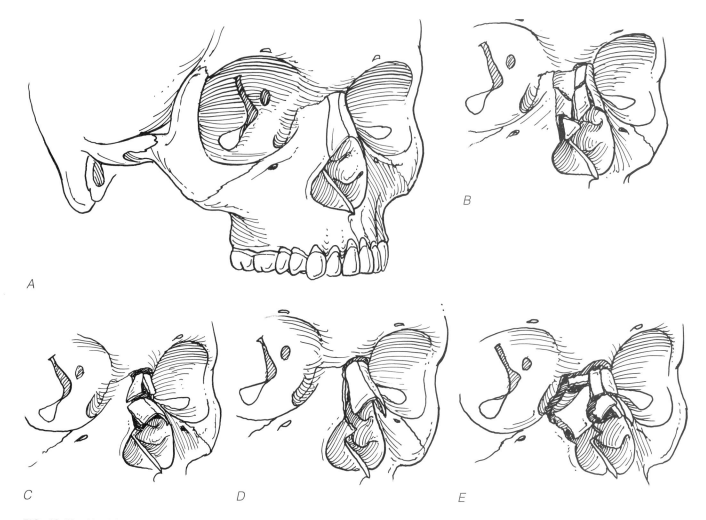

FIG. 43-42. *Nasal fractures. A. Normal skeleton. B. Simple depressed fracture of lateral wall. C. Depressed fracture mid-dorsum. D and E. Complex, comminuted fractures that produce telecanthus.*

feriorly and laterally displaced eye, enophthalmos, and paresthesia of the infraorbital nerve. Malocclusion also can result if the fracture extends along the anterior wall of the maxilla into the dental arch. These fractures require open reduction and internal fixation of the fracture fragments and, if any significant defect exists, reconstruction of the orbital floor.

Orbital Floor Fractures. Orbital floor fractures may occur as a result of a direct blow to the eye. An increase in the infraorbital pressure can result in herniation of intraorbital contents through a fracture in the orbital floor (Fig. 43-45). These "blowout" fractures may involve entrapment of intraorbital fat and occasionally extraocular muscles within the orbital floor defect. These patients typically present with enophthalmos, opacification of the maxillary sinus on radiography, and diplopia, particularly on upward gaze. The orbital floor defect, in effect, increases the orbital volume, allowing the eye to settle posteriorly and inferiorly, resulting in enophthalmos. Diplopia and limitation of upward gaze is the result of entrapment of orbital fat or extraocular muscles within the orbital floor defect. Trauma to the extraocular muscles and resultant edema also can cause diplopia.

The indications for operation on orbital floor fractures have always been controversial. Enophthalmos of 2 mm or more is generally recognized as an indication for operation. It is important to remember, however, that edema after trauma can mask significant enophthalmos. Patients with a normally positioned globe in the immediate posttrauma period may become significantly enophthalmic several weeks later as edema and inflammation subside. We attempt to individualize the decision to operate based on enophthalmos after fully discussing the risks and benefits with each patient. Central to this discussion is the principle that minor degrees of enophthalmos after trauma that are easily correctable can evolve to significant enophthalmos that is difficult to correct once bone and soft tissues are well healed. Entrapment and limitation of extraocular muscles is also a general indication for operation. In some of these patients the limitation of gaze will resolve spontaneously, but as a general rule a floor defect large enough to limit ocular movement will also eventually leave the patient enophthalmic.

Exploration of the orbital floor is performed through an eyelid incision or a transconjunctival incision in the subperiosteal plane. The limits of the floor defect are defined and all periorbita

A

B

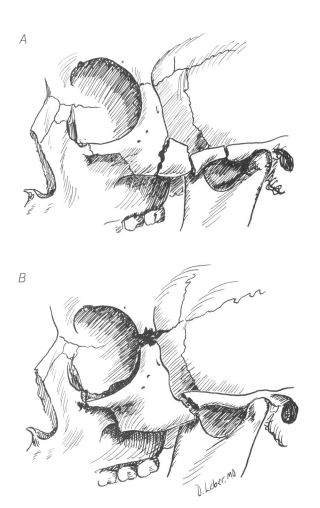

FIG. 43-43. *Zygomatic bone fractures. A. Depressed fracture of the zygomatic arch. This fracture may impinge on the mandible, producing pain (trismus) and difficulty in opening the mouth. B. Displaced fracture of the zygomatic bone. The zygomaticofrontal, zygomaticotemporal, and zygomaticomaxillary sutures are separated. The orbital floor and lateral orbital wall are always involved in this fracture.*

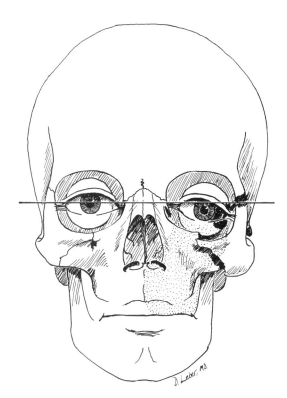

FIG. 43-44. *Fracture-dislocation of the zygoma, with rotation of the fragment, lateral and inferior displacement of the lateral canthus, and subscleral hematomas. Note the surface representation of anesthesia due to infraorbital nerve injury.*

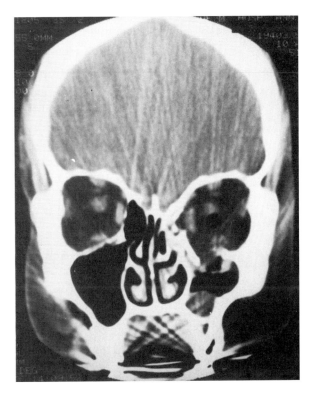

FIG. 43-45. *CT scan of left orbital floor blowout fracture.*

herniated through the fracture are reduced. Most craniofacial surgeons favor repair of floor defects with onlay split calvarial bone grafts. Available data suggest that for moderate and small defects of the orbital floor alloplastic materials also may be safely used. Orbital floor implants are available composed of titanium, hydroxyapatite, silicone, Teflon, and other materials. Any patient with an orbital floor fracture should have a forced duction test performed pre- and postoperatively. Tetracaine is instilled locally to anesthetize the conjunctiva, and then the conjunctiva and insertion of the inferior rectus muscle are grasped with a fine-toothed forceps. Attempting to rotate the globe superiorly will reveal any limitation caused by entrapment. The forced duction test is mandatory as a means of evaluating reduction of entrapped periorbita.

Maxillary Fractures. Maxillary fractures may be classified according to the LeFort classification system (Fig. 43-46). LeFort recorded the pattern of fracture in fresh cadaver skulls subjected to blunt trauma. He noted several characteristic patterns of maxillary fracture. The LeFort I fracture extends from the piriform aperture laterally to the pterygomaxillary fissure. This fracture separates the lower maxilla, hard palate, and max-

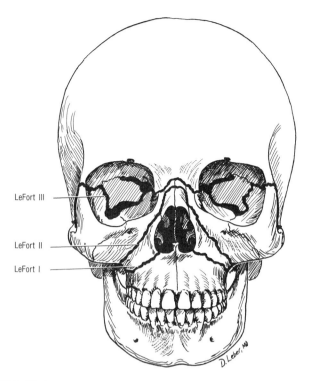

FIG. 43-46. LeFort fracture lines.

illary teeth from the remainder of the skull. The LeFort II fracture extends from the pterygomaxillary fissure superiorly across the anterior maxilla to the nasofrontal junction through the inferior orbital rim. This fracture separates the lower maxilla and nose from the craniofacial skeleton. The craniofacial disjunction or LeFort III fracture separates the entire midface from the cranium by fracturing through the pterygomaxillary fissure and zygomatic frontal sutures, along the floor of the orbit, and through the nasofrontal junction. LeFort fractures are normally treated by placing the patient in intermaxillary fixation and then rigidly fixing the fractures with plates and screws. Typically, 1.5-mm plates are placed on the nasomaxillary and zygomaxillary buttresses in LeFort I fractures. Additional fixation is provided at the nasofrontal junction and zygomatic arches in LeFort III frac-

tures. The intermaxillary fixation may then be released once rigid fixation is established.

Ear Reconstruction

Microtia refers to a congenitally absent or small ear. This condition is often seen with other abnormalities of the first and second branchial arches, including micrognathia, hemifacial microsomia, and lateral facial clefts. The development of middle ear structures in a microtic ear is variable. Hearing is normally decreased in an affected ear. For this reason otitis media in the contralateral ear must be treated aggressively to preserve hearing. Reconstruction of a microtic ear normally begins at age five or six, before the child enters school (Fig. 43-47). The reconstruction is staged beginning with the insertion of a cartilaginous framework sculpted from costochondral cartilage. This stage requires meticulous technique to create a natural-looking ear framework and to avoid hematoma or infection. Subsequent stages include rotation of the native ear lobule and elevation of the ear from the mastoid fascia. A final stage often includes excavation of the concha and reconstruction of the tragus using a composite skin/cartilage graft from the contralateral ear.

Prominent ears are a congenital abnormality, resulting from some combination of an excessively large concha and a poorly developed antihelical fold. These ears tend to project excessively from the lateral skull. Otoplasty for prominent ears is undertaken to recreate an antihelical fold and decrease ear prominence. The Stenstrom technique takes advantage of the natural tendency of cartilage to bend away from any disruption of the perichondrium. When the perichondrium is scored anteriorly along the natural course of the antihelical fold, the ear cartilage will tend to bend posteriorly in this area, recreating the antihelical fold. The Mustarde technique involves placing sutures along the posterior auricular cartilage to recreate the antihelical fold. This cartilage is then fully mobilized and tubed to recreate the antihelical fold. Skin is also sometimes removed from the posterior surface of the ear, and the ear also may be sutured to the mastoid fascia (Fig. 43-48).

Nasal Reconstruction

Nasal defects commonly occur with the excision of squamous and basal cell carcinomas of the nose (Fig. 43-49). Depending on the location and size of these defects, they may be handled

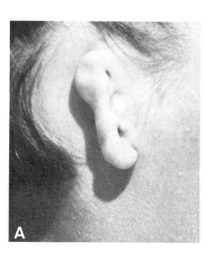
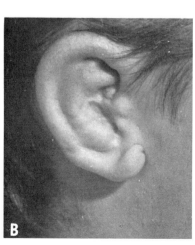

FIG. 43-47. Microtia reconstruction. *A.* Preoperative photograph. *B.* Ear reconstructed using cartilage framework.

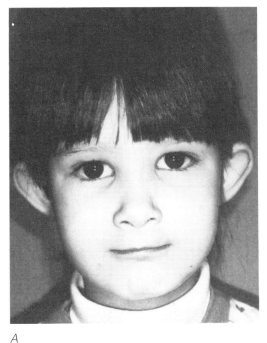
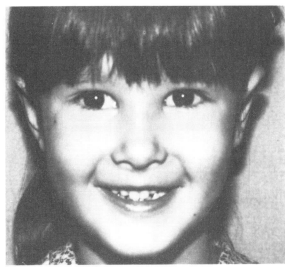

A   B

FIG. 43-48. Prominent ears. *A.* Preoperative photograph. *B.* Postoperative photograph.

by skin grafting or local flaps. Defects of the alar rim may be reconstructed with a composite graft of cartilage and skin from the ear. Total nasal reconstruction remains one of the greatest challenges in plastic surgery. This requires a stable bony framework, often in the form of an iliac bone graft secured to the nasofrontal junction. The lining of the nasal airway may be provided by local flaps in the region of the nasolabial fold or by skin grafts. The nasal contour may be restored with a midline forehead flap, scalp flap, or free-tissue transfer.

Lip Reconstruction

Most defects of the lip encountered by the reconstructive surgeon may be closed primarily. Defects of up to one-third of the lower lip and one-fourth of the upper lip can usually be closed directly without the need for more complex reconstructive techniques. When closing lip defects that cross the vermilion-cutaneous border, it is imperative to align perfectly the vermilion and white roll edge of the vermilion. Any notching of the vermilion tends to catch the eye of an observer and is usually cosmetically unacceptable. A number of local flaps are available for reconstructing larger defects. The Abbe flap, or cross-lip flap, is an extremely useful technique to transfer full-thickness lip (Figs. 43-50 and 43-51).

Eyelid Reconstruction

Full-thickness defects of 25 percent of the upper and lower eyelid often may be closed primarily. When closing lid margins the tarsal plate should be approximated with fine absorbable suture and the gray line of the lid margin accurately approximated. In any laceration medial to the punctum of the lacrimal apparatus a lacrimal injury must be ruled out. Larger defects of the upper lid can be closed by advancing adjacent and lateral eyelid and temporal skin. Lower eyelid skin also can be advanced or rotated

into an upper eyelid defect. At a second operation the flap is completely divided from the lower lid to complete the reconstruction. Large defects of the lower lid also may be closed by advancing lateral eyelid and cheek skin. Conjunctival lining can be provided by a free mucosal graft taken from the nasal septum with or without cartilage.

Eyebrow lacerations usually can be closed primarily with precise realignment of hair follicles (Fig. 43-52). Complete reconstruction of an eyebrow is usually done with thin strips of free scalp grafts or a thin island flap based on the temporal artery (Figs. 43-53 and 43-54).

Eyelid Ptosis. Elevation of the upper eyelid is achieved through contraction of the levator palpebrae superioris muscle and Müller's muscle. The levator muscle is innervated by the oculomotor nerve (IIId cranial nerve) and Müller's muscle receives sympathetic innervation. If either of these muscles functions poorly or not at all, the upper eyelid will fail to elevate adequately, which is known as *ptosis*. Ptosis may be congenital or acquired. Congenital ptosis is usually idiopathic. Acquired ptosis may be a result of dysfunction of the oculomotor nerve or the sympathetic chain. Horner's syndrome includes upper eyelid ptosis, miosis, and decreased sweating on the affected side of the face. Horner's syndrome is seen with disruption of the sympathetic tract and may be a presenting sign of malignancy. Myasthenia gravis can present as eyelid ptosis. Most cases of acquired ptosis are the result of trauma. In these cases disruption or stretching of the levator aponeurosis is usually seen.

Treatment of eyelid ptosis is generally determined by the degree of levator function. Levator function is assessed by immobilizing the frontalis muscle with gentle pressure above the eyebrows. Upper lid excursion is then measured as the patient's gaze moves from inferior to superior. Levator function is classified as excellent (12 to 15 mm), good (8 to 12 mm), fair (5 to

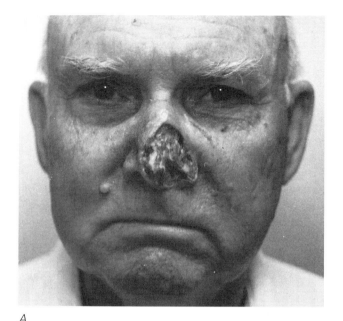

A

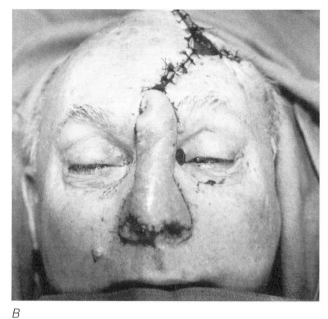

B

C

FIG. 43-49. Nasal reconstruction. *A.* Defect after tumor excision. *B.* Reconstruction with a forehead flap. *C.* Result after flap division and insetting.

7 mm), poor (less than 4 mm). Most cases of congenital ptosis have poor levator function, whereas cases of acquired ptosis generally have fair to good excursion of the upper lid. Minimal ptosis with good levator function can be treated with transconjunctival excision of part of the tarsal plate and Müller's muscle. This is known as the *Fasanella-Servat procedure*. More significant ptosis with fair to good levator function is usually treated by resection of the levator muscle through an upper eyelid incision. The shortened levator muscle is then approximated to the tarsal plate. Resection or plication of the levator muscle is usually accomplished through an upper eyelid skin incision. In cases of severe congenital ptosis with absent levator function, suspension of the upper eyelid to the frontalis muscle usually is required. Fascia lata or alloplastic material may be used for suspension of the lid.

Skull and Scalp Reconstruction

Partial defects of the scalp and calvaria are usually the result of trauma or surgical defects after tumor excision. Acute coverage of small or moderate-sized scalp defects can be accomplished with scalp flaps. Orticochea has described raising the entire scalp as three or four flaps that are then transposed into the defect. By scoring the galea aponeurotica on the undersurface of each flap, increased length can be gained. Large defects can also be closed with split-thickness skin grafts. Split-thickness skin grafts placed on the calvaria provide unstable coverage in the long term, however, and are prone to breakdown. Acute coverage of large, full-thickness defects involving both scalp and calvaria may require free-tissue transfer. The calvaria may be reconstructed with split calvarial or rib grafts that are in turn covered by a free flap. The

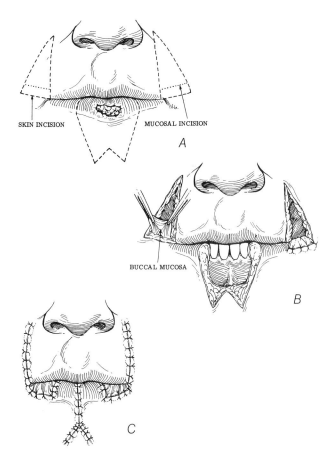

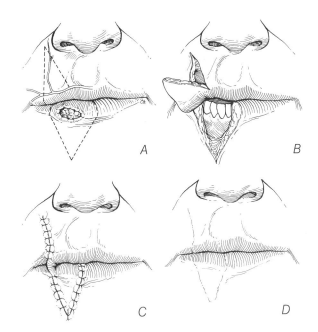

FIG. 43-51. Abbe flap. *A.* Incisions outlined. *B.* Tumor excised and flap developed, based on the labial artery. *C.* Flap healed in place. *D.* Pedicle of flap divided and wound revised.

FIG. 43-50. Bernard procedure. *A.* Outline of skin incisions for removal of tumor and mucosal incisions for excision of nasolabial triangles. *B.* Tumor and nasolabial triangles removed and buccal mucosa turned down into lower lip. *C.* Incisions closed.

Total scalp avulsion is usually the result of hair becoming entangled in machinery. Because the galea is a strong layer that resists separation, scalp avulsions frequently separate between the galea and the periosteum. The avulsed segment usually includes the eyebrow and upper ear. This devastating injury should be treated by microvascular replantation whenever possible. As the scalp is relatively resistant to hypoxia, long delays in treatment do not preclude replantation. Contraindications to scalp replantation include an unstable patient or severe damage to the avulsed scalp.

Facial Reanimation

The facial nerve is both a motor and a sensory nerve. The sensory component of the nerve includes both an afferent division, which is responsible for taste from the anterior two-thirds of the tongue via the chorda tympani nerve, and an efferent division with secretory fibers to the lacrimal gland and, also via the chorda tympani, to the sublingual and submandibular glands.

omentum and latissimus dorsi or serratus anterior muscle are frequent choices for free flaps in reconstruction of the scalp and calvaria. These flaps are thin and broad and easily support a skin graft.

Tissue expansion is a useful technique for reconstructing partial defects of the scalp. By effectively increasing the amount of hair-bearing scalp, areas of burn alopecia or prior skin grafts placed on the scalp may be excised and closed with adjacent hair-bearing scalp.

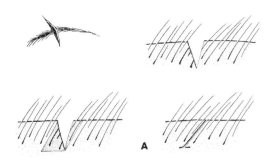

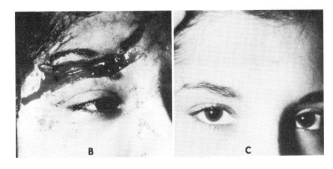

FIG. 43-52. Avoidance of alopecia during repair of eyebrow laceration. *A.* Oblique laceration of eyebrow hairs creates eyebrow alopecia at the wound site unless revised parallel to the hair follicles. *B.* Laceration crossing the eyebrow. Precise realignment of eyebrow elements is important. *C.* Result.

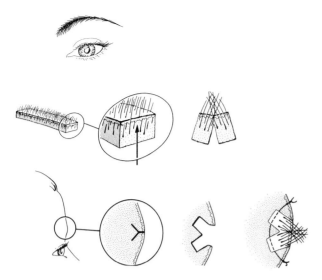

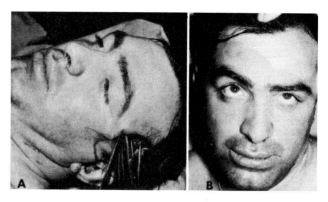

FIG. 43-55. *Facial nerve injury. A. Laceration of temple with bleeding controlled by multiple hemostats. B. Paralysis of left forehead due to injury of temporal branch of facial nerve. The paralysis may have been the result of the laceration or the attempts to achieve hemostasis.*

FIG. 43-53. *Full-thickness graft from scalp for eyebrow reconstruction. The graft is split and interposed in the eyebrow area so that hairs interdigitate and produce an eyebrow effect.*

The motor component innervates the muscles of facial expression and the stapedius muscle in the middle ear. Facial nerve paralysis is seen in a wide variety of disease stages. Congenital facial nerve paralysis is seen in Möbius' syndrome. Bell's palsy is thought to be the result of swelling within the bony canal. It is frequently idiopathic and occurs most commonly in young adults. Penetrating trauma can lacerate the nerve at any point after it exits from the stylomastoid foramen (Fig. 43-55). Facial nerve paralysis can also be seen with fractures of the temporal bone.

A lacerated facial nerve should be explored and repaired as soon as possible. Using microsurgical techniques, the nerve ends are directly coapted whenever possible. Nerve grafts are used for segmental nerve loss when direct repair is not possible. Facial nerve resection as part of a cancer operation also should be re-

constructed with nerve grafts. Planned postoperative radiation therapy does not contraindicate nerve grafting. Fractures of the temporal bone usually do not disrupt the facial nerve. When the facial nerve is affected by temporal bone fractures, partial facial nerve paralysis or late appearance of the facial nerve paralysis indicates that the nerve has not been completely disrupted. Nonoperative management should be pursued in these cases. With immediate and complete facial paralysis after a temporal bone fracture, decompression of the facial nerve within the bony canal should be undertaken.

Paralysis of the facial musculature results in functional problems that include incompetence of the oral and ocular sphincter mechanisms (Fig. 43-56). Paralysis of the orbicularis oculi muscle results in an inability to close the eyelid. This may lead to exposure keratitis. Paralysis of the orbicularis oris muscle can result in oral incompetence and abnormal speech. Facial symmetry and facial expression are also profoundly affected by facial paralysis. When the distal facial nerve–muscle unit is thought to be intact, nerve grafts from the contralateral intact facial nerve or from a partial transection of the ipsilateral hypoglossal nerve may be used to reanimate the affected side of the face (Fig. 43-57). These techniques must be employed within 2 years of the time of injury, as motor endplates degenerate in the absence neural stimulation. Static techniques have long been used to suspend the paralyzed face (Fig. 43-58). These techniques typically involve slings of fascia lata to the eyelids and mouth. More dynamic techniques include transfer of part of the temporalis or masseter musculature to the oral commissure and eyelid. As these muscles are innervated by the Vth cranial nerve, considerable practice is required by the patient to produce a coordinated smile (Fig. 43-59).

Microneurovascular muscle transfers have yielded some of the most promising results in facial reanimation surgery. With these techniques a cross-facial nerve graft is performed and the advancing Tinel's sign followed. Approximately 1 year later a free vascularized muscle flap is performed and its motor nerve anastomosed to the cross-facial nerve graft. The gracilis muscle is the most common donor muscle. The pectoralis minor and latissimus dorsi muscles have also been used. Typically the gracilis muscle would be sutured to the oral commissure and the body of the zygoma in an effort to produce a more normal smile (Fig. 43-60). The advantages of this technique are that facial

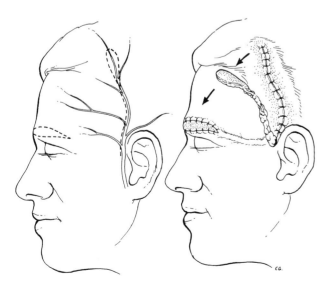

FIG. 43-54. *Eyebrow reconstruction using a hair-bearing island flap from the scalp, based on the superficial temporal artery.*

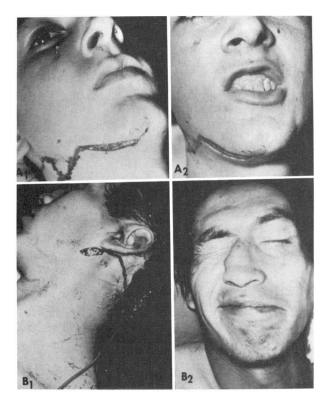

FIG. 43-56. *Facial nerve injury. A1. Laceration of submandibular region. A2. Injury of marginal mandibular branch of facial nerve, producing paralysis of lower lip on the right. B1. Stab wound anterior to mastoid process. B2. Result of complete division of facial nerve on the right side.*

movement is controlled by the contralateral facial nerve and that new vascularized muscle with well-preserved motor endplates is brought to the face. The main disadvantages of the technique are that two long operations are required, donor site scars results, and at least 2 years are usually required before facial movement returns.

Reconstruction After Tumor Extirpation

Surgical extirpation of head and neck tumors can create large complex defects that are potentially very disfiguring. Reconstruction of these defects requires not only restoration of form

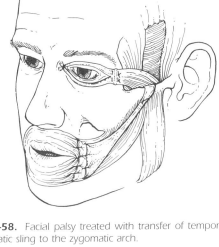

FIG. 43-58. *Facial palsy treated with transfer of temporalis muscle and a static sling to the zygomatic arch.*

but also attention to the functions of speech, oral competence, and alimentation. Through the 1970s large head and neck defects were of necessity reconstructed by regional transposition flaps. The most common and reliable local flaps available to the head and neck included the deltopectoral flap and the pectoralis, latissimus, and trapezius myocutaneous flaps. The advent of microsurgical techniques has revolutionized head and neck reconstruction. Free flaps can provide thin, pliable oral lining, bone, and skin without bulky pedicles or disfiguring donor sites. For this reason free-tissue transfer has become the first choice in reconstruction of most complex head and neck defects.

Intraoral defects require reconstruction with thin, pliable tissue. For small defects split-thickness skin grafting is sometimes adequate. Care must be taken that, with secondary contraction of the skin graft, tongue mobility is maintained. Flaps of tongue tissue occasionally may be employed, but they too may adversely affect tongue mobility and limit speech or swallowing. Large defects of oral lining are usually reconstructed by free-tissue transfer. The free radial forearm flap based on the radial artery provides a flap with relatively thin skin and subcutaneous tissue and a long pedicle. Other available free flaps include scapular and parascapular flaps, based on cutaneous branches of the circumflex scapular artery, and the groin flap, based on the su-

FIG. 43-57. *Facial nerve graft using hypoglossal nerve. A. Normal relationship between descendens hypoglossal and facial nerve. B. Nerve graft from proximal descendens hypoglossi to distal facial nerve.*

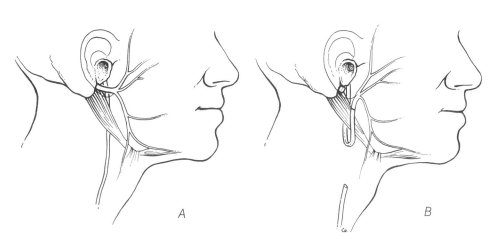

A

B

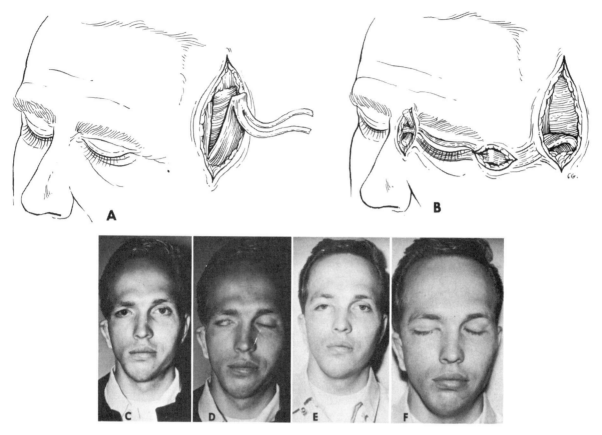

FIG. 43-59. Gillies's procedure to establish motor power for eyelids. *A and B.* Temporalis muscle reflected forward with strips of its own fascia passed through the upper and lower lids to the medial canthal ligament. *C and D.* Preoperative eyelid paralysis. *E and F.* After Gillies's operation.

perficial circumflex iliac artery. Salvage techniques after free-flap failure or for patients thought not to be candidates for free-tissue transfer include deltopectoral and pectoralis major flaps.

Resection of more advanced oral cancers or primary tumors of bone may include defects of the mandible or maxilla. Small defects sometimes may be reconstructed with some combination of a soft-tissue flap and nonvascularized bone graft. Nonvascularized bone grafts do poorly in radiated beds and also poorly tolerate subsequent radiation therapy. When radiation therapy is part of the clinical picture, or for very large defects, free vas-

cularized bone flaps are the procedure of choice. Donor sites include the fibula, based on the peroneal vessels, the lateral border of the scapula, based on circumflex scapular vessels, and the iliac crest, based on the deep circumflex iliac vessels. These free bone flaps may also be taken with an associated skin island to provide tissue for reconstruction of skin or mucosal defects.

The cervical esophagus must often be resected as part of the treatment for a stage T3 or T4 carcinoma of the hypopharynx and larynx. Tubed myocutaneous flaps have been used to reconstruct the cervical esophagus, but they are bulky and prone to

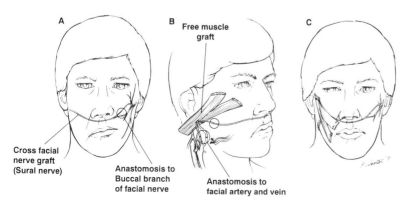

FIG. 43-60. Sequence of cross-facial nerve graft followed by free muscle grafting by microtechniques.

fistula formation. The stomach can also be delivered into the neck and an esophagogastrostomy performed for reconstruction of cervical esophageal defects. A segment of jejunum transferred as a free vascularized flap, however, is our preferred method. This flap is reliable in a radiated wound and also tolerates radiation therapy. It is performed in a single stage and allows early resumption of oral feeding (Fig. 43-61).

Hemangiomas and Vascular Malformations

Hemangiomas are common pediatric tumors that enlarge by cellular proliferation. Historically, hemangiomas have been given a number of names based on their clinical appearance. *Capillary hemangiomas* and *strawberry hemangiomas* have a similar biology. *Cavernous hemangiomas* occur deeper in subcutaneous tissue or muscle and hence appear darker or blue from the skin surface. Hemangiomas usually present within the first month of life and typically undergo a period of proliferation lasting 6 to 18 months. The lesion then begins to involute and this process may continue for several years. The majority of hemangiomas require no treatment. Even large lesions of the face frequently resolve with minimal or no cosmetic sequelae. Treatment is indicated for lesions that obstruct the visual axis, airway, or bilateral external auditory canals. Less commonly hemangiomas may be associated with hemorrhage or platelet consumption (Kasabach-Merritt syndrome), which requires treatment. Treatment modalities include systemic or intralesional steroids. Recent reports have also indicated that interferon-alpha may be effective in rapidly expanding hemangiomas. Invasive treatment generally entails surgical excision for small tumors in areas where a surgical scar does not pose a cosmetic problem.

Vascular malformations are abnormal vascular structures formed during embryogenesis. These lesions are not neoplastic and do not exhibit the rapid cellular proliferation of hemangiomas. Vascular malformations may be predominantly capillary, venous, or lymphatic in composition. Frequently some combination of these components is present. Vascular malformations also may be present as abnormal connections between arteries and veins, known as *arteriovenous malformations*. These may be high-flow lesions that demonstrate bruits or thrills. Arteriovenous malformations can obstruct cervical viscera or massively bleed on dental manipulation if they arise in the head and the neck. Treatment is by intraarterial embolization under radiographic control followed by surgical removal when possible. These lesions can be extensive, and morbidity and mortality can be correspondingly high.

Intradermal capillary malformations are also known as *port-wine stains*. These present at birth and do not undergo resolution with time. Port-wine stains frequently present in the skin area innervated by the trigeminal nerve. Small lesions may be directly excised. Larger intradermal lesions usually benefit from treatment with laser.

Lymphatic malformations often present with some component of venous malformation. Lymphatic malformations most commonly occur in the neck and upper chest. *Cystic hygroma* is a form of lymphatic malformation commonly found in the neck, with large cystic cavities and abnormal venous connections. Treatment of lymphatic malformations is usually by direct surgical excision. Indications for treatment include recurrent infection and airway obstruction. Because these lesions frequently extensively invest vital structures of the neck, it is frequently possible only to debulk the lesion at the time of operation. Involution of cystic hygroma has been observed in some centers.

BREAST

Postmastectomy Breast Reconstruction. Breast cancer is a major public health concern in the United States. Currently most patients with breast cancer are treated by local excision of the cancer followed by radiation or mastectomy and axillary dissection. Even women who have undergone breast-conserving procedures frequently must make a decision about breast reconstruction.

The ideal candidate for breast reconstruction is a woman with a full understanding of the surgical procedures, possible complications, and realistic goals of breast reconstruction. Patients with a favorable prognosis are also usually good candidates for breast reconstruction, although an unfavorable prognosis does not necessarily rule out reconstruction. Possible benefits of breast reconstruction include an improved body image, preservation of feminine identity, elimination of external prostheses, and lessened psychological impact of mastectomy. Available data suggest that breast reconstruction does not delay detection of breast cancer recurrence.

Breast reconstruction often may be performed at the time of the mastectomy. Immediate reconstruction allows the patient to recover from anesthesia with a breast mound in place. Studies suggest that patients who have undergone immediate reconstruction experience less psychological disturbance. Immediate reconstruction requires that the patient undergo a longer initial period of anesthesia. Complications of the mastectomy or reconstruction could also conceivably delay subsequent chemotherapy or radiation therapy. For this reason many reconstructive surgeons prefer to offer immediate reconstruction to patients in whom the likelihood of advanced disease is small. For patients who choose delayed breast reconstruction, the reconstructive procedure usually is performed after chemotherapy or radiation

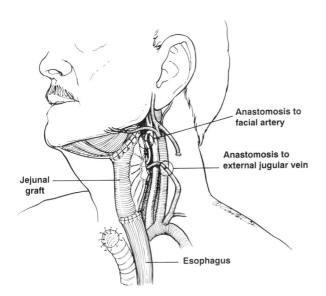

FIG. 43-61. *Free jejunal graft, microtechnique, to replace the pharynx and cervical esophagus.*

Anastomosis to facial artery

Anastomosis to external jugular vein

Jejunal graft

Esophagus

therapy is complete. Advanced age and disease states are not absolute contraindications to reconstruction.

Breast reconstruction techniques may involve autologous or alloplastic materials. Alloplastic materials generally involve some combination of tissue expander and permanent breast prosthesis. Typically a patient choosing reconstruction with an expander/implant would have a tissue expander placed via the original mastectomy incision. Tissue expanders are generally placed in the submuscular position after raising the pectoralis major muscle, the serratus anterior muscle, and the anterior rectus sheath as a unit. Expansion is then carried out postoperatively, allowing for slight overexpansion relative to the desired final breast size. The tissue expander is exchanged for a permanent breast prosthesis during a second surgical procedure. In some patients there is adequate skin after a mastectomy for insertion of an implant large enough to match the contralateral breast without the use of a tissue expander, but this obtains only rarely.

Patients with significant deficiencies in skin and subcutaneous tissue may need to have a latissimus dorsi myocutaneous flap transposed into the surgical defect. The expander/prosthesis may then be positioned beneath the latissimus dorsi flap (Fig. 43-62). Complications following breast reconstruction with a tissue expander or implant include hematoma, infection, exposure of the implant, and capsular contraction. Contraction of the fibrous capsule that forms around a breast implant can cause significant deformity or pain. The true incidence of capsular contraction is unknown but probably ranges from 5 to 20 percent. Capsular contraction may be seen less frequently with textured implants.

Breast reconstruction with autologous tissue offers the patient a warm, natural-feeling breast without the use of alloplastic materials. The abdomen is an excellent source of autologous tissue for breast reconstruction. The entire lower abdominal ellipse of skin and subcutaneous tissue may be lifted as a myocutaneous flap based on perforators from the rectus abdominis muscles. These muscles receive most of their blood supply from the superior epigastric vessels, and care must be taken to preserve these vessels as the rectus abdominis muscle is dissected to the costal margin. The transverse rectus abdominis musculocutaneous (TRAM) flap is then passed under the skin of the upper abdomen and set into the surgical defect. The flap is shaped to match the contralateral breast. Because of the abundant tissue supplied to the TRAM flap a prosthesis is rarely necessary to complete the reconstruction (Fig. 43-63).

In experienced hands, the TRAM flap is extremely reliable and has a low overall complication rate. The incidence of partial flap loss and ventral hernia has been low. The TRAM flap also may be transferred as a free flap pedicled on the inferior epigastric vessels. These are typically anastomosed in the axilla to the thoracodorsal or axillary vessels. The free TRAM flap has the theoretical advantages of improved vascularity of the flap and less disturbance of abdominal wall integrity with a harvest of only a small block of rectus abdominis muscle. The inferior gluteal musculocutaneous unit is less commonly used as a donor site for free-flap breast reconstruction. The inferior gluteal donor site is acceptable but generally provides less tissue and is a more difficult dissection than the TRAM flap.

Nipple reconstruction is usually delayed for at least 6 weeks after breast reconstruction. The nipple itself may be reconstructed using local dermal flaps or grafted tissue from the con-

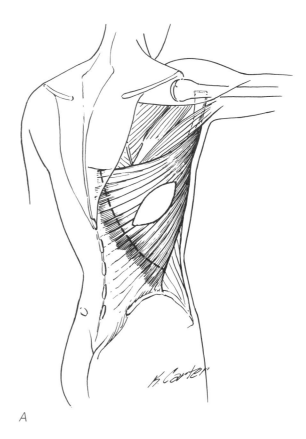

A

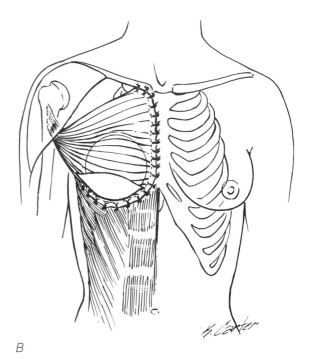

B

FIG. 43-62. *Breast reconstruction using latissimus dorsi musculocutaneous flap. A. A skin island and suitable amount of latissimus dorsi muscle are elevated. B. The musculocutaneous flap is transposed into the anterior chest wall defect and sutured into place. The skin island is positioned to lie along the inferior aspect of the reconstructed breast, without regard for the mastectomy scar. A silicone gel breast prosthesis is placed deep to the latissimus dorsi muscle, providing a breast mound.*

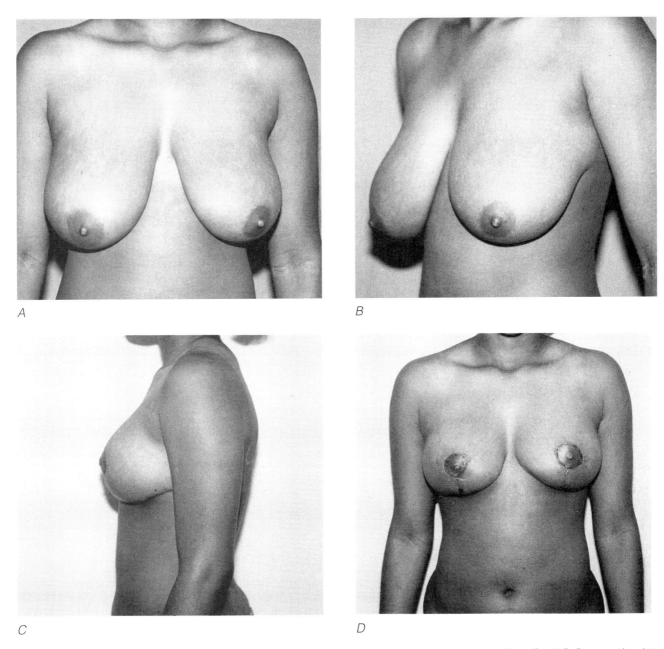

FIG. 43-66. *A* and *B.* Preoperative view of patient for breast reduction. *C* and *D.* Postoperative view after central pedicle technique.

that the nipple is repositioned superiorly and excess breast skin excised. Breast parenchyma is preserved and repositioned.

TRUNK

Chest Wall Defects. Defects of the chest wall have the potential to expose vital organs and compromise respiration. These defects may be seen after tumor extirpation or trauma, or as a result of radiation necrosis. A number of local flaps are available to close chest-wall defects. The pectoralis major muscle may be mobilized to cover defects of the anterior chest wall and sternum. The latissimus dorsi muscle, because of its length and wide arch of rotation, is available to cover most defects of

the back and anterolateral chest wall. The rectus abdominis muscle is frequently transposed into sternal defects. Because of its large surface area the greater omentum is available to resurface large areas of the anterior and lateral chest wall. This flap is particularly useful with extensive radiation injury.

Full-thickness defects of the chest wall may be reconstructed as a single stage with rib grafts or prosthetic materials used for skeletal reconstruction. Alloplastic materials used for skeletal reconstruction of the chest wall include Prolene mesh, Marlex Mesh Gore-Tex, and methyl methacrylate. Prosthetic materials, however, should not be used in radiated wounds.

Sternal Wounds. The infected sternal wound poses a particular challenge in chest-wall reconstruction. The overall infec-

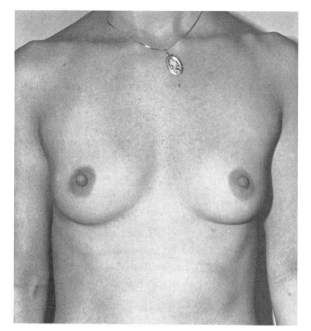

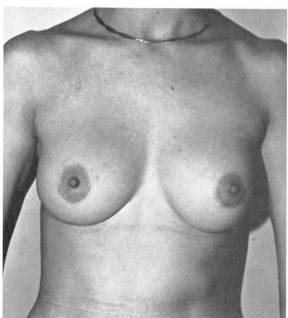

FIG. 43-67. *Augmentation mammaplasty. These breast implants were placed in a subpectoral position (preoperative, top; postoperative, bottom).*

median sternotomy wounds by debridement and closure with muscle flaps, usually in a single stage (Fig. 43-68). This technique has reduced mortality to less than 5 percent and decreased the length of hospitalization significantly. Muscle flaps available for closure of sternal wounds include the pectoralis major and the rectus abdominis muscles, and occasionally the latissimus dorsi muscles. The omentum also has been effectively used in the treatment of infected sternal wounds but requires a laparotomy.

Use of the internal mammary artery as a conduit for coronary artery bypass influences the treatment of sternal wound infections. Blood supply to the ipsilateral pectoralis and rectus mus-

tion rate after median sternotomy for coronary artery bypass procedures is generally reported to be less than 2 percent. Given the large number of these procedures performed annually, however, a significant number of infected sternal wounds require treatment. Historically, the infected sternal wound was treated by debridement and open packing. This yielded mortality rates as high as 50 to 70 percent and long hospitalizations. In the late 1960s and 1970s debridement and reclosure of the sternum over closed irrigation systems reduced the mortality rate of sternal wound infections to 20 percent. Jurkiewicz and associates reported in 1980 their experience with the treatment of infected

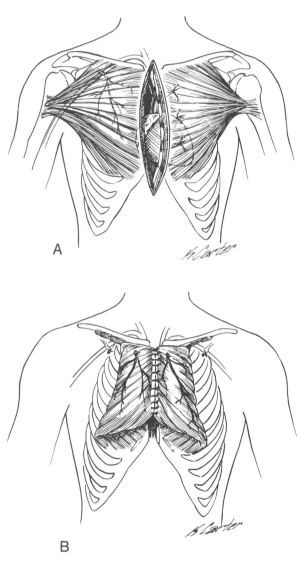

FIG. 43-68. *Pectoralis major muscle coverage of infected sternal wound. A. The infected sternal wound is debrided, exposing the mediastinal structures. The pectoralis major muscle receives blood from perforating branches of the internal mammary artery and from a branch of the thoracoacromial artery. The muscle can survive on either source alone. B. The pectoralis major muscles are separated from their humeral attachments, the thoracoacromial branches are divided, and the muscles are sutured to one another in the midline to cover the defect. Usually enough laxity is present in the chest wall skin to allow direct closure.*

cles are affected by internal mammary artery harvest. In these instances, most surgeons select a muscle flap contralateral to the internal mammary artery graft. More aggressive sternal debridement is usually required in these cases as the ipsilateral sternum is significantly devascularized by internal mammary artery harvest.

Back. Reconstruction of the back is typified by meningomyelocele closure. This variant of spina bifida requires early closure to prevent infection and preserve remaining neural function. These defects are usually closed with some combination of gluteus and latissimus dorsi myocutaneous flap advancement. The latissimus dorsi muscle may be transferred on its thoracodorsal pedicle or reversed and transposed into the defect based on paraspinal perforators. Tissue-expansion techniques have been useful in this disorder when time is not of the essence.

Pressure Sores. Unrelieved pressure over bony prominences results in tissue necrosis if the sustained pressure exceeds the arterial capillary pressure of 32 mmHg. These so-called pressure sores frequently follow spinal cord injuries. They also occur in patients subjected to prolonged anesthesia. *Decubitus ulcers* refer to pressure sores that develop when the patient is recumbent for long periods. These wounds typically occur at the sacrum, the back of the head, and the greater trochanters. Pressure sores that occur over the ischial tuberosities in a sitting patient therefore are not decubitus ulcers. A typical pressure sore involves a cavernous wound overlying a larger area of subcutaneous fat or muscle necrosis. When chronic, these wounds form large bursas lined with granulation tissue.

Small superficial sores may be treated with local care and avoidance of pressure. More extensive sores usually require flap coverage. Flap selection is individualized to the location of the event of recurrence. Sacral sores may be closed with a transverse back flap or gluteus myocutaneous units. Wounds over the ischial tuberosities are often closed with a gluteus myocutaneous flap, posterior thigh flap, or biceps femoris musculocutaneous flap (Fig. 43-69). The tensor fascia lata musculocutaneous flap is often the first choice for closure of greater trochanteric wounds. After flap closure of pressure sores patients are normally kept in air-fluidized or low-air-loss beds for 3 weeks. Mobilization is then begun and the wound carefully observed for any signs of breakdown. Positive nitrogen balance established preoperatively must be maintained in the postoperative period. Behavior patterns must be changed to avoid recurrence. Despite these efforts recurrence rate is high, and recurrence in the young patient with traumatic paraplegia is the rule rather than the exception.

Abdominal Wall. Flaps available for anterior abdominal wall reconstruction are limited. Superiorly or inferiorly based rectus abdominis muscle flaps can reach most of the anterior abdomen, but these muscles are frequently involved in the abdominal wall defect. The tensor fascia lata and rectus femoris muscle flaps may be rotated into the defects of the lower anterior abdomen. Particularly useful for closing wounds of the irradiated perineum are the gracilis muscle and portions of gluteus muscle, usually with overlying skin as musculocutaneous unit.

LOWER EXTREMITY

Difficult wounds of the lower extremity are usually seen in the setting of other disease states, including venous or arterial in-

sufficiency and diabetes. Patients with significant soft tissue defects over the tibia frequently require flap closure. These include patients with type III and IV open tibial fractures. Local gastrocnemius and soleus muscle flaps are preferred for proximal wounds when possible. Wounds of the distal one-third of the leg with exposed bone usually require free-tissue transfer. Posttraumatic chronic osteomyelitis of the tibia also usually requires debridement and muscle flap coverage. Cure rates higher than 90 percent are routinely reported for this difficult problem when muscle flaps are employed. Large defects of the tibia are frequently treated with free vascularized bone flaps. Segmental defects larger than 6 cm may be reconstructed by microsurgical transfer of fibula or iliac crest grafts. This technique typically yields success rates in the range of 80 to 90 percent.

Stasis Ulcers. Patients with venous stasis ulcers should be evaluated for treatment of their venous insufficiency. This may include ligation of incompetent perforators or venous bypass. The majority of patients are treated with compressive garments. Venous stasis ulcers that do not close with conservative care are usually excised and skin grafted. Local flaps are reserved for the most severe stasis ulcers. Free-tissue transfer has not been effective in the treatment of venous stasis ulcers.

Diabetic Ulcers. Recent advances have been made in the care of diabetic foot ulcers and limb salvage. A certain degree of fatalism has always existed concerning the care of diabetic foot ulcers, rooted in the misconception of "small-vessel disease." Historically, diabetic patients have been thought to develop occlusive disease at the level of the arteriole. The concept of small-vessel disease stems from postmortem studies demonstrating proliferative changes and hyaline deposition in vessels of diabetic patients. More recent prospective studies have failed to confirm these findings.

A large number of fasciocutaneous flaps have been described in the foot for closure of diabetic wounds. A number of small series have also reported success with free-tissue transfer for closure of large diabetic foot ulcers. The success of any reconstructive effort in the diabetic foot depends on a thorough vascular evaluation and bypass of flow-limiting lesions. Foot reconstruction may be performed at the time of revascularization. Free flaps have been performed at the time of distal revascularization, and theoretically they may improve patency of distal bypass grafts by providing additional outflow for the graft.

Lymphedema. *Lymphedema*, the abnormal collection of lymph in the interstitial space, is classified as *primary* when it occurs independently of other disease processes or surgery. Primary lymphedema is termed *lymphedema congenitum* when it is present at birth, *lymphedema praecox* when it occurs before the age of 35 years, and *lymphedema tardum* when it presents after the age of 35 years. *Secondary* lymphedema refers to lymphatic obstruction or ablation usually from malignancies, surgery, infection, or radiation.

Treatment of lymphedema is usually nonsurgical. The patient must be instructed to avoid even minor trauma to the extremity and to wear only well-fitting clothing and shoes. Elevation, when possible, and individually fitted compressive garments are the mainstay of treatment. In severe cases, surgical options are limited. Procedures involving skin flaps and skin grafts have been used since the early part of this century. Kondoleon in 1912 described the excision of deep muscle fascia beneath large skin

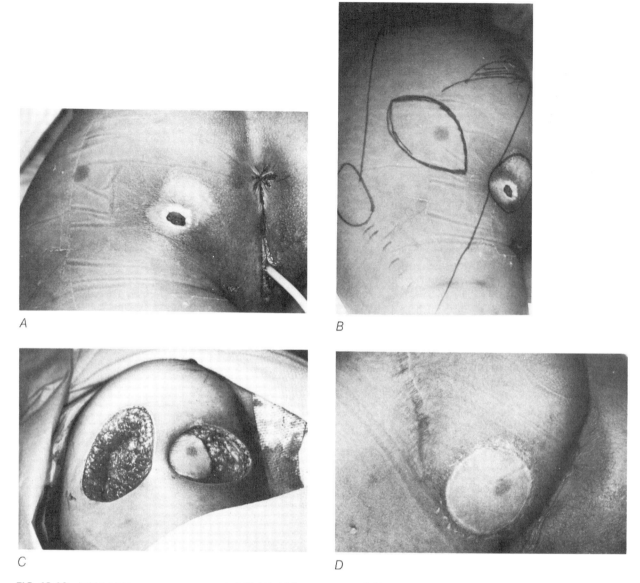

FIG. 43-69. *Ischial pressure sore management. A. Right ischial pressure sore. B. Gluteus maximus island musculocutaneous flap outlined. C. Sore debrided and flap interpolated. D. Wound healed 3 months postoperatively.*

flaps to facilitate lymphatic drainage directly into muscle tissue. This was largely unsuccessful and was modified by Sistrunk in 1918 to include staged subcutaneous excisions of edematous tissue beneath large skin flaps. Charles in 1912 described excision of skin and subcutaneous tissue with immediate regrafting of fascia and muscle of the limb with split- or full-thickness grafts. Full-thickness grafts generally provide a better result than split-thickness grafts, which tend toward unstable coverage, excessive scarring, and hyperkeratotic changes. The Charles technique, in the main, has been abandoned.

A number of procedures have been proposed to bypass or reconstruct the lymphatic system. These include dermal flaps buried in muscle, flaps of omentum placed subcutaneously in the lymphedematous extremity, demucosalized segments of ileum placed over lymph node basins, and microsurgical lymphaticovenous anastomoses. Clinical data and experience remain in-

adequate to demonstrate efficacy in these techniques. None of these procedures has gained widespread acceptance to date. Staged excision of the subcutaneous tissue and excess skin followed by rigorous adherence to use of pressure garments provide the best palliation.

AESTHETIC SURGERY

Facial Aging. Increased laxity of skin and subcutaneous tissues of the face is a normal part of aging. This typically presents as "bags" in the lower eyelids, the appearance of jowls along the jaw line, a deepened nasolabial fold, and excess skin and wrinkling in the face and neck. These changes can be treated effectively by surgical techniques to improve the appearance of the face.

The facelift, or *rhytidectomy*, is designed to excise excess skin and reposition the sagging soft tissue of the face (Fig. 43-70). The procedure may be performed under general or local anesthesia. The face and neck are infiltrated with 0.25% lidocaine with 1:400,000 epinephrine. The standard incision extends from a point in the temporal scalp approximately 6 cm superior to the root of the helix along the anterior margin of the ear around the lobe and along the posterior sulcus of the ear, terminating in hair-bearing scalp. In this manner all but a very fine scar anterior to the ear is hidden by hair-bearing scalp. The skin of the face and neck is then dissected from underlying muscles of facial expression.

A thin facial layer known as the superficial muscular aponeurotic system (SMAS) extends over the facial musculature and is contiguous with the platysma inferiorly and the frontalis muscle and temporal fascia superiorly. The SMAS may be dissected with the skin flap or as a separate layer and tightened by excising redundant SMAS or by plicating it to itself. Tightening the SMAS theoretically gives a more effective lift and longer-lasting results. Additional techniques include dissection in a deeper plane just superficial to the branches of the facial nerve as they exit the parotid gland, or in a subperiosteal plane. After excess SMAS and skin have been excised, the SMAS is sutured to fascia anterior to the ear and over the mastoid process. The skin is then closed. Drains may or may not be used. Ancillary techniques often used with the facelift procedure include suction-assisted lipectomy of the face, direct submental lipectomy through an incision beneath the chin, and tightening the platysma

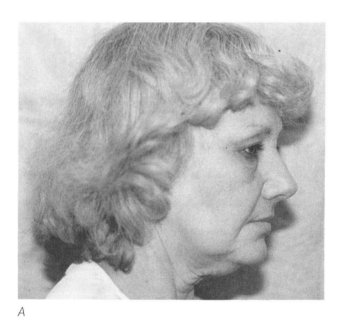

A

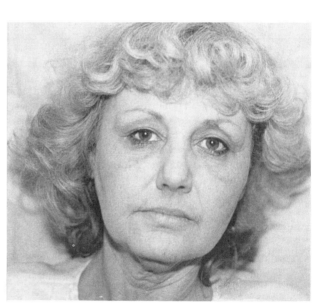

B

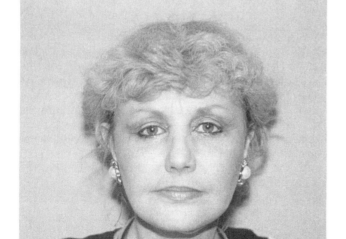

C

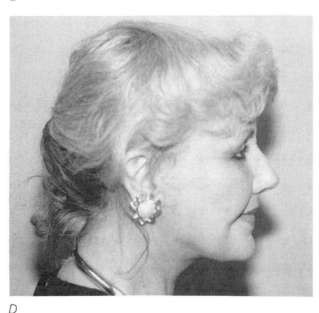

D

FIG. 43-70. *A* and *B*. Preoperative views of a patient with an aging face. *C* and *D*. Postoperative result of facelift and blepharoplasty.

by suturing it laterally or in the midline should there by any diastasis.

Care must be taken to preserve vascularity to the skin flaps. Delayed wound healing may be seen in the posterior auricular incision, especially in patients who smoke. Hematomas sometimes occur and may range from small collections that resolve spontaneously to large hematomas requiring surgical drainage. The overall rate of significant hematoma formation is approximately 4 percent. Facial nerve injury is rare, occurring in less than 1 percent of patients.

As in other surgical specialties, minimally invasive surgery is becoming a standard part of the plastic surgeon's repertoire. Most of the commonly used endoscopic plastic surgery procedures are in the realm of cosmetic surgery. The endoscopic brow lift is one of the most common such procedures. Where previously a coronal incision was used to access the brow musculature and excise lax scalp, now three endoscopic ports are made in the scalp in the temporal and frontal regions (Fig. 43-71). Through these ports the brow musculature can be altered, usually by resection of the corrugator and procerus muscles in the nasofrontal region.

Long-term results in endoscopic aesthetic surgery remain controversial. Difficulty in standardizing pre- and postoperative results contributes to the difficulty. Despite this, patient preference for the limited incision of endoscopic approaches makes the endoscopic brow lift a mainstay of aesthetic surgery.

The fine wrinkles seen in the perioral region are generally not improved by rhytidectomy. These wrinkles may be addressed, however, by dermabrasion or chemical peel. *Dermabrasion* is a technique employing a rotating abrasive cylinder on a hand-held power tool. With this instrument skin surface irregularities such as shallow acne scars and fine wrinkles are removed. Dermabraded skin heals as a superficial partial-thickness

burn. The wound is cared for in an open manner with antibiotic ointment. Pigmentation changes can occur, and it is important to avoid sunlight for several months after the procedure to diminish this risk. Phenol and trichloracetic acid have been used to induce a superficial chemical burn to the face. This technique, known as a *chemical face peel*, has also been used to treat fine wrinkles around the mouth and eyes. When performed by experienced practitioners, the complication rates in chemical face peels are very low. Hypertrophic scarring has been reported. Pigmentation changes are the most common complication.

Similarly, the CO_2 laser also may resurface the face by removing a portion of the epidermis and superficial dermis. Some surgeons feel that this is a more precise technique than dermabrasion or chemical peel.

Eyelid. Facial aging can result in laxity in the soft tissues of the eyelid. The patient may complain of "bags" under the eyes and with excessive upper eyelid skin may actually have the visual field reduced on superior gaze. These changes are the result of excessive eyelid skin, redundant festoons of orbicularis oculi muscle, and prominence of intraorbital fat. The technique of blepharoplasty attempts to restore the eyelids to a more youthful appearance. This technique involves some combination of skin removal and fat excision. Incisions for lower eyelid blepharoplasty may be transconjunctival if no skin excision is planned, or in a subciliary position, immediately below the lower eyelid lashes. The incision for an upper eyelid blepharoplasty is typically in the supratarsal skin fold. The overall complication rate of blepharoplasty is low. Excessive lower lid skin excision in the lower lid may result in ectropion, especially in the elderly patient with poor lower-lid tone. Excessive fat excision results in a sunken or hollow look to the eyes. Blindness, however rare, has been reported in the literature from retrobulbar hemorrhage.

Nasal Deformity. *Rhinoplasty* is undertaken to alter the form of the nose or the function of the nasal airway. Patient complaints frequently include a dorsal nasal hump, broad nasal tip, asymmetry of the tip or dorsum, and nasal airway obstruction. Rhinoplasty may be performed under general or local anesthesia with open or closed technique. An open rhinoplasty involves an incision in the skin at the base of the columella that is then carried inside the nose along the alar rim. Through this incision the skin of the columella and nasal tip is dissected away from the alar cartilages. The surgeon then may reduce or modify alar and tip cartilage under direct vision. Changes in the bony pyramid of the nose are made by using a small osteotome to rasp the dorsum (to reduce any nasal hump) and the infracture of the nasal bones arising from the maxillae (to narrow the nose). The closed technique employs incisions inside the nose near or within the alar cartilages. The surgeon then modifies the nasal cartilages or bony pyramid of the nose as desired (Fig. 43-72). Because the closed technique does not allow these changes to be made under direct vision (Fig. 43-73), many surgeons prefer the open technique for difficult problems of the nasal tip. If nasal airway obstruction is present, the surgeon may elect to resect or modify the nasal septum at the time of rhinoplasty. Excision of hypertrophic inferior turbinates may also improve the nasal airway.

Abdomen, Thighs, and Buttocks. Pregnancy, weight loss, and aging can result in redundancy of abdominal skin. *Abdominoplasty* involves direct excision of a lower abdominal el-

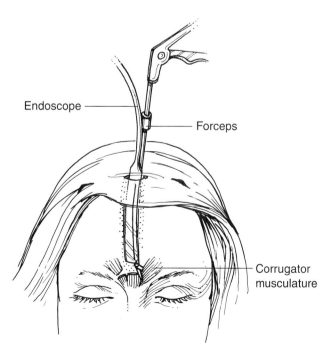

FIG. 43-71. Endoscopic brow lift.

Endoscope

Forceps

Corrugator musculature

lipse of skin to remove excesses of abdominal skin and fat (Fig. 43-74). The umbilicus is repositioned in the superior skin flap as it is advanced over the lower abdomen. If a diastasis recti or ventral hernia is present it may be repaired at the same time. This technique typically leaves an acceptable scar at the level of the pubis that may be concealed under clothing and swimwear.

The most common aesthetic complaint in the region of the abdomen, buttocks, and thighs is localized fat refractory to exercise and diet. For males this fat is typically found in the lower abdomen; females frequently complain of "saddlebags" of the lateral hips and thighs. Suction-assisted lipectomy has proved very helpful for these problems. Direct excision of the redundant skin of the buttocks and thighs is generally reserved for the patient who has undergone massive weight loss, as may be seen after gastric bypass for morbid obesity.

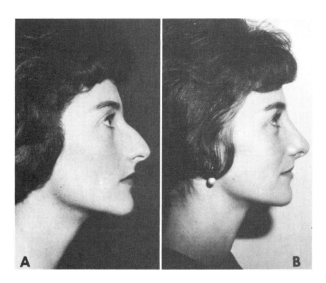

FIG. 43-72. *Aesthetic rhinoplasty. A. Preoperative photograph. B. Postoperative result.*

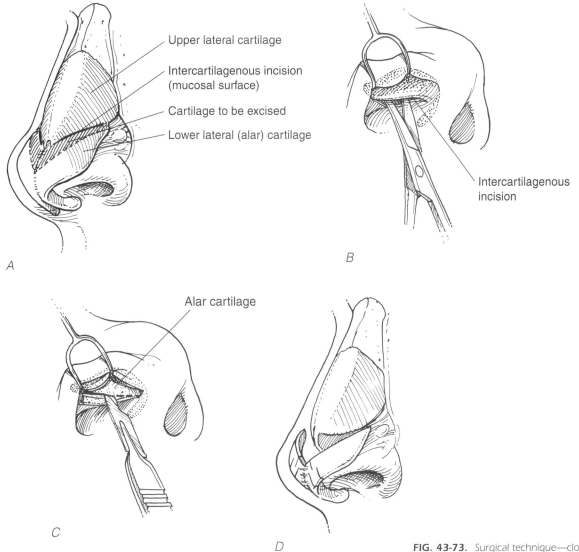

FIG. 43-73. *Surgical technique—closed rhinoplasty.*

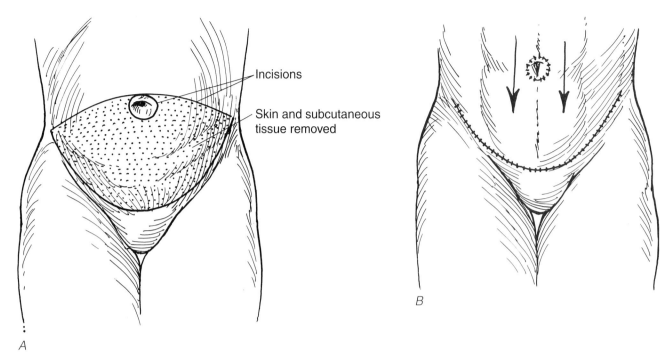

FIG. 43-74. Abdominoplasty. *A.* Excision of lower abdominal ellipse. *B.* Closure with repositioning of umbilicus.

Bibliography

General Principles

Acland RD: *Microsurgery Practice Manual,* St. Louis, CV Mosby, 1980.

American Replantation Mission to China: Replantation surgery in China. *Plast Reconstr Surg* 61:256, 1978.

American Society of Plastic and Reconstructive Surgeons, Ad Hoc Committee on New Procedures: *Commission on Surgical Suction Lipectomy,* Chicago, 1987.

Argenta LC, Marks MW, Pasyk KA: Advances in tissue expansion. *Clin Plast Surg* 12:159, 1985.

Bakamjian VY: A two-stage method for pharyngoesophageal reconstruction with a primary pectoral skin flap. *Plast Reconstr Surg* 36:173, 1965.

Barnett A, Berkowitz RL, et al: Comparison of synthetic adhesive moisture vapor permeable and fine mesh gauze dressings for split-thickness skin graft donor sites. *Am J Surg* 145:379, 1983.

Barton FE (ed): *Selected Readings in Plastic Surgery.* Dallas, University of Texas Southwestern Medical Center, 1992.

Bell E, Ehrlich HP, et al: Development and use of a living skin equivalent. *Plast Reconstr Surg* 67:386, 1981.

Borges AF: Dog-ear repair. *Plast Reconstr Surg* 69:707, 1982.

Davis JS: The story of plastic surgery. *Ann Surg* 113:641, 1941.

Douglas B, Weinberg H, et al: Beneficial effects of ibuprofen on experimental microvascular free flaps: Pharmacologic alteration of the no-reflow phenomenon. *Plast Reconstr Surg* 79:366, 1987.

Feller IA, Deweese MS: The use of stored cutaneous autografts in wound treatment. *Surgery* 44:450, 1958.

Hetter GP: Blood and fluid replacement for lipoplasty procedures. *Clin Plast Surg* 16:245, 1989.

Hoopes JE: Pedical flaps: An overview, in Krizek TJ, Hoopes JE (eds): *Symposium on Basic Science in Plastic Surgery,* vol 15, St. Louis, CV Mosby, 1976.

Hoopes JE, Su CT, Im MJ: Enzymatic responses to skin flap elevation following a delay procedure. *Plast Reconstr Surg* 66:369, 1980.

Hurwitz DJ, Swartz WM, Mathes SJ: The gluteal thigh flap: A reliable, sensate flap for the closure of buttock and perineal wounds. *Plast Reconstr Surg* 68:521, 1981.

Hutchinson J, Tough J, Wyburn G: Regeneration of sensation in grafted skin. *Br J Plast Surg* 2:82, 1949.

Ketchum LD: Pharmacologic alterations in the clotting mechanism: Use in microvascular surgery. *J Hand Surg* 3:407, 1978.

Kraissl CJ: The selection of appropriate lines for elective surgical incisions. *Plast Reconstr Surg* 8:1, 1951.

Magee C, Haury B, et al: A rapid technique for quantitating wound bacterial count. *Am J Surg* 133:760, 1977.

Manchot C: *Die Hautarteriern des Menschlichen Korpeus.* Leipzig, F.C.W. Vogel, 1889.

McCraw JB, Dibbel DG, Carraway JH: Clinical definition of independent myocutaneous vascular territories. *Plast Reconstr Surg* 60:341, 1977.

McGregor IA: The temporal flap in intraoral cancer: Its use in repairing the post-excisional defect. *Br J Plast Surg* 16:318, 1963.

McGregor IA, Jackson IT: The groin flap. *Br J Plast Surg* 25:3, 1972.

McGregor IA, Morgan G: Axial and random pattern flaps. *Br J Plast Surg* 26:202, 1973.

McLean DH, Buncke HJ: Autotransplant of omentum to a large scalp defect, with microsurgical revascularization. *Plast Reconstr Surg* 49:268, 1972.

Mathes SJ, Nahai F: *Clinical Atlas of Muscle and Musculocutaneous Flaps.* St. Louis, CV Mosby, 1979.

Matt RA, McKhann CF: Replantation of severed arms. *JAMA* 189:716, 1964.

Neumann CG: The expansion of an area of the skin by progressive distention of a subcutaneous balloon: Use of the method for securing skin for subtotal reconstruction of the ear. *Plast Reconstr Surg* 19:124, 1957.

Radovan C: Tissue expansion in soft-tissue reconstruction. *Plast Reconstr Surg* 74:482, 1984.

Rees TD, Wood-Smith D, et al: Composite grafts, in *Transactions of the Third International Congress of Plastic and Reconstructive Surgery*. Washington, DC, Excerpta Medica Foundation, 1963.

Russell RC, Roth AC, et al: Reperfusion injury and oxygen free radicals: A review. *J Reconstr Microsurg* 5:79, 1989.

Serafin D, Buncke HJ: *Microsurgical Composite Tissue Transplantation*. St. Louis, CV Mosby, 1979.

Shaw WW, Hidalgo DA: Anatomic basis of plantar flap design: Clinical application. *Plast Reconstr Surg* 78:637, 1986.

Shepard GH: The storage of split-thickness grafts on their donor sites. *Plast Reconstr Surg* 49:115, 1972.

Skiles MS, Chaglassian T: Simple geometric flap for closure of skin defects. *Surg Gynecol Obstet* 149:249, 1979.

Strauch B, Greenstein B, et al: Problems and complications encountered in replantation surgery. *Hand Clin* 2(2):389, 1986.

Stevenson TR, Mathes SJ: Management of foot injuries with free muscle flaps. *Plast Reconstr Surg* 78:665, 1986.

Tanner JC, Vandeput JJ, Olley JF: The mesh skin grafts. *Plast Reconstr Surg* 34:287, 1964.

Tolhurst DE, Haeseker B, Zeeman JJ: The development of the fascio-cutaneous flap and its clinical applications. *Plast Reconstr Surg* 71:597, 1983.

Vanderkolk CA, McCann JC, et al: Some further characteristics of expanded tissue. *Clin Plast Surg* 14(3):447, 1987.

Weiland AJ, Phillips JW, Randolph MA: Bone grafts: A radiologic, histologic, and biomechanical model comparing autografts, allografts, and free vascularized bone grafts. *Plast Reconstr Surg* 74:368, 1984.

Wood RJ, Adson MH, et al: Controlled expansion of peripheral nerves: Comparison of nerve grafting and nerve expansion/repair for canine sciatic nerve defects. *J Trauma* 31(5):686, 1991.

Wood RJ, Peltier GL, Templeman DC: The fat embolism syndrome: A new diagnostic and therapeutic dilemma for the plastic surgeon. *Lipoplasty* 6(1):23, 1989.

Wood RJ, Peltier GL, Twomey JA: Management of the difficult split-thickness donor site. *Ann Plast Surg* 22:80, 1989.

Young CMA: The revascularization of the pedicle skin flaps in pigs: A functional morphologic study. *Plast Reconstr Surg* 70:455, 1982.

Cleft Lip and Palate, Craniofacial Surgery

Bardach J, Morris HL, Olin WH: Late results of primary veloplasty: The Marburg Project. *Plast Reconstr Surg* 73:207, 1984.

Bartkowski SB, Kizystkowa KM: Blowout fracture of the orbit: Diagnostic and therapeutic considerations and results in 90 patients treated. *J Maxillofac Surg* 10:155, 1982.

Bell WH (ed): *Modern Practice in Orthognathic and Reconstructive Surgery*. Philadelphia, WB Saunders, 1992.

Brent B: Auricular repair with autogenous rib cartilage grafts: Two decades of experience with 600 cases. *Plast Reconstr Surg* 90(30):355, 1992.

Brent B: The correction of microtia with autogenous cartilage grafts. I. The classic deformity. *Plast Reconstr Surg* 66:1, 1980.

Brent B: The correction of microtia with autogenous cartilage grafts. II. Atypical and complex deformities. *Plast Reconstr Surg* 66:13, 1980.

Brent B, Byrd HS: Secondary ear reconstruction with cartilage grafts covered by axial, random, and free flaps of temporoparietal fascia. *Plast Reconstr Surg* 72:141, 1983.

Brent B, Upton J, et al: Experience with the temporoparietal fascial free flap. *Plast Reconstr Surg* 76:177, 1985.

David DJ, Sheen R: The surgical correction of Crouzon syndrome. *Plast Reconstr Surg* 85:344, 1990.

Fraser FC: The genetics of cleft lip and palate. *Am J Hum Genet* 22:336, 1970.

Furlow LT, Jr: Cleft palate repair by double opposing Z-plasty. Fourth International Congress on Cleft Palate and Related Craniofacial Anomalies, Acapulco, 1987.

Habib Z: Genetic counseling and genetics of cleft lip and cleft palate. *Obstet Gynecol Surg* 33:441, 1978.

Hagerty RF, Mylin WK: Facial growth and arch symmetry in the surgical prosthetic treatment of cleft lip and palate. *Plast Reconstr Surg* 68:682, 1981.

Hartel J, Kriens O, Kundt G: Incidence of cleft lip, alveolus and palate forms. *J Craniomaxillofac Surg* 19:144, 1991.

LeFort R: Etude expérimental sur les fractures de la mâchoire supérieure. *Rev Chir Paris* 23:201, 1901.

Marchac D, Renier D: *Craniofacial Surgery for Craniosynostosis*. Boston, Little, Brown, 1982.

Marchac D, Renier D: Treatment of craniosynostosis in infancy. *Clin Plast Surg* 14:61, 1987.

Masters FW, Levin JM: Surgical management of the palatal cleft by the V-Y technique (Wardhill-Kilner repair), in Georgiade WC (ed): *Symposium of Management of Cleft Lip and Palate and Associated Deformities*. St. Louis, CV Mosby, 1974.

McCarthy JG, Epstein F: Early surgery for craniofacial synostosis: An 8-year experience. *Plast Reconstr Surg* 73:521, 1984.

McComb H: Primary repair of the bilateral cleft lip nose: A 10-year review. *Plast Reconstr Surg* 77:701, 1986.

McComb H: Primary correction of unilateral cleft lip nasal deformity: A 10-year review. *Plast Reconstr Surg* 75:791, 1985.

McWilliams BJ, Glaser ER, et al: A comparative study of four methods of evaluating velopharyngeal adequacy. *Plast Reconstr Surg* 68:1, 1981.

Maue-Dickson W, Dickson DR: Anatomy and physiology related to cleft palate: Current research and clinical implications. *Plast Reconstr Surg* 65:83, 1980.

Millard DR: Refinements in rotation-advancement cleft lip technique. *Plast Reconstr Surg* 33:26, 1964.

Millard DR: Extensions of the rotation-advancement principle for wide unilateral cleft lips. *Plast Reconstr Surg* 42:535, 1968.

Millard DR, Latham RA: Improved primary surgical and dental treatment of clefts. *Plast Reconstr Surg* 86:856, 1990.

Moore MD: Complications of primary palatoplasty: A twenty-one year review. *Cleft Palate J* 25:156, 1988.

Mulliken JB: Principles and techniques of bilateral complete cleft lip repair. *Plast Reconstr Surg* 75:477, 1985.

Mustarde JC: The correction of prominent ears using mattress sutures. *Br J Plast Surg* 16:170, 1963.

Orticochea M: A review of 236 cleft palate patients treated with dynamic muscle sphincter. *Plast Reconstr Surg* 71:180, 1983.

Proffit WR, White RP: *Surgical-Orthodontic Treatment*. St. Louis, Mosby–Year Book, 1991.

Psillakis JM, Grotting JC, et al: Vascularized outer-table calvarial bone flaps. *Plast Reconstr Surg* 78:309, 1986.

Raulo Y: Treacher Collins syndrome: Analysis and principles of surgery, in Caronni EP (ed): *Craniofacial Surgery*. Boston, Little Brown, 1984.

Rohrich RJ, Byrd HS: Optimal timing of cleft palate closure. Speech, facial growth, and hearing considerations. *Clin Plast Surg* 17:27, 1990.

Stark RB: The pathogenesis of harelip and cleft palate. *Plast Reconstr Surg* 13:20, 1954.

Stenstrom SJ: A natural technique for correction of congenitally prominent ears. *Plast Reconstr Surg* 32:509, 1963.

Stenstrom SJ: A simple operation for prominent ears. *Acta Otolaryngol* 244(suppl):393, 1967.

Tessier P: The definitive plastic surgical treatment of severe facial deformities of craniofacial dysostosis. *Plast Reconstr Surg* 48:419, 1971.

Tessier P: Orbital hypertelorism. I. Successive surgical attempts. Material and methods. Causes and mechanisms. *Scand J Plast Reconstr Surg* 6:135, 1972.

Tessier P, Guiot J, Derome P: Orbital hypertelorism. II. Definitive treatment of orbital hypertelorism (Or.H.) by craniofacial or by extracranial osteotomies. *Scand J Plast Reconstr Surg* 7:39, 1973.

Trier WC, Breyer TM: Primary von Langenbeck palatoplasty with levator reconstruction: Rationale and technique. *Cleft Palate J* 21:254, 1984.

Zide B, Grayson B, McCarthy JG: Cephalometric analysis, Part I. *Plast Reconstr Surg* 68:816, 1981.

Zide B, Grayson B, McCarthy JG: Cephalometric analysis for upper and lower midface surgery, Part II. *Plast Reconstr Surg* 68:961, 1981.

Zide B, Grayson B, McCarthy JG: Cephalometric analysis for mandibular surgery, Part III. *Plast Reconstr Surg* 69:155, 1982.

Head and Neck Reconstruction

Arnold PG, Rangarathnam CS: Multiple-flap scalp reconstruction: Orticochea revisited. *Plastic Reconstr Surg* 69:605, 1982.

Carraway JH: Reconstruction of the eyelids and eyebrows and correction of ptosis of the eyelid, in Smith JW, Aston SJ (eds): *Grabb and Smith's Plastic Surgery*. Boston, Little, Brown, 1991.

Carraway JH, Vincent MP: Levator advancement technique for eyelid ptosis. *Plast Reconstr Surg* 77:394, 1986.

Converse JM, Smith B: Naso-orbital fractures and traumatic deformities of the medial canthus. *Plast Reconstr Surg* 38:147, 1966.

Cruse CW, Blevins K, Luce EA: Naso-ethmoid-orbital fractures. *J Trauma* 20:551, 1980.

Dingman RO, Natvig P: *Surgery of Facial Fractures*. Philadelphia, WB Saunders, 1964.

Duncan MJ, Manktelow RT, et al: Mandibular reconstruction in the radiated patient: The role of osteocutaneous free tissue transfer. *Plast Reconstr Surg* 76:829, 1985.

Furnas H, Lineaweaver WC, et al: Scalp reconstruction by microvascular free tissue transfer. *Ann Plast Surg* 24:431, 1990.

Gruss JS, Mackinnon SE: Complex maxillary fractures: Role of buttress reconstruction and immediate bone grafts. *Plast Reconstr Surg* 78:9, 1986.

Harii K, Ohmori K, Torii S: Free gracilis muscle transplantation with neurovascular anastomoses for the treatment of facial paralysis. *Plast Reconstr Surg* 57:133, 1976.

Hidalgo DA: Fibular free flap: A new method of mandible reconstruction. *Plast Reconstr Surg* 84:71, 1989.

Jones NF, Sekhar LN, Schramm VL: Free rectus abdominis muscle flap reconstruction of the middle and posterior cranial base. *Plast Reconstr Surg* 78:471, 1986.

Jones NF, Grivas A, et al: Studies on enophthalmos. II. The measurement of orbital injuries and their treatment by quantitative computed tomography. *Plast Reconstr Surg* 77:203, 1986.

Jones NF, Crawley WA, et al: Midface fractures: Advantages of immediate extended open reduction and bone grafting. *Plast Reconstr Surg* 76:1, 1985.

Kawamoto HK: Surgery of the jaws, in Lesavoy MA: *Reconstruction of the Head and Neck*. Baltimore, Williams and Wilkins, 1981.

Kazanjian VH, Converse JM: *The Surgical Treatment of Facial Injuries*. Baltimore, Williams and Wilkins, 1974.

LeFort R (Dr Paul Tessier, transl): Experimental study of fractures of the upper jaw, Parts I and II. *Plast Reconstr Surg* 50:497, 1972.

LeFort R: Experimental study of fractures of the upper jaw, Part III. *Plast Reconstr Surg* 50:600, 1972.

Leikensohn JR, Epstein LI, Vasconez LO: Superselective embolization and surgery of noninvoluting hemangiomas and A-V malformations. *Plast Reconstr Surg* 68:143, 1981.

Manktelow RT: Free muscle transplantation for facial paralysis, in Terzis JK (ed): *Microreconstruction of Nerve Injuries*. Philadelphia, WB Saunders, 1987.

Manson PN, Hoopes JE, Su CT: Structural pillars of the facial skeleton: An approach to the management of LeFort fractures. *Plast Reconstr Surg* 66:54, 1980.

McConnell FMS, Hester TR, et al: Free jejunal grafts for reconstruction of pharynx and cervical esophagus. *Arch Otolaryngol* 107:476, 1981.

McGregor IA: Reconstruction of the lower lip. *Br J Plast Surg* 36:40, 1983.

Mulliken JB, Glowacki J: Hemangiomas and vascular malformations in infants and children: A classification based on endothelial characteristics. *Plast Reconstr Surg* 69:412, 1982.

Ord RA, LeMay M, et al: Computerized tomography and B-scan ultrasonography in the diagnosis of fractures of the medial orbital wall. *Plast Reconstr Surg* 67:281, 1981.

Reuther JF, Steinau H, Wagner R: Reconstruction of large defects in the oropharynx with a revascularized intestinal graft: An experimental and clinical report. *Plast Reconstr Surg* 73:345, 1984.

Rubin LR, Lee GW, Simpson RL: Reanimation of the longstanding partial facial paralysis. *Plast Reconstr Surg* 77:41, 1986.

Schwartz WM, Banis JC, et al: The osteocutaneous scapular flap for mandibular and maxillary reconstruction. *Plast Reconstr Surg* 77:530, 1986.

Soutar DS, McGregor IA: The radial forearm flap in intra-oral reconstruction: The experience of 60 consecutive cases. *Plast Reconstr Surg* 78:1, 1986.

Upton J, Mulliken JB, et al: Restoration of facial contour using free vascularized omental transfer. *Plast Reconstr Surg* 66:560, 1980.

White CW: Treatment of hemangiomatosis with recombinant interferon-alfa. *Gen Hematol* 27:15, 1990.

Woods JE: Current management of squamous cell carcinoma of the oral cavity. *Plast Reconstr Surg* 69:361, 1982.

General Reconstruction, Trunk and Extremities

Angell M: Shattuck Lecture: Evaluating the health risks of breast implants: The interplay of medical science, the law, and public opinion. *New Engl J Med* 334(23):1513–1518, 1996.

Arnold PG, Irons G: The greater omentum: Extensions in transportation and free transfer. *Plast Reconstr Surg* 67:169, 1981.

Bostwick J: Breast reconstruction: A comprehensive approach. *Clin Plast Surg* 6:143, 1979.

Bostwick J: *Plastic and Reconstructive Surgery*, St. Louis, Quality Medical Publishing, 1990.

Bostwick J: Repairs in the lower abdomen, groin, or perineum with myocutaneous or omental flaps. *Plast Reconstr Surg* 63:186, 1979.

Bostwick J, Scheflan M: The latissimus dorsi musculocutaneous flap: A one-stage breast reconstruction. *Clin Plast Surg* 7:71, 1980.

Burget GC, Menick FJ: Nasal reconstruction: Seeking a fourth dimension. *Plast Reconstr Surg* 78:145, 1986.

Byrd HS, Cierny G, Tebbetts JB: The management of open tibial fractures with associated soft-tissue loss: External pin fixation with early flap coverage. *Plast Reconstr Surg* 68:73, 1981.

Carlson HE, Spicer TE, Cierny G: Management of open tibial fractures. *Plast Reconstr Surg* 76:719, 1985.

Colen LB: Limb salvage in the patient with severe peripheral vascular disease: The role of microsurgical free tissue transfer. *Plast Reconstr Surg* 79:389, 1987.

Constantian MB: *Pressure Ulcers: Principles and Techniques of Management*. Boston, Little, Brown, 1980.

Courtiss EH, Goldwyn RM: Reduction mammaplasty by the inferior pedicle technique. *Plast Reconstr Surg* 59:500, 1977.

Dingman RO, Argenta LC: Reconstruction of the chest wall. *Ann Thorac Surg* 32:202, 1982.

Dinner MI, Labandter HP, Dowden RV: The role of the rectus abdominis myocutaneous flap in breast reconstruction. *Plast Reconstr Surg* 69:209, 1982.

Ger R: Muscle transportation for treatment and prevention of chronic post-traumatic osteomyelitis of the tibia. *J Bone Joint Surg* 59A:784, 1977.

Gong-Kang H, Ru-Qi H, et al: Microlymphaticovenous anastomosis in the treatment of lower limb obstructive lymphedema: Analysis of 91 cases. *Plast Reconstr Surg* 76:671, 1985.

Goulian D: Dermal mastopexy. *Clin Plast Surg* 3:171, 1976.

Hartrampf CT, Scheflan M, Black PW: Breast reconstruction with a transverse abdominal island flap. *Plast Reconstr Surg* 69:216, 1982.

Hartrampf CT, Scheflan M, Bostwick J: The flexor digitorum brevis muscle island pedicle flap: A new dimension in heel reconstruction. *Plast Reconstr Surg* 66:264, 1980.

Hester TR, Cukcic J: Central breast pedicle and "free hand" technique for alteration of volume and skin envelope of the breast. *Clin Plast Surg* 15(4):613, 1988.

Hurteau JE, Bostwick J, et al: V-Y advancement of hamstring musculocutaneous flap for coverage of ischial pressure sores. *Plast Reconstr Surg* 68:539, 1981.

Jurkiewicz MJ, Bostwick J, et al: Infected median sternotomy wound. *Ann Surg* 191:738, 1980.

Kubayashi MR, Miller TA: Lymphedema. *Clin Plast Surg* 14:303, 1987.

Kernahan DA, Thomson HG, Bauer BS: *Symposium on Pediatric Plastic Surgery*. St. Louis, CV Mosby, 1982.

Larson DL, McMurtrey MJ: Musculocutaneous flap reconstruction of chest-wall defects: An experience with 50 patients. *Plast Reconstr Surg* 73:734, 1984.

Leighton WD, Johnson ML, Friedland JA: Use of the temporary soft-tissue expander in post-traumatic alopecia. *Plast Reconstr Surg* 77:737, 1986.

Leighton WD, Halls MJ, Simon SR: Free microvascular muscle flap with skin graft reconstruction of extensive defects of the foot: A clinical and gait analysis study. *Plast Reconstr Surg* 75:627, 1985.

May JW, Gallico GG, Lupash FN: Microvascular transfer of free tissue for closure of bone wounds of the distal lower extremity. *N Engl J Med* 306:253, 1982.

Mustarde JC, Jackson IT: *Plastic Surgery in Infancy and Childhood*. Edinburgh, Churchill-Livingstone, 1988.

Nahai F: Muscle and musculocutaneous flaps in gynecologic surgery. *Clin Obstet Gynecol* 24:1277, 1981.

Nahai F, Silverton JS, et al: The tensor fascia lata musculocutaneous flap. *Ann Plast Surg* 1:372, 1978.

Pendergrast WJ, Bostwick J, Jurkiewicz MJ: The subcutaneous mastectomy cripple: Surgical rehabilitation with the latissimus dorsi flap. *Plast Reconstr Surg* 66:554, 1980.

Regnault P: Breast ptosis. *Clin Plast Surg* 3:193, 1976.

Reiffel RS, McCarthy JG: Coverage of heel and sole defects: A new sub-fascial arterialized flap. *Plast Reconstr Surg* 66:250, 1980.

Robbins TH: A reduction mammaplasty with the areola-nipple based on an inferior dermal pedicle. *Plast Reconstr Surg* 59:64, 1977.

Russell RC, Pribaz J, et al: Functional evaluation of latissimus dorsi donor site. *Plast Reconstr Surg* 78:336, 1986.

Scheflan M, Nahai F, Bostwick J: Gluteus maximus island musculocutaneous flap for closure of sacral and ischial ulcers. *Plast Reconstr Surg* 68:533, 1981.

Schwartz WM, Mears DC: The role of free-tissue transfers in lower extremity reconstruction. *Plast Reconstr Surg* 76:364, 1985.

Stevenson TR, Rohrich RJ, et al: More experience with the "reverse" latissimus dorsi musculocutaneous flap: Precise location of blood supply. *Plast Reconstr Surg* 74:237, 1984.

Stone HH, Fabian TC, et al: Management of acute full-thickness losses of the abdominal wall. *Ann Surg* 193:612, 1981.

Turpin IM: The modern rhytidectomy. *Clin Plast Surg* 19(2):383–400, 1992.

Yaremchuk MJ, Brumback RJ, et al: Acute and definitive management of traumatic osteocutaneous defects of the lower extremity. *Plast Reconstr Surg* 80:1, 1987.

Aesthetic Surgery

Baker TJ: Patient selection and psychological evaluation. *Clin Plast Surg* 5:3, 1978.

Baker TJ, Gordon HL, Mosienko P: Rhytidectomy. *Plast Reconstr Surg* 59:24, 1977.

Baker TJ, Gordon HL, Mosienko P: Upper lid blepharoplasty. *Plast Reconstr Surg* 60:692, 1977.

Bostwick JB, Eaves FE, Nahai F (eds): *Endoscopic Plastic Surgery*. St. Louis, Quality Medical Publishing, 1995.

Castanares S: Blepharoplasty for herniated intraorbital fat. *Plast Reconstr Surg* 8:46, 1951.

Connell BF: Contouring the neck in rhytidectomy by lipectomy and a muscle sling. *Plast Reconstr Surg* 61:376, 1978.

Courtiss EH: *Male Aesthetic Surgery*. St. Louis, CV Mosby, 1982.

Courtiss EH: Suction lipectomy of the neck. *Plast Reconstr Surg* 76:882, 1985.

Courtiss EH: Suction lipectomy: A retrospective analysis of 100 patients. *Plast Reconstr Surg* 73:780, 1984.

Diamond HP: Rhinoplasty technique. *Surg Clin North Am* 51:317, 1971.

Dingman RO, Natvig P: The deviated nose. *Clin Plast Surg* 4:145, 1977.

Dingman RO, Natvig P: Surgical anatomy in aesthetic and corrective rhinoplasty. *Clin Plast Surg* 4:111, 1977.

Eaves FE, Price CI, Bostwick JB, et al: Subcutaneous endoscopic plastic surgery using a retractor-mounted endoscopic system. *Persp Plast Surg* 7(2):1–22, 1993.

Goldwyn RM: *Long-Term Results in Plastic Surgery*. Boston, Little, Brown, 1980.

Grazer RM, Klingbeil JR: *Body Image: A Surgical Prospective*, St. Louis, CV Mosby, 1980.

Guerrero-Santos J: The role of the platysma muscle in rhytidoplasty. *Clin Plast Surg* 5:39, 1978.

Hamra ST: Composite rhytidectomy. *Plast Reconstr Surg* 90(1):1, 1992.

Lemmon ML, Hamra ST: Skoog rhytidectomy: A five-year experience with 577 patients. *Plast Reconstr Surg* 65:283, 1980.

Meyer R, Kesselring UK: Sculpturing and reconstructive procedures in aesthetic and functional rhinoplasty. *Clin Plast Surg* 4:15, 1977.

Millard DR, Garst WP, et al: Submental and submandibular lipectomy in conjunction with a facelift, in the male or female. *Plast Reconstr Surg* 49:385, 1972.

Mitz V, Peyronie M: The superficial musculo-aponeurotic system (SMAS) in the parotid and cheek area. *Plast Reconstr Surg* 58:80, 1976.

Mosienko P, Baker TJ: Chemical peel. *Clin Plast Surg* 5:79, 1978.

Peek GC: *Techniques in Aesthetic Rhinoplasty*. Philadelphia, JB Lippincott, 1990.

Pitman GH, Teimourian B: Suction lipectomy: Complications and results by surgery. *Plast Reconstr Surg* 76:65, 1985.

Sheen JH: *Aesthetic Rhinoplasty*. St. Louis, CV Mosby, 1978.

Spira M: Lower blepharoplasty: A clinical study. *Plast Reconstr Surg* 59:35, 1977.

Spira M, Dahl C, et al: Chemosurgery: A histological study. *Plast Reconstr Surg* 45:247, 1970.

Stark RB: *Aesthetic Plastic Surgery*. Boston, Little, Brown, 1980.

Vinas JC, Caviglia C, Cortinas JL: Forehead rhytidoplasty and brow lifting. *Plast Reconstr Surg* 57:455, 1976.

CHAPTER 44

Minimally Invasive Surgery

John G. Hunter

HISTORICAL BACKGROUND

PHYSIOLOGY

GENERAL PRINCIPLES OF ACCESS

MINIMALLY INVASIVE GENERAL SURGICAL
    PROCEDURES

SPECIAL CONSIDERATIONS

Minimally invasive surgery describes an area of surgery that crosses all traditional disciplines, from ophthalmology to podiatric surgery. It is not a discipline unto itself but more a philosophy of surgery, a way of thinking. Minimally invasive surgery is to perform major operations through small incisions, often using miniaturized high-tech imaging systems, to minimize the trauma of surgical exposure. Some believe that *minimal access surgery* more accurately describes the small incisions generally necessary to gain access to surgical sites in high-tech surgery, but John Wickham's term *minimally invasive surgery* (MIS) is widely used because it describes the paradox of postmodern high-tech surgery, small holes, big operations—the "minimalness" of the access and the invasiveness of the procedures, captured in three words.

HISTORICAL BACKGROUND

While the term *minimally invasive surgery* is relatively recent, the history of its component parts is nearly a hundred years old. The newest and most popular variety of minimally invasive surgery, laparoscopy, is in fact the oldest. Primitive laparoscopy, placing a cystoscope within an inflated abdomen, was first performed by Kelling in 1901. Illumination of the abdomen required hot elements at the tip of the scope and was dangerous. In the late 1950s Hopkins described the rod lens, a method of transmitting light through a solid quartz rod with no heat and little light loss. Around the same time, thin quartz fibers were discovered to be capable of trapping light internally and conducting it around corners, opening the field of fiber optics and allowing the rapid development of flexible endoscopes. In the 1970s the application of flexible endoscopy grew faster than that of rigid endoscopy except in a few fields such as gynecology and orthopaedics. By the mid-1970s rigid and flexible endoscopes made a rapid transition from diagnostic instruments to therapeutic instruments. The explosion of video surgery in the past 10 years was a result of the development of compact high-resolution charge-couple devices, which could be mounted on the internal end of flexible endoscopes or to the external end of a Hopkins telescope. Coupled with bright light sources, fiber-optic cables, and high-resolution video monitors, the video endoscope has changed our understanding of surgical anatomy and changed the shape of surgical practice.

While optical imaging produced the majority of minimally invasive surgical procedures, other (traditionally radiologic) imaging technologies allowed the development of innovative procedures in the 1970s. Fluoroscopic imaging allowed the adoption of percutaneous vascular procedures, the most revolutionary of which was balloon angioplasty. Balloon-based procedures spread into all fields of medicine, assisting in a minimally invasive manner to open up clogged cylinders. Stents were then developed that were used in many disciplines to keep the newly ballooned segment open. The culmination of fluoroscopic balloon and stent proficiency is exemplified by the transvenous intrahepatic portosystemic shunt (TIPS) (Fig. 44-1).

Minimally invasive surgical procedures using ultrasound imaging have been limited to fairly crude exercises such as fragmenting kidney stones and freezing liver tumors because of the relatively low resolution of ultrasound devices. Newer, high-resolution ultrasound methods with high-frequency crystals may act as a guide while performing minimally invasive resections of individual layers of the intestinal wall.

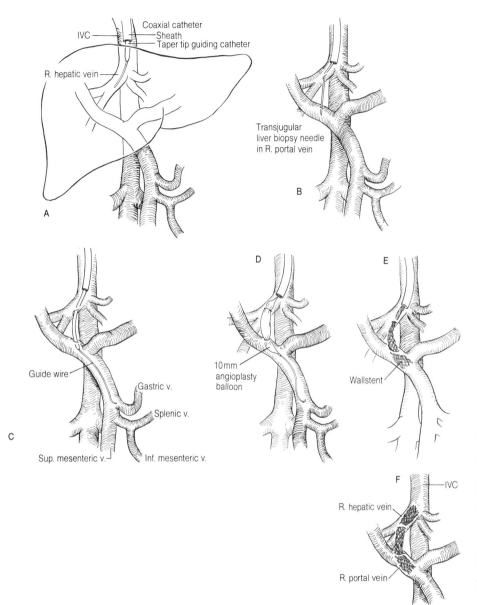

FIG. 44-1. With the transvenous intrahepatic portosystemic shunt (TIPS), percutaneous access to the superior vena cava is followed by the retrograde cannulation of the hepatic veins. Next a needle is advanced through the hepatic parenchyma until the portal venous radical is located. A guide wire is passed across this connection, and after dilation a metallic stent is expanded with a balloon. While not often performed by surgeons, TIPS represents a particularly creative example of minimally invasive surgery. (From: *Hunter JG, Sackier JM (eds): Minimally Invasive Surgery. New York, McGraw-Hill, 1993, chap 28, p 271.*)

Axial imaging, such as computed tomography (CT), has allowed the development of an area of minimally invasive surgery that is not often recognized because it requires only a CT scanner and a long needle. CT-guided drainage of abdominal fluid collections and percutaneous biopsy of abnormal tissues are minimally invasive means of performing procedures that previously required a celiotomy.

The most powerful noninvasive method of imaging that will allow the development of the least invasive—and potentially noninvasive—surgery is magnetic resonance imaging (MRI). MRI is an extremely valuable diagnostic tool, but it is only slowly coming to be of therapeutic value. One obstacle to the use of MRI for minimally invasive surgery is that image production and refreshment of the image as a procedure progresses are slow. Another is that all instrumentation must be nonmetallic when working with the powerful magnets of an MRI scanner. Moreover, MRI magnets are bulky and limit the surgeon's access to the patient. "Open magnets" have been developed that allow

the surgeon to stand between two large MRI coils, obtaining access to the portion of the patient being scanned. The advantage of MRI, in addition to the superb images produced, is that there is no radiation exposure to patient or surgeon. Some neurosurgeons are accumulating experience using MRI to perform frameless stereotactic surgery.

PHYSIOLOGY

With the least invasive of the minimally invasive surgical procedures no significant physiologic alterations occur. Many minimally invasive procedures require no sedation or minimal sedation, and there are few alterations to the cardiovascular, endocrinologic, or immunologic systems. The least invasive of such procedures include stereotactic biopsy of breast lesions and flexible gastrointestinal endoscopy. Minimally invasive procedures that require general anesthesia have a greater physiologic impact because of the anesthetic agent, the incision (even if small), and the induced pneumoperitoneum.

Laparoscopy. The unique feature of endoscopic surgery in the peritoneal cavity is the need to lift the abdominal wall from the abdominal organs. Two methods have been devised for achieving this. The first, used by most surgeons, is the induction of a pneumoperitoneum. Throughout the early twentieth century intraperitoneal visualization was achieved by inflating the abdominal cavity with air, using a sphygmomanometer bulb. The problem with using air insufflation is that nitrogen is poorly soluble in blood and is slowly absorbed across the peritoneal surfaces. Air pneumoperitoneum was believed to be more painful than nitrous oxide pneumoperitoneum. Subsequently, carbon dioxide and nitrous oxide were used for inflating the abdomen. N_2O had the advantage of being physiologically inert and rapidly absorbed. It also provided better analgesia for laparoscopy performed under local anesthesia when compared with CO_2 or air. The disadvantage of N_2O when compared to CO_2 was that it did not suppress combustion. CO_2 suppresses combustion and is rapidly absorbed and therefore is the preferred gas for laparoscopy (Fig. 44-2).

The physiologic effects of CO_2 pneumoperitoneum can be divided into two areas: (1) gas-specific effects and (2) pressure-specific effects. CO_2 is rapidly absorbed across the peritoneal membrane into the circulation. In the circulation, CO_2 creates a respiratory acidosis by the generation of carbonic acid. Body buffers, the largest reserve of which lies in bone, absorb CO_2 (up to 120 L) and minimize the development of hypercarbia or respiratory acidosis during brief endoscopic procedures. Once the body buffers are saturated, respiratory acidosis develops rapidly, and the respiratory system assumes the burden of keeping up with the absorption of CO_2 and its release from these buffers.

In patients with normal respiratory function this is not difficult; the anesthesiologist increases the ventilatory rate or vital capacity on the ventilator. If the respiratory rate required exceeds 20 breaths per minute there may be less efficient gas exchange and increasing hypercarbia. Conversely, if vital capacity is increased substantially there is a greater opportunity for barotrauma and greater respiratory-motion-induced disruption of the upper abdominal operative field. In some situations, it is advisable to evacuate the pneumoperitoneum or reduce the intraabdominal pressure to allow time for the anesthesiologist to adjust for hypercarbia. While mild respiratory acidosis probably is an insignificant problem, more severe respiratory acidosis leading to cardiac arrhythmias has been reported. Hypercarbia also causes tachycardia and increased systemic vascular resistance, which elevates blood pressure and increases myocardial oxygen demand.

The pressure effects of the pneumoperitoneum on cardiovascular physiology also have been studied. In the hypovolemic individual, excessive pressure on the inferior vena cava and a reverse Trendelenburg position with loss of lower-extremity muscle tone may cause decreased venous return and cardiac output. This is not seen in the normovolemic patient. The most common arrhythmia created by laparoscopy is bradycardia. A rapid stretch of the peritoneal membrane often causes a vagovagal response with bradycardia and, occasionally, hypotension. The appropriate management of this event is desufflation of the abdomen, administration of vagolytic agents (e.g., atropine), and adequate volume replacement.

With the increased intraabdominal pressure compressing the inferior vena cava, there is diminished venous return from the lower extremities. This has been well documented in the patient placed in the reverse Trendelenburg position for upper abdominal operations. Venous engorgement and decreased venous return promote venous thrombosis. Many series of advanced laparoscopic procedures in which deep venous thrombosis (DVT) prophylaxis was not used demonstrate the occurrence of pulmonary embolus. This usually is an avoidable complication with the use of sequential compression stockings, subcutaneous heparin, or low-molecular-weight heparin. In short-duration laparoscopic procedures, such as appendectomy, hernia repair, or cholecystectomy, the risk of DVT may not be sufficient to warrant extensive DVT prophylaxis.

The increased pressure of the pneumoperitoneum is transmitted directly across the paralyzed diaphragm to the thoracic cavity, creating increased central venous pressure and increased filling pressures of the right and left sides of the heart. If the intraabdominal pressures are kept under 20 mmHg, the cardiac output usually is well maintained. The direct effect of the pneumoperitoneum on increasing intrathoracic pressure increases peak inspiratory pressure, pressure across the chest wall, and also the likelihood of barotrauma. Despite these concerns, disruption of blebs and consequent pneumothoraces are rare after uncomplicated laparoscopic surgery.

Increased intraabdominal pressure decreases renal blood flow, glomerular filtration rate, and urine output. These effects may be mediated by direct pressure on the kidney and the renal vein. The secondary effect of decreased renal blood flow is to increase plasma renin release, thereby increasing sodium retention. Increased circulating antidiuretic hormone (ADH) levels also are found during the pneumoperitoneum, increasing free water reabsorption in the distal tubules. Although the effects of the pneumoperitoneum on renal blood flow are immediately reversible, the hormonally mediated changes, such as elevated ADH levels, decrease urine output for up to 1 h after the procedure has ended. Intraoperative oliguria is common during laparoscopy, but the urine output is not a reflection of intravascular volume status; intravenous fluid administration during an uncomplicated laparoscopic procedure should not be linked to urine output. Because fluid losses through the open abdomen are elim-

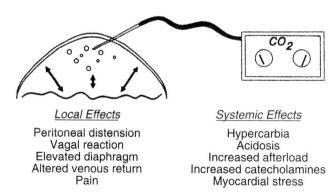

FIG. 44-2. Carbon dioxide gas insufflated into the peritoneal cavity has both local and systemic effects that cause a complex set of hemodynamic and metabolic alterations. (From: *Hunter JG (ed): Baillière's Clinical Gastroenterology: Laparoscopic Surgery, vol 7, 1993, p 758, with permission.*)

inated with laparoscopy, the need for supplemental fluid during a laparoscopic surgical procedure is rare.

The hemodynamic and metabolic consequences of pneumoperitoneum are well tolerated by healthy individuals for a prolonged period and by most individuals for at least a short period. Difficulties can occur when a patient with compromised cardiovascular function is subjected to a long laparoscopic procedure. It is during these procedures that alternative approaches should be considered or insufflation pressure reduced. Alternative gases that have been suggested for laparoscopy include the inert gases—helium, neon, and argon. These gases are appealing because they cause no metabolic effects, but they are poorly soluble in blood (unlike CO_2 and N_2O) and are prone to create gas emboli if the gas has direct access to the venous system. Gas emboli are rare but serious complications of laparoscopic surgery. They should be suspected if hypotension develops during insufflation. Diagnosis may be made by listening (with an esophageal stethoscope) for the characteristic "mill wheel" murmur. The treatment of gas embolism is to place the patient in a left lateral decubitus position with the head down to trap the gas in the apex of the right ventricle. A rapidly placed central venous catheter then can be used to aspirate the gas out of the right ventricle.

In some situations minimally invasive abdominal surgery should be performed without insufflation. This has led to the development of an abdominal lift device that can be placed through a 10- to 12-mm trocar at the umbilicus. These devices have the advantage of creating little physiologic derangement, but they are bulky and intrusive. The exposure and working room offered by lift devices also are inferior to those accomplished by pneumoperitoneum. Lifting the anterior abdominal wall causes a "pinching in" of the lateral flank walls, displacing the bowel medially and anteriorly into the operative field. A pneumoperitoneum, by its well-distributed intraabdominal pressure, provides better exposure. Abdominal lift devices also cause more postoperative pain, but they do allow the performance of minimally invasive surgery with standard (nonlaparoscopic) surgical instruments.

Early it was predicted that the surgical stress response would be significantly lessened with laparoscopic surgery, but this is not always the case. Serum cortisol levels after laparoscopic operations are often higher than after the equivalent operation performed in through an open incision. In terms of endocrine balance, the greatest difference between open and laparoscopic surgery is the more rapid equilibration of most stress-mediated hormone levels after laparoscopic surgery. Immune suppression also is less after laparoscopy than after open surgery. There is a trend toward more rapid normalization of cytokine levels after a laparoscopic procedure than after the equivalent procedure performed by celiotomy.

Thoracoscopy. The physiology of thoracic minimally invasive surgery (thoracoscopy) is different from that of laparoscopy. Because of the bony confines of the thorax it is unnecessary to use positive pressure when working in the thorax. The disadvantages of positive pressure in the chest include decreased venous return, mediastinal shift, and the need to keep a firm seal at all trocar sites. Without positive pressure, it is necessary to place a double-lumen endotracheal tube so that the ipsilateral lung can be deflated when the operation starts. By collapsing the ipsilateral lung, working space within the thorax is obtained.

Extracavitary Minimally Invasive Surgery. Many new minimally invasive surgical procedures are creating working spaces in extrathoracic and extraperitoneal locations. Laparoscopic inguinal hernia repair usually is performed in the anterior extraperitoneal Retzius space. Laparoscopic nephrectomy often is performed with retroperitoneal laparoscopy. Lower extremity vascular procedures and plastic surgical endoscopic procedures require the development of working space in unconventional planes, often at the level of the fascia, sometimes below the fascia, and occasionally in nonanatomic regions. Some of these techniques use insufflation of gas, but many use balloon inflation to develop the space followed by low-pressure gas insufflation or lift devices to maintain the space (Fig. 44-3). These techniques produce fewer and less severe adverse physiologic consequences than does the pneumoperitoneum, but the insufflation of gas into extraperitoneal locations can spread widely, causing subcutaneous emphysema and metabolic acidosis.

Anesthesia. The most important factors in appropriate anesthesia management are related to CO_2 pneumoperitoneum. The laparoscopic surgeon can influence cardiovascular performance by releasing intraabdominal retraction and dropping the pneumoperitoneum. Insensible fluid losses are negligible, and therefore intravenous fluid administration should not exceed a maintenance rate. Minimally invasive surgical procedures usually are outpatient procedures, and short-acting anesthetic agents are preferable. Because the factors that require hospitalization after laparoscopic procedures include the management of nausea, pain, and urinary retention, the anesthesiologist should minimize the use of agents that provoke these conditions and maximize the use of medications that prevent such problems. Critical to the anesthesia management of these patients is the use of nonnarcotic analgesics (e.g., ketorolac) and the liberal use of antiemetic agents.

GENERAL PRINCIPLES OF ACCESS

The most natural ports of access for minimally invasive surgery are the anatomic portals of entry and exit. The nares, mouth, urethra, and anus are used to access the respiratory, gastrointestinal, and urinary systems. The advantage of using these points of access is that no incision is required. The disadvantages lie in the long distances between the orifice and the region of interest.

Access to the vascular system may be accomplished under local anesthesia by "cutting down" and exposing the desired vessel, usually in the groin. Increasingly, vascular access is obtained with percutaneous techniques using a small incision, a needle, and a guide wire, over which are passed a variety of different-sized access devices. This approach, known as the Seldinger technique, is most frequently used by general surgeons for placement of Hickman catheters but also is used to gain access to the arterial and venous system for performance of minimally invasive procedures. Guide-wire-assisted, Seldinger-type techniques also are helpful for gaining access to the gut for procedures such as percutaneous endoscopic gastrostomy, for gaining access to the biliary system through the liver, and for gaining access to the upper urinary tract.

In thoracoscopic surgery, the access technique is similar to that used for placement of a chest tube. In these procedures general anesthesia and split-lung ventilation are essential. A

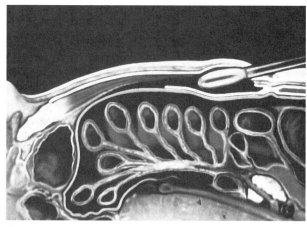

A

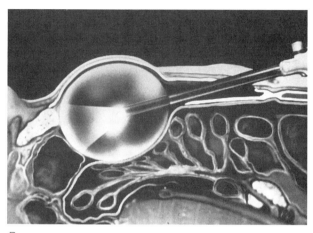

B

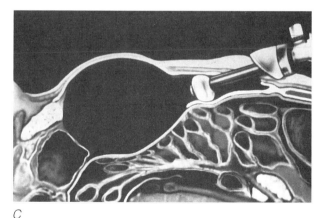

C

FIG. 44-3. *Balloons are used to create extraanatomic working spaces. In this example a balloon is introduced into the space between the posterior rectus sheath and the rectus abdominis muscle. The balloon is inflated in the preperitoneal space to create working room for extraperitoneal endoscopic hernia repair.*

small incision is made over the top of a rib and, under direct vision, carried down through the pleura. The lung is collapsed, and a plastic trocar is inserted across the chest wall to allow access with a telescope. Once the lung is completely collapsed, subsequent access may be performed with direct puncture, view-

ing all entry sites through the videoendoscope. Because insufflation of the chest is unnecessary, simple plastic sheaths that keep the small incisions open are all that is required to allow repeated access to the thorax.

The requirements for laparoscopy are more involved, because the creation of a pneumoperitoneum requires that instruments of access (trocars) contain a valve to maintain abdominal inflation. Two methods are used for establishing abdominal access during laparoscopic procedures. The first, direct puncture laparoscopy, begins with the elevation of the relaxed abdominal wall with two towel clips or a well-placed hand. A small incision is made in the umbilicus, and a specialized spring-loaded (Veress) needle is placed in the abdominal cavity (Fig. 44-4). With the Veress needle, two distinct pops are felt as the surgeon passes the needle through the abdominal wall fascia and the peritoneum. The umbilicus usually is selected as the preferred point of access because in this location the abdominal wall is quite thin, even in obese patients. The abdomen is inflated with a pressure-limited insufflator. CO_2 gas usually is used with maximal pressures in the range of 14 to 15 mmHg. Laparoscopic surgery can be performed under local anesthesia, but general anesthesia is preferable. Under local anesthesia, N_2O is used as the insufflating agent and insufflation is stopped after 2 L of gas is insufflated or when a pressure of 10 mmHg is reached.

After peritoneal insufflation, direct access to the abdomen is obtained with a 5- or 10-mm trocar. The critical issues for safe direct-puncture laparoscopy include the use of a vented stylet for the trocar or a trocar with a safety shield. The trocar must be pointed away from the sacral promontory and the great vessels. For performance of laparoscopic cholecystectomy, the trocar is angled toward the right upper quadrant.

Occasionally the direct peritoneal access (Hasson) technique is advisable. With this technique, the surgeon makes a small incision just below the umbilicus and under direct vision locates the abdominal fascia. Two Kocher clamps are placed on the fascia, and with a curved Mayo scissors a small incision is made through the fascia and underlying peritoneum. A finger is placed into the abdomen to make sure that there is no adherent bowel. A sturdy suture is placed on each side of the fascia and secured to the wings of a specialized trocar, which is then passed directly into the abdominal cavity (Fig. 44-5). Rapid insufflation can

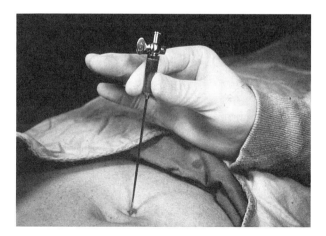

FIG. 44-4. *Insufflation of the abdomen is accomplished with a Veress needle held at its serrated collar with a thumb and forefinger.*

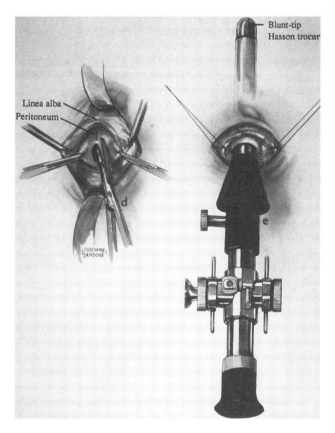

FIG. 44-5. *The open laparoscopy technique involves identification and incision of the peritoneum, followed by the placement of a specialized trocar with a conical sleeve to maintain a gas seal. Specialized wings on the trocar are attached to sutures placed through the fascia to prevent loss of the gas seal.*

make up for some of the time lost with the initial dissection. This technique is preferable for the abdomen of patients who have undergone previous operations, in which small bowel may be adherent to the undersurface of the abdominal wound. The close adherence of bowel to the peritoneum in the previously operated abdomen does not eliminate the possibility of intestinal injury but should make great vessel injury extremely unlikely. Because of the difficulties in visualizing the abdominal region immediately adjacent to the primary trocar, it is recommended that the telescope be passed through a secondary trocar in order to inspect the site of initial abdominal access. This examination usually is performed at the end of the operative procedure.

Secondary punctures are made with 5- and 10-mm trocars. For safe access to the abdominal cavity, it is critical to visualize all sites of trocar entry. At the completion of the operation, all trocars are removed under direct vision and the insertion sites are inspected for bleeding. If bleeding occurs, direct pressure with an instrument from another trocar site or balloon tamponade with a Foley catheter placed through the trocar site generally stops the bleeding within 3 to 5 min. When this is not successful, a full-thickness abdominal wall suture has been used successfully to tamponade trocar site bleeding.

It is generally agreed that 5-mm trocars need no site suturing. Ten-millimeter trocars placed off the midline and above the transverse mesocolon do not require repair. Conversely, if the fascia has been dilated to allow the passage of the gallbladder,

all midline 10-mm trocar sites should be repaired at the fascial level with interrupted sutures. Specialized suture delivery systems similar to crochet needles have been developed for mass closure of the abdominal wall in obese patients, in whom it is difficult through a small skin incision to visualize the fascia. Failure to close lower abdominal trocar sites that are 10 mm in diameter or larger can lead an incarcerated hernia.

Access for Subcutaneous and Extraperitoneal Surgery. There are two methods for gaining access to nonanatomic spaces. For retroperitoneal locations, balloon dissection is effective. This access technique is appropriate for the extraperitoneal repair of inguinal hernias and for retroperitoneal surgery for adrenalectomy, nephrectomy, lumbar discectomy, or para-aortic lymph node dissection. The initial access to the extraperitoneal space is performed in a way similar to direct puncture laparoscopy except that the last layer (the peritoneum) is not traversed. Once the transversalis fascia has been punctured, a specialized trocar with a balloon on the end is introduced. The balloon is inflated in the extraperitoneal space to create a working chamber. The balloon then is deflated, and a Hasson trocar is placed. An insufflation pressure of 10 mmHg usually is adequate to keep the extraperitoneal space open for dissection. Higher gas pressures force CO_2 into the soft tissues and may contribute to hypercarbia. Extraperitoneal endosurgery provides less working space than laparoscopy but eliminates the possibility of intestinal injury, intestinal adhesion, herniation at the trocar sites, and ileus. These issues are important for laparoscopic hernia repair because extraperitoneal approaches protect the small bowel from sticking to the prosthetic mesh.

Subcutaneous surgery, the newest method of access in minimally invasive surgery, uses the creation of working room in nonanatomic spaces. This technique has been most widely used in cardiac, vascular, and plastic surgery. In cardiac surgery, subcutaneous access has been used for saphenous vein harvesting, and in vascular surgery for ligation of subfascial perforating veins (Linton procedure). With minimally invasive techniques the entire saphenous vein above the knee may be harvested through a single incision (Fig. 44-6). Once the saphenous vein is located, a long retractor that holds a 5-mm laparoscope allows the coaxial dissection of the vein and coagulation or clipping of each side branch. A small incision above the knee also can be used to ligate perforating veins in the lower leg.

Subcutaneous access also is used for plastic surgical procedures. Minimally invasive approaches are especially well suited to cosmetic surgery, in which attempts are made to hide the incision. It is easier to hide several 5-mm incisions than one long incision. The technique of blunt dissection along fascial planes combined with lighted retractors and endoscope holding retractors is most successful for extensive subcutaneous surgery. Some prefer gas insufflation of these soft tissue planes. The primary disadvantage of soft tissue insufflation is that subcutaneous emphysema can be created.

Imaging Systems. Two methods of video imaging are widely used. The first of these is flexible video endoscopy. With flexible video endoscopy, a charge-couple device (CCD) is placed on the internal end of a long flexible endoscope. In the second method, thin quartz fibers are packed together in a bundle, and the CCD camera is mounted on the external end of the endoscope. Most standard gastrointestinal endoscopes have the CCD chip at the distal end, but small, delicate choledochoscopes

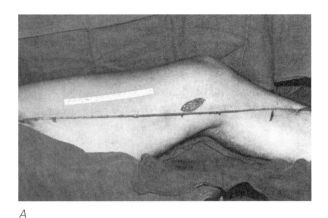

A

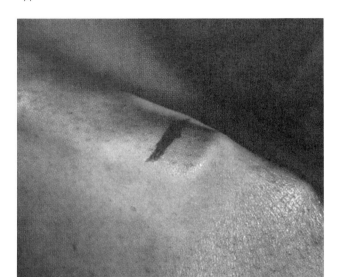

B

FIG. 44-6. *A.* With two small incisions virtually the entire saphenous vein can be harvested for bypass grafting. *B.* The lighted retractor in the subcutaneous space during saphenous vein harvest is seen illuminating the skin. (From: *Bostwick J III, Eaves F III, Nahai F: Endoscopic Plastic Surgery. St Louis, Quality Medical Publishers, 1995, p 542, with permission.*)

and nephroscopes are equipped with fiberoptic bundles. Distally mounted CCD chips were developed for laparoscopy but are unpopular.

Imaging for laparoscopy, thoracoscopy, and subcutaneous surgery uses a rigid metal telescope, usually 30 cm in length. This telescope contains a series of quartz optical rods with differing optical characteristics that provide a specific "character" to each telescope (Fig. 44-7). These metal telescopes vary in size from 2 to 10 mm in diameter. Since light transmission is dependent on the cross-sectional area of the quartz rod, when the diameter of a rod/lens system is doubled, the illumination is quadrupled. Little illumination is needed in highly reflective small spaces such as the knee, and a very small telescope will suffice. When working in the abdominal cavity, especially if blood is present, the full illumination of a 10-mm telescope usually is necessary.

Rigid telescopes may have a flat or angled end. The flat end provides a straight view (0 degrees), and the angled end provides an oblique view (30 or 45 degrees). Angled scopes allow greater flexibility in viewing a wider operative field through a single trocar site; rotating an angled telescope changes the field of view. The use of an angled telescope has distinct advantages for most videoendoscopic procedures, particularly in visualizing the common bile duct during laparoscopic cholecystectomy or visualizing the posterior esophagus or the tip of the spleen during laparoscopic fundoplication.

Light is delivered to the endoscope through a fiberoptic light cable. These light cables are highly inefficient, losing more than 90 percent of the light delivered from the light source. Extremely bright light sources (300 watts) are necessary to provide adequate illumination for video endosurgery.

Video cameras come in two basic designs. The one-chip camera has a black-and-white video chip that has an internal processor capable of converting gray scales to approximate colors. Perfect color representation is not possible with a one-chip camera, but perfect color representation is rarely necessary for endosurgery. The most accurate color representation is obtained using a three-chip video camera. A three-chip camera has red, green, and blue (RGB) input and is identical to the color cameras used for television production. RGB imaging provides the highest fidelity but is probably not necessary for everyday use. An additional feature of new video cameras is digital enhancement.

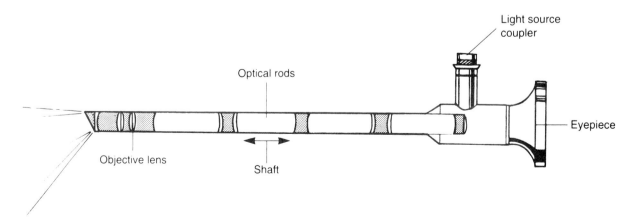

FIG. 44-7. The Hopkins rod lens telescope includes a series of optical rods that effectively transmit light to the eyepiece. The video camera is placed on the eyepiece to provide the working image.

Digital enhancement detects edges, areas where there are drastic color or light changes between two adjacent pixels. By enhancing this difference, the image appears sharper and surgical resolution is improved. Digital enhancement is available on one- and three-chip cameras. Priorities in a video system for minimally invasive surgery are illumination first, resolution second, and color third. Without the first two attributes, video surgery is unsafe.

There has been a recent interest in three-dimensional endoscopy. Three-dimensional laparoscopy provides the additional depth of field that is lost with 2-D endosurgery and allows greater facility for novice laparoscopists performing complex tasks of dexterity, including suturing and knot tying. The advantages of 3-D systems are less obvious to experienced laparoscopists. Additionally, because 3-D systems require the flickering of two similar images, which are resolved with special glasses, the image edges become fuzzy and resolution is lost. The optical accommodation necessary to rectify these slightly differing images negates any advantage offered by the additional depth of field.

Energy Sources for Endoscopic Surgery. Minimally invasive surgery uses conventional energy sources, but the requirement of bloodless surgery to maintain optimal visualization has spawned new ways of applying energy. The most common energy source is radio frequency (RF) electrosurgery using an alternating current with a frequency of 500,000 cycles/s (Hz). Tissue heating progresses through the well-known phases of coagulation (60°C), vaporization and desiccation (100°C), and carbonization (>200°C).

The two most common methods of delivering RF electrosurgery are with monopolar and bipolar electrodes. With monopolar electrosurgery a remote ground plate on the patient's leg or back receives the flow of electrons that originate at a point source, the surgical electrode. A fine-tipped electrode causes a high current density at the site of application and rapid tissue heating. Monopolar electrosurgery is inexpensive and easy to modulate to achieve different tissue effects. A short-duration, high-voltage discharge of current (coagulation current) provides extremely rapid tissue heating. Lower-voltage, higher-wattage current (cutting current) is better for tissue desiccation and vaporization. When the surgeon desires tissue division with the least amount of thermal injury and least coagulation necrosis, a cutting current is used.

With bipolar electrosurgery, the electrons flow between two adjacent electrodes. The tissue between the two electrodes is heated and desiccated. There is little opportunity for tissue cutting when bipolar current is used, but the ability to coapt the electrodes across a vessel provides the best method of small-vessel coagulation without thermal injury to adjacent tissues.

Another method of delivering radio frequency electrosurgery is argon beam coagulation. This is a type of monopolar electrosurgery in which a uniform field of electrons is distributed across a tissue surface by the use of a jet of argon gas. The argon gas jet distributes electrons more evenly across the surface than does spray electrofulguration. This technology has its greatest application for coagulation of diffusely bleeding surfaces, such as the cut edge of liver or spleen. It is of less use in laparoscopic procedures because the increased intraabdominal pressures created by the argon gas jet can increase the chances of a gas embolus.

Gas, liquid, and solid-state lasers have been available for medical application since the mid-1960s. The CO_2 laser (wavelength 10.6 μm) is most appropriately used for cutting and superficial ablation of tissues. It is most helpful in locations unreachable with a scalpel, such as excision of vocal cord granulomas. The CO_2 laser beam must be delivered with a series of mirrors and is therefore somewhat cumbersome to use. The next most popular laser is the neodymium:yttrium-aluminum-garnet (Nd:YAG) laser. Nd:YAG laser light is 1.064 μm (1064 nm) in wavelength. It is in the near-infrared portion of the spectrum and, like the CO_2 laser, is invisible to the naked eye. A unique feature of the Nd:YAG laser is that 1064-nm light is poorly absorbed by most tissue pigments and therefore travels deep into tissue. Deep tissue penetration provides deep tissue heating (Fig. 44-8). For this reason the Nd:YAG laser is capable of the greatest amount of tissue destruction with a single application. Such capabilities make it the ideal laser for destruction of large fungating tumors of the rectosigmoid or tracheobronchial tree. A disadvantage is that the deep tissue heating may cause perforation of a hollow viscus.

When it is desirable to coagulate flat lesions in the cecum, a different laser should be chosen. The frequency-doubled Nd:YAG laser, also known as the KTP laser (potassium thionyl phosphate crystal is used to double the Nd:YAG frequency), provides 532-nm light. This is in the green portion of the spectrum; at this wavelength, selective absorption by red pigments in tissue (such as hemangiomas and arteriovenous malformations) is optimal. The depth of tissue heating is intermediate between those of the CO_2 and the Nd:YAG lasers. Coagulation (without vaporization) of superficial vascular lesions can be obtained without intestinal perforation.

In flexible gastrointestinal endoscopy, the CO_2 and Nd:YAG lasers have largely been replaced by heater probes and endoluminal stents. The heater probe is a metal ball that is heated to a

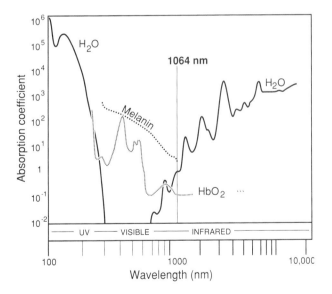

FIG. 44-8. This graph shows the absorption of light by various tissue compounds (water, melanin, and oxyhemoglobin) as a function of the wavelength of the light. The nadir of the oxyhemoglobin and melanin curves is close to 1064 nm, the wavelength of the Nd:YAG laser. (From: Hunter JG, Sackier JM (eds): Minimally Invasive Surgery. New York, McGraw-Hill, 1993, chap 4, p 28.)

temperature (60 to 100°C) that allows coagulation of bleeding lesions without perforation.

A unique application of laser technology provides extremely rapid discharge ($<10^{-6}$ seconds) of large amounts of energy ($>10^3$ volts). These high-energy lasers, of which the pulsed dye laser has seen the most clinical use, allow the conversion of light energy to mechanical disruptive energy in the form of a shock wave. Such energy can be delivered through a quartz fiber and, with rapid repetitive discharges, can provide sufficient shock-wave energy to fragment kidney stones and gallstones. Shock waves also may be created with miniature electric spark-plug discharge systems, known as electrohydraulic lithotriptors. These devices also are inserted through thin probes for endoscopic application. Lasers have the advantage of pigment selectivity, but electrohydraulic lithotriptors are more popular because they are substantially less expensive and are more compact.

Methods of producing shock waves or heat with ultrasonic energy also is of interest. Extracorporeal shockwave lithotripsy creates focused shock waves that intensify as the focal point of the discharge is approached. When the focal point is within the body, large amounts of energy are capable of fragmenting stones. Slightly different configurations of this energy can be used to provide focused internal heating of tissues. Potential applications of this technology include the ability noninvasively to produce sufficient internal heating to destroy tissue without an incision.

A third means of using ultrasonic energy is to create rapidly oscillating instruments that are capable of heating tissue with friction; this technology represents a major step forward in energy technology. An example of its application is the laparoscopic coagulation shears (LCS) device (Harmonic Scalpel), which is capable of coagulating and dividing blood vessels by first occluding them and then providing sufficient heat to weld the blood vessel walls together and to divide the vessel. This nonelectric method of coagulating and dividing tissue with a minimal amount of collateral damage has facilitated the performance of numerous endosurgical procedures. It is especially useful in the control of bleeding from medium-sized vessels that are too big to manage with monopolar electrocautery and require bipolar desiccation followed by cutting.

Balloons and Stents. All minimally invasive procedures, from coronary angioplasty to palliation of pancreatic malignancy, invoke the use of endoluminal balloon dilators and prostheses. Endoluminal balloon dilators may be inserted through an endoscope, or they may be fluoroscopically guided. Balloon dilators all have low compliance—that is, the balloons do not stretch as the pressure within the balloon is increased. The high pressures achievable in the balloon create radial expansion of the narrowed vessel or orifice, usually disrupting the atherosclerotic plaque, the fibrotic stricture, or the muscular band (e.g., esophageal achalasia).

Once the dilation has been attained, it is frequently beneficial to hold the lumen open with a stent. Stenting is particularly valuable in treating malignant lesions and endovascular procedures (Fig. 44-9). Stenting usually is not applicable for the long-term management of benign gastrointestinal strictures, except in patients with limited life expectancy.

A variety of stents are available, but they may be divided into two basic categories, plastic stents and expandable metal stents. Plastic stents came first and are used widely as endo-

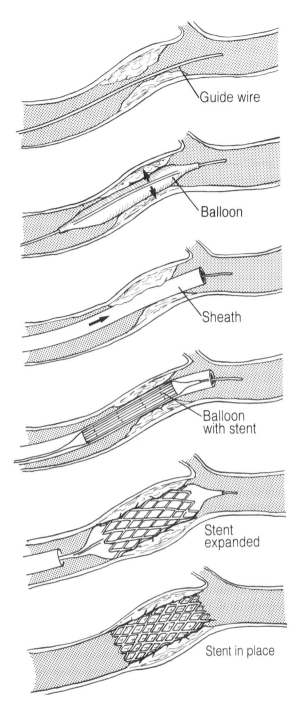

FIG. 44-9. The deployment of a metal stent across an isolated vessel stenosis is illustrated. (From: *Hunter JG, Sackier JM (eds): Minimally Invasive Surgery. New York, McGraw-Hill, 1993, chap 31, p 325.*)

prostheses for temporary bypass of obstructions in the biliary or urinary systems. Metal stents generally are delivered over a balloon and expanded with the balloon to the desired size. These metal stents usually are made of titanium or nitinol. Although great progress has been made with expandable metal stents, two problems remain. The first is the propensity for tissue ingrowth through the interstices of the stent. Ingrowth may be an advantage in preventing stent migration, but such tissue ingrowth may occlude the lumen and cause obstruction anew. This is a particular problem when stents are used for palliation of gastrointestinal malignant growth and may be a problem for the long-term use of stents in vascular disease. Filling the interstices with silastic or other materials may prevent tumor ingrowth but also makes stent migration more likely. Stent designs have incorporated hooks and barbs in an attempt to minimize migration, addressing the second problem.

Hand Instruments. Hand instruments for minimally invasive surgery usually are duplications of conventional surgical instruments made longer, thinner, and smaller at the tip. Certain conventional instruments such as scissors are easy to reproduce with a diameter of 3 to 5 mm and a length of 20 to 45 cm, but other instruments, such as forceps and clamps, cannot provide remote access. Different configurations of graspers were developed to replace the various configurations of surgical forceps and surgical clamps. Standard hand instruments are 5 mm in diameter and 30 cm long, but smaller and shorter hand instruments are now available for pediatric surgery, for microlaparoscopic surgery, and for arthroscopic procedures. A unique laparoscopic hand instrument is the monopolar electrical hook. This device usually is configured with a suction and irrigation apparatus to eliminate smoke and blood from the operative field. The monopolar hook allows tenting of tissue over a bare metal wire with subsequent coagulation and division of the tissue.

Room Setup. Nearly all minimally invasive surgery, whether using fluoroscopic, ultrasound, or optical imaging, incorporates a video monitor as a guide. Occasionally two images are necessary to adequately guide the operation, as in such procedures as endoscopic retrograde cholangiopancreatography (ERCP), laparoscopic common bile duct exploration, and laparoscopic ultrasonography. When two images are necessary, the images should be mounted on two adjacent video monitors or projected on a single screen with a "picture in picture" effect. The video monitor(s) should be set across the operating table from the surgeon. The patient should be interposed between the surgeon and the video monitor; ideally, the operative field also lies between the surgeon and the monitor. In pelviscopic surgery it is best to place the video monitor at the patient's feet, and in laparoscopic cholecystectomy, the monitor is placed at the 10 o'clock position (relative to the patient) while the surgeon stands on the patient's left at the 4 o'clock position. The insufflating and patient monitoring equipment also is ideally placed across the table from the surgeon, so that the insufflating pressure and the patient's vital signs and end tidal CO_2 tension can be monitored.

Trocars for the surgeon's left and right hand should be placed at least 10 cm apart. For most operations it is possible to orient the telescope between these two trocars and slightly retracted from them. The ideal trocar orientation creates an equilateral triangle between the surgeon's right hand, left hand, and the telescope with 10 to 15 cm on each leg. If one imagines the target of the operation (e.g., the gallbladder or gastroesophageal junction) oriented at the apex of a second equilateral triangle built on the first, these four points of reference create a diamond (Fig. 44-10). The surgeon stands behind the telescope, which provides optimal ergonomic orientation but frequently requires that a camera operator (or robotic arm) reach between the surgeon's hands to guide the telescope.

The position of the operating table should permit the surgeon to work with both elbows in at the sides, with arms bent 90

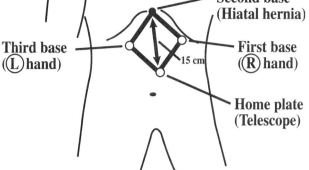

FIG. 44-10. The diamond configuration created by placing the telescope between the left and the right hand, recessed from the target by about 15 cm. The distance between the left and the right hand is also ideally 10 to 15 cm. In this "baseball diamond" configuration, the surgical target occupies the second base position.

degrees at the elbow. It usually is necessary to alter the operating table position with left or right tilt with the patient in the Trendelenburg or reverse Trendelenburg position, depending on the operative field.

Patient Positioning. Patients usually are placed in the supine position for laparoscopic surgery. When the operative field is the gastroesophageal junction or the left lobe of the liver, it is easiest to operate from between the legs. The legs may be elevated in Allen stirrups or abducted on leg boards to achieve this position. When pelvic procedures are performed, it usually is necessary to place the legs in Allen stirrups to gain access to the perineum. A lateral decubitus position with the table flexed provides the best access to the retroperitoneum when performing nephrectomy or adrenalectomy. For laparoscopic splenectomy, a 45-degree tilt of the patient provides excellent access to the lesser sac and the lateral peritoneal attachments to the spleen. For thoracoscopic surgery, the patient is placed in the lateral position.

When the patient's knees are to be bent for extended periods or the patient is going to be placed in a reverse Trendelenburg position for more than a few minutes, deep venous thrombosis prophylaxis should be used. Sequential compression of the lower extremities during prolonged (more than 90 min) laparoscopic procedures increases venous return and provides inhibition of thromboplastin activator inhibitor.

MINIMALLY INVASIVE GENERAL SURGICAL PROCEDURES (TABLE 44-1)

Cholecystectomy. Although flexible endoscopy introduced many general surgeons to video-assisted procedures (e.g., percutaneous endoscopic gastrostomy), it was laparoscopic cholecystectomy that provided the cornerstone around which minimally invasive surgery units were built.

The benefits of laparoscopic cholecystectomy are that it causes little pain and minimal scarring, requires only a short rehabilitation period, and usually can be performed as an outpatient procedure. Common bile duct injury occurs more frequently with laparoscopic cholecystectomy because it frequently

Table 44-1
Laparoscopic Surgical Procedures

Today		Tomorrow
Basic	*Advanced*	*Tomorrow*
Appendectomy	Nissen fundoplication	Intracorporeal anasto-
Cholecystectomy	Heller myotomy	mosis
Hernia repair	Gastrectomy	Cancer surgery
	Esophagectomy	Telepresence surgery
	Enteral access	
	Bile duct exploration	
	Pancreatectomy	
	Colectomy	
	Splenectomy	
	Adrenalectomy	
	Nephrectomy	
	Lymph node dissection	
	Robotics	
	Stereo imaging	
	Telemedicine	
	Laparoscopy-assisted	
	procedures	

is mistaken for the cystic duct. Five steps that help minimize the risk of bile duct injury are: (1) use of an angled (30-degree) scope, (2) maximal cephalic retraction of the gallbladder fundus, (3) lateral retraction of the infundibulum, (4) complete dissection of the gallbladder at its junction with the cystic duct, and (5) liberal use of fluoroscopic cholangiography (Fig. 44-11).

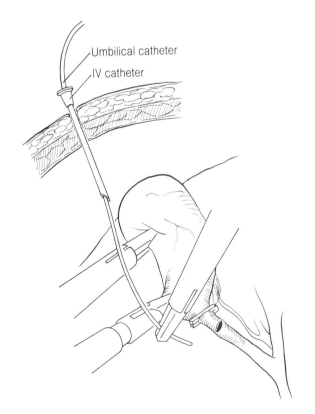

Umbilical catheter
IV catheter

FIG. 44-11. *The percutaneous technique of cholangiography using an intravenous needle and umbilical catheter, which will be held in place by a clip.* (From: *Hunter JG, Sackier JM (eds): Minimally Invasive Surgery. New York, McGraw-Hill, 1993, chap 21, p 223.*)

Appendectomy. The indications for laparoscopic appendectomy depend on the surgeon's confidence in the diagnosis, the age, sex, and weight of the patient, and the stage of appendicitis. Most agree that patients who have right iliac fossa tenderness of uncertain origin might benefit from diagnostic laparoscopy. If uncomplicated appendicitis is found, the appendix should be removed. If the appendix is normal and no other pathology is detected, the appendix should be removed. If a condition is detected that is likely to cause recurrent pain (e.g., terminal ileitis), the appendix should be removed. The appendix is left only if another surgical problem (e.g., acute cholecystitis) is detected. When unsuspected advanced inflammatory conditions of the appendix (gangrene, phlegmon, abscess) are discovered, conversion to a celiotomy, or rarely antibiotic therapy and interval appendectomy, is indicated. The perforated appendix can be treated laparoscopically if the inflammatory reaction is minimal and the base of the appendix is normal.

Additional indications for a selective approach to laparoscopic appendectomy include obese patients and active patients for whom rapid rehabilitation is paramount. The advantages of a nonselective approach to laparoscopic appendectomy were demonstrated in several prospective, randomized trials. In most of these trials, laparoscopic appendectomy resulted in less pain, a more rapid recovery, and an earlier hospital discharge. A meta-analysis of all prospective randomized trials confirmed these findings.

Laparoscopic appendectomy generally requires three ports, at least one of which is 10 mm in diameter. The surgeon needs an assistant to guide the video endoscope. Trocars are placed in the umbilicus (10 to 12 mm) in the suprapubic position (5 mm), and halfway between the umbilicus and the pubis (5 or 10 mm) for the telescope (Fig. 44-12A). Working through the umbilical and suprapubic trocars, the appendix is mobilized and the mesoappendix divided with clips, bipolar electrosurgery, or staples. When the mesoappendix is involved with the inflammatory process, it is impossible to mobilize the appendix; it often is best to make a window next to the base of the appendix, divide the appendix with a stapler, then divide the mesoappendix immediately adjacent to the appendix with clips, stapler, or bipolar coagulation. The appendix is removed through a 10-mm trocar if it is small, or in a specimen bag if it is enlarged.

Inguinal Hernia Repair. Laparoscopic inguinal hernia repair is the most controversial of the minimally invasive procedures, for several reasons: it does not shorten hospitalization; the long-term efficacy of the procedures will take 20 years to evaluate; the technique is different from standard hernia repairs; and the hospital costs are higher than those of open hernia repair.

The early laparoscopic hernia repairs (plication of the internal ring, plug of the hernia sac, and prosthetic "onlay" over the hernia defect) have been abandoned. The two repairs performed today are the transabdominal preperitoneal (TAPP) repair and the totally extraperitoneal (TEP) repair. Although the TEP repair is slightly more difficult, many experienced laparoscopic surgeons prefer it for all but incarcerated hernias and for patients who have had previous lower abdominal operations.

The leading indication for the TEP repair is recurrent hernia. Anterior repair of recurrent hernias is associated with a 20 percent recurrence rate, division of the ilioinguinal nerve, and the possibility of testicular damage. These are the patients for whom the preperitoneal repairs were developed. The TEP repair nearly

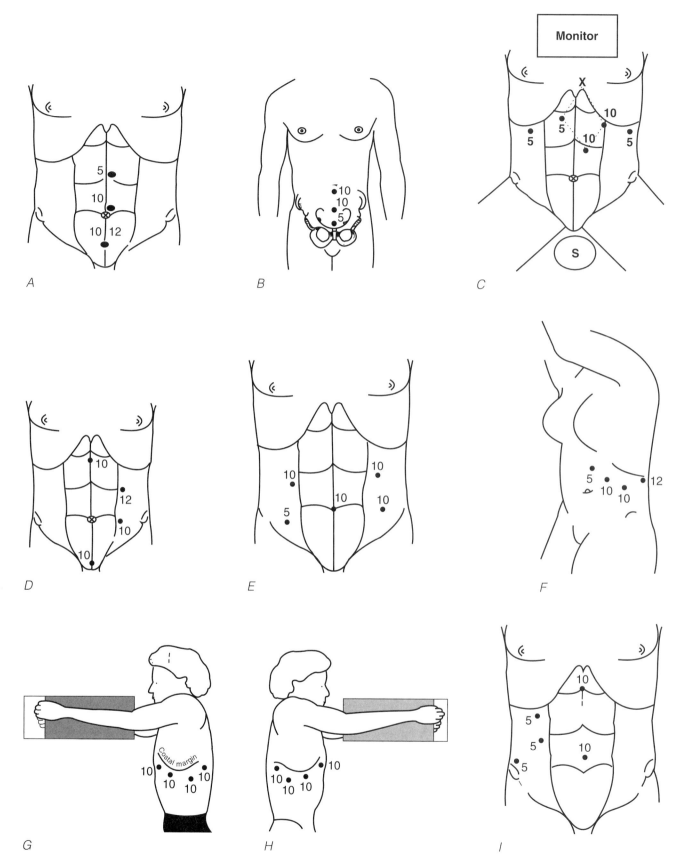

FIG. 44-12. Trocar positions for advanced laparoscopic procedures. *A.* Laparoscopic appendectomy. *B.* Extraperitoneal hernia repair. *C.* Laparoscopic Nissen fundoplication, with the "baseball diamond" positions of trocar, target, monitor, and surgeon (*X* = location of gastroesophageal junction; *S* = location of surgeon). *D.* Right colectomy. *E.* Laparoscopic low anterior resection. *F.* Laparoscopic splenectomy ("hybrid" approach). *G.* Left adrenalectomy. *H.* Right adrenalectomy. *I.* Laparoscopic common bile duct exploration. (From: *Hunter JG: Advanced laparoscopic surgery. Am J Surg 173:14–18, 1997, with permission.*)

reproduces these repairs without the need for the large counterincision to place the mesh into the preperitoneal plane. It appears that the TEP repair will be able to achieve a recurrence rate similar to those of the open procedures, which is less than 5 percent.

Bilateral hernias are a second indication for TEP. The bilateral groin dissection and repair uses the same number and size of incisions as a unilateral repair. The "tension-free" nature of the repair eliminates concerns about a higher recurrence rate associated with simultaneous repair of bilateral hernias. The majority of the expense of laparoscopic herniorrhaphy is related to equipment charges and the time required to establish access. Repair of a contralateral side adds little time or equipment cost. Because of the ease associated with dissection and repair of the contralateral groin after one side has been repaired, a number of surgeons advocate routine dissection of the contralateral groin with simultaneous repair of asymptomatic hernias that are detected.

The preferred TEP approach requires three trocars placed in the lower midline (see Fig. 44-12*B*). A small infraumbilical incision is opened down to the space between either rectus muscle and the posterior rectus sheath. A large balloon dissector is passed immediately to the pubic symphysis and inflated at this level. The balloon does 90 percent of the dissection of Hesselbach's triangle posteriorly. The balloon is removed and a Hasson cannula and 45-degree telescope are replaced. The only remaining dissection separates the spermatic cord from an indirect hernia sac. Small hernia sacs may be reduced entirely and left behind the mesh in the preperitoneal space. Rather than trying to reduce a large sac from the inguinal canal, sufficient sac is mobilized to ensure that no intraperitoneal structures remain within (sliding hernia). A 30-inch nonabsorbable suture is looped around the sac and tied extracorporeally. Extracorporeal knotting should be performed by sliding square knots down with a "knot pusher." Most jamming knots (e.g., Roeder's knot) slip before breaking and have been abandoned. The sac is opened widely distal to the knot and left in the inguinal canal. A large piece of mesh, 10 × 15 cm at a minimum, is placed to cover Hesselbach's triangle, the internal inguinal ring, and the femoral canal. The mesh is fixed to Cooper's ligament, the pubic tubercle, the posterior rectus muscle, and the transversalis fascia lateral to the epigastric vessels. The fixation device should be palpable through the abdominal wall before any tacks are placed. This technique eliminates the possibility of entrapping the genitofemoral or lateral femoral cutaneous nerve within a staple.

Fundoplication. In the landmark study from the Veterans Administration Cooperative Study group it was proved that antireflux surgery better eliminated gastroesophageal reflux (GER) than did medical therapy in patients with severe reflux. These data arrived at the time that laparoscopic fundoplication was in its infancy. The results achieved with laparoscopic antireflux surgery in the 5 years since its inception have been virtually identical to the results of open fundoplication.

The indications for operation is gastroesophageal reflux that requires daily proton-pump inhibitors, symptomatic reflux associated with the complications of stricture, or Barrett's esophagus. Respiratory symptoms (e.g., asthma, cough, hoarseness) associated with well-documented gastroesophageal reflux constitute another indication. Evaluation of patients should be thorough and generally should include esophagogastroduodenoscopy

(EGD), barium swallow, 24-h ambulatory pH, and esophageal motility study (EMS). A gastric emptying study is performed when gastric abnormalities are suspected (e.g., diabetes, vomiting, peptic ulcer disease). Abnormalities in gastric emptying may be addressed with prokinetic agents or concomitant pyloroplasty at the time of laparoscopic fundoplication.

In laparoscopic fundoplication the approach to the field of dissection involves the placement of the primary trocars in a diamond configuration (see Fig. 44-12*C*). The surgeon stands at the base of the diamond. The table height is adjusted so that the surgeon's elbows are kept close to the sides. Intracorporeal knot tying reduces tissue trauma and is preferable to extracorporeal tying.

With laparoscopic fundoplication, it is most important to understand which cases are likely to present difficulty. This group includes patients with previous subdiaphragmatic surgery, obese patients, those with large diaphragmatic hernias (>5 cm), and those with significant esophageal shortening.

Assisted Colectomy. Laparoscopic removal of the colon is an area of rapid growth, but its application in patients with colon cancer has engendered heated debate. Metastatic tumor implantation at the site of the laparoscopic trocars occurs about twice as frequently after laparoscopic colectomy as implantation at the site of incision after open colectomy. Current indications for laparoscopy-assisted colectomy are benign or premalignant disease, colostomy creation, and rectopexy for pelvic floor dysfunction. A creative use of laparoscopy is the mobilization of the splenic and hepatic flexures in procedures being performed primarily in the pelvis. After laparoscopic mobilization of the flexures, almost any operation—e.g., total abdominal colectomy, low anterior resection, or ileoanal pull-through—may be performed through a Pfannenstiel's incision.

The field of dissection usually traverses several quadrants of the abdomen. As the colon is progressively mobilized, it is frequently necessary to change the telescope to other trocar sites, and it may be necessary to add additional trocars. With increasing experience, trocar placement based on triangulation has simplified the approach (see Fig. 44-12*D*, *E*). Additionally, it is necessary to make a counterincision to remove the colon specimen or to create a stoma. The duration of ileus is less than after conventional colectomy.

Splenectomy. The most common indication for laparoscopic splenectomy is immunologic disease (particularly idiopathic thrombocytopenic purpura) in patients with a normal or slightly enlarged spleen. Because of difficulties in getting the spleen into a collection bag, it is wise to restrict laparoscopic splenectomy to spleens that weigh less than 500 g.

The techniques for laparoscopic splenectomy include the supine technique, the left lateral decubitus ("hanging spleen") technique, and the "leaning spleen" position, which is a compromise between the other two. The patient is positioned on the table at a 45-degree tilt, using a bean bag. Four trocars are placed while the table is rolled so that the patient is nearly supine (see Fig. 44-12*F*). It may be necessary to take down the splenic flexure of the colon before placing the last trocar. The splenic artery is identified in the lesser sac by dividing short gastric vessels and rolling the gastric fundus to the right. The splenic artery is ligated (Fig. 44-13). At this point the table is tilted so that the patient moves into the right lateral decubitus position and the spleen allowed to fall anteriorly. The splenophrenic attachments

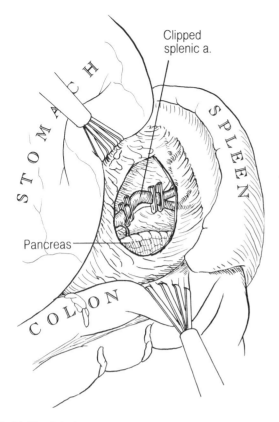

FIG. 44-13. *Splenic artery preligation is not difficult if the greater curvature of the stomach is mobilized with the patient nearly supine. The splenic artery is easily visible at the superior surface of the pancreas and can be secured with a No. 0 silk tie or Hemaclips. (From: Hunter JG, Sackier JM (eds): Minimally Invasive Surgery. New York, McGraw-Hill, 1993, chap 30, p 311.)*

(peritoneal reflection) are divided to allow access to the splenic hilum. In the hilum the splenic vessels are controlled with a linear cutting stapler, or they are individually ligated. Smaller vessels are clipped. The most difficult part of this operation may lie in manipulating the spleen into the retrieval bag. This step is made easier if the bag is opened in the left upper quadrant with the open mouth facing the laparoscope. A strong nylon bag is recommended for retrieving the spleen, as weaker bags may rupture. The neck of the bag is pulled out of a trocar site, and the spleen is morcellated and removed with ring forceps or with mechanized morcellation devices.

Adrenalectomy. Hyperfunctioning adenomas (including pheochromocytoma) are effectively dealt with laparoscopically. When adrenal carcinoma is suspected or the mass is greater than 5 cm, a laparoscopic approach is less appropriate. Similarly, when a search for paragangliomas is indicated or when it is necessary to perform simultaneous bilateral adrenalectomy, a transabdominal or posterior extraperitoneal approach might be warranted. The "no-touch" technique afforded by laparoscopic surgery is ideal for addressing a unilateral pheochromocytoma.

The preferred technique for laparoscopic adrenalectomy is to place the patient in the lateral decubitus position. Four trocars are placed beneath the costal margin, in the epigastrium, the midclavicular line, the anterior axillary line, and the posterior axillary line (see Fig. 44-12*G, H*). On the left side, the surgeon

begins the dissection by rolling the spleen anteriorly by dividing the splenophrenic ligament. Occasionally this is all that is needed to find the adrenal gland. In an obese patient endoscopic ultrasonography may be helpful in locating the adrenal gland. Sticking close to the adrenal gland but being careful not to grasp the gland, the surgeon teases away the retroperitoneal fat with a monopolar electrocautery hook, blunt dissection, and clips. The adrenal vein is located (inferomedially), and two clips are placed on the renal vein side of the adrenal vein. The adrenal vein is placed immediately into a bag and extracted through one of the trocar sites. The dissection on the right side is nearly identical to that on the left side except that a liver retractor is necessary to hold the right lobe of the liver anteriorly. Dissection of the gland away from the inferior vena cava starts inferiorly, allowing identification of the short right adrenal vein, which is divided between clips.

Common Bile Duct Exploration (CBDE). Data from several centers have demonstrated that laparoscopic cholecystectomy with laparoscopic retrieval of bile duct stones is substantially more cost-effective than laparoscopic cholecystectomy followed by endoscopic sphincterotomy and stone retrieval.

Laparoscopic bile duct exploration starts with fluoroscopic cholangiography. A cholangiogram should be performed with a ureteral catheter or a modified ERCP catheter that allows the passage of a guide wire. If stones are detected, a hydrophilic guide wire is passed through the cystic duct into the duodenum. If the common bile duct is small, and the stones are small (<3 mm), the cholangiogram catheter can easily be advanced over the guide wire to a position just above the stones. Intravenous glucagon is given, and a rapid infusion of saline will push small stones into the duodenum. When stones larger than 3 mm are detected or the common bile duct is dilated, it is best to remove the stones through the cystic duct. A helical stone basket frequently is all that is needed to remove small stones (5 mm or less). Larger common bile duct stones usually require an endoscopic approach. The cystic duct is dilated with an 8-mm balloon that has been passed over a guide wire. The balloon is left in place for 5 min while the choledochoscope is set up and an extra 5-mm trocar is placed (see Fig. 44-12*I*). A thin choledochoscope (8 to 10 French) is passed with a rubber shod grasper over the guide wire and into the distal common bile duct. A 2- to 2.5-mm flat wire basket is passed through the operating channel of the choledochoscope and the stone is entrapped. Stones larger than 8 mm in diameter are best dealt with by performing a choledochotomy, stone extraction, and placement of a T tube (choledocholithotomy) (Fig. 44-14). Some use choledocholithotomy as their primary laparoscopic approach to stones of the common bile duct. Most bile duct stones (80 to 90 percent) can be dealt with using these techniques. Laparoscopic CBDE is as effective as endoscopic sphincterotomy and may reduce the risk of postoperative pancreatitis and the long-term and largely unknown sequelae of sphincter destruction.

SPECIAL CONSIDERATIONS

Pediatric Considerations. The advantages of minimally invasive surgery in children may be more significant than in the adult population. Minimally invasive surgery in the adolescent is little different from that in the adult, and standard instrumentation and trocar positions usually can be used. Laparoscopy in

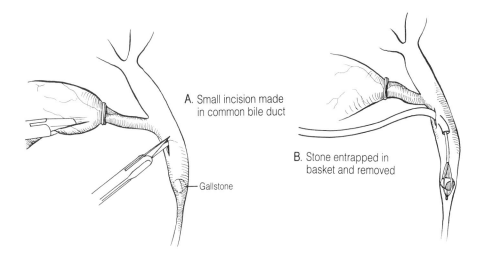

A. Small incision made in common bile duct

B. Stone entrapped in basket and removed

Gallstone

FIG. 44-14. Laparoscopic choledochotomy and bile duct exploration is performed in a nearly conventional fashion. Two notable differences from open surgery are that the gallbladder is left in situ to serve as traction on the common duct and that stay sutures are generally not used as they merely get in the way. Otherwise the technique is nearly identical to that used in open common bile duct exploration. (From: Hunter JG, Sackier JM (eds): Minimally Invasive Surgery. New York, McGraw-Hill, 1993, chap 22, p 241.)

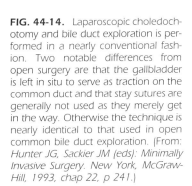

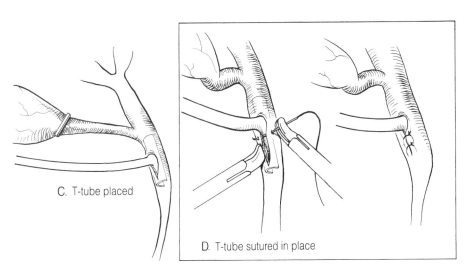

C. T-tube placed

D. T-tube sutured in place

the infant and young child requires specialized instrumentation. The instruments are shorter (15 to 20 cm), and many are 3 mm in diameter rather than 5 mm. Because the abdomen of the child is much smaller than that of the adult, a 5-mm telescope provides sufficient illumination for most operations. The development of 5-mm clippers and bipolar devices has obviated the need for 10-mm trocars in pediatric laparoscopy. Because the abdominal wall is much thinner in infants, a pneumoperitoneum pressure of 8 mmHg can provide adequate exposure. Deep venous thrombosis is rare in children, and prophylaxis against thrombosis is probably unnecessary.

Pregnancy. Concerns about the safety of laparoscopic cholecystectomy or appendectomy in the pregnant patient have been eliminated. The pH of the fetus follows the pH of the mother linearly, and therefore fetal acidosis may be prevented by avoiding a respiratory acidosis in the mother. A second concern was that of increased intraabdominal pressure, but it has been proved that midpregnancy uterine contractions provide a much greater pressure in utero than a pneumoperitoneum. Experiences of well over 100 cases of laparoscopic cholecystectomy in pregnancy have been reported with uniformly good results. Operation should be performed during the second trimester if possible. Pro-

tection of the fetus against intraoperative x-rays is imperative. Some believe it advisable to track fetal pulse rate with a transvaginal ultrasound probe. Access to the abdomen in the pregnant patient should take into consideration the height of the uterine fundus, which reaches the umbilicus at 20 weeks. In order not to damage the uterus or its blood supply, most surgeons feel that the open (Hasson) approach should be used in favor of direct puncture laparoscopy.

Cancer. Minimally invasive techniques have been used for many decades to provide palliation for the patient with an obstruction cancer. Laser treatment, intracavitary radiation, stenting, and dilation are outpatient techniques that can be used to reestablish the continuity of an obstructed esophagus, bile duct, ureter, or airway. Minimally invasive techniques also have been used in the staging of cancer. Mediastinoscopy is still used occasionally before thoracotomy to assess the status of the mediastinal lymph nodes. Laparoscopy also is used to assess the liver in patients being evaluated for pancreatic, gastric, or hepatic resection. New technology and greater surgical skills allow accurate minimally invasive staging of cancer. Occasionally it is appropriate to perform palliative measures (e.g., laparoscopic gastrojejunostomy to bypass a pancreatic cancer) at the time of diagnostic laparoscopy if diagnostic findings preclude attempts at curative resection.

The most controversial role of minimally invasive techniques is that of providing potentially curative surgery to the patient with cancer. It is possible to perform laparoscopy-assisted colectomy, gastrectomy, pancreatectomy, and hepatectomy in patients with intraabdominal malignant disease, as well as thoracoscopic esophagectomy and pneumonectomy in patients with intrathoracic malignant disease. There are not yet enough data to indicate whether minimally invasive techniques provide survival rates or disease-free intervals comparable to those of conventional techniques. It has been proved that in laparoscopy-assisted colectomy and gastrectomy equivalent numbers of lymph nodes to the open procedure can be removed without any compromise of resection margins. A second concern centers around excessive tumor manipulation and the possibility that cancer cells would be shed during the dissection. Alarming reports of trocar site implantation with viable cancer have appeared in the literature.

Considerations in the Elderly and Infirm. Laparoscopic cholecystectomy has made possible the removal of a symptomatic gallbladder in many patients previously thought to be too elderly or too ill to undergo a laparotomy. Operations on these patients require closely monitored anesthesia. The intraoperative management of these patients may be more difficult with laparoscopic access than with open access. The advantage of minimally invasive surgery lies in what happens after the operation. Much of the morbidity of surgery in the elderly is a result of impaired mobilization. In addition, pulmonary complications, urinary tract sepsis, deep venous thrombosis, pulmonary embolism, congestive heart failure, and myocardial infarction often are the result of improper fluid management and decreased mobility. By allowing rapid and early mobilization, laparoscopic surgery has made possible the safe performance of procedures in the elderly and infirm.

Economics of Minimally Invasive Surgery. Minimally invasive surgical procedures reduce the costs of surgery most when length of hospital stay can be shortened. Shorter hospital stays can be demonstrated in laparoscopic cholecystectomy, fundoplication, splenectomy, and adrenalectomy, for example. Procedures such as inguinal herniorrhaphy that are already performed as outpatient procedures are less likely to provide cost advantage. Procedures that still require a 4- to 7-day hospitalization, such as laparoscopy-assisted colectomy, are even less likely to deliver a lower bottom line than their open-surgery counterparts. Nonetheless, with responsible use of disposable instrumentation and a commitment to the most effective use of the inpatient setting, most laparoscopic procedures can be made less expensive than their conventional equivalents.

Bibliography

History

Hopkins HH: Optical principles of the endoscope, in Berci G (ed): *Endoscopy.* New York, Appleton-Century-Crofts, 1976, pp 3–26.

Katzir A: Optical fibers in medicine. *Sci Am* 260(5):120, 1989.

Veritas TF: Coelioscopy: A synthesis of Georg Kelling's work with insufflation, endoscopy, and lufttamponade, in Litynski: *Highlights in the History of Laparoscopy.* Frankfurt/Main, Barbara Bernert Verlag, 1996, pp 3–21.

Physiology, Immunology, Anesthesia

Callery MP, Soper NJ: Physiology of the pneumoperitoneum, in Hunter (ed): *Baillière's Clinical Gastroenterology: Laparoscopic Surgery.* London/Philadelphia, Baillière Tindall, 1993, pp 757–777.

Cullen DJ, Eger EI: Cardiovascular effects of carbon dioxide in man. *Anesthesiology* 41:345, 1974.

Cunningham AJ, Turner J, et al: Transoesophageal echocardiographic assessment of haemodynamic function during laparoscopic cholecystectomy. *Br J Anaesthesia* 70:621, 1993.

Gossot D: Access modalities for thoracoscopic surgery, in Toouli, Gossot, Hunter (eds): *Endosurgery.* New York/London, Churchill-Livingstone, 1996, pp 743–751.

Ho HS, Gunther RA, et al: Intraperitoneal carbon dioxide insufflation and cardiopulmonary functions. *Arch Surg* 127:928, 1992.

Ho HS, Wolfe BM: The physiology and immunology of endosurgery, in Toouli, Gossot, Hunter (eds): *Endosurgery.* New York/London, Churchill-Livingstone, 1996, pp 163–171.

Hunter JG, Staheli J, et al: Nitrous oxide pneumoperitoneum revisited: Is there a risk of combustion? *Surg Endosc* 9:501, 1995.

Schauer PR, Luna J, et al: Pulmonary function after laparoscopic cholecystectomy. *Surgery* 114:389, 1993.

Smith RS, Fry WR, et al: Gasless laparoscopy and conventional instruments: The next phase of minimally invasive surgery. *Arch Surg* 128:1102, 1993.

Wittgen CM, Andrus CH, et al: Analysis of the hemodynamic and ventilatory effects of laparoscopic cholecystectomy. *Arch Surg* 126:997, 1991.

Access

Byron JW, Markenson G, et al: A randomised comparison of Verreìs needle and direct insertion for laparoscopy. *Surg Gynecol Obstet* 177:259, 1993.

Eaves FF: Basics of endoscopic plastic surgery, in Bostwick J, Eaves FF, Nahai F (eds): *Endoscopic Plastic Surgery.* St Louis, Quality Medical Publishing, 1995, pp 59–81.

Fletcher DR: Laparoscopic access, in Toouli, Gossot, Hunter (eds): *Endosurgery.* New York/London, Churchill-Livingstone, 1996, pp 189–196.

Hanney RM, Alle KM, Cregan PC: Major vascular injury and laparoscopy. *Aust N Z J Surg* 65:533, 1995.

Himpens J: Laparoscopic preperitoneal approach to the inguinal hernia, in Toouli, Gossot, Hunter (eds): *Endosurgery.* New York/London, Churchill-Livingstone, 1996, pp 949–959.

Kaiser LR: Video-assisted thoracic surgery: Current state of the art. *Ann Surg* 220:720, 1994.

Lumsden AB, Eaves FF: Vein harvest, in Bostwick J, Eaves FF, Nahai F (eds): *Endoscopic Plastic Surgery.* St. Louis, Quality Medical Publishing, 1995, pp 535–547.

Instrumentation, Energy Sources

Amaral JF, Chrostek C: Comparison of the ultrasonically activated scalpel to electrosurgery and laser for laparoscopic surgery. *Surg Endosc* 7:141, 1993.

Foutch P, Sivak M: Therapeutic endoscopic balloon dilatation of the extrahepatic biliary ducts. *Am J Gastroenterol* 80:575, 1985.

Hoepffner N, Foerster EC, et al: Long-term experience in wall stent therapy for malignant choledochostenosis. *Endoscopy* 26:597, 1994.

Hunter JG: Controversies in laparoscopic cholecystectomy exposure, dissection, and laser versus electrosurgery. *Am J Surg* 165:492, 1993.

Kozarek RA, Ball TJ, et al: Metallic self-expanding stent application in the upper gastrointestinal tract: Caveats and concerns. *Gastrointest Endosc* 38:1, 1992.

Lirici MM, Melzer A, et al: Tissue approximation in minimally invasive surgery. *Endosc Surg* 2:47, 1994.

Margulies DR, Shabot MM: Fiberoptic imaging and measurement, in Hunter, Sackier (eds): *Minimally Invasive Surgery*. New York, McGraw-Hill, 1993, pp 7–14.

McIntyre RC, Stiegmann GV: Intraoperative, endoscopic, and laparoscopic ultrasound, in Hunter, Sackier (eds): *Minimally Invasive Surgery*. New York, McGraw-Hill, 1993, pp 15–21.

Miles WFA, Paterson-Brown S, et al: Laparoscopic contact hepatic ultrasonography. *Br J Surg* 79:419, 1992.

Odell RC: Laparoscopic electrosurgery, in Hunter, Sackier (eds): *Minimally Invasive Surgery*. New York, McGraw-Hill, 1993, pp 33–41.

Prescher T: Video imaging, in Toouli, Gossot, Hunter (eds): *Endosurgery*. New York/London, Churchill-Livingstone, 1996, pp 41–54.

Trus TL, Hunter JG: Principles of laser physics and tissue interaction, in Toouli, Gossot, Hunter (eds): *Endosurgery*. New York/London, Churchill-Livingstone, 1996, pp 103–109.

Voyels CR, et al: Education and engineering solutions for potential problems with laparoscopic monopolar electrosurgery. *Am J Surg* 164:57, 1992.

Laparoscopic Cholecystectomy

Asbun HJ, Rossi RL, et al: Bile duct injury during laparoscopic cholecystectomy: Mechanism of injury, prevention, and management. *World J Surg* 17:547, 1993.

Deziel DJ, Millikan KW, et al: Complications of laparoscopic cholecystectomy: A national survey of 4,292 hospitals and an analysis of 77,604 cases. *Am J Surg* 165:9, 1993.

Hunter JG: Laparoscopic antireflux surgery. *Current Surgery* 51:182, 1994.

NIH Consensus Conference: Gallstones and laparoscopic cholecystectomy. *JAMA* 269:1018, 1993.

Laparoscopic Appendectomy

Bonanni F, Reed J, et al: Laparoscopic versus conventional appendectomy. *J Am Coll Surg* 179:273, 1994.

Frazee RC, Roberts JW, et al: A prospective randomized trial comparing open versus laparoscopic appendectomy. *Ann Surg* 214:725, 1994.

Kum CK, Ngoi SS, et al: Randomized controlled trial comparing laparoscopic and open appendectomy. *Br J Surg* 80:1599, 1993.

Ortega AE, Hunter JG, et al: Laparoscopic Appendectomy Study Group: A prospective randomized comparison of laparoscopic appendectomy with open appendectomy. *Am J Surg* 169:208, 1995.

Semm K: Endoscopic appendectomy. *Endoscopy* 15:59, 1993.

Laparoscopic Inguinal Hernia Repair

Fitzgibbons RJ Jr, Camps J, et al: Laparoscopic inguinal hernia: Results of a multicenter trial. *Ann Surg* 21:3, 1995.

Hoffman HC, Vinton-Traverso AL: Preperitoneal prosthetic herniorrhaphy: One surgeon's successful technique. *Arch Surg* 128:965, 1993.

Phillips EH, Carroll BJ, et al: Laparoscopic preperitoneal inguinal hernia repair without peritoneal incision: Technique and early clinical results. *Surg Endosc* 7:159, 1993.

Stoker DL, Spiegelhalter DJ, et al: Laparoscopic versus open inguinal hernia repair: Randomised prospective trial. *Lancet* 343:1243.

Laparoscopic Fundoplication

Hinder RA, Filipi CJ, et al: Laparoscopic Nissen fundoplication is an effective treatment for gastroesophageal reflux disease. *Ann Surg* 220:472, 1994.

Hunter JG, Swanstrom L, et al: Patterns of dysphagia following laparoscopic antireflux surgery. *Ann Surg* 224:51, 1996.

Hunter JG, Trus TL, et al: A physiologic approach to laparoscopic fundoplication for gastroesophageal reflux disease. *Ann Surg* 223:673, 1996.

Jamieson GG, Baigrie RJ: Indications and evaluation of patients undergoing laparoscopic antireflux surgery, in Toouli, Gossot, Hunter (eds): *Endosurgery*. New York/London, Churchill-Livingstone, 1996, 301–304.

Spechler SJ: The Department of Veterans Affairs Gastroesophageal Reflux Disease Study Group: Comparison of medical and surgical therapy for complicated gastroesophageal reflux disease in veterans. *New Engl J Med* 326:786, 1992.

Waring JP, Hunter JG, et al: The preoperative evaluation of patients considered for laparoscopic antireflux surgery. *Am J Gastroenterol* 90:35, 1995.

Laparoscopy-Assisted Colectomy

Böhm B, Milsom JW, et al: Postoperative intestinal motility following conventional and laparoscopic intestinal surgery. *Arch Surg* 130:415, 1995.

Cirocco W, Schwartzman A, et al: Abdominal wall recurrence after laparoscopic colectomy for colon cancer. *Surgery* 116:842, 1994.

Fowler DL: Laparoscopic right hemicolectomy, in Toouli, Gossot, Hunter (eds): *Endosurgery*. New York/London, Churchill-Livingstone, 1996, pp 665–673.

Franklin ME Jr: Laparoscopic low anterior abdominal perineal resections, in Toouli, Gossot, Hunter (eds): *Endosurgery*. New York/London, Churchill-Livingstone, 1996, pp 685–694.

Reilly WT, Nelson H, et al: Wound recurrence following conventional treatment of colorectal cancer. *Dis Colon Rectum* 39:200, 1996.

Whelan RL, Bessler M, et al: Laparoscopic-assisted sigmoid colectomy, in Toouli, Gossot, Hunter (eds): *Endosurgery*. New York/London, Churchill-Livingstone, 1996, pp 675–683.

Laparoscopic Splenectomy, Adrenalectomy

Böhm B, Milsom JW, et al: Laparoscopic splenectomy: The initial experience at University of California, San Francisco. *Arch Surg* 130:415, 1995.

Cadiere GB, Verroken R, et al: Operative strategy in laparoscopic splenectomy. *J Am Coll Surg* 179:668, 1994.

Delaitre B: Laparoscopic splenectomy: The "hanged spleen" technique. *Surg Endosc* 9:528, 1995.

Gagner M: Laparoscopic adrenalectomy, in Toouli, Gossot, Hunter (eds): *Endosurgery*. New York/London, Churchill-Livingstone, 1996, pp 623–634.

Poulin EC, Thibault C, et al: Laparoscopic splenectomy. *Surg Endosc* 9:172, 1995.

Prinz RA: A comparison of laparoscopic and open adrenalectomies. *Arch Surg* 130:489, 1995.

Vaughan ED Jr: Adrenal surgery, in Marshall FF (ed): *Atlas of Urologic Surgery*, Philadelphia, WB Saunders, 1991.

Laparoscopic Common Bile Duct Exploration

Carroll BJ, Fallas MJ, et al: Laparoscopic transcystic choledochoscopy. *Surg Endosc* 8:310, 1994.

Hunter JG: Laparoscopic transcystic common bile duct exploration. *Am J Surg* 163:53, 1992.

Hunter JG: Laparoscopic cholecystectomy and the common bile duct. *Surg Endosc* 8:285, 1994.

Laycock WS, Hunter JG: Laparoscopic approach to bile duct stones, in Toouli, Gossot, Hunter (eds): *Endosurgery*. New York/London, Churchill-Livingstone, 1996, pp 507–519.

Petelin JB: Laparoscopic approach to common duct pathology. *Am J Surg* 165:687, 1993.

Stoker ME: Common bile duct exploration in the era of laparoscopic surgery. *Arch Surg* 130:265, 1995.

Special Considerations

Georgeson KE: Pediatric laparoscopy, in Toouli, Gossot, Hunter (eds): *Endosurgery*. New York/London, Churchill-Livingstone, 1996, pp 929–933.

Holcomb GW: Diagnostic laparoscopy: Equipment, technique, and special concerns in children, in Holcomb GW (ed): *Pediatric Endoscopic Surgery.* Norwalk, CT, Appleton and Lange, pp 9–19.

Hunter JG, Swanstrom LL, et al: Carbon dioxide pneumoperitoneum induces fetal acidosis in a pregnant ewe model. *Surg Endosc* 9:272, 1995.

Morgenstern L: Ethical considerations in laparoscopic choledocholithotomy, in Berci, Cuschieri (eds): *Bile Ducts and Bile Duct Stones.* Philadelphia, WB Saunders, 1997, pp 161–165.

Morrell DG, Mullins JR, et al: Laparoscopic cholecystectomy during pregnancy in symptomatic patients. *Surgery* 112:856.

Traverso LW, Hargrave K, et al: A cost-effective approach to the treatment of common bile duct stones with surgical versus endoscopic techniques, in Berci, Cuschieri (eds): *Bile Ducts and Bile Duct Stones.* Philadelphia, WB Saunders, 1997, pp 154–160.

Index

Page numbers followed by a "t" indicate tables; numbers followed by an "f" refer to figures.

ISBN 0-07-912318-X

ISBN 0-07-058079-0